HUNTER'S

TROPICAL
MEDICINE

HUNTER'S

TROPICAL MEDICINE

SEVENTH EDITION

G. THOMAS STRICKLAND

M.D., Ph.D., D.C.M.T., F.A.C.P.

Captain, Medical Corps, United States Navy (Retired)
Director, International Health Program
and
Professor of Microbiology and Immunology, Epidemiology
and Preventive Medicine, and Medicine,
University of Maryland School of Medicine,
Baltimore, Maryland
and
Senior Associate, Department of Immunology and Infectious
Diseases, Johns Hopkins School of Hygiene and Public Health,
Baltimore, Maryland

W.B. SAUNDERS COMPANY
Harcourt Brace Jovanovich, Inc.

Philadelphia   London   Toronto   Montreal   Sydney   Tokyo

W. B. SAUNDERS COMPANY
Harcourt Brace Jovanovich, Inc.

The Curtis Center
Independence Square West
Philadelphia, PA 19106

Library of Congress Cataloging-in-Publication Data

Hunter's tropical medicine.—7th ed. / [edited by]
G. Thomas Strickland.

p. cm

Includes bibliographical references and index.

ISBN 0-7216-2970-9

1. Tropical medicine.   I. Hunter, George W.
   (George William).   II. Strickland, G. Thomas.

[DNLM: 1. Tropical Medicine.   WC 680 T857]

RC961.H84 1991

616.9′883—dc20

DNLM/DLC   91-6873

Editor: John Dyson
Developmental Editor: David Kilmer
Designer: Paul Fry
Production Manager: Peter Faber
Manuscript Editors: Constance Burton, Terry Russell, Pam Wight, and Grace Caputo
Illustration Coordinator: Peg Shaw
Indexer: Roger Wall

Hunter's Tropical Medicine, 7th edition   ISBN 0–7216–2970–9

Part Editors

Stephen G. Wright, M.B., D.C.M.T., M.R.C.P.

Senior Lecturer, Department of Clinical Sciences, London School of Hygiene and Tropical Medicine, London, England
PART I: CLINICAL PRACTICE IN THE TROPICS

Thomas P. Monath, M.D.

Chief, Virology Division, U.S. Army Medical Research Institute of Infectious Diseases, Fort Detrick, Frederick, Maryland
PART II: VIRAL INFECTIONS

Michael C. Latham, O.B.E., M.B., M.P.H., D.T.M. & H., F.F.C.M.

Professor and Director, Program in International Nutrition, Division of Nutritional Sciences, Cornell University, Ithaca, New York
PART VIII: NUTRITIONAL PROBLEMS AND DEFICIENCY DISEASES

Jay S. Keystone, M.SC. C.T.M., F.R.C.P.(C).

Associate Professor of Medicine and Microbiology, University of Toronto School of Medicine; Director, Tropical Disease Unit, Toronto General Hospital, Toronto, Canada
PART X: TROPICAL DISEASE IN A TEMPERATE CLIMATE

Contributors

Hassan Abu-Aisha, M.D., F.R.C.P.(E)

Chief, Nephrology Division; Professor of Medicine, College of Medicine, King Saud University, Riyadh, Saudi Arabia
HEAT-ASSOCIATED ILLNESS

M. Farid Abdel-Wahab, M.D., D.T.M. & H.

Professor and Chairman, Department of Tropical Medicine; Cairo University Faculty of Medicine; Dean, Menofia Liver Institute, Shebin El Kom, Egypt.
SCHISTOSOMIASIS

O. O. Akinkugbe, M.D., PH.D., D.SC. (HON.), F.R.C.P.

Professor of Medicine, University of Ibadan; Consultant Physician and Head of Renal and Hypertension Division, University College Hospital, Ibadan, Nigeria
CARDIOVASCULAR DISEASES

Abdul Karem Al-Asaka, M.D.

Chief of Medicine, Security Forces Hospital; Associate Professor of Medicine; King Saud University, Riyadh, Saudi Arabia
HEAT-ASSOCIATED ILLNESS; BRUCELLOSIS

Abdu F. Azad, PH.D., M.P.H.

Professor of Microbiology and Immunology and International Health Program, University of Maryland School of Medicine, Baltimore, Maryland
INJURIOUS ARTHROPODS
TICKS AND MITES IN DISEASE TRANSMISSION

James D. Bales, Jr., M.D., M.SC. C.T.M., F.A.C.P.

Chief, Infectious Diseases Service, Department of Medicine, Letterman Army Medical Center, San Francisco, California
AFRICAN TRYPANOSOMIASIS

Charles B. Beal, M.D.

President, International Health Services, Mountain View; Associate Clinical Professor of Epidemiology and Biostatistics, University of California, San Francisco, School of Medicine, San Francisco, California
GLOBAL EPIDEMIOLOGY OF INFECTIOUS DISEASES

Thomas A. Bell, M.D., M.P.H.

Assistant Professor of Pediatrics and Epidemiology, University of Washington Schools of Medicine and Public Health and Community Medicine, Seattle, Washington
SEXUALLY TRANSMITTED DISEASES
CHLAMYDIAL INFECTIONS: GENERAL PRINCIPLES
NONGONOCOCCAL URETHRITIS AND CERVICITIS
GONOCOCCAL INFECTIONS
CHANCROID

Stephen Berman, M.D.

Associate Professor of Pediatrics, University of Colorado School of Medicine; Director of Health Policy, University of Colorado Health Sciences, Denver, Colorado
VIRAL RESPIRATORY INFECTIONS

Robert E. Black, M.D., M.P.H.

Professor and Chairman, Department of International Health, The Johns Hopkins School of Hygiene and Public Health; Staff, The Johns Hopkins Hospital, Baltimore, Maryland
VIRAL DIARRHEAS

Robert W. Bradsher, M.D.

Director, Division of Infectious Diseases; Associate Professor of Medicine, School of Medicine, University of Arkansas for Medical Sciences; Little Rock, Arkansas
BLASTOMYCOSIS

Joel G. Breman, M.D., D.T.P.H.

Deputy Chief, Malaria Branch, Division of Parasitic Diseases, Center for Infectious Diseases, Centers for Disease Control, Atlanta, Georgia
VIRAL INFECTIONS WITH CUTANEOUS LESIONS

Joel D. Brown, M.D., D.T.M. & H., F.A.C.P.

Chief, Infectious Disease Service, Department of Medicine, Tripler Army Medical Center, Honolulu, Hawaii
PYOMYOSITIS

Alfred A. Buck, M.D., D.P.H., F.A.C.E.

Adjunct Professor of Immunology and Infectious Diseases, Johns Hopkins School of Hygiene and Public Health, Baltimore, Maryland; Visiting Professor of Medicine and Resident Scientist, Ain Shams University Faculty of Medicine, Cairo, Egypt
FILARIAL INFECTIONS: GENERAL PRINCIPLES
FILARIASIS

Danai Bunnag, M.D., D.T.M. & H., F.R.C.P.(T), M.R.C.P.

Head, Department of Clinical Tropical Medicine, Faculty of Tropical Medicine, Mahidol University; Director, Bangkok Hospital for Tropical Diseases, Bangkok, Thailand
INTESTINAL FLUKE INFECTIONS
LIVER FLUKE INFECTIONS
LUNG FLUKE INFECTIONS: PARAGONIMIASIS

Thanongsak Bunnag, M.D., D.P.H., D.T.M. & H., M.P.H. & T.M.

Professor of Tropical Medicine, Faculty of Tropical Medicine, Mahidol University, Bangkok, Thailand
GNATHOSTOMIASIS
ANGIOSTRONGYLUS MENINGITIS
INTESTINAL FLUKE INFECTIONS
LIVER FLUKE INFECTIONS
LUNG FLUKE INFECTIONS: PARAGONIMIASIS

Thomas Butler, M.D.

Professor of Medicine, School of Medicine; Chief of Infectious Diseases, Texas Tech University Health Sciences Center; Physician, University Medical Center, Lubbock, Texas
SPIROCHETAL INFECTIONS: GENERAL PRINCIPLES
RELAPSING FEVER
CAMPYLOBACTER ENTERITIS
YERSINIA ENTEROCOLITICA INFECTIONS
PLAGUE

Robert O. Cannon, M.D., M.P.H.

Medical Epidemiologist, Division of STD/HIV Prevention, Centers for Disease Control; Assistant Professor, Emory University School of Medicine, Atlanta, Georgia
HUMAN T-LYMPHOTROPIC VIRUS TYPE I INFECTION AND
ADULT T-CELL LEUKEMIAS/LYMPHOMAS
HTLV-I–ASSOCIATED MYELOPATHY/TROPICAL SPASTIC
PARAPARESIS (AM/TSP)

Jeffrey D. Chulay, M.D., D.T.M. & H.

Senior Investigator, Virology Division, U.S. Army Medical Research Institute of Infectious Diseases, Ft. Detrick, Frederick, Maryland; Associate Professor of Medicine and Biometrics and Preventive Medicine, Uniformed Services University of the Health Sciences, Bethesda, Maryland.
LEISHMANIASIS

Robert L. Colebunders, M.D.

Visiting Scientist, Division of HIV/AIDS, Center for Infectious Diseases, Centers for Disease Control, Atlanta, Georgia; Institut de Médecine Tropicale "Prince Leopold," Antwerp, Belgium
HUMAN IMMUNODEFICIENCY VIRUS INFECTIONS AND
AIDS

Gordon C. Cook, M.D., D.SC., F.R.C.P., F.R.A.C.P., F.L.S.

Senior Lecturer, Department of Medical Sciences, London School of Hygiene and Tropical Medicine, London, England
CRYPTOSPORIDIOSIS

George Davidson, D.SC.

Professor Emeritus, Department of Entomology, London School of Hygiene and Tropical Medicine, London, England
CONTROL OF ARTHROPODS OF MEDICAL IMPORTANCE

Kevin M. DeCock, M.D., D.T.M. & H., M.R.C.P.

Medical Epidemiologist, Division of HIV/AIDS, Centers for Disease Control, Atlanta, Georgia; Director, Projet RETRO-CI, Abidjan, Côte d'Ivoire, West Africa
HUMAN IMMUNODEFICIENCY VIRUS INFECTIONS AND
AIDS
HUMAN T-LYMPHOTROPIC VIRUS TYPE I INFECTION AND
ADULT T-CELL LEUKEMIAS/LYMPHOMAS
HTLV-I–ASSOCIATED MYELOPATHY/TROPICAL SPASTIC
PARAPARESIS (AM/TSP)

Joseph J. Drabick, M.D., M.A.C.P.

Assistant Professor of Medicine, Uniformed Services University of the Health Sciences, Bethesda, Maryland; Infectious Disease Service, Walter Reed Army Medical Center, Washington, D.C.
PENTASTOMIASIS

Brian O. L. Duke, C.B.E., M.D., SC.D., F.R.C.P.

Distinguished Scientist, Department of Infectious and Parasitic Diseases, Armed Forces Institute of Pathology, Washington, D.C.
LOIASIS
ONCHOCERCIASIS

Richard J. Duma, M.D., PH.D.

Professor of Medicine, Microbiology, and Pathology; Chief, Division of Infectious Diseases, Medical College of Virginia, Virginia Commonwealth University, Richmond, Virginia
FREE-LIVING AMEBIC INFECTIONS

Michael A. Dunn, M.D.

Associate Professor of Medicine, Uniformed Services University of the Health Sciences, Bethesda; Commanding Officer, U.S. Army Medical Research, Institute of Chemical Defense, Aberdeen Proving Ground, Maryland
HEPATOBILIARY DISEASES

Zoheir Farid, M.D., D.T.M. & H., F.A.C.P.

Consultant Physician, U.S. Naval Medical Research Unit No. 3 and Abbassia Fever Hospital, Cairo, Egypt
DIPHTHERIA

Evan R. Farmer, M.D.

Professor of Dermatology, The Johns Hopkins University School of Medicine, Baltimore, Maryland
DERMATOLOGIC DISEASES
DERMATITIS IN TRAVELERS

Susan P. Fisher-Hoch, M.D.

Deputy Branch Chief, Special Pathogens Branch, Division of Viral and Rickettsial Diseases, Centers for Disease Control, Atlanta, Georgia
LASSA FEVER
SOUTH AMERICAN HEMORRHAGIC FEVERS

Alan F. Fleming, M.D., F.R.C.P.

Professor of Pathology, School of Pathology, South African Institute for Medical Research and University of the Witwatersrand, Johannesburg, South Africa
HEMATOLOGIC DISEASES

Émile Fox, M.D., M.SC.C.T.M.

Research Assistant Professor, International Health Program, University of Maryland School of Medicine, Baltimore; WHO Adviser, Kigali, Rwanda
TUBERCULOSIS

Jacob K. Frenkel, M.D., PH.D.

Professor of Pathology, School of Medicine, University of Kansas Medical Center, Kansas City, Kansas
TOXOPLASMOSIS
OTHER TISSUE PROTOZOAN INFECTIONS

Marco Tulio A. Garcia-Zapata, M.SC., M.D., PH.D.

Visiting Professor and Associated Researcher of Nucleo de Medicina Tropical & Nutricáo, University of Brasilia, Brasilia, Brazil
AMERICAN TRYPANOSOMIASIS

Robert Goldsmith, M.D., M.P.H., D.T.M. & H.

Professor of Tropical Medicine, Department of Epidemiology and Biostatistics, University of California, San Francisco, School of Medicine; San Francisco, California
TREMATODE INFECTIONS: GENERAL PRINCIPLES
INTESTINAL FLUKE INFECTIONS
LIVER FLUKE INFECTIONS
LUNG FLUKE INFECTIONS: PARAGONIMIASIS

Brian M. Greenwood, M.D., F.R.C.P.

Director, Medical Research Council Laboratories, Fajara, Banjul, The Gambia, West Africa
MENINGOCOCCAL DISEASE
ACUTE BACTERIAL MENINGITIS

Duane J. Gubler, M.SC., SC.D.

Director, Division of Vector-Borne Infectious Diseases, Center for Infectious Diseases; Centers for Disease Control, Fort Collins, Colorado; Professor, Departments of International Health and Immunology, and Infectious Diseases, The Johns Hopkins School of Hygiene and Public Health, Baltimore, Maryland; Professor, Department of Microbiology, Colorado State University, Fort Collins, Colorado
INSECTS IN DISEASE TRANSMISSION

Richard L. Guerrant, M.D.

Thomas H. Hunter Professor of International Medicine; Head, Division of Geographic Medicine, Department of Medicine, University of Virginia Health Sciences Center, Charlottesville, Virginia
INTESTINAL NEMATODE INFECTIONS: GENERAL PRINCIPLES
INTESTINAL NEMATODES THAT MIGRATE THROUGH SKIN AND LUNG
DIARRHEA IN THE RETURNING TRAVELER

Roderick J. Hay, D.M., F.R.C.P., M.R.C.Path.

Professor of Cutaneous Medicine, United Medical and Dental Schools of Guys and St. Thomas Hospitals; Honorary Consultant Microbiologist, PHLS Mycological Reference Laboratory, London, England
NOCARDIOSIS
ACTINOMYCOSIS
CUTANEOUS MYCOSES
HISTOPLASMOSIS
PARACOCCIDIOIDOMYCOSIS
CRYPTOCOCCOSIS
SYSTEMIC OPPORTUNISTIC MYCOSES

Stephen L. Hoffman, M.D., D.T.M.H.

Director, Malaria Program, Naval Medical Research Institute, Bethesda, Maryland
TYPHOID FEVER

Walter T. Hughes, M.D.

Professor of Pediatrics, School of Medicine, University of Tennessee Center for Medical Sciences; Chairman, Department of Infectious Diseases, St. Jude Children's Research Hospital, Memphis, Tennessee
  PNEUMOCYSTOSIS

Derrick B. Jelliffe, M.D., D.C.H., D.T.M. & H., F.R.C.P.

Director, International Health Program; Professor of Public Health and Pediatrics, School of Public Health and Medicine, University of California, Los Angeles, California
  PROTEIN-ENERGY MALNUTRITION

E. F. Patrice Jelliffe, M.P.H., F.R.S.H.

Lecturer and Researcher, Population and Family Health Division, School of Public Health, University of California, Los Angeles, California
  PROTEIN-ENERGY MALNUTRITION

Elaine C. Jong, M.D.

Associate Professor, Department of Medicine, University of Washington School of Medicine; Director, Travel Medical Service, University of Washington Medical Center, Seattle, Washington
  ADVICE TO TRAVELERS

Benjamin Joseph, M.D., M.S., M.C.H.

Associate Professor of Orthopedics, Kasturba Medical College, Manipal, Karnataka State, India
  ORTHOPEDICS

Irving G. Kagan, PH.D.

Adjunct Professor, Department of Microbiology and Immunology, Emory University School of Medicine; Director, Parasitic Disease Consultants, Atlanta, Georgia
  PARASITIC IMMUNODIAGNOSIS

Samuel G. Kahn, PH.D.

Office of Nutrition, U.S. Agency for International Development, Washington, D.C.
  IRON DEFICIENCY

Jay S. Keystone, M.D., F.R.C.P.(C), M.SC. C.T.M.

Associate Professor of Medicine and Microbiology, University of Toronto School of Medicine; Director, Tropical Disease Unit, Toronto General Hospital, Toronto, Ontario
  TROPICAL DISEASE IN A TEMPERATE CLIMATE: GENERAL
    PRINCIPLES
  DIARRHEA IN THE RETURNING TRAVELER
  EOSINOPHILIA IN TRAVELERS AND IMMIGRANTS

Michael E. Kilpatrick, M.D.

Commanding Officer, U.S. Naval Medical Research Unit 3, Cairo, Egypt
  TOXOCARIASIS

Karen L. Kotloff, M.D.

Assistant Professor of Pediatrics, Division of Infectious Disease and Tropical Pediatrics, University of Maryland School of Medicine, Baltimore, Maryland
  ENTERIC BACTERIAL INFECTIONS: GENERAL PRINCIPLES

F. Marc LaForce, M.D.

Professor of Medicine, University of Rochester School of Medicine and Dentistry, Physician-in-Chief, Department of Medicine, The Genesee Hospital, Rochester, New York
  POLIOMYELITIS

Michael C. Latham, M.D., O.B.E., M.B., M.P.H., D.T.M. & H., F.F.C.M.

Professor and Director, Program in International Nutrition, Division of Nutritional Sciences, Cornell University, Ithaca, New York
  NUTRITIONAL PROBLEMS AND DEFICIENCY DISEASES:
    GENERAL PRINCIPLES
  VITAMIN A DEFICIENCY AND XEROPHTHALMIA
  FLUORIDE, DENTAL CARIES, AND FLUOROSIS
  INFANT FEEDING AND WEANING PROBLEMS

Larry W. Laughlin, M.D., PH.D.

Commanding Officer, Naval Medical Research Institute, Bethesda, Maryland
  URINARY TRACT DISEASES

Myron M. Levine, M.D., D.T.P.H.

Professor of Medicine, Pediatrics, Epidemiology and Preventive Medicine and Microbiology and Immunology; Director, Center for Vaccine Development; Head, Division of Geographic Medicine, Department of Medicine; Head, Division of Infectious Diseases and Tropical Pediatrics, Department of Pediatrics, University of Maryland School of Medicine, Baltimore, Maryland
  SHIGELLOSIS
  DIARRHEA CAUSED BY ESCHERICHIA COLI

Robert N. Longfield, M.D., F.A.C.P.

Assistant Chief, Infectious Disease Service, Brooke Army Medical Center, Fort Sam Houston, Texas
  NONTYPHOIDAL SALMONELLA INFECTIONS
  ANTHRAX

William H. Lyerly, Jr., M.A., M.P.H.

Tropical/Infectious Diseases Officer and HIV/AIDS Coordinator, Health, Population, and Nutrition Division, Bureau for Africa, U.S. Agency for International Development, Washington, D.C.
GLOBAL EPIDEMIOLOGY OF INFECTIOUS DISEASES

Donald W. R. Mackenzie, B.V.SC., PH.D., M.R.C.V.S.

Chief, Mycology Reference Laboratory, Central Public Health Laboratories, London, England
NOCARDIOSIS
ACTINOMYCOSIS
THE MYCOSES: GENERAL PRINCIPLES
SUBCUTANEOUS MYCOSES

Shirley E. Maddison, PH.D.

Formerly, Director, Parasitology Diagnostic Laboratory, Parasitology Division, Center for Infectious Diseases, Centers for Disease Control, Atlanta, Georgia
PARASITIC IMMUNODIAGNOSIS

Andrew M. Margileth, M.D., F.A.A.P., F.A.C.P.

Professor and Vice Chairman, Department of Pediatrics, Uniformed Services University, Bethesda, Maryland
PERTUSSIS
CAT SCRATCH DISEASE

Edward K. Markell, PH.D., M.D.

Clinical Professor of Medicine and Tropical Medicine, University of California, San Francisco, School of Medicine; Clinical Professor of Family, Community and Preventive Medicine, Emeritus, Stanford University, Palo Alto, California
EXAMINATION OF STOOL SPECIMENS
EXAMINATION OF BLOOD, OTHER BODY FLUIDS AND TISSUES, SPUTUM, AND URINE
PRESERVATION AND SHIPMENT OF SPECIMENS

Sheldon M. Markowitz, M.D., F.A.C.P.

Professor, Departments of Medicine and Microbiology and Immunology, Medical College of Virginia School of Medicine, Virginia Commonwealth University; Chief, Infectious Diseases Section, Department of Veterans Affairs Medical Center, Richmond, Virginia
OTHER CLOSTRIDIAL INFECTIONS

Philip D. Marsden, O.B.E., M.D., F.R.C.P., D.T.M. & H.

Titled Professor of Medicine, Nucleo de Medicina Tropical & Nutricáo, University of Brasilia, Brasilia, Brazil
AMERICAN TRYPANOSOMIASIS

Joseph B. McCormick, M.S., M.D.

Chief, Special Pathogens Branch, Division of Viral and Rickettsial Diseases, Center for Infectious Diseases, Centers for Disease Control, Atlanta, Georgia
EBOLA AND MARBURG VIRUS INFECTIONS
CRIMEAN-CONGO HEMORRHAGIC FEVER (CCHF)
DISEASES CAUSED BY HANTAVIRUSES (HEMORRHAGIC FEVER WITH RENAL SYNDROME)

Patrick B. McGreevy, M.SC., PH.D.

Senior Investigator, Division of Experimental Therapeutics, Walter Reed Army Institute of Research, Washington, D.C.
AMERICAN TRYPANOSOMIASIS
LARVAL CESTODE INFECTIONS

Donald E. Meier, M.D.

Consultant Surgeon, Baptist Medical Centre, Ogbomoso, Nigeria; Staff Surgeon, Dallas Veterans Affairs Medical Center, Dallas, Texas
SURGERY

Wayne M. Meyers, M.D., PH.D., D.SC.(HON.)

Chief, Mycobacteriology, Department of Infectious and Parasitic Diseases Pathology, Armed Forces Institute of Pathology, Washington, D.C.
TROPICAL PHAGEDENIC ULCER
LEPROSY
ATYPICAL MYCOBACTERIAL SKIN INFECTIONS
STREPTOCERCIASIS
DIROFILARIASIS
CUTANEOUS LARVA MIGRANS

Karen Midthun, M.D.

Adjunct Assistant Professor of International Health and Pediatrics, The Johns Hopkins University School of Hygiene and Public Health and School of Medicine, Baltimore, Maryland
VIRAL DIARRHEAS

Thomas P. Monath, M.D., F.A.C.P.

Chief, Virology Division, U.S. Army Medical Research Institute of Infectious Diseases, Fort Detrick, Frederick, Maryland
VIRAL INFECTIONS: GENERAL PRINCIPLES
VIRAL FEBRILE ILLNESSES
VENEZUELAN EQUINE ENCEPHALITIS (VEE)
JAPANESE ENCEPHALITIS
ROCIO ENCEPHALITIS
OTHER ARBOVIRAL ENCEPHALITIDES
YELLOW FEVER
KYASANUR FOREST DISEASE

Pedro Morera, M.Q.C.

Professor of Medical Parasitology, School of Medicine, University of Costa Rica, San José, Costa Rica
ABDOMINAL ANGIOSTRONGYLIASIS

J. Glenn Morris, Jr., M.D., M.P.H. & T.M.

Associate Professor of Medicine and Epidemiology and Preventive Medicine, University of Maryland School of Medicine, Baltimore, Maryland
CHOLERA AND OTHER VIBRIOSES

K. Darwin Murrell, M.SC.P.H., PH.D.

Director, Midwest Area, Agricultural Research Service, U.S. Department of Agriculture, Peoria, Illinois
TRICHINOSIS

David R. Nalin, M.D., F.A.C.P.

Director, Clinical Research, Infectious Diseases, Merck, Sharp & Dohme Research Laboratories, West Point, Pennsylvania

ENTERIC BACTERIAL INFECTIONS: GENERAL PRINCIPLES
CHOLERA AND OTHER VIBRIOSES

Ronald C. Neafie, M.S.

Chief, Parasitic Disease Pathology Branch, Department of Infectious and Parasitic Diseases, Armed Forces Institute of Pathology, Washington, D.C.

TROPICAL PHAGEDENIC ULCER
PROTOTHECOSIS
STREPTOCERCIASIS
DIROFILARIASIS
CUTANEOUS LARVA MIGRANS

Ann Marie Nelson, M.D.

Chief, Pathology Unit, Project SIDA, Kinshasa, Zaire; Staff Pathologist, Registry of AIDS, American Registry of Pathology, Armed Forces Institute of Pathology, Washington, D.C.

PROTOTHECOSIS

George S. Nelson, M.D., D.SC., F.R.C.P. F.R.C. PATH., D.A.P. & E., D.T.M. & H.

Emeritus Professor of Parasitology, Liverpool School of Tropical Medicine, Liverpool, England

MISCELLANEOUS FILARIAL INFECTIONS: GENERAL PRINCIPLES
LARVAL CESTODE INFECTIONS

Charlotte G. Neumann, M.D., M.P.H.

Professor of Public Health and Pediatrics, University of California Schools of Public Health and Medicine, Los Angeles, California

INTERACTION OF NUTRITION AND INFECTION

Edward C. Oldfield III, M.D., F.A.C.P.

Head, Infectious Disease Division, Naval Hospital, San Diego; Clinical Associate Professor of Medicine, University of California, San Diego, School of Medicine, San Diego, California

COCCIDIOIDOMYCOSIS
TREATMENT OF THE DEEP MYCOSES

Tomoo Oshima, M.D.

Professor of Parasitology, School of Medicine, Yokohama City University, Yokohama, Japan

ANISAKIASIS

Charles N. Oster, M.D., F.A.C.P.

Chief, Infectious Diseases Service, Walter Reed Army Medical Center, Washington, D.C.

LEISHMANIASIS

B. O. Osuntokun, M.D., PH.D., D.SC., F.R.C.P.

Professor of Medicine (Neurology), College of Medicine, University of Ibadan, Ibadan, Nigeria

NEUROLOGIC DISEASES

Fred P. Paleologo, M.D., F.A.C.P.

Research Area Manager for Infectious Diseases, Naval Medical Research and Development Command, National Naval Medical Center, Bethesda, Maryland

PSITTACOSIS
LYME DISEASE

Mark A. Pallansch, PH.D.

Chief, Enterovirus Section, Division of Viral and Rickettsial Diseases, Centers for Disease Control, Atlanta, Georgia

ACUTE HEMORRHAGIC CONJUNCTIVITIS

Richard D. Pearson, M.D.

Professor of Medicine and Pathology, University of Virginia Health Sciences Center, Charlottesville, Virginia

INTESTINAL NEMATODE INFECTIONS: GENERAL PRINCIPLES
NEMATODES LIMITED TO THE INTESTINAL TRACT
INTESTINAL NEMATODES THAT MIGRATE THROUGH SKIN AND LUNG

Peter L. Perine, M.D., M.P.H.

Professor and Director, Division of Tropical Public Health, Department of Biometrics and Preventive Medicine; Uniformed Services University of the Health Sciences, Bethesda, Maryland

SEXUALLY TRANSMITTED DISEASES
LYMPHOGRANULOMA VENEREUM
NONGONOCOCCAL URETHRITIS AND CERVICITIS
SYPHILIS AND THE ENDEMIC TRIPONEMATOSES
GONOCOCCAL INFECTIONS
CHANCROID
GRANULOMA INGUINALE

J. Philpott, M.D., F.C.F.P.

Attending Physician, Galmi Hospital, Madaova, Niger Republic, West Africa

EOSINOPHILIA IN TRAVELERS AND IMMIGRANTS

Michael F. Rein, M.D.

Professor of Medicine, Division of Infectious Diseases, School of Medicine, University of Virginia Health Sciences Center, Charlottesville, Virginia

TRICHOMONIASIS

Daphne A. Roe, M.D.

Professor of Nutrition, Division of Nutritional Sciences, Cornell University, Ithaca, and Cornell Medical College, New York; Adjunct Professor, State University of New York Health Sciences Center, Syracuse, New York

BERIBERI
SCURVY
RICKETS AND OSTEOMALACIA
PELLAGRA
ARIBOFLAVINOSIS
NUTRITIONAL MACROCYTIC (MEGALOBLASTIC) ANEMIA
DRUG AND NUTRIENT INTERACTIONS

Trenton K. Ruebush II, M.D.

Medical Epidemiologist, Malaria Branch, Division of Parasitic Diseases, Center for Infectious Diseases, Centers for Disease Control, Atlanta, Georgia; on Assignment to Nairobi, Kenya
BABESIOSIS
VECTOR TRANSMISSION OF DISEASES: GENERAL
    PRINCIPLES
ZOONOSES

Jay P. Sanford, M.D., M.A.C.P.

President and Professor of Medicine, Uniformed Services University of the Health Sciences; Dean, F. Edward Hébert School of Medicine, Bethesda, Maryland
TULAREMIA
PSEUDOMONAS INFECTIONS

Joseph D. Schwartzman, M.D.

Associate Professor of Pathology and Medicine, Departments of Pathology and Medicine; University of Virginia School of Medicine; Associate Director of Clinical Microbiology, University of Virginia Hospitals, Charlottesville, Virginia
INTESTINAL NEMATODE INFECTIONS: GENERAL PRINCIPLES
NEMATODES LIMITED TO THE INTESTINAL TRACT
INTESTINAL NEMATODES THAT MIGRATE THROUGH LUNG
    (ASCARIASIS)

Roger Shrimpton, PH.D.

Research Associate and Professor of Nutrition, Division of Nutritional Sciences, Cornell University, Ithaca, New York
ZINC AND OTHER TRACE ELEMENT DEFICIENCIES

William A. Sodeman, Jr., M.D.

Associate Dean for Academic Affairs and Professor of Medicine, Louisiana State University School of Medicine in Shreveport, Shreveport, Louisiana
POISONOUS PLANTS AND FISH
ANIMALS HAZARDOUS TO HUMANS: GENERAL PRINCIPLES
VENOMOUS MARINE ANIMALS
BATS
MOLLUSKS INVOLVED IN DISEASE TRANSMISSION

Alfred Sommer, M.D., M.H.S.

Professor of Ophthalmology, Epidemiology and International Health, The Johns Hopkins School of Medicine and Hygiene and Public Health; Dean, School of Hygiene and Public Health, The Johns Hopkins University; Ophthalmologist, The Johns Hopkins Hospital, Baltimore, Maryland
OPHTHALMOLOGIC DISEASES

Daniel E. Sonenshine, PH.D.

Professor, Department of Biological Sciences, Old Dominion University, Norfolk, Virginia
TICKS AND MITES IN DISEASE TRANSMISSION

Harrison C. Spencer, M.D., M.P.H., D.T.M. & H.

Chief, Parasitic Diseases Branch, Division of Parasitic Diseases, Center for Infectious Diseases, Centers for Disease Control, Atlanta, Georgia
AFRICAN TRYPANOSOMIASIS
DRACUNCULIASIS

John B. Stanbury, M.D.

Emeritus Professor of Experimental Medicine, Massachusetts Institute of Technology, Cambridge, Massachusetts
GOITER AND IRON DEFICIENCY DISORDERS

Mark C. Steinhoff, M.D.

Associate Professor, Department of International Health, The Johns Hopkins School of Hygiene and Public Health; Associate Professor, Department of Pediatrics, The Johns Hopkins School of Medicine, Baltimore, Maryland
PULMONARY DISEASES

Lani S. Stephenson, M.N.S., PH.D.

Associate Professor of International Nutrition, Division of Nutritional Sciences, Cornell University, Ithaca, New York
INTERACTION OF NUTRITION AND INFECTION

G. Thomas Strickland, M.D., PH.D., D.C.M.T., F.A.C.P.

Professor of Epidemiology and Preventive Medicine and Microbiology and Immunology; Professor and Director, International Health Program. University of Maryland School of Medicine, Baltimore, Maryland
PROTOZOAL INFECTIONS: GENERAL PRINCIPLES
MALARIA
HELMINTHIC INFECTIONS: GENERAL PRINCIPLES
SCHISTOSOMIASIS
FEVER IN TRAVELERS

Herbert B. Tanowitz, M.D.

Professor of Medicine and Pathology, Albert Einstein College of Medicine; Associate Director of Parasitic and Tropical Disease Laboratory, Bronx Municipal Hospital Center, Bronx, New York
CESTODE INFECTIONS: GENERAL PRINCIPLES
TAPEWORM INFECTIONS
DISEASES OF IMMIGRANTS

John Tarpley, M.D.

Consultant Surgeon, Baptist Medical Centre, Ogbomoso, Nigeria; Associate Lecturer in Surgery, College of Medicine, University of Ibadan, Ibadan, Nigeria; Assistant Professor of Surgery, The Johns Hopkins University School of Medicine, Baltimore, Maryland
SURGERY

Hugh R. Taylor, M.D., F.R.A.C.S.

Professor and Chairman, Department of Ophthalmology, University of Melbourne; Director of Eye Services, Royal Victorian Eye and Ear Hospital, Melbourne, Victoria, Australia
OPHTHALMOLOGIC DISEASES
CHLAMYDIAL INFECTIONS: GENERAL PRINCIPLES
TRACHOMA AND INCLUSION CONJUNCTIVITIS
ONCHOCERCIASIS

Jean-Claude Theis, M.D., M.C.H., F.R.C.S.

Senior Lecturer, Orthopedic Surgery, University of Otago, Dunedin, New Zealand
ORTHOPEDICS

Frederick L. Trowbridge, M.D., M.SC.

Director, Division of Nutrition, Center for Chronic Disease Prevention and Health Promotion, Centers for Disease Control; Associate Professor, Emory University School of Public Health, Atlanta, Georgia
GOITER AND IRON DEFICIENCY DISORDERS

David A. Warrell, M.A., D.M., D.SC., F.R.C.P.

Professor of Tropical Medicine and Infectious Diseases, Faculty of Medicine, University of Oxford, Oxford, England
RABIES AND RELATED VIRUSES
SNAKES

M. J. Warrell, M.B., F.R.C.P.

RABIES AND RELATED VIRUSES

George Watt, M.D., D.T.M. & H.

Chief, Department of Medicine, Armed Forces Research Institute of Medical Sciences, Bangkok, Thailand
LEPTOSPIROSIS

Louis M. Weiss, M.D., M.P.H.

Assistant Professor of Medicine and Pathology, Albert Einstein College of Medicine, Bronx Municipal Hospital Center, Bronx, New York
DISEASES OF IMMIGRANTS

F. Stephen Wignall, M.D.

Officer-in-Charge, U.S. Naval Environmental and Preventive Medicine Unit 6, Pearl Harbor, Hawaii
BARTONELLOSIS

Robert A. Wirtz, PH.D.

Research Investigator, Division of Entomology, Walter Reed Army Institute of Research, Washington, D.C.; Adjunct Associate Professor, Department of Preventive Medicine and Biometrics, Uniformed Services University of Health Sciences, Bethesda; Department of Microbiology and Immunology, University of Maryland School of Medicine, Baltimore, Maryland
INJURIOUS ARTHROPODS

Charles L. Wisseman, Jr., M.D.

Emeritus Professor of Microbiology and Immunology, University of Maryland School of Medicine, Baltimore, Maryland
RICKETTSIAL INFECTIONS: GENERAL PRINCIPLES
THE TYPHUS GROUP
THE SPOTTED FEVER GROUP
SCRUB TYPHUS
Q FEVER
MISCELLANEOUS RICKETTSIAL INFECTIONS

Murray Wittner, M.D., PH.D.

Professor of Pathology and Parasitology, Albert Einstein College of Medicine; Director of Parasitic and Tropical Disease Laboratory, Bronx Municipal Hospital Center, Bronx, New York
CESTODE INFECTIONS: GENERAL PRINCIPLES
TAPEWORM INFECTIONS
DISEASES OF IMMIGRANTS

Martin S. Wolfe, M.D., D.C.M.T.

Director, Traveler's Medical Clinic; Clinical Professor of Medicine, George Washington University School of Medicine; Clinical Associate Professor of Medicine, Georgetown University School of Medicine, Washington, D.C.
AMEBIASIS
MISCELLANEOUS INTESTINAL PROTOZOA

Stephen G. Wright, M.B., D.C.M.T., M.R.C.P.

Senior Lecturer, Department of Clinical Sciences, London School of Hygiene and Tropical Medicine, London, England
GASTROINTESTINAL DISEASES
BRUCELLOSIS
GIARDIASIS

John L. Ziegler, M.D.

Associate Chief of Staff for Education, and Director, AIDS Clinical Research Center, Veterans Affairs Medicine Center; Professor of Medicine, University of California, San Francisco, School of Medicine, San Francisco, California
MALIGNANT DISEASES

Arie J. Zuckerman, M.D., D.SC., F.R.C.P., F.R.C. PATH.

Dean and Professor of Microbiology, The Royal Free Hospital School of Medicine; Director, WHO Collaborating Centre for Reference and Research on Viral Diseases, London, England
VIRAL HEPATITIS

Preface

Hunter's Tropical Medicine grew out of a World War II Army Medical School tropical and military medicine course taught at the Walter Reed Army Medical Center in Washington, D.C. The first edition, entitled *A Manual of Tropical Medicine,* was published in 1945 by three of the course instructors, Colonel Thomas T. Mackie, Major George W. Hunter III, and Captain C. Brooke Worth. The second edition, by the same authors, was published in 1954. Colonel George Hunter, the "glue" that held the book together, was joined by coauthors from the Louisiana State University School of Medicine, for the third, fourth, and fifth editions published in 1960, 1966, and 1976. I acknowledged Colonel Hunter's contribution by adding his name to the title of the sixth edition, published in 1984. The extensive involvement by members of the Army and Navy and the Public Health Service has continued in the seventh edition. The uniformed services have provided practical experience and research opportunities in tropical and subtropical climates.

The sixth edition of *Hunter's Tropical Medicine* was an entirely new book. Only two chapters were revisions of old ones: "Ticks and Mites in Disease Transmission" by the late Harry Hoogstraal, and "Intestinal Nematode Infections" by Herbert M. Gilles. Almost all the authors were new. Only Charles L. Wisseman, who continues to write the best textbook chapters on rickettsial infections, joined Dr. Hoogstraal as a carry-over from the fifth edition. They and the other 84 contributors helped prepare a complete and detailed textbook of clinical tropical medicine.

In the new seventh edition of *Hunter's Tropical Medicine,* some new chapters have been added: orthopedics in the tropics, human immunodeficiency and leukemia virus infections, cat-scratch fever, and eosinophilia in travelers and immigrants. Some diseases have been promoted from subchapters to separate chapters, e.g., Lyme disease, cryptosporidiosis, African trypanosomi-asis, and American trypanosomiasis. Many chapters were extensively revised; others, on careful review, required only updating.

A major effort has been given to two Parts that were new to the sixth edition: "Clinical Practice in the Tropics" and "Tropical Diseases in a Temperate Climate." These topics are of vital interest to those who either practice medicine in the tropics or see patients who travel or live in developing countries. They provide the outline for courses in clinical tropical medicine in my institution and elsewhere. Stephen G. Wright, from the London School of Hygiene and Tropical Medicine, helped with the first section. Jay S. Keystone from Toronto, who has extensive experience in emporiatrics, assembled a strong and knowledgeable team of experts in traveler's medicine. The chapter "Global Epidemiology of Infectious Diseases," by Charles Beal and William H. Lyerly, Jr., presents organized and condensed information from the Global Epidemiology Working Group and other sources to provide up-to-date (1990) information on the geographic risks of acquiring infectious diseases. With this information the physician can advise travelers on appropriate preventive measures and can formulate a differential diagnosis in a patient who has traveled or lived in the tropics or subtropics.

Certain aspects of *Hunter's Tropical Medicine* have not changed. It remains the most detailed and comprehensive clinical tropical medicine textbook, having extensive sections on parasitic infections, nutritional deficiencies and tuberculosis, and the classic "tropical" diseases. Included also are other diseases either more common or having different presentations in developing countries, e.g., hepatitis virus A, B, C, and D infections, shigellosis; those that have been virtually eliminated from more developed countries but still cause considerable illness elsewhere, e.g., poliomyelitis, measles; and parasitic infections that are not specifically tropical, e.g., trichomoniasis, toxoplasmosis. Also included are infections transmitted by arthropods or with animal reservoirs, e.g., Lyme disease, Rocky Moutain spotted fever.

Hunter's Tropical Medicine is easy to read and use. A complete bibliography and a generous number of illustrations are provided. Medical problems are given a practical clinical approach. In Part I, "Clinical Practice in the Tropics," and Part XI, "Tropical Disease in a Temperate Climate," many of the same diseases are considered, but their manifestations in different locations and patients are dissimilar. It is important that the clinician understand the ecology and laboratory diagnosis of endemic infectious diseases. Hence, *Hunter's Tropical Medicine* has Parts on transmission of diseases and laboratory diagnostic methods for parasitic diseases. Although the book is written primarily for clinicians, it is hoped that nonclinicians and students will find it useful.

A special thanks is due Dr. Thomas P. Monath, who again did an excellent job of subediting the Part on viral infections, and to Drs. Stephen G. Wright, Michael C. Latham, and Jay S. Keystone, who subedited Parts on clinical practice in the tropics, nutritional deficiencies, and tropical diseases in a temperate climate, respectively. Drs. Donald Mackenzie and Roderick J. Hays updated the Part on the mycoses, and Dr. William A. Sodeman, Jr., updated important chapters on animals hazardous to man and mollusks involved in disease transmission. Dr. Edward K. Markell changed topics in this edition to write useful chapters on laboratory diagnostic methods for parasitic diseases.

Some contributors are new to this edition. In some cases, new contributors, after reviewing chapters in the sixth edition, decided that changes other than updating would be detrimental. I wish to thank the following contributors to the sixth edition who either were not involved in the seventh edition or prepared different chapters. In some cases their chapters were considered not to require extensive changes by the seventh edition contributors. These are: Elizabeth Barrett-Connor, John J. Dempsey, William A. Sodeman, Jr., William H. Crosby, Michael S. R. Hutt, Thomas W. Simpson, David R. W. Haddock (deceased), John C. Hume (deceased), Trevor J. Crofts, Glenn W. Geelhoed, E. T. W. Bowen (deceased), David R. Nalin, Zoheir Farid, John G. Bartlett, James W. Bass, Stephen G. Wright, Asim K. Dutt, William W. Stead, Daniel H. Connor, Harrison C. Spencer, P. E. Clinton Manson-Bahr, Herbert M. Gilles, David T. Dennis, Ralph Muller, Dean W. Gibson, Charles D. Mackenzie, Ronald C. Neafie, George S. Nelson, Larry W. Laughlin, Edward K. Markell, Anthony B. Bosworth, Phillip D. Marsden, Derrick B. Jelliffe, E. F. Patrice Jelliffe, S. G. Srikantia, Joseph S. Weiner (deceased), Kenneth J. Collins, Lawrence R. Rubel, Harry Hoogstraal (deceased), Martin S. Wolfe, William Crewe, and Herman Zaiman.

Once again, support from the publishing team at the W. B. Saunders Company was outstanding. My highly respected friend and colleague Albert Meier was replaced by the team of David H. Kilmer, Senior Developmental Editor, and John Dyson, Senior Medical Editor. Copy editor Constance Burton has smoothly and efficiently edited this edition.

G. THOMAS STRICKLAND

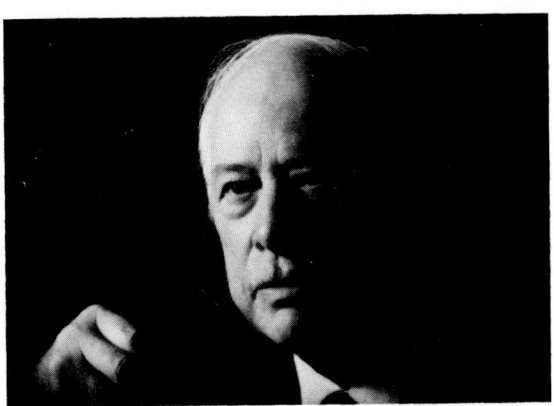

COLONEL GEORGE WILLIAM HUNTER III,
U.S. ARMY (Retired)
1902–1990

Colonel George William Hunter III passed away in San Diego on October 19 of complications from cancer. George was still active at the age of 88. Until recently he lectured on tropical medicine and worked in the University of California in San Diego traveler's clinic.

George Hunter was one of three authors of the first edition of this book, entitled *A Manual of Tropical Medicine,* which was published in 1945. He subsequently was the glue that held the book together as a coeditor of the next four editions. The fifth edition, *Tropical Medicine,* was published in 1976. George provided very useful advice while I was preparing the sixth edition, *Hunter's Tropical Medicine,* which was published in 1984. In the Foreword to that edition he wrote: "It was with the firm conviction that this author would insist on the high standards set by the previous editions that the reins were turned over completely to him." I suspect that he would have been critical but hope that he also would have been proud of the seventh edition.

Colonel Hunter had other accomplishments for which he will be remembered. He was Chief of the Department of Parasitology of the Army Medical School at the Walter Reed Army Institute of Research, where he taught tropical medicine to many military physicians and scientists during and shortly after World War II. At a subsequent post, as Chief of Medical Zoology of the 406th Medical-General Laboratory in Japan, George Hunter had an opportunity that few of us are afforded. He and American and Japanese colleagues were able to investigate and initiate efforts that led to the eradication of schistosomiasis japonica from that country. George Hunter's contribution to the control of schistosomiasis was honored by the Japanese, who erected a statue in his likeness in Kurume.

Contents

PART I
CLINICAL PRACTICE IN THE TROPICS

PART II
VIRAL INFECTIONS

PART III

BACTERIAL INFECTIONS

SECTION A

RICKETTSIAL INFECTIONS

SECTION B

CHLAMYDIAL INFECTIONS

SECTION C

SPIROCHETAL INFECTIONS

SECTION D

ENTERIC BACTERIAL INFECTIONS

SECTION E
BACTERIAL MENINGITIS

SECTION F
SEXUALLY TRANSMITTED BACTERIAL DISEASES

SECTION G
INFECTIONS WITH SMALL PLEOMORPHIC GRAM-NEGATIVE BACTERIA

SECTION H
MISCELLANEOUS BACTERIAL INFECTIONS

SECTION I
MYCOBACTERIAL INFECTIONS

PART IV
THE MYCOSES

PART V
PROTOZOAL INFECTIONS

SECTION A
INTESTINAL AND GENITAL INFECTIONS

SECTION B
INFECTIONS OF THE BLOOD AND
RETICULOENDOTHELIAL SYSTEM

SECTION C
TISSUE INFECTIONS

PART VI
HELMINTHIC INFECTIONS

SECTION A
INTESTINAL NEMATODE INFECTIONS

SECTION B
FILARIAL INFECTIONS

SECTION C
OTHER TISSUE NEMATODE INFECTIONS

SECTION D
TREMATODE INFECTIONS

SECTION E
CESTODE INFECTIONS

PART VII
POISONOUS AND TOXIC PLANTS AND ANIMALS

PART VIII
NUTRITIONAL PROBLEMS AND DEFICIENCY DISEASES

PART IX

VECTOR TRANSMISSION OF DISEASES

PART X
TROPICAL DISEASE IN A TEMPERATE CLIMATE

PART XI
LABORATORY DIAGNOSIS OF PARASITIC DISEASES

PART I

CLINICAL PRACTICE IN THE TROPICS

1. PULMONARY DISEASE

Mark C. Steinhoff

MAGNITUDE OF PROBLEM

In tropical regions, as elsewhere, respiratory infections are the most common illnesses encountered by health workers in clinics and hospital wards. The common mild upper respiratory infections of children are as frequent in tropical regions as in the temperate zones. However, the incidence and mortality of severe lower respiratory tract infections is increased by many fold in the tropics (Fig. 1–1).

Table 1–1 displays a ranking of the important causes of morbidity and mortality for Ghana, showing that childhood pneumonia ranks third, after malaria and measles; and adult pneumonia ranks twelfth—higher than neonatal tetanus, typhoid, meningitis, and hepatitis. These data underscore the importance of pneumonia in all age groups in developing countries. Pneumonia is a major cause of mortality among infants and children who live in developing countries, as it was in North America and Europe 75 to 100 years ago.

The incidence of pneumonia in North America in children less than 5 years of age is estimated at 10 to 50/1000/year; investigations of children in developing countries report pneumonia rates of 100 to 400/1000/year, with the highest rates in the first and second years of life. One study from Gambia noted an annual rate of 165 radiologically proven pneumonias per 1000 children less than 5 years of age. Admissions for respiratory diseases accounted for 17 to 24% of all hospital admissions in 5 African countries, with acute pneumonia exceeding tuberculosis in most of them. The higher incidence and increased severity of pneumonia in these regions may be due to the concatenation of risk factors frequently present in developing countries: low birth weight and malnutrition, changes in weaning practices, vitamin A deficiency, industrial and domestic air pollution, incomplete immunizations, poor access to medical treatment, and crowding and other effects of poverty. It is estimated that the global toll of acute pulmonary infections is 3 to 4 million infant and child deaths per year, or approximately one third of the total global infant and child mortality. The vast majority of these deaths occur in the developing regions.

Virtually all microorganisms can cause lower respiratory tract disease, but only a few, e.g., *Bordetella pertussis* and respiratory syncytial virus, cause syndromes distinct enough to enable diagnosis on clinical grounds. Although the etiologic spectrum of pulmonary infections is wider in developing countries than in developed regions, the availability of diagnostic technology is more limited. If the microbial etiology is known, treatment is straightforward. In the usual clinical situation, however, a treatment decision must be made before the etiologic data are available.

PNEUMONIA

ETIOLOGY. Investigations using pulmonary needle aspiration of children hospitalized with pneumonia have shown that 50 to 60% had bacteria isolated and approximately 20% had viruses isolated. The common bacterial isolates were *Streptococcus pneumoniae, Haemophilus influenzae,* and *Staphylococcus aureus.* Among the viruses, respiratory syncytial virus (RSV) and influenza and parainfluenza viruses accounted for 60% of all viral isolates from lung aspirates, with adenoviruses, enteroviruses, and herpes virus constituting the remainder. Numerous investigations of the virology of lower respiratory tract illness in children show that RSV is the single most important agent (Chapter 17). One study from Papua New Guinea suggests the possible importance of *Pneumocystis carinii* (Chapter 79), *Chlamydia trachomatis* (III B, General Principles), cytomegalovirus (CMV), and *Mycoplasma pneumoniae* in infant pneumonia.

Though clinicians in the tropics recognize epidemics of the influenza syndrome, most hospital and clinic surveys of ill children show low isolation rates of influenza virus. However, seroepidemiologic surveys from Africa confirm the importance of this virus. Data from Kenya and the Gambia over a single epidemic season show primary infection rates of 30 to 50% in children under 5 years of age, with similar rates in older children and adults.

MICROBIOLOGIC DIAGNOSIS. Determining a specific microbiologic etiology for lower respiratory disease is problematic. Sputum for Gram stain and culture is not available from infants and in adults may reveal oral flora that are unrelated to the pneumonia. Blood culture is positive in only 20% of lung aspirate–proven bacterial pneumonias. Needle aspiration of the affected pulmonary tissue is regarded as the diagnostic gold standard, yet it may be falsely negative in up to 20% of blood culture–positive cases.

There is an urgent need for better noninvasive tests for the diagnosis of bacterial pulmonary disease. Detection of bacterial antigen in blood or urine with commercial latex agglutination kits appears to be sensitive and specific in invasive *H. influenzae* type b infections, including pneumonia. The performance of similar commercial tests for *S. pneumoniae* antigens is not satisfactory.

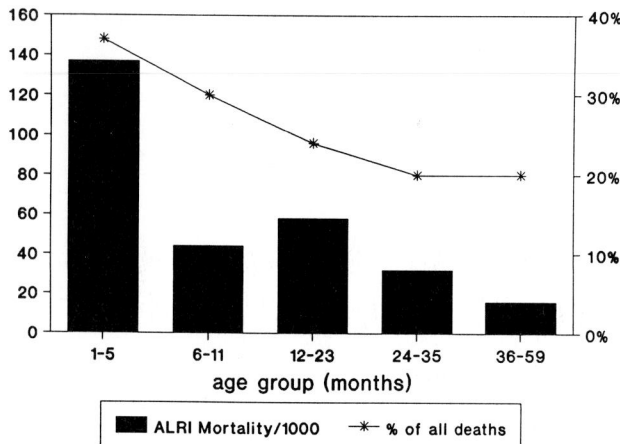

FIGURE 1–1. Acute lower respiratory infection (ALRI)–specific mortality rates, and proportionate mortality of ALRI in Bangladeshi children, by age. The left vertical axis denotes mortality per 1000 per year and the right axis denotes the proportion of all deaths. These data are from Teknaf, Bangladesh. (From Spika JS, et al: Ann Trop Pediatr 9:33, 1989.)

For hospitalized patients, a blood culture and Gram stain of an adequate sputum sample (with ≥25 neutrophils, ≤10 epithelial cells/high-power field) or an antigen detection test is recommended to guide therapy.

RADIOLOGY. Although radiologic investigation may not be available or feasible for every patient, it should be used in the evaluation of hospitalized patients or those who do not improve on standard therapeutic regimens.

INITIAL CLINICAL MANAGEMENT. Since the microbial etiology of pneumonia is rarely ascertained, presumptive treatment must be decided on the basis of the clinical information available at initial presentation. An approach to pneumonia based on age is presented in Table 1–2 to aid initial management (Chapter 17). Since it is not possible to distinguish viral from bacterial disease by clinical signs or simple laboratory tests, antibiotic therapy is advocated for all but mild cases, even though many cases of pneumonia may be caused by viruses. If the bacterial etiology is determined from blood or sputum culture, therapy should be changed to the most appropriate agent.

Newborns and Young Infants. Newborns are most likely to have pneumonia due to enteric or genital tract gram-negative organisms, group B streptococci, or viruses acquired from the mother. Broad-spectrum antibiotic management is required to treat these organisms (Table 1–2). Pneumonia in infants beyond the second month may be caused by the organisms listed previously or by *S. pneumoniae, H. influenzae,* or viruses. Infection with *C. trachomatis* is associated with an afebrile pneumonia syndrome in young infants that will not respond to the foregoing treatment regimen. Erythromycin should be used to treat *C. trachomatis* infections.

Older Infants and Children. Pneumonia in infants and children from 2 months to 5 years is associated with viruses, *S. pneumoniae,* and *H. influenzae.* In this age group, RSV is the most common cause of lower respiratory infections. The differentiation of pneumonia and bronchiolitis caused by RSV is often difficult. Infants and children who are not seriously ill can be adequately treated as outpatients with oral trimethoprim-sulfamethoxazole or amoxicillin. A simplified case management approach to childhood lower respiratory tract infections has been advocated by the World Health Organization (WHO). A simplified version is presented in Figure

TABLE 1–1. Disease Problems of Ghana—Ranked in Order of Days of Healthy Life Lost

Rank Order	Disease	Days of Healthy Life Lost*	Percentage of Total
1	Malaria	32,600	10.2
2	Measles	23,400	7.3
3	Childhood pneumonia	18,600	5.8
4	Sickle cell disease	17,500	5.5
5	Malnutrition (severe)	17,500	5.5
6	Prematurity	16,800	5.2
7	Birth injury	16,400	5.2
8	Accidents	14,900	4.7
9	Gastroenteritis	14,500	4.5
10	Tuberculosis	11,000	3.5
11	Cerebrovascular disease	10,400	3.3
12	Adult pneumonia	9,100	2.9
13	Neonatal tetanus	6,900	2.2
14	Cirrhosis	6,600	2.1
15	Congenital malformations	6,000	1.9
16	Complications of pregnancy	5,900	1.8
17	Hypertension	5,100	1.6
18	Intestinal obstruction	4,900	1.6
19	Typhoid	4,800	1.5
20	Meningitis	4,600	1.5
21	Hepatitis	4,600	1.5
22	Pertussis	4,600	1.5
23	Other birth diseases	4,600	1.5
24	Adult tetanus	4,500	1.4
25	Schistosomiasis	4,400	1.4
	Total of first 25 diseases	270,200	94.9

*Per 1000 persons per year
From Ghana Health Assessment Project Team, 1981.

OUTPATIENT MANAGEMENT ALGORITHM FOR A CHILD WITH COUGH OR DIFFICULTY BREATHING*

Cough or difficult breathing, without other signs of illness
Symptomatic treatment at home

Cough or difficult breathing with rapid respiration (≥50 breaths per minute if 2 to 12 months; ≥ 40 breaths per minute if 1 to 4 years)
Treat with antibiotic at home

Cough or difficult breathing plus chest indrawing (subcostal retractions)
Treat with antibiotic and refer to hospital

*Suggested for use by first-level health workers to manage children 2 months to 5 years of age.

FIGURE 1–2. Suggested treatment algorithm for infants and children 2 months to 5 years of age. (Modified from WHO, 1990.)

1–2. The accuracy of this algorithm in the prediction of physician-diagnosed pneumonia is quite high, with both sensitivity and specificity exceeding 80%. Use of simplified case-management algorithms by village health workers has reduced childhood respiratory mortality by 15 to 50% in community trials in Asia and Africa.

The child with more severe illness should be admitted to the hospital for therapy with chloramphenicol. Infants and children who do not improve with initial therapy may have staphylococci or other bacteria resistant to first-line antibiotic therapy; therefore, a combination of antibiotics (a penicillinase-resistant semisynthetic penicillin plus an aminoglycoside) is required for treatment. All severely malnourished children with pneumonia are at high risk of mortality and also should be treated with this combination of antibiotics. An important aspect of the supportive care of severe pneumonia is the provision of oxygen. Oxygen by nasal catheter or cannula is essential for infants and young children, especially those with pneumonia or bronchiolitis.

Older Children and Adults. The common causes of pneumonia in children older than 6 years and in adults are pneumococci, mycoplasmas, and viruses. Oral ampicillin or amoxicillin or erythromycin is adequate therapy for outpatient management. Severely ill inpatients should receive parenteral therapy designed to treat pneumococci, *H. influenzae,* and staphylococci (Table 1–2).

Lobar Pneumonia

Community-acquired classic pneumococcal lobar pneumonia remains common in the tropics, a situation similar to the preantibiotic era in North America. The typical patient is a previously healthy young adult. In addition to the classic signs of fever, tachypnea, and a cough productive of purulent or rusty sputum, a tender and enlarged liver (in 60%), jaundice (in 20%), myalgia (in 68%), and diarrhea (in 25%) have been described as presenting symptoms in Nigerian patients with lobar pneumonia. Presumptive therapy with penicillin is necessary and adequate for pneumococcal lobar pneumonia. Single-dose, three-dose, and other shortened penicillin regimens have been as effective as the traditional 5- to 7-day course of therapy in adults and older children. In Nigeria, 30% of patients with lobar pneumonia who eventually responded to penicillin therapy remained febrile for 3 or more days.

Pneumococcal strains resistant to penicillin are described from the Pacific, Asia, and Africa. They are more common in patients who have been previously hospitalized or treated with penicillins. Treatment with erythromycin, vancomycin, or rifampin is advised when penicillin-resistant pneumococci are suspected or when penicillin therapy is not successful. Otherwise, if no response is noted with the initial therapy, antibiotics for penicillin-resistant *S. aureus* and gram-negative organisms must be used; a penicillinase-resistant semisynthetic penicillin and chloramphenicol are suggested. Other organisms have been associated with lobar pneumonia, notably *M. tuberculosis* (Chapter 61), *Klebsiella* species, and *S. aureus. Mycoplasma pneumoniae* was present in 17% of lobar pneumonia cases in Nigeria.

TABLE 1–2. Suggested Initial Therapy for Acute Pneumonia, by Age Group

Age Group	Common Agents	Initial Empirical Therapy	
		Outpatient	*Inpatient*
0–2 months	Enteric bacilli Group B streptococcus *S. pneumoniae* H. influenzae C. trachomatis *S. aureus* Viruses	Not appropriate*	Ampicillin plus aminoglycoside PRSP† if *S. aureus suspected* Erythromycin if *C. trachomatis* suspected
3 months–5 years	*S. pneumoniae* H. influenzae *S. aureus* Viruses	TMP/SMX‡ or amoxicillin	Chloramphenicol PRSP plus aminoglycoside if *S. aureus* suspected
6 years–adult	*S. pneumoniae* H. influenzae *S. aureus* Mycoplasma Viruses	Ampicillin, or amoxicillin, or erythromycin	Penicillin G PRSP if *S. aureus* suspected

*Most young infants with pneumonia should be admitted for parenteral therapy.
†PRSP = penicillinase-resistant synthetic penicillin (e.g., methicillin, cloxacillin, flucloxacillin)
‡TMP/SMX = trimethoprim-sulfamethoxazole.

Atypical Pneumonia

Atypical pneumonia describes a syndrome that is distinct from the acute lobar pneumonia syndrome. Usually, an older child or young adult presents with an illness of gradual onset and with constitutional symptoms of fever and malaise that are more marked than the respiratory symptoms; cough is often minimal with little sputum production. The causes of the atypical pneumonia syndrome include *M. tuberculosis* (Chapter 61), mycoplasmas, influenza viruses A and B, adenovirus, and RSV. *Chlamydia* pneumonia (III B, General Principles) and *Legionella pneumophila* (III B, General Principles) have been reported in this syndrome in developed societies and may also be important in developing regions. Erythromycin or trimethoprim-sulfamethoxazole is the recommended empirical therapy for adults with mild illness. Older children and adults who develop pneumonia after an influenza-like syndrome should be managed with penicillinase-resistant penicillin because of the possibility of staphylococcal disease.

DIFFERENTIAL DIAGNOSIS. The spectrum of differential diagnoses of pneumonia of the nonlobar type is very broad in trcpical regions; the major causative organisms are discussed below (also see Chapter 17 for viral causes).

Bacteria. *Salmonella typhi* not infrequently causes a bronchitis and also has been associated with a nonspecific bronchopneumonia (Chapter 38). The pneumonic form of plague should be considered when a severe, rapidly progressive bronchopneumonia is encountered in the regions endemic for *Yersinia pestis* in Asia and Africa. The bronchopneumonia may occur without buboes, is characterized by watery and bloody sputum, and has a high fatality rate unless antibiotic therapy is begun early in the course of disease with streptomycin or tetracycline (Chapter 47). A sputum Gram stain can be useful for diagnosis. About half of patients with leptospirosis have pulmonary disease with cough, hemoptysis, and patchy bronchopneumonia on radiograph (Chapter 35). Pulmonary disease caused by the soil saprophyte *Pseudomonas pseudomallei* is infrequently seen in residents or travelers in Southeast Asia. Melioidosis may present as an acute upper lobe pneumonitis or as chronic cavitary disease (Chapter 56.2).

Protozoa. Parasitic infections may be associated with pulmonary findings. Falciparum malaria infrequently causes a pneumonia-like syndrome of high fever and bloody sputum, with patchy infiltrates on radiography (Chapter 73). Hepatic abscess caused by *Entamoeba histolytica* may be associated with pneumonitis or pleural effusion due to sympathetic inflammation or to direct extension through the diaphragm. One should consider amebiasis when confronted with right-sided lower lobe disease or right-sided pleural fluid of obscure origin. (Fig. 1–3; Chapter 68). Although reported more frequently from developed countries, *Pneumocystis carinii* has been associated with illness in malnourished and immunosuppressed patients in tropical countries. It is characterized by nonspecific clinical findings and a diffuse alveolar or interstitial pneumonitis on radiograph (Chapter 79).

Helminths. Metazoan parasites may cause pulmonary

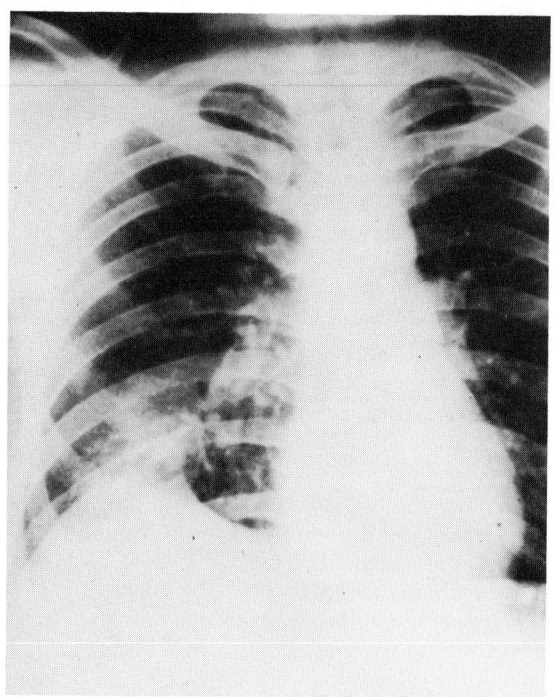

FIGURE 1–3. Amebic liver abscess with pulmonary extension. (Courtesy of Dr. E. Barrett-Connor.)

disease by at least 3 mechanisms: (1) during the obligatory migration of larvae from the gut through the pulmonary capillaries to the alveoli and back to the gut, (e.g., ascariasis, strongyloidiasis, and hookworm infections); (2) by passage through the pulmonary vasculature as part of a blood-borne stage of the parasite's life cycle (e.g., schistosomiasis, filariasis); and (3) by residence of the adult or cyst form in pulmonary tissue (e.g., paragonimiasis, echinococcosis).

Pulmonary paragonimiasis is often asymptomatic but in the endemic regions of West Africa, Asia, and the Americas may present with chronic persistent cough with intermittent hemoptysis. Sputum or feces may reveal *Paragonimus westermani* eggs (Fig. VID–2C and Chapter 99), and radiographs may demonstrate peripheral or cystic nodular lesions (Figs. 1–4 and 99–5).

The lung is second only to the liver as the most common site for the hydatid cysts of *Echinococcus granulosus*. These may be associated with chronic cough, dyspnea, and hemoptysis. Chest radiograph classically reveals one or more round "cannonball" shadows (Figs. 1–5 and 101–8). Peripheral eosinophilia may or may not be present (Chapter 101.2).

Measles-associated Pneumonia. Up to 25% of all childhood pneumonia in developing countries may be associated with measles, and pneumonia is the most frequent complication of measles infection (Chapter 16.1). Pneumonia occurring with the measles rash is likely to be primary measles giant-cell pneumonia. Pneumonia that has its onset after the rash has faded may be associated with bacteria (e.g., *S. pneumoniae*, *H. influenzae*, *S. aureus*, *Klebsiella*, *Pseudomonas*, and other gram-negative bacilli) or viruses (e.g., herpes simplex, adenovirus). Because of the high case-fatality of measles-associated pneumonia and the probability of bacte-

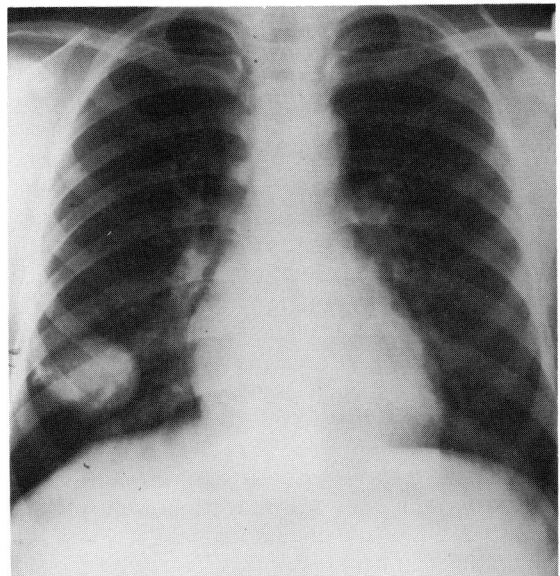

FIGURE 1–4. Pulmonary paragonimiasis. (Courtesy of Dr. E. Barrett-Connor.)

rial etiology, these children should be admitted for inpatient therapy with broad-spectrum antibiotics.

Eosinophilic Pneumonia Syndromes. Tropical pulmonary eosinophilia is associated with the host response to filarial infections *(Wuchereria bancrofti* and *Brugia malayi);* it is seen mostly in the Indian subcontinent, although it has also been reported from Africa and the Americas. The disease occurs more often in males and is characterized by a persistent cough and wheezing of insidious onset associated with a striking eosinophilia (Chapter 85.4). There is usually little systemic disturbance, but low-grade fever is common. The cough is often worse at night and is not productive of sputum. Physical examination reveals minimal pulmonary findings, hepatosplenomegaly, and generalized lymphadenopathy. Radiography shows diffuse coarse interstitial

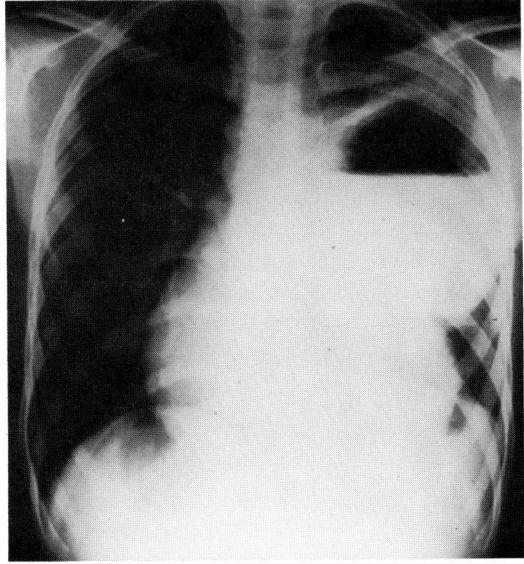

FIGURE 1–5. Ruptured pulmonary hydatid cyst. (Courtesy of Dr. E. Barrett-Connor.)

infiltrates and hilar lymphadenopathy. The absolute eosinophil count often exceeds 4000/mm³. This syndrome must be distinguished from other eosinophilic pulmonary syndromes; this is generally not difficult, given the geographic regions of occurrence and the rapid clinical and radiologic response to therapy with diethylcarbamazine.

The migration of parasite larvae from pulmonary capillaries to alveoli may be associated with a short-lived syndrome of pulmonary symptoms, transient radiologic infiltrates, and moderate peripheral eosinophilia, sometimes referred to as Löffler's syndrome. *Ascaris, Necator,* or *Ancylostoma* larvae may be present in sputum (Chapters 83 and 84.1). Immunocompromised hosts may have severe pulmonary disease and eosinophilia caused by *Strongyloides stercoralis* (Chapter 84.2). Acute infections with *Schistosoma mansoni* and *S. japonicum* may produce an acute eosinophilic syndrome caused by the passage of schistosomula through the pulmonary vasculature, with diffuse nodules on radiography (Chapter 96). The migration of the ascarid larvae of *Toxocara canis* and *T. cati* in pulmonary tissue as a manifestation of visceral larva migrans may be associated with hepatosplenomegaly, transient reticular radiographic infiltrates, and eosinophilia (Chapter 91).

Pneumonia in HIV-infected Persons

Because HIV depletes CD4+ helper T lymphocytes and is associated with functional abnormalities of B lymphocytes, opportunistic pneumonia is a frequent occurrence in HIV-infected persons (Chapter 15.1). In North America, these pulmonary infections constitute most of the AIDS-defining illnesses and cause a major proportion of mortality. There are meager data on the causes of opportunistic infections in tropical settings with limited diagnostic facilities. *M. tuberculosis* reactivation or infection is frequently reported in AIDS patients in Africa (Chapter 61.1). Unlike North America, where *P. carinii* pneumonia occurs in up to 80% of all AIDS patients, this organism has been described less frequently in people with AIDS in Africa and Asia. An increased incidence of pneumonia due to *S. pneumoniae* and *H. influenzae* has been reported in patients with AIDS in North America as well as increased rates of CMV infection, cryptococcosis, and pulmonary and systemic infection with the *Mycobacterium avium-intracellulare* complex. An aggressive diagnostic evaluation with sputum induction by inhalation of saline mist, bronchoscopic procedures, arterial blood gases, and lung biopsy may not be feasible in many developing country settings. Presumptive therapy for the bacterial causes should be instituted in AIDS patients who present with the sudden onset of pulmonary symptoms (Chapter 15.1). A more gradual onset of pulmonary symptoms should prompt diagnostic efforts and therapy for *M. tuberculosis* (Chapter 61.1) or *P. carinii* infection (Chapter 79).

BRONCHIECTASIS

Bronchiectasis remains common in the developing tropical regions, where the most frequent causes are infectious. Bronchiectasis may be a sequela of childhood measles or pertussis, may occur as a complication of bacterial pneumonia, or may be caused by compression of an airway by enlarged lymph nodes. Although in North America cystic fibrosis is the most common cause of bronchiectasis, cystic fibrosis appears to be rare in most tropical countries.

Chronic cough productive of purulent sputum is the usual clinical presentation of this syndrome. Repeated episodes of acute pneumonia and evidence of chronic pulmonary disease (e.g., generalized wasting and clubbing of fingers) are often encountered. Plain chest radiographs may or may not be abnormal, and bronchographic studies are the definitive diagnostic test. Therapy consists of physiotherapy for drainage of sputum, antibiotic management of exacerbations, and surgery for localized disease.

ASTHMA

Although a common chronic illness in developing regions, asthma is often underdiagnosed and frequently undertreated. Nonproductive recurrent cough, especially in the evening, is an important symptom for the clinical diagnosis. The pathophysiology and clinical management of asthma in the tropics do not appear to be unique. Therapy with corticosteroids, sympathomimetics, methylxanthines, and the cromones must be tailored to the local availability and cost of these agents.

PLEURAL EFFUSION

Pleural effusions may be seen more frequently in developing regions than in developed regions, and the etiologic spectrum is more varied. A common etiology is *M. tuberculosis,* either as pleural disease without pulmonary parenchymal involvement or as part of more widespread pulmonary disease (Chapter 61). Pleural effusion or empyema is a common complication of pneumonia due to *Streptococcus pneumoniae, S. pyogenes, Staphylococcus aureus,* and *Klebsiella pneumoniae.* A right-sided pleural effusion may be associated with amebic hepatic abscess (see Fig. 1–3). Any syndrome associated with edema may also cause a pleural effusion: Cardiac failure, cirrhosis of the liver, hypoproteinemia, endomyocardial fibrosis, and neoplastic disease should also be considered in tropical settings. Thoracentesis and pleural biopsy are the mainstays of diagnosis, and the results dictate treatment.

PREVENTION OF PNEUMONIA

Economic development with improved nutrition and better access to medical services, including immunizations, will be accompanied by a decreased incidence and mortality of pneumonia. In the interim, improved clinical management and immunization are the foundation of control programs.

Immunization

VIRUSES. Routine measles vaccination at 9 to 12 months of age is likely to prevent a sizable proportion of childhood pneumonia deaths. Immunization with newer measles vaccines at 6 to 9 months of age would probably prevent a still larger proportion of pneumonia. When safe and effective vaccines for respiratory syncytial and parainfluenza viruses become available, they will be useful in the prevention of childhood morbidity and deaths in the developing world.

BACTERIA. New acellular pertussis vaccines will be used to control this disease in developing countries. A randomized double-blind trial of a 14-valent pneumococcal polysaccharide vaccine in adults in Papua New Guinea demonstrated an 85% reduction in pneumococcal pneumonia, proved by positive blood culture or lung aspirates, as well as a 44% reduction in all pneumonia mortality. A 13-valent pneumococcal vaccine was evaluated in novice miners in South Africa, whose incidence of pneumonia was 90/1000/year. These studies showed a 50% reduction in radiologic pneumonia and an 80% decrease in bacteremia and pneumonia caused by serotypes included in the vaccine. The South African data led to the licensure of pneumococcal vaccine for high-risk adults and older children in the United States.

A randomized double-blind evaluation of pneumococcal vaccine in over 3000 six- to 36-month-old children in Papua New Guinea demonstrated an estimated 59% reduction in deaths ascribed to pneumonia and a reduction in overall mortality of 19%. Further studies of the currently licensed pneumococcal vaccine are warranted. Even though there are geographic and temporal variations of the serotypes seen in developing regions, a high proportion of reported serotypes is included in the current vaccine, which includes 23 serotypes. The development of a protein-conjugated pneumococcal polysaccharide vaccine that would be immunogenic in infants is a priority.

Although pneumonia can be caused by any of the 6 serotypes or untypable *H. influenzae* organisms, type b is the cause of up to 60 to 70% of all *H. influenzae* pneumonias. *H. influenzae* type b protein-conjugated polysaccharide vaccines have been proved safe and efficacious against meningitis and are licensed for universal use in children in North America and Europe. The use of these vaccines to prevent a major proportion of *H. influenzae* pneumonia would also benefit children in developing regions by preventing meningitis and other invasive infections caused by this bacterium.

Vitamin A

Some authorities advocate vitamin A (200,000 IU by mouth × 2 doses in children >1 year) for all children with measles in regions where vitamin A deficiency is common (Chapter 107.1). This may reduce postmeasles pneumonia morbidity and mortality.

BIBLIOGRAPHY

Barker J, Gratten M, Riley I, et al: Pneumonia in children in the Eastern Highlands of Papua New Guinea: A bacteriological study of patients selected by standard clinical criteria. J Infect Dis 159:348–352, 1989.

Barrett-Connor E: Parasitic pulmonary disease. Am Rev Respir Dis 126:558–563, 1982.

Campbell H, Lamont AC, O'Neill KP, et al: Assessment of clinical criteria for identification of severe acute lower respiratory tract infections in children. Lancet 1:297–299, 1989.

Cherian T, John TJ, Simoes E, et al: Evaluation of simple clinical signs for the diagnosis of acute lower respiratory tract infection. Lancet 2:125–128, 1988.

Cherian T, Simoes EAF, Steinhoff MC, et al: Bronchiolitis in tropical south India. Am J Dis Child 144:1026–1030, 1990.

Cockshott P, Middlemiss H (eds): Clinical Radiology in the Tropics. Edinburgh, Churchill Livingstone, 1979, pp 149–174.

Datta N, Kumar V, Kumar L, Singhi S: Application of case management to the control of acute respiratory infections in low-birth-weight infants: a feasibility study. Bull WHO 65:77–87, 1987.

Ghana Health Assessment Project Team: A quantitative method of assessing the health impact of different diseases in less developed countries. Int J Epidemiol 10:73–80, 1981.

Kaschula ROC, Druker J, Kipps A: Late morphologic consequences of measles: A lethal and debilitating lung disease among the poor. Rev Infect Dis 5:395–404, 1983.

Macfarlane JT, Adegboye DS, Warrell MJ: Mycoplasma pneumoniae and the aetiology of lobar pneumonia in northern Nigeria. Thorax 34:713–719, 1979.

McLeod DT, Latif A, Neill P, Lucas S: Pulmonary diseases in AIDS patients in central Africa. Am J Respir Dis 137:119–121, 1988.

McGregor IA: The epidemiology of influenza in a tropical (Gambian) environment. Br Med Bull 35:15–22, 1979.

Management of the Young Child with an Acute Respiratory Infection. Geneva, WHO, 1990.

Metselaar D: Machakos project studies; agents affecting health of mother and child in a rural area of Kenya. X. Haemagglutination inhibiting antibodies against influenza A (H2N2) and influenza B virus in sera from children living in the Machakos district of Kenya. Trop Geogr Med 30:523–530, 1978.

Oppenheim B, Koornhof HJ, Austrian R: Antibiotic resistant pneumococcal disease in children at Baragwanath Hospital, Johannesburg. Pediatr Infect Dis 5:520–524, 1986.

Pinkston P, Vijayan VK, Nutman TB, et al: Acute tropical pulmonary eosinophilia. Characterization of the lower respiratory tract inflammation and its response to therapy. J Clin Invest 80:216–225, 1987.

Reeder MM, Palmer PED: The Radiology of Tropical Diseases with Epidemiological, Pathological and Clinical Correlation. Baltimore, Williams & Wilkins, 1981.

Respiratory Infections in Children: Management in Small Hospitals. Geneva, WHO, 1988.

Riley ID, Andrews M, Howard R: Immunization with a polyvalent pneumococcal vaccine. Lancet 1:1338–1340, 1977.

Riley ID, Lehmann D, Alpers MP: Pneumococcal vaccine prevents death from acute lower respiratory tract infections in Papua New Guinean children. Lancet 2:877–881, 1986.

Shann F: Etiology of severe pneumonia in children in developing countries. Pediatr Infect Dis J 5:247–252, 1986.

Shann F, Walters S, Pifer LL, et al: Pneumonia associated with infection with pneumocystis, respiratory syncytial virus, chlamydia, mycoplasma, and cytomegalovirus in children in Papua New Guinea. Br Med J 292:314–317, 1986.

Spika JS, Munshi MH, Wojtyniak B, et al: Acute lower respiratory infections: a major cause of death in children in Bangladesh. Ann Trop Paediatr 9:33–39, 1989.

Steinhoff MC: Pathogenesis and prevention of childhood pneumonias in developing regions. Lancet 2:1228, 1989.

Sutton DR: One day treatment for lobar pneumonia. Thorax 25:241–244, 1970.

Teklu B, Rigatto M, Bovornkitti S: Geographic variation in respiratory disease. In Weatherall DJ, Ledingham JGG, Warrell DA (eds): Oxford Textbook of Medicine. Oxford, Oxford University Press, 1987, pp 15.171–15.177.

Teklu B, Warrell DA, Femi-Pearse D: The lung. In Parry EHO (ed): Principles of Medicine in Africa. 2nd ed. Oxford, Oxford University Press, 1984, p 761.

Wall RA, Corrah PT, Mabey DCW, Greenwood BM: The etiology of lobar pneumonia in the Gambia. Bull WHO 64:553–558, 1986.

Warrell DA, Fawcet IW, Harrison BDW, et al: Bronchial asthma in the Nigerian Savanna region. Q J Med 174:325–347, 1975.

2. CARDIOVASCULAR DISEASE

O.O. Akinkugbe

The pattern of cardiovascular diseases varies between developed and developing countries (Fig. 2–1). Although ischemic heart disease still accounts for the highest mortality in the former, hypertension, rheumatic heart disease, and the cardiomyopathies constitute most cardiovascular pathology in adults in the tropics. Cardiovascular morbidity also varies between children and adults, even in the same tropical setting. In Nigeria, for example, congenital heart disease is by far the most common cardiovascular disease in the pediatric population (Fig. 2–2).

It is important to know which cardiovascular conditions occur most frequently in a specific area of clinical practice. Chagas' disease needs to be considered in the rural environment of South and Central America. Pulmonary hypertension can be caused by restrictive cardiomyopathy in a Rwandan laborer, filariasis in a young Sri Lankan, bilharziasis in an Egyptian farmer, and rheumatic mitral stenosis in a child from an urban slum.

For the majority of those who live between the extremes of starvation and affluence, diseases caused by infection pose major threats. Cardiovascular diseases of infectious origin are much more common in developing than in developed countries. But as the burden of infection is overcome, the so-called diseases of affluence, notably ischemic heart disease, will take their place unless a conscious effort is made to forestall them through preventive measures.

CONGENITAL HEART DISEASE

INCIDENCE AND ETIOLOGY. In the pediatric age group in practically all developing countries, congenital heart disease (CHD) accounts for over 70% of cardiologic cases. Data from hospital records and community-based deliveries suggest an incidence of 6.6 per 1000 live births in the tropics, as opposed to 8.0 in the developed world.

The most frequently diagnosed acyanotic malformations are ventricular septal defect (VSD), patent ductus arteriosus (PDA), pulmonary stenosis (PS), atrial septal defect (ASD), and coarctation of the aorta (CA), in that order. Of the cyanotic group the tetralogy of Fallot (TF) is the most common. With the exception of PDA and ASD (both of which show a female predilection) and VSD (which shows no gender bias), the other common defects are more prevalent in males. In areas of Latin America, Africa, and Asia that are above 1000 meters in altitude, PDA and pulmonary hypertension are more common.

CLINICAL MANIFESTATIONS AND PROGNOSIS. Many children are born at home. Neonatal surgery is seldom available, and thus infants with the more severe forms of CHD do not survive. The clinical features of these cardiac defects are similar to those reported elsewhere in the world except that concomitant

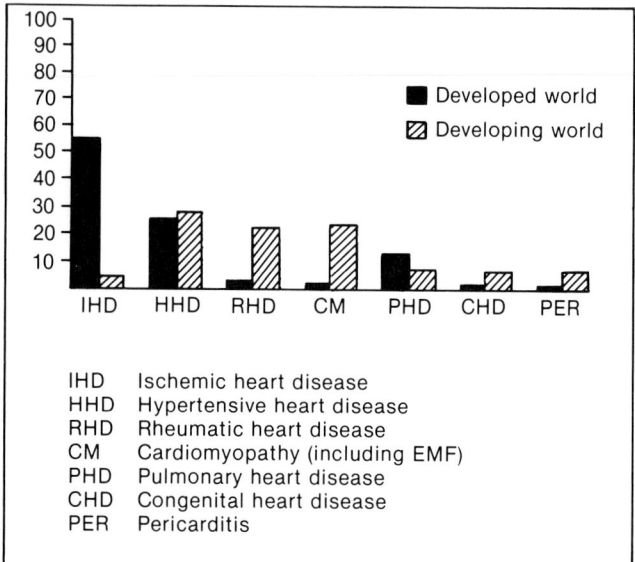

FIGURE 2–1. Profile of cardiovascular diseases in the context of developed and developing countries. Percentages indicate proportion of cardiac pathology for relevant environment.

growth retardation is much more striking in tropical countries. Etiologic factors in CHD include intrauterine rubella and perinatal asphyxia. The low prevalence of CA and aortic stenosis in these communities has been linked with hypocalcemia.

HYPERTENSIVE CARDIOVASCULAR DISEASE

INCIDENCE AND ETIOLOGY. Hypertension is the most serious cardiovascular problem worldwide. It affects both rich and poor and is present almost everywhere. The few communities in which the blood pressure does not rise with age are isolated, small, and diminishing in number. Their members are often unacculturated and consume little or no salt. The highest incidence of hypertension is found among groups with the highest salt intake, e.g., Japanese fishermen. Even when racially similar groups are compared, e.g., New Guinea tribes, salt intake correlates with blood pressure, independent of body build or fatness. More recently, careful multicenter "inter-salt" studies have shown that the salt-hypertension association is more complex; that large amounts of salt must be consumed over a considerable time to cause sustained hypertension; and that the diet

must be practically devoid of salt to lower the blood pressure consistently in mild hypertension. Moreover, there is marked individual variation in the ability to handle salt. Many black hypertensive populations have a delayed excretory capacity for salt.

Renal disease appears to account for about 20% of hypertension in developing countries and is particularly likely to be the cause of severe hypertension in the younger age groups. There is no convincing evidence of an etiologic relationship between urinary schistosomiasis and hypertension.

CLINICAL MANIFESTATIONS, DIAGNOSIS, AND TREATMENT. A low incidence of atherosclerotic heart disease makes the other target organs—the kidney and brain—more commonly susceptible than the heart to the more devastating effects of severe hypertension. Hypertensive heart failure may be easily confused with chronic rheumatic heart disease or dilated cardiomyopathy, as the dysfunctional heart readily becomes fibrotic and dilated.

The goal of treating patients with hypertension is to prevent morbidity and mortality attributable to high blood pressure. This may involve the use of nonpharmacologic and pharmacologic therapy. The success of the therapeutic alliance depends on motivation and effective communication. Projects for the community control of hypertension in developing countries have been started in pilot areas as part of integrated programs for the control of noncommunicable diseases. The emphasis is on primordial and primary prevention in these communities.

RHEUMATIC HEART DISEASE

EPIDEMIOLOGY. Streptococcal pharyngitis, rheumatic fever (RF), and rheumatic heart disease (RHD) can occur anywhere. RHD would appear to be the leading form of acquired heart disease in the tropics in those between 5 and 15 years of age.

Fortunately, most children are not susceptible to the development of RF following an untreated episode of streptococcal throat infection. Perhaps 6 out of 100 children will do so if challenged repeatedly; about half of them will be left with heart murmurs that permit a retrospective diagnosis. Genetic factors may be important in determining those who develop RF. When a prevalence of chronic RHD of over 2% is encountered, an RF experience of over 4% is implied. Such percentages indicate that the population at risk has been saturated with streptococcal infection.

Bacteriologic and serologic surveys from many parts of the world confirm the ubiquity of streptococcal disease. Antistreptolysin (ASO) surveys show that children living in crowded and poor conditions begin to experience streptococcal infections in infancy. Throat culture surveys in primary school children often show more than 30% with beta-hemolytic streptococcus carriage. M-typing of these organisms has shown regional differences, but in some studies the majority of isolates could be typed (an indication of virulence), with more than one type detected in children from a single classroom.

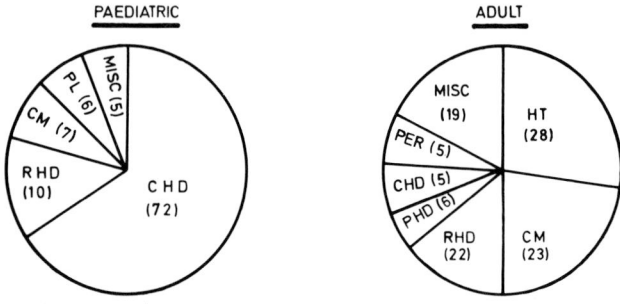

FIGURE 2–2. Cardiovascular morbidity in Nigeria. (See Figure 2–1 for key to abbreviations.)

Infection with one M type does not confer immunity against others of the more than 60 identified. Consequently, repeated infection is almost inevitable. When such exposure and infection start in the first few years of life, RF and RHD often appear so early that valve calcification and stenosis are commonly seen in children and young adults.

PATHOGENESIS. That pharyngitis frequently precedes RF has been recognized for over a century; the importance of the streptococcus in the development of RF has been known for 50 years. However, it is only in recent years that it became apparent that the Group A beta-hemolytic streptococcus is the sole etiologic agent of RF. Streptococcal pharyngitis is followed by RF, whereas streptococcal pyoderma is not. There are some M types (5, 14, 24) that appear to be especially likely to cause RF. The role of host (including genetic) factors is not entirely clear, but there appears to be no ethnic group either particularly prone or unusually resistant to RF. Good antibiotic prophylaxis programs work well everywhere, one reason for implicating the streptococcus as the sole agent of the disease.

PATHOLOGY. Although the rheumatic cardiac nodule, or Aschoff body, is considered the pathognomonic lesion of RHD, nonspecific changes such as lymphocytic interstitial exudation and myocardial fibril fragmentation predominate during the acute illness. The pericardial surface has a fibrinous exudate, and serosanguineous pericardial effusion is common. Adhesions subsequently form, but chronic constrictive pericarditis does not occur even though pericardial calcification occasionally results. The endocardial involvement is most common in the mitral and aortic areas, with the tricuspid valve involved less often and the pulmonary valve rarely. Fibrinous deposits are organized via granulation and fibrosis, which lead to regurgitation and/or stenosis of the affected valve(s). Persistence of the Aschoff body is more common in patients who subsequently develop mitral stenosis.

CLINICAL MANIFESTATIONS. There is a belief that RF in the tropics is clinically different from that in the temperate zones because severe carditis is more common and arthritis is less frequent. A prospective study in Nigeria supports this, whereas a similar study in India does not. The earlier the onset of RF, the more likely the patient is to have carditis and the less likely he is to have arthritis. Sixty years ago, carditis and chorea were more common signs of RF in the United States than was arthritis. American students were taught that "rheumatic fever licks the joints but bites the heart"; this may still be true in tropical Africa.

Symptomatology. In developing countries a child suffering from joint pain or swelling may be considered to have a hemoglobinopathy (sickle cell disease, Chapter 5), particularly if the symptoms are accompanied by fever. Although the child with carditis and congestive heart failure is unlikely to be misdiagnosed, first presentation in hospital is usually delayed. In the tropics, many children have parasitic diseases that directly or indirectly place a burden on the heart. In such children, rheumatic carditis is an additional burden that can cause cardiac decompensation. In developing countries, many children with rheumatic carditis and congestive failure are likely to be experiencing their second or later episode of RF and are chronically, rather than acutely, ill.

There may be genuine racial differences in the response to streptococcal infection beyond the differences due to socioeconomic factors and age of onset. To the clinician the important point is that in the tropics the child presenting with RF is likely to have carditis, with or without mitral insufficiency, and not likely to have migratory polyarthritis. Chorea is not common (with an incidence of less than 5%); subcutaneous nodules and erythema marginatum are also rare.

Cardiac Failure. The incidence of cardiac failure reported in different series is extremely variable, ranging from below 5% to over 90%. When cardiac failure is present, there are obvious changes clinically and on the chest film. In addition to the murmur of mitral regurgitation, the child may have murmurs of aortic and tricuspid valve involvement, evidence of pulmonary hypertension, inappropriate tachycardia, and signs and symptoms of pericarditis. The electrocardiogram (ECG) and echocardiogram are useful in confirming the presence of complications such as arrhythmias and pericardial effusion.

Left Atrial Enlargement. The involvement of the atrial wall in the rheumatic process in childhood is a reasonable explanation for the prominence of the left atrium and its appendage (LAA) in RHD. The LAA enlargement can be easily appreciated on the chest film (Fig. 2–3). The enlarging left atrium can protect the lungs against mitral regurgitation, so that some patients with mitral incompetence of rheumatic origin may not complain of significant dyspnea until they develop atrial fibrillation. This discrepancy between dramatic physical findings (i.e., very large hyperactive heart with a loud murmur and third heart sound) and minimal symptoms can exist for some years in a patient with moderate mitral insufficiency.

Chorea. As mentioned previously, chorea is not a common manifestation of RF. It usually occurs, by itself

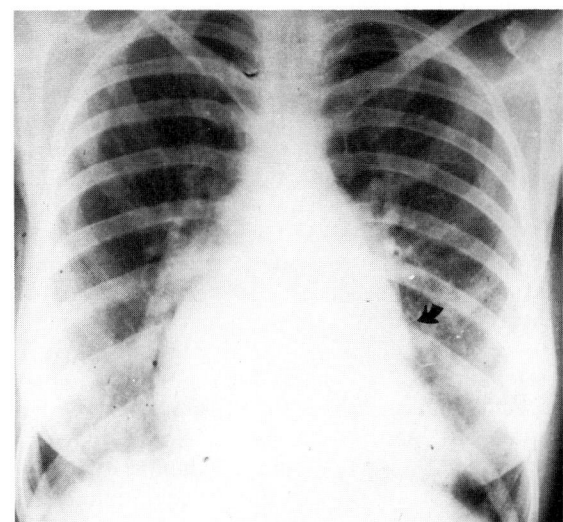

FIGURE 2–3. Posteroanterior chest film in patient with mitral insufficiency due to rheumatic heart disease. Arrow points to prominent left atrial appendage.

or with carditis but not with arthritis, several months after the streptococcal infection. After puberty it occurs more frequently in girls. It may be associated with a normal temperature or normal erythrocyte sedimentation rate (ESR), and the ASO titer may be normal. This "pure" chorea does not respond to the usual treatment for RF and responds poorly to sedatives (diazepam, chlorpromazine).

DIAGNOSIS. The major criteria for the diagnosis of RF in the tropics are carditis, chorea, subcutaneous nodules, erythema marginatum, and migratory arthritis. However, there are children who have RF with fever, tachycardia, and severe migratory polyarthropathy without definite joint swelling. An elevated white blood cell count or ESR or a positive C-reactive protein test is diagnostically helpful in such situations. The finding of first-degree AV block on the electrocardiogram is also useful.

Preceding Streptococcal Infection. Current criteria for the diagnosis of RF stress the importance of establishing whether there had been an antecedent streptococcal infection. A history of sore throat is of some help. A history of scarlet fever is specific, though unusual, but a negative culture does not exclude RF. The demonstration of a high and rising streptococcal antibody titer is the most important laboratory confirmation of streptococcal infection (250 Todd units in adults, 300 Todd units in children). The ability to culture and identify beta-hemolytic streptococcus and to perform the ASO test is expected of all but the most rudimentary laboratories. However, these investigations are more often than not unavailable to doctors practicing in developing countries. Increased reliance has to be placed on clinical skills and a high index of suspicion. The possibility of RF must always be considered in any child or young adult with fever, sore throat, and a heart murmur.

DIFFERENTIAL DIAGNOSIS. Deciding whether a patient with established valvular heart disease has RF is usually not too difficult, even in the absence of a typical history. Mitral stenosis, with or without regurgitation, is usually due to RF. Mitral valve disease in association with aortic valve disease is almost certainly rheumatic in origin. The presence of tricuspid valvular abnormalities with mitral disease suggests a rheumatic origin. Atrial fibrillation in a young patient with valvular heart disease favors a diagnosis of RHD or endomyocardial fibrosis (EMF). In patients with mitral incompetence, the larger the left atrium, the more likely a rheumatic etiology. Patients with giant left atria (>40 mm diameter) are almost always in atrial fibrillation, have mitral incompetence, and frequently have RHD. The following conditions must always be excluded in the differential diagnosis of rheumatic fever: typhoid fever (Chapter 38), bacterial septicemias, infective endocarditis, tuberculosis (Chapter 61), sickle cell anemia (Chapter 5), nonspecific pancarditis with effusion, undulant fever (Chapter 50), serum sickness, leukemia, rheumatoid arthritis, and systemic lupus erythematosus. A high index of suspicion, a careful history, and a critical assessment of the character of the fever, the arthritis, the murmur, and other cardiac abnormalities will serve to distinguish RF from these various conditions.

TREATMENT AND PROPHYLAXIS

Rest. Patients with active RF should be at rest. Those with congestive heart failure and severe carditis or arthritis will wish and need to stay in bed. Those with less serious symptoms will be at modified rest. The duration of disease activity, although masked by therapy, ranges from 2 to 4 months or as long as 6 to 12 months when chorea is a feature.

Anti-inflammatory Drugs. Aspirin has been used to treat RF since 1876 and is still the mainstay of therapy. For children, 100 mg/kg/day in 5 divided doses is standard. For adults, 6 to 8 gm/day should be given, increasing this cautiously until side effects (salicylism) limit the dose. The fever, joint symptoms, and tachycardia should respond promptly. The C-reactive protein test should rapidly become negative, but the sedimentation rate (ESR) is usually much slower to respond.

Corticosteroids should be used in patients with severe carditis, at a dose of 40 to 60 mg/day for adults and 2 mg/kg/day for children, even though controversy surrounds their presumed efficacy and the distinct possibility exists of rebound carditis on withdrawal of the steroids. The rationale for steroids is the prevention of valvular damage in the early stages of the disease. Steroids should be tapered off within a few weeks. Patients with mild carditis can be treated with either salicylates or steroids. A reasonable program is to start with steroids, reducing them during the third week while starting salicylates. Congestive heart failure is treated with steroids plus diuretics and digitalis.

Antistreptococcal Therapy. A most important part of the original therapy is the administration of an antistreptococcal dose of antibiotic. This should be given even if the throat cultures taken on admission are negative. Usually the most effective antistreptococcal therapy is 1.2 million units of dibenzyl penicillin as a single intramuscular injection for adults (600,000 to 900,000 units for children). Erythromycin, 250 mg four times daily for 10 days, is satisfactory therapy for individuals with penicillin sensitivity, but erythromycin plus aspirin frequently causes gastrointestinal symptoms. Sulfonamides are bacteriostatic, not bactericidal, and should not be used to treat streptococcal infection.

Prophylactic Therapy. Prophylaxis against further episodes of RF is mandatory in a patient diagnosed as having RF or RHD. The best prophylaxis is 1.2 million units of dibenzyl penicillin G once-monthly in adults (600,000 units in children weighing less than 27 kg). Less reliable are sulfadiazine, 1.0 gm once daily (0.5 gm in children weighing less than 27 kg); buffered penicillin G tablets, 250,000 units twice daily; or erythromycin, 250 mg twice daily. If sulfadiazine is used, the white blood cell count should be checked every few weeks for the first several months. In children with carditis, prophylaxis should be continued indefinitely, certainly into adult life. In those without evidence of residual carditis, it should be continued into adult life.

PROGNOSIS, LATE MANIFESTATIONS, AND CONTROL. Death from acute RF is unusual but can occur in severe congestive cardiac failure or with arrhythmias. Prognosis depends on the amount of residual cardiac damage and on recurrence of active disease. A child who has had RF and experiences another episode of untreated streptococcal infection is very likely to develop RF again. A child left with badly damaged valves may do well for a short while but will eventually develop pulmonary hypertension and become symptomatic.

Surgery. Valve replacement is not available in many parts of the developing world. Even where it is available, the cost of the surgery and subsequent care is beyond the reach of most patients, and those patients with replaced valves often do poorly. The reasons for this poor outcome include the following: (1) Artificial valves may become infected and require replacement; (2) anticoagulation is often indicated in patients with artificial valves but is impossible in many areas of the developing world; and (3) porcine replacement valves have generally not worked well in children. Whenever possible, surgeons in cardiac centers in developing countries favor valvuloplasty. Children with significant mitral and/or aortic insufficiency from RF are unlikely to have a normal life span in most developing countries, and the majority having both lesions die young, principally from heart failure.

The child who develops mitral stenosis as the principal cardiac lesion after an attack of RF is much more likely to benefit from surgery (closed valvotomy). Here the problem is one of diagnosis, since mitral stenosis may escape detection unless it is specifically suspected. Dyspnea, hemoptysis, early age of onset, a sudden cerebrovascular accident, or the appearance of atrial fibrillation is a more important clue. A loud first heart sound is the auscultatory hint to listen carefully for the opening snap and apical diastolic rumble. Embolic manifestations frequently precede the appearance of atrial fibrillation. Echocardiography, when available, is diagnostic.

Prevention. Treatment of streptococcal pharyngitis is the key to prevention of RF. In an area where streptococcal infection and RF are common, it is better to overtreat nonstreptococcal causes of sore throat than to let RF develop.

In several areas of the developing world where there are good antistreptococcal treatment and RF prophylaxis programs, the incidence of RF has declined sharply over the past decade, despite lack of improvement in living conditions, indicating that when specific therapy is available, a disease can be controlled without social change. Such observations place a burden on physicians to prevent and control this major cause of cardiac disability and death.

INFECTIVE ENDOCARDITIS

The majority of cases of infective endocarditis occur in patients with congenital or acquired cardiac defects. The clinical course of bacterial endocarditis may be acute, subacute, or chronic depending on the pathogenicity of the organisms and the response of the host.

ETIOLOGY. The usual causative organisms are *Streptococcus viridans* and *Staphylococcus aureus*. Less common are *Staphylococcus albus, Streptococcus faecalis, Escherichia coli, Klebsiella* and *Pseudomonas* spp.,

and rarely, fungal and atypical organisms such as *Chlamydia, Coxiella,* and *Brucella*. Not infrequently the offending organism remains elusive despite repeated blood cultures. Persistently negative cultures may be due to previous indiscriminate use of antibiotics for unexplained fever. Unusual primary sites of infection include the skin (sepsis), scalp, muscle (pyomyositis), and bone (osteomyelitis). Some of the lesions (cutaneous vasculitis, focal and diffuse glomerulonephritis) have an immunologic basis.

CLINICAL MANIFESTATIONS. Generally the mitral, aortic, pulmonary, and tricuspid valves are affected in that order of frequency. In acute infective endocarditis (usually due to *S. aureus*) there is extensive valvular damage with a rapidly progressive illness. The more common subacute form is characterized by low-grade fever, the presence of cardiac murmurs, and a raised ESR. There may also be arthralgia, anorexia, lassitude, weight loss, splenomegaly, finger clubbing, unexplained cardiac failure, or one of the consequences of peripheral embolization. The telltale Osler's nodes are not common in the tropics, nor are café-au-lait spots easily discernible on dark skin. Investigations often show a mild to moderate normochromic normocytic anemia with moderate polymorphic leukocytosis. Hematuria may be present, and occasionally there is evidence of renal impairment. Chest films, ECGs, and echocardiograms are sometimes useful in monitoring progress.

Unexplained fever, heart failure that is out of proportion to the severity of the heart lesion or that is resistant to conventional therapy, persistent anemia, and hemoptysis should prompt a high index of suspicion.

TREATMENT AND PREVENTION. Patients with valvular heart disease should be protected with prophylactic antibiotics at certain periods, e.g., during dental surgery, urogenital instrumentation, or abdominal operations. For definitive therapy, the choice of antibiotic should be bactericidal and parenteral; preferably, more than one should be used. When the causative organism is difficult to pinpoint, it may be necessary to commence therapy with a combination of gentamicin with penicillin, amoxicillin, or floxacillin. The long-term prognosis is often determined by the late consequences of residual valve damage.

THE CARDIOMYOPATHIES

Two important varieties of heart disease have been identified in the tropics over the past four decades—idiopathic cardiomegaly and endomyocardial fibrosis. Both are now grouped as the cardiomyopathies and on the basis of their effects on ventricular structure and function have been classified into dilated, restrictive, and hypertrophic forms. When the cause of heart muscle disease is known or there is some association with systemic disease, the disorder is classified under specific heart muscle disease and designated by the etiology—viral, nutritional, alcoholic, toxic, and so forth.

DILATED CARDIOMYOPATHY

Incidence and Etiology. This accounts for at least 10% (in children) and 30% (in adults) of acquired heart diseases in many parts of tropical Africa. Subclinical viral myocarditis has been implicated in its pathogenesis in children. In adults, however, the majority have a background of undiagnosed or untreated hypertension with one or more superimposed factors: alcohol, malnutrition, thiamine deficiency, anemia, multiparity and viral (e.g., coxsackie, echo) and protozoal infections (e.g., *Toxoplasma gondii*).

Pathology. Macroscopically the hearts are pale and flabby, with hypertrophy and dilatation of all chambers. Occasionally, only the left ventricle and atrium are involved. The atrioventricular rings are dilated and the trabeculae carneae flattened into a lacelike pattern, and there are focal areas of ventricular endocardial fibrosis. Mural thrombi may be present in the atrial appendage or ventricular apex in up to 50% of adults with this disease. Microscopically the cardiac muscle fibers are hypertrophied, there are scattered areas of myocytolysis, replacement fibrosis, and lymphocytic collections. The coronary arteries are normal.

Clinical Manifestations. Only about 10% of children with this condition present with asymptomatic cardiomegaly. The rest exhibit fever, cough, tachypnea, signs of biventricular failure, an apical impulse and a ventricular gallop with evidence of mitral regurgitation. In adults there is also evidence of congestive cardiac failure with signs of gross biventricular enlargement, functional atrioventricular incompetence, murmurs, and pulmonary hypertension in the absence of systemic hypertension. These patients are prone to systemic and pulmonary embolism and cardiogenic shock.

Laboratory Findings. Chest x-ray shows cardiomegaly, pulmonary artery and venous hypertension, and edema. Various forms of arrhythmia may be evident on the electrocardiogram (atrial fibrillation, atrial or ventricular extrasystoles), or there may be both right and left ventricular hypertrophy. With time, heart failure supervenes with consequent clockwise rotation of the precordial leads and dominant S waves in V5 and V6.

Hemodynamic studies are useful in confirming primary heart muscle disease. There is reduction in the cardiac output and an increase in the end-diastolic pressures of both ventricles. Angiographic and echocardiographic studies show a large, dilated, poorly contractile left ventricle without septal hypertrophy or cavity obliteration. The coronary vessels are patent.

Association with Pregnancy. Dilated cardiomyopathy is occasionally seen in pregnancy, when it may present as heart failure toward term and up to 6 months post partum in women with no previous history of heart disease. The pathogenesis in some of these cases of peripartal heart disease is linked to volume overload from excessive salt consumption. It is also possible that previous myocardial damage is triggered into failure as a result of the metabolic demands of pregnancy and the puerperium.

RESTRICTIVE CARDIOMYOPATHY (EMF)
Etiology. This includes endomyocardial fibrosis and Loeffler's eosinophilic endomyocardial disease. EMF is typically found in the hot and humid areas of the tropics. Its etiology is obscure, but malnutrition, serotonin (from consumption of plantain or banana), vitamin E defi-

ciency, filariasis, lymphatic obstruction, and allergy all are suspected causes.

Pathology. Structurally there is dense deposition of fibrous tissue in the walls of one or both ventricles, with involvement of the inflow tract and posterior cusp of the AV valves. This leads to restriction in ventricular filling with consequent decrease in cardiac output, simulating massive pericardial effusion or constrictive pericarditis.

Clinical Manifestations. The clinical features of right- and left-sided EMF are as shown in Figure 2–4. The chest x-ray shows, with (R) EMF, a globular heart with oligemic lung fields. In (L) EMF there is either a normal cardiac silhouette or an enlarged left atrium with changes suggestive of pulmonary congestion, edema, and hypertension.

Laboratory Findings and Diagnosis. The ECG of (R) EMF shows low-voltage complexes in the event of a pericardial effusion. The rhythm is sinus, or there may be atrial fibrillation, and an rSr pattern may be seen in leads V1–V4. In (L) EMF there may be atrial fibrillation and evidence of left atrial or ventricular hypertrophy.

Definitive diagnosis of EMF can be made by cardiac catheterization and angiocardiography. The pressure tracing in (R) EMF shows the "dip and plateau" configuration, indicating a restrictive filling defect. With angiocardiography there is a small right ventricle with irregular margins and dilated outflow tract. With (L) EMF, angiography shows a reduction in cavity size and obliteration of the apex.

Apart from the initial febrile illness with facial edema, progressive edema, and evidence of carditis as described, patients with EMF often have such extracardiac features as cyanosis, finger clubbing, oral gingival or periorbital pigmentation, parotid enlargement, and retarded growth.

HYPERTROPHIC CARDIOMYOPATHY (HCM)
This is a much less common form of cardiomyopathy in the tropical setting. There is marked hypertrophy of the left and sometimes the right ventricular muscle, without obvious cause, predominantly involving the sep-

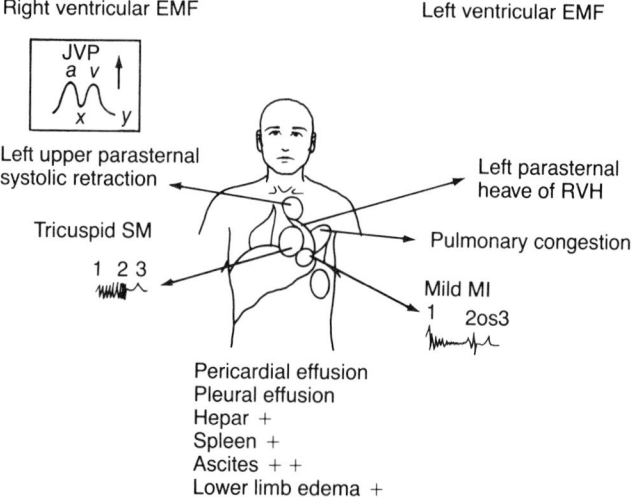

FIGURE 2–4. The clinical features of right and left restrictive cardiomyopathy (EMF). (From Akinkugbel OO, and Falase AO: Cardiovascular Disease. Oxford, Blackwell Scientific Publications, 1987.)

tum. This may occur with or without outflow obstruction. HCM is thought to be inherited as an autosomal dominant trait, with incomplete penetrance.

TREATMENT. Treatment of all these forms of cardiomyopathy is as for congestive heart failure: diuretics as necessary, digitalis in the presence of fast atrial fibrillation, and amiodarone in suppressing troublesome ventricular arrhythmias. Peripheral vasodilators may be indicated in severe heart failure to "unload" the left ventricle and its inotropic effects. Thromboembolic events may call for the use of anticoagulants. For EMF, a loop diuretic may need to be combined with thiazides to obtain effective results. Where the facilities exist for open heart surgery, resection of the fibrous tissue in one or both ventricles has been undertaken with prosthetic replacement of the AV valve. Beta-blocking agents are useful in angina associated with HCM.

CHAGAS' DISEASE

Chagas cardiomyopathy has supplanted rheumatic fever (RF) as the most common form of heart disease and the leading cause of cardiac death in young adults in parts of South and Central America, particularly Chile, Argentina, and Mexico (Chapter 75).

ACUTE MYOCARDITIS. This is usually associated with fever, lymphadenopathy, and inflammation at the site of inoculation. The heart is enlarged, and there may be systolic murmurs due to cardiac dilatation. A gallop rhythm may be associated with heart failure. The electrocardiogram may be normal, although T-wave changes and first-degree atrioventricular block are common. The higher degrees of AV block or the appearance of congestive heart failure (CHF) are poor prognostic signs in the acute phase.

CHRONIC MYOCARDITIS. CHF is the most common form of presentation. Syncope is a frequent early symptom, and sudden death is not unusual. Patients may also have dysphagia or constipation due to aperistalsis. A pancarditis is present, but right-sided heart failure predominates. The heart is enlarged (Fig. 75–14), and in addition to the presence of regurgitant systolic murmurs, the second heart sound may be abnormally split.

Electrocardiographic Findings. Conduction and rhythm abnormalities are the outstanding clinical features of chronic Chagas' disease. Atrioventricular blocks of all degrees, bundle branch block, intraventricular block, and premature ventricular contractions are often present in some combination on the ECG. Premature ventricular contractions (often multifocal) are the most common arrhythmia, and right bundle branch block with left anterior hemiblock is the most common conduction abnormality.

Cardiac Aneurysm. Another distinctive feature of Chagas' heart disease is the predilection for the formation of cardiac "aneurysms," usually located at the apex of the left ventricle, which predispose these patients to arterial embolization. Post-mortem findings show these aneurysms as herniations of endocardium at the cardiac apex.

DIAGNOSIS. Chagas' disease often occurs where RHD, other forms of cardiomyopathy, and schistosomal cor pulmonale also exist. Typically, the patient with this infection is young and is from a rural area. Patients may have the symptoms of CHF or complain of dysphagia or abnormal bowel function. Most have an abnormal heart rhythm and an enlarged heart. There may be Stokes-Adams attacks and evidence of arterial embolization. In contrast, conduction disturbances other than atrial fibrillation are less common in chronic RHD.

PERICARDIAL DISEASE

Pericarditis of infectious origin is secondary either to septicemia or to infection of the structures contiguous to the heart.

Pericarditis in the tropics is typified by few reported cases of viral etiology and an increased prevalence of pyogenic and tuberculous involvement. The incidence of pericardial disease due to uremia, connective tissue diseases (e.g., systemic lupus erythematosus), and malignancy is not as high as that reported for more developed countries.

PYOGENIC PERICARDITIS. Pyogenic pericarditis is more common in infants and children. In infants in particular, a pericardial rub may not be heard, and the electrocardiogram may not show ST-T changes (although the voltages will generally be low). The diagnosis should be considered in children with clinical deterioration following soft tissue infection, osteomyelitis, or post-measles bronchopneumonia. The presence of a pericardial rub and ST-segment elevation on the ECG is helpful, but the appearance of a globular cardiac shadow on the chest film of a child with evidence of cardiac tamponade is the traditional diagnostic confirmation of effusive pericarditis. Echocardiography, if available, is the best noninvasive method of determining the presence of pericardial fluid collection.

Pericardiocentesis will yield purulent fluid. Unless inhibited by antibiotic therapy, the organism can be cultured. Since the most common responsible bacterium is the staphylococcus, therapy must include a bactericidal penicillinase-resistant antibiotic. Appropriate antibiotic therapy plus surgical drainage usually results in cure of a condition that is otherwise universally fatal.

TUBERCULOUS PERICARDITIS. Tuberculous pericarditis is an indolent disease, usually occurring in adults, that may sometimes present in an acute fibrinous form. Most patients will have a pleural effusion, pulmonary infiltrate, and/or hilar adenopathy, but the pleurae, lungs, and mediastinum may all be radiologically normal. A positive tuberculin skin test is a helpful diagnostic aid, but a negative test does not exclude the diagnosis. The pericardial fluid is usually serosanguineous, and lymphocytes predominate on cell count. Tubercle bacilli are usually not recovered. In exceptional cases a pericardial biopsy will confirm the diagnosis, revealing tubercle bacilli or caseating granulomas. As is often the case in nonpulmonary tuberculosis, a therapeutic trial may be required to establish the diagnosis (Chapter 61).

AMEBIC PERICARDITIS. Although sometimes confused with tuberculous pericarditis, amebic pericarditis is much less common and is rarely seen in nontropical areas. It deserves discussion, particularly since the well-known dictum that "amebic pericarditis has never been observed unassociated with amebic liver abscess" can be misleading.

Pathophysiology. Suppurative amebic pericarditis is probably always due to rupture of an amebic liver abscess into the pericardium (Chapter 68). However, such an abscess is likely to be in the left lobe of the liver and may escape clinical detection. Therefore, the patient with amebic pericarditis may have cardiac tamponade without obvious clinical evidence of liver disease (Fig. 2–5).

Diagnosis and Treatment. Rapid diagnosis and treatment are lifesaving in a disease that is otherwise fatal. The diagnosis of amebic pericarditis is not likely to be made fortuitously because these patients usually do not experience diarrhea or have amebae in the stool, nor is the organism likely to be seen in the pericardial aspirate. The pericardial fluid can be either purulent or a mixture of blood and pus. In amebic pericarditis, neutrophils predominate in the pericardial fluid, in contrast to tuberculous pericarditis, in which lymphocytes are predominant.

Diagnosis is established by performing a serologic test (e.g., IHA test) for amebiasis on either blood or pericardial/pleural aspirate. Treatment with metronidazole is the same as for liver abscess except that the pericardium should be surgically drained. Adequate pericardial drainage may obviate the need for laparotomy and subdiaphragmatic drainage.

ATHEROSCLEROTIC HEART DISEASE

In the early 1970s in Ibadan, Nigeria, only 10 cases of myocardial infarction were seen among 8000 necropsies over a 10-year period. Four of these were due not to atherosclerosis but to coronary embolism. In the past two decades, reports indicate a rising incidence in ischemic heart disease in developing countries, particularly in the urban setting with a rapidly changing social and dietary lifestyle. Attendant risk factors include the high consumption of saturated fats, cigarette smoking, sedentary habits, and lack of exercise. Hypertension and diabetes are also well-recognized predisposing factors. Cardiologic practice in many parts of the developing world would thus appear to be going through a transition phase of two populations of cardiac patients—one with congestive heart failure from diseases associated with infection and hypertension, and the other with complaints of chest pain from coronary heart disease.

ISCHEMIC HEART DISEASE (IHD). This may lead to sudden death, or less commonly, to congestive heart failure (CHF). An antecedent history of angina is often lacking, and CHF patients often have the symptoms associated with fluid retention. Physical signs may be few and definitive diagnosis hampered by the paucity of investigative facilities (ECG, myocardial enzymes). Particular attention should be paid to controlling the blood pressure, as there is ample evidence to show that hypertension worsens the prognosis in blacks with end-organ damage.

It should be stressed that IHD is not an unavoidable concomitant of socioeconomic development. The recent decline in IHD mortality in many industrialized societies has been related to the effective reduction of risk factor levels through the adoption of healthier lifestyles. The developing world can borrow a leaf from their book by avoiding or minimizing known risk factors and thus forestall the development of overt disease.

SCHISTOSOMAL COR PULMONALE

Chronic cor pulmonale is heart disease secondary to disease of the respiratory system, e.g., fibrosis, emphysema, pneumonia. Dyspnea is the cardinal presenting feature and is due to the increased work of breathing resulting from the mechanical effects of lung disease with right heart overload. In its chronic form, its differential diagnosis includes mitral stenosis and thromboembolic pulmonary hypertension.

In the context of tropical pathology, attention will be focused on schistosomal cor pulmonale, which is a major cause of cardiac morbidity and mortality in certain parts of the tropics (Chapter 96).

PATHOPHYSIOLOGY. Schistosoma seldom seriously injure the heart directly. An adult worm in a coronary artery at autopsy is rare. Ova in the myocardium can elicit a granulomatous response and, when present in large numbers, can produce myocarditis. This granulomatous myocarditis does exist in serious infection, but references to nonspecific "toxic" or "allergic" schistosomal myocarditis are suspect. Some of the antischistosomal drugs used in the past have been cardiotoxic. Moreover, "toxic" schistosomal myocarditis has been reported principally in areas where Chagas' disease is also present. The major way in which schistosomiasis

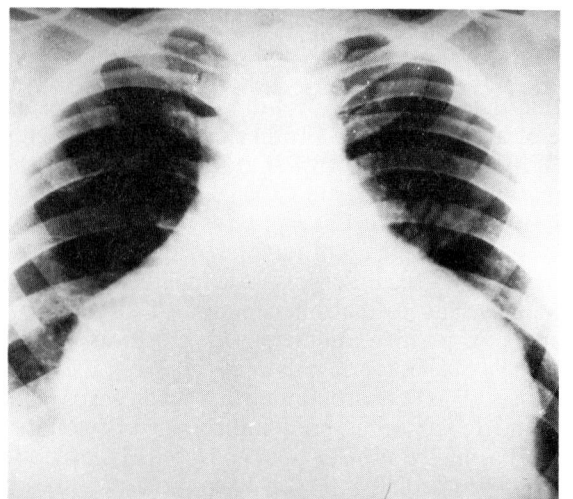

FIGURE 2–5. Posteroanterior chest film in patient with amebic pericarditis without evidence of liver abscess clinically or by scan. He received corticosteroids for "fever of unknown origin." Pulmonary oligemia is also evident.

causes cardiovascular disease is through the production of cor pulmonale.

Of patients dying with schistosomal hepatic fibrosis, about 15% have right ventricular hypertrophy. Although ova are routinely found in the lungs of patients with *Schistosoma haematobium* infection, cor pulmonale is rare. It is also unusual in *S. mansoni* infection without hepatic involvement. The reason for this is unclear, but the association between pulmonary hypertension and hepatic cirrhosis of other etiologies suggests that factors other than ova deposition in the pulmonary arterioles play a role. The patient with schistosomal pulmonary hypertension routinely shows evidence of portal hypertension as well. Both sexes are involved, with men outnumbering women. Presumably, this predilection is due to the greater exposure of men to repeated and prolonged infection.

CLINICAL MANIFESTATIONS. In endemic areas, where infection occurs early in life, clinical features of schistosomal cor pulmonale can be present in children below the age of 10 years. The usual patient is a young farmer who complains of dyspnea on exertion. He may also experience exertional dizziness or syncope and oppressive chest or epigastric discomfort (right ventricular angina). Cough and wheezing are common. Hemoptysis is rare but ominous. Exertional palpitation is a frequent complaint. Premature atrial contractions may be present, but atrial fibrillation is unusual before the age of 40. The presence of syncope and the absence of hemoptysis and atrial fibrillation are important points in the diagnostic differentiation from RHD.

Physical examination of the patient with schistosomal cor pulmonale should be conclusive. The noncardiac findings are those of portal hypertension with hepatosplenomegaly and venous collaterals.

Inspection of the cardiovascular system shows visible neck vein activity, with a prominent *a* wave in early cases and a large *v* wave if tricuspid regurgitation is present. When the patient lies back, pulsations along the left upper sternal border indicate the presence of an enlarged pulmonary artery. On palpation, right ventricular heave and loud pulmonary valve closure may be felt. If tricuspid and/or pulmonary regurgitation has occurred, appropriate thrills may be felt.

Auscultation confirms the presence of a loud pulmonary closure. If there are no murmurs, a right atrial S4 can be heard in the epigastrium (corresponding to the *a* wave in the neck) along with an ejection sound along the left sternal border. If present, the systolic murmur of tricuspid regurgitation should not be confused with that of a ventricular septal defect (which is usually rougher). The diastolic blow of pulmonary regurgitation secondary to the pulmonary hypertension with dilatation of the pulmonary artery sounds similar to the murmur of aortic regurgitation. The tricuspid valve flutters in the flow produced by the pulmonary regurgitation and produces a rumble that can be mistaken for tricuspid or mitral stenosis.

LABORATORY FINDINGS. The electrocardiogram (Fig. 2–6) shows normal sinus rhythm and right ventricular hypertrophy. The chest film (Fig. 2–7) reveals the cardiac silhouette of right ventricular hypertrophy and

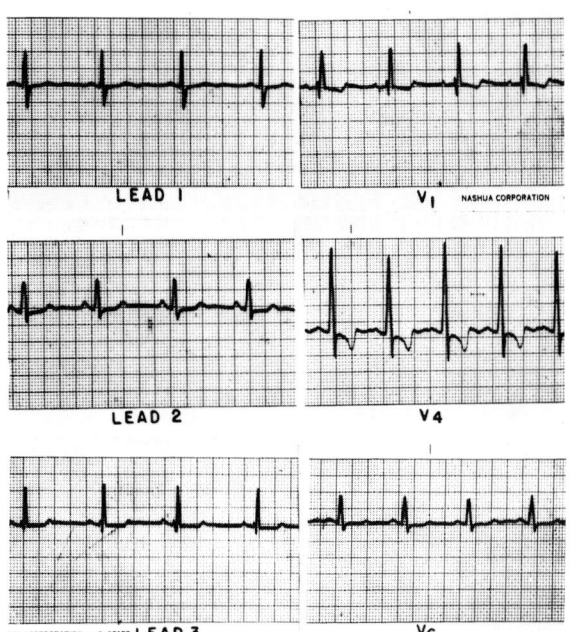

FIGURE 2–6. Electrocardiogram of patient with bilharzial cor pulmonale, showing a vertical axis and right ventricular hypertrophy and strain.

a large pulmonary artery (PA). Sometimes, granulomas are visualized on the roentgenogram, being most noticeable in the lower lung fields. As the pulmonary artery becomes aneurysmal, pulmonary regurgitation becomes inevitable. Huge pulmonary arteries are commonly seen in farmers who continue to work in the fields during the progression of pulmonary hypertension. At cardiac catheterization, these patients have lower PA pressures and higher right ventricular diastolic pressures than do patients with a lesser degree of PA enlargement.

TREATMENT AND PROGNOSIS. Since schistosomal cor pulmonale is a complication of hepatosplenic schistosomiasis and since patients with pulmonary hypertension of any cause do poorly, it is not surprising that patients with schistosomal cor pulmonale do not do well. Cardiac catheterization can be hazardous. If angiographic demonstration of the pulmonary vasculature is

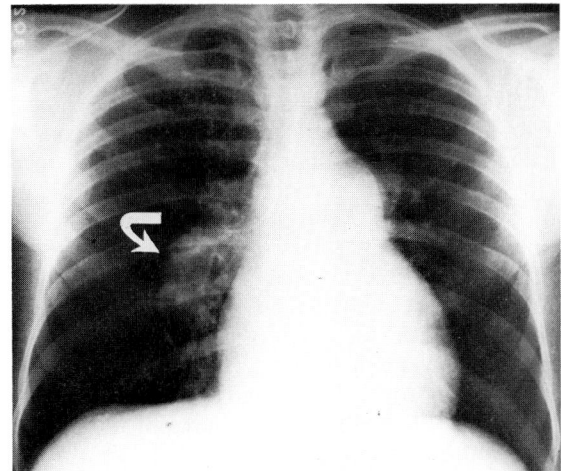

FIGURE 2–7. Chest film in patient with bilharzial cor pulmonale. Arrow points to dilated right pulmonary artery.

desired, it is better done selectively. Treatment is also associated with some risks, since dead or dying worms can embolize to the lungs and complete the obstructive process. Thrombus in situ, particularly of the right pulmonary artery, also occurs. Dissection of the aneurysm provokes sudden hemoptysis, chest pain, and death. Some other patients die suddenly without obvious cause, possibly from arrhythmias. If a patient with schistosomal cor pulmonale can leave the fields and hard labor, he may live longer. But the poor farmer with schistosomiasis usually is not able to afford to do this.

PRIMARY ARTERITIS OF THE AORTA

This clinically distinctive arteritis of unknown etiology occurs in all continents but most often in Asia, Africa, and Latin America. It is most common in Oriental women and has been frequently reported by Japanese investigators since its first description by Takayasu in 1908.

There is no definite association between this disease and infection, but there is some evidence implicating mycobacteria. Histologically, however, the disease does not resemble tuberculous infection but rather a nonspecific, nonatherosclerotic panarteritis. Current thinking favors an autoimmune etiology.

CLINICAL MANIFESTATIONS AND DIAGNOSIS. Early symptoms of this arteritis include fever, weight loss, night sweats, and erythema nodosum. The tuberculin test may be positive. Such findings in a young Oriental woman, coupled with the presence of tenderness and/or bruits over the carotid arteries plus a very high sedimentation rate, clinically suggest the diagnosis of Takayasu's arteritis.

Later in the disease, when "pulselessness" is apparent, the diagnosis is obvious. Patients complain of visual or neurologic symptoms and sometimes note claudication in their arms. Pulses are difficult to feel in the arms and neck, and the retinal arteries are nonpulsatile. The femoral arteries usually are easily felt. Unless there is considerable involvement of the descending thoracic aorta, the pressure in the legs is usually high. Involvement of the carotid arteries below the carotid sinus also results in systemic hypertension. The renal arteries may be involved, producing stenosis and hypertension. Because of the high pressure in the ascending aorta and involvement of the aortic valve, patients with primary arteritis can develop aortic regurgitation. The combination of an aortic regurgitation murmur with weak rather than bounding pulses in the arms is a distinctive finding in this disease.

TREATMENT AND PROGNOSIS. Treatment consists of surgical correction of the lesion when feasible, but early involvement of the coronary or renal arteries carries a poor prognosis. Steroids have not been effective except in the early febrile phases of the Takayasu variety. Antituberculous drugs should be considered in patients with positive tuberculin skin tests, because of the possibility of an active tuberculous infection.

AORTIC AND VENTRICULAR ANEURYSMS

AORTA. Aneurysms of the aorta may be saccular, fusiform, or dissecting. They may give rise to pressure symptoms depending on their size and location. Abnormal pulsation may be visible over the chest wall, but the diagnosis is best made on chest or abdominal x-ray confirmed by angiography.

A dissecting aneurysm usually results from a tear in the aorta such that blood leaks into the media, dissecting the aortic wall for a variable length. It becomes rapidly fatal if it eventually ruptures outside the aortic wall. The clinical picture of dissection is that of severe chest pain extending rapidly to the back, groin, and legs. Ischemia or infarction of organs may occur from blockage of arteries to the brain, the kidneys and gastrointestinal tract, or the limbs. Serial chest x-ray shows enlargement of the aorta, and an angiogram determines the site and extent of the dissection. Treatment, when possible, is by resection and graft replacement.

VENTRICLE. In many tropical areas, ventricular aneurysms are of the subvalvular type, affecting more the mitral and aortic valve rings. Most of these patients are symptomless, but a few complain of palpitations or chest pain radiating to the neck and arm; some may have symptoms due to pressure on neighboring structures. Emboli may arise from these aneurysms, giving rise to angina or pain over the spleen or kidneys. Physical signs may be confined to congestive heart failure, but there is sometimes a pansystolic mitral incompetence murmur with an audible third heart sound.

The chest x-ray shows an enlarged heart with an unusual bulge on the left cardiac border caused by the aneurysm. A left ventricular angiogram demonstrates its location and size. The only effective treatment is open heart surgery: resection of the aneurysm combined with valve replacement.

NUTRITIONAL HEART DISEASE

PROTEIN-CALORIE MALNUTRITION. Protein-calorie malnutrition can lead to hearts with interstitial edema or with gradual disappearance of all pericardial fat and consequent atrophy. Clinically the cardiac output is reduced, and there is ECG evidence of S-T segment elevation and low-voltage, flat, or inverted T waves. There may also be sudden cardiac arrest or fibrillation (Chapter 106).

BERIBERI HEART DISEASE. With deficiency in dietary thiamine, the beriberi heart may develop, characterized by peripheral vasodilatation, high-output biventricular myocardial failure, and sodium retention. In its extreme form, cardiomegaly is associated with marked dyspnea, restlessness, and cyanosis. This condition improves rapidly when large doses of thiamine (50 mg) are given orally or parenterally. The skin temperature falls, and the gross cardiac picture reverses itself to near-normal within a few days (Chapter 107.2).

ALCOHOL AND HEART DISEASE

This is a form of cardiomyopathy that results from the direct toxic effect of alcohol on the heart in the relatively malnourished, thiamine-deficient individual. Certain additives in beer (e.g., cobalt) may complicate the picture. Patients have a long history of heavy alcohol intake and complain of palpitations followed by features of left- or right-sided heart failure. A chest x-ray shows a globular enlarged heart with evidence of pulmonary congestion. A wide variety of ECG abnormalities have been described, including arrhythmias (atrial and ventricular extrasystoles, atrial fibrillation, sinus tachycardia), abnormal P waves, low-voltage QRS complex, prolonged Q-T interval, and bizarre forms of T waves (dimpled, spinous, cloven, flat, or negative). The blood pressure is normal, and there is no evidence of coronary or valvular heart disease.

Congestive heart failure is managed along conventional lines; complete abstinence from alcohol is mandatory. Some patients respond well to thiamine or vasodilator drugs.

CARDIOVASCULAR SYPHILIS

Syphilitic involvement of the heart and arteries has become unusual in the industrialized world, but autopsy series from elsewhere (e.g., Khartoum) show syphilis accounting for over 10% of all cardiovascular deaths, just as it did in Europe a century ago. It has a male preponderance, and the common age spectrum is 10 to 40 years (Chapter 32.1). Aneurysms may occur in the ascending or thoracic aorta or less commonly in the abdominal aorta above the renal vessels. Pathologically there is endarteritis obliterans of the vasa vasorum of large vessels, leading to medial necrosis and disruption of the elastic tissue in the relevant part of the aorta.

Diagnostic clues include a history of chancre, angina in a young man with mild to moderate aortic insufficiency, and tell-tale neurologic stigmata (in about 40% of patients). Standard tests (e.g., the VDRL) may be negative in about a third of patients with cardiovascular syphilis, but the FTA/ABS test is almost always positive.

Distinct clinical syndromes associated with cardiovascular syphilis include (1) asymptomatic uncomplicated aortitis, (2) aortic incompetence, (3) aneurysms (fusiform or saccular, but not dissecting), and (4) coronary ostial stenosis.

Although treatment with penicillin is routinely given, it is difficult to know what purpose it serves, since the disease is chronic and the changes irreversible. Conversely, in very rare instances, treatment has been associated with the dramatic enlargement of a small aneurysm.

BIBLIOGRAPHY

Akinkugbe OO, Falase AO: In Clinical Medicine in the Tropics Series: I. Cardiovascular Disease. Oxford, Blackwell Scientific Publications, 1987.

Amorim DS: Chagas' disease. In Yu PN, Goodwin IF (eds): Progress in Cardiology, Vol. 8. Philadelphia, jLea & Febiger, 1979, pp 235–279.

Basta LL, El-Din HE, Mokhtar A, et al: Clinical and hemodynamic study of patients with bilarzial pulmonary hypertension. Ain Shams Med J. 23:101, 1972.

Braithwaite AF: Cardiac disease at autopsy in the Bahamas. CAREC Surveillance Report 10: 1, 1984.

Cheever AW, Kamel IA, Elwi AM, et al: Schistosoma mansoni and S. haematobium infections in Egypt. III. Extrahepatic pathology. Am J Trop Med Hyg 27:55, 1978.

Ikeme AC: Idiopathic cardiomegaly in Africa. In Akinkugbe OO (ed): Cardiovascular Disease in Africa. Basel, Ciba Geigy, 1976, pp 15–23.

Ishikawa K: Survival and morbidity after diagnosis of occlusive thromboaortopathy (Takayasu's disease). Am J Cardiol 47:1026, 1981.

Okoroma EO, Ihenacho HNC, Anyanwu CH: Rheumatic fever in Nigerian children. Am J Dis Child 135:236, 1981.

Olsen EGI, Spry CIF: The pathogenesis of Loeffler's endomyocardial disease and its relationship to endomyocardial fibrosis. In Yu PN, Goodwin, JF (eds): Progress in Cardiology, Vol. 8. Philadelphia, Lea & Febiger, 1979, pp 281–303.

Shaper AG: Cardiovascular disease in the Tropics. I. Rheumatic heart. Br Med J 3:683, 1972.

Shaper AG: Cardiovascular disease in the Tropics. II. Endomyocardial fibrosis. Br Med J 3:743, 1972.

Stollerman GH: Rheumatic fever. In Braunwald E (ed): Heart Disease, 3rd ed. Philadelphia, WB Saunders, 1988, pp 1706–1717.

Vaughan JP: A brief review of cardiovascular disease in Africa. Trans R Soc Trop Med Hyg 71:226, 1977.

3. GASTROINTESTINAL DISEASES

Stephen G. Wright

COMMON SYNDROMES OF GASTROINTESTINAL DISEASE IN THE TROPICS

Gastrointestinal problems are common in medical practice in the tropics and subtropics. The principal syndromes are acute diarrhea (less than 2 weeks' duration), chronic diarrhea (greater than 2 weeks' duration), abdominal pain, and abdominal distention.

Diarrhea

This is one of the most common presentations. The majority of patients are children, but individuals of all ages can be affected. Increased frequency of bowel action and altered consistency of the stools are the usual symptoms. The duration of diarrhea is a guide to the range of conditions that must be considered. Most acute infections of the gut have resolved or are resolving within 2 weeks. Diarrhea that wakens the patient at night should always prompt thorough investigation, as it suggests an underlying organic cause.

ACUTE DIARRHHEA. Intoxications, viral and bacterial pathogens, and Cryptosporidium cause diarrhea of shorter duration (Table 3–1). In a large study from Bangladesh, rotavirus was the most common cause of diarrhea in children under 2 years of age (Chapter 18.2). The presence of systemic upset suggests an invasive bacterial infection, though this may also be a feature in rotavirus illness.

TABLE 3–1. Causes of Diarrhea Lasting Less Than 2 Weeks

Viruses
Rotavirus
Norwalk agent
Adenoviruses
Coronaviruses
(Probably more agents yet to be defined)

Bacteria
Intoxication—Staphylococcal enterotoxin
        Clostridium perfringens enterotoxin
        Bacillus cereus enterotoxin
        Botulism (uncommon)
Infection—*Escherichia coli* (enterotoxigenic, enteropathic,
    enteroinvasive)
    Vibrio cholerae
    Vibrio parahaemolyticus
    Campylobacter enteritis
    Salmonella species (nontyphoid)
    Shigella species
    Yersinia enterocolitica

Protozoa
Cryptosporidium species (immunocompetent host)

Watery Diarrhea. Large-volume stools indicate a small bowel etiology, with cholera and enterotoxigenic *Escherichia coli* often implicated (Chapter 41.1). Diarrhea induced by accumulation of malabsorbed solutes in the gut lumen also produces large-volume stools, and in children low stool pH may be an indicator of this. Toxin-induced secretory diarrhea will continue unaffected by food intake, whereas solute-induced diarrhea is reduced by reduced food intake. The passage of much rectal gas and frothy stools is an indication of malabsorption of carbohydrate in the small intestine and fermentation of unabsorbed substrates by colonic bacteria. *Cryptosporidium* is the only parasite to cause short-lived and self-limiting diarrhea. Both small and large bowel can be involved, but the stools are nondysenteric. This infection in patients with impaired immune responses causes prolonged diarrhea.

Dysentery. Diarrhea with blood in the stools indicates inflammation and ulceration of the colonic wall. In acute illnesses, bacterial infection is usually the cause; the presence of pus cells in fecal smears supports this possibility. Colicky abdominal pain is more common with this group of infections, and tenderness over the colon, particularly the sigmoid colon, is often found. Amebic dysentery does not usually present acutely as a cause of dysenteric diarrhea.

CHRONIC DIARRHEA. Weight loss is the main clinical feature that separates functional disorders of intestinal motility and hypolactasia in the adult (in whom it is not solely responsible for significant weight loss) from disorders causing malabsorption (Table 3–2) or inflammatory and malignant disease of the gastrointestinal tract. When there is continuing diarrhea without systemic upset or weight loss, disorders of intestinal motility need to be considered.

Small Bowel Disorders. The passage of frequent, pale, offensive stools suggests malabsorption. Stool weight is a useful clinical indicator, greater than 200 gm/24 hours being abnormal. Pancreatic disease in the tropics is not uncommon and often is unrelated to alcohol ingestion. Calcific pancreatitis can occur, even in young children.

TABLE 3–2. Causes of Diarrhea Lasting More Than 2 Weeks

Specific Infections
Cryptosporidiosis (immunodeficient)
Giardia lamblia
Amebic dysentery
Trichinella spiralis (rare)
Capillaria philippinensis (limited geographic distribution)
Strongyloides stercoralis (uncommon)

Malabsorption Syndromes
Giardiasis
Chronic calcific pancreatitis
Tropical sprue
Intestinal tuberculosis
Celiac disease (rare in indigenous populations)

Diarrhea in AIDS
Mild to moderate to severe

Tuberculosis is a cause of intestinal strictures that may cause malabsorption (Chapter 58). Immunoproliferative small intestinal disease (IPSID), also known as alpha-chain disease, occurs widely throughout the tropics and should be considered as a cause of malabsorption. Hyperpigmentation, gross weight loss, finger clubbing, and edema are prominent clinical features in advanced cases (Chapter 11).

The acquired immunodeficiency syndrome (AIDS) commonly causes chronic diarrhea in patients in the tropics and the subtropics (Chapter 15.1). Clinicians in Uganda described "slim disease," manifested as continuing diarrhea with weight loss, as a recognized presentation of AIDS. Several intestinal parasites (e.g., *Cryptosporidium, Isospora belli, Microsporidia*) are commonly found in association with other infectious agents (e.g., cytomegalovirus, nontyphoidal salmonellae, *Shigella, Mycobacterium avium-intracellulare,* and *M. tuberculosis*) in the gut of patients with AIDS.

LARGE BOWEL DISORDERS. Inflammatory bowel disease due to Crohn's disease and ulcerative colitis is widely recognized throughout the temperate world; there are increasing numbers of case reports of these diseases in migrants from tropical areas and in indigenous tropical residents. Although this should be considered in patients with diarrheal disease, abdominal pain, weight loss, and mucosal abnormalities in the small or large intestine, specific infectious causes of inflammatory disease, e.g., amebiasis or tuberculosis, must first be rigorously excluded before nonspecific inflammatory diseases are diagnosed. Proctocolitis is a relatively common finding in homosexuals and patients with AIDS, though a specific infection is not always found. *Cryptosporidium* and cytomegalovirus are two well-recognized causes. Leishmaniasis in its visceral form can involve the intestine, and in AIDS severe infections occur. There has been a report of a rectal lesion due to *Leishmania.*

Abdominal Pain

The range of causes is as wide as it is in temperate regions (Table 3–3). Both gastric and duodenal peptic ulcers are common in the tropics. Malignant lesions of

TABLE 3–3. Causes of Abdominal Pain

Peptic ulceration (gastric or duodenal; benign or malignant, including gastric lymphoma)
Chronic pancreatic disease
Complications of heavy ascaris infection
Sickle cell disease with abdominal crisis
Intussusception
Intestinal volvulus
Incarcerated or strangulated hernia
Pelvic inflammatory disease
Ectopic pregnancy
Appendicitis

the stomach, e.g., carcinoma and lymphoma, occur. Therefore, full investigation with endoscopic biopsy should be undertaken where indicated, if facilities exist. Chronic pancreatitis can be a cause of persisting epigastric pain. Pancreatic calcification may be seen on plain radiographs of the abdomen, and marked changes may be present on ultrasound scans. This disease occurs in children as well as adults.

Adult ascaris worms can migrate into the biliary and pancreatic ducts to cause upper abdominal pain as well as biliary tract obstruction or pancreatitis (Fig. 83–3; Chapter 83). A massive knotted bolus of worms can also cause intestinal obstruction and may be associated with volvulus of the intestine.

Sickle cell disease is common in many parts of the tropics and in migrants and their children moving from those areas to temperate regions (Chapter 5). Acute abdominal pain with physical signs as a manifestation of sickle cell crisis can be difficult to distinguish from acute appendicitis or other causes of acute abdominal pain. Intussusception is fairly common in the tropics. Pelvic inflammatory disease and ectopic pregnancy secondary to infection-induced damage to the fallopian tubes should also be considered in females with acute lower abdominal pain. Appendicitis is well recognized in the tropics.

Abdominal Distention

Abdominal distention can be caused by a wide range of diseases (Table 3–4). Ascites is frequently encountered, and examination of ascitic fluid is essential for diagnosis. Tuberculosis (Chapter 61) and chronic liver disease are among the most common causes. It should be remembered that spontaneous bacterial peritonitis may complicate ascites due to chronic liver disease

TABLE 3–4. Causes of Abdominal Distention

Fluid—Ascites *due to* chronic liver disease (cirrhosis, hepatosplenic schistosomiasis)
intra-abdominal tuberculosis
intra-abdominal malignancy
disease of the heart or pericardium
lymphatic disease (chylous ascites)
Mass effect—Huge ovarian cyst
Dissemination of hydatid cysts into the peritoneal cavity
Gaseous distention—Hypolactasia
Bowel motility disorders
Toxic dilatation of the colon

(Chapter 4). Hepatosplenic schistosomiasis is a common cause of ascites in endemic areas (Chapter 96). Intra-abdominal malignancy may present with ascites, and cytologic examination of fluid may show cancer cells. Chylous ascites is uncommon. Heart disease due to endomyocardial fibrosis, rheumatic heart disease, and constrictive pericarditis can cause ascites as part of severe heart failure (Chapter 2). Huge ovarian cysts can present with massive abdominal distention, but the central location of the swelling, presence of a fluid thrill, and absence of shifting dullness help to distinguish this from ascites. Occasionally, patients who have peritoneal dissemination of hydatid material from a ruptured hepatic cyst are seen with a massively distended abdomen in which numerous small lumps can be felt (Chapter 101.2). Eosinophilia is usual in these cases. Ultrasound scanning is especially useful in visualizing the numerous peritoneal cysts. Ultrasound is also particularly valuable in the investigation of intra-abdominal conditions.

Gaseous distention of the abdomen is a common complaint. It may relate to hypolactasia, which can be primary or secondary. It may be part of the irritable bowel syndrome. When abdominal distention develops acutely in a very ill patient with dysenteric diarrhea, toxic dilatation of the colon must be considered. This complication can occur in the course of any of the colitides related to infection and nonspecific ulcerative colitis or Crohn's disease.

The Acquired Immunodeficiency Syndrome and the Gastrointestinal Tract

The acquired immunodeficiency syndrome (AIDS) due to infection with the human immunodeficiency virus (HIV) is commonly associated with gut disease, most often due to infections but also due to Kaposi's sarcoma and intestinal lymphoma (Chapter 15.1). Gut involvement is summarized in Table 3–5.

ESOPHAGITIS. This is a common manifestation of AIDS, and *Candida albicans* is the most frequent cause (Chapter 66.6). It presents with dysphagia and is usually associated with florid oral candidiasis. Cytomegalovirus (CMV), *herpes simplex,* and much less commonly, *Torulopsis glabrata* can also produce esophagitis.

TABLE 3–5. Gut Involvement in AIDS

Infection	Esophagitis	*Candida albicans*
		Cytomegalovirus
		Herpes simplex
		Torulopsis glabrata
	Enteritis	Mild, nonspecific CMV
		Salmonellosis
		Campylobacter
		Tuberculosis (*M. tuberculosis* and atypical organisms, esp. *M. avium-intracellulare*)
		Cryptosporidium
		Isospora belli
		Microsporidia
		Leishmania (possible)
	Pancreatitis	CMV
		Toxoplasma gondii
Malignancy	Any location	Kaposi's sarcoma
		Intestinal lymphoma

ENTERITIS. Chronic diarrhea may be the presenting feature in AIDS, and "slim disease" described from Uganda is one manifestation of this. A wide range of viral bacterial and parasitic pathogens have been isolated from the intestines of infected patients with diarrhea, and often more than one pathogen may be found. However, a recent study showed that 50% of patients with chronic diarrhea had no detectable gut pathogen.

Mycobacterial infections of the gut are fairly common; it should be noted that the clinical features and findings on investigation are similar to those seen in non–HIV infected patients (Chapter 61.1). Bearing in mind how common tuberculosis is in the tropics, gastrointestinal manifestations of tuberculous disease may become more common because of AIDS. The disease responds to standard antituberculous therapy, but there are indications that reactions to these drugs may be more common. It will be important for clinicians to document their experience in treating these cases, particularly with regard to duration of therapy and occurrence of relapses. Short-course chemotherapy in these cases will require careful assessment. Atypical mycobacteria also cause intestinal tuberculosis in AIDS (Chapter 61.2). Colitis is recognized in AIDS, though it may be less common in Africa. Cytomegalovirus and *Cryptosporidium* are two causes.

PANCREATITIS. The pancreas may be infected with CMV. *Toxoplasma gondii* has also been identified in the pancreas. Pancreatitis and other abnormalities, e.g., swelling of the gland, are common. Abnormal endocrine and exocrine functions have been suggested, but studies from Uganda have failed to show defects in exocrine function.

MALIGNANCY. Kaposi's sarcoma is the most common malignancy seen in AIDS and can occur anywhere in the gut (Chapter 11). Multicentric tumors are found. Lymphomas also occur.

DISEASES OF THE GASTROINTESTINAL TRACT COMMON TO THE TROPICS

Gastrointestinal diseases are among the most common encountered in the tropics. Table 3–6 lists some of those that are frequently found in the tropical and temperate regions of the world.

Cancrum Oris

Gangrenous necrosis of the soft tissues of the lips and cheeks is the main feature of this condition. It is common in malnourished children. Measles and anemia are other predisposing conditions. The sequence of events is that an ulcer on the lip, perhaps due to herpes, becomes secondarily infected with the anaerobic bacteria *Fusiformis fusiformis* and *Borrelia vincentii*. An area of soft tissue necrosis spreads from the original ulcer, with these bacteria growing in the tissue at the extending margin. In most cases, there is an obvious line of demarcation between healthy and gangrenous tissues. Treatment with penicillin will control the infection, but

TABLE 3–6. Occurrence of Gastrointestinal Diseases in the Tropics

More Common in the Tropics	Less Common in the Tropics
Pyloric stenosis due to duodenal ulcer	Gastric ulcer
Gastrointestinal infections	Hemorrhage and perforation as complications of duodenal ulcer
Tuberculosis of the abdomen and intestine	
Malabsorption due to	Gluten-sensitive enteropathy
Giardiasis	Mesenteric vascular occlusion
Tropical sprue	Diverticulosis
Chronic calcific pancreatitis	Nonspecific ulcerative colitis
Malnutrition	Crohn's disease
Alpha-chain disease	Ischemic colitis
Hypolactasia	
Capillariasis	
Strongyloidiasis	
Specific inflammatory bowel disease	
Intestinal obstruction due to	
Ascariasis	
Intestinal volvulus	
Intussusception	

necrotic tissues will slough and surgical reconstruction is needed to correct the deformities.

Esophageal Disease

ESOPHAGITIS. Chemical burns of the esophagus are common in the tropics as a result of drinking corrosive substances, e.g., Lysol, sodium hydroxide, sulfuric acid, and nitric acid, either with suicidal intent or by accident. Two Nigerian proprietary medicines contain corrosive substances.

Severe pain, shock, esophagitis, and perforation of the esophagus are immediate effects of drinking such corrosive agents. There is a high mortality rate; those who survive often develop fibrous strictures, which cause dysphagia and necessitate periodic dilatation.

ESOPHAGEAL VARICES. Esophageal varices are relatively common in the tropics. The causes can be classified as prehepatic, hepatic, and posthepatic. Increased blood flow through the hepatic portal vein in the tropical splenomegaly syndrome and portal vein thrombosis are prehepatic causes. Cirrhosis, schistosomal hepatofibrosis, veno-occlusive disease of the liver, and Indian childhood cirrhosis are hepatic causes, whereas constrictive pericarditis and chronic congestive cardiac failure due to rheumatic heart disease and endomyocardial fibrosis are posthepatic causes. Bleeding from varices is a life-threatening complication, and management comprises restoration of circulating volume with blood transfusions and prevention of further bleeding by measures such as balloon tamponade, vasopressin (Pitressin) infusion, and obliteration of bleeding varices by endoscopic sclerotherapy. Surgical decompression by shunting procedures is a very difficult undertaking.

MEGAESOPHAGUS. This is irreversible dilatation of the esophagus that may occur in chronic *Trypanosoma cruzi* infections owing to destruction of ganglion cells of the autonomic plexuses in the esophageal wall (Chapter 75). Contractile activity is lost, and the patients complain of dysphagia. Aspiration pneumonia may also occur. There is no specific treatment for megaesophagus, but pneumonia will require antibiotic treatment.

Peptic Ulcer Disease

DISTRIBUTION AND INCIDENCE. Gastric ulcer and duodenal ulcer occur in indigenous populations throughout the tropics and subtropics, although information about their incidences is incomplete.

Gastric ulcer is relatively rare in Africa and Asia. An increased incidence of gastric ulcer has been reported from the highland regions of Papua New Guinea, but most of the ulcers found were prepyloric, conforming to the pattern of duodenal ulcer. The incidence of gastric ulcer increases with age in developed countries; thus, the low incidence in the tropics may be related to shorter life expectancy in indigenous populations.

Duodenal ulcer is particularly common in West Africa, northern Tanzania, Ethiopia, southern and northeastern India, and Afghanistan. It is relatively common in the hilly areas of northwestern India. The ratio of duodenal ulcer to gastric ulcer in the tropics is higher than in developed countries.

ETIOLOGY. Repeated observations have linked the presence of organisms first referred to as *Campylobacter pyloridis* but now called *Helicobacter pylori* with gastric ulcer, duodenal ulcer, and antral gastritis. They have been found in Gram-stained biopsies of inflamed and ulcerated tissue. Reports from Africa, India, and Malaya have identified these organisms in symptomatic patients with dyspepsia both with and without ulceration. There have also been suggestions that *H. pylori* may contribute to cases of "epidemic hypochlorhydria." The exact role of these organisms in the pathogenesis of gastroduodenal inflammation and ulceration has yet to be defined, and it should be noted that a proportion of normal individuals also carry these organisms without having dyspepsia.

CLINICAL MANIFESTATIONS, COMPLICATIONS, AND THERAPY. Epigastric pain after eating is a usual symptom, with the pain usually relieved by taking antacids. Symptoms wax and wane with time. Management consists of relieving pain and promoting healing. Drugs that have antimicrobial action against *H. pylori* have caused healing in patients with gastritis and peptic ulceration.

The main complications are hemorrhage, perforation, and, most commonly, pyloric stenosis. Projectile vomiting, absence of bile staining of the vomitus, and the presence of food residue from meals eaten on the previous day are features that suggest the presence of pyloric stenosis. Partial gastrectomy (Polya type) is indicated to relieve the stenosis and to reduce gastric acid secretion.

Intestinal Infection

Gastrointestinal infection is a major cause of morbidity and mortality in the tropics and subtropics. Children are most often and most seriously affected. Dehydration is the main cause of death, whereas deterioration of nutritional state is the main cause of morbidity. The mortality rate among infants and young children from dehydrating diarrheal disease in the tropics is 55 per 1000 per year, compared with a rate of 0.4 per 1000 per year in Europe.

ETIOLOGY AND DISTRIBUTION. Rotavirus is the most common gut pathogen found worldwide in children under 2 years of age (Chapter 18.2). When all age groups are considered, enterotoxigenic strains of *Escherichia coli* are the most common pathogens (Chapter 41.1), responsible for almost one third of episodes of diarrhea in a large study from Bangladesh and the second most common pathogen in children under 2 years (Table 3–1 and 3–2). *Campylobacter* species have a worldwide distribution and are relatively common causes of infectious diarrheal disease wherever they are looked for. Salmonellosis is the most common cause of food poisoning in developed countries. Varying incidences of salmonellosis have been reported from countries in the tropics (Chapter 39). Shigellae are common worldwide and cause diarrhea in all age groups (Chapter 37). *Escherichia coli* O:157 causes a dysenteric illness very similar to shigellosis. The last 2 decades have seen the spread of cholera due to the El Tor biotype; most African countries have now had epidemics (Chapter 40). *Vibrio parahaemolyticus* is one of the few organisms limited in geographic distribution, with most cases in Japan and the countries of Southeast Asia. Sporadic cases occur in other areas (Chapter 40.1).

TRANSMISSION AND EPIDEMIOLOGY. Infection occurs by the ingestion of organisms in food and water contaminated by feces from a man or animal excreting the organism. This contamination is associated with inadequate public sanitation and low standards of personal hygiene. Defecation near pools and streams that are sources of water for domestic use is common, and simple sewage disposal systems often empty feces into the domestic water supply of the next house. Person-to-person spread of infection also occurs.

Seafoods such as shellfish, mussels, and crabs transmit viruses causing gastroenteritis, cholera and *V. parahaemolyticus*. Flies carry bacteria from feces to food on their mouth parts and legs. Low standards of kitchen hygiene in homes and public eating places also encourage transmission of intestinal infection. Precooked food kept warm for long periods, e.g., food bought from roadside food peddlers, may transmit a number of gut pathogens and contain enterotoxin formed by staphylococci growing in warmed food. Poultry and eggs are important sources of nontyphoid salmonellae. Salmonellae are harbored in the gut of chickens.

An important and avoidable source of intestinal infection in infants results from misguided attempts at bottle-feeding with powdered milk solution instead of breast-feeding. Unsterilized bottles and nipples and contaminated water all contribute to the considerable risk of gut infection.

Most intestinal infections occur in children; 40% of all cases occur in those under 2 years old; 60% occur in children under 9 years of age. Lower socioeconomic groups are most often affected. Malnutrition is a predisposing factor, and diarrhea is prolonged in malnourished children. Reduced gastric acid secretion as a result of malnutrition, surgery, or atrophic gastritis is also a predisposing factor. There is some evidence to suggest that specific infections may cause gastritis and reduced acid secretion, e.g., *H. pylori*.

PATHOGENESIS AND PATHOLOGY. Diarrhea can be defined as an increase in the water content of stools. Physiologically, the cause may be that (1) the small intestine secretes more fluid than it reabsorbs; (2) solute absorption in the small intestine is impaired so that the osmotic load retains fluid in the gut lumen; (3) the volume of fluid entering the colon exceeds its capacity for water absorption; (4) water- and electrolyte-reabsorbing capacity of the colon is reduced as a result of enterotoxigenic infection such as cholera; or (5) the water-reabsorbing capacity and motility of the colon are altered by localized or generalized colonic inflammation and ulceration. Protein-rich fluid is also lost through inflamed and ulcerated mucosa in any area of the gut. Infectious agents produce diarrhea by causing one or more of these effects.

Enterotoxin-Producing Bacteria. *Vibrio cholerae* typifies those bacterial pathogens that cause diarrhea through the actions of enterotoxins. The cholera vibrio adheres to proximal small bowel epithelial cells but does not invade the mucosa. The cholera enterotoxin is secreted and binds to the GM_1 ganglioside component of the epithelial cell surface. A subunit of the bound toxin is transported into the cell, where it activates the enzyme adenyl cyclase located in the basolateral regions of the cell. Increased amounts of cyclic adenosine monophosphate (cyclic AMP) are produced. This inhibits absorption of sodium, chloride, and water by villous epithelial cells and stimulates sodium-dependent secretion of chloride and possibly bicarbonate by crypt cells (Chapter 40). This is not the sole mechanism causing net fluid secretion in cholera. There is also evidence that local neurohumoral mechanisms are involved.

Enterotoxigenic *E. coli* produce 2 enterotoxins, designated heat-labile enterotoxin and heat-stable enterotoxin (Chapter 41.1). The former activates adenylate cyclase, and the heat-stable enterotoxin activates guanylate cyclase to produce cyclic guanosine monophosphate. There are some differences in the physiologic changes that ensue, but the result is net secretion of isotonic fluid. The enterotoxin of *Staphylococcus aureus* is thought to act through adenylate cyclase stimulation, and the *Shigella* enterotoxin may have a similar effect in the proximal small intestine. *Salmonella* enterotoxin causes intracellular accumulation of cyclic AMP with net secretion of isotonic fluid mediated by local synthesis of prostaglandins.

Colonic function in infectious diarrhea has not had the intense examination given to the small intestine. Recent work in cholera has shown defects in epithelial function, and new insights into the absorptive functions have shown the colonic epithelium to be actively involved in substrate absorption.

Invasive Bacteria. *Shigella*, *Salmonella*, and *Campylobacter* species are enteroinvasive organisms. *Campylobacter* can invade the mucosa at any site in the small or large intestine, whereas *Shigella* and *Salmonella* invade the colonic mucosa and terminal ileum. Histologically, the changes comprise epithelial ulceration, tissue edema, and acute inflammation.

Intestinal Protozoa. *Giardia lamblia*, *Cryptosporidium*, and *Entamoeba histolytica* frequently cause diarrhea; *Balantidium coli* infections are rare. Direct mucosal damage, malabsorption of nutrients, and secondary bacterial colonization contribute to diarrhea in giardiasis (Chapter 69). Histologic changes in the proximal small bowel are nonspecific, although trophozoites may be found in the intervillous spaces. *Cryptosporidium* causes a short-lived, self-limiting diarrheal illness in immunocompetent persons. The mechanisms involved are poorly understood (Chapter 70).

Diarrhea in amebic dysentery results from ulceration where amebas invade the colonic mucosa (Chapter 68). The cecum and rectum are favored sites of invasion. Amebas are found in the tissues at the edges of the ulcers. Necrosis of tissue around the amebas is usual, although there may be acute inflammatory responses in the mucosa due to secondary bacterial infection.

Balantidium coli is usually a parasite of pigs, but in communities where there is close contact with pigs, it is known to invade the mucosa in man to cause dysenteric diarrhea (Chapter 71.1).

CLINICAL MANIFESTATIONS AND COMPLICATIONS. Vomiting and diarrhea are the most common symptoms in gastrointestinal infection. The onset of symptoms can vary from a few hours after ingesting food containing *Staphylococcus aureus* enterotoxin, to several days after ingesting bacterial pathogens, to 2 or more weeks in giardiasis.

Profuse watery diarrhea suggests infection causing net secretion of fluid in the small intestine. *Vibrio cholerae*, enterotoxigenic *E. coli*, rotavirus, and *Campylobacter* are the common causes of watery diarrhea. Frequent bowel actions with small volumes of stool and the passage of blood suggest colonic infection. Continuous central abdominal pain often precedes the onset of diarrhea in *Campylobacter* infections. Colicky abdominal pain is common in many gut infections, but the patient with cholera usually has no pain. Fever, chills, and generalized myalgia are usually associated with infection by invasive organisms. Diarrhea that persists for weeks with offensive yellow stools may indicate giardiasis. Irregular bowel movements with stools that vary in consistency and contain blood and mucus are characteristic of amebic dysentery.

Dysentery. Patients infected with invasive organisms are often ill-looking and febrile. Most patients have generalized abdominal tenderness with increased bowel sounds. The findings on rectal examination may be abnormal in patients with dysenteric diarrheas, e.g., an edematous, roughened mucosa and blood on the examiner's glove. A smear from the material on the glove should be made for immediate microscopy. Proctosigmoidoscopy should be performed in all patients with dysentery. This should be done with great care. Diffuse inflammation, ulceration, and bleeding of the rectal mucosa are usual in invasive bacterial infections, but scrapings should always be taken and examined for amebae.

Dehydration. The most important physical signs to be elicited concern the assessment of hydration (Part III, Section D, General Principles); the patient should be weighed at first presentation, as weight gain or loss can be a valuable guide to the effectiveness of rehydration. Severe dehydration is most common in cholera and enterotoxigenic *E. coli* infection.

Sequelae of Diarrhea. Dehydration is the most important cause of death in infants and children with gastrointestinal infection. The nutritional state of children often deteriorates because of anorexia, malabsorption of nutrients, and the common practice of not feeding children with diarrhea. Hypolactasia is a sequela of many gut infections and one that may be a cause of persisting diarrhea. Hemorrhage, perforation, and toxic dilatation of the colon may complicate diarrhea caused by invasive organisms. A hemolytic-uremic syndrome can complicate *Shigella dysenteriae* and *E. coli* O:157 infections (Chapter 37 and 41.1). Reactive arthritis and Reiter's syndrome can follow *Shigella, Salmonella, Campylobacter,* and *Yersinia* infections. Chronic diarrhea in children is the subject of considerable attention. Frequently, no specific pathogen can be related either to antecedent diarrheal disease or to continuing diarrhea. A child with persistent diarrhea is more likely to be malnourished. Cow's milk protein intolerance has been shown to be one cause of persisting diarrhea in Europe, and it may also contribute to this relatively common entity in the tropics.

DIAGNOSIS. The range of laboratory tests and expertise needed to make a specific microbiologic diagnosis in most patients with intestinal infection requires facilities not often available in the tropics. Some simple tests can be useful in most circumstances. It is important to examine the stool sample for blood. Flecks of blood-stained mucus should be mounted in saline for direct microscopic examination for motile trophozoites of *E. histolytica* (Chapter 122). A smear of fluid stools should always be examined by direct microscopy for amebic trophozoites and trophozoites and cysts of *G. lamblia.* The presence of any cellular exudate in the smear should also be noted. The presence of polymorphonuclear leukocytes suggests infection with enteroinvasive bacteria, whereas a predominance of red cells is found in amebic dysentery. A proctosigmoidoscopy should be performed in patients with dysentery. Ulcerated or bleeding areas of mucosa should be scraped and the material examined immediately for amebic trophozoites (Chapter 68).

TREATMENT AND PROGNOSIS. The mortality from dehydrating diarrheal diseases will decline if measures to correct and maintain hydration are started as early as possible.

Oral Rehydration. Oral rehydration with glucose electrolyte solution (ORS) has markedly reduced mortality from dehydrating diarrhea in communities in the tropics (Part III, Section D, General Principles). Local lay persons can distribute ORS and teach others how to make up and give the solution. The standard formula recommended by the World Health Organization is sucrose 40 gm, sodium chloride 3.5 gm, trisodium citrate dihydrate 2.9 gm, and potassium chloride 1.5 gm made up to 1 liter with clean water. The trisodium citrate has replaced sodium bicarbonate because the former gives better stability to the powdered mixture. An oral rehydration mixture made with rice flour as the carbohydrate source is also very effective.

Antimicrobial Agents. Antimicrobial drugs have a limited role in the treatment of gut infections. Giardiasis (Chapter 69) and amebiasis (Chapter 68) will require specific treatment with metronidazole or tinidazole. Antibiotics should also be given to those patients who have fever, abdominal pain, toxicity, tenesmus, and frequent stools containing mucus and blood, the symptoms and signs of infection with enteroinvasive organisms. Erythromycin is the drug of choice for *Campylobacter* infection, but the choice of agent for shigellosis and salmonellosis can be difficult because antibiotic resistance is common. Tetracycline treatment reduces the duration of diarrhea and fecal excretion of vibrios in cholera. The newer quinoline antibiotics are currently believed to have efficacy against all the foregoing enteroinvasive bacteria.

Symptomatic Therapy. Intestinal sedatives cannot be recommended in the treatment of infectious diarrhea. These drugs reduce intestinal motility but do not affect the pathologic processes. The reduced frequency of bowel movements causes fluid stagnation in the gut lumen, encouraging proliferation of organisms. The forward motion of fluid along the gut washing out organisms and toxins is lost.

The adverse effects of diarrhea on nutrition can be lessened by maintaining breast-feeding in infants and by the early reintroduction of feeding. Management of persistent diarrhea is rather empirical but comprises continued feeding despite the persistent diarrhea. Energy-rich, low-osmolality foods should be given. Frequent small-volume feeds may allow better absorption of nutrients than less frequent, large-volume feeds. Vitamin and mineral supplements should be given. Where the possibility of cow's milk protein intolerance exists, withdrawal of cow's milk may be tried. There is no evidence that the routine use of antibiotics has any role in management.

PREVENTION AND CONTROL. Providing clean drinking water and proper sewage disposal reduces the incidence of gut infections. Tube wells are one means of providing clean water. The construction of acceptable latrines will help to break the cycle of fecal-oral transmission of gut pathogens. Health education regarding the importance of good sanitary practices and breast-feeding should be given by trained members of the community.

Vaccination has been of considerable value in controlling many communicable diseases in man but hitherto has contributed little to the control of gut infections. Cholera vaccination has been used extensively, but the present parenteral preparation gives limited protection for a relatively short time. Oral immunization is the obvious route for vaccination against enteric pathogens. A variety of candidate vaccines are being tried. Rotavirus vaccines are currently under trial. Mutant and modified strains of other pathogens such as *Salmonella typhi* and *Vibrio cholerae* are also being assessed for antigenicity and protective efficacy.

Control of epidemics of gastrointestinal infection includes finding the source(s) of infection, detection of cases, and treatment, when necessary, to prevent transmission of the disease.

Malabsorption

Conditions that cause malabsorption in the tropics are listed in Table 3–7.

TROPICAL ENTEROPATHY. Minor degrees of malabsorption occur in patients following diarrhea due to many causes and in residents of the tropics. Impaired absorption of D-xylose is the usual abnormality, and there are minor abnormalities of the jejunal mucosa. This is referred to as tropical enteropathy and is the usual state in most tropical residents. It is not a stage in the development of other conditions such as tropical sprue. It may be noted that immunoproliferative small intestinal disease occurs in those in the underprivileged strata of society, whose intestines are exposed to more infectious insults and who may therefore have more "marked" tropical enteropathy. An abnormal jejunal microflora has been found in some of these patients who remain symptomatic after leaving the tropics.

TROPICAL SPRUE

Definition. Tropical sprue (TS) has been defined as impaired absorption of 2 or more unrelated test substances with no recognized underlying cause. The diagnosis of TS is therefore made by the exclusion of other conditions. A disadvantage of this definition is that it includes no measure of the severity of intestinal dysfunction and so it includes patients with minor abnormalities of absorption who do not develop severe weight loss and the hematologic complications that are so common in TS. The variability of the clinical presentations and the absence of a diagnostic test make the study of this condition difficult and raise the query that TS studied in the different endemic areas may not be the same disease process.

Distribution and Incidence. The endemic areas are Central and Southeast Asia, Puerto Rico, Cuba, Haiti, the Dominican Republic, Guatemala, Costa Rica, and Venezuela. Tropical sprue occurs in the Middle East but is rare in Africa. Epidemics of TS have occurred in India.

Both indigenous and expatriate populations are sus-

TABLE 3–7. Causes of Malabsorption in the Tropics

Tropical sprue
Chronic calcific pancreatitis
Parasitic infections
Giardiasis
Cryptosporidiosis
Strongyloidiasis
Capillariasis
Hypolactasia
Malnutrition
Alpha-chain disease
Intestinal tuberculosis

ceptible to TS in endemic areas. Upper and lower socioeconomic groups develop the condition. Black troops from West Africa serving in India were resistant to TS, whereas among Indian troops the incidence of TS was higher in vegetarians. Children are not commonly affected in endemic TS, although in epidemics they often develop it. Tropical sprue may follow a rapidly progressive course in women who are folate-deficient in late pregnancy or the puerperium.

Etiology and Pathogenesis. It is probable that several factors act together to cause TS. Patients often give a history of an acute gastrointestinal infection at the start of their illness, but no particular organism has been incriminated. Some persons affected in epidemic TS were found to be "resistant" to the condition in a second epidemic, suggesting that a single agent might have initiated both epidemics. If TS is simply a postinfective malabsorption syndrome, it is surprising that the condition is so uncommon in children, who have intestinal infections most often.

Gut Bacterial Flora. The jejunum is normally bacteriologically sterile. An abnormal jejunal microflora has been found in patients with TS studied in India and Puerto Rico and in Europeans with TS acquired in Asia and studied later in London. This microflora comprised enterobacteria, with higher yields of organisms from cultures of jejunal biopsy specimens than from aspirated jejunal fluid, suggesting that the organisms are adherent to the mucosa. Bacteria-free filtrates from cultures of these organisms produced net fluid secretion and mucosal changes in isolated loops of intestine in experimental animals. This abnormal microflora may therefore produce 1 or more toxins that damage the intestinal mucosa, impairing digestive and absorptive functions. Treatment with tetracycline usually eradicates the bacteria and is often associated with resolution of symptoms and intestinal abnormalities. Reduced gastric acid secretion, which has been found in Indians with TS, and incoordinate to-and-fro movements of intestinal contents with prolonged intestinal transit may be factors that promote and maintain colonization.

Folic Acid Deficiency. This occurs with increasing frequency in patients whose symptoms have been present for longer than 3 months. Women who have folate deficiency due to pregnancy and breast-feeding seem particularly susceptible to developing TS. Folic acid alone will cure a proportion of patients with TS. These observations indicate that folate deficiency may be important in the pathogenesis of TS. Folic acid is a vital cofactor in deoxyribonucleic acid (DNA) synthesis and therefore in the processes of cell replication. Two tissues with the highest folate requirements are the bone marrow and the intestinal epithelium. There is a similarity between erythropoiesis and the renewal of villous epithelial cells by crypt cell division. Both processes involve a stem cell compartment containing dividing cells that mature and enter the functional compartment. When folate deficiency is established in tropical sprue, disordered epithelial cell renewal may be analogous to disordered erythropoiesis. At this stage, the effects of folate deficiency on the gut may be the dominant abnormality. The cells of both the intestinal epithelium and the bone marrow are turning over rapidly, and so both tissues will be competing for available folate.

Malnutrition. Body wasting, hypoproteinemia, and depletion of vitamins and trace elements occur in severe TS, indicating malnutrition secondary to anorexia and malabsorption; however, malnutrition alone is not a primary cause of TS.

Immune Response. The prominent infiltrate of plasma cells and lymphocytes in the jejunal mucosa in TS suggests that immunologically mediated events may be occurring. These may be unrelated to the mucosal damage but may be evoked by antigens derived from the jejunal microflora and contribute to tissue damage.

Pathology. Impaired absorption of fat, D-xylose and vitamin B_{12} is usual. Secondary hypolactasia is common in expatriates of European stock with TS. Red cell folate levels decline with increasing duration of symptoms, and serum vitamin B_{12} levels may be reduced. These changes are associated with macrocytosis in the peripheral blood and, later, megaloblastic anemia. Plasma albumin levels decline, and there is depletion of trace elements, e.g., magnesium and zinc. Protein-losing enteropathy contributes to the low plasma albumin levels.

Nonspecific changes comprising thickening of mucosal folds and dilatation of small bowel loops are seen in small bowel radiologic studies (Fig. 3–1).

Jejunal biopsies are abnormal. A ridged or convoluted mucosa is usually seen on dissecting microscopy (Fig. 3–2). Light microscopy shows reduced villous height with deeper crypts containing increased numbers of cells in mitosis (Fig. 3–3). There is a prominent infiltrate of plasma cells and lymphocytes in the lamina propria and of lymphocytes in the surface epithelium. A completely atrophic mucosa is rarely seen in TS. The jejunal biopsy of an asymptomatic tropical resident is abnormal by North American standards but can be distinguished from TS by the greater degree of abnormality in TS.

Clinical Manifestations. The patient usually recalls an acute attack of diarrhea at the beginning of his illness, after which his bowel habit does not return to normal. Typically, the patient has several bowel actions in the early part of the day and the need may wake him from sleep in the early morning. The stools are soft, bulky, pale, and foul-smelling. Bowel actions are often accompanied by the passage of foul-smelling flatus. Abdominal distention and discomfort are commonly noticed. Appetite and energy decline, and the patient loses weight (Fig. 3–4). Patients with symptoms of several months' duration may have a sore tongue and mouth. Examination shows evidence of weight loss with mucosal pallor and glossitis in some patients. Abdominal distention and increased bowel sounds are often present. Rectal examination and sigmoidoscopy are normal.

Complications. The complications of TS are those of continuing diarrhea and malabsorption. Dehydration with electrolyte depletion is common among those patients with watery stools. Depletion of trace elements, e.g., zinc and magnesium, is common in patients having TS for several months. These deficiencies may contribute more to the clinical picture in severe TS than is appreciated at present. Low serum magnesium and calcium levels can cause tetany.

Severe megaloblastic anemia is most often caused by folic acid deficiency, with vitamin B_{12} deficiency being a less common cause. In a few of these patients, the hematologic features predominate, and gastrointestinal symptoms may be minimal or even absent. Subacute combined degeneration of the spinal cord has been seen in one patient with this form of tropical sprue.

Diagnosis. This depends on the results of intestinal absorption tests together with abnormalities of the jejunal biopsy (Figs. 3–2 and 3–3) and a history of residence in endemic areas. Some other causes of malabsorption are listed in Table 3–7 together with those conditions that can cause malabsorption in any area of the world.

Treatment

Diet. Provision of an adequate diet can cure TS. One third of a group of Indian patients were cured by diet alone. A low-lactose diet may control symptoms due to hypolactasia. Some patients are intolerant of fat, and thus a low-fat diet may be necessary. Avoidance of alcohol and foods seasoned with herbs and spices may also help alleviate symptoms.

Antibiotics and Folic Acid. Tetracycline, 250 mg 4 times daily for 1 to 3 months, is often effective; courses of up to 6 months' duration have been used in patients with prolonged TS. Physiologic doses of folic acid, 200 µg per day, will cure TS when there is folate deficiency, but it is usual to give 5 mg daily for a month or more. Tetracycline and folic acid are often given concurrently. A deficiency of vitamin B_{12}, if present, will need correction.

Prognosis. Within 3 months of starting treatment,

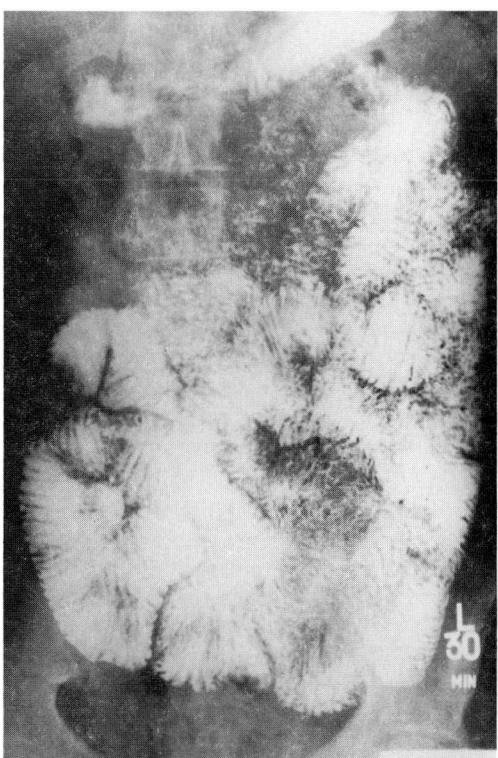

FIGURE 3–1. Widened loops of small bowel with thickened mucosal folds in a patient with tropical sprue. These are nonspecific signs and also occur in malabsorption due to giardiasis and celiac disease.

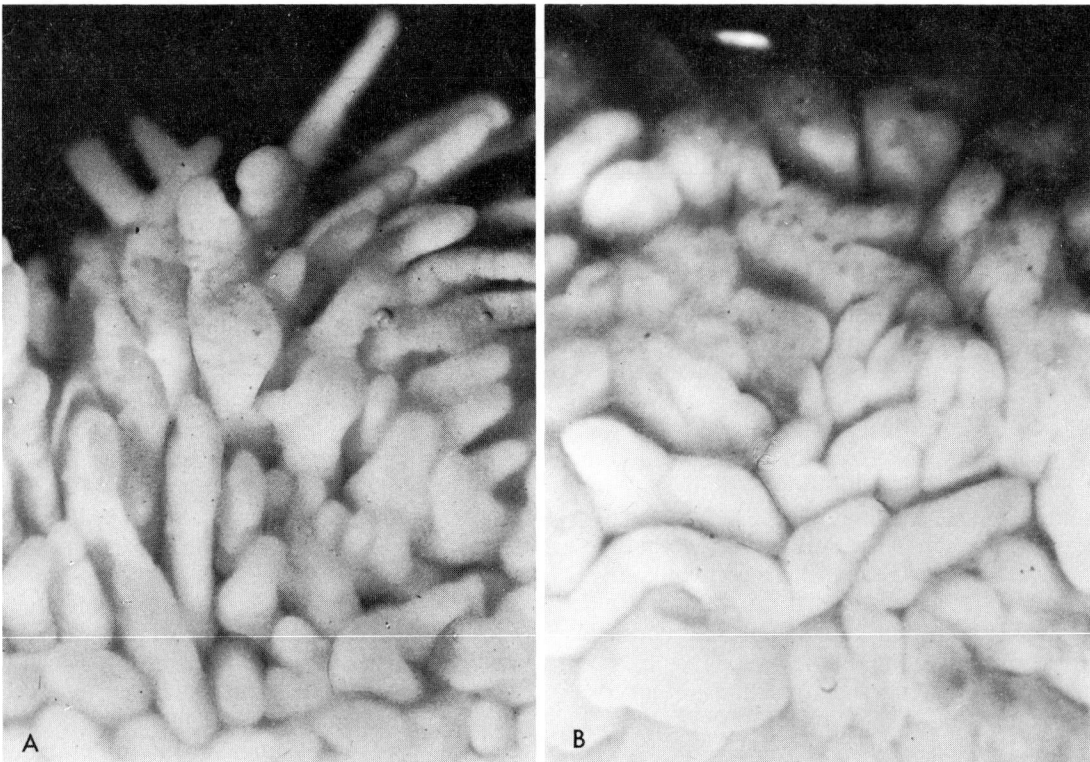

FIGURE 3–2. Dissecting microscopy of jejunal biopsies (× 60). *A*, Normal leaf- and finger-shaped villi. *B*, Thick, ridge-shaped, and convoluted villi from a patient with tropical sprue.

most patients show considerable improvement (Fig. 3–4), and intestinal absorption and mucosal changes will have improved or returned to normal. Some patients notice an improvement in symptoms within 2 or 3 days of starting treatment. Symptoms and impaired absorption persist in a minority of patients despite all combinations of treatment, in which case the original diagnosis of TS must be reconsidered to ensure that no other cause has been overlooked.

The prognosis in tropical sprue is now excellent, and most patients are completely cured. Deaths from TS were reported in the earlier part of this century and in epidemic TS before treatment could be given. The recurrence rate following cure is not known.

PARASITES AND MALABSORPTION. *Giardia lamblia, Cryptosporidium, Isospora belli, Strongyloides stercoralis,* and *Capillaria philippinensis* have all been associated with malabsorption. There is reasonable evidence for this association with giardiasis, although only a quarter of infected patients have gastrointestinal symptoms and less than half of those have malabsorption. Capillariasis causes a severe diarrheal illness with malabsorption and dehydration in well-defined areas in the Philippines and Thailand (Chapter 82.3). Strongyloidiasis is an occasional cause of malabsorption, although this has been disputed (Chapter 84.2).

Helminths and the Gut. The availability of upper gastrointestinal endoscopy has led to the reporting of series of cases in which ascaris worms have been found in the bile or the pancreatic ducts. Some of these patients had fibroscopic endoscopy for nonspecific colicky upper abdominal pain. A few had more severe upper abdom-

inal pain, jaundice due to bile duct obstruction, and ascending biliary tract sepsis and septicemia. Worms can also be demonstrated in these ectopic sites by ultrasound scanning. The nutritional effects of ascariasis, the world's most common helminthic infection, continue to be debated.

MALNUTRITION. Diarrhea in malnourished patients is caused by increased susceptibility to infections and abnormalities of digestion and absorption (Chapter 109.1). Mucosal changes found in jejunal biopsy specimens range from mucosal atrophy in kwashiorkor to relatively normal appearances with reduced crypt cell replication in marasmus. An abnormal jejunal bacterial flora has been found in malnourished children with and without diarrhea, although net fluid secretion and reduced glucose absorption were found only in those with diarrhea. Brush border sucrase and lactase levels are reduced, but these increase after refeeding. Each of these functional abnormalities may contribute to diarrhea by the osmotic effects of a high solute load drawing water into the gut lumen. Steatorrhea can be caused by maldigestion of fat due to reduced secretion of pancreatic lipase and by defective fat absorption due to epithelial damage in the jejunum. Protein digestion and absorption are surprisingly well maintained owing to the considerable reserve capacity possessed by the gut. The practical importance of these changes concerns diets to be used in refeeding programs. Animal fats may be poorly tolerated, but vegetable fats can be used as a palatable source of calories in the diet.

CHRONIC CALCIFIC PANCREATITIS. Chronic calcific pancreatitis is a relatively common cause of

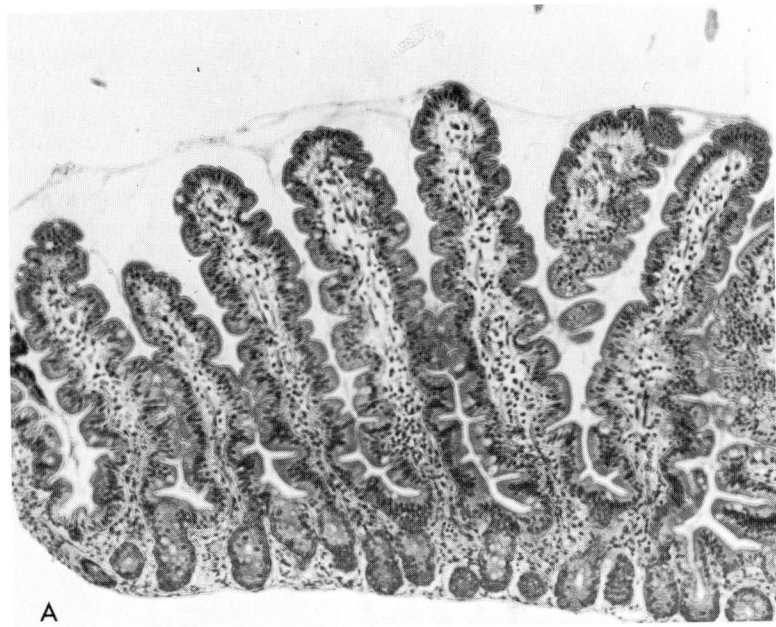

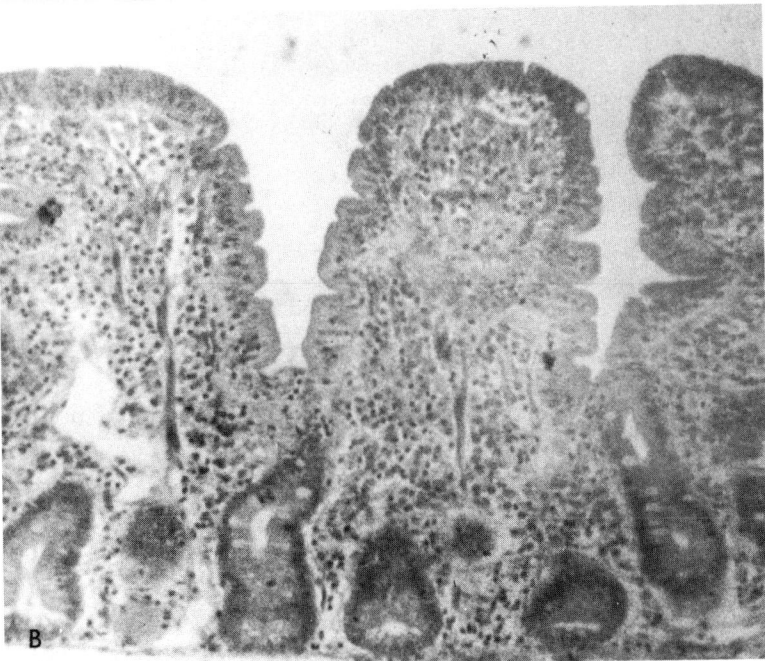

FIGURE 3–3. Histologic appearance of jejunal biopsies (H & E stain). *A*, Normal mucosa. *B*, Abnormal changes in a patient with tropical sprue of 4 months' duration.

malabsorption in East and West Africa and on the Indian subcontinent. Calcific disease causing pain has been reported in children as young as 6 years. Presenting features include recurrent upper abdominal pain, diarrhea with steatorrheic stools, weight loss, and sometimes diabetes mellitus. There are no specific physical signs. Pancreatic calcification is seen on a radiograph of the abdomen in about 50% of cases. Steatorrhea, normal D-xylose absorption, and a normal jejunal biopsy are the usual findings.

Exocrine pancreatic function is abnormal, with reduced secretion of pancreatic enzymes and bicarbonate. There is extensive destruction of glandular acini with marked fibrosis. Diabetes mellitus results from the destruction of insulin-secreting cells. Stones may form in both small and large pancreatic ducts, and removing the

stones may reduce symptoms. The cause is unknown, but viral infections, malnutrition, and the toxic effects of cyanide in cassava have all been suggested. Management consists of relief of pain, control of steatorrhea with pancreatic supplements, and insulin for diabetes mellitus.

HYPOLACTASIA. Lactose is a disaccharide and cannot be absorbed intact from the gut. The brush border enzyme lactase hydrolyzes it into glucose and galactose, monosaccharides that are absorbed separately. Lactose is an important source of calories in breast milk, and lactase levels are high at birth. Congenital absence of lactase is extremely rare. In the majority of the world's population, lactase synthesis declines under genetic control over the few years after breast-feeding ceases. Most of the indigenous popula-

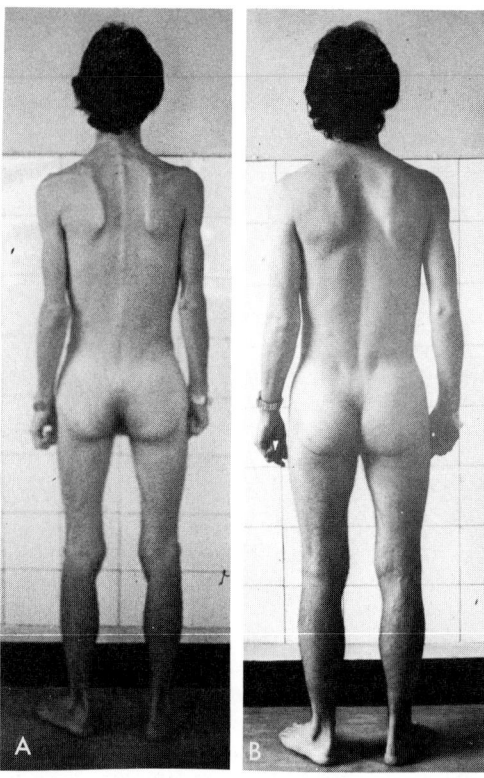

FIGURE 3–4. *A,* Patient with tropical sprue of 14 weeks' duration acquired during overland travels in Asia. *B,* The same patient 6 weeks after finishing a 6-week course of tetracycline and folic acid.

tions of Africa, Asia, and South America conform to this pattern. Persistence of high lactase levels into adult life is usual among Europeans and North Americans of European ancestry and in Bedouins, Yemenis, the Tutsi of Uganda and Rwanda, and the Punjabis. Lactase is a noninducible enzyme, and therefore, enzyme levels cannot be increased by substrate feeding.

Clinical Manifestations. Nausea, abdominal pain, colic, abdominal distention, flatulence, and diarrhea after drinking milk or taking food containing dairy products are usual symptoms in persons with lactose intolerance from hypolactasia. Some who have hypolactasia as judged by an abnormal lactose tolerance test do not develop symptoms after drinking milk. Many persons are aware of their intolerance and avoid dairy products, whereas others who are intolerant learn this only when they follow a low-lactose diet. The osmotic effects of undigested lactose draw fluid into the gut lumen, causing diarrhea, and lactose is broken down by colonic bacteria, producing other osmotically active molecules, lactic acid, and gas. Children pass acid stools containing reducing sugars. As little as 12.5 gm of lactose, 250 ml of milk, produces symptoms in some patients, whereas others who have hypolactasia according to the formal test have few symptoms after ingesting 25 gm or more.

Diagnosis. A lactose tolerance test can be done. Capillary blood glucose levels are measured fasting and 15, 30, 60, 90, and 120 minutes after drinking 50 gm of lactose dissolved in 400 ml of water. Children are given 2.0 gm/kg of body weight. An increase in blood glucose

level of less than 1.1 mmol/L (20 mg/dl) over the fasting value indicates hypolactasia. Brush border lactase levels can be measured in jejunal biopsy samples. Typical symptoms usually accompany the lactose tolerance test in patients with hypolactasia.

Treatment. Avoidance of lactose relieves symptoms arising from this condition. Gut infection may cause hypolactasia during the first year of life, when breast milk is essential for adequate nutrition. Enzyme levels will recover at this age, so that it is vital that the flow of milk be maintained until full breast-feeding can be resumed.

INTESTINAL TUBERCULOSIS. Several mechanisms can cause malabsorption in intestinal tuberculosis (Chapter 61), one or more of which can be involved in a patient. Mucosal atrophy has been found in jejunal biopsy specimens. Stricture formation in the small bowel and fistulas between adjacent loops of intestine allow colonization with anaerobic bacteria that deconjugate bile salts to cause steatorrhea and utilize vitamin B_{12}. Mucosal damage in the ileum causes bile salt malabsorption and depletion of the bile salt pool. Bile salts in the colon cause diarrhea. Fever, night sweats, weight loss, diarrhea, and abdominal signs, such as a tender mass or ascites, suggest intestinal tuberculosis. Laparoscopy is a valuable technique that allows diagnosis of this infection, often with definitive proof from histologic sections of biopsies. Standard chemotherapy has been used with excellent results, including regression of strictures, so that surgical intervention for relief of tuberculous strictures should not be undertaken until chemotherapy has been given an adequate trial.

ALPHA-CHAIN DISEASE. Alpha-chain disease (αCD) is a relatively common cause of diarrhea associated with wasting, edema, hypoproteinemia, malabsorption, and villous atrophy in countries of the Mediterranean littoral, the Middle East, and Pakistan (Chapter 11). There are case reports from South America. The geographic distribution is much wider than the condition's earlier name, Mediterranean lymphoma, implied. Jejunal biopsies show gross mucosal atrophy with a dense infiltrate of lymphocytes of the B-cell series in the mucosa. These cells produce large amounts of alpha chains, which are found in high concentrations in intestinal secretions, plasma, and urine. The etiology and pathogenesis of this condition are unknown, but it is tempting to speculate that the proliferation of cells represents an inappropriate and uncontrolled response to an antigen derived from the gut lumen. No specific infectious agent has been incriminated, but some patients respond well to treatment with tetracycline alone.

GLUTEN-SENSITIVE ENTEROPATHY. This condition is uncommon in the tropics, although cases have been reported from the Sudan and among Asians living in Britain. Diarrhea with pale, offensive stools, weight loss, and sometimes anemia due to folate deficiency are usual presentations. Absorption of D-xylose and fat is usually impaired, but vitamin B_{12} absorption is normal. Severe mucosal atrophy is found in jejunal biopsy samples. Symptoms, functional abnormalities and morphologic changes resolve when gluten is withdrawn from the diet. Definitive diagnosis is obtained by observing relapse of symptoms, functional impairment, and mucosal changes when gluten is reintroduced into the diet. Lifelong exclusion of gluten from the diet is required.

The usual infant feeding practices in the tropics, with prolonged breast-feeding and delayed introduction of mixed feeding, may protect against this condition. British pediatricians have reported a decline in the frequency of diagnosis of gluten-sensitive enteropathy in recent years, which they attribute to the use of similar feeding practices by mothers in Britain.

Protein-Losing Enteropathy

A relatively small amount of protein is normally lost into the gut each day. Acute invasive infections of the gastrointestinal tract will cause mucosal inflammation and ulceration, with increased protein loss into the gut. When there is extensive inflammation of the gut, the protein loss may be clinically significant. Protein-losing enteropathy occurs in (1) children with persistent diarrhea after measles; (2) intestinal tuberculosis; (3) obstruction of intestinal lymphatics as a result of tuberculous adenitis, malignancy, or filariasis; (4) granulomatous polyps (caused by *Schistosoma mansoni* infection); and (5) intestinal capillariasis.

Inflammatory Disease of the Large Bowel

The incidence of specific inflammatory disease of the large bowel in the tropics is far greater than that of nonspecific inflammatory bowel disease.

BACTERIAL INFECTIONS

Invasive Organisms. *Salmonella, Shigella, Campylobacter,* and *Yersinia* infections can all involve the colon, causing diarrhea with blood and pus in the stools. Fever, diarrhea, colicky abdominal pain, dysentery, and tenesmus are presenting features that suggest colonic infection clinically. Generalized abdominal tenderness is a usual physical sign, and the colonic mucosa is abnormal, with inflammation and ulceration seen on proctosigmoidoscopy. An exudate of mucopus is present, and the mucosa bleeds where the instrument makes contact with it. Microscopy of fecal smears shows an exudate of pus cells with a few red cells. Culture of stool samples or rectal swabs gives the bacteriologic diagnosis. Specific antibiotic treatment is indicated in patients with marked symptoms and signs.

Antibiotic-Associated Pseudomembranous Colitis (AAPC). AAPC was first described in patients who had been given lincomycin (Chapter 55.5). During the course of treatment, these patients developed fever and diarrhea. Sigmoidoscopy showed an inflamed mucosa with pseudomembranous plaques adhering to the mucosa. Subsequently, AAPC has been reported in association with a range of antibiotics, including penicillin, ampicillin, co-trimoxazole, and metronidazole. The cause of AAPC is colonic overgrowth with *Clostridium difficile,* which secretes a cytotoxin that causes the pathologic changes. With the widespread use of antibiotics in the tropics, it would be surprising if cases did not occur. Management consists of replacement of lost fluids and

oral vancomycin, which is not absorbed from the gut. Metronidazole is a cheaper alternative.

PARASITIC INFECTIONS. Amebic dysentery must always be considered in the differential diagnosis of patients with inflammatory bowel disease (Chapter 68). As with most infectious diseases, there is a range of severity of disease. This varies from mild cases, in which the patient reports a change in bowel habit, with stools that vary in consistency and often contain some blood-stained mucus, to severe cases, in which the patient is febrile and toxic and is passing uniformly blood-stained stools. Mucosal changes seen at sigmoidoscopy vary from the typical appearances of flask-shaped ulcers, with a sloughing base and a surrounding area of mucosal erythema scattered in an otherwise normal mucosa in those mildly affected, to a diffusely ulcerated bleeding mucosa in severe cases. More severe illness is usually associated with more extensive colonic involvement. Fecal smears and scrapes from the rectal mucosa should be examined for motile trophozoites of *E. histolytica.* Specific treatment with metronidazole or tinidazole produces rapid clinical improvement.

Postdysenteric ulcerative colitis has been described in patients who have been successfully treated for amebic dysentery. Diarrhea with blood and mucus in the stools is usual, and on sigmoidoscopy, an ulcerative colitis is found. Stool examinations for amebas and bacterial pathogens are negative. Histologic changes comprise ulceration of the epithelium, an infiltrate of lymphocytes and plasma cells in the mucosa, and, where full-thickness biopsies are obtained, destruction of smooth muscle layer. Goblet cell depletion and glandular atrophy are not seen. Barium enemas show mucosal ulceration. It has been suggested that sulfasalazine produces remission in these patients.

INTESTINAL TUBERCULOSIS. This can affect any part of the gastrointestinal tract, but the ileocecal region is an area of predilection (Chapter 61). Fever, night sweats, and loss of weight over a period of weeks or even months are symptoms that suggest tuberculosis, whereas abdominal pain, swelling of the abdomen due to ascites, diarrhea, and the presence of an abdominal mass raise the question of abdominal involvement. Abdominal tuberculosis is a common cause of ascites in the tropics. About half of the patients with intestinal tuberculosis have open pulmonary disease, and therefore, the patient's chest should be examined carefully. Tuberculin tests are usually strongly positive in those patients who are adequately nourished but are frequently negative in those whose nutritional state has deteriorated. Sputum and gastric washings should be examined for tubercle bacilli. Ascitic fluid should be aspirated for examination, as tubercle bacilli can be found in the fluid; a high protein content with an exudate of lymphocytes suggests a tuberculous etiology. Peritoneal biopsies should be taken when diagnostic paracentesis is performed. Radiographic contrast studies of the gut show a range of changes, including mucosal ulceration, stricture formation, segmental narrowing, and fistula formation. Laparotomy may be the only means of establishing the diagnosis in some patients. Where facilities for investigation are inadequate, it may be necessary to treat the patient on the basis of a clinical diagnosis.

NONSPECIFIC INFLAMMATORY BOWEL DISEASE. Cases of nonspecific inflammatory bowel disease, both ulcerative colitis and Crohn's disease, continue to be reported from the tropics, with a progressive increase in the total number of countries from which these reports come. The specific causes of intestinal inflammation must always be considered first. In particular, Crohn's disease should not be diagnosed in a patient who lives or has lived in the tropics without first excluding abdominal tuberculosis. In addition, amebiasis can be confused with ulcerative colitis.

Both the specific and the nonspecific causes of intestinal inflammation and ulceration can be complicated by hemorrhage, intestinal perforation, and toxic dilatation.

ENTERITIS NECROTICANS. This rare condition occurs worldwide in premature infants. It is a relatively common condition among children in the highland region of Papua New Guinea, where it seems to be associated with communal pig feasting. Infection with *Clostridium perfringens* Type C occurs by ingestion of organisms. The beta-toxin (Chapter 55.4) is produced in the gut lumen, causing gross thickening, discoloration, or necrosis of the affected gut. The jejunum and ileum are usually affected, but colonic involvement also occurs. Fever, abdominal pain, and bloody diarrhea are usual presenting features; thickened loops of intestine may be palpable. Active immunization against *C. perfringens* Type C beta-toxin has produced a dramatic decline in the incidence of this condition in New Guinea.

Stenosing Lesions of the Colon and Rectum

Stenosing lesions of the bowel can be caused by amebiasis, schistosomiasis, tuberculosis, and lymphogranuloma venereum. The last involves the rectum.

AMEBOMA. The cecum is the most common site for ameboma formation, but any part of the colon may be affected. Occasionally, multiple amebomas occur in the same patient. Persisting diarrhea with blood in the stools and localized abdominal pain are the usual features, and 1 or more tender masses may be palpable in the abdomen. The lesion itself consists of granulation tissue with areas of necrosis and fibroblast proliferation. Amebas are often difficult to find, but serologic tests for amebiasis are positive in over 90% of cases. Rapid resolution follows specific treatment, and surgical excision is not required.

SCHISTOSOMIASIS. Granulomatous lesions of the colon due to schistosomiasis can cause narrowing of the bowel. Early lesions are reversible with antischistosomal treatment. The rare fibrotic strictures that form require surgical removal.

Intestinal Obstruction

MEGACOLON. Colonic involvement with Chagas' disease causes chronic constipation and fecal impaction and can predispose to volvulus of the sigmoid colon. These megalesions are irreversible.

ASCARIS OBSTRUCTION. Small bowel obstruction by a large mass of tangled *Ascaris lumbricoides* worms is a relatively common cause of obstruction in children in the tropics.

OTHER CAUSES OF INTESTINAL OBSTRUCTION. Overall strangulated inguinal hernia is probably the most common cause of intestinal obstruction. Volvulus of the small intestine is common in some areas of India and East and South Africa, whereas volvulus of the sigmoid colon is relatively common in South and Central Africa, Brazil, western India, and Pakistan.

Intussusception

This is a relatively common cause of acute abdominal pain in adults in Africa. Cecocolic intussusception is usual in these cases. Amebomas, Burkitt's lymphoma, and schistosomal granulomas may be at the apex of the intussusception. Colicky abdominal pain, vomiting, bloody diarrhea, and a palpable abdominal mass are usual clinical features. This condition is uncommon in adults in temperate regions. Among children in the tropics, intussusception is ileoileal or ileocecal, the types found in the temperate regions of the world. The incidence of this condition in childhood is similar worldwide.

Umbilical Hernia

This is a common condition in children of school age in tropical Africa and rarely causes symptoms. The majority of these hernias regress spontaneously.

Rectal Prolapse

This is a relatively common condition in the tropics. Contributing factors include recurrent diarrheal disease, malnutrition, and hyperinfection with *Trichuris trichiura*.

BIBLIOGRAPHY

Adams EB, MacLeod IN: Invasive amebiasis. 1. Amebic dysentery and its complications. Medicine 56:315, 1977.
Banwell JG, Hutt MSR, Leonard PJ, et al: Exocrine pancreatic disease and the malabsorption syndrome in tropical Africa. Gut 8:388, 1967.
Blaser MJ: Gastric campylobacter-like organisms, gastritis and peptic ulcer disease. Gastroenterology 93:371, 1987.
Cook GC: Tropical Gastroenterology. Oxford, Oxford University Press, 1980.
Ferguson A: Diagnosis and treatment of lactose intolerance. Br Med J 283:1423, 1981.
Gledhill T, Leicester RJ, Addis B, et al: Epidemic hypochlorhydria. Br Med J 290:1383, 1985.
Guerrant RL (ed): Diarrhoeal Disease. London, Ballière's Clinical Tropical Medicine and Communicable Diseases, 1989.
Reid NW: Diarrhoea, a failure of colonic salvage. Lancet 2:481, 1982.
Speelman P, McGlaughlin R, Kabir I, Butler T: Differential clinical features and stool findings in shigellosis and amoebic dysentery. Trans R Soc Trop Med Hyg 81:549, 1987.
Stoll BJ, Glass RI, Huq MI, et al: Surveillance of patients attending a diarrhoeal disease hospital in Bangladesh. Br Med J 285:1185, 1982.

4. HEPATOBILIARY DISEASES

Michael A. Dunn

IMPORTANCE OF LIVER DISEASE. From ancient times, when the liver was regarded as the core of being by the Babylonians, to the present, when the profound influence of liver cell function on nearly all biochemical events is becoming clear, liver diseases have attracted great interest. This interest is intensified for students of tropical medicine for three reasons.

Increased Morbidity and Mortality. In nearly all tropical regions, there is an impression that morbidity and death from liver disease are much greater than in other geographic areas. With few exceptions, verification of this impression is difficult, because rigorous population-based data for prevalence and attack rates of most liver diseases are lacking. The personal experience of clinicians and pathologists working in tropical areas supports the idea that most liver diseases are more prevalent in the tropics (Table 4–1). This predominance of liver disease in the tropics is easy to understand in the case of parasitic infections that require specific conditions for their transmission, e.g., schistosomiasis, hydatid disease, and clonorchiasis. It is also easy to account for the high prevalence of those diseases that are more easily transmitted under conditions of poor sanitation, crowding, and close personal contact, e.g., hepatitis A, B, and C and amebiasis. There remains a group of poorly understood liver diseases, such as veno-occlusive disease, nonspecific portal fibrosis, and Indian childhood cirrhosis, whose prevalence is certainly greater in the tropics but whose causes and pathogenic mechanisms are poorly defined.

Unknown Etiology. The second reason liver diseases attract interest in the tropics is that speculation on general causes and effects in liver disease is stimulated by the coexistence of attractive potential etiologic agents and unexplained end results. Perhaps the most intensely discussed topic in this regard has been the unproved concept of nutritional cirrhosis or chronic liver disease of any form resulting from dietary deficiency. One motivation that has fueled this discussion is the long debate on the mechanisms that cause cirrhosis in persons with chronic alcoholism in nontropical countries. The weight of evidence suggests that alcoholic liver disease is a direct result of the hepatotoxicity of alcohol and its metabolic products. However, the multiple effects of alcohol on nutrient absorption and metabolism make it difficult to prove or exclude a nutritional component in the evolution of alcoholic cirrhosis. In this context, the frequent occurrence of cirrhosis in nonalcoholic residents of tropical areas where nutrition is marginal has been used to support the idea of dietary deficiency as a cause of chronic liver disease. Although the concept of overall nutritional deficiency or lack of specific critical nutrients remains attractive to some workers as a possible cause of cirrhosis, the support for this proposal is as lacking in the tropics as it is elsewhere.

Focal Distribution. The third factor that leads to interest in liver diseases in the tropics is the strikingly localized occurrence of some unique problems. This may be based on the limited geographic range of a parasite; for example, the occurrence of cholestasis and hepatomegaly in a resident of northeastern Thailand can nearly always be explained by infection with the biliary fluke *Opisthorchis viverrini* (Chapter 98.1), which affects nearly half the population of Thailand's northernmost province. Geographic prevalence also applies strikingly to some forms of nonparasitic disease, e.g., the hemosiderosis occurring in African Bantus, whose method of food preparation and brewing in cast-iron pots subjects them to an extraordinary load of absorbable iron.

GEOGRAPHIC DISTRIBUTION. Investigation of the causes of liver disease is more heavily influenced by geography than that of the causes of disease of any other major organ system. This results both from lack of specificity of the clinical manifestations of most liver diseases and from localized distribution of several important problems. The geographic ranges of the diseases covered in this chapter and a notation of other chapters dealing with liver diseases are shown in Table 4–1. Within broad geographic ranges, specific information can be very useful. For example, nearby pairs of villages and settlements in Egypt, the Caribbean, and Brazil have been shown to have very high prevalences and nonexistence of *Schistosoma mansoni* infection. Length of residence and habits of visitors to these regions are important as well: Anyone visiting the Nile delta who has had minimal water contact is unlikely to have hepatic schistosomiasis but may have viral hepatitis. A middle-

TABLE 4–1. Liver Diseases Prevalent in the Tropics

Condition	Geographic Distribution
Noninfectious	
Bantu siderosis	Southern Africa
Veno-occlusive disease	Southern Africa, India, Middle East, Caribbean
Indian childhood cirrhosis	Indian subcontinent, Malaysia, Sri Lanka
Infectious	
Viral	
Hepatitis (A; B; C; D) (Chapter 19)	
Yellow fever and other viral hemorrhagic fevers (Chapter 22)	
Rickettsial, Bacterial, Spirochetal	
Q Fever, brucellosis (Chapters 26 and 50)	
Syphilis, leptospirosis (Chapters 32.1 and 35)	
Protozoal	
Amebiasis, malaria (Chapters 68 and 73)	
Visceral leishmaniasis, toxoplasmosis (Chapters 76.1 and 78)	
Helminthic	
Ascariasis, visceral larva migrans (Chapters 83 and 94)	
Capillariasis, schistosomiasis (Chapters 82.3 and 96)	
Clonorchiasis, opisthorchiasis (Chapters 98.1 and 98.2)	
Fascioliasis, dicroceliasis, hydatid disease (Chapters 97.1 and 97.4)	

aged lifelong resident of Haiti with acute hepatitis is unlikely to have hepatitis A, but this would be the most likely cause of acute hepatitis in a northern European visitor to the same country. In inhabitants of developing countries acute hepatitis in children is frequently caused by hepatitis A infection; acute hepatitis in adolescents and adults is often due to hepatitis B or C virus (Chapter 19). Although a specific cause of liver disease cannot often be assigned on geographic grounds, a knowledge of the liver diseases prevalent in any location weighs heavily in directing clinical evaluation of a given illness.

CARDINAL MANIFESTATIONS OF LIVER DISEASES

The limited number of clinical responses to a wide variety of causes of liver injury is the same in both tropical and nontropical regions. Specific comments on some of these major findings are relevant.

Subclinical Liver Injury

The majority of the viral, bacterial, and parasitic infections discussed elsewhere in this text have the capacity to cause laboratory evidence of liver injury, not necessarily with direct invasion of the organ. In most cases, there are no clinical manifestations. In some infections, such as those with endotoxin-producing gram-negative bacteria, biochemical evidence of cholestasis can be followed by clinically recognizable jaundice that resolves as soon as the primary infection subsides. The main concern in dealing with multisystem infections that cause incidental minor liver injury is to maintain diagnostic and therapeutic focus on the primary problem and to follow the subclinical liver abnormalities to resolution. The orderly evaluation of persistently abnormal biochemical tests, including appropriate serologic tests, imaging procedures, and liver biopsy, is the same in tropical and nontropical areas. A heightened suspicion is in order in tropical residents for chronic active hepatitis, many of the causes of granulomatous hepatitis, secondary syphilis, and the inadvertent use of hepatotoxic drugs.

Hepatomegaly

Hepatomegaly in a person of average size is suggested on physical examination by a liver span in the right midclavicular line of more than 12 cm in a man or more than 10 cm in a woman. These limits are not absolute; their accuracy depends on individual skill and consistency in percussion and palpation, and imaging procedures sometimes fail to confirm the liver span measured on physical examination. In general, however, the same examiner will measure liver spans consistently. The character of a palpable liver edge on physical examination can be helpful when a definite finding exists, such as pulsations, tenderness, obvious coarse nodularity, or hardness. Findings such as fine nodularity often are not borne out under direct vision at surgery or autopsy.

Point tenderness over an expanding amebic abscess is a very important finding that calls for therapeutic needle aspiration (Chapter 68).

ULTRASOUND EVALUATION. Reports from many tropical centers over the last ten years emphasize the increasing importance of gray-scale ultrasound examination in the evaluation of hepatomegaly. This diagnostic method has become the most widely used supplement to physical examination in most tropical areas for several reasons. In initial investment and operating costs, ultrasound is within the economic reach of many centers in the developing world, whereas computerized axial tomography is not. It has supplanted most isotopic imaging procedures in these same areas, where cost and timely delivery of isotopes are limiting factors. A major disadvantage of ultrasound over other imaging methods is its dependence on operator skill and experience for accuracy. With an experienced operator, however, accuracy of diagnosis is high for solid masses such as hepatocellular carcinomas, cystic masses such as pyogenic and amebic abscesses, hydatid cysts that often have distinctive echogenic walls and daughter cysts (Fig. 101–9), dilated intrahepatic bile ducts, and the distinctive echogenic patterns of cirrhosis and schistosomal liver fibrosis (Figs. 4–1 and 96–16). Ultrasonography has now provided the first accurate estimates of the prevalence and severity of Symmers' periportal fibrosis in schistosome-infected populations. Serial examinations promise to be a noninvasive method of following the progression or stabilization of this key manifestation of the disease.

BLOOD TESTS. Serum biochemical tests of aminotransferase and other enzyme activities are not often helpful in choosing the most likely cause of either diffuse hepatomegaly or a focal lesion. Plasma protein patterns are mainly useful in confirming that chronic liver disease exists. Positive serologic tests for antibody to hepatitis A and B viruses are usual in most tropical areas. The high prevalence of hepatitis B surface antigenemia in many of these areas limits the confidence with which one can implicate hepatitis B as the cause of a given case of liver injury without tissue confirmation (Chapter 19.2). The most useful tests that help to confirm a specific diagnosis are an α-fetoprotein level of more than 400 ng/ml, which strongly suggests hepatocellular carcinoma, and a positive serologic test for invasive amebiasis. Practical experience with current serologic tests for schistosomiasis and echinococcosis suggests that they are of limited value in assessing individual patients (Chapter 125).

DIAGNOSIS. History, physical examination, and an imaging procedure such as gray-scale ultrasonography will help to determine whether hepatomegaly is focal or diffuse. In the case of focal lesions, imaging results and supplementary laboratory tests will aid in selecting medical therapy, diagnostic or therapeutic needle aspiration, or surgical therapy for abscesses, tumors, or cysts. If diffuse hepatomegaly is not simply part of an obvious multisystem illness such as malaria, visceral leishmaniasis, lymphoma, or right heart failure, strong consideration should be given to obtaining tissue by needle biopsy for accurate diagnosis and appropriate therapy.

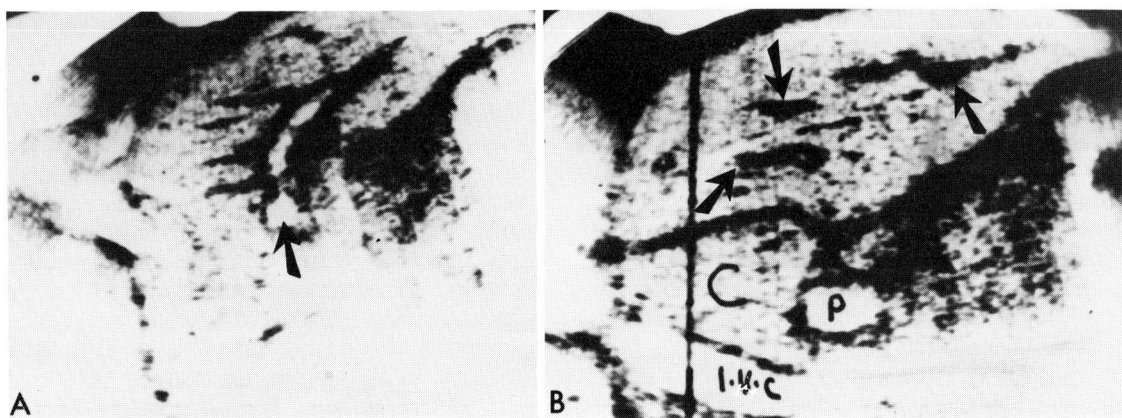

FIGURE 4–1. Gray-scale sonograms showing pipe-stem fibrosis in a patient with hepatosplenic schistosomiasis. Both panels are parasagittal sections with the left edge cephalad. *A,* The arrow points to a sonolucent portal vein branch within the liver surrounded by an accumulation of highly echogenic fibrous tissue, with strands of fibrous tissue radiating into the surrounding less echogenic parenchyma. *B,* Similar fibrous tissue around the intrahepatic portion of the main portal vein (P) as well as additional echogenic deposits of fibrous tissue in the parenchyma (*arrows*). The caudate lobe (C) and inferior vena cava (I.V.C.) are labeled. (Courtesy of Professor M. Farid Abdel Wahab, Cairo University Faculty of Medicine.)

Jaundice

The common mechanisms that govern the excretion and retention of bilirubin, bile salts, and other organic compounds have particular relevance to several tropical diseases. The normal daily production of unconjugated bilirubin is taken up in hepatocytes and conjugated to glucuronic acid prior to excretion into the bile ducts. In the event of failure of this excretion pathway, conjugated bilirubin that refluxes from hepatocytes into plasma can be filtered and excreted in the urine. The jaundice that occurs in a severe episode of malaria illustrates these principles. The hemolysis that results from heavy parasitemia or the severe hemolysis that sometimes results from administration of primaquine to persons with glucose-6-phosphate dehydrogenase deficiency (Chapter 5) overwhelms the bilirubin uptake and conjugation capacity of even a normal liver. If liver blood flow falls below that required to maintain normal cellular perfusion, bilirubin conjugation and excretion are directly impaired. Finally, if acute renal failure occurs in a malaria attack, the only remaining pathway for bilirubin excretion is blocked and jaundice intensifies.

Jaundice can be expected in those diseases that cause hemolysis with overloading of unconjugated bilirubin, e.g., malaria (Chapter 73) and the congenital and drug-induced hemolytic anemias (Chapter 5). Any viral or bacterial illness that affects hepatic uptake and excretion of bilirubin may also cause jaundice, which can become especially prominent when renal impairment blocks the secondary pathway for bilirubin excretion, as in leptospirosis.

DIAGNOSIS. Evaluation of the biliary tract for evidence of mechanical obstruction is appropriate in the event that jaundice is accompanied by hepatomegaly, chills, fever, or abdominal pain. Once again, gray-scale ultrasonography is the most convenient and reliable screening method to detect dilated bile ducts proximal to a mechanical obstruction. When required, direct contrast imaging by endoscopic retrograde cholangiography or fine-needle percutaneous cholangiography is performed, especially when surgical relief of mechanical duct obstruction is being planned. A stool examination may suggest that helminthic infection is responsible for bile duct obstruction. *Fasciola, Dicrocoelium, Ascaris,* and *Clonorchis* can cause mechanical obstruction while alive; dead adult ascaris and clonorchis in the ductal system can become a nidus for stone formation as well. Cholangiocarcinoma (Chapter 11) is a late complication of infection with clonorchis and opisthorchis biliary flukes.

Acute Hepatic Failure

Fortunately, massive necrosis of a previously normal liver is a rare event. As in nontropical areas, a few persons with hepatitis A or B, some immunologically deficient patients with opportunistic viral or fungal infection, and some victims of toxin ingestions such as phosphorus or carbon tetrachloride, will die of acute hepatic insufficiency. Of specific interest is that acute hepatic failure occurs in some persons with Rocky Mountain spotted fever, yellow fever, and some of the other hemorrhagic fevers (Chapter 22). In all these cases, intensive physiologic support with attention to correction of hypoxia, hypoglycemia, cerebral edema, and hemorrhagic tendencies is needed to promote recovery. When recovery occurs, liver structure and function return to normal.

Chronic Liver Injury

The bulk of morbidity and death from liver disease is associated with chronic liver injury, with permanent distortion of architecture and disturbance of normal circulation. The number of functioning hepatocytes in persons dying of chronic liver disease is usually more than sufficient to sustain life; failure of adequate circulation to these cells is of prime importance in the chronic liver failure of cirrhosis. Liver cirrhosis requires two components: (1) distortion of normal architecture and blood flow by an excessive deposition of fibrous tissue, and (2) the presence of regenerative nodules of liver cells. Because the cells within these regenerative nodules are not adequately perfused, their contribution to overall liver function is impaired.

The symptoms, findings, and supportive therapy of patients with cirrhosis in the tropics are the same as those for persons in other areas. A number of other chronic liver diseases occur in tropical areas; they sometimes cause changes such as portal hypertension without leading to the regenerative nodule formation of cirrhosis. Among these diseases are portal fibrosis and hepatic schistosomiasis (Chapter 96).

Assignment of a specific etiology to explain the manifestations of chronic liver disease in a tropical population can be both difficult and critically important in planning control measures. Perhaps the most important current example of this problem is the occurrence of chronic liver failure in persons with *Schistosoma mansoni* infection. The normal liver architecture seen with schistosomal liver fibrosis (Fig. 4–1) should not be associated with any manifestations of chronic liver disease other than presinusoidal portal hypertension. When they occurred, hepatic encephalopathy, hemostatic defects, jaundice, and ascites were viewed as end stages of schistosomiasis in persons with this infection, without any clear explanation. We now know that the majority of schistosome-infected persons who present with these signs of chronic liver failure have coexisting hepatitis B infection, with chronic active hepatitis and cirrhosis on histologic examination. It appears that a large proportion of the morbidity and death once attributed to schistosomiasis is at least in part due to coexisting hepatitis B disease, based on similar data from Brazil and Egypt. It is not yet clear whether these observations simply represent the additive effects of two common diseases or whether chronic schistosome infection and chronic hepatitis B infection, both immunosuppressive states, might predispose to mutual morbidity. The practical implications of answering this question are great; eradication of schistosomiasis has been a costly and largely unsuccessful venture in economically undeveloped regions. On the other hand, hepatitis B vaccination is currently expensive but may afford lifelong protection against the morbidity once attributed to schistosomiasis alone. Clearer definition of the possible interactions between these two conditions will be critical in planning efforts directed at either one.

GEOGRAPHIC LIVER DISEASES

Portal fibrosis, idiopathic cirrhosis, Bantu siderosis, Indian childhood cirrhosis, and veno-occlusive disease are all tropical clinical problems that are not addressed in detail elsewhere in this text.

Portal Fibrosis

The normal portal tract contains a supporting framework of connective tissue, composed mainly of a family of structural proteins, the collagens. Portal tracts contain collagen Types I and III, which are associated with nearly all interstitial supporting tissues, and additional collagens associated with basement membrane structures. Fibrosis can be defined as a net increase in the collagen content of an organ, which usually occurs in such a way as to distort normal architecture and circulation. In the case of hepatic schistosomiasis, the primary disturbance is disruption of normal portal inflow by extensive portal fibrosis. In cirrhosis, regenerative nodules of liver cells further disrupt normal architecture and circulation.

An incidental finding in many biopsy and autopsy liver specimens from tropical centers, especially in Africa, is an increase in portal tract connective tissue. As with all other examples of liver fibrosis, this increase includes all the collagen types normally present in the portal tract; there are no new or distinctive collagens associated with portal fibrosis. The degree of fibrosis present is usually not sufficient to interfere with normal circulation; clinically manifest portal hypertension is not usually a problem; and serum biochemical tests are normal. There is no evidence of inflammation or liver cell necrosis adjacent to the portal tract, as would be the case in chronic hepatitis. The finding is not present in nontropical residents of African descent, so that it appears to be acquired rather than inherited, in much the same way as the occurrence of the blunted-villus intestinal histology of asymptomatic tropical residents. Its cause is unknown; there is no evidence that it progresses to significant parenchymal liver disease; and no therapy other than reassurance is needed.

Idiopathic Cirrhosis

The frequency of the finding of liver cirrhosis on autopsy in most tropical countries is considerably greater than it is in nontropical regions. In most cases, the architectural pattern is macronodular or mixed macronodular and micronodular. Before the development of serum and tissue markers for hepatitis B virus infection, no clear-cut cause could be assigned to the majority of these cases. As autopsy material is studied more intensively with the full range of hepatitis B tissue markers, the bulk of previously unexplained cirrhosis seems to be attributable to chronic hepatitis B infection in many tropical areas (Chapter 19.2). There remain a substantial number of cases of unexplained cirrhosis in the tropics. Their assessment appears to await development of reliable tissue assays for other viral etiologic agents.

Bantu Siderosis

Among the Bantu residents of southern Africa, there is a high prevalence of cirrhosis associated with iron overload. Use of cast-iron vessels for cooking and brewing beer leads to oral ingestion of huge quantities of absorbable iron that exceed the regulatory capability of the normal intestinal control mechanisms that limit iron absorption. Hepatic iron stores in Bantus with cirrhosis match those of persons with idiopathic hemochromatosis. The disease differs from inherited hemochromatosis in several important respects, however. There is extensive reticuloendothelial as well as parenchymal iron deposition in the liver in Bantu siderosis. Once cirrhosis develops, its rate of progression to liver failure and death is considerably more rapid than that of hemochromatosis, which tends to remain clinically stable over many years. The strong association of excessive alcohol consumption in concert with the iron loading makes primary assignment of alcohol or iron as the key injuring agent problematic. Although iron deposits in other tissues may sometimes occur in a similar pattern to that of idiopathic hemochromatosis, their extent and the occurrence of clinically significant organ damage such as diabetes and heart failure are much less common in Bantu siderosis than they are in idiopathic hemochromatosis.

Indian Childhood Cirrhosis

This important disease of children on the Indian subcontinent and in Malaysia, Burma, and Sri Lanka is a rapidly progressive illness of unknown cause that usually leads to death from hepatic failure within a year of the initial manifestations of liver injury. Its onset can resemble that of acute hepatitis, or it can present with failure to thrive and well-developed evidence of chronic liver failure and portal hypertension.

There is no correlation of risk for this disease with any known infectious agent, toxin, dietary deficiency, or social class. There is positive family history in one third of the cases. The histologic appearance of liver biopsy specimens is distinctive, with focal intralobular inflammation and necrosis, Mallory's alcoholic hyaline, rapidly progressive fibrosis involving the whole lobular structure, and development of a micronodular cirrhosis with relatively little regenerative activity. There is striking cytoplasmic copper overload, with liver copper contents as high as those of Wilson's disease or biliary cirrhosis. Rhodamine stains for copper and orcein stains for copper-binding protein are positive. Unlike Wilson's disease, however, there are no Kayser-Fleischer corneal rings or basal-ganglion abnormalities, and serum ceruloplasmin levels are normal. There is no established therapy for Indian childhood cirrhosis. However, an initial controlled trial suggests that administration of penicillamine to children who had not yet developed jaundice or ascites led to marked clinical improvement in about half the cases, and prolonged survival compared with that of control patients. As with penicillamine therapy for primary biliary cirrhosis, potential mechanisms might include copper removal, inhibition of collagen crosslinking, or poorly understood anti-inflammatory effects.

Veno-Occlusive Disease

Postsinusoidal hepatic outflow tract obstruction can occur at any level from the hepatic venules to the right heart. In a number of tropical regions, particularly the Middle East, Jamaica, India, and southern Africa, a common cause of hepatic outflow tract obstruction is occlusion of the small intrahepatic venules. In nearly all locations where veno-occlusive disease occurs, it has been associated with ingestion of pyrrolyzidine alkaloids, plant-derived compounds found in herbal teas as well as in contaminated grain. Depending on the opportunity for toxin exposure, veno-occlusive disease is predominantly a pediatric problem. Clinical findings include rapidly progressive ascites (Fig. 4–2), tender hepatomegaly, clinically evident portosystemic collaterals, wasting, anorexia, and death from liver failure or variceal bleeding. There are a few reports of spontaneous resolution of the illness with restoration of normal liver function and development. A key finding on most adequate liver biopsy specimens is marked proliferation of the intima of the small hepatic venules. Presence of organized clots in larger hepatic veins can sometimes be seen in veno-occlusive disease, but they are more commonly found with more distal outflow tract obstructions such as the Budd-Chiari syndrome of hepatic vein thrombosis, membranous webs of the hepatic vein or vena cava, or constrictive pericarditis.

Evaluation should include an attempt to define the level of obstruction in order to exclude treatable alternative problems, such as vena cava webs and right-sided

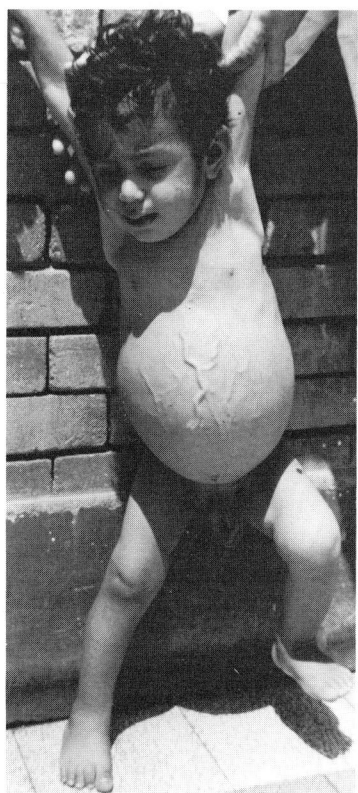

FIGURE 4–2. Egyptian child with acute onset of severe ascites and hepatomegaly due to veno-occlusive disease. In Egypt, the disease occurs more frequently in male children younger than 5 years old from rural areas. They often have some evidence of malnutrition. Note distended collateral veins across the abdomen. (Courtesy of Professors I. M. Fayad and M. Safouh, Cairo University Faculty of Medicine.)

obstruction to cardiac inflow. When available, right heart and vena caval catheterization with pressure measurements and injection of contrast medium into the hepatic vein ostia is useful for this purpose. In theory, relief of the postsinusoidal portal hypertension by construction of a side-to-side portosystemic shunt might benefit patients who could tolerate extensive surgery, as has been proposed for therapy of the Budd-Chiari syndrome. However, at present, there is no basis of experience to recommend such a procedure in veno-occlusive disease.

HIV Infection (AIDS)

The AIDS pandemic has had a devastating impact on health in many tropical areas (Chapter 15.1). Liver involvement by Kaposi's sarcoma, lymphoma, and the usual opportunistic infections is evident in many patients, with hepatomegaly, abnormal hepatic blood tests, and liver biopsy abnormalities each present in at least two thirds of those with overt disease. The biopsy findings are generally either nonspecific or attributable to infectious or malignant processes that are clinically evident elsewhere. Death from liver failure is not a usual outcome of AIDS. An unusual syndrome of cholestasis in AIDS patients has been attributed to biliary tract infection with cytomegalovirus or cryptosporidia, leading to stenosis at the papilla of Vater and sclerosing cholangitis. Endoscopic sphincterotomy is often helpful in relieving itching and jaundice and minimizing recurrence of superimposed bacterial cholangitis.

BIBLIOGRAPHY

Abdel-Wahab MF, Esmat G, Milad M, et al: Characteristic sonographic pattern of schistosomal hepatic fibrosis. Am J Trop Med Hyg 40:72, 1989.

Bassily S, Farid Z, Higashi GI, et al: Chronic hepatitis B antigenemia in patients with hepatosplenic schistosomiasis. J Trop Med Hyg 82:248, 1979.

Bras G, Brooks SEH, Walter DC: Cirrhosis of the liver in Jamaica. J Pathol Bacteriol 82:503, 1961.

Burke DS, Snitbhan R, Johnson DE, Scott RM: Age-specific prevalence of hepatitis A virus antibody in Thailand. Am J Epidemiol 113:245, 1981.

Higginson J, Gerritsen T, Walker ARP: Siderosis in the Bantu of South Africa. Am J Pathol 29:779, 1953.

Homeida M, Ahmed S, Dafalla A, et al: Morbidity associated with Schistosoma mansoni infection as determined by ultrasound: A study in Gezira, Sudan. Am J Trop Med Hyg 39:196, 1988.

Lebovics E, Dworkin BM, Heier SK, Rosenthal WS: The hepatobiliary manifestations of human immunodeficiency virus infection. Am J Gastroenterol 83:1, 1988.

Lyra LG, Reboucas F, Andrade ZA: Hepatitis B surface antigen carrier state in hepatosplenic schistosomiasis. Gastroenterology 71:641, 1976.

Nayak LC, Ramalingaswami V: Indian childhood cirrhosis. Clin Gastroenterol 4:333, 1975.

Safouh M, Shehata A, Elwi A: Hepatic vein occlusion disease in Egyptian children. Arch Pathol 79:505, 1965.

Safouh M, Shehata AH: Hepatic vein occlusion disease of Egyptian children. J Pediatr 67:415, 1965.

Schiff L, Schiff ER (eds): Diseases of the Liver, 6th ed. Philadelphia, JB Lippincott, 1987.

Schneiderman DJ, Cello JP, Laing FC: Papillary stenosis and scleros-
ing cholangitis in the acquired immunodeficiency syndrome. Ann Intern Med 106:546, 1987.

Tandon BN, Tandon RK, Tandon HD, et al: An epidemic of veno-occlusive disease of the liver in central India. Lancet 2:271, 1976.

Tanner MS, Bhave SA, Pradhan AM, Pandit AM: Clinical trials of penicillamine in Indian childhood cirrhosis. Arch Dis Child 62:1118, 1987.

Wright R, Alberti KGMM, Karran S, Millward-Sadler GH (eds): Liver and Biliary Disease, 2nd ed. Philadelphia, WB Saunders, 1986.

5. HEMATOLOGIC DISEASES

Alan F. Fleming

ANEMIA

Definition and Prevalence

The World Health Organization has proposed levels of hemoglobin concentration considered normal for age, sex, and pregnancy status (Table 5–1). There is no evidence of racial differences in hemoglobin concentration in the absence of recognized genetic or environmental factors: A population of black Americans may have a mean hemoglobin 0.5 gm/dl lower than a population of white Americans matched for age, sex, and socioeconomic status, but this difference can be explained by a higher frequency of a gene for α^+-thalassemia.

Anemia is possibly the most common manifestation of disease in the tropics. Anemia is most prevalent during pregnancy and the first 5 years of life, periods during which it is estimated that about half the world's population is anemic (Table 5–2).

Anemia of Infection

MALARIA. Anemia is an inevitable and serious complication of malaria, especially with *Plasmodium falciparum* infection (Chapter 73).

Mechanisms. The intracellular development of parasites results in the intravascular rupture of red cells, but anemia is always greater and persists longer than can be explained by the number of parasitized red cells. Following infection there is lymphoid and macrophage hyperplasia, with enhancement of phagocytic activity. The spleen becomes enlarged, and both nonparasitized and parasitized red cells are pooled and phagocytosed.

In addition, an autoimmune hemolysis probably contributes to the anemia in about 15% of those who have minimal immunity. It is postulated that the passive

TABLE 5–1. Hemoglobin Concentrations Below Which Anemia is Likely in Populations Living at Sea Level

	Hemoglobin (gm/L)
Newborn infants	140
6 months–6 years	110
6–14 years	120
Adult males	130
Adult females—nonpregnant	120
Adult females—pregnant	110

TABLE 5–2. Estimated Prevalence of Anemia by Geographic Region, Age, and Sex (Circa 1980)*

	Children						Women						Men		
	0–4 Years			5–12 Years			15–49 Years						15–49 Years		
							Pregnant			All					
		Anemic			Anemic			Anemic			Anemic			Anemic	
	Number	No.	%	Number	No.	%	Number	No.	%	Number	No.	%	Number	No.	%
Africa	85.7	48.0	56	96.6	47.3	49	17.9	11.3	63	106.4	46.8	44	116.8	23.4	20
South Asia	212.0	118.7	56	278.4	139.2	50	41.7	27.1	65	329.4	91.0	58	386.3	123.6	32
East Asia	16.1	3.2	20	25.4	5.6	22	2.7	0.5	20	46.9	8.4	18	55.8	6.1	11
Europe	33.4	4.7	14	55.0	2.7	5	5.7	0.8	14	117.5	14.1	12	147.2	3.0	2
North America	19.6	1.6	8	27.5	3.6	13	3.4	—	—	64.2	5.1	8	76.3	3.1	4
Developing regions	395.0	183.2	51	456.8	208.3	46	71.0	41.9	59	539.5	255.7	47	621.2	162.2	26
Developed regions	86.1	10.3	12	130.7	9.1	7	14.8	2.0	14	285.5	32.7	11	346.5	12.0	3
World	445.1	193.5	43	587.6	217.4	37	85.8	43.9	51	825.0	288.4	35	967.7	174.2	18

*Population data in millions.

China excluded. Anemia is defined as hemoglobin concentration below WHO reference values for age, sex, and pregnancy status.

Modified from DeMaeyer E, Adiels-Tegman M: World Health Statistics Q 38:302, 1985.

absorption of a complex of soluble antigen released at schizogony and specific IgG subclass 1, with the fixation of complement, render the red cells susceptible to phagocytosis. Both the circulating soluble antigens and the immune hemolytic process can persist for several weeks after the elimination of parasites.

Bone marrow dysfunction is an important cause of anemia. This has been demonstrated morphologically as dyserythropoiesis and functionally as ineffective erythropoiesis and is probably caused by products of the parasites acting on the erythroblasts.

Clinical Manifestations. The anemia of malaria in children and others who are nonimmune may be profound; hemoglobin concentrations less than 2 gm/dl are not uncommon. The red cells show anisocytosis, with both microcytes and macrocytes; during recovery, in the second week, macrocytosis and polychromasia predominate. In the first 2 days, there is a neutrophilic leukocytosis, but later there is a moderate neutropenia. From the second week, there is often considerable neutrophilic leukocytosis, with the release into blood of young forms (shift to the left), with toxic granulation and vacuolation of the cytoplasm, especially if there are complicating bacterial infections; rarely, there is a myeloid leukemoid reaction. There is a monocytosis, frequently with vacuolated cytoplasm or cytoplasm containing malarial pigment. The lymphocyte count is raised, with numerous transformed cells with dark blue–staining cytoplasm (on Romanovsky stains), large nuclei with nucleoli, and occasional plasma cells. There is invariably a moderate thrombocytopenia during the acute phase of malaria.

In immune adults, recurrent malaria causes a constant moderate hemolysis with compensatory erythroid hyperplasia; the mean hemoglobin in such a population is around 2 gm/dl lower for both sexes at all ages than in populations not exposed. There is moderate anisocytosis, with some macrocytes and microcytes and occasional polychromatic red cells. This balance is disturbed in two conditions, pregnancy and (less commonly) hyperreactive malarial splenomegaly (HMS).

Malaria in Pregnancy. Malaria is more severe in pregnant than in nonpregnant women (Chapter 73). Pregnant women with low immunity or none to *P. falciparum,* for example, in southern Africa, present with severe acute malaria, often complicated by cerebral malaria, renal failure, blackwater fever, profound anemia, and disseminated intravascular coagulation. There are high rates of abortion, premature delivery, and perinatal and maternal mortality.

In areas where malaria is hyper- or holoendemic and adults have high levels of immunity, the frequency of palpable splenomegaly approximately doubles in pregnant women of all gravidae classes, the peak frequency of palpable spleens being reached before 16 weeks of gestation (Fig. 5–1). In primigravidae and possibly in gravidae 2, the frequency and density of malaria parasitemia increase also, to a peak in the second trimester. However, parasite densities are not as great as those in childhood, and patients either are asymptomatic or have only minor complaints. The chief pathologic finding is extravascular hemolysis leading to anemia, most commonly in the second trimester (Fig. 5–1). Compensatory erythroid hyperplasia increases demands for folic acid so that the hemolytic anemia frequently is complicated

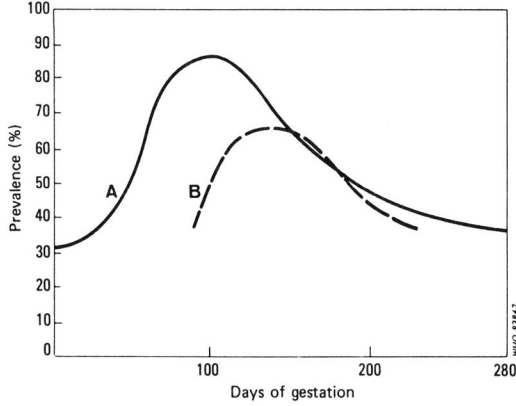

FIGURE 5–1. Prevalence of *P. falciparum* parasitemia *(A)* and hemolytic anemia associated with splenomegaly *(B)* in pregnancy. (From Brabin BJ: Bull WHO 61:1005, 1983. Reprinted by permission.)

by megaloblastic erythropoiesis. Anemia is often profound and life-threatening, but in the majority of patients there is a rapid response to antimalarials and folic acid. In about 25%, the hypersplenism of HMS makes a major contribution, and the hematocrit response to treatment is slow. In about 5%, there is an immune hemolysis, so that the hematocrit constantly falls, necessitating frequent transfusions of blood unless corticosteroids are given.

Hyperreactive Malarial Splenomegaly (HMS). In the great majority of the population exposed to endemic malaria, the spleen diminishes in size (although still remaining larger than the typical size in nonmalarial areas) once a degree of immunity has been acquired during childhood. A small proportion of adults have HMS. This is characterized by splenomegaly, hypersplenism, a polyclonal B-lymphocyte proliferation, high IgM levels, and raised titers of antimalarial antibodies (Chapter 73). There is pooling in the spleen of granulocytes, platelets, and red cells up to one third of the total red cell volume, and an expansion of the plasma volume. There is a pancytopenia as a consequence of pooling, destruction in the spleen, and dilution of the circulating red cells, granulocytes, and platelets. The lymphocyte count is usually in the range of 1.0 to 4.0 $\times$ 10^9/L, but in about 15% of patients the peripheral blood lymphocyte count is from 40 to 100 $\times$ 10^9/L, and the condition may be mistaken for chronic lymphatic leukemia.

The condition is associated with *P. falciparum* epidemiologically; there is an almost total protection afforded by sickle cell trait, suggesting that malarial antigens play an essential role in etiology; there is a slow but complete recovery with the administration of antimalarial prophylactics. The etiology of HMS is obscure, but it seems likely that B-cell proliferation in response to malarial antigens is excessive owing to either an abnormal population of T-helper cells or the escape from control T-suppressor cells (Chapter 73).

VISCERAL LEISHMANIASIS. *Leishmania donovani* infects macrophages throughout the reticuloendothelial system. There is a progressive hyperplasia of macrophages and lymphocytes, massive production of IgG antibodies, and hepatosplenomegaly (Chapter 76.1). Spleen size, hypersplenism, and pancytopenia are all directly related to the duration of the infection. Other mechanisms of hemolysis have been postulated, but hypersplenism is certainly the main factor. The picture may be complicated by megaloblastic erythropoiesis secondary to high demands for folic acid. Neutropenia may be profound and complicated by severe secondary infections, especially in children. Thrombocytopenia can lead to spontaneous epistaxis and bleeding from mucosal surfaces. Monocyte and lymphocyte counts are raised, occasionally to leukemoid levels. The bone marrow is generally hyperplastic. In chronic kala-azar there may be hypoplasia and myelofibrosis with continued hypersplenism.

AFRICAN TRYPANOSOMIASIS. Infection by *Trypanosoma brucei rhodesiense* or *T. b. gambiense* is followed by proliferation of macrophages and lymphocytes, high production of IgM antibodies, splenomegaly,

and hypersplenism (Chapter 74). Anemia and granulocytopenia are usually moderate but may be more severe with *T.b. rhodesiense* infections. Lymphocyte and monocyte counts are raised. Thrombocytopenia is sometimes severe in acute infections.

HELMINTH INFECTIONS

Mechanisms. Helminths cause several hematologic changes: (1) Invasive infections stimulate the production and release of eosinophils. In those nematodes causing intestinal infections, eosinophilia is pronounced only during the invasive migrating phase (Table 5–3). (2) Chronic intestinal hemorrhage associated with hookworm infection may lead to iron deficiency. Other less common or less severe causes of chronic hemorrhage and iron deficiency are *Trichuris trichiura* in the gut, *Schistosoma mansoni* and *S. japonicum* in the colon, and *S. haematobium* in the bladder. (3) *S. mansoni* and *S. japonicum* can cause fibrosis of the liver, congestive splenomegaly, and hypersplenism. (4) Infections of the small intestine may deprive the host of nutrients; *Diphyllobothrium latum* occasionally causes megaloblastic anemia from vitamin B_{12} deficiency.

Hookworm. Approximately 1 billion individuals are infected by hookworm (Chapter 84.1). In the majority, infections are mild, but in 50 million to 100 million, the intensity is sufficient to cause anemia, making hookworm second only to malaria as an infectious cause of anemia.

Ecology. In much of Africa east and north of the Niger River, generally only men and boys work in the fields, where they become heavily infected, with resultant iron-deficiency anemia. In the remainder of Africa, women perform agricultural work and can be heavily infected. The women often are accompanied by small children, who play on the ground; the surface area exposed is large and the hookworm loads are heavy in proportion to body weight and stores of iron, so that young children can present with Löffler's syndrome, abdominal pain, diarrhea, eosinophilia, and florid anemia from acute or subacute intestinal hemorrhage.

Pathophysiology. The daily loss of blood into the gut is 0.03 to 0.05 ml for each *Necator americanus* worm and 0.15 to 0.23 ml for each *Ancylostoma duodenale* worm. In the iron-sufficient subject, iron loss is equivalent to approximately 0.5 mg per ml of blood; about 40% of the iron in the gut is reabsorbed. As iron deficiency develops, reabsorption increases to about 60% and the iron content of the blood is less. As *N. americanus* produces fewer ova (9000 per day per female) than does *A. duodenale* (30,000 per day per female), a daily iron loss of 1 mg/1000 ova/gm of feces is a reasonable estimation of the burden of a hookworm infestation, regardless of species.

Progress to iron deficiency depends on three factors: (1) the dietary intake of bioavailable iron, (2) the size of the iron stores in the body, and (3) the hookworm load (Chapter 108.1). Where the diet is a poor source of bioavailable iron and the population has a high frequency of nutritional deficiency (e.g., India, Mauritius, Mexico), almost any degree of hookworm infection will contribute to negative iron balance or deficiency. In populations with moderately good intake of iron (e.g.,

TABLE 5–3. Host Reactions to Helminthic Infections

	Eosinophilia	Chronic Hemorrhage/ Iron Deficiency	Portal Hypertension/ Hypersplenism	Altered Nutrition
Nematodes	*Necator americanus** *Ancylostoma duodenale** *Strongyloides stercoralis** *Ascaris lumbricoides** *Toxocara* species *Trichinella spiralis* *Wuchereria bancrofti* *Brugia malayi* *Loa loa* *Onchocerca volvulus* *Dracunculus medinensis*	*N. americanus* *A. duodenale* *Trichuris trichiura*		*S. stercoralis* *A. lumbricoides*
Trematodes	*Schistosoma haematobium* *S. mansoni* *S. japonicum*	*S. haematobium* *S. mansoni* *S. japonicum*	*S. mansoni* *S. japonicum*	
Cestodes	*Cysticercus cellulosae* *Echinococcus* species			*Taenia solium* *T. saginata* *Diphyllobothrium latum*

*Eosinophilia during the invasive phase.

Central America, southern United States, Fiji), a threshold of about 5000 ova/gm of feces, equivalent to a loss of about 5 mg of iron per day, has to be reached before iron deficiency develops. In populations with a high intake of bioavailable iron (e.g., western Nigeria), hookworm loads of more than 20,000 ova/gm of feces with hemorrhage of 100 to 200 ml/day are needed before the males go into negative balance. Iron depletion and anemia will always develop more rapidly in infected women and children than in men, because of their smaller reserves.

The iron-deficiency anemia of hookworm can be profound (e.g., Hb 2.0 gm/dl) and life-threatening; it can be distinguished clinically or hematologically from nutritional iron-deficiency anemia only in a few details. Many patients show a loss of skin pigmentation (melanin) in addition to the pallor of anemia. In communities where heavy hookworm loads are required to induce iron deficiency, the loss of protein and zinc can lead to hypoalbuminemia and diminished serum zinc concentrations. The combination of eosinophilia and hypochromic anemia should alert the clinician to the probability of hookworm infection.

Trichuriasis. Infestation by *Trichuris trichiura* (whipworm) is extremely common wherever young children come into contact with warm, moist, and polluted soil (Chapter 82.2). Blood loss is about 5 μl per worm, or 0.25 ml/1000 ova/gm of feces. The majority of infections are harmless, but if there are more than 500 worms (16,000 ova/gm of feces), the daily loss of blood may be 4 ml and of iron about 2 mg per day. This is sufficient to cause iron-deficiency anemia in young children, which commonly occurs in Southeast Asia and Central America.

Schistosomiasis

Urinary Schistosomiasis. Established infections with *S. haematobium* in the bladder cause hematuria, with a blood loss of up to 125 ml per day, and a mean loss of iron up to nearly 40 mg per day (Chapter 96). This loss of iron is usually short-lived, and the associated anemia is generally normocytic. Ureteral obstruction can lead to pyelonephritis, erythroid hypoplasia, and neutrophilic leukocytosis. However, high prevalences of iron deficiency anemia associated with *S. haematobium* are found on the coastal plain of eastern Africa from Somalia to South Africa, affecting adolescent boys especially.

Intestinal Schistosomiasis. *S. mansoni* is the most frequent cause of anemia in Egypt (Chapter 96). The anemia may have three mechanisms: (1) Ova lodged in the colon may lead to formation of polyps, from which there is chronic loss of blood and of iron up to 8 mg per day. (2) Ova carried to the liver result in hepatic fibrosis, leading to portal hypertension, and progressive splenomegaly with hypersplenism. This may cause anemia, granulocytopenia, and thrombocytopenia; pancytopenia may be profound. (3) Acute hemorrhage from esophageal varices can cause acute anemia, with a diminution of the size of the spleen.

AIDS

Epidemiology. It was estimated in 1990 that about 10 million people are already infected with the human immunodeficiency virus Type 1 (HIV-1) and that HIV-2 is also epidemic in West Africa (Chapter 15.1). By 1991, there will be 500,000 to 3 million new cases of AIDS and 1 million to 5 million cases of the AIDS-related complex (ARC). The most seriously affected areas include the Caribbean, East and Central Africa from Uganda to Zimbabwe and from Congo to the east coast, and West Africa from Senegal to Benin. Highest incidence figures reported during 1987 were 54 per 100,000 per year in French Guyana and 45 in Congo, compared with fewer than 10 per 100,000 population per year in the United States. Transmission is predominately by heterosexual contact; women are infected about as frequently as men, and vertical transmission to the newborn is common. Transmission by blood transfusion accounts for about 10% of cases, making the largest relative contribution during childhood.

Hematologic Manifestations. The hematologic implications of the epidemic of HIV and AIDS are twofold. First, there is the impact on blood transfusion practices, where up to 20% of potential donors are HIV-infected.

Second, AIDS must now be considered in the differential diagnosis of any cytopenia in tropical Africa and America.

Hematologic complications are features of advanced disease only. Pathogenesis is complex and includes dysregulation of immunity, hypergammaglobulinemia, autoimmunity, dysregulation of T-cell and other controls of cell proliferation, retroviral invasion of marrow cells, and responses to opportunistic or other infections.

Anemia is observed in 70 to 90% of AIDS and in around 15% of ARC patients. Usually the hemoglobin is about 10.0 gm/dl, but anemia may be profound. The red cells are normocytic and normochromic but commonly show anisocytosis and poikilocytosis. The reticulocyte count is usually normal or low. Associated with hypergammaglobulinemia there are rouleaux and often a positive direct Coombs' test with various antibody specificities, but hemolysis is not significant in most patients.

About 60% of patients with AIDS and 30% with ARC have leukopenia. Granulocytopenia is usually associated with a shift to the left of the neutrophils. Atypical lymphocytes with dark blue–staining cytoplasm and large nuclei with nucleoli occur with lymphopenia. Monocytes are frequently vacuolated.

About 30% of patients with AIDS have thrombocytopenia, and about 45% develop a lupus anticoagulant at some stage. The combination of these two is of clinical importance, because it leads to excessive hemorrhage on accidental trauma or following surgery.

Bone marrow examinations generally show nonspecific changes. Cellularity may be low, normal, or increased. Myeloid hyperplasia is usual. There is often a striking plasmacytosis and aggregates of lymphocytes. The iron in macrophages may be increased, a consequence either of inflammation following secondary infections or of alcoholism associated with a way of life that also carries a high risk of exposure to HIV.

Treatment. Therapeutic options are limited in developing countries. Anemia may require transfusion with concentrated red cells. The effects of leukopenia can be countered by antibiotics, with varying success. Steroids are not recommended for the long-term treatment of thrombocytopenia associated with AIDS. Intravenous IgG is often effective in the control of hemorrhage or in preparation for invasive procedures but is prohibited by cost and unavailability. The platelet count rises following splenectomy in many patients, but the operation could be foolhardy without adequate surgical facilities, antipneumococcal vaccine, long-term penicillin prophylaxis, and antimalarial prophylactics.

Nutritional Anemias

IRON DEFICIENCY. The iron of food is in three main forms: (1) heme iron, (2) nonheme iron, and (3) extraneous iron (Chapter 108.1).

Heme in animal food (meat, poultry, and fish) is absorbed most readily as an intact metalloporphyrin by cells of the duodenal mucosa, and the iron is utilized. The nonheme iron of animal foods (with the exception of eggs, which contain phospholipids that block absorption) also has a high bioavailability, as absorption is enhanced by amino acids derived from the digestion of protein. Diets rich in animal protein generally meet the daily physiologic requirements for iron (Table 108–2). Iron deficiency is infrequent in communities whose members have survived as hunter-gatherers, e.g., the Hadza in Tanzania and the !Kung Bushmen in the Kalahari desert, and among pastoralists such as the Masai in Kenya, who eat meat and drink blood. Nearly 50% of the iron in breast milk is absorbed, and deficiency is uncommon in breast-fed infants.

In contrast, nonheme iron of vegetable foods has low bioavailability. Absorption is inhibited by bulk, fiber, phytates, phosphates, polyphenols, and tannin. Ascorbic acid and amino acids are the main enhancers of absorption of nonheme iron, but sources of these are expensive or may not be eaten because of religious beliefs, e.g., the vegetarian diet of Hinduism. Much of the world's population subsists on diets based on the cereal staples, rice, wheat, maize, sorghum, and millet, from which sufficient iron cannot be absorbed to meet physiologic requirements, especially during early childhood, adolescence, menstruation, and pregnancy (Table 108–4). Chronic hemorrhage and loss of iron from hookworm, schistosomal, and whipworm infection coincide frequently with low intake of bioavailable iron and contribute to the worldwide high prevalence of iron deficiency.

Iron deficiency is the most common nutritional disorder in all populations and has been estimated to occur in 30 to 50% of pregnant women and preschool children in tropical America, Africa, northern India, and western Asia and in up to 99% of pregnant women in southern India. Iron deficiency is the most common cause (with malaria) of anemia in tropical countries (Table 5–2).

FOLIC ACID DEFICIENCY

Folate Metabolism. The core molecule of folic acid, pteroylglutamic acid, does not exist free in nature. In its active forms (folates) it is conjugated, reduced, and condensed (Chapter 107.7). Folates may be monoglutamates, such as N5 methyl tetrahydrofolate in serum, or may be conjugated to form the polyglutamates found intracellularly. Folates are reduced to dihydro- or tetrahydrofolates by dihydrofolate reductase, which in mammals is a liver enzyme. Finally, the molecule is condensed with one-carbon radicals, for example, methyl, methenyl, methylene, or formyl. Folates are essential cofactors in the transfer of one-carbon radicals in the synthesis of purines, pyrimidines, and nucleic acids. They are involved in amino acid intraconversions, e.g., histidine to glutamic acid, homocysteine to methionine, and glycine to serine. Folates are required in the conversion of uridine to thymidine in the synthesis of DNA. Folates are necessary, therefore, for all dividing cells, and the highest turnover is in tissues of rapid cell division, e.g., the bone marrow and the gastrointestinal tract.

Folate Sources and Requirements. Folates are widespread, and dietary sources are varied. Liver, kidney, and other meats, yeast products, eggs, yams, sweet potatoes, other tubers, plantain, bananas, mangoes, fresh green and red peppers, locust beans, and green

TABLE 5–4. Daily Dietary Requirements for Folates and Vitamin B$_{12}$

Nutrient	Group	Daily Dietary Requirement (µg)
Folate	0–6 months	40–50
	7–12 months	120
	1–12 years	200
	≥13 years	400
	Pregnant women	800
	Lactating women	600
Vitamin B$_{12}$	0–12 months	0.3
	1–3 years	0.9
	4–9 years	1.5
	≥10 years	2.0
	Pregnant women	3.0
	Lactating women	2.5

From World Health Organization, 1972.

leaf vegetables are all rich sources of folates. The grains, including rice, maize, sorghum, and millet, and roots, e.g., cassava, are poor sources. Folates are deconjugated and absorbed actively as monoglutamates in the jejunum. The liver is the main storage organ, but body stores normally are sufficient for only about 3 weeks. Folates are secreted in bile, urine, and breast milk. Physiologic requirements for folate are highest during periods of rapid growth, pregnancy, and lactation (Table 5–4).

Causes of Folate Deficiency. Deficiency of folate can follow (1) inadequate intake, (2) malabsorption, (3) high physiologic requirements, (4) high demands following hemolysis or other pathologic processes, and (5) disturbances of metabolism (Table 5–5).

Reduced Dietary Intake. Reduced dietary intake of folate may reflect a shortage of food but is frequently a result of inappropriate selection or preparation of food.

TABLE 5–5. Causes of Folate Deficiency

Inadequate intake	Excessive boiling of bottle feeds
	Goat's milk feeding of infants
	Inappropriate weaning food (PEM)
	Anorexia (recurrent infections)
	Prolonged cooking, reheating
	Seasonal food shortages
	Prolonged storage of food
	Famine
	Taboos
	Food fads
	Alcoholism
Malabsorption	Diarrhea in infancy
	Other enteric infections
	Systemic infections (pneumonia, tuberculosis)
	Acute tropical sprue
	Nontropical sprue
High physiologic demands	Premature infants
	Growth in infancy and adolescence
	Pregnancy
	Lactation
Pathologic high demands	Sickle cell disease
	Other chronic hemolytic diseases
	Recurrent malaria
	Burkitt's lymphoma
	Choriocarcinoma
Disturbed metabolism	Pyrexia
	Overdosage of pyrimethamine, trimethoprim, methotrexate

Folates are water soluble and heat labile and so are leached out by boiling and destroyed by prolonged cooking. Soups or relishes added to bulky staple food, e.g., maize-porridge, often contain foods that were originally folate rich, e.g., spinach, peppers, meat, or fish. Prolonged boiling and reheating for each day's meal reduces active folate. For example, the frequency of folate deficiency is high in Indians, intermediate in Malays, and low in Chinese in Singapore, reflecting precisely their cooking practices. There are seasonal variations in the availability of folate and in the frequency of megaloblastic anemias in many countries. For example, folate deficiency is increasingly common in the late dry season and into the early rainy season in Nigeria, but the lifting of the new yam crop in August is followed almost immediately by a dramatic decline of megaloblastic anemia in pregnancy.

Decreased Utilization. Infectious diseases disturb the folate balance through several mechanisms: (1) prolonged anorexia following intercurrent infections, e.g., malaria; (2) depressed absorption due not only to enteric infections but also to severe systemic diseases, including pneumonia, tuberculosis, and malaria; and (3) erythroid hyperplasia following malaria, which is a major cause of severe folate deficiency in pregnancy. This mechanism, however, does not seem to be important in childhood. The enzyme dihydrofolate reductase is inactive at 39C, a probable mechanism for acute megaloblastic arrest of erythropoiesis complicating infectious diseases of childhood and pregnancy.

In Africa, subjects with sickle cell disease are invariably folate deficient when seen for the first time—the result of high demands due to constant erythroid hyperplasia and the effects of intercurrent infections.

Metabolic Inhibitors. The 2-4 diaminopyrimidines, pyrimethamine and trimethoprim, are distant analogues of folic acid and are competitive inhibitors of dihydrofolate reductase. Their usefulness as antimalarials and antibiotics is due to their greater affinity for the enzymes of protozoa and bacteria than for those of man. However, overdosage can occur and lead to megaloblastic anemias. This has been observed in infants receiving adult dosages of pyrimethamine and with self-medication with pyrimethamine plus co-trimoxazole.

Folate deficiency in infancy and childhood is seen commonly in association with prematurity, inappropriate bottle feeding with either boiled milk or goat's milk, inappropriate weaning foods such as paps from maize or cassava, diarrhea, intercurrent infections, and hemoglobinopathies. For example, folate deficiency contributed to one third of all anemias in children aged 3 months to 3 years in the north of Nigeria. One third of all Nigerian children with protein-energy malnutrition studied were also folate deficient.

Folate deficiency commonly complicates the course of pregnancy (because of nutritional deficiencies and high demands of pregnancy) and occurs following malarial hemolysis. Megaloblastic erythropoiesis was observed in 55% of all primigravidae in northern Nigeria; it contributed to over 75% of severe anemias in Nigeria and to 66% in India.

Hematologic Manifestations. Folate deficiency is manifest as a macrocytic, megaloblastic anemia. The mean corpuscular hemoglobin concentration (MCHC) remains normal, but both the mean cell volume (MCV) and the mean cellular hemoglobin (MCH) are raised. The reticulocyte count is low or normal, unless raised when the primary lesion is hemolysis. The leukocyte count is most variable; the neutrophil count is often low with the characteristic hypersegmentation. However, with concurrent infections it may be raised, with release of early precursor cells from the bone marrow, to give a leukemoid reaction. The platelet count is also reduced, and in some instances patients may have purpura. The peripheral blood film shows considerable anisocytosis and macrocytosis with a few microcytes. In acutely developing anemias there is no poikilocytosis, but in more long-standing deficiencies there is ovalocytosis and poikilocytosis; polychromasia is more pronounced with hemolytic anemias, and there can be numerous nucleated red cells with megaloblastic features.

Smears of bone marrow aspirates show megaloblastic erythropoiesis and giant metamyelocytes. When there is underlying hemolytic disease, changes are apparent earlier in the red cell than in the granulocyte series; in purely nutritional deficiencies, however, giant metamyelocytes may be the first feature. In the majority of patients, megaloblastic erythropoiesis is due to folate deficiency; with the history and the presence of diseases known to deplete folate stores (Table 5–5), a diagnosis of folic acid deficiency can be made with a high degree of certainty. When there is doubt, folate deficiency and vitamin B$_{12}$ deficiency must be distinguished by the assay of folate in serum and red cell, and vitamin B$_{12}$ in serum, using either bioassay or isotope dilution techniques. If these assays are not available, the hematologic response to physiologic doses (folic acid 50 μg/day or vitamin B$_{12}$ 1 μg/day) can be followed with daily estimates of reticulocyte count and hemoglobin.

VITAMIN B$_{12}$. The cobalamins that are known collectively as vitamin B$_{12}$ are synthesized by microorganisms and found exclusively in animal food, not in vegetables (Chapter 107.7). Many of the functions of vitamin B$_{12}$ remain obscure, but it is essential in conjunction with folate for the synthesis of purines and pyrimidines, and in particular for the conversion of uridine to thymidine in the synthesis of DNA. It is required by the cells of the central nervous system, such that deficiency leads not only to megaloblastic anemia but also to subacute combined degeneration of the spinal cord.

Dietary Sources. Dietary sources of vitamin B$_{12}$ are liver and other animal tissues, eggs, and milk. Fecal contamination of well water is a major source of vitamin B$_{12}$ in some impoverished vegetarian communities. Daily requirements are small (Table 5–4). Absorption depends on release of vitamin B$_{12}$ in the stomach and binding to the intrinsic factor (IF) secreted by parietal cells. The IF-B$_{12}$ complex is absorbed by mucosal cells of the ileum, and the vitamin B$_{12}$ is transported actively to the portal circulation. Transport is by transcobalamin II protein. The major store is in the liver; it is normally sufficient for about 2 years.

Causes of Vitamin B$_{12}$ Deficiency. Deficiency of vitamin B$_{12}$ can result from (1) inadequate intake, (2) gastric disease leading to a failure to secrete IF, (3) disease of the ileum, and (4) competition by the fish tapeworm *Diphyllobothrium latum* (Chapter 100.1).

Dietary Deficiency. A nutritional deficiency of vitamin B$_{12}$ is difficult to achieve, as daily requirements are extremely low (Table 5–4) and are met by the smallest intake of animal food, including milk and milk products, or bacterially contaminated water. Women in southern India can be deficient as a consequence of low intake, malabsorption caused by chronic sprue, and the increased demands of pregnancy; the deficiency may be manifest in their infants, who are fed with vitamin B$_{12}$– free breast milk. Prisoners have developed severe vitamin B$_{12}$ deficiency and megaloblastic anemia when fed for long periods on unrelieved vegan diets.

Malabsorption. Malabsorption of vitamin B$_{12}$ in tropical countries is less often the result of addisonian pernicious anemia (a disease seen more commonly in those of northern European descent) than it is of disease of the ileum. Malabsorption can follow infection with *Giardia lamblia* or can follow severe enteritis. The fish tapeworm is transmitted by eating raw or undercooked freshwater fish, and infections have been reported on the shores of African lakes and elsewhere in the tropical world. However, fewer than 1 in 1000 of those infected progress to deficiency; megaloblastic anemia is more likely to be due to coincidental folate deficiency.

Clinical Manifestations. The clinical presentation of vitamin B$_{12}$ deficiency differs from that of folate deficiency in that there is a greater likelihood of neurologic complications and hyperpigmentation of the skin, best seen on the soles and the palms and across the knuckles. However, these complications can occur also with folate deficiency when it is long-standing.

The hematologic picture of vitamin B$_{12}$ deficiency is indistinguishable from that of folate deficiency; owing to the greater chronicity of vitamin B$_{12}$ depletion, there is more likely to be poikilocytosis and thrombocytosis. The deficiency of vitamin B$_{12}$ is confirmed by a low serum vitamin B$_{12}$ concentration. In many tropical communities the reference range of serum vitamin B$_{12}$ is high (150 to 2500 pg/L) compared with Caucasian reference ranges, owing partly to genetically determined higher cobalamin-B$_{12}$ binding. Malabsorption of vitamin B$_{12}$ can be confirmed by measuring the absorption of radioactive cobalt-labeled vitamin. Malabsorption due to gastric disease is distinguished from that due to ileal disease, as it is reversed by the addition of intrinsic factor (Schilling test).

ANEMIA IN PROTEIN-ENERGY MALNUTRITION. Children with protein-energy malnutrition (PEM) usually have a moderate anemia (Hb 7.5 to 10.0 gm/dl), which is normocytic and normochromic with low or normal reticulocyte counts (Chapter 106). The bone marrow is cellular and normoblastic. Erythropoietin levels are normal, and the mechanism of anemia appears to be an impairment of erythropoiesis due to decreased reaction of erythroid progenitor cells to erythropoietin. In kwashiorkor, but not in marasmus, there is a moderate shortening of red cell survival besides.

Anemia is more severe if there are complications, such as infections, which are common because of the impairment of immune mechanisms frequently associated with PEM. In some communities, e.g., West Africa, up to one third of children with PEM are folic acid deficient; iron deficiency in early childhood is a common complication of PEM in almost any community.

Genetically Determined Anemias

BALANCED POLYMORPHISMS. There have been numerous mutations during human evolution causing inherited abnormalities in red blood cell hemoglobin, enzymes, and membranes. Some of these variations rendered the red blood cells a less perfect environment for the development of malarial parasites. Any gene conferring partial protection against malaria also would confer great survival advantage; the genetic advantage of heterozygous inheritance would lead to increased gene frequency in each generation until a balance was reached between the genetic disadvantage of ill health and homozygous inheritance. This is illustrated most clearly by HbS gene.

In its original global distribution before the transatlantic slave trade and modern travel, the HbS gene occurred at high frequency only in Africa and other parts of the world where *P. falciparum* malaria was endemic (Fig. 5–2). Subjects with sickle cell trait (HbAS) have a distinct survival advantage in regions where malaria is hyper- or holoendemic (Chapter 73); e.g., in Garki in the north of Nigeria the incidence of HbAS in newborns was 24%; this proportion rose to 29% by 5 years, at which level it remained in all older age groups. The proportion of newborns with sickle cell anemia (HbSS) was 2%, but survival after 4 years was extremely unusual. The advantage of HbAS over the normal (HbAA) was the result of lower frequencies of *P. falciparum* parasitemia and, more importantly, lower

densities between the ages of 6 months and 4 years. The partial protection against intense *P. falciparum* infection was shown clearly by the hospital observations that almost no one with sickle cell trait died from cerebral malaria.

Mechanisms for limiting parasitemia have been demonstrated in vitro. In long-term cultures of *P. falciparum* at low oxygen tension, as experienced in the last 12 hours of the erythrocyte cycle in vivo, there is an inhibition of growth of mature parasites in red cells containing HbS compared with red cells containing HbA only. This inhibition could be accounted for by the jelling of deoxygenated HbS molecules. Another postulated mechanism involves the consumption of oxygen by the early parasite forms in circulating red cells, leading to sickling, and the preferential removal by the reticuloendothelial system of the parasitized sickled red cells. The protection of sickle cell trait extends to beyond early childhood: There are reduced parasitemia during pregnancy, protection against hyperreactive malarial splenomegaly, and less inhibition by malaria upon the antibody response to pneumococcal vaccine. Subjects with HbSS have the same limitation of *P. falciparum* parasitemia, but parasitemia is likely to precipitate hemolytic and infarctive crises, with high morbidity and mortality.

Genes that reach polymorphic frequency include hemoglobin S (Fig. 5–2); the hemoglobins C, D, and E (Fig. 5–3); beta-thalassemias (Fig. 5–7); alpha-thalassemias (Fig. 5–9); certain forms of glucose-6-phosphate dehydrogenase (G6PD) deficiency; (Fig. 5–10); and some types of congenital elliptocytosis (Fig. 5–11). Although their geographic coincidence with malaria provides evidence that the other genetically determined abnormalities of red cells confer protection against malaria, the extent and mechanisms of the protection have not been demonstrated as clearly as with HbS.

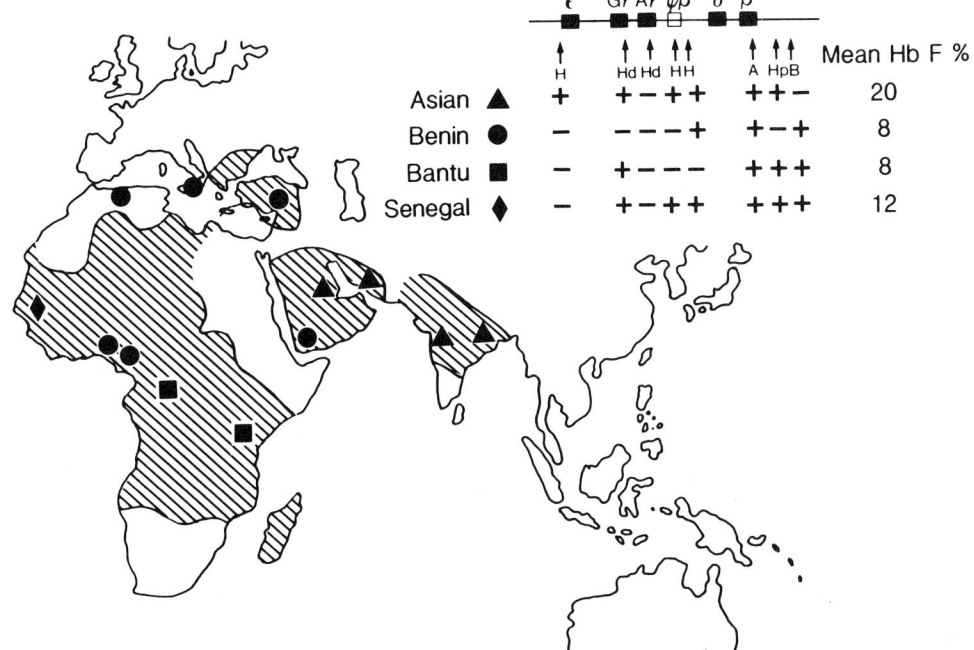

FIGURE 5–2. Areas of the Old World where HbS gene frequency is greater than 0.02. Distribution of beta-chain haplotypes.

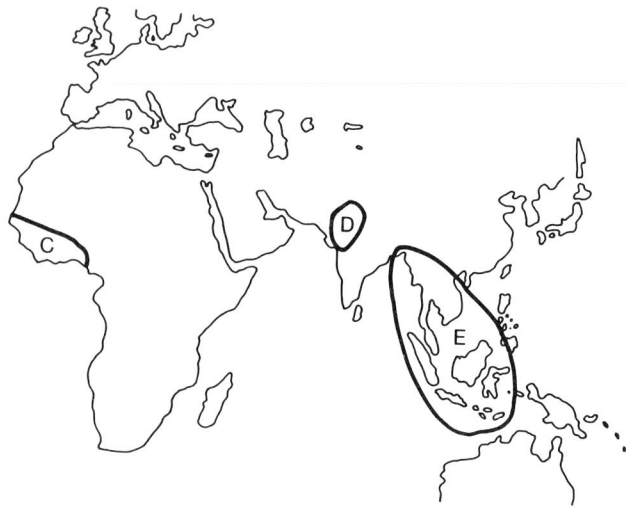

FIGURE 5–3. Areas of the Old World where HbC, HbD (Punjab or Los Angeles), and HbE reach polymorphic frequencies.

SICKLE CELL DISEASE

Definition. Sickle cell disease results from the inheritance of two abnormal allelemorphic genes, at least one of which is the sickle cell gene, controlling the synthesis of the beta-chains of hemoglobin. The most common form of sickle cell disease is sickle cell anemia or homozygous HbSS, but other forms include HbSC, HbS/β-thalassemia, and other doubly heterozygous conditions. HbSS is the most severe but is scarcely distinguished from HbS/β⁰-thalassemia. HbSC is less severe, and HbS/β⁺-thalassemia is relatively mild. The main description of sickle cell disease refers to HbSS as seen in Africa, unless stated otherwise.

Pathophysiology. All pathology of sickle cell disease is derived from one mutation causing the substitution of the hydrophobic amino acid valine for the hydrophilic amino acid glutamic acid at position 6 on the β-chain of the adult hemoglobin (HbA) molecule. When deoxygenated, the sickle hemoglobin (HbS) has reduced solubility compared with HbA. Molecules of HbS jell, that is, they adhere to each other to form long chains with 14 molecules in cross section. These polymers become aligned in parallel, so distorting the red cell into the characteristic sickle form. At first, sickling is reversible with reoxygenation, but repeated sickling and unsickling leads to loss of cell membrane components, a decline in intracellular water and K^+, a rise in intracellular Ca^{2+}, and the formation of the irreversibly sickled cell. Sickled cells are rigid and have a tendency to adhere to each other and to endothelium. The pathology of sickle cell disease results from hemolysis and infarction from the blocking of small blood vessels. Secondary effects include increased susceptibility to infections and retardation of growth and development.

Clinical Manifestations

Hemolysis and Anemia. In the steady state the Hb concentration is usually in the range from 6.0 to 10.0 gm/dl in HbSS and HbS/β⁰-thalassemia, and from 11.0 to 14.0 gm/dl in HbSC disease. There is constant moderate jaundice, with a serum bilirubin level of 35 to 140 μmol/L (2 to 8 mg/dl). About one quarter of patients

over 15 years of age have pigment gallstones, but cholelithiasis is almost invariably asymptomatic.

There is a constant erythroid hyperplasia that leads to expansion of the bone marrow cavity and bossing of the bones of the skull (Fig. 5–4). The forehead is rounded, with an exaggeration of the line of the supraorbital sulcus. Expansion of the maxilla causes a forward protrusion of the upper incisors (gnathopathy). Bossing of the vault of the skull is less common but can be dramatic, so that the head is grossly enlarged and the outer table is so thin as to be easily depressed on palpation. A radiograph of the skull can demonstrate the bossing and shows a hair-on-end picture of the bone marrow cavity of the vault (Fig. 5–5). As gross bossing is reversible with long-term antimalarial prophylaxis and as it is not observed in black Americans with sickle cell disease, it is probably due largely to the additional hemolysis of malaria.

The steady state can be interrupted by anemic crises, which may be caused by malaria, acute splenic sequestration, folate deficiency, or bone marrow aplasia.

Acute *P. falciparum* malaria can cause severe hemolytic crisis and profound anemia. Anemic cardiac failure with malaria is probably the most common cause of death in tropical Africa in children with HbSS not under medical supervision.

A splenic sequestration crisis is characterized by an acutely enlarging spleen with sequestration of a large proportion of the red cell mass and a catastrophic decline of the Hb by at least 2.0 gm/dl, but with an elevated reticulocyte count and erythroid hyperplasia in the bone marrow. This is believed to be precipitated by infection and a consequent alteration of the surface of the red

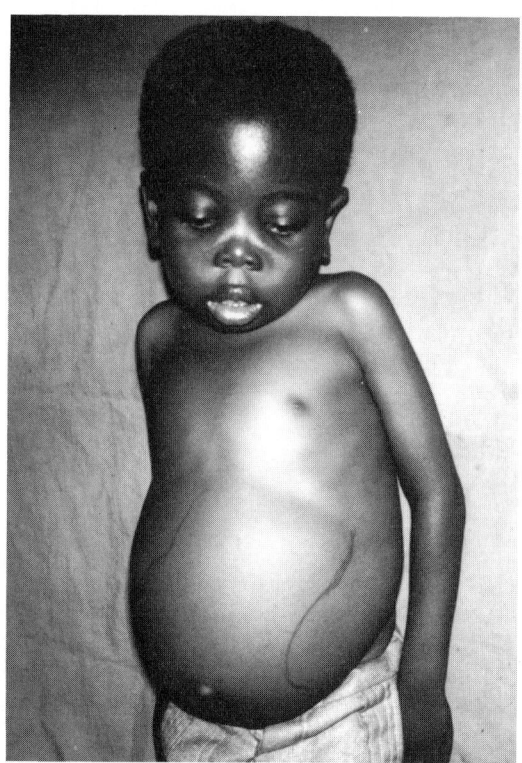

FIGURE 5–4. African child with HbSS having prominent frontal bossing and splenomegaly.

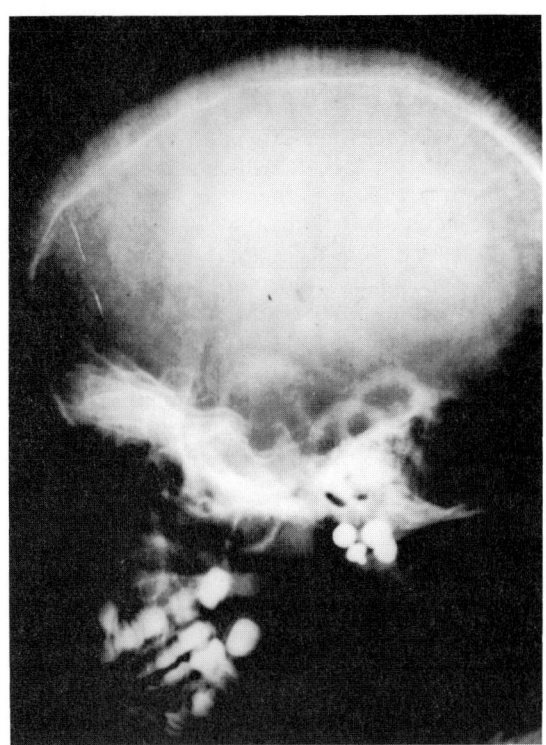

FIGURE 5–5. Skull radiograph of an African with HbSS, showing expansion of the vault with the "hair-on-end" appearance from erythroid hyperplasia.

cell membrane. It occurs most often in patients aged 6 months to 2 years but can be seen in older individuals who retain splenic function or who are pregnant. Its frequency in Africa is not defined, but in Jamaica it is the single most common cause of death in early life.

Megaloblastic erythropoiesis with anemic crisis can interrupt the steady state as a consequence of any of the other causes of folate deficiency (Table 5–5) superimposed on the constant high demands due to erythroid hyperplasia of sickle cell disease. In West Africa, megaloblastic erythropoiesis is almost inevitable during pregnancy and occurs in over 10% of nonpregnant patients with HbSS disease who have not been receiving supportive therapy.

Any acute infection can depress erythropoiesis to some extent in an otherwise normal subject, usually without any significant clinical manifestations. However, such depression can be catastrophic in HbSS disease, in which the steady-state Hb level depends on a rate of erythropoiesis 6 or 8 times normal. Many acute infections are followed by rapid declines in Hb and reticulocyte counts, but parvovirus causes epidemics of severe aplastic crises among the populations with HbSS disease. The incidence of parvovirus infections in Africa is unknown, but it has been well documented in the Caribbean.

Infarctive Crises. Infarction of sickled red cells in the small blood vessels of the small bones of the hands and feet is followed by tissue necrosis and an acute, painful, nonpitting, swelling of the dorsa and digits, the so-called hand-foot syndrome (Fig. 5–6). This is the most common first clinical presentation, occurring in about 90% of

children between the ages of 6 months and 2 years diagnosed as having HbSS disease in tropical Africa. In less than 10% of crises there is a superimposed osteomyelitis, often with *Salmonella* as the infecting organism.

After about 2 years of age, the site of bone infarction shifts from the hands and feet to the long bones of the limbs. Pain is experienced most often around the large joints but can be present in any part of the limbs or bony skeleton. Pain has an acute onset and varies in severity from mild, lasting perhaps only a few minutes, to extremely severe, characteristically lasting 5 days. On physical examination there is usually only mild pyrexia and no more than warmth and tenderness at the site of infarction. However, the paucity of signs should not lead to an underestimation of the severity of the patient's condition. Bone pain crisis is the first presentation in up to 40% of patients in tropical Africa; the most frequently recognized precipitating factors are malaria and various bacterial infections, but in many no inciting factors are identified. Bone pain crises usually resolve within 1 week, but their course may be complicated by fat or bone embolism to the lungs, brain, kidney, or other tissues or by osteomyelitis.

Chest Pain. Acute pain in the chest can result from pneumonia, pulmonary infarction, infarction into the thoracic cage, or rarely, angina pectoris. The first two conditions are often impossible to distinguish, and as one may precede and precipitate the other, many clini-

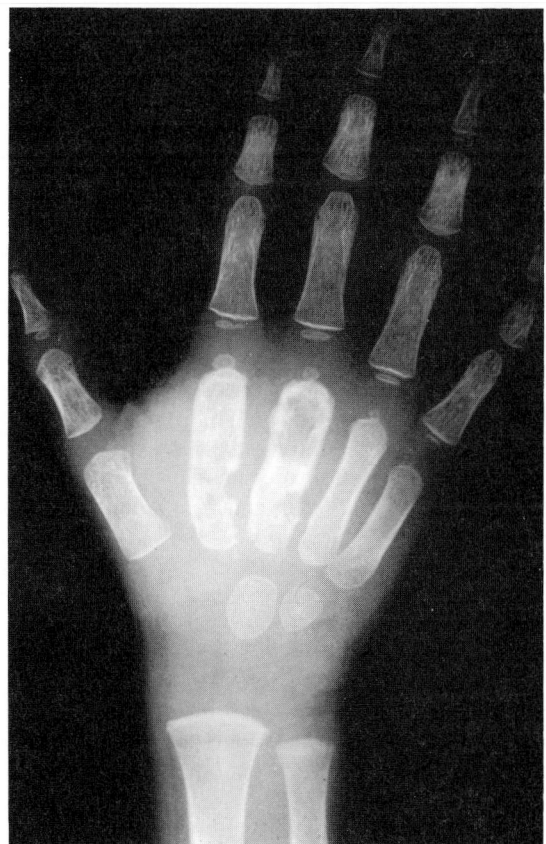

FIGURE 5–6. Multiple osteolytic lesions in the second and third carpal bones due to bone infarctions in an African child with HbSS.

cians refer to the complex as acute pulmonary episodes. The cumulative frequency of acute pulmonary disease in African patients is over 30%.

Abdominal Pain. Over two thirds of patients give a history of mild recurrent abdominal pain, and over 10% require admission to the hospital at some time because of severe abdominal pain. The pain of the acute abdominal crisis of sickle cell disease is usually central or epigastric. There may be vomiting and constipation: Bowel sounds are reduced or absent, and x-ray reveals gas and fluid levels. The etiology is obscure, but the probable cause is infarction in the mesenteric vessels. Usually there is spontaneous recovery in about 5 days. Other causes of acute abdominal pain include splenic infarction, infarction in the lumbar spine, duodenal ulceration (usually in males over 25 years), cholecystitis, obstruction of cystic or bile ducts, acute pancreatitis, and abdominal crises unrelated to sickle cell disease.

Infarctions Elsewhere. Infarction can occur in any tissue and may be followed by a wide range of symptoms, signs, and pathology. For example, intracranial infarctions are fortunately uncommon but cause severe paralyses and alterations of cerebral function. Infarction into the skin around the ankles is followed by sickle cell ulcers; infarction into the corpora cavernosa results in priapism; and infarction in the kidneys causes hematuria and scarring.

Infections. Patients with sickle cell disease have a greater than normal susceptibility to bacterial infections as a result of (1) hyposplenism, which follows recurrent splenic infarction and fibrosis (autosplenectomy); (2) constant activation of the alternative pathway of complement by free hemoglobin in plasma, causing depletion of factor C3 and hence a deficit of opsonization; (3) colonization by bacteria of dead infarcted tissue; and (4) breaches in mucosal surfaces from infarction. Other possible mechanisms include defects of cell-mediated immunity and high levels of free iron being available for the metabolic processes of invading organisms.

Patients with HbSS disease are particularly susceptible to *Streptococcus pneumoniae*, *Salmonella*, and other gram-negative organisms as well as *Haemophilus influenzae* type B. The major infectious cause of morbidity and mortality in temperate countries is the pneumococcus, whereas in tropical Africa it is *P. falciparum*. Pneumococcal septicemia, pneumonia, and meningitis occur most frequently below the age of 2 years and have a greater than 50% mortality in the absence of appropriate treatment. Other organisms commonly isolated from bacteremic children with HbSS disease include *Klebsiella*, *Salmonella*, *Pseudomonas aeruginosa*, *Escherichia coli*, *Staphylococcus* species, and *Streptococcus faecalis*.

At some stage, nearly 10% of patients develop an acute osteomyelitis at the site of bone infarction. In tropical Africa, organisms infecting bones are *Salmonella* (usually *S. typhi*) in 50%, other coliforms in about 45%, and *Staphylococcus pyogenes* in 20%; mixed infections are common.

Growth and Development. Before puberty, height and weight are well below average for age. The shortening is more evident in the trunk than in the legs. The limbs are characteristically long and thin, the abdomen protuberant, and the thorax barrel-shaped; the head and face show bossing (Fig. 5–4). After age about 11 years, skeletal maturation is slow and fusion of epiphyses may be delayed until after age 20 years. This allows subjects with HbSS disease to catch up on their growth during and after puberty, and some men may be excessively tall (over 190 cm, 6 ft, 3 in).

Puberty is delayed. Menarche occurs in girls with HbSS disease later than normal. These females tend to be immature emotionally and to have prolonged dependence on parents. First pregnancies often are delayed until well after the age of 20 years. In contrast, in some cultures the girls may be forced into marriage before they are physically or emotionally prepared for childbirth. Men are often impotent as a result of priapism leading to fibrosis.

Pregnancy. Women with the milder forms of sickle cell disease, e.g., HbSC disease, HbS/β+-thalassemia, or sickle cell anemia with favorable genetic or environmental factors, are likely to survive to adulthood and to be fertile. Women with sickle cell disease who are not under medical care are liable to develop extremely severe anemia during the second trimester of pregnancy, associated with malaria and folate deficiency. Other common complications include acute sequestration crises, bone pain crises near the time of delivery, preeclampsia during labor, operative deliveries necessitated by pelvic disproportion, bacterial infections, and wound sepsis. Maternal mortality remains high in Africa.

HIV and Sickle Cell Disease. There is a close geographic coincidence between regions where the HbS gene is frequent and those where the HIVs are epidemic (Chapter 15.1). HIV seropositivity may be as high as 20% among blood donors, and as a consequence, 5 to 20% of patients with sickle cell disease have become infected through blood transfusion in some cities. The highest rates of infection have occurred where there has not been active maintenance of health but merely treatment of sickle cell crises, often with blood transfusions. Patients with sickle cell disease who are infected with HIV present most commonly with generalized lymphadenopathy. Other common features are failure to gain (or loss of) weight, chronic lower respiratory tract infections, persistent watery diarrhea, oral candidiasis, and herpes zoster. Both onset of HIV-related disease following transfusion (even less than 2 months) and progression to death seem to be rapid in the small series studied so far.

The advent of HIV and AIDS has made it more important than ever that (1) there be investment in maintenance of health of patients with sickle cell disease (Table 5–6), and (2) blood transfusions be carefully controlled. Transfusions should be given only to save life wherever it is not possible to exclude HIV-infected units from the blood bank. The relative size of this problem is clear when it is remembered that 120,000 infants are born with sickle cell disease in Africa each year, compared with only 400 born with hemophilia.

Prognosis. In rural Africa, where there is poor hygiene, no mosquito avoidance, and no modern medicine, less than 2% of children with sickle cell disease live beyond 4 years of age. However, there are both inherited and environmental factors that vastly improve the prognosis.

Genetic Factors. The type of sickle cell disease is important: HbSS and HbS/β⁰-thalassemia carry the worst prognosis; HbSC is less severe, and HbS/β⁺-thalassemia is a relatively mild condition.

There are numerous polymorphisms of the β-globin gene cluster, referred to as the β-globin haplotypes. Four β-globin haplotypes are associated with the βˢ mutation. The Senegal haplotype is found on the western seaboard of West Africa (Fig. 5–2). The Benin haplotype is prevalent in West Africa, whence it has spread probably to the Mediterranean basin, southwest Arabia, and Turkey. The Bantu haplotype is common in East and Central Africa. The Asian haplotype is prevalent around the Arabian Sea, including eastern Arabia and the Indian subcontinent. These haplotypes are linked to determinants of levels of HbF persisting in SS anemia beyond infancy. The highest level of HbF (mean, 20%) is associated with the Asian haplotype. The Senegal haplotype has a higher HbF (mean, 12%) than do the other African haplotypes, Benin and Bantu (both average 8%). High levels of HbF lead to less gelling and sickling, longer red cell survival, and higher total Hb, hematocrit, MCV, and MCH. There is less infarction, less autosplenectomy, and generally milder disease.

Coincidental inheritance of homozygous α⁺-thalassemia (present in approximately 7% of the population of tropical Africa) with SS disease decreases the total Hb per red cell (low MCH); there are fewer sickled cells, longer red cell survival, increased red cell counts, lower reticulocyte counts, and lower serum bilirubin along with fewer complications.

Environmental Factors. The genetic differences explain the wide variation in severity of sickle cell disease even within one family. However, the environmental factors are of far greater importance. Prognosis is improved greatly when families are able and willing to care for their children by protecting them from malaria, ensuring cleanliness and good hygiene, obtaining all immunizations, providing adequate nutrition, and seeking medical care. The role of health professionals is to support families in their attempts to maintain the health of their members born with this disorder. With proper care, patients with sickle cell disease lead full and active lives.

Maintenance of Health. Emphasis must be placed on maintaining the steady state in sickle cell disease through early diagnosis, education, and supportive care at sickle cell clinics, hospitals, and obstetric units (Table 5–6).

Diagnosis. Policies should be formulated and implemented for the widespread neonatal diagnosis of sickle cell disease. All pregnant women should be screened (by Serjeants' HbS solubility test—*not* by commercial kits or the sickling test) followed by Hb electrophoresis on cellulose acetate at alkaline pH if HbS is present. All infants born of women carrying at least one S gene should be tested at birth by electrophoresis on cellulose acetate at alkaline pH followed by electrophoresis on citrate agar at pH 6 to 6.5 if an abnormality is detected.

TABLE 5–6. Maintenance of Health in Sickle Cell Disease

Early diagnosis	Laboratory techniques—HbS solubility
	—Hb electrophoresis
	Screening—pregnant women
	—newborn of mother with S gene
	—anemic children
	—siblings of patients
	Clinical awareness
Education	Parents and patients
	Health professionals
	General public
Sickle cell clinics	Prevent infection—prophylactic antimalarials
	—immunization
	—prophylactic penicillin
	Nutrition—folic acid supplements
	—general nutritional advice
	Advice—avoid cold, fatigue, dehydration, excessive alcohol
	—no useless treatment
	—attend clinic regularly
	—report when ill
	—report when pregnant
Hospital	Prompt treatment of crises
Obstetrics	Supervision of pregnancy, delivery, puerperium
	Family limitation to ≤3 viable children

Such a scheme would detect infants with HbSS, but would miss HbSC and HbSβ-thal in infants who inherit the S gene from the father. In populations in which β-thalassemia is common, pregnant women should be screened with the one-tube osmotic fragility test. However, HbC can be detected only by electrophoresis, which is not cost-effective in prenatal screening.

Health Education. The condition should be explained to the parents and patients, preferably in their first language verbally and by the use of pamphlets. Discussions at subsequent visits to the clinic reinforce the importance of disease prevention and health maintenance. Education should be extended to all medical and paramedical staff and to the general public.

Preventive Care. The most important intervention is the lifelong protection against malaria (Chapter 73). Patients should receive curative chloroquine at their initial clinic visit and at the first visit following any break in attendance. Proguanil is used frequently in Africa as prophylaxis: 25 mg/day during the first year of life, 50 mg/day for children 1 to 4 years of age, 100 mg/day for those over 5 years, and 200 mg/day for adults. Compliance in taking one white tablet (proguanil) and one yellow tablet (folic acid) has been excellent. Oral prophylactic penicillin is highly effective in preventing pneumococcal infection in the United States and the United Kingdom but has not received a trial in tropical Africa. There are obvious problems of cost and logistics, but a controlled trial of oral penicillin prophylaxis in Africans with sickle cell disease is needed.

Another essential function of the sickle cell clinic is to provide a place where patients can report when sick, so that they can be assessed rapidly and admitted to the hospital, if necessary, without becoming lost in the mass of patients attending the acute pediatric or medical outpatients' clinics.

Management of Crisis

General Measures. Whenever a patient with sickle cell disease is seriously ill, a minimum of laboratory studies includes Hb (or hematocrit), reticulocyte count, total and differential white cell count, thick film for malaria, and urinalysis. If the patient has fever (<39C) or if pneumonia, meningitis, or acute osteomyelitis is suspected, the blood should be cultured. A Gram stain and a sputum culture are required when there is an acute pulmonary disease. A lumbar puncture should be performed when there is even minimal meningism. Feces should be examined by microscopy and culture if there is diarrhea. Radiography of the chest is indicated when there is high fever (<39C) or suspected pneumonia. Serum should be tested for anti-HIV if there has been possible exposure, e.g., through blood transfusion, or if the clinical presentation suggests HIV-related disease.

It should be assumed that malaria is contributing to the crisis, and treatment should be started before results of microscopy of the blood are available (Chapter 73). Antimalarial prophylaxis and supplements of folic acid should be started or continued.

Treatment of Anemic Crises. The administration of antimalarials, folic acid, and antibiotics, if indicated, will arrest the decline of hematocrit and will be followed by recovery in most patients. Blood transfusion should be avoided whenever possible because of its dangers, including those of transmitting HIV-1, HIV-2, hepatitis B virus, and other infections. Transfusion is indicated (1) when there is incipient or established cardiac failure, which can develop when the Hb is less than 4.0 gm/dl; (2) when there is acute sequestration crisis, with Hb less than 6.0 gm/dl and falling rapidly; (3) when obstetric delivery is imminent and the Hb is less than 8.0 gm/dl; (4) following acute hemorrhage, when blood pressure and oxygenation cannot be restored by crystalloids or colloids; and (5) preceding or during emergency major surgery.

HbAA blood donors should be selected and HbAS blood transfused only in an emergency and in the absence of suitable HbAA blood. Except for treating hemorrhage, concentrated red cells, *not* whole blood, should be transfused, 10 ml/kg body weight administered over 4 to 6 hours, preceded by intramuscular furosemide 1.0 mg/kg body weight when there is cardiac failure.

Other Indications for Blood Transfusions. Emergency exchange blood transfusions have been advocated in the treatment of acute cerebrovascular accident, severe priapism, acute chest syndrome, and acute abdominal crisis. There is no convincing evidence that this treatment is advantageous, and it is contraindicated where HIV is epidemic. Elective exchange blood transfusions have been recommended to precede major surgery or contrast radiography. In every case, the potential benefit must outweigh the risks, including those of infection and alloimmunization. The blood selected must be HbAA-, HIV-, and HBV-negative and closely matched antigenically to the recipient. At least twice the patient's volume of blood is exchanged by an isovolemic procedure, with the aim of reducing the HbS to below 20% and giving a final Hb concentration of 14.0 to 15.0 gm/dl.

Hypertransfusion regimens have been proposed (1) in the management of pregnancy; (2) for 3 months following prosthetic joint surgery; (3) for 3 years following

cerebrovascular accidents; (4) for recurrent life-threatening chest crises; and (5) when recurrent infarctive crisis prevents a normal life. There is no evidence that randomized pregnant women and their fetuses do better on a hypertransfusion regimen, and this is not recommended as routine in the management of sickle cell disease in developing countries. Decisions to administer hypertransfusion treatment must be made on an individual basis for both pregnant and nonpregnant patients; however, such programs should not be embarked upon unless (1) an adequate supply of suitable HbAA blood is ensured; (2) blood infected by HIV or HBV can be excluded effectively; and (3) chances of alloimmunization can be kept to a minimum.

Treatment of Infarctive Crises. The principles of management are the control of pain, the maintenance of hydration and acid-base balance, and the treatment of infection. The physician must assess the severity of pain and prescribe analgesics at fixed dosages and regular intervals and not delegate decisions as to the control of pain to others, e.g., nurses. Mild pain can be controlled by acetaminophen (paracetamol), moderate pain by dihydrocodeine tartrate, and severe pain by opiates. Patients should be encouraged to drink fluids if they are able to do so. More seriously ill patients may need nasogastric fluid or, if bowel sounds cannot be heard, intravenous fluid.

Treatment of Acute Infections. Antibiotics should be given only when they are needed, and then they must be administered quickly and in adequate dosage.

When a patient has fever higher than 39C not accounted for by malaria, an acute pulmonary episode, or suspected meningitis, treatment should be started. Cefuroxime sodium 150 mg/kg/24 hr, or large doses of ampicillin or penicillin plus chloramphenicol, are recommended. The initial treatment of acute osteomyelitis should be cloxacillin plus chloramphenicol.

Prenatal Diagnosis. There are several constraints preventing the large-scale application of prenatal diagnosis in developing countries. These include (1) the lack of trained staff and facilities for collection of chorionic villous biopsies or fetal blood samples; (2) the complexity and expense of gene analysis; (3) a lack of comprehension by most couples at risk; and (4) the illegality or ethical nonacceptance of therapeutic abortion. However, recent advances in the techniques of chorionic villous biopsy, DNA extraction, selective amplification of DNA fragments by polymerase chain reaction, and restriction endonuclease analysis allow for the prenatal diagnosis of sickle cell disease and β-thalassemia during the first trimester of pregnancy. Since the new methods do not require radioactive isotopes and can be completed within 2 days of obtaining the samples, and the cost has been reduced by half, it is possible that some centers in developing countries will be able to provide prenatal diagnosis of the hemoglobinopathies in the near future.

BETA-THALASSEMIAS. Depressions of synthesis of the β-chains of hemoglobin, conditions known collectively as the β-thalassemias, occur commonly throughout a broad belt from the Mediterranean to Oceania and on the Atlantic seaboard of West Africa (Fig. 5–7). Within

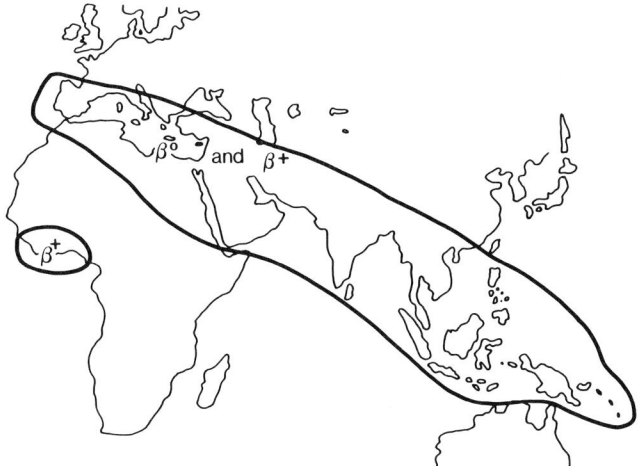

FIGURE 5–7. Areas of the Old World where various forms of β-thalassemia reach polymorphic frequencies.

this area, between 2% and 30% of the population are carriers of the abnormal genes, but β-thalassemia is seen sporadically in all racial groups. As much as 3% of the world's population, or 150 million individuals, mostly in Asia, carry genes for β-thalassemia.

By 1989, there were nearly 60 known mutations leading to β-thalassemia. Of these, three are deletions of the β-gene, and 51 are point mutations affecting rates of β-chain synthesis at any stage from initiation of transcription to translation, to mRNA function and mRNA processing (Table 5–7). About 20 alleles account for 90% of β-thalassemia genes. In general, each population tends to have a different group of mutations, with a few common alleles and a variable number of rare ones.

The genes are expressed either as complete suppression of β-globin synthesis ($β^0$-thalassemia genes) or partial suppression ($β^+$-thalassemia genes) (Table 5–7).

Clinically the thalassemias are classified according to their severity. *Thalassemia major* is a severe disorder in which the patient is dependent on blood transfusion for survival beyond early childhood. *Thalassemia intermedia* is characterized by anemia and splenomegaly, requiring blood transfusion only at irregular intervals. *Thalassemia minor* is the symptomless state, with moderate anemia only.

Beta-Thalassemia Major. Major disease arises from the homozygous or compound heterozygous inheritance of $β^0$-or most $β^+$-thalassemia genes. About 50,000 infants are born each year with β-thalassemia major.

Etiology and Pathophysiology. As production of γ-globin declines in the first 6 months of postuterine life, it is not replaced with β-globin in infants with β-thalassemia. The excess of α-globin chains form intracellular inclusions, which cause both ineffective erythropoiesis and hemolysis, especially from phagocytosis of erythrocytes in the spleen. There is gross erythroid hyperplasia with massive expansion of the bone marrow cavities (Fig. 5–8). Splenic hypertrophy leads to hypersplenism with further sequestration of red cells, granulocytes, and platelets and expansion of plasma volume. The absorption of iron is increased and it is poorly utilized in hemoglobin synthesis, so that iron accumulates in tissues. Some red cell precursors normally retain the ability to produce HbF ($α_2 γ_2$); the synthesis of these cells is increased in the hypertrophic bone marrow and they survive preferentially in the blood. As δ-chain synthesis is normal, there is a relative and absolute increase in HbA$_2$ ($α_2 δ_2$).

Clinical Manifestations. Infants fail to thrive and have intermittent fevers, pallor, and splenomegaly. With no treatment, or only intermittent blood transfusions, there is severe retardation of growth and development throughout childhood. There is progressive enlargement of the spleen. Hypersplenism occurs and worsens the anemia and may cause hemorrhage as a complication of thrombocytopenia. There is gross bossing of all the bones of the skull, with poorly formed teeth and blockages of sinuses. Secondary infection of the middle ear may cause deafness. Skull x-ray shows thinning of the outer table and spicules of bone in the expanded marrow cavity (i.e., hair-on-end appearance) (Fig. 5–5). Changes in the long bones are associated with pathologic fractures (Fig. 5–8). Severe drops in Hb concentration follow either infection or folic acid depletion.

The accumulation of iron leads to progressive hemosiderosis. This may cause cardiac arrhythmias, pericarditis, and congestive heart failure. There can be complex endocrine disorders also, including diabetes mellitus, hypoparathyroidism, hypothyroidism, adrenal insufficiency, and hypogonadism. Hemosiderosis leads to progressive hepatic cirrhosis and liver failure. There is bronze discoloration of the skin.

Other biochemical changes include hyperuricemia and secondary gout as well as depletion of ascorbate and vitamin E.

Without treatment, children die usually within the first 2 years from anemic heart failure. With intermittent treatment with blood transfusion, they are likely to succumb to overwhelming infection in childhood. If they survive beyond the age of puberty, the most common cause of death is cardiac failure from hemosiderosis.

Hematology. The hemoglobin is usually 2.0 to 8.0 gm/dl at the time of presentation. The MCH and MCV are reduced. The peripheral blood film is grossly abnormal, and characteristically there is considerable anisocytosis with macrocytes and microcytes, numerous target cells, poikilocytosis, fragmented red cells, marked hypochromia, nucleated red cells that may show megaloblastic change, and basophilic stippling. The reticulocyte count is usually only slightly elevated. White cell counts may be high from infection or low from hypersplenism. Platelets may be decreased owing to hypersplenism. There is erythroid hyperplasia, often with megaloblastosis, and an excess of iron in the bone marrow.

Bilirubin levels, both conjugated and unconjugated, are high. There is an ahaptoglobulinemia. The serum iron and serum ferritin levels are raised. Patients with homozygous $β^0$-thalassemias have only HbF and HbA$_2$ and no HbA on Hb electrophoresis. Patients with $β^+$-thalassemias have 30 to 90% HbF, the rest being HbA except for less than 4% HbA$_2$.

The clinical observations, peripheral red cell appearances, and Hb electrophoretic patterns are diagnostic.

TABLE 5–7. Molecular Basis of the Beta-Thalassemias

Mutant Class	Mechanisms of Action	Expression
Transcriptional	Substitutions in promoter regions upstream (5′) from β-gene slowing transcription	β⁺
RNA processing	(a) *Splice junction changes,* preventing splicing of exons following removal of introns	β⁰
	(b) *Consensus changes,* around splice junctions destroying sequences important but not essential for splicing	β⁺
	(c) *Alternative splice sites* created by intron substitutions leading to abnormal mRNA	β⁰ or β⁺
	(d) *Cryptic splice sites* activated by exon substitutions leading to abnormal mRNA: concurrent amino acid substitutions	β⁺HbE, Hb-Knossos
Cap site	Substitutions at 5′ end or cap site reducing transcription, slowing capping reducing mRNA stability	β⁺
RNA cleavage + polyadenylation	Substitution of 3′ end reducing RNA cleavage, leading to elongated unstable mRNA	β⁺
Nonfunctional mRNA	(a) *Frameshift:* deletion/addition 1–4 nucleotides in exons throwing code out of phase with early chain termination from new stop codon	β⁰
	(b) *Nonsense:* exon mutation to stop codon, and early chain termination	β⁰
Mis-sense	Amino acid substitutions creating highly unstable β-globins, rapidly degraded (e.g., β-Indianapolis)	β⁰
Deletions	(a) β gene	β⁰
	(b) δβ genes	(δβ)⁰thal:HPHF
	(c) γδβ genes	(γδβ)⁰thal
	(d) γ gene	γthal
Crossover	Mispaired synapsis with unequal crossing over between δ and β genes, forming δβ fusion genes that produce Hb-Lepore(s)	δβ (Lepore)

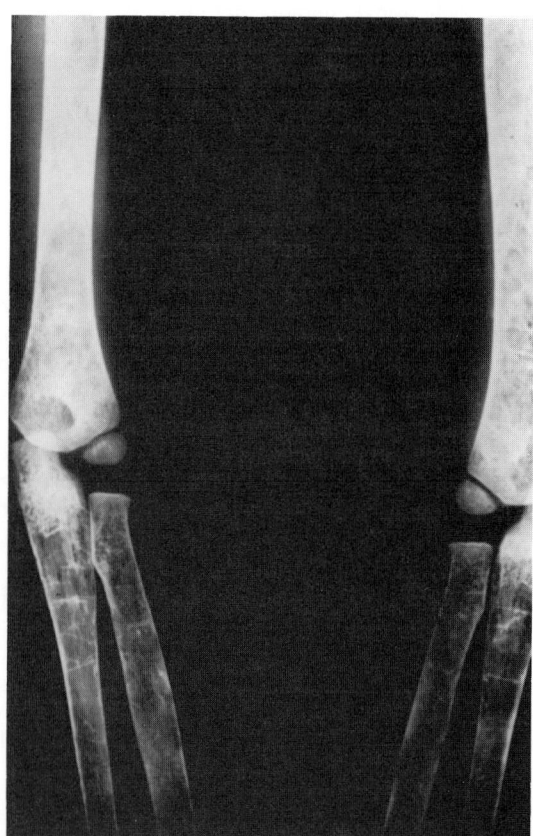

FIGURE 5–8. Massive expansion of the bone marrow cavities due to erythroid hyperplasia has caused loss of calcification and cystic changes in x-ray of femur, tibia, and fibula with β-thalassemia major.

Treatment. The symptomatic treatment of β-thalassemia major depends upon high blood-transfusion regimens, deferoxamine as an iron chelator, and splenectomy to counteract hypersplenism.

Blood Transfusion. Shortly after the diagnosis is made, a hypertransfusion regimen should be implemented, with the aim of maintaining the hemoglobin above 12.0 gm/dl. This may mean transfusion every 6 or 8 weeks. Washed or frozen red cells are preferred, since they cause fewer reactions from antileukocyte antibodies. This treatment effectively suppresses the patient's own abnormal erythropoiesis and allows for normal growth and development.

However, as each milliliter of red cell contains 1 mg of iron, accumulations of iron in the body are inevitable. Hemosiderosis suppresses the normal adolescent growth spurt and secondary sexual development and may cause other endocrine disorders. Death is usual in the second or third decade of life from progressive damage to the heart.

Iron Chelation. Deferoxamine is the only effective agent for enhancing the excretion of iron. A wide variety of routes of administration and dosages have been advocated for treating iron overload. One treatment regimen is to give deferoxamine, 6 to 12 gm daily, by intravenous indwelling catheter. Iron overload can be prevented by the subcutaneous infusion of 2 gm daily, starting at the same time as the high-transfusion regimen. All regimens are troublesome and expensive.

Splenectomy. Increasing requirements for blood transfusions, along with leukopenia and thrombocytopenia, suggest hypersplenism and are, if severe, indications for splenectomy. The operation should be delayed until after the age of 5 years and should be followed by lifelong penicillin prophylaxis, and antimalarial prophylaxis in endemic areas.

Despite their limited success, these regimens have revolutionized the symptomatic treatment and outlook for patients with β-thalassemia major. However, about 25 units of blood are needed for each patient per year. The total cost per patient is $5000 to $8000 (US) per year. These are impossible burdens for the health resources of developing countries. The future lies in prevention through prenatal diagnosis and therapeutic abortion of affected fetuses.

Prevention. There are two approaches to prevention of β-thalassemia major.

Health Education. In the first approach, carriers are identified and given genetic counseling about either the choice of marriage partner, or in the case of couples already married, the chances of infants being affected. This approach has not been conspicuously successful.

Prenatal Diagnosis and Abortion. The second approach is prenatal diagnosis by chorion biopsy at 10 weeks of pregnancy, followed by therapeutic abortion of fetuses with major disease. The recognition of major disease is more complex with β-thalassemia than with HbSS disease because of the multiplicity of mutations; a knowledge of the mutations present in the population and of those being carried by the two parents is necessary. Prenatal diagnosis is well established in Greece, Cyprus, and Sardinia. Techniques are becoming simpler and cheaper. The need for the widespread application of prenatal diagnosis is essential because of the severity of the disease and the limitations and cost of treatment.

Beta-Thalassemia Intermedia

Etiology. Intermediate disease arises from the inheritance of HbEβ-thal, HbCβ-thal, various δβ-thalassemias, or Hb-Lepore disorders or from some homozygous β-thalassemias coinciding with α-thalassemias, homozygous β+-thalassemia in West Africa, or the coinheritance of genes for enhanced HbF production.

About 40,000 infants are born each year into the largest group, which is HbEβ-thal in Southeast Asia (Figs. 5–3 and 5–7).

Clinical Manifestations. The spectrum of disease ranges from those who have only moderate anemia to those with Hb levels of 5.0 to 7.0 gm/dl, splenomegaly, folate deficiency, skeletal deformities, iron overload progressing with age, recurrent leg ulcers, gallstones, and increased susceptibility to infections.

Treatment. These patients need regular surveillance. For patients with more severe anemia, folic acid supplements are indicated, and antimalarial prophylaxis will be required in endemic areas. Blood transfusions should be given to treat anemic crises, and regular transfusion regimens may have to be instigated for patients with growth retardation and serious bone deformities. Some develop hypersplenism and require splenectomy. Antibiotics are necessary to counteract infections.

Beta-Thalassemia Minor.
The heterozygous inheritance of any of the β-thalassemia genes is usually symptom-free, but rarely there is mild splenomegaly. The Hb is generally 9.0 to 11.0 gm/dl, but in pregnancy it is often 2.0 gm/dl lower. The MCH and MCV are low. Red cells show anisocytosis, microcytosis, hypochromia, and occasional target cells. Sometimes basophilic stippling is seen in a few cells. The changes in the red cells are characteristically more than would have been expected from the Hb concentration. The bone marrow shows moderate erythroid hyperplasia. The frequency of iron deficiency reflects that of the general population. The HbA_2 is elevated to 4 to 6%, and this is the most valuable diagnostic observation. HbF is up to 3% in about half the subjects. Osmotic fragility is reduced; the one-tube osmotic fragility test is useful in population and antenatal screening.

Partial protection against *P. falciparum* parasitemia has been demonstrated in Liberia.

Persistent anemia during pregnancy in women with β-thalassemia minor causes a degree of fetal hypoxia, compensatory placental hypertrophy, intrauterine growth retardation, low urinary estriol excretion, and an increased frequency of fetal distress during delivery. The resulting high frequency (about 12%) of 1-minute Apgar scores of 3 or less is not associated with any appreciable increase in infant mortality.

δβ-Thalassemias. These are much less common than β-thalassemias. They arise from either gene deletion or crossing over between δ- and β-genes leading to the production of Hb-Lepore.

Homozygous (δβ)⁰-Thalassemia. This is characterized by an Hb of 8.0 to 10.0 gm/dl, moderate splenomegaly, and HbF of 100%. Anemia is more severe with infection and pregnancy. Heterozygotes are symptom-free; they have 5 to 20% HbF and normal HbA_2.

Homozygous δβ(Lepore). This presents generally as thalassemia intermedia. Electrophoresis shows only Hb-Lepore. Heterozygotes have a thalassemic blood picture and 5 to 15% Hb-Lepore.

Hereditary Persistence of Hemoglobin F (HPHF). This is a group of conditions that are seen most commonly in Africa. Defective synthesis of β- and δ-chains is almost wholly compensated for by the continued synthesis of γ-chains. Homozygotes are not anemic but have a mild thalassemic red cell appearance and 100% HbF. Heterozygotes have no clinical or hematologic abnormality except HbF 20 to 30%, distributed homogeneously in all red cells.

γδβ-Thalassemias. These conditions are rare, arising from deletions of γ- and δ- as well as β-genes. Homozygous inheritance is obviously incompatible with fetal survival. Heterozygotes have severe hemolytic disease of the newborn. Those who survive have a thalassemia minor with normal HbF and HbA_2.

ALPHA-THALASSEMIAS

Pathophysiology. The conditions that arise from genetically determined reductions in production of α-globin chains are known as the α-thalassemias. The α-globin genes are duplicated on chromosomes 16, so that the normal individual has four active genes (αα/αα). Most α-thalassemias are the result of deletions of one (−α or α+-thalassemia) or both genes (−− or α⁰-thalassemia). Some α+-thalassemias are nondeletional mutations effectively inactivating one α-gene through (1) abnormal splicing, (2) the synthesis of unstable α-chains, (3) interference with polyadenylation of mRNA, or (4) the slow synthesis of elongated chains (e.g., Hb-Constant Spring, which is present in 2 to 5% of the population of Thailand).

There are three genotypes that result in clinically asymptomatic states: (1) heterozygous α^+-thalassemia ($-\alpha/\alpha\alpha$); (2) homozygous α^+-thalassemia ($-\alpha/-\alpha$); and (3) heterozygous α^0-thalassemia ($--/\alpha\alpha$). There are two genotypes that cause symptomatic disease: (1) the double heterozygous α^+-thalassemia/α^0-thalassemia ($-\alpha/--$), in which 3 out of 4 genes are inactive, causing HbH disease; and (2) homozygous α^0-thalassemia ($--/--$), causing the Hb-Barts hydrops syndrome. The pathophysiology of these conditions depends on the excess of γ-chains in fetal life combining to form tetramers (γ_4) called Hb-Barts, and the excess of β-chains in postuterine life combining to form tetramers (β_4) called HbH. The hemoglobins have excessively high oxygen affinity, causing tissue hypoxia. HbH is also unstable, being precipitated as inclusion bodies, causing hemolysis.

Clinical Manifestations

Asymptomatic States. The gene frequency (about 0.26) for α^+-thalassemia is remarkably uniform throughout tropical Africa, making this by far the most common variant of hemoglobin synthesis; 38% of the population is heterozygous and 7% homozygous. The condition is wholly asymptomatic; hematologic changes are minimal and include slight anemia, reductions in MCV and MCH, and slight microcytosis on blood film appearance. Hb-Barts can be detected in trace amounts in only 10% of heterozygotes at birth and is about 2.5% of total Hb in all homozygotes. Only by DNA analysis or by measuring rates of globin-chain synthesis can α^+-thalassemia be diagnosed with certainty.

In Africa, α^+-thalassemia is significant because of (1) the high gene frequency accounting for an average reduction of Hb of 0.5 gm/dl in blacks in comparison with Caucasians; (2) causing a trimodal distribution of the proportion of HbS in subjects with sickle cell trait (i.e., mean HbS is 27% in α^+-thalassemia homozygotes, 35% in heterozygotes, and 41% in those with normal α-globin synthesis); (3) the amelioration of HbSS disease by α-thalassemia; and (4) the probability that α-thalassemia affords slight partial protection against malaria.

Heterozygous α^0-thalassemia is hematologically identical to homozygous α^+-thalassemia; each has two active globin genes. About 30 million subjects in Southeast Asia and southern China are carriers for α^0-thalassemia.

Hemoglobin-H Disease. The most common genotype leading to HbH disease is α^+-thal/α^0-thal, but the disorder arises also from α^0-thal/Hb-Constant Spring in Southeast Asia and homozygous inheritance of severe nondeletion α^+-thalassemias in Saudi Arabia. About 56,000 affected infants are born each year in Thailand alone. The condition presents with a variable degree of anemia and splenomegaly. The course is usually mild, but rarely children have significant growth retardation and skeletal changes. Severe hemolytic anemic crises are associated with infection, pregnancy, and exposure to oxidant drugs. Patients survive into adult life, often with progressive pancytopenia due to hypersplenism.

At birth, there is up to 25% Hb-Barts; after the first year of life, there is 5 to 40% HbH, with HbA and low levels of HbA_2. The hemoglobin is 7.0 to 10.0 gm/dl in the steady state; the peripheral blood film shows a typical thalassemic picture. The reticulocyte count is usually slightly raised. There are numerous inclusion bodies of precipitated HbH in the preparation of red cells stained with cresyl blue. Following splenectomy, these inclusions are much more numerous.

Patients should be seen in medical clinics at regular intervals. They should be warned against the use of oxidant drugs and advised to report when unwell or pregnant. Splenectomy may become necessary with progressive hypersplenism.

Hemoglobin Barts Hydrops Syndrome. The homozygous inheritance of α^+-thalassemia occurs commonly in Southeast Asia, Greece, and Cyprus (Fig. 5–9). About 20,000 affected infants are delivered each year. The infants are stillborn at 28 to 40 weeks of gestation or die shortly after delivery. They are pale and edematous and have massive hepatosplenomegaly. The placenta is enlarged and friable. The Hb is 6.0 to 8.0 gm/dl, and the blood picture is typically thalassemic. Electrophoresis reveals about 80% Hb-Barts and about 20% embryonic Hb-Portland ($\zeta_2\gamma_2$).

The mother frequently suffers from pre-eclampsia or even eclampsia. Both parents will have the mildly abnormal hematologic findings of α^0-thalassemia trait.

There is a strong case to be made for the identification of couples at risk, the prenatal diagnosis by chorion biopsy, and the termination of pregnancies with affected infants. This would avoid the obstetric complications and psychologic trauma of delivery of stillborn hydropic infants.

GLUCOSE-6-PHOSPHATE DEHYDROGENASE DEFICIENCY

Pathophysiology. About 90% of glucose in red cells is degraded by the Embden-Meyerhof pathway to produce ATP and release energy for cellular metabolic processes. The remaining 10% is degraded via the hexose monophosphate shunt (pentose shunt), with the

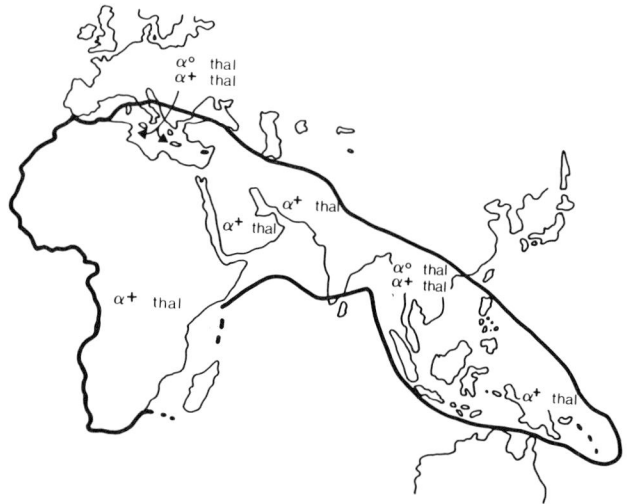

FIGURE 5–9. Areas of the Old World where the different forms of α-thalassemia reach polymorphic frequencies.

TABLE 5–8. Variants of Glucose-6-Phosphate Dehydrogenase

Class	G6PD Activity	Clinical Presentation	Polymorphic Variants
I	Near-absent	Congenital nonspherocytic hemolytic disease	—
II	Severe <10%	Intermittent hemolysis	Mediterranean, Mali, Union
III	Moderate 10–60%	Less severe intermittent hemolysis	A⁻, Canton, Mahidol
IV	Normal activity 60–150%	None	B (the normal enzyme), A, Gambia
V	Increased activity >150%	None	—

reduction of nicotinamide adenosine dinucleotide phosphate (NADP) to NADPH, which is the main H donor in other enzymatic reactions, including the maintenance by glutathione reductase of glutathione (GSSG) in its reduced form (GSH). GSH protects components of the red cells from auto-oxidation. Failure of the system leads to oxidation of hemoglobin to methemoglobin or to the intracellular precipitation of globin as Heinz bodies, and oxidation of lipids in the membrane. A common cause of failure and consequent hemolysis is the congenital deficiency of activity of glucose-6-phosphate dehydrogenase (G6PD), the first enzyme of the hexose monophosphate shunt.

Over 300 variants of G6PD have been identified by thermostability, chromatography, and kinetic properties. They have been classified according to clinical manifestations and enzyme activity (Table 5–8). The main discussion is confined to those enzymes that achieve polymorphic frequency in large populations. The most common, or normal, enzyme is GdB of class IV (normal activity). Variants with normal activity include GdA, common throughout Africa. Variants with moderately reduced activity (class III) include GdA⁻, the common deficient enzyme of Africa (Fig. 5–10). The most common variant with severely deficient activity (class III) is Gd^{Mediterranean}.

The inheritance of G6PD synthesis is sex-linked. The male who inherits an abnormal gene (XY) will have all red cells containing the variant enzyme, as will the homozygous female ($\overline{XX}$). Heterozygous females ($\overline{X}$) will have, on average, half of all red cells with the variant and half with the normal enzyme.

Geographic Distribution and Malaria. The first evidence that G6PD deficiency confers some advantage against malaria is the worldwide coincidence between populations in which deficient enzymes are frequent and areas of the world where *P. falciparum* malaria is, or was until recently, endemic (Fig. 5–10). The Old World can be divided broadly into three zones. In the first zone, from the Mediterranean basin to the Indian subcontinent, Gd^{Mediterranean} with severely defective activity is highly prevalent: The frequency in males is around 10% in Iran and 14% in Bengal. In the second zone, covering Southeast Asia and southern China, there is great heterogeneity of enzyme variants, including variants of both severely deficient activity (Gd^{Mediterranean}, Gd^{Union}) and moderately deficient activity (Gd^{Mahidol}, Gd^{Canton}). G6PD deficiency of all types is found in 12 to 15% of males in Indochina. The common deficient enzyme of the third zone, sub-Saharan Africa, is GdA⁻ with moderately deficient activity. Frequency is highest at 32% of males among the Luo in the Lake Victoria region of Kenya; frequency declines as one moves west or south from Lake Victoria, enzyme deficiency being found in 22 to 23% of males in Nigeria and Cameroon; 16 to 18% in Togo, Ghana, and Mali; 6% in the Gambia; and 12% in Zambia. The variant GdA with normal activity is found in the same populations at slightly greater frequency, e.g., 25% of males in Nigeria; Gd^{Mali} (severe deficiency) and Gd^{Gambia} (normal activity) reach polymorphic frequency locally.

Within these broad areas, micromapping has shown clear correlations between the frequencies of G6PD deficiencies and the intensity of transmission of malaria, e.g., in Sardinia, Greece, East Africa, and Papua New Guinea. Field studies have not shown consistently any parasitologic advantage, except that Nigerian girls heterozygous for GdB/GdA⁻ had significantly lower *P. falciparum* parasite densities. Long-term cultures of *P. falciparum* in vitro have shown impaired growth of the parasites in deficient, compared with normal, red cells; in some studies oxidative stress was required to make this difference apparent, however. Malarial parasites are highly susceptible to oxidative damage, and it is likely that parasite development is severely impeded by an excess of oxidant radicals in G6PD-deficient cells. However, parasites that survive passage through G6PD-deficient red cells become adapted to this environment after several cycles, adaption being associated with

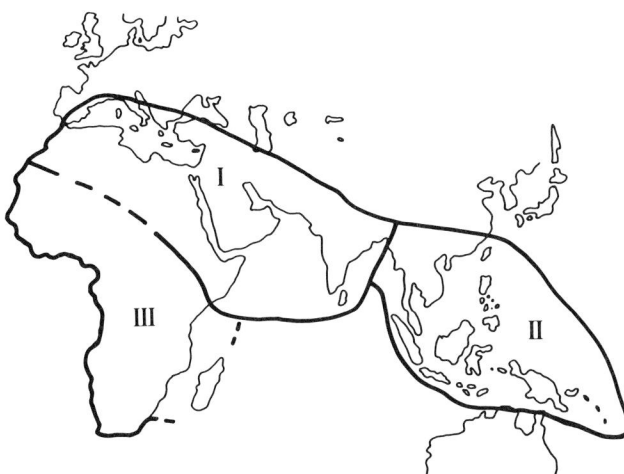

FIGURE 5–10. Areas of the Old World where glucose-6-phosphate dehydrogenase (G6PD) deficiency reaches polymorphic frequency. Zone I, Gd^{Mediterranean}; Zone II, Gd^{Mediterranean}, Gd^{Canton}, Gd^{Union}, Gd^{Mahidol}; Zone III, Gd A⁻.

expression of the parasites' own G6PD. This adaption is impeded by passage through G6PD-normal cells, which may explain why the parasitologic advantage is observed only, or is greater, in heterozygous females, whose blood contains an approximately equal mixture of G6PD-deficient and normal red cells.

Clinical Manifestations. Severe or moderately severe G6PD deficiency is associated with the following clinical hemolytic conditions: (1) neonatal jaundice, (2) infection-induced hemolysis, (3) favism and other food-induced hemolysis, and (4) drug-induced hemolysis. Hemolysis is both more frequent and more severe with enzymes of class II (e.g., Gd^{Mediterranean}) than with class III (e.g., GdA$^-$) (Table 5–8), and in male hemizygotes and female homozygotes than in female heterozygotes.

Enzymes of class I are associated with chronic nonspherocytic hemolytic anemia, but as these are rare everywhere in the world they will not be discussed further.

Neonatal Jaundice. Severe jaundice with serum bilirubin above 250 μmol/L (15 mg/dl) on about the fourth day of life is seen commonly in hospitals throughout the Mediterranean basin, Asia, tropical Africa, and the Caribbean, although accurate estimates of prevalence are not available. Etiology is often multiple, the three most common identified factors being sepsis, prematurity, and G6PD deficiency. Other less common causes include fetomaternal ABO incompatibility, the resorption of hematomas, rhesus incompatability, and intrauterine infections. GdA$^-$ is rarely the sole identified cause of neonatal jaundice in Africa but is almost always associated with sepsis, prematurity, or maternal ingestion of modern or traditional oxidative medications. GdA$^-$ is not a major cause of neonatal jaundice in black Americans in the absence of prematurity or exposure to oxidant drugs. The contribution made to neonatal jaundice by G6PD deficiency varies widely in different populations: Estimates have been 33 to 80% in West Africa, 21% in Jamaica, 15 to 25% in Chinese populations, 31 to 64% in Thailand, 9% in Sardinia, and 82% in Greece.

Jaundice is the result of both hemolysis and poor hepatic function, especially in premature infants. The infant's blood picture is most variable; changes include anisocytosis, spherocytosis, polychromasia, and numerous nucleated red cells. Anemia is usually in the midrange (Hb<13.0 gm/dl). Serum bilirubin levels may rise rapidly to above 300 μmol/L, especially with Gd^{Mediterranean}.

Management. Treatment while serum bilirubin levels are less than 300 μmol/L is by UV phototherapy, if necessary by exposure to sunlight as long as the infant is cooled and the eyes are protected. When the serum bilirubin is above 300 μmol/L, there is a danger that kernicterus will develop with permanent damage to the brain. Treatment is by double-volume exchange transfusion using blood compatible with both mother and infant.

Prevention. Neonatal jaundice is largely preventable by good prenatal care, nontraumatic obstetric delivery, and hygienic precautions in the puerperium, so reducing the frequency of prematurity, sepsis, and hematomas.

Oxidant drugs should not be prescribed during pregnancy unless absolutely essential and unless there are no alternatives.

Infection-Induced Hemolysis. Jaundice due to both hemolysis and hepatocellular failure may complicate the course of pneumonia, infectious hepatitis, typhoid, paratyphoid, and other septicemias in G6PD-deficient subjects. The clinical severity of this complication will be greater if there is pre-existing anemia, impaired hepatic or renal function, and the simultaneous administration of oxidant drugs. A patient may enter into a vicious circle of impaired renal function, superimposed urinary tract infection, hemolysis, administration of an oxidant drug, more intravascular hemolysis, hemoglobinuria, tubular obstruction, and renal failure.

Favism and Other Food-Induced Hemolysis. Acute hemolysis may be precipitated by the ingestion of the fava bean *(Vicia faba),* commonly in the Mediterranean basin, North Africa, and western and eastern Asia. Fresh beans in the spring are more potent than dried or frozen beans, but the chemical trigger to hemolysis has not been identified. Hemizygous males and homozygous females for Gd^{Mediterranean} and other severely deficient enzymes are affected most, but mild hemolysis is seen in heterozygous females. Children aged 2 to 6 years are affected most commonly, and hemolysis has been observed in breast-fed infants of mothers who have eaten fava beans.

Acute hemolysis starts 24 to 48 hours after the ingestion of the beans. There is pallor, jaundice, and hemoglobinuria. The anemia may be severe, and patients may progress to acute renal failure. There is no specific treatment; blood transfusion will be indicated in the most profound anemias. Further episodes are prevented by avoiding eating beans or inhaling the pollen.

Similar but milder hemolytic episodes have been described following eating red suya, peppered kebab-like roast meat, in Nigeria.

Drug-Induced Hemolysis. The ingestion of certain oxidant drugs (Table 5–9) by G6PD-deficient subjects will be followed by intravascular hemolysis after 2 or 3 days. There is pallor, jaundice, and hemoglobinuria. Peripheral red cells show Heinz bodies. Once the oldest red cells, with the lowest G6PD activity, are destroyed, the hemolysis is generally self-limiting. Anemia is worst at about 7 to 8 days, after which there is a reticulocyte response and the Hb rises. Hemolysis and anemia can be prolonged with the more severely deficient enzyme activity or with higher dosage of the drug.

Often it is not necessary to withdraw the drug, and it is possible to continue with treatment when this is essential; for example, in the treatment of leprosy with dapsone, the patient has a clinically unimportant compensated hemolysis. In some patients, hemolysis and anemia may be more severe or complicated by hemolysis triggered by infection or renal failure; the only specific treatment is withdrawal of the drug. Prevention is by avoiding prescribing oxidant drugs (Table 5–9), especially during pregnancy.

Diagnosis. G6PD activity of red cells can be measured by several methods depending on the production of NADPH. The level of activity in young red cells is

TABLE 5–9. Drugs and Chemicals Associated with Hemolysis in G6PD-Deficient Subjects

	Strong Association	Weak Association*
Antimalarials	Primaquine, pamaquine, pentaquine	Chloroquine
Sulfonamides	Sulfanilamide, sulfacetamide, sulfapyridine, sulfamethoxazole	Sulfamethoxypyridazine, sulfadimidine
Sulfones	Thiazolesulfone, diaminodiphenylsulfone (DDS, dapsone)	
Nitrofurans	Nitrofurantoin	
Antipyretic/analgesic	Acetanilid	
Others	Nalidixic acid, naphthalone, niridazole, phenylhydrazine, toluidine blue, trinitrotoluene, methylene blue, phenazopyridine	Chloramphenicol, Vitamin K analogues

*Significant hemolysis occurs only in subjects with variants with severely deficient activity, or in neonates, or with greater than therapeutic dosage. (Adapted from Luzzatto L, Mehta A: *In* Scriver CR, et al (eds): The Metabolic Basis of Inherited Disease. Vol 2, ed 6. New York, McGraw-Hill, 1989. Reprinted by permission.)

higher than in old cells, so that immediately after an acute hemolytic episode, total activity may be in the normal range. The problem can be overcome by centrifuging the red cells and measuring separately the activity in the red cells from the top (young cells) and from the bottom (older cells) of the column. Alternatively, measurement of activity can be delayed until about 6 weeks after any episode of acute hemolysis.

CONGENITAL ELLIPTOCYTOSIS. Several inherited abnormalities of spectrin or other proteins of the cytoskeleton of the red cells cause the cells to have an oval or elliptical shape and a membrane more rigid than normal. Up to 30% of populations from peninsular Malaya to Papua New Guinea have a form of congenital elliptocytosis (also referred to as ovalocytosis) (Fig. 5–11). These red cells have been shown to be resistant to invasion by *P. falciparum* in vitro. In vivo, frequencies and densities of both *P. falciparum* and *P. vivax* have been found to be lower in children aged 2 to 4 years with elliptocytosis than in those with normal red cells. Congenital elliptocytosis in Southeast Asia and Oceania is not associated with any clinical symptoms or anemia.

A similar blood picture is seen in up to 3% of populations in West Africa (Fig. 5–11). Reduced invasion by *P. falciparum* of African elliptical red cells has been demonstrated in vitro. Severe anemia has been observed in some African subjects with elliptocytosis, but this could be coincidental.

Pathophysiology of Anemia

Anemia has three grades of severity: (1) compensated anemia, when the Hb is generally above 7.0 gm/dl; (2) uncompensated anemia, when the Hb is usually below 7.0 gm/dl; and (3) anemic heart failure, which may develop when the Hb falls below 4.0 gm/dl. The Hb level is not the only determinant of the severity of anemia. Compensation will be less effective and the pathology of anemia more advanced with (1) increasing age, children being better able to withstand anemia than adults; (2) rapidly developing anemia, more chronic disease allowing time for the compensating mechanisms to become effective; (3) hypervolemia of splenomegaly or pregnancy; and (4) intense muscular activity, e.g., obstetric delivery.

COMPENSATED ANEMIA. Individuals with mod-

erate anemia are breathless only on exertion. Their maximal work capacity and ability to sustain work are directly related to their degree of anemia. Productivity, earnings, and ability to look after home and children are all reduced. The family, the community, and the national economy all suffer.

The major compensatory mechanism at this stage is a rise in the intraerythrocyte concentration of 2,3-diphosphoglycerate, which has the function of fixing hemoglobin in the deoxygenated state and hence making oxygen more readily available for uptake by the tissues. Cardiac output is increased on exertion by a more rapid heart-rate.

UNCOMPENSATED ANEMIA. Individuals with more severe anemia are breathless even at rest and are wholly unable to perform their usual work. It is at this stage that many patients in developing countries seek medical advice. Cardiac output is increased by both a large stroke volume and a rapid heart rate. Anemia of this severity is not by itself a cause of death but is commonly contributory, as patients are less able to withstand other conditions, e.g., hemorrhage or infection. Over half of maternal deaths in some countries are associated with Hb less than 7.0 gm/dl.

ANEMIC HEART FAILURE. The myocardium is no longer able to increase its work when its oxygenation becomes further impaired. The jugular venous pressure

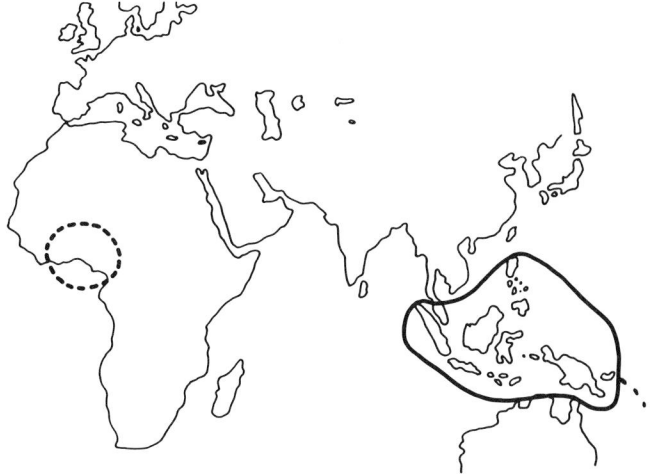

FIGURE 5–11. Areas of the Old World where congenital elliptocytosis is common.

is raised. Pulmonary edema, peripheral edema, or ascites may develop. Without appropriate treatment, anemic heart failure is commonly fatal. Twenty percent of maternal deaths were due to anemia in Nigeria and India before the introduction of blood transfusions.

ASSOCIATED CAUSES OF MORBIDITY. The morbidity of anemia is often made worse by the morbidity of the primary cause of the anemia, e.g., malaria and hemoglobinopathies. Iron deficiency further reduces work capacity through diminished activity of iron-dependent oxidative enzymes. Both iron and folate deficiencies may be associated with impaired cell-mediated immunity and increased susceptibility to some infections.

ANEMIA IN PREGNANCY. Maternal anemia has adverse effects on the infant besides being a cause of maternal morbidity. With even moderate anemia, there is a degree of fetal hypoxia and a compensatory placental hypertrophy. This compensation is often inadequate, and there is intrauterine growth retardation. Maternal malaria causes additional growth retardation through parasitization of the placenta (Chapter 73). Anemia, folate deficiency, and malaria all cause premature delivery and hence further lowering of the birthweight. In pregnancies complicated by severe anemia due mainly to malaria and folate deficiency, perinatal mortality can be over 35%, and about half of all surviving infants can have very low birthweight (<2000 gm). These small infants have immature immune systems and poor reserves of iron and folate and show high frequencies of neonatal jaundice, infections, malnutrition, and anemia.

ANEMIA IN CHILDHOOD. Children in the tropical environment enter a vicious circle. Infections, e.g., malaria and measles, depress immunity and so lead in particular to secondary infections of the respiratory and intestinal tracts. Infections can cause malnutrition through the mechanisms of repeated periods of anorexia, malabsorption, and disturbances of metabolism. PEM and deficiencies of iron and folate further reduce immune responses. Nutritional anemias and anemias of infection are outcomes of this vicious circle. Children with hemoglobinopathies enter the circle readily, as they have impaired immunity and folate deficiency.

Treatment of Anemia

The first principle of treatment of the anemic patient is to diagnose the causes of the anemia. Where diagnostic facilities are inadequate and treatment should not be delayed, it is often necessary to direct initial therapy against the causes that are known to be most probable from previous experience or research. The initial management of anemia in pregnancy or childhood in the tropics is likely to include the treatment of malaria (Chapter 73), antibiotics as indicated from clinical findings, oral iron (Chapter 108.1) and folic acid (Chapter 107.7).

When anemia has a treatable cause, blood transfusion is necessary only when the patient is in danger of dying of anemic heart failure during the approximately 5 days it takes for the Hb to rise following appropriate medication. Since the advent of HIV, it is even more important that strict criteria for blood transfusion be applied. Blood transfusion is indicated when (1) there is incipient or established heart failure due to anemia; (2) obstetric delivery is imminent and the Hb is below 6.0 gm/dl; or (3) emergency major surgery is essential, the Hb is below 8.0 gm/dl, and a blood loss of more than 500 ml is anticipated. Cardiac overload is avoided by giving concentrated red cells (*not* whole blood) 10 ml per kg body weight, transfusing slowly over 4 to 6 hours, and by administering a rapidly acting diuretic, e.g., intramuscular furosemide 0.1 mg/kg body weight, before the transfusion.

The role of blood transfusion in congenital anemias has been discussed earlier. Other absolute indications include: (1) exchange blood transfusions for neonatal jaundice with serum bilirubin above 300 μmol/L, and (2) whole blood transfusion for acute hemorrhage of more than 30% of the total blood volume, when blood pressure and oxygenation cannot be maintained by crystalloids or colloids.

Prevention of Anemia

The prevention of anemia in pregnancy and childhood ought to be followed by significant reductions in maternal, infancy, and childhood morbidity and mortality rates. Prevention of anemia has an essential role in AIDS control programs through reducing the need to transfuse blood.

ANEMIA IN PREGNANCY. Measures to be taken at prenatal clinics include (1) therapeutic antimalarials at first attendance followed by prophylactics throughout pregnancy, and (2) supplements of iron and folic acid. At family planning clinics, first pregnancies can be delayed until growth is completed and subsequent pregnancies spaced in time.

JAUNDICE AND ANEMIA IN INFANCY. During pregnancy, maternal anemia and malaria should be prevented, and oxidant drugs avoided where the frequency of G6PD deficiency is high. At delivery, small women should be supervised carefully and birth trauma and infant hemorrhages avoided by assisted deliveries. Placenta–infant transfusion should be allowed before cutting the umbilical cord so that the infant retains the hemoglobin-iron. Perinatal sepsis must be prevented by cleanliness. Breast feeding is to be encouraged for all infants. Iron and folic acid supplements should be given to the premature infant after 2 weeks. When infants have diarrhea, breast feeding should be continued with oral dehydration therapy and folic acid supplements. Hemoglobinopathies should be diagnosed shortly after birth.

ANEMIA IN CHILDHOOD. Prevention of anemia in childhood starts with the prevention of anemia and malaria in pregnancy. Breast feeding should be encouraged for up to 2 years. Weaning foods should be rich in energy, protein, bioavailable iron, and folate. At the maternal-child health clinics, children should be weighed and measured and malnutrition, malaria, and hemoglo-

TABLE 5–10. Leukocyte Counts (× 10⁹/L) : Means and 95% Confidence Limits

	Total Counts		Neutrophils		Eosinophils		Monocytes		Lymphocytes	
	Mean	*Range*	*Mean*	*Range*	*Mean*	*Range*	*Mean*	*Range*	*Mean*	*Range*
Caucasians										
Age 12 hours	22.8	13.0–38.0	15.5	6.0–28.0	0.5		1.2		5.5	2.0–11.0
1 year	11.4	6.0–17.5	3.5	1.5–8.5	0.3		0.6		7.0	4.0–10.5
6 years	8.5	5.0–14.5	4.3	1.5–8.0	0.3		0.5		3.5	1.5–7.0
Adults	7.4	4.5–11.0	4.4	1.8–7.7	0.2	0–0.4	0.3		2.5	1.0–4.8
Pregnancy	9.0	5.2–16.1	6.8	2.3–13.7						
Black Africans										
Adults	5.1	2.6–10.2	2.8	1.1–7.1	0.5	0–2.0	0.2	0–1.3	1.7	0.7–4.5

binopathies identified. Schedules of immunizations should be followed strictly.

ANEMIA IN THE COMMUNITY. Preventive measures should not be confined to the prenatal, family planning, pediatric, and hemoglobinopathy clinics but introduced in the community and at primary health care posts. Transmission of infections can be reduced (e.g., by mosquito control, introduction of clean water, disposal of waste, and immunization) and nutrition improved (e.g., through education and encouragement of gardening, poultry-keeping, fish-farming, and breast feeding). Primary health care workers and traditional birth attendants can be trained to administer regimens of antimalarials and hematinic supplements to pregnant women, premature infants, infants with severe diarrhea, and children with hemoglobinopathies.

LEUKOCYTES

The reference ranges for total and differential leukocyte counts in peripheral blood vary with age, sex, pregnancy state, and race. These differences need to be appreciated, especially by physicians working in the tropics, where half the population may be aged less than 15 years, women are seen frequently with complications of pregnancy, and Caucasian reference ranges are inappropriate for the community.

Variations and Distributions

NEUTROPHILS

Age. At birth, there is a transient high neutrophilic leukocytosis (Table 5–10) and a high count of nonsegmented cells (up to 1.8 × 10⁹/L); this declines, however, and lymphocytes are more numerous than neutrophils in the blood after 24 hours. The percentage and absolute number of neutrophils increase with age until adult life, when they are normally 40 to 75% of the total count in Caucasians (Table 5–10).

Sex. Women aged 18 to 47 years have counts on average 0.66 × 10⁹/L higher than men. They show cyclical changes with two peaks coinciding with peaks of estrogen secretion and a fall following menstruation.

Pregnancy. The total leukocyte and neutrophil counts rise during pregnancy to plateau in the second trimester (Table 5–10). There is a shift to the left, and up to 3% are metamyelocytes or myelocytes. There is a high neutrophilic leukocytosis during labor, when the total

count may reach $40.0 \times 10^9/L$ even in the uninfected individual. Counts return to nonpregnant levels by the sixth day following delivery.

Race. Black Africans and individuals of black African descent, Arabs, and Yemeni Jews normally have a relative neutropenia during adult life according to Caucasian standards (Table 5–10).

Total body neutrophils are the same in all races, but Caucasians have a greater number in circulation and black Africans have larger bone marrow storage pools. The neutrophil count rises to the same level in both races following provocation either artificially by hydrocortisone or naturally by infection. This racial difference is not present at birth but is apparent by 6 months of age. It is probably genetically determined, but hypersplenism may contribute where malaria is endemic.

Response to Infections. The usual response to infections is an increase in neutrophil release and production by the bone marrow, especially in older children and adults (Table 5–11). Total counts may be as high as 40.0 × 10⁹/L with 95% neutrophils. There can be numerous immature nonsegmented cells released into the blood. The cytoplasm of these cells often contains numerous azurophilic primary granules (toxic granulation). Degenerative changes can occur as well. The nuclei may show irregular staining, pyknosis, and vacuoles and Döhle bodies (condensed RNA). Overwhelming infections, including typhoid and other gram-negative septicemias, lead to leukopenia, especially in elderly and debilitated individuals.

EOSINOPHILS

Age. Eosinophil counts are relatively high at birth and decline steadily with age during childhood. The eosinophil count in the normal adult uninfected by helminths is less than 0.4 × 10⁹/L (Table 5–10).

Pregnancy. The eosinophil count declines during pregnancy, and these cells vanish almost entirely from the blood during delivery, even when there is an initially high eosinophilia.

Eosinophilia. Eosinophilia is associated with three groups of conditions that raise serum IgE concentrations: (1) helminth infections (Table 5–3), (2) type I allergic conditions, and (3) miscellaneous conditions (Table 5–11). Symptom-free individuals in tropical countries frequently exhibit eosinophilia due to subclinical infections with helminths (Table 5–10). Counts are higher in rural populations and in poorer socioeconomic groups.

BASOPHILS. The basophil count in the peripheral blood is normally low, and small changes cannot be detected except by modern automated differential cell

TABLE 5–11. Reactive Causes of Leukocytosis

Neutrophilia	Viral infections (e.g., poliomyelitis)
	Bacterial infections (e.g., staphylococci, streptococci, gram-negative sepsis)
	Tissue damage (e.g., trauma, burns, cardiac infarction)
	Hemorrhage
	Hemolysis
	Malignancy
	Miscellaneous (e.g., drug reactions, chemicals, renal failure)
	Pregnancy and delivery
Eosinophilia	Helminth infections (e.g., during larval migration of *Ascaris*, and tissue invasion by *Schistosoma*, *Toxocara*)
	Type I allergic disease (e.g., rhinitis, bronchial asthma, dermatitis, food and drug reactions)
	Viral and other infections during convalescence
	Miscellaneous (e.g., post splenectomy, familial, lead ingestion, pulmonary aspergillosis, rheumatoid arthritis)
	Malignancy (e.g., Hodgkin's disease, cytotoxic therapy)
Monocytosis	Protozoal infections (e.g., malaria)
	Rickettsial infections
	Subacute/chronic bacterial infections (e.g., tuberculosis, brucellosis)
Lymphocytosis	Infection in childhood generally
	Protozoal infections (e.g., malaria, toxoplasmosis)
	Viral infections (e.g., measles, influenza, rubella, hepatitis, chickenpox, infectious mononucleosis)

counters. A raised count is highly suggestive of myeloproliferative disease, but slight increases may occur with allergic responses. Counts are diminished by stress, corticosteroids, and some acute infections as well as during pregnancy.

MONOCYTES. The monocyte count is normally highest in the first 2 weeks of life (Table 5–10). Counts do not alter during pregnancy but fall at the time of delivery. Counts are lower in symptom-free black Africans and Arabs than in Caucasians.

Monocyte counts are high during viral, protozoal, rickettsial, and subacute or chronic bacterial infections (Table 5–11). Erythrophagocytosis, vacuolation, or malarial pigment may be seen following malaria and may be of diagnostic importance if parasitemia has been cleared naturally or by self-medication. Exceptionally high counts are seen occasionally with tuberculosis.

LYMPHOCYTES

Age. The lymphocyte count in the peripheral blood is highest in the first year of life and declines slowly during childhood (Table 5–10).

Pregnancy. The total lymphocyte count is slightly lower during pregnancy. Of much greater importance is the alteration of function and depression of cell-mediated immunity that is a physiologic response during pregnancy.

Racial or Environmental Differences. Symptom-free Africans and inhabitants of the Arabian peninsula have a relative lymphocytosis that is due to their neutropenia (Table 5–10). T cells, B cells, and null cells are intermingled in the blood in approximate proportions of

80%, 10 to 15%, and 5 to 10%, respectively, and CD4 and CD8 T cells are in a ratio of 2:1 in adults in industrialized countries. Inhabitants of the tropics have lower T-cell and higher B-cell counts, B-cell counts being highest in rural inhabitants. Recurrent malaria and other infections probably account for the shift of balance from T cells to B cells.

Response to Infections. Peripheral blood lymphocytosis is seen more commonly as a response to infection in childhood than in adult life (Table 5–11). Absolute lymphocyte counts are high during protozoal disease, especially malaria; activated lymphocytes with basophilic cytoplasm, large nuclei containing nucleoli, and plasma cells (Türk's cells) are seen commonly. Atypical lymphocytes, often with large nuclei and slate gray cytoplasm, are more characteristic of viral infections.

Leukemias

Contrary to what has been believed in the past, the leukemias are not uncommon in tropical countries. In fact, because of the large populations being served, individual doctors are likely to see far more patients with leukemia than they would in practice in a developed country. There are epidemiologic differences in the distribution by age and sex, problems of clinical presentation and diagnosis, and limitations to the management of patients are unique for developing countries (Chapter 11).

ACUTE LYMPHOBLASTIC LEUKEMIAS. The identification of cell-surface markers has led to the classification of acute lymphoblastic leukemias (ALL) according to their probable cell of origin. Malignant change in pre-B cells leads to common or cALL, in early T cells to T-ALL, in early B cells to B-ALL, and in primitive blast or stem cells to null-ALL.

Epidemiology. ALL is seen most often in childhood, although it may occur at any age. There are three epidemiologic patterns in the world (Table 5–12). First, where both clinical and laboratory facilities are inadequate, the rate of diagnosis of leukemias is extremely low. Second, where facilities have been established, there emerges a peak of frequency of ALL between 5 and 14 years, with T-ALL being the most common

TABLE 5–12. Epidemiologic Patterns of Childhood Acute Lymphoblastic Leukemia (ALL)

Pattern	Socioeconomic Status	Incidence of ALL	Examples
I	Low	Low <0.1/10^5/yr	Tropical Africa generally
II	Intermediate	Uncommon <1/10^5/yr T-ALL peak 5–14 yr	North Africa Arabs in Gaza Strip Blacks and Colored in South Africa Nigeria, Kenya
III	High	High 2–3/10^5/yr cALL peak 2–5 yr	Whites in the Americas, Europe, Australasia, South Africa Japanese

subtype. Third, cALL has a peak incidence between 2 and 5 years of age in white children in Europe, the Americas, Australasia, and South Africa. A similar peak has emerged recently in Asia, including Japan, Taiwan, and Malaysia, associated with improvements in socioeconomic status. It is probable that much of the difference between pattern I and pattern II can be accounted for by improved diagnosis following development of specialized centers but without any significant changes in the lifestyle of the general population (Table 5–12). On the other hand, it is accepted that the rarity of cALL, e.g., in tropical Africa, is actual. It has been hypothesized that pre-B cells have a high rate of spontaneous mutation during fetal life and that a second event leading to the "epidemic" of cALL in countries of pattern III is a result of high socioeconomic status, with late exposure of either the mothers or their infants to an unidentified leukemogenic agent or agent(s).

Males are affected about twice as often as females.

Clinical Presentation. The symptoms and signs of ALL are the consequences of anemia, hemorrhage and thrombosis, loss of immunity and infection, and malignant infiltration (lymphadenopathy, hepatosplenomegaly, and bone pain or tenderness). Presentation is essentially the same as in temperate countries. The diagnosis may be overlooked in a tropical pediatric clinic, where the majority of all acutely ill patients have anemia, infection, lymphadenopathy, and hepatosplenomegaly.

Diagnosis. The total leukocyte count is 20 to 50 × 10^9/L in about 70% of patients but is normal or low in the remainder. Lymphoblasts are present in the peripheral blood, and 70 to 95% of nucleated cells in the bone marrow are blasts. Anemia is always present, and thrombocytopenia is usual.

The peripheral blood picture may resemble ALL during lymphocytic responses to acute infections, especially malaria in early childhood. Other conditions that may mimic ALL include miliary tuberculosis, measles, pertussis, chickenpox, syphilis, and infectious mononucleosis (see Table 5–11). These leukemoid reactions are differentiated from ALL by positive diagnosis of the infection, by recovery with appropriate antimicrobial treatment or spontaneously, and by the absence of blastic infiltration of the bone marrow.

ALL is classified on Romanovsky staining and light microscopy into three types:

1. L1—The blast is small and uniform; the nucleus is regular in shape and staining; nucleoli are absent or inconspicuous; and the cytoplasm is scanty and pale-blue staining.

2. L2—Cell size, nuclear shape and staining, and nucleoli are more variable, and the cytoplasm is more abundant. L1 and L2 may be cALL, T-ALL, or null-ALL.

3. L3—The cell is large and uniform; the nucleus has uniformly granular chromatin; nucleoli are conspicuous; the cytoplasm is deep-blue staining, and there are prominent vacuoles in the cytoplasm and the nucleus. L3 cells are blasts of B-ALL and indistinguishable from Burkitt's lymphoma cells (Fig. 11–9).

L2 ALL can be distinguished from M1 acute myeloid leukemias (AML) by the Sudan black or peroxidase stain, which is negative with ALL and positive with AML. T-ALL cells stain positive with acid phosphatase.

Treatment and Prognosis. Supportive treatment should be given in the absence of specific treatment or while awaiting transfer to a specialized center. Anemia and thrombocytopenia can be countered with appropriate transfusions of concentrated red cells and platelets. All patients should receive curative followed by prophylactic antimalarials where malaria is endemic. Antibiotics should be given as indicated. Survival averages about 20 weeks without specific therapy.

Long-term remissions, which are probably cures, are achieved now in over 50% of children in centers specializing in the treatment of ALL in childhood. Regrettably, the benefits of these advances are not available to most children in developing countries. First, cytotoxic agents are expensive, and supplies are likely to be intermittent and insufficient; radiotherapy is available in only a few centers and liable to failure from lack of maintenance. Second, many features carrying poor prognosis have high prevalence; these include late presentation, poor subsequent attendance, high leukocyte and low platelet counts, mediastinal masses, and T-cell rather than cALL markers.

ACUTE MYELOBLASTIC LEUKEMIAS. The French-American-British (FAB) classification of AML on Romanovsky stain is as follows: M1, AML with predominantly myeloblasts that have few or no granules in the cytoplasm; M2, AML with blasts that have granules and Auer rods, and some promyelocytes; M3, promyelocytic leukemia; M4, myelomonocytic leukemia; M5, monocytic leukemia; and M6, erythroleukemia.

Epidemiology. In the Western world, there is a gradually rising age-specific incidence of AML from childhood to old age; ALL is around four times more common in childhood than AML. In tropical Africa, AML and ALL have equal frequency in children below the age of 15 years, owing in part to the low incidence of ALL but also probably to a true high incidence of AML. It has been postulated that there are two forms of AML in tropical Africa. One is associated with low socioeconomic status, childhood, presentation with chloromas and a male to female (M:F) ratio of 2:1. The second type conforms to the pattern of the Western world, being seen most often in adults, affecting males and females equally, and showing no association with low social class.

Exposure to benzene is known to increase the probability of developing AML. Unofficial vendors siphoning gasoline into motor vehicles in Nigeria have high frequencies of anemia, neutropenia, and thrombocytopenia. It may be predicted that they will show a greater than normal frequency of AML.

Alkylating agents have a leukemogenic effect. In tropical countries, Burkitt's lymphoma, other non-Hodgkin's lymphomas, Hodgkin's disease, multiple myeloma, and chronic lymphatic leukemia (CLL) all occur in the young or relatively young and are treated almost exclusively by cytotoxic drugs, especially alkylating agents, e.g., cyclophosphamide. It can be expected that some patients will develop AML.

Clinical Presentation. AML in Africa cannot be distinguished clinically from ALL, or from acute leukemias in general, except for the one feature of chloroma. About 25% of East African and 10% of West African patients present with a solid tumor, usually around the face and most commonly in the orbit. Chloromas are most frequent in male children. The tumors are histologically myeloblastic tissue: The name chloroma is derived from a characteristic green color of the freshly cut surface, which fades on exposure to air but may be renewed by adding a reducing agent such as ascorbic acid.

Diagnosis. The only infection that can cause a blood picture resembling any of the types of AML is severe pulmonary or extrapulmonary tuberculosis, when a monocytic or myelomonocytic leukemoid reaction may be present (Table 5–11).

L2 ALL and M1 AML are differentiated by Sudan black or myeloperoxidase reaction, which is positive with AML. The esterase reaction is positive with myelomonocytic (M4) and strongly positive with monocytic (M5) leukemias.

Treatment and Prognosis. Supportive treatment should be given as for ALL. Without specific treatment, survival is on average about 2 months.

Modern treatment involves marrow ablation followed by bone marrow transplant, the financial and technical resources for which are simply not available in developing countries. Useful and enjoyable life can be prolonged, however, by regimens of cytotoxic drugs given in rotation so as not to cause intolerable depression of normal bone marrow activity. Average survival in one center in Nigeria was about 9 months.

CHRONIC GRANULOCYTIC LEUKEMIA. Over 90% of chronic granulocytic leukemias (CGL) show the Philadelphia (Ph[1]) chromosome, an anomaly that consists of a translocation of part of chromosome 22 to, most often, chromosome 9. There are also Ph[1]-negative adult CGL and juvenile CGL, which is an embryonic malignancy.

Epidemiology. The epidemiology of CGL appears to be uniform throughout the world, with a gradually increasing age-specific incidence from late childhood. Peak frequency is in the fifth decade in Europe and North America. In developing countries with younger populations, more patients are seen under the age of 40 years than over, and CGL occurs frequently in childhood, e.g., in Nigeria 10% and in Sudan 19% of childhood leukemias.

Clinical Presentation. Onset is insidious, and presentation is usually with gross hepatosplenomegaly, some lymphadenopathy, emaciation, and anemia.

Diagnosis. The leukocyte count is up to $500 \times 10^9/L$ with predominantly mature neutrophils (sometimes eosinophils and, rarely, basophils) and metamyelocytes, myelocytes, promyelocytes, and a few blast cells. The distribution of cells in the bone marrow is similar, and usually this investigation contributes little to the diagnosis.

Chronic granulocytic leukemoid reactions can occur with tuberculosis, meningococcal meningitis, septicemia, severe megaloblastic anemia in pregnancy, eclampsia, acute hepatic necrosis, amebic liver abscess, burns, mercury poisoning from skin-lightening ointments, and severe hemorrhage (Table 5–11). CGL is differentiated by there being (1) often a gap in the progressive leukocyte count, i.e., numerous myelocytes and neutrophils but few metamyelocytes; and (2) low leukocyte alkaline phosphatase reaction. Leukemoid reactions do not show the hiatus in progression from blast to mature neutrophil, have strongly positive leukocyte phosphatase reactions, and are associated with features of the primary disease.

Treatment and Prognosis. Supportive treatment should include curative followed by prophylactic antimalarials in malaria-endemic areas. Modern treatment has tended to be increasingly aggressive with the aim of achieving long-term remission, but for most centers in tropical countries, this approach is not advisable.

CGL can be effectively controlled and active life prolonged by regimens of busulfan alone or preferably busulfan plus mercaptopurine, with allopurinol during the remission-induction period. Response is monitored easily by the total and differential leukocyte count, with the aim of keeping the total below $20 \times 10^9/L$. Patients survive on average 3 years, but active life of over 10 years can be achieved. Blastic transformation to AML or ALL is the usual terminal event.

CHRONIC LYMPHATIC LEUKEMIA. The majority of CLLs arise from mature B cells, but T-CLL occurs as well, especially in Asia. Other variants include prolymphocytic leukemia and hairy-cell leukemia.

Epidemiology. In Europe and North America, CLL is seen rarely under the age of 40 years; above that age there is a rapidly rising age-specific incidence and an M:F ratio of 2:1. The pattern in tropical Africa is very different. CLL is as frequent below as above 45 years, the youngest patients being in the second decade. Below 45 years, the M:F ratio is 1:2, and there is an increasing frequency in women up to the end of their reproductive life.

CLL in younger adults is seen exclusively in rural populations or those of low socioeconomic status. Above the age of 45 years, the M:F ratio is 2:1, as in the Western world.

It is hypothesized that recurrent malaria and other infections greatly enlarge the B-cell pool and so increase the probability of mutation. The greatest enhancement of the B-cell pool occurs in those living in poor hygienic conditions and in grand multiparae, whose cell-mediated immunity has been depressed repeatedly during pregnancy. A second mutagenic event could follow infection by an unidentified virus, whose transmission is greater with overcrowding, and whose proliferation is more rapid with depression of immunity by malaria and pregnancy. The human T-cell lymphotropic virus type 1 (HTLV-1) is endemic in much of sub-Saharan Africa and the Caribbean (Chapter 15.2). It is associated causally with adult T-cell leukemia-lymphoma (ATL). HTLV-1 also shows a higher than expected prevalence in patients with B-CLL, but the mechanism of this association is not understood and it does not contribute to the frequency of CLL in younger adults.

Clinical Presentation. The onset is gradual. The condition may be discovered incidentally, or patients may present with hepatosplenomegaly, lymphadenopathy, and emaciation. The clinical picture is the same in the developed countries as in the tropics, except that splenomegaly is often much more pronounced where malaria is endemic.

Diagnosis. The lymphocyte count is raised usually above $40 \times 10^9/L$. The predominant cell is a mature lymphocyte. In malarial regions, two populations of lymphocytes can be identified in the peripheral blood, one identical with cells infiltrating the bone marrow and presumably the malignant clone, and the other looking like reactive lymphocytes and presumably the result of a response to malaria. The raised lymphocyte count of HMS may be confused with that of CLL.

Treatment and Prognosis. All patients living where malaria is endemic should receive curative antimalarials at the time of diagnosis, followed by lifelong prophylaxis. It has been shown that proguanil alone reduces spleen size and leukocyte count, supporting the view that CLL and malaria interact. Specific therapy is not always required. Chlorambucil 10 mg/day should be given for about 4 to 6 weeks and then in maintenance doses to keep the total leukocyte count below $20 \times 10^9/L$. This regimen can be monitored safely with limited facilities. Average survival after diagnosis is about 4 years.

HEMOSTASIS

REFERENCE VALUES

Age. Vitamin K is not detectable in umbilical cord blood, and in infants the vitamin K–dependent coagulation factors (factors II [prothrombin], VII, IX, and X) are only 25% to 70% of adult values. The prothrombin times (PT) and partial thromboplastin times (PTT) of cord-blood plasma are moderately prolonged compared with values for adult plasma. In preterm infants the PT can be up to 4 seconds longer than the adult range (11 to 14 seconds) and the PTT up to 15 seconds longer than the adult range (23 to 35 seconds). These factors decline further to reach a nadir of 5% to 20% of adult activity at 48 to 60 hours of life. Early feeding and colonization of the intestines by vitamin K–producing microorganisms normally supply sufficient vitamin for the infant liver to synthesize the coagulation factors and correct the defect by 72 to 120 hours of life. However, a few infants, especially those who are preterm, may progress to hemorrhagic disease of the newborn.

Other hemostatic functions at birth do not differ from adult values to any clinically significant degree.

Pregnancy. There are profound changes in the hemostatic mechanisms during pregnancy, which are probably beneficial at the time of parturition and separation of the placenta.

Platelets. There is a progressive decline of platelet count with period of gestation to around 80% of nonpregnant adult values (150 to $400 \times 10^9/L$), reflecting the expansion of plasma volume. Platelet function is unchanged, except for a great availability of phospholipid platelet factor 3.

Coagulation. The coagulability of the blood increases throughout pregnancy. The factors of the rapidly acting extrinsic pathway (thromboplastin of the uterus itself, factors VII and X), plasma phospholipid, and fibrinogen show rises greater than the factors of the slowly but massively acting intrinsic pathway (factors XII, XI, IX, and VIII). Hypercoagulability is enhanced by a fall in antithrombin III activity. The PT, PTT, and clotting time are accelerated. Fibrin monomers are detected in plasma in about half of normal pregnancies. Any tendency toward disseminated intravascular coagulation (DIC) is counteracted to some degree by a decline in about one half of factor XIII activity.

Fibrinolysis. Plasminogen levels double during pregnancy in parallel with fibrinogen. However, spontaneous fibrinolytic activity of plasma is progressively reduced during the second and third trimesters to reach zero at term, owing to the action of the placenta in suppressing plasminogen-activator release from maternal endothelial cells. Only small quantities of fibrinogen/fibrin degradation products (FDPs) are present during the third trimester.

Parturition and the Puerperium. The potentials for coagulation and fibrinolysis, which are latent during normal pregnancy, are released at parturition. Vascular constriction and uterine contraction are major factors in the control of hemorrhage once the placenta has separated. There is deposition of fibrin over the whole inner surface of the uterus, followed by decreased plasma fibrinogen, platelets, and factors II, V, and VIII. Plasminogen activators are released from the inhibitory effect of the placenta, and FDPs reach a maximum 1 to 4 hours post partum.

Platelet numbers and their activity rise in the first week of puerperium. Platelet, coagulation, and fibrinolytic values return to nonpregnant levels by 2 weeks.

ENVIRONMENTAL AND POSSIBLE GENETIC VARIATIONS

Platelets. Platelet counts at birth have not been found to differ between ethnic groups or geographic location. Symptom-free adults living in malaria-endemic areas have a mild thrombocytopenia, e.g., 73 to $370 \times 10^9/L$ in male blood donors in northern Nigeria, in comparison with the internationally accepted reference range of 150 to $400 \times 10^9/L$. The most likely explanation is increased pooling of platelets in subclinically enlarged spleens.

Adhesion. Ristocetin-induced platelet agglutination (RIPA) in vitro depends on the receptor sites for the von Willebrand factor involved in platelet adhesion to collagen. RIPA is greatly reduced or even absent in rural nonelite Nigerians, whereas elite Nigerians show agglutination intermediate between that of nonelite Nigerians and that of Europeans. Inhibition of RIPA in Nigerians is due to plasma factors—probably high concentrations of macroglobulins, including IgM and fibrinogen. Platelet adhesion measurement has been reported to be less in black than in white South Africans.

Aggregation and Release. The platelets of inhabitants of tropical countries can show a relative resistance to aggregation induced by ADP and thrombin in vitro. This is due also to inhibition by plasma factors, probably macroglobulins. In contrast, platelet factor 3 is reported to be more readily available, possibly owing to a younger population of circulating platelets when there is enhanced splenic pooling.

Coagulation. In general, PTT, PT, and thrombin times (TT) do not show racial or geographic differences. However, subpopulations of adults can be identified, e.g., in Africa and Papua New Guinea, who have prolonged PT and TT, probably as the result of subclinical hepatic disease.

Fibrinogen levels are high in nonelite populations in the tropics (e.g., 2.0 to 8.4 gm/L in rural northern Nigerians) compared with elite groups and Caucasians. The higher levels are probably the result of more intense and more frequent muscular exercise.

In Africans, factor VIII coagulant activity is greater than 150% and factor VIII–related antigen is up to 460% of the values of pooled European plasma. These are likely to be genetically determined differences, as no variations are seen in different social classes of Nigerians.

Fibrinolysis. High plasminogen-activator levels and high spontaneous fibrinolytic activity are reported in nonelite groups of South Africa, Kenya, Nigeria, and Papua New Guinea. These are likely to be the normal response to active life and prolonged muscular exercise, as urbanization in Africans and rising social class in black Americans are associated with declining fibrinolytic activity.

Hemorrhage, Atheroma, and Thrombosis. Intercurrent malaria and other infections leading to hypersplenism and high plasma concentrations of IgM and other macroglobulins, diets low in saturated fatty acids and high in fiber, and frequent muscular exercise are associated with low platelet counts, diminished platelet adhesion, early disaggregation of platelets, and active spontaneous fibrinolysis. There is no apparent impairment of hemostasis in response to trauma, but these qualities of the blood of nonelite groups in rural areas of the tropics are likely to contribute importantly to the low incidence of atheroma and thrombotic disease.

ACQUIRED DISORDERS OF HEMOSTASIS

The congenital disorders of hemostasis are better known by members of the medical profession, but the acquired disorders are much more common and of greater clinical importance in communities in the tropics.

Purpuras. There are three groups of disorders leading to disturbances of the initiation of hemostasis and to purpura: vascular disorders, diminished platelet function, and thrombocytopenia. The bleeding time is a simple, highly sensitive, and specific test for deficiencies in the initiation of hemostasis.

Vascular Purpuras. The endothelium may be damaged as a result of infections, through (1) direct toxicity, e.g., viremias and septicemias; (2) early immune reactions following the common childhood infections, e.g., rubella; and (3) late immune reactions leading to Henoch-Schönlein purpura or purpura fulminans. Idiosyncratic reactions to drugs, such as any antibiotic, are relatively common causes of vascular purpura.

Defective Platelet Function. Purpura due to disordered platelet aggregation can complicate the course of uremia and the acute leukemias or can result from large doses of salicylates.

Thrombocytopenia. The platelet count may be decreased either by diminished production or by increased destruction or consumption. Thrombocytopenia may be part of primary or secondary aplastic anemias. Specifically, platelet formation by the bone marrow is defective, most commonly as a result of exposure to drugs, e.g., co-trimoxazole, or chemicals, e.g., benzene in gasoline siphoned by illicit vendors of fuel for motor vehicles. Acute infective causes include typhoid and other septicemias. Thrombocytopenia can be a clinically important complication of the bone marrow depression of chronic inflammatory disease, e.g., tuberculosis. Rarely there is purpura with severe megaloblastic anemia. Platelet destruction by immune mechanisms includes idiopathic thrombocytopenic purpura and reactions to quinine and other drugs.

A form of immune thrombocytopenia called *onyalai* is endemic to southern and central Africa, the highest frequency (about 1% of all hospital admissions) being reported in northern Namibia. It occurs at all ages and in both sexes. It is characterized by hemorrhagic bullae of the mucous membranes of the mouth and by other manifestations of purpura. There is gross thrombocytopenia associated with IgG and IgM antibodies. The condition is usually self-limiting but can become chronic. There is a mortality of up to 10% in the acute phase. Increased pooling and destruction of platelets is a feature of hypersplenism from any cause, e.g., acute malaria, HMS, and portal hypertension following hepatic fibrosis of *S. mansoni* or hepatic cirrhosis. A moderate thrombocytopenia is an invariable feature of acute malaria, but purpura is unusual; recovery follows resolution of the parasitemia. Platelet consumption is a common feature of DIC.

Thrombocytopenia can be recognized by the absence or near-absence of platelets on a well-spread and stained film of the peripheral blood, as a confirmation of, or instead of, the platelet count.

Hypoprothombinemia. Deficiencies of factors II, VII, X, and IX occur together as a result of vitamin K deficiency, hepatic disease, and anticoagulant therapy. The PT is prolonged, as is the TT.

Vitamin K Deficiency. The vitamin is not available in hemorrhagic disease of the newborn or if the bowel has been sterilized by antibiotics. The fat-soluble vitamin is not absorbed in conditions of malabsorption. Parenteral vitamin K reverses the defect within 1 hour.

Hepatic Disease. The PT is prolonged frequently in patients with hepatic cirrhosis or fibrosis or in acute hepatic failure. Hemorrhage may follow trauma or surgery. Vitamin K should be administered but is usually ineffective, and replacement therapy with cryosupernate or plasma may be necessary. (Cryosupernate is the plasma fraction removed from cryoprecipitate.)

Disseminated Intravascular Coagulation. Three groups of conditions can lead to the uncontrolled activation of coagulation mechanisms: (1) endothelial damage triggering the intrinsic coagulation cascade; (2) release of thromboplastins into the blood, triggering the extrinsic coagulation pathway; and (3) procoagulant venoms.

Etiology. Endothelial damage and DIC are features

of the hemorrhagic fevers resulting from the viral infections of yellow fever, Lassa fever, dengue, Ebola viruses, Rift Valley fever, and Marburg virus. Other infections that may be complicated by DIC include septicemias (especially meningococcal and gram-negative bacterial) and *T. b. rhodesiense.* Severe *P. falciparum* parasitemia is only rarely further complicated by DIC. Other causes of extensive endothelial damage include heat stroke, hypotensive shock, diabetic ketosis, eclampsia, and the hemolytic uremic syndrome.

Excessive thromboplastins are released in the circulation following abruption of the placenta, amniotic fluid embolus, retention of a dead fetus, trauma, acute hemolysis (e.g., ABO incompatibility, hemolytic disease of the newborn), acute hepatic necrosis, burns, and certain malignancies (e.g., adenocarcinoma of the prostate, promyelocytic leukemia). The likelihood and severity of DIC are greater during pregnancy, owing both to obstetric accidents and to the hypercoagulability of the blood.

Snakebite. The venoms of various snakes contain powerful procoagulants (Chapter 103.5). The most important in Asia include the vipers *Echis carinatus* and *Vipera russelli* and the pit viper *Calloselasma rhodostoma.* In Africa, incoagulable blood results from the bite of *Echis carinatus.* The venom of the puff adder (*Bitis arientans*) damages endothelium and may be complicated by thrombocytopenia, DIC, and spontaneous hemorrhage. Bites of *Naja nigricollis* (the spitting cobra) cause necrosis of tissue, which, when extensive, may be complicated by DIC. The venom of the boomslang (*Dispholidus typus*) contains procoagulants and spontaneous hemorrhage starts around 2 days after envenomation, but the snake is not aggressive and bites are rare except in snake handlers.

The snakes of tropical America with procoagulant venoms include *Bothrops atrox* and *Bothrops jararaca.* Australian species are *Notechis scutatus* (tiger snake), *Oxyuranus scutellatus* (taipan), and *Tropidechis carinatus* (rough scaled snake).

Pathology. The activation of the coagulation cascade causes (1) consumption of platelets and coagulation factors, including fibrinogen; (2) widespread deposition of fibrin with microvascular obstruction; and (3) activation of plasmin, with fibrinolysis and digestion of coagulant factors. As a result of consumption of clotting factors, hypofibrinogenemia, fibrinolysis, and circulating FDPs, the blood is partially or wholly incoagulable. There are spontaneous hemorrhages, which may be massive.

In subacute DIC, vascular obstruction causes death of tissue, which may lead to circulatory collapse and renal failure. Chronic DIC is characterized by microangiopathic hemolytic anemia resulting from the rupture of red cells when forced across fibrin strands.

Diagnosis. In acute disease the patient will show the features of the primary condition, complicated by purpura or hemorrhage. In some the condition is so serious that the blood fails to clot at all following collection. The TT, PT, and PTT or kaolin-cephalin clotting time are all prolonged, and FDPs are present at high concentrations in plasma. Subacute or chronic DIC is diagnosed when there are thrombocytopenia, FDPs in plasma, and schistocytes in the peripheral blood.

Treatment. The primary condition should be diagnosed and treated. Appropriate therapy of bacterial infections, protozoal infections, and snakebite leads to a rapid cessation of DIC.

Transfusion of whole blood or red cells may be required to maintain blood volume and oxygenation. Cryoprecipitate, fresh frozen plasma, or platelets may be necessary to replace the missing factors.

In subacute or chronic conditions for which there is no effective treatment, e.g., virus infections, it may be necessary to control the coagulation process with intravenous heparin 100 U/kg body weight/4 hours; treatment is monitored by repeated estimates of the clotting time, which should be kept at about 15 minutes.

CONGENITAL DEFECTS OF COAGULATION.
The inherited abnormalities of clotting are not more rare in tropical countries than they are in the temperate zone. For example, the most common, hemophilia A (factor VIII deficiency), has a frequency of about 2 per 100,000 in Nigeria and in Europe. Hemophilia B (factor IX deficiency) and von Willebrand's disease are also not uncommon.

The clinical manifestations show no geographic differences, except that practices of circumcision are obviously important.

The best specific treatment for bleeding episodes and surgical procedures are factor VIII concentrates for hemophilia A and factor IX concentrates for hemophilia B. These are now treated so as to inactivate viruses, removing the risk of transmission of HIV, hepatitis, or other viral diseases. They have long shelflife but are expensive and not often available in developing countries.

Cryoprecipitate can be prepared cheaply and simply even in small hospitals, by separating donor plasma and freezing at −20C overnight. The cryoprecipitate can be stored at −20C for up to 6 months and is effective in the treatment of hemophilia A, von Willebrand's disease, DIC, and the bleeding of uremia. Desmopressin is a preferred treatment of patients with von Willebrand's disease.

The supernatant plasma from the cryoprecipitate (cryosupernate) can also be stored at −20C for up to 6 months. Cryosupernate or fresh frozen plasma is effective in controlling bleeding in patients with hemophilia B and hypoprothrombinemia unresponsive to vitamin K.

BIBLIOGRAPHY

Brabin BJ: An analysis of malaria in pregnancy in Africa. Bull WHO 61:1005–1016, 1983.
DeMaeyer E, Adiels-Tegman M: The prevalence of anaemia in the world. World Health Stat 38:302–316, 1985.
Dupuy E, Fleming AF, Caen P: Platelet function, factor VIII, fibrinogen, and fibrinolysis in Nigerians and Europeans, in relation to atheroma and thrombosis. J Clin Pathol 31:1094–1101, 1978.
Facer CA: Direct antiglobulin reactions in Gambian children with *P. falciparum* malaria. III. Expression of IgG subclass determinants and genetic markers and association with anaemia. Clin Exp Immunol 41:81–90, 1980.

Fleming AF: Haematological manifestations of malaria and other parasitic diseases. Clin Haematol 10:983–1011, 1981.

Fleming AF: Iron deficiency in the tropics. Clin Haematol 11:365–388, 1982.

Fleming AF: Possible aetiological factors in leukaemias in Africa. Leuk Res 12:33–43, 1988.

Fleming AF: The presentation, management and prevention of crisis in sickle cell disease in Africa. Blood Rev 3:18–28, 1989.

Fleming AF: Tropical obstetrics and gynaecology. Anaemia in pregnancy in tropical Africa. Trans R Soc Trop Med Hyg 83:441–448, 1989.

Fleming AF: Chronic lymphatic leukaemia in tropical Africa: a review. Leukemia Lymphoma 1:169–173, 1990.

Greaves MF: Speculations on the cause of childhood acute lymphoblastic leukemia. Leukemia 2:120–125, 1988.

International Committee for Standardization of Haematology: Recommendations for neonatal screening for haemoglobinopathies. Clin Lab Haematol 10:335–345, 1988.

Kulozik AE, Lyons J, Kohne E, et al: Rapid and non-reactive prenatal diagnosis of β thalassaemia and sickle cell disease: application of the polymerase chain reaction (PCR). Br J Haematol 70:455–458, 1988.

Lux SE, Becker PS: Disorders of the red cell membrane skeleton: hereditary spherocytosis and hereditary elliptocytosis. *In* Scriver CR, Beaudet AL, Sly WS, Valle D (eds): The Metabolic Basis of Inherited Disease. Vol 2. 6th ed. New York, McGraw-Hill, 1989, pp 2367–2408.

Luzzatto L, Mehta A: Glucose-6-phosphate dehydrogenase deficiency. *In* Scriver CR, Beaudet AL, Sly WS, Valle D (eds): The Metabolic Basis of Inherited Disease. Vol 2. 6th ed. New York, McGraw-Hill, 1989, pp 2237–2265.

Migasena S, Gilles HM: Hookworm infection. Baillière's Clin Trop Med Comm Dis 2:617–627, 1987.

Perkocha LA, Rodgers GM: Hematologic aspects of human immunodeficiency virus infection: laboratory and clinical considerations. Am J Hematol 29:94–105, 1988.

Phillips RE, Looareesuwan S, Warrell DA, et al: The importance of anaemia in cerebral and uncomplicated falciparum malaria: role of complications, dyserythropoiesis and iron sequestration. Q J Med 58:305–323, 1986.

Serjeant GR: Sickle Cell Disease. Oxford, Oxford University Press, 1985.

Weatherall DJ, Clegg JB, Higgs DR, Wood WG: The hemoglobinopathies. *In* Scriver CR, Beaudet AL, Sly WS, Valle D (eds): The Metabolic Basis of Inherited Disease. Vol 2. 6th ed. New York, McGraw-Hill, 1989, pp 2281–2339.

World Health Organization: Nutritional anaemias. Technical Report Series 503. Geneva, World Health Organization, 1972.

6. URINARY TRACT DISEASES

Larry W. Laughlin

Urinary tract disease is frequently occult and underreported in developing countries. Therefore, clinical reports are sparse, focus on clinically obvious disease, and usually cannot be extrapolated to the general population.

Common urinary tract problems of the temperate, developed world also occur in the tropics. Disease frequency, individual impact, and outcome will vary in the tropics based on environmental factors, sociocultural practices, and economic status (Tables 6–1 and 6–2). Differences among ethnic and racial groups are nearly always due to one of these determinants, although genetically determined susceptibility may influence outcome following exposure to environmental insults, e.g., poststreptococcal glomerulonephritis. In addition, a few genetic disorders that occur more frequently in the tropics, e.g., sickle cell disease, may be associated with renal disorders.

Clinical features of the renal syndromes encountered in the tropics are, for the most part, similar to those seen in temperate zones; unusual features relate mainly to those environmental or etiologic factors that are peculiar to tropical countries (Tables 6–1 and 6–2). However, many patients seek medical care at advanced stages of disease.

ACUTE NEPHRITIS SYNDROMES

DEFINITION. Acute nephritis is the sudden onset of glomerular inflammation, and to a much lesser extent tubular inflammation, most often caused by immune injury. Although this process is frequently transient, it is usually severe enough to allow red blood cells and plasma proteins to pass into the urinary tract. Gross or microscopic hematuria, red blood cell casts, and proteinuria are hallmarks of this syndrome. Clinical manifestations center around the acute reduction in glomerular filtration rate (GFR), oliguria, salt and water retention, and progressive azotemia. Patients present with abrupt-onset hypertension and its attendant complications, facial and peripheral edema, hematuria, and proteinuria.

ACUTE POSTSTREPTOCOCCAL GLOMERULONEPHRITIS. This prototypical acute nephritis is the delayed sequela of pharyngeal or cutaneous infection with particular "nephritogenic" strains of group A beta-hemolytic streptococci (types 1–4, 12, 25, 49, 57, 59–61).

Epidemiology. Of all cases of acute glomerulonephritis, streptococcal infection can be associated with approximately 25% of adult cases and more than 75% of childhood cases. During circumscribed epidemics, such as have occurred in Africa, the Caribbean, and the Middle East, virtually 100% of cases are streptococcus-related. Because of the hot, humid climate of the tropics and prevalent poor hygiene, skin infections, particularly impetigo and secondarily infected scabies, cause poststreptococcal glomerulonephritis more commonly than in temperate developed regions.

Histopathology. Poststreptococcal glomerulonephritis is characterized histopathologically by diffuse exudative and proliferative lesions of the glomerular tufts, resulting from the deposition of specific streptococcal antigen-antibody complexes and activation of the complement cascade. Low levels of C3 occur; deposits of C3 and IgG are demonstrated by specific immunofluorescence as electron-dense "humps" on the epithelial side of the glomerular basement membrane, consistent with complement-mediated immune complex injury.

NONSTREPTOCOCCAL GLOMERULONEPHRITIS. Some patients with a clinically identical illness show no evidence of an antecedent streptococcal infection. The natural history of nonstreptococcal glomerulonephritis is not well understood but presumably involves infections that are currently prevalent in the tropics. Pneumococcal pneumonia, typhoid fever, diphtheria, leptospirosis, syphilis, toxoplasmosis, varicella, hepatitis B, mononucleosis, measles, mumps, falciparum

TABLE 6–1. Differences Between Common Renal Diseases in North America and the Tropics

Disease	North America	Tropics
Acute glomerulonephritis	Decreasing frequency	Frequency stable
	Detection high	Detection low
	Throat infections	Skin infections
Nephrotic syndrome	Minimal change	Proliferative
	Steroid-sensitive	Steroid-resistant
	Uncommon in adults	Common in adults and children (*P. malariae, S. mansoni*, amyloidosis)
Acute renal failure	Uncommon	Common (trauma, severe infection, dehydration, snake venom, agrichemicals)
	Prognosis good	Prognosis poor (paucity of emergency medical care)
Chronic renal failure	Uncommon	Common (poor detection, more infectious etiologies)
	Prognosis good (dialysis)	Prognosis poor (dialysis/transplant and other support not widely available)
Urinary tract infection	Common	Probably common (poor detection)
	Few complications	Frequent complications

malaria, and enteroviral, adenoviral, and togaviral infections have been incriminated.

DIFFERENTIAL DIAGNOSIS. Unless the patient has received specific antibiotic therapy, *Streptococcus pyogenes* can often be isolated from the pharynx or from skin lesions. Streptococcal exoenzyme titers may be discriminating when positive, but titers are not always elevated and the assays not always available in the tropics. Infective endocarditis must also be considered, although the presence of a low-grade fever is usually distinguishing. Systemic lupus erythematosus and other autoimmune connective tissue disorders (Henoch-Schönlein anaphylactoid purpura, polyarteritis nodosa, Goodpasture's syndrome) can be differentiated only with specific immunologic tests during the course of disease. Mesangiocapillary glomerulonephritis and focal glomerulonephritis with recurrent hematuria must also be excluded.

LABORATORY TESTS. Blood agar cultures for *Streptococcus* must be taken from the pharynx and all suspicious skin lesions immediately. For the throat, rough brushing with two untreated cotton-tipped wooden swabs for a minimum of 10 seconds each will yield the best results. Skin lesions should be washed and lightly debrided, then cultured near the edge of the scabbed area, elevating the crusted edge where possible. Streptococcal skin lesions may appear uninflamed, without purulence, or nearly healed. Streptococcal exoenzyme titers, including antistreptolysin O (ASO), antistreptokinase (ASK), antideoxyribonuclease B

TABLE 6–2. Uniquely Tropical Renal Disease Seen in Endemic Populations

Urinary schistosomiasis (*S. haematobium*):
  Gross hematuria, hydronephrosis, bladder polyps, and calcification
Schistosomal nephrotic syndrome (*S. mansoni*):
  Proteinuria, edema, hypoproteinemia, and hyperlipidemia
Salmonella bacteriuria (*Salmonella* spp.):
  Chronic fever, with urinary schistosomiasis only
Malarial nephrotic syndrome (*P. malariae*):
  Proteinuria, edema, hypoproteinemia, and hyperlipidemia
Bladder stones: Bladder infection and obstruction, hematuria, nutritional association, low-protein diets, young boys
Chyluria: Lymphatic obstruction:
  Chronic bancroftian filariasis, tuberculosis, malignancy
Renal tuberculosis (*Mycobacterium tuberculosis* and *M. bovis*):
  Painless hematuria, culture-negative pyuria, fever

(ADNase B), antinicotinyl adenine denucleotidase (ANADase), and antihyaluronidase (AH), are often helpful in diagnosis. ASO titers are usually highest in pharyngeal infections and absent in cutaneous infections, whereas AH, ADNase, and ANADase responses are most evident in cutaneous infections. Urinary sediment, erythrocyte sedimentation rate, and serum complement levels will be abnormal but diagnostically nonspecific; however, they can be used to follow the progression and resolution of acute disease. By far the most clinically profound diagnostic test is the renal biopsy, which provides the best evidence to distinguish between transient self-resolving nephritis and disease associated with progressive renal failure.

TREATMENT AND PROGNOSIS. Treatment is supportive. Salt and fluid restriction and diuretics will frequently suffice for mild hypertension and edema. Circulatory overload manifest as severe hypertension, hypertensive encephalopathy, and congestive heart failure must be treated immediately with antihypertensive drugs and digitalis. Profound oliguria may require dialysis and/or treatment with ion exchange resin, especially if significant hyperkalemia exists. Immunosuppressive therapy, e.g., steroids and cytotoxic agents, is not useful. Penicillin or erythromycin antibiotic therapy is customary; it will eradicate persisting streptococcal infection but will have no impact on the renal disease. Prognosis in those from developed countries is variable, relating to whether the patient is a child or an adult and whether the case was sporadic or epidemic, epidemic disease in children having the most favorable outcome and sporadic disease in adults having the worst prognosis. However, mortality rates are less than 1%, and only 2% show residual renal abnormalities. Comparable data from the tropics are unavailable; collective wisdom suggests similar trends but higher acute mortality rates in patients with cardiocirculatory and electrolyte complications because of the unavailability of intensive medical care.

NEPHROTIC SYNDROME

DEFINITION AND ETIOLOGY. Nephrotic syndrome is characterized by generalized edema (most

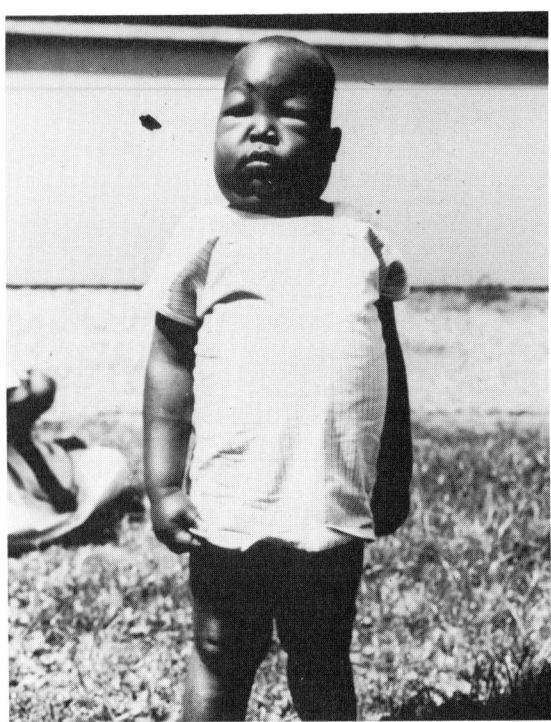

FIGURE 6–1. African child with the nephrotic syndrome with edema. (Courtesy of Dr. Philip Marsden.)

clinically evident in the face), proteinuria of greater than 3.5 gm/day, hypoproteinemia, and hyperlipidemia (Fig. 6–1). The primary renal lesion results from glomerular basement membrane injury due to immunologic, toxic, or vascular pathologic processes, all producing increased capillary permeability with striking losses of protein into the glomerular filtrate. Etiology usually cannot be determined clinically. Exact diagnosis depends on immunopathologic evaluation of renal biopsy findings in the context of the patient's medical and environmental background.

QUARTAN MALARIA NEPHROSIS. *Plasmodium malariae* infection has long been associated with nephrotic syndrome in Africa. Renal biopsy reveals specific malaria antigen in complex with IgG, IgM, and C3. Studies from Nigeria suggest that certain glomerular lesions are morphologically specific for "quartan malarial nephrotic syndrome" (Figs. 6–2 and 6–3). Reports from the Ivory Coast and Senegal confirm the frequency of the lesion on biopsy but fail to support the contention that the findings are pathognomonic for quartan malaria, suggesting instead nonspecific trapping of IgM in the glomerulus. There is, however, acceptance by most investigators that quartan malaria may be followed by the nephrotic syndrome and that this probably occurs through the deposition of immune complexes rather than other immunologic mechanisms such as antigenic resemblance between basement membrane and malarial products.

SCHISTOSOMA MANSONI NEPHROSIS. Typical nephrotic syndrome may also occur with *Schistosoma mansoni* infection. Renal biopsy specimens show specific deposits of schistosomal polysaccharide, IgG, IgM, and C3. Immune complex glomerulonephritis has been in-

duced in animals experimentally infected with *S. mansoni*. Pathologic changes are more likely to occur in the presence of large worm burdens and may parallel the development of portal obstruction with collateral circulation.

MISCELLANEOUS INFECTIONS. Immune complexes are present in low concentrations in the serum of many apparently healthy inhabitants of the tropics, reflecting the frequency and variety of chronic infections. Intravascular deposition of specific complexes in many infectious diseases, e.g., kala-azar, lepromatous leprosy, toxoplasmosis, and hepatitis B, can be readily demonstrated. Skin-lightening creams may produce membranous nephropathy. There is little evidence, however, that these individual cases are important in the overall prevalence of the nephrotic syndrome in the tropics.

PATHOLOGY AND PATHOGENESIS. Histologic examination of a satisfactory biopsy specimen may show changes consistent with minimal-change glomerular disease (lipoid nephrosis), focal glomerulosclerosis, membranous glomerulopathy, or proliferative glomerulonephritis; the last condition may be further characterized as acute exudative, mesangial, extracapillary (crescentic), or mesangiocapillary (membranoproliferative).

Biopsies of African children with the nephrotic syndrome have revealed a rather distinct lesion that may be diffuse or focal; it is distinguished by an irregular thickening of the glomerular capillary wall, which displays a twisted plexiform or double-outline appearance (Fig. 6–2). On electron microscopy, lacunae may be noted in the basement membrane (Fig. 6–3).

After the glomerular injury and protein leak are established, the remainder of clinical disease follows expected physiologic changes. Sustained heavy proteinuria, the hallmark of nephrosis, is eventually followed by hypoproteinemia via processes of excessive urinary losses, increased renal catabolism, and inadequate hepatic synthesis of albumin. The resulting decreased plasma oncotic pressure leads to fluid migration into tissue spaces, i.e., edema. Hepatic lipoprotein synthesis increases, probably stimulated by low plasma oncotic pressure, resulting in hyperlipidemia. This lipid aberration probably contributes to the accelerated atherosclerosis seen in nephrotic syndrome patients. Urinary losses of functionally important plasma proteins besides albumin have medical impact ranging from misleading thyroid function tests to anemia, vitamin D deficiency, trace mineral deficiency, hypercoagulable states, and increased susceptibility to infections because of the loss of specific protective immunoglobulins.

LABORATORY FEATURES. Gross proteinuria, frequently above 5 gm/day, is the hallmark of nephrotic syndrome. Plasma albumin may fall below 1.0 gm/dl; hyperlipidemia involves cholesterol, triglycerides, and phospholipids but with variability in each component. Renal biopsy with immunopathologic staining provides the most precise functional diagnosis and is rarely contraindicated.

Differential permeability of the glomerular membrane, with selective loss of smaller protein and lipid molecules, is thought to reflect a better prognosis than

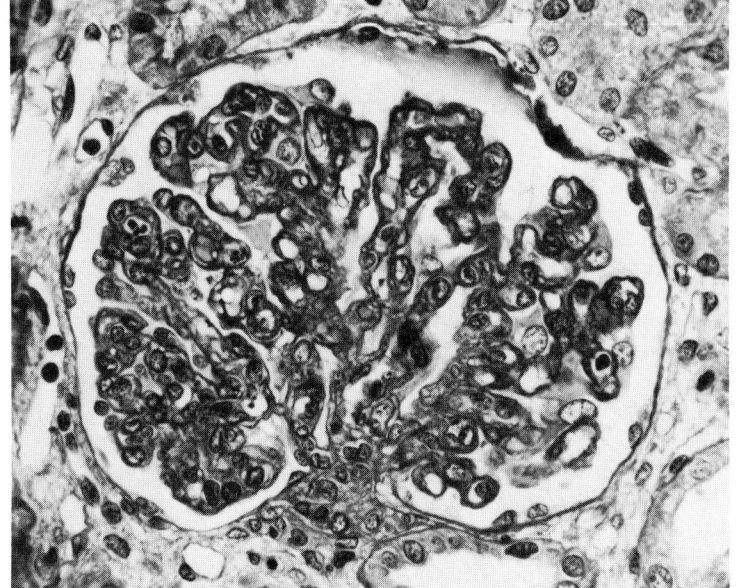

FIGURE 6–2. Renal biopsy from West African child with the nephrotic syndrome. Glomerulus showing the changes of "tropical nephropathy." There is irregular thickening of the capillary wall, which has a twisted, plexiform appearance. (Courtesy of Dr. Renee Habib.)

does a pattern of generalized protein excretion. This distinction can be made, when laboratory facilities permit, by correlation of plasma and urinary protein electrophoretic patterns. The ratio of urinary IgG to transferrin is a useful index, with values less than 0.15 denoting high selectivity of protein loss and a generally favorable prognosis.

CLINICAL MANAGEMENT. Generalized "soft" edema, particularly evident in the face, is the clinical sine qua non of nephrotic syndrome. As this extravascular fluid accumulation intensifies, ascites and pleuropericardial effusions accumulate, to become difficult management problems in late-stage disease. Pharmacologic diuresis is tempting to the clinician but can be dangerous and is rarely of long-term benefit. Albumin infusion is similarly deceptive; most administered proteins will be excreted within 48 hours. Generally, treatment of edema should be reserved for severe refractory anasarca or profound postural symptoms.

Hyperlipidemia is nearly constant, but not absolutely associated with increased morbidity or mortality. Most lipid-reducing agents are either too toxic or so poorly tolerated that treatment is rarely indicated.

Thromboembolic complications are common. Renal vein thrombosis is most often noted, with a striking clinical syndrome of flank/loin pain, gross hematuria, reduced GFR, asymmetry of renal size, scalloping of the ureters (due to collateral circulation), and evidence of pulmonary embolic disease. Oral anticoagulation is required.

The precise role of immunosuppressive therapy in nephrotic syndrome is unknown. Relating most directly to classification by renal biopsy, nephrosis either progresses to chronic renal failure or spontaneously remits. Immunosuppressive agents speed the process of spontaneous recovery but probably do not increase the absolute number of resolved cases. However, steroids probably reduce the amount of protein lost in the urine

FIGURE 6–3. Electron micrograph of glomerulus from African child with the nephrotic syndrome. The basement membrane is irregular and contains many lacunae. (Courtesy of Dr. Renee Habib.)

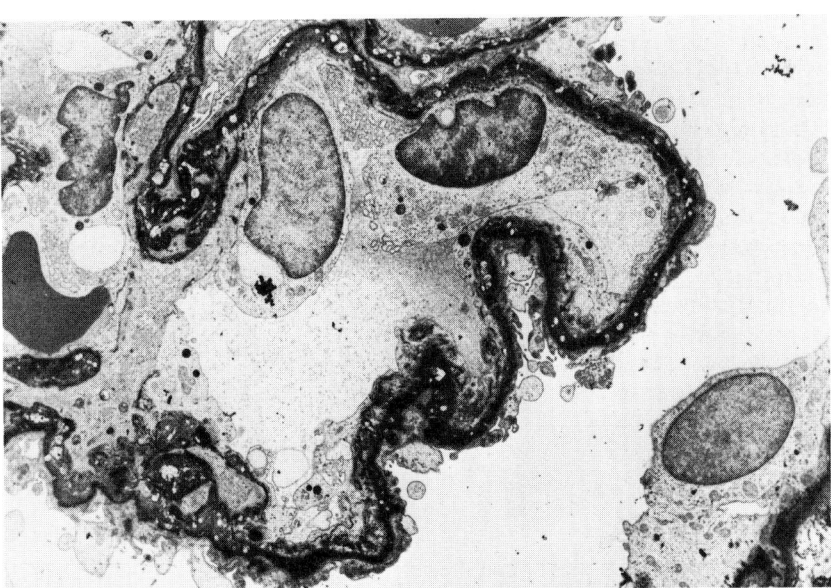

in unremitting disease. Therefore, most patients with nephrotic syndrome are given at least a trial of immunosuppressive drugs; the positive impact on outcome may not outweigh the negative complications of long-term steroid treatment.

DIFFERENTIAL DIAGNOSIS. Systemic conditions associated with the nephrotic syndrome are primary or secondary amyloidosis, diabetes mellitus, myelomatosis, and renal vein thrombosis. Quartan malaria *(Plasmodium malariae* infection) (Chapter 73.2) has been associated with the nephrotic syndrome in Nigeria, Uganda, other regions of West and Central Africa, and Guyana. *S. mansoni* infection (Chapter 96) in Brazil has been causally linked to the nephrotic syndrome through demonstration of specific antigens in the glomerular immune complex deposits. Secondary amyloidosis associated with chronic tuberculosis (often extrapulmonary) (Chapter 61) or lepromatous leprosy (Chapter 62) accounts for a variable proportion of cases in tropical countries.

TREATMENT AND PROGNOSIS IN CHILDREN. In temperate climates, most children (90% or more) show minimal glomerular lesions on biopsy, have a selective pattern of protein loss, and respond well to steroid therapy. This is not true of some tropical situations. Studies in the Sahel region of Africa have revealed structural glomerular lesions in most children with the nephrotic syndrome, even the very young, who might be expected to have minimal-lesion disease. A typical example may be seen in the biopsy of a West African child with the nephrotic syndrome; changes characteristic of "tropical nephropathy" include irregular capillary wall thickening (Fig. 6–2). Even so, corticosteroid therapy is usually recommended along with appropriate dietary and symptomatic management. Cyclophosphamide therapy has not been successful in West African cases, and azathioprine may adversely affect survival. Despite therapeutically induced remission, more of these children develop renal failure than do those from temperate climates. The natural history of the disease in Africa and elsewhere in the tropics requires much more investigation.

TREATMENT AND PROGNOSIS IN ADULTS. Many studies from tropical countries attest to the surprisingly high prevalence of the nephrotic syndrome in young adults. Proliferative glomerulonephritis predominates in reported renal biopsies, although minimal-lesion and membranous glomerulopathies may be more common in some areas, as in the Ryukyu Islands. In Singapore, more than 30% of glomerulonephritis cases, some associated with the nephrotic syndrome, are related to specific deposition of IgA complexes. Corticosteroid or other immunosuppressive therapy is not likely to be effective in other than minimal-lesion glomerulopathy; membranous or proliferative glomerular disease is usually not altered and requires symptomatic management as the disease runs its course.

ACUTE RENAL FAILURE

DEFINITION AND ETIOLOGY. Acute renal failure occurs when there is a sudden loss of the kidneys' contribution to body metabolism, associated with ineffective salt and water homeostasis, deficient hydrogen ion excretion, and accumulation of nitrogenous waste products in the plasma. The syndrome, manifested usually by acute oliguria and occasionally anuria, has many causes and always represents a medical emergency.

PREVALENCE IN THE TROPICS. Acute renal failure is a common clinical emergency in most tropical countries. Common to all areas are the frequency of trauma and infections and the delay in initiating effective antibiotic therapy or fluid replacement. Trauma, often with crush injuries, is becoming increasingly common with industrialization. In underdeveloped countries, a major cause of acute renal failure is untreated septic abortion; it may also complicate typhoid fever, leptospirosis (Weil's disease), pyomyositis, coliform septicemia, cholera, yellow fever, viral hemorrhagic fevers, and falciparum malaria (Chapter 73). Blackwater fever, characteristically seen in partially immune expatriates in areas of endemic malaria and thought to be precipitated by quinine administration, is now extremely rare. Reports from South India emphasize the frequency of the hemolytic-uremic syndrome in children with bacillary dysentery (Chapter 37); in Vellore, such cases accounted for nearly 40% of acute renal failure in patients under the age of 15 years.

PATHOLOGY AND PATHOGENESIS. The causes of acute renal failure are usually classified as prerenal, renal, and postrenal. Hypovolemia with poor renal perfusion due to prerenal pathologic events (e.g., severe hemolysis or hemorrhage, extensive trauma or burns, various forms of septicemia, and severe dehydration from gastrointestinal disease or environmental conditions) may result in acute tubular necrosis, usually reversible with proper acute care. Examination by light microscopy of renal biopsies from such cases shows interstitial edema and dilated tubules containing casts, with varying degrees of tubular epithelial necrosis. Acute renal failure may be caused by direct injury to the kidneys (e.g., from poisoning by nephrotoxic chemicals carelessly introduced into the environment, certain drugs and local plant products, or snake venom), with acute tubular necrosis of greater severity. Postrenal causes include obstruction of urinary flow by bilateral renal calculi, bilateral ureteral schistosome granulomas, bladder stones, and malignant growths or other causes as well as neurogenic mechanisms.

CLINICAL MANAGEMENT. Patients seen during the early oligemic phase have care focused on the treatable underlying disease, hypovolemia, and shock or infection. The ensuing oliguric phase, generally associated with tubular necrosis, may last from a few days to more than a month. During this time, progressive uremia with hyperkalemia, acidosis, and overhydration becomes life-threatening and requires meticulous monitoring of fluid balance and nutrient intake. Peritoneal dialysis or hemodialysis may be lifesaving but is highly dependent upon sophisticated support systems frequently unavailable in the tropics. Gastrointestinal hemorrhage and intercurrent infection are the most important complications. The diuretic phase usually begins 10 to 14 days after onset but may be delayed. Beginning with functional nephrons, healing may continue until improved tubular function leads to an outpouring of urine rich in sodium and chloride, which usually lasts about 10 days. Obligatory loss of water may produce severe deficits of electrolytes during this period, in sharp contrast to accumulations during the oliguric phase. Prognosis is influenced by careful monitoring, competent management, and the underlying disease process.

CHRONIC RENAL FAILURE

DEFINITION. Chronic renal failure is the result of slow but progressive destruction of renal tissue by a variety of pathologic processes. The "end-stage" kidney is characterized by an inadequate number of functional nephrons with failure of glomerular and tubular function, loss of homeostasis, and progressive uremia.

ETIOLOGY AND PREVALENCE IN THE TROPICS. Owing to the relatively quiet onset, the infrequent availability of autopsy and biopsy material, and poor population health statistics in the tropics, the relative importance of different diseases as causes of chronic renal failure is difficult to estimate. Chronic glomerulonephritis, representing the end stage of the various histologic types, appears to predominate. In Kampala, Uganda, about 5% of necropsies (excluding infants) showed some form of progressive glomerulonephritis. Similar findings have been reported from Nigeria and New Guinea. These figures reflect the frequency of acute glomerulonephritis and the nephrotic syndrome in these populations. Chronic pyelonephritis appears to be an unimportant cause of chronic renal failure in Africa. Renal vascular disease and diabetes mellitus are uncommon causes except in certain groups, e.g., the Indian immigrant population in South Africa. Amyloidosis is the most common cause of death in lepromatous leprosy in some areas, but it is relatively rare in the general population.

Hydronephrotic atrophy and chronic pyelonephritis are well-known complications of *Schistosoma haematobium* infection, caused by inflammation and scarring (Figs. 6–4, 96–18 and 96–19) from deposition of eggs in the tissues of the lower urinary tract (Chapter 96). The frequency of obstructive uropathy that proceeds to end-stage renal disease in these cases increases with worm burden and with age. Although long-term studies on infected patients are generally inadequate, *S. haematobium* infection must account for many cases of chronic renal failure in areas of endemicity.

Chronic obstructive uropathy due to urethral stricture or neglected prostatic hyperplasia in men or advanced pelvic carcinoma in women is apparently as common in the tropics as in temperate climates.

CLINICAL MANAGEMENT. Tropical patients with end-stage renal disease do not display unusual or unique clinical features but do present formidable problems in management. Long-term dialysis and transplantation programs are inadequate in almost all developing countries. Therapy usually consists of symptomatic management of hypertension, azotemia, and anemia, with correction of obstruction and treatment of infection as

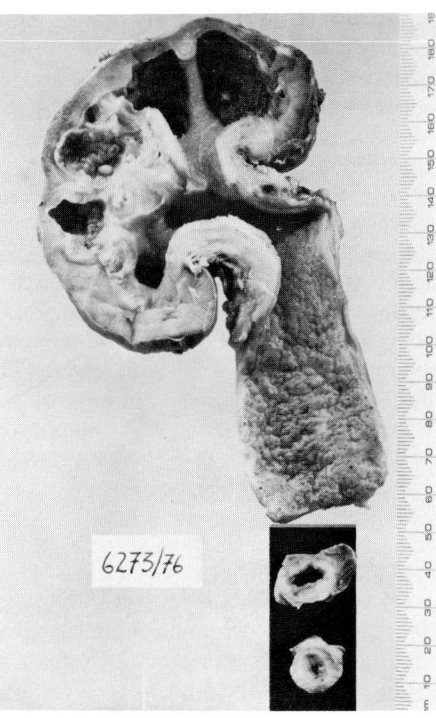

FIGURE 6–4. Hydronephrotic atrophy of kidney associated with thickening of the ureteric wall due to *Schistosoma haematobium* infection.

feasible. Specific measures in the management of the azotemic patient include: (1) judicious protein restriction and perhaps alkalinizing therapy for correction of acidosis, and (2) restriction of sodium intake to 25 to 35 mEq/day, with water intake between 1800 and 3500 ml/day. Therapeutic goals are necessarily limited, but proper therapy will improve the quality of life and often add months of useful activity. However, renal failure is nearly always progressive, even when there are no serious complications. The terminal stage is often defined as the point at which the plasma creatinine level exceeds 10 ml/dl. Experience in a modern hospital setting suggests that about 20% of patients with terminal renal failure stabilize and exhibit improvement with careful management, but 80% will not survive beyond 5 months without dialysis, with half of these succumbing within 2 months.

HEMATURIA

ETIOLOGY. Symptomatic recurrent hematuria in the tropics is usually associated with grossly visible pathologic lesions (e.g., tumors, stones) or is the result of schistosomiasis haematobia (Chapter 96). Gross hematuria rarely results from microscopic abnormalities of the kidney or lower urinary tract.

PATHOGENESIS AND PREVALENCE. Hematuria that results from diffuse renal disease, sometimes grossly visible but usually microscopic, is almost always accompanied by proteinuria. That resulting from local diseases of the genitourinary tract is rarely associated with protein excretion in excess of a few hundred milligrams daily, whereas in diffuse disorders of the kidney, the proteinuria may approach 10 gm/day. One of the diffuse renal diseases that produce episodic painless hematuria is IgA nephropathy of Berger, characterized by deposits of IgA in the mesangium, with resultant mesangial proliferation. An unusually high prevalence of this entity, said to be provoked by upper respiratory infections or undue physical exertion, has been reported from Singapore. Painless hematuria is seen in sickle cell disease, probably resulting from small renal infarctions (Chapter 5). Gross bleeding associated with trauma, hemorrhagic cystitis, stones, genitourinary tumors, and hemorrhagic disorders such as thrombocytopenic purpura is common. Gross painless hematuria, a classic sign of urinary schistosomiasis, is regional in distribution (Chapter 96). Diagnosis rests upon standard urologic procedures, usually including cystoscopy.

CHYLURIA

Frequently found in conjunction with hematuria, chyluria is the draining of lymphatic material directly into the urinary tract, resulting in a characteristic milky-tan urine. Chyluria is usually intermittent, asymptomatic, and caused by chronic bancroftian filariasis; it requires no specific therapy (Chapter 85.1). Its pathogenesis is obstructed lymphatic ducts and retrograde duct engorgement and dilation, with rupture or fistula formation into the urinary tract, frequently the renal pelvis. Rarely, chyluria may be severe, with massive urinary lipid excretion resulting in uncontrollable weight loss and renal colic from ureteral fibrin clots. In such cases surgical repair of the fistula, if it can be located, is curative; otherwise, a fat-restricted diet can be instituted to ameliorate symptoms. Diagnosis is established by Sudan III staining of the urine to identify fat globules or by allowing the urine to stand for 72 hours to separate into a top creamy layer, a red bottom deposit, and a cloudy intermediate layer that may clot. Other uncommon causes of chyluria are echinococcosis, urinary schistosomiasis, tuberculosis, and neoplastic infiltration of the retroperitoneal spaces.

URINARY CALCULI

Urinary tract stones may be asymptomatic, associated with infection, or manifested by episodes of excruciatingly severe colic and gross hematuria. They consist of crystalline aggregates of urinary salts or acids, precipitated within the urinary tract as a result of excessive excretion or changes in the physiochemical milieu of the urine. The primary distinction must be made on the basis of chemical composition, which often provides a clue to the underlying metabolic or endocrine disturbance; however, useful separation can be made clinically between stones of renal origin and primary bladder stones.

BLADDER STONES. These occur endemically among children in some less developed agricultural countries such as Thailand, Indonesia, Yemen, and the Sudan. Malnutrition, vitamin A deficiency, and low-protein diets are common in these areas but cannot be specifically incriminated. It is clear, however, that improved socioeconomic conditions result in amelioration of the problem.

The radiologic curiosity "fetal head" calcification of the bladder is sometimes seen in patients with chronic urinary schistosomiasis (Fig. 96–21). Submucosal deposition of schistosome eggs with calcification leads to a thin layer of calcification involving the entire bladder.

KIDNEY STONES. Collective wisdom indicates that North Americans and Europeans living in the tropics have increased rates of ureteral stone formation, attributed to unaccustomed dehydration and consequent urinary concentration. A curious situation exists in Fiji, where renal calculi are uncommon except among immigrant Indians, who suffer from so-called curry kidney, attributed locally to excessive ingestion of curries, pickles, and spices. Epidemiologic or physiologic studies to substantiate these impressions have yet to be reported.

URINARY TRACT INFECTION

DEFINITION AND EPIDEMIOLOGY. Urinary tract infections in the tropics, as elsewhere, are common, more frequent in women than in men, and strongly associated with structural abnormalities, e.g., congenital malformations, stasis, stones, foreign bodies, or diseases that disrupt bladder mucosal integrity (bladder carcinoma, urinary schistosomiasis). While there is a paucity of pertinent epidemiologic and postmortem pathologic studies, it is believed that urinary tract infections seldom lead to chronic pyelonephritis and renal failure, although they undoubtedly contribute heavily to morbidity. Asymptomatic bacteriuria, universally defined as quantitative counts of more than 10^5 organisms/ml in freshly voided specimens, is a largely unacknowledged entity in the tropics, as the required bacteriologic culture methods are available only in the most modern medical centers.

ETIOLOGY AND PATHOGENESIS. Urinary tract infections are much more common in women than in men, probably owing to anatomic differences (i.e., urethral length and vulnerability to coital trauma) and childbearing. Acute and chronic pyelonephritis may follow infection of the lower urinary tract, depending on the presence of vesicoureteral reflux, obstruction, stones, congenital abnormalities, and other acquired or hereditary factors. As elsewhere, gram-negative bacterial organisms are most commonly isolated, usually from intestinal flora but sometimes introduced from the environment.

Salmonella Bacteriuria. Chronic *Schistosoma haematobium* infection usually results in disruption of bladder mucosa and/or some degree of urinary obstruction with stasis. Under these circumstances, salmonella bacteriuria (with or without bacteremia) is seen in unexpectedly high rates. The pathogenesis of this entity is complex (Chapter 96). Curative therapy requires both antischistosomal and antibacterial agents.

Renal Tuberculosis. Tuberculosis is extraordinarily

prevalent in most underdeveloped countries of the tropics. Genitourinary tuberculosis is one of the common extrapulmonary manifestations of the disease. It results from hematogenous spread, usually with a delayed reactivation of lesions in the renal parenchyma (Chapter 61). Involvement of the prostate, seminal vesicles, and epididymides may occur secondarily in the male, whereas involvement of the female pelvic organs is usually the result of direct spread to the fallopian tubes. Sterile pyuria in a patient with chronic fever, frequency, dysuria, or hematuria should suggest the possibility of renal tuberculosis. Appropriate cultures obtained from early-morning urine specimens will confirm the diagnosis.

BIBLIOGRAPHY

Abu-Romeh SH, van der Meulen J, Cozma MC: Renal diseases in Kuwait. Experience with 244 renal biopsies. Int Urol Nephrol 21:25, 1989.

Adu D, Anim-Addo Y, Foli AK, et al: Acute renal failure in tropical Africa. Br Med J 1:890, 1976.

Andrade ZA, Rocha H: Schistosomal glomerulopathy. Kidney Int 16:23, 1979.

Boonpucknavig V, Sitprija V: Renal disease in acute *Plasmodium falciparum* infection in man. Kidney Int 16:44, 1979.

Cooke RA, Champness LT: Amyloidosis in Papua New Guinea. Med J Aust 2:1177, 1970.

Coovadia HM, Adhikari M, Morel-Maroger L: Clinico-pathological features of the nephrotic syndrome in South African children. Q J Med 189:77, 1979.

Date A, Raghavan R, John TJ, et al: Renal disease in adult Indians: a clinicopathological study of 2827 patients. Q J Med 64:729, 1987.

Date A, Unni JC, Raghupathy P, et al: The pattern of medical renal disease in children in a south Indian hospital. Ann Trop Paediatr 4:207, 1984.

De Geus A: Chyluria in immigrants from Surinam. Neth J Med 28:482, 1985.

Dolev E, Bass A, Nussinowitz N: Frequent occurrence of renal calculi in tuberculous kidneys in Israel. Urology 26:544, 1985.

Edwards BD, Eastwood JB, Shearer RJ: Chyluria as a cause of haematuria in patients from endemic areas. Br J Urol 62:609, 1988.

Hendrickse RG: Epidemiology and prevention of kidney disease in Africa. Trans R Soc Trop Med Hyg 74:8, 1980.

Hendrickse RG, Adeniyi A: Quartan malarial nephrotic syndrome in children. Kidney Int 16:64, 1979.

Houba V: Immunological aspects of renal lesions associated with malaria. Kidney Int 16:3, 1979.

Hutt MSR: Renal disease in a tropical environment. Trans R Soc Trop Med Hyg 74:17, 1980.

Hutt MSR, White RHR: A clinicopathological study of acute glomerulonephritis in East African children. Arch Dis Child 39:313, 1964.

Hutt MSR, Wing AJ: Renal failure in the tropics. Br Med Bull 27:122, 1971.

Kaiser C, Doehring-Schwerdtfeger E, Abdel-Rahim IM, et al: Renal function and morphology in Sudanese patients with advanced hepatosplenic schistosomiasis and portal hypertension. Am J Trop Med Hyg 40:176, 1989.

Kibukamusoke JW, Hutt MSR, Wilks NE: The nephrotic syndrome in Uganda and its association with quartan malaria. Q J Med 36:393, 1967.

Lyrdal F, Hofvander Y: Urinary bladder stones. Their occurrence in children in South-East Asia. Trop Doct 18:102, 1988.

Ngu JL, Youmbissi TJ: Special features, pathogenesis and aetiology of glomerular diseases in the tropics. Clin Sci 72:519, 1987.

Nseka M, Tshiani KA: Chronic renal failure in tropical Africa. E Afr Med J 66:109, 1989.

Poon-King T, Svartman M, Mohammed I, et al: Epidemic acute nephritis with reappearance of M type 55 streptococci in Trinidad. Lancet 1:435, 1973.

Prathap K, Looi LM: Morphological patterns of glomerular disease in renal biopsies from 1000 Malaysian patients. Ann Acad Med Singapore 11:52, 1982.

Segasothy M, Cheong K, Kong BCT, et al: Further evidence of analgesic nephropathy in Malaysia. Med J Malaysia 41:377, 1986.

Singh R, Singh MM, Lahiri VL, et al: Tuberculosis as a continuing cause of secondary amyloidosis. J Indian Med Assoc 85:328, 1987.

Sinniah R: Renal disease in Singapore with particular reference to glomerulonephritis in adults. Singapore Med J 21:583, 1980.

Sitprija V: Renal involvement in malaria. Trans R Soc Trop Med Hyg 64:695, 1970.

Van Reen R: Idiopathic urinary bladder stones of childhood. Aust NZ J Surg 50:18, 1980

Whittle HC, Abdullahi MT, Fakunle F, et al: Scabies pyoderma and nephritis in Zaria, Nigeria. Trans R Soc Trop Med Hyg 67:349, 1973.

7. DERMATOLOGIC DISEASES

Evan R. Farmer

With the exception of certain infectious diseases involving the skin, the spectrum of diseases seen in the tropics is the same as that seen in temperate and cooler climates, although with different rates of prevalence. A skin disease that is common or easily recognizable in the temperate zones may be markedly altered in its morphologic appearance and natural history by exposure to the heat and humidity of the tropics, malnutrition, lack of appropriate therapy, and concomitant diseases.

The skin is the major part of the body that is directly exposed to the environment, and consequently, it must be able to adapt to a wide range of climatic conditions, provide a barrier to numerous noxious chemicals and microorganisms, and withstand the physical stress that we constantly impose upon it. These factors will vary from community to community, and it is important that the clinician understand the customs, living conditions, occupations, and environment of the population that is being treated. These factors will modify the morphologic appearance of the skin disease and may require modification of standard therapy if the desired outcome is to be achieved.

Studies on the prevalence of the various skin diseases in the tropics are usually limited to the patient population that presents to a large skin clinic, most frequently found at a university or teaching hospital in a major city. These studies are therefore biased toward patient self-selection and severity of disease and may not give an accurate reflection of the prevalence of disease in the community. They can, however, be used as a rough guideline and suggest that diseases such as scabies, other insect bites, pyoderma, and dermatitis constitute a large part of dermatologic practice in the tropics.

APPROACH TO THE PATIENT

HISTORY. A good history is the initial and best foundation on which to establish the diagnosis. Practice in the tropics often involves large numbers of patients per clinician, thus limiting the amount of history that can be obtained. Therefore, the following basic information should be recorded as accurately as possible:

1. *Duration of the disease:* This should be noted from the onset of the earliest symptom but, in many cases, will be vague, such as several weeks, months, or years.

2. *Initial body site(s) involved.*

3. *Description of the earliest lesion:* What did the earliest lesion look like before it was scratched, treated, or evolved, e.g., pustule, vesicle?

4. *Distribution of the lesions.*

5. *Recurrences:* Are the current lesions part of a cyclic phenomenon, possibly with disease-free intervals?

6. *Associated symptoms:* Are there any associated systemic symptoms, e.g., fever, arthritis, diarrhea?

7. *Prior therapy:* What measures has the patient used to alleviate the skin disorder, since this may modify the appearance and natural history of the lesion?

8. *Cutaneous symptoms:* Whether the skin lesions itch or are painful may be helpful in differential diagnosis, but these symptoms rely on subjective sensations and may be misleading. For example, some patients with scabies do not have itching, and an occasional patient with herpes zoster does not complain of pain.

PHYSICAL EXAMINATION. When examining the patient, it is best to have him completely undressed, so that the entire skin surface may be studied. In many cases, clues to the diagnosis will be found on sites remote from the patient's main concern. Natural sunlight gives the best color rendition to the lesions, incandescent lighting the second-best, and fluorescent lighting the poorest. Turning the patient tangential to the light source will cast shadows from raised lesions, accentuating them and making them more perceptible, particularly on dark-colored skin. The use of a magnifying glass to appreciate the fine detail of a given lesion or to help locate a minute lesion such as a scabietic burrow cannot be overemphasized. Examination of the hair, nails, and mucous membranes may also provide valuable clues. A general physical examination cannot usually be performed for lack of time or facilities.

DEFINITIONS. Since the differential diagnosis of skin disease is based on the morphology of the lesions, it is important to be able to accurately categorize the various primary skin lesions, their pattern or relationship to each other, and their distribution over the body surface. Because the terms used in describing skin lesions are relatively unique to dermatology, the following definitions are listed.

1. A *macule* is an area of altered skin color without a change in texture, elevation, or depression.

2. A *papule* is a solid elevation of skin less than 10 mm in diameter.

3. A *plaque* is a raised, solid area of skin with a flat surface resembling a plateau. This lesion may be formed by thickening of the skin or confluence of papules.

4. A *nodule* is a solid lesion measuring greater than 10 mm in diameter and may vary in location from subcutaneous tissue to the skin surface.

5. A *vesicle* is a fluid-filled cavity elevated above the skin surface and measuring less than 10 mm in diameter. The terms *bulla* or *blister* may be used when the lesion is greater than 10 mm in diameter.

6. A *pustule* is a fluid-filled cavity also containing white blood cells (pus) that is elevated above the skin surface.

7. A *wheal* is a transient, localized area of edema that may or may not have an alteration in color.

8. An *ulcer* is a localized area of loss of the epidermis leaving raw, denuded skin.

9. *Scale* is thickened stratum corneum that is usually gray to white and is normally found on top of a primary lesion such as a papule or a plaque.

10. A *crust* is composed of dried serum and white blood cells and is usually formed following the rupture of vesicles or pustules or covering the surface of an ulcer.

By using various combinations of these terms, most skin lesions can be described with a minimum of words. For example, a viral exanthem may be red and have both macular and papular components and can be briefly described as an "erythematous maculopapular eruption."

DISTRIBUTION. Once the basic lesion is identified, it is helpful to note the pattern of the lesions—whether they are randomly distributed, grouped in clusters, or take on a geometric arrangement such as linear or annular (ring-shaped). Finally, the distribution of the lesions over the body surface should be noted, particularly whether the lesions are generalized, localized to various body sites, or follow the distribution of the dermatomes.

LABORATORY AIDS. The following simple tests may be performed with a minimum of equipment and are useful in confirming a diagnosis or ruling out a diagnosis from the differential list:

1. A *potassium-hydroxide (KOH) preparation* is useful in the diagnosis of fungal diseases and is made by gently scraping scales with the edge of a scalpel blade or the edge of a glass slide onto a second glass slide, adding a drop or two of 10 to 20% KOH in water, and covering with a coverslip. The slide is gently warmed with a match or candle until the preparation just begins to boil. After cooling, the slide is examined with a microscope with the condenser in the down position or the diaphragm partially closed, and the hyphae and spores of fungi can be easily seen.

2. A *smear* is useful in the diagnosis of viral or bacterial diseases and can be made by scraping the base of a lesion with a scalpel blade and transferring the serum and cellular debris to a glass slide. After fixation by either heat or alcohol, the specimen may be stained with a variety of stains, depending on the suspected disease. If stains are not readily available, the fixed specimen may be stored and stained at a later date or sent to another facility.

3. *Skin snips* are useful in the diagnosis of onchocerciasis (Chapter 87) and may be performed with either a razor blade or a special instrument designed for this purpose. Using the razor blade method, the skin is first cleaned with an antiseptic solution and then pinched up between two fingers or lifted with a needle; then, a small piece of skin (usually 2 to 3 mm in size) is quickly sliced off. This examination is usually done without anesthesia and is well tolerated by the patient. The specimen is then placed on a glass slide, covered with saline, and gently teased apart with forceps or needles. After it is covered with a coverslip, the specimen is

examined under low power with a microscope for motile microfilariae.

4. A *skin biopsy* is useful in the diagnosis of most skin diseases and can be processed at a later time if facilities are not readily available. A representative lesion is selected, cleaned thoroughly with an antiseptic solution, and infiltrated with a local anesthetic such as 1 to 2% Xylocaine. If the lesion has an annular configuration and appears to be enlarging, the advancing border is the best place to biopsy; otherwise, the center of the lesion, if it is not necrotic, usually yields the best results. The specimen may be obtained with a punch biopsy instrument or an ellipse may be made with a scalpel. It is important to take the specimen down to and including the subcutaneous tissue. Sutures may be used to close the site if it is larger than 4 mm in diameter. The specimen may be divided into several pieces if cultures are desired. The specimen for histologic study should be placed in 10% buffered formalin or another suitable fixative. Once in the fixative, it may be stored indefinitely and processed at any time.

DERMATOLOGIC DISEASES

The most frequently encountered dermatologic diseases discussed in this chapter can be grouped according to their morphologic characteristics (Table 7–1), as this form of classification is helpful in establishing a differential diagnosis.

Macules

POSTINFLAMMATORY HYPERPIGMENTA-TION/HYPOPIGMENTATION. The development of

TABLE 7–1. Dermatologic Diseases in the Tropics

Macules	Nodules	Papules
Hypopigmented	Leprosy	Scabies
Postinflammatory	Kaposi's sarcoma	Tungiasis
Vitiligo	Myiasis	Flea bites
Tinea versicolor	Chromomycosis	Onchocerciasis
Pityriasis alba	Sporotrichosis	Cutaneous larva
Leprosy	Maduromycosis	migrans
Onchocerciasis	Paracoccidioidomycosis	Lichen planus
Pinta		Secondary syphilis
Hyperpigmented	**Vesicles**	Leprosy
Postinflammatory	Dermatitis	Myiasis
Mongolian spots	Erythema multiforme	Kaposi's sarcoma
Malnutrition	Herpes simplex	Erythema multiforme
Pellagra	Herpes zoster	Dermatitis
	Pemphigus foliaceus	
		Ulcers
		Leishmaniasis
		Leprosy
		Buruli ulcer
		Tropical ulcer
		Cancrum oris
		Primary syphilis
		Sporotrichosis
		Pustules
		Pyoderma
		Herpes simplex
		Herpes zoster
		Paracoccidioidomycosis

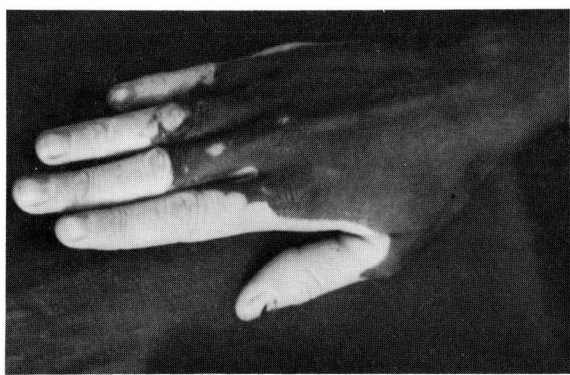

FIGURE 7–1. Vitiligo. Acral depigmentation is well developed in this Ethiopian woman.

hyperpigmentation, hypopigmentation, or various combinations of altered skin color is common. Such alterations are frequent sequelae of any inflammatory process that occurs in the skin. Thermal burns, in particular, leave markedly abnormal areas of pigmentation. Lichen planus, lupus erythematosus, and erythema multiforme tend to leave deeply pigmented macules once the initial inflammatory eruption has resolved, and the diagnosis of these diseases may be suspected by the history of the eruption and the pattern of hyperpigmentation. Whether the patient will develop hyperpigmentation or hypopigmentation following any given inflammatory process cannot be predicted, although the darker the patient's normal skin color, the more likely hyperpigmentation will develop. The diagnosis of postinflammatory hyperpigmentation/hypopigmentation is based on the history of a prior inflammatory process at that site. In the case of burns, scarring may be an associated finding. Hyperpigmentation may be treated with daily applications of 1 to 2% hydroquinone, but the results tend to be less than satisfactory. These topical hydroquinone preparations should not be used longer than 6 months as they may cause acquired ochronosis, which results in further unwanted pigmentation. Cosmetic cover-up of hypopigmentation can be achieved with frequent applications of aniline dyes. With the passage of time measured in months, areas of postinflammatory altered pigmentation tend to return toward the normal skin color, but complete resolution is unusual.

VITILIGO. Vitiligo is a common idiopathic disorder characterized by depigmented, white macules that gradually enlarge and coalesce over time. No prior inflammatory process is known to occur. Approximately 30% of patients with vitiligo have at least one affected family member. The typical depigmented lesion is surrounded by a hypopigmented or tan border, which blends into the adjacent normal skin (Fig. 7–1). No scaling or scarring develops. Hairs within the lesion may become white or retain their normal pigmentation. The lesions tend to develop around the orifices, over the extensor bony surfaces, particularly the elbows, knees, and digits, and along the lower back. They may also involve most of the body surface, may be confined to a single dermatome, and may also occur at sites of trauma. The natural history is unpredictable, although the lesions tend to progressively enlarge. Spontaneous resolution can occur. The diagnosis is established by the lack of a prior inflammatory process and by the characteristic skin lesions. Since vitiligo in the tropics may carry a social stigma because of similarities to leprosy and other diseases, most patients wish to be treated. Cosmetic cover-up may be achieved with repeated applications of aniline dyes. Repigmentation may be achieved in some cases by the use of oral trimethylpsoralen, 0.6 to 0.8 mg/kg, followed 2 hours later by exposure of the affected areas to 15 minutes of midday sunlight. The time of exposure should be increased by 5 minutes each treatment until persistent and faint erythema remains at 24 hours. The treatments should be at least twice weekly but not on consecutive days. Repigmentation usually requires 30 to 50 treatments to appear, and complete repigmentation may require up to 300 treatments. If treatment is discontinued prior to complete repigmentation, loss of the pigment tends to occur. PUVA (methoxsalen 0.3 mg/kg and ultraviolet-A irradiation) administered in a UVA irradiator is more effective and easier to control but is not readily available owing to the cost of the equipment. Also, eye protection from UVA exposure must be ensured to prevent retinal damage.

TINEA VERSICOLOR. Tinea versicolor is a common chronic superficial mycosis caused by *Pityrosporum orbiculare* and is characterized by asymptomatic, well-defined, scaly macules of variable color, most of which tend to be hypopigmented (Fig. 64–8). In some areas of the tropics, up to 50% of the population may be affected, mainly adolescents and young adults. The scaly macules tend to coalesce, forming large patches, particularly on the trunk. Other sites of predilection include the neck, shoulders, and proximal aspects of the extremities. No known susceptibility factors have been established, except that patients taking immunosuppressive agents, particularly corticosteroids, have a higher incidence of the disease. The diagnosis is established by the characteristic lesions and by the demonstration of spores and hyphae using the KOH test. The lesions are difficult to treat because of the high recurrence rate. If the disease is localized, topical therapy with 2.5% selenium sulfide or 1% clotrimazole may be used. For topical treatment failures, extensive disease, or follicular infection, a 5- to 7-day course of systemic ketoconazole is usually effective. Once the fungus is removed, the residual hypopigmentation takes a few months to recover.

PITYRIASIS ALBA. Pityriasis alba is a chronic, idiopathic disorder characterized by ill-defined, hypopigmented, scaly macules that tend to occur on the face, neck, shoulders, and extremities. The lesions usually appear in childhood, persist for months to years, and spontaneously disappear by late adolescence. The lesions may initially have mild erythema and be pruritic, but these features quickly disappear. Many of the patients with pityriasis alba also have atopic dermatitis, but a definite cause-and-effect relationship has not been established. The diagnosis is based on the characteristic lesions, distribution of the lesions, occurrence in childhood, and a negative KOH test for spores and hyphae. Since the condition is often mistaken for vitiligo, tinea versicolor, or leprosy, the patient needs additional re-

assurance regarding the diagnosis. Mild topical corticosteroids or bland emollients seem to be equally effective in the treatment of this disorder.

LEPROSY. Leprosy is a chronic disease caused by *Mycobacterium leprae* that predominantly affects the skin and peripheral nerves but may eventually involve all internal organs except the central nervous system (Chapter 62). The clinical characteristics depend on the degree of immunologic competence that is developed by the patient against the microorganism. In general terms, the greater the resistance, the more localized the disease; conversely, an absence of resistance leads to widespread disease. The initial lesions may appear anywhere on the body surface but tend to develop on the buttocks, neck, trunk, or extremities. The individual lesion is a fairly well-defined, hypopigmented macule that may be slightly erythematous (Fig. 62–6). Loss of sensation of pain or temperature discrimination, or anhidrosis in the cutaneous lesions may develop. Thickening of the peripheral nerves and its sequelae may be present or may develop at a later time. This stage of leprosy is termed *indeterminate* leprosy, as it may last unchanged for years, spontaneously disappear, or evolve into the other forms of leprosy. If the well-developed clinical features of sensory loss and peripheral nerve thickening are not present, the diagnosis can still be established by a skin biopsy demonstrating a perineural infiltrate of lymphocytes and mononuclear cells and, occasionally, an acid-fast bacillus within a peripheral nerve. Most cases show only a perivascular and periadnexal infiltrate, and the diagnosis can only be suspected. If the diagnosis is not established on the first clinic visit, repeat examinations at 3- to 6-month intervals may be helpful. The other clinical forms of leprosy will be discussed in the sections on papules, nodules, and ulcers.

ONCHOCERCIASIS. Onchocerciasis is a chronic disease caused by *Onchocerca volvulus* and characteristically affects the skin, subcutaneous tissue, and eyes (Chapter 87). The helminth is transmitted to man by the bite of the Simulium black fly, and there is an incubation period of approximately 1 year. In Central and South America, the lesions tend to occur on the upper half of the body, whereas in Africa, the lesions predominate on the lower half of the body. The initial lesions appear as pruritic edematous papules or nodules. Fever and arthralgias may be associated findings. The pruritus is so intense that excoriations and secondary bacterial infection are common. After several years, the initial lesions resolve, leaving characteristic skin changes consisting of spotty depigmentation (white spots) with associated atrophy or wrinkling (Fig. 87–6). These lesions are located on the shins, groin, or lower abdomen and have been termed leopard spots. During this late stage, there is no itching and the organisms are located deep in the dermis. The diagnosis may be confirmed in the early stages by a skin snip and, in the late depigmented stage, by a skin biopsy.

PINTA. Pinta is an endemic, nonvenereal, treponematosis caused by *Treponema carateum* and characterized in its late stages by depigmented patches (Chapter 32.4). The disease is confined to Central and South America and occurs predominantly in infants, children, and adolescents. The initial lesion is a slightly scaly papule, which evolves into a round or oval scaly plaque (Fig. 32–9). The lesions vary in size from a few millimeters in diameter to over 20 cm. Initially erythematous in color, the lesions gradually lose their pigment. With resolution, the lesion evolves into a depigmented patch. The most frequently involved sites include the lower extremities, face, neck, arms, and chest. The diagnosis is established by the occurrence of characteristic lesions in a patient from an endemic area, a positive serologic test, or the demonstration of the organism from the lesion with darkfield microscopy.

MONGOLIAN SPOTS. A mongolian spot is a blue-black macule or patch that is frequently found in dark-skinned people. The lesion may be single or multiple, may occur on the lumbosacral area or buttocks, or may be widespread. They are usually present at birth or appear shortly thereafter and tend to disappear by 5 years of age. Occasional persistence into adulthood has been observed. The diagnosis is established by the characteristic lesions. No treatment is necessary.

MALNUTRITION. The skin changes associated with protein-calorie malnutrition (kwashiorkor) are quite characteristic and in most cases diagnostic (Chapter 106). The basic change is depigmentation in association with edema and desquamation (scaling). In severe cases, large areas of erosion of the skin occur. The appearance and texture of the skin have been termed "enamel paint," "flaky paint," and "crazy paving" dermatosis (Fig. 106–3). Sites of predilection include areas of trauma such as the diaper area, elbows, knees, and ankles. In contrast to pellagra, the dermatosis seldom involves sun-exposed skin. The changes may also affect the hair, with black hair becoming brown or red and brown hair turning blond. The nails become thin and soft. The diagnosis is based on the dietary history and the characteristic skin and hair changes.

PELLAGRA. Pellagra is a clinical syndrome caused by a deficiency of niacin and usually associated with a staple diet of maize; it is characterized by dermatitis, diarrhea, and dementia (Chapter 107.6). The skin lesions tend to appear over the sun-exposed parts, particularly the dorsa of the hands and the forearms, neck, and shins. The initial lesions are erythematous and may progress to vesiculation and crusting (Fig. 107–11). With time, the skin becomes hyperpigmented, with associated fine scale. The areas of involvement are well defined; the lesions around the neck have been termed "Casal's necklace" (Fig. 107–10). The mucous membranes of the mouth and genitalia are inflamed and may develop ulcerations. The diagnosis is established by a dietary history, characteristic skin and mucous membrane lesions (diarrhea and dementia may not always be present), and the therapeutic response to niacin.

Papules

SCABIES. Scabies is a skin disease caused by infestation with and sensitization to the itch mite *Sarcoptes scabiei* var. *hominis* and is characterized by intense itching and burrows (Chapter 105.2). The disease is exceedingly common and widely distributed throughout the tropics and affects both sexes and all age groups. The pathognomonic burrow is the only skin lesion caused by the mite and results from tunnelling or burrowing of the female mite into the stratum corneum to lay her eggs (Figs. 7–2 and 105–9). The burrow appears as a 1- to 3-mm whitish, threadlike, elevated channel with a grayish speck at one end representing the location of the female mite. The sites of predilection for the burrows include the finger webs, flexor surface of the wrist, elbows, nipples, genitalia, and anterior axillary folds. Urticarial papules, excoriations, and nodule formation are the result of sensitization to the mite and vigorous scratching. These lesions may be located anywhere on the body but tend to spare the head, except in infants. Secondary bacterial infection of the skin, i.e., impetigo, is a frequent complication and may mask the appearance of the underlying scabies. A rare variant of scabies, termed Norwegian scabies, is characterized by infestation, with literally millions of mites covering the body surface. This causes intense scaling and crust formation and is most frequently found in patients with lepromatous leprosy or mental retardation. For some unknown reason, these patients do not have itching. With this exception, the diagnosis of scabies is established by the history of intense pruritus, especially at night, distribution of the skin lesions, and the presence of the pathognomonic burrow. The mite can be teased out from the end of the burrow with a needle, placed on a glass slide, and examined under the microscope.

Treatment consists of killing the mites and ova and treating the secondary bacterial infection. The treatment of choice is 1% hexachlorobenzene (lindane), which should be applied to the entire body after a thorough shower and left on for 24 hours. A second application for an additional 24 hours increases the cure rate. This treatment should be repeated in 1 week. Undergarments and bed linen should be washed in hot water. Other forms of therapy include 10% crotonotoluide, 25% benzyl benzoate, and 6% sulfur ointment. The secondary bacterial infection should be treated with a full course of systemic antibiotics such as penicillin, dicloxacillin, or erythromycin.

TUNGIASIS. Tungiasis is a skin disease caused by the burrowing flea *Tunga penetrans* and is characterized by pruritic papules at the site of penetration (Chapter 105.2). The female flea burrows into the skin to lay eggs beneath the toenails and soles and along the sides of the foot (Fig. 105–5). The genitalia, buttocks, and hands may occasionally be affected. The lesions appear as small papules with a central black dot or pore that gradually enlarges and becomes inflamed and painful. Secondary bacterial infection is a common complication. The diagnosis is established by teasing out the flea with a sterile needle and examining it under a magnifying glass or microscope. The lesions may be treated by removing the insects with a sterile needle or an application of chloroform or turpentine. Secondary bacterial infection should be treated with systemic antibiotics.

FLEA BITES. Flea bites are a common problem throughout the tropics and are caused by infestation with *Pulex irritans*. Fleas that are generally host-specific

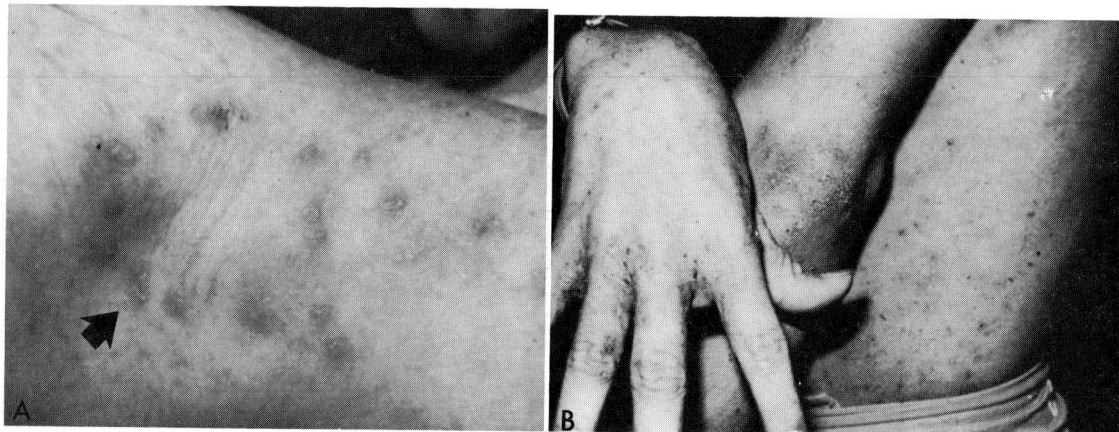

FIGURE 7–2. Scabies. *A.* The arrow points to a typical burrow in the axilla of a child. Nodules and papules are also present. *B,* The typical distribution of the papules and excoriations in scabies: web spaces, elbows, and flanks. (*A,* Courtesy of Dr. Antoinette Hood: *B,* Courtesy of Dr. Stanford Lamberg.)

to other animals e.g., dog, cat, or rat, may also infest man because of close contact with the animals or during the first few weeks following removal of the animals from the environment. Flea bites tend to involve the exposed surfaces of skin but may involve the entire cutaneous surface during heavy infestation. The individual lesions are small, discrete papules with central puncta that may evolve into vesicles or pustules. There may be an erythematous ring or wheal surrounding each lesion. The lesions tend to cluster in groups of 3, probably caused by bites from a single flea. Excoriations and secondary bacterial infections are common sequelae. Bites from other insects provoke similar cutaneous lesions, and the diagnosis of the specific offending insect can be made by demonstrating the organism or suspected from the history and distribution of the lesions.

Therapy consists of killing the fleas with an insecticide and treatment of the secondary bacterial infection. The source of fleas in the environment should also be treated. Itching may be alleviated by the use of topical corticosteroids, calamine lotion, or systemic antihistamines.

ONCHOCERCIASIS. The early lesions of onchocerciasis present as pruritic edematous papules, which may evolve into areas of edema or nodules. Lichenified papules and secondary bacterial infection develop as a result of scratching.

CUTANEOUS LARVA MIGRANS. This disorder, also known as creeping eruption, is caused by the migration in the skin of the larvae of certain nematodes, commonly *Ancylostoma braziliense, Ucinaria stenocephala* and *Ancylostoma caninum* (Chapter 94). Following penetration of the larvae into human skin, a progressive, pruritic, serpiginous, elevated cord develops, which later becomes erythematous (Fig. 94–1). The lesion may advance at a rate of up to 5 cm per day. The cord may be several centimeters in length but is usually only a few millimeters in diameter. The diagnosis is established by the characteristic appearance of the lesion. The lesion may be treated by local application of liquid nitrogen or ethyl chloride to the advancing end of the cord. Topical chemical agents such as piperazine ointment and thiabendazole are also useful.

LICHEN PLANUS. Lichen planus is a disease of

unknown cause characterized by pruritic, flat-topped, violaceous papules that tend to favor the flexor surfaces of the skin, mucous membranes, nails, and genitalia. The disease occurs worldwide, affects both sexes, and most commonly affects the 30- to 60-year-old age group. The basic lesion is a papule measuring 3 to 8 mm in diameter, with angulated borders, a flat top, and thin, delicate, white lines, termed Wickham's striae, on the surface. The individual papules may coalesce to form plaques and characteristically form a linear pattern, usually following trauma. Healed lesions develop marked hyperpigmentation without scarring. A number of variations in the types of lesions may occasionally occur, e.g., annular, hypertrophic, atrophic, or ulcerative. A number of drugs, e.g., antimalarials, para-aminosalicylic acid, gold, streptomycin, tetracycline, and hydrochlorothiazide, may cause a clinical eruption similar to lichen planus.

The diagnosis of lichen planus is based on the appearance of the characteristic papule and the absence of drug ingestion known to cause a similar eruption. The differential diagnosis also includes psoriasis and secondary syphilis. Psoriasis may be excluded by a skin biopsy and secondary syphilis by a serologic test. Lichen planus may be treated with either topical corticosteroids or a 2- to 6-week course of systemic corticosteroids. Antihistamines are helpful for the pruritus. In most cases the lesions are self-limited, but they may persist for years, and relapses may occur.

SECONDARY SYPHILIS. Syphilis is a chronic infectious disorder caused by *Treponema pallidum,* usually transmitted by sexual contact, and characterized by 3 stages of disease (Chapter 32.1). The second stage usually occurs 6 to 8 weeks after the appearance of the chancre, and the lesions tend to involve the skin and mucous membranes, but internal organs may be affected at times. The basic lesion is a firm, slightly elevated papule that varies in color from pink to reddish brown (copper penny). The lesions may be widespread but commonly affect the palms and soles (Fig. 7–3). Annular forms of lesions commonly affect the face, particularly at the angles of the mouth and the nares (Fig. 32–2). Macular lesions, hair loss, moist erythematous patches

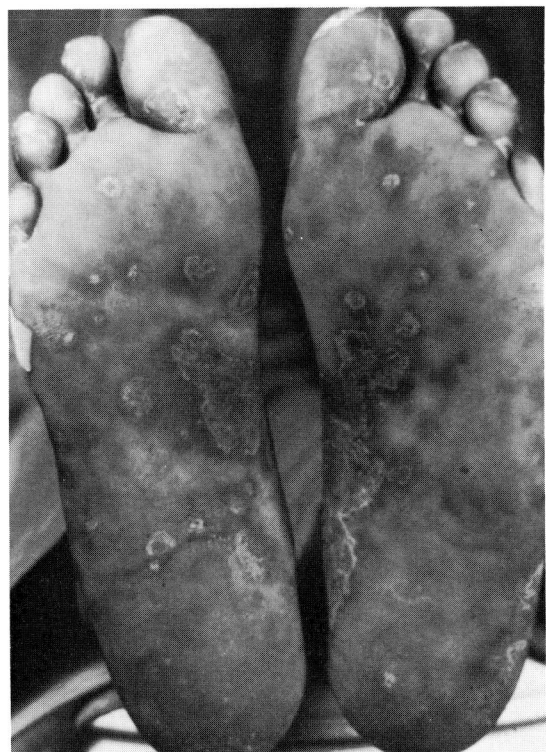

FIGURE 7–3. Secondary syphilis. Brown keratotic papules and plaques on the soles are characteristic lesions of secondary syphilis.

on the mucous membranes, fever, and generalized lymphadenopathy are frequent associated findings. The diagnosis is suspected on the basis of the clinical lesions and is confirmed by either a positive darkfield demonstration of the spirochetes or a positive serologic test for syphilis. The treatment of choice is long-acting penicillin, but erythromycin or tetracycline may be used in patients allergic to penicillin.

LEPROSY. Papular lesions may develop as part of any of the forms of leprosy, with the exception of indeterminate leprosy. For example, in tuberculoid leprosy, the lesions usually evolve from a papule into a plaque or an annular lesion that is hypopigmented, dry, and anesthetic (Fig. 62–7). The well-defined border of each lesion is elevated in comparison with the center. Peripheral nerves are thickened and tender, with occasional abscesses (Fig. 62–8). In the borderline forms of leprosy, the lesions are similar to those of tuberculoid leprosy, except for being less well defined at the edges and having centers elevated above the borders (Fig. 62–9). The lesions are more numerous than in tuberculoid leprosy but are still asymmetrically distributed over the body surface. The peripheral nerves are enlarged and tender as in tuberculoid leprosy. In lepromatous leprosy, the patient may have a variety of types of lesions, including papules, plaques, or nodules (Fig. 62–11). The lesions are numerous, symmetrically distributed over the body surface, and less well defined at the edges than the lesions of borderline leprosy. The mucous membranes and internal organs may be involved. The peripheral nerves are slightly thickened.

MYIASIS. Myiasis is the result of infestation by larvae from several types of flies (Chapter 105.2). The site of infestation is usually the skin but can also be mucous membranes, the gastrointestinal tract, and the urinary tract. The larvae are deposited on the skin by the adult fly via clothing or soil or are carried there by other insects. Depending on the species, the larvae may penetrate normal skin or may invade through an open wound. The initial lesion appears as an edematous, pruritic papule, which may enlarge into a nodule or may develop into a migratory lesion. The patient characteristically notes movement or "something alive" within the lesion. The larvae may also protrude through the top of the lesion and be observed by the clinician (Fig. 105–6). The diagnosis is established by the characteristic skin lesion. The larvae may be extracted through the dilated opening by pressing on the sides of the lesion and grasping the insect with fine forceps. Excision biopsy is rarely necessary.

KAPOSI'S SARCOMA. Kaposi's sarcoma is a multicentric neoplasm characteristically presenting as multiple vascular papules, nodules, or plaques in the skin and internal organs. The incidence of the disease varies worldwide, but in the tropics it is particularly common in Kenya, Tanzania, and Zaire. In non-African cases, the disease occurs most frequently in the fifth through the seventh decades, whereas in Africa, it has a peak in the first decade, few cases in the second decade, and then a gradually rising incidence throughout adult life. It is predominant in males at a ratio of 9 to 1. Kaposi's sarcoma is frequently one of the manifestations of the acquired immunodeficiency syndrome (AIDS). The lesions are purple to dark blue and are usually associated with edema of the affected extremity (Fig. 11–4). The diagnosis is established by skin biopsy. Both chemotherapy and radiotherapy have been somewhat effective in treatment.

ERYTHEMA MULTIFORME. Erythema multiforme is an acute, self-limiting, recurrent eruption characterized by annular or "target" lesions. The lesions predominate on the extremities, but the mucous membranes are also frequently involved. In severe cases, fever, weakness, fluid loss, and anorexia may develop. The etiology is unknown, but many cases have been associated with viral infections (particularly herpes simplex) and drug ingestion (particularly sulfonamides). The diagnosis is established by the presence of the characteristic target lesions and confirmed by a skin biopsy. Since the episodes are usually self-limited, supportive care is all that is required in most cases. Therapy of underlying infections and discontinuance of suspected drugs should be promptly instituted. Occasional severe cases may require hospitalization and the use of systemic corticosteroids.

DERMATITIS. The term dermatitis (eczema) simply means inflammation of the skin and does not imply a specific cause. Most cases can usually be categorized as contact dermatitis, atopic dermatitis (eczema), or seborrheic dermatitis. The lesions present as patches of erythema, which evolve into erythematous grouped papules and small vesicles. The lesions are characteristically pruritic, and excoriations with secondary bacterial infection are quite common. The diagnosis of a specific type of dermatitis is made by history of contactants, body

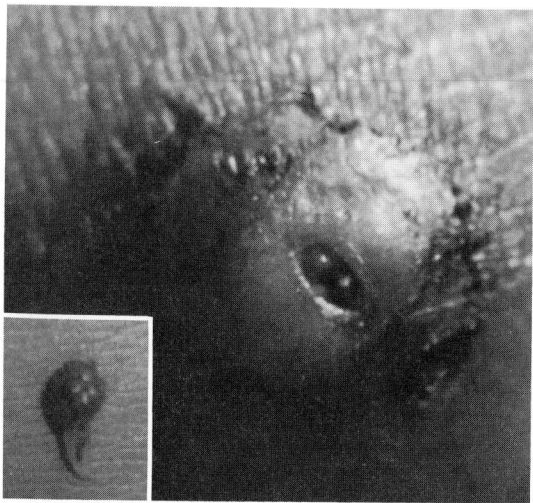

FIGURE 7-4. Myiasis. Nodular lesion of myiasis demonstrates a central pore with the larva protruding. *Inset,* Intact larva has been extracted from the lesion.

sites of lesions, and association with asthma or hay fever in the patient or close relatives. The treatment for most types of dermatitis includes removal of offending contactants; treatment of secondary bacterial infection, if present; cool baths or local cool water compresses, depending on the extent of the disease; topical or systemic corticosteroids (the latter for short-term use only); lubrication of the skin to decrease dryness once the vesicular stage has resolved; and education of the patient as to the cause of his disease and possible aggravating factors.

Nodules

LEPROSY. Patients with leprosy, particularly at the lepromatous end of the spectrum, may develop numerous widespread asymptomatic nodules. These nodules are filled with histiocytes laden with numerous bacilli. Some patients at the lepromatous end of the spectrum may also acutely develop tender erythematous nodules on the legs, arms, and back in association with fever, malaise, iritis, hepatitis, arthritis, and orchitis (Fig. 62–14). This syndrome is one of the reactional phases in leprosy and is termed erythema nodosum leprosum. It is thought to be the result of an antigen-antibody complex reaction.

KAPOSI'S SARCOMA. Kaposi's sarcoma may also present as violaceous vascular nodules.

MYIASIS. Some of the well-developed lesions of myiasis present as erythematous pruritic nodules, which, to the patient, have the sensation of movement (Fig. 7–4).

CHROMOMYCOSIS. Chromomycosis is a chronic granulomatous disease of the skin and mucous membranes tending to affect agricultural workers and is caused by infection by various pigmented fungi (Chapter 65.3). The legs are most frequently involved. Following inoculation of the spores, usually from vegetation or through open wounds, an erythematous nodule develops, which subsequently ulcerates (Fig. 65–4). The lesions then become verrucous, with compact scaling and crust formation (Fig. 65–5). With time, the affected extremity becomes swollen and develops an elephantoid appearance. The diagnosis can be made by a skin biopsy demonstrating the characteristic spores or by fungal culture. Treatment for small lesions consists of surgical removal or destruction, and that for extensive disease consists of systemic antifungal agents such as amphotericin B.

SPOROTRICHOSIS. Sporotrichosis is a chronic granulomatous disease of the skin and lymphatic vessels caused by infection with *Sporotrichum schenckii* (Chapter 65.2). It is worldwide in distribution, predominantly affecting agricultural workers and gardeners. The extremities are most frequently involved, followed by the face and trunk. Following inoculation of the spores, an erythematous nodule develops, which subsequently ulcerates. New lesions then appear along the course of the regional lymphatic vessels, giving the disease its characteristic appearance (Fig. 7–5). In rare cases, the infection disseminates to involve the bones and lungs. The diagnosis can be established by demonstrating the

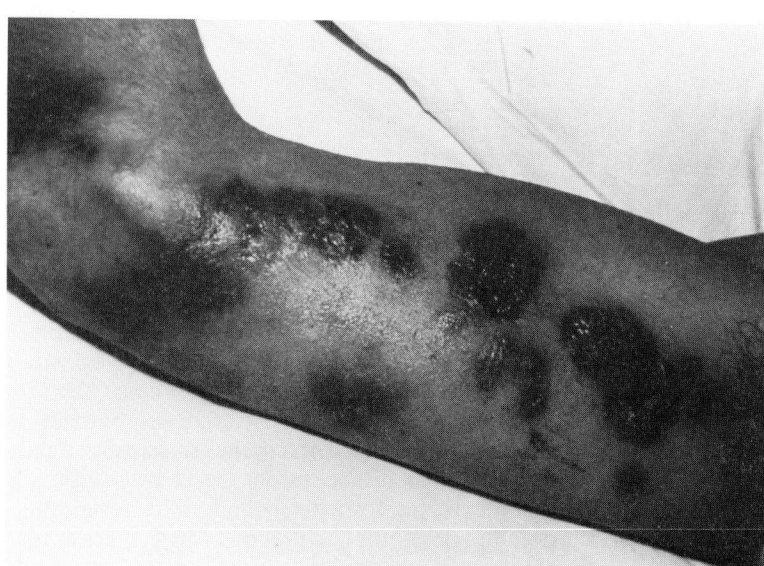

FIGURE 7-5. Sporotrichosis. Ulcerative nodular lesions are arranged in a linear fashion on the arm extending to the axilla in this South African man. (Courtesy of Dr. Michael Radowsky.)

spores in a skin biopsy or by fungal culture. Potassium iodide remains the treatment of choice and is usually given as a saturated solution in a beverage 3 times daily before meals.

MADUROMYCOSIS. Maduromycosis (mycetoma, Madura foot) is a chronic granulomatous disease of skin and underlying bone caused by infection by various fungi, including *Madurella, Allescheria,* and *Cephalosporium* (Chapter 65.1). The foot is the most common site involved, but other areas may be affected as well. The lesions are characterized by nodules, abscesses, draining sinuses, scarring, and deformity (Fig. 12–3). Infection of the bone results in periostitis and cavity formation, with eventual destruction of the bone. Surprisingly, pain is not a marked feature, unless secondary bacterial infection develops. The diagnosis may be established by the characteristic radiographic findings, demonstration of the organism in the pustular exudate, or demonstration of the organism by skin biopsy or by fungal culture. Treatment, except for the secondary bacterial infection, has not been particularly successful, and amputation may be required.

Ulcers

LEISHMANIASIS. Cutaneous leishmaniasis is a chronic granulomatous disease of the skin and mucous membranes caused by infection by parasites of the genus *Leishmania* (Chapter 76). It can generally be divided into two types—Old World (Oriental sore) or New World (American leishmaniasis). Both types are transmitted by the *Phlebotomus* sandfly. The lesions are most frequently found on the face and other unclothed parts of the body (Fig. 7–6) and begin as small papules, which enlarge into ulcerative nodules. In the Old World type, the lesions tend to heal spontaneously in about a year (Fig. 76–10), but a few patients may have a number of relapses (recidivans type). In the New World type, in addition to the localized ulcerative nodule, mucous membrane lesions may develop, probably by hematogenous or lymphatic spread. These mucous membrane lesions are ulcerative and may cause extensive destruction of the nose and mouth (Fig. 76–14). Other clinical forms of leishmaniasis occur, including post–kala-azar skin eruption (Fig. 76–7) and disseminated anergic leishmaniasis. The diagnosis of leishmaniasis may be established by the demonstration of the organisms from a Giemsa-stained smear (taken from the depth of an incision of the lesion), by a skin biopsy, or by culture.

LEPROSY. Ulcers usually develop in patients with leprosy as the result of trauma rather than as an innate characteristic as seen in leishmaniasis. Because of nerve involvement by the leprosy bacillus, with subsequent impairment of the senses of pain and temperature discrimination, patients do not withdraw from noxious stimuli and therefore unknowingly develop tissue destruction. Blisters from improperly fitting shoes and from touching hot objects are the most common examples. These ulcers develop most frequently on the hands and feet and may become extensive and secondarily infected through neglect due to the lack of pain. The other features of leprosy are usually well developed by this time, and the diagnosis can be established.

BURULI ULCER. A Buruli ulcer develops from the toxin produced by *Mycobacterium ulcerans* (Chapter 63). The disease is common in Uganda and Zaire and predominantly affects children. The lesion, most frequently found on the legs, begins as a small nodule, which rapidly breaks down to form a large necrotic ulcer (Fig. 63–1). Characteristically, the lesions are painless, and there is no regional lymphadenopathy. The diagnosis can be established by a skin biopsy demonstrating the organisms or by culture.

TROPICAL ULCER. Tropical ulcer (phagedenic ulcer) is a rapidly growing, painful ulcer usually found on the legs of malnourished children (Chapter 33). The lesion usually begins, following minor trauma or pyoderma, as a small ulcer that rapidly enlarges. Its borders are well defined and elevated, and the cavity is cup-shaped. The ulcer develops its maximum size in about 2 weeks. The ulcer is painful and tender, in contrast to Buruli ulcer, but lymphadenopathy is minimal unless secondary bacterial infection develops. Bacteriologic studies have implicated *Bacillus fusiformis* and *Treponema vincenti* as possible etiologic agents. Fibrosis subsequently develops, but healing may be delayed for years. In addition to secondary infection, squamous cell carcinoma may develop as a late complication. The diagnosis is made by the clinical presentation and the exclusion of other causes for ulceration such as Buruli ulcer, pyoderma, and stasis dermatitis. Systemic penicillin or tetracycline, balanced diet high in calories and proteins, and cleansing of the ulcer are helpful in therapy. Reconstructive surgery may be needed for chronic lesions.

CANCRUM ORIS. Cancrum oris is a disorder characterized by rapidly developing necrotic ulceration of the face, occurring predominantly in malnourished children, and is thought to be due to infection by *Treponema vincenti* and *Bacillus fusiformis* (Fig. 12–5). Many of

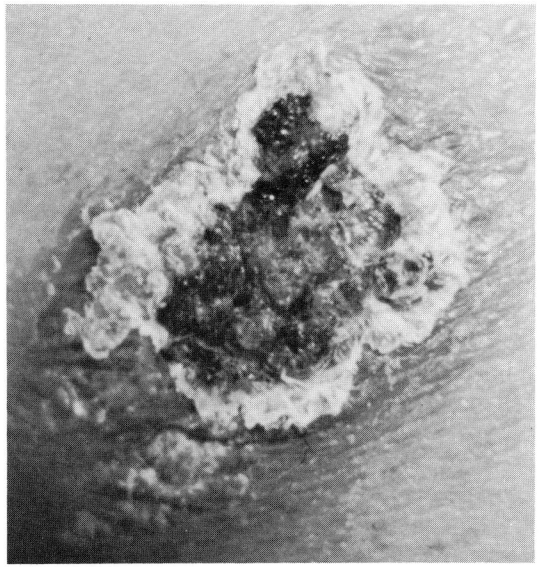

FIGURE 7–6. Leishmaniasis. This shallow ulcer on the arm of a Peruvian woman has a peripheral collar of scale and crust.

these children also have malaria, measles, kala-azar, or other systemic diseases. The ulceration is usually unilateral and tends to involve the mouth. Large defects may quickly develop, and death may occur in untreated patients. The lesions are quite painful, with variable systemic symptoms. The diagnosis is made by the characteristic clinical appearance and the exclusion of other diseases such as bacterial abscesses, actinomycosis, and maduromycosis. Systemic penicillin is the treatment of choice, along with cleansing of the lesion and a balanced diet high in calories and protein. Reconstructive surgery may be required for repair of extensive defects.

PRIMARY SYPHILIS. The primary lesion of syphilis is an indurated, painless, oval or round ulcer called a chancre. The border is well defined, and the base is characteristically clean. The most common sites are the genitalia, anus, and mouth. The lesion is usually single, and there is associated regional lymphadenopathy. Spirochetes can be easily demonstrated by darkfield microscopy of the exudate. The lesions of secondary syphilis may appear before the chancre has resolved.

SPOROTRICHOSIS. The lesions of sporotrichosis characteristically present as ulcerative nodules, but the ulcerative feature may predominate.

Vesicles

DERMATITIS. Dermatitis, particularly contact dermatitis, may have vesicles as a prominent feature of the skin lesions in addition to the erythematous macules and papules. The vesicles are usually small, less than 5 mm in diameter, but at times may be much larger. They usually contain clear, pale yellow fluid, rarely become pustular, and do not contain red blood cells. The distribution of the lesions helps to suggest a cause for the dermatitis. For example, lesions arranged in a linear fashion are frequently found in plant contact dermatitis. Rupture of the vesicles creates a break in the skin barrier, and secondary bacterial infection is a frequent complication.

ERYTHEMA MULTIFORME. Severe erythema multiforme may have vesicles as a component of the skin lesions. These are usually in the center of the cutaneous annular lesions. The mucous membrane lesions are more difficult to recognize as being vesicular because they easily rupture and present as raw, denuded areas. The vesicles vary in size, frequently becoming bullae up to 2 to 3 cm in diameter. As in the case of dermatitis, rupture of the vesicles predisposes the patient to secondary bacterial infection.

HERPES SIMPLEX. This is a viral infection of skin, mucous membranes, the nervous system, and, occasionally, internal organs caused by the herpes simplex group of viruses. The disease is common, worldwide in distribution, and affects both sexes and all age groups. Primary infection usually occurs in childhood and may present as a painful vesicular stomatitis with fever and lymphadenopathy, spontaneously resolving in 7 to 14 days. The lesions are small, clear vesicles, occasionally pustules, that rupture easily, leaving raw, denuded areas on the mucosal surfaces and crusted lesions on the skin.

Primary infection may also occur in the genital region, usually in adolescents and adults, with a similar clinical presentation and time course. The primary infection may also be subclinical. Once the primary infection has resolved, the virus goes into a latent state in the regional ganglia, where it seems to remain for years. The virus may be reactivated under a variety of conditions including fever, trauma, or emotional stress. Following reactivation, the virus travels down the peripheral nerves to the skin, presenting as grouped, painful vesicles on an erythematous base. Lesions that appear on the lips or around the mouth are called fever blisters, and those on the genitalia are called herpes genitalis. The lesions in both areas spontaneously resolve in 7 to 14 days unless secondarily infected. The lesions tend to recur at the same sites at variable and unpredictable intervals. Patients who are immunosuppressed, have atopic dermatitis, or are neonates are at high risk of having disseminated herpes simplex involving all of the skin surface and internal organs. The lesions appear as small vesicles without a tendency to group together. The patient is febrile and toxic and has a high morbidity and high rate of mortality.

The diagnosis of herpes simplex infection is made by the clinical presentation and confirmed by either viral culture, a twofold rise in serologic titers of anti-herpes simplex antibodies, or more simply, by a Giemsa-stained smear made from the base of the vesicle demonstrating balloon cells (enlarged nucleus) and giant cells, both of squamous cell origin.

Systemic acyclovir is the drug of choice in the treatment of herpes simplex infections. For localized lesions, such as fever blisters in the immunocompetent patient, the drug may be given orally in a 5-day course. For prevention of frequently recurring lesions, acyclovir may be given in a lower dose on a daily basis. In the immunocompromised patient or in patients with disseminated disease, a much higher oral dose or intravenous administration should be used. Drying lotions such as calamine lotion are helpful in symptomatic management of the individual lesions. Secondary bacterial infections should be treated with systemic antibiotics.

HERPES ZOSTER. Herpes zoster is a painful vesicular disorder caused by herpesvirus varicellae and characterized by grouped vesicles on an erythematous base in a dermatomal distribution. The disorder is worldwide in distribution, affects both sexes, and is seen predominantly in adults. The causal virus, which is the same virus that causes varicella, resides in a latent state in ganglia following an attack of varicella. For unknown reasons, the virus becomes reactivated, travels down the peripheral nerves, and infects the skin, causing blisters. The most frequent sites of involvement include the trigeminal and thoracic dermatomes. Characteristically, the lesions are unilateral, crossing the midline no more than 1 to 2 cm. Disseminated herpes zoster is analogous to disseminated herpes simplex infection occurring in immunosuppressed patients. In contrast to herpes simplex, recurrent episodes of herpes zoster are rare. The lesions of herpes zoster normally resolve in 7 to 14 days, but there may be persistent pain for months, especially in elderly patients. The diagnosis of herpes zoster is made by the characteristic lesions in a dermatomal distribution and may be confirmed by viral culture or a Giemsa-stained smear made from the base of a vesicle. If taken within 4 days after the appearance of the lesions, the smear will show balloon cells and giant cells identical to those seen in herpes simplex. Systemic acyclovir is the drug of choice in the treatment of herpes zoster. It may be given orally in the immunocompetent patient and should be administered intravenously in the immunocompromised patient. Secondary bacterial infection should be treated with systemic antibiotics. Drying agents such as calamine lotion are helpful in the management of individual lesions. Analgesics may be required for the pain.

PEMPHIGUS FOLIACEUS. Pemphigus foliaceus is a disorder of unknown cause characterized by flaccid blisters that rupture easily, forming eroded areas with peripheral rolls of epidermis (Fig. 7–7). The disorder is uncommon, except in Brazil, where it is endemic, frequently affects children, and is known as "fogo selvagem" because of its burning sensation. In other parts of the world, pemphigus foliaceus tends to affect adolescents and adults. The lesions are widespread over the body surface, and the patients are not usually febrile or toxic unless a secondary bacterial infection develops. The diagnosis is made by the characteristic skin lesions and may be confirmed by skin biopsy. The treatment of choice is systemic corticosteroids, which may be required for prolonged periods.

Pustules

PYODERMA. Pyoderma is infection of the skin caused by group A beta-hemolytic *Streptococcus, Staphylococcus aureus,* or a mixed flora of both microorganisms with additional pathogens. The infection may develop on normal skin but more commonly appears as a complication of wounds or other skin diseases. Malnutrition and poor hygiene are prime predisposing factors in its development. Specific names are given for the various clinical presentations of pyoderma. *Impetigo*

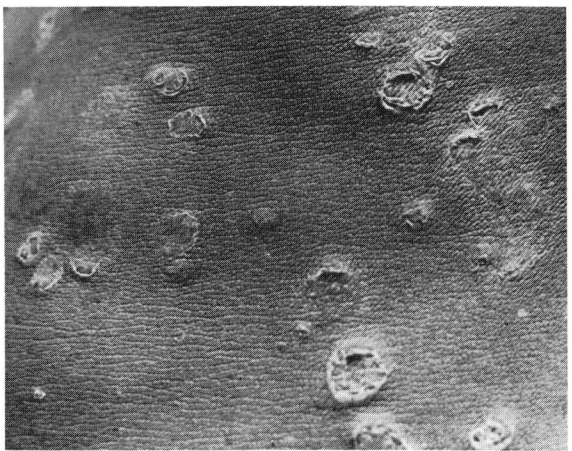

FIGURE 7–7. Pemphigus foliaceus. Ruptured flaccid bullae with peripheral rolls of epidermis are scattered on the trunk of an Ethiopian boy.

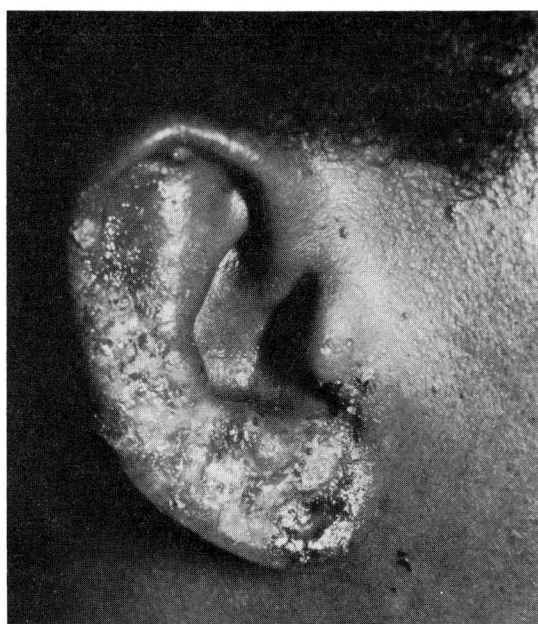

FIGURE 7–8. Pyoderma. Yellow, crusted lesions are present on the pinna, developing as a complication of allergic contact dermatitis to nickel contained in earrings. (Courtesy of Dr. Robert Weiss.)

presents as small pustules or vesicles that evolve into yellow crusts that heal without scarring (Fig. 7–8). *Bullous impetigo,* more common in young children, is characterized by large bullae (blisters) that, upon rupture, develop brown crusts instead of the yellow crusts of impetigo. *Ecthyma* is a deep infection of the skin presenting as ulcers covered by a brown, hemorrhagic crust. The lesions of ecthyma may begin as pustules, as in impetigo, or directly in a previous open wound and are most frequently located on the legs. In contrast to impetigo, the lesions of ecthyma heal with scarring. *Folliculitis* is characterized by pustules developing within the openings of the hair follicles. These papules evolve into yellow crusts similar to those in impetigo. If the infection is in the deep portion of a hair follicle, forming an abscess, the term *furuncle* is used. A *carbuncle* refers to a localized aggregation of furuncles. *Erysipelas* is a skin infection caused by the sudden appearance of an erythematous plaque that enlarges peripherally. Small vesicles may appear at its advancing edge. In contrast to the previous forms of pyoderma, patients with erysipelas are systemically sick with fever, chills, and malaise. Recurrent attacks of erysipelas, particularly on the extremities, leads to lymphatic obstruction and the development of lymphedema. The diagnosis of the various forms of pyoderma is established by the clinical morphology and may be confirmed by bacterial culture. Systemic antibiotics are the treatment of choice, in conjunction with cleansing of the skin with soap and removal of the crusts. Penicillin or one of the semisynthetic penicillins should be used in full dosage for 10 to 14 days, depending on the sensitivities of the microorganisms. Erythromycin, lincomycin, or clindamycin may be substituted in patients allergic to penicillin.

PARACOCCIDIOIDOMYCOSIS. This is an infection of the skin, mucous membranes, and internal organs caused by the fungus *Paracoccidioides brasiliensis* (Chapter 66.4). It is endemic in South America and occurs in both sexes and all age groups. The initial site of infection in most cases is thought to be the oral cavity. Irrespective of the initial inoculation site, the organism follows the same pathway in the host. It travels in sequence to the lymphatic vessels, lymph nodes, vena cava, right heart, lung, and left heart and then hematogenously to the skin and mucous membranes. The skin lesions are most frequently found on the face and scalp, particularly around orifices. They have a variable appearance, consisting of papules, nodules, ulcers, crusts, and abscesses. Multiple hemorrhagic puncta are a characteristic feature. The diagnosis is made by the location and morphology of the skin lesions and the chest radiographic findings and may be confirmed by culture or by skin biopsy. Long-acting sulfonamides and amphotericin B have been effective in treatment.

HERPES SIMPLEX. Herpes simplex, particularly of several days' duration, may present as pustules and crusts on an erythematous base.

HERPES ZOSTER. Herpes zoster, like herpes simplex, may present as pustules rather than vesicles. Otherwise, the clinical characteristics are similar to the vesicular phase.

BIBLIOGRAPHY

Elpern DJ: The dermatology of Kauai, Hawaii, 1981–1982. Int J Dermatol 24:647–52, 1985.

Gupta AK, Anderson TF: Psoralen photochemotherapy. J Am Acad Dermatol 17:703–734, 1987.

Hodes RM, Kloos H: Health and medical care in Ethiopia. N Engl J Med 319:918–924, 1988.

Leigh IM: Management of non-genital herpes simplex virus infections in immunocompetent patients. Am J Med 85:34–38, 1988.

Nethercott JR, Choi BC: Erythema multiforme (Stevens-Johnson syndrome)—chart review of 123 hospitalized patients. Dermatologica 171:383–396, 1985.

Phillips JI, Isaacson C, Carman H: Ochronosis in black South Africans who used skin lighteners. Am J Dermatopathol 8:14–21, 1986.

Scully C, el-Kom M: Lichen planus: review and update on pathogenesis. J Oral Pathol 14:431–458, 1985.

8.   NEUROLOGIC DISEASES

B.O. Osuntokun

Neurologic problems are common in tropical areas and contribute substantially to mortality and morbidity. Diseases of the nervous system that are often seen in developed countries are also encountered in the tropics, albeit less frequently. Bacterial meningitis, cerebral malaria, tetanus, and cerebrovascular disease are leading causes of death and disability. Tropical countries are not homogeneous with regard to disease patterns, but certain features of neurologic illness are common to many areas. Important factors determining the pattern of neurologic illness include a high prevalence of infectious disease, poverty, ignorance, and malnutrition; a large proportion of children in the population; and a relative paucity of the degenerative diseases of old age.

Many of the common neurologic disorders in the tropics are diseases of the socially and economically disadvantaged.

Certain diseases, e.g., trypanosomiasis, rabies, poliomyelitis, and leprosy, are confined to or are much more common in the tropics; other neurologic diseases are rarer in the tropics than in temperate climates (Table 8–1).

The reactions of the nervous system to disease are relatively limited; many different pathogenic agents produce well-defined clinical syndromes, e.g., acute meningoencephalitis, hemiplegia, and paraplegia. In medical practice in the tropics, the differential diagnosis of the neurologic clinical syndromes is wider because it includes disorders of the nervous system that may be encountered anywhere as well as those that are almost always confined to the tropics. Generally, diagnostic facilities are less available than in temperate areas. The physician's objectives of prevention and early diagnosis and treatment are often unattainable because of inadequate primary care, late presentation, and poor public health services. High mortality rates and permanent neurologic damage are commonplace in the tropics.

ACUTE CONFUSIONAL STATES

The common causes of acute confusional state (acute organic brain syndrome) in adults are shown in Table 8–2.

ACUTE INFECTIONS. Confusion, disorientation in time and space, clouding of consciousness, agitation, and hallucinations are seen as a result of severe febrile illness, e.g., malaria (Chapter 73), pneumonia (Chapter 1), or typhoid fever (Chapter 38). In these states, there is no macroscopic evidence of brain inflammation. Similar findings may mark the onset of meningitis (Chapter 43), encephalitis, or a metabolic encephalopathy. Lumbar puncture may be necessary to distinguish these conditions from meningitis.

ACUTE METABOLIC AND TOXIC ENCEPHALOPATHIES. Certain metabolic disorders and toxins cause confusion, coma, and, sometimes, recurrent convulsions. However, in contrast to acute infectious encephalitis, fever is usually absent and the cerebrospinal fluid is normal. The delay in seeking or obtaining medical care contributes to the increased frequency of these problems in developing countries.

DEHYDRATION. Severe dehydration from diarrhea is common in children; usually, there is a balanced loss of water and electrolytes. In perhaps 5 to 10% of those with severe dehydration, excessive loss of electrolytes or replacement with water results in hyponatremic dehydration with circulatory failure, shock, and osmotic swelling of the brain, causing headaches, seizures, and coma. The intravenous administration of full-strength normal saline solution or even 3% NaCl is needed in severe cases, but correction of hyponatremia should be done cautiously to avoid precipitating the syndrome of

TABLE 8–1. Differences in the Incidence of Neurologic Illness in the Tropics and in Europe and North America

More Common in Tropics	Less Common in Tropics
Pyogenic meningitis	Subacute combined degeneration
Tuberculous meningitis	Multiple sclerosis
Arbovirus encephalitis	Prolapsed disk syndromes
Tetanus	Neurologic syndromes associated with malignancy, Meniere's
Poliomyelitis	disease, and trigeminal neuralgia
Rabies	Degenerative disorders of old age, e.g., Parkinson's disease,
Nutritional neuropathy	Alzheimer's disease
Neurologic complications of malaria, trypanosomiasis, relapsing fever, amebiasis, hemoglobinopathies, hepatic failure, hydatid disease, cysticercosis, schistosomiasis, and Burkitt's lymphoma	
Pyomyositis	

acute central pontine myelinosis. Less commonly in the tropics, severe hypernatremia with plasma sodium levels above 150 mEq/L results from diarrhea, causing coma and seizures. These patients need to be treated with intravenous hypotonic solutions.

HEPATIC FAILURE. In countries with poor sanitation, viral hepatitis has a high incidence. In a few, it assumes a fulminant form, causing liver failure, particularly in pregnant women. Some herbal toxins also cause acute liver failure. The outlook is grave, but full recovery without permanent liver damage is possible if the patient is treated with intravenous glucose solutions, neomycin (1 gm orally every 6 hours to sterilize the gut), and laxatives or lactulose and is protected from secondary infection. Intravenous cimetidine may diminish gastrointestinal bleeding, a frequent complication in these patients.

Chronic liver damage by cirrhosis is a common cause of hepatic coma and may be initiated by hemorrhage, alcohol consumption, infection, hypovolemia and electrolyte imbalance due to diarrhea, too-aggressive use of diuretics, or excessive removal of ascitic fluid. Mental changes, flapping tremor, and fetor hepaticus are danger signals in these patients. Precipitating causes need to be corrected and treatment for hepatic coma started.

HYPOGLYCEMIA. Patients in the tropics may be particularly liable to hypoglycemia owing to malnutrition and liver damage, which cause low hepatic glycogen stores. They also have difficulty obtaining emergency treatment. Common causes of hypoglycemia include (1) alcoholic intoxication; (2) viral hepatitis and hepatoma; (3) excessive insulin therapy for diabetics, who may have irregular food intake and energy output; (4) the vomiting sickness of Jamaica caused by the unripe akee fruit that contains hypoglycin A and B; (5) acute falci-

parum malaria; and (6) protein-energy malnutrition. A high index of suspicion is necessary in patients with these problems, and intravenous glucose should be given promptly if hypoglycemia is likely.

REYE'S SYNDROME. An encephalopathy with fatty degeneration of the liver is increasingly being recognized in children. It is a significant cause of death where its association with aflatoxin and administration of acetylsalicylic acid has been established. There is an acute onset, with vomiting, convulsions, coma, and decerebrate posturing. Pallor, hypoxia, hepatomegaly, hypoglycemia, elevated blood ammonia, and abnormal results on liver function tests also occur. Progressive coma and death ensue in many; survivors may have mental retardation, paralyses, and seizures. Intensive care with correction of hypoglycemia, acidosis, hypoxia, and electrolyte imbalance improves the outlook.

CENTRAL NERVOUS SYSTEM (CNS) INFECTIONS

Syndromes associated with infections of the CNS include acute encephalitis, acute meningitis (Chapter 43), chronic meningoencephalitis, and brain abscess. Important points in differentiating these syndromes are changes in mental status, the presence or absence of nuchal rigidity, and pleocytosis of the cerebrospinal fluid (CSF). Fever with the relevant symptoms and signs suggests an infectious etiology.

ACUTE ENCEPHALITIS. Acute encephalitis implies inflammation of the brain, which can be accompanied by meningeal inflammation. Viruses are often responsible, and pathologically they produce chromatolysis of neurons followed by necrosis and neuronophagia, microglial proliferation (Fig. 21–6), perivascular inflammation (Figs. 21–1 and 21–5), and inclusion bodies in nerve (Fig. 21–2) or glial cells.

Acute encephalitis usually begins as a nonspecific, febrile illness followed by involvement of the central nervous system, with increasing headache, mental disturbance, and sometimes delirium. Drowsiness, coma, and seizures may ensue. Focal pyramidal and brain stem disturbances and hyperpyrexia sometimes occur. If the meninges are involved, nuchal rigidity will be present. Permanent disabilities, e.g., mental retardation and spasticity, are not infrequent. Differentiation from bacterial meningitis by lumbar puncture is essential. In viral

TABLE 8–2. Common Causes of Acute Confusional State (Acute Organic Brain Syndrome) in Adults

Systemic Disorders	Intracranial Disorders
Alcohol ingestion	Purulent meningitis
Hypoglycemia (often associated with alcohol ingestion)	Head injury (post-traumatic states)
Lobar pneumonia	Cerebral malaria
Hemorrhage or shock with peripheral circulatory failure	Encephalitis
Typhoid fever	Subdural hematoma
Renal failure	Cerebrovascular accident
Hepatic failure	Epilepsy (postictal state)
Hypovitaminosis	

encephalitis, there may be very few, and sometimes no, cells in the CSF. In viral meningitis, there is usually an increase in CSF protein concentration and lymphocytes (10 to 1000 cells/mm³), but the glucose content is normal (50 to 75 mg/dl).

Important causes of encephalitis in the tropics include arboviruses (Chapter 21), poliomyelitis (Chapter 18.1), cerebral malaria (Chapter 73), rabies (Chapter 21.1) and African and American trypanosomiasis (Chapters 74 and 75). An acute encephalitic state with seizures is often due to cerebral malaria and, less frequently, to relapsing fever (Chapter 34). Sometimes, infections with helminths may involve the brain and cause acute encephalitis. This may occur in trichinosis (Chapter 90), cysticercosis (Chapter 101.1), and toxocariasis (Chapter 91), and, rarely, after treatment of onchocerciasis (Chapter 87) or loiasis (Chapter 86) with diethylcarbamazine. *Angiostrongylus cantonensis* causes eosinophilic meningitis (Chapter 93.1).

All the postinfectious or postvaccination types are also found in the tropics. Measles is widespread and virulent, and encephalitis sometimes ensues (Chapter 16.1); vaccination at 9 months of age is now part of the worldwide program of expanded immunization against the major childhood infections (poliomyelitis, tetanus, whooping cough, diphtheria, tuberculosis), but there are major problems of cost and cold storage. Encephalomyelitis and peripheral neuropathy following vaccination against rabies using the Semple type vaccine may be as frequent as 1 in 500. Neurologic complications would disappear if human diploid cell vaccine were in universal use.

CHRONIC MENINGOENCEPHALITIS. Chronic meningoencephalitis is characterized by a gradual evolution and relentless progression over weeks, months, or years. The earliest symptoms are usually intellectual deterioration progressing to organic dementia, affective changes (particularly depression), and headache. Motor and sensory changes, tremors, convulsions, and urinary and fecal incontinence appear in the course of the disease; disturbances of consciousness and, finally, coma are terminal signs. The CSF usually shows increased protein and lymphocytic cells. In areas where African trypanosomiasis (Chapter 74) exists, it must be considered the most common cause of chronic meningoencephalitis, and lumbar puncture must be performed. In kuru, now almost extinct because abolition of cannibalism has interrupted the transmission of the disease among the Fore-speaking people of New Guinea (Part II, General Principles), there is predominantly cerebellar symptomatology in the early stages, followed by mental changes and death in a few months; the CSF is normal. General paresis, a form of neurosyphilis, is a chronic meningoencephalitis resulting in gradual but progressive loss of cortical function, leading to organic dementia (Chapter 32.1). Fortunately, it is a rare complication of syphilis, meningovascular neurosyphilis being more common in the tropics. Subacute sclerosing panencephalitis, a sequela to measles infection characterized by psychomotor and developmental deterioration, myoclonus, and periodic EEG changes, is rare in tropical Africa despite the high prevalence of measles.

INTRACRANIAL TUMORS AND SPACE-OCCUPYING LESIONS

Signs and symptoms of raised intracranial pressure, e.g., headache, vomiting, and diminished vision; progressive focal neurologic signs; mental changes, including dementia; epilepsy; and endocrine changes due to pituitary or hypothalamic involvement are characteristic of CNS space-occupying lesions. Intracranial neoplasms have not been extensively investigated in many areas of the tropics because of a lack of neurosurgical facilities and postmortem examinations but are probably as common as in temperate regions. Meningiomas may be relatively more common and gliomas less common in Africa than in Europe and North America. Tuberculomas may account for up to 10% of cerebral tumors diagnosed in the tropics, detection being aided by their intracranial calcification (Chapter 61). Pituitary tumors are relatively easily diagnosed when simple radiology is available. The possibility of a brain abscess, a hydatid cyst, or a hematoma should always be seriously considered as a nonmalignant cause of intracranial masses.

BRAIN ABSCESS. This may be more common than in temperate climates because of the frequency of neglected otitis media and chronic suppurative lung disease in the tropics. The symptoms and signs of cerebral tumor are present, but these evolve rapidly over days rather than weeks. Drowsiness is seen at an early state, and signs of infection such as fever and leukocytosis are found but may not be prominent. A primary source of sepsis in ears, lungs, paranasal sinuses, or heart valves is found in over 70% of patients. A brain abscess may present as meningitis secondary to rupture into the subarachnoid space. The role of anaerobic bacteria has been emphasized, and metronidazole has been employed in treatment in conjunction with antibiotics and surgery. In Europe and the United States, neurosurgical drainage and abscess removal after accurate localization by computed axial tomography (CAT) has improved the gloomy prognosis. Prolonged chemotherapy and drainage may be required when this advanced technology is not available.

PARASITIC LESIONS OF THE CNS. Parasitic infections may present as intracranial masses (sometimes progressing rapidly), as focal or generalized epilepsy, as acute encephalopathies, or as organic dementia (Table 8–3). In the spinal cord, paraplegia due to cord compression or a transverse myelitis is the usual presentation. Diagnosis may be difficult, because although a space-occupying lesion is suspected from radiographic studies, the parasitic nature may not be revealed until exploratory operation. Parasitic infection elsewhere in the body, positive serologic tests, and eosinophilia may be helpful diagnostic clues. Surgery is usually the treatment, but sometimes, as in cysticercosis, the cysts are multiple and inoperable. Specific drugs generally are not useful, but in suspected schistosomiasis of the brain or spinal cord (Chapter 96) or amebic brain abscess (Chapter 68), schistosomicidal or amebicidal drugs should be given as soon as the diagnosis is made. Mebendazole and albendazole have been used in treating hydatid disease, and praziquantel is efficacious in treating cere-

TABLE 8–3. Parasitic Diseases Causing Lesions in the Nervous System

Disease	Parasite	Remarks
Amebic brain abscess	*Entamoeba histolytica*	Cerebral abscess—rare, usually fatal.
Primary amebic meningoencephalitis	*Naegleria* or *Acanthamoeba* species	Meningitis due to free-living ameba. Probable infection via nose while bathing—usually fatal.
Trypanosomiasis	*Trypanosoma gambiense/rhodesiense*	Encephalitis
Trichinosis	*Trichinella spiralis*	Epilepsy (usually) and encephalitis (sometimes) with focal features.
Angiostrongyliasis	*Angiostrongylus cantonensis*	Eosinophilic meningitis, granulomatous lesions in brain.
Gnathostomiasis	*Gnathostoma spinigerum*	Cerebral and cord lesions, and eosinophilic meningitis.
Schistosomiasis	*Schistosoma japonicum* *Schistosoma mansoni*	Epilepsy: CNS granulomas. Transverse myelitis, spinal cord granulomas, and anterior spinal arteritis—uncommon.
Paragonimiasis	*Paragonimus westermani*	Epilepsy. CNS granulomas (3%).
Cysticercosis	*Taenia solium*	Multiple cerebral cysts. Epilepsy is most common manifestation; may cause organic dementia, hydrocephalus, or focal signs.
Hydatid disease	*Echinococcus granulosus*	Space-occupying lesions in brain or spinal cord (2%).
Dracontiasis	*Dracunculus medinensis*	Cord compression due to extradural location—rare.
Coenuriasis	*Coenurus cerebralis*	Cerebral tumor—rare, usually fatal. Cord compression, paraplegia—rare.

bral cysticercosis (Chapter 101.1) and paragonimiasis (Chapter 99).

HEAD INJURY AND INTRACRANIAL HEMATOMA. Head injury is frequent in the tropics. In many places, automobile and motorcycle accidents are the main cause, but assault and falls, e.g., from coconut trees, are also common. Subdural hematoma must be considered in coma and "stroke," for a history of injury may not be obtained. Head injury is a significant cause of epilepsy in the tropics.

COMA

The diagnosis and management of coma are basically the same worldwide. However, the usual causes of coma are rather different in many parts of the tropics (Table 8–4).

It is important to diagnose inflammatory conditions of the nervous system by examination of the CSF and to consider cerebral malaria, as specific therapy can be crucial.

EPILEPSY

Epilepsy is a significant medicosocial problem in developing countries. It is more common than in developed countries; estimates of the prevalence of chronic epilepsy vary from 5 to 40 per 1000 population. Birth injuries due to primitive midwifery, residua of repeated febrile convulsions, meningitis, encephalitis, and parasitic infections partially explain the increased prevalence of chronic epilepsy. Febrile convulsions are frequent because of the great number of febrile illnesses, including malaria, suffered by children in the tropics. Prolonged febrile convulsions may lead to permanent neurologic damage and chronic epilepsy. Severe and prolonged convulsions should be treated with anticonvulsants (i.e., diazepam, phenobarbital, or paraldehyde) and by cold sponging and antipyretics. Children under 18 months of age with recurrent febrile convulsions in whom antipyretic measures fail to prevent seizures should be given at least a year's treatment with phenobarbital or valproic acid, although it has been established that the adverse effects of phenobarbital on cognition may outlast by several months the period of administration of the drug. Cerebral malaria and meningitis must be considered as possible causes of febrile convulsions.

Sufferers from epilepsy in tropical countries have serious social difficulties. Ignorance, prejudice, and erroneous beliefs about the nature of the illness lead to exclusion from school, loss of marriage prospects, and even divorce. Epilepsy is sometimes believed to be due to bewitchment or diabolic possession and is considered infectious by breath, saliva, or flatus. Thus, there is concealment of the illness, recourse to traditional healers, social isolation, and depression. Treatment is often sporadic, increasing the danger of status epilepticus. Burns from falling on open fires are a particular hazard. Management is often difficult because of the lack of drugs and the patient's inability to appreciate the need for prolonged treatment. Repeated explanations to the patient and the relatives are necessary to obtain cooperation.

CEREBROVASCULAR DISEASE

Cerebrovascular disease (CVD) is becoming as prevalent as in developed countries and is now a leading cause of mortality and morbidity in developing countries. Indeed, it is said to be the most common certified cause of death in Jamaican adults, accounting for 12% of all deaths in those over 15 years of age. There are fewer older people (with increased risk of CVD) in the tropics, but in many areas, such as West Africa, the West Indies, and Southeast Asia, hypertension is prevalent and predisposes to CVD. Although hypertension

TABLE 8–4. Causes of Coma in the Tropics, with Incidence in the Tropics Compared with That in Temperature Regions

More Common	As Common	Less Common
Cerebral malaria	Diabetic ketoacidosis	Sedative
Bacterial meningitis	Hypoglycemia	intoxication
Arbovirus encephalitis	Uremia	
Hepatic failure	Alcohol poisoning	
Hyperpyrexia	Head injury	
Poisoning with	Cerebrovascular	
insecticides	accident	
Trypanosomiasis		

is the most important factor, diabetes mellitus is also a contributor.

Rheumatic heart disease is extremely common in the tropics; severe cardiac valvular involvement occurs at an early stage and causes cerebral emboli (Chapter 2), as do tropical cardiomyopathies and Chagas' disease (Chapter 75). Nonembolic ischemic cerebrovascular disease is the most common variety of CVD. The following are frequently observed in CVD in the tropics: (1) Hemorrhage strokes occur in young people with hypertension. (2) Cerebrovascular occlusions and subarachnoid hemorrhage are complications of sickle cell disease. (3) Arteriovenous congenital malformations are more common than berry aneurysms as the cause of subarachnoid hemorrhage in Malaysia and Thailand. (4) In Japan and areas of Southeast Asia, an aortic arch syndrome known as Takayasu's arteritis, or pulseless disease, is a cause of cerebral infarction (Chapter 2). (5) Meningovascular syphilis is a significant cause of ischemic CVD in some parts of the tropics (Chapter 32.1). (6) Malignant trophoblastic disease in women of childbearing age is a great imitator of stroke and may, in fact, present as cerebral hemorrhage.

The best way to prevent CVD is to detect and treat hypertension. The relatively high incidence of CVD in tropical Africa exists in parallel with a relatively low incidence of coronary heart disease.

NEUROLOGIC COMPLICATIONS OF HEMOGLOBINOPATHIES. In those diseases in which the erythrocytes sickle under hypoxic conditions, the central nervous system may be affected by microcirculatory obstruction and profound anemia (Chapter 5). Neurologic disturbances may be precipitated by crisis, childbirth, blood transfusion, or general anesthesia. Lesions found at autopsy include diffuse microcirculatory stasis, large vessel obstruction, dural sinus thrombosis, pericapillary hemorrhages, subarachnoid hemorrhage, and subdural hematoma.

Patients in crisis may be mentally disturbed, and the EEG often shows generalized abnormalities even when there are no overt neuropsychiatric symptoms. There may be drowsiness proceeding to coma, meningismus, and convulsions. Less commonly, hemiparesis due to vascular occlusion, subarachnoid hemorrhage, paraparesis, and cranial nerve palsies occur. Patients with hemoglobin SS disease are susceptible to pneumococcal meningitis because of depressed immune responses; polyvalent pneumococcal vaccine may be given prophylactically. Sudden blindness due to occlusion of the central artery of the retina is rare; chronic retinopathy is more common.

Patients with major thalassemia syndromes have an increased prevalence of strokes, convulsions, recurrent focal cerebral ischemia, and proximal myopathy.

CRANIAL NERVE DISORDERS

OPTIC ATROPHY. The etiology of optic atrophy is often obscure, with the disorder being referred to as tropical nutritional amblyopia. Occasionally, there is some improvement in the early stages after treatment with B complex vitamins. It may be associated with tropical ataxic neuropathy, beriberi, and pellagra. Bilateral retrobulbar neuritis is seen in Nigeria and may be associated with transverse myelitis (the syndrome of neuromyelitis optica), although multiple sclerosis is rare. Other causes of optic atrophy are meningitis, trypanosomiasis, onchocerciasis, syphilis, epidemic dropsy due to argemone oil, and methanol poisoning resulting from illicit alcohol production. Drugs used in the tropics that occasionally cause optic atrophy include quinine, chloramphenicol, isoniazid, para-aminosalicylic acid, and tryparsamide.

OPHTHALMOPLEGIA. A self-limiting, painful ophthalmoplegic syndrome of unknown etiology with an acute onset, spontaneous remission, and a tendency to recur has been described from parts of the tropics, including India, Zimbabwe, and West Africa. It responds to steroid therapy and must be differentiated from ophthalmoplegia due to berry aneurysms. The syndrome has been reported from temperate climates but appears to be more common in tropical areas. Elapid snakebites can cause ptosis and ophthalmoplegia, the former being an early sign of envenomation, requiring treatment with antivenin (Chapter 103.5).

FACIAL NERVE PARALYSIS. Lower motor neuron paralysis is usually due to Bell's palsy; middle ear disease and diabetes should be considered as well.

EIGHTH NERVE DISTURBANCES. Nerve deafness may follow pyogenic (Chapter 43) and tuberculous (Chapter 61) meningitis and may accompany tropical ataxic neuropathy. Meniere's disease is rarely seen in tropical countries, but vestibular neuronitis is not uncommon. Hearing loss may follow the use of quinine, chloroquine (in large doses), aminoglycoside antibiotics, and furosemide.

MISCELLANEOUS. Acute bulbar palsy may be due to poliomyelitis (Chapter 18.1), diphtheria (Chapter 57), or elapid snakebite (Chapter 103.5). Nasopharyngeal carcinoma is common in Malaysia, Hong Kong, and parts of Kenya and sometimes causes multiple lower cranial nerve paralyses (Chapter 11). Trigeminal neuralgia is rare in most tropical countries. Burkitt's lymphomas can cause polyneuritis cranialis (Chapter 11).

SPINAL CORD DISEASE

Paraparesis and tetraparesis are the most common manifestations of spinal cord disease. They may be of gradual or sudden onset and may be associated with sphincter disturbances, sensory changes, and radicular, motor, and sensory signs. The prognosis is often poor because of late presentation, pressure scores, urinary infections, and lack of specialized medical facilities. The common causes of spinal cord syndrome are tuberculous osteitis, intra–spinal canal neoplasms, tropical "nutritional" myelopathy, myelopathy associated with retroviral infections (human T-cell lymphotrophic virus-1, human immunodeficiency virus) (Chapter 15), trauma, and spondylitic myelopathy.

TUBERCULOSIS OF THE SPINE. This is a leading cause of paraplegia of subacute or insidious onset. A spinal deformity is usually obvious, but occasionally *Mycobacterium tuberculosis* involves the spinal cord meninges without bone involvement and causes an arachnoiditis (Chapter 61).

TRAUMA TO THE SPINE. This often occurs in automobile and motorcycle accidents. Falling out of trees while gathering coconuts is a tropical hazard. Falls while carrying heavy loads on the head sometimes cause paraplegia with injury at the C4–C5 level.

OTHER CAUSES. Burkitt's lymphoma is the most common childhood malignancy in tropical Africa and often causes either paraplegia due to involvement of the spinal cord or a meningoencephalitis. Other tumors causing paraplegia are neurofibroma, meningioma, schwannoma, ependymoma, astrocytoma, and ganglioneuroma. Neuroplastic involvement of the cord may be secondary to primary lesions in the prostate, breast, thyroid, or liver or to Hodgkin's lymphoma or multiple myeloma. Neuromyelitis optica with paraplegia is sometimes found, although, as stated, multiple sclerosis is a rarity. Transverse myelitis has been associated with

Schistosoma mansoni infection (Chapter 96), and *Gnathostoma spinigerum* can cause an eosinophilic myeloencephalitis with pain and paralysis (Chapter 92). Fluorosis may cause spinal cord compression in parts of India (Chapter 108.3), and congenital atlantoaxial dislocation with quadriplegia is mysteriously frequent in India, Sri Lanka, and Thailand. Less common causes of spinal cord disease include epidural abscess, cysticercosis, dermoid cyst, and *Histoplasm duboisii* infection in Africa.

TROPICAL ATAXIC NEUROPATHY/MYELOPATHY. A myeloneuropathy resembling the syndrome first described among Jamaicans at the end of the nineteenth century has been reported from most parts of Africa including Nigeria, Senegal, Kenya, Uganda, and Natal. The syndrome includes myelopathy with or without visual and hearing impairment. Because ataxia is prominent, the disorder is often referred to as tropical ataxic neuropathy (Fig. 8–1). In Nigeria, Tanzania, and Mozambique, strong circumstantial evidence has accrued in the last three decades suggesting that the syndrome of tropical ataxic neuropathy is causally related to chronic cyanide intoxication of dietary origin, riboflavin deficiency, and possible low plasma ceruloplasmin levels. Epidemics of spastic paraparesis linked to cassava cyanide poison have been described in Tanzania, Mozambique, and Zaire.

The syndrome of tropical ataxic neuropathy (TAN) comprises myelopathy with predominant involvement of the posterior columns, bilateral optic atrophy, perceptive deafness, and symmetric peripheral polyneuropathy, with evidence of more diffuse degenerative lesions in the neuraxis consisting of cerebellar degeneration,

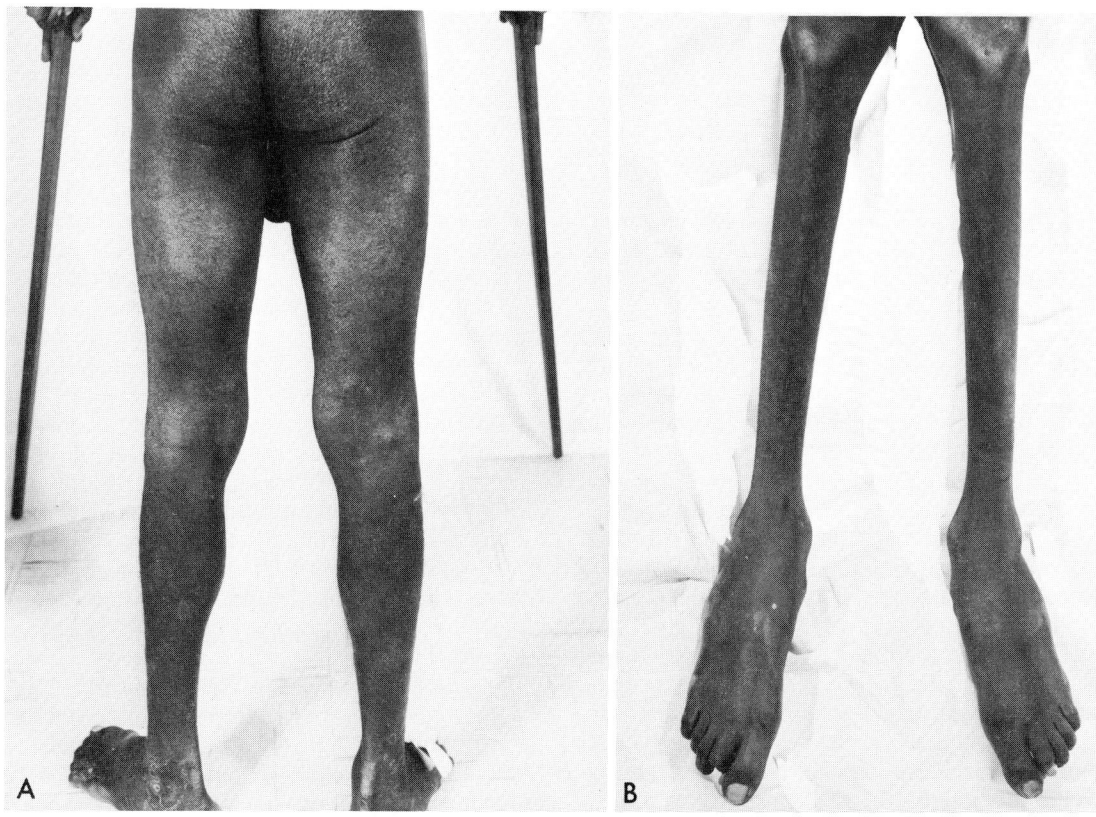

FIGURE 8–1. *A* and *B,* Patient with ataxic neuropathy.

parkinsonism, motor neuron disease, dementia, and schizophreniform psychosis in various combinations. The cerebrospinal fluid is normal. The disease affects all age groups and the sexes equally but is rare in the first decade of life. Familial cases accounted for 40% of patients in one series, but there was no evidence of genetically determined predisposition. Patients subsisted mainly on a cassava diet, and the cyanide content of food items of cassava derivatives was high. Plasma levels of thiocyanate (a detoxification product of cyanide) and cyanide and urinary thiocyanate excretion were high. The levels fell when the patients were fed on a hospital diet low in cassava and rose again when they reverted to cassava meals. Levels of free cyanide in blood were raised. Sulphur-containing amino acids were absent in the plasma of 60% of the patients and were greatly reduced in others. The levels of serum and tissue (hepatic) cyanocobalamin (another product of cyanide detoxification) were high. Total serum and hepatic B_{12} levels were normal, however.

Neuroepidemiologic studies in Nigeria showed correlation of the prevalence of the disease with the intensity of cassava cultivation, frequency of cassava meals, and plasma thiocyanate levels. Those who handled cassava roots, such as cassava farmers and processors, appeared to have the highest risk of developing the disease.

Cassava diet has been incriminated as a cause of some form of diabetes mellitus in young people in the tropics. The evidence is tenuous. No increase in frequency of glucose intolerance or diabetes mellitus has been seen in the cassava-associated TAN.

Some tropical staple foods contain cyanogenetic glycosides, particularly cassava (manioc) but also sorghum, maize, and millet. These neuropathic syndromes occur particularly, but not exclusively, in individuals whose main diet consists of cassava. The actual intake of cyanogens depends on methods of cooking and preparation. Soaking the root and discarding the water markedly lowers cyanogen content, as does pressing it into a farina.

Tropical ataxic neuropathy is not explained by cyanide poisoning in all areas; vitamin deficiencies may play a part. The prognosis for complete recovery is poor. Treatment with vitamin B12 and other B vitamins has not been beneficial. If possible, the patient should stop eating cassava or at least should receive instructions on the safest way of preparing it. Smoking and alcohol may increase cyanide sensitivity and should be prohibited in these patients. Prevention involves replacement of cassava as a staple, ensuring proper preparation of the root drop, and cultivating strains with a low cyanide content. Early detection of minimal neuropathy may enable dietetic correction and prevention of serious disease.

Tropical Spastic Paraparesis. Throughout the tropics, geographic isolates of another type of spinal cord syndrome have been described and referred to as tropical spastic paraparesis (TSP). Clusters of the disease have been reported in many countries, including islands in the Caribbean, Colombia, the Seychelles, Ivory Coast, Senegal, and Ethiopia. The disorder is characterized by chronic spastic myelopathy of slow onset and progression accompanied initially by lumbalgias, foot dysesthesias, increased urinary frequency, and constipation. The predominant pyramidal tract involvement leads to spastic gait with hyperreflexia and Babinski sign. The syndrome is now established as causally related to human T-cell lymphocytic virus-1 (HTLV-I), an association first reported from Martinique and subsequently well documented among the Japanese (Chapter 15.3). CSF pleocytosis and elevated protein are present in 15% to 40% of patients. HTLV-I virus has been isolated from the CSF. It is distinguished from cassava-induced TAN, in which spasticity is less obvious and perceptive deafness and optic atrophy are more frequently present. Acute-onset HTLV-I–associated myelopathy following blood transfusion HTLV-I infection, HTLV-I–associated subacute meningoencephalitis, and polymyositis are also known to occur. HTLV-I–associated myelopathy may be associated with adult T-cell leukemia, vasculitis, uveitis, pulmonary alveolitis, monoclonal gammopathy, Sjögren's syndrome, and cryoglobulinemia.

Myelopathy Associated with Human Immunodeficiency Virus (HIV). HIV-associated myelopathy is characterized neuropathologically by vacuolar demyelination resembling subacute combined degeneration of vitamin B12 deficiency (Chapter 15.1). Although it may occur alone, it is often associated with HIV dementia or the HIV-associated minor cognitive motor syndrome. The latter is characterized by symptoms and signs such as forgetfulness, slowness of thinking, reduced concentration, gait and hand clumsiness, and slowness of psychomotor response. In HIV-associated dementia, psychomotor slowing, apathy, and impaired memory are severe enough to interfere with social and occupational functioning and positive frontal release signs (snout, sucking, grasp, palmomental reflexes) may be present. The frequency of HIV-associated myelopathy in patients with the AIDS syndrome may be as high as 20%. Symptoms and signs predominate in the lower limbs, but the upper limbs may be involved. There is usually no sensory level. Myelography (a spinal MRI and CT where available) is normal. CSF abnormalities include mononuclear pleocytosis, raised protein concentration, and HIV isolation. Table 8–5 shows that the range of neuropsychiatric manifestations in HIV infection is protean.

Obscure Tropical Paraplegias. The cause of as much as 20% of paraplegias in the tropics remains obscure. These cases are labeled tropical spastic paraplegia. Many of these cases progress, and many become arrested, but few improve. The disease is usually of insidious onset, afflicting individuals below the age of 40 years and presenting as spastic paraparesis with or without "posterior column" deficit. Many cases have normal myelography and are unrelated to retroviral infections, probably representing an autoimmune mechanism. In some patients, adhesions around the cord are detected radiologically or found at operation. This is known as adhesive arachnoiditis.

Spinal Cord Adhesive Arachnoiditis. This condition is common in parts of India, Sri Lanka, the West Indies, South America, and Africa. It is seen in Europe but is rare and diminishing in incidence. The patient has a subacute or chronic transverse myelitis or ascending radiculomyopathy. There may be paralysis, paresthesias,

TABLE 8–5. Neuropsychiatric Associations with Human Immunodeficiency Virus Infection

HIV-Associated Cognitive Motor Complex
HIV-1–associated dementia
HIV-1–associated myelopathy
HIV-1–associated minor cognitive motor syndrome

HIV-Associated Mental and Behavioral Disorders
Delirium
Acute psychotic disorders
Affective disorders
Adjustment disorders
Acute stress reactions
Suicide

Other HIV-Associated CNS Disorders
Progressive encephalopathy of childhood
Meningitis (aseptic)

HIV-Associated Peripheral Nervous System Disorders
Inflammatory polyneuropathy
Predominantly sensory neuropathy
Myopathy

Neuropsychiatric Disorders due to Opportunistic Processes in HIV-Infected Subjects
Progressive multifocal leukoencephalopathy
Cerebral toxoplasmosis
Cryptococcal meningitis
Cytomegalovirus encephalopathy
Cytomegalovirus neuropathy
CNS tuberculosis
Herpes zoster/simplex encephalitis
Varicella zoster radiculitis
Other syndromes due to opportunistic infections
Primary CNS lymphoma

bladder disturbances, muscle wasting, and sensory root pain. In rare cases, ascending paralysis leads to respiratory paralysis. The CSF shows an elevated protein level and minimal pleocytosis. There may be a spinal block syndrome. Myelography shows filling defects, fragmentation of the dye, or a total block over several segments. The etiology is usually unknown, but some cases are due to tuberculosis or syphilis, and some follow pyogenic meningitis, trauma, spinal anesthesia, or the intrathecal injection of radiopaque dyes for myelography. Laminectomy is often necessary to confirm the diagnosis and exclude tumor. Division of adhesions or decompression rarely benefits the patient. Any suspicion of schistosomiasis as a cause of paraplegia should lead to prompt chemotherapy.

Lathyrism. Lathyrism is a spastic paraplegia associated with the consumption of large amounts (e.g., 200 to 300 gm) of the chickpea *Lathyrus sativus*. The toxic factor in the pea is an unusual amino acid, β-oxalyl-aminoalanine. This substance can be destroyed by boiling in a large volume of water or by parboiling before cooking. Heavy consumption of the chickpea takes place during severe food shortages, and lathyrism has occurred in India, Algeria, and Ethiopia. In lathyrism, there is fairly sudden onset of an upper motor neuron type of paralysis of the legs, which is usually permanent. At autopsy, demyelination of the lateral spinal cord is found. No specific therapy is known.

DISEASES OF PERIPHERAL NERVES

In a large proportion of cases of peripheral neuropathy (30% to 60%), no specific etiology is found. How-

ever, the common causes include leprosy, nutritional deficiencies, Guillain-Barré syndrome, metabolic and toxic conditions (especially diabetes mellitus), drugs, and trauma. As a nosologic entity, leprosy is the most common cause of neuropathy in the world, affecting 15 million people, most of them resident in the tropics (Chapter 62). In certain areas, neuropathy is widespread and associated with malnutrition and exposure to toxic factors. There are many classifications of peripheral neuropathy. Asbury described five main patterns according to the clinical features. Some diseases, e.g., diabetes, appear in more than one pattern.

SYNDROME OF ACUTE ASCENDING MOTOR PARALYSIS WITH VARIABLE DISTURBANCE OF SENSORY FUNCTION. Acute idiopathic polyneuritis (Landry's syndrome, Guillain-Barré syndrome) may follow viral or bacterial infection. Death results in 10 to 15% of patients owing to respiratory paralysis. Vital capacity should be monitored and respiratory assistance given if it falls below 1 L in an adult. Rarely, the syndrome follows viral hepatitis or diphtheria. Plasma exchange, where the facilities are available, is now accepted as efficacious in treament of the Guillain-Barré syndrome if the patient is seen early and the disease severe enough to warrant respiratory assistance. Acute motor paralysis has also occurred following exposure to triorthocresyl phosphate, sometimes a contaminant of cooking oil in the tropics, e.g., in Morocco.

SYNDROME OF SUBACUTE SENSORIMOTOR PARALYSIS. When symmetric, this is often associated with calf tenderness and absent deep tendon reflexes. In the tropics, this may be due to alcoholism or beriberi (Chapter 107.2), may be associated with pellagra, or may occur following shigellosis or typhoid fever. Certain drugs, e.g., isoniazid, dapsone, nitrofurantoin, and nitrofurazone, can also be responsible. The incidence of diabetes is increasing in the tropics and is often undiagnosed or poorly controlled. It is a leading cause of this syndrome, and neuropathy is sometimes asymmetric.

SYNDROME OF CHRONIC SENSORIMOTOR POLYNEUROPATHY. Tropical ataxic neuropathy, leprosy, uremia, beriberi, and diabetes are acquired causes of this syndrome. Carcinomatous neuropathic syndromes are reported less often in the tropics than in temperate zones, partly because of the low incidence of carcinoma of the bronchus. Genetic causes are rare but include peroneal muscular atrophy.

SYNDROME OF CHRONIC RELAPSING POLY-NEUROPATHY. This is rare but may respond to corticosteroids; acute intermittent porphyria is rare, but porphyria cutanea tarda is not uncommon in South Africa and may be associated with a neuropathy.

SYNDROME OF MONONEUROPATHY OR MULTIPLE NEUROPATHIES. Pressure neuropathies include a radial palsy following drunken slumber. Cervical and lumbar disk root pressure due to prolapsed intervertebral disks is diagnosed less often than in developed countries. Leprosy causes inflammatory destruction of individual nerves, such as the ulnar and median nerves (Chapter 62).

Adverse reactions to drugs include polyneuropathies.

Among the drugs commonly used in the tropics that can cause nerve damage are quinine, chloroquine, isoniazid, metronidazole, clioquinol (Entero-Vioform), phenytoin, arsenicals, streptomycin, para-aminosalicylic acid, ethambutol, and pentamidine. Intramuscular quinine injections have caused sciatic palsies by local damage.

THE BURNING FEET SYNDROME. The burning feet syndrome is a distressing affliction that occurs in the nutritional, alcoholic, and drug-induced (isoniazid) and diabetic neuropathies; in the sensory neuropathies associated with HIV infection; and, often, in patients without any objective signs of peripheral nerve dysfunction. The pathogenesis of pain in the peripheral neuropathies is not well understood. Pain may occur when the degeneration affects predominantly the large fibers in the peripheral nerves subserving modalities of proprioception (vibration, joint position sense), which should predispose to pain or dysesthesia, as well as the small fibers subserving perception of pain. Pain in diabetic neuropathies may diminish with normalization and stabilization of blood glucose levels, as hyperglycemia is a major factor in the pathogenesis of pain. The use of sorbinil (an aldose reductase inhibitor that theoretically should lower tissue sorbitol concentration by inhibiting conversion of glucose to sorbitol) may, or may not, relieve pain. Drugs beneficial in the symptomatic treatment of painful neuropathies include imipramine, carbamazepine, phenytoin, and intravenous lidocaine (5 mg/kg body weight), which may bring relief of pain for 3 to 21 days after a single injection. Recently, mexiletine, an analogue of lidocaine (which can be given by mouth 150 mg daily for 3 days, then 300 mg daily for 3 days, then 10 mg/kg body weight daily), was found to be efficacious in treatment of chronic painful diabetic neuropathy.

Anecdotal reports regarding the beneficial effects in herpetic neuralgia and the painful neuropathy of HIV infection of a cream containing 0.075% capsaicin (trans-8-methyl-N-vanillyl-6-nonenamide) have been made. Capsaicin is a naturally occurring substance derived from plants of the family Solanaceae that apparently selectively affects unmyelinated C sensory fibers. It has no effect on discriminatory senses such as touch, pressure, or vibration at the site of application. It causes a release and subsequent depletion of substance P, thereby impeding the conduction and transmission of peripheral pain impulses.

PRIMARY MUSCLE DISEASES

PYOMYOSITIS. Muscle diseases are not uncommon (Table 8–6). The most common type is pyomyositis, widely reported in tropical Africa (Chapter 58). It affects young adults; the abscesses are either intra- or intermuscular and may be multiple. Staphylococci and coliforms are the organisms most frequently isolated. The muscle groups usually involved are the quadriceps femoris, hamstrings, gastrocnemii, erector spinae, latissimus dorsi, and trapezius. Treatment with drainage and antibiotics achieves cure in about 95% of cases.

OTHER CAUSES. Of the genetic myopathies, Du-

TABLE 8–6. Etiology of Primary Muscle Diseases as Seen in Ibadan, Nigeria

Disease	No. of Cases	Percentages
Pyomyositis	372	67.5
Genetic	76	13.8
Duchenne type	31	
Limb-girdle	28	
Facioscapulohumeral	12	
Dystrophia myotonica	5	
Polymyositis/dermatomyositis	60	10.9
Myasthenia gravis	32	5.8
Other*	11	2.0
Total	551	100.0

*Includes thyrotoxic, hypocalcemic and McArdle's myopathy in 6, 4, and 1 cases, respectively.

From Osuntokun BO: J Neurol Sci 12:417, 1971. Reprinted by permission.

chenne, limb-girdle, facioscapulohumeral, and dystrophia myotonica are the types commonly seen. Autoimmune disease is rarely reported in Africans; however, polymyositis is occasionally encountered, and, like migraine, it shows a female preponderance. It may be associated with lymphoma, rheumatoid arthritis, multiple myeloma, and retroviral infections.

PSYCHIATRIC DISEASE IN THE TROPICS

There are relatively few psychiatrists and mental hospitals in the tropics, and the general physician has to cope with many psychiatric problems. It is probable that psychiatric disease is as big a problem in the tropics as in temperate zones. Mental oddity is well tolerated in most simple farming communities, and there is often good family support for the mentally ill. Mental illness is often attributed to supernatural influences or witchcraft, and therefore, traditional healers are consulted rather than "Western medicine men."

Schizophrenia is probably as common as in Europe but may have a better prognosis because of better family support. Depressive illness often presents with somatic symptoms. Failure to have children often causes depression in women, who complain of abdominal pains. Acute, agitated, transient hallucinatory states are sometimes precipitated by fear of bewitchment. Recovery frequently occurs after sedation for a few days. Organic causes are frequently responsible for acute psychotic states and must always be excluded. Neurosis is perhaps more common in urban dwellers and students than in farmers, and societies in a state of rapid social change with increasing urbanization are subject to considerable mental stress. On migration to the town, there may be unemployment, loss of family support, and unfulfilled aspirations. New ideas and concepts are thrust upon the individual, and the conflicts with ingrained beliefs can be traumatic. Students are under great pressure to succeed and thus often develop tension headache, inability to concentrate, poor memory, and reduced visual acuity—the West African brain fag syndrome. There is considerable fear of heart disease; the palpitations or chest pain of an anxiety state may be attributed to heart disease. Classic hysterical syndromes, sometimes epidemic in schools, are probably more common than in Europe or the United States.

KORO, LATAH, AND RUNNING AMOK. Three mental states peculiar to the tropics are koro, latah, and running amok. These are mainly seen in the Far East. In koro, the patient believes that his penis is withdrawing into his abdomen and that if this should happen, death will result. Latah is a fright neurosis with hysterical elaborations, including coprolalia, echolalia, and compulsive movements. In running amok, which usually occurs in Malaya, the victim runs wild and attacks those around him with murderous intent. It is suggested that this is a Malay form of suicide.

EXPATRIATE PSYCHONEUROSIS. Expatriate workers in the tropics and their wives may be under stress and are prone to neurotic illness, depression, and alcoholism. Frequently, there are frustrations, dissatisfaction with living and working conditions, worries about children and parents at home, heat intolerance, and boredom. Proper selection of personnel, enlightened management, reasonable leave arrangements, and organized recreation can help prevent these problems.

PREVENTION OF NEUROLOGIC DISEASE

Treatment of neurologic disease is often unsatisfactory, and recovery is sometimes slow and incomplete. Children are often victims and may be disabled for life. There is need and scope for preventive measures in tropical neurology. Improved primary care facilities would permit earlier diagnosis and treatment of meningitis, malaria, and metabolic derangements. Early oral rehydration in gastroenteritis prevents hyponatremia and hypernatremia. Improved midwifery could diminish birth injuries and neonatal and postpartum tetanus. There are many problems associated with vaccination in the tropics, including cost, the cold chain, lack of trained personnel, and depression of the immune response by concurrent infection or malnutrition. However, tetanus, poliomyelitis, measles, and selective meningococcal vaccination would considerably lessen neurologic illness. Detection and treatment of hypertension would diminish cerebrovascular disease. Health education is important in preventing and understanding epilepsy, tetanus, rabies, and other diseases that may affect the nervous system.

BIBLIOGRAPHY

Asbury AK, Gilliatt RW (eds): Peripheral Nerve Disorders: A Practical Approach. London, Butterworths, 1984.
Anonymous: Schizophrenia in different cultures. Br Med J 1:1271, 1980.
Bharucha NE, Bharucha EP, Dastur HD, Schoenberg BS: Pilot survey of the prevalence of neurologic disorders in the Parsi Community of Bombay. Am J Prev Med 3:293, 1983.
Dalal PM: Strokes in the young in West Central India. Adv Neurol 25:339, 1979.
Gout O, Cressain A, Bolgert F, et al: Chronic myelopathies associated with human T-lymphocytic virus type I. Arch Neurol 46:255, 1989.
Gray F, Gherardi F, Scaravilli F: The neuropathology of the acquired immune deficiency syndrome. Brain 111:245, 1988.
Howlett WP, Nrya Wm, Mmuni KA, Missalek WR: Neurological disorders in AIDS and HIV disease in the northern zone of Tanzania. AIDS 3:289, 1989.
Lambo TA: Stroke—a world-wide health problem. Adv Neurol 25:1, 1979.
Mesulam MM: Schizophrenia and the brain. N Engl J Med 322:842, 1990.
Ndekei DM: Psychiatric phenomenology across countries. Psychol Med 16:33, 1986.
Osuntokun BO, Adeuja AOG, Schoenberg BS, et al: Neurological disorders in Nigerian Africans: a community-based study. Acta Neurol Scand 75:13, 1987.
Pavlakis SG, Prohovnik I, Piomelli S, DeVivo DC: Neurologic complications of sickle cell disease. Adv Pediatr 36:247, 1989.
Roman GC, Spencer PS, Schoenberg BS: Tropical myeloneuropathies. The hidden endemias. Neurology 35:1158, 1985.
Sartorius N, Jablensky A, Korten A, et al: Early manifestation and first contact incidence of schizophrenia in different cultures. Psychol Med 16:909, 1986.
Shorvon SD, Palmer PJ: Epilepsy in developing countries. Epilepsia 29(Suppl):536, 1988.
Spillane J: Tropical Neurology. London, Oxford Medical Publications, 1973.
Swift CR, Asuni T: Mental Health and Disease in Africa. Edinburgh, Churchill Livingstone, 1975.
Vejjajiva A: Parasitic diseases of the nervous system in Thailand. Clin Exp Neurol 15:92, 1978.
Wadia NH: Myelopathy complicating atlanto-axial dislocation. Brain 90:449, 1967.
White NJ, Looareesuwan S, Phillips RE: Single dose phenobarbitone prevents convulsion in cerebral malaria. Lancet 2:64, 1988.
WHO Collaborative Study: Assessment of depressive disorders. Psychol Med 10:743, 1980.
WHO Study Group: Peripheral Neuropathies. Technical Report Series 654. Geneva, World Health Organization, 1980.

9. OPHTHALMOLOGIC DISEASES

Hugh R. Taylor and Alfred Sommer

THE MAGNITUDE OF BLINDNESS. Blindness remains one of the major disabilities affecting man. The vast majority of blind people live in developing areas (Table 9–1). In the developed countries, blindness most commonly occurs in the elderly and is usually caused by conditions that are, by and large, poorly understood and for which preventive treatment is not entirely satisfactory. In many ways, the rate of blindness in developed countries represents a baseline of unavoidable blindness about which relatively little can be done with the available technology and forms of treatment.

Blindness in the developing areas presents a totally different picture. Superimposed on the baseline of "unavoidable blindness" is a tremendous overburden of "unnecessary blindness." Millions of people in the developing areas are blinded by diseases that are either preventable or treatable. What is needed is a proper awareness of the problem and a rejection of the myth that only ophthalmologists are competent to deal with ocular disease. Trained field workers are crucial for the control of blinding infections, malnutrition, and filariasis; for primary care of simple trauma and acute glaucoma; and for the recognition and referral of cases of chronic glaucoma, cataracts, and the more complicated of the diseases requiring surgery.

The eye is made up of tissues that have similarities to tissues elsewhere in the body, and the eye responds to

TABLE 9–1. Distribution and Characteristics of Blindness on a World Scale

	Developing World	Developed World
Number of blind (in millions)*	38.9–51.6	3.4–5.5
Blindness rate*	11–14/1000	3–5/1000
Major causes	Trachoma	Senile degeneration
	Cataract	Glaucoma
	Xerophthalmia	Cataract
	Onchocerciasis	Diabetes
	Corneal scarring	Congenital diseases
Primary anatomic area	Anterior segment	Posterior segment
Age at onset	All ages	Predominantly elderly
Percentage preventable	80%	20%
Etiology	Usually well known	Poorly understood

*WHO Prevention of Blindness Programme, 1987; (acuity less than 6/60).

inflammation and injury in much the same way as other organs do. Inflammation of the eye produces pain, redness, swelling (and often discharge), and heat and is frequently attended by at least a partial loss of function. Whether from trauma or infection, ocular inflammation often leads to scarring. Since the eye depends on transparency of the ocular media (cornea, aqueous, lens, and vitreous) for normal function, it can be rendered useless by a relatively small, axially located scar or other opacity. Infection in the eye needs to be treated like infection elsewhere, with appropriate hygienic and antibiotic therapy. Foreign bodies usually must be removed from the eye, as is the case in other parts of the body.

There are, however, a number of specific conditions that involve only the eye. These conditions include cataract, glaucoma, and macular degeneration, which will be discussed in later sections of this chapter.

THE OPHTHALMIC EXAMINATION. In ophthalmology, as in other fields of medicine, the most important steps in assessing a patient's problem involve taking a careful and appropriate history and performing a proper examination. It is important to elicit a history of the onset, duration, and characteristics of the presenting complaint, together with a review of the patient's general health and individual and family history. Specific information concerning vision—such as blurring, flashes or floaters, double vision, visual field loss, and night blindness—should be sought, and questions about ocular discharge, pain, and discomfort should be asked.

A basic part of the ophthalmic examination is the assessment of visual acuity, which is traditionally measured with a letter test chart, placed 6 meters away from the patient. The acuity of small children can be assessed by determining their ability to fixate upon and follow a target, such as a light, with one eye at a time while the other eye is covered.

Simple observation of the eye will often give much information, especially in terms of the presence and site of infection or trauma, the alignment and movement of the eyes, or their possible displacement (Figs. 9–1 and 9–2). Careful examination of the front of the eye with a hand light will reveal gross corneal or conjunctival disease, including xerophthalmia, trachoma, foreign bodies, or corneal ulcers. It also reveals much about the anterior chamber and lens, the presence of blood or pus in the eye, acute glaucoma, and significant lens opacities (cataract). Whenever possible, the front of the eye should be examined with some magnification, such as a

×2 or ×3 loupe, or a direct ophthalmoscope using the +10 diopter lens. The diagnosis of mild trachoma requires examination of the conjunctiva on the undersurface of the upper lid, which is accomplished by everting the eyelid (Fig. 9–3). The pupils can also be examined with a hand light, taking note of their size, shape, and response to light. It is usually easier to examine the pupils in a somewhat darkened room. A direct ophthalmoscope is essential for examining the back of the interior eye, to search for abnormalities of the optic disk, macular region, blood vessels, and other areas.

DIFFERENTIAL DIAGNOSIS OF THE PAINFUL, RED EYE

The painful, red eye is one of the most common ocular problems. Many such patients have conjunctivitis, but all should be examined carefully, because a number of serious eye conditions can present with a similar picture. In almost every case, the correct diagnosis can be made from the history and a simple ocular examination.

The most important conditions that present as a painful, red eye are conjunctivitis, keratitis (including keratoconjunctivitis), corneal trauma and foreign bodies, anterior uveitis, and acute angle–closure glaucoma (Table 9–2).

CONJUNCTIVITIS. Conjunctivitis is the most common cause of red eyes bilaterally. It is usually infective, although conjunctivitis may be allergic or traumatic. It is commonly bilateral, and a unilateral red eye increases the likelihood of other diagnoses. Infectious conjunctivitis usually has an acute onset, which is accompanied

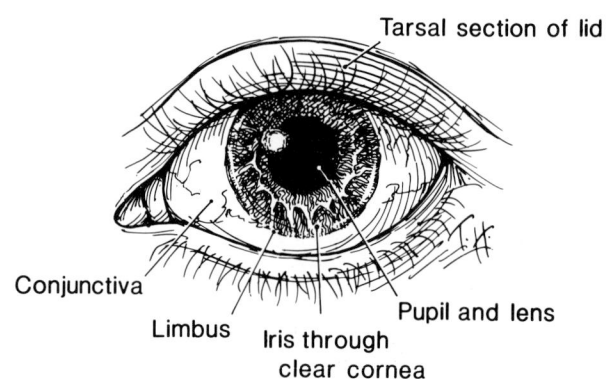

FIGURE 9–1. The front of the eye, showing the important landmarks.

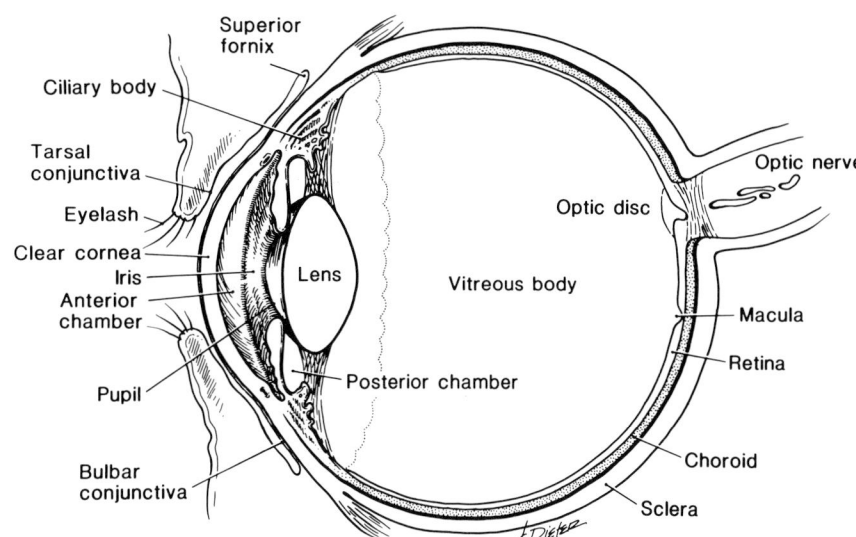

FIGURE 9–2. Cross-sectional diagram of the eye.

by ocular discharge. In viral and chlamydial conjunctivitis, the discharge is usually thin and watery. With bacterial conjunctivitis or secondary bacterial infection, the discharge is mucopurulent or purulent. A frankly purulent discharge is especially common in gonococcal infections. Mucopurulent and purulent discharges frequently accumulate on the eyelashes and lid margins, causing the lids to stick together.

The most consistent sign of conjunctivitis is conjunctival injection. The superficial and tortuous vessels of the conjunctiva appear dilated and bright red or pink, giving rise to the common term "pink eye." The conjunctival injection of the globe (bulbar conjunctiva) is most prominent in the fornices and is less marked at the limbus (the junction of the cornea and the sclera). The conjunctiva underneath the eyelids (tarsal conjunctiva) is frequently brick red. With severe inflammation, red blotches of subconjunctival hemorrhage may occur. These are seen more frequently in pneumococcal con-

junctivitis and in some viral conjunctivides, such as epidemic hemorrhagic conjunctivitis. In severe inflammation, pseudomembranes, or even true membranes, may be present. These are seen as dirty gray sloughs on the tarsal conjunctiva. In viral and chlamydial conjunctivitis, follicles are frequently present (Fig. 28–2). Giant, fleshy papillae may occur in allergic conjunctivitis. A detailed description of trachoma and inclusion conjunctivitis is provided in Chapter 28.

Visual acuity is usually not affected in conjunctivitis. The cornea is clear and bright, the pupil is circular and reacts normally, and the anterior chamber is clear and of normal depth.

Bacterial conjunctivitis usually requires specific antibiotic treatment. Antibiotics, such as chloramphenicol, may be given topically as 0.5% drops every 1 or 2 hours during the day and as 1.0% ointment at night. Alternatively, and especially in children, antibiotic ointment, such as 1.0% tetracycline, may be used 4 times a day and continued for 1 week. Patients should be cautioned to keep their eyes clean by washing away accumulated discharge. They should wash their hands carefully and not share towels or clothes with others, to avoid spreading the infection.

Neonatal gonococcal conjunctivitis is a medical emergency. The infant should be hospitalized and intravenous crystalline penicillin administered in a dose of 50,000 U/kg/day in two doses for 7 days. Saline irrigation of the eyes should be performed immediately and then at hourly intervals for as long as necessary to eliminate the purulent discharge.

Chlamydial conjunctivitis should be treated with systemic erythromycin. For neonates, a dose of 50 mg/kg/day in four divided doses should be used for 2 weeks. In adults, doxycycline (100 mg/day for 2 weeks) is preferred, although erythromycin should be used in pregnant women.

Viral conjunctivitis does not respond to antibiotics: therefore, this form of treatment is usually contraindicated. Significant symptomatic relief can be obtained with the use of cold compresses and local vasoconstric-

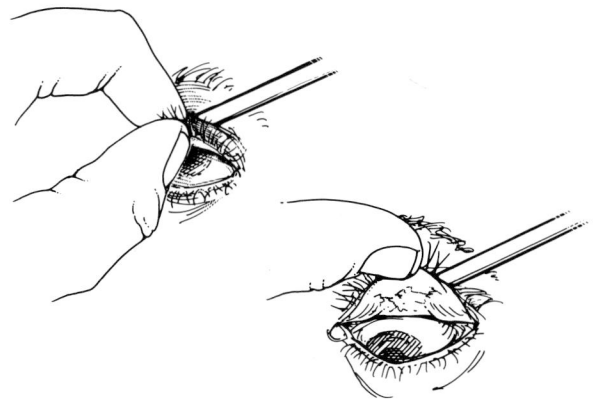

FIGURE 9–3. Eversion of the upper eyelid. With the patient looking down to relax the upper eyelid, gently grasp the eyelashes and lift the lid margin forward and upward over a probe placed above the tarsal plate. The tarsal plate is about 0.5 inch high, and its upper edge corresponds to the superior lid fold. The lid can be kept everted by holding the lashes against the brow. When the patient blinks, the lid will return to its normal position.

TABLE 9–2. Differential Diagnosis of the Painful Red Eye

	Acute Conjunctivitis	Keratitis	Anterior Uveitis	Acute Angle–Closure Glaucoma
Occurrence	Very common	Common	Uncommon	Uncommon
Age	All ages, especially the young	All ages	Adolescents and adults	Elderly
Onset	Gradual	Sudden (trauma) or gradual	Gradual	Sudden
Pain	Itching, irritation	Moderate to severe	Moderate	Severe, with nausea
Vision	Normal	Blurred	Blurred	Marked reduction, with halos
Injection	Conjunctiva, bright red	Ciliary* or diffuse	Ciliary	Ciliary, purple
Discharge	Moderate to marked, watery to purulent	Variable, mild to marked	None	None
Cornea	Clear and bright	Abrasion, opacity, foreign body	Clear; keratic precipitates	Steamy
Pupil	Normal	Variable	Small, irregular, sluggish	Large, oval, unresponsive
Intraocular pressure	Normal	Normal	Usually normal	Markedly elevated

*Ciliary injection—a ring of redness at the limbus because of inflammation of the ciliary body and iris.

tors, which also can be used for patients with allergic conjunctivitis. Topical steroids should never be used without the direct supervision of an ophthalmologist.

KERATITIS AND CORNEAL ULCERATION. These are common causes of painful, red eyes and are usually uniocular. Severe photophobia is often the main symptom, and the vision is usually blurred. Secondary uveitis may develop and cause ciliary injection. Ciliary injection shows a ring of redness, which is most intense around the limbus, and is a sign of inflammation of the ciliary body and iris. A history of trauma can often be elicited. At other times, a corneal ulcer and, more especially, keratitis may occur as a result of viral or severe bacterial conjunctivitis, in which case the signs of conjunctivitis may coexist. Sometimes, corneal ulcers develop spontaneously, especially with herpetic keratitis and in young children with vitamin A deficiency; in Africa it is particularly common following measles.

The most important diagnostic sign is the appearance of a corneal defect—either an opacity, which will obscure underlying iris details, or a surface defect, which will distort the surface reflex. If an ulcer penetrates the cornea, the globe may collapse and the intraocular contents may be expelled, or the hole in the cornea may be plugged with a knuckle of iris, which then shows as dark tissue in the base of the ulcer. A small ulcer, such as a dendritic ulcer caused by herpes simplex, is best seen if fluorescein is instilled and the eye is observed with a blue light. Large infective ulcers frequently are filled with white sloughed material and other debris. At times, pus may accumulate in the anterior chamber as a hypopyon.

Most corneal ulcers are medical emergencies. Proper management frequently requires a microbiologic diagnosis of the infectious agent, using isolation cultures. Intensive systemic and local antibiotics are used. The local antibiotics may be given by both the topical and the subconjunctival routes. Doses of some commonly used subconjunctival antibiotics are penicillin, 1 megaunit; ampicillin, 100 mg; methicillin, 100 mg; carbenicillin, 100 mg; and gentamicin, 20 mg. The volume injected is usually 0.5 ml. These patients should be under the care of an ophthalmologist.

If a characteristic dendritic figure can be seen on the cornea and if the cornea has decreased sensation, a presumptive diagnosis of herpetic keratitis can be made. Dendritic ulcers are most appropriately treated with topical antiviral agents, such as idoxuridine (IDU) ointment applied 4 times daily for at least 1 week, although simple debridement and patching of the eye are very effective, especially for large, single lesions. A mydriatic, such as 5% homatropine 3 times a day, should be used until the ulcer has healed.

Again, as with conjunctivitis, steroids should not be used in patients with corneal ulcers and keratitis.

CORNEAL NECROSIS. A number of systemic conditions are associated with corneal ulceration and necrosis, including collagen vascular diseases, leukemia, and granulomatoses. In developing countries, nutritional keratopathy (xerophthalmia, keratomalacia) is the most common cause of childhood blindness (Chapter 107.1). In many Asian countries, measles is an important precipitating event for xerophthalmia. Even in well-nourished Western children, measles causes a mild, superficial, self-limiting keratitis, which does not require therapy. In much of Africa, however, measles itself is considered an important blinding condition. The mechanism is not entirely clear. In many instances it represents precipitation of acute xerophthalmia, as in Asia. In others it appears to represent secondary herpetic infection, which also accounts for accompanying stomatitis and skin ulcers. In still others, corneal damage is a chemical keratitis or bacterial infection secondary to the common practice of placing herbal and other traditional medicines in the eyes of measles patients.

CORNEAL TRAUMA. With trauma, ocular signs and symptoms are usually unilateral and the onset is sudden. A history of trauma or foreign bodies is usually present. Conjunctival foreign bodies cause pain and a feeling of having "something in the eye." Conjunctival vascular "injection" and some watering of the eye are usually present. A foreign body may be seen with a simple external examination. At other times, however, conjunctival foreign bodies lodge behind the upper eyelid and are not seen until the lid is everted, at which time they can be easily removed.

A corneal foreign body usually produces more severe pain and photophobia. After some time, it will often cause a secondary inflammation with ciliary-limbal injection. Most corneal foreign bodies can be removed fairly easily with a cotton-tipped swab, but if this is not possible, the case should be referred to an ophthalmologist. Frequently, patching the eye for 24 hours after the removal of a foreign body will give symptomatic relief and hasten healing of the corneal epithelium. A single application of antibiotic ointment should be used prophylactically.

In tropical environments in particular, corneal abrasions from plant matter, whether or not they leave a foreign body behind, carry a high risk of subsequent fungal infection. These can be notoriously difficult to treat and should be watched for closely.

Chemical burns to the eyes are best treated with immediate, thorough, and copious irrigation. Ideally, sterile saline solution should be used, but rather than delay irrigation, tap water should be used if saline is not available. The damage caused by an acid burn can usually be determined immediately. Because alkali continues to penetrate the eye, alkaline burns are frequently much more severe than initially realized. All chemical burns should be assessed by an ophthalmologist.

Conjunctival hemorrhages, which may be traumatic or spontaneous, require no treatment and will resolve in 1 to 2 weeks. Minor conjunctival lacerations do not require suturing and will heal in a few days. Topical antibiotics are usually given until the eye has healed.

All cases of penetrating trauma to the eye and lacerations to the globe, including corneal lacerations and intraocular foreign bodies, are medical emergencies that require prompt referral to and careful assessment by an ophthalmologist.

ANTERIOR UVEITIS. Anterior uveitis is a relatively uncommon cause of a sore, red eye. The term is used to describe inflammation of the anterior uveal structures—the iris and the ciliary body. "Anterior uveitis" is usually preferable to the terms describing inflammation in each of these structures individually, i.e., iritis, cyclitis, and iridocyclitis, because at least some inflammation is almost always present in both these tissues. Uveitis may occur as a primary event, either in isolation or in association with some underlying systemic disease. It also may occur as a result of other ocular pathology. Secondary uveitis is commonly seen with corneal trauma and ulceration.

Primary anterior uveitis has a gradual onset, with moderate to severe pain and some blurring of vision. It may be unilateral or bilateral, and the patient may have a history of similar episodes. Ciliary injection is the most important feature. This injection decreases with distance from the limbus, and the conjunctiva of the fornices and lids is not inflamed. There is usually no discharge.

The other important sign in anterior uveitis is a pupillary change. The pupil is usually small and reacts poorly to light. Frequently, the pupil is irregular because of adhesions, called posterior synechiae, between the pupillary margin and the lens. On examination with a slit lamp, keratic precipitates or inflammatory cells may be seen on the back of the cornea and also inflammatory cells and an aqueous "flare" in the anterior chamber. In severe cases, these changes may be recognized during the examination of the front of the eye with an ophthalmoscope, using the +10 diopter lens.

Uveitis may occur as an isolated ocular condition, but it also is often associated with underlying systemic infections such as arthropathy, collagen diseases, and other systemic illnesses. For this reason, patients with anterior uveitis, especially those with recurrent episodes, should be examined in detail to exclude the possibility of such an underlying condition.

Treatment involves cycloplegia and mydriasis obtained with topical drops, such as atropine. One percent atropine drops may be given 3 times a day. A systemic analgesic, such as aspirin, will often give symptomatic relief. Topical steroids are frequently indicated, but they should be given only at the direction of an ophthalmologist. In severe uveitis and in chronic uveitis, secondary cataracts and secondary glaucoma may develop. These conditions require specific treatment.

ACUTE ANGLE–CLOSURE GLAUCOMA. Acute angle–closure glaucoma is a relatively uncommon cause of a painful, red eye, although its diagnosis is of great importance because (without prompt treatment) irreversible blindness can result. Acute angle–closure glaucoma is characterized by a sudden increase in intraocular pressure when the drainage channels for the intraocular fluid (aqueous humor) are obstructed. The persistence of elevated intraocular pressure can cause permanent and total loss of vision within 1 to 2 days. The condition is most frequent in Asian populations.

Acute angle–closure glaucoma usually starts with sudden and severe ocular pain, often severe enough to cause nausea and vomiting. Vision is markedly reduced, and the patient often complains of seeing halos, or colored rings, around lights. On examination, there may be ciliary injection, but the most striking features are the "steamy" or hazy cornea and the greatly increased intraocular pressure. The corneal changes are due to corneal edema. Intraocular pressure can be assessed by gently palpating the globe through the closed upper lid and comparing the degree of resilience of the affected eye with that of the other eye or with that of the eye of a person with normal vision. Increased intraocular pressure causes the eye to feel firmer, or hard.

The anterior chamber is usually very shallow in angle-closure glaucoma, and the iris appears to be almost touching the cornea. The pupil is frequently found to be semidilated and unreactive, and it may have an irregular or vertically oval shape.

Medical attempts to reduce intraocular pressure in such patients should be started without delay. Hyperosmotic agents, such as oral glycerin, 3 ml/kg, should be given, followed by frequent use of 2 to 4% topical pilocarpine drops, 1 drop every 15 minutes for 4 doses, then every half hour for 1 hour, and then every 1 to 2 hours, and oral carbonic-anhydrase inhibitors, such as acetazolamide, 500 mg orally or intravenously. These patients require referral to an ophthalmologist. An iridectomy or iridotomy may be necessary to prevent further episodes. Pilocarpine 1 to 2% should be initiated twice daily in the fellow eye to reduce the risk of an acute attack until definitive surgical prophylaxis.

CHRONIC DISEASES

Cataracts, glaucoma, and macular degeneration are major causes of blindness in aged populations of both developed and developing countries.

CATARACT. Opacification of the lens interferes with transmission of clear images to the retina by both decreasing and scattering the light rays as they pass through. To the examiner, the pupillary area may look opaque and whitish or dark greenish-brown on handlight illumination, and fundus details will be obscured when viewed with the direct ophthalmoscope. Aside from cataracts of rare congenital causes and those that result from chronic inflammation, most cataracts are lumped together under the heading "senile." These are undoubtedly of multifactorial origin. Because the precise causes of such cataracts are as yet unknown, preventive measures do not now exist. Cataracts can be surgically removed, however, with a high degree of technical success and likelihood of return of useful vision.

In general, cataracts are the leading cause of blindness in developing countries. Visually disabling cataracts appear to occur earlier in life in some cultures than in others. More importantly, surgical therapy is commonly unavailable to large segments of the population. Some countries are overcoming the paucity and maldistribution of ophthalmologists by conducting intensive rural "cataract camps"; others are doing so by training properly supervised paramedical personnel to remove cataracts. Because the potential for intraoperative complications and postoperative infections is high under these circumstances, these approaches require careful consideration and detailed organization. However, as no other recourse exists, these methods require further development and extension.

Merely removing an advanced cataract can improve vision, but removal alone will not restore reading acuity. Some form of aphakic correction, most commonly spectacles or intraocular lenses, is also required.

GLAUCOMA. There are two major forms of glaucoma—acute and chronic. As already discussed, the acute form, with its red, injected, painful eyes, is the more dramatic. Chronic open-angle glaucoma, however, is much more common and is the more important cause of blindness.

Chronic elevation of intraocular pressure, at levels below those reached in acute angle–closure glaucoma, results in progressive destruction of the optic nerve. After many years (usually 10 to 20), this painless, asymptomatic destruction of the optic nerve results in loss of visual field, detectable by careful visual-field examination. Antiglaucoma therapy may delay or prevent further damage, but it cannot replace the vision that has already been lost. Unfortunately, patients are usually unaware of the problem until late in the course of the disease, when central acuity is finally involved and little vision or optic nerve remains to be saved.

Glaucoma is the classic disease in which screening methods have played an important role. Unfortunately, the simplest technique, that of demonstrating by tonometry that the intraocular pressure is greater than 21 mm Hg, is far from infallible. Half of those with established glaucomatous field loss will have a normal pressure on a single casual screening test, and only 1 in 20 or 30 persons with an elevated pressure will already have field loss. The higher the pressure, however, the greater the likelihood of having, or soon developing, field loss. Screening is improved by combining tonometry with examination of the optic disk (by direct ophthalmoscopy or, preferably, with a slit lamp and contact lens). Deep, large, asymmetric optic-disk cupping, equal to or greater than 0.6 disk diameter, or loss of nerve-fiber–layer striations, suggests glaucomatous damage.

Ultimately, diagnosis requires demonstration of classic changes in the visual fields.

Treatment consists of lowering the intraocular pressure below 21 mm Hg or to whatever level prevents further damage. A number of topical medications may accomplish this: Beta blockers such as betaxolol and timolol have the fewest side effects and are often the first agents of choice, though they are also the most expensive. An alternative initial agent is dipivylepinephrine (Propine), an epinephrine-like agent with fewer local side effects than epinephrine itself. Like beta blockers, epinephrine primarily works by decreasing aqueous formations. Pilocarpine, a parasympathomimetic agent, increases aqueous drainage and has had the most extensive use. It is usually the least expensive agent but requires application 4 times a day and results in severe miosis, which may degrade vision, particularly at night. As one agent proves inadequate, even at maximum dosage, others may be added to the regimen. Oral carbonic-anhydrase inhibitors, such as acetazolamide, are often effective and have an additive effect to that of the topical agents.

Glaucoma management requires careful monitoring of pressure and visual field and frequent adjustment of dosage and regimen, while compliance of patients with the treatment plan is generally poor.

When visual-field loss continues, even on "maximum" medical therapy, the patient requires filtering surgery. A small channel is produced through the tough outer coats of the eye, so that some of the aqueous may percolate out of the eye into the subconjunctival space, where it is absorbed. Such artificial channels are at least temporarily successful, after one or more operations, in 85% of Caucasian patients. Because of their greater tendency for scarring, which closes the new channel, black patients do not fare so well.

Despite the potential for preventive measures, glaucoma is an especially difficult clinical problem in tropical countries; screening and diagnostic procedures are time-consuming and complex, and medical therapy is expensive, requires careful monitoring, and usually is attended by poor compliance. Although results of surgery are less than ideal, when available, surgery is probably the only practical treatment for patients who live in depressed rural communities of developing countries.

MACULAR DEGENERATION. In temperate climates, macular degeneration is the first or second leading cause of blindness. Because it is difficult to diagnose without a dilated-pupil fundus examination and is virtually impossible to treat, macular degeneration has received little attention in the tropics.

Of the many disease processes that can cause macular destruction, two are paramount—diabetes and age-related macular degeneration (AMD).

As its name implies, AMD comes on with aging, and at least some cases appear to be familial. Whether one or more causes are involved is unknown. Early in the disease, scattered, white, deep-retinal dots, known as drusen, can be seen concentrated in the macular area. Some, but not all, persons with these signs eventually develop progressive degeneration of their retinal pigment epithelium and the underlying choroid. Loss of vision is gradual, unpredictable, and almost always confined to loss of fine reading acuity. Such patients rarely develop "black blindness" (total loss of vision) and can usually care for themselves. In some, a net of new blood vessels pushes its way up from the choroid, and these vessels lie above or below the pigment epithelium. Such nets occasionally can be treated with a laser, perhaps delaying the sudden and dramatic loss of vision that can accompany leakage of fluid or blood. In any event, the benefits of therapy are far from dramatic, even when available.

Diabetic retinopathy includes a wide, complex spectrum of changes. Because few long-time diabetics survive in the rural, depressed communities of developing countries, diabetic retinopathy is of most concern in the developed countries and in increasingly affluent urban communities elsewhere. Again, the major treatable component of the disease is the growth of neovascular membranes, in this instance out into the vitreous from the surface of the optic nerve or retina. Photocoagulation, by either white light or laser therapy, provides substantial benefit to some groups of patients with this condition. It also benefits patients with fluid accumulation in the macula (macular edema) if they are treated early.

BIBLIOGRAPHY

Buck AA (ed.): Onchocerciasis. Symptomatology, Pathology, Diagnosis. Geneva, World Health Organization, 1974.

Diabetic Retinopathy Study Research Group: Photocoagulation treatment of proliferative diabetic retinopathy: The second report of diabetic retinopathy study findings. Ophthalmology 85:82, 1978.

Dawson CR, Jones BR, Tarizzo ML: Guide to Trachoma Control. Geneva, World Health Organization, 1981.

Early Treatment Diabetic Retinopathy Study Research Group: Photocoagulation for diabetic macular edema. Early Treatment Diabetic Retinopathy Study Report Number 1. Arch Ophthalmol 103:1796–1806, 1985.

Fraunfelder F, Roy FH: Current Ocular Therapy. Philadelphia, WB Saunders, 1980.

Gass JDM: Stereoscopic Atlas of Macular Diseases. Diagnosis and Treatment. St. Louis, CV Mosby, 1977.

Guidelines for Programmes for the Prevention of Blindness. Geneva, World Health Organization, 1979.

Kolker AE, Hetherington J: Becker-Shaffer's Diagnosis and Therapy of the Glaucomas. St. Louis, CV Mosby, 1976.

Methods of Assessment of Avoidable Blindness. Geneva, World Health Organization, WHO Offset Publication No. 54, 1980.

Newell FW: Ophthalmology, Principles and Concepts. St. Louis, CV Mosby, 1978.

Sommer A: Field Guide to the Detection and Control of Xerophthalmia. Geneva, World Health Organization, 1982.

Sommer A: Nutritional Blindness. New York, Oxford University Press, 1982.

Vaughan D, Asbury T: General Ophthalmology. Los Altos, California, Lange Medical Publications, 1980.

World Health Organization: Conjunctivitis of the Newborn. Geneva, World Health Organization, 1986.

10. SEXUALLY TRANSMITTED DISEASES

Peter L. Perine
and Thomas A. Bell

DEFINITION AND ETIOLOGY. In the golden era of microbiology in the late nineteenth and early twentieth centuries, the microbial causes of five diseases clinically recognized as being transmitted predominantly by sexual intercourse—syphilis (hard chancre), gonorrhea, chancroid (soft chancre), lymphogranuloma venereum, and granuloma inguinale—were identified. Only syphilis and gonorrhea were recognized as major public health problems and became known as the major venereal diseases; the others were of "minor" public health concern. After World War II, new diagnostic techniques and clinical and epidemiologic studies in North America and Europe established that more than a dozen other microbial species could be sexually transmitted and were potentially pathogenic. Most have probably affected human beings since antiquity, but others may be newly evolved species. Among the latter are human immunodeficiency viruses (HIV) 1 and 2, agents of the current pandemic of the acquired immunodeficiency syndrome (AIDS).

Recognizing that multiple microorganisms cause symptomatic infections at the same anatomic site, most venereologists prefer a syndromic approach to the diagnosis of sexually transmitted diseases (STDs) (Table 10–1). Treatment regimens should be chosen with the recognition that several pathogens may be simultaneously infecting the same genital site and that several drugs may be required (Tables 10–2 to 10–4).

DISTRIBUTION AND PREVALENCE. Epidemiologic data on STDs in developing countries are limited and based largely on sporadic prevalence surveys for gonorrhea, HIV, and syphilis in urban clinics and hospitals. Reported STDs thus compose only a fraction of all infections in the relevant populations. Many symptomatic persons attempt self-treatment or consult pharmacists or traditional medical practitioners before seeking care in a bona fide health care facility. Delays inherent in this process may allow the development of complications and atypical clinical features caused by partial treatment.

Certain demographic and socioeconomic conditions promote the transmission of STDs. Persons 15 to 30 years of age are the most sexually active and constitute a large proportion of the populations of most developing countries. A ubiquitous trend of rural to urban migration is associated with loss of social constraints on sexual activity outside traditionally sanctioned relationships. Such migration usually results in an excess of men in urban areas and of women in rural areas. Such imbalances promote sharing of sexual partners. Lack of employment in cities often leads women, and occasionally

TABLE 10–1. Selected Syndromes and Complications, With Corresponding Sexually Transmitted Etiologic Agents*

Syndrome or Complication	Sexually Transmitted Etiologic Agent
Acquired immunodeficiency syndrome (AIDS)	Human immunodeficiency virus (HIV) 1 and 2
Adult T-cell lymphoma/leukemia; tropical spastic paraparesis, chronic progressive myelopathy	Human T-cell lymphotropic viruses (HTLV) 1 and 2
Salpingitis	*N. gonorrhoeae, C. trachomatis, M. hominis*
Infertility	
Postsalpingitis, postpartum, postabortion	*N. gonorrhoeae, C. trachomatis, M. hominis*
Spontaneous abortion, fetal wastage	Herpes simplex virus, *T. pallidum, N. gonorrhoeae, U. urealyticum, C. trachomatis*
Postepididymitis	*N. gonorrhoeae, C. trachomatis*
Congenital and perinatal infections	
TORCHES complex†	Cytomegalovirus (CMV), herpes simplex virus, *T. pallidum*
Other infant and childhood morbidity	
Sepsis, death	Group B streptococcus, herpes simplex virus
Eye infection	*C. trachomatis, N. gonorrhoeae*
Pneumonia	*C. trachomatis, T. pallidum,* CMV, *U. urealyticum*
Otitis media	*C. trachomatis*
Neurologic impairment	CMV, herpes simplex virus, *T. pallidum*
Male urethritis	*N. gonorrhoeae, C. trachomatis, U. urealyticum*
Epididymitis	*N. gonorrhoeae, C. trachomatis*
Lower urogenital tract infection in women	
Female urethritis	*N. gonorrhoeae, C. trachomatis*
Vulvitis	*C. albicans,* herpes simplex virus
Vaginitis	*T. vaginalis, C. albicans, G. vaginalis*
Cervicitis	*N. gonorrhoeae, C. trachomatis,* herpes simplex virus
Venereal warts, genital carcinomas	Human papillomaviruses
Genital ulceration	Herpes simplex virus, *T. pallidum, H. ducreyi, C. granulomatis, C. trachomatis* (LGV)
Proctitis	*N. gonorrhoeae,* herpes simplex virus, *C. trachomatis, E. histolytica*
Acute arthritis with genital infection	*N. gonorrhoeae, C. trachomatis*
Hepatitis	Hepatitis A and B viruses, CMV

*For each of the syndromes and complications, a variable proportion are not sexually transmitted, and some cannot yet be ascribed to pathogenic etiologic agents.

†TORCHES complex refers to congenital infections caused by toxoplasmosis, rubella, cytomegalovirus, herpes simplex virus, and syphilis.

men, into prostitution and thereby promotes a large reservoir of STDs in the community. Tourists and others who contact an STD in one locale can rapidly spread it to another, as well as internationally.

Most STD statistics in developing tropical countries deal only with the traditional infections that usually are treated in a primary health care system. Uniform criteria are seldom used to diagnose STDs. Reported cases usually include only syphilis, gonorrhea, and AIDS, and these are often substantially underreported. Gonorrhea is usually the most prevalent STD and is present in one third to one half of patients in public venereology clinics in developing countries. Gonorrhea is underdiagnosed in women because accurate diagnosis requires a more

sophisticated examination than can be done in many primary care clinics. A more accurate picture of the prevalence of gonorrhea in women comes from studies of obstetric patients, in whom the prevalence of asymptomatic endocervical gonorrhea ranges from 1 to 12%, *Chlamydia trachomatis* infection from 5 to 10%, latent syphilis from 1 to 20%, and HIV-1 infection from 0 to 14%.

In large African cities, the annual incidence of gonorrhea may be 3000 to 10,000 cases per 100,000 population. The emergence of penicillinase-producing *Neisseria gonorrhoeae* in 1976 in eastern Asia and western Africa was followed by its rapid spread to almost all areas of the world (Chapter 44). In much of Africa and

TABLE 10–2. Diseases Caused by Sexually Transmitted Viruses

Viral Agents	Diagnostic Test	Disease or Syndrome
Human immunodeficiency viruses 1 and 2	Serology, PCR,* tissue culture	Acquired immunodeficiency syndrome
Human T-lymphotropic virus 1 and 2	Serology, tissue culture, PCR	T-lymphocyte leukemia and lymphoma; tropical spastic paresis; myelopathy
Herpes simplex virus	Serology, culture	Genital herpes; aseptic meningitis, neonatal herpes with associated mortality or neurologic sequela; spontaneous abortion and premature delivery; cervical cancer
Hepatitis A virus	Serology	Hepatitis in homosexual men
Hepatitis B virus	Serology	Acute, chronic, and fulminant hepatitis; hepatocellular carcinoma
Cytomegalovirus	Serology, culture	Congenital birth defects; heterophil-negative infectious mononucleosis; cervicitis
Human papillomaviruses	PCR	Condylomata acuminata, laryngeal papilloma in young children; cervical dysplasia

*Polymerase chain reaction technique, which is based on the identification of part or all of the genome of a specific pathogen in tissues or fluids.

TABLE 10–3. Diseases Caused by Sexually Transmitted Bacteria

Pathogen	Diagnostic Test	Disease or Syndrome
Neisseria gonorrhoeae	Gram stain; cultures	Urethritis, epididymitis, proctitis, pharyngitis, conjunctivitis, endometritis, perihepatitis, bartholinitis, amniotic infection, bacteremia, premature rupture of membranes, salpingitis, tubal scarring resulting in infertility, ectopic pregnancy, and recurrent salpingitis
Chlamydia trachomatis	Direct FA; tissue culture; serology	Urethritis, epididymitis, cervicitis, proctitis, salpingitis, inclusion conjunctivitis, trachoma, infant pneumonia, otitis media, lymphogranuloma venereum, perihepatitis, bartholinitis, fetal and neonatal mortality
Mycoplasma hominis	Culture	Postpartum fever, salpingitis
Ureaplasma urealyticum	Culture	Urethritis, chorioamnionitis
Treponema pallidum	Darkfield microscopy; serology	Venereal and endemic syphilis (closely related strains cause yaws)
Gardnerella vaginalis	Culture	Vaginitis
Haemophilus ducreyi	Culture; Gram stain	Chancroid
Calymmatobacterium granulomatis	Biopsy	Granuloma inguinale (donovanosis)
Shigella, Campylobacter sp.	Culture	Enterocolitis in homosexual men
Group A beta-hemolytic streptococcus	Culture	Neonatal sepsis and meningitis

Asia, these strains constitute 30 to 60% of the isolates of *N. gonorrhoeae*. Once introduced, they tend to increase rapidly to prevalence rates of 10 to 30% within 3 to 5 years. Their rapid spread is promoted in part by inadequate treatment and the common practice of self-prophylaxis with oral penicillins, but penicillinase plasmids also spread between strains of *N. gonorrhoeae* and even between genera. The morbidity associated with some STDs in the tropics, such as secondary infertility following gonococcal or chlamydial salpingitis, is often used as a surrogate measure of the prevalence of these diseases.

Syphilis is common in eastern, central, and southern Africa, where it is a major cause of fetal wastage (Chapter 32.1). The relative scarcity of venereal syphilis in western Africa and parts of Asia and Oceania may reflect cross-immunity conferred by nonvenereal endemic syphilis or yaws acquired during childhood. Genital ulcers caused by herpes simplex virus and *Haemophilus ducreyi* are increasing worldwide. Chancroid is common in eastern Africa, especially among prostitutes (Chapter 45). Granuloma inguinale is endemic to the southeastern coast of India and to Papua New Guinea (Chapter 46).

THE GENITAL EXAMINATION. Any patient presenting with a history of sexual exposure and genitourinary symptoms may have acquired an STD and deserves a thorough physical examination, which should include speculum examination of the cervix and vagina for women and anoscopy for either sex when warranted by the patient's sexual practices. Some lesions of the genitalia, such as carbuncles, fixed drug eruptions, and the autoimmune Behçet syndrome, are not acquired sexually. The nongenital erogenous areas of the body should not be neglected in the examination; the oropharynx may be the first or only site infected in persons with gonorrhea or primary syphilis.

Lymph node enlargement is an important and common feature of primary syphilis, herpes genitalis, lymphogranuloma venereum (Fig. 29–1), chancroid, and HIV infection. The enlarged nodes may be tender (herpes genitalis, lymphogranuloma venereum, chancroid) or relatively painless (syphilis, HIV) and may be localized to the inguinal area irrespective of constitutional symptoms such as fever.

The anorectum is a frequent site of infection for several STD pathogens. *N. gonorrhoeae* can be isolated from the anus of about half the women with endocervical infection. This results from anal intercourse or, more often, contamination from vaginal secretions. The presence of an STD pathogen in the rectum of a man usually results from homosexual exposure.

Uncircumcised men may be more susceptible to infection with certain STDs, such as balanitis caused by *Trichomonas vaginalis*. The foreskin may be more susceptible to trauma during coitus and provide a portal of entry for such pathogens as *H. ducreyi, C. trachomatis*, and HIV. Studies in Africa suggest that circumcised men have a lower risk for HIV than do uncircumcised men and that genital ulcers facilitate HIV transmission.

TABLE 10–4. Diseases Caused by Sexually Transmitted Pathogens Excluding Viruses and Bacteria

Pathogen	Diagnostic Test	Disease or Syndrome
Fungi		
Candida albicans	Microscopy, culture	Vulvovaginitis, balanitis
Protozoa		
Trichomonas vaginalis	Microscopy, culture	Vaginitis, urethritis, balanitis
Entamoeba histolytica	Microscopy	Amebiasis in homosexual men
Giardia lamblia	Microscopy	Giardiasis
Ectoparasites		
Phthirus pubis	Microscopy	Pubic louse infestation ("crabs")
Sarcoptes scabei	Microscopy	Scabies

The panoply of STD pathogens includes several strains of human papillomavirus (HPV), which are associated with but do not necessarily cause cancer of the cervix, vulva, and anus. Many flat warts cannot be seen without a colposcope. The atypical aggressive Kaposi's sarcoma occurring in homosexual men infected with HIV may also be caused by a sexually transmitted agent (Chapter 11).

URETHRAL DISCHARGE/URETHRITIS

ETIOLOGY. Almost all urethritis in men is sexually transmitted. In Europe and North America, the relative importance of *N. gonorrhoeae* (Chapter 44) and *C. trachomatis* (Chapter 30) as causes depends on socioeconomic status, with the former infection being more frequent among poorer men. In developing countries, *N. gonorrhoeae* seems to be much more common, for reasons that remain conjectural. Studies of the etiology of urethritis in developing countries involve a selection bias toward cases that are more severe and thus more likely to be caused by *N. gonorrhoeae*. In populations with endemic trachoma, ocular infections with "trachoma" serovars of *C. trachomatis* exist simultaneously with "genital" infections with "genital" serovars; the effects of these two kinds of infection on each other are not understood. Other causes of urethritis include *Ureaplasma urealyticum* and *Trichomonas vaginalis* (Chapter 72). Frequently claimed but unproven noninfectious causes are consumption of ethanol, physical or emotional stress, allergy, and exposure to spermicides. In North America, many cases of urethritis, especially those caused by *C. trachomatis*, are asymptomatic but may be detected by finding pus in the first aliquot of urine (Fig. 44–3).

CLINICAL MANIFESTATIONS. Urethritis usually has an incubation period of 3 to 7 days if caused by *N. gonorrhoeae*, and 1 to 3 weeks if caused by *C. trachomatis*. Thus, chlamydial urethritis often appears as a "postgonococcal urethritis" when the latter has been treated with a drug ineffective against the former. Both organisms, and especially *C. trachomatis*, may cause asymptomatic infection. Either organism may ascend the reproductive tract. In males, *N. gonorrhoeae* may cause prostatitis, epididymitis, or orchitis, while *C. trachomatis* probably causes only epididymitis. Epididymitis and orchitis are often difficult to distinguish from testicular torsion; a surgical opinion should be sought if the diagnosis is uncertain.

REITER'S SYNDROME. *C. trachomatis* infection is a precipitating cause of Reiter's syndrome, which consists of asymmetric large-joint arthritis, nongonococcal urethritis, conjunctivitis, and keratoderma blennorrhagica. Other causes include intestinal pathogens such as *Shigella, Campylobacter,* and *Yersinia enterocolitica*. The condition is more common in men, most of whom have the histocompatibility antigen HLA-B27.

ACUTE URETHRAL SYNDROME. In women, the analogue of urethritis is the acute urethral syndrome. Its definition is more problematic than that of urethritis in males. Like cystitis, its cause is not necessarily a sexually transmitted infection, although many cases may be caused by coital trauma. Symptoms are similar to those in males, except that the urethral discharge is rarely noted by the patient.

The acute urethral syndrome in women is not caused by conventional urinary tract pathogens such as *Escherichia coli* and *Staphylococcus saprophyticus*. Some cases are caused by the same organisms that cause urethritis in males—*N. gonorrhoeae, C. trachomatis,* and *T. vaginalis*. Anatomic abnormalities may also be a cause.

CERVICITIS

ETIOLOGY. Cervicitis is often confused with normal anatomic features of the cervix. During adolescence, when the prevalence of sexually transmitted diseases in females may be high, the endocervical columnar epithelium is exposed on the portio vaginalis of the cervix. Pregnancy and oral contraceptives also cause such ectropion of the cervix; such epithelium is neither ectopic nor eroded. True erosions, or ulcers, on the cervix may be caused by herpes simplex virus, *Treponema pallidum,* or *Haemophilus ducreyi. Trichomonas vaginalis* may cause small hemorrhages in the squamous epithelium of the ectocervix—colpitis macularis ("strawberry cervix")—and may be difficult to detect without colposcopic magnification (Chapter 72).

CLINICAL MANIFESTATIONS AND DIAGNOSIS. Mucopurulent cervicitis is manifested by the presence of yellow or green endocervical secretions, friability of the columnar epithelium of the endocervix when it is swabbed, or redness of the exposed endocervical epithelium. A Gram-stained smear of the endocervical secretions that contains increased numbers of polymorphonuclear leukocytes is also an indicator of mucopurulent cervicitis. The upper limit of the normal concentration of leukocytes in such a smear is not well defined, and many studies have found a poor correlation between infection with *C. trachomatis* or *N. gonorrhoeae* and the presence of endocervical leukocytosis. A commonly used criterion for a normal smear is that it contain less than 10 leukocytes per × 1000 microscopic field in the 3 most concentrated fields where the cells are in monolayers. Contamination by vaginal secretions may make smears uninterpretable. Mucopurulent cervicitis is an insufficiently sensitive indicator of infection with *C. trachomatis* or *N. gonorrhoeae* to obviate the need to test women for these organisms by more specific means, such as isolation.

COMPLICATIONS. *C. trachomatis* and *N. gonorrhoeae* may ascend from the cervix to the upper genital tract. Many women with chlamydial cervicitis have asymptomatic endometritis, and some may have asymptomatic salpingitis (Chapter 30). *N. gonorrhoeae* infection has similar sequelae but is more often symptomatic (Chapter 44). Both organisms may also cause perihepatitis (Fitz-Hugh–Curtis syndrome). Both are important causes of infertility in developed countries and probably in developing countries, too. Both may be transmitted to infants at birth.

VAGINAL DISCHARGES

Vaginal discharge is usually the complaint that causes symptomatic women to seek care at an STD clinic. A normal physiologic vaginal discharge (leukorrhea) occurs in response to high estrogen levels and thus may occur at ovulation, in the immediate premenstrual period, in pregnancy, or with oral contraceptive use. This discharge is usually not pruritic; its odor is not offensive; and it rarely contains leukocytes. Normal leukorrhea may leave a brown stain on the underwear. Vaginal discharge is rare in prepubescent girls, in whom its presence may indicate sexual abuse.

A pathologic vaginal discharge may be malodorous and accompanied by vulvovaginal irritation or itching. The two most common causes are *Candida* spp. and *Trichomonas vaginalis,* which can be diagnosed by microscopic examination of the discharge (Fig. 72–1). Chronic or recurrent candidal vaginitis is common in diabetic women (Chapter 64.3). Trichomoniasis may be accompanied by severe vulvar itching, edema of the labia, and a copious vaginal discharge (Chapter 72).

"Nonspecific" vaginitis ("bacterial vaginosis") is a microbiologically complex disturbance of the vaginal flora, in which commensal bacteria, especially *Lactobacillus* spp. are replaced by *Gardnerella vaginalis* and anaerobic bacteria. The diagnosis is a clinical one and requires the presence of a vaginal pH greater than 4.5, coating of the vaginal epithelial cells with coccobacilli ("clue" cells), and the presence of a putrid odor.

GENITAL ULCERATIONS

Genital ulcerations are common worldwide. In Africa and Asia, the most common cause is chancroid (Fig. 45–1), followed by syphilis and herpes genitalis. In some countries, genital ulcers may be as common as gonorrhea. Both syphilis and herpes genitalis can infect a child during pregnancy or at delivery and thereby cause serious and potentially fatal complications.

Syphilis is sexually transmissible only during its primary and secondary stages, although an untreated mother may infect her fetus during any subsequent pregnancy (Chapter 32.1). The prevalence of venereal syphilis decreased greatly after long-acting penicillins were introduced as a single-dose treatment in the late 1940s. During the past decade, however, syphilis has increased in several African nations and in the major metropolitan areas of the United States. The reasons for this increase are not clear. The prevalence of HIV is also high in these populations; perhaps coinfections with HIV and its destruction of the immune system prolongs the duration of primary and secondary syphilitic lesions and thereby increases the period of infectivity (Chapter 15.1). In developed countries, the increase is related to the exchange of sexual favors for "crack" cocaine.

PELVIC INFLAMMATORY DISEASE

DEFINITION AND INCIDENCE. The endocervix is the most common site of gonococcal and chlamydial infection in women, and the infection remains minimally symptomatic until ascending infection extends to the fallopian tubes. This causes endometritis, salpingitis, oophoritis, or pelvic peritonitis; the syndrome of pelvic inflammatory disease (PID) includes these entities. Factors predisposing to PID are the surgical trauma of dilatation and curettage, surgical abortion, normal parturition, intrauterine contraceptive devices, and vaginal douching.

PID is the major complication of gonococcal and chlamydial cervicitis. It is often the first sign of gonococcal infection and may occur early in the course of the disease (Chapter 44). *N. gonorrhoeae* is isolated from 10 to 40% of cases of PID in Asia and Africa, but *C. trachomatis* may be as common a cause. In recent studies, infertile women with tubal obstruction had significantly higher titers of chlamydial antibodies than did fertile women. Gonococcal and chlamydial damage to fallopian tube cilia may promote secondary infection by other bacteria, such as anaerobes, which are normally cleared from the upper genital tract if they gain access. Thus, tubal aspirates or abscesses often contain a mixture of aerobic and anaerobic bacteria.

PATHOLOGY. Both fallopian tubes are usually infected, but the damage may be unequal. Some women with PID develop chronic fibrosis of both tubes, pyosalpinx, or tubo-ovarian abscess. Extension of acute infection into the peritoneum with peritonitis and abscess formation is frequently confused with acute appendicitis or ruptured tubal pregnancy. The correct diagnosis can usually be established by laparoscopy with aspiration of tubal material, and a test of urine or blood for chorionic gonadotropin.

CLINICAL MANIFESTATIONS AND MANAGEMENT. Subacute salpingitis produces symptoms of intermittent lower abdominal pain, low backache, painful menstruation, dyspareunia, or abnormal uterine bleeding. About half of affected women note an increase in vaginal discharge as well as fever. Lateral motion of the cervix produces acute tenderness, and bimanual examination reveals thickening or tenderness of either or both fallopian tubes. Male sexual partners of women with PID may have gonococcal or chlamydial urethritis but mild or no symptoms. Male sexual partners of women with PID should be treated for both gonococcal and chlamydial organisms before they resume sexual relations, even when they have no symptoms or signs of infection.

Women with gonococcal PID usually are more symptomatic than those with nongonococcal, nonchlamydial infection, but they usually respond more rapidly to antimicrobial therapy. Those with nongonococcal, nonchlamydial PID are more likely to have tubo-ovarian abscesses that require surgical drainage.

Although a variety of specific immune responses is generated against gonococci and chlamydiae during an episode of PID, the diseases tends to recur, perhaps because women are repeatedly exposed to infection. In a Swedish study, the proportions of women who had tubal infertility after one, two, and three or more episodes of laparoscopically proven salpingitis were 11%, 23%, and 54%, respectively. The rate was about

10% higher in each group for women who were older than 25 years. These women also had a risk of ectopic pregnancy 7- to 10-fold higher than that of women who had never had PID.

SEXUALLY TRANSMITTED DISEASES IN MALE HOMOSEXUALS

Homosexual and bisexual men are at increased risk for several STD pathogens, including enteric pathogens transmitted by fecal-oral contact, such as anilingus. In North America and Europe, homosexual men are still the group with the highest rate of AIDS (especially if they have multiple sexual partners and practice receptive anal intercourse), although users of illicit intravenous drugs cause an increasing proportion of cases (Chapter 15.1). Exclusively homosexual women have negligible risks for STDs.

Clinical manifestations of systemic STDs in homosexual men do not differ from those of the same disease transmitted by other routes. The most common sites of infection are the oropharynx, anus, and rectum. Specimens for detection of *N. gonorrhoeae* and *C. trachomatis* should be taken from these sites if the patient's sexual practices indicate such exposure. Proctosigmoidoscopic examination for gonococcal and chlamydial proctitis and primary syphilis should be done on men who practice receptive anal intercourse. Culture for enteric pathogens and appropriate serologic tests should be done if symptoms are compatible with bacterial dysentery, hepatitis, amebiasis, or giardiasis.

Venereal warts in the anus and rectum are common in homosexual men and are difficult to treat with cryotherapy or fulguration. These warts are usually caused by HPV types 6, 11, 16, and 18.

PREVENTION AND CONTROL. At a primary care clinic or a private practice, every reasonable effort should be made to ensure that all sexual partners of a patient with syphilis, urethritis, or PID are adequately treated before resuming coitus. Similarly, the parents of infants with gonococcal or chlamydial conjunctivitis should be treated. The reservoir of STDs in a community is dynamic. It includes prostitutes and their clients and others, such as barmaids, users of illicit drugs, truck drivers, and military personnel, whose employment or activities involve them with prostitutes. Persons at high risk may take oral antibiotics prophylactically or in inadequate doses before or after coitus. Such practices select resistant strains of *N. gonorrhoeae,* thus complicating both diagnosis and treatment.

Limited resources inevitably require that STD control activities be focused on priority groups. Pregnant women are given high priority because careful antenatal examination, laboratory screening tests for STDs, and appropriate antenatal treatment should prevent the congenital and perinatal transmission of syphilis, *N. gonorrhoeae,* and *C. trachomatis.*

Much of the STD control effort today is devoted to education and other activities to prevent transmission, especially by members of the STD "core-transmitter" group. This curriculum includes such subjects as the signs and symptoms of prevalent STDs, the importance of sexual partner referral, and avoidance of sexual contact until therapy has been completed for patients and their sexual partners. The AIDS epidemic has focused attention on the advantages of mutually exclusive sexual relationships and the use of condoms and vaginal sponges and suppositories containing compounds such as nonoxynol-9, which kills HIV and most other STD pathogens. Persons planning to travel to developing countries should be advised of the risk of STDs in areas where special problems exist and be made aware that national governments are often reluctant to publicize the extent of STDs in their countries.

BIBLIOGRAPHY

Arya OP, Alergant CD, Annels EH, et al: Management of non-specific urethritis in men. Evaluation of six treatment regimens and effect of other factors, including alcohol and sexual intercourse. Br J Vener Dis 54:414, 1977.

Berger RE, Alexander ER, Monda GD, et al: *Chlamydia trachomatis* as a cause of acute "idiopathic" epididymitis. N Engl J Med 289:301, 1978.

Brunham RC, Paavonen J, Stevens CE, Kiviat N, et al: Mucopurulent cervicitis—the ignored counterpart in women of urethritis in men. N Engl J Med 311:1, 1984.

Cates W, Farley TM, Rowe PJ: Worldwide patterns of infertility: Is Africa different? Lancet 2:596, 1985.

Centers for Disease Control: Quality Assurance Guidelines for STD Clinics—1986. Atlanta, U.S. Department of Health and Human Services, 1986.

Fransen L, Nsanze H, Klauss V, et al: Ophthalmia neonatorum in Nairobi, Kenya. The roles of *Neisseria gonorrhoeae* and *Chlamydia trachomatis.* J Infect Dis 153:862, 1986.

Hira SK, Bhat GJ, Chikamata DM, et al: Syphilis intervention in pregnancy: Zambian demonstration project. Genitourin Med 66:159, 1990.

Holmes KK, Handsfield HH, Wang SP, et al: Etiology of nongonococcal urethritis. N Engl J Med 292:1199, 1975.

Meheus AZ, Van Dyck E, Ursi JP, et al: Etiology of genital ulcerations in Swaziland. Sex Transm Dis 10:33, 1980.

Muir DG, Belsey MA: Pelvic inflammatory disease and its consequences in the developing world. Am J Obstet Gynecol 138:913, 1980.

Perine PL, Handsfield HH, Holmes KK, Blount JH: Epidemiology of sexually transmitted diseases. Annu Rev Public Health 6:85, 1985.

Piot P, Plummer FA, Mhalu FS, et al: AIDS: An international perspective. Science 239:573, 1988.

Plummer FA, D'Costa LJ, Nsanze H, et al: Epidemiology of chancroid and *Haemophilus ducreyi* in Nairobi, Kenya. Lancet 2:1293, 1983.

Quinn TC, Mann JM, Curran JW, Piot P: AIDS in Africa: An epidemiologic paradigm. Science 234:955, 1986.

Reiners J, Collet M, et al: Chlamydia antibodies and tubal infertility. Int J Epidemiol 18:261, 1989.

Stamm WE, Wagner KF, Amsel R, et al: Causes of the acute urethral syndrome in women. N Engl J Med 303:409, 1980.

Veeravahu M, Smyth RW, Clay JC: Detection of leukocyte esterase in urine: A new screening test of nongonococcal urethritis compared with two microscopic methods. Sex Transm Dis 14:180, 1987.

Weström L: Incidence, prevalence and trends of acute pelvic inflammatory disease and its consequences in industrialized countries. Am J Obstet Gynecol 138:880, 1980.

World Health Organization: Conjunctivitis of the Newborn. Prevention and Treatment at the Primary Health Care Level. Geneva, WHO, 1986.

World Health Organization: Control of Sexually Transmitted Diseases. Geneva, WHO, 1985.

Yorke JA, Hethcote HW, Nold A: Dynamics and control of the transmission of gonorrhea. Sex Transm Dis 5:51, 1978.

11. MALIGNANT DISEASES

John L. Ziegler

From 1850 until 1950, the enthusiasm and energy of most doctors working in the tropics and subtropics were directed toward the problems of infectious, parasitic, and nutritional diseases. Although these problems still dominate the day-to-day practice of rural tropical medicine, methods of control have greatly improved, and more emphasis is now being placed on the importance of noninfectious diseases in these regions. The concept that cancer is a disease of civilization is erroneous; certain types of malignancy are much more common in the tropics than in temperate climates. In those localized areas where age-specific rates are available, overall cancer incidence is the same as in industrial countries. In Africa, the decline in rates in older people is accounted for by the greater reluctance of elderly people, particularly those living in rural areas, to seek medical advice or to be admitted to the hospital. It is also evident that cancer incidence will be less in countries with a pyramidal age structure with fewer people in the older, most susceptible age groups.

Age-specific or proportional cancer rates of indigenous populations of most tropical countries and the rates found in Europe or North America differ markedly. Some cancers vary in frequency between, or even within, countries or regions in the tropics. Difference in incidence may be explained by environmental and geographic factors, cultural practices, or the socioeconomic level of particular communities. Some etiologic factors, such as nutrition, are influenced by all these. Increasing organization and industrialization are beginning to alter the cancer pattern in the big cities of many tropical countries, particularly among the upper socioeconomic groups, in whom the pattern is beginning to resemble that in Europe or North America.

The average annual incidence rates per 100,000 population for a variety of tumors in different parts of the world are shown in Table 11–1. These data are derived from Cancer Registries serving defined populations with good medical facilities. Certain tumors, e.g., carcinoma of the lung, rectum, colon, prostate, kidney (excluding nephroblastoma), endometrium, pancreas, and breast, are less common in the tropics than in Europe or North America. In urbanized areas, there is evidence that some of these tumors are increasing in incidence. Other tumors, e.g., carcinoma of the liver, cervix, and penis, Burkitt's lymphoma, Kaposi's sarcoma, choriocarcinoma, esophageal carcinoma, gastric carcinoma and nasopharyngeal carcinoma, occur in tropical regions much more frequently than in the West. The features of these tumors will be discussed according to the WHO rubric of classification, emphasizing those tumors that are common or have unusual features in the tropics.

Acquired immunodeficiency syndrome (AIDS) is being reported from many tropical countries (particularly central and eastern Africa and Brazil) with increasing frequency since 1982 (Chapter 15.1). AIDS has altered both the incidence and the clinical manifestations of Kaposi's sarcoma and non-Hodgkin's lymphoma and may affect the pattern of other malignancies as well.

CARCINOMA OF THE ORAL CAVITY AND PHARYNX

DEFINITION. Squamous cell carcinomas arising in the buccal mucosa, gingival mucosa, palate, tongue, floor of the mouth, and hypopharynx are considered together because they form a very high proportion of malignant tumors in parts of the Indian subcontinent and the Far East.

EPIDEMIOLOGY AND ETIOLOGY. Cancer of the mouth and pharynx is the most common malignant tumor in India and Bangladesh, accounting for over half of tumors in males in many areas. These tumors are also common in Malaysia and some other countries of the Far East, particularly those with immigrant populations from the Indian subcontinent (Table 11–1). Within these areas, however, differences in the anatomic distribution of the tumors are related to local cultural practices. Factors that are associated with high incidence rates in India include (1) the chewing of tobacco or betel "quid" and (2) the use of alcohol. Betel quid consists of the young leaves of the betel vine, sliced betel nut,

TABLE 11–1. Average Annual Cancer Incidence per 100,000 Population, All Ages*

	USA (Conn)	UK (Oxford)	Colombia (Cali)	India (Bombay)	Singapore	Nigeria (Ibadan)	Zimbabwe (Bulawayo)	S. Africa (Natal)
Male								
Oropharynx and tongue	12.7	4.7	3.3	19.5	12.6	0.8	1.0	5.1
Esophagus	6.6	4.9	2.2	6.1	6.3	0.4	15.2	24.3
Stomach	17.5	28.8	25.2	4.7	7.5	3.9	2.7	6.6
Colon	32.0	20.0	2.1	1.9	1.4	0.6	1.9	1.1
Liver	4.9	1.3	1.9	0.3	5.5	5.9	20.9	20.1
Lung	50.6	84.5	7.3	6.2	6.2	0.7	12.3	26.3
Prostate	40.3	27.5	8.8	1.9	0.3	2.5	3.1	7.6
Penis	3.7	1.0	1.7	1.2	0.8	0.1	1.0	3.9
Bladder	23.5	15.5	4.4	1.0	0.8	1.4	5.0	2.2
Skin (not melanoma)	—	34.0	17.4	0.7	2.5	1.0	2.7	2.3
Female								
Cervix	12.2	20.9	46.1	14.4	14.6	8.2	7.5	35.2
Endometrium	19.0	27.6	3.8	0.7	2.6	0.0	0.6	2.8
Breast	77.4	66.7	15.7	10.9	5.2	7.6	3.2	7.2

*Modified from Cancer Incidence in Five Continents, Vols. I and II. Berlin, Springer, UICC, 1966.

and variable quantities of tobacco, aromatic spices, and slaked lime. In some areas, tobacco chewing is prevalent without the use of additional substances. The "bidi" is a locally made, cheap cigarette containing uncured tobacco. Oral cancers are related to the use of betel and tobacco chewing; cancer of the hypopharynx is associated with bidi smoking.

In Andhra Pradesh in Southeast India, a high incidence of palatal cancer is attributed to the habit of smoking cheroots, known as chutta, which are smoked with the lighted end inside the mouth adjacent to the palatal mucosa.

CLINICAL AND PATHOLOGIC MANIFESTATIONS. The clinical features of these tumors are similar to those seen elsewhere in the world. In high-incidence populations, precancerous lesions have been recognized and are characterized clinically by areas of leukoplakia and histologically by epithelial dysplasia. Eventually, foci of carcinoma in situ develop, and local invasion of tissues follows. These squamous cell carcinomas show varying degrees of differentiation. Spread to cervical lymph nodes is usually a late phenomenon.

TREATMENT AND PREVENTION. Successful management of these tumors involves (1) prevention, (2) early detection, and (3) prompt treatment with surgery and/or radiotherapy. Preventive measures include education regarding the hazards of betel chewing and cigarette smoking. Early detection is facilitated by a high index of suspicion in indigenous areas, with routine oral examination of populations at risk. Excisional biopsies of precancerous lesions and suspicious tumors should be performed on detection. Wider extirpative surgery (with preoperative or postoperative radiotherapy) should be considered in patients with larger lesions. Preoperative chemotherapy may reduce inoperable tumors to resectable size. Finally, topical or systemic chemoprophylactic agents are being used experimentally to treat precancerous lesions.

NASOPHARYNGEAL CARCINOMA (NPC)

DEFINITION. This tumor, formerly called lymphoepithelioma, is now recognized to be a squamous cell carcinoma, usually poorly differentiated in type. Tumors arise from the epithelium overlying nasopharyngeal lymphoid tissue.

EPIDEMIOLOGY AND INCIDENCE. NPC is uncommon in Europe and North America, although it has a high incidence in Alaskan Indians. The highest incidence rates are found in the Far East, including the Guangzhou area of China, Hong Kong, and Malaysia. Throughout these Far Eastern countries, the tumor is much more common in the Chinese populations than, for example, in the Malays or Indians living in the same environment. Three regions of high incidence of NPC have been reported in Africa—Tunisia, areas in western Sudan, and some highland areas of Kenya.

ETIOLOGY. The epidemiologic features in the Far East can best be explained on the basis of environmental factors acting on a susceptible population of southern Chinese stock. It has been shown that there is an unusual

HLA type, known as Sin 2 (Singapore), in many patients. Factors suggested as exogenous carcinogens include inhalation of smoke in chimneyless huts in Kenya, ingestion of nitrosamines in certain foods, and the use of wood as a cooking fuel. None of these factors is common to all high-incidence areas.

The isolation of Epstein-Barr virus (EBV) from tumor cells from patients with NPC points strongly to a viral etiology. The oropharyngeal epithelium contains receptors for EBV and is the primary site of infection and viral replication. Elevated antibody titers to EBV have been found in patients from all high-incidence areas, from China to the Sudan. The difference between antibody titers in patients and controls is most significant for IgA viral capsid antibodies. EBV genome has also been demonstrated in the nuclei of the malignant epithelial cells. This evidence is similar to that incriminating EBV in the etiology of Burkitt's lymphoma, although it must be stressed that the geographic features of these two tumors are quite different.

PATHOLOGY. NPC cells contain large vesicular nuclei with nucleoli, and the tumor may be mistaken histologically for histiocytic lymphoma. Lymphocytic infiltration of the tumor, sometimes marked, may be present, and epithelioid cell granulomas and eosinophils may be seen among the tumor cells.

CLINICAL MANIFESTATIONS. Most patients present with symptoms and signs of lymph node metastases and seldom complain of local nasal symptoms. The lymphadenopathy may be gross and is sometimes bilateral, affecting particularly the upper cervical groups (Fig. 11–1). In such cases, nasopharyngoscopy may reveal slight thickening of the nasopharynx, asymmetry of the wall, or narrowing of the eustachian tube. Other patients may have local symptoms with bleeding and discomfort. When the base of the skull is invaded, cranial nerve palsies may develop, and in late cases, intracranial pressure is raised.

DIAGNOSIS. This depends on clinical awareness and appropriate removal of tissue for histologic examination. In China, attempts have been made to screen susceptible populations by cytologic examination of the nasopharynx, but it is too early to assess the value of this procedure.

TREATMENT. Because of its anatomic location, NPC is not amenable to surgical resection; radiotherapy is the treatment of choice. Treatment with alkylating agents, e.g., cyclophosphamide, nitrogen mustard, has met with some success but does not supplant radiation therapy. Experimental therapy with interferon has produced tumor regression, encouraging further trial.

ESOPHAGEAL CARCINOMA

DEFINITION. Tumors arising from the lining of the esophagus occur throughout the world but show over 100-fold differences in incidence rates.

EPIDEMIOLOGY AND ETIOLOGY. In Africa, esophageal cancer is most common in Zimbabwe, with a recorded rate of 75.6 per 100,000 males in Bulawayo. Other areas of high incidence include parts of Zambia,

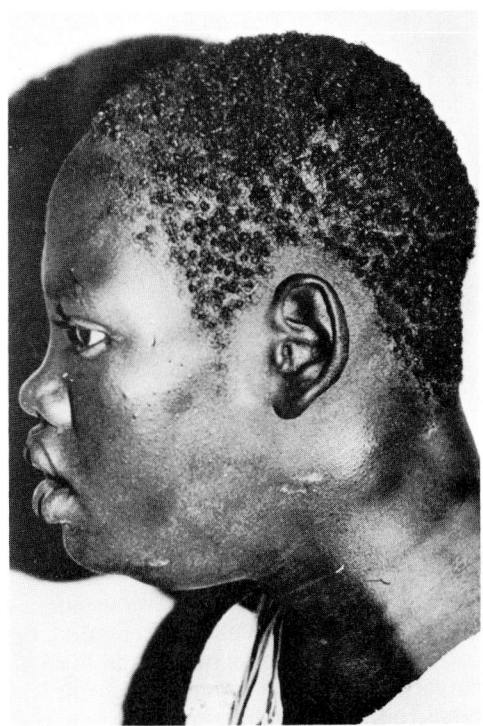

FIGURE 11–1. Enlarged cervical lymph nodes in a patient with nasopharyngeal carcinoma. (Courtesy of M. A. O. Malik, Khartoum.)

Malawi, western Kenya near Lake Victoria, and the Transkei in South Africa (Table 11–1). There is a high-incidence area around the Caspian Sea, where two unusual features occur: an increasing incidence gradient from west to east and a unique female predominance. Finally, esophageal cancer is particularly common in the Linhsien area of China, with rates of over 200 per 100,000 population on record.

Because of the restricted nature of the high-incidence areas, many believe that dietary and nutritional factors are responsible. Thus far, alcohol, particularly vagaries in local brewing practices, fungal toxins, the swallowing of pyrolyzed substances from opium pipes, pickled foods, and other nutritional factors have been implicated.

CLINICAL MANIFESTATIONS, TREATMENT, AND PREVENTION. Precancerous dysplastic lesions have been identified in high-risk populations through cytologic and direct visual screening techniques. In China, approximately 1 in 100 individuals at risk has had esophageal cancer diagnosed in this manner.

The typical mode of presentation is dysphagia, first to solids and later to all foods, with weight loss. Aspiration pneumonia is common in more advanced cases. Early detection and surgery have been the mainstays of successful treatment, with radiotherapy reserved for inoperable cases. Improved radiotherapeutic approaches using "superfractions" and radiosensitizers, e.g., misonidazole, show promise in the management of advanced tumors. Chemotherapy cannot be advocated except on an experimental basis, since responses to most agents are infrequent and transitory.

STOMACH CARCINOMA

DEFINITION. The majority of stomach cancers are adenocarcinomas of the intestinal differentiated or anaplastic variety.

EPIDEMIOLOGY AND ETIOLOGY. Throughout most of the tropical and subtropical world, carcinoma of the stomach is less common than in temperate areas (Table 11–1). However, high rates have been recorded around Mount Kilimanjaro in Tanzania and Kenya and near Lake Kivu in Zaire. In South America, there is a high incidence in the mountainous regions of Colombia, with lower rates near the coast. High rates have also been reported from Chile. Outside the tropics, the highest rates occur in Japan, Finland, and Iceland. The association with mountainous areas in the tropics is apparent. In Colombia, very high concentrations of nitrate have been found in the soil. It has been shown that carcinogenic nitrosamines may be formed in the stomach of patients taking high concentrations of nitrates, particularly if they have achlorhydria with bacterial overgrowth in the stomach. The local production of oxidative free radicals from inflammatory cells may augment the carcinogenic effect. In Chile, nitrate concentrations may be related to the high production of fertilizers.

In high-incidence areas, the histologic type is more frequently intestinal, developing in long-standing chronic atrophic gastritis. The anaplastic variety may be related to different etiologic factors.

CARCINOMA OF THE COLON

DEFINITION. Adenocarcinomas of the large bowel are common in Western countries. Although most tumors arise from adenomatous polyps, some occur de novo.

EPIDEMIOLOGY AND ETIOLOGY. The incidence rates of carcinoma of the colon and rectum show a very close relationship with Western influences (Table 11–1). Colorectal cancer rates are low in the tropics. The only industrialized, urbanized country without high rates is Japan. Migration from low- to high-incidence areas is associated with an increase in tumor rate.

These differences can best be explained by dietary factors. Low-incidence areas are associated with a high intake of unrefined carbohydrate and fiber and a low intake of animal fat and protein and refined carbohydrate. This diet increases bowel transit times and stool bulk and decreases the levels of steroid derivatives, anaerobic bacteria, and pH of the stool. In high-incidence areas, carcinogenic or cocarcinogenic factors may be produced in the large bowel by the action of certain anaerobic bacteria. One hypothesis holds that the long transit time and small stool bulk in developed countries prolong contact of these substances with the bowel wall, increasing the likelihood of a carcinogenic mutation. Recent evidence indicates a role for genetic factors, possibly heritable, in colorectal carcinogenesis.

There is a close relationship between the incidence of

carcinoma of the large bowel and adenomatous polyps in populations throughout the world; these benign tumors are exceedingly rare in Africans.

HEPATOCELLULAR CARCINOMA

DEFINITION. Hepatocellular carcinoma (HCC) arises from the parenchymal cells of the liver and must be distinguished from cholangiocarcinoma (bile duct carcinoma), which arises from intrahepatic bile ducts. HCC shows some of the largest variations in geographic incidence throughout the world (Table 11–1).

EPIDEMIOLOGY. Incidence rate surveys have shown that throughout large areas of the tropics and subtropics HCC is 10 to 100 times more common than in Western countries. In Africa, this high frequency is confined to the indigenous black populations of the sub-Sahara, although within these regions there are marked local variations. The tumor is most common in rural areas, with the incidence decreasing among the more affluent urban populations. The highest rates recorded were 103.8 per 100,000 in the male population of Lorenço Marques, Mozambique, although recent surveys suggest that the rates are declining.

High rates are also seen in the Far East, particularly in the coastal belt of China, Taiwan, Hong Kong, Malaysia, and Singapore. Proportional rates indicate that HCC is more common in southern India and Sri Lanka than in northern India and that the tumor is common in Papua New Guinea and Fiji. In all high-incidence areas, there is a male dominance, varying from 3 to 6 times the rate in females.

ETIOLOGY. Throughout the world, the majority of hepatocellular carcinomas develop in cirrhotic livers. HCC occurs most frequently as the macronodular type in endemic areas. Infection with hepatitis B virus is a major cause of macronodular cirrhosis. In all high-incidence areas, the carrier rate of hepatitis B surface antigen is high. In virtually all patients with HCC from endemic areas, serologic markers of active hepatitis B infection are present. The virus may act by producing a form of cirrhosis in which the regenerating cells are susceptible to other carcinogenic influences, although a direct oncogenic effect is also possible.

Aflatoxin, a highly potent hepatocarcinogen, is derived from the fungus *Aspergillus flavus,* which grows on ground nuts and some cereals. Aflatoxin contamination of foodstuffs has correlated with the incidence of HCC in Kenya and the Transkei. This epidemiologic evidence suggests that aflatoxin is directly or indirectly implicated in the etiology of liver cancer.

PATHOLOGY. Hepatocellular carcinomas may form one large mass or be composed of multiple variably sized tumor nodules (Fig. 11–2). If HCC arises in a noncirrhotic liver, it usually forms a single large mass. Necrosis and hemorrhage, often with hemoperitoneum, are common features. The portal and the hepatic veins may be involved and filled with tumor. At postmortem examinations, metastases to the lungs and bone are common. Histologically, most hepatocellular carcinomas are described as trabecular and resemble, to a varying

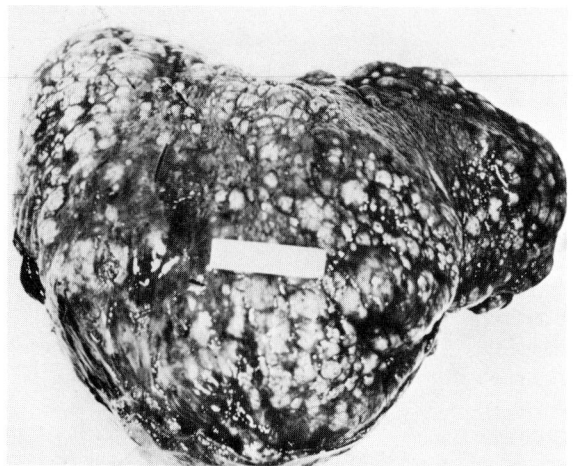

FIGURE 11–2. Multiple nodules of liver cell carcinoma, involving both lobes, in a cirrhotic liver.

extent, liver parenchymal cells and sinusoids. A useful diagnostic feature in the well-differentiated tumors is the absence of reticulin fibers or stromal fibrosis. Other histologic varieties include an adenoid form with pseudoglandular formation, a pleomorphic variety, and a clear cell type.

CLINICAL MANIFESTATIONS. HCC in temperate climates usually occurs in older people with established cirrhosis and is heralded by weight loss, pain, or jaundice. In high-incidence areas of the tropics, the tumor frequently occurs in younger people, even under the age of 10. Age-specific rates increase with age; the most common ages at presentation are in the 30s and 40s. Most patients present with advanced tumors, wasting, and ascites but without prior symptoms related to the underlying cirrhosis. The disease progresses very rapidly; prognosis is not related to histologic type. Ascites, often bloody, may be present, and hemoperitoneum is often found at postmortem examination. On examination, one or more discrete, hard masses may be palpated in the liver; marked jaundice is not common. In endemic areas, the diagnosis of HCC is virtually certain in a patient with a large hepatic mass and a positive alpha-fetoprotein determination.

TREATMENT AND PROGNOSIS. Partial hepatectomy is the treatment of choice if 1 or more tumor nodules are localized to a single lobe and the patient is a reasonable operative candidate. The surgical mortality rate varies from 30 to 70%. HCC is usually radioresistant, and damage to surrounding normal liver precludes this approach. Hepatic artery ligation or embolization has been advocated by some, but this method affords only temporary benefit. Chemotherapy with a variety of agents has been attempted with disappointing results. At present only doxorubicin (Adriamycin), 60 to 75 mg/ M^2 intravenously every 3 weeks, has resulted in consistent but modest tumor regression. Drug toxicity, particularly cardiac toxicity, is dose-limiting.

Prognosis in HCC in the tropics is most dependent on performance status, weight loss, and elevation of bilirubin. Nearly all patients with HCC die within 6 to 12 months of diagnosis.

CARCINOMA OF THE PENIS

DEFINITION. Malignant tumors of the penis arise on the prepuce or glans and are usually well-differentiated squamous cell carcinomas that metastasize eventually to the regional inguinal lymph nodes.

EPIDEMIOLOGY AND ETIOLOGY. The incidence of penile carcinoma is related to socioeconomic and cultural conditions affecting circumcision. Uncircumsized men in poor hygienic conditions have the highest rates of penile carcinoma. Low rates are found among Jews and Muslim groups; the condition is uncommon in Western countries. Significant differences exist between tribes in East Africa that practice pubertal circumcision and those that do not. Recent evidence points to a role for papillomaviruses in anogenital malignancies.

CLINICAL AND PATHOLOGIC FEATURES. As noted previously, the majority of penile carcinomas are well-differentiated squamous types. They present as papillary or ulcerative lesions and, in the rural tropics, may be advanced before treatment is sought. Large tumors may be present without lymph node involvement, which occurs late; enlarged inguinal nodes are often present owing to secondary infection. Diagnosis is usually not difficult, except in slow-growing verrucous carcinomas, which may resemble condylomata acuminata (venereal warts). These viral lesions may occasionally undergo malignant change. Treatment is surgical.

BLADDER CARCINOMA

DEFINITION. In industrialized countries, the majority of urothelial neoplasms are transitional cell in type and often arise in the trigone. In tropical and subtropical regions, squamous and, to a lesser extent, adenocarcinoma or anaplastic cell types predominate. Premalignant changes, such as leukoplakia and squamous metaplasia, are common findings in the bladder urothelium.

EPIDEMIOLOGY AND ETIOLOGY. Transitional cell carcinomas of the bladder in industrialized regions have been associated with occupational carcinogens. In Egypt, the Sudan, Malawi, and Zimbabwe, over 50% of bladder cancers are squamous in type and are often well differentiated and highly keratinizing. The high incidence rates are in areas where *Schistosoma haematobium* is endemic and are related to the prevalence and intensity of this infection in the population and the degree of vesical damage it causes (Chapter 96). Squamous carcinoma of the bladder is also seen in Jamaica and Uganda, where it is associated with obstructive uropathy due to long-standing urethral strictures. Secondary and recurrent bacterial infections may play an etiologic role in the development of squamous metaplasia and carcinoma.

CLINICAL MANIFESTATIONS. Patients with bladder cancer present with hematuria, pain, and a suprapubic mass. In regions endemic for *S. haematobium*, these symptoms are often obscured by manifestations of chronic bilharzial cystitis. Therefore, the majority of patients present with advanced tumors (Fig. 11–3).

TREATMENT AND PROGNOSIS. Treatment consists of cystectomy, which may be curative, and urinary tract diversion. The 5-year survival rate is about 65% in patients with carcinoma in stages I to III. Radiation therapy, whether preoperative or postoperative, has not proved beneficial. Chemotherapy is still in experimental stages, although some of the newer drugs, such as *cis*-platinum and etoposide, cause regression of tumors.

KAPOSI'S SARCOMA

DEFINITION. Although this tumor was first described by Kaposi in Eastern Europe in 1872, it was thought to be a rarity. It was not until the 1950s that this sarcoma was discovered to be endemic in sub-Saharan Africa. The tumor arises from angioformative cells, usually starts on the skin, and is often multifocal.

EPIDEMIOLOGY. The high incidence of Kaposi's sarcoma is confined to tropical Africa; it is not common in other similar tropical regions, e.g., Papua New Guinea. Within Africa, surveys indicate that there is an epicenter of high incidence in central and eastern Zaire and in western Uganda. The tumor occurs in the southern Sudan but is rare in the Saharan region. Kaposi's sarcoma occurs in parts of South Africa, but the incidence declines to the extreme south. Within this vast area, there are some local variations, suggesting environmental rather than ethnic factors. An unusual feature is the male predominance that increases with age.

ETIOLOGY. No adequate explanation exists for the geographic distribution or the sex incidence. The tumor appears to be more common in hot and humid areas with high rainfall. The distribution is quite different from that of Burkitt's lymphoma, however, and does not appear to be related to another disease such as malaria. Kaposi's sarcoma is associated with an increased risk of developing malignant lymphoma. More recently, the incidence is increasing among transplant recipients and patients on immunosuppressive drugs, an

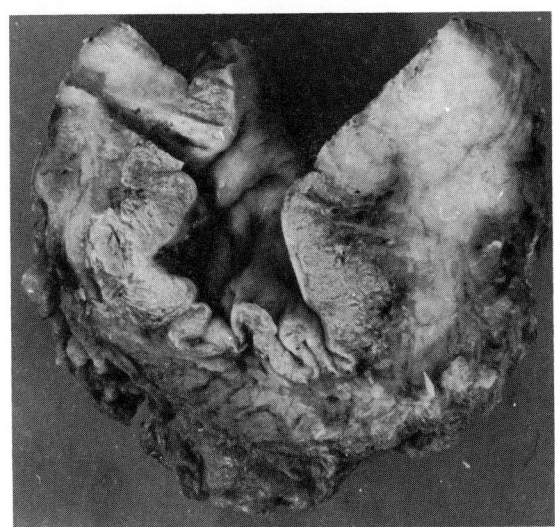

FIGURE 11–3. Invasive squamous cell carcinoma in a bladder with heavy *Schistosoma haematobium* infection.

observation that implies an etiologic relationship with immune deficiency.

The epidemic of AIDS has focused much investigative attention on Kaposi's sarcoma (Chapter 15.1). This tumor predominates in homosexual men who become infected with the causative agent of AIDS—human immunodeficiency virus, or HIV. Although HIV itself is not present in the tumor cells, other etiologic cofactors have been postulated. HIV is also prevalent in central and eastern Africa, and many victims develop a severe, aggressive form of Kaposi's sarcoma.

CLINICAL MANIFESTATIONS. Four clinical types of Kaposi's sarcoma have been described. Nodular skin lesions are the most common presentation in Africa. The tumors are multifocal and develop as small, raised lesions on the extremity (Fig. 11–4A). Most patients with this form of the disease have a benign course and a normal life span. Lesions respond to radiation therapy or treatment with an alkylating agent and occasionally undergo spontaneous regression.

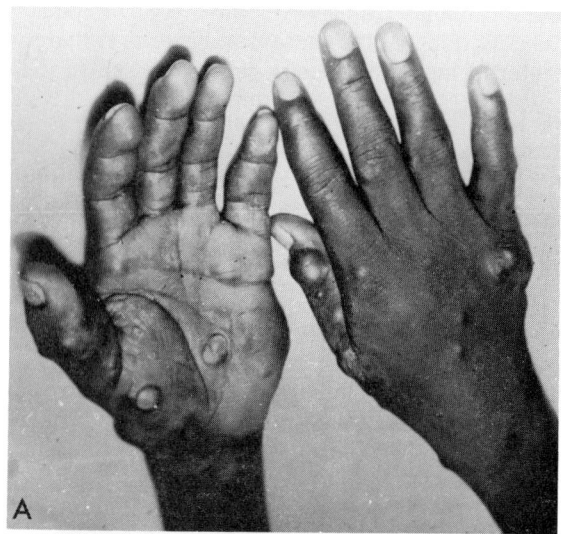
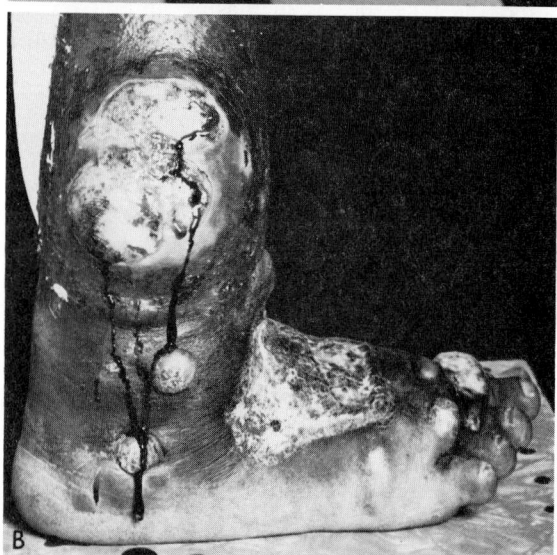

FIGURE 11–4. *A,* Nodular form of Kaposi's sarcoma on the hands of an African male. *B,* Florid form of Kaposi's sarcoma on the lower leg. Nodular lesions are also present, and there is some lymphedema. (*A,* Courtesy of Dr. E. H. Williams.)

Florid skin lesions are rapidly growing, often fungating skin tumors and may complicate the nodular variety or present as the initial lesion (Fig. 11–4B). Spread to deep tissues and bone may occur, and the tumor may metastasize to local lymph nodes.

Infiltrative skin lesions are characterized by growth involving deeper structures in the skin and underlying tissues. Clinically, the tumor forms plaques and becomes indurated and edematous.

The lymphadenopathic type is common in children, who present with widespread lymphadenopathy that is usually mistaken for lymphoma. The disease is rapidly progressive, with involvement of many internal organs; conjunctival and mucosal nodules are not infrequent. In contrast to patients who present with skin lesions, the incidence in males and females in childhood cases is nearly the same.

African patients who acquire Kaposi's sarcoma in association with HIV infection often develop a combination of lymphadenopathic and aggressive nodular disease. Visceral involvement, particularly lung and gastrointestinal tract, is common. These patients respond temporarily to chemotherapy (usually vincristine, vinblastine, or dactinomycin) but their ultimate prognosis is related to the severity of the underlying immunodeficiency.

PATHOLOGY. Kaposi's sarcoma arises from primitive vasoformative mesenchymal cells. The tumor is composed of interlacing bundles of spindle cells, with vascular slits between the cells that often contain erythrocytes (Fig. 11–5). Unless ulceration has occurred, the tumor is usually situated in the dermis, with a tumor-free zone under the epithelium. Occasionally, involution is present, with atrophy of cells, fibrosis, and infiltration by plasma cells and lymphocytes. The tumor cells often contain eosinophilic droplets that stain with PAS. This common pattern is called a "mixed" cell type or Kaposi's sarcoma with slit formation.

Some tumors have a more monomorphic pattern with less of a vasoformative element. This variety is common in the florid clinical type and is more difficult to distinguish from other forms of soft tissue sarcoma such as leiomyosarcoma and fibrosarcoma. A rare variant is the pleomorphic type that is anaplastic with more cellular variation. It is associated with a poor prognosis. The histology of the highly malignant childhood lymphadenopathic variety is usually of the typical "mixed" pattern.

DIAGNOSIS. The clinical features of the typical nodular form in an endemic area rarely cause diagnostic difficulties. Occasionally, a single lesion may be mistaken for a non-neoplastic lesion such as pyogenic granuloma, a *Tunga penetrans* mass, or a chronic infection. Larger fungating lesions may be confused with other soft tissue sarcomas or, on the sole of the foot, with malignant melanoma.

TREATMENT AND PROGNOSIS. Kaposi's sarcoma responds to radiotherapy and chemotherapy. When localized to an extremity, 800 cGy in a single dose may be curative in 30 to 40% of patients. Deeper lesions require higher dosage. Patients with widespread disease (beyond the confines of reasonable radiation

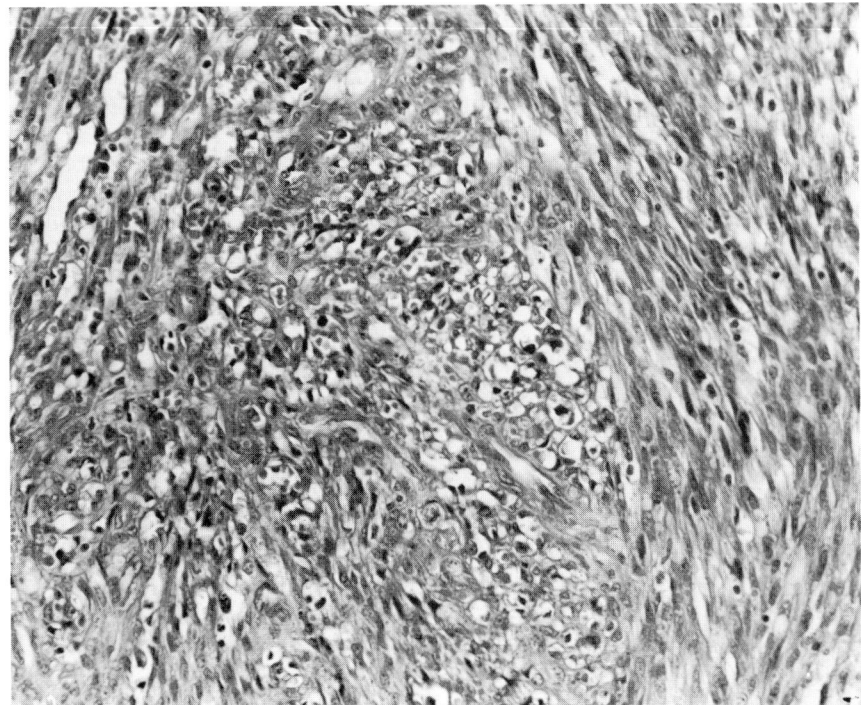

FIGURE 11–5. Typical "sievelike" pattern of interlacing bundles of angioformative spindle cells. From a patient with Kaposi's sarcoma. (H & E stain, × 250.)

ports) will respond to single-agent chemotherapy. In this setting, vinblastine, 0.1 mg/kg/week, is the treatment of choice. Patients with more aggressive tumors, e.g., florid, infiltrative, or lymphadenopathic, may respond favorably to a variety of drug combinations. One such regimen is Adriamycin, 30 mg/M² intravenously day 1, imidazole carboxamide (DTIC), 750 mg intravenously day 1; and bleomycin, 15 units intravenously days 1 and 8. This combination is repeated every 21 days. Prognosis varies with histologic type, clinical manifestations, and response to treatment. Patients on immunosuppressive drugs may improve after these drugs are withheld. Patients with AIDS may respond temporarily, but intensive chemotherapy tends to worsen the immune deficiency, leading to opportunistic infection.

CARCINOMA OF THE SKIN

DEFINITION. The incidence of squamous and basal cell carcinomas of the skin shows variations throughout the world. However, the etiologic factors in populations with a similar overall incidence may be quite different.

EPIDEMIOLOGY AND ETIOLOGY. In white races, there is a correlation between the incidence of squamous and basal cell carcinoma and exposure to ultraviolet light, the risk being increased in fair-skinned white individuals and being highest in albinos of any race. Prolonged residence in the tropics increases the risk of development of these tumors. In the poor, rural, tropical areas of the world, squamous cell carcinoma is also common. These tumors arise in ulcers, sinuses, or scars, the last often from old burns (Fig. 11–6). Malignant change in poorly treated tropical ulcers accounts for up to 10% of all malignant tumors in some groups in sub-Saharan Africa. By contrast, black or brown

populations living in good socioeconomic conditions, e.g., in the West Indies and in large parts of India, rarely have skin cancer, since pigmentation gives protection from solar irradiation. Localized areas of high incidence related to specific cultural practices have been reported from India; these include the Kangri cancer, caused by the holding of a clay pot containing burning

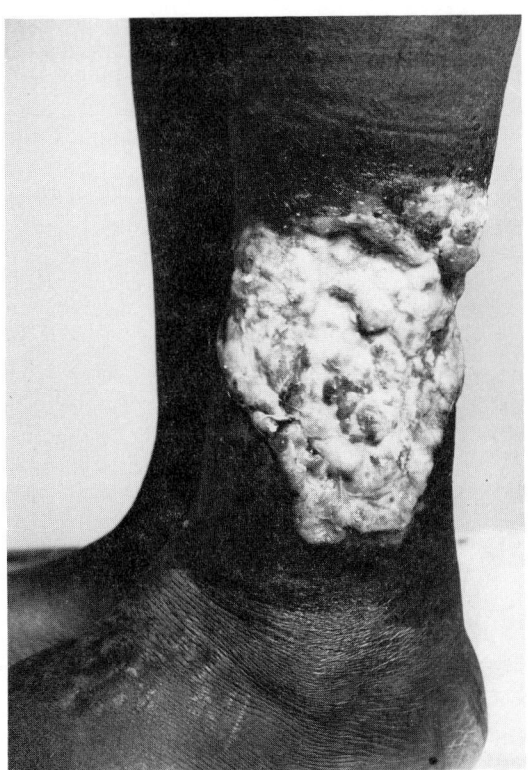

FIGURE 11–6. Malignant change (squamous cell carcinoma) arising in the scar of an unhealed tropical ulcer.

embers against the abdomen or thigh for warmth, and the dhoti cancer, occurring on the trunk and groin and related to constant irritation from a loincloth. The lowest incidence of skin cancer is found in dark-skinned races living in good socioeconomic conditions.

CLINICAL AND PATHOLOGIC MANIFESTATIONS. In the tropics, the main clinical and diagnostic problems are malignancies in such predisposing lesions as ulcers and scars. Many patients present with advanced infiltrating lesions that have raised and everted edges. Most tropical ulcers occur on the shin, and invasion may involve the underlying tibia, sometimes causing pathologic fractures. The majority of tumors are well-differentiated squamous cell carcinomas; diagnosis requires biopsy. The rare anaplastic spindle cell carcinomas are difficult to differentiate from sarcomas.

MALIGNANT MELANOMA

EPIDEMIOLOGY AND ETIOLOGY. The incidence and anatomic distribution of malignant melanomas in different populations are determined by ethnic factors related to skin pigmentation and by environmental factors such as exposure to sunlight or trauma. In dark-skinned races, malignant melanoma develops almost exclusively in areas with little pigment, e.g., the palms, soles, and mucosa (Fig. 11–7). The tumors arise from small centers of melanocytes that are focally distributed and occur near the junction of pigmented and nonpigmented skin. These tumors are common in barefoot black populations.

CLINICAL FEATURES. Clinical suspicion of melanomas in dark-skinned individuals should be aroused by the presence of any tumor on the nonpigmented areas of the hand or foot. Pigmented tumors present no diagnostic problems, but an amelanotic melanoma may be mistaken for a squamous cell carcinoma. Some tumors metastasize early to regional lymph nodes, whereas others may produce large fungating lesions without

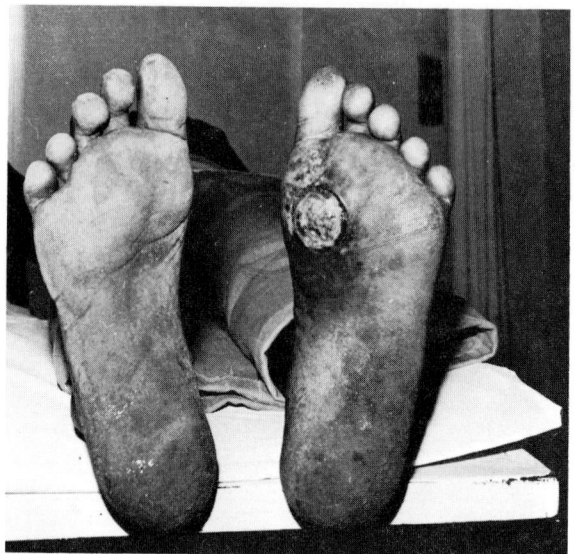

FIGURE 11–7. Malignant melanoma on the sole of the foot in an adult African. (Courtesy of Dr. E. H. Williams.)

metastases. Occasional patients present with lymph node metastases and a primary lesion that is very small or undetectable.

TREATMENT AND PROGNOSIS. Extirpative surgery remains the best treatment. Chemotherapy (with the possible exception of dacarbazine) is unsuccessful, and malignant melanoma responds only partially to radiation therapy. Removal of the draining lymph nodes does not reduce the recurrence rate or influence prognosis.

LEUKEMIA AND MALIGNANT LYMPHOMA

LEUKEMIA. Age-specific incidence rates for the various types of leukemia are not available from many parts of the tropics, although overall rates appear to be less than in the West (Chapter 5). In sub-Saharan Africa, there is a low incidence of acute lymphoblastic leukemia of young children; acute myeloid leukemia in older children and in adults is not common. Chronic myeloid and chronic lymphatic leukemia occur throughout the world and have no specific features. Clinically, hyperreactive malaria splenomegaly (HMS) may sometimes be associated with an absolute lymphocytosis; in such cases, HMS may mimic chronic lymphatic leukemia. The patients with HMS are usually younger, and the splenomegaly and lymphocytosis respond to prolonged malarial prophylaxis (Chapter 73.2).

MYELOMATOSIS. Most reports from the tropics suggest that myelomatosis is less common than in Europe or North America. However, it is probable that there is considerable underdiagnosis of this condition. An unusual clinical feature of myeloma in Africa is the frequency with which it presents as an isolated bone tumor causing pain or pathologic fracture. These bone lesions frequently affect the limbs, preceding general symptoms.

HODGKIN'S DISEASE. Hodgkin's disease in the tropics has some unusual clinical and histologic features. It occurs more frequently in the younger age groups. The rates for males in Uganda for ages 5 to 15 are higher than those in the United States and the United Kingdom; nearly half the patients are under age 20 years at the time of diagnosis, and some are under age 5 years. Histologically, the "mixed" and "lymphocyte-depleted" varieties that have a poor prognosis are proportionally more common than in the West.

Patients with Hodgkin's disease frequently seek medical attention with advanced (stage III or IV) disease, often at a facility lacking radiotherapy. The treatment of choice is therefore combination chemotherapy. The regimen commonly known as MOPP (nitrogen mustard, Oncovin, prednisone, and procarbazine in combination) has yielded cure rates of 75%.

BURKITT'S LYMPHOMA

DEFINITION. Although several clinicians had noted the occurrence of a peculiar sarcoma of the jaw affecting young African children, it was not until 1958 that Burkitt described the clinicopathologic entity that now bears his name (Fig. 11–8). He pointed out that these children often had tumors in other sites and that jaw involvement was not always present. Later, Davies, O'Conor, and Wright showed that this was a form of malignant lymphoma and that it was histopathologically and cytologically a specific entity. There is little doubt that the tumor has been endemic in sub-Saharan Africa for at least 100 years.

EPIDEMIOLOGY. During the 1960s, Burkitt showed that the tumor is limited to sub-Saharan Africa and is absent in high-altitude regions. It also does not occur in Zanzibar, although it is present in the adjacent coastal regions of Tanzania. The distribution of the tumor suggested an insect vector, since it occurs only in those areas where the mean temperature does not fall below 16 C or the annual rainfall below 75 cm. Burkitt's lymphoma was later shown to be endemic in New Guinea, where it was also altitude-, temperature-, and rainfall-related. A few cases have been reported from other developing countries in the Middle East, Brazil in South America, and Malaysia in the Far East. In none of these, however, do the rates approach those in Africa. Cytologically similar tumors are seen very rarely in most other parts of the world.

ETIOLOGY. Like most tumors, Burkitt's lymphoma has multiple causes. The geographic distribution corresponds closely with the prevalence and intensity of *Plasmodium falciparum* malaria. This could explain its absence from Zanzibar, where malarial control has been established for many years.

In 1964, Epstein and colleagues isolated a hitherto unknown herpesvirus, now known as the Epstein-Barr virus (EBV), from a tissue culture of Burkitt's lymphoma cells. Subsequently, it was shown that patients with Burkitt's lymphoma had higher mean antibody titers to EBV than controls in the same area, although antibodies were present in most children in endemic areas. Prospective studies in the West Nile region of Uganda revealed that children who later developed the tumor had unusually high titers to EBV for up to 15 months before the tumor was clinically manifest. Further evidence that EBV is directly implicated in the etiology of Burkitt's lymphoma is the finding of viral antigens in tumor cells and of EBV genomes in nuclear DNA. Moreover, when added to a tissue culture of human lymphocytes, the virus can transform the cells so that they develop malignant characteristics. How can these two pieces of evidence for the involvement of malaria and EBV be linked? It is known that malaria has profound effects on the immunologic system, particularly if there are recurrent attacks in infancy and early childhood. Among these effects is immunosuppression. In experimental animals, concurrent malaria may enhance the effect of oncogenic viruses. It is hypothesized that EBV infection in such individuals, particularly if it occurs at a very early age, may induce the tumor.

A specific chromosomal translocation (q^{8-14}) is known to occur in Burkitt's lymphoma. This genetic accident transfers a known oncogene called c-*myc* to an area of high promotional activity (i.e., near a region of immunoglobulin genes). Other oncogenes are also activated in Burkitt's lymphoma cells in tissue culture, and the inactivation of cancer "repressor" genes may also occur. The present etiologic paradigm in Burkitt's lymphoma proposes a B-cell proliferation driven by EBV and augmented by malaria-induced immunosuppression. Among these proliferating B cells, genetic accidents confer a growth advantage on certain resistant clones. A polyclonal proliferation then progresses to oligoclonal and finally to monoclonal, exhibiting increasing characteristics of malignant change in the process. This scenario does not exclude the possibility that other as yet undetermined factors such as genetic susceptibility or other infections may play some role in the genesis of the tumor. It is of interest that most of the sporadic cases of Burkitt's lymphoma seen in temperate climates do now show an association with EBV.

PATHOLOGY. Burkitt's lymphoma is a specific cytologic type of non-Hodgkin's malignant lymphoma arising from B lymphocytes of follicular origin. The histopathology is similar in all sites, modified only by the structure of the organ affected, e.g., bone or soft tissues. The tumor cells are uniformly immature lymphocytes (Fig. 11–9A) containing basophilic cytoplasm. The nucleus usually contains 2 or 3 nucleoli. Scattered through the tumor are large, pale macrophages that contain nuclear debris. Tumor imprints stained with Giemsa should be made at the time a biopsy is done (Fig. 11–9B).

CLINICAL MANIFESTATIONS. In endemic areas, Burkitt's lymphoma is predominantly a disease of the young. It is rarely seen before age 2 years, but 60% of patients are between the ages of 4 and 8; less than 10% of cases occur after age 15. Within the endemic zones, the prevalence may differ among ethnic groups. There is usually a slight male predominance.

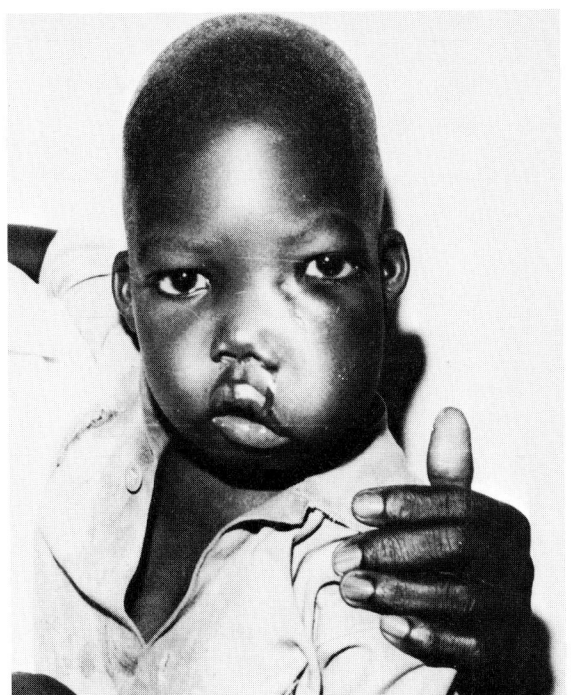

FIGURE 11–8. Left maxillary tumor in a child with Burkitt's lymphoma. (Courtesy of Dr. E. H. Williams.)

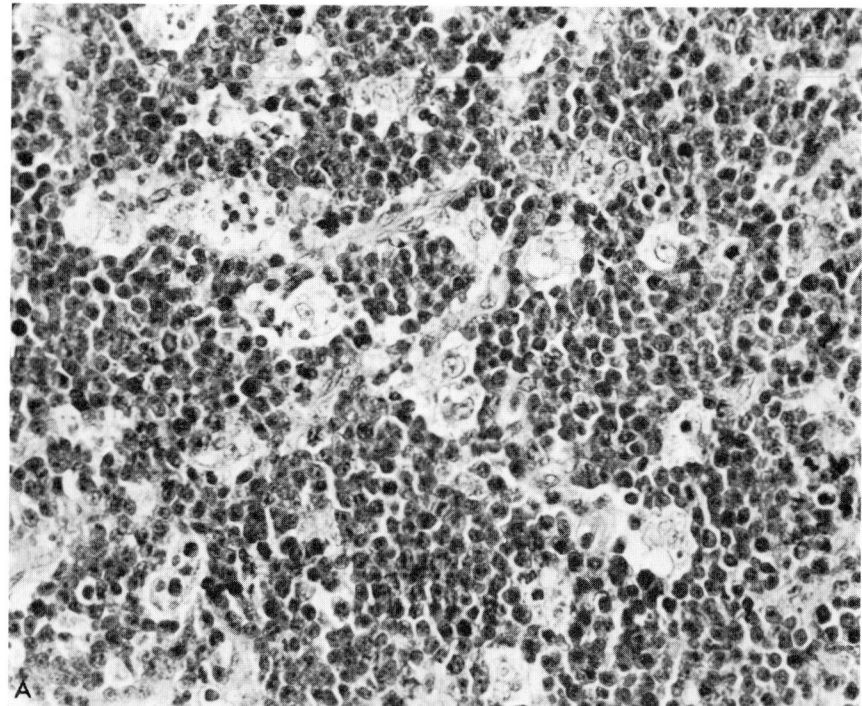

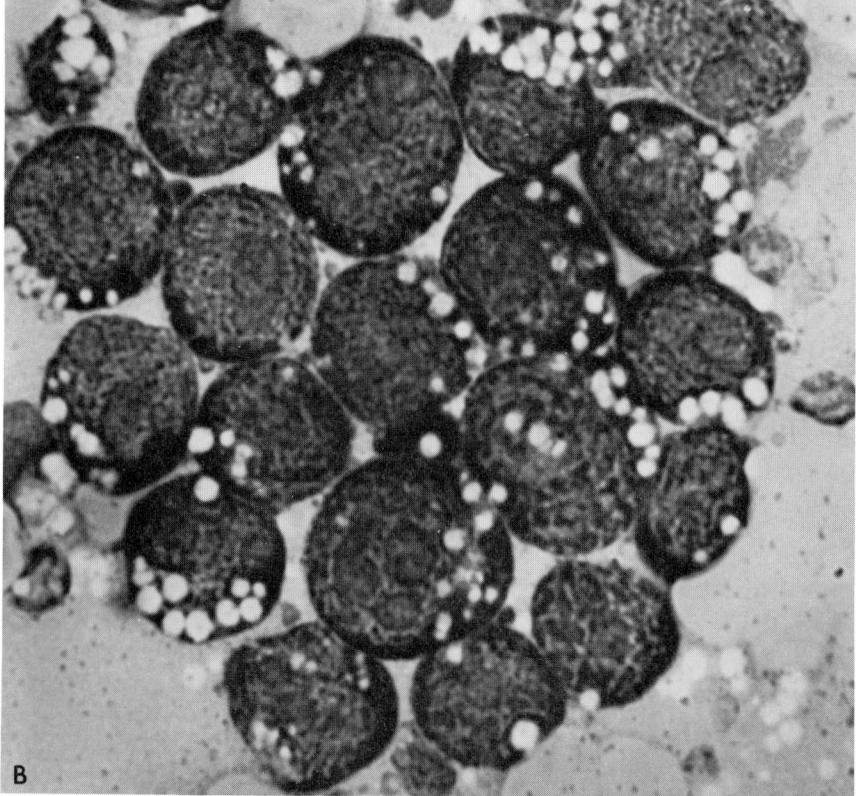

FIGURE 11–9. *A,* Burkitt's lymphoma with typical "starry sky" appearance due to the presence of large, pale macrophages in a background of small, immature malignant lymphocytes. *B,* Imprint smear from Burkitt's lymphoma tumor showing lymphocytes with immature but regular nuclei, containing 2 or 3 nucleoli, and deeply basophilic, vacuolated cytoplasm. (Giemsa stain.) (Courtesy of Professor D. H. Wright.)

Over half the patients are first seen because of jaw tumors; these may affect one or more quadrants of the mandible or maxilla (see Fig. 11–8). Most other patients present with intra-abdominal swellings due either to involvement of the retroperitoneal lymph nodes or to ovarian tumors. A common feature in these cases is the development of flaccid paraplegia. This may result from interference with spinal cord blood supply or from

vertebral metastases. Other unusual presenting sites are the salivary glands, testis, bone, soft tissue, and thyroid.

DIAGNOSIS. In children presenting with a jaw tumor in an endemic area, clinical suspicion of Burkitt's lymphoma will nearly always be confirmed by biopsy. Secondary neuroblastoma may cause a jaw tumor, and orbital embryonal rhabdomyosarcoma must be considered in children with exophthalmos. Intra-abdominal

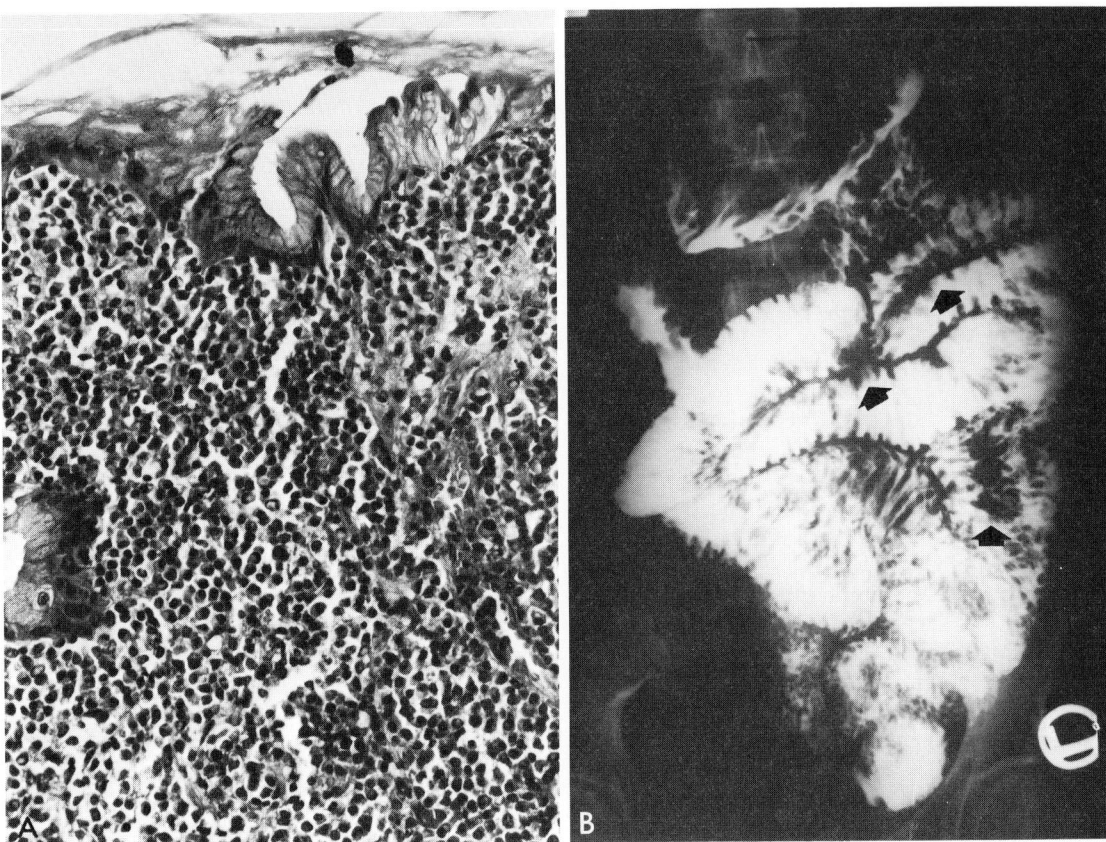

FIGURE 11–10. *A,* Complete absence of intestinal villi and heavy lymphoplasmacytic infiltration throughout entire thickness of mucosa in immunoproliferative small intestinal disease (H & E stain, × 30). *B,* Diffuse nodular lesions of primary intestinal lymphoma with coarsening of mucosal folds and thickening of bowel wall in proximal jejunum, leading to separation of adjacent segments. (From Vessal K, et al: Am J Radiol 135:491, 1980.)

masses may be mistaken for nephroblastoma or soft tissue sarcoma. Pott's disease can cause paraplegia in children, but in high-incidence areas of Burkitt's lymphoma the latter is a more frequent cause of spinal cord dysfunction.

TREATMENT. Burkitt's lymphoma is often curable with chemotherapy. A variety of regimens have proved successful; one that is easily administered consists of cyclophosphamide, methotrexate, and vincristine. In remote areas, high doses of cyclophosphamide (40 mg/kg intravenously) are effective in inducing remissions. Central nervous system involvement, often a manifestation of relapse, may require intrathecal chemotherapy with methotrexate, 15 mg instilled weekly.

PRIMARY (MEDITERRANEAN) INTESTINAL LYMPHOMA

DEFINITION. Primary intestinal lymphoma (PIL) must be differentiated from involvement of the gut by a pre-existing malignant lymphoma that extends into the bowel. Two forms of PIL occur. One particularly affects the lymphoid tissues of the ileum, appendix, and colon in adults over age 50 and shows no specific or geographic prevalence. The second type is associated with malabsorption, atrophy of intestinal villi, and predominant involvement of the lower duodenum and jejunum; it occurs in younger age groups from low socioeconomic

areas. This type is more common in the tropics and may be associated with alpha heavy-chain disease.

EPIDEMIOLOGY. Although PIL and alpha-chain disease were shown to be related in Israel in 1966, similar cases had been described in Peru in 1963. In Israel, the condition occurred predominantly among Jews of non-European stock who had migrated to Israel. The tumor syndrome was later described from Iraq, Iran, Lebanon, Egypt, Greece, and Syria, leading to the concept of a "Mediterranean lymphoma." However, the syndrome is also seen in mixed-blood "coloreds" of South Africa, in Central America, and in some countries of sub-Saharan Africa. That the rates in Israel appear to be declining is attributed to improved socioeconomic conditions in the immigrant groups.

ETIOLOGY AND PATHOLOGY. PIL occurs in teenagers and young adults of low socioeconomic status, usually living in the tropics or subtropics. The development of lymphoma is preceded and accompanied by diffuse changes in the small intestinal mucosa. These pathologic features are characterized by a diffuse lymphoplasmacytic cellular infiltrate of the lamina propria of the duodenum and jejunum associated with marked villous atrophy (Fig. 11–10*A*). With the development of lymphoma, proliferative tumor cells may form nodular or diffuse infiltrates in the gut wall. At a later stage, regional lymph nodes may be involved. The neoplastic lymphoma cells have been variably called "malignant cells," "large cell lymphocytic lymphoma," "reticulum cells," and "histiocytes." The frequent association with alpha-chain disease, which sometimes precedes the development of overt lymphoma, has led to the use of such terms as "immunocytic enteropathy" and "alpha-chain disease with lymphoplasmacytic neoplasia."

CLINICAL MANIFESTATIONS. In areas of high incidence, immunoproliferative small intestinal disease should be suspected in young adults of either sex who present with malabsorption, weight loss, and diffuse abdominal pain and who have clubbing of the fingers and toes. With the development of lymphoma, these features become exacerbated, abdominal masses can be palpated, and intestinal obstruction or perforation may occur. In such patients, radiographic examination of the small bowel may show a spruelike pattern with diffuse infiltrative or stenotic lesions (Fig. 11–10*B*). Alpha chains may be detected in serum. Diagnosis can be confirmed by a small bowel biopsy, although it can be difficult to decide whether the infiltrate of plasma cells in the mucosa represents a true neoplastic change.

TREATMENT. Management of predisposing lymphoproliferative small bowel disease has not been well studied. The development of frank lymphoma requires chemotherapy. The regimen of cyclophosphamide, vincristine, and prednisone has produced temporary remissions.

HISTIOCYTIC MEDULLARY RETICULOSIS

This is a very rare tumor in temperate climates but has been reported as occurring with undue frequency in parts of sub-Saharan Africa, e.g., Uganda, Zambia, and Malawi.

Clinically, these patients present with fever, anemia, splenomegaly, and wasting; slight lymphadenopathy and hepatomegaly may be present. The anemia is hemolytic in type, but the direct Coombs' test is usually negative. It occurs predominantly in teenagers and young adults and is nearly always mistaken for a systemic infection such as typhoid fever or malaria. Diagnosis can be made by liver biopsy that shows atypical and pleomorphic malignant histiocytes with erythrophagocytosis in the hepatic sinusoids or bone marrow. Results of chemotherapy have been disappointing; most patients die within 3 months of diagnosis.

BIBLIOGRAPHY

Ackerman LV, Murray JF (eds): Symposium on Kaposi's Sarcoma. Unio Internationalis Contra Cancrum. Basel, S. Karger, 1962.
Alpert ME, Hutt MSR, Davidson CS: Primary hepatoma in Uganda. A prospective clinical and epidemiological study of 46 patients. Am J Med 46:794, 1969.
Anthony PP: Primary carcinoma of the liver: A study of 282 cases in Ugandan Africans. J Pathol 110:37, 1973.
Burkitt DP: Large bowel cancer: An epidemiologic jigsaw puzzle. J Natl Cancer Inst 54:3, 1975.
Burkitt DP, Wright DH (eds): Burkitt's Lymphoma. Edinburgh, E & S Livingstone, 1970.
Burton GJ: Parasites. *In* Schottenfeld D, Fraumeni JF (eds): Cancer Epidemiology and Prevention. Philadelphia, WB Saunders, 1982.
Cheever AW: Schistosomiasis and neoplasia. J Natl Cancer Inst 61:13, 1978.
Chevlen EM, Aurvad HK, Ziegler JL, et al: Cancer of the bilharzial bladder. Int J Radiat Oncol Biol Phys 5:921, 1979.
Cook P, Burkitt DP: Cancer in Africa. Br Med Bull 27:14, 1971.
de-Thé G, Geser A, Day NE, et al: Epidemiological evidence for the causal relationship between Epstein-Barr virus and Burkitt's lymphoma from Ugandan prospective studies. Nature 274:756, 1978.
Eidelmann S, Parkins A, Rubin CE: Abdominal lymphoma presenting as malabsorption: A clinicopathological study of nine cases in Israel and a review of the literature. Medicine 45:111, 1966.
Hirayama T (ed): Cancer in Asia. Gann Monograph on Cancer Research No. 18. Baltimore, University Park Press, 1976.
Hutt MSR, Burkitt DP: Geographical distribution of cancer in East Africa: A new clinicopathological approach. Br Med J 2:719, 1965.
Lewis MG: Malignant melanoma in Uganda. Br J Cancer 21:483, 1967.
Schmauz R, Jain DK: Geographical variation of cancer of the penis in Uganda. Br J Cancer 25:25, 1978.
Serck-Hanssen A, Purohit GP: Histiocytic medullary reticulosis. Br J Cancer 22:506, 1968.
Templeton AC (ed): Tumours in a Tropical Country. New York, Springer-Verlag, 1973.
Vessal K, Dutz W, Kohout E, et al: Immunoproliferative small intestinal disease with duodenojejunal lymphoma: Radiologic changes. Am J Radiol 135:491, 1980.
Wynder EL, Shiagmatsu T: Environmental factors of cancer of the colon and rectum. Cancer 20:1520, 1967.
Ziegler JL, Magrath IT, Gerber P, et al: Epstein-Barr virus and human malignancy. Ann Intern Med 86:323, 1977.
Ziegler JL: Burkitt's lymphoma. N Engl J Med 305:735, 1981.
Ziegler JL, Beckstead JH, Volberding PA, et al: Non-Hodgkin's lymphoma in 90 homosexual men. Relationship to generalized lymphadenopathy and acquired immunodeficiency syndrome. N Engl J Med 311:565, 1984.
Ziegler JL, Dorfman RL (eds): Kaposi's Sarcoma. Pathophysiology and Clinical Management. New York, Marcel Dekker, 1987.

12. SURGERY

John Tarpley
and Donald E. Meier

Compared with the 51 surgeons per 100,000 persons in the United States, the developing world struggles with a surgical manpower shortage. Colombia has 7 surgeons per 100,000 and the Philippines, 1.5 per 100,000. West African nations have only 0.5 surgeon per 100,000, which is 1% of the rate in the United States. In developing countries, physicians with minimal or no surgical training, or even nonphysicians, perform surgery. Surgical specialist opinion and referral are capital city and teaching hospital luxuries, and professional isolation is the norm. Patients in tropical areas expect the general surgeon to have expertise in orthopedics, urology, plastic surgery, and obstetrics and gynecology, a situation comparable to that of pre–World War II rural America. A 1988 survey of physicians practicing surgery in Africa revealed an operative case frequency very different from that of colleagues in the developed world (Table 12–1). Because of unreliable epidemiologic studies and deficient diagnostic capabilities, comparisons between disease occurrence frequencies in the developing and developed worlds are of limited value, but differences do occur (Table 12–2).

TABLE 12–1. The Five Most Frequently Performed Elective and Emergency Major Procedures in Sub-Saharan Africa

Elective Procedures
Inguinal herniorrhaphy
Laparotomy
Hysterectomy
Prostatectomy
Repeat (elective) Cesarean section
Emergency Procedures
Cesarean section
Laparotomy (acute abdomen, bowel obstruction)
Incarcerated/strangulated hernia
Trauma
Ruptured ectopic gestation

PRACTICAL ASPECTS OF SURGERY IN DEVELOPING COUNTRIES

The essentials for a tropical surgical service are basic equipment, sterile supplies, and anesthesia. Infrastructural components include water, electricity, anesthesia equipment and supplies, sterilization capability, a dynamic supply system, and adequate personnel. Laboratory, transfusion, radiology, and histopathology services are desirable but not essential to the tropical surgeon, whose most reliable diagnostic tools are clinical experience and judgment predicated on history, physical examination, and, at times, surgical exploration.

WATER. Public utilities, even where available, may not supply water reliably. Entrapment and holding systems (cisterns), wells, and pumps for rivers or ponds can serve as primary sources or as supplements to public sources of water.

ELECTRICITY. Hospitals in the developed countries maintain back-up generators to ensure uninterrupted electrical supply during blackouts and power failures. In developing countries, hospital generators may serve either as the sole source of electricity or as a supplement to public power. "Browns" (low-voltage periods) and unstable current damage or destroy electrical equipment, notably those types with compressors; therefore, on-line stabilizers and protective circuit-breaking systems are recommended.

STERILIZATION TECHNIQUES. Four techniques of sterilization can be utilized to meet differing needs: soaking in an antiseptic solution, boiling, steam autoclaving, and gassing (ethylene oxide). A steam autoclave, powered by electricity, gas, wood, coal, or kerosene, is preferred for sterilizing instrument sets. Since disposable drapes and linens are expensive rarities, surgical linens require a steam autoclave. Soaking solutions sterilize scissors, blades, and needles without the attendant dulling or rusting of steam autoclaving. Boiling, which does not kill spores, is not routinely employed but can serve as a "flash" technique for a dropped instrument. Commercially available (Anpro) small ethylene oxide ampule systems allow repeated sterilization of rubber and plastic tubes, catheters, drains, and electrical cords and of instruments such as diathermy pencils and power drills.

ANESTHESIA. Anesthetic options range from vocal-hypnotic-acupuncture through local-regional-conduction to dissociative and general anesthesia techniques. The choice of a particular method depends on the patient, the procedure, the availability of drugs and trained personnel, and the preference of the patient and surgeon. Of prime importance in all anesthetic techniques is airway management. The Eleven Golden Rules (after Maurice King) demand adherence regardless of the level of medical sophistication (Table 12–3).

Most elective operations below the diaphragm can be performed under spinal anesthesia. Surgery on the hand and upper extremity can be done with an axillary block or intravenous regional technique. Local anesthetics with or without supplemental sedation can be used in many cases, including herniorrhaphy, in selected patients. General anesthesia capability necessitates additional equipment and personnel. Inhalational anesthetic systems that are technologically appropriate for the tropics continue to be developed. Drawover techniques, exemplified by the ubiquitous ether vaporizer EMO (Epstein Macintosh Oxford), do not require compressed gases, electricity, or bulky anesthetic systems and have been modified for use with halothane. Since halothane has a cardiodepressant action, however, it should be given with oxygen enrichment. Portable oxygen concentrators can supply up to 6 L oxygen/minute to supplement these drawover systems (Fig. 12–1). Air compressors employed in combination with Boyle's type units can provide freshly compressed air as the carrier gas, thus eliminating the need for expensive and hard-to-find nitrous oxide.

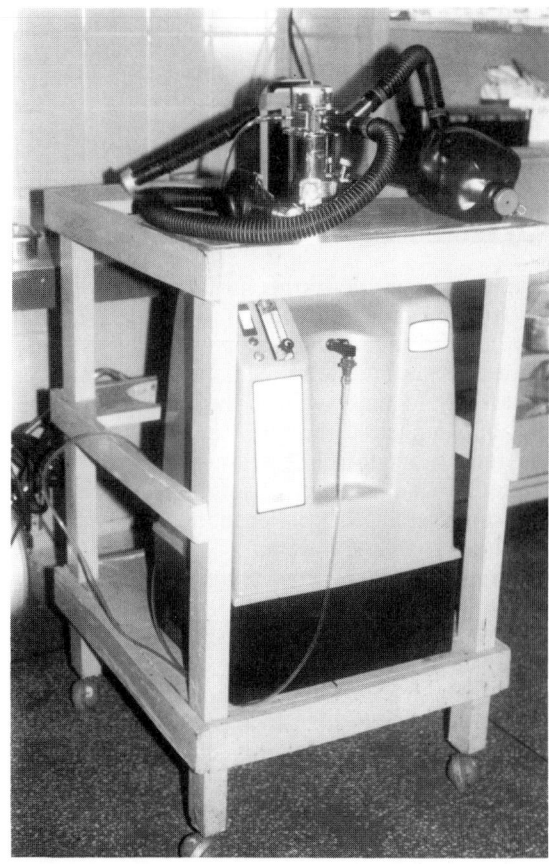

FIGURE 12–1. Drawover vaporizer and oxygen concentrator: inhalational general anesthesia without commercial gas cylinders.

TABLE 12–2. Frequency in Detection and Treatment of Diseases in the Tropics

System	Frequent	Less Frequent
Extremities	Trauma, pyomyositis, pyarthrosis, osteomyelitis	Rheumatoid arthritis, osteoporosis, sarcoma
Skin	Burns, pyoderma, melanoma of sole, Marjolin's ulcer, keloids, hypertrophic scars, tropical ulcer, cutaneous larva migrans, tinea capitis, scabies	Psoriasis, actinic skin carcinoma, atopic dermatitis, mucocutaneous lymph node syndrome (Kawasaki's)
Head and neck	Scrofula, cancrum oris, Burkitt's tumor	Streptococcal pharyngitis
Pulmonary	Tuberculosis, empyema thoracis	Bronchogenic carcinoma, emphysema, cystic fibrosis
Airway	Postmeasles laryngotracheobronchitis	Asthma
Cardiac	Rheumatic valvular disease, congestive heart failure secondary to anemia, cardiomyopathy: hypertensive, endomyocardial fibrosis, Chagas' disease (South America)	Atherosclerotic coronary artery disease
Vascular	Hypertension, cerebrovascular accidents, trauma, elephantiasis	Atherosclerotic peripheral vascular disease, carotid atherosclerosis, thrombophlebitis, pulmonary embolism, venous insufficiency
Endocrine	Endemic goiter, diabetes mellitus (adult-onset)	Diabetes mellitus (juvenile-onset)
Upper gastrointestinal tract	Gastric outlet obstruction (peptic ulcer disease, stomach carcinoma), carcinoma of the esophagus (Kenya, Zambia), megaesophagus (South America)	Esophageal varices (Africa)
Abdominal wall	Umbilical hernia, groin hernia, strangulated groin hernia	
Hepatobiliary	Hepatocellular carcinoma, hepatitis A and B, amebic liver abscess, hepatic schistosomiasis	Cholelithiasis (Africa), pancreatitis, alcoholic hepatitis
Small bowel	Typhoid enteritis, intussusception, ascariasis	Regional enteritis
Lower gastrointestinal tract	Appendicitis, sigmoid volvulus, megasigmoid (South America)	Ulcerative colitis, colon carcinoma, diverticular disease of the colon, ischemic colitis
Obstetrics and gynecology	Cephalopelvic disproportion, obstetric fistula, carcinoma of cervix, carcinoma of ovary, pelvic inflammatory disease with tubal obstruction, secondary infertility, ruptured ectopic gestation	Endometriosis, carcinoma of the endometrium
Blood	Hemoglobinopathies (SS,SC), nutritional and hookworm anemia, hyperreactive malarial splenomegaly, G6PD deficiency, anemia secondary to malaria, neonatal hyperbilirubinemia	Hemophilia, ITP
Breast	Carcinoma of the breast, abscess	Fibrocystic changes
Genitourinary	Postgonococcal urethral stricture, benign prostatic hypertrophy, carcinoma of the prostate, renal and ureteric calculi (Arabs of Sudan and Yemen), hydrocoele, nephrotic syndrome (focal glomerulosclerosis)	Renal and ureteric calculi (most of sub-Saharan Africa), testicular carcinoma, nephrotic syndrome (minimal change)
Neurology	Polio, leprosy, cerebral malaria, neonatal tetanus, tetanus, tuberculous spondylitis, peripheral neuropathy (idiopathic, nutritional, toxic), meningitis	Alzheimer's disease, alcoholic brain syndromes
Nutrition	Malnutrition, vitamin A deficiency	Obesity, food faddism, anorexia nervosa

Ketamine, a neuroleptic agent, provides a dissociative anesthesia and is invaluable to the tropical surgeon. Airway monitoring is mandatory. Although ketamine does not provide muscle relaxation, it may serve as the sole anesthetic agent, as an induction agent, or as one part of a balanced technique when combined with a muscle relaxant, control of the airway, and controlled ventilation. Intramuscular ketamine safely anesthetizes children for dressing or cast changes, burn wound care, herniorrhaphy, or with repeated injections, for even longer procedures such as clubfoot operations. For adults, intravenous ketamine is especially useful as a short-duration anesthetic for dressing changes or incision and drainage procedures. Diazepam comedication decreases emergence phenomena. Since ketamine does not lower the blood pressure, it is useful for induction of general anesthesia in emergency situations.

Emergency intra-abdominal procedures present an anesthetic problem. Gastric decompression to minimize the risk of aspiration is obligatory before delivery of any anesthetic in such situations. Intrathecal (spinal) anesthesia can be used for emergency procedures below the diaphragm, but hypovolemia must be corrected before anesthesia, since the spinal technique abolishes the sympathetic tone of the lower extremities, increases the capacitance, and produces hypotension. A general anesthetic with a controlled airway is safer in emergency situations if appropriate equipment, agents, and personnel are available.

EQUIPMENT AND SUPPLIES. Equipment decisions are based on the surgeon's needs in relation to the hospital's capability to acquire and maintain technologically appropriate materials. In some operating rooms a fly swatter is technologically more appropriate than an electrocautery. Operating room essentials include an adjustable table, a lighting system, suction, and instrument sets. Nonessential but useful are an electrocautery, a fiberoptic headlight, and a table-mounted self-retaining retractor for upper abdominal surgery.

While conditions vary from hospital to hospital, expense, erratic availability, pilferage, and deterioration complicate the maintenance of an adequate central store for supplies and drugs. The tropical surgeon must decide which supplies and drugs are essential and then purchase

TABLE 12–3. The Eleven Golden Rules of Anesthesia

1. Perform an adequate history and physical examination.
2. Perform surgery on fasting patients. For abdominal emergencies, empty the stomach with a nasogastric tube and use a crash induction.
3. Place the patient on a tilt-top table.
4. Check the anesthetic equipment BEFORE you begin.
5. Always have suction capability available.
6. Keep the airway clear and open.
7. Be prepared to control the patient's ventilation. (Have an Ambu type bag available.)
8. Have a good IV line (optional in some instances of local anesthesia or IM ketamine).
9. Monitor the patient frequently.
10. Have someone around to help.
11. Be ready with equipment and agents to manage resuscitation from a cardiopulmonary arrest.

them locally, import them, or improvise from local materials. Nylon fishing line can substitute for monofilament suture and carpet or sewing thread for multifilament suture. Plastic food storage bags serve as barrier-protection gloves when handling dressings, examining wounds, and performing digital rectal examinations. For centuries, worn sheets and cloth have been converted into rolled bandages. Towels can be cut to serve as lap packs. Organization, frugality, improvisation, repeated use of disposables, and local manufacture can improve the supply system.

PERSONNEL. The tropical surgeon must recruit, train, and motivate available personnel—physicians, nurses, technicians—to perform at the highest level possible given the local conditions. Anesthetic personnel constitute a striking example. An estimated 200 anesthesiologists served Nigeria's 108 million people in 1988. The general surgeon along with a personally trained nurse or technician is the anesthesia department in most tropical hospitals. Small group identity with each member's sense of responsibility, worth, and importance is key in developing a viable surgical service.

TRANSFUSION SERVICE. The prevalence of anemia in the population served, the quality and utilization of antenatal obstetric care, and the incidence of major trauma determine the volume of blood required for transfusion. Anemias may be due to chronic or acute blood loss or may be of nutritional, hemolytic, hemoglobinopathic, or unknown origin. The blood bank is heavily utilized by the obstetric unit because of multiparity, short intervals between parturitions, poor nutrition, and peripartum hemorrhage. Poor vehicle maintenance, reckless driving habits, and a fatalistic mindset contribute to high incidences of traffic accidents with attendant blood loss. Penetrating trauma from guns, knives, or explosives, especially in areas of political unrest and warfare, produces a major demand for transfusion. The transfusion service is principally a blood typing and collecting station and not a blood storage facility, since transfusions usually involve on-the-spot donor recruitment and immediate transfusion. Local customs and beliefs often inhibit blood donation. Establishing and maintaining a blood bank in such locales is always difficult and often impossible.

"Walking" blood banks, wherein volunteers in an institution, organization, or community are typed and recorded, provide a measure of supply, especially in emergency situations.

Potential transmission of hepatitis and HIV is a major consideration in determining blood banking policies worldwide. Unfortunately, even in highly endemic areas, many centers screen neither for hepatitis nor for HIV. In the developed world only a few cases of post-transfusion hepatitis are now caused by hepatitis B virus (HBV), one case per 2000 units transfused. Hepatitis C virus (HCV), now detectable with screening, accounted for 80% of non-A, non-B post-transfusion hepatitis prior to 1990. The prevalence of post-transfusion hepatitis in developing countries is unknown but high, and HBV remains a major threat (Chapter 19.2). The technology for screening for HBV antigens is appropriate, but the expense and erratic availability of test sera often preclude routine use. HIV virus is a threat for transmission by transfusion throughout the world (Chapter 15.1). Easy to use and affordable, the newer test kits can now distinguish HIV-1 and HIV-2. It is hoped that HVB, HBC, and HIV screening of all blood for transfusion will become the norm in the developing world. Transmission of malaria parasites by transfusion is common; Chagas' disease can also be transmitted in blood products. Alternatives to transfusion are few, since hemoglobin substitutes and volume expanders other than crystalloid solutions are not usually available. Autotransfusion has been much touted but infrequently practiced in most tropical medical centers. Patients with ruptured ectopic pregnancies, vascular injuries, and splenic or hepatic injuries without bowel contamination are the most appropriate candidates for simultaneous autotransfusion. Galley pot collection and gauze sieving of blood in the peritoneal cavity with retransfusion have been performed with varying results, enthusiasm, and recommendations. Modern autotransfusion systems are impractical because of initial expense, high cost of disposable components, and infrequency of use with attendant unfamiliarity. For some elective procedures with an anticipated transfusion requirement, patients can donate a unit of blood at weekly intervals for 2 or 3 weeks prior to their operation, take hematinics and follow a good diet in the interim, and then receive their own banked blood at the time of operation. This delayed autotransfusion has only limited application, however, since most transfusion requirements occur in emergencies or in debilitated patients.

LABORATORY. Finances, personnel, maintenance, utilization, and physician oversight determine the level at which a laboratory functions. The tropical surgeon must decide which laboratory procedures are desirable, endeavor to secure these in the simplest and most dependable way, and then assume responsibility for quality control if the hospital staff includes no qualified laboratory supervisor. Laboratory results are often unreliable, and the surgeon must remember to treat the patient and not the laboratory report.

RADIOLOGY AND ENDOSCOPY. Outside of teaching hospitals and certain urban medical centers, the tropical surgeon rarely encounters radiologists, functioning fluoroscopic units, or interventional techniques. Ultrasound offers an affordable diagnostic capability.

Sonography is relatively inexpensive, noninvasive, portable, and easy to maintain. It is, however, quite operator-dependent. The accuracy, dependability, and reproducibility are proportional to the interest and competence of the operator, be it the physician or a locally trained technician. Sonography is especially useful in assessing the pelvis and for obstetrics but also can provide the surgeon with important anatomic information about the biliary tree, the liver, the pancreas, and the kidneys; it can detect ascites, distinguish solid from cystic masses, and localize intra-abdominal abscesses.

Endoscopic training and equipment have become more widespread, and esophagogastroduodenoscopy with flexible fiberoptic instrument systems is sometimes found even in peripheral areas. Initial cost plus equipment maintenance, however, limits the availability of this valuable diagnostic tool.

HISTOPATHOLOGY. Frozen-section capability is generally unavailable. Unless specimens are processed locally, the processing time for histopathologic reports may be measured in months. Decisions relating to diagnosis, adequacy of resection margins, or institution of chemotherapy (e.g., antitubercular or antineoplastic) must therefore be made on clinical grounds alone or deferred for unacceptably long periods.

DIFFERENCES IN SURGICAL PRACTICE BETWEEN TROPICAL AND TEMPERATE SETTINGS

Surgery in the tropics is better distinguished from surgery in the temperate zones by measuring sociologic, economic, philosophic, cultural, and material differences than by using variances in disease spectra.

PATIENT PROFILES

Age. Most tropical countries have a pyramidal age structure. The "graying of the West" phenomenon is not apparent in the developing world, where half the population is younger than twenty years of age.

Nutrition. Overnutrition and its resultant medical complications warrant research and funding in developed countries. Undernutrition afflicts many in the tropics, where surgical patients usually have no access to intravenous hyperalimentation. Enteral formulas are unavailable commercially, but "homemade" substitutes can be prepared by hospital personnel or family members from locally available agricultural products such as soya beans.

Presentation. In developing countries, patients usually seek Western-type medical care at a tertiary level and only after exhausting traditional and spiritual attempts at healing. "Imported" medical care is perceived as foreign, incomprehensible, and expensive; therefore, the patient is frequently first seen in advanced stages of illness. For example, most women with breast cancer arrive with regional or disseminated disease, and the duration of illness in patients with peritonitis is usually measured in days, not in hours.

Expectations. Many tropical residents lead an economically marginal life and hold a fatalistic outlook. Residual deformity and loss of range of motion are the accepted results of a fracture. Although malpractice

does occur, litigation is not yet a major factor in surgical decision-making. Controversies over active and passive euthanasia do not surface in most developing countries. Grossly deformed neonates may be adjudged expendable, since families cannot afford vast expenditures for corrective surgery with uncertain results.

Body Image. Reincarnation figures prominently in the metaphysics of many traditional religions. Belief that physical deformities in this life will accompany one into the next passage leads many to resist a stoma or an ablative procedure such as amputation, even when the alternative is death.

Preoperative Status. Although surgical patients often present late and with advanced disease, on the whole they are younger and more active and have fewer pulmonary complications. They are frequently anemic, but this is usually well tolerated. They seldom have severe atherosclerosis and thus have fewer adverse effects from brief periods of hypotension. Few operative candidates are immunocompromised by steroids, concomitant cancer chemotherapy, or cyclosporine.

Compliance and Follow-up. Distance, inconvenience, expense, and lack of perceived need limit follow-up for subsequent treatment, evaluation, or physiotherapy. Many patients reappear only when a problem arises. The physician's awareness of treatment results or even survival is often incomplete or inaccurate. The surgeon may elect to lengthen a patient's hospital stay for rehabilitative purposes when compliance with clinic follow-up is unlikely.

DISEASE PROFILES. Trauma is a major cause of death in the tropics. Parturition significantly threatens women during their childbearing years and is often the leading cause of death, either from bleeding or from infection, during that period. Infectious diseases overshadow degenerative and geriatric problems. As many as 40% of children die before their fifth birthday from causes such as diarrhea and dehydration, pneumonia, malaria, measles, malnutrition, and trauma. Hemoglobinopathies, malaria, and tuberculosis are ubiquitous problems that, along with the aforementioned childhood diseases, compromise potential surgical patients. Osteomyelitis is a scourge. Helminthic problems contribute only a small percentage to the surgical practice, exceptions being schistosomiasis in Africa, China, and Brazil.

Cancer occurs as a problem of greater magnitude than was previously supposed. Coronary artery disease and atherosclerotic peripheral vascular disease are diagnosed less frequently in the tropics but may increase as Western dietary habits and lifestyles are adopted and as clinical suspicion increases and detection improves. Diabetes and hypertension increasingly confront both the internist and the surgeon. Degenerative joint diseases, the sequelae of trauma, infection, and aseptic necrosis from hemoglobinopathy, debilitate many. Most are managed with anti-inflammatory and analgesic agents and only occasionally with surgical fusion. Prosthetic joint replacement is almost unknown.

PROCEDURE PROFILES. Trauma, infection, obstetric emergencies, and elective cases fill the operating schedule, with much of the surgeon's time spent in responding to emergencies. Operating rooms in developing countries often have poor illumination and climate control, with attendant dust and flying insects. Operative cases tend to be short-duration, frequent, and simple.

SURGEON PROFILES. Sociologic variables affecting tropical surgery manpower are currently in a flux. Populations are increasing markedly, but gross national products and amounts budgeted for health care remain small. Many developing countries have established medical schools and are producing graduates who, because they cannot find suitable postgraduate training locally, must look elsewhere. Since undeveloped nations are unable to support their local medical institutions and provide the infrastructure necessary for basic medical care, many of the better trained national physicians emigrate from their economically depressed home areas to developed nations or to the oil-rich areas of the Middle East, thus effecting a medical "brain drain." In the United States, 18% of all physicians are foreign medical graduates. The demand for surgical services in the developing world has increased while the supply has at best remained static.

AN OVERVIEW OF SURGICAL PRACTICE IN THE TROPICS

GENERAL SURGERY. Trauma, infections, abdominal problems including groin hernias, and neoplasms constitute the four major areas of general surgery.

Endocrine procedures are generally limited to the thyroid; vascular procedures are for trauma only; and transplants are not performed.

Trauma. Trauma can be blunt, penetrating, or thermal. The proximity of a medical facility to major highways will determine the volume of accident victims treated. Some of the world's highest traffic fatality rates are reported from tropical countries. A surgeon's daily chores include wound care and wound coverage, especially for open fractures of the tibia and machine injuries of the hand (Chapter 13). Recently described muscle, myocutaneous, and fasciocutaneous flap techniques that do not require a microscope appreciably expand the surgeon's options in dealing with wound coverage problems (Fig. 12–2).

Bites. Human, animal, snake, spider, and insect bites plus scorpion stings present local and systemic problems. Human bites are often underrated and mismanaged. Many bites are near hand joints, with possible joint violation. Infections frequently occur. A common offender is *Eikenella corrodens,* a gram-negative rod that is sensitive to penicillin. The hand joints should be examined closely and opened if there is any suspicion of violation, then irrigated and left unsutured. The patient should be admitted, given antibiotics, and have the extremity elevated. Dog and cat bites often inoculate *Pasteurella multocida,* which is sensitive to ampicillin or penicillin. Rabies is a major concern with dog and wild animal bites (Chapter 21.1).

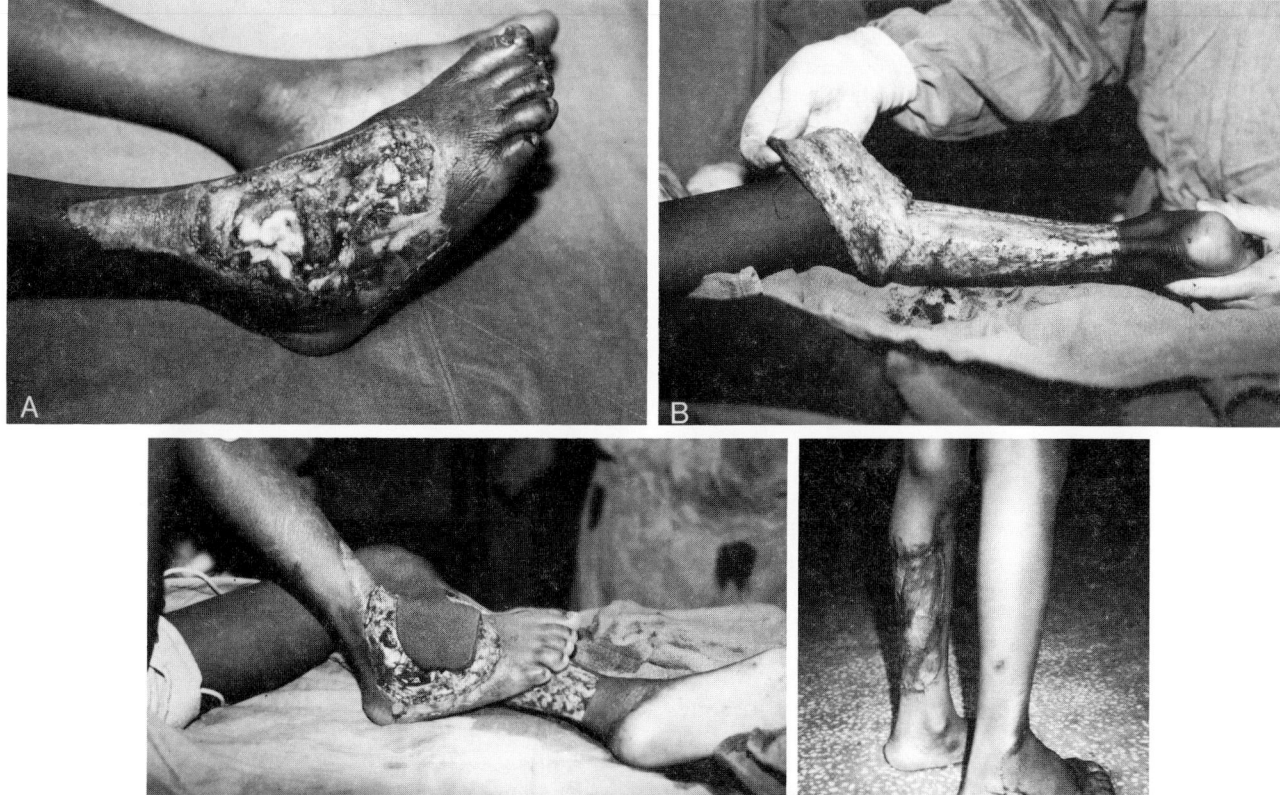

FIGURE 12–2. A 5-year-old boy's right foot traumatized by a taxi. *A,* Preoperative view with exposed ankle joint, tarsal joints, and soft tissue defect. *B,* Fasciocutaneous flap elevated from the left calf. *C,* Cross-leg flap placed to cover right foot defect. *D,* Postoperative result: full coverage and function.

Poisonous snakebites vary in incidence and type by topography and locale (Chapter 103.5). Considerations are local and systemic. Wound excision and fasciotomy may be required to treat local and vascular compartment problems. Procaine infiltration, ice, and analgesics can relieve the pain of scorpion sting and envenomation. Hypersensitivity reactions constitute the threat to individuals stung by bees and wasps; resuscitative measures should include epinephrine administration in cases of anaphylaxis. Spider bites from the black widow spider produce generalized muscle spasms, whereas brown recluse spider bites produce a local ulcer with ischemic necrosis (Chapter 105.3).

Abscesses. Abscesses of the skin, subcutaneous tissue, muscles (pyomyositis; Chapter 58), bones (osteomyelitis), joints (pyarthrosis), thorax (empyema), and pericardial sac occur frequently and require drainage. *Staphylococcus aureus* is the most frequent etiologic agent. Multiple abscesses are common and may occur either synchronously or metachronously. Early and wide drainage, preferably with antibiotic coverage, minimizes the hematogenous spread of infection. Hand infections pose a special difficulty, since most patients delay seeking medical care. Even after drainage, antibiotics, elevation, and physiotherapy, residual hand deformity is the rule.

Mycoses. Subcutaneous and deep mycotic infections occur throughout the tropics. The clinically important mycoses include mycetoma, aspergillus granuloma, phycomycosis, histoplasmosis, and chromoblastomycosis. Mycetoma (Madura foot) is a clinically defined lesion with three cardinal signs: swelling (chronic inflammation), multiple sinuses, and discharge of granules. The disease is common in the thorny semidesert zones lying on either side of the fifteenth parallel north of the equator (Fig. 13–10). The actinomycetoma can be treated with antibiotics (Chapter 65.1). Surgical treatment options include observation, local excision through healthy tissue, and amputation.

Abdominal Surgery. Abdominal problems can be infectious, congenital, mechanical, obstructive, vascular, inflammatory, neoplastic, or a combination of these. Appendiceal perforation, strangulated bowel (intestinal obstruction, hernia, volvulus), typhoid perforations of the ileum, and perforation of duodenal ulcers are leading causes of secondary bacterial suppurative peritonitis and carry a high mortality rate because of frequent sepsis due to delays in seeking medical care. Groin hernias constitute a major cause of intestinal obstruction (Fig. 12–3). Since many persons seek care only for complications of a hernia, strangulation and peritonitis are common, sometimes causing fatalities. Appendicitis often progresses to perforation with abscess or peritonitis by the time the patient seeks treatment.

Volvulus of the small bowel is associated with, and similar to, closed-loop obstruction secondary to adhesions. Though volvulus of the stomach and cecum seldom occur, sigmoid volvulus is a frequent abdominal problem and, in areas of East Africa, constitutes the leading cause of intestinal obstruction. The patients present with marked abdominal distention and tympany to percussion but without peritonitis unless strangulation or perforation has occurred. Although colonoscopic or

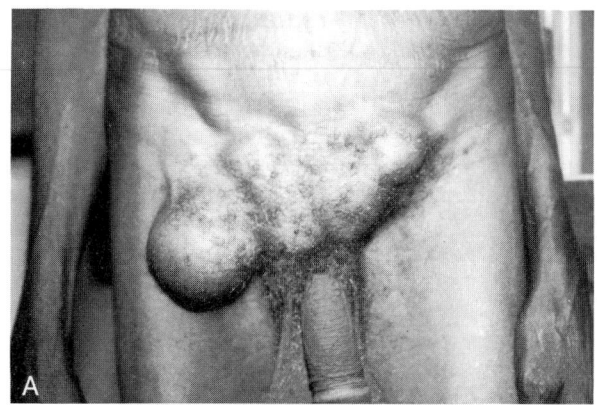

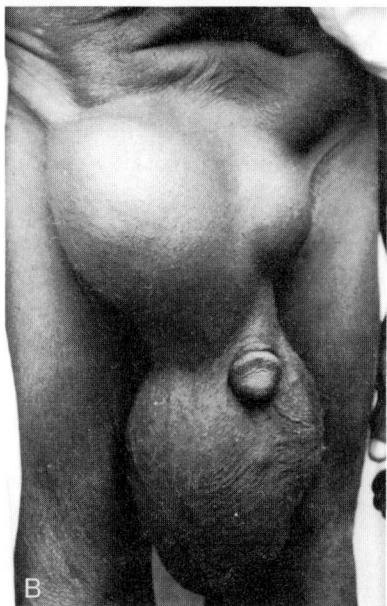

FIGURE 12–3. *A,* Femoral and inguinal hernias. *B,* Inguinoscrotal hernias.

sigmoidoscopic deflation can be attempted, operation is the usual treatment since the colon is often strangulated. If the bowel is viable, a rectal tube can be guided safely into place, the loop deflated, and the volvulus manually reduced. After a bowel preparation an interval sigmoid resection should be performed, since recurrence is likely. When the sigmoid is strangulated, resection of the dead bowel with the creation of an end colostomy and mucus fistula or Hartmann's pouch is recommended. Not infrequently a loop of small bowel will be caught up in the twist of the sigmoid colon mesentery, producing a concomitant closed-loop obstruction and strangulation of the small bowel, the so-called compound volvulus or "knotting of the bowel." A small bowel resection and reanastomosis must then be performed, in addition to correction of the colonic volvulus.

Although perforation and bleeding may complicate peptic ulcer disease, the leading operative indication for this condition in the developing world is gastric outlet obstruction (Chapter 3). Mesenteric vascular diseases are not common. Although not diagnosed frequently in blacks, inflammatory bowel diseases (regional enteritis, ulcerative colitis) are now seen in patients with AIDS but may prove to be infectious, not idiopathic. Enteritis necroticans (pig-bel), a particular problem in the highlands of New Guinea, is a necrotizing enteritis produced by a *Clostridium perfringens* toxin (Chapter 55.4). Surgery may be required to remove necrotic bowel.

Operative hepatobiliary and pancreatic diseases are not often encountered in sub-Saharan Africa although they are frequent in the East (see later under Schistosomiasis and Ascaris).

Bezoars are concretions formed in the stomach; they are trichobezoars if they consist of hair and phytobezoars if they are composed of vegetable fibers. Bezoars are seen in edentulous patients with deficient mastication, in some young females, in patients after partial gastrectomy, and in psychiatric patients. Bezoars may occlude the stomach, produce a mass, and limit nutrition, or they may cause intestinal obstruction, ulceration, bleeding, or perforation. Although enzymatic dissolution of phytobezoars can be tried, the treatment for most patients is operative removal with subsequent counseling.

Skin Tumors. Melanoma arising from the sole of the foot and Marjolin's ulcer, a squamous cell carcinoma developing in an area of chronic inflammation, are two common skin tumors (Chapter 11). Marjolin's ulcer, the most frequently encountered carcinoma in many rural hospitals, arises from burn scars, osteomyelitis sinus tracts, and neglected tropical ulcers.

OBSTETRICS–GYNECOLOGY. Lack of antenatal care, obstructed labor, eclampsia, peripartum hemorrhage, ruptured ectopic gestations, and infertility are all problems for the tropical obstetrician. Most deliveries are performed in the patient's home with traditional birth attendants (TBAs) or older women supervising the delivery. Young age at first pregnancy, dietary deficiencies, and small stature increase the incidence of cephalopelvic disproportion. Not only does prolonged labor lead to increased chance of infection and fetal and maternal loss, but also it can produce ischemia of the genital canal and adjacent tissues with eventual pressure necrosis and creation of an obstetric fistula. The incidence of vesicovaginal fistula in a community is an inverse indicator of the local level of obstetric care. Most obstetric fistulas are vesicovaginal fistulas that produce a continuous urine leak through the vagina; the result is odor and skin excoriation problems and social problems of exclusion and desertion or divorce by the husband. The majority can be repaired through a vaginal approach utilizing local tissues. Some larger fistulas and those with urethral loss may require labial flaps or a gracilis muscle flap, or both, to provide adequate support and to promote continence.

Close spacing between successive children, multiparity, and inadequate nutrition compromise the obstetric patient's health, resilience, and hemoglobin level. In areas where society demands many children and places a high priority on the production of a son and heir, the infertile woman or couple is an obstetric challenge. Gonorrhea and other sexually transmitted diseases, conflicts between traditional and Western mores and practices, and increasing criminal abortions affect the tropical obstetrician's practice. The tropical gynecologist routinely sees patients with fistulas, prolapse, myomata, and neoplasms; for the last-named there is rarely access to radiotherapy.

ORTHOPEDICS. Musculoskeletal problems in the tropics are ubiquitous (Chapter 13). Categories include trauma, congenital conditions (talipes equinovarus), developmental abnormalities (rickets, genu varus and valgum), bacterial infections (osteomyelitis, pyarthrosis), viral infections (poliomyelitis), hemoglobinopathies (bone crisis, avascular necrosis) (Chapter 5), and degenerative diseases. Trauma victims and osteomyelitis patients often fill the majority of beds on a tropical surgical ward.

UROLOGY. Urologic problems may be congenital, infectious, obstructive, or neoplastic.

Congenital. Undescended testes, hypospadias, posterior urethral valves, and torsion of the testis (cord) are congenital-anatomic problems. Histologic changes are noted in undescended testes by 18 months; hence, groin or retroperitoneal exploration by 18 months maximizes the chances for spermatogenesis after successful orchiopexy. Children with hypospadias should not be circumcised, because the foreskin can be utilized later for a flap repair before school entry. Posterior urethral valves are diagnosed during the early months of life in males from the history of difficulty in initiating urination and a very weak urinary stream. A voiding cystourethrogram is the definitive diagnostic test. Treatment consists of valve destruction, either endoscopically or through a perineal approach. Torsion of the testis in a male with a tender scrotum-testis can be excluded only by direct observation. In societies in which procreation is nearly mandatory, all males without progeny who present with a swollen, tender scrotum-testis should undergo scrotal exploration for diagnosis. Although the ipsilateral testis with torsion often is unsalvageable, the contralateral testis can be protected by suturing the tunica albuginea testis to the tunica dartos at 3 sites with either absorable or unabsorbable suture, the goal being to produce scar fixation at several points.

Obstructive. Renal and ureteric stones are not prevalent among blacks, but Arabs in the Sudan and Yemen have frequent stone problems. Lithotomy is indicated for obstruction complicated by pain, progressive renal damage, or persistent infection. Since endoscopic and ultrasonic techniques are generally not available, open operation is the usual procedure. Lower tract obstructions in older men generally result from benign prostatic hypertrophy, prostatic carcinoma, or urethral stricture secondary to prior gonococcal urethritis. Benign prostatic hypertrophy is treated by prostatectomy, usually open rather than transurethral. Urethral stricture can be managed by repeated bougienage, suprapubic tube cystostomy, or urethroplasty.

Neoplastic. Cancers of the kidneys, bladder, prostate, and penis (squamous cell carcinoma) are generally seen at an advanced, nonoperative stage (Chapter 11). Prostate carcinoma can be successfully palliated with orchiectomy or estrogen administration.

Infectious. Pyelonephritis can lead to a perinephric abscess, which should be drained (Chapter 6). Urinary tuberculosis should be considered in patients with acid pyuria or sterile pyuria (Chapter 61). Infection by *Schistosoma haematobium* may produce granulomas of the ureters and bladder and result in bleeding, obstructive uropathy, pyelonephritis, or carcinoma of the bladder (Chapters 11 and 96). Fournier's gangrene is a spontaneous gangrene of the skin of the scrotum and penis. The pathogenesis remains speculative. Multiple organisms have been cultured, including *Clostridium perfringens*. The onset is sudden and painful, often in the dependent scrotum, and is accompanied by fever and toxemia. A partial- or full-thickness slough of the scrotum occurs after a few days, frequently exposing the testes. Penicillin, local wound care, and at times, split skin grafts, constitute the treatment.

EAR–NOSE–THROAT AND DENTAL SURGERY. Foreign bodies, neoplasms, infections, allergic conditions, maxillofacial trauma, and congenital anomalies are all seen in a tropical surgical practice. Tuberculous cervical adenitis (Fig. 12–4), Ludwig's angina, dental abscesses, and otitis media with or without mastoiditis are common infections of the head and neck. Croup and laryngotrachiobronchitis, especially as a complication of measles, may so compromise a child's airway that tracheostomy is mandatory. If nursing care, suctioning, and humidification are deficient, serious complications may accompany tracheostomy. Cancrum oris, or noma, usually seen in malnourished children, is a destructive, necrotic process (Fig. 12–5) that can produce oronasocutaneous fistulas and ankylosis of the temporomandibular joint. Once infarction, infection, and inflammation respond to debridement, penicillin, and diet, the resultant fibrosis and tissue defects present a formidable reconstructive challenge. Myocutaneous flaps such as the pectoralis major island flap can be utilized to repair these complex problems. Dental care, often extractive rather than preservative and preventative in nature, is not found in many rural areas.

PLASTIC SURGERY. Wound care occupies a significant percentage of the tropical surgeon's time as he attempts to deal with large, infected, neglected wounds with a minimum of equipment and supplies.

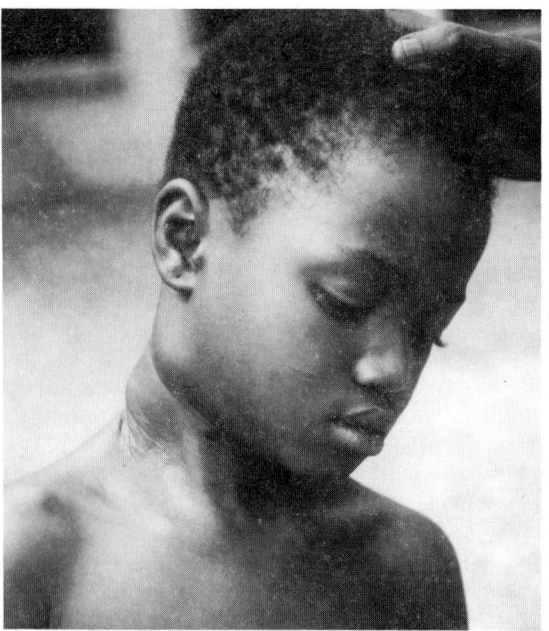

FIGURE 12–4. Tuberculous cervical lymphadenitis (scrofula) in an 8-year-old Yoruba boy.

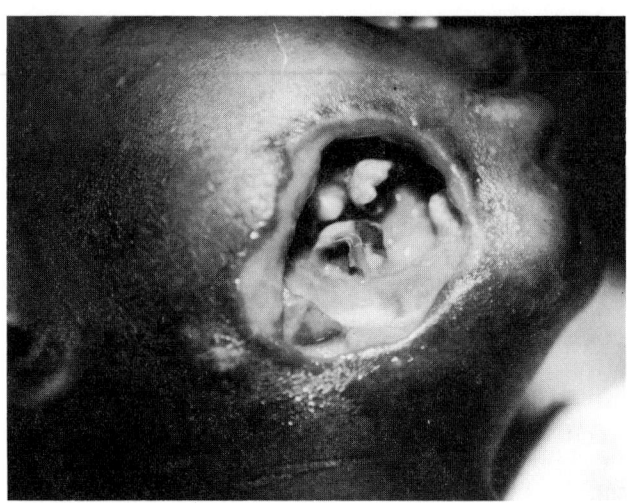

FIGURE 12–5. Cancrum oris (noma). Gangrenous stomatitis with soft tissue and bone defect producing an orocutaneous fistula in a 5-year-old malnourished boy.

Burn Care. Thermal burns occur daily and often receive inadequate initial treatment, with resultant high mortality from renal failure and burn wound sepsis. In acute burn survivors, residual contractures and hypertrophic scarring are often crippling. Skin-grafting capability for burn wound care is essential. Grafts may be taken freehand or with a drum or electric dermatome. The meshing technique of Tanner is recommended to allow expansion of the graft and to improve graft "take."

Hand Surgery. Burns of the hands are especially debilitating, but improved functional results can be obtained with early tangential excision and grafting, proper splinting, and conscientious physiotherapy. Nonthermal hand injuries are also common and require prompt debridement and adequate coverage to encourage primary healing and to avoid fibrosis and contractures. The technique of groin-flap coverage is particularly helpful in dealing with hand injuries.

Cleft Lip and Palate. A common congenital abnormality is cleft lip with or without a palatal defect. Parents, disturbed by the neonate's deformity, want immediate repair. Counseling is indicated, since lip repairs traditionally are not undertaken until "10 weeks of age, 10 pounds of weight, and with a hemoglobin level of at least 10 g/dl." Palatal repair is delayed until about 1 year of age but should be performed before speech develops in order to prevent a nasalized speech pattern.

NEUROSURGERY. The imaging techniques, hardware, and personnel to detect and treat tumors, arteriovenous malformations, and various congenital abnormalities are rarely available.

Head Trauma. Tropical neurosurgery focuses on trauma. Without benefit of sophisticated diagnostic equipment, head injury victims who have deterioration in their level of consciousness or who develop lateralizing neurologic signs should undergo exploration through burr holes and drainage of an epidural or subdural hematoma, if found. Patients with open, depressed skull fractures require operation for debridement, hemostasis, elevation, and closure and coverage of the dura.

Spinal Injuries. Spinal injuries, which often ensue from vehicular accidents or falls from trees, are a major cause of morbidity and mortality. Spinal cord injury rehabilitation programs are almost nonexistent in developing countries, and if the para- or quadriplegic patient survives the in-hospital period of stabilization by traction, he often will succumb to urinary or decubitus ulcer–related sepsis after discharge to his home. Tuberculosis is also a common cause of paralysis. If deterioration in neurologic function in a patient with Pott's disease is recent or if it continues while the patient is receiving adequate antituberculous chemotherapy, drainage of the paraspinal abscess with spine stabilization should be considered (Chapters 13 and 61).

PEDIATRIC SURGERY. Special concerns in tropical pediatric surgery include the congenital anomalies of imperforate anus, bowel atresia, esophageal atresia, and abdominal wall defects. These anomalies are apparent at birth, and parents may seek no treatment for such neonates and refuse surgical intervention if it is offered. Hirschsprung's disease, urinary tract abnormalities, and pediatric tumors, on the other hand, are usually detected after the child has been named and officially recogized as a family or clan member; thus surgical help is sought although stomas are refused. Intussusception is the leading cause of intestinal obstruction in children 3 months to 2 years of age. Hydrostatic reduction is not routinely employed because of the uncertainty of adequate reduction as well as the scarcity of barium, film, and fluoroscopy units. Operative reduction is the usual management for intussusception, and a nonviable intussusceptum is common.

CARDIOTHORACIC SURGERY. Pump oxygenators and the technological and financial support they require might be found in one or two medical centers in a developing country. Rheumatic fever with resultant valvular problems, congestive failure, congenital heart diseases, endomyocardial fibrosis, and other cardiomyopathies, e.g., Chagas' heart disease, and the pericardial problems of constriction (tuberculosis) and effusion (pyopericardium) are the major problems facing the cardiologist and cardiac surgeon (Chapter 2). Atherosclerosis with coronary artery disease, conduction abnormalities, and aneurysm formation is uncommon. The noncardiac thoracic surgeon deals primarily with tuberculosis (Chapter 61), thoracic empyema (especially postmeasles), and hemoptysis from destroyed lung, bronchiectasis, or lung abscess. Lung cancer is not as great a health problem as it is in developed countries, although it is increasing along with cigarette smoking. Hydatid cyst of the lung is focally prevalent in some areas with animal husbandry utilizing dogs (Chapter 1).

OPHTHALMOLOGY. Eighty percent of the world's cases of preventable blindness occurs in patients living in the developing world. Blindness results from trauma, trachoma (Chapter 28), onchocerciasis (Chapter 87), corneal scarring, xeropathia (dryness/vitamin A deficiency) (Chapter 107.1), and cataracts (Chapter 9). A nation may have one or more major eye treatment centers, but only a select population have access to such care. Most people with treatable eye diseases never see an ophthalmic surgeon.

SPECIFIC TOPICS OF SHARED INTEREST TO PHYSICIANS AND SURGEONS

TETANUS (Chapter 55.1). Even with expanded immunization programs, the majority of tropical residents remain unprotected from tetanus. Certain injuries are more tetanus-prone than others, but without prior immunization and appropriate wound care even trivial injuries are potentially lethal. Initial treatment for all patients with tetanus includes thorough wound debridement. A large neglected wound of the extremity may require amputation, and tetanus secondary to a septic abortion may necessitate a hysterectomy. Active and passive immunization should accompany debridement in the initial treatment. In the absence of intensive care units and ventilators, the management choices for patients with severe tetanus are (1) sedation without control of the airway; (2) sedation with control of the airway (oro- or nasotracheal tube, tracheostomy) without paralysis; and (3) sedation, control of the airway, paralysis, and manual ventilation.

In each option, competent individual nursing care for monitoring, suctioning, and turning the patient is the primary requisite. Most deaths from tetanus result from asphyxia, aspiration, or pneumonia. A tube gastrostomy can be utilized to meet the accelerated nutritional needs of these patients without rendering the gastroesophageal sphincter incompetent as a nasogastric tube does.

TYPHOID (Chapter 38). Hemorrhage from and perforation of ileal ulcers are potentially fatal complications of typhoid fever. After prolonged periods of fever, catabolism, undernutrition, and immunosuppression, the patient often develops secondary bacterial suppurative peritonitis (Fig. 12–6). A properly randomized, prospective study to evaluate the comparability of operative versus nonoperative treatment for these exceedingly ill patients has not been reported. Published data support resuscitation followed by operative intervention to limit further contamination and to cleanse the peritoneal cavity. Simple two-layer closure in a transverse axis with chromic catgut and silk is adequate for one or two perforations. Multiple perforations require segmental resection with attempted retention of the ileocecal valve. Copious irrigation of the entire peritoneal cavity

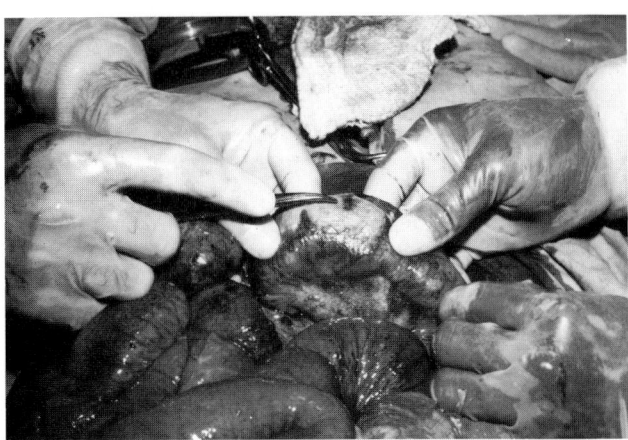

FIGURE 12–6. Perforation of the ileum in typhoid fever with secondary bacterial suppurative peritonitis.

with saline is recommended. Operative mortality continues in the 30% range.

LEPROSY (Chapter 62). Patients with Hansen's disease may require surgical intervention to prevent or treat complications of the feet, hands, and eyes. Ulcers of the feet with or without accompanying osteomyelitis of the underlying bones demand bed rest, debridement, antibiotics, adequate footwear, and a change of lifestyle. Occasionally, ulcers necessitate a below-knee amputation. Tendon transfers to improve the pinch or intrinsic muscle function of a hand or to counter a drop-foot gait enhances limb function and rehabilitation (Chapter 13).

The eyes of patients with Hansen's disease deserve special attention. With facial nerve damage, the orbicularis oculi muscles become paretic and the lids do not close completely (lagophthalmos), leading to corneal exposure, desiccation, and irritation. An insensitive cornea risks irreversible damage. Timely tarsorrhaphy or a temporalis muscle transplant procedure preserves vision (Chapter 9).

TUBERCULOSIS (Chaper 61). This ubiquitous disease with protean manifestations remains a scourge amid economically deprived, overcrowded, and underfed populations. Pulmonary tuberculosis with cavities, empyema, and destroyed lung remains the primary problem from *Mycobacterium tuberculosis*. Tuberculous adenitis, (see Fig. 12–4), abdominal and hepatic tuberculosis, Pott's disease with or without neurologic deficit (Chapter 13), urinary tuberculosis, and tuberculous arthritis are important differential diagnoses for the surgeon to consider in patients with failure to thrive, masses, or fever. Gastrointestinal tuberculosis, especially of the ileum and cecum, and tuberculous peritonitis must be considered along with neoplasms in patients with weight loss, ascites, and abdominal masses. Even tuberculosis of the skin and breast can be confused with cancer.

The diagnosis of pulmonary tuberculosis depends on symptoms, radiology, and positive bacteriology. Smears for acid-fast organisms are the bacteriologic standard; culture capability for subgrouping and drug sensitivity testing is not ordinarily available. Multiple drug chemotherapy is the primary treatment (Chapter 61). The surgeon obtains material for diagnosis (bronchoscopy, lymph node biopsy) and treats complications. Tube thoracostomy is employed to treat pneumothorax, empyema, and pyopneumothorax. Elective resections are employed for bronchostenosis, bronchiectasis, destroyed lung, giant emphysematous bullae, resistant organisms, and recalcitrant patients with sputum-positive, localized open cavities. Elective pericardiectomy may be required in patients with constrictive pericarditis. Emergency thoracotomy with lobectomy or pneumonectomy is required in cases of life-threatening hemoptysis, a not unusual sequela of smoldering inflammation. Thoracoplasty procedures are not routine for residual pleural space conditions, but the Eloesser flap permits patients with space problems to go without a tube.

SCHISTOSOMIASIS (Chapter 96). Granuloma formation with bleeding or with fibrosis and stricture occurs in the lower gastrointestinal tract and in the genitourinary tract. Intestinal polyps sometimes occur and require removal either by surgery or during colonoscopy because

of bleeding. Schistosomiasis is the world's leading cause of portal hypertension. Deposition of schistosomal ova in small portal venules increases resistance to flow at the hepatic level, specifically a presinusoidal block. Treatment options for life-threatening variceal bleeding include medical management (vasopressin), balloon tamponade, injection sclerotherapy, variceal ligation, esophageal transection, and portal decompression. Because of better liver function, patients with schistosomiasis do better following shunt surgery than do those who bleed from alcoholic cirrhosis. Repeated hemorrhage, however, remains a frequent complication.

Urinary schistosomiasis can cause an obstructive uropathy with progressive renal failure. Intraluminal obstruction of the distal ureter and damage to the ureteric muscle with loss of peristalsis produce hydronephrosis. Preoperative assessment entails detection and treatment of active infection, assessment of renal function, and definition of anatomic lesions by radiologic methods. Operative options for an abnormal distal ureter include ureteroneocystostomy and ureteric reconstruction (Boari flap or ileal ureter). Cystoplasty utilizing sigmoid, cecal, or ileal bowel segments may be indicated in patients with a contracted bladder and can be combined with a ureteric replacement. Urinary schistosomiasis has an association with carcinoma of the bladder (Chapter 11). Since such patients are often first seen with advanced disease, obstruction, and renal failure, few are candidates for total cystectomy. Urinary diversion, most frequently with a ureterocolostomy to avoid a stoma and appliance, sometimes provides palliation.

HYDATID CYST (Chapter 101.2). Surgical resection remains the treatment of choice for most patients with cystic hydatid disease (*Echinococcus granulosus* infection). Hypertonic saline solution or 0.1% cetrimide is recommended as the operative scolicide in preference to formalin. The operative goal is removal of the cyst without (1) fluid leakage, which may cause toxic or anaphylactic reaction; (2) spillage of scoleces or germinal epithelium, which may produce new cysts; or (3) bleeding and secondary infection. Alveolar hydatid disease of the liver (*E. multilocularis* infection) requires a partial hepatectomy for treatment. Surgical resection, when possible, is recommended for polycystic hydatid disease (*E. vogeli* infection).

AMERICAN TRYPANOSOMIASIS (Chapter 74). The "megasyndromes" cause either dysphagia from megaesophagus or constipation from megacolon. Treatment is symptomatic: excision of a spastic cardia, esophagectomy creating an intestinal conduit as esophageal replacement, or sigmoid resection for megasigmoid.

FILARIAL ELEPHANTIASIS (Chapter 85). Bancroftian, Malayan, and Timorian filariasis can produce secondary lymphedema and the chronic obstructive signs of elephantiasis involving the subcutaneous tissues of the scrotum and the lower extremities. Scrotal elephantiasis can be treated with excision of redundant tissue and placement of the testes in upper thigh adductor pockets or in a newly constructed scrotum. More than 20 operative procedures for the relief of chronic lower extremity lymphedema are extant, in itself an indication that none is superior. Operations for edematous extremities should be recommended only with hesitancy. The procedure employed most often at present is that of Charles (1912), in which the involved skin and lymphedematous subcutaneous tissue are excised down to deep fascia, and the fascia then skin-grafted.

ASCARIASIS (Chapter 83). In the former decades, small bowel obstruction was frequently attributed to a heavy ascaris worm burden. Recent reviews attest that, while obstruction can occur, its incidence is low. In the patient exhibiting signs of partial bowel obstruction with a putty-like mass palpable on abdominal examination, a nonoperative trial of intravenous fluids and nasogastric suction is warranted to allow the obstruction to decompress; after the acute episode, vermicides are given to relieve the patient of the worm load. In the unusual instance of total intestinal obstruction, a history of recent antihelminthic use implies that the dead or dying worms have converted a partial obstruction into a complete obstruction requiring surgical intervention. Options during laparotomy include milking the worm mass bolus into the cecum and right colon, enterotomy with manual worm removal and decompression, and, in rare instances, resection of compromised bowel.

Whereas intestinal obstruction requires a sizeable nematode biomass, a single ascaris in the common bile duct can precipitate biliary tract obstruction with secondary jaundice or cholangitis. Biliary ascariasis is difficult to diagnose preoperatively without radiology and endoscopic retrograde cholangiopancreatography. When infection is suspected, nonoperative management (intravenous fluids, nasogastric suction, antibiotics, and antispasmodics, with antihelminthic administration after the acute attack has subsided) can be successful. If a trial of nonoperative management is unsuccessful (deepening jaundice, increasing fever, peritonitis, increasing colic), common duct exploration will be required for operative removal of the worm(s) and any associated calculi. Ascaris has also been incriminated as a cause of volvulus, intussusception, appendicitis, intestinal perforation, granulomatous peritonitis, pancreatitis, pyogenic cholangitis, acute cholecystitis, and perforation of the bile ducts. Considering the prevalence of this ubiquitous nematode, the actual number of patients who suffer surgical complications from ascariasis is extremely small.

ESOPHAGOSTOMIASIS (HELMINTHOMA). Reported from northern Ghana and Uganda, the nematode *Oesophagostomum*, a hookworm relative, can provoke an inflammatory reaction of the bowel in man when larvae are ingested and penetrate the bowel mucosa. Tumor-like masses, granulomas, and abscesses may ensue, usually in the cecum and right colon, though the stomach, ileum, and even the abdominal wall may be involved. The disease may mimic appendicitis by the right lower quadrant presentation or may be confused with carcinoma or inflammatory lesions such as ameboma, ileocecal tuberculosis, or pyomyositis of the abdominal wall. Most helminthomas will subside with nonoperative treatment, although complications (abscesses, intestinal obstruction, peritonitis) or uncertainty of diagnosis may require exploration.

AIDS. AIDS has serious ramifications for the surgeon practicing in the tropics, where seropositivity for HIV in hospitalized adults may approach 50% in some countries, supplies are short, reuse of equipment is the rule, open wards are crowded, and serotyping is unavailable. Tropical wards and operating rooms float in a sea of secretions. Observing "Universal Precautions" is the ideal, since *all* blood and body secretions of *all* patients are considered potentially infectious for HIV as well as HBV and other blood-borne pathogens.

CONCLUSION

The surgeon working in developing countries faces demands on his endurance, ingenuity, intelligence, and patience. He is often the local expert in all surgical specialities and may be so professionally isolated that the only available consultant is a textbook or an atlas. The successful surgeon must be well founded in basic surgical principles with a thorough knowledge of anatomy. Surgical diseases vary somewhat from one area of the world to another, but the general conditions of underdevelopment or developmental heterogeneity provide strikingly similar obstacles. The primary challenge lies not in knowing what to do with surgical problems per se but in establishing the infrastructure needed to deliver adequate surgical care.

BIBLIOGRAPHY

Adeloye A (ed): Davey's Companion to Surgery in Africa. 2nd ed. Edinburgh, Churchill Livingstone, 1987.

Badoe EA, Archampong EQ, Jaja MOA (eds): Principles and Practice of Surgery including Pathology in the Tropics. Accra, Ghana Publishing Corp., 1986.

Bewes P: Surgery. Nairobi, African Medical and Research Foundation, 1984.

Binford CH, Connor DH (eds): Pathology of Tropical and Extraordinary Diseases. Washington, DC, Armed Forces Institute of Pathology, 1976.

Bitar R, Tarpley J: Intestinal perforation in typhoid fever: a historical and state-of-the-art review. Rev Infect Dis 7:257–271, 1985.

Centers for Disease Control: Update: Universal precautions for prevention of transmission of human immunodeficiency virus, hepatitis B virus, and other bloodborne pathogens in health-care settings. MMWR 37:377–382, 387–388, 1988.

Ezi-Ashi TI, Papworth DP, Nunn JF: Inhalational anaesthesia in developing countries: Part I, The problems and a proposed solution. Anaesthesia 38:729–735, 1983.

Ezi-Ashi TI, Papworth DP, Nunn JF: Inhalational anaesthesia in developing countries: Part II, Review of existing apparatus. Anaesthesia 38:736–747, 1983.

King M (ed): Primary Anaesthesia. Oxford, Oxford University Press, 1986.

King M (ed): Primary Surgery. Vol 1, General Surgery. Oxford, Oxford University Press, 1988.

King M (ed): Primary Surgery. Vol 2, Trauma. Oxford, Oxford University Press, 1987.

MacGowan WAL: Surgical manpower worldwide. Bull Am Coll Surg 72:5–7, 1987.

Meier DE, Imediegwu O, Tarpley JL: Perforated typhoid enteritis–operative experience with 108 cases. Am J Surg 157:423–427, 1989.

Schwartz SI, Adesola AO, Rob CG (eds): Tropical Surgery. New York, McGraw-Hill, 1971.

Tobin GR: Myocutaneous and muscle flaps: refinements and new applications. Curr Probl Surg 23:315–393, 1986.

Wasunna AEO: Surgical manpower in Africa. Bull Am Coll Surg 72:18–19, 1987.

Zacharin RF: Obstetric Fistula. Vienna, Springer-Verlag, 1988.

13. ORTHOPEDICS

Jean Claude Theis
and Benjamin Joseph

Most employment in developing countries requires manual labor. Thus, injury or chronic disease of the musculoskeletal system leading to severe disability will compromise the lives and livelihoods of those concerned, since medical insurance and rehabilitative facilities are nonexistent.

SPECTRUM OF ORTHOPEDIC DISEASES IN THE TROPICS

Diseases of the musculoskeletal system are a common cause of morbidity in developing countries. As the spectrum of diseases is different from that in developed countries, it is essential for orthopedic surgeons to be familiar with the epidemiology of orthopedic disorders in the tropics (Table 13–1). Certain diseases related to poverty, poor hygiene, and malnutrition, e.g., bone and joint infections, poliomyelitis, and leprosy, are confined to or much more common in developing countries. Other orthopedic conditions related to advanced age and sedentary lifestyle, e.g., osteoporosis and degenerative arthritis, are rarer in the tropics than in temperate climates.

Congenital dislocation of the hip is virtually unknown among black Africans, whereas other races (Caucasians, North American Indians, Eskimos, and Mongolians) have a very high incidence. Genetic and environmental factors account for these differences. Owing to natural selection, spina bifida cystica and cerebral palsy are rare conditions in tropical countries. Children born with myelodysplasia die in the neonatal period from meningitis and tetanus. Cerebral palsy is relatively uncommon because neonates with a low Apgar score do not survive because resuscitation facilities are usually not available. On the other hand, the prevalence of congenital talipes equinovarus is much higher in developing countries. There appear to be racial and geographic variations in the incidence of Perthes' disease. It is rare among Africans but common in rural parts of southwest India. The highest incidence is found in urban areas of England.

Infection of the musculoskeletal system is the most common cause of orthopedic disability in developing countries. Salmonella osteomyelitis, rarely seen in developed countries or in individuals with normal hemoglobin, is common in children with sickle cell disease. Chronic osteomyelitis following compound fractures or hematogenous osteomyelitis is prevalent in most of the tropical countries as a result of inadequate and delayed treatment. Bone and joint tuberculosis is a major problem in Africa, Asia, and Oceania. In these continents the incidence has been estimated at 25 to 35 per 100,000 per year. For comparison, in developed countries the incidence is much less and varies between 0.3 and 3 per 100,000 per year. Poliomyelitis has become an exclusively tropical disease, as it has been virtually eradicated from developed societies by immunization. In India alone, 150,000 new cases are reported yearly, and the incidence has been estimated at 20 to 30 per 100,000 per year. The incidence of leprosy is highest in Africa and India, where the disease affects 1 to 4% of the population in certain areas.

Sickle cell disease (HbSS, SC) is endemic in many African and Caribbean countries and may lead to orthopedic complications.

Primary osteoarthritis of the hip is rarely seen among Chinese and Indians, whereas the same condition is very common in the knee and is probably associated with squatting. Rheumatoid arthritis is seldom seen among the black population of rural South Africa but is not uncommon in those living in urban areas. Osteoporosis is rare in the tropics, most likely because of continuous physical activity until late in life.

The rarity of hallux valgus in Indians and Africans is probably due to the fact that closed footwear is not common. Nevertheless, hallux varus, a very rare condition in developed countries, is frequently encountered in unshod persons (Figure 13–1).

A clear idea of epidemiologic aspects of trauma in the tropics is also important. There is a higher incidence of road traffic and industrial accidents because of a total lack of or neglect of safety regulations. Trauma due to gunshot and knife wounds as well as explosions is more common because of frequent political unrest. Many spinal injuries are secondary to falls from trees. Nonunion, malunion, and osteomyelitis following compound fractures are frequent problems.

PRACTICAL CONSIDERATIONS

The principles of orthopedic surgery in developing countries are the same as in developed countries: prevention, treatment, and rehabilitation. However, orthopedic practice depends largely on the patient and the available facilities.

Patients with orthopedic problems are slow to seek medical assistance and present with major deformities of the limbs. Surgery should aim at improvement of function, as cosmesis is less important than in developed societies. Established treatment methods are not necessarily appropriate in tropical countries on account of social and cultural factors. For example, total hip and knee replacements are of little use in many rural areas, as they are not designed to flex beyond 90 degrees,

TABLE 13–1. Prevalence of Musculoskeletal Diseases and Injuries in the Tropics

More Common	Less Common
Osteomyelitis	Degenerative arthritis
Tuberculosis	Rheumatoid arthritis
Poliomyelitis	Osteoporosis
Leprosy	Back pain
Pyomyositis	Secondary bone tumors
Fungal infections	Congenital hip dislocations
Sickle cell disease	Spina bifida cystica
Congenital talipes equinovarus	Sports injuries
Neglected trauma	

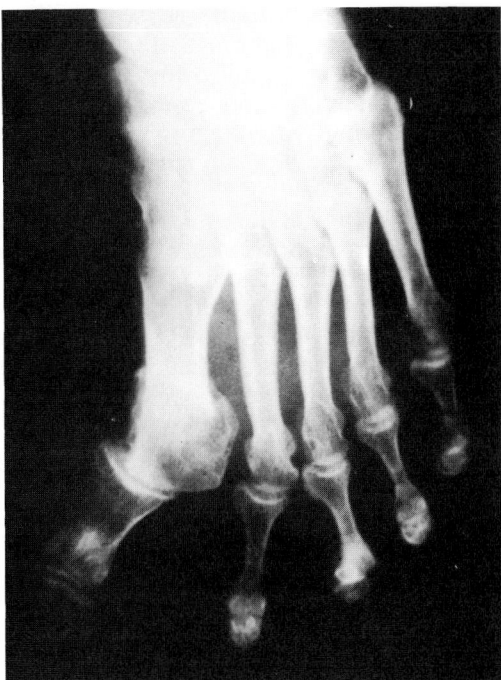

Figure 13–1. X-ray showing a hallux varus deformity in an unshod foot.

which is insufficient for squatting. Available facilities vary, and orthopedic practice must be adapted to the local conditions.

RADIOLOGY. If radiodiagnostic facilities are not available, the surgeon must rely on clinical signs in the assessment of orthopedic patients. It is possible to determine clinically if a fracture is reduced by checking the bony landmarks and comparing the length of the fractured limb with the opposite one.

ANESTHESIA. Local and regional (epidural or spinal) anesthesia is appropriate for most of the common orthopedic procedures because it is cheap, safe, and reliable. When a fully trained anesthetist is not available, the anesthetic can be administered by the surgeon or a trained nurse.

ASEPSIS AND ORTHOPEDIC IMPLANTS. Asepsis in the operating room must be the main concern if orthopedic implants are used. Sterilization facilities and operating room ventilation are often poor and subject to regular breakdowns. Treatment of orthopedic disorders is further complicated by the fact that the vast majority of implants and instrumentation used in reconstructive procedures are expensive and often in short supply. Therefore, closed treatment of fractures is preferred to internal fixation. The importance of preparing the patient for the operation should be emphasized.

REHABILITATION. Physiotherapy services very often are nonexistent, and it depends on the surgeon to organize them. Orthoses and prostheses can be made locally at a reasonable cost.

CONGENITAL MALFORMATIONS

Congenital talipes equinovarus or clubfoot is the most common congenital foot deformity in the tropics. The deformity (varus/equinus of the hindfoot and adduction/inversion of the forefoot) is rigid in the intrinsic and mobile in the extrinsic type. The rigid type, associated with calf wasting, is probably due to neuromuscular imbalance. In the mobile type, owing to a postural malposition in utero, the calf muscles are normal. Before treatment, the spine should be examined to exclude myelodysplasia.

Although in some parts of the tropics children with clubfeet do not receive medical attention until they are several months old, in areas where health care is more advanced infants are seen soon after birth.

The treatment of the deformity in infancy consists of serial manipulation and maintenance of the correction by strapping, splints, or casts. In planning the treatment it is necessary to adopt a schedule that entails the fewest possible appointments at the clinic; these visits also have to be spaced appropriately, as patients often must travel great distances. It has been the authors' practice to use plaster casts after each manipulation, changing them only at fortnightly intervals. If the feet do not respond to these measures by 3 to 6 months of age, soft tissue release operations are done without undue delay so that treatment can be completed by the time the child is ready to walk. The use of corrective footwear after surgery may be appropriate only in urban areas.

Treatment of children presenting later includes initial soft tissue release operations and possibly bony procedures such as calcaneal osteotomy or calcaneocuboid fusion. In children older than 12 to 14 years, triple fusion is done to obtain a plantigrade foot. Occasionally the young adult presents with a clubfoot deformity. In this case it is debatable whether surgery should be performed, as the foot may become painful following the operation. Weight bearing in adulthood is generally good, allowing an acceptable and pain-free gait.

TUMORS OF THE MUSCULOSKELETAL SYSTEM

Unless there is pain, tumors of the soft tissue and bone often attain a large size before the patient seeks treatment (Fig. 13–2). All types of benign bone tumors occur in the tropics and seldom pose problems in treatment.

GIANT CELL TUMORS. Giant cell tumors of bone are seen frequently in some tropical countries. They affect adults between the ages of 20 and 40. The tumor arises from supporting connective tissue of the marrow and is characterized by multinuclear giant cells. The majority develop in the lower end of the femur, the upper end of the tibia, and the lower end of the radius. In the tropics, patients present late with a painful large swelling around the joint. The x-ray shows an osteolytic lesion involving the epiphyseal end of the bone, with thinning and expansion of the overlying cortex. Giant cell tumors are classified as benign, but 30% recur after treatment. Occasionally they metastasize and may become malignant. After the diagnosis has been established by biopsy the tumor is treated by curettage of the lesion and bone grafting if it has not breached the cortex. If the tumor recurs or if it has already breached

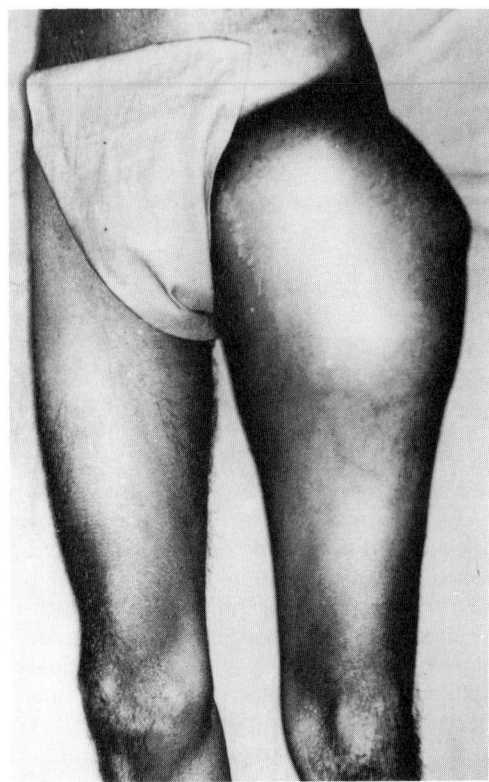

Figure 13–2. Patient with a large synovial sarcoma of the hip.

the cortex at the time of presentation, excision of the involved segment of bone with massive bone grafting is performed, sacrificing the involved joint. In lesions involving expendable bones such as the metatarsals or fibula, primary excision is indicated.

MALIGNANT BONE TUMORS. Treatment of malignant bone tumors like osteosarcoma and Ewing's tumor is extremely frustrating. The patients often present late and even those who are seen early in the course of the disease can seldom afford the prohibitively expensive multidrug chemotherapy used in developed countries.

There is also little role for limb saving surgery in these conditions as custom made prostheses for resected bones are not available. The mainstay of treatment is ablative surgery, although amputation may often be refused by the patient.

POLIOMYELITIS (Chapter 18.2)

It is estimated that there are about 90,000 individuals in Uganda alone with residual paralysis following poliomyelitis. This suggests that the total number of cases worldwide would run into several million. The vast majority of these patients are in tropical countries.

Although the orthopedic surgeon is usually called upon to treat the residual permanent paralysis and its sequelae, it is imperative that he be aware of both preventive measures and treatment in the acute stage of the disease.

EARLY TREATMENT. An important aspect of treatment in the acute stage is correct posturing. This minimizes fixed deformities and contractures. The joints should be put through a full range of passive movement daily. This should be maintained for 6 weeks. Progressive recovery of muscle power occurs over the next 12 months. During this period appropriate calipers are provided to support the paralyzed limb and prevent deformities.

TREATMENT OF RESIDUAL PERMANENT PARALYSIS. The basic principles of treatment include correction of deformities, restoration of muscle power, stabilization of joints, and orthotic management.

Correction of Deformities. The two main causes of deformities in poliomyelitis are faulty posture and muscle imbalance. As a consequence of either factor, various deformities can develop with contractures of tendons and fascia. In long-standing cases, adaptive bony changes also occur. In the early stages, correction of the deformities may be achieved by release of the contracted fascia and tenotomy or lengthening of tendons. In the older child, bone surgery is often necessary in addition to these procedures.

Hip Deformity. The most common hip deformities are flexion, abduction, and external rotation. If these deformities are severe and bilateral, bipedal gait is impossible until the contractures are released. The main offending structure is the iliotibial band, which can be released quite easily at its proximal attachment. In a patient with long-standing and severe deformity it may be necessary to release the glutei and rectus femoris from the ilium. In severe cases, any residual deformity after a radical release can be treated by a corrective osteotomy of the femur at the subtrochanteric level.

Knee Deformity. The common deformities of the knee include genu valgum and flexion deformity. Minor degrees are due to a contracted iliotibial band. This is released just proximal to the knee along with the lateral intermuscular septum. If the flexion deformity at the knee is more marked, the hamstring tendons need to be lengthened surgically or by serial wedging of plaster casts.

Ankle and Foot Deformities. Various deformities around the ankle and foot are seen following poliomyelitis. Balancing of muscle power and stabilization of joints are required to correct most of these deformities. The equinus deformity of the ankle can be corrected by lengthening the Achilles tendon combined with capsulotomy of the ankle joint in severe cases.

Restoration of Muscle Power. If a neighboring tendon can be spared without jeopardizing function, it can be transferred to replace the paralyzed muscle. Such tendon transfers additionally remove the deforming force at the joint. For example, in patients with paralyzed peronei and tibialis anterior muscles, an equinovarus deformity develops owing to unopposed action of tibialis posterior and triceps surae. Transfer of the tibialis posterior to the dorsum of the foot not only restores the power of dorsiflexion but also removes the deforming varus force.

Prior to planning tendon transfers, careful assessment of muscle power of every muscle is carried out. Since postoperative muscle re-education is necessary, tendon transfers are usually deferred until the child is over 7 years of age.

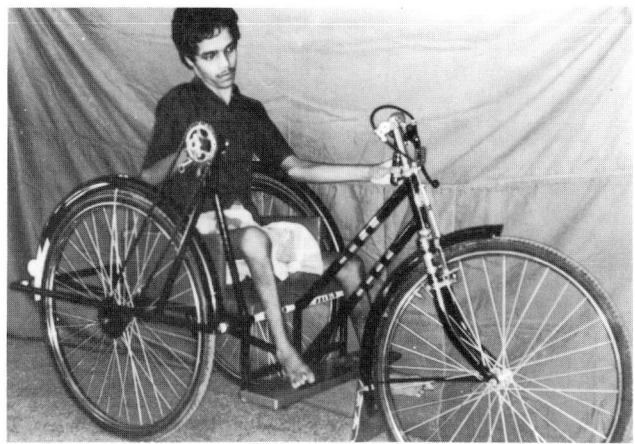

Figure 13–3. Hand-propelled tricycle used in the rehabilitation of patients with severe poliomyelitis.

Stabilization of Unstable Joints. The majority of stabilization operations are done for instability around the foot and ankle and (less commonly) for shoulder paralysis. Most of these procedures are applicable only when the child is approaching skeletal maturity. The advantages of stability of joints, particularly the more proximal joints, should be weighed against the disadvantage of loss of mobility. A fused shoulder may be an asset for a manual laborer, whereas it may be a hindrance to a housewife who cannot comb her hair.

Orthotic Management. Orthotic appliances for poliomyelitis can be fabricated from inexpensive, locally available cheap materials with minimal equipment. Below-knee calipers (ankle-foot orthosis, AFO) are used for instability of the foot and ankle. Above-knee calipers (knee-ankle-foot orthosis, KAFO) are used when the quadriceps muscle is weak. A pelvic band is added (hip-knee-ankle-foot orthosis, HKAFO) when the hip is also very weak.

All children with weak limbs in whom a deformity might develop should be encouraged to wear calipers until their growth is complete even if they can walk without support. Once skeletal maturity has been attained, unstable joints of the foot should be stabilized so that below-knee calipers can be discarded. In patients who need bilateral calipers, a walking aid is also required. Bilateral calipers are of little use to those with weakness of the upper limbs, as they will be unable to use crutches. These patients require a wheelchair (Fig. 13–3).

BONE AND JOINT TUBERCULOSIS (Chapter 61)

The majority of the 15 million to 20 million individuals with active tuberculosis live in developing countries. Estimates of the proportion with bone and joint tuberculosis vary from 5 to 10%, indicating at least 750,000 active cases of bone and joint tuberculosis. Approximately 50% are spinal, 15% in the hip, 15% in the knee, 10% in other joints, and 10% in bone without joint involvement. Most cases occur in adolescents and young adults. The incidence is unknown for most tropical countries but is probably similar to the Asian immigrant population of Great Britain—35 per 100,000 per year.

Musculoskeletal tuberculosis arises following hematogenous spread from a primary focus. Pathology of the bone lesions is similar to that of other tissues. Osteoclastic activity is not a particular feature of bone tuberculosis, although monocytes have the ability to resorb bone.

In the absence of diagnostic facilities, management is often based on clinical suspicion. An elevated ESR and bone destruction characterized by severe regional osteoporosis with little surrounding sclerosis and swelling of soft tissue on x-ray is characteristic of tuberculosis. Antituberculous chemotherapy should be started (Chapter 61).

TUBERCULOSIS OF THE SPINE. Spinal tuberculosis is common in developing countries and may lead to severe disabilities. Most of those infected are young adults and children. The thoracic and lumbar vertebrae are most frequently involved, and paraplegia or other neurologic involvement is present in 30 to 40% of patients when they first seek medical assistance.

The characteristic lesion involves the vertebral bodies with destruction of the intervening disk (Fig. 13–4). As destruction proceeds, kyphosis develops. Soft tissue abscesses, composed of debris and lined by tuberculous granulation tissue, form. These may remain paravertebral, spread to the extradural space, or track to form a distinct abscess in paraspinal, psoas, buttock, or thigh muscles (Fig. 13–5). Paraplegia with active disease is caused by an extradural tuberculous abscess and formation of a kyphosis.

Back pain, stiffness, kyphosis, and occasionally paraparesis or paraplegia in a young child or adult is usually

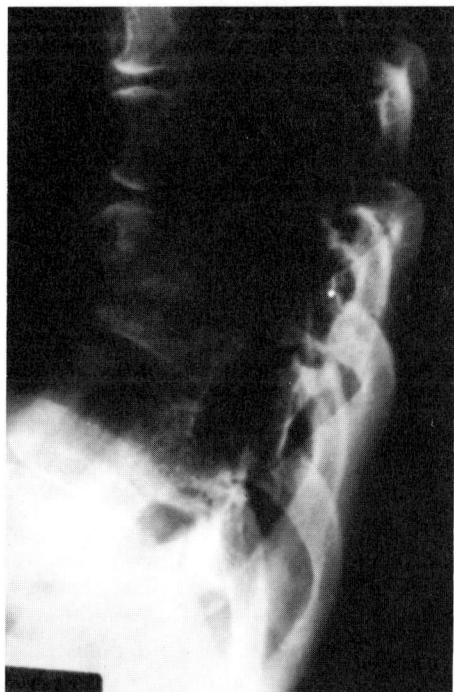

Figure 13–4. X-ray showing vertebral body destruction and secondary kyphosis in the thoracic spine due to tuberculosis. (Courtesy of Professor A.K. Jeffery, Otago University, Dunedin.)

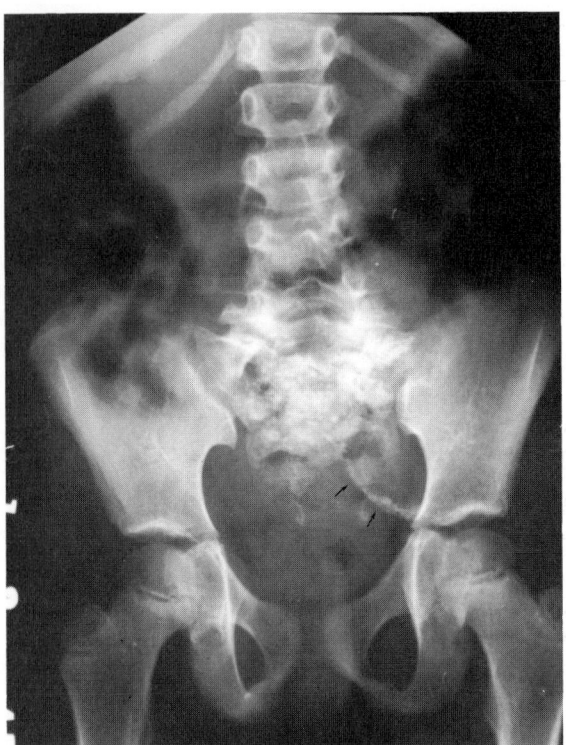

Figure 13–5. X-ray showing a calcified buttock abscess following tuberculosis of the sacrum in a child. (Courtesy of Professor A.K. Jeffery, Otago University, Dunedin.)

due to tuberculous disease. Radiologic evidence of vertebral body destruction or paravertebral abscess formation makes the diagnosis virtually certain. In the absence of other diagnostic possibilities, antituberculous treatment should be started.

Other methods of treatment, including surgery, are supplementary to antituberculous chemotherapy. A Medical Research Council Working Party reported no differences between in-patient rest in bed for 6 months followed by outpatient treatment (91% healed) and outpatient treatment from the start (89% healed) in the presence of triple-drug chemotherapy of 18 months' duration. In a similar study it was shown that aggressive surgery, varying from simple debridement to radical anterior excision of the tuberculous focus and bone grafting, did not improve the results significantly compared with the ambulant treatment.

Ten percent of spinal tuberculosis is complicated by paraplegia. The distinction between paraplegia of early and late onset is less important than it formerly was. The real distinction is between paraplegia arising in the presence of active disease in the vertebral bodies and that arising from healed disease, which is always of late onset. Many lesions associated with active disease will respond to conservative treatment. However, pressure on the front of the dura mater by caseous material is the most common cause of paraplegia, and surgical relief of that pressure usually leads to a rapid resolution of the paralysis. Surgery is indicated in rapidly progressive paresis, slowly progressive paresis despite adequate chemotherapy, total paralysis not responding to 3 weeks of adequate chemotherapy, and "cord tumor–like" syn-

drome. The spine can be decompressed by a radical anterior resection or anterolateral decompression when adequate facilities are lacking. Laminectomy, although still performed by some surgeons, is no longer recommended. Paraplegia in patients with healed disease is more difficult to treat. The paralysis is attributed to stretching of the spinal cord over the angle at the back of the affected bodies, the so-called internal gibbus, leading to chronic ischemia. Surgery, if indicated, should be performed only in specialized centers.

TUBERCULOUS ARTHRITIS. Although any synovial joint can be affected by tuberculosis, the hip and knee are the most common sites. In developing countries, diagnosis often relies on clinical judgment. A painful, swollen, and stiff joint with radiologic evidence of localized osteoporosis or joint destruction is most likely due to tuberculosis (Fig. 13–6). A good clinical response to antituberculous chemotherapy is a valuable diagnostic test.

Standard chemotherapy in all active cases is the keystone of treatment. Orthopedic management depends upon the stage of disease. Early disease presents with regional osteoporosis, minimal joint space loss, and minimal bone destruction. Advanced disease is characterized by total joint space loss, severe bone destruction, and instability or subluxation. Early in the disease a good range of movement is normally preserved. Treatment consists of early mobilization and protected weight bearing. Later, when there is marked muscle wasting and joint stiffness, immobilization in a position of func-

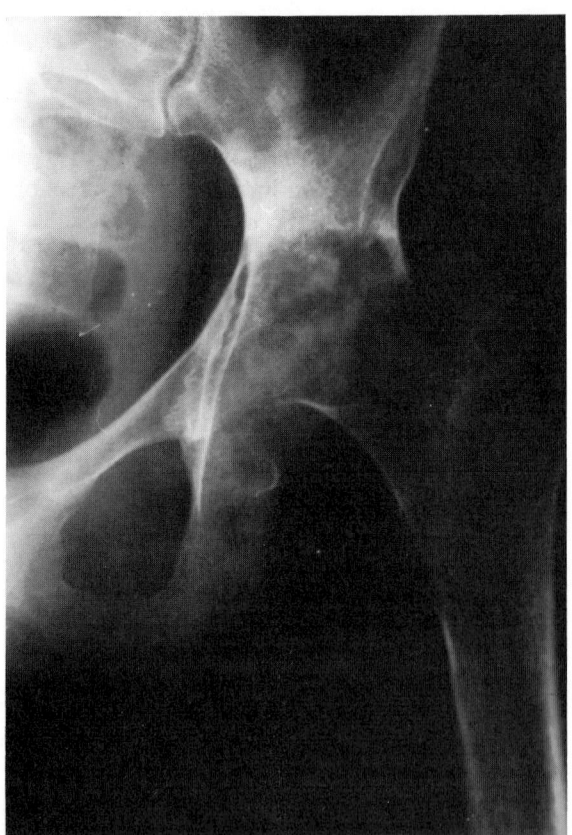

Figure 13–6. X-ray showing destruction of the hip due to tuberculosis. (Courtesy of Professor A.K. Jeffery, Otago University, Dunedin.)

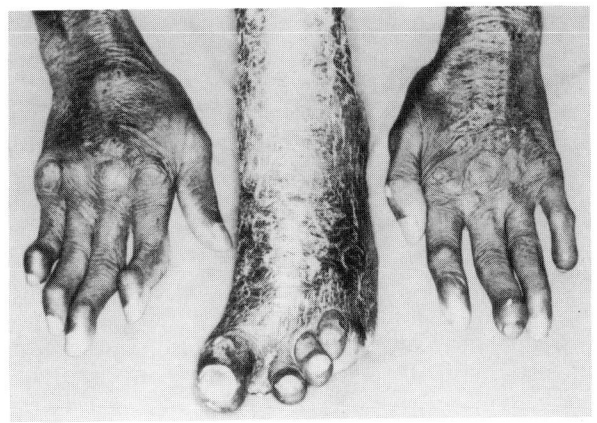

Figure 13–7. Finger and toe deformities in a patient with leprosy.

tion is the accepted treatment. Either the joint will ankylose spontaneously or a painful, unstable, and deformed joint will result. In that case, two options are available: surgical arthrodesis or joint excision arthroplasty. The latter procedure should be performed only in adults. Arthrodesis is unacceptable in many countries, and excision arthroplasty (hip and elbow) may relieve pain with preservation of an acceptable range of movement. Unstable knees and ankles are best treated by arthrodesis.

ORTHOPEDIC ASPECTS OF LEPROSY (Chapter 62)

Leprosy is a chronic disease of the peripheral nerve due to infection by *Mycobacterium leprae*. The bacilli multiply in the Schwann cells, leading to a chronic granuloma that slowly infiltrates the nerve. This causes edema and ischemia, gradually resulting in fibrosis of the nerve. Pain is present in the early stages; later a sensory neuropathy is followed by paralysis. The small nerve fibers of the skin, bone, and vessels are also involved, explaining the chain of events leading to neurotrophic complications, e.g., skin ulceration and bone and joint destruction. Hands and feet are commonly involved, and secondary bone infection leads to further damage (Fig. 13–7).

The orthopedic management of leprosy varies from simple procedures such as neurolysis to complex reconstructive procedures and amputation, according to the stage of disease (Table 13–2).

NEUROLYSIS AND TRANSPOSITION OF THE ULNAR NERVE AT THE ELBOW. There is a predilection for *M. leprae* to involve the ulnar nerve near the elbow, where it is located subcutaneously in an osteofibrous canal. A palpable localized fusiform swelling of the infected nerve occurs at this site. Transposition of the ulnar nerve to the front of the elbow in the initial stage results in immediate pain relief in most cases. Occasionally the epineurium needs to be incised to drain an abscess.

TREATMENT OF HAND DEFORMITIES. Clawing of the ring and little fingers from involvement of the ulnar nerve is the most common deformity. Median nerve paralysis, resulting in wasting of the thenar muscles, is less common, and radial nerve paralysis is uncommon. Sometimes more than one nerve is involved, resulting in a useless hand. If paralysis is long-standing, the deformity may become fixed owing to joint contracture. This must be corrected by physiotherapy or surgery before tendon transfer. Reconstructive hand surgery in leprosy needs special orthopedic expertise.

MANAGEMENT OF NEUROPATHIC FOOT

Prevention. The patient must be made to understand the significance of lost "protective feeling." He must be educated to inspect his feet regularly so that trivial injuries can be recognized and treated early. Protective footwear is essential but often not well accepted in the tropics.

Foot Drop. The choice is between an orthosis (double-iron or ankle-foot orthosis) or transfer of the tibialis posterior tendon through the interosseous membrane into the dorsum of the foot.

Plantar Ulcers. These develop as a result of abnormal weight bearing secondary to change in the architecture of the foot. They are localized over the metatarsal heads (owing to clawing of the toes) or in the midsole (owing to collapse of the tarsal bones). Very often there is underlying infection (osteomyelitis or septic arthritis), explaining the chronicity of the problem. Treatment of the infection must be surgical and consists of extensive debridement and excision of all infected tissues (including bone). The wound is left open and packed regularly until it granulates; at this stage a well-padded, below-knee walking plaster cast is applied for 6 to 8 weeks.

Useless Foot. Syme's (above-ankle) amputation is indicated where a good heel pad is available and prosthetic facilities are poor. For all other cases, a below-knee amputation is preferred.

SALMONELLA OSTEOMYELITIS (Chapters 38 and 39)

Bone and joint complications after *Salmonella* infections are relatively rare. However, there is an association between these infections and sickle cell disease. In these

TABLE 13–2. Orthopedic Evaluation and Guide to Management in Leprosy

	Nerve Macroscopy	Sensory Function	Motor Function	Skin	X-rays	Treatment
Stage 1	Edema Thickening	Pain Paresthesia Hypoesthesia	Normal or weakness	Normal	Normal	Prevention Neurolysis
Stage 2	Abscess Necrosis	Pain ± Anesthesia	Weakness or paralysis	Ulcers ±	Osteoporosis	Tendon transfers
Stage 3	Fibrosis	Pain 0 Anesthesia	Paralysis	Ulcers +	Acroosteolysis Charcot joints Osteomyelitis	Ablative procedures Amputations

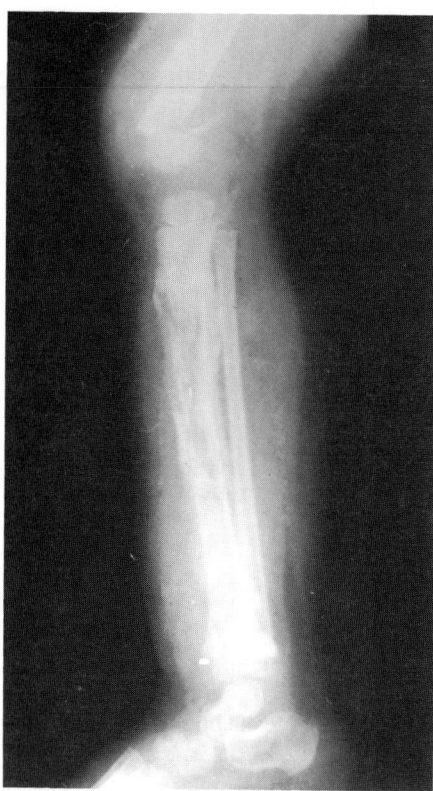

Figure 13–8. X-ray showing destruction of the midshaft of the tibia due to salmonella osteomyelitis in a child.

patients, multiple sites of infection are common, involving hands, feet, and long bones. Many species have been identified, but *S. choleraesuis* is particularly prone to cause bone infections. Children under 5 years of age have the highest incidence of salmonella osteomyelitis and clinically present with painful and swollen limbs associated with pyrexia and toxemia. An aseptic bone infarct in a patient with sickle cell disease may have a similar presentation. Most patients seek medical assistance late in the illness, with a soft tissue abscess, discharging sinuses, or pathologic fractures. Radiographs (Fig. 13–8) show extensive bone destruction and sequestration of the diaphysis surrounded by periosteal new bone formation.

Acute infections respond well to chloramphenicol (80 mg/kg/day) and immobilization. The presence of an abscess, causing poor clinical response, requires surgical exploration. Chronic osteomyelitis, characterized by multiple recurrences despite adequate surgical debridement, is best treated by extensive "guttering." In this technique the entire medullary canal is deroofed, followed by a split-skin graft once adequate granulation tissue has formed. However, amputation is often the final outcome.

MISCELLANEOUS INFECTIONS

PYOMYOSITIS (Chapter 58). No accurate figures are available for the incidence of pyomyositis. It is common in tropical countries but rare elsewhere. Many patients present with a fully developed intramuscular

abscess. The route of bacterial spread is presumed to be hematogenous from skin and other lesions. Over 90% of cases are caused by *Staphylococcus aureus*, the remainder being caused by *Streptococcus* species. Trauma has been suggested as a potential predisposing factor. The majority of abscesses occur in the lower limbs and trunk. Many patients have multiple abscesses. Pyomyositis is occasionally associated with guinea worm (*Dracunculus medinensis*) infection.

Local signs usually predominate, but occasionally patients have systemic symptoms. The management is based upon surgical drainage and antibiotic therapy. Abscesses draining up to 5 liters of pus have been described.

SMALLPOX OSTEOMYELITIS. Although smallpox has been eradicated, patients with residual deformities secondary to variola osteomyelitis or arthritis are occasionally encountered (Fig. 13–9). Deformities are due to damage to the epiphyseal plate resulting in a growth disturbance. In some instances, bony ankylosis of the joints occurs. Treatment entails correction of bony deformities.

FUNGAL INFECTION OF BONES AND JOINTS. Mycetoma is endemic in Sudan and some parts of India (Chapter 65.1). It usually involves the foot and less commonly the hand (Fig. 13–10). The lesions extend deep into subcutaneous tissues and eventually invade bone. They suppurate, and pus drains through multiple sinuses. The pus contains granules of various colors depending upon the etiologic agent. The causative agent may be among at least 6 actinomycetes (false fungi) or 16 species of true fungi. The lesion spreads slowly, but treatment is difficult. Often the infected foot requires amputation.

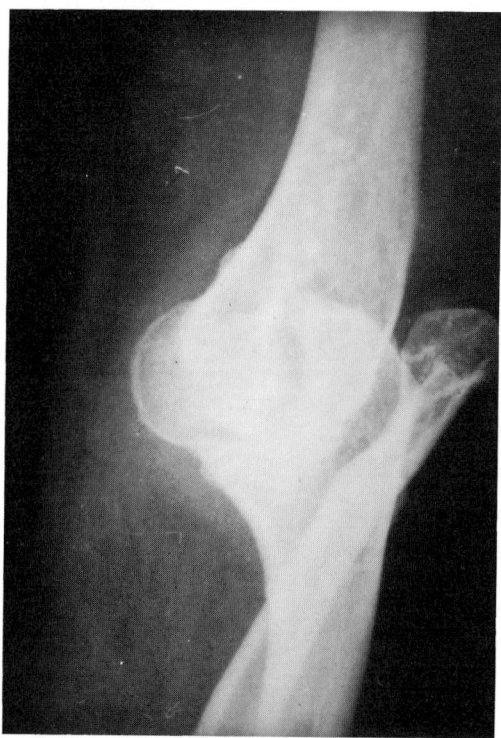

Figure 13–9. X-ray showing a dislocation of the radial head following variola arthritis in childhood.

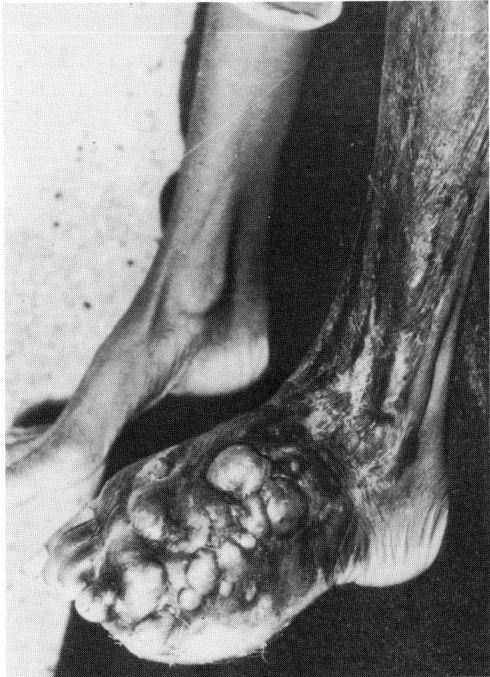

Figure 13–10. Granulomatous tumor of the foot due to mycetoma infection.

ORTHOPEDIC COMPLICATIONS OF SICKLE CELL DISEASE (Chapter 5)

With the exception of salmonella osteomyelitis, avascular necrosis of the hip is the main orthopedic problem in sickle cell disease. Avascular necrosis of the femoral head is a disabling complication predominantly affecting children and adolescents. The disease varies in incidence from 1 to 3% and seems to be more common in sickle cell SC disease. The severity of hip symptoms varies with the amount of femoral head necrosis and collapse. The prognosis in children is better than in adults, as the epiphysis is remodeled following revascularization. Treatment is symptomatic, but in an adult, resection arthroplasty (excision of the femoral head and neck) may be performed if the hip is stiff and painful.

TRAUMA MANAGEMENT IN DEVELOPING COUNTRIES

The incidence of major traffic accidents is increasing in developing countries because of construction of paved roads, increasing number of motor vehicles, and absence of safety precautions.

Mortality and morbidity of multiply injured patients is high because of isolation and lack of organized ambulance service, which results in delayed treatment. If the patient has severe head, chest, or abdominal injuries, his chances of survival are poor unless he is evacuated to a major medical center.

Lack of safety regulations leads to frequent industrial accidents, resulting in crush injuries and traumatic amputations of fingers and hands. The incidence of flexor tendon injuries due to knife and machete wounds is high. These injuries, especially the machete type, often are associated with damage to neurovascular structures

and bone. Treatment is difficult, and the results are disappointing.

Gunshot and explosion injuries frequently occur during civil unrest. Half the wounds result in fractures, which are often followed by wound infections and osteomyelitis. Damage to neurovascular structures is common, occurring in one third of cases. Low-velocity gunshot wounds, not producing damage to vital structures, should be left open to heal. High-velocity wounds or those with possible damage to vital structures should be explored, debrided, and left open. Additionally, tetanus and antibiotic prophylaxis must be given. Fractures are best stabilized with external fixation followed by secondary wound closure. Skin grafting or reconstructive plastic surgery procedures may be indicated.

Falls from trees (coconut) are a frequent cause of spinal injuries. Fractures are managed with bed rest followed by plaster immobilization. Management of spinal injuries with para- or quadriplegia is very difficult in developing countries because of insufficient nursing and rehabilitation facilities. The morbidity and mortality are very high in these patients. Fractures of the neck of the femur and distal radius in the elderly is very rare in developing countries because the incidence of osteoporosis is low.

The treatment of fractures in developing countries should be conservative. Internal fixation devices are often not available or are in short supply and should not be used unless expertise and clean surgical facilities are available. Closed stable fractures are treated in plaster. If the fracture is unstable, traction or external

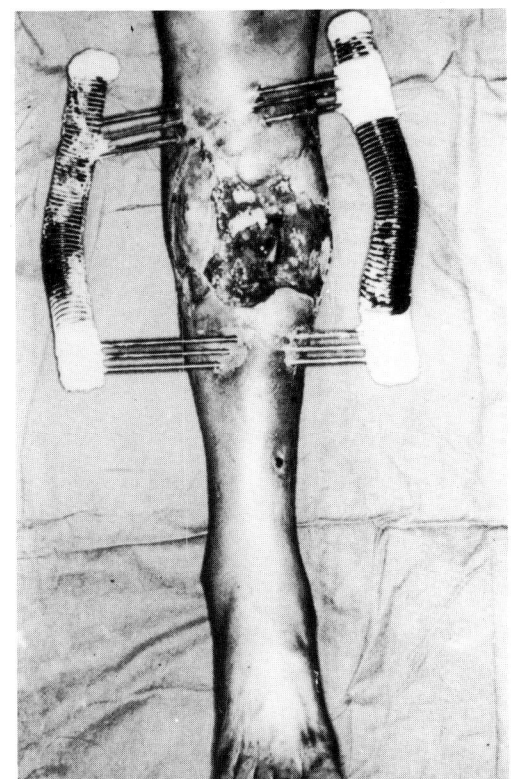

Figure 13–11. A locally fabricated external fixator made of PVC (polyvinyl chloride) tubing and dental acrylic used to treat an open fracture of the tibia.

fixation is used. Locally made external fixators are cheap and usually satisfactory (Fig. 13–11). Open fractures with minor skin and soft tissue damage are debrided and treated in the same way as a closed fracture. In patients with major soft tissue and neurovascular damage, amputation is often the only alternative. Infection and nonunion after compound fractures are common complications and lead to secondary amputation in many cases. Malunion interfering with function should be treated by osteotomy if facilities are available.

BIBLIOGRAPHY

Adeyokunnu AA, Hendrickse RG: Salmonella osteomyelitis in childhood. Arch Dis Child 55:175–184, 1980.
Brand PW: Paralytic claw hand with special reference to paralysis in leprosy and treatment by the sublimis transfer of Stiles and Bunnell. J Bone Joint Surg 40B:618–632, 1948.
Chacko V, Joseph B, Mohanty SP, Jacob T: Management of spinal cord injury in a general hospital in rural India. Paraplegia 24:330–335, 1986.
Donovon WH, Carter RE, Bedbrook GM, et al: Incidence of medical complications of spinal cord injury. Patients in specialized compared with nonspecialized centers. Paraplegia 22:282–290, 1984.
Ebong WW: Legg-Calve-Perthés' disease in Nigerians. Int Surg 62:217–218, 1985.
Griffiths DL, Seddon HJ, Roaf R: Pott's Paraplegia. Oxford, Oxford University Press, 1956.
Hodgson AR, Stock FE, Fang HSY, Ong GB: Anterior spinal fusion. Br J Surg 48:172–178, 1960.
Huckstep RL: Poliomyelitis: A Guide for Developing Countries, Including Appliances and Rehabilitation for the Disabled. Edinburgh, Churchill Livingstone, 1975.
Iwegbu CG, Fleming AF: Avascular necrosis of the femoral head in sickle cell disease. J Bone Joint Surg 67B:28–32, 1985.
Kelsey JL: Epidemiology of Musculoskeletal Disorders. Vol 3. In Lilienfeld AM (ed): Monographs in Epidemiology and Biostatistics. New York, Oxford University Press, 1982.
MRC Working Party in Tuberculosis of the Spine: J Bone Joint Surg 60B:168–177, 1978; 67B:103–110, 1985.
Reddy CRRM, Rao PS, Rajakumari K: Giant-cell tumors of bone in South India. J Bone Joint Surg 56A:617–619, 1974.
Sim-Fook L, Hodgson AR: A comparison of foot forms among non–shoe and shoe-wearing Chinese population. J Bone Joint Surg 40A:1058–1062, 1958.
Tuli SM, Mukherjee SK: Excision arthroplasty for tuberculous and pyogenic arthritis of the hip. J Bone Joint Surg 63B:29–32, 1981.

White AA, Feagin JA: The management of the foot in leprosy. Clin Orthop 85:115–121, 1972.
Zancolli EA: Claw hand caused by paralysis of the intrinsic muscles: a simple surgical procedure for its correction. J Bone Joint Surg 39A:1076–1080, 1957.

14.   HEAT-ASSOCIATED ILLNESSES

Hassan Abu-Aisha
and Abdul Karim Al-Aska

PATHOPHYSIOLOGY

The physiologic responses to heat stress in man are controlled by a sensitive and efficient thermoregulatory system (Fig. 14–1). Optimal body temperature is a balance of environmental temperature, relative humidity, endogenous production of heat, and effective loss of body heat. The majority of the heat load is lost through radiation, conduction, and convection (65%); evaporation from the skin and lungs accounts for 30%; only minor loss is through urine and feces (5%).

Optimal thermal balance can work effectively within certain limits. In hot climates, several factors can throw the system off balance. Radiation from the body to the environment is inhibited when the ambient temperature rises to 30 C. Under such circumstances, sweating becomes the most important means of heat loss by evaporation. Evaporation is severely hampered by high humidity. Thus, the combination of high ambient temperatures and increased relative humidity sets the stage for the development of heat illness. Under such circumstances individuals at high risk for heat illnesses (see below) are likely to suffer most.

ADAPTATION TO HEAT EXPOSURE. Repeated exposures to heat result in several physiologic changes that help the individual tolerate higher than usual environmental temperatures. The acclimatization thus achieved is largely a process of changes in sodium and water balance as well as a gradual increase in metabolic efficacy in energy utilization. Initial exposure to increas-

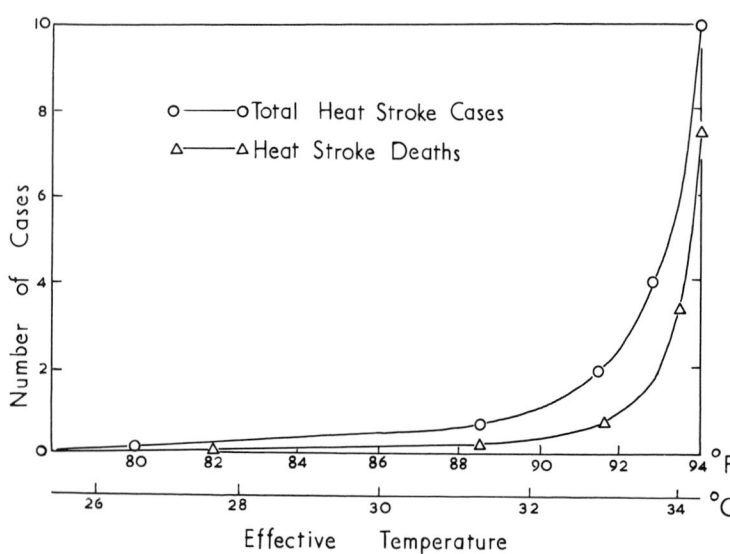

FIGURE 14–1. Incidence of heat stroke cases and deaths with increased effective temperature in hot, humid gold mines in South Africa. (From Wyndham CH: J S Afr Inst Min Metall 66:125, 1965. Reprinted by permission.)

ing ambient temperature results in profuse sweating and contraction of the extracellular fluid (ECF) volume. Blood is shunted to the skin and to the active muscle mass, leading to a further decrease in the ECF volume. The circulatory response to this decline in effective blood volume is a decrease in stroke volume and tachycardia. The renal blood flow eventually decreases, and the renin-angiotensin-aldosterone system is activated. The baroreceptors will also detect the hypovolemia and stimulate the release of antidiuretic hormone (ADH). Thus the kidney will activate the conservation of sodium and water, and the cardiac output will improve. The improved peripheral circulation results in more sweating and better heat dissipation.

More exposures to heat result in more efficient sweat glands that produce sweat of a high water content and low electrolyte concentration at lower environmental temperatures. Heat is therefore dissipated more effectively with a lower electrolyte loss. After long-term acclimatization the volume of sweat produced by a given workload is decreased (but still greater than in the unacclimatized person). This is presumably because of increased metabolic efficiency, possibly due to a greater number of mitochondria and higher glycogen content in muscles that help convert anaerobic to aerobic energy utilization.

The spectrum of heat-associated illnesses is summarized in Table 14–1. In clinical practice the most important of these are heat stroke, heat exhaustion, and heat cramps.

HEAT STROKE

Heat stroke (sunstroke) is characterized by excessive core temperature (usually 40 C or above) and severe central nervous system dysfunction. It is the least common of heat-related illnesses but carries by far the highest morbidity and mortality.

PATHOGENESIS. Heat stroke results from failure of the heat regulatory mechanisms to maintain a tolerable core temperature. The excessive heat load is usually from environmental sources, but occasionally it may be produced endogenously by the body. In either case, the

TABLE 14–1. Classification of Heat Illnesses

Heat stroke (heat apoplexy, siriasis, heat pyrexia, sunstroke)
Due to environmental heat overload—
    As a sequel to severe heat exhaustion
    Direct heat effect
Due to excessive exertion
Heat exhaustion
Due to excessive heat load and—
    Predominant water depletion
    Predominant salt depletion
    Anhidrotic heat exhaustion
Heat cramps
Due to excessive heat load and—
    Electrolyte depletion
    Muscle fatigue (lactic acid accumulation)
Other heat illnesses
    Heat edema
    Heat syncope
    Heat-and-friction skin damage (prickly heat)

TABLE 14–2. Drugs that Increase the Risk for Heat Stroke

Diuretics
Anticholinergics
Antiparkinsonism agents
Phenothiazines
Tricyclic antidepressants
Barbiturates
Monoamine oxidase (MAO) inhibitors
Antihistamines
Thyroid hormones
Hallucinogens (e.g., LSD)
Beta-adrenergic blockers
Methyldopa
Guanethidine

For mechanisms of production of heat-related problems by drugs, see Lomax P: Drug-induced changes in the thermoregulatory system. *In* Khogali M, Hales JRS (eds): Heat Stroke and Temperature Regulation. New York, Academic Press, 1983, pp 197–211.

heat dissipation mechanisms may be inefficient or hindered by other factors. For example, hypovolemia, hypotension, and peripheral vasoconstriction result in reduced blood flow to the sweat glands, thereby severely hampering heat loss by evaporation. Causitive pathologic conditions, e.g., cardiovascular diseases and diabetes mellitus, lead to heat intolerance.

Factors that favor excessive endogenous heat production include extreme exercise and fevers. Athletes and marchers may develop heat stroke and so may many patients with high-grade fevers or those who use drugs that affect temperature regulation (Table 14—2). Environmental factors include heat waves, high relative humidity, and overcrowding. Table 14–3 summarizes the risk factors that predispose to heat stroke.

EPIDEMIOLOGY. Heat stroke may be limited to isolated cases, or small groups of victims, or it may occur in epidemics, depending on the prevalence of the predisposing factors. Sporadic cases arise when there is occupational exposure requiring physical exertion in an environment that favors the development of heat stroke. Examples are the cases reported among gold miners in South Africa. Military troops are at risk, especially early in their training, when acclimatization is incomplete. Epidemics of heat stroke may strike crowds of people gathered in confined areas when the ambient temperature is high, the relative humidity high, and the air speed low. These conditions prevail in the pilgrimage to Makkah (Haj) when it occurs in the summer.

Epidemics have also occurred during heat waves in St. Louis and Kansas City, Missouri, where those at

TABLE 14–3. Factors Predisposing to Heat Stroke

In Healthy Persons
Lack of acclimatization
Salt and water depletion
Acute infection or fever
Obesity
Extremes of age (infants and elderly)
Commonly Associated Disease States
Cardiovascular problems: cardiac insufficiency, atherosclerosis
Endocrine disorders: diabetes mellitus, thyrotoxicosis, Addison's disease
Acute or chronic alcoholism
Malnutrition
Impaired sweat production
Drugs Increasing the Risk (See Table 14–2)

highest risk are elderly persons of low socioeconomic status. Marathon runners and recreational runners may also suffer from heat stroke. No gender-related or racial differences in susceptibility have been consistently observed. However, in the Makkah pilgrimage, different races seem to have different prevalence rates. These are probably accounted for by variation in acclimatization and prevalence of other risk factors in each group rather than by racial differences.

Precise statistics for the morbidity and mortality of heat stroke are not available because of the irregular occurrence of the condition, the poor certification, and the multiplicity of confounding factors. The most reliable figures are perhaps those from the South African gold mines because they refer to a population that remains fairly steady in size, composition, and exposure over the working year. Cases occur at rates of 0.3/1000/year at environmental temperatures of 32 C (90 F) wet bulb, and 4.0/1000/year at 34.4 C (94 F) wet bulb. The increase in the incidence rises exponentially with the rise in the environmental temperatures (Fig. 14–1).

PATHOLOGY. Hyperthermia per se causes widespread tissue damage. At about 42 C there may be denaturation of enzymes, liquification of membrane lipids, mitochondrial damage, and alterations of phospholipids and stability of lipoproteins. Cellular and organ damage produces contributory pathologic processes, e.g., hypoxia, congestion, and endotoxemia.

Multiorgan system involvement is the rule, the degree of involvement depending on individual variations and the heat load quantum. Brain tissue is by far the most vulnerable to hyperpyrexia, and central nervous system damage has invariably been found in all heat stroke victims examined at autopsy. The most frequent findings are edema of the brain tissue and the meninges, with congestion and petechial hemorrhages in the periventricular areas. Cellular destruction occurs especially in the cerebellum, where degeneration of the Purkinje cell layer is the most common finding.

Hemorrhages, degeneration, and necrosis are also observed in the heart, kidneys, lungs, and other organs. The liver is affected early in the course of heat stroke. Prominent changes usually are congestion with polymorphonuclear cell infiltration.

Hematologic injury occurs in severe cases: Petechial hemorrhages and ecchymosis with generalized coagulopathy are usually signs of grave outcome. Electron microscopy has shown that the primary event initiating the coagulopathy is direct thermal injury to vascular endothelium, with subsequent platelet aggregation and activation of the coagulation cascade.

Evidence of skeletal muscle necrosis has been found in a large percentage of patients with heat stroke induced by strenuous physical activity, but is rarely seen in patients with environmental heat injury.

CLINICAL MANIFESTATIONS. The onset is usually acute. Collapse and loss of consciousness often occur without warning. Some patients may develop prodromal symptoms over a period of minutes to hours. These include malaise, dizziness, headache, anorexia, nausea and vomiting, abdominal pain, diarrhea, muscle cramps, mental confusion, ataxia, and paresthesia.

The syndrome of heat stroke has classically been described by the triad of hyperthermia (40 C or more), severe CNS disturbance, and hot, dry skin with absence of sweating. The most constant of these features are the first two. The rectal temperature may range from 40 C to 43.8 C. In our experience, 70% of patients at the Makkah pilgrimage had rectal temperature of 41 C or higher.

For practical purposes it is best to devide heat stroke into environmental and exertion-induced types.

Environmental Heat Stroke. This usually occurs under adverse environmental conditions, when the ambient temperature and the relative humidity are high and the air speed is very low. The clinical picture is usually that of an epidemic affecting elderly patients who often have other diseases such as circulatory disturbances. Table 14–4 shows the differences between environmental and exertion-induced heat stroke.

Exertion-Induced Heat Stroke. This usually affects young individuals who perform unusually severe exercise. They often have more profound disease than do those with environmental heat stroke, including a high prevalence of vital organ damage (Table 14–4).

Systemic involvement in heat stroke is summarized under several headings.

Neurologic Manifestations. These can be divided into three groups according to the time of onset: in the acute stage, during convalescence, or as late sequelae. When first seen, heat stroke victims are usually in coma or have profound disorientation. Pupillary findings can be misleading: wide, dilated, "fixed" pupils may occur even in victims who recover. It is not uncommon to see nuchal rigidity, particularly in elderly patients with environmental heat stroke, but the diagnosis of meningitis must always be considered in such cases. Seizures may occur in 60% of patients, and they may be noted for the first time during the cooling period.

Cardiovascular Manifestations. The usual cardiovascular signs reflect a high-output state. Tachycardia with a wide pulse pressure and often a low blood pressure is usually noted. The central venous pressure is usually normal or elevated; severe hypovolemia is not a usual finding. The electrocardiographic findings are nonspecific.

Lung Involvement. Pulmonary involvement is a fre-

TABLE 14–4. Differences Between Environmental and Exertional Heat Stroke

	Environmental	Exertional
Characteristics		
Age	Older	Younger
Epidemiologic factors	Epidemic form	Isolated cases
Predisposing illness	Frequent	Rare
Clinical Features		
Core temperature	Very high	High
Sweating	Often absent	May be present
Rhabdomyolysis	Rare	Common
DIC	Rare	Common
Acute renal failure	Rare	Common
Hyperuricemia	Mild	Marked
Enzyme elevation	Mild	Marked

Modified from Hart GR, Anderson RJ, Crumpler CP, et al: Epidemic classical heat stroke. Clinical characteristics and course of 28 patients. Medicine 61:189–197, 1982. © by Williams & Wilkins, 1982.

TABLE 14–5. The Incidence of Heat Stroke and Mortality Rate at the Makkah Pilgrimage When It Coincided with the Summer Months in 1983–1986*

Year	Date of Peak Pilgrimage Activities	Number of Foreign Pilgrims	Number of Heat Stroke Cases	Incidence per 100,000	Mortality (%)
1983	16 September	1,050,000	1365	130	12
1984	5 September	919,000	1058	115	13
1985	25 August	851,000	2087	245	10
1986	14 August	856,000	594	69†	8

*Kindly supplied by Dr. Adnan Jamjoum, Hajj Health-services Centre, Jeddah, Saudi Arabia.
†Vigorous preventive measures taken.

quent finding in severe cases. Of 52 consecutive cases of heat stroke at Makkah, 12 (23%) were diagnosed as adult respiratory distress syndrome (ARDS), and 9 of these patients died. The direct thermal injury and the presence of disseminated intravascular coagulopathy (DIC) seem to be the most important factors in the development of ARDS.

Bleeding Tendencies. Bleeding tendencies with petechiae and ecchymosis are found in severe cases. DIC, as defined by thrombocytopenia, elevated fibrinogen degradation products (FDP), and hypofibrinogenemia, is a major cause of severe hemorrhage and death during the convalescent phase. The combination of DIC and ARDS usually indicates a grave prognosis.

Metabolic and Hepatic Disturbances. Metabolic abnormalities noted during heat stroke include substantial increases in liver and muscle enzymes, hyperglycemia, hypomagnesemia, hypocalcemia, and hypophosphatemia. The latter two may be due to sequestration of calcium and phosphorus in the injured muscles.

Hepatocellular injury with marked elevation in the serum transaminases and bilirubin may occur. The hepatic enzymes usually peak by 48-72 hours following exposure and fall rapidly over the next week. Transaminase levels greater than 1500 IU in the first 24 hours after cooling indicate a poor prognosis.

Renal Involvement. Acute rhabdomyolysis with myoglobinuria and renal insult is more common in exertional than in environmental heat stroke. The myoglobin insult to the kidneys is more profound when there is an associated hypovolemic state. In exertional heat stroke, victims are usually volume-contracted, have hyperuricemia, and excrete large quantities of uric acid. The intravascular volume contraction is largely due to a shift of fluid to the interstitial space under the effect of strenuous exercise. Proteins also tend to move in the same direction. The vasodilation induced by heat is usually not enough to oppose these effects, and the result is reduced renal perfusion and tubular injury.

The combination of hypovolemia, myoglobinuria, and hyperuricosuria may lead to acute tubular necrosis, and DIC may result in glomerular injury. Severe renal failure necessitating dialysis may thus be produced, and the prognosis is usually grave.

PROGNOSIS. Experience from the Makkah pilgrimage health studies has shown that about 90% of environmentally induced heat stroke victims recover. Table 14–5 shows the outcome of patients seen over 4 successive years at Makkah. Poor prognostic features include a prolonged cooling time, the presence of severe coag-

ulation abnormalities, the presence of ARDS, persistent oliguria with renal failure, and SGOT values greater than 1000 IU.

PREVENTION. There are five lines of action that can reduce the occurrence of heat illnesses.

Define the Upper Limits of "Safe" Environmental Temperatures. Industrial workers should not continue to work under extreme heat conditions. Bell and Watts (1971) have made comprehensive recommendations. Because heat stress may be induced by many different combinations of air temperature, radiant temperature, relative humidity, and air speed, an index of equivalence—the corrected effective temperature (CET)—is often used to express limiting thermal environments. Conditions become unsafe for moderate activities above a CET of 30 to 33 C. Another thermal index is the wet bulb globe temperature (WBGT). This is the sum of 70% of the wet bulb temperature, 20% of the BLACK globe temperature, and 10% of the dry bulb temperature. These values are very similar to CET values. Outdoor activity is to be avoided when the WBGT exceeds 29.4 C (85 F).

Preventive Cooling Measures. Open areas that are at risk of becoming too hot in certain seasons should be shaded by trees wherever possible. It has been estimated that one large tree cools as much as do five 10,000-BTU air conditioners. An example of such a preventive effort is the attempt to shade the mountainous area of Arafat in Saudi Arabia, where about a million pilgrims gather in an area of 10 square kilometers.

In urban communities, adequate ventilation or air conditioning will reduce the heat load. Some coal miners have worn special jackets packed with ice to face the severe heat underground.

Artificial Acclimatization. Tolerance to heat can be raised by progressively exposing a subject to a high heat load. Steady-state conditions are achieved after 7 to 12 days. Athletes, miners, and military troops may use the procedure to improve their heat tolerance. At the same time, refractory, heat-intolerant individuals can be identified.

Salt and Water. Regular water replacement at frequent intervals is required during heat exposure to maintain efficient evaporative cooling.

Extra salt intake is usually not necessary except for totally unacclimatized persons. If salt supplements are necessary, increased amounts of water must be taken simultaneously. Excessive salt intake may lead to hypokalemia during early acclimatization.

Health Education. Several simple roles should be

taught to those who are likely to face heat stress: (1) Clothing must be light and porous. (2) Light head covers or umbrellas to provide shade in exposed areas. (3) An abundant water supply must be available. (4) Alcohol and heavy meals should be avoided, especially during the day. (5) Well-ventilated, cooled quarters should be available for sleeping and for part of the working day. (6) Regular exertion *before* exposure helps provide a degree of heat acclimatization.

TREATMENT. Early recognition and prompt treatment of heat stroke reduce the mortality rate. The standard measures for handling an unconscious or confused patient should be taken. The most important therapeutic measure is to cool the patient. In the past it was often recommended to immerse the patient in an ice-water bath and briskly massage the body to prevent the cutaneous vasoconstriction that may impede core heat dissipation. This method is not practical in the face of large numbers of individuals such as may be seen with environmental heat stroke, and there is the danger of aspiration to the comatose patients. Iced-saline lavage of the stomach was tried in attempts to reduce core temperature, but we do not recommend such methods today. The best and simplest way to achieve cooling seems to be by spraying water at a reasonable room temperature (20 to 25 C) and fanning the subject vigorously. Ice cold water should be avoided, as it induces vasoconstriction and heat loss by evaporation is thus greatly reduced.

As the patients are usually delirious, violent, and possibly incontinent, special cooling devices have been designed to meet the various problems. Weiner and Khogali devised a body-cooling unit with controlled water and air temperatures; this proved to be effective in combating heat stroke in the Haj season in Saudi Arabia. A simplified cooling bed using the same principle of evaporation (sponging by water and fanning) was devised by our group in 1986; this proved to be as effective as the Weiner-Khogali body cooling unit but less expensive and much simpler to use (Fig. 14–2).

Whichever method of cooling is used, it is important to slow down when the rectal temperature drops to 39 C. Overcooling may be associated with shivering, convulsions, vomiting, diarrhea, and hypotension.

Intravenous diazepam (10 to 20 mg) or chlorpromazine (25 to 50 mg) has been used successfully for sedation and to prevent shivering.

The question of how much intravenous fluid a patient needs has recently been objectively studied. Al-Harthi and coworkers have shown that most patients are *not* dehydrated when first seen. Rapid infusion of normal saline or similar infusion fluids may have serious effects on the circulation, since the heart is often injured by the heat insult and may not be able to pump an extra load of fluids. It is recommended that patients not receive more than 1 liter of intravenous fluids over the first 3 hours unless there are distinct signs of fluid depletion.

Dantrolene sodium, which is useful in arresting malignant hyperthermia, has been shown experimentally to prevent hyperthermia after exertion. It may have a prophylactic value in exertional heat stroke but seems to have no role in environmental heat stroke. Salicylates, corticosteroids, and beta-blocking agents have no role in the management of heat stroke.

HEAT EXHAUSTION

This is the most common clinically significant heat-associated illness. It may be divided into three categories.

HEAT EXHAUSTION WITH PREDOMINANT WATER DEPLETION. This syndrome is characterized by marked thirst, fatigue, weakness, and impairment of judgment. In severe cases there may be delirium and coma. The body temperature is usually normal in the early stages but later rises, and the patient may develop heat stroke.

HEAT EXHAUSTION WITH PREDOMINANT SALT DEPLETION. Excessive sweating in a hot environment may lead to salt depletion. The early symp-

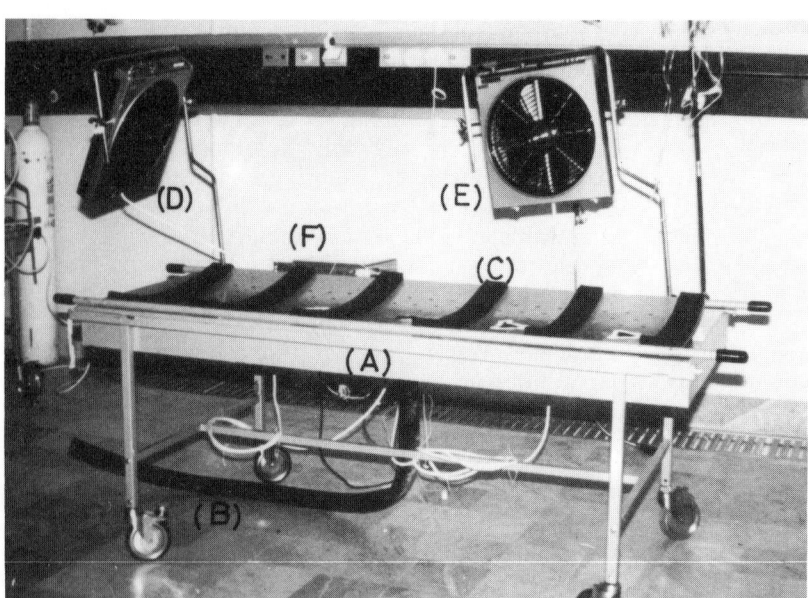

FIGURE 14–2. The King Saud University Cooling Bed (KSU-CB). Stainless steel pan (A); drain pipe (B); rubber strips fixed on steel stretcher (C); electric fans adjustable in 3 dimensions (D and E); and panel for temperature probes and a single electricity outlet for the whole unit (F).

toms are headache, nausea, vomiting, and giddiness. As the condition worsens the patient becomes restless and weak and may show changes in personality. The body temperature may be normal or high.

Some patients will benefit from being placed in a cool place and having fluid and electrolyte replacement. Oral fluids will be sufficient in most cases, but some individuals may need intravenous fluids and/or active cooling, as described for heat stroke.

ANHIDROTIC HEAT EXHAUSTION. This syndrome usually occurs in persons who suffer impairment of perspiration as a result of blockage of sweat ducts secondary to miliaria (prickly heat) and other diffuse skin diseases such as acute sunburn, exfoliative dermatitis, and congenital ectodermal dysplasia. These individuals are unable to perform even a small amount of work in the heat. Attempting to do so may precipitate heat stroke. The diagnosis becomes apparent in patients with diffuse skin diseases and anhidrosis who have heat exhaustion syndrome or heat stroke.

HEAT CRAMPS

These are painful muscle contractions commonly involving the lower limbs. Unacclimatized subjects are affected by heat cramps, usually caused by muscle fatigue rather than by heat injury. Studies on workers in mines, however, have shown that electrolyte depletion resulting from profuse sweating may cause heat cramps without undue muscle fatigue. Heat cramps respond well to rest and replacement of electrolytes; the condition may require mild analgesics.

HEAT SYNCOPE

Fainting is common in unacclimatized persons exposed to a hot environment. It is precipitated by prolonged standing, sudden cessation of exercise, or stooping. Heat syncope occurs because peripheral vascular pooling, augmented by heat-induced cutaneous vasodilation, reduces venous return to the heart. The resulting reduced cardiac output may lead to orthostatic hypotension and syncope, usually without accompanying fever. Such patients usually recover when placed in the head-low position in a cool place.

HEAT EDEMA

Travelers to the tropics may have swelling of the feet and ankles; the edema is usually mild and disappears within a few days. It is probably due to vasodilation in the legs combined with venous stasis during prolonged sitting or standing. The edema may be a manifestation of the expansion of the ECF space due to increased secretion of aldosterone and antidiuretic hormone in the first few days of acclimatization. Enquiry should be made as to whether the edematous patient has overdosed himself with salt and water as a "precaution"

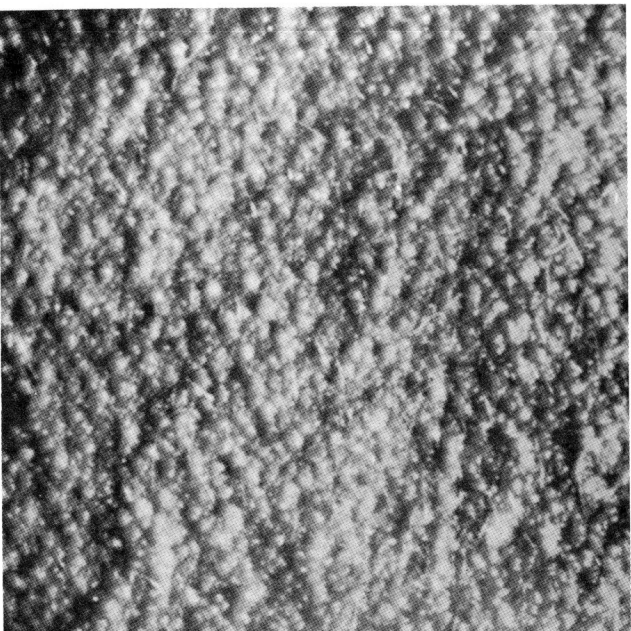

FIGURE 14–3. An enlarged picture of human skin showing miliaria profunda. Notice the goose flesh–like appearance. (From Horne GO, Mole RH: Trans R Soc Trop Med Hyg 44:465, 1951 Reprinted by permission.)

against the hot climate; excessive intakes should be discouraged.

PRICKLY HEAT

This is one of the most common skin problems in hot climates, causing considerable irritation and discomfort. The most serious consequence of prickly heat, however, is anhidrotic heat exhaustion. Prickly heat results from acute (miliaria rubra) or chronic (miliaria profunda) blockage of sweat ducts as a result of maceration of the stratum corneum, which is most likely caused by continuous wetting of the skin from sweating in hot and humid environments. Areas covered by clothing and subject to friction are usually involved. The rash of miliaria rubra is an erythematous epidermal vesicular eruption that is pruritic and accompanied by a prickling sensation ("prickly heat") when sweating is provoked. Miliaria profunda, occurring subsequently, is characterized by dermal vesicles without erythema or pruritus; the appearance is that of goose flesh (Fig. 14–3). Secondary bacterial and fungal infections are frequent sequelae. Treatment consists of removal to a cool environment and application of topical antimicrobial and keratolytic agents as indicated. Any associated heat illness must be treated at once.

BIBLIOGRAPHY

Al-Aska A, Abu-Aisha H, Yaqub B, et al: Simplified cooling bed for heat stroke. Lancet 1:381, 1987.
Al-Harthi S, Akhtar J, and Al-Nozha, M: Hemodynamic changes and intravascular hydration state in heat stroke. Ann Saudi Med 9:378–383, 1989.

Bacon C, Scott D, Jones P: Heat stroke in well-wrapped infants. Lancet 1:422–425, 1979.

Bell CR, Watts AJ: Thermal limits for industrial workers. Br J Ind Med 28:259, 1971.

Dreosti AO: Pathological reactions produced by work in hot and humid environment in the Witwatersrand Gold Mines. S Afr J Med Sci 2:29, 1937.

Escourron P, Freund PR, Rowell LB, Johnson DG: Splanchnic vasoconstriction in heat-stressed men: role of renin-angiotensin system. J Appl Physiol Respir Environ Exercise Physiol 52:1438–1443, 1982.

Hart GR, Anderson RJ, Crumpler CP, et al: Epidemic classical heat stroke: clinical characteristics and course of 28 patients. Medicine 61:189–197, 1982.

Jardon OM: Physiologic stress, heat stroke, malignant hyperthermia—a prospective. Milit Med 147:8, 1982.

Jones TS, Liang AP, Kilbourne EM, et al: Morbidity and mortality associated with the July 1980 heat wave in St. Louis, and Kansas City, Mo. JAMA 247:2327–2331, 1982.

Kassimi FA, Al-Mashhadani S, Abdullah AK, Akhtar J: Adult respiratory distress syndrome and disseminated intravascular coagulation complicating heat stroke. Chest 90:571–574, 1986.

Kew M, Bersohn I, Seftel H: The diagnostic and prognostic significance of the serum enzyme changes in heat stroke. Trans R Soc Trop Med Hyg 65:325, 1971.

Khogali M, Weiner JS: Heat stroke: Report on 18 cases. Lancet 2:276, 1970.

Khogali MK, Hales JRS (eds): Heat Stroke and Temperature Regulation. Sydney, Academic Press, 1983.

Lee DHK: Epidemic heat effects. JAMA 247:3354–3355, 1982.

Malamud N, Haymaker W, Custer RP: Heat stroke: A clinicopathological study of 125 fatal cases. Milit Surg 99:397, 1946.

Nadel ER: Circulatory and thermal regulations during exercise. Fed Proc 39:1491, 1980.

Pattengle PG, Holloszy JO: Augmentation of skeletal muscle myoglobulin by a program of treadmill running. Am J Physiol 213:783, 1967.

Shibolet S, Lancaster MC, Danon Y: Heat stroke: A review. Aviat Space Environ Med 47:280–300, 1976.

Smith NJ: The prevention of heat disorders in sports. Am J Dis Child 138:786–790, 1984.

Weiner JS, Khogali M: A physiological body-cooling unit for treatment of heat stroke. Lancet 1:507–509, 1980.

Wheeler M: Heat stroke in the elderly. Med Clin North Am 60:1289, 1976.

Whitworth J, Wolfman M: Fatal heat stroke in long distance runners. Br Med J 287:948, 1983.

Wyndham CH: A survey of the causal factors in heat stroke and of their prevention in the gold mining industry. J S Afr Inst Min Metal 66:125, 1965.

Yaqub B, Al-Harthi S, Al-Orainey I, et al: Heat stroke at the Mekkah Pilgrimage: clinical characteristics and course of 30 patients. Q J Med 59:523–530, 1986.

Yaqub B: Neurologic manifestation of heat stroke at the Mecca Pilgrimage. Neurology 37:1004–1006, 1987.

PART II

VIRAL INFECTIONS

GENERAL PRINCIPLES

Thomas P. Monath

Viruses are small, obligatory intracellular infecting agents with unique mechanisms of replication and a simple structure, consisting of a core of genetic material (RNA or DNA) enclosed by a protein shell (capsid) and sometimes by an additional lipid bilayer–protein envelope. The structural characteristics of viruses—i.e., type and strandedness of the nucleic acid, morphologic appearance or symmetry of the capsid as determined by electron microscopy, size and shape of the intact viral particle, and presence or absence of an envelope—are used to classify viruses into families. Further groupings into genera are made on the basis of antigenic relationships, nucleic acid homology, and other criteria. The major characteristics and taxonomic status of the viruses included in this part are shown in Table II–1.

INFECTIVITY. Viruses gain access to the host by way of the respiratory, gastrointestinal, or genitourinary tract or through the skin by the bite of an animal or insect vector. Once in the host, they interact with susceptible cells; initial steps in infection include attachment to and penetration through the plasma membrane and freeing of the viral nucleic acid from its protein coat. Normal synthetic processes of host cells are inhibited and shifted over to viral synthesis. Mechanisms by which different virus groups replicate their genetic material, assemble their protein components into mature viral particles, and escape from host cells are complex and vary widely. Host cells may or may not be adversely or irreversibly affected by the infection. However, virulent viruses (those with which we are mainly concerned here) generally produce damage to cells in specific organ systems and capably resist available host defenses.

DISEASE PATTERNS. A number of patterns of disease are evident. In localized infections, such as influenza or rotaviral gastroenteritis, viral replication and cell damage occur at the site of viral entry and in adjacent tissues of the same organ, e.g., lung or intestine. A more common pattern is represented by viruses that multiply at the site of entry and in regional lymphatic tissue draining the site and then disseminate widely by the blood stream to other sites of replication, including the target organ, or organs, that manifest clinical and pathologic responses. Examples of such viruses cited in this part of the text are poliovirus; the viral exanthems, e.g., smallpox and measles; and the arboviruses. A third and extremely important pattern is that of abortive or inapparent infection, mediated by attenuation of the virus strain or by host defense factors that prevent full clinical expression of the disease. In-

dividuals with abortive or inapparent infections may nevertheless shed organisms into the environment and thereby spread virus, e.g., polio, to others. *Slow viral infections* (of which kuru is an example) are characterized by long incubation periods and a slow, progressive course. Still other patterns of virus-host interaction exist, including (1) induction of chromosomal aberrations and teratogenic effects, (2) cellular transformation and tumor induction, and (3) chronic latent infections. Although of major medical importance, examples of these disease patterns are generally not unique to tropical medicine; an exception may be Burkitt's lymphoma associated with Epstein-Barr virus (Chapter 11).

IMMUNITY. Various host defense mechanisms that are not specific for the infecting virus play an early role in viral clearance and recovery; these include interferon alpha and beta, natural killer cells, complement, and macrophages. Viral antigens stimulate specific immune responses by the infected host, both circulating antibodies and cell-mediated immunity. These responses bring about recovery from infection and natural protection from reinfection. Both live attenuated and inactivated vaccines have been developed for a number of viral diseases; in fact, vaccine development has its greatest realized and potential impact on viral infections of the developing world, e.g., smallpox, yellow fever, rabies, measles, and dengue. The immune response is, however, a double-edged sword; antibody or cell-mediated injury to host cell tissues may occur in some viral infections, e.g., in patients with dengue hemorrhagic fever/shock syndrome or in children immunized with killed measles vaccine and later naturally infected with measles virus.

THERAPY. Because of the unique replicative mechanisms of viruses and their dependence on host cell biosynthetic processes, development of specific therapeutic and chemoprophylactic measures has been difficult. Breakthroughs in this area are occurring, and future progress will dictate new approaches to rapid and specific early diagnosis. Already some drugs are useful, e.g., adenosine arabinoside for certain herpesvirus infections and ribavirin for bunyaviral and arenaviral infections. The synthesis of human interferon by means of DNA recombinant technology and of human antibodies by means of hybridoma technology will open new avenues for the treatment and prevention of viral infections.

RELEVANCE IN THE TROPICS. A limited number of viral diseases are described in this part. The overall basis for inclusion is relevance to tropical medicine, because of either (1) geographic restriction of the disease or high incidence in tropical regions or (2) recognition of clinical manifestations or epidemiologic features of a disease that are peculiar to the tropics. To

TABLE II–1. Some Major Characteristics of Viruses Responsible for Clinical Disease in the Tropics

	Family	Genus	Examples	Nucleic Acid	Presence of Envelope	Morphology	Diameter (nm)
Immunodeficiency Infections (Chapter 15.1)	Retroviridae	Lentivirus	HIV-1 HIV-2	RNA, single strand	+	Spherical	100–120
Leukemia Infections (Chapters 15.2 and 15.3)	Retroviridae	Oncovirus	HTLV-I	RNA, single strand	+	Spherical	100–120
Infections with Cutaneous Lesions (Chapter 16)	Paramyxoviridae	Morbillivirus	Measles	RNA, single strand	+	Roughly spherical	125–250
	Poxviridae	Orthopoxvirus	Variola Vaccinia Monkeypox	DNA, double strand	+	Brick or ovoid shape	200–250 250–350
Respiratory Infections (Chapter 17)	Orthomyxo-viridae	Influenzavirus	Influenza	RNA, single strand	+	Roughly spherical	80–120
Enteroviral Infections (Chapter 18)	Picornaviridae	Enterovirus	Poliovirus Coxsackievirus Echovirus Enterovirus 70 Hepatitis A	RNA, single strand	–		22–30
	Reoviridae	Rotavirus	Rotavirus	RNA, double strand, segmented	–	Spherical	70
	Hepadnaviridae (Chapter 19)		Hepatitis B	DNA, double strand	+	Spherical (Dane particle)	42
Febrile Illnesses (Chapter 20)	Togaviridae	Alphavirus	Chikungunya O'nyong nyong Sindbis	RNA, single strand	+	Spherical	45–75
	Flaviviridae	Flavivirus	West Nile fever Dengue	RNA, single strand	+	Spherical	37–50
	Bunyaviridae	Bunyavirus	Bunyamwera Group C viruses Oropouche	RNA, single strand, segmented	+	Spherical	90–100
		Phlebovirus	Sandfly fever viruses	RNA, single strand, segmented	+	Spherical	90–100
	Reoviridae	Orbivirus	Orungo	RNA, double strand, segmented	–	Spherical	70
	Rhabdoviridae	Vesiculovirus	Vesicular stomatitis	RNA, double strand, segmented	+	Bullet-shaped	75 × 185
Encephalitides (Chapter 21)	Rhabdoviridae	Lyssavirus	Rabies Mokola Duvenhage	RNA, double strand, segmented	+	Bullet-shaped	75 × 185
	Togaviridae	Alphavirus	Venezuelan equine encephalitis	RNA, single strand	+	Spherical	45 × 75
	Flaviviridae	Flavivirus	Japanese encephalitis Rocio	RNA, single strand	+	Spherical	37–50
Hemorrhagic Fevers (Chapter 22)	Flaviviridae	Flavivirus	Yellow fever	RNA, single strand	+	Spherical	37–50
	Bunyaviridae	Nairovirus	Crimean-Congo hemorrhagic fever	RNA, single strand, segmented	+	Spherical	90–100
	Arenaviridae	Arenavirus	Lassa Machupo Junin	RNA, single strand, segmented	+	Spherical or pleomorphic	110–130
	Filoviridae	Filovirus	Marburg Ebola	RNA, single strand	+	Bizarre, rod-shaped	75–80 × 130–4000

be most useful to the clinician, diseases are arranged by the predominant syndrome or organ system affected. This arrangement presents certain problems, since many viruses produce two or more syndromes or significant disease in two or more organ systems, but it is widely used in other texts and will be familiar to the practitioner.

The principal importance of most viral diseases included in this part lies in their capacity to spread in epidemic form, by means of direct interhuman transmission; vehicles, e.g., water; or arthropod vectors. In terms of human suffering and economic losses, the devastating effects of epidemics of measles, dengue, viral hemorrhagic fever, and other viral diseases have been repeatedly illustrated. The physician involved in primary clinical care usually provides the first line of defense, since clinical suspicion or diagnosis of individual patients with these diseases in the community may lead to public health intervention and containment of an outbreak. It is expected that, by providing a source of up-to-date, readily accessible knowledge about transmissible viral infections, the bridge between clinical and preventive medicine will be broadened.

The most important development in medicine and virology since the publication of the last edition is the emergence of acquired immunodeficiency disease syndrome (AIDS) as a global pandemic, having its greatest impact on populations in tropical areas, especially Central Africa. The causative agents, the human immunodeficiency viruses HIV-1 and HIV-2, are estimated to have infected 10 million people worldwide (Chapter 15.1). The unique tropism for T lymphocytes and macrophages, with eventual destruction of the infected host's immune functions, results in a mortality rate exceeding 85% due to opportunistic infections and various cancers. The insidious nature of the disease, with its prolonged incubation period during which infected individuals unwittingly spread the virus by various means, has assured a rapid expansion of the pandemic. The pattern of spread of HIV in tropical areas differs from that in North America and Europe. In the tropics, transmission is principally by heterosexual contact and from infected mother to infant, with important ancillary spread by uncontrolled blood transfusion, reused needles and syringes, and ritual scarification. In addition to its medical importance, AIDS creates enormous political, social, and economic problems for countries in the developing world.

Another human retrovirus, human T-cell leukemia virus (HTLV-I), was first associated with a relatively rare adult T-cell leukemia in Japan and subsequently with an encephalomyelopathy (tropical spastic paraparesis). Although the full spectrum of disease associated with this agent and its mode(s) of spread remains uncertain, it is clear that latent infection is widespread and highly prevalent among healthy populations in the tropics.

KURU

DEFINITION. Kuru is a fatal, slowly progressive, transmissible spongiform encephalopathy of primitive New Guinean tribesmen.

ETIOLOGY AND HISTORY. Kuru was first studied by Gajdusek and Zigas in 1956. The name means trembling or shivering in the language of the Fore tribe of New Guinea and refers to a major clinical feature of the disease. In 1959, similarities were shown between the pathologic changes of Kuru and scrapie, a transmis-

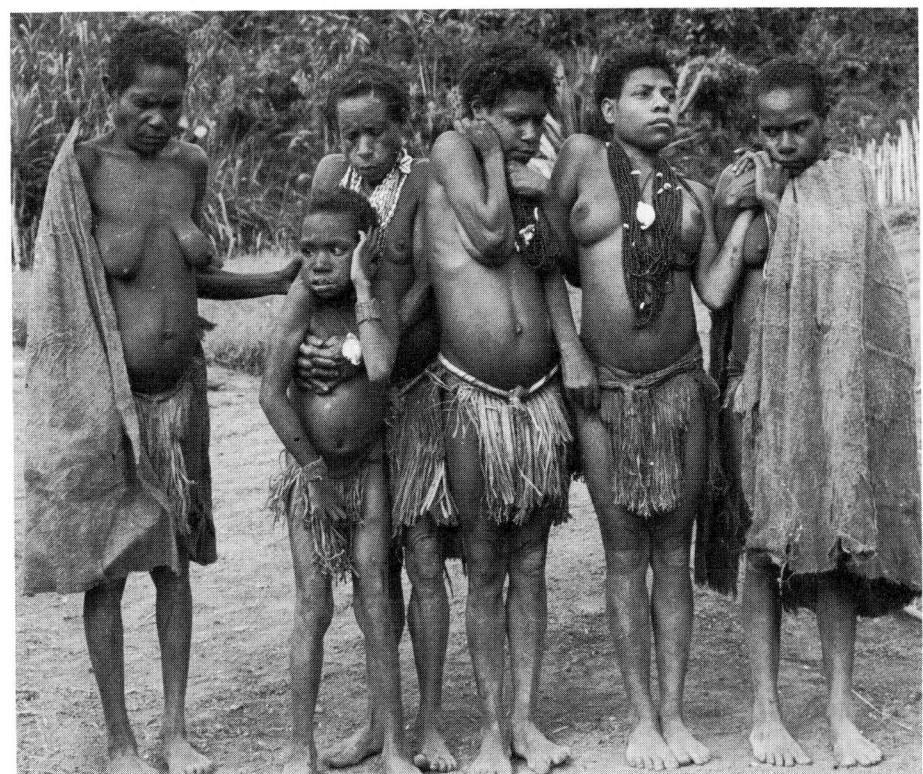

FIGURE II–1. Six kuru patients from one village in the South Fore. Their postural instability may be seen from the activity of muscle groups in their legs and feet. To maintain their posture and also damp down involuntary movements, their arms are held closely and firmly against each other. The girl shows a left convergent strabismus. (Courtesy of Dr. Carleton Gajdusek, National Institutes of Health, and Am J Med 26:447, 1959.)

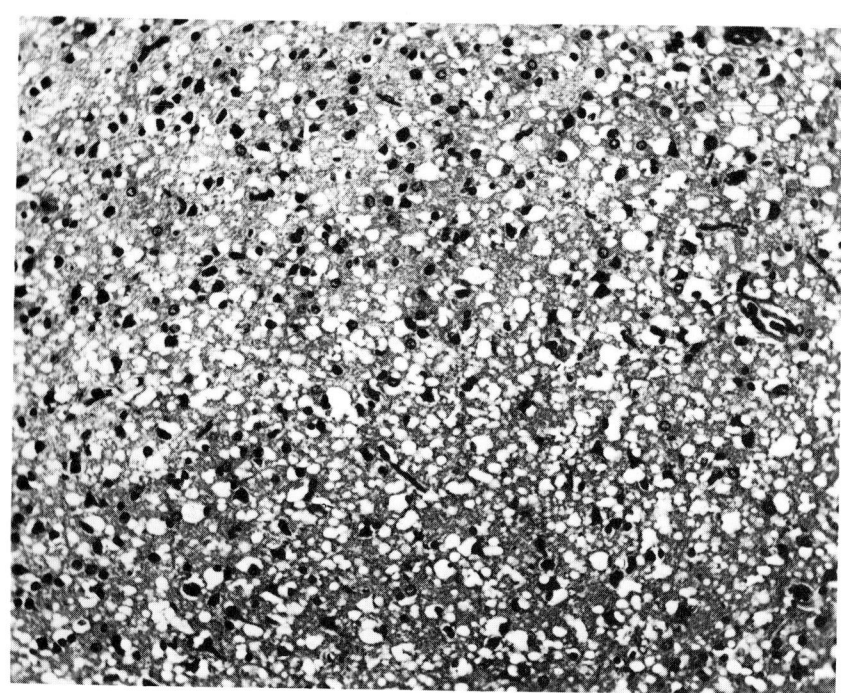

FIGURE II–2. Basal ganglion showing diffuse spongiform changes in patients dying of kuru (× 180). (Courtesy of Armed Forces Institute of Pathology, Photograph Neg. No. 71-5785.)

sible disease of sheep; this observation led to the successful transmission of kuru to chimpanzees inoculated intracerebrally with affected human brain tissue. A long incubation period (at least 18 months) characterized these experiments.

The etiologic agent, presumed to be a virus or viruslike organism, is of extremely small size and is highly resistant to inactivation by 80 C heat, ultraviolet light, ionizing radiation, and many disinfectants, including formaldehyde and beta-propiolactone; however, hypochlorite, iodide, and phenolic disinfectants; autoclaving; and potassium permanganate are effective in inactivation. Nucleases do not affect transmissibility, and the agent appears to lack demonstrable nucleic acid. Kuru shares many characteristics with other spongiform encephalopathies, including Creutzfeldt-Jakob disease, scrapie, and transmissible mink encephalopathy.

DISTRIBUTION, PREVALENCE, TRANSMISSION, AND EPIDEMIOLOGY. The disease occurs among the Fore cultural group in the highlands of eastern New Guinea. In the 1950s kuru accounted for nearly 50% of deaths (over 200/year) in the Fore tribe. Children and adult females were principally affected (Fig. II–1). Study of the disease led to the conclusion that transmission occurred during the practice of ritual cannibalism, probably by self-inoculation of infective tissues through skin abrasions or mucosae. Experimental studies have excluded oral ingestion as a mode of infection, and the disease is not contagious. Infected brain tissues contain up to 10^8 LD_{50} organisms/gm. Since

1960 cannibalistic practices have been gradually discontinued, resulting in disappearance of new cases.

PATHOLOGY AND PATHOGENESIS. Brains show spongiform changes due to vacuolation of astroglial and neuronal cell processes (Fig. II–2), diffuse neuronal degeneration and proliferation of glial elements, and absence of inflammatory cells. Lesions are most intense in the cerebellum.

CLINICAL MANIFESTATIONS. The incubation period is prolonged, up to 20 years. Onset is gradual, with shivering tremor of the trunk, head, and limbs; cerebellar ataxia; dysarthria; dysphagia; and progressive cachexia and debilitation leading to death, usually within 3 to 9 months. Dementia is not a prominent feature.

PROGNOSIS AND TREATMENT. The disease is progressive and fatal. No specific therapy is known.

DIAGNOSIS AND PREVENTION. Diagnosis is by clinical features, the restricted geographic and racial distribution, and histopathology. Since the Fore people have abandoned cannibalistic practices, kuru has now been effectively eliminated among tribal members.

BIBLIOGRAPHY

Gajdusek DC: Unconventional viruses and the origin and disappearance of Kuru. Science 197:943, 1977.
Gajdusek DC, Zigas V: Kuru: Clinical, pathological and epidemiological study of an acute progressive degenerative disease of the central nervous system among natives of the Eastern Highlands in New Guinea. Am J Med 26:442, 1957.

15. HUMAN IMMUNODEFICIENCY AND LEUKEMIA VIRUS INFECTIONS

15.1. HUMAN IMMUNODEFICIENCY VIRUS INFECTION AND AIDS

Kevin M. De Cock
and Robert L. Colebunders

Human immunodeficiency virus (HIV) infection causes progressive impairment of cellular immunity and is associated with a wide spectrum of disease manifestations. The acquired immunodeficiency syndrome (AIDS) is the most advanced stage of this infection and is characterized by severe immunodeficiency and the presence of opportunistic infections or malignancies. Most developed countries have adopted the revised Centers for Disease Control (CDC) surveillance case definition for AIDS (Table 15–1). Many of the criteria in the CDC case definition are impractical for use in the developing world for lack of diagnostic facilities. The World Health Organization (WHO) has therefore proposed a clinical case definition of AIDS for use in Africa (Table 15–2).

Two retroviruses, human immunodeficiency virus type 1 (HIV-1) and human immunodeficiency virus type 2 (HIV-2) cause infection and AIDS in humans.

HISTORY. Since its recognition in 1981 in homosexual men in the United States, AIDS has rapidly emerged as a problem of global public health importance. Consideration of HIV infection in a textbook of tropical medicine is justified by the international distribution of the infection, the high burden of disease in certain developing countries, the regional variations in disease expression, the potential for interaction with certain endemic tropical diseases, and the broad implications that AIDS holds for health and development in the tropics.

In June 1981, CDC published a report of pneumonia due to *Pneumocystis carinii* in several previously healthy homosexual men in Los Angeles. Shortly thereafter, Kaposi's sarcoma was described in a group of homosexual men in New York, some of whom were also suffering from *Pneumocystis* pneumonia. Subsequent surveillance for this new syndrome revealed cases in other groups, including intravenous drug users, persons with hemophilia, blood transfusion recipients, recent immigrants into the United States from Haiti, and the heterosexual partners and children of those at risk for AIDS. The clinical manifestations were more diverse than those described in the first reports and included other unusual infections and tumors, but fundamental to these clinical manifestations was profound cellular immunodeficiency without obvious explanation.

As awareness of this new syndrome increased, clinicians frequently reported other, lesser manifestations of altered immunity in persons at risk for AIDS. These were collectively referred to as AIDS-related complex (ARC) and included fevers and sweats, weight loss, generalized lymphadenopathy, and autoimmune thrombocytopenia. These epidemiologic and clinical observations suggested that (1) AIDS was the end stage of an infection whose epidemiology in the United States was reminiscent of that of hepatitis B, and (2) for every overt case of AIDS there were probably numerous mild or subclinical infections.

In 1983 and 1984, respectively, workers at the Institut Pasteur (Paris) and at the National Cancer Institute (Washington) isolated the retrovirus that was identified as the causative agent of AIDS. The term HIV now replaces earlier names for the AIDS virus, such as lymphadenopathy-associated virus (LAV), human T-lymphotropic virus type III (HTLV-III), and AIDS-associated retrovirus (ARV). A serologic test for antibody to this virus, essential for the screening of blood for transfusion, became widely available in 1985.

After AIDS was recognized in the United States, cases affecting the same risk groups began to be recognized in other parts of the world, particularly Western Europe. In the early 1980s, cases of AIDS were identified in Africans seeking medical care in Europe; these patients lacked the previously identified risk factors. Investigations demonstrated that an epidemic of AIDS in heterosexuals was occurring in parts of Central Africa. Retrospectively, the emergence of the epidemic was demonstrated by increasing numbers of cases of certain indicator diseases in various locations from the mid-1970s onward, and by the testing of stored serum (Table 15–3).

In 1986 French workers discovered another human retrovirus, now called HIV-2, in persons with AIDS who were serologically negative for HIV-1. The initial cases described were from Guinea Bissau and Cape Verde Islands, but this infection has since been recognized in several other West African countries. Isolated cases have also been described in Europe and North America.

ETIOLOGY.

Classification. Two distinct retroviruses, HIV-1 and HIV-2, cause HIV infection in humans. The fundamental property of retroviruses is the possession of the enzyme reverse transcriptase. Within the retrovirus family, the HIVs are classified as lentiviruses, a group of agents that includes visna, which causes degenerative neurologic disease in sheep. A number of retroviruses closely related to HIV have been isolated from various species of monkeys, including macaques, mangabeys, and African green monkeys. Collectively these agents are referred to as simian immunodeficiency virus (SIV). Macaques and mangabeys have developed an illness resembling human AIDS (simian immunodeficiency syndrome, SIAIDS) following infection with SIV.

Early published work suggested the occurrence in West Africa of two human viruses distinct from HIV-1, referred to as lymphadenopathy-associated virus type II (LAV-II), and human T-lymphotropic virus type IV (HTLV-IV). It is now accepted that HTLV-IV is not a distinct human virus, the isolation of this agent having been the result of laboratory contamination with SIV. The isolate LAV-II is now called HIV-2; HIV-1 and

TABLE 15–1. CDC 1987 Revision of Case Definition for AIDS for Surveillance Purposes

For national reporting, a case of AIDS is defined as an illness characterized by one or more of the following "indicator" diseases, depending on the status of laboratory evidence of HIV infection, as shown below.

I. **Without Laboratory Evidence Regarding HIV Infection**

If laboratory tests for HIV were not performed or gave inconclusive results and the patient had no other cause of immunodeficiency listed in Section I.A below, then any disease listed in Section I.B indicates AIDS if it was diagnosed by a definitive method.

A. **Causes of immunodeficiency that disqualify diseases as indicators of AIDS in the absence of laboratory evidence for HIV infection**

1. high-dose or long-term systemic corticosteroid therapy or other immunosuppressive/cytotoxic therapy ≤3 months before the onset of the indicator disease

2. any of the following diseases diagnosed ≤3 months after diagnosis of the indicator disease: Hodgkin's disease, non-Hodgkin's lymphoma (other than primary brain lymphoma), lymphocytic leukemia, multiple myeloma, any other cancer of lymphoreticular or histiocytic tissue, or angioimmunoblastic lymphadenopathy

3. a genetic (congenital) immunodeficiency syndrome or an acquired immunodeficiency syndrome atypical of HIV infection, such as one involving hypogammaglobulinemia

B. **Indicator diseases diagnosed definitively**

1. candidiasis of the esophagus, trachea, bronchi, or lungs
2. cryptococcosis, extrapulmonary
3. cryptosporidiosis with diarrhea persisting >1 month
4. cytomegalovirus disease of an organ other than liver, spleen, or lymph nodes in a patient >1 month of age
5. herpes simplex virus infection causing a mucocutaneous ulcer that persists longer than 1 month; or bronchitis, pneumonitis, or esophagitis for any duration affecting a patient >1 month of age
6. Kaposi's sarcoma affecting a patient <60 years of age
7. lymphoma of the brain (primary) affecting a patient <60 years of age
8. lymphoid interstitial pneumonia and/or pulmonary lymphoid hyperplasia (LIP/PLH complex) affecting a child <13 years of age
9. *Mycobacterium avium* complex or *M. kansasii* disease, disseminated (at a site other than or in addition to lungs, skin, or cervical or hilar lymph nodes)
10. *Pneumocystis carinii* pneumonia
11. progressive multifocal leukoencephalopathy
12. toxoplasmosis of the brain affecting a patient >1 month of age

II. **With Laboratory Evidence for HIV Infection**

Regardless of the presence of other causes of immunodeficiency (I.A), in the presence of laboratory evidence for HIV infection, any disease listed above (I.B) or below (II.A or II.B) indicates a diagnosis of AIDS.

A. **Indicator diseases diagnosed definitively**

1. bacterial infections, multiple or recurrent (any combination of at least two within a 2-year period), of the following types affecting a child <13 years of age:

septicemia, pneumonia, meningitis, bone or joint infection, or abscess of an internal organ or body cavity (excluding otitis media or superficial skin or mucosal abscesses), caused by *Haemophilus, Streptococcus* (including pneumococcus), or other pyogenic bacteria

2. coccidioidomycosis, disseminated (at a site other than or in addition to lungs or cervical or hilar lymph nodes)

3. HIV encephalopathy (also called "HIV dementia," "AIDS dementia," or "subacute encephalitis due to HIV")

4. histoplasmosis, disseminated (at a site other than or in addition to lungs or cervical or hilar lymph nodes)
5. isosporiasis with diarrhea persisting >1 month
6. Kaposi's sarcoma at any age
7. lymphoma of the brain (primary) at any age
8. other non-Hodgkin's lymphoma of B-cell or unknown immunologic phenotype and the following histologic types:
   a. small noncleaved lymphoma (either Burkitt or non-Burkitt type)
   b. immunoblastic sarcoma (equivalent to any of the following, although not necessarily all in combination: immunoblastic lymphoma, large-cell lymphoma, diffuse histiocytic lymphoma, diffuse undifferentiated lymphoma, or high-grade lymphoma)

Note: Lymphomas are not included here if they are of T-cell immunologic phenotype or their histologic type is not described or is described as "lymphocytic," "lymphoblastic," "small cleaved," or "plasmacytoid lymphocytic"

9. any mycobacterial disease caused by mycobacteria other than *M. tuberculosis,* disseminated (at a site other than or in addition to lungs, skin, or cervical or hilar lymph nodes)
10. disease caused by *M. tuberculosis,* extrapulmonary (involving at least one site outside the lungs, regardless of whether there is concurrent pulmonary involvement)
11. *Salmonella* (nontyphoid) septicemia, recurrent
12. HIV wasting syndrome (emaciation, "slim disease")

B. **Indicator diseases diagnosed presumptively**

Note: Given the seriousness of diseases indicative of AIDS, it is generally important to diagnose them definitively, especially when therapy that would be used may have serious side effects or when definitive diagnosis is needed for eligibility for antiretroviral therapy. Nonetheless, in some situations, a patient's condition will not permit the performance of definitive tests. In other situations, accepted clinical practice may be to diagnose presumptively based on the presence of characteristic clinical and laboratory abnormalities.

1. candidiasis of the esophagus
2. cytomegalovirus retinitis with loss of vision
3. Kaposi's sarcoma
4. lymphoid interstitial pneumonia and/or pulmonary lymphoid hyperplasia (LIP/PLH complex) affecting a child <13 years of age
5. mycobacterial disease (acid-fast bacilli with species not identified by culture), disseminated (involving at least one site other than or in addition to lungs, skin, or cervical or hilar lymph nodes)
6. *Pneumocystis carinii* pneumonia
7. toxoplasmosis of the brain affecting a patient >1 month of age

III. **With Laboratory Evidence Against HIV Infection**

With laboratory test results negative for HIV infection, a diagnosis of AIDS for surveillance purposes is ruled out *unless:*

A. all the other causes of immunodeficiency listed above in Section I.A are excluded; **AND**

B. the patient has had either:

1. *Pneumocystis carinii* pneumonia diagnosed by a definitive method, **OR**

2. a. any of the other diseases indicative of AIDS listed above in Section I.B diagnosed by a definitive method, **AND**

   b. a T-helper/inducer (CD4) lymphocyte count <400/mm^3.

From CDC: Revision of the CDC surveillance case definition for acquired immunodeficiency syndrome. MMWR 36:1-15S, 1987.

TABLE 15–2. World Health Organization Clinical Case Definition of AIDS for Use in Africa

AIDS in an adult is defined by the existence of at least two major signs associated with at least one minor sign, in the absence of known causes of immunosuppression such as cancer or severe malnutrition or other recognized etiologies.

Major Signs
Weight loss >10% body weight
Chronic diarrhea >1 month
Prolonged fever >1 month (intermittent or constant)

Minor Signs
Persistent cough >1 month
Generalized pruritic dermatitis
Recurrent herpes zoster
Oropharyngeal candidiasis
Chronic progressive and disseminated herpes simplex infection
Generalized lymphadenopathy

The presence of Kaposi's sarcoma or cryptococcal meningitis is in itself sufficient for the diagnosis of AIDS.

From WHO: Acquired immunodeficiency syndrome (AIDS). Workshop on AIDS in Central Africa, Bangui, 22–25 October 1985. Wkly Epidemiol Rec 60:342, 1985; and Colebunders RL, Francis H, Izaley L, et al: Evaluation of a clinical case definition of acquired immunodeficiency syndrome in Africa. Lancet 1:492–494, 1987.

HIV-2 are the only lentiviruses currently known to infect humans. The possibility that other human retroviruses are circulating, particularly in Africa, and are capable of causing disease requires study.

Genomic Organization

HIV-1. All retroviruses share similar major structural genes *gag, pol,* and *env,* but in addition, HIV-1 contains a number of regulatory genes, making a total of at least 8 identifiable genes. As is common among retroviruses, the termini of the HIV genome are flanked by repetitive sequences called long terminal repeats (LTRs), which are involved in integration and expression of the HIV proviral genome (the DNA copy of the retroviral RNA transcribed using the reverse transcriptase).

The major structural genes *gag, pol,* and *env* code, respectively, for the viral core proteins (*gag*); the reverse transcriptase, protease, and endonuclease (*pol*); and the surface glycoproteins (*env*). The protein products of these major genes are of diagnostic importance, since they elicit antibody responses recognized by Western

TABLE 15–3. Historical Aspects of HIV Infection and AIDS

Year	Event
1959	Collection of a serum sample in Zaire subsequently shown to be positive for HIV-1.
1969	Possible AIDS case in the United States.
1970	HIV seroprevalence of 0.1% (shown on retrospective testing of stored sera) among pregnant women in Kinshasa.
1976	HIV seroprevalence of 0.8% (shown on retrospective testing of stored sera) among villagers in Equateur Province of Zaire. HIV-1 isolated from one stored serum specimen in 1986.
1975–1980	Cases suggestive of AIDS in Central Africa and the United States.
1981	Recognition of *Pneumocystis carinii* pneumonia and Kaposi's sarcoma in American homosexuals.
1983	Isolation of HIV-1.
1985	Licensure of ELISA for HIV testing.
1986	Isolation of HIV-2.

blot analysis (Fig. 15–1; see below). The *gag* gene encodes for a 55 kd protein (p55) that is broken down enzymatically into p24, p18, and p15. *Env* codes for a heavily glycosylated precursor, gp160, which is cleaved by a kinase to form gp120 (the protein giving the virus its spiked surface) and gp41 (the transmembrane glycoprotein). Several other genes exist having regulatory functions that have been characterized to varying degrees. These include *tat,* controlling the level of other viral gene expression by regulating production of a protein messenger; *rev* (previously called *art,* or *trs*), enhancing viral structural protein synthesis by transactivation; *nef* (previously called 3 *orf*), acting to downregulate viral replication; *vif* (previously called *sor*), of uncertain function but perhaps one related to viral transmission; and *VPR* (previously called R) and VPU, whose function also is unknown. The *tat* and *rev* genes appear to be essential for virus replication.

HIV-2. The genomic organization of HIV-2 is considered the same as for HIV-1, but with an additional central open reading frame, VPX, whose function is not known. HIV-2 does not contain the VPU gene. In terms of sequence homology, HIV-1 and HIV-2 are approximately 40% homologous, with the most highly variable regions occurring within the *env* genes. HIV-2 is more closely related to SIVmac, with which it is 80% homologous. The variability in the envelope between HIV-1 and HIV-2 is of practical importance, since it may result in diagnostic tests for HIV-1 infection without recognizing infection due to HIV-2; it is also of theoretical importance for future vaccine development, since type-specific vaccines may be too specific to prevent all HIV infections.

DISTRIBUTION. By 30 November 1988, AIDS had been reported to WHO from 142 countries or territories, for a global total of 129,385 cases. The distribution of cases by region was as follows: Africa, 13.4%; the Americas, 72.4%; Asia, 0.2%; Europe, 13.1%; and Oceania, 0.9%. For various reasons, these global surveillance data underestimate the actual number of cases, which is likely to be in excess of 275,000. The data are more useful as an indicator of the countries where the disease has occurred than they are of the number of cases.

In considering the international distribution of AIDS, a useful model has been to categorize the world into 3 broad patterns. The first comprises countries having *well-defined risk groups.* Heterosexual and perinatal transmissions may occur and are increasing in some countries but are not the dominant mode of spread. Overall, HIV infection rates are low in the general population—usually well under 1%. Since most countries in this category are economically developed, screening of blood for transfusion generally was introduced early, and blood transfusion is no longer a significant route of infection. Examples of countries in this category are the United States and Canada, most countries in Western Europe, and some in South America. In Western Europe and North America, the highest rates of HIV infection are found in homosexual men, intravenous drug users, and persons with hemophilia (Table 15–4). Variable rates are found in female pros-

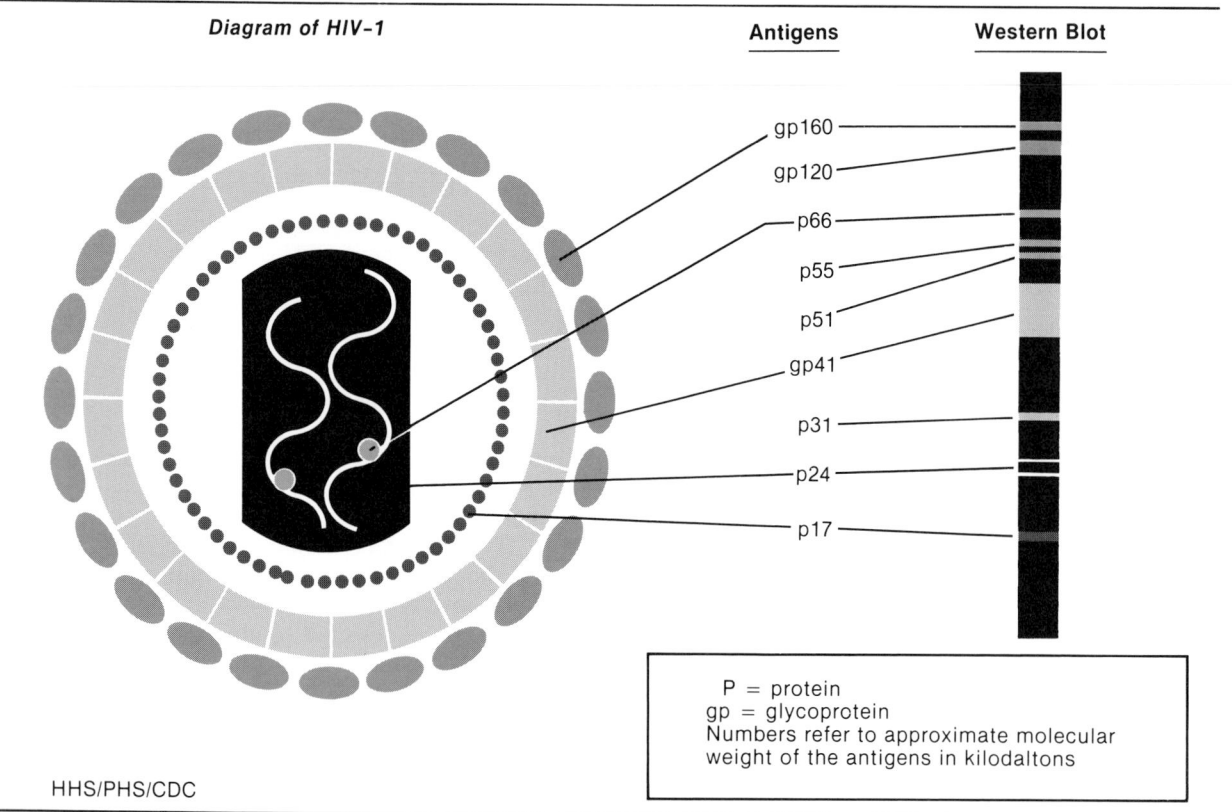

FIGURE 15–1. Schematic representation of HIV-1. The virus consists of an outer envelope and an inner core containing the genetic material. Viral protein products coded for by individual genes elicit specific antibody responses in the infected host, which can be demonstrated on Western blot (see text). Envelope proteins are gp160, gp120, and gp41, coded for by the *env* gene; *gag* gene products are the core proteins p55, p24, and p17. The reverse transcriptase and endonuclease proteins, coded for by the *pol* gene, are p66 and p31.

titutes, the highest infection rates in the latter occurring among those who also inject intravenous drugs.

The second category includes countries *with extensive heterosexual transmission*. Most nations in this group have fragile economies, and lack the infrastructure to guarantee universal screening of blood for transfusion or to undertake widespread intervention. Disease surveillance tends to be poor, and accurate data on numbers of cases are limited. Because heterosexual transmission is the dominant mode of spread and women have many children, pediatric AIDS is a rapidly emerging problem. Countries in this category are in the Caribbean and sub-Saharan Africa.

HIV infection rates in the general population of capital cities in Central and East Africa range from about 2% to 25%, the highest figures being reported in the sexually active age groups. Infection rates are lower in West Africa, but rates similar to those found in some cities of East and Central Africa are beginning to be reported from certain West African cities. Among the countries for which data are available, Cape Verde Islands, Guinea Bissau, and Senegal have the highest HIV-2 infection rates. Although the modes of spread of HIV-2 have been less intensively studied, these would be expected to be the same as for HIV-1. For instance, the highest rates of infection have been reported among female prostitutes.

The third category comprises countries with *little or no HIV transmission*. They are currently in Eastern Europe, the Middle East, North Africa, and Asia. When cases do occur, they are most often imported infections or the result of transmission from contact with persons from outside. These countries vary in their economic development. They have the opportunity to undertake preventive action before they face an epidemic of HIV infection. When it does occur, AIDS may be in either heterosexual or homosexual persons, depending on the relevant high-risk behavior.

Within some countries, more than one epidemiologic pattern may be present, and patterns may be changing. Thus, in certain cities of the United States, especially in underprivileged areas, the epidemiology of HIV infection may share some features with the African situation. In some countries with little or no HIV transmission, the situation may change rapidly. In Bangkok, Thailand, for example, HIV infection has spread rapidly in a group of intravenous drug users. These observations show that the epidemic of HIV infection is a mosaic of microepidemics, each with its different epidemiologic characteristics, all contributing to the global epidemic of AIDS.

EPIDEMIOLOGY

Transmission. HIV infection is transmitted sexually, through contact with blood, and perinatally from mother to offspring. The epidemiology of hepatitis B virus in the developed world has provided a useful model for studying the spread of HIV. However, hepatitis B is considerably more infectious, and unlike hepatitis B, HIV is not spread by close personal contact within

TABLE 15–4. HIV Antibody Prevalence in Selected Populations in Developing and Developed Countries

Type of Population	Country: City	Year	No. Tested	Percentage HIV-1 (+)	Percentage HIV-2 (+)
General population	Cameroon	1986	1273	1	
	Central African Republic: Bangui	1986	1263	4	
	Zaire: Kinshasa	1987	9640	3	
Hospital staff	Rwanda: Kigali	1984	150	19	
	Zaire: Kinshasa	1987	1938	7	
Blood donors	Rwanda: Kigali	1984	180	18	
	Senegal	1987–88	4194	0.02	0.6
	Zambia: Lusaka	1986	207	18	
	Zaire: Kinshasa	1987	8701	7.7	
	United States			0.01–0.07	
Pregnant women	Ivory Coast: Abidjan	1987	311	3	
	Uganda: Kampala	1986	1011	14	
	Zaire: Kinshasa	1987	6000	5.6	
	Kenya: Nairobi	1987	2265	2.7	
	United States: Massachussets,	1986–87	30708	0.2	
	New York (Bronx)	1987	820	2.4	
Prostitutes	Cameroon: Meiganga	1986	221	8	
	Kenya: Nairobi	1987	286	61	
	Zaire: Kinshasa	1985	377	27	
	Senegal	1988	1165	0.9	10.8
Homosexual men	United States: San Francisco	1987	6680	70	
	Italy: Milan	1988	2657	22	
	Argentina: Buenos Aires	1987	348	60	
Intravenous drug users	United States: New York (Brooklyn)	1985	553	54	
	Italy: Palermo	1988	684	68	
	Thailand: Bangkok	1988		16	
Persons with hemophilia	United States: 10 treatment centers	1986	541	75	
	Brazil: Rio de Janeiro	1987	213	94	

families or other closed groups without sexual or blood contact. The epidemiology of hepatitis B in Africa or Asia is not representative of that of HIV.

Sexual Transmission. HIV may result from heterosexual and homosexual intercourse; male-to-female transmission is perhaps more efficient than that from female to male. Among homosexual men, important risk factors are a greater number of sex partners and the practice of receptive anal intercourse. For heterosexuals, concomitant sexually transmitted diseases, particularly genital ulcers, are important factors enhancing acquisition and transmission of HIV. In Africa, sexual contact with prostitutes, and being a prostitute, are risk factors; female prostitutes constitute an important reservoir of HIV infection.

Transmission with Blood. HIV infection can result from contact with infected blood and blood products and from contaminated needles. The groups most heavily affected by these routes of infection have been persons with hemophilia, the recipients of blood transfusions, and intravenous drug users who share injection equipment. The transfusion of contaminated blood almost always results in HIV infection in the recipient, perhaps because this is invariably associated with transfer of a high virus load.

In the developing world, the use of unsterilized needles and other contaminated cutting or piercing instruments may be an important (although difficult to quantify) mode of spread. HIV infection has been accidentally transmitted in industrialized countries through needlesticks, but documented episodes of this nature have been rare. In the United States, the HIV transmission rate was only 0.42% in persons exposed percutaneously to HIV-contaminated blood in the context of health care work.

Perinatal Transmission. The exact timing of transmission is uncertain, although most infections probably occur in utero. Estimates of the likelihood of an infected mother transmitting the virus to her offspring range from about 25% to 50%. Individual case reports, most concerning women transfused in the postpartum period, suggest that HIV can be transmitted by breast milk, although the frequency is unclear. Isolated instances of HIV transmission through breast milk do not warrant altering public health policy on breast feeding in the developing world.

The documented rates of HIV transmission to the sex partners of infected persons, ranging from 9% in wives of persons with hemophilia in the United States to 52% of wives of AIDS patients in Zaire, may (at least in part) reflect increased infectivity of the index case as immunodeficiency progresses. This may also explain the different rates of perinatal transmission observed in different studies, immunosuppressed mothers apparently transmitting HIV infection to their children more efficiently. Observations in Zaire suggest that mothers with advanced AIDS are more likely to transmit HIV to their children than are other infected women. Progressive immunosuppression may lead to increased levels of viremia, with a resulting increase in infectivity to sex partners and to the fetus.

Transmission in Africa. In sub-Saharan Africa, heterosexual transmission is the driving force behind the epidemic of HIV infection. Although heterosexually transmitted cases are increasing in Western Europe and North America, the spread of HIV infection among heterosexuals has been slower and has frequently been concentrated among intravenous drug users and their sex partners. HIV infection in heterosexuals may have been introduced earlier in Africa than in industrialized countries. Greater numbers of sex partners, more contact with female prostitutes, a higher background rate of other sexually transmitted diseases (particularly genital ulcers), and biologic differences, e.g., exposure to other infections activating the immune system, are suggested but unproven causes of increased HIV transmission in Africa.

HIV infection is not transmitted through casual contact or through routes other than those mentioned previously. Transmission by insect vectors has not been documented and is excluded as a significant means of spread by epidemiologic evidence; age-specific infection and disease rates, with the sexually active age groups most affected, are quite unlike those of vector-borne infections such as malaria.

Prevalence of Infection with HIV

Western Europe and North America. The highest rates of HIV infection are found in homosexual men, intravenous drug users, and persons with hemophilia (Table 15–4). Variable rates are found in female prostitutes, the highest occurring in those who also inject intravenous drugs. As discussed earlier, rates of infection in heterosexual partners of HIV-infected persons vary, perhaps in part with the immune status of the index case.

Africa. HIV-1 infection rates in the general population of capital cities in Central and East Africa range from about 2% to 25%, the highest figures being reported in the sexually active age groups. Rates are highest in female prostitutes, one study in East Africa having documented HIV infection in 88% of a cohort of lower socioeconomic class prostitutes. Infection rates are lower in West Africa, but higher rates are beginning to be reported from certain cities there as well.

HIV-2 infection rates are reported to be highest in Cape Verde Islands, Guinea Bissau, and Senegal, although fewer systematic studies have been done than for HIV-1 infection. The highest rates of infection have been reported among female prostitutes. Isolated cases of HIV-2 infection have been found outside of West Africa, either in persons previously resident there or in those sexually exposed to such persons.

PATHOGENESIS. HIV has been demonstrated by virus culture or detection of reverse transcriptase in

whole blood, plasma, semen, vaginal fluids, urine, cerebrospinal fluid, saliva, tears, breast milk, lymph nodes, bone marrow, brain, and lung tissue. Epidemiologic evidence, however, suggests that blood, blood products, semen, and vaginal or cervical fluids are the most important sources of HIV in the transmission of infection.

Cellular Infection. It is uncertain whether infection usually results from entry into the host of cell-free or cell-associated virus, or both. The HIV envelope glycoprotein, gp120, binds specifically to the CD4 receptor that is found on the surface of a subset of T lymphocytes and some other members of the macrophage-monocyte cell line. After entry into the cell, a double-stranded DNA copy is made from the viral RNA using the viral reverse transcriptase, and this DNA copy becomes integrated into the host genome. The infection may remain quiescent in this fashion for a long period, the factors that determine virus expression being poorly understood. Infection of macrophages, including infection of glial cells in the central nervous system, may provide an important mechanism for long-term persistence of infection. Transcription of viral RNA off the proviral template by the host cell RNA transcriptase appears to be regulated in part by elements of the viral LTRs. In vitro studies suggest that lymphocyte activation, as by infectious stimuli and specific cytokines, enhances viral gene expression. Appearance of further infectious virus follows by budding from the host cell (Fig. 15–2).

Immunodeficiency. The fundamental pathologic defect in AIDS is collapse of the immune system, to which depletion of lymphocytes bearing the CD4 receptor appears to be central. The extraordinary degree of T4 lymphocyte depletion in AIDS is greatly out of proportion to the number of HIV-infected cells, raising questions concerning the pathogenesis of the disease. Suggested mechanisms of immunodeficiency include a direct cytopathic effect of the virus; formation of syncytia involving infected and noninfected lymphocytes; autoimmune reaction destroying both infected and normal cells; infection and early death of stem cells; and abnormalities of certain lymphokines that modulate immune function.

Natural History of HIV Infection. HIV antigen may appear transiently in the serum following acute infection, to reappear in some cases when immunosuppression is advanced. Seroconversion for antibody to HIV usually occurs within 6 to 12 weeks after infection, but in isolated instances has been delayed for many months. In advanced disease, HIV antibody levels may fall again.

AIDS Incubation Period. The period between the acquisition of HIV infection and the development of AIDS is widely variable. Estimation of mean or median incubation periods is difficult, because patients diagnosed thus far may have atypically short incubation periods compared with other infected, currently healthy persons. Estimated mean incubation periods are from 6 to 8 years for adults. The development of AIDS is much more rapid in infancy; many perinatally infected children become ill in the first year of life. Informative data have been gathered among homosexual men who participated in hepatitis B vaccination studies in San Francisco in the late 1970s. HIV testing of stored serum specimens linked

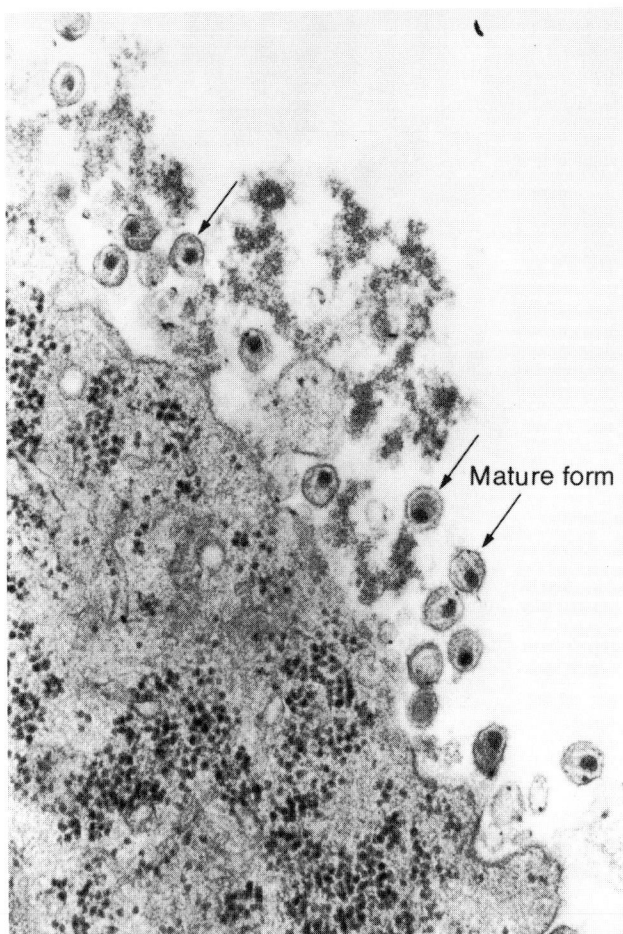

FIGURE 15–2. HIV particles. This electron micrograph shows mature virus particles budding off the surface of a lymphocyte.

with follow-up of these subjects has shown that 5% progressed to AIDS within 3 years of HIV infection, 10% within 4 years, 23% within 6 years, 37% within 8 years, and 48% within 10 years. Of those who do not have AIDS after this time, most have other manifestations of altered immunity; only about 15% remain completely healthy (but nevertheless infected) after 7 or 8 years of infection. The possibility that ultimately most or all HIV-infected persons will develop AIDS cannot be excluded.

There is no evidence that the natural history of HIV infection is different in the various adult risk groups. Longitudinal follow-up of asymptomatic HIV-infected persons in Kishasa, Zaire, showed progression to AIDS at a rate of 1.3/100 person years among healthy seropositive subjects, and progression to AIDS-related complex at a rate of 10.4/100 person years. The natural history of HIV infection does not appear to differ by geographic region, although outcome may vary depending on the availability of medical care.

Course of HIV-2 Infection. The data concerning natural history and disease progression quoted above relate to infection with HIV-1. Most workers believe that HIV-2 infection also causes AIDS, but its natural history may vary from that of HIV-1 infection. Definitive prospective studies on the natural history of HIV-2 infection are currently lacking.

CLINICAL MANIFESTATIONS. The spectrum of clinical manifestations associated with HIV infection ranges from the asymptomatic carrier state to fatal disease with opportunistic infections, malignancies, degenerative neurologic disease, and general inanition. Important geographic differences exist in disease presentation, which to some extent reflect variation in the frequency of opportunistic organisms in the environment but often remain unexplained, even when varying diagnostic facilities in hospitals are taken into account.

Classification Systems. Different classifications have been proposed for the spectrum of diseases associated with HIV; the most widely used are the ones proposed by CDC and by the Walter Reed Institute of Research (Tables 15–5 and 15–6). Their purpose is to facilitate communication concerning the spectrum of HIV disease.

Acute Retroviral Syndrome. Acute infection with HIV may cause a syndrome that resembles infectious mononucleosis, sometimes associated with an acute meningoencephalitis. This acute retroviral syndrome, which most often occurs 2 to 6 weeks after infection, has been recognized in the tropics as well as in the industrialized world and may sometimes allow retrospective determination of the timing of infection.

AIDS-Related Complex. After acute infection, a person remains asymptomatic for months or years. The symptoms of HIV infection that precede the development of AIDS have been grouped under the heading AIDs-related complex (ARC), a term less used than previously. Progressive immunodeficiency is most commonly heralded by weight loss, fever, night sweats, diarrhea, lymphadenopathy, prurigo, varicella zoster infection, and oral candidiasis. Less common findings are hairy leukoplakia in the mouth (asymptomatic whitish plaques on the side of the tongue that cannot be rubbed off), and idiopathic thrombocytopenic purpura. In women, amenorrhea is frequent.

AIDS, Slim Disease, and Diarrhea. Most AIDS patients have severe weight loss, which is generally progressive and may exceed 30% of total body weight. In Africa, gastrointestinal manifestations are particularly

TABLE 15–5. Classification System for Human Immunodeficiency Virus Infection

Group I	Acute infection
Group II	Asymptomatic infection*
Group III	Persistent generalized lymphadenopathy*
Group IV	Other disease
Subgroup A	Constitutional disease
Subgroup B	Neurologic disease
Subgroup C	Secondary infectious diseases
Category C-1	Specified secondary infectious diseases listed in the CDC surveillance definition AIDS†
Category C-2	Other specified secondary infectious diseases
Subgroup D	Secondary cancers†
Subgroup E	Other conditions

*Patients in Groups II and III may be subclassified on the basis of a laboratory evaluation (based on whether hematologic and/or immunologic laboratory studies have been done and whether results are abnormal in a manner consistent with the effects of HIV infection).

†Includes those patients whose clinical presentation fulfills the definition of AIDS used by CDC for national reporting.

From MMWR 35:334, 1986.

TABLE 15–6. The Walter Reed Staging Classification for HIV Infection

Stage	HIV Antibody and/or Virus	Chronic Lymphadenopathy	T-Helper Cells/mm	Delayed Hypersensitivity	Thrush	Opportunistic Infections
WR0	–	–	>400	NORMAL	–	–
WR1	+	–	>400	NORMAL	–	–
WR2	+	+	>400	NORMAL	–	–
WR3	+	+/–	<400	NORMAL	–	–
WR4	+	+/–	<400	P	–	–
WR5	+	+/–	<400	C AND/OR THRUSH		–
WR6	+	+/–	<400	P/C	+/–	+

The essential criteria for assignment to each stage are indicated by squares/rectangles.
P = Partial defect.
C = Complete defect.
From Redfield RR, Wright DC, Tramont EC: The Walter Reed staging classification for HTLV-III/LAV infection. N Engl J Med 314:131–132, 1986. Reprinted by permission.

frequent in AIDS patients. The most common such symptom is persistent diarrhea, observed in 40% to 80% of African AIDS patients. Profound weight loss and persistent diarrhea, often accompanied by chronic fever, have been referred to as enteropathic AIDS, or "slim," a vivid reference to the extreme weight loss (Fig. 15–3). The natural history of this disease is one of relentless weight loss, punctuated by chronic diarrhea that waxes and wanes. Other opportunistic complications may supervene, but many patients die literally from wasting, without an obvious specific infection.

Diarrhea in AIDS is frequently intermittent, watery or semiliquid, and without mucus or blood. Although careful parasitologic examination of the stool may show

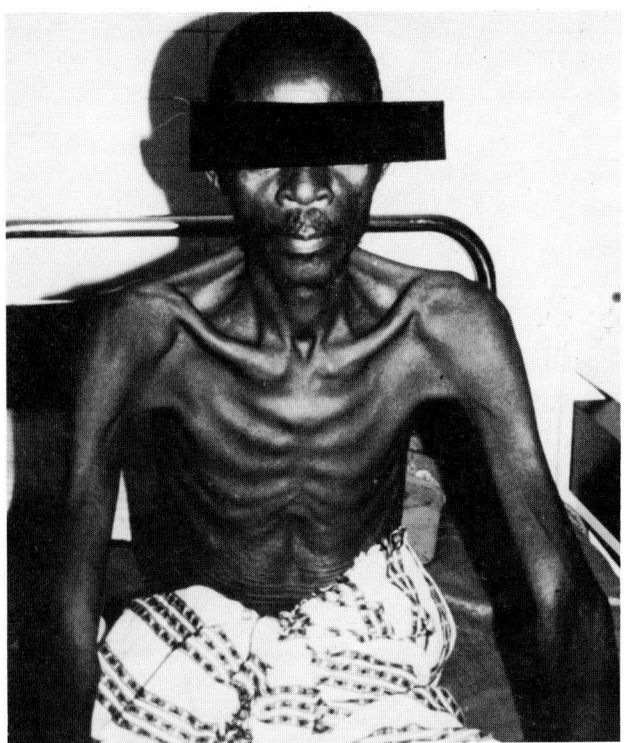

FIGURE 15–3. African AIDS: a patient with AIDS from the Ivory Coast. Profound weight loss, chronic diarrhea, fever, and oral candidiasis are the most common manifestations of AIDS in Africa. In Uganda, the term "slim" has been widely used to describe the disease. Weight loss exceeds that seen in almost all other diseases.

parasites in one quarter to one half of patients, most often the diarrhea remains unexplained. The most common pathogens identified are *Cryptosporidium* species, and *Isospora belli*. Cryptosporidiosis may cause secretory diarrhea, sometimes with life-threatening fluid loss.

Other Gastrointestinal Lesions. Oral candidiasis, hairy leukoplakia, acute necrotizing ulcerative gingivitis, and lesions of Kaposi's sarcoma are the most important oral manifestations in HIV-infected patients. In persons who do not have other immunosuppressive conditions and are not taking antibiotics, oral candidiasis is a strong predictor of HIV disease. The infection may take several forms, the most easily recognized being pseudomembranous candidiasis, presenting as whitish plaques that can be removed by scraping. Erythematous candidiasis gives an erythematous, atrophic appearance to the tongue or palate, with loss of papillae on the tongue. Oral involvement may also result from varicella zoster and herpes simplex infection as well as from malignant disease, such as non-Hodgkin's lymphoma. Enlargement of the parotid gland is a rare sign in adults but is more common in children.

Patients with oral candidiasis who complain of dysphagia frequently have esophageal candidiasis. Dysphagia may also result from herpetic or cytomegaloviral involvement of the esophagus. Kaposi's sarcoma of the gastrointestinal tract is most often asymptomatic but may cause dysphagia, hemorrhage, or symptoms of obstruction. Both Kaposi's sarcoma and non-Hodgkin's lymphoma can occur anywhere in the gastrointestinal system; symptoms depend on location. Another gastrointestinal complication is infection of the small intestine with atypical mycobacteria, causing lesions that resemble Whipple's disease. Cytomegalovirus infection may result in colitis.

Fever. Nearly all AIDS patients develop prolonged fever during their illness. This may be caused by opportunistic infections, tuberculosis or malignancies. Salmonellosis, often with septicemia, frequently recurs in HIV-infected patients. In many, however, the cause of the fever cannot be found.

Pulmonary Manifestations

Pneumocystosis. Many AIDS patients present with pulmonary symptoms. In industrialized countries, *P. carinii* pneumonia is the most frequent opportunistic infection complicating HIV infection. The frequency of *P. carinii* in African AIDS is uncertain. It is probably underdiagnosed; however, even in European countries, African patients with AIDS have a lower frequency of *Pneumocystis* infection than do European patients. The most common findings in *Pneumocystis* pneumonia are shortness of breath, nonproductive cough, bilateral lower zone shadowing on chest X-ray, and hypoxemia (Chapter 79). Differential diagnoses include infections with *Mycobacterium tuberculosis* or one of the atypical mycobacteria, most commonly *M. avium-intracellulare,* cytomegalovirus pneumonia, cryptococcal lung disease, and pulmonary Kaposi's sarcoma.

Tuberculosis. Tuberculosis is a more frequent complication of HIV infection in developing countries because of the higher background rate of tuberculosis in the general population (Chapter 61.1). Most cases result from reactivation of prior infection with *M. tuberculosis* and not from infection with atypical mycobacteria. In patients with pulmonary tuberculosis, cough is generally productive. HIV seroprevalence in tuberculosis patients in African cities with high rates of HIV infection has been 25% to 40%; high rates are also found in selected tuberculosis populations in some industrialized countries, where tuberculosis attributable to underlying HIV infection has increased. Extrapulmonary tuberculosis, particularly affecting lymph nodes, is more frequent in HIV-seropositive than in HIV-seronegative patients. Although controlled clinical trials are currently lacking, response to treatment for tuberculosis in HIV-positive patients is frequently favorable, emphasizing the importance of diagnoses. Just as a high index of suspicion should exist for tuberculosis in HIV-positive patients, so should the possibility of underlying HIV infection be considered in patients with tuberculosis. HIV-positive patients with tuberculosis often have delayed hypersensitivity to tuberculin; in a recent study in Abidjan, 70% of HIV-positive patients with pulmonary tuberculosis were tuberculin skin test positive.

Neurologic Manifestations. Neurologic disease in AIDS can result from specific opportunistic infections but also is caused by the direct effect of HIV on the nervous system.

HIV Subacute Encephalopathy. Direct involvement of the nervous system by HIV is the cause of the subacute encephalopathy ("AIDS-dementia") recognized in about a third of patients with advanced AIDS. Progressive loss of intellectual function occurs, initially manifested as slowing and loss of concentration. Physical impairment may follow, with ataxia, spasticity, and incontinence. Rarely, these neurologic changes dominate the clinical picture before the onset of more typical opportunistic diseases. Myelopathy, autonomic neuropathy, peripheral neuropathy, and myopathy probably also result directly from HIV infection.

Opportunistic Infections of the CNS. The most frequent infectious diseases affecting the central nervous system in patients with AIDS are cryptococcal meningitis, cytomegalovirus retinitis, and toxoplasmosis. The symptoms and signs of cryptococcosis (Chapter 66.5) and toxoplasmosis (Chapter 78) are most often those of a chronic meningitis and of a space-occupying lesion,

respectively. Signs of a space-occupying lesion can also be caused by cerebral non-Hodgkin's lymphoma. Cryptococcal meningitis occurs in 5% to 10% of AIDS patients in Africa. The symptomatology is broad, and classic signs of meningitis are not always found. Symptoms and signs range from characteristic headache, photophobia, and neck stiffness to subtle changes in mood and behavior. Both cryptococcosis and toxoplasmosis are probably underdiagnosed complications of AIDS in developing countries. In Europe, 17% of African patients with AIDS had cerebral toxoplasmosis.

Cutaneous Manifestations. A wide variety of skin manifestations have been described in AIDS.

Pruriginous Dermatitis. About 20% of African patients with AIDS develop so-called pruriginous dermatitis (Fig. 15–4). Itchy papules that weep on scratching eventually leave hyperpigmented, scarlike macules. The trunk and the extensor surfaces of the limbs are most affected. The histologic appearance of the lesions is nonspecific and simply shows hyperkeratosis and chronic inflammation. The etiology of this condition, which also has been seen in Haitian AIDS patients, is unknown. In Africa, pruriginous dermatitis is highly predictive of HIV infection; 87% of cases in one published series were shown to be HIV positive.

Varicella Zoster. Approximately 10% of African patients with AIDS give a history of varicella zoster infection. This condition was predictive of underlying HIV infection in about 90% of consecutive cases in one series reported from Kinshasa. Varicella zoster infection may be an early manifestation of HIV-related disease.

Genital Ulcers. Chronic or recurrent genital ulcerations are found in about 6% of African patients with AIDS (Chapter 10). In homosexual men, genital and anorectal ulcerations are common and are most often caused by herpes simplex infection.

Kaposi's Sarcoma. The skin is the most frequent organ involved by Kaposi's sarcoma (Chapter 11). Other dermatologic manifestations observed in patients with HIV infection are seborrheic dermatitis, molluscum contagiosum, fungal infection of the nails, and psoriasis, which may be particularly troublesome. Certain changes, such as angular cheilitis and hair thinning, may result from nutritional deficiencies. Some patients show striking changes of premature aging.

Kaposi's sarcoma occurs in up to 40% of homosexual men with AIDS but is less common in other groups. The reason for this high prevalence in homosexuals, or for the recent decline in incidence of Kaposi's sarcoma observed in this group, remains unclear. Kaposi's sarcoma occurs in 4% to 10% of cases of AIDS in Africa, a frequency not greatly different from that found in nonhomosexual Western AIDS patients. Among African patients with AIDS, males are affected 3 to 4 times more frequently than females. Whether a similar geographic distribution of AIDS-related Kaposi's sarcoma occurs in Africa as is described for the classic form of the tumor is unknown.

Kaposi's sarcoma is probably of endothelial origin and histologically shows abnormal vascular spaces with interweaving bundles of spindle cells. In contrast to the relatively indolent classic form of Kaposi's sarcoma,

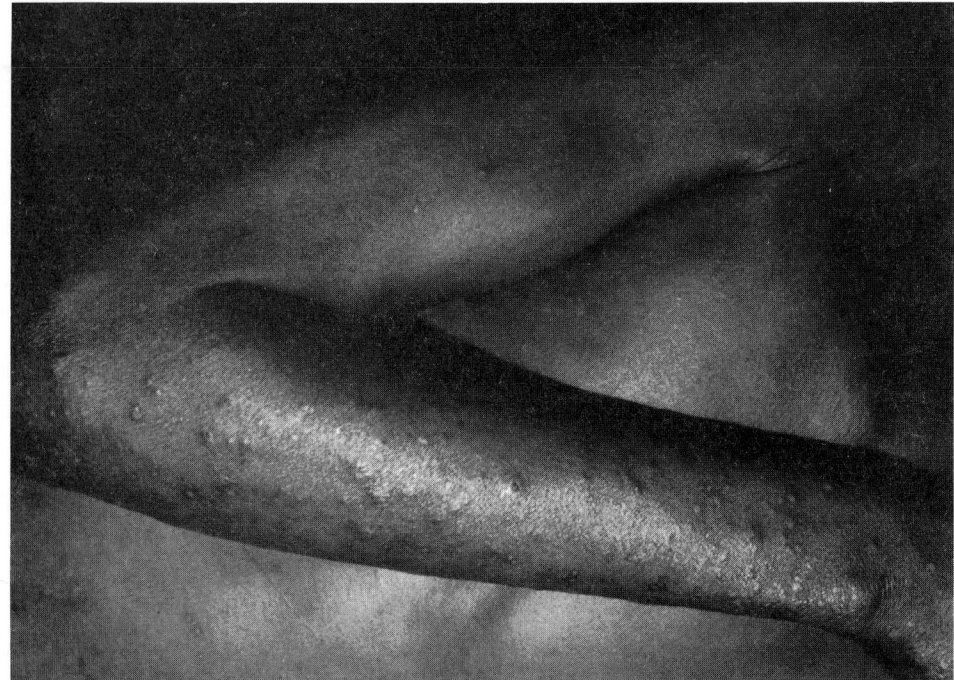

FIGURE 15–4. Pruriginous dermatitis. A condition of unknown cause, it is seen in many African AIDS patients and is highly predictive of HIV infections. Initially, itchy papules, which eventually leave a hyperpigmented, macular rash, appear. Scratching probably affects the appearance of the lesions. Histologic features are nonspecific.

AIDS-related Kaposi's sarcoma is aggressive and carries a poor prognosis.

The appearance is of nodules or plaques on the skin, violaceous in Caucasians but darker in blacks. All parts of the skin may be involved, and lesions can be disfiguring and disabling (Figs. 15–5 and 15–6). Widespread systemic involvement can occur; lymph nodes and the alimentary tract, including the mouth, are most frequently affected. Lung involvement is well recognized and may be confused with other pulmonary complications of AIDS. In some cases, the appearance of the tumor is more like that of the classic form, some patients having features of both aggressive and classic lesions.

Lymphoma. In Europe and the United States, an increased incidence of non-Hodgkin's lymphoma has been seen in patients with AIDS. These high-grade malignancies are generally of B-cell origin and include some Burkitt-like lesions. They are frequently localized at extranodal sites and may involve the central nervous system. Response to chemotherapy is generally poor. Whether Hodgkin's disease occurs more frequently than expected in patients with HIV infection is controversial, but the disease is more aggressive in these persons. Lymphoma occurs as a complication of AIDS in Africa, although its frequency is uncertain.

RELATION TO ENDEMIC TROPICAL DISEASES. The effect of HIV infection on the major endemic tropical diseases is not yet clear. Nevertheless, concern exists that certain of the latter may act as opportunistic infections complicating AIDS, and that HIV infection may alter the clinical presentation or response to treatment of certain tropical infections.

Malaria. Malaria does not act as an opportunistic disease, and there is no evidence thus far that malarial illness is clinically different in HIV-positive persons than in HIV-negative persons. In Kinshasa, Zaire, an indirect association between malaria and HIV infection was demonstrated in children with malarial anemia who received transfusions of unscreened blood.

Leishmaniasis. Individual case reports, mainly from southern Europe, suggest that visceral leishmaniasis (due to infection with *Leishmania donovani*) can be a manifestation of AIDS. Symptomatic HIV infection has not become widespread in areas where leishmaniasis is endemic, and the importance of this particular association remains to be determined.

Mycobacterial Infections. As mentioned earlier, human tuberculosis is frequent in HIV-positive persons and in AIDS patients. Reactivation of tuberculosis in HIV-positive persons may have a severe adverse effect on tuberculosis control, especially in Africa, and tuberculosis incidence may rise. Leprosy might also be ex-

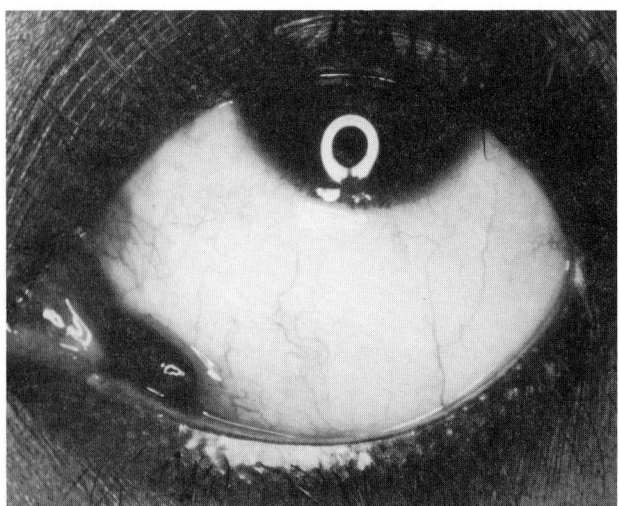

FIGURE 15–5. Kaposi's sarcoma affecting the lower eyelid. Kaposi's sarcoma may appear anywhere on the body. Careful examination of the whole skin and all mucous membranes is required for detection of the typical lesions. These are red-violet when involving the mucosa, and brown-violet on black skin. Occasionally, external lesions are absent despite extensive visceral involvement.

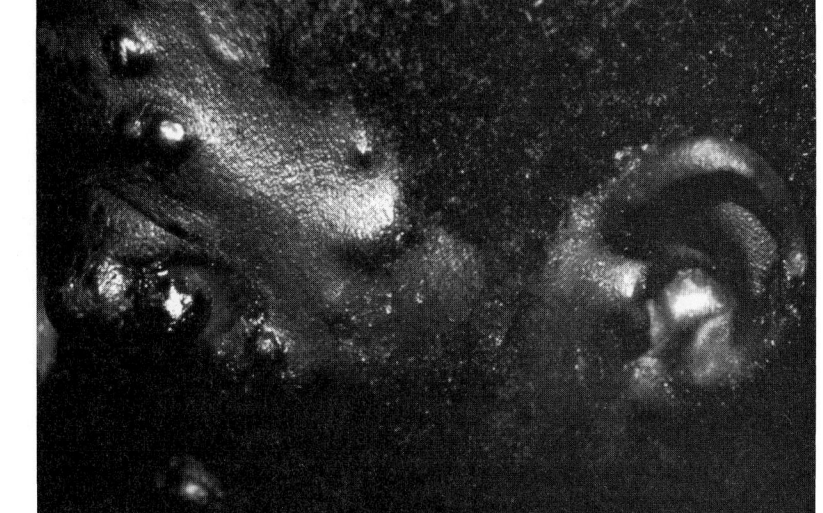

FIGURE 15–6. Kaposi's sarcoma nodules on the face. Extensive nodular involvement of the face is seen in this patient with disseminated Kaposi's sarcoma secondary to HIV infection. AIDS-related Kaposi's sarcoma in Africa does not always produce these aggressive appearances; it sometimes resembles the classic variety of the tumor.

pected to act as an opportunistic infection, and the clinical expression of disease due to *Mycobacterium leprae* could be altered toward the lepromatous end of the clinical spectrum (Chapter 62). However, data from populations in which both HIV infection and leprosy are prevalent are lacking.

Other Parasitic Infections. No information is available concerning the interaction between HIV infection and schistosomiasis, filariasis, or trypanosomiasis.

HIV-2 INFECTION. Controversy exists over the pathogenicity of HIV-2 infection. It clearly can cause AIDS that is indistinguishable from that associated with HIV-1 infection, but some workers believe that it does so less frequently. Individual reports have claimed that the latency period for HIV-2 is longer than for HIV-1, but data from long-term cohort studies are not yet available.

AIDS IN CHILDREN

Transmission. AIDS in children is emerging as an important problem in areas where heterosexual transmission causes many women of reproductive age to be infected. Most children are infected perinatally. Transfusion of infected blood or blood products and exposure to contaminated needles account for the remaining cases. Infection through breast milk is thought to be relatively uncommon.

Low Birth Weight. Infants born to seropositive mothers often have low birth weight, short body length, and reduced head circumference for gestational age. It is uncertain to what extent these signs reflect HIV infection in the child, and to what extent poor health in the HIV-infected mother. Low birth weight may be an important contributing factor to the increased infant mortality rate observed in children born to HIV-infected mothers.

Congenital Abnormalities. An embryopathy with recognizable facial abnormalities has been reported by some workers in the United States but remains to be further substantiated.

Clinical Manifestations. These are nonspecific, e.g., failure to thrive and delay in psychomotor development. Lymphadenopathy, hepatosplenomegaly, and parotid swelling are common. Some features, e.g., chronic diarrhea, oral candidiasis, and *P. carinii* pneumonia, are similar to those in adults. Kaposi's sarcoma occurs but is rare. Children with AIDS seem to suffer more frequent bacterial infections than do adult AIDS patients. Measles may be particularly severe in HIV-infected children. Cases of severe measles without a rash have been described.

Lymphoid Interstitial Pneumonitis. A condition described in pediatric patients but rarely seen in adults with AIDS is lymphoid interstitial pneumonitis, characterized by lymphoid infiltration of the lung with symptoms of respiratory insufficiency. The etiology is unknown.

DIAGNOSIS

Clinical Classification. AIDS is a clinical diagnosis; proof of HIV infection requires laboratory-based serologic tests. In developing countries, facilities are often inadequate for diagnosing opportunistic diseases that would fulfill the CDC case definition (see Table 15–1). For this reason, the WHO clinical case definition of AIDS may be helpful (see Table 15–2). In Kinshasa, Zaire, evaluation of this clinical case definition against HIV seropositivity demonstrated a sensitivity of 62%, a specificity of 94%, and a positive predictive value of 74% for diagnosing symptomatic HIV infection in hospitalized patients. Very similar results (sensitivity 55%, specificity 85%, positive predictive value 73%) were obtained in an evaluation of the case definition in Uganda. The positive predictive value of the case definition (i.e., proportion of persons meeting the clinical case definition who actually are HIV seropositive) increases with the prevalence of HIV infection in the population under consideration (Fig. 15–7). The weakness of the WHO case definition is its limited sensitivity for diagnosing HIV-associated disease.

Serologic Tests. Ideally, a clinical diagnosis should be confirmed by serology. Serologic tests for HIV infection are based on the demonstration of antibody to HIV in serum. The most common test system used is enzyme-linked immunosorbent assay (ELISA), which is both sensitive and specific. However, false positive ELISA tests do occur, and the predictive value of the test is highest when the prevalence of HIV infection is high. It is customary to test positive specimens by a supplemen-

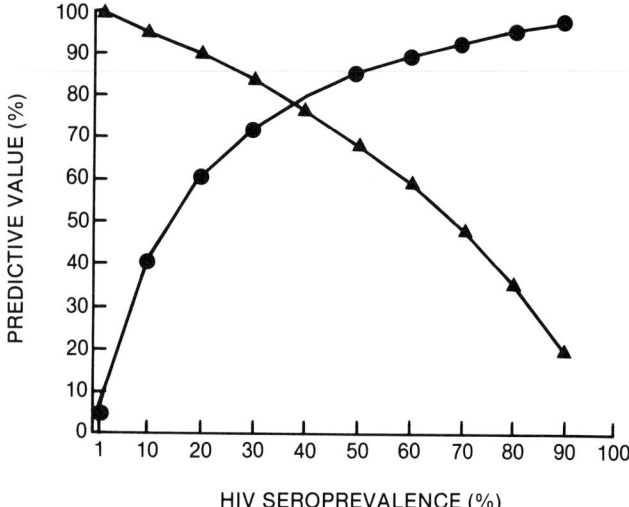

FIGURE 15–7. Positive and negative predictive value of WHO clinical case. Definition for AIDS in Africa by HIV seroprevalence. The predictive value of the clinical case definition (proportion of people meeting the case definition who are HIV-positive) increases with the prevalence of HIV infection. The clinical case definition has been useful but suffers from lack of sensitivity. Whenever possible, clinical diagnosis of AIDS should be accompanied by serologic diagnosis of HIV infection.

tal ("confirmatory") test, e.g., Western blot or radioimmunoprecipitation assay (RIPA). Western blots depend on the demonstration of specific antibody in the test serum binding to individual viral proteins, coded for by specific viral genes, that have been electrophoretically separated and transferred to a solid surface (see Fig. 15–1).

Tests are available for the detection of HIV antigen in serum. A potential application of such tests is in identifying HIV infection before the appearance of antibody detectable by conventional ELISAs (the so-called window period). This could be of particular importance to blood banks. Antigen tests have thus far not been widely used in clinical practice and have not been extensively evaluated.

Viral Isolation. The most specific test to demonstrate HIV infection is viral culture, an investigation that is generally limited to research. The presence of virus that has been cultured in a suitable medium can be demonstrated either by tests to show viral antigen or reverse transcriptase activity, or directly by the use of molecular probes. A new technique is gene amplification using the polymerase chain reaction (PCR). Integrated proviral genome can be demonstrated in the host lymphocyte genetic material after amplification and identification with specific probes.

Diagnostic Difficulties and Needs. ELISA, Western blot, RIPA, and PCR can specifically diagnose HIV-1 and HIV-2 infection. However, serologic cross-reactivity between HIV-1 and HIV-2 antibody–positive specimens is common, and more specific diagnostic methods are required. ELISA systems based on synthetic peptides representing a fraction of the transmembrane glycoprotein of the two viruses are being evaluated.

All diagnostic tests are expensive, and many require technological resources unsuitable for developing coun-

tries. Low-cost, simple, rapid diagnostic tests for HIV infection, including both screening and secondary tests, are urgently needed.

TREATMENT. Although AIDS remains a progressive and incurable disease, much can be done for the physical treatment and social provision for persons with AIDS.

Treatment of Opportunistic Infections. The treatment of specific opportunistic diseases is outlined in Table 15–7, and in specific chapters dealing with individual diseases.

Some opportunistic diseases are currently untreatable, such as infection with *M. avium* complex (Chapter 61.2), cryptosporidiosis (Chapter 70), and progressive multifocal leukoencephalopathy. Other conditions, such as non-Hodgkin's lymphoma and Kaposi's sarcoma (Chapter 11), respond to varying degrees, often poorly. Some opportunistic infections, such as cryptococcal meningitis (Chapter 66.5), central nervous system toxoplasmosis (Chapter 78), and probably also *P. carinii* (Chapter 79), are treatable but may require maintenance therapy to prevent relapse.

Antiviral Chemotherapy. Several antiviral drugs have been evaluated, of which only one, zidovudine (also called azidothymidine, AZT), has been demonstrated to improve prognosis in AIDS. Zidovudine is phosphorylated in the host cell and inhibits HIV replication either by interfering with reverse transcriptase activity or by terminating viral nucleic acid chain synthesis. The major side effect of zidovudine is bone marrow suppression leading to anemia and leukopenia. The drug is extremely expensive and does not produce a cure. Lifelong therapy is required. Although zidovudine currently is recommended only for patients with AIDS, its effects earlier in the course of HIV infection are being assessed.

Symptomatic Treatment. Treatment of diarrhea or prurigo should be tried after specific causes have been ruled out. Psychologic and social support is essential to the person with AIDS. Integral to this are involvement of the patient's family or friends, honesty concerning the nature of the infection and illness, and advice concerning avoidance of transmission of HIV to others.

PREVENTION AND CONTROL. Without a cure or effective vaccine for HIV infection and AIDS, prevention of transmission of HIV infection is fundamental to AIDS control. Prevention requires attention to the three major routes of infection: sexual, blood contact, and from mother to child.

Surveillance. Public health surveillance for AIDS and HIV infection is essential in all countries for assessment of the magnitude of the epidemic and for the timely implementation and evaluation of intervention efforts.

Interruption of Sexual Transmission. This requires extensive health education concerning the threat posed by HIV. Such education needs to start with children of school age and become universal, to persuade people to restrict unprotected sexual activity to mutually monogamous long-term relationships.

Targeted education, aimed at those who are especially at risk, will also be required to prevent noninfected persons from having unprotected sexual intercourse with

TABLE 15–7. Therapy and Prophylaxis for Infectious Diseases in AIDS Patients

Infections	Drug	Usual Daily Adult Dose	Interval	Route	Minimum Duration
Therapy					
Pneumocystis pneumonia	Trimethoprim-sulfamethoxazole *or*	20 mg/kg trimethoprim 100 mg/kg sulfamethoxazole	Every 6–8 hours	Oral	14–21 days
	Pentamidine isethionate	4 μg/kg	Daily	Intravenous (or intramuscular)	14–21 days
Toxoplasmosis	Pyrimethamine Sulfadiazine *and* Folinic acid	100–200 mg loading dose, then 75–100 mg/day 6–8 gm/day 10–15 mg/day	Daily Daily Daily	Oral Oral Oral	6 weeks 6 weeks 6 weeks
Cryptosporidiosis	No drug known to be effective				
Isosporiasis	Trimethoprim-sulfamethoxazole	10 mg/kg 50 mg/kg	Every 6 hours	Oral	3 weeks
Oral candidiasis	Nystatin *or*	300,000 units	Every 8 hours	Oral	7–14 days
	Ketoconazole	200 mg	Daily	Oral	7–14 days
Esophageal candidiasis	Ketoconazole	200 mg	Daily	Oral	7–14 days
Cryptococcosis	Amphotericin 5-Flucytosine	0.5–1 mg/kg 75–100 mg/kg	Daily 6 hourly	Intravenous Oral	6 weeks
Mucocutaneous herpes simplex (mild)	Acyclovir	1 gm	5 times/day	Oral *or*	7 days
Mucocutaneous herpes simplex (severe)	Acyclovir	15 mg/kg	Every 8 hours	Intravenous	10 days
Visceral herpes simplex	Acyclovir	30 mg/kg	Every 8 hours	Intravenous	10 days
Varicella zoster	Acyclovir	3–4 gm *or* 30 mg/kg	5 times/day *or* Every 8 hours	Oral *or* Intravenous	7–10 days 7–10 days
Mycobacterium avium-intracellulare infection	No drug known to be effective				
Mycobacterium tuberculosis infection	Isoniazid *and*	300 mg	Daily	Oral	At least 6 months after culture conversion
	Rifampicin *and*	600 mg	Daily	Oral	At least 6 months after culture conversion
	Pyrazinamide	20–30 mg/kg	Daily	Oral	First 2 months of therapy
Prophylaxis					
Pneumocystis pneumonia	Trimethoprim-sulfamethoxazole *or*	5 mg/kg 20 mg/kg	12 hourly	Oral	Lifelong
	Pyrimethamine Sulfadoxine *or*	25 mg 500 mg	Once weekly	Oral	Lifelong
	Pentamidine *or*	4 mg/kg	Once monthly *or*	Intravenous *or*	Lifelong
	Pentamidine	Uncertain	Once weekly	Aerosol	Lifelong
Toxoplasmosis	Pyrimethamine Sulfadiazine	25–50 mg 2–4 gm	Daily	Oral	Lifelong
Cryptococcosis	Amphotericin *or*	100 mg	Once weekly	Intravenous	Lifelong
	Ketoconazole	400 mg	Daily	Oral	Lifelong
Tuberculosis	Isoniazid	300 mg	Daily	Oral	Indications not established

those who are infected. Proposed strategies include reducing the number of sex partners, avoiding high-risk partners, using condoms and spermicides (spermicides may have an antiviral effect, thus enhancing the effectiveness of condoms as protection against HIV infection), and widespread HIV testing and counseling. Prevention of sexual transmission may usefully be integrated into control programs for other sexually transmitted diseases. The problem of prostitution, important in the spread of all sexually transmitted diseases, and in some areas inextricably linked to intravenous drug use, must be faced, as must that of HIV transmission in other special situations such as imprisonment.

Interruption of Blood and Needle Transmission. Reliable screening tests can eliminate blood transfusion as a means of HIV transmission, although cheaper and simpler tests are required for the developing world. Unnecessary transfusions and injections must be avoided. Scrupulous adherence to the use of sterile needles for medical purposes is required; in developing countries, greater attention must be given to the sterilization of contaminated medical equipment and to the provision of clean needles and syringes. Traditional surgical practices, such as circumcision and birth attendance, must also be modified.

Attempts must be made to eliminate intravenous drug abuse; treatment programs must be established for addicts; and innovative ventures should be undertaken to ensure that those who do inject drugs use sterile needles and equipment.

Interruption of Perinatal Transmission. This can be lowered through reducing sexual HIV transmission to women of childbearing age, counseling infected women to avoid pregnancy, and, under certain circumstances, considering termination of pregnancy.

Interruption of Transmission to Infants and Children. Recommendations concerning breast feeding and vaccination of infants born to HIV-infected mothers will vary with the economic development of the country of residence. In developing countries, breast feeding should be encouraged for all infants, and routine vaccinations should be given. Baccille Calmette-Guérin (BCG) should not be given to persons symptomatic for HIV infection. In industrialized countries, or where safe and effective alternatives to breast feeding exist, HIV-infected women should be advised not to breast-feed their infants.

Recommendations in the United States for vaccination of children born to HIV-positive mothers are to use diptheria, tetanus, and pertussis (DTP) vaccine; live measles, mumps, and rubella (MMR) vaccines; and *Haemophilus influenzae* type b conjugate vaccine (HbCV) in standard fashion; and to replace oral, attenuated poliovirus vaccine (OPV) with inactivated poliovirus vaccine (IPV). For persons with symptomatic HIV infection, pneumococcal and influenza vaccines are recommended. Hepatitis B vaccine seems less effective in HIV-infected adults than in those not infected. Data on the use of hepatitis B vaccine in HIV-infected children are lacking, and the usual recommendations for the prevention of hepatitis B should be followed. In countries where the risk of tuberculosis is low, BCG should not be given to persons with HIV infection.

BIBLIOGRAPHY

Centers for Disease Control: AIDS. Recommendations and Guidelines. Reprinted from Morbidity and Mortality Weekly Report. (Available from CDC.)

Institute of Medicine, National Academy of Science: Confronting AIDS. Washington, DC, National Academy Press, 1986.

Institute of Medicine, National Academy of Science: Confronting AIDS. Update 1988. National Academy Press, Washington, DC, 1988.

Piot P, Mann JM (eds): AIDS and HIV infection in the tropics. Clin Trop Commun Dis 3:1–171, 1988. (Whole issue devoted to AIDS in the tropics.)

Piot P, Plummer FA, Mhalu FS, et al: AIDS: An international perspective. Science 239:573–579, 1988.

Quinn TC, Mann JM, Curran JW, Piot P: AIDS in Africa: An epidemiologic paradigm. Science 234: 955–963, 1986.

Sande M, Volberding PA: Medical management of AIDS. Infect Dis Clinics North Am 2:21, 1988. (Whole issue devoted to management of patients with AIDS.)

Scientific American: What science knows about AIDS. October 1988. (Whole issue devoted to AIDS.)

15.2   HUMAN T-LYMPHOTROPIC VIRUS TYPE I INFECTION AND ADULT T-CELL LEUKEMIA/LYMPHOMA

Robert O. Cannon
and Kevin M. De Cock

HUMAN T-LYMPHOTROPIC VIRUS TYPE I INFECTION

DEFINITION. Human T-lymphotropic virus type I (HTLV-I), the first human retrovirus discovered, is a type C retrovirus that preferentially infects T lymphocytes. HTLV-I causes two divergent diseases: adult T-cell leukemia/lymphoma (ATL) and HTLV-I–associated myelopathy/tropical spastic paraparesis (HAM/TSP). ATL is characterized by skin lesions, lymphadenopathy, hepatosplenomegaly, and hypercalcemia, and it usually has a rapidly progressive course resistant to treatment. HAM/TSP is a degenerative neurologic disease characterized by progressive bilateral leg weakness and spasticity, spastic bladder, and minimal sensory deficits.

INTRODUCTION AND HISTORY. For several decades, retroviruses have been recognized as the etiologic agents of certain malignancies and immune system disorders in various animal species, but human retroviruses remained undiscovered. Then in 1978, HTLV-I was isolated in the United States from a patient with an atypical variant of a cutaneous T-cell lymphoma.

ATL was first recognized as a distinct clinicopathologic condition in southern Japan, the first case descriptions being published in 1977. In 1982, ATL was described in black patients from the West Indies. Serum specimens from most ATL patients in both Japan and the Caribbean contained HTLV-I antibodies, and the virus was isolated from the lymphocytes of some of the patients.

HAM/TSP, initially described in 1956 as a subgroup of Jamaican neuropathy with predominantly spastic symptoms, was shown to be associated with the presence of HTLV-I antibodies in natives of Martinique, West Indies, in 1985 and native Japanese in 1986.

Because of concern about the disease-causing potential of HTLV-I, screening of donated blood began nationwide in Japan in 1986 and recommendations for screening were issued in the United States in 1988.

EPIDEMIOLOGY

Distribution. The epidemiology of HTLV-I infection is incompletely understood. Evidence of endemic HTLV-I is well documented for southern Japan and the Caribbean basin, but there is accumulating serologic evidence of HTLV-I or a related virus in certain populations of the Pacific basin (including Australia, Papua New Guinea, and the Marshall Islands), Central and South America, the United States, southern Italy, Israel, the Seychelles Islands, and parts of sub-Saharan Africa.

Prevalence. In the well-studied areas, HTLV-I seroprevalence in the general population ranges from 5% (Jamaica) to 15% (southern Japan). In these areas, the seroprevalence increases with age until about age 65; seroprevalence among older age groups reaches 15% in Jamaica and 30% in southern Japan. Women over the age of 20 have a higher seroprevalence rate than do men, and the difference in rates increases with age.

In the Caribbean basin and the United States, HTLV-I seroprevalence is more frequent in blacks than in other ethnic groups. In the United States, groups of intravenous drug users and their sex partners have the highest HTLV-I seroprevalence rates. The HTLV-I seroprevalence rate in blood donors in the United States is 0.025%.

Transmission. HTLV-I may be transmitted in one of four ways: from mother to child, through blood transfusion, by sexual contact, or through sharing of needles and syringes. No evidence exists for transmission by insects or casual contact.

Mother-to-child transmission is thought to occur predominantly through breast feeding; in Japan, approximately 25% of breast-fed infants of seropositive mothers become infected. Perinatal transmission also may occur transplacentally or at birth, though infrequently; perhaps 1% or less of infants born to infected mothers acquire the disease this way. Passively transferred maternal antibody disappears by 12 to 18 months of age.

Transmission through transfusion of blood products is strongly associated with cellular components, since serum components and plasma do not appear to transmit infection. A greater than 60% seroconversion rate among recipients of cellular components of seropositive blood has been reported in Japan. Recipients of cell-free blood products, such as men with hemophilia, do not have increased HTLV-I seroprevalence rates. An estimated $\geq 10^7$ transfused cells are necessary to transmit HTLV-I infection.

Sexual transmission may be inefficient; however, male-to-female heterosexual transmission appears to be more efficient than the reverse. The efficacy of transmission by contaminated needles and syringes is unknown.

BIOLOGY. HTLV-I is a member of the oncovirus subgroup of retroviruses with an RNA genome that contains at least 3 structural genes *(gag, env,* and *pol)* and 2 regulatory genes *(tax* and *rex).* The structural genes, *gag* (virus core) and *env* (virus envelope), encode the dominant immunogenic proteins; the detection of antibodies to these proteins is the basis of serologic diagnosis of HTLV-I infection.

HTLV-I preferentially infects mature CD4$^+$, helper/inducer T lymphocytes (although cells with other functional phenotypes may be infected), as does human immunodeficiency virus (HIV). Like HIV, HTLV-I can incorporate its genome into the genome of the host cell. Unlike HIV infection, HTLV-I infection does not result in reduced numbers of CD4$^+$ cells, although infected cells may show reduced helper and suppressor cell function in vitro.

HTLV-I is not closely related to HIV-1 or HIV-2 and rarely is associated with marked immunosuppression unless ATL occurs. HTLV-I is closely related serologically to human T-lymphotropic virus type II (HTLV-II). Very little is known about the epidemiology of HTLV-II, and it has not been etiologically associated with any disease. There is increasing evidence that HTLV-II is the most prevalent HTLV type among intravenous drug users in the United States (30% or more of some groups of urban black intravenous drug users may be infected). Recently, endemic (8% seroprevalence) HTLV-II infection has been documented among a group of Guaniyi Indians in Panama. Infected persons were not intravenous drug users, and there was no clustering of seropositivity in family units. HTLV-II has been isolated from two patients with hairy cell leukemia; however, most patients with the disease are serologically negative for HTLV-II.

ATL and HAM/TSP rarely occur in the same person. The reasons are unknown but may include the host's immunologic response to infection or differences in virus strains. By disrupting the host immune function, HTLV-I infection may affect the development and course of diseases other than ATL and HAM/TSP. Concurrent HTLV-I infection in HIV-infected persons may alter the expression of HIV disease. In a few persons, some B-cell malignancies are associated with HTLV-I infection. In these persons, malignant transformation of B cells occurred in cells producing HTLV-I antibody.

DIAGNOSIS. The most sensitive screening assay for HTLV-I antibody is an enzyme immunoassay (EIA) that uses whole disrupted virus. Particle agglutination is used extensively in Japan. Indirect immunofluorescent antibody tests are being developed. The EIA test is sufficiently sensitive but insufficiently specific. Tests used to confirm the presence of HTLV-I antibodies include Western blot (WB) and radioimmunoprecipitation assay (RIPA). WB appears to be the supplementary test most sensitive to antibody to *gag* protein products p19 and p24, whereas RIPA appears to be most sensitive to antibody to the *env* glycoprotein gp46 and the *env* precursor gp61/68. A positive serum specimen demonstrates immunoreactivity to the *gag* gene product p24 and to an *env* gene product (gp46 and/or gp61/68) by WB and/or RIPA. Neither the EIA nor the supplementary tests distinguish between antibodies to HTLV-I and HTLV-II. Persons with reactive serum are assumed to be infected with HTLV-I, HTLV-II, or a closely related virus. EIA tests for HTLV-I show very little, if any, cross-reactivity with antibodies to HIV-1 or HIV-2, and vice versa.

TREATMENT. There is no specific treatment for HTLV-I infection. Antiviral agents, e.g., zidovudine (AZT), have no in vitro activity against HTLV-I, have not been used in treatment of HTLV-I infection, and cannot be recommended.

PREVENTION AND CONTROL. No vaccine currently exists to prevent HTLV-I infection. Once acquired, HTLV-I infection probably is lifelong because the viral genome is integrated into the host cell DNA.

All body fluids, such as breast milk, blood, and semen and cervical fluid, that contain cellular components from HTLV-I–infected persons should be considered potentially infectious. To prevent mother-to-child transmission, infected women may be advised not to breast-feed when realistic alternatives are available. However, in developing countries, where there are few acceptable alternatives to breast feeding, and where, as elsewhere, the risk of HTLV-I–associated disease is low, breast feeding cannot be reasonably prohibited. Screening of donated blood for HTLV-I should be of low priority in the developing world. No firm recommendations can be given for preventing sexually transmitted HTLV-I infection because the efficiency of this mode of transmission and the consequences of infection are not known. Intravenous drug abuse should be discouraged.

ADULT T-CELL LEUKEMIA/LYMPHOMA

EPIDEMIOLOGY. Although ATL occurs in persons less than 30 years of age, it is primarily a disease of the 40- to 65-year group. The median age at onset is 40 to 50 years. The lifetime risk of ATL among HTLV-I–infected persons is estimated at 2% to 4%; the latency period between infection and development of disease may be several decades. On the island of Kyushu in southern Japan, where the age-adjusted HTLV-I seroprevalence rate is 12.7%, the annual incidence of ATL is 3.5 cases per 100,000 persons under 40 years of age and 5.7 per 100,000 among persons aged 40 and older. The age-adjusted annual incidence of ATL in Jamaica is estimated at 1 to 3 cases per 100,000 persons. ATL occurs with the same frequency in men and women. ATL is the most common hematopoietic neoplasm in Jamaica and southern Japan.

PATHOGENESIS. There is strong evidence that HTLV-I is the etiologic agent of ATL. Antibodies to HTLV-I are present in most (>90%) ATL patients. HTLV-I proviral DNA is monoclonally integrated into the DNA of all malignant cells but not other host cells, which implies cell proliferation from a singly infected and transformed cell. HTLV-I can be isolated from malignant cells of most ATL patients. HTLV-I immortalizes normal lymphocytes in vitro, and these transformed lymphocytes have properties of leukemic cells.

Neither the viral factors that contribute to malignant cell transformation nor the differences in host response that contribute to development of disease have been determined. Unlike other transforming retroviruses, HTLV-I does not contain an oncogene. HTLV-I may initiate transformation by activating interleukin-2 recep-

tors and/or by stimulating increased production of lymphokines, including interleukin-2.

PATHOLOGY. In persons with ATL, CD4+ malignant cells frequently are observed in the peripheral blood as circulating lymphocytes with irregular multilobulated nuclei. These circulating cells have scant, agranular cytoplasm, occasionally with vacuoles. The chromatin of the nucleus is condensed with a vesicular to coarse pattern, and the nucleus may contain up to 3 usually inconspicuous nucleoli.

Malignant cell infiltrates are diffuse rather than nodular, and the underlying structure usually is preserved. From patient to patient, however, there is considerable cytomorphologic pleomorphism. The histologic patterns of ATL are not readily classified into any group of lymphomas. The system proposed by the Japanese Lymphoma Study Group may be useful; in this system tumors are subclassified as small cell, medium-sized cell, mixed cell, pleomorphic, or other. Malignant lymphocytes may infiltrate multiple sites, including the spleen, liver, and meninges, but only very rarely the mediastinum. No recognized histologic pattern correlates with a given clinical outcome.

Infiltrative skin lesions contain malignant cells in dense dermal nodules. Lytic bone lesions usually contain areas of fibrosis and increased osteoclastic activity rather than malignant cells. When malignant infiltration of the bone marrow occurs, it is always diffuse rather than paratrabecular. In the primary pulmonary disease of ATL, both leukemic infiltrates and diffuse fibrosis have been observed.

CLINICAL MANIFESTATIONS. Persons with ATL show several different clinical patterns.

Acute Disease. For those with the more acute pattern (the most common form), initial symptoms often include fever, rash, cough, malaise, weakness, and abdominal distention and pain. These patients often have tachypnea and dyspnea, which may progress to pulmonary failure. Opportunistic pathogens, such as *Pneumocystis carinii,* cytomegalovirus, *Cryptococcus,* and *Candida,* and various bacterial and mycobacterial agents also have been associated with pulmonary disease, especially in patients receiving combination chemotherapy. Central nervous system abnormalities, due to leptomeningeal involvement, manifest as meningeal signs or an altered level of consciousness. Lymphadenopathy, skin lesions, and hepatosplenomegaly frequently occur. When present, lymphadenopathy is usually widespread. The skin lesions may appear as papules, nodules, tumors, generalized maculopapular rashes, parapsoriatic rashes, or generalized or localized erythroderma. Generally, the cutaneous lesions are not pruritic.

Hypercalcemia, occasionally in association with lytic bone lesions, occurs in up to 75% of patients with the acute pattern. Liver function tests often are abnormal. Although some patients initially may have a lymphoma-like syndrome, most eventually become leukemic, often with marked leukocytosis and lymphocytosis; 10% or more of the lymphocytes may contain multilobulated nuclei. Eosinophilia may develop, but usually anemia and thrombocytopenia are either absent or mild. Glucose and protein in cerebrospinal fluid (CSF) are usually normal, but there may be a minimal increase in the number of cells (mostly lymphocytes). Patients with the acute form of ATL have a median survival period of approximately 1 year.

Chronic Disease. Patients with the more chronic form of ATL (perhaps one third or fewer of all patients with ATL) may have lymphadenopathy and skin lesions, although these manifestations are less extensive than in acute ATL. Patients with chronic ATL do not have hepatosplenomegaly. Bone marrow involvement, if present, is mild. There may be minimally elevated numbers of circulating leukemic cells. Serum calcium levels are normal. The proportion of persons with chronic ATL who progress to the acute form is unknown, but it may be substantial.

DIAGNOSIS. There is no conventional single test or sign that allows an unequivocal diagnosis of ATL. It is more difficult to diagnose chronic ATL than acute ATL because the former lacks many of the distinctive features of the latter. Acute ATL can be diagnosed confidently for persons with a diffuse T-cell non-Hodgkin's lymphoma, skin lesions, hypercalcemia, leukemic cells, and reactive HTLV-I serologic test results. Patients with less acute illness, however, may be difficult to differentiate from persons with a cutaneous T-cell lymphoma such as mycosis fungoides or Sézary syndrome. Typical cutaneous T-cell lymphoma lesions spread less rapidly and less extensively than those of ATL, and they are typically bandlike and sparsely infiltrated compared with the dense nodules of ATL. Also, patients with cutaneous T-cell lymphoma rarely have metabolic bone disease, lymphocytic invasion of the leptomeninges, and opportunistic infections; when present, these conditions suggest the diagnosis of chronic ATL. T-cell chronic lymphocytic leukemia and peripheral T-cell lymphoma also may be quite difficult to differentiate from chronic ATL. The differential diagnosis of ATL, therefore, may rely on the combination of clinical, pathologic, serologic, and epidemiologic features.

TREATMENT. Aggressive combination chemotherapy, similar to that used for B-cell lymphomas, is recommended for patients with acute ATL. Prolonged remissions are rare, however, and treated persons are at an increased risk for developing opportunistic infections. Hypercalcemia unresponsive to conventional therapy may respond to chemotherapy, only to become refractory to all interventions later. Patients with hypercalcemia have a shorter median survival period (3 to 5 months) than do those without hypercalcemia (12 to 15 months). No therapy is advocated for patients with chronic ATL because known regimens are unsuitable and because a good prognosis is possible without therapy.

15.3. HTLV-I—ASSOCIATED MYELOPATHY/ TROPICAL SPASTIC PARAPARESIS

Robert O. Cannon
and Kevin M. De Cock

EPIDEMIOLOGY. The median age of onset for HAM/TSP, as for ATL, is 40 to 50 years. For approximately 80% of persons with HAM/TSP, onset occurs after age 30; only a few become ill after age 60. HAM/TSP most often occurs in women; in Japan, 70% of cases are female. The lifetime risk of HAM/TSP among HTLV-I–infected persons is very low (perhaps 1% or less), and the latency period may be shorter than for ATL. HAM/TSP (but not ATL) has been associated with blood transfusions. In Japan, 24% of HAM/TSP patients (versus approximately 2% of the general population) have a history of blood transfusion. In these patients, the median interval between transfusion and onset of disease is 4 years, and it ranges from 3 months to more than 25 years. In Kagoshima, Japan, where HTLV-I is endemic, the prevalence rate is between 6 and 8 cases per 100,000 persons. HAM/TSP is the most common form of paraplegia in some areas of the tropics and in Japan.

PATHOGENESIS. Evidence for an association between HAM/TSP and HTLV-I includes the high prevalence of HTLV-I antibodies in HAM/TSP patients (60% to 100%), the demonstration of intrathecal synthesis of HTLV-I antibody, the finding in some patients of multilobulated cells (like those that occur with ATL) in the peripheral blood and cerebrospinal fluid (CSF), and the isolation of HTLV-I from peripheral blood lymphocytes and CSF mononuclear cells.

The pathogenic mechanisms of the disease are unknown but may be related to modulation of the immune system by activated T lymphocytes, indirect effects of cytokines, or cell-mediated immune responses directed against neural tissue; they also may be the result of viral neurotropism (though the virus has not been found at lesion sites). In Japan, an association has been noted between certain histocompatibility antigen haplotypes and HAM/TSP.

PATHOLOGY. The neuropathology of HAM/TSP is mainly axonal degeneration and myelin loss in the pyramidal tracts of the spinal cord. Changes are most severe at the thoracic and lumbar levels and less so in the posterior columns and in the spinothalamic and spinocerebellar tracts. A chronic meningomyelitis, predominantly at the spinal cord level but also involving the midbrain, the cerebellum, and the cerebrum, is typical. Although the degree of inflammation varies from patient to patient, perivascular lymphocytic infiltration, fibrosis, and hyaline arteriolar thickening are usually observed in the affected parts of the nervous system.

CLINICAL MANIFESTATIONS. HAM/TSP is characterized by leg weakness, usually more proximal than distal, and difficulty walking. Stiffness and sensations of heaviness and numbness of the legs often are reported. Initially, the weakness may be asymmetric. Onset is usually gradual but may be rapid. Mild arm weakness also may be present. Low back pain that often radiates into the legs is frequent, as is bladder incontinence (often an early condition) and constipation (often a later condition). Sensations of burning or pins and needles in the feet occur less commonly and may be more prominent than objective sensory signs. Patients also may complain of vague visual or auditory problems. Men may become impotent.

Physical examination of patients with HAM/TSP reveals upper motor neuron involvement with spastic paraparesis, hyperreflexia of the legs (in 90% to 100% of patients) and often of the arms (in 80%), and extensor plantar responses. Some patients may have a slight loss of vibratory perception in the feet; proprioception is less frequently impaired. Measures of higher mental functions are normal. Infrequently, HAM/TSP patients may exhibit cerebellar signs, optic atrophy, deafness, nystagmus, and depressed or absent ankle jerk.

HAM/TSP usually progresses over a decade or longer, but progression may be rapid, especially in older persons; patients eventually become unable to walk even with crutches.

Reports of the prevalence of CSF pleocytosis in HAM/TSP patients have varied considerably (from 16% to 60% of patients). If present, pleocytosis is lymphocytic and mild with rarely more than 100 cells/mm³ of CSF. Multilobulated cells may be present in the CSF. Elevated CSF protein (40 to 60 mg/dl) and immunoglobulin G levels (often with oligoclonal bands) occur in approximately half of all persons with HAM/TSP. Spinal myelograms are normal. In one series, 62% of patients had abnormalities of their somatosensory evoked potentials.

DIAGNOSIS. The differential diagnosis of HAM/TSP includes spinal cord compression, chronic progressive myelopathies (such as multiple sclerosis and subacute combined degeneration of the cord), and other conditions. Persons with arachnoiditis and other forms of spinal cord compression have abnormal myelograms, unlike persons with HAM/TSP. Intracranial nerve signs and a clinical course characterized by exacerbations and remissions are characteristic of multiple sclerosis but not of HAM/TSP. Multiple sclerosis lacks the meningeal inflammation of HAM/TSP. Subacute combined degeneration of the cord is dominated by sensory symptoms and signs uncharacteristic of HAM/TSP. Tropical ataxic neuropathy, frequently confused with HAM/TSP in the tropics, is primarily a proprioceptive myeloneuropathy often involving the optic and eighth nerves and only occasionally mild pyramidal signs (Chapter 8). Tropical ataxic neuropathy has been linked to the ingestion of cyanide glucosides, derived from inadequately dried cassava, among persons deficient in the amino acids essential for cyanide detoxification (methionine and cystine). Unlike HAM/TSP patients, those with tropical ataxic neuropathy may respond to nutritional and vitamin therapy.

TREATMENT. Researchers in Japan have reported that some persons with HAM/TSP improve when treated with corticosteroids or interferon. It has been suggested that treatment early in the course of HAM/TSP may be more effective than treatment later.

BIBLIOGRAPHY

Blattner WA: Retroviruses. *In* Evans AS (ed): Viral Infections of Humans: Epidemiology and Control. 3rd ed. New York, Plenum Publishing, 1989, pp. 545–592.
Knowles DM: The human T-cell leukemias: Clinical, cytomorphological, immunophenotypic, and genotypic characteristics. Hum Pathol 17:14, 1986.
Kuefler PR, Bunn PA: Adult T-cell leukemia/lymphoma. Clin Hematol 15:695, 1986.
Proceedings: Retroviruses in the nervous system. Ann Neurol 23(Suppl):1, 1988.
Roman GC, Vernant J-C, Osame M (eds): HTLV-I and the Nervous System. (Neurology and Neurobiology, Vol 51.) New York, Alan R. Liss, 1989.

16. VIRAL INFECTIONS WITH CUTANEOUS LESIONS

Joel G. Breman

16.1. MEASLES

DEFINITION. Measles (rubeola) is an acute, highly transmissible viral illness, usually of childhood, characterized by fever, a generalized maculopapular rash, cough, coryza, and conjunctivitis. The disease takes a heavy toll in many areas of the tropics because almost all unvaccinated children are afflicted before they reach 5 years of age and the case fatality rates range from 1% to 5% or greater.

ETIOLOGY AND HISTORY. Measles is a paramyxovirus. The virus has an outer envelope of glycoproteins and lipids and an internal core of single-stranded RNA. Measles virus strains are genetically stable and are the same throughout the world. This genotypic stability is due in part to the genome's having a single strand of RNA. The virus was first grown in human and monkey tissue culture by Enders and Peebles in 1954. Characteristic cytopathic effects occur in cell culture, i.e., formation of multinucleated giant cells, vacuolization in the syncytial cytoplasm, and the presence of eosinophilic intranuclear and intracytoplasmic inclusion bodies. These changes can be neutralized by measles antibody.

Measles virus is fragile under certain environmental conditions. Half the infectivity is lost every 2 hours at 37 C. The virus loses titer rapidly when exposed to light, while drying on fomites, and at pH 5. Lyophilization renders the virus more stable at higher temperatures, an important factor in vaccine preparation. Infective virions survive readily in droplet nuclei and can thus be spread effectively as an aerosol.

The clinical features of measles were described clearly by Rhazes, an eminent Persian physician (860–932 AD), who also quoted others who wrote on measles in the seventh century. The infective nature of the disease was considered by the British clinicians Sydenham in 1675 and Home in 1758. It was, however, Panum who, during his trip to the Faröe Islands in 1846, first clearly observed the epidemiologic characteristics of measles and later described these in a classic monograph. Panum reported person-to-person transmission, a 14-day incubation period, and lifelong immunity after infection.

The importance of measles in developing areas of the world was publicized by Morley and colleagues in the 1960s. They studied childhood illness in Imesi, Nigeria, a community of about 1800 persons. The mean age of measles patients was 15 months, the case-fatality rate was 7%, and the epidemics occurred in the dry season. Morley showed that the clinical and epidemiologic features of measles in Africa were similar to those observed in Scotland in the late 1800s. This was evidence against the theory that measles virus could mutate and become more virulent in Africa, a widely held view at the time.

Vaccine trials in Upper Volta in the early 1960s paved the way for mass vaccination campaigns against measles and smallpox in West and Central Africa. With the impetus of the eradication of smallpox, worldwide control of measles, diphtheria, pertussis, tetanus, poliomyelitis, and tuberculosis is now one of the major goals of the World Health Organization (WHO) coordinated Expanded Program on Immunization. The United States and several European countries have goals to eliminate indigenous measles.

DISTRIBUTION AND INCIDENCE. Measles is present throughout the world. Although the severity of measles in Africa and South America has been widely known for almost three decades, it is only more recently that the public health importance of this disease in Asia has been recognized. The number of cases and their geographic and age distribution depend on the size and density of the susceptible population, the birth rate, immigration of susceptible persons, contact patterns of the population, and previous exposure to measles or measles vaccine. Except among isolated populations, measles can be considered a universally acquired disease. If immunization is not given over a 5- to 10-year-period, the average incidence of measles in children approximates the birth rate minus the death rate due to other causes—up to the age when most children have acquired the disease. In developing countries with high birth rates (up to 50 per 1000 persons per year), the measles incidence was between 20 and 30 cases per 1000 persons per year before measles immunization activities. Only a small fraction of these cases, perhaps no more than 5% to 10%, were ever reported.

TRANSMISSION AND EPIDEMIOLOGY. Humans are the only reservoirs and vectors of measles. Both sexes are equally affected. It is transmitted person to person via respiratory droplets and droplet nuclei laden with measles virus; airborne transmission also may occur.

The disease is one of the most contagious infections. Approximately 90% of susceptible persons in close contact with a patient will develop measles. The required contact includes sleeping in the same room or sitting near someone with measles, as in a classroom, dispensary, or bus. Indeed, nosocomial transmission to both inpatients and outpatients has been reported. The most infectious period is during the pre-eruptive stage of illness; hence, the diagnosis can be missed easily when patients are shedding the largest quantities of virus.

The highest measles incidence, like that of most respiratory diseases, occurs in late winter and early spring in both temperate and tropical climates. Why this occurs is not understood, although in the tropics it has been ascribed to increased travel and more social contact during the "dry season" of winter and spring. Additionally, the pharyngeal membranes become dry and raw during these periods and may be more receptive to all respiratory pathogens.

To sustain measles transmission in a closed unvaccinated population (birth rate 20 to 40 per 1000 persons per year), at least 200,000 persons are needed to provide an adequate number of new susceptibles.

Developing Countries. With the beginning of vaccination programs, the mean age of measles onset in unvaccinated sub-Saharan African and South American populations was between 1 and 3 years in large cities and 2 and 4 years in rural areas, where close contact with other population groups was less frequent. In developing countries, young children are carried almost everywhere by their mothers and have close exposures to other children during the many daily social exchanges. In isolated populations, such as nomad groups or islanders, measles may occur throughout all age groups during an epidemic if the last exposure to the disease was many years previously. Recent studies have demonstrated an association between severity of measles and overcrowded conditions and intensity of exposure.

Maternal measles antibody is generally protective for an infant until 6 months of age. Children who develop the disease at less than 1 year are particularly vulnerable to the complications and to death from measles.

In large urban areas, an unvaccinated population will have endemic measles throughout the year, with peaks of measles activity at least once a year, usually in the spring. In small towns and villages there will be large outbreaks in an unvaccinated population every 2 to 3 years. This occurs most often after the disease is introduced into the newly susceptible infant group, born since the last outbreak. Large population centers are often responsible for seeding villages with measles.

Developed Countries. The mean age of attack is over 5 years because of the nature of social contact. Transmission often occurs at school, and the disease is also propagated at home. As the incidence of measles decreases in the United States, outbreaks have occurred in students between 10 and 14 years and also in special population groups, e.g., military recruits, nursery school members, and immigrants. Importations have become of greatest importance as the national incidence approaches zero. In some developed countries, there have been outbreaks in nursery care facilities (crèches). These groups have become more important epidemiologically, and special strategies are required to keep them free from measles.

PATHOGENESIS AND PATHOLOGY. Measles is a systemic infection. Virus particles enter lymphoid tissue in the respiratory tract of persons having close (usually face-to-face) contact with a patient. In the pharynx, virus is ingested by cells of the tonsils, adenoids, and lymph nodes. Hyperplasia of the reticuloendothelial (RE) system occurs. The virus multiplies and disseminates via the blood stream. Large multinucleated giant cells are observed in the RE system (Fig. 16–1), as well as in the pharyngeal and bronchial mucosa.

Immunosuppression. Leukopenia occurs during the incubation period. With the onset of the prodome, virus can be found in the throat, tears, nasal secretions, urine, and blood. At this time, anergy develops in the form of suppressed dermal reactions to many skin test antigens. Anergy may last up to 1 month and may be due to destruction of lymphocytes in which measles virus grows. Pre-existing tuberculosis may be exacerbated as a result of the suppression of delayed hypersensitivity.

Pathologic Findings. Koplik spots appear on the buccal mucous membrane after 2 or 3 days. These nucleocapsid-containing bluish white spots are above the molars and surrounded by erythema. Until recently, they were considered pathognomonic for measles, but other viral infections can cause similar lesions. Nucleocapsid structures can also be found in the early macular lesions of the skin as well as in the Koplik spots. An acute mononuclear inflammatory reaction occurs in the macules, beginning at the time circulating antibody is detectable in the skin or blood.

Immunity. IgG and IgM antibodies become detectable at about the time the rash begins. The IgM antibody level peaks at about 10 days after the appearance of the rash and is no longer detectable after 1 month; the IgG titer peaks at about 30 days and then drops by 2 to 4 fold at 6 months following the illness, after which antibody levels remain stable. Although humoral antibody levels are an important indicator of protection, cellular immunity undoubtedly plays an important role in clearing the virus. Immunity to measles is lifelong.

CLINICAL MANIFESTATIONS

Acute Illness. The incubation period of measles is about 10 to 12 days, with a range of from 8 to 18 days. The classic signs of cough, conjunctivitis, and coryza begin almost simultaneously, with a concurrent temperature rise to 38 to 40 C. Diarrhea is a frequent sign of measles in young children, especially those who are poorly nourished. Measles is an excellent example of the synergism between infection and poor nutrition. This is most often manifested by rapidly developing protein-calorie malnutrition associated with chronic diarrhea if treatment is not prompt.

The relatively nonproductive cough increases in severity as the rash develops to its fullest. The cough lasts the entire illness, about 7 to 10 days. The illness may be more prolonged in younger, more debilitated children. Coryza and nonpurulent conjunctivitis, occasionally accompanied by photophobia, continue to day 6 to 8 of the illness. Koplik spots begin on day 2 and usually remain 4 days or less. They must be searched for toward the back of the buccal mucosa, above or to the side of the molars. The maculopapular rash of measles begins on about the third day of illness (range 1 to 7 days). It first appears on the upper face and head and then spreads inferiorly during the next 2 or 3 days (Fig. 73–5K). The child is most ill during day 2 to 4 of the rash, until the elevated temperature (40 to 41 C) subsides. In black children, the sandpaper-like texture of the skin can be used in diagnosis, particularly at the start of the illness.

When the rash is totally coalescent, desquamation may occur. This begins toward the end of the first week of illness and can last through the following week (Fig. 16–2). Anorexia and malaise are common throughout the illness, and generalized lymphadenopathy may be present in severe cases. For most patients, the signs and symptoms begin to abate rapidly when the temperature falls on day 4 or 5. Recovery is usually complete within 10 to 14 days after onset of illness.

Complications. Case-fatality rates from measles vary, depending on the age and nutritional status of the

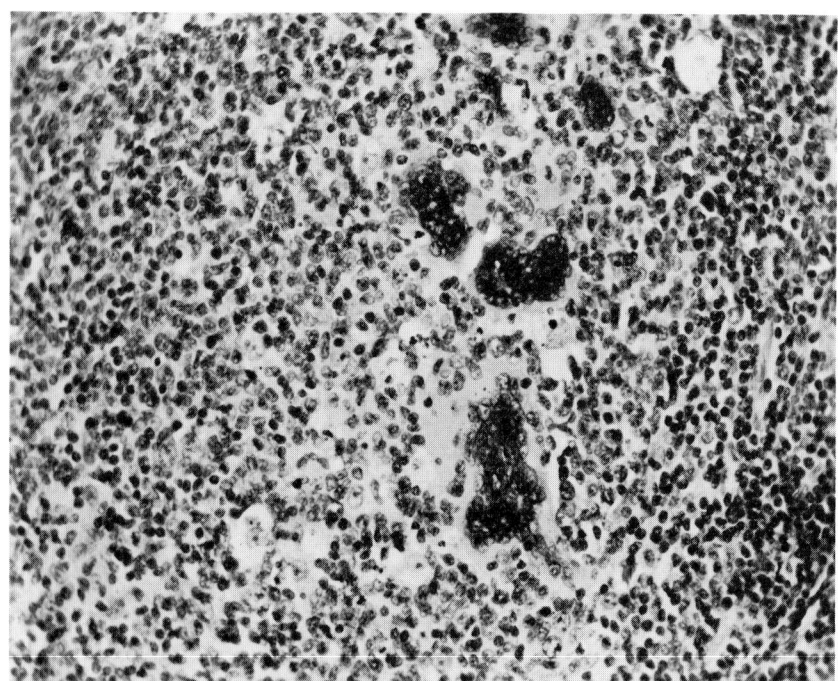

FIGURE 16–1. Lymph node from patient with measles showing Warthin-Finkeldey giant cells in reactive center (× 260). (Courtesy of Armed Forces Institute of Pathology, Photograph Neg. No. 57-1921.)

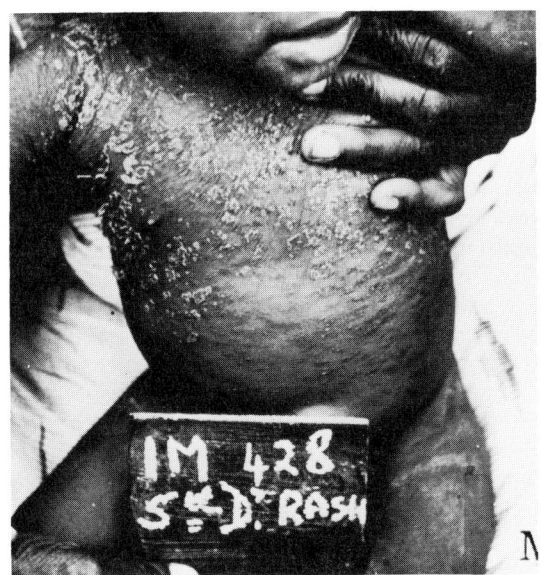

FIGURE 16–2. Desquamation on fifth day of rash due to measles in black child. (Courtesy of Institute of Child Health, D. Morley.)

patient and the type and severity of intercurrent infection. In developed countries, the case-fatality rate is probably about 1:1000 patients. In West Africa, Asia, and South America it has been reported as high as 25% but is usually between 1 and 5%. High rates are usually reported from hospitals where the most severe cases are treated. Death is usually due to bacterial pneumonia (caused by *S. pneumoniae* or *H. influenzae*), diarrhea, or malnutrition. A rare primary interstitial pneumonia with widespread giant cell infiltration can be caused by measles; this complication occurs most frequently in association with other debilitating diseases or in immunocompromised individuals, e.g., with leukemia.

The most frequent complication is otitis media, which should be suspected when fever is prolonged. Pneumonia, due to either the measles virus or a superimposed bacterial infection, is a frequent and life-threatening complication. Laryngitis or laryngotracheitis may cause airway obstruction and requires prompt tracheostomy if respiration is severely impaired. Mastoiditis due to chronic otitis media can occur if antibiotics are not used. Acute ("postinfectious") encephalitis occurs in 0.1 to 0.4% of all cases. It usually begins on day 2 to 6 after the onset of rash. The course varies between mild and rapidly fulminant, with death occurring within 24 hours in the latter instance. About 15% of patients with acute encephalitis die, and 25% later develop mental retardation, seizures, or behavioral and learning disorders. Neurologic involvement is probably more prevalent than is indicated by the incidence of overt postinfectious encephalitis; electroencephalographic changes and cerebrospinal fluid pleocytosis during the acute illness as well as subtle neurologic residua (behavioral changes) have been described in association with classic measles.

Stomatitis is frequent and may interfere with eating. Severe debilitating diarrhea and chronic malnutrition as a consequence of measles are common and contribute to stunted growth and death. Cancrum oris, a painful oral lesion developing concurrently with measles, is a frequent complication. Xerophthalmia and keratomalacia leading to blindness may occur when there is vitamin A deficiency due to measles-induced malnutrition. There is now overwhelming evidence that children with corneal scarring typical of vitamin A deficiency have a history of measles immediately preceding eye damage. Electrocardiographic alterations may occur, but clinically important myocarditis is rare. Measles acquired during the first trimester of pregnancy may result in fetal death; however, congenital abnormalities (as seen in rubella) are not reported.

Subacute sclerosing panencephalitis is a poorly understood late complication of measles. Progressive behavioral changes and intellectual deterioration are usually associated with motor incoordination. Death frequently occurs within 6 months of symptom onset. Among the typical laboratory findings are an extremely high serum measles antibody titer and antibody in the cerebrospinal fluid.

As with many viral illnesses, measles is generally more severe in infants and older persons.

DIAGNOSIS. The diagnosis is straightforward when several children in a community have fever, cough, conjunctivitis, coryza, and a morbilliform rash without a prior history of measles or vaccination.

Differential Diagnosis. Common diseases to consider in the differential diagnosis are drug eruptions (penicillin- and sulfonamide-containing drugs in particular), rubella, and enteroviruses (ECHO 9 and 16 and coxsackieviruses 4, 6, and 9). Rubella has a briefer and milder course, with more prominent posterior cervical and generalized lymphadenitis. Other diseases with a maculopapular eruption that can resemble measles are meningococcemia, scarlet fever, typhus and tick fevers, and infectious mononucleosis. However, none of these syndromes has the triad of cough, conjunctivitis, and coryza or the descending morbilliform eruption.

In the tropics, papulovesicular eruptions may occasionally be confused with measles. These most often include insect bites or impetigo due to *Staphylococcus* or *Streptococcus*. It is wise to recall that secondary syphilis may mimic just about any rash, but this is not usually a childhood disease.

Laboratory Diagnosis. During the prodromal and early phase of illness associated with rash, large multinucleated ("giant") cells may be demonstrated in stained smears of sputum or urine. Serologic testing of acute and convalescent sera for measles antibodies is the best method for confirmation of the diagnosis, but this may not always be possible. A significant rise in titer 3 weeks after the initial infection is confirmatory. Detection of measles antibody within 1 to 2 days of disease onset indicates previous contact with measles or vaccine and the need to seek another cause for the illness. Measles virus may be isolated from either the blood or the nasopharyngeal secretions during the initial days of infection, but isolation of virus is rarely indicated for making the diagnosis. In measles encephalitis, the cerebrospinal fluid contains elevated protein levels and up to 1000 mononuclear cells per mm^3.

TREATMENT AND PROGNOSIS. There is no specific treatment for measles. Alert supportive care is needed, as complications such as pneumonia and diarrhea may present abruptly, especially in younger children. Rest, hydration, adequate nutrition, antipyretics, antitussives, and meticulous attention to prevention of bacterial complications are advised. The eyes should be carefully rinsed daily with sterile saline solution or, lacking this, with clean water. There should be daily examination for otitis media, bacterial pneumonia, and skin infections. Antibiotics must be given at once if these complications occur. WHO and UNICEF recommend high-dose vitamin A supplementation (200,000 IU) for all children diagnosed with measles in communities where vitamin A deficiency is a recognized problem and where the case fatality rate from measles is ≥1%. In the rare case of postmeasles encephalitis, general supportive care is needed, including anticonvulsant drugs. Gamma globulin and corticosteroids have been assessed but offer no advantage in the treatment of clinical measles or its complications.

PREVENTION AND CONTROL

Immunization. Passive immunization with gamma globulin (0.25 mg/kg, maximum dose 15 ml) is effective in preventing measles if given within 6 days of exposure. This is recommended to protect pregnant women, immunosuppressed patients (0.5 mg/kg, maximum dose 15 ml), and others at high risk, e.g., those with tuberculosis, but is rarely possible in tropical countries. Measles vaccine is one of the safest and most effective of the vaccines. Ninety-five percent or more of susceptible persons will develop HI antibodies after immunization with a potent vaccine. HI antibodies fall off relatively slowly after 1 or 2 years and persist for more than 15 years after vaccination. The rate of seroconversion among malnourished children is generally good. Protection following vaccination is probably lifelong. Recent promising trials with the Edmonston-Zagreb strain of measles vaccine may enable successful immunization of infants 4 to 5 months old or younger.

Measles antibody is transferred transplacentally. Maternal antibody may last as long as 1 year in some infants, and its presence will interfere with development of seroconversion after vaccination. The age at which maternal antibody disappears varies somewhat in different areas of the world; many children in tropical countries lose maternal antibody 3 to 6 months earlier than those in developed countries. There are probably multiple reasons for this, none completely understood, although the local epidemiology of measles may play an important role.

Because the case-fatality rates are so high in young children in developing countries, it is advised that they be vaccinated as soon as feasible after 9 months of age. The practice in some areas is to immunize children during outbreaks. Children who are immunized at less than 9 months of age should receive a second immunization to increase assurance of protection. In developed countries, in which the average age for measles is above 5 years and the case-fatality rates are relatively low, vaccination should begin at 12 to 15 months of age.

Measles vaccination should be integrated into a permanent community and nationwide immunization program that is part of an effective primary health care system. Adequate record keeping and follow-up should assure that all childhood immunizations are given. Emphasis on maintenance vaccination is important so that newborns, immigrants, and other susceptible persons are protected after the initial campaigns. When mass vaccination campaigns are employed, it is essential to provide routine services to maintain or improve coverage after the short-term activities associated with campaigns. Nosocomial transmission can be averted through immunization of all susceptible outpatients and selected inpatients; hospital staff at all times should take full advantage of the opportunity to immunize children.

Other Measures. Quarantine is usually ineffective in controlling measles, since transmission most often occurs before the onset of rash and before a diagnosis is made.

BIBLIOGRAPHY

Aaby P, Bukh J, Hoff G, et al: High measles mortality in infancy related to intensity of exposure. J Pediatr 109:40, 1986.

Foster A, Sommer A: Corneal ulceration, measles and childhood blindness in Tanzania. Br J Ophthalmol 71:331, 1987.

Gordon JE, Jansen AAJ, Ascoli W: Measles in rural Guatemala. J Pediatr 66:779, 1965.

Halsey NA: The optimal age for measles vaccination in developing countries. *In* Halsey NA, de Quadros CA (eds): Recent Advances in Immunization. A Bibliographic Review. Washington, DC: Pan American Health Organization (Publication 451), 1983.

Halsey NA, Boulos R, Mode F, et al: Response to measles vaccine in Haitian infants 6 to 12 months old. Influence of maternal antibodies, malnutrition and concurrent illnesses. N Engl J Med 313:544, 1985.

Hinman AF, Brandling-Bennett DA, Bernier RH, et al: Current features of measles in the United States: feasibility of measles elimination. Epidemiol Rev 2:153, 1980.

Hopkins DR, Koplan JP, Hinman AR, et al: The case for global measles eradication. Lancet 2:1596, 1982.

John TJ, Joseph A, George TI, et al: Epidemiology and prevention of measles in rural south India. Indian J Med Res 72:153, 1980.

Khanum S, Uddin N, Garelick H, et al: Comparison of Edmonston-Zagreb and Schwarz strains of measles vaccine given by aerosol or subcutaneous injection. Lancet 1:150, 1987.

Klein-Zabban ML, Foulon G, Gaudebout C, et al: Frequence des rougeoles nosocomiales dans un centre de protection maternelle et infantile d'Abidjan. Bull WHO 65:197, 1987.

Koster FT, Curlin GC, Aziz KMA, et al: Synergistic impact of measles and diarrhea on nutrition and mortality in Bangladesh. Bull WHO 59:901, 1981.

Krugman S: Further attenuated measles vaccine: Characteristics and use. Rev Infect Dis 5:477, 1983.

Markowitz LE, Preblud SR, Orenstein WA, et al: Patterns of transmission in measles outbreaks in the United States, 1985–1986. N Engl J Med 320:75, 1989.

Morley D: Severe measles in the tropics. Br Med J 1:297, 1969.

Morley D, Woodland M, Martin WJ: Measles in Nigerian children. J Hyg (Cambr) 61:115, 1963.

Scrimshaw NS, Salomon JB, Bruch HA, et al: Studies of diarrheal disease in Central America. VIII. Measles, diarrhea and nutritional deficiency in rural Guatemala. Am J Trop Med Hyg 15:625, 1966.

Walsh JA: Selective primary health care: Strategies for control of disease in the developing world. 4. Measles. Rev Infect Dis 5:330, 1983.

16.2 POXVIRUSES: VARIOLA, VACCINIA, MONKEYPOX, TANAPOX

VARIOLA (SMALLPOX)

DEFINITION. Before its eradication, smallpox was an acute exanthematous viral infection having a 2- to 4-day febrile prodrome followed by a characteristic rash. Variola major was the most severe form of the disease with death occurring in about 20% of patients, whereas variola minor (alastrim) had a case-fatality rate of less than 2%. Cases of endemic smallpox have not occurred anywhere in the world since October 1977, and the disease was declared eradicated by the World Health Organization (WHO) in May 1980. This was the result of an intensified program to eradicate smallpox that began in 1967 and was coordinated by WHO.

DISTRIBUTION. Smallpox was a widespread disease. In 1947, 85 countries reported cases; in 1967, when the intensified global eradication program began, 47 countries still reported smallpox and 33 of these were endemic. Whereas two thirds of the endemic countries were in Africa, 75% of the cases occurred in India, which then had a population of close to 500 million people. More than 131,000 cases were reported worldwide in 1967, but reporting efficiency was probably less than 1%; 10 to 15 million cases may have actually occurred that year. The last case of endemic smallpox occurred in October 1977 in Merka, Somalia. In August 1978, two cases occurred in Birmingham, England, but these were associated with a laboratory in which variola virus was kept.

TRANSMISSION AND EPIDEMIOLOGY. Humans were the only reservoirs and vectors of smallpox, a critical factor favoring eradication. The disease was usually spread by respiratory droplets. The secondary attack rates among close unvaccinated household contacts was 25 to 40%, indicating that the disease was not as contagious as influenza, measles, or chickenpox. This observation, coupled with the relatively long 2-week incubation period, showed that the disease was less explosive than previously thought. Prompt, carefully planned, and sustained intervention could interrupt transmission in a relatively short time, even in populations in whom the immunity level was low, and under the most difficult field conditions.

Smallpox afflicted persons of all ages and both sexes. Higher attack rates occurred in younger children, but only because they were more often unvaccinated.

There were fluctuations of cases during the year, but most countries had distinct seasonal patterns. Incidence of the disease in the tropics was highest in the dry season.

CLINICAL MANIFESTATIONS

Usual Syndrome. The incubation period for smallpox was 10 to 12 days (range 7 to 17 days). Fever (as high as 39 to 41 C) and severe headache, backache, and malaise occurred during the 2- to 4-day prodrome. This was followed by the eruption, which began on the face and upper extremities. Most lesions evolved through similar stages, i.e., macules, papules, vesicles, and pus-

tules, over an 8- to 15-day period; they grew to about 0.5 cm in diameter and were fixed to the deep layers of the skin. The pustules umbilicated, dried, and began to desquamate between day 6 to 10 of rash, followed by the crusting or scab stage. All crusts were usually separated by the end of week 3.

The rash was concentrated mainly on the periphery, a cardinal point of differentiation between smallpox and chickenpox. In the severe form, lesions occurred on the palms of the hands and soles of the feet. Fever usually dropped 2 to 3 days after the onset of rash, but rose again 4 to 6 days later before leveling off during the desquamation and recovery phase. After desquamation, the lesions were hypopigmented, then darkened over the next several months. Disfigurement due to pitting, or pock marking, was most common over facial areas with heavily concentrated sebaceous glands. The hyperpigmentation gradually faded and the pitting may have flattened out. There were clinical variations, from very mild disease to hemorrhagic forms, but these were the exceptions.

Immunity. Complement fixation (CF), HI, and neutralizing antibody titers rose within the first 5 to 10 days after infection; CF and HI antibodies began to drop after 30 to 60 days but were sometimes detected for many months or years. Neutralizing antibody titers continued to rise for 4 to 8 weeks and, as a rule, persisted for several years. Cellular immunity probably played the major protective role in orthopoxvirus infections. Second attacks of smallpox were virtually unknown.

DIAGNOSIS. During large outbreaks, smallpox was easily diagnosed because the clinical presentation was typical and several cases were often seen at about the same time. As the disease became rarer, the diagnosis on clinical grounds alone became more difficult.

Differential Diagnosis. More than 95% of the diagnostic problems have been related to confusing chickenpox with smallpox.

Other common conditions that have been confused with smallpox include drug reactions, insect bites, secondary syphilis, and measles. Monkeypox (described below) is an infrequent disease that cannot be distinguished from smallpox on clinical grounds, but is different epidemiologically.

Despite the characteristic clinical picture of measles (see Figs. 16–2 and 73–5K), it is occasionally confused with smallpox. This is usually because of the high case-fatality rates measles causes in developing countries.

Laboratory Diagnosis. As smallpox has been eradicated, the diagnosis of a highly suspect case will probably turn out to be one of the other diseases mentioned above or another illness that causes a rash. If the diagnosis is in doubt and smallpox cannot be excluded, scrapings of skin lesions and serum specimens should be collected and sent with advance notification to a suitably equipped WHO Collaborating Center (Viral Exanthems and Herpesvirus Branch, Division of Viral Diseases, Center for Infectious Diseases, Centers for Disease Control, Atlanta, Georgia 30333, USA; Laboratory of Smallpox Prophylaxis, Research Institute of Viral Preparations, Moscow, USSR). Testing is by electron microscopy, viral culture, biochemical identification of virus, and serologic analysis.

TREATMENT AND PROGNOSIS. There is no specific treatment for smallpox. Supportive care is essential to assure survival of patients and to prevent disfiguring complications. Topical idoxuridine (IDUR) (Dendrid, Herplex, Stoxil) should be used for corneal involvement.

Case-fatality rates were about 20% for those who had the "ordinary" type of rash caused by variola major in Asia and was about 10% in West and Central Africa. Less than 2% of persons died of variola minor, a form recently seen in South and East Africa and in Brazil. Residual pitting scars developed on the face in about two thirds of those with variola major.

PREVENTION AND CONTROL

Vaccination. Smallpox vaccine is one of the most effective immunizing agents. The current vaccines are made from vaccinia virus. When the accelerated WHO smallpox eradication program began in 1967, fewer than one third of the vaccine batches in use met these standards.

Within 4 years, the WHO program switched from the mass vaccination strategy, whereby the goal was to cover 80% of the entire population in a country, irrespective of the location of smallpox cases, to that of vigorous and prompt case detection and containment. Selective epidemiologic surveillance and containment were used throughout all endemic areas in Africa and Asia by the mid-1970s. Tens of thousands of surveillance workers actively searched for cases in high-risk areas until every last focus was identified and eliminated. The last case of endemic smallpox occurred in South America (Brazil) in 1971, in Asia (Bangladesh) in 1975, and in Africa (Somalia) in 1977.

In 1980, with the eradication of smallpox, WHO recommended discontinuing vaccination. This came after a careful 2-year study by the International Commission for the Certification of Smallpox Eradication, charged with evaluating whether smallpox eradication had been achieved. The risk of complications from the vaccine, although small, completely outweighed the nonexistent risk from endemic smallpox. However, laboratories working with orthopoxviruses should have their personnel vaccinated and apply strict measures to assure containment of variola virus strains. The real danger to laboratory workers was shown by laboratory-associated cases of smallpox that occurred in England in 1973 and 1978. As of 1989, there were 2 WHO collaborating center laboratories still retaining smallpox virus (the Soviet Union and the United States). Strict containment of these strains is the responsibility of national authorities and WHO.

Surveillance. The eradication of smallpox has been one of the greatest public health achievements and an example for other programs. During the posteradication period, WHO has promoted surveillance for human monkeypox and other diseases resembling smallpox to ensure that eradication has been achieved and to maintain public confidence. Research is still in progress on variola virus and the closely related orthopoxviruses to better define the biology and ecology of these agents.

VACCINIA

Vaccinia is an orthopoxvirus that is genetically distinct from variola virus (Table 16–1). Jenner's original vaccine is thought to have been cowpox, but the exact origin of the strains of vaccine used subsequently and of vaccinia virus is obscure. Vaccinia virus is widely used in biomedical research. However, its traditional role has been to protect against smallpox. Current research with vaccinia concerns its possible role as a carrier of other antigens. Indeed, there have been at least 35 strains of vaccinia virus studied during this century, and several have been used as vaccines against smallpox. In addition to an incomplete pedigree of many of these vaccine strains, there are known differences in pathogenicity in biologic systems, in adverse effects following vaccination in humans, and in genetic composition. The Lister strain and the New York City Board of Health strains of vaccinia are among the most extensively studied for adverse effects in people and are considered safe for vaccination; thus, they have been recommended as seed strains for vaccine production. With the increased use of vaccinia virus as a vector of foreign genes, it is important to develop guidelines for using standard vaccinia strains in modern research.

SMALLPOX VACCINATION. The vaccination can be given by the multiple puncture method or by the Ped-O-Jet injector, a needleless vaccination apparatus. The bifurcated needle for vaccine administration was widely used during the WHO eradication program and gave higher rates of effective immunization (and used less vaccine) than other methods. The needle is dipped into reconstituted vaccine, and a drop stays between the needle's prongs. The needle is pushed rapidly into about a 0.25-cm radius area in the dermis of the upper arm; 15 punctures are advised for a primary vaccination or a revaccination. Until abandonment of vaccination, revaccination every 3 years was recommended, although protection following immunization against smallpox lasted at least 10 years.

Vaccination Complications. Vaccination has few complications, but since smallpox is now eradicated, it is not justified except for those at special risk, such as laboratory investigators working with variola or other orthopoxviruses pathogenic for humans. Important complications are postvaccinal encephalitis, generalized vaccinia, autoinoculation of the eye, eczema vaccinatum, and painful local reactions at the site of vaccination. The rate of all complications from smallpox vaccination was about 750 per 10 million primary vaccinations. About four cases of encephalitis and one death occurred

TABLE 16–1. Members of the Genus Orthopoxvirus

Virus	Host
Camelpox	Camels
Cowpox	Bovines or rodents
Ectromelia	Mice
Monkeypox	Squirrels or monkeys
Turkmenia rodentpox	Wild rodents
Vaccinia	Unknown
Variola	Humans

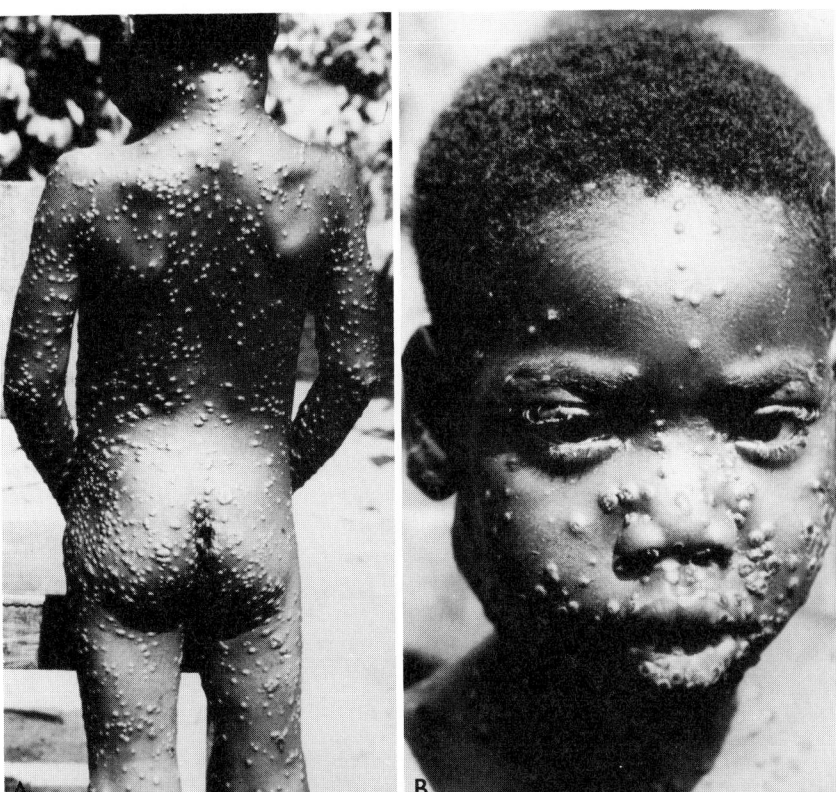

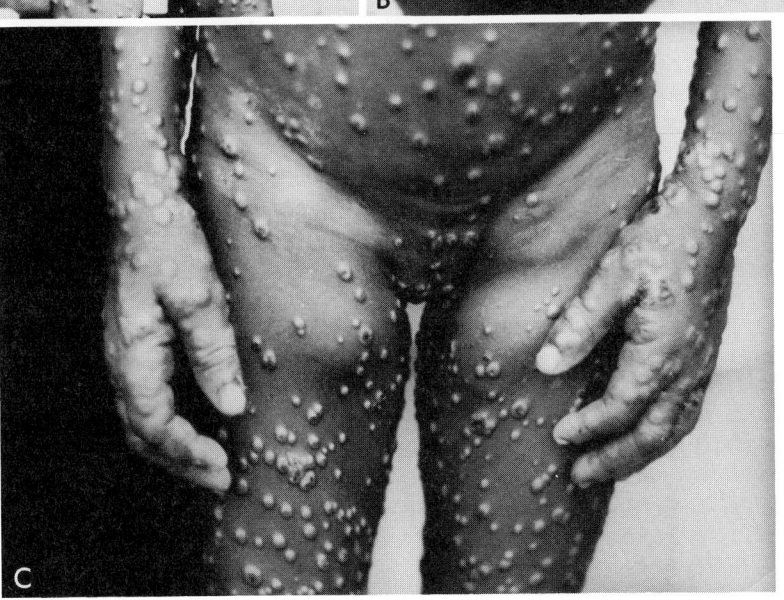

FIGURE 16–3. Monkeypox on eighth day of rash. *A*, The eruption resembles smallpox. *B*, Lesions on eyelid, nares, and lips. *C*, Note inguinal lymphadenopathy and dense concentration of lesions on hands. (Courtesy of World Health Organization, M. Szczeniowski.)

per 10 million primary vaccinations. The rates of complications are much lower for persons being revaccinated.

Vaccinia immune globulin (VIG) is used for severe vaccination complications, e.g., eczema vaccinatum, progressive or severe generalized vaccinia, or vaccinia of the eye, at a dose of 0.6 ml/kg of body weight, given intramuscularly. Other drugs are not beneficial, except for IDUR, mentioned earlier in regard to autoinoculation of the eye.

Smallpox vaccine has not been shown to be effective for warts or herpetic lesions, conditions for which the vaccine has been erroneously used.

MONKEYPOX

Monkeypox virus is genetically distinct from other orthopoxviruses. Human monkeypox was first discovered in Zaire in 1970.

EPIDEMIOLOGY AND TRANSMISSION. Before 1989, more than 400 cases of human monkeypox were reported from West and Central Africa and over 95% of them occurred in Zaire. This disease resembles smallpox clinically (Fig. 16–3). Detection of the first cases was worrisome because they were found in areas where smallpox transmission had been eliminated. The causative agent is called monkeypox because the virus was

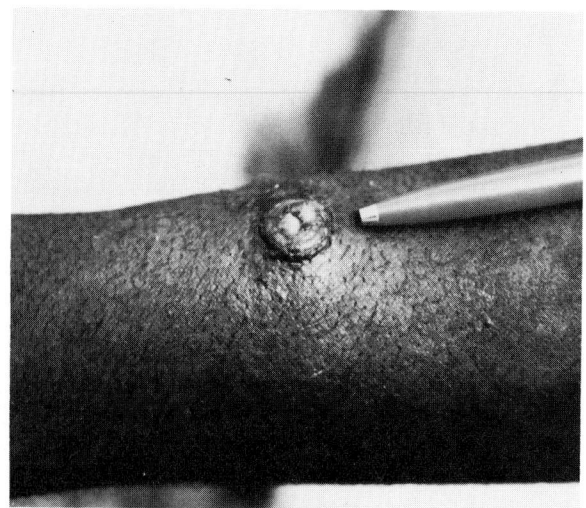

FIGURE 16–4. Solitary tanapox lesion on arm, 10 days after onset. (Courtesy of World Health Organization, M. Szczeniowski.)

first isolated from nonhuman primates in laboratories between 1958 and 1968. The virus has recently been isolated from a squirrel captured in the wild; however, the natural cycle of monkeypox virus is unknown. This disease does not represent a danger to the smallpox eradication program because of its infrequent occurrence and poor transmission rates.

CLINICAL MANIFESTATIONS. The major clinical and epidemiologic differences between smallpox and monkeypox are (1) pronounced postauricular, submandibular, cervical, and inguinal lymphadenopathy in a large majority of patients with monkeypox, not noted with smallpox (Fig. 16–3C); (2) occurrence of monkeypox cases in small forest villages in West and Central Africa, whereas smallpox was cosmopolitan; (3) predominance of children with monkeypox (median age of 4 years), whereas smallpox would affect unvaccinated persons of all age groups; (4) relatively poor interhuman transmission of monkeypox; the secondary attack rate in susceptible family contacts is about 10% as compared with 25 to 40% for smallpox; and (5) interhuman spread to a fourth generation is rare with monkeypox; smallpox spread was by continuous person-to-person transmission. The case-fatality rate for monkeypox has been about 10%, the same rate as seen previously with smallpox in this area. Vaccination protects against monkeypox.

Field and laboratory research continues on monkeypox and closely related poxviruses in order to find the natural cycle of monkeypox virus, to confirm that there is no animal reservoir of smallpox, and to monitor other poxvirus diseases that might menace humans in the future.

TANAPOX

Tanapox is an unclassified poxvirus that is not a member of the orthopoxvirus group. It causes a single or, rarely, two papulovesicular lesions, usually on the extremities (Fig. 16–4). Persons with this disease have

been found only in Kenya (the Tana River Valley) and Zaire. The virus is difficult to culture; clinical, epidemiologic, and serologic information is needed to confirm the diagnosis. The natural reservoir and vector are unknown, although it is speculated that mosquitoes may be involved because more cases seem to occur during the rainy season in populations living along the banks of flooding rivers.

BIBLIOGRAPHY

Breman JG, Kalisa Ruti, Steniowski MV, et al: Human monkeypox, 1970–1979. Bull WHO 58:665, 1980.
Breman JG, Arita IA: The confirmation and maintenance of smallpox eradication. N Engl J Med 303:1262, 1980.
Esposito JJ, Murphy FA: Infectious recombinant vectored virus vaccines. *In* Bittle JL, Murphy FA (eds): Vaccine Biotechnology: Advances in Veterinary Science and Comparative Medicine (Vol 33). San Diego, Academic Press, 1988, pp 196–247.
Fenner F, Henderson DA, Arita I, et al: Smallpox and Its Eradication. Geneva, WHO, 1988.
Fenner F, Wittek R, Dumbell K: The Orthopoxviruses. San Diego, Academic Press, 1989.
Foege WH, Millar JD, Lane JM: Selective epidemiologic control in smallpox eradication. Am J Epidemiol, 93:311, 1971.
Jezek Z, Szczeniowski M, Paluku KM, et al: Human monkeypox: Clinical features of 282 patients. J Infect Dis 156:293, 1987.
Khodakevich L, Szczeniowski M, Mambu-ma-Disu, et al: The role of squirrels in sustaining monkeypox virus transmission. Trop Geogr Med 39:115, 1987.
Lane JM, Ruben FL, Neff JM, et al: Complications of smallpox vaccination, 1968. N Engl J Med, 281:1201, 1969.

17. VIRAL RESPIRATORY INFECTIONS

Stephen Berman

Acute viral respiratory infections are the most frequent type of self-limited childhood illness throughout the world. A small percentage of these infections progress to severe and even fatal disease (Chapter 1). In children less than 5 years living in the developing world, approximately 1 in 400 cases of respiratory syncytial virus (RSV) infection and 1 in 600 cases of parainfluenza virus infection result in death (Table 17–1). More than 4 million children under the age of 5 years die of pneumonia annually. This number represents 30% of the 14.25 million childhood deaths that occur in the developing world each year. The relative importance and interactive role of viruses and bacteria related to this high respiratory mortality rate are unclear. The most important viral respiratory pathogens are RSV; parainfluenza viruses 1, 2, and 3; influenza viruses A and B; and adenovirus. RSV is the most frequent cause of lower respiratory infection during infancy and early childhood, whereas influenza is the most important pathogen in older groups.

The viral respiratory pathogens infect and disrupt the epithelial lining of the respiratory tract. The inflammatory response produces increased airway secretions, vascular engorgement, and smooth muscle contraction. This results in airway obstruction. It is uncertain whether

TABLE 17–1. Frequency With Which Viral Pathogens Result in Severe Disease and Death

Clinical Severity of ARI*	Relative Frequencies of Viral Infections by Clinical Severity	
	RSV	Parainfluenza Viruses
Upper respiratory infection (common cold)	300	500
Lower respiratory infection not needing hospitalization	100	100
Lower respiratory infection needing hospitalization	10	10
Death	1 (0.24%)	1 (0.16%)

From Institute of Medicine: New Vaccine Development, Establishing Priorities. Volume II: Diseases of Importance in Developing Countries. Washington, DC, National Academy Press, 1986.

*Acute respiratory infection.

viral infection predisposes to secondary bacterial pneumonia. The site and severity of the viral infection determine the clinical manifestations. The clinical manifestations are used to classify respiratory infections into clinical syndromes.

CLINICAL SYNDROMES

Acute viral infections are classified into clinical syndromes that reflect lower, middle, or upper respiratory tract involvement. When multiple areas of the respiratory tract are infected, there is considerable overlap. Acute viral respiratory infections initially present with upper respiratory tract findings because the portal of entry is the nose, mouth, or eyes. Progression of the infection to the middle and lower tract usually occurs within 2 to 4 days. Any viral respiratory agent can produce any of the clinical syndromes. The three syndromes can be manifested initially by nonspecific symptoms of cough, fever, malaise, and anorexia.

LOWER RESPIRATORY TRACT SYNDROMES. The viral lower respiratory tract syndromes are pneumonia and bronchiolitis, which usually present as rapid breathing and retractions. Pneumonia (inflammation of the pulmonary interstitial space or alveoli) is often associated with auscultatory findings of rales or crepitations. Brochiolitis (inflammation of the small airways or bronchioles) presents as wheezing due to airway obstruction. Rales or crepitations may also be heard in cases with bronchiolitis because of atelectasis distal to bronchiolar mucus plugging.

MIDDLE RESPIRATORY TRACT SYNDROMES. The viral middle respiratory syndromes are acute laryngitis, laryngotracheobronchitis (LTB, croup), and tracheobronchitis. Laryngitis presents with hoarseness. Laryngotracheobronchitis presents with hoarseness, barking cough, and stridor. Tracheobronchitis is difficult to diagnose and is associated with the auscultatory finding of rhonchi, a harsh respiratory sound. Rhonchi are often difficult to clinically distinguish from sounds related to nasal congestion or discharge transmitted from the upper airway. Older children and adults with tracheobronchitis may cough up purulent sputum, but this finding is not present in young children.

UPPER RESPIRATORY TRACT SYNDROMES. The viral upper respiratory syndromes are acute rhinitis, pharyngitis, tonsillitis, sinusitis, and otitis media. Rhinitis (inflammation of the nasal mucosa) presents with nasal congestion and discharge. The discharge is frequently purulent for several days. Pharyngitis and tonsillitis present with sore throat. The pharynx and tonsils appear injected and may have exudate. Sinusitis and otitis media may initially be related to a primary viral infection but usually indicate secondary bacterial infection. Sinusitis presents with cough, fever, purulent nasal discharge, and bad breath. Headache and pain over the face are more common in older patients than in children with sinusitis. In the absence of ear discharge, otitis media, or inflammation of the middle ear space, is diagnosed best with pneumatic otoscopy.

ETIOLOGY

RSV causes 15 to 20%, parainfluenza viruses 7 to 10%, influenza viruses 5%, and adenovirus 2 to 4% of lower respiratory infections seen in children in both outpatient and inpatient settings (Table 17–2).

RSV. RSV is the most frequent cause of pediatric lower respiratory infections in developing countries. In children under 5 years, RSV infections are 2 to 4 times more frequent than other viral respiratory agents. Although RSV infections occur throughout childhood, the incidence is highest in the first 2 years of life. Primary RSV infection in the first 6 months of life often results in severe lower respiratory illness with bronchiolitis or pneumonia, or both. Subsequent reinfection usually produces less severe illness because infection provides partial immunity. Transmission of RSV is by contact or droplet spread, the nose, eyes, and mouth being the portals of entry. RSV can survive on hard surfaces and be transmitted by fomites.

In most developing countries, RSV appears to have characteristic epidemic peaks of activity that recur at yearly intervals. However, the seasonal pattern of these peaks varies in different areas of the world. In temperate climates the peaks occur during the winter months. In tropical areas the peaks follow no common pattern and can occur during wet or dry seasons. An epidemic of bronchiolitis and pneumonia that primarily affects infants is a strong indication of RSV activity in the community.

INFLUENZA VIRUSES. Influenza viral infections have a worldwide distribution and tend to produce illness in older children and adults. The incubation period for influenza is 18 to 72 hours. Person-to-person transmission is principally by small-particle aerosols generated by coughing and sneezing. Onset is abrupt, with fever, chills, generalized malaise, myalgias, and headache. Fever and systemic symptoms subside within several days, at which time respiratory symptoms, including cough, nasal obstruction and discharge, and pharyngitis, increase. Symptoms subside over 4 to 5 days, but cough may persist for weeks. Patients with underlying cardiac

TABLE 17–2. Epidemiologic Characteristics of Viral Agents

Characteristic	RSV	Parainfluenza Type 2	Parainfluenza Types 1 and 3	Influenza	Adenovirus
Highest age-specific infection rate	<1 yr	<1 yr	1–5 yrs	>5 yrs	1–5 yrs
Most common lower respiratory clinical syndrome	Bronchiolitis Pneumonia (tachypnea, wheezing, rales)	Bronchioliitis Pneumonia (tachypnea, wheezing, rales)	Croup LTB (stridor, sore throat)	Tracheobronchitis Pneumonia (high fever, headache, sore throat, myalgias, tachypnea, rales)	Pneumonia (fever, tachypnea, rales)
Activity pattern	Epidemic peak	Variable	Variable	Epidemic peak	Endemic

and pulmonary disease are at high risk for fatal infection. Influenza is the only respiratory viral infection known to predispose to the development of secondary bacterial pneumonia.

Influenza occurs in an epidemic form, usually at intervals of 2 to 3 years. Pandemics, resulting from the appearance of new antigen subtypes, occur at longer intervals (10 to 15 years). In the 1969 influenza A (Hong Kong H3N2) epidemic in Belém, Brazil, absenteeism in all establishments rose from 10.7% during the first 6 weeks of the year to 40.8% during the next 6 weeks. During this period there was an excess mortality of 45%.

PARAINFLUENZA VIRUSES. There are 3 serotypes of parainfluenza viruses. Parainfluenza virus types 1 and 3 are the most frequent cause of croup. Parainfluenza 2 is the second most common cause (after RSV) of pediatric bronchiolitis and pneumonia. Transmission of parainfluenza viruses is by contact or large droplets as well as by fomites. There is considerable variation in the pattern of activity for parainfluenza in developing countries. While epidemic peaks of activity are noted in some countries, in others the virus appears to be endemic. Infection with one serotype provides no protection against infection with another serotype; as with RSV, protection against reinfection with the same strain is incomplete.

ADENOVIRUS. Adenoviral infections occur throughout the developing world. This virus causes respiratory infections throughout all age groups. Although adenovirus usually causes a self-limited lower respiratory infection, the infection can progress to necrotizing bronchiolitis. If this severe infection does not result in death, survivors have severe chronic lung disease. Transmission is similar to that of RSV. Usually adenoviral infections have an endemic activity pattern, occurring throughout the year.

DIAGNOSIS

Viral respiratory agents can be diagnosed by tissue culture isolation or rapid diagnostic techniques. Tissue culture isolation is expensive to maintain and technically difficult. Specimens should be collected by nasal pharyngeal aspirate and transported in viral transport media. Specimens should be inoculated as soon as possible, as RSV is quite labile. The best isolation results are obtained when multiple cell lines, such as HEP2, MDCK, MRC, and LLCMK2, are used. Clinical usefulness is limited because tissue culture isolation takes 2 to 14 days.

Rapid viral diagnostic techniques have greater clinical usefulness because results can be available in hours. However, the identification of a viral agent does not rule out a mixed viral-bacterial infection. The three methods currently available are immunofluorescence, enzyme immunoassay (EIA), and monoclonal antibody tests (Table 17–3). Although rapid diagnostic techniques are very effective in identifying RSV infections, they are less sensitive in diagnosing the other respiratory viruses. EIAs are being developed for viruses other than RSV, but they are not currently available commercially because of low sensitivity and low specificity.

PATHOGENESIS

Complex interactions between the host, viral and bacterial agents, and environmental factors produce respiratory disease. Knowledge of the pathogenesis of acute respiratory infections in developing countries has been complicated by the number of potential pathogens, by the need for sophisticated laboratories for diagnosis, by a potentially large number of host risk characteristics, and by diverse social, cultural, and environmental factors. The incidence and severity of acute lower respiratory infections relate to four pathogenic interactions: (1) the effectiveness of the host defenses against the respiratory viral pathogens; (2) the degree of selectivity with which the inflammatory response destroys the pathogen while minimizing lower airway obstruction and damage to lung tissue; (3) the integrity of repair mechanisms that determine the rate of tissue recovery; and (4) the

TABLE 17–3. Rapid Viral Diagnosis

Method	Specimen	Viruses	Sensitivity	Specificity	Commercial Reagents	Comments
Immunofluorescence	NPA*	RSV, PI, Ad, I, M	RSV: 80–90%	—	Yes	UV microscope needed
Enzyme immunoassay (EIA)	NPA	RSV	73–90%	—	Yes	
Monoclonal tests	NPA	Adenovirus	57–87%	—	Yes	

*Nasopharyngeal aspirate.

ability of the host to maintain adequate respiratory function.

The effectiveness of the host defenses against the viral pathogen is impaired by factors that promote pathogen transmission and increase the size of infecting dose, promote replication and spread, and inhibit host defenses. Large family and household size, crowding, inadequate sanitation, and poor personal hygiene facilitate transmission and increase the size of the infecting dose. Increasing birth order also appears to be an important risk factor for severe viral lower respiratory infection. Indoor smoke pollution from biomass fuels alters the integrity of the respiratory mucosal lining, disrupts mucociliary function, and promotes viral penetration and spread.

The inflammatory response produced by the child's immune system on the lung tissue can be more significant than the direct toxic effects of the pathogen. The immune defense mechanisms that fight infection are the same mechanisms of inflammation that damage functioning lung tissue. Factors that exaggerate the inflammatory response beyond what is needed to control the pathogen are counterproductive. The most obvious example of this occurs in a child with asthma or other allergies. Coexisting parasitic infections that have a migratory phase through the lung may also increase the inflammatory response and cause more severe disease. Smoke pollution may increase the inflammatory response and/or make the lung tissue more susceptible to damage.

The severity of a respiratory infection will be affected by the underlying state of the lung. If the lung is exposed to another infection before it has fully recovered from an earlier insult, the damage is likely to be considerably more extensive. Therefore, it is important to understand factors that limit tissue repair and the subsequent recovery of respiratory functions. These include protein-calorie malnutrition; deficiencies in vitamin A and elemental minerals such as iron, copper, and zinc; and underlying disease of the lungs or heart. Conditions that predispose to frequent recurrent infections (such as crowding and smoke pollution) will also affect recovery rates.

Several factors affect the ability of the host to maintain adequate respiratory function in the presence of acute respiratory infection. Age is a significant factor. Prematurity is associated with muscle weakness and fatigue that predispose the host to respiratory failure. Malnutrition impairs respiratory function by causing muscular weakness, blunting of the hypoxic response, and decreasing respiratory drive. Infants have a compliant chest wall that leads to inefficient respiratory function; in addition, the upper airway of infants is more susceptible to obstruction than that of adults. The respiratory drive center of young infants is more sensitive than that of older infants and children. RSV infection is often associated with apnea in young infants, especially premature infants.

PREVENTION AND CONTROL

IMMUNIZATION. Advances in the prevention of viral respiratory infection in childhood await the successful development of effective vaccines against RSV and parainfluenza. Early attempts at formaldehyde inactivation and more recently developed attenuated vaccines have not been effective. Successful prophylaxis for these agents requires a better understanding of the immunology of mucosal infections and the chemistry of glycoprotein antigens. Oral adenovirus types 4 and 7 vaccines have been developed and tested on military recruits, but their benefit in children has not been assessed. Influenza vaccine, usually containing both type A and type B virus, is widely used in developed countries for persons with chronic illness and advanced age. The use of influenza vaccine in developing countries is limited by the high cost, the need for frequent revaccination because of antigenic shift, and the fact that the target population is the elderly rather than the young.

CHEMOTHERAPY. Two specific antiviral therapies are currently available—amantadine and ribavirin. Oral amantadine (adult dose: 200 mg total, 100 mg twice daily for 5 days) is effective treatment for influenza if given early in the disease course. It also may be used prophylactically. Ribavirin is an aerosolized drug used to treat severe RSV infections. It is currently recommended for hospitalized patients with high-risk conditions, including bronchopulmonary dysplasia and other chronic lung diseases, congenital heart disease, and immunocompromised states. The drug must be delivered with a special small-particle aerosol generator unit. Its use in developing countries is limited because of the very high cost of the drug, technical difficulties in drug delivery, and lack of data from developing countries on preventing death.

CASE MANAGEMENT. Good case management remains the most feasible strategy to reduce the mortality of viral respiratory infections. Upper respiratory infections and tracheobronchitis are almost always caused by viral agents, with the exception of acute otitis media, sinusitis, and streptococcal pharyngitis. Middle respiratory tract infections are also usually caused by viral agents. The exceptions to this are acute epiglottitis caused by *Haemophilus influenzae* and croup caused by *Corynebacterium diphtheriae*. Unfortunately, clinical signs, laboratory tests, and chest x-rays cannot reliably distinguish viral from bacterial lower respiratory infections. High fever cannot be used to discriminate between viral and bacterial disease because fever occurs as frequently with documented viral infections as with bacterial infections. The child's response to an antipyretic such as acetaminophen will not distinguish between these two types of infection. While wheezing is more often associated with viral infections, especially RSV and parainfluenza viruses, it can be caused by *H. influenzae* and *Chlamydia* infections. Also, the possibility of a mixed viral-bacterial infection in a wheezing child always exists.

These limitations on the ability to distinguish viral from bacterial disease actually simplify the clinical approach to the management of acute respiratory infections. Any patient with evidence of a lower respiratory infection should be treated with antibiotics. Indications of a lower respiratory infection are respiratory rate greater than 60 for infants under 2 months of age, greater than 50 for infants 2 to 12 months of age, and greater than 40 for children 1 to 5 years of age; retractions; grunting respirations; cyanosis; and wheezing, rales, or crepitations. Signs of respiratory distress that require hospitalization include respiratory rate greater than 70, severe retractions with decreased air exchange unresponsive to bronchodilators, cyanosis, or stridor at rest. Chest x-rays can be helpful but are expensive and usually available only in a hospital setting. Findings suggestive of a bacterial infection are lobar or segmental consolidation or pleural fluid. Findings suggestive of a viral infection are hyperexpansion, peribronchial thickening, and streaky perihilar infiltrates. The finding of diffuse or patchy infiltrates (bronchopneumonia) can be associated with viral or bacterial disease. Microbiology studies are not useful in the primary care setting because a management decision must be made prior to obtaining the results of these tests. In the hospital setting, blood and pleural fluid cultures provide information that is useful for selecting appropriate antibiotic therapy. Viral tissue culture and rapid viral diagnostic techniques are most useful in epidemiologic studies but are rarely helpful in the management of individual cases.

BIBLIOGRAPHY

Berman S, McIntosh K: Selective primary health care: Strategies for control of disease in the developing world. Acute respiratory infections. Rev Infect Dis 7:674, 1985.

Gwatkin DR: How many die? A set of demographic estimates of the annual number of infant and child deaths in the world. Am J Public Health 70:1286, 1980.

Hall CB, Powell KR, Schnabel KC, et al: Risk of secondary bacterial infection in infants hospitalized with respiratory syncytial viral infection. J Pediatr 113:266, 1988.

Hendersen FM, Collier AM, Clyde WA, et al: Respiratory syncytial-virus infections, reinfections and immunity. N Engl J Med 300:530, 1979.

Institute of Medicine: New Vaccine Development. Establishing Priorities. Vol II: Diseases of Importance in Developing Countries. Washington, DC, National Academy Press, 1986.

Leventhal JM: Clinical predictors of pneumonia as a guide to ordering chest roentgenograms. Clin Pediatr 21:730, 1982.

Putto A, Ruuskanen O, Meurman O: Fever in respiratory virus infections. Am J Dis Child 140:1159, 1986.

Shann F, Hart K, Thomas D: Acute lower respiratory tract infections in children: possible criteria for selection of patients for antibiotic therapy and hospital admission. Bull WHO 62:749, 1984.

Smith JJ, Lemen RJ, Taussig LM: Mechanisms of viral-induced lower airway obstruction. Pediatr Infect Dis J 6:837, 1987.

Wald ER, Dashefsky B, Green M: In re ribavirin: A case of premature adjudication. J Pediatr 112:154, 1988.

World Health Organization: Global medium-term programme 13.7. Acute respiratory infections. Document TRI/ARI/MTP/83.1. Geneva, World Health Organization, 1983.

18.   ENTEROVIRAL INFECTIONS

18.1.   POLIOMYELITIS

F. Marc LaForce

DEFINITION. Poliomyelitis is an acute viral infection that is frequently asymptomatic but occasionally results in central nervous system invasion and clinical syndromes characterized by asymmetric lower motor neuron palsies. Killed and live poliomyelitis vaccines have eradicated the disease in many developed countries; however, poliomyelitis remains an important public health problem in most developing countries.

ETIOLOGY AND HISTORY. Poliomyelitis is caused by a RNA virus belonging to the family Picornaviridae. Three antigenic types, 1, 2, and 3, have been described.

Poliomyelitis was first described clinically in 1840 by Heine, a German orthopedist, and the natural history of the illness was outlined in 1890 by Medin, a Swedish pediatrician—hence, the origin of the term Heine-Medin disease for poliomyelitis. Poliomyelitis was formerly a very important public health problem in the United States, where, during this century, the overall incidence increased during each decade until the 1950s, when the introduction of killed vaccine reversed this trend.

The infectious nature was proved in 1908 when Landsteiner and Popper successfully transmitted the disease to primates by intracerebral inoculation of human spinal cord homogenates. Progress toward control was slow until 1949, when Enders, Weller, and Robbins showed that polioviruses could be grown in vitro in cells not of neural origin. This discovery proved to be the key that facilitated definitive virologic, pathogenetic, and sero-epidemiologic studies by which the distribution and pathogenesis of the disease became understood. In 1953 Salk showed that formalin-inactivated poliovirus (IPV) was immunogenic. A large field trial using IPV demonstrated efficacy, and the vaccine was licensed in 1955. A few years later, Sabin introduced a live attenuated vaccine (OPV). The impact of these two vaccines was phenomenal. Within 20 years, the average number of United States cases fell from 15,000 per year to fewer than 10.

DISTRIBUTION AND INCIDENCE. Poliomyelitis viruses are distributed worldwide. Man is the sole reservoir of poliomyelitis, although primates have long been used for experimental transmission studies. In temperate zones, the disease is more common during summer months, whereas the seasonality is less striking in tropical countries.

The reported incidence of the disease is largely determined by two factors: (1) use of poliomyelitis vaccine and (2) efficiency of case reporting. Use of IPV and OPV in the United States resulted in a drop in incidence rate from 15 to 20 cases per 100,000 population in the early 1950s to less than 0.01 case per 100,000 population since 1972. Thus, within a single generation, poliomyelitis went from a dread disease whose yearly victims crowded rehabilitation centers to one that most current American medical students have never seen.

Until recently, poliomyelitis was not considered an important public health problem in developing countries, an impression supported by the low incidence rates reported from these countries. The usual reason given was that children were infected with poliovirus early in life, when they were partially protected by maternal antibody and at low risk of paralytic disease, and therefore developed solid immunity. The validity of this assumption is now being seriously questioned as more careful surveys of paralyzed children in developing tropical countries are showing that poliomyelitis is a far more important public health problem than was formerly believed.

The clinical sequelae of paralytic poliomyelitis are distinctive, and when observed, can be attributed to this disease with a high degree of certainty. Thus, by studying cases of paralysis in school-aged children, it is possible to determine the prevalence of paralysis due to poliomyelitis and to estimate the annual incidence of this disease in recent years. For example, Nicholas and coworkers reported on lameness due to poliomyelitis in Ghanaian school children. In an area where poliomyelitis was not believed to be a problem, more than 7 per 1000 children were lame because of this disease. The annual incidence was estimated to be 28 per 100,000 population, a figure comparable to incidence rates in the United States prior to the development of poliomyelitis vaccine. Lame surveys in developing countries have all shown prevalence rates higher than originally suspected. Thus, the axiom that a low attack rate of paralytic poliomyelitis followed infection with poliovirus at an early age was not correct. Previously cited low incidence rates were more a reflection of incomplete reporting. For example, surveys in India suggest an annual incidence rate of about 20 per 100,000 population, or more than 150,000 new cases yearly. These data have re-emphasized the importance of early introduction of poliomyelitis vaccine in immunization programs.

TRANSMISSION AND EPIDEMIOLOGY. Polioviruses are spread predominantly by the fecal-oral route, although respiratory tract spread can occur. Thus, the age-specific attack rate is largely determined by the level of sanitation. Poor hygienic practices result in early exposure to poliomyelitis viruses. Under such circumstances, poliomyelitis is "infantile"; i.e., more than 95% of new cases occur in children between 6 months and 4 years of age. This age distribution characterizes new cases in all countries without effective vaccination programs.

The epidemiology of poliomyelitis in the United States has traced a fascinating course. At the turn of the century, virtually all new cases were in children under age 5 years. Over the next 40 years, a gradual shift in new cases to older age groups occurred, as sanitation improved and exposure to wild polioviruses was delayed. Associated with this shift to an older age group was a gradual increase in the yearly attack rate. This observation has been the cornerstone of our understanding of the epidemiology of poliomyelitis in developed countries, i.e., that the ratio of paralytic to inapparent cases increases as the patient's age at time of infection increases. Therefore, the age distribution of primary infections is an important determinant of the average annual incidence of paralytic disease. Convincing epidemiologic evidence exists to support this hypothesis, although this issue is still somewhat controversial. In recent years, use of poliomyelitis vaccine has virtually eliminated the disease in the United States, and virtually all the 10 or so yearly cases are caused by vaccine strains.

PATHOGENESIS AND PATHOLOGY. Ingestion of poliovirus by a susceptible person is followed by viral multiplication in the oropharyngeal and intestinal mucosa. A transient viremia disseminates virus to other tissues, and in most individuals the infection is contained at this stage. In a few persons, continued viral replication results in a major viremia. In still fewer individuals, persistent viremia is followed by true central nervous system invasion. The mechanisms by which neural tissue is invaded remain unclear, although the preponderance of evidence suggests a hematogenous route. The most characteristic histologic feature of poliomyelitis is that the main site of attack is the gray matter of the anterior horn of the spinal cord (Fig. 18–1). Some pathologic changes are reversible; these account for the frequent return of motor function after onset of disease.

CLINICAL MANIFESTATIONS AND COMPLICATIONS. The incubation period of poliomyelitis is between 9 and 12 days. Clinical manifestations are quite variable and range from inapparent infection to fatal bulbar paralysis.

Inapparent, Abortive, and Nonparalytic Infections. About 95% of poliomyelitis infections are subclinical and *inapparent*. These are recognized only by laboratory studies. About 5% of infections are characterized by fever, headache, sore throat, and myalgia. These poliomyelitis infections are called *abortive* and are indistinguishable from other viral infections. They are recognized as being caused by poliovirus only if laboratory studies are done. About 1% of infections result in the syndrome called *nonparalytic poliomyelitis*. These patients have an aseptic meningitis syndrome with fever, meningismus, myalgia, and headache. All recover without therapy.

Paralytic Infections. A few patients develop true paralysis *(paralytic poliomyelitis)*. They usually experience fever, myalgia, and meningismus, and most complain of severe muscle and back pain. Hypesthesia is sometimes noted. The distribution of paralysis in the limbs is asymmetric, with legs more commonly involved than arms and proximal muscles involved more frequently than distal muscles. The paralysis may become more severe for 2 or 3 days, but progression invariably stops after the temperature returns to normal. Cranial nerves are involved in some patients and are associated with a variety of clinical syndromes collectively called bulbar poliomyelitis. These infections carry a much higher mortality rate and are more common in older individuals.

Severe fatigue, tonsillectomy, and pregnancy all predispose to paralytic poliomyelitis. Children with immunodeficiency states are particularly prone to poliomyelitis, especially following OPV immunization.

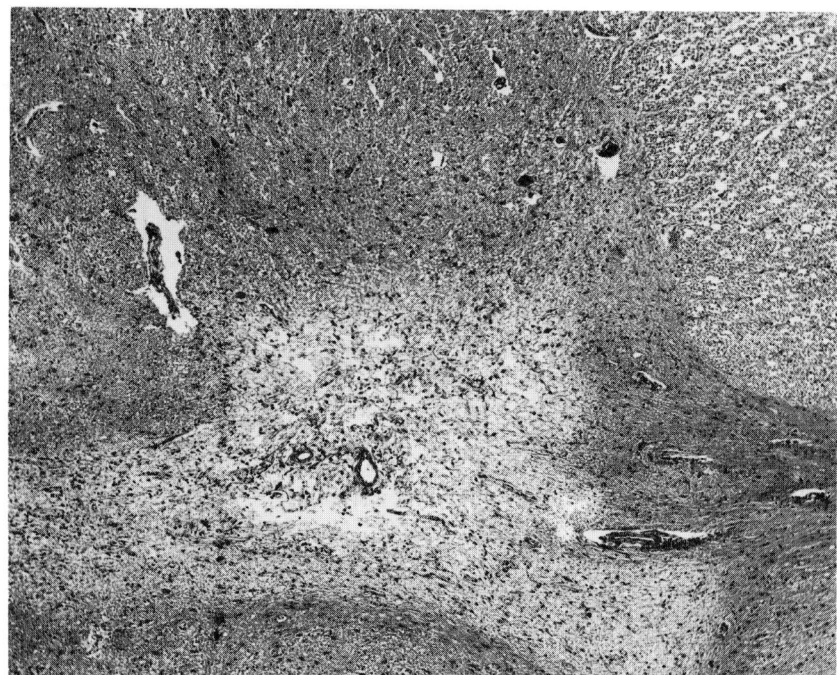

FIGURE 18–1. Loss of the anterior horn cells of the spinal cord in the late stages of poliomyelitis (× 35). (Courtesy of Armed Forces Institute on Pathology, Photograph Neg. No. 74-9520.)

Injections and other trauma are important factors predisposing to paralysis, particularly in developing countries. The history in such cases is very characteristic. Usually a young child is acutely ill with fever. The child is brought to a health center where an injection is given, and within 1 week paralysis develops in the injected limb. Epidemiologic studies have implicated a variety of agents, such as diphtheria-pertussis-tetanus (DPT) immunization, antibiotics, antimalarials, and antipyretics. The association between injections and paralysis has been confirmed experimentally. The mechanism by which this phenomenon occurs is not well understood, although the best evidence to date suggests that trauma initiates a reflex dilatation of blood vessels at the corresponding spinal cord level and facilitates entry of virus at that level.

DIAGNOSIS. The diagnosis of poliomyelitis is most often made on clinical grounds. Few diseases are likely to be confused with acute poliomyelitis. Sudden lower motor neuron dysfunction and hypo- or areflexia with few or no sensory changes are characteristic findings. More unusual forms of poliomyelitis, such as poliomyelitis encephalitis, cannot be diagnosed on clinical grounds.

Laboratory Diagnosis. This requires isolation of a poliovirus from pharyngeal secretions or stool and the demonstration of a fourfold or greater rise in neutralizing antibody to the isolated strain in acute and convalescent serum specimens. In the absence of a virus isolate, a serologic diagnosis can be made by testing acute and convalescent serums against types 1, 2, and 3 polioviruses.

Differential Diagnosis. Guillain-Barré syndrome can be confused with poliomyelitis. Usually patients with Guillain-Barré syndrome have a symmetric ascending paralysis with sensory changes. Spinal fluid in patients with this syndrome is usually normal, except for elevated protein levels, whereas pleocytosis is frequently seen in those with acute poliomyelitis. Paralysis may increase over a 2-week period in Guillain-Barré syndrome, whereas extension of paralysis beyond 3 or 4 days is unusual in poliomyelitis.

TREATMENT AND PROGNOSIS. There is no specific treatment for poliomyelitis. More specifically, antibiotics, gamma globulin, and vitamins are all without effect. Management is symptomatic and supportive.

In the early phase of illness, bed rest is mandatory in order to properly treat patients and to minimize the extent of paralysis. The application of wet heat to painful muscles often produces considerable relief. Bed rest is no longer necessary later, when severe discomfort is absent.

Physiotherapy. This is the mainstay of treatment and should be begun 3 to 4 days after cessation of fever and when progression of paralysis has ceased. Physiotherapy will not prevent the atrophy that follows anterior horn cell denervation, but it will result in fewer deformities by ensuring that those motor units with regenerating axons stay in good condition. An added benefit is the psychologic one of helping the child and parents come to terms with the disease. With a little training, parents can become important partners in this therapy.

Other Treatment. Patients with bulbar paralysis often require special treatment facilities. Repeated aspiration causing pneumonia is common in these patients. Finally, decreased diaphragmatic or intercostal muscle function may necessitate respirator assistance.

Prognosis. Except for bulbar poliomyelitis, the prognosis in most cases is good. Full return of function is less likely in patients with severely paralyzed muscles than in those who are mildly paralyzed. Data from developing countries show that about 9% of children die during the acute phase of the illness, another 15% recover completely, and 75% have some residual deformity. The overall impact of poliomyelitis on mortality may not become apparent until much later.

Late Denervation Syndromes. Over the last few years a postpoliomyelitis syndrome has been described in which patients with old poliomyelitis sequelae develop new muscle weakness. Muscle biopsies and electromyographic studies suggest that the syndrome is the result of progressive denervation of previously reinnervated muscle fibers. No treatment exists for this syndrome.

PREVENTION AND CONTROL. The only method of controlling poliomyelitis is vaccination. Both IPV and OPV have been used with great success.

Live Attenuated Vaccine. In developing countries the first dose of OPV is given at birth, with 3 subsequent doses given at monthly intervals beginning at 6 weeks of age. A booster dose at 18 months is also recommended. This vaccine results in local (IgA) and systemic (IgG) antibody. OPV is contraindicated in immunosuppressed persons but can safely be used during pregnancy. It is the only vaccine to be used in epidemics, since liberal use of OPV blocks circulation of wild polioviruses by interfering with intestinal colonization. The main disadvantage of OPV is that paralysis can occur in the immunized person or a contact. This is a rare event, occurring about once in every 520,000 first doses received, and becomes a public health problem only when incidence rates drop to extremely low levels as a result of vaccination. Such a situation has arisen in the United States, where laboratory testing of poliomyelitis isolates has shown that no United States case since 1979 has been caused by wild poliovirus. The 10 or so yearly cases occur for the most part in OPV vaccine recipients, their contacts, or infants with undiagnosed immunodeficiency syndromes. The occurrence of these vaccine-associated cases and their attendant medicolegal problems has resulted in a reconsideration of poliomyelitis vaccination policy by the Institute of Medicine. It is likely that when enhanced inactivated polio vaccine (E-IPV) is available as a combined E-IPV/DPT vaccine, United States vaccination policy will change to a strategy that begins with E-IPV (thus eliminating the possibility of vaccine-induced cases of poliomyelitis) but that also includes OPV (to ensure the benefit of gut immunity).

The current recommendation of the World Health Organization's Expanded Program on Immunization is to introduce OPV into routine immunization programs as soon as the cold chain and availability of vaccine warrant introduction. A radically different strategy is that of a yearly two-dose mass vaccination campaign, whereby all children less than 5 years of age are given OPV. This strategy has been successful in Brazil.

Formalin-Inactivated Vaccine. Newer production methods have resulted in the manufacture of a more potent IPV, so-called enhanced IPV or E-IPV. This vaccine has shown high seroconversion rates after 2 doses and has been shown to be effective in preventing cases under field conditions in Senegal. In this study, vaccine efficacy was closely linked to the number of doses of E-IPV received, with protection going from 36% after 1 dose to 89% after 2 doses. The vaccine is more heat-stable than OPV and offers the advantage of being given simultaneously with DPT vaccine.

BIBLIOGRAPHY

Cashman NR, Maselli R, Wollmann RL, et al: Late denervation in patients with antecedent paralytic poliomyelitis. N Engl J Med 317:7, 1987.
Institute of Medicine: An Evaluation of Poliomyelitis Vaccine Policy Options. Publication no. IOM 88-04. Washington, DC, National Academy of Sciences, 1988.
International Symposium on Poliomyelitis Control: J Infect Dis 6(Suppl 2):S301, 1984.
Nathanson N, Martin JR: The epidemiology of poliomyelitis: enigmas surrounding its appearance, epidemicity, and disappearance. Am J Epidemiol 110:672, 1979.
Nicholas DD, Kratzer JH, Ofosu-Amaah S, et al: Is poliomyelitis a serious problem in developing countries?—the Danfa experience. Br Med J 1:1009, 1977.
Paul JR: A History of Poliomyelitis. New Haven, Yale University Press, 1971.
Robertson SE, Traverso HP, Drucker JA, et al: Clinical efficacy of a new enhanced-potency, inactivated poliovirus vaccine. Lancet 1:897, 1988.

18.2. VIRAL DIARRHEAS

Karen Midthun
and Robert E. Black

The term "viral diarrheas" has been used to describe acute, self-limited illnesses characterized by diarrhea and often by vomiting for which bacterial enteropathogens could not be identified. Although these illnesses were presumed to be due to viral infections, until recently not a single virus could be implicated as an important cause of diarrhea. However, since 1972, two groups of viruses have been found to be major etiologic agents of diarrhea. One group, the rotaviruses, are responsible for a high proportion of the serious sporadic diarrheas of young children. The other group, the Norwalk-like viruses, commonly cause epidemic as well as endemic diarrhea. More recently, other groups of viruses have been found in the feces of persons with diarrhea. There is sufficient information to implicate one group of adenoviruses as etiologic agents of diarrhea, but the role of other viruses is still being defined.

ROTAVIRUS DIARRHEA

DEFINITION. Rotavirus diarrhea is an acute infectious disease, characterized by watery diarrhea and vomiting, occurring primarily in children less than 2 years of age.

ETIOLOGY AND HISTORY. Rotavirus in human disease was first identified in 1973 by Australian workers using thin-section electron microscopic studies of duodenal mucosa biopsy specimens taken from children with diarrhea. Subsequently, researchers in several countries detected viral particles by direct electron microscopic examination of feces from children with diarrhea. The term "rotavirus," derived from the Latin word *rota* (wheel), was suggested by the appearance of the virus as a wheel with spokes radiating from a hub. Initially, it was also called infantile gastroenteritis virus, orbivirus, duovirus, and reovirus-like agent. Rotavirus is accepted as an etiologic agent of diarrhea because (1) it can be found in the stools of patients with diarrhea significantly more often than in the stools of appropriately selected control subjects without diarrhea; (2) viral particles have been found in histopathologically damaged jejunal mucosa of patients with diarrhea; (3) the virus will cause disease when given to a variety of experimental animals, including rhesus monkeys, and to human volunteers; and (4) humans and experimental animals demonstrate serologic response to infection with rotavirus.

Rotaviruses are classified as a genus in the family Reoviridae and are etiologic agents of diarrhea in many animal species as well as in humans. They are spherical, are 70 nm in diameter, and have an inner and an outer capsid (Fig. 18–2). They have a double-stranded RNA genome with 11 segments and possess 3 important antigenic specificities: group, subgroup, and serotype. Most rotaviruses share the common group antigen and are classified as group A rotaviruses. Six serotypes of human rotavirus have been described. Several rotaviruses that do not share the common group antigen have been discovered and are classified as non–group A (groups B–F) or "pararotaviruses." This discussion will focus on group A rotaviruses. Rotavirus particles remain structurally stable after exposure to heat (37 C for 1 hour) or ambient temperature (for 24 hours), ether, and mild acids but are disrupted by acid treatment at a pH of less than 3. Proteolytic enzymes such as trypsin, pancreatin, and elastin enhance viral infectivity and are essential for growth of human rotaviruses in cell cultures.

DISTRIBUTION AND INCIDENCE. Rotaviruses have a worldwide distribution and are considered important agents of diarrhea in studies from every area of the world. In developed countries, they are the single most important pathogen causing severe childhood diarrhea. Hospital-based studies of at least 1 year's duration in several developed countries indicated that approximately 40% of diarrheal episodes in young children were associated with rotavirus. Two-family surveillance studies in developed countries showed that 10 to 23%

of diarrheal episodes in infants and young children were related to rotavirus. Hospital-based studies from 12 developing nations revealed that approximately 30% (range 14 to 46%) of cases of diarrhea in children under 5 years (mostly under 2 years) were associated with rotavirus. In contrast, a review of 6 studies from developing countries of children at an outpatient clinic, or children with diarrhea identified by prospective community surveillance, indicated that only 11% (range 3 to 19%) of episodes were associated with rotavirus. In hospital-based studies of young children in developing countries, rotavirus either was the most frequent enteropathogen identified or was second to bacterial agents, particularly enterotoxigenic and enteropathogenic *E. coli*. This pre-eminence of rotavirus among children hospitalized with diarrhea in developed and developing countries is undoubtedly related to the greater degree of dehydration with rotavirus diarrhea than with most other types of childhood diarrhea.

In temperate climates, rotavirus diarrhea is very seasonal, with the highest prevalence in cold weather. During winter, rotavirus can often be found in 70 to 80% of childhood diarrheas. In summer, it is detected infrequently. In tropical areas, the rotavirus seasonality is less clear. According to most studies from tropical countries, rotavirus diarrhea can be found throughout the year; however, there is often some seasonal variation, with higher incidence during the cooler and drier months. Although this apparent variation is due partly to the decreased number of cases caused by bacterial pathogens during the cool season, there appears to be a slight seasonal increase in the absolute number of children with rotavirus diarrhea during the cool months in some tropical areas.

Since few population-based studies of rotavirus diarrhea have been done in developing countries, little information is available on the incidence of the disease. In some community-based studies in rural Bangladesh, the incidence of rotavirus diarrhea reached a peak in the second 6 months of life and was high between 3 and 23 months of age; no rotavirus was noted in children more than 24 months old (Fig. 18–3). In the same area,

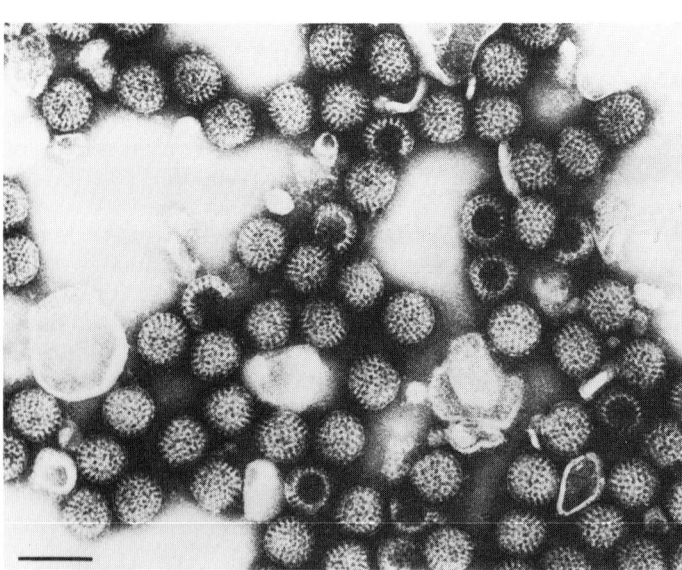

FIGURE 18–2. Rotavirus particles in a stool filtrate from an 11-month-old child with diarrhea. The particles appear to have a double-shelled capsid, and occasional "empty" particles are seen. (Electron micrograph by Dr. A. Z. Kapikian.) (Bar represents 100 nm.)

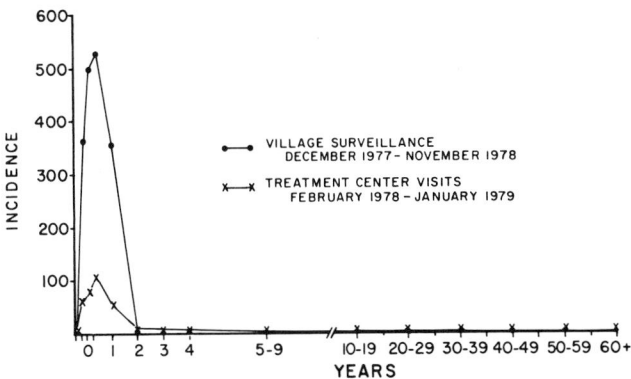

FIGURE 18–3. Annual age-specific incidence of rotavirus diarrhea per 1000 persons assessed by village surveillance and by treatment center visits. (From Black RE, et al.: Lancet 1:141, 1981.)

treatment center visits for rotavirus diarrhea also reached a peak for children 6 to 11 months of age, whereas those for older children and adults were low. This and other incidence studies from communities in rural Bangladesh and Guatemala suggest that rotavirus diarrhea occurs once or twice in children during the first 2 years of life.

TRANSMISSION AND EPIDEMIOLOGY. Rotavirus diarrhea is primarily an endemic problem, although clear-cut epidemics have been reported in a variety of settings such as primary schools, day-care nurseries, hospitals, and nursing homes. Community-wide epidemics involve primarily young children, although all age groups have been affected in outbreaks occurring in isolated areas. Several large outbreaks of non–group A rotavirus diarrhea affecting adults have been described in China.

Hospitalized Patients and Neonates. Of particular interest is the problem of nosocomial spread of rotavirus among patients and medical staff and the frequent demonstration of rotavirus in the feces of hospitalized newborns. In one hospital in Canada, 20% of the rotavirus diarrhea cases were nosocomial. In a hospital in the United States, 17% of pediatric patients admitted for nondiarrheal disorders developed rotavirus diarrhea while in the hospital. The infection was transmitted from patient to patient by the medical staff. Outbreaks of rotavirus infections have been well documented in hospital newborn nurseries. In these outbreaks, up to 57% of newborns were infected within the first few days after birth, but relatively few (6 to 28%) had diarrhea. Furthermore, when diarrhea occurred, it was usually mild. Some studies have shown that breast-fed neonates had a lower incidence of infection and excreted less virus during infection than did bottle-fed neonates. Transmission of rotavirus is especially common in special-care nurseries, but even well neonates housed in communal nurseries at one Australian hospital had a tenfold higher rate of nosocomial rotavirus diarrhea than did neonates who were rooming-in with their mothers at the same institution. The most important factor favoring transmission of rotavirus was proximity to other newborns and frequency of handling by unrelated adults.

Adult Infections. Adults are also susceptible to rota-

virus diarrhea. Illnesses, which are usually mild, are often associated with exposure to infected children either in the hospital or at home. Studies of the adult household contacts of children with rotavirus diarrhea revealed a high rate of infection; but fewer than one third of infected adults developed diarrhea. Also, adults may experience rotavirus diarrhea when traveling in developing countries. Ten studies of traveler's diarrhea showed that 0 to 36% (median of 4%) of diarrheal illnesses were associated with rotavirus. However, the etiologic significance is unclear, since patients with rotavirus were frequently infected with other pathogens and a high proportion of asymptomatic controls were also infected with rotavirus.

Serology. Seroepidemiologic studies in both developing and developed countries show an initial high prevalence and titer of serum antibody in infants, which falls by 6 months of age. By age 2 years, nearly all children have serum rotavirus antibody; titers remain elevated until late adulthood. The initial titers represent maternal antibodies, and the rise in early childhood is due to one or more rotaviral infections. Furthermore, evidence from a Bangladesh longitudinal study indicates that many transient infections not associated with diarrhea stimulate an increase in serum antibodies.

Transmission. Rotavirus infection spreads by the fecal-oral route. When given orally, infectious particles from diarrheal feces have reproduced the disease in volunteers. The usual mode of transmission is probably by direct person-to-person contact or contact with contaminated objects. The virus is relatively resistant to adverse environmental conditions and can remain on surfaces for prolonged periods. It also maintains structural integrity in water, and water-borne transmission is a possibility. The respiratory symptoms associated with rotaviral diarrheal illnesses, the rapid acquisition of serum antibody during the first few years of life regardless of hygienic conditions, and the failure to document fecal-oral spread in a few large outbreaks have led to speculation that transmission can take place via airborne droplets. However, there is no evidence of airborne transmission and no indication that rotavirus multiplies with production of infectious particles in any tissue other than small bowel enterocytes.

PATHOGENESIS AND PATHOLOGY. Electron microscopy (EM) first demonstrated viral particles in duodenal mucosal enterocytes obtained by biopsy of children with acute diarrhea. This and subsequent biopsy studies revealed shortening and blunting of villi, flattening of epithelial cells, and infiltration of the lamina propria with mononuclear cells. Abnormalities varied from mild to severe and tended to be patchy.

However, most knowledge of the pathophysiology of rotavirus diarrhea has come from a series of studies in animals, particularly gnotobiotic colostrum-deprived calves infected with human rotavirus. Denuding of villi and flattening of epithelial cells were observed in the upper small intestine shortly after the onset of diarrhea. At this time, the lower small intestine was intact, although rotavirus antigen could be found in the epithelial cells. The morphologic changes spread in a cephalocaudal direction and involved the lower small intestine after

7 hours of diarrhea. The changes were confined to the small intestine. Forty hours after onset of diarrhea, the intestine appeared relatively normal.

Secretion. The diarrhea in rotaviral infections results from disordered electrolyte transport in the small bowel. There is a net secretion of water, sodium, and chloride that results from the transient replacement of the absorptive villous cells with immature crypt cells, which retain some of their secretory characteristics. Rotaviral diarrheal stools contain 30 to 40 mEq/L of sodium, and the sodium concentration does not increase with higher rates of stool loss. Stool potassium losses also range from 30 to 40 mEq/L.

Malabsorption. In addition to the structural changes in the bowel mucosa, rotavirus infection results in decreased brush border disaccharidase activity. Children with rotavirus diarrhea may have increased fecal reducing substances, indicating some sugar malabsorption during illness. Furthermore, in one study the rate of stool output and degree of metabolic acidosis were related to the carbohydrate content of the stool, suggesting that sugar malabsorption plays a role in the metabolic acidosis and perhaps a secondary role in determining the diarrheal fluid loss.

Since the diet of children under the age of 2 years is often based on milk, lactose malabsorption during and following the illness is of particular concern. On the basis of the lactose–breath hydrogen test, 15 (29%) of 51 children studied on the fifth to nineteenth day after onset of rotavirus diarrhea were classified as malabsorbers of lactose. There was significantly more lactose malabsorption (60%) in children who continued to excrete rotavirus until the day of study compared with children whose stools had become rotavirus-negative. Follow-up studies of subjects originally diagnosed as malabsorbers showed marked improvement. It is likely that during rotavirus diarrhea the incidences of lactose malabsorption and intolerance are related to the amount of lactose in the diet. Experimental studies in lambs suggest that normal or slightly reduced dietary levels of lactose are well tolerated during rotavirus diarrhea.

CLINICAL MANIFESTATIONS AND COMPLICATIONS. The incubation period for rotavirus diarrhea ranges from 1 to 5 days but is usually less than 48 hours. The illness is characterized by the abrupt onset of watery diarrhea and vomiting. Vomiting is present in up to 90% of patients, may precede the onset of diarrhea, and usually stops within the first 2 days of the disease. Low-grade fevers have been found in 50 to 100% of cases. Some studies, but not all, have demonstrated a higher prevalence of upper respiratory tract symptoms in children with rotavirus diarrhea compared with those having other types of diarrhea.

In developing countries, the majority of children with rotavirus diarrhea have a mild self-limited illness lasting 3 to 8 days. However, dehydration develops in a substantial proportion. Many hospital-based studies note that children with rotavirus diarrhea have more frequent and severe dehydration than do children with other types of diarrhea. Furthermore, several community-based studies demonstrate that rotavirus diarrhea is associated with the highest rate of dehydration of all types of diarrhea except cholera.

Severe, life-threatening dehydration occurs in only a small percentage of children with rotavirus diarrhea but is nonetheless an important cause of mortality among children under 2 years in developing countries. In Bangladesh it was estimated that 42% of the deaths from watery diarrhea in this age group were due to rotavirus and that another 35% were caused by enterotoxigenic *E. coli.* These two illnesses alone were thought to result in an annual mortality rate of 6.5 per 1000 children. Occasional deaths from rotavirus diarrhea have also been documented in developed countries. In a 5-year study in Canada, 21 deaths in children 4 to 30 months of age were attributed to rotavirus.

Although most rotaviral illnesses resolve within 10 days, a small percentage have a much longer duration. Viral shedding in the stool frequently continues for 10 days after onset of illness, sometimes for 3 weeks, and is associated with a higher prevalence of lactose malabsorption, suggesting persistent viral replication with continued mucosal injury. Children with primary immunodeficiency syndromes can also develop chronic symptomatic diarrhea with prolonged shedding of rotavirus.

Complications. Children with rotavirus diarrhea may have dehydration with commensurate elevations in blood urea nitrogen, urine and plasma specific gravity, and hematocrit. A metabolic acidosis, usually partially compensated, is a common finding. Serum electrolytes are usually normal, but low sodium and potassium levels are common; hypernatremia also occurs. Peripheral white blood counts are usually normal. Fecal leukocytes are present at rates (9 to 31%) similar to those found in cases of nonrotavirus diarrhea but are significantly less common than in diarrhea associated with invasive bacterial pathogens.

Single cases of Reye's syndrome, encephalitis, and aseptic meningitis following rotavirus diarrhea have been reported, but a causal relationship is unclear. Other central nervous system disorders such as altered mental status and seizures are probably due to hypoglycemia or electrolyte abnormalities. A temporal association of rotavirus infection with intussusception, Henoch-Schönlein purpura, hemolytic-uremic syndrome, sudden infant death syndrome, Kawasaki syndrome, and exanthem subitum has been noted, but its significance remains to be determined. A recent study has shown a strong association between rotavirus and necrotizing enterocolitis and hemorrhagic gastroenteritis in neonates.

DIAGNOSIS

Differential Diagnosis. The watery diarrheal illness due to rotavirus can be partially distinguished from diarrhea due to bacteria (e.g., enterotoxigenic or "enteropathogenic" *E. coli, Vibrio cholerae*) by its characteristic early vomiting and fever. Epidemiologic clues are its relative restriction to children under age 2 years and its greater prevalence during the cool season. There are no features of this illness that would distinguish it from other viral diarrheas such as those due to Norwalk-like agents or to adenovirus.

Laboratory Diagnosis. Demonstration of the virus in the feces or an increase in serum antibodies to rotavirus establishes the diagnosis. Stools from the first to fourth day of illness are optimal for rotavirus detection, although shedding may continue for 3 weeks or longer. The original diagnostic test was examination of a stool suspension by electron microscopy. This method detects only relatively large amounts of virus, i.e., at least 10^5 virions/ml of feces; however, most children with rotavirus diarrhea have concentrations of virus above this threshold of sensitivity. A number of other methods have been developed to detect rotavirus in feces. These include enzyme-linked immunosorbent assay (ELISA), reverse passive hemagglutination assay (RPHA), latex agglutination (LA), RNA electrophoresis, complement fixation (CF), free viral immunofluorescence (IFA), counterimmunoelectrophoresis (CIC), and radioimmunoassay (RIA). Of these methods, the ELISA is probably the most commonly used because it is both sensitive and easy to perform. Commercial kits are available for the ELISA, RPHA and the LA, and RNA electrophoresis assays. Human rotavirus can be isolated in cell culture from approximately 75% of stool specimens known to contain virus by other test procedures. However, cell culture for the detection of rotavirus in stool specimens is impractical and has poor sensitivity when compared with other methods.

With rotavirus infection, antibodies have been detected as soon as day 3 of illness, with peak antibody titers occurring on days 14 to 21. IgM antibody peaks in the serum 5 to 10 days after infection, and IgG and IgA antibodies become detectable later. A variety of serologic methods are available, but the complement fixation assay and the ELISA are the most practical and widely used.

TREATMENT AND PROGNOSIS

Oral Rehydration. The most important principle of therapy of watery diarrhea, including that caused by rotavirus, is replacement of water and electrolytes that are lost in the diarrheal stool. This is necessary to prevent (or correct) dehydration and electrolyte imbalance. Most patients, even those with dehydration, can be managed with an oral sugar-electrolyte solution (General Principles, Section III D). The oral solution recommended by the World Health Organization can be prepared by adding the following to 1 liter of water: sodium chloride 3.5 gm, trisodium citrate dihydrate 2.9 gm (or sodium bicarbonate 2.5 gm), potassium chloride 1.5 gm, and glucose 20 gm. The result is a solution consisting of sodium 90 mmol/L, potassium 20 mmol/L, citrate 23 mmol/L (or bicarbonate 30 mmol/L), and glucose 111 mmol/L. The volume of fluid administered should be appropriate to the size of the patient, the degree of dehydration, and the rate of stool loss and should include water, breast milk, or other dilute fluids in addition to the solution. Several comparative studies of rotavirus diarrhea also indicate that sucrose (40 gm/L) can be substituted for glucose in the oral rehydration solution with only minimal loss of efficacy. Vomiting, although frequent, rarely prevents successful use of the oral solution.

Although oral intake during diarrhea may slightly increase the stool volume, there is little evidence that it prolongs illness or complicates fluid therapy except in rare cases. Diarrhea has been found to be an important cause of malnutrition, and withdrawal of breast milk and other food during illness may be one reason for this adverse consequence. Thus, during diarrhea, children should continue to receive breast milk and other staple foods such as rice. Milk or lactose formula should be diluted to one-third to one-half the usual concentration during the first several days of illness.

Intravenous Fluids. Patients with severe dehydration, excessive vomiting, or other infrequent complications should be treated with intravenous fluid replacement. With prompt and appropriate treatment, mortality is negligible (General Principles, Section III D).

PREVENTION AND CONTROL. Preventive measures should include sanitary waste disposal, avoidance of feces-contaminated water and objects, and hygienic practices such as handwashing. However, as noted earlier, the rapid acquisition of serum antibody during the first 2 years of life, regardless of hygienic conditions, suggests that there may be routes of transmission other than the fecal-oral one.

Neonates presumably have maternally derived rotavirus-specific serum antibodies. In addition, breast-fed infants may derive some added protection. In animals, colostrum usually contains rotavirus antibody and prevents rotavirus disease in neonates. Human colostrum has specific rotavirus-neutralizing antibodies, and antirotavirus IgA antibody persists in breast milk for as long as 9 months after delivery.

Children over age 2 years and adults have substantial resistance to rotavirus diarrhea. Natural immunity probably follows one or more illnesses in early childhood and repeated asymptomatic exposures to the virus. Although serum antibodies correlate with resistance to illness, the role of local intestinal immunity has not been determined in humans. In animals, antibody in the small intestine is the major correlate of resistance. Sequential rotavirus illnesses in children have been described, but the serotypes of the rotaviruses causing initial infection and reinfection have not been determined in many instances. Recently, monoclonal antibodies that identify the serotype of rotavirus-positive stool specimens by ELISA have been produced. Such an ELISA will make it possible to serotype large numbers of human rotavirus strains to define the extent and duration of homotypic or heterotypic immunity to rotavirus illness.

Because of the importance of the rotavirus as a cause of morbidity and mortality throughout the world, there is considerable interest in developing a vaccine. Two live attenuated rotavirus vaccine candidates, derived from bovine or simian hosts, have shown efficacy in certain geographic locations but not in others. The consensus at present is that a polyvalent rotavirus vaccine will be needed to protect against the different serotypes of rotavirus, analogous to poliovirus vaccine. Efforts toward identifying and testing such vaccine candidates are currently under way.

DIARRHEA DUE TO NORWALK-LIKE VIRUSES

DEFINITION. The Norwalk agent and a series of other 27 nm viruses cause diarrhea and vomiting of abrupt onset and short duration.

ETIOLOGY AND HISTORY. The prototype virus of this group, the Norwalk agent, was discovered in an outbreak occurring in Norwalk, Ohio. Half the students and teachers in an elementary school developed vomiting and diarrhea. Since no enteropathogens could be detected by direct methods, a bacteria-free filtrate of one patient's feces was administered orally to adult volunteers. The illness produced was identical to the disease seen in the school epidemic. In further studies in adult volunteers, it was found that the same agent can cause a spectrum of symptoms. In some, diarrhea occurred without vomiting, whereas others had vomiting without diarrhea. Most had both manifestations. The virus can be visualized by immune electron microscopy (IEM) and has been said to resemble a calicivirus because of its size and physical properties (Fig. 18–4). The fine ultrastructure of the virion is difficult to visualize by IEM, and final classification awaits determination of the virus nucleic acid.

Volunteer studies using bacteria-free stool filtrates from other outbreaks of diarrhea have also reproduced disease similar to that induced by the Norwalk agent. IEM studies further identified 27 nm viral particles in outbreaks and sporadic cases. The group of Norwalk-like viruses includes at least four distinct serotypes: Norwalk, Hawaii, Snow Mountain, and Ditchling agents. Several other strains, including Montgomery County, Wollan, cockle, Taunton, and Parramatta agents, either are antigenically related to one of the four serotypes or are uncharacterized. The Norwalk-like viruses are similar in size (27 nm) and in buoyant density in cesium chloride (1.36 to 1.41 gm/cm³). They have been difficult to classify further because they do not grow in cell culture, and their nucleic acid content is unknown.

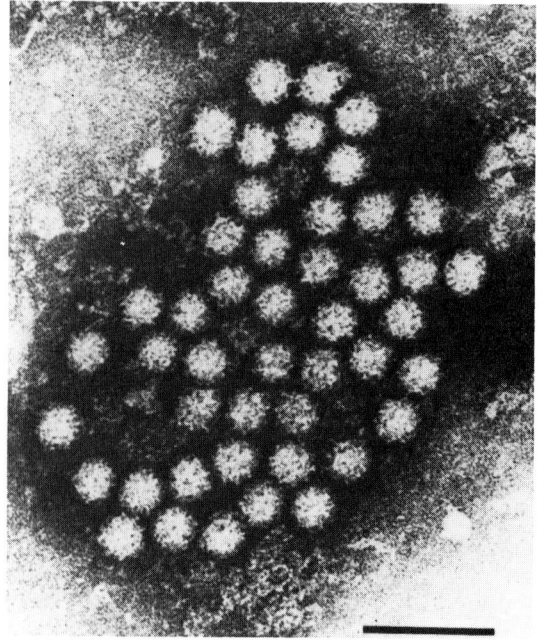

FIGURE 18–4. Immune aggregate of Norwalk virus in stool from an adult volunteer who developed diarrhea after ingesting a filtrate of a rectal swab specimen from an adult who was affected by a diarrhea outbreak in Norwalk, Ohio. (Electron micrograph by Dr. A. Z. Kapikian.) (Bar represents 100 nm.)

DISTRIBUTION AND PREVALENCE. At present, information on the distribution and prevalence of these agents is limited to the Norwalk agent, which has an RIA and an ELISA available for epidemiologic studies. Such assays have also been developed for the Snow Mountain agent, but its seroepidemiology has not yet been studied. In the United States, Norwalk virus has been responsible for approximately one third of gastroenteritis outbreaks in which no bacterial pathogen could be identified. These outbreaks have occurred at all times of the year and in all age groups but primarily affect older children and adults. They have occurred in recreational camps, in communities with contaminated drinking or swimming water, on cruise ships, in schools, in nursing homes, and in families. Some adults who have had diarrhea after traveling to developing countries have had serologic responses to Norwalk virus.

Seroepidemiologic studies indicate that infection with Norwalk virus is worldwide. In developed countries the prevalence of serum antibody increases gradually during childhood, and the majority of adults have antibody. The importance of 27 nm viruses as a cause of endemic childhood diarrhea in developing countries is unknown. However, acquisition of antibody to Norwalk virus in Bangladesh, Ecuador, and the Philippines occurs early in life, suggesting that these infections may cause diarrheal illnesses in young children. A prospective study in rural Bangladesh found a high incidence of increased serum titers of Norwalk antibody among children in their second and third years and demonstrated that children who seroconverted had a higher incidence of diarrhea than those who did not. It was estimated that Norwalk virus may cause 1 to 2% of episodes of diarrhea during a child's first 5 years. Since there are several 27 nm viruses that are not detected using the Norwalk RIA, other viruses in this group may also cause childhood diarrhea.

TRANSMISSION AND EPIDEMIOLOGY. Norwalk-like viruses are transmitted by the fecal-oral route. Virus has been identified in vomitus, suggesting the possibility that aerosolization of virus during vomiting results in airborne spread. Transmission via a common source such as feces-contaminated water and food (primarily shellfish) has been reported frequently, and secondary transmission by person-to-person contact is relatively common.

PATHOGENESIS AND PATHOLOGY. Volunteers ingesting Norwalk or Hawaii viruses develop histologic abnormalities in the proximal small bowel, including broadening and blunting of the villi, mononuclear cell infiltrate, and cytoplasmic vacuolization of epithelial cells. The virus has not been detected within mucosal cells, presumably because of its small size and the patchy distribution of the lesions. The mucosal changes in the small bowel return to normal within 2 weeks. The gastric and rectal mucosa remains normal during infection.

During experimentally induced Norwalk virus illness, small intestinal brush border enzymes are decreased; malabsorption of fat and xylose has been demonstrated. These alterations may persist for several days after diarrhea has stopped and may occur during asymptomatic infections. The role of these changes vis-à-vis nutrient malabsorption and chronic diarrhea remains to be clarified.

CLINICAL MANIFESTATIONS AND COMPLICATIONS. The incubation period for Norwalk disease averages between 24 and 48 hours. Illness is usually mild and lasts between 24 and 60 hours. The majority of patients and experimentally infected volunteers have nausea, vomiting, or diarrhea or a combination of these. Additional symptoms may include anorexia, fever, headache, myalgias, and abdominal cramps. In naturally occurring outbreaks, it has been observed that vomiting is more common than diarrhea in children, whereas the opposite is true of adults. Stools are usually loose and watery and without blood, mucus, or leukocytes.

DIAGNOSIS. The illness cannot be distinguished from other viral diarrheal illnesses, such as that due to rotavirus. However, Norwalk-like viruses should be considered as possible etiologic agents in vomiting or diarrhea in an older child or adult, especially when other individuals with the same exposure history develop gastrointestinal illness.

Laboratory diagnosis is by identification of viral particles in stool obtained early in the illness or by demonstration of a serologic response to viral antigen. Diagnostic tests, which include IEM, RIA, and ELISA, are still research procedures, since reagents are generally not available.

TREATMENT AND PROGNOSIS. Treatment consists of replacement of fluids and electrolytes as indicated for rotavirus diarrhea. Inasmuch as most illnesses are mild and self-limited, the prognosis is excellent.

PREVENTION AND CONTROL. Interruption of fecal-oral transmission is the primary means of prevention. Volunteer studies have demonstrated that short-term homologous resistance to disease develops after Norwalk agent infection. The occurrence of long-term immunity is less clear, and the protective mechanisms are unknown. These uncertainties and the inability to grow the viruses in tissue culture have prevented development of a vaccine.

OTHER VIRAL AGENTS ASSOCIATED WITH DIARRHEA

ENTEROVIRUSES. Prior to the discovery of rotavirus and the Norwalk-like agents, enteroviruses were occasionally associated with diarrhea, but most studies found a similar prevalence of enteroviruses in control subjects as in patients with diarrhea. Of these, the echoviruses were the most frequently implicated, and some ill individuals were found to develop a serum antibody rise against the virus during diarrheal illnesses.

ADENOVIRUSES. Enteric adenoviruses are the second most common cause, after rotavirus, of viral diarrhea in infants and young children. Adenoviruses are classified into 6 groups (A–F) and are composed of 41 distinct serotypes. Enteric adenoviruses belong to group F and include two serotypes, types 40 and 41. Enteric adenoviruses appear to have a worldwide distribution.

Epidemiology. Hospital-based and outpatient studies in several developed countries have shown that 4 to 10% of diarrheal episodes in infants and young children are associated with enteric adenoviruses. The importance of enteric adenoviruses as etiologic agents of diarrhea in developing countries is not clear. Studies from South Africa and Brazil detected enteric adenoviruses in 6.5% and 2%, respectively, of children with acute gastroenteritis. Most cases of diarrhea caused by adenovirus occur in children under 2 years. In contrast to rotavirus, enteric adenovirus infections show no seasonal variation. Outbreaks of diarrhea caused by enteric adenoviruses have occurred among young children in closed communities. The mode of transmission has not been clearly documented but is presumably by the fecal-oral route.

Clinical Manifestations. Disease develops after an incubation period of 8 to 10 days and is characterized by watery diarrhea that lasts for an average of 10 days. Vomiting, fever, and dehydration may occur but are usually mild. Secondary lactose malabsorption has been reported. Respiratory symptoms were common in one study but rare in others. Enteric adenoviruses have not been detected in the respiratory secretions of children with adenovirus diarrhea.

Diagnosis. The diagnosis of diarrhea secondary to enteric adenovirus requires the identification of the virus in the stool specimen. Adenoviruses in stool can be detected by IEM (Fig. 18–5) or genus-specific ELISA. However, additional tests are necessary to identify these adenoviruses as enteric adenoviruses (group F, types 40 and 41), since non–group F adenoviruses can also be shed in the feces. IEM and type-specific ELISA to identify group F adenoviruses are available in research

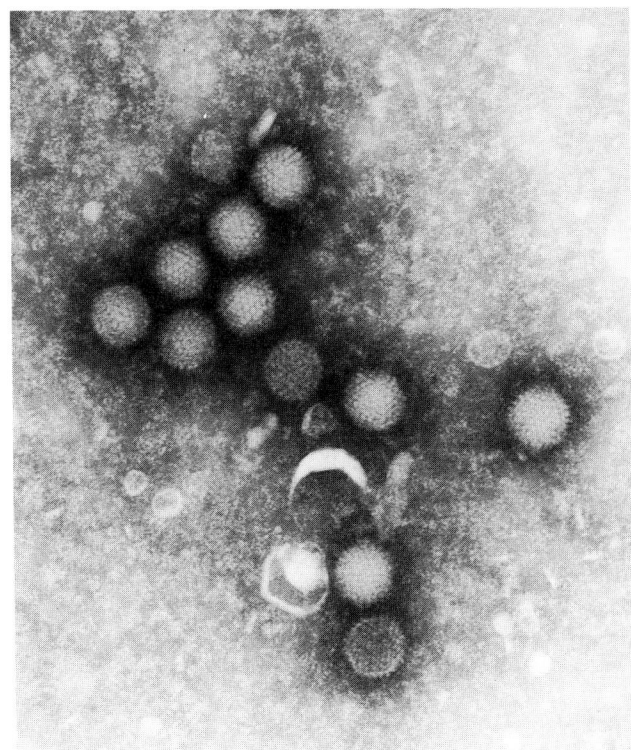

FIGURE 18–5. Adenovirus particles in a stool filtrate from a patient with diarrhea ($\times$ 142,500). (Electron micrograph by Dr. A. Z. Kapikian.)

laboratories. The recent development of monoclonal antibodies to the enteric adenoviruses should make the type-specific ELISA more widely available, facilitating further clinical and epidemiologic studies of diarrhea caused by enteric adenoviruses. Group F adenoviruses differ from groups A–E adenoviruses in that the former will not grow in the conventional cell cultures used to propagate the latter. Thus, a presumptive diagnosis of enteric adenovirus can be made if the adenovirus infection detected by EM or genus-specific ELISA fails to grow in conventional cell cultures.

ASTROVIRUSES. Astrovirus particles were first noted by EM in the stool of an infant with diarrhea. They are 28 nm diameter, star-shaped particles with a worldwide distribution. Several studies have identified astrovirus as a cause of gastroenteritis primarily in young children and the elderly. Outbreaks have occurred in pediatric wards, day care centers, and nursing homes. The incubation period is 3 to 4 days and the illness is mild, usually resolving within 1 to 2 days. A study in England demonstrated that over 80% of children between the ages of 5 and 10 years had serum antibody to astrovirus. Thus, it appears that infection with astrovirus is widespread, but its relative importance as a cause of diarrhea is unclear. Astrovirus has been propagated in cell culture, and monoclonal antibodies to it have been made. These advances should allow further characterization of astroviruses.

CORONAVIRUSES. Coronaviruses cause diarrhea in neonatal animals of several species, but they are not confirmed as causing diarrhea in man. These particles are pleomorphic, measure 120 to 230 nm in diameter, and have a distinctive 20 to 28 nm fringe composed of regularly spaced knobs on very thin stalks. They were first observed in patients with tropical sprue but were also noted in the stools of normal controls. One laboratory detected similar particles in stools collected during 3 outbreaks of diarrhea among adults in the United Kingdom and propagated 1 strain in human embryo intestinal organ cultures, although serial passage could not be accomplished. Coronavirus-like particles have also been detected by EM in the stools of infants and young children with acute nonbacterial gastroenteritis and in some cases of acute hemorrhagic gastroenteritis and necrotizing enterocolitis in neonates.

CALICIVIRUSES. Calicivirus particles of human origin were first noted by EM in the stools of children with diarrhea. They are 30 nm in diameter, and there are characteristic cuplike depressions on the surface of some particles. They have been identified as the etiologic agents of gastroenteritis outbreaks among infants, schoolchildren, and the elderly. At least 3 different serotypes have been identified and an RIA blocking test has been developed, which should allow seroepidemiologic investigations to determine the overall importance of human caliciviruses in diarrheal disease. Of interest, a recent study has demonstrated a one-way serologic cross-relatedness between some human caliciviruses and the Norwalk agent. This lends support to the belief that Norwalk virus may be a calicivirus.

OTHER VIRAL AGENTS. A variety of other virus-like particles have been observed by EM in diarrheal stool. These include one that has been called the mini-reovirus. It looks similar to the rotavirus but is smaller, measuring only 30 nm. Its importance as a cause of diarrhea is unknown.

Further research is needed to determine the siginicance of these other virus-like agents. Although the majority of diarrheal episodes can now be associated with a bacterial or viral enteropathogen, there remains an important minority of episodes for which no etiologic agent can be found.

BIBLIOGRAPHY

Albert MJ: Enteric adenoviruses. Arch Virol 88:1, 1986.

Banatvala JE, Chrystie IL, Totterdell BM: Rotaviral infections in human neonates. J Am Vet Med Assoc 173:527, 1978.

Birch CJ, Heath RL, Gust ID: Use of serotype-specific monoclonal antibodies to study the epidemiology of rotavirus infection. J Med Virol 24:45, 1988.

Bishop RF, Davidson GP, Holmes IH, et al: Virus particles in epithelial cells of duodenal mucosa from children with acute nonbacterial gastroenteritis. Lancet 2:1281, 1973.

Black RE, Merson MH, Rahman ASMM, et al: A two-year study of bacterial, viral, and parasitic agents associated with diarrhea in rural Bangladesh. J Infect Dis 142:660, 1980.

Black RE, Merson MH, Huq I, et al: Incidence and severity of rotavirus and *Escherichia coli* diarrhoea in rural Bangladesh: Implications for vaccine development. Lancet 1:141, 1981.

Black RE, Merson MH, Taylor PR, et al: Glucose vs sucrose in oral rehydration solutions for infants and young children with rotavirus-associated diarrhea. Pediatrics 67:79, 1981.

Black RE, Brown KH, Becker S, et al: Longitudinal studies of infection and physical growth of children in rural Bangladesh. II. Incidence of diarrhea and association with known pathogens. Am J Epidemiol 115:315, 1982.

Black RE: Epidemiology of travelers' diarrhea and relative importance of various pathogens. Rev Infect Dis 12:573, 1990.

Brandt CD, Kim HW, Rodriguez WJ, et al: Pediatric viral gastroenteritis during eight years of study. J Clin Microbiol 18:71, 1983.

Brandt CD, Kim HW, Rodriguez WJ, et al: Adenoviruses and pediatric gastroenteritis. J Infect Dis 151:437, 1985.

Chiba S, Yokohama T, Nakata S, et al: Protective effect of naturally acquired homotypic and heterotypic rotavirus antibodies. Lancet 2:417, 1986.

Ciba Foundation Symposium 128: Novel Diarrhea Viruses. Chichester, John Wiley and Sons, 1987.

Cubitt WD, Blacklow NR, Herrmann JE, et al: Antigenic relationships between human caliciviruses and Norwalk virus. J Infect Dis 156:806, 1987.

Dai G, Sun M, Liu S, et al: First report of an epidemic of diarrhoea in human neonates involving the new rotavirus and biological characteristics of the epidemic virus strain (KMB/R85). J Med Virol 22:365, 1987.

Dolin R, Treanor JJ, Madore HP: Novel agents of viral enteritis in humans. J Infect Dis 155:365, 1987.

Espejo RT, Calderon E, Gonzalez N, et al: Rotavirus gastroenteritis in hospitalized infants and young children in Mexico City. Rev Lat Am Microbiol 20:239, 1978.

Flewett TH, Bryden AS, Davies H, et al: Epidemic viral enteritis in a long-stay children's ward. Lancet 1:4, 1975.

Flores J, Perez-Schael I, Gonzalez M, et al: Protection against severe rotavirus diarrhoea by rhesus rotavirus vaccine in Venezuelan infants. Lancet 1:882, 1987.

Foster SO, Palmer EL, Gary GW Jr, et al: Gastoenteritis due to rotavirus in an isolated Pacific island group: an epidemic of 3439 cases. J Infect Dis 141:32, 1980.

Gary GW, Kaplan JE, Stine SE, et al: Detection of Norwalk virus antibodies and antigen with a biotin-avidin immunoassay. J Clin Microbiol 22:274, 1985.

Gerna G, Passarani N, Battaglia M, et al: Human enteric coronaviruses: antigenic relatedness to human coronavirus OC43 and possible etiologic role in viral gastroenteritis. J Infect Dis 151:796, 1985.

Greenberg HB, Valdesuso J, Kapikian AZ, et al: Prevalence of antibody to the Norwalk virus in various countries. Infect Immun 26:270, 1979.

Hieber JP, Shelton S, Nelson JD, et al: Comparison of human rotavirus diseases in tropical and temperate settings. Am J Dis Child 132:853, 1978.

Hrdy DB: Epidemiology of rotaviral infection in adults. Rev Infect Dis 9:461, 1987.

Hung T, Chen G, Wang C, et al: Waterborne outbreak of rotavirus diarrhoea in adults in China caused by a novel rotavirus. Lancet 1:1139, 1984.

Kapikian AZ, Flores J, Hoshino Y: Rotavirus: the major etiologic agent of severe infantile diarrhea may be controllable by a "Jennerian" approach to vaccination. J Infect Dis 153:815, 1986.

Kaplan JE, Gary GW, Baron RC, et al: Epidemiology of Norwalk gastroenteritis and the role of Norwalk virus in outbreaks of acute nonbacterial gastroenteritis. Ann Intern Med 96:756, 1982.

Konno T, Suzuki H, Katsushima N, et al: Incidence of temperature and relative humidity on human rotavirus infection in Japan. J Infect Dis 147:125, 1983.

Madore HP, Treanor JJ, Pray KA, et al: Enzyme-linked immunosorbent assays for Snow Mountain and Norwalk agents of viral gastroenteritis. J Clin Microbiol 24:456, 1986.

Murphy AM, Albrey MB, Crewe EB: Rotavirus infections of neonates. Lancet 2:1149, 1977.

Perez-Schael I, Daoud G, White L: Rotavirus shedding by newborn children. J Med Virol 14:127, 1984.

Resta S, Luby JP, Rosenfeld CR, et al: Isolation and propagation of a human enteric coronavirus. Science 229:978, 1985.

Richmond SJ, Wood DJ, Bailey AS: Recent respiratory and enteric adenovirus infection in children in the Manchester area. J R Soc Med 81:15, 1988.

Rodriguez WJ, Kim HW, Arrobio JO, et al: Clinical features of acute gastroenteritis associated with human reovirus–like agent in infants and young children. J Pediatr 91:188, 1977.

Rotbart HA, Nelson WL, Glode MP, et al: Neonatal rotavirus-associated necrotizing enterocolitis: case control study and prospective surveillance during an outbreak. J Pediatr 112:87, 1988.

Santosham M, Burns B, Nadkarni V, et al: Oral rehydration therapy for acute diarrhea in ambulatory children in the United States: a double-blind comparison of four different solutions. Pediatrics 76:159, 1985.

Schreiber DS, Blacklow NR, Trier JS: The mucosal lesion of the proximal small intestine in acute infectious nonbacterial gastroenteritis. N Engl J Med 288:1318, 1973.

Suzuki H, Sato T, Kitaoka S, et al: Epidemiology of rotavirus in Guayaquil, Ecuador. Am J Trop Med Hyg 35:372, 1986.

Uhnoo IG, Wadell G, Svensson L, et al: Importance of enteric adenoviruses 40 and 41 in acute gastroenteritis in infants and young children. J Clin Microbiol 20:365, 1984.

Uhnoo I, Olding-Stenkvist E, Kreuger A: Clinical features of acute gastroenteritis associated with rotavirus, enteric adenoviruses, and bacteria. Arch Dis Child 61:732, 1986.

Vesikari T, Isolauri E, Delem A, et al: Clinical efficacy of the RIT 4237 live attenuated bovine rotavirus vaccine in infants vaccinated before a rotavirus epidemic. J Pediatr 107:189, 1985.

Wyatt RE, Yolken RH, Urrutia JJ, et al: Diarrhea associated with rotavirus in rural Guatemala: A longitudinal study of 24 infants and young children. Am J Trop Med Hyg 28:325, 1979.

Wyatt RG, James HD Jr, Pittman AL, et al: Direct isolation in cell culture of human rotaviruses and their characterization into four serotypes. J Clin Microbiol 18:310, 1983.

18.3. ACUTE HEMORRHAGIC CONJUNCTIVITIS

Mark A. Pallansch

DEFINITION. Acute hemorrhagic conjunctivitis (AHC) is a highly contagious epidemic disease characterized by painful conjunctivitis, subconjunctival hemorrhages, and, in rare cases, neurologic symptoms.

ETIOLOGY AND HISTORY. AHC first appeared almost simultaneously in 1969 in Ghana and Indonesia; within 3 years, epidemics swept through North and East Africa, India, and Asia, with scattered outbreaks extending into parts of Europe. From this first pandemic, two novel enteroviral agents were isolated. Enterovirus 70 (EV70) was isolated in 1971 in Japan and shown to be a new enterovirus, unrelated serologically to other picornaviruses. The second virus was an antigenic variant of coxsackievirus A24 (CA24v) and was first isolated from Southeast Asia during epidemics in 1970. Although EV70 has been responsible for most cases, AHC caused by CA24v or adenovirus 11 is clinically nearly indistinguishable from ACH caused by EV70. In 1980 a new pandemic due to EV70 began in Asia, and by 1981 epidemics appeared for the first time in South and Central America, the Caribbean, and the southern United States. CA24v was subsequently introduced into the Western Hemisphere in 1986 during renewed worldwide activity of this virus, and continuing outbreaks have persisted in the Caribbean and Central America through 1988.

DISTRIBUTION AND PREVALENCE. The distribution is worldwide, covering most tropical and semitropical areas. Infections seem favored in hot, humid, crowded conditions with a low level of sanitation, and outbreaks have occurred primarily in coastal towns and cities. Morbidity estimates are imprecise, although it is estimated that tens of millions of cases occurred in Africa and Asia between 1969 and 1972. In a study conducted in Ghana, a low prevalence of neutralizing antibodies was found in sera collected before the 1969 epidemic, and prevalence rates of 50 to 60% were detected after the epidemic. The disease remains endemic in many tropical areas. The incidence of neurologic manifestations has been estimated at 1 case per 10,000 to 15,000 persons with AHC.

TRANSMISSION AND EPIDEMIOLOGY. AHC is highly contagious and is spread by contaminated fingers, towels, and clothing and possibly as well by respiratory droplets. Transmission by flies is possible but conjectural. As with many enterovirus infections, secondary spread within households occurs readily and seems facilitated by the presence of young household members. Iatrogenic transmission (in eye clinics) is also of importance. The origin of these viral agents is problematic. Studies on the viral genome of EV70 isolates have confirmed that all isolates are related and extrapolation of differences over time predicts that a common ancestor arose in the mid-1960s. It is possible that EV70 is a human virus that escaped from some segregated population, whence it was spread by pilgrims to other parts of the world. The origin of CA24v also is conjectural. The possibility that the agent has an animal reservoir has received some attention, and neutralizing antibodies have been found in cattle and sheep in West Africa. Evolution from an insect picornavirus might also be considered.

CLINICAL MANIFESTATIONS AND COMPLICATIONS. The incubation period is 12 to 48 hours, followed by acute onset of lacrimation, severe pain, chemosis and periorbital edema, photophobia, conjunc-

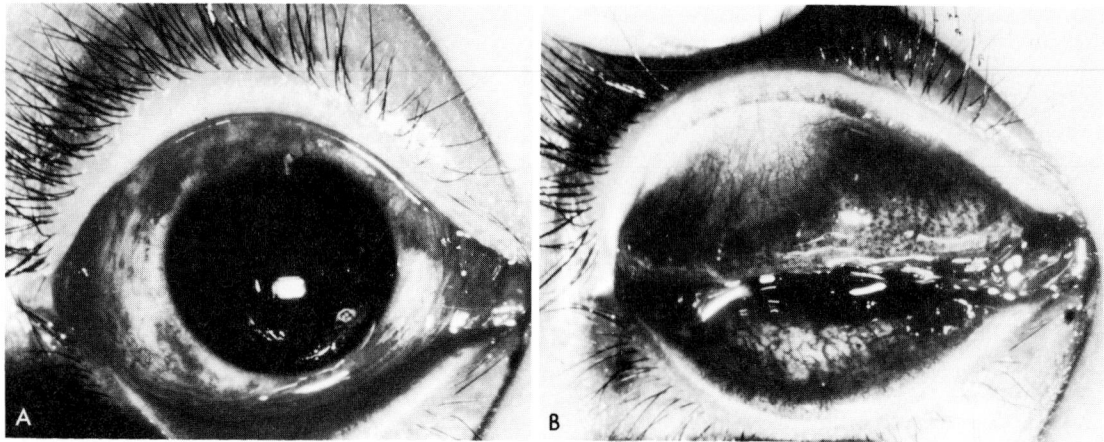

FIGURE 18–6. Subconjunctival hemorrhage *(A)* and inflammation and eyelid edema *(B)* 2 days after onset of acute hemorrhagic conjunctivitis due to enterovirus 70. (From Hung T-P, Kono R: Handbook of Clinical Neurology, Vol. 38. Amsterdam, North-Holland Publishing Co, 1979. Reprinted by permission.)

tival hyperemia, and, in 10 to 100% of patients in various series, mild to severe subconjunctival hemorrhages (Fig. 18–6). The disease begins in one eye and rapidly spreads to the other. Preauricular lymphadenopathy, a scant purulent discharge, punctate epithelial keratitis, and conjunctival follicular hypertrophy are variably present. Secondary bacterial infection may complicate recovery. Recent studies during outbreaks of AHC due to CA24v have indicated that upper respiratory symptoms may be more common with this virus than during infection with EV70.

As previously stated, limited reports indicate that AHC may be followed by a neurologic syndrome characterized by generalized malaise, occasional fever, and bilateral lumbosacral radiculomyelitis (severe bilateral root pain and signs of asymmetric lower motor neuron dysfunction, including weakness, hypotonia, and diminished reflexes especially involving the proximal muscles of the lower extremities). Sensory function is preserved. The syndrome is more common in adults than in children, and full recovery is the rule. Isolated unilateral facial palsy has also been described.

DIAGNOSIS. The clinical diagnosis is relatively straightforward in the setting of an epidemic with prominent subconjunctival hemorrhage. EV70, coxsackievirus A24, and adenovirus 11 may produce an identical clinical illness, and outbreaks may be of mixed etiology. Specific diagnosis depends upon virus isolation from conjunctival swabs or serologic testing. Eye swab specimens may be collected in transport medium (tryptose phosphate broth containing 0.5% gelatin) and shipped on ice as rapidly as possible to a competent virus laboratory. Virus isolation of CA24v is readily accomplished in human embryonic lung fibroblast cell cultures or other cell lines of human origin. Since 1982, isolation of EV70 has been difficult and therefore rare regardless of the cell types employed for isolation. Prior to this time, isolation of EV70 was often obtained in a variety of human and primate cell lines. Diagnosis of EV70 and CA24v infection may also be made by demonstrating a rise in neutralizing antibody titers. In addition, tests are available to measure specific IgG, IgA, and IgM antibodies to EV70 and CA24v using a capture ELISA.

Specific diagnosis of the neurologic syndrome is often complicated by the absence of virus isolation and lack of diagnostic serologic results. The presence of antibodies in cerebrospinal fluid in these patients and a recent history of AHC is presumptive evidence for an etiologic association.

TREATMENT AND PROGNOSIS. AHC is a self-limited disease, and full recovery occurs within 10 to 14 days. Treatment is symptomatic and includes astringent eye drops and cold soaks. Steroid and antibiotic preparations should be avoided unless bacterial superinfection is suspected, in which case cultures should be obtained and antibiotic therapy instituted.

PREVENTION AND CONTROL. Spread of AHC within familial groups and eye clinics may be limited by scrupulous hand washing and disinfection of fomites.

BIBLIOGRAPHY

Hierholzer JC, Hatch MH: Acute hemorrhagic conjunctivitis. *In* Darrell RW (ed): Viral Diseases of the Eye. Philadelphia, Lea & Febiger, 1985, pp 165–196.
Kono R: Apollo 11 disease or acute hemorrhagic conjunctivitis: A pandemic of a new enterovirus infection of the eyes. Am J Epidemiol 101:383–390, 1975.
Kono R, Miyamura K, Tajiri E, et al: Neurologic complications associated with acute hemorrhagic conjunctivitis virus infection and its serologic confirmation. J Infect Dis 129:590–593, 1974.
Quarcoopome CO, Hosaka A, Uchida Y, et al: Clinico-epidemiological studies of acute hemorrhagic conjunctivitis in Ghana. Jpn J Ophthalmol 23:119–125, 1979.
Wadia NH, Wadia PN, Katrak SM, et al: Neurologic manifestations of acute haemorrhagic conjunctivitis. Lancet 2:528–529, 1981.
Wulff H, Anderson LJ, Pallansch MA, et al: Diagnosis of enterovirus 70 infection by demonstration of IgM antibodies. J Med Virol 21:321–327, 1987.

19. VIRAL HEPATITIS

Arie J. Zuckerman

DEFINITION. Human viral hepatitis is caused by at least five different viruses: hepatitis A (infectious or epidemic hepatitis), hepatitis B (formerly referred to as serum hepatitis), and non-A, non-B hepatitis (a more recently identified type that is caused by at least two—probably by several—different viruses). Recently, a serologic marker for one of the agents causing non-A, non-B hepatitis, named hepatitis C, has been developed and is commercially available. The delta agent (hepatitis D) is a defective virus requiring certain helper functions coded for by the hepatitis B virus. As a consequence, delta hepatitis is found only in close association with hepatitis B infections. All known types are endemic throughout the world.

Infection results in acute inflammation of the liver. Inapparent or subclinical infections and infections without jaundice are common. However, the clinical picture ranges from an asymptomatic infection to mild anicteric illness to acute disease with jaundice to severe prolonged jaundice to acute fulminant hepatitis. Hepatitis A virus does not persist in the host, nor is there evidence of progression to chronic liver damage. However, both hepatitis B and the parenterally transmitted forms of non-A, non-B hepatitis may be associated with persistent infection, prolonged carrier state, and progression to chronic liver disease, which may be severe. In addition, there is substantial evidence of an etiologic association between hepatitis B virus and hepatocellular carcinoma.

Hepatitis A and hepatitis B can be differentiated by sensitive laboratory tests for specific antigens and antibodies, and the viruses have been characterized. Hepatitis C and hepatitis D can be diagnosed by serologic tests. On the other hand, there are as yet no precise virologic criteria or specific laboratory tests for the other parenterally transmitted and enteric forms of non-A, non-B hepatitis (hepatitis E).

PATHOLOGY. The pathologic features that are constant in all types of acute viral hepatitis (i.e., A, B, and non-A, non-B) consist of parenchymal cell necrosis and histiocytic periportal inflammation. The reticulin framework of the liver is usually well preserved, except in some cases of massive and submassive necrosis.

The liver cells show necrotic changes that vary in form and intensity. The necrotic areas are usually multifocal, but necrosis frequently tends to be zonal, with the most severe changes occurring in the centrilobular areas. Individual hepatocytes are frequently swollen and may show ballooning, but they can also shrink. Shrunken cells give rise to acidophilic bodies. Characteristic hepatocytes with eosinophilic "ground-glass" cytoplasm are found in hepatitis B, as are orcein-staining cells. Dead or dying rounded liver cells are extruded into the perisinusoidal space. There are variations in the size and staining quality of the nuclei. Fatty changes in the liver are conspicuous by their absence.

A monocellular infiltration, which is particularly marked in the portal zones, is the characteristic mesenchymal reaction. This is accompanied by some proliferation of bile ductules.

Kupffer cells and endothelial cells proliferate, and the Kupffer cells often contain excess lipofuscin pigment. In the icteric phase of the average case of hepatitis, the walls of the hepatic vein tributaries may be thickened and are frequently infiltrated, with proliferation of the lining cells in the terminal hepatic veins. Cholestasis may occur in the early stages of viral hepatitis, and plugs of bile thrombi may be found in the bile canaliculi.

Spotty or focal necrosis with the associated mesenchymal reaction may also be found in anicteric hepatitis, but on the whole the lesions tend to be less severe than in the icteric type of illness. At the other extreme, there is rapid massive necrosis of the liver cells in fulminant hepatitis.

Repair of the liver lobules occurs by regeneration of hepatocytes; frequent mitoses, polyploidy, atypical cells, and binucleated cells are found. There is gradual disappearance of the mononuclear cells from the portal tracts, but elongated histiocytes and fibroblasts may remain. The outcome of acute viral hepatitis may be complete resolution or fatal massive necrosis. Chronic persistent or chronic aggressive hepatitis, resolution with scarring, and cirrhosis may follow acute hepatitis B and the parenterally transmitted forms of non-A, non-B hepatitis.

BIOCHEMICAL TESTS OF LIVER FUNCTION. The serum levels of aspartic and alanine aminotransferase are elevated, as are levels of other enzymes released by the damaged liver cells. Usually the levels of alanine aminotransferase are higher than those of aspartic aminotransferase, a difference particularly marked in non-A, non-B hepatitis. Elevation of these enzymes may be the only abnormality found in individuals with asymptomatic and anicteric infections who were tested because of known exposure. Bilirubin is found in the urine, and conjugated serum bilirubin levels are raised in most symptomatic infections. The leukocyte count is usually normal, but some atypical lymphocytes are frequently found.

CLINICAL MANIFESTATIONS. Differences between the clinical syndromes of acute hepatitis A, acute hepatitis B, and non-A, non-B hepatitis become apparent on analysis of large numbers of well-documented cases, but these differences are not reliable for the diagnosis of icteric disease in individual patients.

Hepatitis A is frequently heralded by a variety of nonspecific symptoms such as fever, chills, headache, fatigue, malaise, and aches and pains. A few days later, these progress to anorexia, nausea, vomiting, and right upper quadrant abdominal pain, followed by passage of dark urine and clay-colored stools and the development of jaundice of the sclera and skin. With the appearance of jaundice, there is usually a rapid subjective improvement in symptoms. The jaundice usually deepens during the first few days and persists for 1 or 2 weeks. The feces then darken and the jaundice diminishes, at first rapidly and then more slowly, over an additional period of 2 weeks or so. Convalescence may be prolonged, and complete recovery in adults usually takes place within a few months. In children, the prodromal features may be mild or even absent, although anorexia, when present, tends to be severe. The icteric or posticteric phase in children is short. There is no evidence of progression of hepatitis A to chronic liver disease. The prodromal phase of hepatitis B and of some types of non-A, non-B hepatitis is often prolonged and more insidious. Low-grade fever, arthralgias, and skin rashes, particularly in hepatitis B, are not uncommon. The clinical features of the icteric phase are similar for all types of acute viral hepatitis.

The mortality rate is low, approximately 1 death in 500 to 1000 cases, with the exception of hepatitis B following blood transfusion. High mortality rates for hepatitis occurring during pregnancy have been reported from India, the Middle East, and North Africa. The infection was often considered to be caused by hepatitis A virus, but is now known to be associated with the epidemic form of non-A, non-B hepatitis (hepatitis E).

DIAGNOSIS. The various types of viral hepatitis cannot be differentiated on clinical and biochemical grounds, but specific serologic tests are now available for hepatitis A, B, and C and infection with the delta hepatitis virus.

TREATMENT. There is no specific treatment for any of the types of acute viral hepatitis. Treatment is largely supportive and is directed toward regeneration of liver cells by rest and the provision of a well-balanced diet.

BIBLIOGRAPHY

World Health Organization: Technical Report Series on Viral Hepatitis, No. 512 (1973), No. 570 (1975), No. 602 (1977), No. 691, Geneva, 1983.
Zuckerman AJ (ed): Viral hepatitis. Clin Trop Med Comm Dis 1:281–458, 1986.
Zuckerman AJ (ed): Viral Hepatitis and Liver Disease. New York, Alan R. Liss, 1988.

19.1. HEPATITIS A

EPIDEMIOLOGY. Hepatitis A is endemic in all parts of the world, but the exact incidence is not known because of the high proportion of asymptomatic and anicteric infections, differences in surveillance, and differing patterns of disease. The degree of underreporting is very high. Serologic surveys have shown that although the prevalence of hepatitis A in industrialized countries, particularly those in northern Europe and North America as well as Australia, is decreasing, the infection is virtually universal in most other regions.

Incubation Period. The incubation period of hepatitis A is between 3 and 5 weeks, with a mean of 28 days. Subclinical and anicteric infections are very common, particularly in children.

Mode of Spread. Hepatitis A virus is spread by the fecal-oral route, usually by person-to-person contact, and the infection is particularly common in conditions of poor sanitation and overcrowding. Common source outbreaks result most frequently from fecal contamination of drinking water and food, but water-borne transmission is not a major factor in the industrialized countries and in areas where a piped water supply has been adequately treated and chlorinated. On the other hand, many food-borne outbreaks have been reported, which can be attributed to the shedding of large amounts of virus in the feces of infected foodhandlers during the incubation period. The source of the outbreak can often be traced to uncooked food or food that has been handled after cooking. Food-borne outbreaks have become important epidemiologically in developed countries. The consumption of raw or inadequately cooked shellfish cultivated in polluted water is also associated with a high risk of infection with hepatitis A virus. Hepatitis A is frequently contracted by travelers to areas of high endemicity. Hepatitis A is very rarely transmitted by blood and blood products, and rarely by the parenteral route, although this has been achieved experimentally in volunteers and in susceptible nonhuman primates.

Age Incidence and Seasonal Pattern. All age groups are susceptible to infection. In developing countries, the highest incidence is observed in children of school age. In some countries, virtually everyone is infected early in life. In North America and in many countries in northern Europe most cases occur in adults, frequently after travel abroad. In temperate zones, the characteristic seasonal trend is for an increased incidence in the autumn and early winter, falling progressively to a minimum in midsummer, but recently this seasonal trend has disappeared in some countries. In many tropical countries, the peak of reported infection tends to occur during the rainy season, with low incidence in dry periods.

CHARACTERISTICS OF HEPATITIS A VIRUS. In 1973, small cubic virus particles (Fig. 19–1) were identified by immune electron microscopy (IEM) in feces obtained from experimentally infected adult volunteers during the early acute phase of hepatitis A. The availability of the viral antigen resulted in the identification of the specific antibody and the development of serologic tests for hepatitis A.

Numerous virus particles are found during the incu-

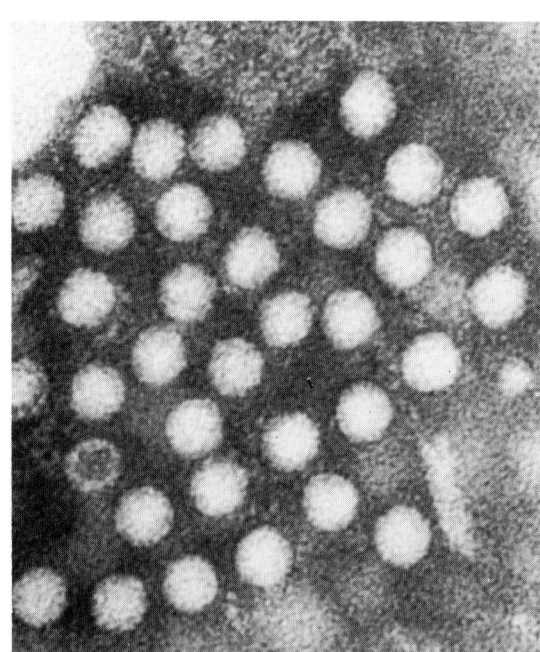

FIGURE 19–1. Hepatitis A virus particles in a fecal extract obtained from a patient during the late incubation period of the infection. The particles measure 25 to 27 nm in diameter and possess cubic symmetry (× 300,000).

bation period in experimentally infected susceptible chimpanzees, beginning as early as 9 days after exposure. Shedding of the virus usually continues until peak elevations of serum aminotransferase levels are reached. Similar observations have been made in the course of experimental and natural infection in man. The virus is also detected during the acute phase of illness, but the number of virus particles decreases rapidly after the onset of clinical jaundice. Prolonged virus excretion and a persistent carrier state have not been demonstrated.

Molecular Biology. Hepatitis A virus is unenveloped, containing a linear genome of single-stranded RNA, 32 to 35 S, approximately 7500 nucleotides in length, and coding for 3 major polypeptides with molecular weights of 27,000, 29,000, and 33,000. A fourth truncated VP4 polypeptide of only 17 amino acids has been reported. There is no information so far on the arrangement of the individual polypeptides on the viral capsid. The organization of the genome of hepatitis A virus is similar to that of the picornavirus; it has been classified as enterovirus type 72, although there are substantial differences between hepatitis A and the established four genera of the picornavirus family, for example, by an unusually low GC content of 38%.

The genome of hepatitis A virus is a linear, single-stranded RNA with a positive polarity. Cloning and sequencing data indicate that the genome consists of 7478 nucleotides with a polyadenylic tract at the 3′ terminus and a small covalently bound protein at the 5′ terminus. The available sequences do not provide evidence for the existence of a poly(C) tract in the vicinity of the 5′ terminus, which is characteristic of picornaviruses.

A single open reading frame extends from nucleotide 710–750 at the 5′ terminus to about 60 nucleotides in advance of the 3′ terminal poly(A) tract. This sequence can encode a protein with molecular weight of about 250,000. The predicted amino acid sequence compared with analogous regions of other picornaviruses suggests that the 5′ region of the genome codes for the three major structural proteins of the virus, including the fourth small VP4. A polymerase is probably coded in the 3′ region. Dipeptide cleavage sites, which are present in poliovirus, are not found in hepatitis A virus, but a detailed description of the post-translational processing of the proteins of hepatitis A virus is not available yet.

Physical Properties. Hepatitis A virus is exceptionally stable; the virus is ether-resistant, stable at pH 3.0, and relatively resistant to inactivation by heat. Hepatitis A virus retains its physical integrity and biologic activity at 60 C for 10 hours and is inactivated at 100 C for 5 minutes. The virus is inactivated by ultraviolet irradiation and by treatment with 1:4000 concentration of formaldehyde solution at 37 C for 72 hours. There is also evidence that hepatitis A virus is inactivated by chlorine at a concentration of 1 mg/L for 30 minutes.

Culture Characteristics. The successful propagation in 1979 of hepatitis A virus in primary monolayer and explant cell cultures and in continuous cell strains of primate origin was a major advance and opened the way to the preparation of hepatitis A vaccines. The viral antigen is detectable by immunofluorescence, radioimmunoassay, an indirect quantitative autoradiographic plaque assay, and complementary DNA-RNA hybridization.

The virus, which does not induce cytopathic changes, replicates in several types of cell cultures of primate origin. The virus tends to induce persistent infections in cell cultures. The virus remains largely cell-associated in most infected cell cultures. However, primary isolation of wild virus is difficult, and several weeks elapse before intracellular antigen is detectable in the cytoplasm of infected cells. Virus isolation is not a practical diagnostic technique in most laboratories.

Adaptation occurs after passage with more rapid production of intracellular antigen and with higher final yields. Virus adapted to growth in cell culture may become attenuated.

The virus replicates in vivo in the liver; there is only one report that replication may also occur in experimental infection in the mucosa of the small intestine.

Serotypes and Antigens. Only one serotype of hepatitis A has been identified in human volunteers infected experimentally, in patients from different outbreaks of hepatitis A, and in naturally and experimentally infected chimpanzees. This has been confirmed by viral cross-neutralization tests and by the protective efficacy of pooled human immunoglobulin obtained from different geographic regions. However, strain-specific differences exist, at least at the level of the nucleotide sequences of viral RNA from different strains of hepatitis A virus. The RNA genome of the virus, like that of other picornaviruses, is subject to relatively high rates of spontaneous mutation.

Note, however, that the topographic nature of the antigen of the surface of the virus has not been fully defined, although recent evidence using monoclonal antibodies suggests that it is associated with the principal surface polypeptide, VP1, which plays a dominant role in the formation of immunogenic and neutralization epitopes. It is believed that secondary or higher orders of protein structure may play essential roles in this antigenic site, since it has not been possible to detect this predominant antigen in virus preparations disrupted with detergent.

PATHOPHYSIOLOGY. The mechanisms underlying liver injury in hepatitis A are not understood. The initial noncytopathic phase, during which virus replicates and is released, is followed by decreased virus multiplication. Inflammatory cell infiltration suggests that immune mechanisms are involved in pathogenesis.

DIAGNOSIS. Specific diagnosis of hepatitis A can be established by demonstrating the virus in feces by enzyme immunoassay or radioimmunoassay or by EM. Isolation of the virus in cell cultures is not yet feasible for routine diagnosis.

Specific antibodies to hepatitis A virus are always demonstrable by enzyme immunoassay or radioimmunoassay at the onset of the disease. The antibodies persist indefinitely. The diagnosis of a recent episode of hepatitis A is most conveniently and reliably established by the demonstration of hepatitis A antibody of the IgM class, which is detectable for up to 4 months after infection, as shown in Figure 19–2.

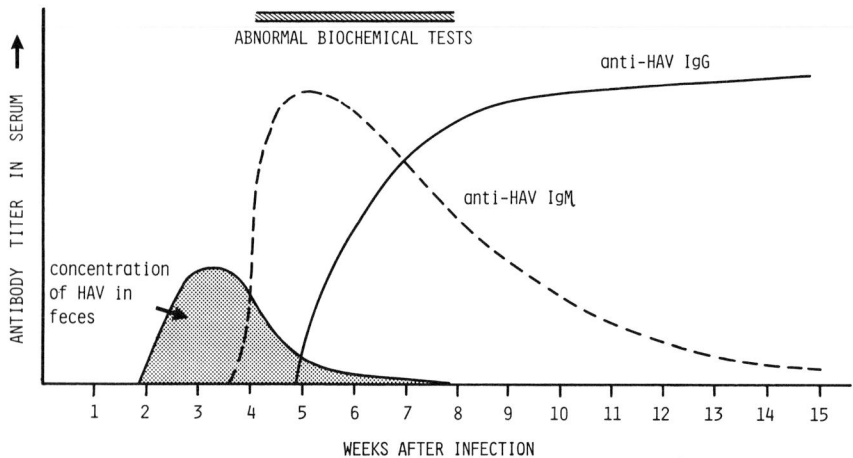

TYPICAL COURSE OF HEPATITIS A

FIGURE 19–2. Typical course of hepatitis A. (From McCollum RW, Zuckerman AJ: J Med Virol 8:1, 1981. Reprinted by permission.)

PREVENTION AND CONTROL. Control of the infection is difficult. Since fecal shedding of the virus is at its highest during the late incubation period and prodromal phase of the illness, strict isolation of cases is not a useful control measure. Spread of hepatitis A is reduced by simple hygienic measures and the sanitary disposal of excreta.

Passive Prophylaxis. Normal human immunoglobulin, containing at least 100 IU/ml of anti-HAV, given intramuscularly before exposure to the virus or early during the incubation period will prevent or attenuate a clinical illness. The dosage should be at least 2 IU of anti-HAV/ kg body weight, but in special cases such as pregnancy or in patients with liver disease the dosage may be doubled (Table 19–1). Immunoglobulin does not always prevent infection and excretion of hepatitis A virus, and inapparent or subclinical hepatitis may develop. The efficacy of passive immunization is based on the presence of hepatitis A antibody in the immunoglobulin, but the minimum titer of antibody required for protection has not yet been established. Immunoglobulin is used most commonly for close personal contacts of patients with hepatitis A and for those exposed to contaminated food. Immunoglobulin has also been used effectively for controlling outbreaks in institutions such as homes for the mentally handicapped and in nursery schools. Prophylaxis with immunoglobulin is recommended for persons without hepatitis A antibody who are visiting highly endemic areas. After a period of 6 months the administration of immunoglobulin for travelers should be repeated, unless it has been demonstrated that the recipient has developed his own hepatitis A antibodies.

Immunization. Live attenuated and killed hepatitis A vaccines are under clinical evaluation. Vaccines produced by recombinant DNA techniques are under development.

BIBLIOGRAPHY

Deinhardt F, Abb J: Hepatitis A. Clin Trop Med Commun Dis 1:303–319, 1986.

Krugman S, Giles JP, Hammond J: Infectious hepatitis: Evidence for two distinctive clinical, epidemiological and immunological types of infection. JAMA 200:365–373, 1967.

Lemon SM: Type A viral hepatitis. New developments in an old disease. N Engl J Med 313:1059–1067, 1985.

19.2. HEPATITIS B

EPIDEMIOLOGY. The discovery in 1965 of Australia antigen (now referred to as hepatitis B surface antigen) and the demonstration by Blumberg and his colleagues of its association with hepatitis B have led to rapid and unabated progress in the understanding of this complex infection.

In the past, hepatitis B was diagnosed on the basis of infection occurring approximately 60 to 180 days after the injection of human blood or plasma fractions or the use of inadequately sterilized syringes and needles. The development of specific laboratory tests for hepatitis B confirmed the importance of the parenteral routes of transmission, and infectivity appears to be especially related to blood. However, several factors have altered the epidemiologic dogma that hepatitis B is spread exclusively by blood and blood products. These include the observations that under certain circumstances the virus is infective by mouth, that it is endemic in closed institutions and institutions for the mentally handicapped, that it is more prevalent in adults in urban communities and in poor socioeconomic conditions, that there is a huge reservoir of carriers of markers of hepatitis B virus in the human population, and that the

TABLE 19–1. Passive Immunization with Normal Immunoglobulin for Travelers to Highly Endemic Areas

Persons	Period < 3 Months	Period > 3 Months
<25 kg	50 IU anti-HAV (0.5 ml)	100 IU anti-HAV (1.0 ml)
25–30 kg	100 IU anti-HAV (1.0 ml)	250 IU anti-HAV (2.5 ml)
>50 kg	200 IU anti-HAV (2.0 ml)	500 IU anti-HAV (5.0 ml)

carrier rate and age distribution of the surface antigen vary in different regions.

There is much evidence for the transmission of hepatitis B by intimate contact and by the sexual route. The sexually promiscuous, particularly male homosexuals, are at very high risk. Hepatitis B surface antigen has been found in blood and in various body fluids such as saliva, menstrual and vaginal discharges, seminal fluid, colostrum and breast milk, and serous exudates, and these have been implicated as vehicles of transmission of infection. The presence of the antigen in urine, bile, feces, sweat, and tears has been reported occasionally but has not been confirmed. It is not surprising, therefore, that contact-associated hepatitis B is of major importance. Transmission of the infection may result from accidental inoculation of minute amounts of blood or fluid contaminated with blood during medical, surgical, and dental procedures; immunization with inadequately sterilized syringes and needles; intravenous and percutaneous drug abuse; tattooing; ear and nose piercing; acupuncture; laboratory accidents; and accidental inoculation with razors and similar objects that have been contaminated with blood. Additional factors may be important for the transmission of hepatitis B infection in the tropics; these include traditional tattooing and scarification, bloodletting, ritual circumcision, and repeated biting by blood-sucking arthropod vectors. Investigation of the role that biting insects may play in the spread of hepatitis B has yielded conflicting results. Hepatitis B surface antigen has been detected in several species of mosquitoes and in bedbugs that were either trapped in the wild or fed experimentally on infected blood, but no convincing evidence of replication of the virus in insects has been obtained. Mechanical transmission of the infection, however, is a possibility.

Perinatal Transmission. Clustering of hepatitis B virus also occurs within family groups but does not appear to be related to genetic factors and does not reflect maternal or venereal transmission. The mechanisms of intrafamilial spread of the infection are not known. Transmission of hepatitis B virus from carrier mothers to their babies can occur during the perinatal period and appears to be an important factor in determining the prevalence of the infection in some regions, particularly in China and Southeast Asia. The risk of infection in the infant may reach 50 to 60%, although it varies from country to country and appears to be related to ethnic groups. The risk is greatest if the mother has a history of transmission of infection to previous children or has a high titer of hepatitis B surface antigen and/or e antigen. There is also a substantial risk of perinatal infection if the mother had acute hepatitis B in the second or third trimester of pregnancy or within 2 months after delivery. Although hepatitis B virus can infect the fetus in utero, this appears to be rare, and it is generally associated with antepartum hemorrhage and tears in the placenta. The mechanism of perinatal infection is uncertain, but it probably occurs during or shortly after birth as a result of a leak of maternal blood into the baby's circulation or of its ingestion or inadvertent inoculation. Most children infected during the perinatal period become persistent carriers.

The Carrier State. The carrier state is defined as persistence of the hepatitis B surface antigen in the circulation for more than 6 months. The carrier state may be lifelong and may be associated with liver damage varying from minor changes in the nuclei of hepatocytes to chronic active hepatitis and cirrhosis. Several risk factors have been identified in relation to development of the carrier state. It is more frequent in males, more likely to follow infections acquired in childhood than those acquired in adult life, and more likely to occur in patients with natural or acquired immune deficiencies. A carrier state becomes established in approximately 5 to 10% of infected adults. In countries where hepatitis B infection is common, the highest prevalence of the surface antigen is found in children aged 4 to 8 years, with steadily declining rates among older age groups. The e antigen has been reported to be more common in young carriers than in adult carriers of hepatitis B, whereas the prevalence of e antibody appears to increase with age.

Survival of hepatitis B virus is ensured by the reservoir of carriers, estimated to number over 300 million worldwide. The prevalence of carriers, particularly among blood donors, in northern Europe, North America, and Australia is 0.1% or less, and in central and Eastern Europe, up to 5%; in southern Europe, the countries bordering the Mediterranean, and parts of Central and South America the frequency is even higher; and in some parts of Africa, Asia, and the Pacific region as many as 20% or more of the apparently healthy population may be carriers. There is an urgent need to define the mechanisms that lead to the carrier rate in endemic areas and to introduce methods of interruption of transmission. The management of the carrier state is a complex issue with personal, social, and economic implications.

CHARACTERISTICS OF HEPATITIS B VIRUS (HBV). Electron microscopic examination of serum containing hepatitis B surface antigen reveals small spherical particles measuring about 22 nm in diameter, tubular forms of varying length but with a diameter of approximately 22 nm, and large double-shelled or solid particles approximately 42 nm in diameter (Fig. 19–3). The large particles contain a core or nucleocapsid about 28 nm in diameter. The 42 nm particle (referred to in the past as the Dane particle) is the hepatitis B virus, whereas the small particles and the tubules are noninfectious surplus virus coat protein.

Molecular Biology. The core of the virus contains a DNA-dependent polymerase that is closely associated with a DNA template. Double-stranded circular DNA has been isolated from circulating virus and also from cores extracted from the nuclei of infected hepatocytes. The molecular weight of the DNA is about 2.3×10^6. The DNA measures approximately 3200 nucleotides in length and contains a single-stranded gap varying from 600 to 2100 nucleotides.

The entire DNA of hepatitis B virus has been cloned in *Escherichia coli,* in yeast (*Saccharomyces cerevisiae*), and also in several strains of mammalian cells.

Initial studies of HBV were hampered by the inability to cultivate the virus in vitro and were essentially limited

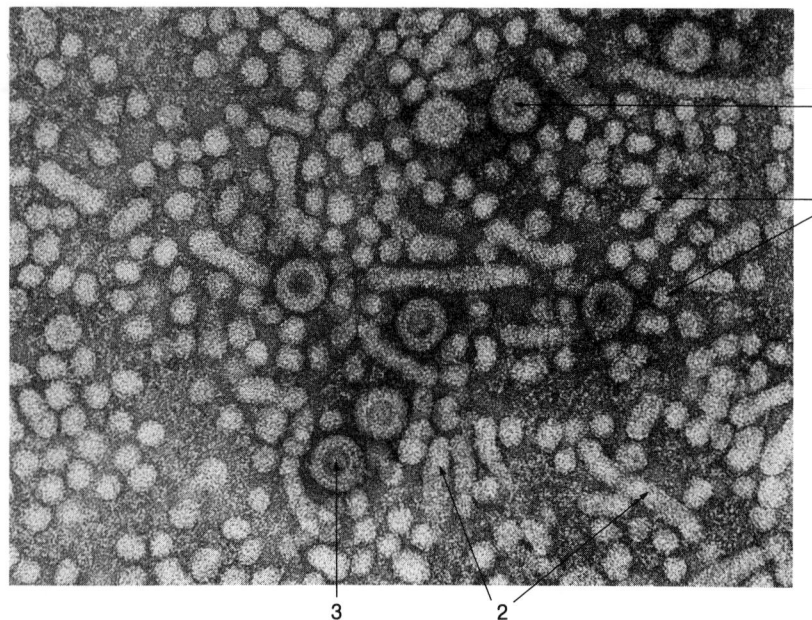

FIGURE 19–3. Electron micrograph showing the complex morphology of hepatitis B virus in serum: (1) Small spherical particles of hepatitis B surface antigen about 22 nm in diameter, (2) tubular structures of the surface antigen, and (3) large spheroidal particles about 42 nm in diameter. This is the complete virus particle, which may be solid or double-shelled ($\times$ 252,000).

to biochemical analysis of purified virions and viral antigens and to serologic and histologic investigations of clinical infections. Molecular cloning of the viral genome provided better analytical methods and resulted in the determination of the entire nucleotide sequence. Analysis of the nucleotide sequence revealed four open reading frames, regions of the genome that code for proteins.

Prior to the sequencing of the HBV genome, the amino acid sequence of both the amino and the carboxyl termini of the major hepatitis B surface antigen (HBsAg) polypeptide had been determined, and it was therefore possible to locate the gene for this polypeptide within one of the open reading frames. Part of the open reading frame was not represented in the HBsAg polypeptide and was designated pre-S, as it was assumed that these sequences were cleaved off a larger precursor polypeptide after translation. The pre-S region is therefore subdivided into pre-S1 and pre-S2. Sequences in pre-S2 appear to encode a viral-cell receptor, but the function of the pre-S1 region, which is variable between the different HBV subtypes, is not yet established.

The product of the C gene is the hepatitis B core antigen (HBcAg). Both the core polypeptide expressed in *E. coli* and the native polypeptide from the virus particle may be converted by proteolytic digestion to e antigen. Hepatitis B e antigen may exist as two or three antigenically distinct polypeptides of slightly different size, and the precise relationship of these to one another and to HBcAg remains to be determined. The protein kinase activity detected in the hepatitis B virion resides in the core antigen, which appears to be self-phosphorylating.

The largest open reading frame overlaps the other three and codes for the polymerase responsible for the replication of the viral genome. Viral DNA replication proceeds via an RNA intermediate; domains within the putative translation product of this gene share amino acid homology with the reverse transcriptase of retroviruses and with the polymerases of caulimonviruses,

plant DNA viruses that also replicate via an RNA intermediate. The replication of hepatitis B virus, and indeed that of the related hepatitis B viruses of animals, the hepadnaviruses, are thus strikingly different from that in other DNA viruses.

The predicted gene product of the X gene is a small polypeptide of approximately 150 amino acids. Evidence has recently been obtained that this gene is expressed during infection resulting in antibody response, particularly in patients with chronic active hepatitis and hepatocellular carcinoma. This gene appears to have a transactivating function.

Antigens. The morphologic complexity of hepatitis virus is surpassed by the antigenic heterogeneity of the surface antigen reactivities. Careful serologic analysis has shown that the hepatitis B surface antigen particles share a common group-specific antigen a and generally carry at least two mutually exclusive subdeterminants, d or y and w or r. The subtypes are the phenotypic expressions of distinct genotype variants of hepatitis B virus.

Four principal phenotypes are recognized, adw, adr, ayw, and ayr, but other complex permutations of these subdeterminants and new variants have been described, all apparently on the surface of the same physical particles. The major subtypes have differing geographic distribution. For example, in northern Europe, the Americas, and Australia, subtype adw predominates. Subtype ayw occurs in a broad zone that includes northern and western Africa, the eastern Mediterranean, Eastern Europe, northern and central Asia, and the Indian subcontinent. Both adw and adr are found in Malaysia, Thailand, Indonesia, and Papua New Guinea, whereas subtype adr predominates in other parts of Southeast Asia, including China, Japan, and the Pacific Islands. The subtypes provide useful epidemiologic markers of hepatitis B virus.

Variants of hepatitis B virus have been described in Senegal, Italy, France, and Taiwan. Some of these variants share a few epitopes with the envelope of the

TABLE 19–2. Interpretation of Results of Serologic Tests for Hepatitis B

HBsAg	HBeAg	Anti-HBe	Anti-HBc *IgM*	Anti-HBc *IgG*	Anti-HBs	Interpretation
+	+	−	−	−	−	Incubation period
+	+	−	+	+	−	Acute hepatitis B or persistent carrier state
+	+	−	−	+	−	Persistent carrier state
+	−	+	+/−	+	−	Persistent carrier state
−	−	+	+/−	+	+	Convalescence
−	−	−	−	+	+	Recovery
−	−	−	+	−	−	Infection with hepatitis B virus without detectable HBsAg
−	−	−	−	+	−	Recovery with loss of detectable anti-HBs
−	−	−	−	−	+	Immunization without infection. Repeated exposure to antigen without infection, or recovery from infection with loss of detectable anti-HBc

From Zuckerman AJ: Priorities for immunisation against hepatitis B. Br Med J 284:686, 1979.

prototype hepatitis B virus, but no cross-reactivity with the core and e antigen. There is no anti-HBc response and no cross-protection from anti-HBs (the surface antibody). A hepatitis B escape mutant virus has been described more recently.

SEROLOGIC DIAGNOSIS OF INFECTION WITH HEPATITIS B VIRUS. Sensitive and specific laboratory tests such as enzyme immunoassay and radioimmunoassay are now available for the detection of specific serologic markers of infection with hepatitis B virus.

Progressive Course of Hepatitis B Antigens and Antibodies. A simplified guide to the interpretation of the test results is shown in Table 19–2. During the incubation period, hepatitis B virus infection leads to the appearance of hepatitis B viral DNA and a specific antigen, hepatitis B surface antigen, in the plasma. This occurs 2 to 8 weeks before biochemical evidence of liver dysfunction or the onset of jaundice. The antigen persists during the acute illness and is usually cleared from the circulation during convalescence. Next to appear in the circulation is a specific viral DNA polymerase associated with the core or nucleocapsid of the virus. At about the same time another antigen, the e antigen, becomes detectable, again preceding elevation of serum aminotransferase levels. The e antigen is a distinct soluble antigen that is located within the core and correlates closely with the number of virus particles and relative infectivity. Antibody to the hepatitis B core antigen is found in the serum 2 to 4 weeks after the appearance of the surface antigen; it is always detectable during the early acute phase of the illness. Core antibody of the IgM class becomes undetectable within some months of the onset of uncomplicated acute infection, but IgG core antibody persists for many years, possibly for life. The next antibody to appear in the circulation is directed against the e antigen. There is evidence that, in general, the presence of anti-e indicates relatively low infectivity of serum. Antibody to the surface antigen component, i.e., hepatitis B surface antibody, is the last marker to appear, late during convalescence (Fig. 19–4).

The open reading frame of the S gene of HBV codes for the surface antigen of the virus (HBsAg), while the region upstream codes for two proteins designated pre-S1 and pre-S2. The presence of pre-S proteins in serum has been found to be associated with high HBV replication, and pre-S proteins have also been found in the liver. The presence of pre-S1 proteins in the serum and in the liver correlates closely with HBV DNA, and on cessation of viral replication pre-S1 is no longer detectable. Anti–pre-S2 has received much more attention because antibodies to pre-S2 have been reported as markers of viral clearance and recovery, and indeed, complete clearance of pre-S2 antigen after interferon therapy predicated elimination of all markers of HBV from serum. Furthermore, anti–pre-S2 antibodies neutralize the infectivity of HBV, and experimental immunization with a pre-S2 peptide has protected against challenge infection.

These antibodies may be relevant to the clearance of

FIGURE 19–4. Diagram showing serologic course of uncomplicated acute hepatitis B with recovery. (From McCollum RW, Zuckerman AJ: J Med Virol 8:1, 1981. Reprinted by permission.)

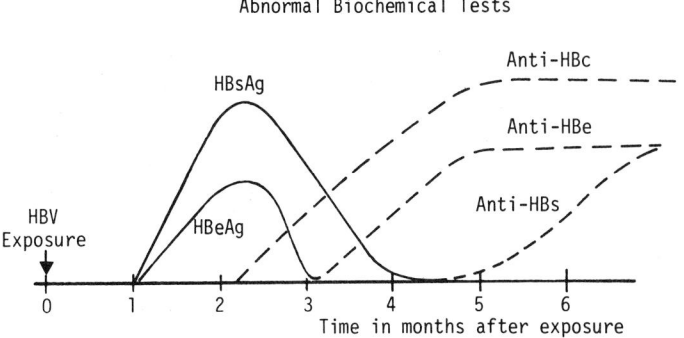

circulating hepatitis B virions and the termination of the infection; their absence in patients with chronic active hepatitis may explain why the infection persists. Cell-mediated immunity is also important in terminating hepatitis B infection and, under certain circumstances, in promoting liver damage and generating autoimmunity.

THE DELTA VIRUS. Delta antigen and antibody are serologic reactivities that are detected in carriers of hepatitis B surface antigen. Delta antigen is distinct from known antigenic determinants of hepatitis B virus and is localized in the nuclei of liver cells of patients with chronic hepatitis B infection. Most patients develop anti-delta. Delta antigen appears to be a distinct agent that requires helper function of hepatitis B virus.

Distribution and Transmission. The epidemiology of delta infection seems to have three patterns: (1) endemic and associated with nonparenteral spread in Italy, other Mediterranean countries, and the Middle East; (2) endemic-epidemic in remote areas of northern South America; and (3) sporadic and associated with parenteral transmission in almost all other geographic areas examined. Nonpercutaneous transmission probably also occurs.

In 1981 an outbreak was studied among Amerindians inhabiting villages southwest of Maracaibo, Venezuela. The disease, characterized by severe hepatitis and a high mortality, especially among children and adolescents, was shown to be due to delta agent. The clinical and epidemiologic features of this outbreak were similar to those in previous (unpublished) reports of "Labréa hepatitis" (black fever) in the upper Amazon River basin along the Purus and Juruá Rivers in Brazil.

Anti-delta appears to be associated with continuing viral replication; however, other recognized markers of infectious hepatitis B virus production are absent. The presence and persistence of high-titer anti-delta in a symptomless carrier of the surface antigen may be a useful indicator of underlying chronic liver disease.

Delta virus (HDV) has been transmitted to susceptible chimpanzees, and evidence was obtained that the infectivity of the delta-associated agent appears to be distinct from, but dependent upon, the replication of hepatitis B virus.

Biology. Physical characterization of delta activity in the serum of an experimentally infected chronic chimpanzee carrier of hepatitis B surface antigen revealed that delta antigen was associated with a discrete subpopulation of particles. The predominant morphologic form was a 35- to 37-nm particle that shared determinants with hepatitis B surface antigen. The delta antigen particles were fully precipitated by anti-HBs. Low molecular weight circular RNA (molecular weight about 500,000) is found in the delta virus. The hepatitis D virus appears to require helper functions of hepatitis B virus for its expression and replication. The apparent encapsulation of the delta antigen with hepatitis B surface antigen could represent one such helper function of hepatitis B virus, to provide that agent a mode of transmission and access to hepatocytes.

Clinical Manifestations. Acute coinfection with hepatitis B virus and the delta virus results in typical acute hepatitis. A proportion of patients will remain as carriers of both viruses, although HDV infection in some instances can suppress HBsAg RNA. Superinfection with delta of a symptomless carrier of hepatitis B results usually in a second episode of clinical hepatitis, which may progress to chronic liver disease. Superinfection in a hepatitis B carrier with liver disease leads to reactivation and progression of liver damage and often to fulminant hepatic failure.

HEPATITIS B, CHRONIC LIVER DISEASE, AND HEPATOCELLULAR CARCINOMA. The outcome of acute hepatitis B may be complete resolution, massive necrosis, chronic hepatitis, or resolution with scarring and cirrhosis. Therefore, chronic liver disease following hepatitis may be the result of necrosis, collapse of the reticulum framework, formation of scars or nodular hyperplasia, and/or various immunologic and host factors.

Chronic Active Hepatitis. There is evidence that liver damage in hepatitis B is related to the immune response by the host. Patients with active chronic hepatitis with persistent hepatitis B antigens are usually male and are older than patients without the surface antigen. Autoantibodies are usually absent from the serum, and multisystem involvement is not present. A proportion of patients with cryptogenic cirrhosis have evidence of persistent hepatitis B infection. In addition, there is an etiologic association between hepatitis B infection, macronodular cirrhosis, and hepatocellular carcinoma.

Hepatocellular Carcinoma. In many parts of the world, hepatocellular carcinoma is one of the most common human cancers, particularly in young men (Chapter 11). Compelling evidence exists for the implication of hepatitis B virus in the etiology of this important cancer. There are epidemiologic and geographic observations of a strong correlation between hepatitis B infection and primary liver cancer. A relatively constant risk exists of developing hepatocellular carcinoma in both endemic and nonendemic areas among male persistent carriers of hepatitis B surface antigen. Infection precedes and may accompany the development of cancer, usually in a patient with chronic liver damage or macronodular cirrhosis associated with hepatitis B virus. Hepatitis B antigens are present in the malignant tissue, and there is covalent integration of the genome of hepatitis B virus into the DNA of the tumor cells. Several cell lines derived from hepatocellular carcinomas secrete hepatitis B surface antigen in culture. DNA is integrated into the genome of these cells, as are RNA molecules containing specific sequences of hepatitis B virus, and at least one of these cell lines has been shown to be heterotransplantable. Finally, chronic liver damage and primary liver cancer have been found in several animal species infected with viruses that are phylogenetically related to human hepatitis B virus.

ANTIVIRAL TREATMENT OF CHRONIC HEPATITIS B INFECTION

Interferon. Interferon is being evaluated in several centers for the treatment of chronic hepatitis B. A number of reports indicate that the administration of human alpha-interferon, both in man and in persistently infected chimpanzees, inhibits replication of hepatitis B virus in about half of those treated.

Adenine Arabinoside. Adenine arabinoside (ara-A, vidarabine) acts as an analogue of the deoxyribonucleoside of adenine and has significant antiviral activity against several DNA viruses. Several small studies have been carried out in patients with chronic liver disease. Most patients had an immediate loss of DNA polymerase, which was followed by a rebound in many when treatment was stopped. A similar temporary effect was found in infected chimpanzees treated with adenine arabinoside. Further trials with this potent drug and with its monophosphate derivative have been discontinued in view of toxic side effects.

The Flavinoid (+)-Cyanidanol-3. The use of this drug for the treatment of acute viral hepatitis has shown what appear to be marginal and mainly subjective beneficial effects.

PREVENTION AND CONTROL

Passive Immunization. Hepatitis B immunoglobulin is prepared from pooled plasma with high titer of hepatitis B surface antibody; it may confer temporary passive immunity under certain defined conditions. The major indication for the administration of hepatitis B immunoglobulin is a single acute exposure to hepatitis B virus, such as occurs when blood containing surface antigen is inoculated, ingested, or splashed onto mucous membranes and the conjunctiva. The optimal dose has not been established, but doses in the range of 250 to 500 IU have been effective. Hepatitis B immunoglobulin should be administered as soon as possible after exposure, preferably within 48 hours; usually 3 ml (containing 200 IU of anti-HBs/ml) is given to adults. It should not be administered 7 days or later following exposure. It is generally recommended that two doses be given 30 days apart.

Results with the use of hepatitis B immunoglobulin for prophylaxis in babies at risk of infection with hepatitis B virus are encouraging if the immunoglobulin is given within 12 hours of birth; the chance of the baby's developing the persistent carrier state is reduced by about 70%. More recent studies using combined passive and active immunization indicate an efficacy approaching 90%. The dose of hepatitis B immunoglobulin recommended in the newborn is 1 to 2 ml (200 IU of anti-HBs/ml).

Active Immunization. Immunization against hepatitis B is required for groups that are at an increased risk of acquiring this infection. These include individuals requiring repeated transfusions of blood or blood products, those who need prolonged inpatient treatment, patients in whom frequent tissue penetration or repeated access to the circulation is required, patients with natural or acquired immune deficiency, and patients with malignant diseases. Viral hepatitis is an occupational hazard among health care personnel and the staff of institutions for the mentally retarded and in some semiclosed institutions. High rates of infection with hepatitis B occur in narcotic drug addicts and drug abusers, homosexuals, and prostitutes. Individuals working in highly endemic areas are also at an increased risk of infection. Women in areas where the carrier state in that group is high are another segment requiring immunization, in view of the increased risk of transmission of the infection to their offspring. Young infants, children, and susceptible persons living in certain tropical and subtropical areas where socioeconomic conditions are poor and the prevalence of hepatitis B is high should also be immunized.

The failure to grow hepatitis B virus in tissue culture has directed attention to the use of other preparations for active immunization. Since hepatitis B surface antigen leads to the production of protective surface antibody, purified 22 nm spherical surface antigen particles have been developed as vaccines. These vaccines have been prepared from the plasma of symptomless carriers (Fig. 19–5). Trials on protective efficacy in high-risk groups have demonstrated the value of the vaccines and their safety. There is no risk of transmission of the acquired immune deficiency syndrome (AIDS) or any other blood-borne infection by vaccines derived from plasma that meet the WHO Requirements of 1981, 1983, and 1987. Local reactions reported after immunization have been minor, occurring in less than 20% of immunized individuals, and consisting of slight swelling and reddening at the site of inoculation. Temperature elevations of up to 38C were observed in only a few individuals.

Indications for Immunization Against Hepatitis B. The current indications for the use of hepatitis B vaccines in low-prevalence areas are summarized below. The recommendations for immunization against this infection in intermediate- and high-prevalence regions also include universal immunization of infants.

1. All health care personnel in frequent contact with blood or needles. Groups at the highest risk in this category include:
   A. Personnel, including teaching and training staff, directly involved over a period of time in patient care in residential institutions for the mentally handicapped where there is a known high risk of hepatitis.
   B. Personnel directly involved in patient care over a period of time, working in units giving treatment to patients with a known high risk of hepatitis B infection.
   C. Personnel directly involved in patient care working in hemodialysis, hemophilia, and other centers regularly performing maintenance treatment of patients with blood or blood products.
   D. Laboratory workers regularly exposed to increased risk from infected material.
   E. Health care personnel working in areas where there is a high prevalence of hepatitis B infection, if they are to be directly involved in patient care.
   F. Dentists and ancillary dental personnel with direct patient contact.
2. Patients
   A. Patients on first entry into those residential institutions for the mentally handicapped where there is a known high incidence of hepatitis B.
   B. Patients treated by maintenance hemodialysis.
   C. Patients requiring major surgery who are likely to need a large number of blood transfusions and/ or treatment with blood products.
3. Contacts of patients with hepatitis B
   A. The spouses and other sexual contacts of those with acute hepatitis B or those who are carriers

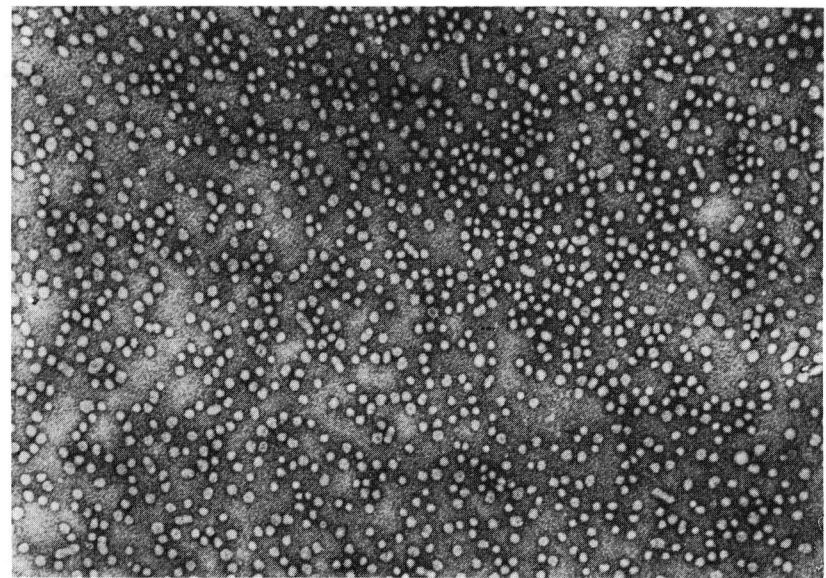

FIGURE 19–5. Hepatitis B small particle vaccine after purification of the surface antigen from pooled plasma obtained from carriers and inactivation of the purified antigen with formalin ($\times$ 80,000).

of hepatitis B virus, and other family members in close contact.

4. Other indications for immunization
  A. Infants born to mothers who are persistent carriers of hepatitis B surface antigen (HBsAg) or who are HBsAg-positive as a result of recent infection, particularly if hepatitis B e antigen is detectable, or infants of HBV-positive mothers without antibody to e antigen (anti-e). The optimal time for immunoglobulin to be given at a contralateral site is immediately at birth or within 12 hours.
  B. Health care workers who are accidentally pricked with needles used for patients with hepatitis B. The vaccine may be used alone or in combination with hepatitis B immunoglobulin as an alternative to passive immunization with hepatitis B immunoglobulin only.
5. Immediate protection
  A. Whenever immediate protection is required, as, for example, in infants born to HBsAg-positive mothers (see earlier) or following transfer of an individual into a high-risk setting or after accidental inoculation, active immunization with the vaccine should be combined with simultaneous administration of hepatitis B immunoglobulin at a different site. It has been shown that passive immunization with up to 3 ml (200 IU of anti-HBs/ml) of hepatitis B immunoglobulin does not interfere with an active immune response. A single dose of hepatitis B immunoglobulin (usually 3 ml for adults, 1 to 2 ml for the newborn) is sufficient for healthy individuals. If infection has already occurred at the time of the first immunization, virus multiplication is unlikely to be inhibited completely; however, severe illness and, most important, the development of the carrier state of HBV may be prevented in many individuals, particularly in infants born to carrier mothers.
6. The immune response to the current hepatitis B vaccines is poorer in immunocompromised persons and in the elderly. For example, only about 60% of patients undergoing treatment by maintenance hemodialysis develop anti-HBs. It is suggested, therefore, that patients with chronic renal damage be immunized as soon as it appears likely that they will ultimately require treatment by maintenance hemodialysis or receive a renal transplant. Consideration should be given to the use of blood from healthy immunized donors with high titers of anti-HBs for the routine hemodialysis of such patients who respond poorly to immunization against hepatitis B.
7. Other groups at risk of hepatitis B include the following:
  A. Individuals who frequently change sexual partners, particularly promiscuous male homosexuals and prostitutes.
  B. Narcotic and intravenous drug abusers.
  C. Staff at reception centers for refugees and immigrants from areas where hepatitis B is very common, such as Southeast Asia.
  D. Although they are at lower risk, long-term prisoners and staff of custodial institutions, members of ambulance and rescue services, and selected police personnel should also be considered for immunization.
  E. Military personnel are included in some countries.

Polypeptide Vaccines. Hepatitis B polypeptide vaccines containing specific hepatitis B antigenic determinants of the major nonglycosylated peptide I of the surface antigen with a molecular weight of 22,000 to 24,000 and its glycosylated form, a polypeptide with a molecular weight in the same range, have been prepared (Fig. 19–6). The individual polypeptides of the surface antigen are immunogenic, and the purified 25,000 (designated as p25) and 30,000 (p30) molecular weight polypeptides are effective antigens. Clinical trials of the polypeptide micelle vaccine are in progress.

Production of Hepatitis B Vaccines by r-DNA Techniques. Recombinant DNA techniques have been used for expressing hepatitis B surface antigen and core antigen in prokaryotic cells (*Escherichia coli* and *Bacillus*

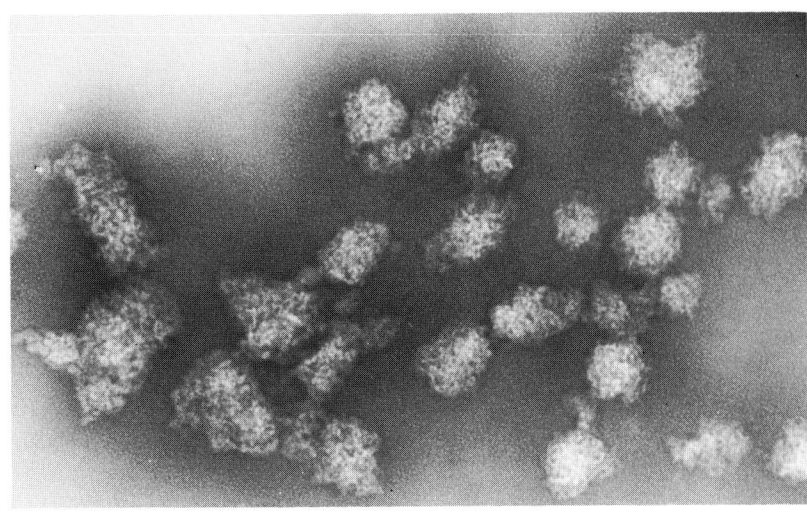

FIGURE 19–6. Hepatitis B polypeptide vaccine in micelle form. The diameter of the micelles ranges from 60 to 200 nm. Note the large surface area of the micelles, which, together with the altered distribution of the antigenic sites and the absence of host-derived proteins, probably accounts for the vigorous antibody response induced (× 100,000).

subtilis) and in eukaryotic cells, such as mutant mouse LM cells, HeLa cells, COS cells, CHO cells, and yeast cells (*Saccharomyces cerevisiae*).

Recombinant yeast hepatitis B vaccines have undergone extensive evaluation by clinical trials. These vaccines are safe, antigenic, and free from side effects (apart from minor local reactions in a proportion of recipients). The immunogenicity is similar to that of the plasma-derived vaccine. Recombinant yeast hepatitis B vaccines have now been licensed for use in many countries.

Hybrid Virus Vaccines. Potential live vaccines using recombinant vaccinia viruses have been constructed for hepatitis B and also for herpes simplex, rabies, and other viruses. Foreign viral DNA is introduced into the vaccinia DNA by the construction of chimeric genes. This is accomplished by homologous recombination in cells, since the large size of the genome of vaccinia virus (185,000 base pairs) precludes in vitro gene insertion. A chimeric gene consisting of vaccinia virus promoter sequences ligated to the coding sequence for the desired foreign protein is flanked by vaccinia virus DNA in a plasmid vector.

The recloned vaccinia virus containing hepatitis B surface antigen sequences has been used successfully for "priming" experimental animals. At present, however, there is no accepted laboratory marker of attenuation or of virulence of vaccinia virus for man, either in the host directly inoculated with the virus or after several passages in the same species. Alterations in the genome of vaccinia virus that are concomitant with the selection of recombinants may alter the virulence of the virus. Changes in host range or tissue tropism of vaccinia viruses may occur as a result of their genetic modification; these could be caused by changes in the virus envelope as a result of the incorporation of gene products of the foreign viral genes inserted into the vaccinia virus.

The advantages of recombinant vaccinia virus as a vaccine include low cost, ease of administration by multiple pressure or by the scratch technique, vaccine stability, long shelf life, and the possible use of polyvalent antigens. The known adverse reactions with vaccinia virus vaccines are well documented; their incidence and severity must be carefully weighed against the adverse reactions associated with the existing vaccines that a new recombinant vaccine might replace. There are also reports of spread of current strains of vaccinia virus to contacts, and this may present difficulties. Other recombinant viruses as vectors are being explored, in particular the oral adenovirus vaccines that have been in use for 20 years.

Novel Hepatitis B Vaccines Using Hybrid Particles. More recent developments include the use of the envelope proteins of hepatitis B virus (hepatitis B surface antigen) in a particulate form by expressing the proteins in mammalian cells. In-phase insertions of variable length and sequence of another virus (poliomyelitis virus type I) were made in different regions of the S gene of hepatitis B virus. The envelope proteins carrying the surface antigen and the insert are assembled with cellular lipids in the cultured mammalian cells after transfection. The inserted polio neutralization peptide was found to be exposed on the surface of the hybrid envelope particles, and it induced neutralizing antibodies against poliovirus in mice immunized experimentally. This approach may be useful for studying the biologic activity of other peptides incorporated into the surface of an organized multimolecular complex. The expression and secretion of hybrid envelope particles by established cell lines may thus provide an efficient system for the production of potential new vaccines.

Another potentially excellent carrier vehicle for human and veterinary vaccines, in addition to hepatitis B, is the core particles of hepatitis B virus (Fig. 19–3). The advantage of the core structure as a particle includes its ability to induce antibody with approximately 100-fold greater efficiency than for the surface antigen particle, and an ability to augment T-helper cell function. The feasibility of this approach was recently demonstrated with synthetic and biosynthetic peptides of foot-and-mouth disease virus (FMDV) after fusion to hepatitis B core.

Chemically Synthesized Hepatitis B Vaccines. The development of chemically synthesized polypeptide vaccines offers many advantages in attaining the ultimate goal of producing chemically uniform, safe, and cheap viral immunogens. These would replace many current vaccines, which often contain large quantities of irrelevant microbial antigenic determinants, proteins, and other material besides the essential immunogen required for the induction of a protective antibody. The preparation of antibodies against viral proteins using fragments of chemically synthesized peptides mimicking viral amino acid sequences is now a possible and attractive alternative approach to immunoprophylaxis.

Successful mimicking of determinants of HBsAg using chemically synthesized peptides in linear and cyclical forms has been reported by several groups of investigators. Peptides have been synthesized that retain biologic function and appropriate secondary structure, even though they have a limited sequence homology with the natural peptide or are much smaller.

Various other studies also confirm that selected overlapping peptides corresponding to relevant epitopes of hepatitis B surface antigen may be useful as synthetic vaccines when combined with adjuvants.

BIBLIOGRAPHY

Gerety RJ: Recombinant hepatitis B vaccines. In Zuckerman AJ (ed): Viral Hepatitis and Liver Disease. New York, Alan R. Liss, 1988, pp 1017–1024.

Harrison TJ, Chen J-Y, Zuckerman AJ: Hepatitis B virus and hepatocellular carcinoma. Clin Trop Med Commun Dis 1:395–409, 1986.

Howard, CR: Hepatitis B–associated Delta agent. Clin Trop Med Commun Dis 1:411–423, 1986.

Rizzetto M, Gerin JL, Purcell RH: The hepatitis delta virus and its infection. Prog Clin Biol Res 234:1, 1987.

Thomas HC, Lever AML: Treatment of chronic hepatitis B virus infection. Clin Trop Med Commun Dis 1:377–393, 1986.

Thomas HC, Scully LJ: Antiviral therapy in chronic hepatitis B virus infection. Br Med Bull 41:374–380, 1986.

Zuckerman AJ: Who should be immunised against hepatitis B? Br Med J 289:1243–1244, 1984.

Zuckerman AJ: Immunization against hepatitis B. Clin Trop Med Commun Dis 1:425–440, 1986.

Zuckerman AJ: The development of novel hepatitis B vaccines. Bull WHO 65:265–275, 1987.

Zuckerman AJ, Sun TT, Linsell A, Stjernsward J: Prevention of primary liver cancer. Lancet 1:463–465, 1983.

19.3. NON-A, NON-B HEPATITIS (NANB)

The availability of specific laboratory tests for the diagnosis of hepatitis A, hepatitis B, and hepatitis D has revealed a new type of unrelated viral hepatitis. There is epidemiologic, clinical, and experimental evidence of more than two forms of non-A, non-B hepatitis that are transmitted by the parenteral and enteric routes. Recently, a serologic marker that identifies some cases of non-A, non-B hepatitis has been described, and the virus has been tentatively named hepatitis C virus.

ENTERICALLY TRANSMITTED NON-A, NON-B HEPATITIS. An epidemic strain of non-A, non-B hepatitis virus(es) is transmitted by contaminated water in the subcontinent of India. There is ample serologic evidence that this form of epidemic hepatitis is not caused by the recognized serotype of hepatitis A, and by exclusion this infection may be regarded as a type of non-A, non-B hepatitis. A prospective study of the epidemic form of non-A, non-B hepatitis in the Kashmir Valley revealed that the infection was more frequent in pregnant women than in the general population and that there was a high incidence of fulminant hepatitis during pregnancy. In India, an endemic form of hepatitis, which epidemiologically appeared to be due to hepatitis A, would also be difficult to explain in the face of the apparent solid immunity of the population to hepatitis A.

Many outbreaks of epidemic non-A, non-B hepatitis that are enterically transmitted have been reported from India, south central USSR, Nepal, Burma, other regions in Central and Southeast Asia, the Middle East, North Africa, West Africa, and Mexico as well as in travelers returning from these regions. The infection is acute and self-limiting and occurs predominantly in young adults. It is often less severe than infection with HBV or HBV and HDV. The incubation period is 30 to 40 days. It is more severe in pregnant women, in whom it is associated with high mortality (10 to 20%), especially during the last trimester of pregnancy. The infection is spread by the ingestion of contaminated water and probably by food, but secondary cases appear to be uncommon. Studies by electron microscopy suggest that the virus measures about 32 nm in diameter, with a degraded particle measuring 27 nm in diameter. Serologic tests are under development.

In a study in the United States, an estimated 25% of sporadic cases of hepatitis were considered to have been due to virus(es) of non-A, non-B hepatitis; drug addiction and administration of blood appeared to be predisposing factors. In Denmark, 14% of consecutive patients hospitalized with hepatitis were diagnosed as having non-A, non-B hepatitis.

There also appears to be yet another endemic form of non-A, non-B hepatitis that is clearly not the result of water-borne infection and is not necessarily or commonly associated with apparent parenteral transmission. A 3-year community survey of viral hepatitis in West London revealed that, by excluding hepatitis A or B, Epstein-Barr (EB) virus, or cytomegalovirus by sensitive serologic tests, 13% of the patients suffered from sporadic non-A, non-B hepatitis. Neither drug addiction nor administration of blood or blood products appeared to be important factors in the transmission of the infection in the British study. In addition, although cases among household contacts were significantly less common than in hepatitis A, a history of close personal contact was found in a few patients, as was the case in studies in Costa Rica and Egypt.

PARENTERALLY TRANSMITTED NON-A, NON-B HEPATITIS. It appears that some cases of enterically transmitted non-A, non-B hepatitis are caused by the newly recognized hepatitis C virus; 58% of 59 cases of sporadic acute hepatitis were serologically positive at some stage after the clinical onset.

Epidemiology. Parenterally transmitted non-A, non-B hepatitis has been found in every country in which it has been sought; it shares a number of features with hepatitis B. This form of hepatitis has been most commonly recognized as a complication of blood transfusion; in countries where all blood donations are screened for hepatitis B surface antigen by very sensitive techniques, non-A, non-B hepatitis may account for as much as 90% of all cases of post-transfusion hepatitis. Outbreaks of non-A, non-B hepatitis have also been reported after the administration of blood clotting factors VIII and IX. Non-A, non-B hepatitis has occurred in hemodialysis and other specialized units, among drug addicts, and after accidental inoculation with contaminated needles and other sharp objects. Occasionally, maternal-to-infant transmission has been reported.

Clinical Manifestations. Although, in general, the illness is mild and often subclinical or anicteric, severe hepatitis with jaundice does occur and the infection is a significant cause of fulminant hepatitis. There is considerable evidence that the infection may be followed in many patients, and in experimentally infected chimpanzees, by prolonged viremia and the development of a persistent carrier state. Studies of the histopathologic sequelae of acute non-A, non-B hepatitis infection revealed that chronic liver damage, which may be severe, may occur in as many as 40 to 50% of patients.

Etiology. Clinical, epidemiologic, and experimental studies in several laboratories indicate that non-A, non-B hepatitis may be caused by two, and possibly more, infectious agents. Clinical evidence is based on the observation of multiple attacks of hepatitis in individual patients. Epidemiologically, short-incubation (2 to 5 weeks) and long-incubation (5 to 10 weeks or longer) forms of non-A, non-B hepatitis have been described. The incubation period, however, does not appear to be a reliable index for differentiating the two non-A, non-B types of hepatitis, and it is likely that differences in the incubation period reflect differences in the infective dose. Experimental evidence for the existence of at least two distinct non-A, non-B hepatitis viruses has been obtained from cross-challenge experimental transmission studies in chimpanzees, but final confirmation must await the development of specific laboratory tests and the identification and characterization of the virus(es).

The Viruses. Recent investigations have isolated a cDNA clone derived from a blood-borne non-A, non-B viral hepatitis genome. They have developed an assay for detecting antibodies to this virus, named hepatitis C virus. This test reacts with serum from patients with post-transfusion non-A, non-B hepatitis and with serum from chimpanzees that developed hepatitis after being experimentally infected with NANB inoculum. This new virus has the characteristics of either a togavirus or a flavivirus.

Diagnosis. The diagnosis of non-A, non-B hepatitis has been until recently a diagnosis of exclusion. However, an as yet unknown proportion of cases can now be diagnosed by using the newer serologic tests for detecting hepatitis C virus (HCV). Both radioimmunoassays and an ELISA are available for detecting HCV antigen. These tests are now being used to screen blood transfusions, to diagnose cases of post-transfusion hepatitis that are negative for markers for HAV and HBV, and in epidemiologic studies to determine the prevalence of HCV infection in sporadic cases of NANB hepatitis in various areas of the world.

BLOOD TRANSFUSION SCREENING. Several "nonspecific" (surrogate) tests have been recommended for screening units of blood. Two large studies were conducted to assess the role of anti-HBs detected in blood donor units in the subsequent development of non-A, non-B hepatitis. Although the studies did show a higher incidence of hepatitis in recipients of anti-HBs–positive blood, subsequent reports indicated that it was related not to the presence of anti-HBs per se but to the higher frequency of anti-HBs in commercial blood. Others, however, failed to confirm the association between anti-HBs in donor blood and the increased risk of non-A, non-B hepatitis in recipients.

The Transfusion-Transmitted Viruses (TTV) Study Group proposed that units of blood that were positive for anti-HBc were associated with a 2- to 3-fold greater risk of non-A, non-B hepatitis in recipients than were units without anti-HBc. This was confirmed more recently by a study that suggested that by excluding anti-HBs–positive donors, 54% of non-A, non-B cases could be prevented, with a donor unit loss of only 4%.

However, the nonspecific indicator that has received greatest attention is serum alanine aminotransferase (ALT) levels in blood donors. Several studies have shown that the risk of non-A, non-B post-transfusion hepatitis is directly related to the serum ALT level of the donor. It was concluded that exclusion of blood units with serum ALT levels of 53 IU/L or more would prevent 29% of post-transfusion hepatitis with a loss of only 1.6% of donor units. This method is thus better than screening for anti-HBc, since the corrected efficacy of anti-HBc as a screening test was slightly less than that of ALT and the number of blood units lost would be twice those which would be if ALT were used. But the sensitivity of the test for ALT is only 26%, and despite the high specificity, the predictive value is only 42%. Thus, almost 60% of blood with an elevated ALT level will not transmit non-A, non-B hepatitis. ALT levels vary with age, sex, alcohol use, and geographic region and would therefore not be useful as a surrogate marker of non-A, non-B hepatitis.

BIBLIOGRAPHY

Alter HV: Transfusion-associated non-A, non-B hepatitis. The first decade. *In* Zuckerman AJ (ed): Viral Hepatitis and Liver Disease. New York, Alan R. Liss, 1988, pp 537–542.

Dienstag JL: Non-A, non-B hepatitis. 1: Recognition, epidemiology, and clinical features. Gastroenterology 85:439–462, 1983.

Editorial: Will the real hepatitis C stand up? Lancet 2:307–308, 1989.

Gerety R, Iwarson S: Non-A, non-B hepatitis. Clin Trop Med Commun Dis 1:441–458, 1986.

Khuroo MS: Study of an epidemic of non-A, non-B hepatitis. Possibility of another human hepatitis virus distinct from post-transfusion non-A, non-B type. Am J Med 70:252, 1980.

Kuo G, Choo Q-L, Alter HJ, et al: An assay for circulating antibodies to a major etiologic virus of human non-A, non-B hepatitis. Science 244:362–364, 1989.

Ramalingaswami V, Purcell RH. Waterborne non-A, non-B hepatitis. Lancet 1:571–573, 1988.

Tsiquaye KN, Amini S, Kessler H, et al: Ultrastructural changes in the liver in experimental non-A, non-B hepatitis. Br J Exp Pathol 62:41, 1981.

20. VIRAL FEBRILE ILLNESSES

Thomas P. Monath

20.1. DENGUE (AND DENGUE HEMORRHAGIC FEVER)

DEFINITION. Classic *dengue fever* ("breakbone fever") is an acute self-limited illness with diphasic fever, headache, arthralgia, myalgia, rash, lymphadenopathy, and leukopenia caused by four distinct serotypes of dengue virus, a mosquito-borne flavivirus. *Dengue hemorrhagic fever* (DHF) (Philippine, Singapore, or Thai hemorrhagic fevers) is distinguished from classic dengue by hemorrhagic manifestations, thrombocytopenia with concurrent hemoconcentration and, in severe cases, circulatory failure, shock (*dengue shock syndrome*, DSS), and death in a proportion of cases. DHF and DSS result from infection with the same four serotypes of dengue virus; immunopathologic mechanisms are postulated to play a role in the genesis of these diseases.

ETIOLOGY AND HISTORY. The clinical syndrome was first described in 1780 as "breakbone fever" by Benjamin Rush in Philadelphia. The term "dengue" was first applied in 1828 during an epidemic in Cuba. In earlier times the similar diseases dengue and chikungunya were often confused. Throughout the eighteenth, nineteenth, and twentieth centuries, dengue has caused recurrent epidemics worldwide. *Aedes aegypti* was first implicated as the vector in 1905. In 1907, the virus was demonstrated in human plasma by filtration and transmission to human volunteers. Prototype dengue types 1 and 2 viruses were isolated, characterized, and adapted to mice by Albert Sabin and his colleagues in 1944 to 1945; dengue types 3 and 4 viruses were first recovered in 1956 in the Philippines. Although hemorrhagic phenomena were described in earlier epidemics, DHF gained nosologic status (as Philippine hemorrhagic fever) in 1954 and subsequently became endemic and epidemic in many areas of tropical Asia. In 1981 DHF occurred in epidemic form in the Caribbean for the first time.

The four dengue viruses (types 1 to 4) are antigenically closely related and constitute a distinct subgroup within the flavivirus genus (group B arboviruses) of the family Flaviviridae. Dengue serotypes are distinguishable by complement fixation (CF) and neutralization tests using hyperimmune antisera or by immunofluorescence tests using monoclonal antibodies. Despite the antigenic closeness of these viruses, cross-protection in humans is incomplete and short-lived.

Dengue virions are small (40 nm) spherical particles composed of a lipoprotein envelope and nucleocapsid of single-stranded RNA genome with positive polarity. Three structural proteins are associated with the virion; the major envelope (E) glycoprotein is exposed on the virion surface and contains type-specific and group-reactive antigens. At least 7 nonvirion proteins are also formed during infection, of which at least one (NS1) is present on the surface of infected cells and may play a significant role in immunologic responses of the host.

Many strains of dengue are nonpathologic or only minimally pathologic for suckling mice unless adapted by repeated passage. A variety of mammalian cell lines may be used for isolation and assay, but use of mosquito cells or intrathoracic inoculation of living mosquitoes is the most sensitive procedure.

DISTRIBUTION AND INCIDENCE. The distribution of dengue corresponds roughly to that of the principal vector, *Ae. aegypti,* and includes tropical and subtropical regions of the Americas, Africa, Asia, and Australia. *Ae. aegypti*–infested areas of the southern United States have experienced dengue in the remote past and remain receptive to summertime introduction and spread of the disease. During and after World War II, *Ae. aegypti* became more widely distributed and more prevalent in Asia. In the 1980s *Ae. aegypti* reinvaded Brazil, Ecuador, Paraguay, and Bolivia, with resulting large epidemics. All 4 serotypes have long been endemic in Asia. Dengue viruses 2 and 3 were known in the Americas as early as 1942; dengue virus 1 first appeared in the Caribbean in 1977 and dengue virus 4 in 1981. Dengue viruses 1, 2, and 4 have been isolated in West Africa, and types 2 and 3 have been isolated in East Africa.

Dengue fever epidemics involve many thousands of cases and are characterized by attack rates as high as 75 to 80%. Immunity is serotype-specific and long-lasting (probably for life). Repeated outbreaks of dengue in a geographic area are the result of introduction of new serotypes or recurrence of infection with the same serotype affecting segments of the population previously spared, e.g., those born after the last epidemic.

The incidence of dengue fever and DHF has increased dramatically in the past 30 years, owing to expanding urbanization and *Ae. aegypti* populations and to increased opportunities for movement of viremic travelers by airplane. Dengue hemorrhagic fever is a perennial epidemic problem in parts of Southeast Asia, where it is a ranking cause of pediatric hospitalization. In the decade from 1976 to 1985, 965,000 cases of DHF and over 14,000 deaths were officially reported from Thailand, Indonesia, Vietnam, and Burma alone; these incidence data are widely accepted as a gross underestimate. DHF appeared for the first time in epidemic form in the Western Hemisphere in Cuba in 1981. All 4 serotypes are associated with DHF. Infection with dengue virus 2 appears to be especially likely to produce DHF. The ratio of DHF to classic dengue cases is between 1:100 and 1:500.

TRANSMISSION AND EPIDEMIOLOGY. The transmission cycle is simple, involving humans as the viremic host and the *Ae. aegypti* mosquito as the vector. In certain areas, other vectors may play a role in transmission (*Ae. albopictus* in Asia; *Ae. scutellaris,* and the *Ae. scutellaris* complex, including *Ae. polynesiensis* in the South Pacific). The extrinsic incubation period in mosquitoes is 8 to 11 days (time between ingestion of infectious blood and ability to transmit); mosquitoes remain infective for life. *Ae. aegypti* breeds in peridomestic containers, such as water storage jars, flower pots, tin cans, and discarded tires. Its flight range is limited (100 m); interrupted probing and feeding are common, and 1 mosquito may infect a number of household members.

Age, sex, and race do not influence susceptibility to classic dengue fever, but DHF in Asia is predominantly a disease of children. In tropical areas, dengue outbreaks coincide with the monsoon or rainy season. Dengue virus has been shown experimentally to be passed vertically in *Aedes,* but the epidemiologic significance of transovarial transmission is uncertain. A jungle cycle of dengue (analogous to yellow fever), involving forest mosquitoes and wild monkeys, has been documented in Malaysia and in West Africa. The role of enzootic dengue as a source of human infections is presently unknown.

PATHOLOGY AND PATHOGENESIS. After inoculation of dengue virus by the bite of an infected mosquito, the virus replicates in regional lymph nodes and is disseminated via the lymph and blood to other tissues, especially the reticuloendothelial system and skin, which sustain viral growth and seed the blood with virus. Microscopic changes in skin lesions of patients with classic dengue fever include perivascular edema, endothelial cell swelling, and mononuclear cell infiltration.

Dengue Hemorrhagic Fever. The pathogenesis and pathophysiology of DHF are incompletely defined. Patients with shock have increased capillary permeability, resulting in rapid internal shifts of extracellular fluid from the plasma to interstitital spaces. Coupled with volume depletion due to inadequate intake and increased gastrointestinal and insensible fluid losses, this increased permeability results in hemoconcentration, hypovolemia, reduced tissue perfusion and oxygenation, acidosis, and widespread cell damage. Pathologic changes associated with these events include pleural and peritoneal effusions, petechial hemorrhages, widespread diapedesis of erythrocytes, and edema of retroperitoneal tissues.

The immunologic status of the host is believed to be an important component in determining the course of dengue infection and development of DHF. The presence of non-neutralizing antibodies to a heterologous dengue serotype has been shown to increase attachment of dengue virus–antibody complexes to Fc receptor–bearing lymphoid cells and thereby to enhance dengue viral growth in lymphoid cells (so-called immune enhancement). Immune clearance of infected cells could result in release of vascular permeability factors, tissue thromboplastin, or complement-activating substances, which may play a role in the genesis of capillary leakage and activation of coagulation cascades. Although DHF may occur in cases of primary dengue infection, there is a strong association with superinfection in individuals with prior exposure to another serotype or (in infants) with the presence of maternal antibodies. It is possible that dengue virus strains differ in virulence and propensity to induce the hemorrhagic syndrome, either in cases of primary infection or in the induction of immunopathologic alterations.

Other Pathologic Findings. Pathologic changes in fatal cases of DHF are not extensive or impressive and do not reflect the profound physiologic disturbances or cause of death. Pathologic findings other than those already mentioned include megakaryocytic arrest in the bone marrow; active proliferation and lymphocytolysis of germinal centers in lymph nodes and spleen; focal midzonal necrosis, fatty changes, swelling, and hyaline necrosis of Kupffer cells and the appearance of Councilman bodies in the liver; and glomerulonephritis (probably due to immune complex deposition). Hemorrhages are generally minor and not life threatening; occasionally, major gastrointestinal bleeding may be clinically significant and appears to be more frequent in adolescents and adults.

CLINICAL MANIFESTATIONS AND COMPLICATIONS

Classic Dengue. The incubation period is usually 5 to 8 days, followed by abrupt onset of fever, chills, headache, eye pain, and lumbosacral aching. A transient, generalized erythematous flushlike rash may be present during the first 24 to 48 hours (Fig. 20–1). Generalized myalgia and arthralgia increase in severity. Other symptoms appearing on the second to the fourth day include anorexia, nausea, vomiting, respiratory symptoms, marked lassitude, cutaneous hyperesthesia, and altered taste. The physical examination may reveal relative bradycardia and generalized lymphadenopathy. Marked leukopenia, i.e., as few as 1500 cells/mm³, and neutropenia are typical, and thrombocytopenia may occur on the third to eighth day. On the third to fifth day, the fever abates and a morbilliform rash appears on the trunk, spreading centripetally to involve the face and extremities, and sometimes accompanied by a brief (12 to 24 hour) recrudescence of fever (Fig. 20–2). Hemorrhagic phenomena, particularly petechial hemorrhages and epistaxes, may occur during the course of the illness; in the absence of hemoconcentration these patients do not meet the criteria for having DHF.

Dengue Hemorrhagic Fever. A positive tourniquet test or spontaneous hemorrhages, thrombocytopenia

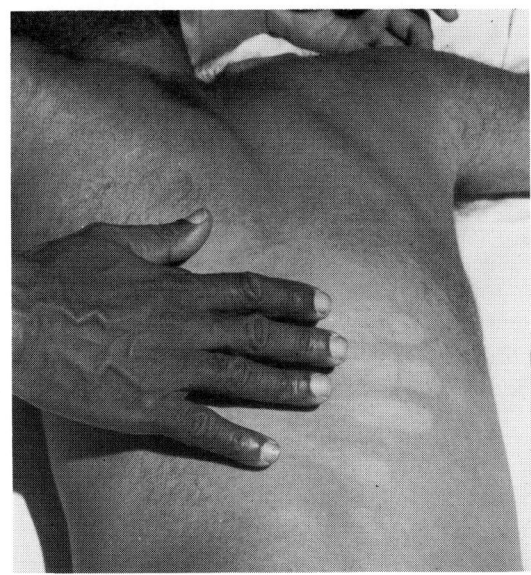

FIGURE 20–1. Pressure blanching of erythematous, macular rash of dengue. (Courtesy of Dr. Telford H. Work.)

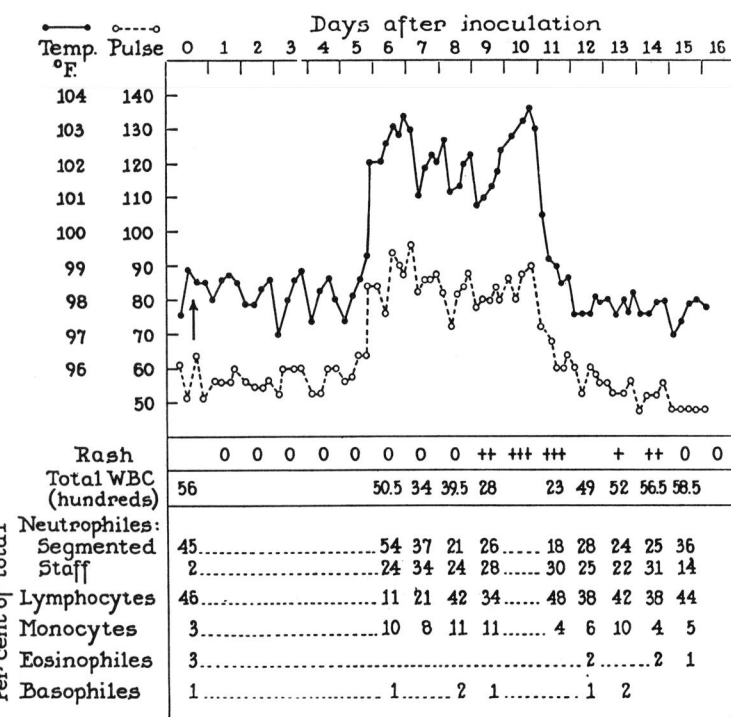

Days after inoculation

	Days after inoculation
Rash	0 0 0 0 0 0 0 ++ +++ +++ + ++ 0 0
Total WBC (hundreds)	56 ...... 50.5 34 39.5 28 ...... 23 49 52 56.5 58.5
Neutrophiles: Segmented	45 .... 54 37 21 26 ...... 18 28 24 25 36
Staff	2 .... 24 34 24 28 .... 30 25 22 31 14
Lymphocytes	46 .... 11 21 42 34 .... 48 38 42 38 44
Monocytes	3 .... 10 8 11 11 .... 4 6 10 4 5
Eosinophiles	3 .... 2 .... 2 1
Basophiles	1 .... 1 ...... 2 1 .... 1 2

(Per cent of total)

FIGURE 20–2. Graphic representation of temperature and pulse rate of a human volunteer inoculated experimentally with the Hawaiian strain of dengue virus by means of the bites of 8 infected *Aedes aegypti* mosquitoes; arrow indicates day on which the patient was bitten. Time of appearance of rash is also indicated as well as total and differential blood counts. (From Sabin AB: *In* Rivers TM, Horsfall FL Jr: Viral and Rickettsial Infections of Man, 3rd ed. Philadelphia, JB Lippincott, 1959. Used by permission of the National Foundation.)

(≤ 100,000 cells/mm³), *and* evidence of hemoconcentration (increase in hematocrit by 20% or more) constitute the minimal criteria for a diagnosis of DHF (Fig. 20–3). In severe cases, patients develop the shock syndrome; i.e., rapid deterioration occurs on the second to fifth day of a typical dengue illness (the time of defervescence), with restlessness, abdominal pain, and signs of hypotension (cold, clammy extremities, diaphoresis, circumoral cyanosis, collapse). The blood pressure is low and the pulse pressure narrowed, the pulse is rapid and weak, and the respiratory rate is increased. Petechiae, ecchymoses, and other spontaneous hemorrhages may appear. Enlargement and tenderness of the liver have been noted in some, but not all, outbreaks. Laboratory findings include hypoproteinemia, reduced plasma osmolarity, elevated hematocrit, thrombocytopenia, hyponatremia, and mildly elevated serum aspartate aminotransferase and urea nitrogen levels. Evidence for disseminated intravascular clotting, prolonged prothrombin and partial thromboplastin times, and reduced fibrinogen and clotting factors II, V, VII, IX, and XII are found in up to 25% of patients with shock. Metabolic acidosis may be present. Without treatment, up to 50% of such patients die. Patients with less severe illness or those successfully treated recover rapidly after a 1- to 2-day period of acute illness.

Other Manifestations. There are isolated reports, requiring further confirmation, of myocarditis and encephalopathy associated with dengue infections.

PROGNOSIS AND THERAPY. After recovery from classic dengue, convalescence may be prolonged for several weeks and associated with weakness; depression; and occasional cardiac symptoms, e.g., palpitations, ventricular extrasystoles, and bradycardia; but without recurrent rheumatic complaints. The case-fatality rate in severe DHF/DSS is high (up to 50%) in patients who are not hospitalized and treated promptly,

but with good medical management less than 5% of these patients die.

Treatment of classic dengue is symptomatic, e.g., acetaminophen, bed rest, and oral (rarely parenteral) fluid replacement. In cases of DHF without shock,

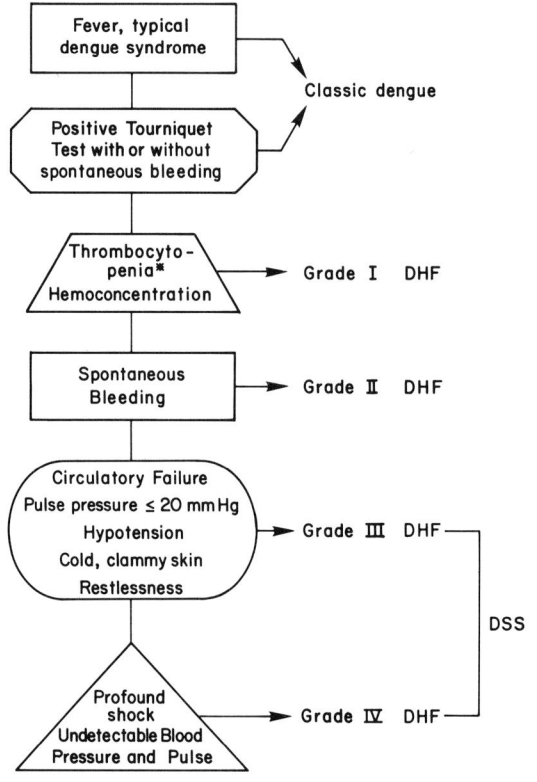

* Platelet count ≤ 100,000 /mm³
  Hematocrit increased by 20% or more

FIGURE 20–3. Algorithm for the diagnosis and grading of dengue, dengue hemorrhagic fever (DHF), and dengue shock syndrome (DSS).

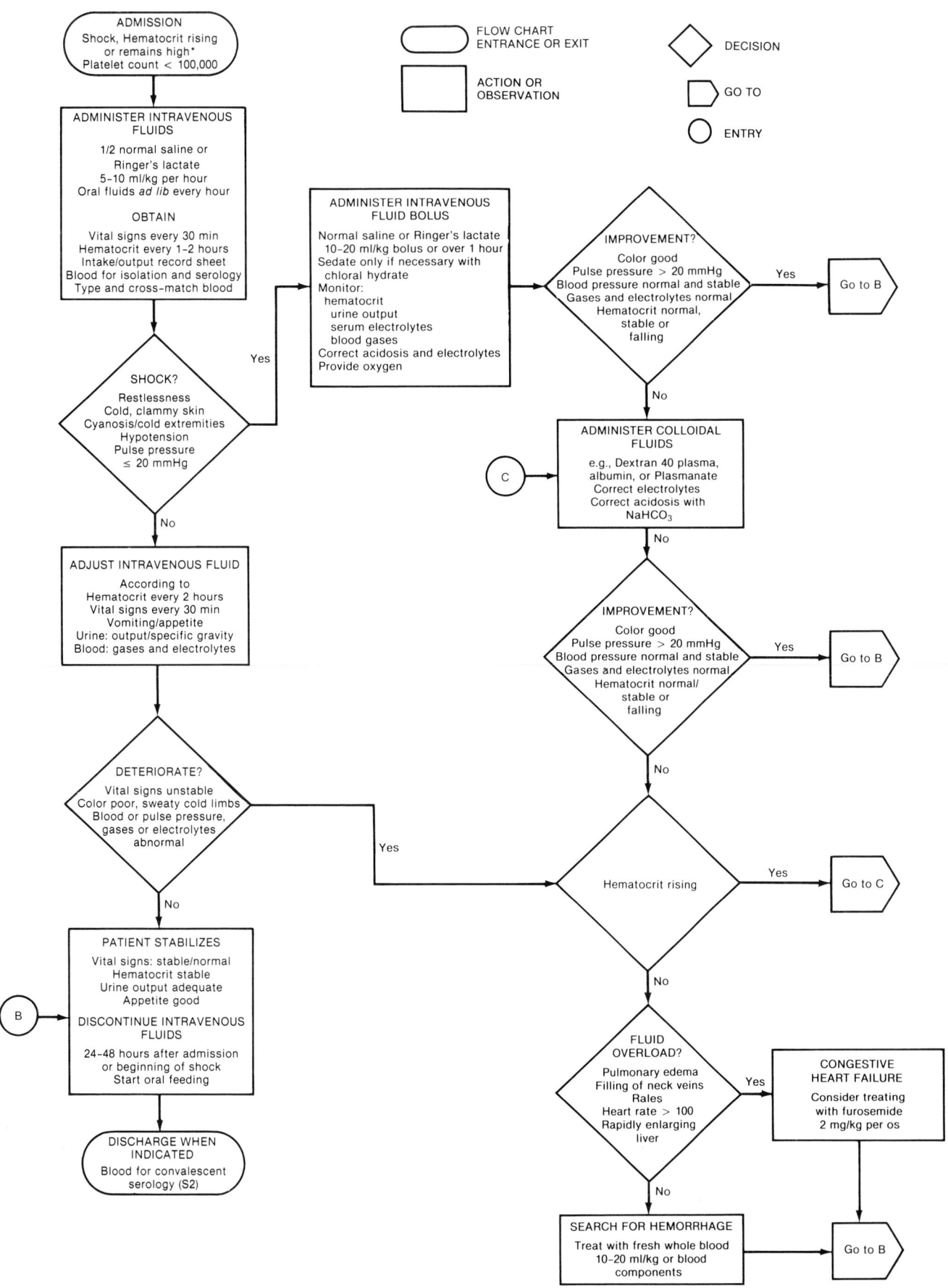

FIGURE 20–4. Algorithm for the treatment of hospitalized patients with dengue hemorrhagic fever. (From Dengue Haemorrhagic Fever: Diagnosis, Treatment, and Control. Geneva, WHO, 1986. Reprinted by permission.)

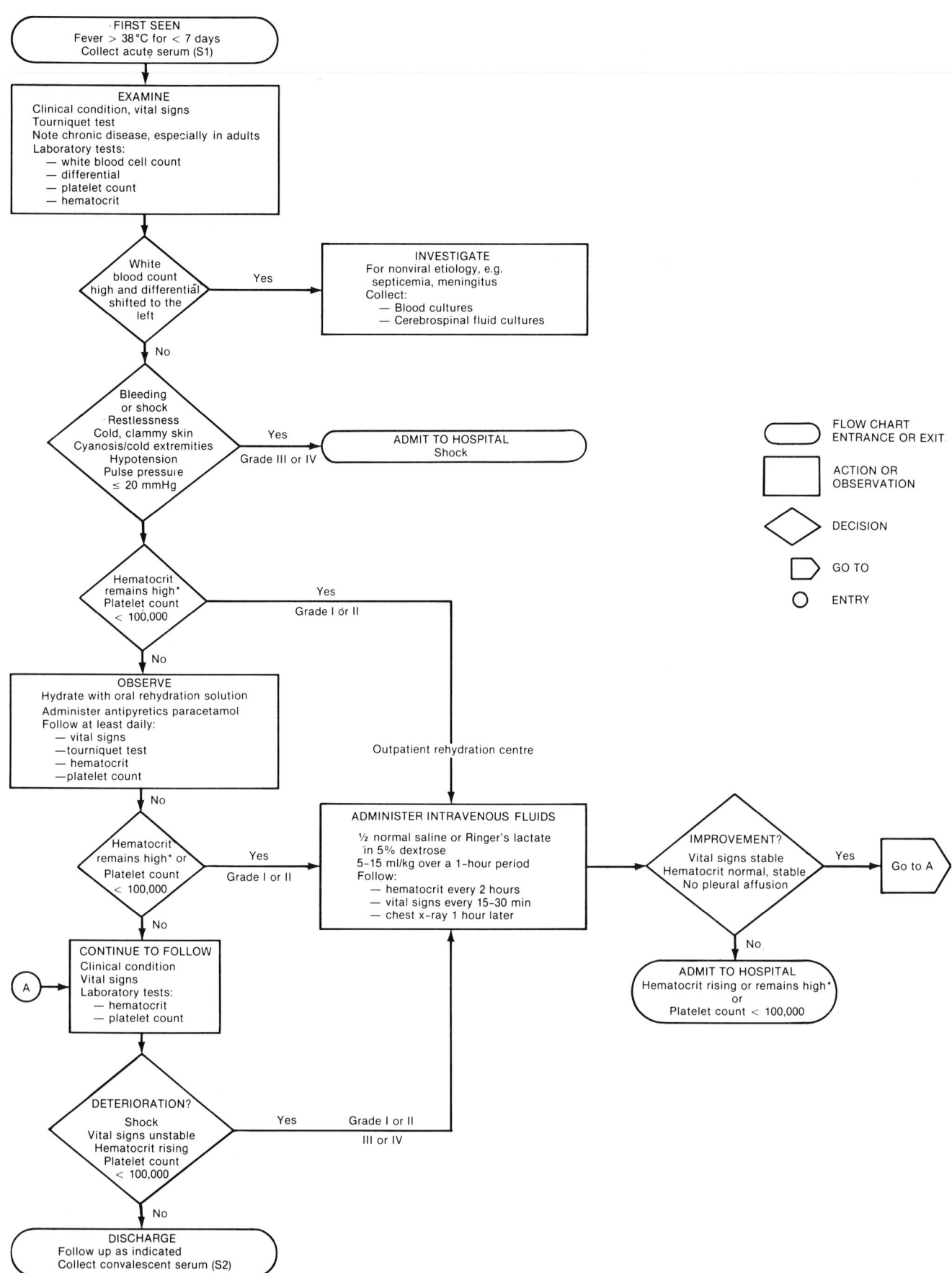

FIGURE 20–5. Algorithm for the treatment of outpatients with dengue hemorrhagic fever. (From Dengue Haemorrhagic Fever: Diagnosis, Treatment, and Control. Geneva, WHO, 1986. Reprinted by permission.)

dehydration and hemoconcentration may be managed by oral or intravenous fluid replacement in the hospital (Fig. 20–4) or on an outpatient basis (Fig. 20–5). Acetaminophen should be used to control fever, as salicylates are contraindicated because of the bleeding diathesis. The early recognition of DHF with shock, followed by intensive care in the hospital and proper management, is essential to reduce the potential lethality of this infection. Immediate replacement of fluids, e.g., with normal saline, Ringer's lactate, plasma, or plasma expanders, is necessary. Whole blood transfusions are required only in the case of documented major hemorrhage. Careful and repeated estimation of volume depletion is essential and is obtained by measuring vital signs, urine output, and hematocrit or serum protein concentration; in severe cases monitoring central venous pressure or pulmonary capillary wedge pressure may be required, especially if signs of cardiac decompensation appear. Oxygen should be given to patients in shock. Blood gases and serum electrolytes should be monitored; acidosis should be treated by vigorous attempts to reverse shock and improve tissue perfusion and (if arterial pH is below 7.2) by administration of parenteral sodium bicarbonate ($NaHCO_3$). Because the acid-base disturbance in DHF/DSS is usually a mixed respiratory alkalosis and metabolic acidosis (both of which lower the plasma HCO_3 concentration), $NaHCO_3$ should be administered only after determination of blood pH. To avoid fluid overload, parenteral fluid therapy should be stopped when the hematocrit drops to approximately 40% and clinical signs and urine output improve (generally after 24 to 72 hours). If there is laboratory evidence of disseminated intravascular coagulation and intractable bleeding not manageable by administration of fresh blood or fresh or fresh-frozen plasma, consideration may be given to intravenous infusion of heparin.

Corticosteroids have been used to treat DHF/DSS; however, comparative therapeutic trials have yielded conflicting results. A double-blind evaluation in Indonesia showed that hydrocortisone (50 mg/kg) given as a single dose had no value over physiologic treatment alone.

DIAGNOSIS

Virus Isolation. Diagnosis may be achieved by isolation of the virus from serum obtained during the acute phase of illness, generally the first 3 to 5 days after onset. Serum should be aseptically collected and kept at refrigerator temperatures (wet ice) for delivery to a virus laboratory within 24 to 48 hours or should be frozen on dry ice if a longer delivery time is anticipated. Virus isolation is attempted by inoculation of cell cultures, e.g., *Aedes albopictus, Ae. pseudoscutellaris,* or LLC-MK2 cells, and observing these for development of cytopathic effect, plaques, or immunofluorescent antigen. Alternatively, live mosquitoes, e.g., *Toxorhynchites* or *Ae. aegypti,* may be intrathoracically inoculated and examined for virus by immunofluorescence after incubation for 7 to 14 days. Dengue virus serotypes are identified by complement fixation or neutralization tests using hyperimmune antisera or by immunofluorescence with type-specific monoclonal antibodies.

Serology. Serologic diagnosis is achieved by demonstrating a rise in hemagglutination inhibition, CF, or neutralizing antibody titers in appropriately timed paired sera. For this purpose both an acute serum and a convalescent serum drawn 10 to 14 days later are required. In patients with primary dengue infection and no previous exposure to related flaviviruses, e.g., yellow fever, St. Louis encephalitis, and West Nile fever, the serologic responses are relatively type-specific, whereas persons with prior dengue or nondengue flaviviral exposure have a more rapid, high-titered, and broadly cross-reactive antibody response. The IgM antibody-capture enzyme-linked immunosorbent assay (ELISA) has improved dengue serodiagnosis. By day 5 after infection, patients with primary or superinfection have detectable IgM antibodies. These antibodies wane relatively rapidly, so that by 2 to 3 months, the majority of patients are seronegative; thus, tests on a single serum sample may indicate recent infection (however, some patients have persisting IgM antibodies, and further studies are required to determine the duration of detectable immunity by this method). IgM antibodies are relatively specific for dengue (minimal cross-reactions with heterologous flaviviruses), but do not readily distinguish infections with the individual dengue serotypes.

PREVENTION AND CONTROL. Live attenuated vaccines against dengue types 1, 2, and 4 have been prepared in Thailand and the United States, and several of these have been successfully tested in human volunteers. Considerable effort and years of research will be necessary before these vaccines can be applied to the control of dengue. Because of the potential for severe disease in individuals sequentially exposed to wild dengue viruses, it will be necessary to simultaneously immunize against all or multiple serotypes. Considerable progress has been made on the molecular structure of flaviviruses in general, and dengue viruses in particular. Dengue viral genes for protective antigens of the envelope and NS1 proteins have been cloned and expressed in several recombinant systems, including vaccinia, baculovirus, and bacteria, and these approaches offer promise for development of diagnostic reagents and vaccines.

Prevention of dengue fever outbreaks can be achieved by reducing vector mosquito populations (principally *Ae. aegypti*) through elimination of breeding sites and use of larvicides. Emergency control of dengue or DHF epidemics requires the use of ground or aerial ultra-low-volume sprays of an effective mosquito adulticide. Such emergency measures have generally been undertaken without studies to determine efficacy, and recent research indicates that ultra-low-volume adulticides have little impact on *Ae. aegypti* adults resting indoors.

BIBLIOGRAPHY

Dengue Haemorrhagic Fever: Diagnosis, Treatment, and Control. Geneva, World Health Organization, 1986.

Dengue in the Caribbean, 1977. Pan American Health Organization, Scientific Publication No. 375, Washington, DC, 1979.

Gubler DJ: Dengue. *In* Monath, TP (ed): The Arboviruses: Epidemiology and Ecology, Vol II. Boca Raton, FL, CRC Press, 1988, pp 223–260.

Halstead SB: Dengue hemorrhagic fever—a public health problem and a field for research. Bull WHO 58:1, 1980.

Halstead, SB: Pathogenesis of dengue: Challenges to molecular biology. Science 239:476, 1987.

Halstead SB, Nimmannitya S, Margiotta MR: Dengue and chikungunya virus infection in man in Thailand, 1962–1964. II. Observations on disease in out-patients. Am J Trop Med Hyg 18:972, 1969.

Sabin A: Research on dengue during World War II. Am J Trop Med Hyg 1:30, 1952.

20.2. WEST NILE FEVER

DEFINITION. West Nile fever is an endemic and epidemic mosquito-borne flaviviral disease clinically resembling dengue. It may produce encephalitis, especially in the elderly.

ETIOLOGY AND HISTORY. The virus was first isolated from a febrile Ugandan in 1937. It is a flavivirus, antigenically related most closely to Murray Valley encephalitis, St. Louis encephalitis, and Japanese encephalitis viruses. West Nile virus is pathogenic for suckling and weanling mice inoculated intracerebrally and intraperitoneally, chick embryos, hamsters, and a wide variety of cell cultures. Strains vary in pathogenicity; antigenic differences have also been shown between strains from India and those from Africa and the Middle East, and variation occurs even within these regions. West Nile virus has occasionally been recovered from horses with encephalitis in Egypt and France. Laboratory infections occur, and aerosol transmission is well documented in laboratory experiments.

DISTRIBUTION AND INCIDENCE. The virus is widely distributed in the Old World, including Africa, Europe, the Middle East, the Soviet Union, and tropical Asia. Sporadic human disease has been found in Egypt, Uganda, Nigeria, France, and India. Epidemics occurred in Israel between 1951 and 1957, involving hundreds of cases; an attack rate of 64% was documented in 1 outbreak in a military camp. An epidemic was reported in southern France (the Camargue) in 1962. The largest outbreaks on record have occurred in South Africa (in 1974 in the highveld of the Transvaal and Orange Free State and in 1983 to 1984 in the Pretoria area). In the 1974 outbreak, it was estimated that 18,000 persons were infected with the virus in a population of 30,000, but morbidity is not known, and inapparent infections are common. Antibody surveys indicate high prevalence rates (up to 70%) in hyperendemic areas, but cross-reactions with other flaviviruses complicate interpretation of these data.

TRANSMISSION AND EPIDEMIOLOGY. In tropical, endemic areas, e.g., South India and Egypt, infection is generally acquired during childhood; disease in juveniles frequently escapes detection or is subclinical or mild. Accumulated immunity prevents epidemics from affecting the adult population. In more temperate or arid zones, e.g., Israel and South Africa, summertime epidemics have affected all age groups; in these areas the virus may be periodically reintroduced or transmitted enzootically at low levels until ecologic conditions favor amplified spread. West Nile virus is transmitted between mosquito vectors and wild bird reservoir hosts; humans and equines are dead-end hosts. Domestic fowl may play a role in the cycle and may suffer fatal illness.

The principal vectors are *Culex univittatus* (Egypt, South Africa, Israel), *Cx. modestus* (Israel, France), and *Cx. vishnui* complex in India; other species of *Culex* (including *Cx. pipiens*) play secondary roles. Recrudescence of West Nile virus and survival over the winter in temperate areas or across the dry season in the tropics have not been fully elucidated. Possible mechanisms include survival in hibernating adult *Culex* mosquitoes, survival in ticks (isolations of the virus have been made from ticks in Egypt and the Soviet Union), and reintroduction by migrating birds. Transovarial transmission of the virus in mosquitoes has been demonstrated in the laboratory, but not in species implicated in natural transmission.

PATHOLOGY AND PATHOGENESIS. In the few fatal cases of encephalitis studied, histopathologic changes were similar to those of Japanese encephalitis.

CLINICAL MANIFESTATIONS AND COMPLICATIONS. The disease is similar in many respects to dengue and Sindbis fever; in the mixed 1974 epidemic in South Africa, Sindbis fever and West Nile fever could not be clinically distinguished, but this may be due to superficial observations. The incubation period is 3 to 6 days and is followed by sudden onset. Young children experience high fever (occasionally biphasic), lasting 1 to 6 days. Rash appears toward the end of the febrile period, is maculopapular and nonirritating, and is most conspicuous on the trunk and limbs. Gastrointestinal symptoms, e.g., vomiting, abdominal pain, and diarrhea, are not uncommon. In adults, fever is less severe and rash and gastrointestinal symptoms less frequent. Acute pancreatitis has been described in association with West Nile virus infection and may explain some of the gastrointestinal complaints associated with the disease. Headache, periocular pain, myalgia, and arthralgia are prominent. Lymphadenopathy and conjunctival injection may be present. Convalescence may be prolonged and associated with lassitude and depression. Meningoencephalitis was first reported during the Israeli epidemics in the 1950s and affected primarily elderly persons. Subsequently, however, severe cases of central nervous system infection have been reported in younger patients, including several fatalities in children in India. Among patients experimentally infected with West Nile virus as a treatment of cancer, clinical signs of encephalitis appeared in 4.5%. Myocarditis has been an occasional complication.

PROGNOSIS AND THERAPY. The typical disease is self-limited, with full recovery expected, although convalescence may be prolonged in adults. In patients with encephalitis, the case-fatality rate is uncertain; of 49 elderly patients in one Israel study, 12 had meningoencephalitis and 4 died. Neurologic residua are not described (but probably occur in some patients). Therapy for the benign form is symptomatic. Management of the cerebral infection is as described for Venezuelan equine encephalitis (Chapter 21.2).

DIAGNOSIS. The virus may be isolated from serum during the acute febrile phase or during the incubation period (1 or 2 days before onset). Serodiagnosis is performed by standard tests (hemagglutination inhibition, complement fixation, neutralization) on paired sera. Cross-reactions with other flaviviruses may complicate diagnosis.

PREVENTION AND CONTROL. No vaccine is available. Emergency mosquito adulticide spraying may be considered in the event of an epidemic.

BIBLIOGRAPHY

Goldblum N, Sterk VV, Paderski B: West Nile fever. The clinical features of the disease and the isolation of West Nile virus from the blood of nine human cases. Am J Hyg 59:89, 1954.

Hayes CG: West Nile fever. *In* Monath, TP (ed): The Arboviruses: Epidemiology and Ecology, Vol V. Boca Raton, FL, CRC Press, 1988, pp 59–88.

Marburg K, Goldblum H, Sterk VV, et al: The natural history of West Nile fever. I. Clinical observations during an epidemic in Israel. Am J Hyg 64:259, 1956.

McIntosh BM, Jupp PG, Dos Santos I, et al: Epidemics of West Nile and Sindbis viruses in South Africa with *Culex univittatus* Theobold, as vectors. S Afr J Sci 72:295, 1976.

20.3. CHIKUNGUNYA FEVER

DEFINITION. Chikungunya is a self-limited epidemic and endemic dengue-like disease caused by a mosquito-borne alphavirus. The name represents the Swahili word meaning "that which bends up," a reference to the severe joint pains associated with the illness.

ETIOLOGY AND HISTORY. The virus belongs to the alphavirus genus of the family Togaviridae. Viral particles are spherical, are 60 nm in diameter, have a single-stranded RNA core and a lipid-containing envelope, develop in the cytoplasm, and bud from the plasma membranes of infected cells. The virions possess hemagglutinating activity. Chikungunya virus is pathogenic for intracerebrally inoculated infant mice, hamsters, and rats and for a variety of cell cultures, including Vero, BHK-21, LLC-MK2, primary chick and duck embryo. HeLa, and BSC-1. The virus is antigenically most closely related to o'nyong nyong virus and more distantly to other members of the Semliki Forest virus complex, e.g., Mayaro, Ross River, and Getah viruses.

The virus was first isolated from humans and mosquitoes during an epidemic in Tanzania in 1952. The first description of the clinical disease was probably made in 1779, when Batavia (the former name for Jakarta) suffered an outbreak. In this and other instances, the disease historically has been confused with dengue. The virus is probably of African origin, from where it has spread to tropical Asia and possibly America. Historical evidence indicates that extensive epidemics of chikungunya occurred in Egypt, East Africa, India, Indonesia, and the Caribbean in the eighteenth and nineteenth centuries. Since 1952, virologically documented epidemics have occurred in sub-Saharan Africa, India, Southeast Asia, and the Philippines.

DISTRIBUTION AND INCIDENCE. The distribution of disease outbreaks is mentioned above. The virus is endemically established in West, Central, East, and South Africa, where it is also maintained as a mosquito-borne zoonosis in nonhuman primate populations. Endemic transmission also occurs in parts of Southeast Asia, but the presence of an enzootic cycle is uncertain.

Epidemics are sustained by a human-mosquito-human cycle involving *Aedes aegypti,* and mixed chikungunya-dengue and chikungunya-yellow fever outbreaks are described. Morbidity in chikungunya epidemics has rarely been documented, but hundreds or even thousands of cases are typical. The outbreak in Tanzania (1952) affected as many as 40% of residents of some communities.

TRANSMISSION AND EPIDEMIOLOGY. The ecology of chikungunya virus is analogous to that of yellow fever. A forest cycle involves enzootic and epizootic transmission between subhuman primates and mosquitoes. In southern Africa, *Ae. furcifer-taylori* and possibly *Mansonia africana* are the principal vectors. The virus has been isolated from treehole-breeding *Ae. africanus* in Uganda and the Central African Republic and from *Ae. luteocephalus* and *Ae. vittatus* in Senegal. These sylvatic vectors are responsible for monkey-monkey, monkey-human, and interhuman transmission in rural areas. The presence of a forest cycle in Asia has not been documented. An urban cycle involving human-human spread by the peridomestic mosquito *Ae. aegypti* is responsible for explosive epidemics in Africa and Asia. The occurrence of epidemics is related to a variety of factors, some of which have been identified. The coincidence of epidemic transmission of chikungunya, dengue, and yellow fever in some cities suggests that the density and longevity of *Ae. aegypti* are important factors. Intrinsic biologic variables within mosquito species may also determine the distribution and rate of transmission, because experimental studies have documented genetically determined intraspecific differences in vector efficiency between mosquito populations. A most important factor is background immunity in the human population. In endemic areas of Africa, the prevalence of chikungunya immunity may approach 100% in adults, and children under 10 years have the highest incidence of disease. Outbreaks occur in urban areas at 5- to 10-year intervals, sufficient to allow for accumulation of susceptible childhood populations.

PATHOLOGY AND PATHOGENESIS. Fatal infections are extremely rare, and there are few data on the pathologic findings in the human disease. Joint biopsies have been reported in two cases; one showed normal synovium and the other pannus formation, inflammation, and germinal center formation. Skin biopsy in another case with rash showed perivascular mononuclear cell infiltration and capillary damage. The pathogenesis in experimentally infected mice includes encephalitis, myositis, and myocarditis typical of alphavirus infections; an unusual feature is the occurrence of intestinal and subcutaneous hemorrhages in infant mice caused by infection with some virus strains.

CLINICAL MANIFESTATIONS AND COMPLICATIONS. The incubation period is 2 to 6 days. In adults the predominant symptom is pain in one or more joints; the onset of pain is exceedingly abrupt. Accompanying symptoms include myalgia, fever, headache, nausea and vomiting, and abdominal pain. The acute phase lasts 3 to 10 days. The fever may be biphasic, with a 1- or 2-day remission occurring after an initial pyrexia of 1 to 6 days. Respiratory symptoms and especially sore throat, with injection and swelling of the fauces and cervical lymphadenopathy, occur in a high proportion of cases. In the early phase of illness, the skin is flushed, and just before or accompanying defervescence, a macular or maculopapular rash appears on the trunk and extensor surfaces of the extremities. The face, soles, and palms may sometimes be involved. Lesions are not infrequently pruritic. The conjunctivae are reddened, and the affected joints may be swollen and red. Multiple joints are affected, predominantly small joints of the hands, wrists, feet, and ankles. Residual arthralgia and joint stiffness may last weeks or months after recovery; periarticular nodules may be present and neuritic pains are described. In young children, joint symptoms are less evident and residual arthralgia is rare. Febrile convulsions are common in children less than 3 years of age.

Minor abnormal bleeding phenomena, including a positive tourniquet test, petechiae, and hemorrhagic rash, are described. These findings occur with approximately the same frequency as in classic dengue fever. Cases with shock are rarely reported.

Clinical laboratory abnormalities are few; leukopenia and thrombocytopenia and transient elevations in levels of serum aminotransferases may be present, but are not invariable features of the disease. Acute phase reactants (prolonged erythrocyte sedimentation rate and presence of C-reactive protein) are a feature of the acute stage of illness.

PROGNOSIS AND THERAPY. Rare deaths associated with hemorrhagic phenomena, shock, myocarditis, and encephalopathy are described. The residual arthritis, with morning stiffness, swelling, and pain on movement, may persist for weeks or months (rarely for as long as 1 year). An association between chronic arthritic symptoms and HLA-B27 haplotype has been reported.

Treatment is symptomatic, consisting of bed rest and nonaspirin analgesics (because of the hemorrhagic diathesis) during the acute phase. In children, dehydration and febrile convulsions may require specific corrective measures. The residual arthritis should be treated with physical therapy and anti-inflammatory agents (salicylates, sulindac).

DIAGNOSIS. Viremia titers in human blood often exceed 6 dex during the early phase of clinical infection. Diagnosis depends on isolation of the virus from serum (by inoculation of baby mice or Vero cell cultures), demonstration of viral antigen in serum, or a rise in antibody titer between appropriately timed acute and convalescent phase sera. Hemagglutination-inhibiting IgM and neutralizing antibodies appear late in the first week and complement-fixing antibodies in the second week after onset.

Differential Diagnosis. The differential diagnosis may be difficult in areas where dengue fever occurs (Chapter 20.1). In children, maculopapular rash, conjunctival injection, and arthralgia are more frequent in chikungunya than in dengue. In adults, features that distinguish chikungunya from dengue are the exceedingly sudden onset of arthralgia and the relative absence of an altered sense of taste in the acute phase and of bradycardia,

depression, weakness, and fatigue in the convalescent phase. The febrile period is usually shorter in chikungunya than in dengue. Headache and retro-orbital and lumbosacral pain are more prominent in dengue. The residual joint symptoms may mimic those seen in rheumatoid arthritis. Other conditions that might be confused with chikungunya are o'nyong nyong fever (Chapter 20.4), rubella, measles, Sindbis fever (Chapter 20.5), epidemic polyarthritis, West Nile fever (Chapter 20.2), Coxsackievirus infections, and rickettsioses (Chapters 23 to 27).

PREVENTION AND CONTROL. A live attenuated vaccine has been tested in a small number of volunteers and appears to be safe and effective. Vaccination would be of little public health interest, but may be useful for military personnel, laboratory workers, and other specialized groups.

In urban areas prone to repeated outbreaks, reduction of *Ae. aegypti* breeding (as discussed for dengue and yellow fever) would limit the potential for spread. Emergency vector control (use of aerial or ground ultra-low-volume sprays) could be used to abort *Ae. aegypti*-borne outbreaks.

BIBLIOGRAPHY

Carey DE: Chikungunya and dengue. A case of mistaken identity? J Hist Med Allied Sci 26:243, 1971.

Deller JJ, Russell PK: Chikungunya disease. Am J Trop Med Hyg 17:107, 1968.

de Moor PP, Steffens FE: A computer-simulated model of an arthropod-borne virus transmission cycle with special reference to chikungunya virus. Trans Roy Soc Trop Med Hyg 64:927, 1970.

Halstead SB, Nimmannitya S, Margiotta MR: Dengue and chikungunya virus infection in man in Thailand, 1962–1964. II. Observations on disease in out-patients. Am J Trop Med Hyg 18:972, 1969.

Lumsden WHR: An epidemic of virus disease in southern Province, Tanganyika Territory, in 1952–53, II. General description and epidemiology. Trans Roy Soc Trop Med Hyg 49:33, 1955.

Peters CJ, Dalrymple JM: Alphaviruses. In Fields BN (ed): Virology. New York, Raven Press, 1990, pp 713–762.

Robinson MC: An epidemic of virus disease in southern Province, Tanganyika Territory, in 1952–53. I. Clinical features. Trans Roy Soc Trop Med Hyg 49:28, 1955.

Tomori O, Fagbami A, Fabiyi A: The 1974 epidemic of chikungunya fever in children in Ibadan, Nigeria. Trop Geogr Med 27:413, 1975.

20.4. O'NYONG NYONG FEVER

DEFINITION. O'nyong nyong is an acute nonfatal alphaviral disease with clinical features similar to those of dengue and chikungunya. It is mosquito-borne and has occurred in epidemic form in East Africa.

ETIOLOGY AND HISTORY. O'nyong nyong was first described and the virus first isolated in 1959 when an extensive epidemic began in Uganda and eventually involved Tanzania, Malawi, and Zambia. A clinically similar epidemic occurred in 1905 to 1906 in the Sudan and Uganda. The term "o'nyong nyong" was used by the Acholi tribe in 1959 to describe the severe joint pains associated with the disease. The disease was last described in 1962 when an outbreak occurred in the

Hoima District, Uganda. Since 1962, the virus has been isolated only once in East Africa.

The virus is a member of the alphavirus genus of the family Togaviridae. It has not been studied extensively but undoubtedly shares physicochemical and ultrastructural properties with other alphaviruses. It is a member of the Semliki Forest virus complex (which includes chikungunya, Mayaro, Ross River, Bebaru, Getah, and Una viruses). Chikungunya-immune sera neutralize o'nyong nyong virus, but the reverse is not observed. Hence, heterologous (chikungunya) cross-reactive antibodies may confuse serodiagnosis. The unadapted virus is difficult to isolate in infant mice; such mice may show patchy alopecia, runting, and occasional paralysis. Cytopathic effect is observed in BHK and HeLa cells, and plaques form in infected Vero and LLC-MK2 cell cultures.

DISTRIBUTION AND INCIDENCE. The outbreaks of 1959 to 1962 in Uganda, Tanzania, and Malawi affected an estimated 2 million people, with attack rates of nearly 100% in some population groups. Because all age groups were involved, investigators concluded that the disease was new to the region. Few cases occurred in Europeans. O'nyong nyong has not reappeared in epidemic form. Antibodies have been found in Ethiopia, Mozambique, Nigeria, Ghana, Liberia, Senegal, Upper Volta, Ivory Coast, and the Central African Republic. An isolation (from sentinel mice) is reported from Senegal.

A closely related unregistered virus (named Igbo-Ora) occurs in West and Central Africa. A single clinical case is described from Nigeria, and an outbreak of undetermined size affected 4 villages in Ivory Coast in 1984. The clinical illness was similar to o'nyong nyong or chikungunya.

TRANSMISSION AND EPIDEMIOLOGY. The virus is transmitted by *Anopheles funestus* and *An. gambiae* mosquitoes, which are endophilic and highly anthropophilic. It is the only well-documented anopheline-borne epidemic viral disease of humans. The distribution of the disease in the affected region of East Africa was similar to that of malaria. The vertebrate reservoir is unknown. On epidemiologic grounds it is probable that viremia in humans is of sufficient degree to infect *Anopheles* vectors and that interhuman transmission occurs.

PATHOLOGY AND PATHOGENESIS. These are unknown.

CLINICAL MANIFESTATIONS AND COMPLICATIONS. The incubation period is 8 days or more. Onset is sudden and is sometimes accompanied by rigors and epistaxis. The syndrome consists of joint pains, rash, and lymphadenitis. Fever was not found in as many as one third of the patients; this is most likely due to infrequent recordings made during the epidemics of 1959 to 1962, but it is probable that high fever is unusual. A saddleback fever curve has not been described. Unlike those in chikungunya, the joint pains in o'nyong nyong are usually symmetric and generalized and range in severity from vague or mild to excruciating discomfort that prevents sitting or standing. The morbilliform rash is unusually pruritic, appears on the fourth to seventh day after onset, and often begins on the face and neck, spreading downward. Rash persists for 4 to 7 days and is not followed by desquamation (a feature sometimes seen in dengue). Enlargement of lymph glands is striking; the postcervical adenopathy is especially noteworthy. Headache is a universal symptom. Retro-orbital pain and backache are frequent. Anorexia, nausea, vomiting, abdominal pain, photophobia, conjunctival injection, edema of eyelids, cough, and coryza are also described. Bradycardia has not been observed. Leukopenia (neutropenia) occurs in the acute phase. The acute phase lasts 5 to 7 days; residual weakness, fatigue, and joint discomfort may prolong convalescence, but the protracted arthritis seen in chikungunya has not been observed. Despite early suspicions, no increase in abortions or congenital malformations occurred during or after the epidemics of 1959 to 1962.

PROGNOSIS AND THERAPY. The disease is self-limited. Therapy is symptomatic, consisting of rest, fluids, and analgesics.

DIAGNOSIS. Virus may be isolated from serum during the acute phase of the disease. The difficulties of virus isolation in mice have been mentioned; near-blind or blind passages are frequently required. It is likely that another technique, e.g., use of mammalian or mosquito cell cultures or intrathoracic inoculation of mosquitoes with subsequent examination by immunofluorescence, would be a more sensitive and practical means of virus isolation. Serologic diagnosis depends upon demonstration of a rising titer of hemagglutination-inhibiting, complement-fixing, or neutralizing antibodies in appropriately time paired sera. Cross-reactions with chikungunya antigen may present problems; antibody titers are higher to the infecting than to the heterologous antigen.

PREVENTION AND CONTROL. No vaccine is available. In the event of an outbreak, use of insecticides to control anopheline vectors could be tried to interrupt transmission.

BIBLIOGRAPHY

Corbet PS, Williams MC, Gillett JD: O'Nyong nyong fever: An epidemic virus disease in East Africa: IV. Vector studies at epidemic sites. Trans Roy Soc Trop Med Hyg 55:463, 1961.
Shore H: O'Nyong nyong fever: An epidemic virus disease in East Africa. III. Some clinical and epidemiological observations in the Northern Province of Uganda. Trans Roy Soc Trop Med Hyg 55:361, 1961.

20.5. SINDBIS FEVER

DEFINITION. Sindbis is a nonfatal endemic-epidemic mosquito-borne alphaviral disease with clinical features resembling those of West Nile and dengue fevers.

ETIOLOGY AND HISTORY. The virus belongs to the alphavirus genus, family Togaviridae. It is a member of the western equine encephalitis antigenic complex and was originally isolated from *Culex univittatus* mosquitoes collected in Egypt in 1952. The virus is pathogenic for intracerebrally and intraperitoneally inoculated infant mice, embryonated chicken eggs, and a variety of primary and continuous cell cultures. Human disease has been recorded in Uganda, South Africa, and Australia; an epidemic occurred in South Africa in 1974.

A similar disease in Sweden (Ockelbo disease), Finland (Pogosta disease), and Karelia in the Soviet Union (Karelian fever) is now known to be caused by an antigenic subtype of Sindbis virus. Molecular characterization and antibody tests distinguish at least 2 major groupings: virus strains from the Palearctic-Ethiopian region and those from the Asian-Australian region. A closely related virus, Barmah Forest virus, has been reported to cause febrile disease with arthralgia (but no rash) in several patients in New South Wales, Australia.

DISTRIBUTION AND INCIDENCE. On the basis of serosurveys and virus isolations from mosquitoes and birds, the virus has a wide dissemination including Africa, Asia, Australia, the Middle East, Eastern Europe, Scandinavia, and the Soviet Union. Sporadic human illness has been recognized in Uganda, South Africa, Scandinavia, the Soviet Union, and Australia. Immunity rates of 10 to 45% occur in endemic areas. In 1974, an outbreak occurred following heavy rains in an arid region of the Transvaal and Orange Free State, South Africa; approximately 4000 persons (16%) of those tested were infected; morbidity estimates are lacking, but hundreds of clinical cases may have occurred. An epidemic of West Nile fever (Chapter 20.2) occurred concurrently.

TRANSMISSION AND EPIDEMIOLOGY. Sindbis virus is transmitted by mosquitoes, which acquire the infection from viremic wild birds. Viremia in humans is of low grade, insufficient to infect vector mosquitoes. In Africa and the Arabian Peninsula, *Cx. univittatus*, which is highly ornitho- and anthropophilic, is the principal vector. This mosquito breeds in semipermanent collections of water with aquatic vegetation. In Australia, *Cx. annulirostris* is the probable vector. Sindbis virus has also been isolated from *Cx. tritaeniorhynchus* (Malaysia), *Cx. pseudovishnui* (Sarawak), *Cx. bitaeniorhynchus* (Philippines), *Cx. antennatus* (Egypt), and *Cx. theileri* (South Africa); from *Aedes, Anopheles,* and *Mansonia* in Australia and Uganda; from wild and domestic birds in India, Czechoslovakia, South Africa, and Egypt; and from sentinel mice in Nigeria. The Sindbis subtype causing disease in Sweden has been recovered from *Culiseta morsitans, Cx. pipiens torrentium,* and *Aedes* spp.

PATHOLOGY AND PATHOGENESIS. No fatal human cases are recorded. In mice the infection is pantropic; necrosis and inflammation have been observed in brain tissue, dermal connective tissue, skeletal muscle, periarticular connective tissue, bone marrow, brown fat, thymus, and myocardium.

CLINICAL MANIFESTATIONS AND COMPLICATIONS. The incubation period is unknown. Patients frequently first note the sudden appearance of rash, but this may be preceded by fever, lassitude, headache, joint pains, and myalgia for 1 or 2 days. The exanthem is most severe over the buttocks, legs, palms, and soles

and rarely involves the head. Lesions are papular or vesicular, occur in crops, last up to 10 days, leave brownish discolorations, and are pruritic. In 1 case in Australia, the vesicular rash was hemorrhagic and recurred several times over a period of months. Vesicles or small ulcerated lesions occasionally appear in the oropharynx, and a sore throat may be noted. Fever is of low grade, lasting several days. Muscle aches and tenderness, pains and swelling of multiple joints, mild headache, periocular pain, paresthesias, and shooting neuritic pains are described, but conjunctivitis, lymphadenitis, and respiratory symptoms are generally absent. Blood counts are normal, but the sedimentation rate may be elevated. Signs of meningeal irritation, jaundice, and myocardial damage (electrocardiographic changes) are reported, but rare.

PROGNOSIS AND THERAPY. The disease is self-limited and generally mild. Treatment is symptomatic.

DIAGNOSIS. The virus may be isolated from acute phase serum and has also been recovered from vesicular fluid and throat swabs. Standard serologic tests (HI, CF, neutralization, IgM antibody-capture ELISA) are applicable to diagnosis; paired acute and convalescent sera should be obtained.

Differential Diagnosis. The most difficult element in the differential diagnosis is distinction from West Nile fever, which may occur in simultaneous outbreaks (Chapter 20.2). Laboratory tests are required to distinguish these conditions. Other conditions that must be considered are chikungunya, o'nyong nyong, rickettsial infections, measles, rubella, and coxsackievirus infections.

PREVENTION AND CONTROL. No vaccine is available. In the event of an outbreak, adult mosquito control measures may be considered.

BIBLIOGRAPHY

Guard RW, McAuliffe MJ, Stallman ND, Bramston BA: Haemorrhagic manifestations with Sindbis infection: A case report. Pathology 14:89, 1982.

Malherbe H, Strickland-Cholmley M, Jackson AL: Sindbis virus infection in man. Report of a case with recovery of virus from skin lesions. S Afr Med J 37:547, 1963.

McIntosh BM, McGillivray GM, Dickinson, DB, et al: Illness caused by Sindbis and West Nile viruses in South Africa. S Afr Med J 39:291, 1964.

Niklasson B, Espmark A, LeDuc JW, et al: Association of a Sindbis-like virus with Ockelbo disease in Sweden. Am J Trop Med Hyg 33:1212, 1984.

20.6. EPIDEMIC POLYARTHRITIS

DEFINITION. Epidemic polyarthritis is a self-limited epidemic and endemic dengue-like disease caused by a mosquito-borne alphavirus (Ross River virus).

ETIOLOGY AND HISTORY. Epidemics were first described in Australia in 1928; many cases occurred in soldiers stationed in northern Australia during World War II. During a widespread epidemic in 1956, serologic evidence for an alphaviral etiology was obtained. In

1963 Ross River virus, a new alphavirus, was isolated from *Aedes vigilax* mosquitoes and, on serologic grounds, was associated with the human illness. Subsequent serologic confirmation and isolation of Ross River virus from the blood of typical patients have established the etiology. Epidemics were confined to Australia until 1979, when the disease appeared in the Central and South Pacific. Ross River virus is a member of the antigenic complex comprising Semliki Forest, Mayaro, chikungunya, and Getah viruses, to which it is most closely related. The virus is pathogenic for infant mice inoculated intraperitoneally and intracerebrally; mice develop a typical illness with hind limb paralysis. Strain differences in pathogenicity have been noted. A possible association with a neuromuscular syndrome in horses has been noted.

DISTRIBUTION AND INCIDENCE. The disease is endemic and epidemic in northern and eastern Australia, where cases occur annually in the summer and fall (between January and May). The largest outbreak in Australia occurred in 1983 to 1984, involving 1196 confirmed cases in New South Wales. Outbreaks have also occurred at intervals in western Australia. Antibodies or indigenous cases have been found in Papua New Guinea, the Solomon Islands, the Moluccas, New Caledonia, Wallis and Futuna islands, Tonga, and Iryan Jaya. In 1979 and 1980 the disease appeared for the first time outside Australia. Explosive epidemics in the Fijian Islands, American Samoa, and Rarotonga (in the Cook Islands) involved thousands of cases. Infection rates of more than 90% and clinical attack rates of greater than 40% were documented in certain areas. Attack rates are highest in adults 20 to 50 years of age. Children have significantly milder clinical symptoms than adults. An excess of cases in females was noted.

TRANSMISSION AND EPIDEMIOLOGY. Human infection is acquired by mosquito bites. In Australia, *Ae. vigilax, Culex annulirostris,* and *Ae. normanensis* are implicated vectors. The vertebrate reservoir-host(s) involved in virus circulation are uncertain, but a role for large marsupials (kangaroos and wallabies) is suspected. In the Pacific, studies in Rarotonga showed *Ae. polynesiensis* to be responsible for transmission. By use of the sensitive mosquito inoculation technique, viremia was documented in nearly half the patients studied during the acute phase of illness, and viremic titers were shown to be sufficient to infect vectors. It is likely that a human-mosquito-human cycle was responsible for these explosive island outbreaks. *Ae. aegypti* and *Ae. albopictus* have been shown experimentally to be efficient vectors, raising the specter of spread of the disease to populous areas of Hawaii and the Americas.

PATHOLOGY AND PATHOGENESIS. No fatal human cases are recorded. Synovial fluid obtained from patients early in the disease has shown cell counts of 1500 to 15,000/mm³ with a marked predominance of actively phagocytic macrophages and monocytes. The fluid contained viral antigen and normal C3 and C4 levels; antibodies were absent. The observations suggest viral replication in joint tissues and phagocytosis by macrophages during the early phase of disease, with no evidence of immune complex disorder. Additional evidence for a role for the monocyte-macrophage class of cells and for genetic determinants in the infection was provided by a study that showed an increased risk of disease in association with the HLA-DR7 antigen. The pathogenesis of the persistent or relapsing joint disorder in some patients is unknown; however, long duration of IgM antibodies has been noted, suggesting the possibility of persistent viral infection.

CLINICAL MANIFESTATIONS AND COMPLICATIONS. The incubation period is 3 to 9 days. Onset is usually abrupt with low-grade fever, chills, myalgia, and arthralgia. Approximately 20% of the patients develop maculopapular (occasionally vesicular) pruritic rash, most marked on the extremities and trunk. Some patients experience a rash without arthralgia. Knees, ankles, wrists, and small joints of the hands and feet are most prominently affected by pain and swelling. Headache, eye pain, paresthesias, sore throat, and lymphadenopathy are described. Gastrointestinal complaints are uncommon. Recovery from the acute disease is rapid, but joint pains often persist for several weeks. Some patients experience relapsing or persistent arthritic symptoms for long periods, i.e., up to 1 year.

PROGNOSIS AND THERAPY. Although joint symptoms may be prolonged, no instances of progression to chronic or deforming arthritis are known. Treatment consists of rest and analgesics.

DIAGNOSIS. The epidemic disease may be confused with dengue (Chapter 20.1) or chikungunya (Chapter 20.3). Sporadic cases are difficult to diagnose and may mimic rubella, other viral infections with arthritis (e.g., infectious mononucleosis), rheumatic fever, rheumatoid arthritis, or systemic lupus erythematosus. Examination of the joint fluid may be helpful in distinguishing the last two (noninfectious) conditions, which are characterized by more numerous neutrophils in the synovial fluid. Fluorescent antibody cytologic examination of joint fluid may provide a rapid diagnosis. Attempts to isolate virus from blood by mouse inoculation have been generally unsuccessful, but recent studies using intrathoracic inoculation of mosquitoes showed a high rate of virus isolation from blood during the acute phase of illness. Serologic diagnosis is most generally applicable. Hemagglutination-inhibiting antibodies appear early, and most patients have detectable titers by the time they present with illness (providing a useful rapid presumptive diagnosis). Complement-fixing antibodies appear during the second week of illness. IgM antibodies detected by antibody-capture enzyme-linked immunosorbent assay (ELISA) appear within a few days after onset and may last for up to 4 months.

PREVENTION AND CONTROL. No vaccine is available. Mosquito control measures may be considered.

BIBLIOGRAPHY

Aaskov JG, Mutaika JU, Lawrence GW, et al: An epidemic of Ross River virus infection in Fiji, 1979. Am J Trop Med Hyg 30:1053, 1981.

Doherty RL: Arthropod-borne viruses in Australia and their relation to infection and disease. Prog Med Virol 17:136, 1974.

Fraser JRE, Cunningham AL, Clarris BJ, et al: Cytology of synovial effusions in epidemic polyarthritis. Aust NZ J Med 11:168, 1981.

Kay BH, Aaskov JG: Ross River virus (epidemic polyarthritis). *In* Monath TP (ed): The Arboviruses: Epidemiology and Ecology, Vol IV. Boca Raton, FL, CRC Press, 1988, pp 93–112.

Rosen L, Gubler DJ, Bennett PH: Epidemic polyarthritis (Ross River) virus infection in the Cook Islands. Am J Trop Med Hyg 30:1294, 1981.

20.7. MAYARO FEVER

DEFINITION. Mayaro virus disease is an acute self-limited dengue-like illness of the neotropics, transmitted by mosquitoes and caused by an alphavirus of the same name. Synonyms include Uruma fever and Uruma virus disease.

ETIOLOGY AND HISTORY. Mayaro virus was first isolated in 1954 from five febrile patients in Trinidad. Outbreaks were recognized in 1955 in Pará, Brazil, and in a remote area of eastern Bolivia. In 1977 to 1978, a large epidemic that occurred in the rural village of Belterra, Pará, Brazil, was carefully studied. Mayaro virus is an alphavirus (family Togaviridae), placed within the Semliki Forest virus antigenic complex. The unadapted virus is pathogenic for infant mice and hamsters by the intracerebral and intraperitoneal routes, for embryonated hens' eggs, and for a variety of cell cultures (HeLa, BHK-21, Vero, primary chick and duck embryo).

DISTRIBUTION AND INCIDENCE. Human cases of Mayaro fever have been documented in Trinidad, Surinam, Brazil, and Bolivia, and the virus has been isolated from mosquitoes in Brazil, Panama, and Trinidad; from lizards and a marmoset in Brazil; and from a migrating bird captured in Louisiana. Antibodies have been found in human populations of Peru, Colombia, Panama, and Guyana. Sporadic overt infections are undoubtedly frequent and go unrecognized in forested endemic areas of northern and eastern South America, where antibody prevalences of up to 60% have been found. Mayaro virus infection was one of the most frequently encountered diseases among settlers along the Trans-Amazon highway in Brazil. The potential for epidemics has been clearly illustrated, especially when immunologically virgin groups enter forested areas, e.g., Okinawan colonists in Bolivia and Dutch military personnel on patrol in Surinam. Annual infection rates in the Dutch soldiers varied between 1.6 and 5.3%. In the 1954 to 1955 outbreak in Bolivia, Mayaro virus was responsible for 10 to 15% of 200 cases of jungle fever. In Brazil, the epidemic in 1955 involved 50 persons; the outbreak in 1977 affected 800 persons in a population of 4000. It is estimated that 80% of infected persons develop clinical illness.

TRANSMISSION AND EPIDEMIOLOGY. Humans acquire the disease by the bite of infected mosquitoes. Wild vertebrates are involved in both amplification and enzootic maintenance of the virus, but the possibility that viremic humans may infect vector mosquitoes is not excluded (viremic titers of greater than 10^5/ml have been documented). *Haemagogus* mosquitoes appear to be of principal importance as epidemic

vectors. In the Belterra outbreak, *Hg. janthinomys* was clearly responsible for transmission to humans and to sylvan marmosets (the probable amplifying sylvan host). The epidemiology of Mayaro virus disease is thus analogous to that of jungle yellow fever, and, in fact, both viruses simultaneously affected the Belterra population. However, vector and wild vertebrate species other than *Haemagogus* and nonhuman primates may also play a role in the enzootic maintenance cycle. The virus has been isolated from lizards; a wild bird; *Coquillettidia mansonia, Culex,* and *Sabethes* mosquitoes; and *Gigantolaelaps* mites. Antibodies have been found in birds, rodents, and marsupials. The possibility that Mayaro virus could orally infect and be transmitted by *Aedes aegypti* or *Ae. albopictus* deserves study, because of the potential for urbanization of the disease in the Americas.

PATHOLOGY AND PATHOGENESIS. No fatal human infections have been reported, and the pathogenesis of the disease syndrome in humans is unknown. In mice, necrosis of skeletal muscle, periosteum, and perichondrial tissues has been demonstrated; similar lesions might account for the myalgia and arthralgia of the human disease.

CLINICAL MANIFESTATIONS AND COMPLICATIONS. The maximum incubation period has been estimated to be 7 to 12 days. Onset is abrupt, with fever, chills, headache, and dizziness. Arthralgia and rash are the most prominent symptoms. The wrists, fingers, ankles, and toes are most commonly affected, but larger joints may also be involved. Joint swelling occurs in 20% of the cases. Fever subsides after 2 to 4 days. Arthralgia, which may be incapacitating, generally subsides after 4 or 5 days, but may persist with decreasing severity for up to 2 months. The rash, which is present in two thirds of patients, is maculo- or micropapular, generally appears on the fifth day after onset, and fades within 3 or 4 days. Rash is more common in children and is more intense on the trunk and limbs than on the face and hands. Other features include headache, nausea, vomiting, diarrhea, dizziness, inguinal lymphadenopathy, leukopenia, mild albuminuria, and slight thrombocytopenia.

PROGNOSIS AND THERAPY. No fatalities are recorded. The acute illness may be severe and incapacitating, but is of short duration. Persistent arthralgia, lasting up to 2 months, has been described in a few cases. Treatment is symptomatic.

DIAGNOSIS. Diagnosis is made by virus isolation from blood or a rising titer of hemagglutination-inhibiting, complement-fixing, or neutralizing antibodies in appropriately timed paired sera.

PREVENTION AND CONTROL. An inactivated vaccine produced in human diploid cells has been preliminarily studied in mice but is not yet available for use. For casual visitors to jungle areas of northern and eastern South America, advice should be given regarding avoidance of mosquito bite and use of repellents and protective clothing. Emergency ultra-low-volume-spray mosquito control measures in human settlements and surrounding forested areas might be effective in instances of a circumscribed outbreak.

BIBLIOGRAPHY

Hoch AL, Peterson NE, LeDuc JW, et al: An outbreak of Mayaro virus disease in Belterra, Brazil, III. Entomological and ecological studies. Am J Trop Med Hyg 30:689, 1981.

LeDuc JW, Pinheiro FP, Travassos da Rosa APA: An outbreak of Mayaro virus disease in Belterra, Brazil. II. Epidemiology 30:682, 1981.

Pinheiro FP, Freitas RB, Travassos da Rosa JF, et al: An outbreak of Mayaro virus disease in Belterra, Brazil. I. Clinical and virological findings. Am J Trop Med Hyg 30:674, 1981.

20.8. GROUP C VIRUS FEVERS

DEFINITION. Ten viruses of this antigenic group cause similar, nondescript, self-limited, sporadic febrile illness in the New World tropics (Table 20–1).

ETIOLOGY AND HISTORY. These viruses belong to serogroup C, genus *Bunyavirus,* family Bunyaviridae. The *Bunyavirus* genus comprises more than 150 serologically interrelated viruses belonging to 16 antigenic groups, including group C. Virus particles are spherical, are 90 to 100 nm in diameter, and contain a single-stranded RNA genome. The genome is in 3 segments, which allows for genetic reassortment and explains the evolutionary diversity of this group. Virus replication occurs in the cytoplasm of infected cells. Virus particles are susceptible to lipid solvents. The first virus in group C to be isolated (Murutucu virus) was recovered from a sentinel monkey near Belém, Brazil, in 1954. There are now 13 recognized group C viruses, of which 10 have been associated with human illness: Oriboca, Caraparu, Murutucu, Restan, Nepuyo, Ossa, Apeu, Marituba, Itaqui, and Madrid viruses. The group C viruses hemagglutinate goose erythrocytes. They replicate and may be assayed in many cell cultures and are pathogenic for infant mice by the intraperitoneal and intracerebral routes.

DISTRIBUTION AND INCIDENCE. The geographic distribution of the group C viruses is shown in Table 20–1. Disease in humans is sporadic, and fewer than 50 cases have been diagnosed by virus isolation from adult patients with undifferentiated illness who were inhabiting or working in forested areas. Oriboca and Caraparu viruses have been most frequently implicated in human infections. Disease is undoubtedly underrecognized; hemagglutination-inhibiting antibodies have been found in as many as 38% of residents in some areas, and up to 4.3% of persons residing for as long as 6 months along the Trans-Amazon Highway developed antibodies. The annual incidence of infection among Dutch soldiers in Surinam was 2.5%. No epidemics have been recorded, however, even in such susceptible groups.

The group C viruses are transmitted by forest mosquitoes, principally *Culex (Melanoconion)* spp. Forest rodents, marsupials, and possibly bats are the principal viremic hosts.

PATHOLOGY AND PATHOGENESIS. No fatal human cases have been recognized. The viruses produce encephalitis and hepatitis in laboratory mice.

CLINICAL MANIFESTATIONS AND COMPLICATIONS. Illness begins abruptly. Symptoms and signs include fever (occasionally biphasic) lasting up to 5 days, chills, generalized malaise, headache, photophobia, backache, myalgia, nausea, conjunctival congestion, and dizziness. Rash is not reported. Severely ill patients may be prostrate. The peripheral white cell count is normal or depressed; other clinical laboratory tests have not been performed. A prolonged convalescence with weakness and fatigue may follow the acute phase.

DIAGNOSIS. This is made by virus isolation from blood or serum and specific identification of the agent. Serologic diagnosis is also possible, but cross-reactions between the group C viruses may render interpretation difficult.

PROGNOSIS AND THERAPY. Illness is benign and recovery is complete. Treatment is symptomatic.

PREVENTION AND CONTROL. No vaccines or other specific preventive measures are available. Avoidance of mosquito bites by use of bed nets and repellents may be recommended to casual visitors to tropical forests.

BIBLIOGRAPHY

Gibbs CJ Jr, Bruckner EA, Schenker S: A case of Apeu virus infection. Am J Trop Med Hyg 13:108, 1964.

Pinheiro FP, Bensabath G, Andrade AHP, et al: Infectious diseases along Brazil's Trans-Amazon Highway; surveillance and research. Bull PAHO 8:111, 1974.

Shope RE, Woodall JP, Travassos da Rosa A: The epidemiology of diseases caused by viruses in group C and Guama (Bunyaviridae). *In* Monath TP (ed): The Arboviruses: Epidemiology and Ecology, Vol III. Boca Raton, FL, CRC Press, 1988, pp 37–52.

20.9. OROPOUCHE VIRUS DISEASE

DEFINITION. Oropouche virus disease (febre de Mojui) is an acute undifferentiated febrile illness transmitted by *Culicoides* midges in Trinidad and the Amazon region of Brazil.

ETIOLOGY AND HISTORY. Oropouche virus is the only important human pathogen belonging to the Simbu serogroup of the genus *Bunyavirus,* family Bunyaviridae. It was originally isolated from the blood of a forest worker in Trinidad in 1955. In 1961, the virus was responsible for a large epidemic in Belém, Brazil. Between 1967 and 1981, 15 major outbreaks occurred in cities and towns of the Amazon region.

**TABLE 20–1. Group C Viruses
Known to Cause Human Disease**

Virus	Known Geographic Distribution
Apeu	Brazil
Caraparu	Brazil, Panama, Trinidad, Guianas
Itaqui	Brazil
Madrid	Panama
Marituba	Brazil
Murutucu	Brazil, French Guiana
Nepuyo	Brazil, Trinidad, Central America, Mexico
Oriboca	Brazil, Trinidad, Guianas
Ossa	Panama
Restan	Trinidad, Surinam

Oropouche virus is pathogenic for infant mice and for infant and adult hamsters by the intracerebral and intraperitoneal routes of inoculation, for adult mice and guinea pigs inoculated intracerebrally, and for embryonated hens' eggs. A variety of cell cultures are useful for growth and assay of the virus, including BHK-21, Vero, LLC-MK2, and MA-111.

DISTRIBUTION AND INCIDENCE. The virus has been isolated and associated with human disease in Trinidad and northern Brazil, and antibodies have been found in monkeys in Colombia (Magdalena Valley). The epidemic of 1961 affected an estimated 11,000 residents of Belém. Subsequent outbreaks in Brazil (Bragança, 1967; Belém, 1968; Baiáo, 1972; Itupiranga, 1975; Santarém, 1975; Tomé-Acú, 1978; Belém, 1979–1980; Manaus, 1980–1981; and Mazagao, 1980) were responsible for at least 250,000 infections. Human infection rates during outbreaks have been as high as 15 to 40%. All ages and both sexes are equally affected. The illness to infection ratio is believed to be high (63%). Most cases occurred in children and young adults, and there was no sex predilection. Nearly 400 virus isolations have been made from the blood of patients.

EPIDEMIOLOGY AND TRANSMISSION. The virus was repeatedly recovered from *Culicoides paraensis* midges during the Santarém and Tomé-Acú outbreaks in Brazil. *C. paraensis* has also been shown to transmit Oropouche virus in laboratory experiments. These midges, which feed indoors and out, readily pass through mosquito screens, breed in decomposing vegetation, are abundant in areas of towns affected during epidemics and are believed to be the principal urban vector, with viremic humans serving as vertebrate hosts. The virus has also been recovered from *Aedes serratus* and *Coquillettidia venezuelensis* mosquitoes. *Culex quinquefasciatus* mosquitoes have also been suspected of transmitting Oropouche virus in the urban environment; compared with *Culicoides,* however, these mosquitoes are not only less abundant, but also significantly less competent biologic vectors.

The maintenance cycle in the tropical forest is uncertain. Antibodies have been found in monkeys and birds, and virus isolations have been made from sloths. The vectors involved in enzootic transmission are unknown.

PATHOLOGY AND PATHOGENESIS. No fatal human cases are recorded. The virus produces encephalitis in the laboratory mouse. Monkeys and sloths develop viremia but no signs of illness.

CLINICAL MANIFESTATIONS AND COMPLICATIONS. The illness is similar in children and adults. Onset is abrupt, with fever to 40 C, headache, generalized malaise, and myalgia. Gastrointestinal complaints are frequent, i.e., anorexia, nausea, vomiting, diarrhea, and epigastric pain. Physical findings are few, i.e., fever and conjunctival injection, and there is no rash or lymphadenopathy. The peripheral leukocyte count is usually decreased. The acute illness lasts for 2 to 7 days. Some patients are severely ill and may be prostrate or require hospitalization, but no fatalities have been recorded. Cases with aseptic meningitis have been described. A prolonged convalescence may follow the acute phase, with weakness, fatigue, and other nonspe-

cific complaints. Relapses, with fever, headache, and myalgia, may occur during the second and third weeks after onset; virus has not been recovered from such patients.

DIAGNOSIS. The specific diagnosis is made by isolation of the virus from serum or whole blood during the acute illness or by demonstration of a rise in hemagglutination-inhibiting, neutralizing, immunofluorescent, or enzyme-linked immunosorbent assay (ELISA) antibodies in paired acute and convalescent sera.

PROGNOSIS AND THERAPY. The disease is self-limited. Analgesics, antipyretics, and antiemetics may be used to control symptoms. In view of the teratogenic potential of other Simbu group viruses in domestic livestock and experimental animals, follow-up studies of pregnant women should be conducted during future outbreaks.

PREVENTION AND CONTROL. No vaccine is available. Emergency vector control, aimed at adult *Culicoides paraensis* midges, may be warranted during epidemics in the Amazon region.

BIBLIOGRAPHY

LeDuc JW, Pinheiro FP: Oropouche fever. *In* Monath TP (ed): The Arboviruses: Epidemiology and Ecology, Vol IV. Boca Raton, FL, CRC Press, 1988, pp 1–14.
Pinheiro FP, Travassos da Rosa APA, Travassos da Rosa JF, et al: An outbreak of Oropouche virus disease in the vicinity of Santarem, Para, Brazil. Trop Med Parasit 27:213, 1976.
Pinheiro FP, Travassos da Rosa APA, Travassos da Rosa JF, et al: Oropouche virus. I. A review of clinical, epidemiological, and ecological findings. Am J Trop Med Hyg 30:149, 1981.

20.10.   RIFT VALLEY FEVER

DEFINITION. Rift Valley fever is an acute viral infection of sheep, cattle, and human beings in Africa. The human disease may be characterized by a nonspecific influenza-like syndrome or, in severe cases, by encephalitis, retinitis, or hemorrhagic fever.

ETIOLOGY AND HISTORY. Rift Valley fever virus is a member of the family Bunyaviridae, genus *Phlebovirus* (Chapters 20.8 and 20.11). Various tests have shown serologic relationships between Rift Valley fever and a number of other phleboviruses, especially Gordil, St. Floris, Arumowot, Punta Toro, and Frijoles. As is the case for other bunyaviruses, the RNA genome of Rift Valley fever virus is segmented, allowing for possible genetic reassortment of viruses in nature. Oligonucleotide mapping of Rift Valley fever virus strains from different parts of Africa has demonstrated variation. The virus has a wide host range; it grows to high titer in a variety of cell lines and is pathogenic for infant and adult mice, hamsters, and rats by the intracerebral and intraperitoneal inoculation routes. Inbred rat strains show differing susceptibility to visceral and encephalitic infection with the virus and can be used to study variation in virulence among geographic virus strains.

The disease in sheep, cattle, and humans was first described and a virus etiology proved in 1931 in Kenya;

an earlier outbreak (in 1912) in Kenya is retrospectively attributed to Rift Valley fever virus. In 1944, the virus was isolated from wild-caught mosquitoes in Uganda. Epizootics in southern and East Africa in the 1950s, 1960s, and early 1970s were associated with human cases, which were characterized as self-limited undifferentiated febrile illnesses. The first recognition of severe and fatal infections (hemorrhagic fever) occurred in South Africa in 1975. In 1977 to 1978, the first large human epidemic was recorded in the Nile Delta of Egypt; many cases were complicated by hemorrhagic fever, encephalitis, or retinitis. In 1987 and 1990 epizootic-epidemics occurred in southern Mauritania and Madagascar, respectively.

DISTRIBUTION AND INCIDENCE. Rift Valley fever virus is widely distributed throughout sub-Saharan Africa. The virus has been isolated in Burkina Faso, the Central African Republic (where it was first called Zinga virus), Guinea, Kenya, Mozambique, Namibia, Nigeria, Senegal, Mauritania, South Africa, Sudan, Tanzania, Uganda, Zaire, Zambia, and Zimbabwe. Serologic evidence suggests virus activity in many other countries. Epizootics affecting livestock have been most frequent in South Africa, Zambia, Zimbabwe, Kenya, Tanzania, and Uganda, but have been associated with a relatively low incidence of human disease. In contrast, the outbreaks in Egypt (1977–1978) and Mauritania (1987) were characterized by high attack rates in livestock and humans and by severe human disease. In the Egyptian epidemic, more than 18,000 human cases and 598 deaths were officially reported, but other estimates indicate an incidence of at least 200,000 cases. In the Mauritanian epidemic, approximately 1000 human cases and 50 deaths may have occurred in the epicenter (the town of Rosso).

TRANSMISSION AND EPIDEMIOLOGY. Infection of domestic livestock during epizootics is the result of transmission by mosquitoes. A wide variety of mosquito species belonging to 5 genera have yielded virus isolations. Cattle and sheep develop high-titer viremias and serve as source of infection for mosquitoes. Outbreaks coincide with periods of heavy rainfall and high vector density. Direct contact, mechanical transmission by biting and nonbiting insects, or milk-borne spread may also play a role in animal infection.

Transmission to humans may occur by the bite of infected vectors or by direct contact with carcasses, tissues, and organs of animals dying of the disease; butchers, ranchers, veterinarians, and others with frequent exposure to animals are at highest risk of infection. Aerosol infection may also occur under both natural and laboratory conditions.

In Egypt, where many persons acquired Rift Valley fever without direct exposure to animals, arthropod-borne infection was considered a probable means of transmission. Virus isolations were made from *Culex pipiens* mosquitoes. Humans develop high-titer viremias, raising the possibility of human-mosquito-human transmission. Virus can also be recovered from the throat, and interhuman spread by contact or aerosol transmission and mechanical spread by flies and fomites must be considered.

The Egyptian epidemic was the result of introduction of the virus from an enzootic focus, and the virus has not persisted. The enzootic maintenance cycle of Rift Valley fever virus in sub-Saharan Africa has only recently been elucidated. The primary cycle involves floodwater *Aedes* spp. which maintain the virus by transovarial transmission over the long dry season, and domestic livestock, which serve as amplifying hosts during the rains. An important geologic feature of the enzootic focus is the *dambo,* a shallow depression that collects ground water and serves as a breeding site for *Aedes.* During years of prolonged and excessive rainfall, the initial emergence of *Aedes* vectors is followed by successive waves of secondary vectors, species of *Anopheles* and *Culex,* which further amplify the rate of virus transmission and cause recognized epizootics. Identification of dambos and monitoring of changes in ground water and vegetation by means of aerial and satellite photography have provided new approaches to predictive surveillance.

PATHOGENESIS AND PATHOLOGY. Rift Valley fever virus is highly hepatotropic. The most extensive lesions are seen in newborn lambs and are characterized by massive hepatic necrosis. Councilman-like bodies and intranuclear eosinophilic inclusions are also described. Lymphocyte necrosis in lymph nodes, widespread serosal and visceral hemorrhages, and renal glomerular and tubular changes are present. These pathologic features are also seen to a lesser degree in adult sheep and in cattle. Laboratory rodents provide useful models of the hepatitis and encephalitis associated with human Rift Valley fever.

Only limited pathologic studies of human cases have been reported. Changes include severe hepatic necrosis and hemorrhages, myocardial fiber degeneration, and interstitial pneumonitis.

CLINICAL MANIFESTATIONS AND COMPLICATIONS

In Animals. The disease in sheep and cows is characterized by fever, listlessness, leukopenia, vomiting, melena, and blood-stained nasal discharge. Mortality is 90% or higher in newborn lambs, 20 to 30% in adult sheep, and usually 10% or less in cattle. Abortions are common. Horses are refractory to disease, and infection in water buffalo, camels, and goats is usually inapparent or mild.

In Humans. The incubation period is 3 to 6 days. The onset is sudden. Uncomplicated illness (observed in 98% of cases) is characterized by fever, chills, headache, lumbosacral pain, generalized myalgia, anorexia, nausea, and vomiting. Upper respiratory tract symptoms are absent. Physical findings include relative bradycardia and conjunctival injection. Clinical laboratory tests may show an initial leukocytosis followed by leukopenia; results of liver function tests are normal. The disease runs its course in 4 to 7 days and recovery is complete.

Complications. Rift Valley fever may be complicated (in 1% of cases) by hemorrhagic manifestations and jaundice; the clinical features of this syndrome resemble those of yellow fever. In another 1% of cases, signs of meningoencephalitis and elevated cerebrospinal fluid lymphocyte counts develop 5 to 15 days after onset of fever and may result in permanent neurologic deficits. Fatalities are recorded in patients with both the hemorrhagic and, more rarely, the encephalitic forms.

Ocular complications are not uncommon and take the form of macular, paramacular, and extramacular retinal lesions; hemorrhages; and vasculitis. Central visual loss may be permanent.

There is no evidence at present for or against an increased risk of abortion in humans.

DIAGNOSIS. During the acute phase of illness, Rift Valley fever virus may be isolated from blood by inoculation of cell cultures or mice. A serologic diagnosis is made by testing paired acute and convalescent phase sera by hemagglutination inhibition, complement fixation, IgM antibody-capture ELISA, or indirect fluorescent antibody tests. IgM antibodies are locally produced in the central nervous system in patients with encephalitis and may be measured in cerebrospinal fluid.

TREATMENT AND PROGNOSIS. Treatment of Rift Valley fever is symptomatic. Drugs that are potentially hepatotoxic or may exaggerate the bleeding diathesis should be avoided. In patients with jaundice and hemorrhage, measures to counteract shock may be required.

The case-fatality rate in Egyptian hospitalized patients (many of whom had severe complications of the disease) was 14%.

An antiviral drug, ribavirin, as well as interferon and interferon inducers, and passive antibody have demonstrated efficacy in murine models of Rift Valley fever, but remain to be tested in humans.

PREVENTION AND CONTROL. Both inactivated and live attenuated vaccines have been developed for use in livestock. Formalin-inactivated cell culture–propagated vaccine has also been used to protect laboratory and field workers and military troops; there have been several thousand recipients of this vaccine. Adequate serologic responses occur in over 95% of vaccinated persons, with only a few minor local reactions. However, 1 possible case of Guillain-Barré syndrome has been reported to follow immunization. Research on genetically engineered vaccines is under way in several laboratories.

Mosquito control measures are indicated in the setting of epidemic-epizootics. Public health measures also include advice to the general public and to high-risk groups to avoid contact with sick or dead sheep and cattle. Surveillance, animal quarantine, and animal vaccinations are important in preventing spread of the disease.

BIBLIOGRAPHY

Abdel-Wahab KSE-D, El Baz LM, El Tayeb EM, et al: Rift Valley fever virus infections in Egypt: Pathological and virological findings in man. Trans Roy Soc Trop Med Hyg 72:392, 1978.

Daubney R, Hudson JR, Garnham, PC: Enzootic hepatitis or Rift Valley fever: An undescribed disease of sheep, cattle and man from East Africa. J Pathol Bacteriol 34:545, 1931.

Klingberg MA (ed): Rift Valley fever. In Contributions to Epidemiology and Biostatistics, Vol 3. Basel, S. Karger, 1981.

Meegan JM, Bailey CL: Rift Valley fever. In Monath TP (ed): The Arboviruses: Epidemiology and Ecology, Vol IV. Boca Raton, FL, CRC Press, 1988, pp 51–76.

20.11. SANDFLY FEVERS

DEFINITION. Sandfly fevers (pappataci fever, phlebotomus fever) are acute, self-limited, undifferentiated febrile illnesses caused by viruses belonging to the phlebotomus fever serogroup and transmitted by sandflies.

ETIOLOGY AND HISTORY. At least 38 registered viruses belong to the phlebotomus fever serogroup and constitute the *Phlebovirus* genus of the family Bunyaviridae. Of these, 8 viruses have been recovered from infected persons (sandfly fever Naples, sandfly fever Sicilian, Chagres, Candiru, Punta Toro, Toscana, Alenquer, and Rift Valley fever) (Chapter 20.10). Some of these viruses, including sandfly fever Naples and Sicilian and Punta Toro viruses, do not produce illness in most laboratory animals (unless adapted by repeated passage), and cell cultures, e.g., Vero or BHK-21, are more useful than animals for primary isolation and assay.

The clinical disease was delineated and transmission of the causative agent by *Phlebotomus papatasi* was described by the Austrian Military Commission in Dalmatia in 1909, but the viruses (Naples and Sicilian serotypes) were not isolated until 1943 to 1944. During the 1960s and 1970s, a large number of other phlebotomus fever serogroup viruses were isolated, mainly in the neotropics. The history of sandfly fever is closely tied to military campaigns.

DISTRIBUTION AND INCIDENCE. The distribution of Naples and Sicilian viruses overlaps that of the vector, *P. papatasi* (Fig. 20–6). Sporadic cases, mainly in children, occur in these endemic areas. Serologic studies show acquisition of high titers of antibody early in life, and most infections escape medical attention. The disease has assumed great importance when large numbers of nonimmune persons (military troops, refugees) enter endemic areas. Nearly 20,000 cases were reported in United States soldiers during World War II (1.8 cases/1000 troops stationed overseas); British Middle East Forces suffered an incidence of 21.5 cases/1000 troops in 1942.

Chagres and Punta Toro viruses have been isolated in Panama and Candiru virus in Brazil. The maximum prevalence of antibodies to Chagres and Punta Toro viruses in residents of Panama is 17 and 35%, respectively. Only sporadic cases of illness have been recognized. Toscana virus occurs in the Mediterranean region; outbreaks have been reported in Italy, and sporadic cases have been recognized among foreign travelers and military personnel in Italy and Cyprus. Alenquer virus occurs in Brazil.

EPIDEMIOLOGY AND TRANSMISSION. *P. papatasi* is the principal vector of Naples and Sicilian viruses. These nocturnal biting midges avidly feed on humans and are closely associated with human habitation. They breed in organic debris and loose soil near houses; adults rest during the day in dark areas and crevices in and around dwellings. Only the adult females bite; they are small (2 to 3 mm) and readily pass through bed nets and screens. Sandfly fever viruses are transovarially transmitted in their vector species. This mechanism probably accounts for virus maintenance, al-

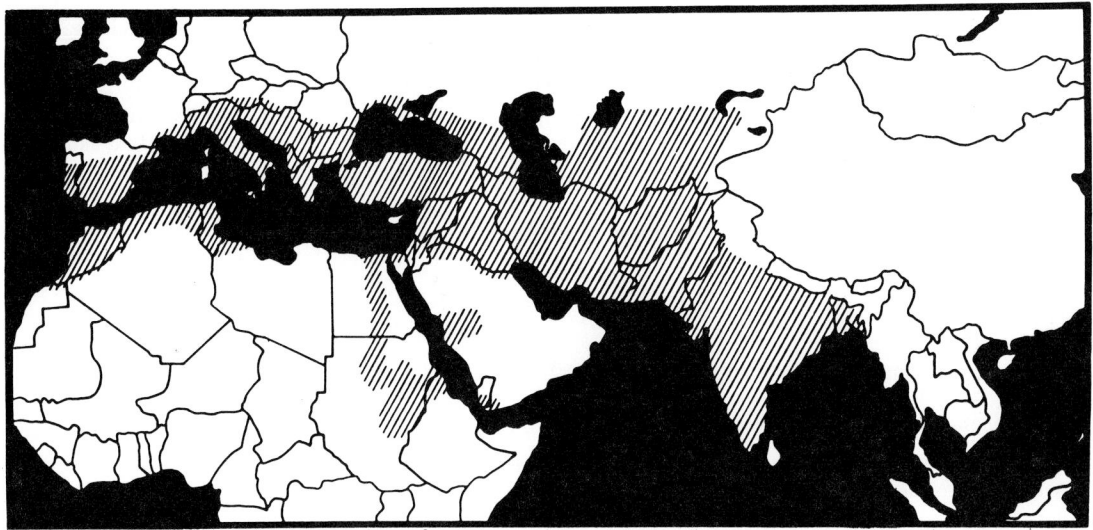

FIGURE 20–6. Distribution of *Phlebotomus papatasi,* which closely parallels areas affected by sandfly fever. (From Tesh RB, Saidi S, Gajdamovic SJ, et al: Bull WHO 54:663, 1976. Reprinted by permission.)

though horizontal transmission involving viremic humans or wild vertebrates may play a secondary role. Sandfly abundance and activity may be quite focal and strongly influenced by rainfall. In some endemic areas high rates of viral infection (1:150 infected female sandflies) are found, with a high relative risk of human infection.

Punta Toro and Chagres viruses have been isolated from the Panamanian sandflies, *Lutzomyia trapidoi* and *L. ylephilator.* Both male and female sandflies have yielded virus, indicating transovarial transmission of these viruses. *L. trapidoi* is a highly anthropophilic species. Toscana virus has been recovered from both male and female *P. perniciosus* in Italy and Portugal.

PATHOLOGY AND PATHOGENESIS. No fatal human cases are reported. Mice inoculated intracerebrally develop encephalitic lesions.

CLINICAL MANIFESTATIONS AND COMPLICATIONS. Illness begins abruptly after an incubation period of 3 to 6 days. Symptoms include fever, generalized malaise, headache, retro-orbital pain, photophobia, gastrointestinal symptoms (nausea, vomiting), and myalgia. There is no rash or lymphadenopathy. The total white blood cell count is typically depressed, principally because of a neutropenia.

The acute febrile illness lasts approximately 3 days but may be followed by a period of weakness, fatigue, and depression lasting 1 to 2 weeks.

Homologous immunity is probably lifelong; however, neutralizing antibody titers wane significantly after 20 years. Infection with Naples virus does not confer protection against the Sicilian serotype or vice versa. Because both viruses occur together in endemic areas, clinical reinfections are reported.

The clinical disease associated with the neotropical sandfly fever viruses is probably similar, but descriptions are incomplete.

DIAGNOSIS. Specific diagnosis depends on serologic tests (hemagglutination inhibition, ELISA, neutralization) on paired sera or isolation of the virus from blood,

although it may be suspected on clinical and epidemiologic grounds.

PROGNOSIS AND THERAPY. The disease is self-limited. Treatment is symptomatic.

PREVENTION AND CONTROL. No vaccines have been developed. Use of residual insecticides has resulted in effective control of *P. papatasi*–transmitted sandfly fever. Visitors to forested areas of the New World tropics may be advised to use repellents to protect against the bites of sandflies. Oral ribavirin is an effective prophylactic agent in experimental sandfly fever.

BIBLIOGRAPHY

Hertig M, Sabin AB: Sandfly fever. *In* Preventive Medicine in World War II, Vol VII. Office of the Surgeon General, Department of the Army, Washington, DC, 1964, pp 109–174.

Srihongse S, Johnson C: Human infections with Chagres virus in Panama. Am J Trop Med Hyg 23:690, 1974.

Tesh RB, Saidi S, Gajdamovic SJ, et al: Serological studies on the epidemiology of sandfly fever in the Old World. Bull WHO 54:663, 1976.

Tesh RB: *Phlebotomus* fevers. *In* Monath TP (ed): The Arboviruses: Epidemiology and Ecology, Vol IV. Boca Raton, FL, CRC Press, 1988, pp 15–28.

20.12. OTHER ARBOVIRUS INFECTIONS

Thirty-three arboviruses not described in other sections of the text have been associated with human disease in the tropics. Table 20–2 lists and classifies these agents and shows their geographic distribution and vector-host relationships. Only sporadic disease in humans has been described, and in some cases there are only single case reports. For some viruses, e.g., Orungo and Tataguine, which are presumably transmitted by *Anopheles* mosquitoes, high prevalences of antibodies are found in human populations. Infections may frequently be inapparent, or mild undifferentiated illness may escape attention, especially in children.

TABLE 20–2. Tropical Arboviruses That Are Rarely Diagnosed or Cause Undifferentiated Febrile Illness at Low Frequency*

Region	Virus	Taxonomic Status (Family/Antigenic Group or Genus)	Cycle of Transmission	Specific Distribution	Notable, Clinical Manifestations	Comment
Tropical America†	Bussuquara	Flaviviridae/Flavivirus	*Culex* spp.—?host	Panama, Brazil, Colombia		
	Catu	Bunyaviridae/Guama	*Culex portesi*—rodent	Brazil, Trinidad, Fr. Guiana		
	Changuinola	Reoviridae/Changuinola	Phlebotomine fly—?host	Panama		
	Cotia	Poxviridae	?Mosquito—host	Brazil, Fr. Guiana		
	Guama	Bunyaviridae/Guama	*Culex*—rodent	Brazil, Trinidad, Guianas, Panama		
	Guaroa	Bunyaviridae/Bunyamwera	?*Anopheles*—?host	Colombia, Brazil, ?Panama		
	Ilheus	Flaviviridae/Flavivirus	Mosquito—bird	Widespread	Encephalitis in some cases	
	Tacaiuma	Bunyaviridae/Anopheles A	Mosquito—mammal	Brazil		
	Vesicular stomatitis	Rhabdoviridae/Vesiculovirus	?Mosquito or sandfly—mammal; ?mammal—mammal	Widespread	Vesicles in mouth, nose	Disease in cows, horses
	Wyeomyia	Bunyaviridae/Bunyamwera	*Wyeomyia*—?host	Colombia, Panama, Trinidad, Brazil, Fr. Guiana		
Africa‡	Bangui	Bunyaviridae/Bunyavirus-like	Unknown	Central African Republic (CAR)	Rash	
	Banzi	Flaviviridae/Flavivirus	*Culex*—rodent	S. Africa, Kenya, Tanzania		
	Bunyamwera	Bunyaviridae/Bunyamwera	Mosquito (esp. *Aedes* spp.)–?host	Uganda, Nigeria, Kenya, Cameroon, CAR, S. Africa		
	Bwamba	Bunyaviridae/Bwamba	?*Anopheles*–?host	Uganda, Nigeria, CAR, Kenya	Rash in some cases	Has occurred in small outbreaks
	Dugbe	Bunyaviridae/Nairovirus	Tick–cattle	Nigeria, CAR, Uganda, Senegal	Rash in some cases	
	Ilesha	Bunyaviridae/Bunyamwera	?*Anopheles*—?host	Nigeria, CAR, Cameroon, Uganda		
	Lebombo	Reoviridae/Orbivirus	Mosquito—rodent	Nigeria, S. Africa		
	Le Dantec	Rhabdoviridae	?	Senegal		
	Nairobi sheep disease	Bunyaviridae/Nairovirus	*Rhipicephalus* (tick)—sheep/goats	S.E., and Central Africa		Also in India
	Nyando	Bunyaviridae/Ungrouped	*Anopheles*—?host	Kenya, CAR		
	Orungo	Reoviridae/Orbivirus	?*Anopheles*—humans	Uganda, Nigeria, CAR, Senegal	See Chapter 20.12	See Chapter 20.12
	Quaranfil	?Arenaviridae	*Argas* (tick)—birds	Eygpt, S. Africa, Nigeria		Virus also in Iran and Afghanistan
	Semliki Forest	Togaviridae/Alphavirus	*Aedes*—?birds	Widespread		Epidemics reported in CAR; equine encephalitis in Senegal
	Shokwe	Bunyaviridae/Bunyamwera	*Aedes*—rodents	S., W., and E. Africa		
	Shuni	Bunyaviridae/Simbu	*Culicoides* and ?mosquitoes—?ruminants	Nigeria, S. Africa		
	Tataguine	Bunyaviridae/Unassigned	*Anopheles*—humans	Senegal, Cameroon, CAR, Nigeria, Ethiopia	Rash	Hyperendemic in W. Africa
	Thogoto	Orthomyxoviridae	Ticks—ruminants	Egypt, Kenya, Nigeria, CAR	1 fatal case with optic neuritis, encephalitis	Antigenically related virus in Sicily, Iran
	Usutu	Flaviviridae/Flavivirus	*Culex*—birds	Sub-Saharan Africa	Rash	
	Wesselsbron	Flaviviridae/Flavivirus	Mosquito—?host	S. and W. Africa	Disease and abortion in sheep, cattle	
	Zika	Flaviviridae/Flavivirus	*Aedes*—monkeys	Widespread		Also in S.E. Asia

TABLE 20—2. Tropical Arboviruses That Are Rarely Diagnosed or Cause Undifferentiated Febrile Illness at Low Frequency* *Continued*

Region	Virus	Taxonomic Status (Family/Antigenic Group or Genus)	Cycle of Transmission	Specific Distribution	Notable, Clinical Manifestations	Comment
Tropical Asia,† Australia	Chandipura	Rhabdoviridae/Vesiculovirus	?*Phlebotomus*—?rodent	India	Rash	
	Kunjin	Flaviviridae/Flavivirus	*Culex*—birds	New Guinea, Australia		
	Nairobi sheep disease (Ganjam)	See above	See above	India		
	Sepik	Flaviviridae/Flavivirus		New Guinea		Antigenically related to Wesselsbron
	Wanowrie	Ungrouped	Tick—?host	India, Iran, Egypt	Hemorrhage	
	Zika	See above	See above	S.E. Asia		

*See text for more commonly diagnosed tropical arboviruses.
†Piry virus occurs in Brazil. Clinical laboratory infections, but no natural disease, have been reported.
‡Bhanja, Kemerovo, and Chandipura viruses (known human pathogens) have been isolated in Africa but have not been associated with human disease there. Germiston virus occurs in Africa. Clinical laboratory infections, but no natural infections, are reported with this virus.

Orungo virus was questionably incriminated in several epidemics in Nigeria. Illness was characterized by fever, vomiting, myalgia, headache, conjunctivitis, skin tenderness, leukopenia, and a papular rash. Antibody to the virus has been found in monkeys and sheep. Virus isolates have been made from *Anopheles* spp., *Culex perfuscus,* and *Aedes dentatus* mosquitoes.

The viruses listed in Table 20–2 should be considered in the differential diagnosis for patients with febrile illnesses acquired in the tropics. The common clinical feature of infections with most of these agents is undifferentiated febrile illness. Thogoto virus has been isolated from a patient with meningoencephalitis and optic neuritis.

Diagnosis has been made most often by virus isolation from blood or serum, but serologic tests are also useful.

BIBLIOGRAPHY

Fabiyi A, Tomori O, El Bayoumi MSM: Epidemic of a febrile illness associated with UgMP-359 virus in Nigeria. W Afr Med J 23:9, 1975.

21. VIRAL ENCEPHALITIS

21.1. RABIES AND RELATED VIRUSES

D. A. Warrell
and M. J. Warrell

DEFINITION. Rabies is a zoonosis of wild and domestic mammals that may be transmitted to humans, usually by the bite of a rabid dog. Virus-bearing saliva is also infective through broken skin and intact mucosas. Rare routes of transmission include inhalation of aerosolized virus and transplantation of infected corneal grafts. In humans, rabies encephalitis is almost invariably fatal. The disease is enzootic in mammals throughout most parts of the world, involving different species of carnivores and bats in different regions. The problem of human rabies is most severe in tropical developing countries where the disease is uncontrolled in domestic dogs. Rabies virus and 6 other morphologically and immunologically related viruses compose the genus *Lyssavirus* of the Rhabdoviridae. Apart from rabies, only three of these, Mokola, European bat Lyssavirus, and Duvenhage, have caused disease in humans.

ETIOLOGY. Rabies virus is a rhabdoid or rod-shaped virus approximately 180×80 nm (Fig. 21–1). The nucleocapsid contains a single negative strand of RNA, nucleoprotein, phosphoprotein, and an RNA transcriptase required for production of positive messenger RNA. The envelope contains lipid, matrix protein, and a glycoprotein, which forms the spiky surface projections. Repeated intracerebral passage in animals of "street virus" from naturally infected species results in a "fixed virus" of uniformly shortened incubation period and reduced pathogenicity, which is used in vaccine production. Strains of rabies virus from different vector species have been identified using monoclonal antibodies. In the laboratory, rabies can be isolated and cultivated by intracerebral inoculation of suckling mice, in mouse neuroblastoma cell cultures, and via other continuous cell lines. The virus is inactivated by heat (56C for 1 hour), ultraviolet light, detergents and soap solution, ethanol, iodine, quaternary ammonium compounds, chloroform, and acetone. The 6 rabies-related viruses have been isolated from shrews, bats, rodents, other mammals, and insects in Africa and Europe (Table 21–1). Two human infections caused by Mokola virus and 4 indistinguishable from rabies, caused by Duvenhage and the related European bat lyssavirus viruses, have been reported. These infections may not be detected by routine diagnostic rabies immunofluorescent antigen detection tests.

DISTRIBUTION AND INCIDENCE. Rabies is enzootic worldwide, except for Australia, Antarctica, most of Scandinavia, and a number of islands including the British Isles, Iceland, New Guinea, Borneo, New Zealand, Japan, and Taiwan. Human rabies is generally under-reported. An annual mortality of 50,000 in India now seems probable. Peak annual mortalities in Sri

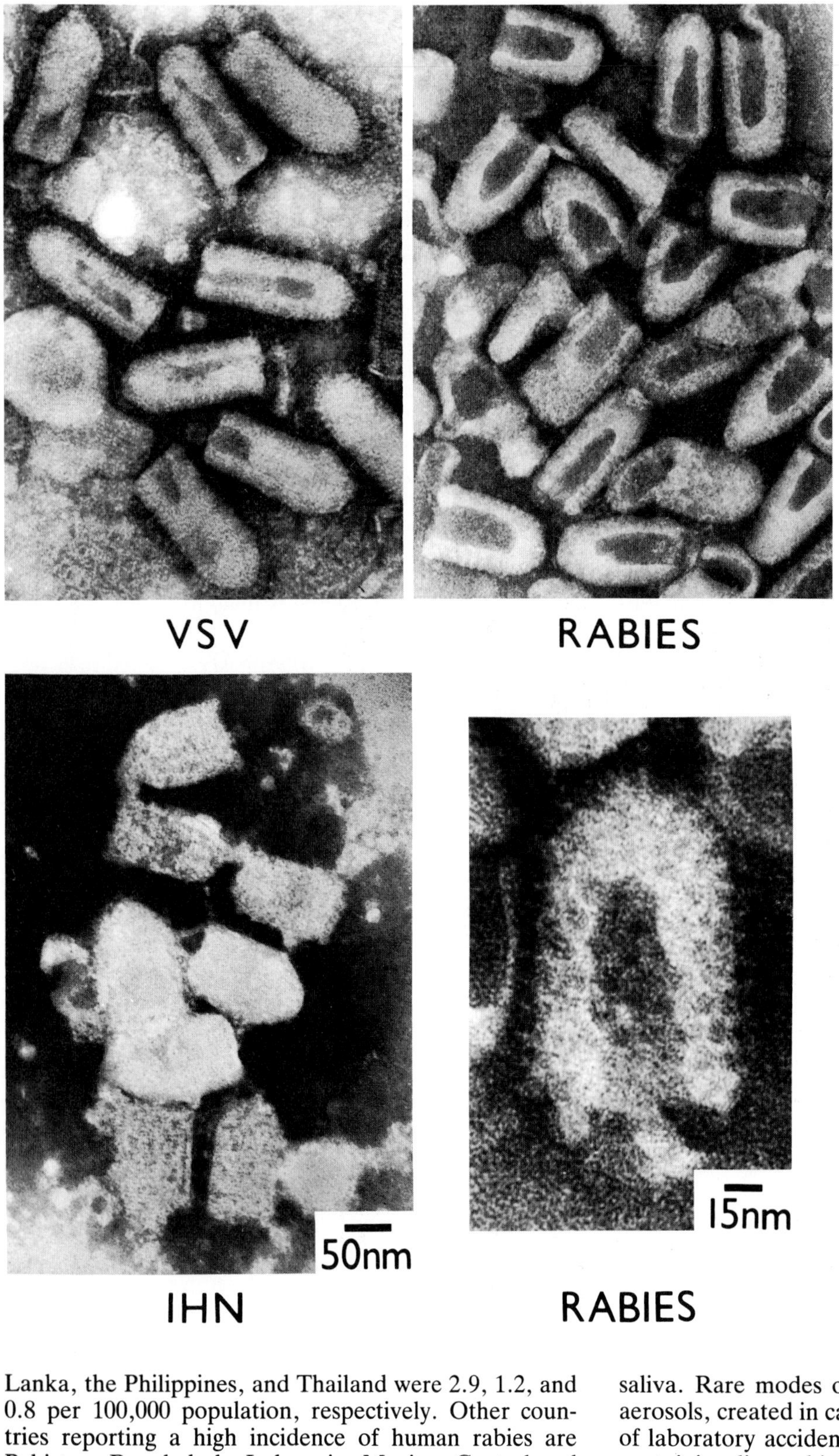

VSV   RABIES

IHN   RABIES

FIGURE 21–1. Rhabdoviruses. VSV = vesicular stomatitis virus; IHN = infectious hematopoietic necrosis virus of fish. (Courtesy of G. J. Smale.)

50nm

15nm

Lanka, the Philippines, and Thailand were 2.9, 1.2, and 0.8 per 100,000 population, respectively. Other countries reporting a high incidence of human rabies are Pakistan, Bangladesh, Indonesia, Mexico, Central and South America, and China. In the United States, there have been about 50 cases in the last 30 years.

TRANSMISSION AND EPIDEMIOLOGY. Human rabies usually results from inoculation of virus-bearing saliva through the skin by the bite of a rabid dog. Scratches, abrasions and other wounds, and intact mucosal membranes can be contaminated with infected saliva. Rare modes of infection are inhalation of virus aerosols, created in caves inhabited by bats or as a result of laboratory accidents; accidental injection of vaccines containing live rabies virus (rage de laboratoire); and transplantation of infected corneal grafts. In the 7 cases of transplant rabies, the donors had died of unsuspected rabies. The major reservoir and vector of urban rabies is the domestic dog. Sylvatic rabies occurs predominantly in skunks, foxes, raccoons, and insectivorous bats in North America; foxes in the Arctic; mongooses in some Caribbean islands; vampire bats in Latin America

TABLE 21–1. Rabies-Related Viruses

Lyssavirus Serotype	Virus	Source	Geographic Range	Human Disease (No. of Cases)
2	Lagos bat	Fruit bat, cat	Nigeria, Central African Republic, South Africa, Zimbabwe	
3	Mokola	Shrew, mouse, cat, dog	Nigeria, Cameroon, Central African Republic, Zimbabwe	
		Human	Nigeria	Pharyngitis (1) Fatal encephalitis (1)
4	Duvenhage	Insectivorous bat, human	South Africa	Fatal furious rabies (1)
4	European bat lyssavirus	Insectivorous bat	Germany, Denmark, Holland, Russia, Poland, Spain	
		Human	Finland, Russia	Fatal furious rabies (3)
	Obodhiang	Mosquito	Sudan	—
	Kotonkan	Midge	Nigeria	—

Data from King J, Crick J: *In* Campbell JB, Charlton KM (eds): Rabies. Boston, Kullver Academic Publ., 1988, p 179.

and Trinidad; wolves, jackals, and small carnivores in Africa and Asia; and foxes, wolves, raccoon dogs, and insectivorous bats in Europe. Each species forms its own ecologic compartment with a distinct strain of rabies virus. Transmission between sylvatic and urban populations and between different species occurs when, for example, wild Canidae come into towns, scavenging for food, or when a carnivore eats or is bitten by a sick bat. In countries such as the United States, where control of rabies in domestic animals has been successful, wild animals such as skunks and raccoons now constitute the main threat for spread to humans. Vampire bats *(Desmodontinae)* are confined to Southern Texas, Mexico, Central and South America, and some Caribbean islands such as Trinidad and Margarita. While taking their blood meals from cattle they transmit "derriengue," a form of paralytic rabies responsible for the loss of 1 to 2 million cattle per year. In Trinidad, 89 human cases of vampire bat–transmitted paralytic rabies were identified between 1925 and 1935; others have been described from Mexico, Guyana, Brazil, Bolivia, and Argentina. Insectivorous and frugivorous bats in North America, India, and Europe have also been responsible for human cases of rabies, Duvenhage, and European bat Lyssavirus infection. It has been suggested that infection by rabies-related viruses, such as Kotonkan virus in domestic herbivores in Nigeria and Mokola virus in cats and dogs in Zimbabwe, may have conferred some protection against rabies.

PATHOGENESIS AND PATHOLOGY. After entering a susceptible host, the virus envelope fuses with the plasma membrane and the ribonucleoprotein enters the cytoplasm. Local replication usually occurs in striated muscle near the site of the bite, but there may be direct invasion of nerve cells. Postsynaptic nicotinic acetylcholine receptors at neuromuscular junctions and in the central nervous system (CNS) are important binding sites. After it is inside peripheral nerves, the virus is carried in the flow of axoplasm at the rate of about 3 mm/hour to the dorsal root ganglia where replication may be responsible for prodromal paresthesia at the site of the bite (see below). On reaching the CNS, there is massive viral replication on membranes of neurons and glial cells and direct transmission of virus from cell to cell. Free virus spreads within extracellular spaces such as the cerebrospinal fluid (CSF).

Passive centrifugal spread of virus from the CNS in the axoplasm of many efferent nerves, including those of the autonomic nervous system, spreads the virus to the salivary glands (whence it is shed and in the case of infected animals spread by the bite) and to lacrimal glands and a variety of other tissues. In animals, centrifugal spread to the skin is detectable before development of symptoms. In human victims of rabies, histopathologic changes may be surprisingly mild. In furious rabies, the midbrain and medulla are mainly involved and in paralytic rabies, the spinal cord. The brain, spinal cord, and peripheral nerves may show ganglion cell degeneration, perineural and perivascular mononuclear cell infiltration (Fig. 21–2), neuronophagia, and formation of glial nodules. Negri bodies, the characteristic intracytoplasmic inclusion bodies, contain viral components, mainly ribonucleoprotein and fragments of cellular organelles such as ribosomes (Fig. 21–3). They are most numerous in pyramidal cells of the hippocampus, in Purkinje cells of the cerebellum, and in the medulla and ganglia. The spongiform encephalopathy found in skunks and foxes is probably an immunologic response to infection. Extraneural changes include focal degeneration of salivary and lacrimal glands, pancreas, adrenal medulla, and lymph nodes and an interstitial myocarditis with round cell infiltration, which may explain the cardiac arrhythmias and other cardiovascular abnormalities sometimes observed in patients.

IMMUNOLOGY. Immunity to infection was thought to depend largely on neutralizing antibody induced by viral glycoprotein. Recent experiments show that nucleoprotein antigens can stimulate protective immunity in the absence of neutralizing antibody. In unvaccinated patients with rabies encephalomyelitis, no antibody response is detectable in serum or cerebrospinal fluid for about 7 days after the first symptom, suggesting immune evasion or immune suppression by rabies virus. Intrathecal production of rabies IgG is detectable in patients whose survival is prolonged by intensive care. After symptoms of encephalitis have developed, the role of antibody is uncertain. In experimental animal models, low levels of antibody may produce "early death," perhaps by enhancing viral replication. Low levels of interferon are sometimes detectable in human victims but large amounts have been found in animal brains.

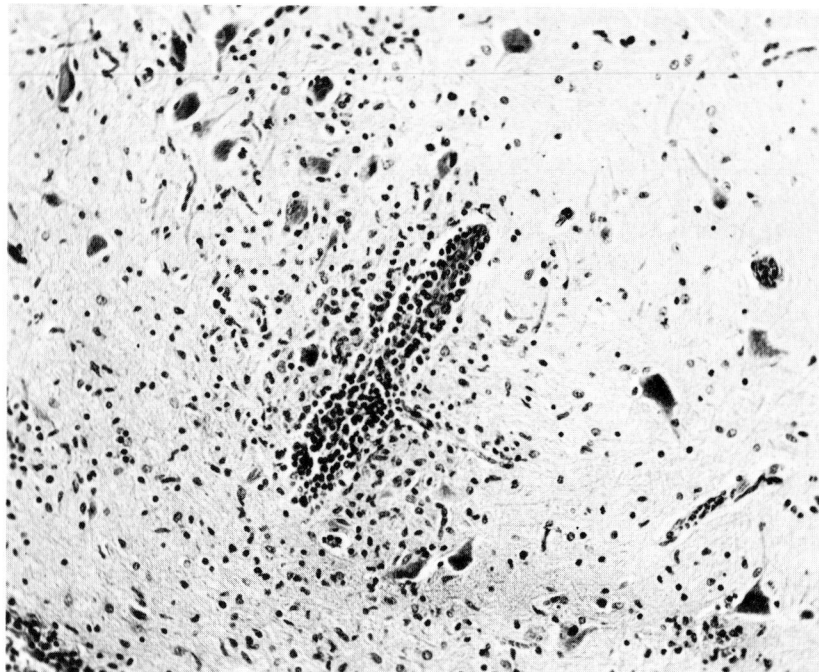

FIGURE 21–2. Perivascular cuffing by lymphocytes, histiocytes, and plasma cells in the brain stem of a patient dying of rabies (× 165). (Courtesy of Armed Forces Institute of Pathology, Photograph Neg. No. 73–12328.)

CLINICAL MANIFESTATIONS AND COMPLICATIONS

In Animals. In dogs, the incubation period is usually between 2 weeks and 4 months (extreme range 5 days to 14 months). The illness may start with 2 to 3 days of prodromal symptoms, such as a change in behavior, fever, and intense irritation at the site of the bite. Dogs with the less common but more familiar furious form of the disease become aggressive, wander away from home, and may develop convulsions, dysphagia, pharyngeal paralysis causing an altered bark, and hypersalivation. Those with paralytic or "dumb" rabies hide themselves away and develop paralysis of the jaw, neck, and hind limbs. Dysphagia and drooling of saliva may raise the

suspicion of a foreign body stuck in the throat. Virus may be excreted in the saliva for 2 or 3 days before there are signs of rabies and the animal usually dies within the next 7 days. A small proportion of infected animals recover and may continue to excrete virus for long periods. Horses, cats, Mustelidae, and Viverridae usually exhibit furious symptoms, whereas paralytic disease is the rule in foxes and bovines. Hydrophobia is not seen in animals but inability to drink is a common symptom of rabies.

In Humans. The incubation period is usually between 20 and 90 days (extreme range 4 days to more than 20 years). Relatively short incubation periods are observed after facial and severe multiple bites, transmission by

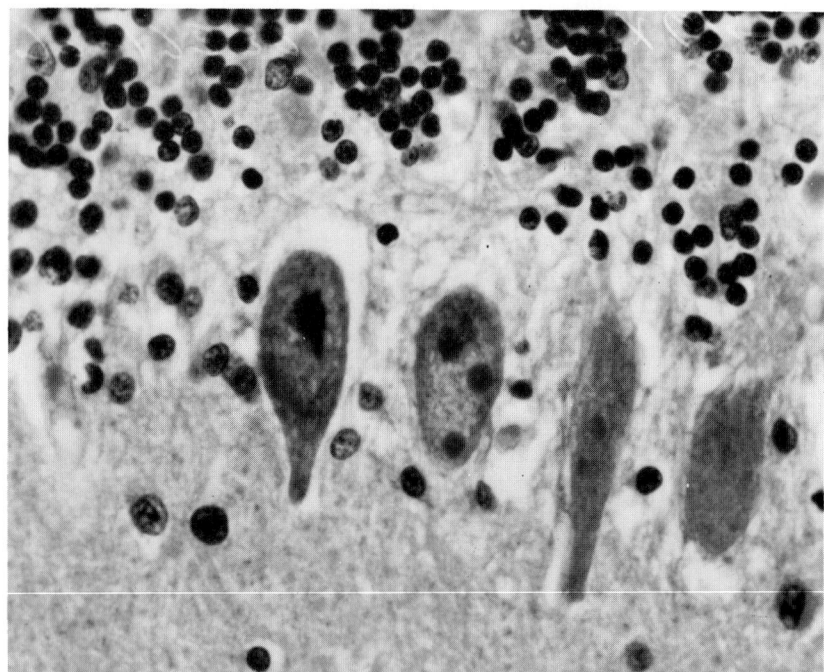

FIGURE 21–3. Negri bodies in Purkinje cells of the cerebellum of a patient dying of rabies (× 615). (Courtesy of Armed Forces Institute of Pathology, Photograph Neg. No. 73–12332.)

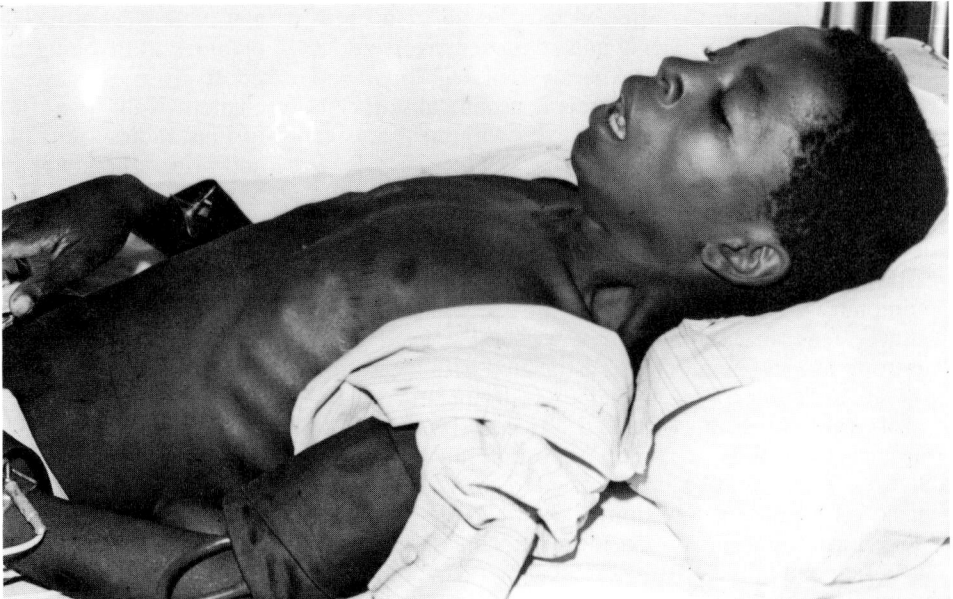

FIGURE 21–4. Hydrophobic spasm in a Nigerian boy with furious rabies. Note forceful contraction of the diaphragm (depressing the xiphisternum) and sternocleidomastoid muscles. (Copyright D. A. Warrell.)

corneal grafts, and accidental inoculation of live virus (rage de laboratoire). The prodromal symptom most suggestive of rabies encephalitis is paresthesia, especially itching, at the site of the healed bite wound. Other early symptoms include fever, mood changes, and nonspecific upper respiratory tract or gastrointestinal symptoms. The 2 distinct clinical forms of rabies, furious (agitated) and paralytic (dumb), may be determined by the strain of rabies virus or the immune response. Furious rabies is the commoner presentation. After a few days of prodromal symptoms, the pathognomonic symptom and sign of hydrophobia or aerophobia develops (Fig. 21–4). A forceful jerky inspiratory spasm is provoked either by attempts to drink water or by a draft of air on the face. Both reflexes are associated with a compelling but inexplicable terror. The spasms involve the diaphragm and accessory muscles of inspiration, particularly the sternomastoids; the head is thrown back; the arms are raised; and a generalized extension response may ensue, resulting in opisthotonus and generalized convulsions with cardiac or respiratory arrest. Splashing water on the skin, irritation of the respiratory tract, or, by conditioning, the sight, sound, or even the mention of water may provoke a hydrophobic spasm. Patients also experience episodic generalized arousal during which they become wild, hallucinated, and sometimes aggressive. During lucid intervals, they cerebrate normally and are aware of their terrible predicament. Neurologic abnormalities include meningism, cranial nerve lesions, upper motor neuron lesions, fasciculation, and involuntary movements. Generalized hyperesthesia or hyperacusis is described. Hypersalivation (Fig. 21–5), lacrimation, sweating, fluctuating blood pressure and body temperature, and inappropriate secretion of antidiuretic hormone or diabetes insipidus suggest disturbances of the hypothalamus or autonomic nervous system. Lesions of the amygdaloid nuclei result in increased libido, priapism, and spontaneous orgasms. Without intensive care, most patients die within a few days of developing hydrophobia. About one third of patients die during a

hydrophobic spasm, whereas the others lapse into coma with abnormalities of respiratory rhythm, such as periodic or cluster breathing with prolonged apneic periods.

Paralytic rabies is less distinctive than furious rabies and is undoubtedly underdiagnosed. All the reported cases of rabies transmitted by vampire bats in Latin America and the Caribbean were of this type, as were the cases of rabies caused by vaccination with live virus and inhalation of fixed virus. It may develop in patients and experimental animals who have a low but unprotective level of immunity. After the usual prodromal symptoms, especially fever, headache, and local paresthesia, flaccid paralysis develops (usually in the bitten limb) and ascends symmetrically or asymmetrically, with pain

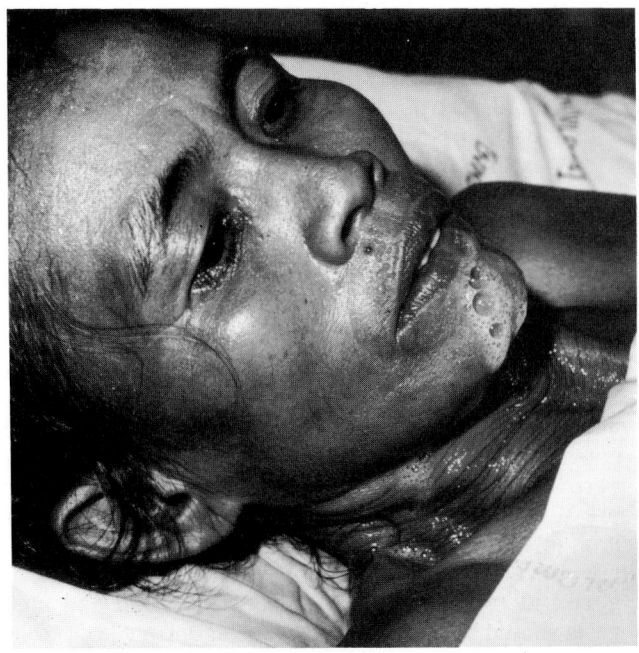

FIGURE 21–5. Sweating and hypersalivation in a Thai woman with furious rabies. (Copyright D. A. Warrell.)

and fasciculation in the affected muscles and mild sensory disturbance. Paraplegia and sphincter involvement then develop and finally fatal paralysis of deglutitive and respiratory muscles. Hydrophobia is usually absent. Patients may survive for a month even without intensive care.

Patients with rabies whose lives are prolonged by intensive care may develop a wide range of complications, including aspiration pneumonia, pneumothorax, respiratory failure, cardiac arrhythmias, hypotension, pulmonary edema, myocarditis with congestive cardiac failure, generalized convulsions, cerebral edema, polyneuropathy, and hematemesis associated with ulceration or tears in the mucosa of the upper gastrointestinal tract.

Infections by Rabies-Related Viruses. Two cases of Mokola virus infection were reported in children in Nigeria. A 3½-year-old girl presented with febrile convulsions and mild congestion of the pharynx. The CSF was entirely normal and so the original description of "aseptic meningitis" was incorrect. She recovered in 48 hours. The other patient, a 6-year-old girl, was admitted to the hospital drowsy and with generalized flaccid paralysis and died 3 days later. The original South African case of Duvenhage virus infection was clinically indistinguishable from furious rabies. The recent Finnish case of Duvenhage-like, European bat lyssavirus infection had ascending paralysis followed by hyperexcitability and spasms. Two Russian girls died of bat-transmitted furious rabies. Virus was isolated from only 1, and this was also in the European bat lyssavirus group.

PROGNOSIS AND TREATMENT. In patients who develop signs of rabies encephalomyelitis, the prognosis remains virtually hopeless. One patient who inhaled fixed virus developed paralytic rabies despite pre-exposure immunization, but survived with severe neurologic sequelae. This case is the only fully documented human survival from the infection, but the diagnosis was serologic. One patient in the United States and one in Argentina who had been given postexposure duck embryo and suckling mouse brain rabies vaccine, respectively, developed severe neurologic symptoms from which they recovered after intensive care. In neither case could rabies virus be demonstrated, but a diagnosis of rabies encephalitis rather than postvaccinal encephalitis was based on very high titers of rabies antibody in the CSF. Two Indian patients, who had received postexposure prophylaxis with Semple vaccine, developed symptoms of furious rabies, but recovered after intensive care. There was no virologic confirmation. Intensive care is the only known method for prolonging the lives of patients with rabies encephalomyelitis. Life-threatening complications such as cardiac arrhythmias, cardiac and respiratory failure, raised intracranial pressure, convulsions, fluid and electrolyte disturbances, and hyperpyrexia can be prevented or treated. Immunosuppressive agents, including corticosteroids, rabies hyperimmune serum, antiviral agents, and interferon, have not proved effective. If intensive care is not possible or is considered inappropriate, heavy sedation and analgesia should be given to relieve the agonizing symptoms.

DIAGNOSIS
Differential Diagnosis. Rabies should be suspected in any patient who develops neurologic symptoms a week or more after being bitten by an animal. However, in up to 16% of cases no history of exposure can be elicited. Rabies is often misdiagnosed. In patients with furious rabies, the alteration in mood, hallucinations, and bizarre behavior may raise suspicions of psychiatric disease, hysteria, or malingering. Other patients are sent to otolaryngologists because of their upper respiratory tract symptoms. Rabies phobia or pseudohydrophobia is usually manifest as a caricature of popular conceptions of rabies with an emphasis on aggression and spitting. The interval between the mammal bite and the appearance of symptoms is usually short. The spasms of tetanus may resemble hydrophobia, especially if they involve the pharyngeal muscles (hydrophobic tetanus), and this disease can also complicate an animal bite (Chapter 54). Severe tetanus is distinguished by its shorter incubation period (usually less than a week), by the presence of trismus, and the persistence of muscular rigidity between spasms. Tetanus does not cause an encephalitis and the CSF is usually normal. The combination of severe brain stem encephalitis with full consciousness in rabies is rare in other encephalitides, but has been described in serum sickness. In a case of an anaphylactic reaction to an insect sting, paroxysms of muscle spasms, tachycardia, sweating, and rage were attributed to brain stem dysfunction analogous to the "rage reaction" produced experimentally in animals by diencephalic damage or stimulation. Various poisons, drugs, and plant toxins can produce syndromes of muscle spasm, agitation, hallucinations, psychiatric disturbances, signs of autonomic nervous system stimulation, and convulsions. These include strychnine, phenothiazines, atropine-like compounds, and cannabis. Delirium tremens may also be included in a differential diagnosis of furious rabies. Paralytic rabies should be considered in patients with rapidly ascending (Landry type) flaccid paralysis, suspected Guillain-Barré syndrome, and transverse myelitis. In the many tropical developing countries where Semple-type and suckling mouse brain rabies vaccines are still used, the most important differential diagnosis is postvaccinal encephalomyelitis. This usually develops within 2 weeks of the first dose of vaccine, but a delayed onset cerebral type with psychiatric symptoms has been described in Japan. Poliomyelitis is distinguished by the lack of sensory abnormalities. Herpes simiae (B virus) encephalomyelitis, transmitted by monkey bites, has an incubation period of only a few days. Vesicles may be found in the monkey's mouth and at the site of the bite. The diagnosis can be confirmed virologically and the patient treated with acyclovir.

Laboratory Diagnosis. In humans, rabies encephalitis can be confirmed during life by immunofluorescence of skin and brain biopsies, but the corneal impression smear technique is too often falsely negative to be useful. Early in the illness, rabies virus can be isolated from saliva, brain, CSF, and even spun urine, but not from blood. Virus can be identified in neuroblastoma cell cultures in 2 to 4 days and in 2 to 3 weeks using intracerebral inoculation of suckling mice. The presence of rabies antibody in CSF or serum is diagnostic of rabies encephalitis unless the patient has been vaccinated or given rabies immune globulin. In postvaccinal encephalomyelitis, rabies neutralizing antibody leaks across the blood-CSF barrier but a very high titer (as in 2 of the patients thought to have recovered from rabies) suggests rabies encephalitis. The most reliable method for distinguishing rabies from postvaccinal encephalomyelitis while the patient is alive is by demonstrating rabies antigen by immunofluorescence in skin or brain biopsies. In rabies encephalitis, pleocytosis was absent in 40% of patients in the first week, and 13% in the second week of illness. The average pleocytosis is about 75 lymphocytes/μl, but rarely exceeds a few hundred cells. A neutrophil leukocytosis of 20,000 to 30,000/μl is commonly found in the blood. In the mammal responsible for the bite, rabies can be confirmed within a few hours by immunofluorescence of acetone-fixed brain or spinal cord impression smears, a technique that has replaced the classic Seller's stain for Negri bodies, which is less specific. A simple enzyme-linked immunosorbent assay (ELISA) test can be used if fluorescent microscopy is not available, and a sensitive avidin-biotin peroxidase method has recently been developed for use with formalin-fixed histologic sections. Rapid examination of CNS tissue in animals suspected of being rabid is now preferred to observing them in isolation for 10 days.

PREVENTION AND CONTROL

Local Measures. Bite wounds (Fig. 21–6), scratches, or abrasions that may have been contaminated by infected saliva should be scrubbed with soap or detergent and generously rinsed under running water for at least 5 minutes. Foreign material and dead tissue should be removed under anesthesia. Wounds should be irrigated with a virucidal agent such as 20% soap solution, povidone iodine, 0.1% aqueous iodine, or 40 to 70% alcohol. Quaternary ammonium compounds, hydrogen peroxide, and mercurochrome are not recommended. Suturing should be avoided or delayed wherever possible as it may inoculate virus deeper into the tissues. The risk of other viral, bacterial, fungal, and protozoal infections associated with mammal bites should be considered and in particular tetanus prophylaxis may be required. Dicloxacillin and cephalexin are recommended antimicrobials for mammal bite wounds.

PROPHYLAXIS

Postexposure (Table 21–2). Specific prophylaxis includes the use of both active immunization with vaccine and passive immunization with hyperimmune serum. Tissue culture vaccines are now the vaccines of choice, but nervous tissue vaccines (e.g., Semple and suckling mouse brain) are still the most widely used throughout the tropical rabies endemic area. These vaccines are of variable potency and carry a risk of neuroparalytic reactions. Currently available tissue culture vaccines include human diploid cell strain vaccine (introduced in 1973), purified Vero cell rabies vaccine, and purified chicken embryo cell vaccine. These vaccines are given by intramuscular injection (deltoid muscle or anterolateral aspect of the thigh but not the gluteal region) on days 0, 3, 7, 14, and 30. The initial dose should be doubled or tripled and given at several different sites, if there has been a delay of more than 48 hours in starting postexposure prophylaxis; if passive immunization was

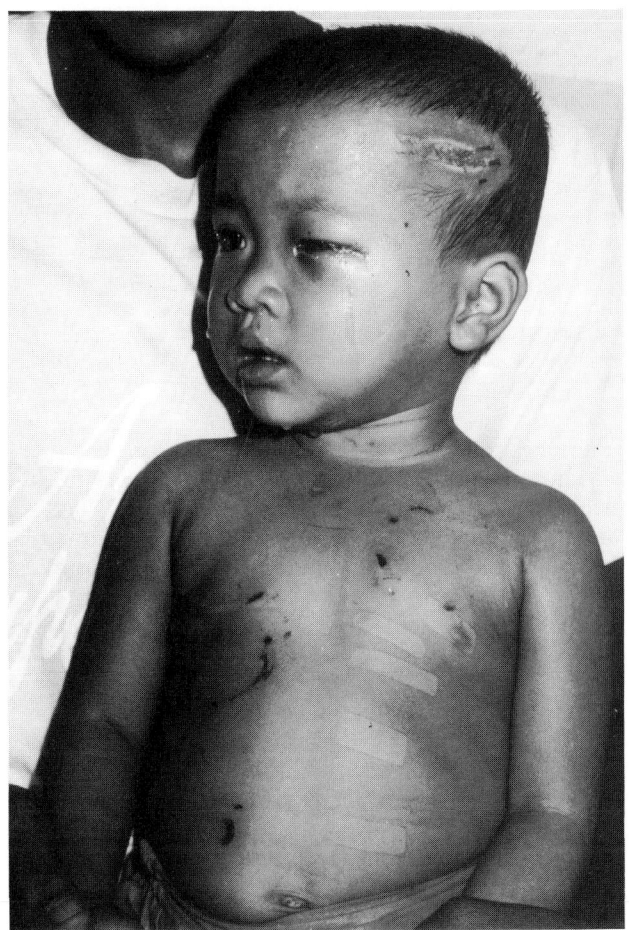

FIGURE 21–6. Multiple bite wounds of the trunk, face, and scalp inflicted by a rabid dog on a 3-year-old Thai boy. (Copyright D. A. Warrell.)

given 24 hours or more before active immunization; if patients are elderly, have chronic diseases such as hepatic cirrhosis, or are likely to be immunodeficient, immunosuppressed, or severely malnourished; and if hyperimmune serum is not available. An abbreviated regimen consists of two injections at different sites on day 0, followed by single injections on days 7 and 21. The most economical regimen with proven efficacy consists of intradermal injections of 0.1 ml (one tenth of the usual intramuscular dose) given at 8 sites (deltoids, suprascapular, abdominal, and thighs) on day 0; 4 sites on day 7; and single sites on days 28 and 90.

Passive immunization consists of equine antirabies serum (40 IU/kg body weight) or, preferably, human rabies immune globulin (20 IU/kg). This should be given at the same time as the first dose of vaccine but at a different site. Approximately half the dose should be infiltrated around the bite wound unless this is on a digit, and the rest given intramuscularly.

Those who have received pre-exposure vaccination do not require passive immunization if they are then exposed to rabies. A booster course of tissue culture vaccine is required (e.g., intramuscular injections on days 0, 3, and 7).

Pre-exposure. Immunization with safe tissue culture vaccines is recommended for high-risk groups such as

TABLE 21–2. Specific Postexposure Prophylaxis for Use in a Rabies-Endemic Area

Nature of Exposure	Circumstances of Bite and Species Involved	Treatment
Minor Exposure Licks of the skin Scratches or abrasions Minor bites	(a) Unprovoked attack by cat or dog	*Start vaccine:* stop treatment if animal remains healthy for 10 days or if brain fluorescent antibody test proves negative: administer serum on positive diagnosis and complete the course of vaccine
	(b) Attack by wild animal, or domestic cat or dog unavailable for observation	*Serum and vaccine*
Major Exposure Licks of mucosa Major bites (multiple or on face, head, finger, or neck)	(a) or (b) above	*Serum and vaccine:* stop if domestic cat or dog remains healthy for 10 days, or if any animal's brain fluorescent antibody test proves negative

veterinarians, health care personnel, laboratory workers, dog catchers, zoologists, other field workers, foresters, cave explorers, and those whose work involves walking and cycling in urban and rural areas of India, Southeast Asia, and Latin America. In the areas with a high prevalence of canine rabies there may be a case for including rabies vaccine in the expanded program of immunization for children. Three doses are given on days 0, 7, and 28, either intramuscularly or a tenth of the dose intradermally. A single booster given 1 year later may produce sustained immunity for 5 to 8 years. Alternatively, a booster dose can be given every 2 years if the neutralizing antibody levels fall and continued protection is needed. People working with rabies virus in laboratories should have their antibody titer checked every 6 months and further booster injections given when indicated. A failure of pre-exposure vaccination by the intradermal route was found in American Peace Corps workers who were immunized in the tropics while taking chloroquine for antimalarial prophylaxis. The intradermal course should therefore be completed before starting chloroquine administration or the vaccine should be given in the full dose intramuscularly.

Efficacy of Postexposure Prophylaxis. Combined active and passive immunization can reduce the risk of rabies from about 15 to 60% in untreated cases to less than 5% with nervous tissue vaccines. The risk varies with the biting species and the site and severity of the bites and is highest following head bites by rabid wolves. Prophylaxis may fail if nervous tissue vaccine of uncertain potency is used, if vaccination is delayed for more than about a week, if wound cleaning and passive immunization are neglected, and if the vaccinee is not normally immunoresponsive. Failure of tissue culture vaccines is exceptionally rare. Conventional rabies vaccines may not be effective against the rabies-related viruses, Mokola, Duvenhage, and European bat lyssavirus, because of antigenic differences from rabies.

Complications of Rabies Vaccines. Tissue culture vaccines cause only mild local or transient influenza-like symptoms in a small minority of vaccinees. However, in the United States, 10% of booster injections were associated with mild immune complex disease 3 to 13 days later. Neuroparalytic accidents complicate 1 in 220 courses of Semple vaccine and 1 in 27,000 courses of suckling mouse brain vaccine according to recent reports. Clinical forms include Guillain-Barré syndrome

(especially after suckling mouse brain vaccine), mononeuritis multiplex, dorsolumbar transverse myelitis, and encephalitis. The overall mortality is 10 to 20%. If symptoms of a neuroparalytic reaction develop, vaccination with nervous tissue vaccines should be stopped immediately, corticosteroids should be given in high dosage, and the postexposure course should be continued with tissue culture vaccine.

Control of Animal Rabies. Domestic dogs, including strays, are responsible for urban rabies. The size of stray dog populations is determined by the amount of food, water, and shelter available. Muzzling, restricting movement of owned dogs, and killing strays were effective in eradicating rabies from some islands and peninsulas (e.g., Britain, Japan, and West Malaysia). However, in many tropical endemic zones, attempts to eliminate stray dogs are difficult, unpopular, and inefficient. In several large cities in South America, intense mass vaccination programs, aimed at immunizing 60 to 80% of the entire dog population, including strays, were dramatically effective in reducing the incidence of canine rabies and eliminating human disease. Control of wildlife rabies by reducing populations of important species such as foxes in Europe and skunks in Canada were of limited benefit, costly, and at odds with current principles of ecology and conservation. However, the use of oral live attenuated rabies vaccines in baits has reduced the prevalence of fox rabies in Switzerland and West Germany, and recombinant vaccines have produced promising preliminary results in raccoons in the United States and in cattle in South America.

BIBLIOGRAPHY

Baer GM, Bridbord K, Hui FW, et al: Research towards rabies prevention. Rev Infect Dis 10:S573, 1988.

Bernard KW, Fishbein DB, Miller KD, et al: Pre-exposure rabies immunization with human diploid cell vaccines: Decreased antibody responses in persons immunized in developing countries. Am J Trop Med Hyg 34:633, 1985.

Callaham M: Controversies in antibiotic choices for bite wounds. Ann Emerg Med 17:1321, 1988.

Campbell JB, Charlton KM (eds): Rabies. Boston, Kluwer, 1988.

Dietzschold B, Wang H, Rupprecht CE, et al: Induction of protective immunity against rabies by immunization with rabies virus ribonucleoprotein. Proc Natl Acad Sci USA 84:9165, 1987.

Grauballe PC, Baagøe HJ, Fekadu M, et al: Bat rabies in Denmark. Lancet 1:379, 1987.

Helmick CG, Tauxe RV, Vernon AA: Is there a risk to contacts of patients with rabies? Rev Infect Dis 9:511, 1987.

Hurst EW, Pawan JL: An outbreak of rabies in Trinidad. Without history of bites, and with the symptoms of acute ascending myelitis. Lancet 2:622, 1931.

Kaplan C, Turner GS, Warrell DA (eds): Rabies: The Facts, 2nd ed. Oxford, Oxford University Press, 1986.

Lentz TL, Hawrot E, Donnelly-Roberts D, Wilson PT: Synthetic peptides in the study of the interaction of rabies virus and the acetylcholine receptor. In Bridget TP, et al (eds): Psychological, Neuropsychiatric and Substance Abuse Aspects of AIDS. New York, Raven Press, 1988.

Murphy FA: Rabies pathogenesis. Brief review. Arch Virol 54:279, 1977.

Suntharasamai P, Warrell MJ, Warrell DA, et al: New purified Vero-cell vaccine prevents rabies in patients bitten by rabid animals. Lancet 2:129, 1986.

Turner GS: Immune response after rabies vaccination: Basic aspects. Ann Inst Pasteur Virol 136E:435, 1985.

Warrell DA: The clinical picture of rabies in man. Trans R Soc Trop Med Hyg 70:188, 1976.

Warrell DA, Davidson NMcD, Pope HM, et al: Pathophysiologic studies in human rabies. Am J Med 60:180, 1976.

Warrell MJ, Looareesuwan S, Manatsathit S, et al: Rapid diagnosis of rabies and post-vaccinal encephalitides. Clin Exp Immunol 71:229, 1988.

Warrell MJ, Nicholson KG, Warrell DA, et al: Economical multiple-site intradermal immunisation with human diploid-cell-strain vaccine is effective for post-exposure rabies prophylaxis. Lancet 1:1059, 1985.

WHO Expert Committee on Rabies, 7th Report. WHO Tech Rep Ser 709, 1984.

Wunner WH, Dietzschold B: Rabies virus infection: Genetic mutations and the impact on viral pathogenicity and immunity. Contrib Microbiol Immunol 8:103, 1987.

21.2. VENEZUELAN EQUINE ENCEPHALITIS (VEE)

Thomas P. Monath

DEFINITION. VEE ("peste loca") is an acute viral disease transmitted from horses to humans by a variety of mosquito vectors. The human disease most often is grippelike, but severe and fatal encephalitis occurs in a small proportion of those infected, especially children.

ETIOLOGY AND HISTORY. VEE is the most important arboviral disease in tropical America. The disease probably occurred in northern South America in the 1920s, but its etiology was first established in 1938 when the virus was isolated from the brain of a dead horse in Venezuela. Numerous outbreaks, many of considerable magnitude, have been reported since 1935 in northern South America. VEE virus is a togavirus belonging to the alphavirus genus. Antigenic variations of VEE virus strains correlate with important differences in geographic distribution, epidemiology, and virulence. The use of sensitive serologic and biochemical techniques has allowed recognition of 6 subtypes (I to VI) of VEE virus; subtype I has been divided into at least five variants and subtype III into 3 variants. Only 2 closely related subtype I variants (AB and C) are associated with epidemics and equine epizootics, whereas the others are enzootic viruses with reduced pathogenicity for horses. Although human infections with the enzootic viruses are not uncommon, clinical disease in humans has been sporadic and infrequently recognized. The specific enzootic subtypes that have been associated with natural disease in the tropics are subtype ID in Panama, subtype II (Everglades virus) in southern Florida, subtype IIIA (Mucambo virus) in Brazil and Surinam, and subtype IIIB (Tonate virus) in French Guiana. The disease associated with these viruses is usually grippelike and self-limited, but severe and fatal cases are described.

VEE virus may be isolated and assayed in a variety of laboratory hosts, including mice, hamsters, and avian or mammalian cell cultures.

DISTRIBUTION AND INCIDENCE. VEE has occurred in epidemic form in Trinidad, Guyana, Venezuela, Colombia, Ecuador, and Peru; on 1 occasion (1969–1971) the virus was introduced into Guatemala and spread to Mexico, Texas, Honduras, Nicaragua, and Costa Rica, but subsequently retreated again to South America. No epizootic virus isolations have been recorded since 1973. Enzootic virus subtypes are more widely distributed in tropical and subtropical regions of the Americas from Florida to Argentina.

Outbreaks have varied in size, but some major examples serve to illustrate their potential. In an epidemic lasting more than 2 years (1962–1964) in Venezuela, there were 23,283 human cases, including 960 with major neurologic syndromes and 156 deaths. In Ecuador in 1969, 20,000 to 30,000 horses died, and an estimated 31,000 human cases occurred; 1% of these were fatal.

Infection rates for the grippelike disorder have been similar for all age groups and both sexes or have been higher in adult males, whereas the incidence of encephalitis is highest in children. Outbreaks occur during the rainy months and are most intense in tropical coastal regions with distinct wet-dry seasons. Equine epizootics precede the appearance of human cases. A high proportion of the surviving equine population usually has immunity, and up to 10 years may be required for accumulation of enough susceptible animals to sustain another epizootic.

TRANSMISSION AND EPIDEMIOLOGY. Equines are the principal amplifier hosts for the epidemic strains of VEE virus, which are transmitted by a wide variety of mosquito vectors, including *Psorophora, Aedes,* and *Mansonia* spp. (Fig. 21–7). Transmission to humans is by mosquitoes previously infected from a viremic equine blood meal. Although VEE virus has been recovered from the serum and throat washings of human patients, people play a minor (if any) role as a source of infection for mosquitoes, and no epidemiologic evidence exists for contact or aerosol person-to-person transmission.

The basic cycle of transmission of the enzootic VEE virus subtypes involves wild forest rodents and *Culex (Melanoconion)* mosquitoes in forest and swamp habitats.

PATHOLOGY AND PATHOGENESIS. Pathologic correlations with the grippelike illness seen most frequently in adults have not been reported. Cases of encephalitis represent the most severe end of the clinical spectrum. Two fundamental pathologic processes are common to the arboviral encephalitides: (1) neuronal and glial cell damage (manifested by necrosis, degeneration, and neuronophagia) mediated by intracellular

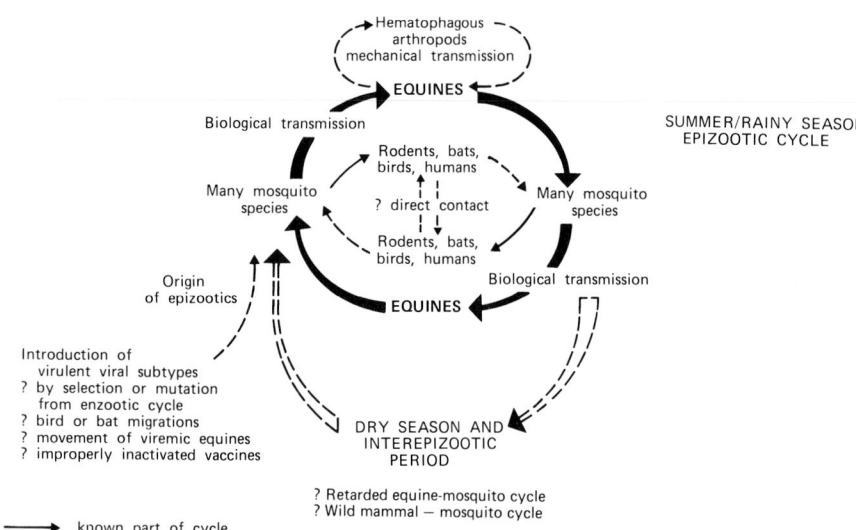

FIGURE 21–7. Transmission cycle of epizootic subtypes of Venezuelan equine encephalitis virus.

viral infection; and (2) an inflammatory reaction involving migration of immunologically active cells, i.e., lymphocytes, macrophages, and microglia, into the perivascular spaces and brain parenchyma. In the few human cases of VEE that have been studied, lesions (principally congestion, perivascular cuffing and hemorrhage, glial nodule formation, and focal necrosis) are most prominent in the substantia nigra and basal ganglia, but also affect the deep cerebral white matter and cerebral cortex. In the congenitally infected fetus, there is massive and widespread necrosis, hemorrhage, and resorption of brain tissue, resulting in cystic changes and hydranencephaly.

After the bite of an infected mosquito, the virus replicates in extraneural tissues. Virus shed into the circulating blood may breach the blood-brain barrier, possibly by passive diffusion, and invade the neuroparenchyma. The sites of extraneural replication (and injury) in humans are uncertain, but in horses and laboratory rodents, skeletal muscle and hematopoietic and lymphoid tissues have been implicated. Acute VEE deaths in hamsters have been related to virus-induced depression of the reticuloendothelial system, necrosis of Peyer's patches, and endotoxic shock. Impaired glucose tolerance and insulin release have been described in experimental animals as long as 1 year after VEE infection, but there are no reports of a diabetogenic effect in humans.

CLINICAL MANIFESTATIONS AND COMPLICATIONS

Febrile Illness. Inapparent infections are rare; most, if not all, persons infected with the epizootic strains develop an overt febrile illness, usually mild and nonspecific. Typically, VEE appears as a grippelike disease with sudden onset 2 to 5 days after exposure. Fever, chills, malaise, headache, myalgia, lumbosacral pain, nausea, and vomiting occur initially and may be followed by diarrhea and sore throat. Physical findings include fever, tachycardia, lethargy, pharyngitis, conjunctival congestion, facial hyperemia, muscle tenderness, and, rarely, lymphadenopathy. A proportion of patients ex-

hibit somnolence, photophobia, and mild confusion, but no progression or localization of neurologic signs occurs. The duration of illness is generally 2 or 3 days with a prolonged convalescent phase of lethargy and weakness lasting 1 or 2 weeks. A biphasic febrile and symptomatic form has been described.

Neurologic Illness. The severe neurologic syndrome is seen in approximately 4% of infected children under 15 years of age and rarely in adults. Central nervous system (CNS) manifestations include nuchal rigidity, stupor, coma, delirium, seizures, cranial nerve palsies, nystagmus, pathologic reflexes, and spastic paralysis. Involuntary movement disorders, tremors, and visual field defects are unusual or absent. Leukopenia with a decrease in lymphocytes or both granulocytes and lymphocytes is a frequent finding on days 1 to 3 after onset. Eosinopenia and abnormal vacuolated monocytes have been described. Cerebrospinal fluid (CSF) mononuclear pleocytosis ($\leq$500 cells/mm^3) with a normal glucose concentration is usual. Elevated serum aspartate aminotransferase and lactate dehydrogenase levels have been reported.

PROGNOSIS AND TREATMENT. Non-neurologic infections are self-limited, with return to full activity within several weeks after onset. The overall fatality rate of encephalitic infections is approximately 20%, but it is age dependent. In the 0- to 5-year age group the fatality rate is 35%, but it falls to 6 to 9% in older children and young adults. A prolonged convalescence is not uncommon, with asthenia, recurrent headaches, forgetfulness, and poorly defined complaints lasting up to 1 month after recovery. Long-term sequelae have been noted in children following encephalitic illness. Dysarthria, motor disorders, pathologic reflexes, abnormal electroencephalograms, and affective disorders are described.

No specific chemotherapeutic agent is known. Antipyretics and analgesics will help to relieve the fever, headache, and myalgia in patients without CNS disease. In encephalitic patients, supportive and competent nursing care will reduce mortality. Control of high fever by sponging and administration of antipyretics orally or rectally is recommended. Prompt administration of anticonvulsants (intravenous diazepam for acute control and phenytoin for more prolonged control) should be used to prevent protracted seizures. Dehydration caused by fever, vomiting, and insufficient oral intake may be severe, and fluid and electrolyte balance must be restored and maintained by intravenous infusions. Management of airways in semicomatose and comatose patients is essential. Blood gas levels should be monitored and respiratory assistance provided if hypoxia occurs. Prevention and treatment of secondary bacterial infections may be required; good pulmonary toilet and care of urinary catheters are mandatory. If clinical signs suggest cerebral edema or if the CSF pressure is high (≥ 400 mm H_2O), measures to reduce brain swelling are indicated. There is no evidence that corticosteroids have either a salutary or an adverse effect on the course of the viral infection, and the only indication for their use is reduction of edema.

DIAGNOSIS. The mild form of illness resembles other systemic infections and will be suspected only in the setting of an epidemic. In cases with encephalitis it is important to distinguish treatable causes of CNS infection, i.e., bacterial, fungal, and mycobacterial, from VEE and other viral disease. The geographic and epidemiologic setting, e.g., occurrence of equine cases, and examination and culture of the CSF are essential elements of the diagnostic procedure. Specific diagnosis of VEE may be made by isolation of the virus from blood or throat swab (taken during the viremic phase, 1 to 3 days after the symptomatic onset) or by serologic tests. An acute phase serum and a second serum taken 10 to 14 days later are necessary to demonstrate a rise in antibody titer. Hemagglutination-inhibiting, IgM antibody-capture enzyme-linked immunosorbent assay, and neutralizing antibodies appear within the first week after onset, and complement-fixing antibodies are found during the second week.

PREVENTION AND CONTROL. VEE outbreaks in horses and humans may be prevented by mass vaccination of equines, thereby reducing or eliminating the susceptible primary vertebrate host population. During epizootics, equines can be vaccinated in unaffected areas juxtaposed to or threatened by the epizootic. Large-scale (usually aerial), ultra-low-volume applications of insecticides to kill infected mosquitoes may be justified in areas already affected or immediately threatened.

Attenuated live (TC-83) and formalin-inactivated (C-84) vaccines are used to protect laboratory workers but are not licensed for use in the general public; their safety has not been assessed in children, who are the principal target population.

BIBLIOGRAPHY

Dietz WH, Peralta PH, Johnson KM: Ten clinical cases of human infection with Venezuelan equine encephalomyelitis virus, subtype 1D. Am J Trop Med Hyg 28:329, 1979.

Johnson KM, Martin DH: Venezuelan equine encephalitis. Adv Vet Sci Comp Med 18:79, 1974.

Leon CA, Jaramillo R, Martinez S, et al: Sequelae of Venezuelan equine encephalitis in humans: A four year follow-up. Int J Epidemiol 4:131, 1975.

Venezuelan Encephalitis. Pan American Health Organization, Scientific Publication No. 243, Washington, DC, 1972.

Walton TE, Grayson MA: Venezuelan equine encephalomyelitis. In Monath TP (ed): The Arboviruses: Epidemiology and Ecology, Vol IV. Boca Raton, FL, CRC Press, 1988, pp 203–231.

21.3. JAPANESE ENCEPHALITIS

Thomas P. Monath

DEFINITION. Japanese encephalitis (formerly known as Japanese B encephalitis) is an acute mosquito-borne flaviviral infection of the central nervous system. Japanese encephalitis virus also causes epizootics of clinical encephalitis in equines, and it produces abortion and stillbirth in swine, an important economic problem in parts of Asia.

ETIOLOGY AND HISTORY. In 1924 the virus was first isolated from brain tissue in patients with fatal cases in Japan. It is a flavivirus closely related to St. Louis encephalitis, West Nile, Rocio, and Murray Valley encephalitis viruses. Serologic cross-reactivity may lead to confusion in certain serologic tests. The virus may be isolated and assayed in a variety of cell cultures and in laboratory mice.

DISTRIBUTION AND INCIDENCE. The disease is endemic in tropical areas of south and southeastern Asia (e.g., southern Thailand, Malaysia, Indonesia, and the Philippines); sporadic cases are reported without epidemics. In contrast, subtropical and temperate zones of Asia are prone to recurrent epidemics of considerable magnitude. China reports the occurrence of over 10,000 cases annually; northern Thailand, 2000 to 5000 cases; and northeastern India has had repeated outbreaks with many thousands of cases. Case-fatality rates of 25 to 95% have been described, but the higher rates reflect under-recognition of nonfatal cases. Where the disease is endemic or causes annual epidemics, a high proportion of the adult population has antibodies, and children under 15 years old are principally affected by the disease. Where Japanese encephalitis has struck areas without a high prevalence of background immunity, e.g., northern India in 1978, however, all age groups have been affected; and in Japan, where school children have been protected by vaccination campaigns targeted at this age group, an excess of cases in the elderly has emerged. The overall inapparent:apparent infection ratio is approximately 300:1, but varies with age; the very young and very old are at highest risk of overt encephalitis. In temperate areas, Japanese encephalitis is a summertime disease, whereas in the tropics it occurs year-round, with peak incidence related to fluctuations in vector density (Fig. 110–2). Japanese encephalitis is predominantly a rural disease, and the incidence in males is usually higher than in females.

In some areas, i.e., Japan, Korea, and Taiwan, the incidence has declined dramatically in the last 25 years. This decrease is attributed to mass vaccination, anti-mosquito campaigns, use of agricultural pesticides in

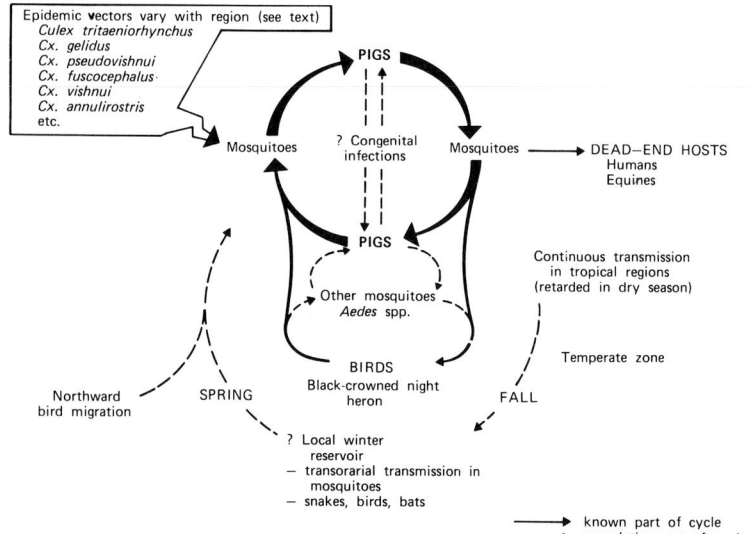

FIGURE 21–8. Transmission cycle of Japanese encephalitis virus.

rice-growing areas, and changes in agricultural practices and pig husbandry.

TRANSMISSION AND EPIDEMIOLOGY. The natural cycle involves *Culex* mosquito vectors and vertebrates susceptible to viremic infection, including wild birds, especially ardeid birds, and swine (Fig. 21–8). Humans and equines are incidental dead-end hosts. The vector species varies with geographic area; *Culex tritaeniorhynchus,* a rice-paddy breeder, is of principal importance in northern Asia. In many tropical regions of southern Asia this species also plays a prominent role, but other mosquitoes are also implicated as follows: *Cx. fuscocephalus* and *Cx. annulus* in Taiwan, *Cx. gelidus* and *Cx. fuscocephalus* in Thailand, *Cx. gelidus* in Malaysia and Indonesia, and the *Cx. "vishnui"* complex in India. Survival during winter and springtime recrudescence in temperate areas may be due to transovarial viral transmission in *Aedes* and *Culex* mosquitoes.

PATHOLOGY AND PATHOGENESIS. After the bite of an infected mosquito, the virus replicates in extraneural tissues and is shed into the blood stream, from where it may cross the blood-brain barrier. In a small proportion of infected persons, invasion or damage to the brain parenchyma results in clinical encephalitis. Gross pathologic findings include congestion, edema, and focal hemorrhage of meninges and brain tissue. Microscopic changes include perivascular mononuclear cell cuffing (Fig. 21–9), widespread neuronal degeneration and necrosis, and neuronophagia, especially in the cerebral cortex and basal ganglia. Necrosis of Purkinje cells in the cerebellum is a prominent feature.

CLINICAL MANIFESTATIONS AND COMPLICATIONS. Many infections are inapparent or so mild as to escape notice. The spectrum of illness includes febrile headache, aseptic meningitis, and meningoencephalitis. The incubation period ranges between 4 and

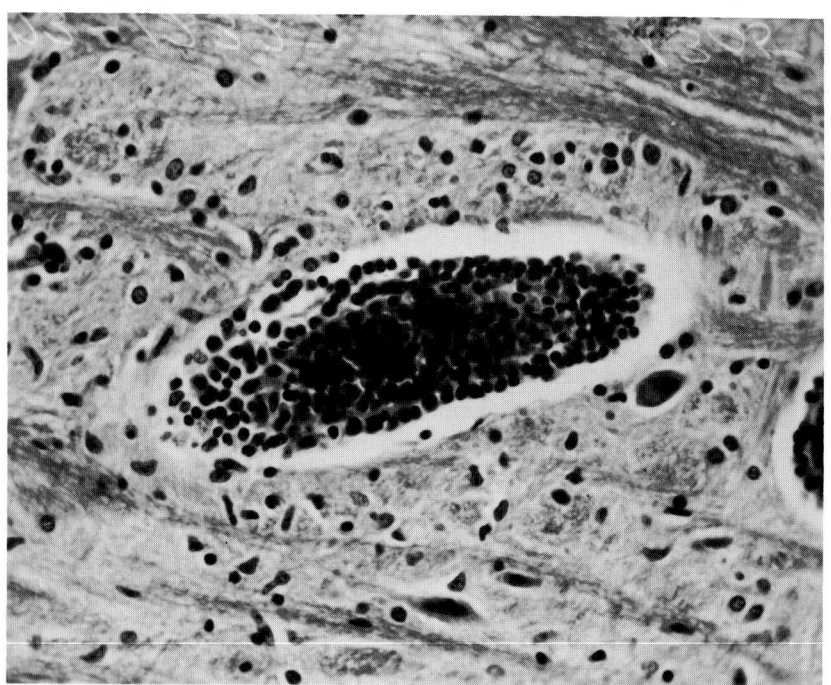

FIGURE 21–9. Perivascular cuffing by lymphocytes in brain of patient dying of Japanese encephalitis (× 305). (Courtesy of Armed Forces Institute of Pathology, Photograph Neg. No. 73-12327.)

14 days, followed by an abrupt onset with fever, headache, and respiratory and gastrointestinal symptoms. This nonspecific stage is followed within 2 or 3 days by an acute phase with meningeal irritation, impaired consciousness, convulsions (especially in children), muscular rigidity, masklike facies, ataxia, coarse tremor, involuntary movements, cranial nerve deficits, paresis, hyper- or hypoactive deep tendon reflexes, and pathologic reflexes. Weight loss, dehydration, and changing neurologic signs are often striking findings. In patients with mild involvement, fever subsides on the sixth or seventh day and neurologic signs resolve by the end of the second week after onset. In severe cases, hyperpyrexia, progressive neurologic dysfunction, cardiorespiratory complications, and coma result in death between the seventh and tenth day, or the patient undergoes a prolonged recovery, sometimes complicated by bacterial infections and leaving permanent sequelae. Atypical forms with predominance of bulbar or myelitic disturbances occur.

Early in the illness there is a low-grade leukocytosis and granulocytosis. The cerebrospinal fluid (CSF) has increased albumin concentration and white blood cells (generally $\leq 500/mm^3$), predominantly lymphocytes.

Transplacental infection has been described, resulting in fetal death and abortion. The clinical attack and case-fatality rates both appear to be lower in persons with a background of immunity to dengue viruses.

PROGNOSIS AND TREATMENT. Approximately 25% of cases with encephalitis prove fatal. A poor prognosis is indicated by prolonged high fever, frequent or severe convulsive seizures, a high protein content in the CSF, and early appearance of respiratory depression. Sequelae correlate with severity of illness during the acute phase and are especially frequent in children. Mental impairment, emotional lability, choreoathetosis, tremor, parkinsonism, autonomic disturbances, motor paralysis, and pathopsychologic syndromes, including schizophrenia, follow in at least half of the surviving cases.

Treatment is supportive (Chapter 21.2).

DIAGNOSIS. In many patients who die during the first week after onset, the virus may be isolated from the brain or viral antigen may be demonstrated by immunofluorescence. Virus may be isolated from CSF during the early phase of the acute illness; in such cases, fulminating infection is present, and prognosis is poor. Isolations from blood are uncommon. IgM, hemagglutination-inhibiting, and neutralizing antibodies appear during the first week and complement-fixing antibodies during the second week after onset. Studies have shown measurement of IgM antibodies in spinal fluid by the enzyme-linked immunosorbent assay (ELISA) to be especially useful. More than 75% of cases have detectable CSF IgM at the time of admission to hospital; moreover, presence of IgM in the CSF indicates local antibody formation associated with brain infection and is not seen in persons with asymptomatic infections with Japanese encephalitis virus.

PREVENTION AND CONTROL. Inactivated, partially purified suckling mouse brain or tissue culture vaccines commercially produced in Japan, Korea, and China are used principally in preschool and school age children. Reactogenicity is low, and there are no reports of demyelinating postvaccinal accidents. A minimum of 2 doses of the Japanese inactivated mouse brain vaccine spaced 7 to 14 days apart is required for protection. Limited production and supply have precluded the use of these vaccines in many areas of Asia. Live attenuated vaccines have undergone successful trials in China.

A small number of severe and even fatal infections have occurred in expatriates living in or visiting Asian countries. It may be advisable to immunize those at high risk who are going to travel in an epidemic zone or prolonged exposure in rural, rice-growing areas. Vaccine is not currently available in the United States. Advice regarding vaccination and vaccine supply is available from the Centers for Disease Control.

Emergency (epidemic) control may be obtained by ground-operated or aerial ultra-low-volume applications of organophosphate insecticides, thereby reducing adult *Culex* vector populations.

BIBLIOGRAPHY

Burke DS, Leake CJ: Japanese encephalitis. *In* Monath TP (ed): The Arboviruses: Epidemiology and Ecology, Vol III. Boca Raton, FL, CRC Press, 1988, pp 63–92.

Halstead SB: Arboviruses of the Pacific and Southeast Asia: Japanese encephalitis. *In* Feigin RD, Cherry JD (eds): Textbook of Pediatric Infectious Diseases. Philadelphia, WB Saunders, 1987, pp 1502–1510.

Hammon W McD, Kitaoka M, Downs WG (eds): Immunization for Japanese Encephalitis. Baltimore, Williams & Wilkins, 1971.

Ketel WB, Ognibene AJ: Japanese B encephalitis in Vietnam. Am J Med Sci 261:271, 1971.

Weaver OM, Haymaker W, Pieper S, et al: Sequelae of the arthropod-borne encephalitides. V. Japanese encephalitis. Neurology 8:887, 1958.

21.4. ROCIO ENCEPHALITIS

Thomas P. Monath

DEFINITION. Rocio encephalitis is an acute flaviviral infection of the central nervous system; the disease has been found only in southeastern Brazil. There is no associated morbidity in domestic animals.

ETIOLOGY AND HISTORY. In 1975, Rocio encephalitis was first described in Brazil, where a series of severe outbreaks occurred in the coastal region of São Paulo State. Rocio virus was isolated from brain tissue of patients with fatal encephalitis. The virus is serologically related most closely to mosquito-borne flaviviruses in the antigenic complex that includes St. Louis, Japanese, and Murray Valley encephalitis and West Nile viruses. Rocio virus grows to high titer and forms plaques in a variety of mammalian cell cultures and is highly pathogenic for laboratory mice.

DISTRIBUTION AND INCIDENCE. The disease is presently known only in a 1000-km² area of coastal plain south of Santos, São Paulo State, Brazil. In 1975 and 1976, approximately 1000 cases occurred with attack rates of up to 38/1000 population. The highest incidence was in young adult males engaged in outdoor work in impoverished rural agricultural areas. Children under 15 years were also affected frequently. No cases of Rocio encephalitis have been confirmed since 1977 (although a few are strongly suspected on serologic grounds). On the basis of complement-fixing or IgM antibodies in residents of the coastal counties, indicating recent infection, continued virus transmission seems to be occurring, but at a low level.

TRANSMISSION AND EPIDEMIOLOGY. The disease ecology is not well defined. Humans and domestic animals are probably dead-end hosts, incidental to the transmission cycle. Wild birds are believed to be important viremic hosts and mosquitoes are thought to be the vector, but the species involved remain unknown. A single isolate has been made from *Psorophora ferox* mosquitoes, but *Aedes scapularis* is the prime suspect vector.

PATHOGENESIS AND PATHOLOGY. A small number of patients with fatal encephalitis have been studied. Microscopic analysis revealed leptomeningitis and parenchymal lesions, i.e., lymphocytic perivascular infiltrates and glial nodule formation most marked in the midbrain, pons, and medulla, but also in the dentate nucleus of the cerebellum and anterior horn of the spinal cord.

CLINICAL MANIFESTATIONS AND COMPLICATIONS. After an incubation period of 7 to 14 days, the disease begins abruptly with fever, generalized malaise, and headache. Other nonspecific signs and symptoms include nausea, vomiting, abdominal distention, and pharyngeal and conjunctival redness. Myalgia is an infrequent complaint. Neurologic manifestations include stiff neck, stupor, coma, disturbed gait and balance, hyperreflexia, and pathologic reflexes. Tremor is present in 15% of the patients. Paralysis, sensory deficits, cranial nerve abnormalities, and convulsions are less frequent. The mean number of cells (predominantly lymphocytes) in the cerebrospinal fluid was 242, with a maximum of 3500 cells/mm³. During the acute illness, the peripheral white blood cell count was moderately elevated in 50%, normal in 36%, and depressed in 14% of patients.

PROGNOSIS AND TREATMENT. In the absence of good supportive care the case-fatality rate has been as high as 15 to 20%; it fell to approximately 4% with prompt hospitalization and good nursing care and medical management. Neuropsychiatric residua, including persistent motor and cerebellar deficits, behavioral disturbances, and retardation, were noted in 20% of survivors, both children and adults.

DIAGNOSIS. As in most other acute viral infections of the central nervous system, the clinical features do not allow specific etiologic diagnosis. Rocio encephalitis should be suspected on the basis of geographic origin, but because the distribution of Rocio virus may not be limited to southeastern Brazil, the diagnosis should be considered in cases of encephalitis elsewhere in tropical America. Diagnosis is made by demonstration of a rise in specific complement-fixating or neutralizing antibodies to Rocio virus or, in fatal infections, by virus isolation from brain tissues. The IgM enzyme-linked immunosorbent assay has been shown to be a useful diagnostic

tool. Cross-reactivity between flavivirus antigens in tests for antibody complicate serologic diagnosis, since human infections with other viruses related to Rocio, e.g., St. Louis encephalitis and Ilheus, are prevalent in Brazil.

PREVENTION AND CONTROL. No vaccine is available. Until the ecology and vector relationships of Rocio virus are understood, specific preventive and control measures cannot be formulated accurately; however, because the disease is almost certainly mosquito borne, adulticide sprays should be used to control future epidemics.

BIBLIOGRAPHY

Iversson LB: Rocio encephalitis. *In* Monath TP (ed): The Arboviruses: Epidemiology and Ecology, Vol IV. Boca Raton, FL, CRC Press, 1988, pp 78–92.

Lopes OS, Sacchetta LA, Coimbra TLM: Emergence of a new arbovirus disease in Brazil. I. Isolation and characterization of the etiological agent, Rocio virus. Am J Epidemiol 107:444, 1978.

Monath TP: Arthropod-borne encephalitides in the Americas. Bull WHO 57:513, 1979.

Tiriba A da C, Miziara AM, Lorenco R, et al: Encefalite humana primaria epidemica por arbovirus observada no litoral sul do estado de São Paulo. Rev Assoc Med Brasil 22:415, 1976.

21.5. OTHER ARBOVIRAL ENCEPHALITIDES

Thomas P. Monath

Although found principally in temperate areas of North America, *St. Louis* (Fig. 110–1), *eastern equine,* and *western equine encephalitis viruses* are also present in tropical America. Human infections associated with forest exposures are frequent (Fig. 21–10), but disease is recognized rarely and no epidemics have occurred. Twelve human cases of St. Louis encephalitis have been recorded from Argentina, Brazil, Surinam, Panama, Trinidad, and Jamaica. Western and eastern equine encephalitis outbreaks in Argentina and Uruguay have resulted in large numbers of equine cases. On 2 occasions, western equine encephalitis epizootics in the area of Viedma, Argentina, have been associated with small numbers of human cases. Eastern equine encephalitis (South American serotype) is enzootic and epizootic in the Amazon region, north coastal South America, Panama, and Trinidad; equine epizootics occur without recognized human involvement. In some Caribbean islands, i.e., Cuba and the Dominican Republic, the North American serotype has been responsible for epidemics affecting both horses and humans.

Murray Valley encephalitis is a severe disease caused by a flavivirus closely related to Japanese encephalitis, West Nile, and St. Louis encephalitis viruses. Infrequent small epidemics affect southeastern Australia; between 1951 and 1984, 104 cases and 30 deaths were reported. Risk factors include male sex, young age, and old age. The principal epidemic vector is *Culex annulirostris*; birds, and possibly wild mammals, play a role in transmission. The virus also occurs in northern and western Australia and in New Guinea; sporadic human cases have been reported from these areas. The closely related

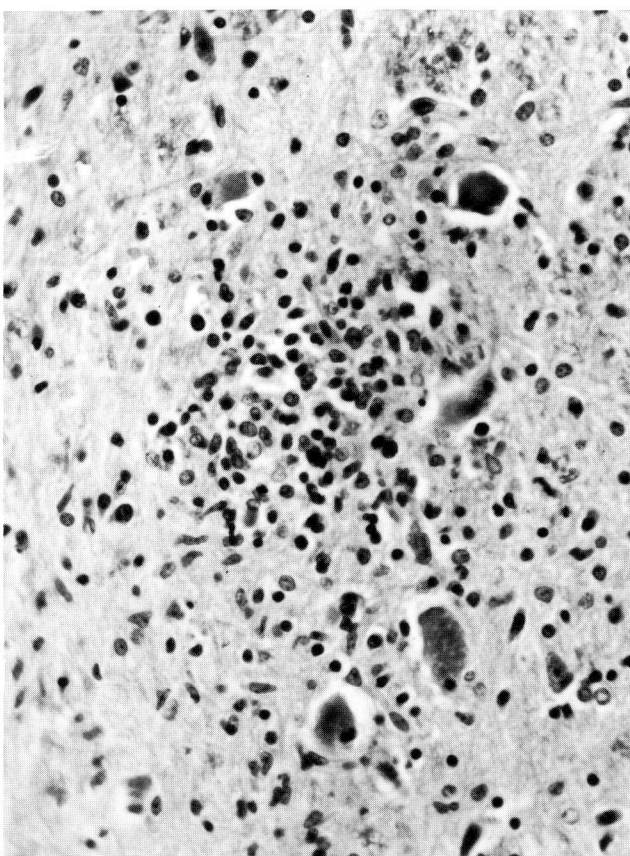

FIGURE 21–10. Glial nodule in dentate nucleus of brain from patient dying of western equine encephalitis virus infection. Reactive cells are astrocytes and microglia (rod cells) (× 265). (Courtesy of Armed Forces Institute of Pathology, Photograph Neg. No. 73–12319.)

Kunjin virus occurs in Australia, New Guinea, and Kalimantan; the first recognized human case (severe encephalitis) was reported in southeastern Australia in 1984. The clinical similarity and close antigenic relationship to Murray Valley encephalitis suggest that Kunjin encephalitis has been under-reported.

Arboviruses that are principally associated with other syndromes may occasionally cause encephalitis. These include *Sindbis* (Chapter 20.5) and *West Nile viruses* (Chapter 20.2), which are responsible for both endemic and epidemic infections in Africa and are typically characterized by a dengue-like febrile illness with rash.

Patients with *Rift Valley fever* (Chapter 20.10) may present with nondescript febrile illness, hemorrhagic fever, or an encephalitic illness. The predominant syndrome in *Kyasanur forest disease* (Chapter 22.8) is hemorrhagic fever, but meningoencephalitis may be a component of the disease spectrum. Other tropical arboviruses possibly associated with encephalitis include *Semliki Forest virus* (a mosquito-borne alphavirus in Africa), *Ilheus* (a mosquito-borne flavivirus in South and Central America), and *Thogoto* (a tick-borne member of the Orthomyxoviridae family in Africa). In an outbreak of *Oropouche virus disease* (Chapter 20.9) in Brazil, 22 patients with aseptic meningitis were found. The presenting syndrome was that of headache, stiff neck, vomiting, and lethargy; some patients had diplo-

pia, nystagmus, and disturbances of equilibrium. Toscana virus, a sandfly-transmitted member of the genus *Phlebovirus,* family Bunyaviridae, in the Mediterranean region (Portugal, Italy, Cyprus), has been associated with meningitic illness (Chapter 20.11).

BIBLIOGRAPHY

Hart KL, Keen D, Belle EA: An outbreak of eastern equine encephalomyelitis in Jamaica, West Indies. I. Description of human cases. Am J Trop Med Hyg 13:331, 1964.
Monath TP (ed): St. Louis Encephalitis. Am Pub Health Assoc, Washington, DC, 1980.

22. VIRAL HEMORRHAGIC FEVERS

22.1. YELLOW FEVER

Thomas P. Monath

DEFINITION. Yellow fever is an acute mosquito-borne flaviviral infection characterized, in its severe form, by fever, jaundice, hemorrhage, and albuminuria. The disease is endemic and epidemic in tropical regions of the Americas and Africa, where it remains a major public health problem. Yellow fever does not occur in Asia.

ETIOLOGY AND HISTORY. Yellow fever was first recognized as a nosologic entity in the New World in the seventeenth century, but its origins probably were in Africa. For over 200 years, it was responsible for devastating epidemics and economic losses. In 1881, Dr. Carlos J. Finlay of Havana, Cuba proposed that yellow fever was transmitted by mosquitoes. Major Walter Reed and his colleagues proved Finlay's theory in 1900 and showed that the transmissible agent was filterable. The virus was finally isolated in 1927 by inoculation of the blood of a Ghanaian man (Asibi) into rhesus monkeys.

Yellow fever virus is the prototype of the flavivirus taxonomic group, which is composed of a variety of other medically important, antigenically related viruses, including several that also cause hemorrhagic fevers (Omsk hemorrhagic fever, Kyasanur Forest disease, dengue). The yellow fever virus (and other flaviviruses) is a spherical, enveloped, RNA-containing particle approximately 38 nm in size. Virions develop by budding from intracytoplasmic membranes and accumulate in cisternae of the endoplasmic reticulum. The virus shares antigenic sites with other flaviviruses, and serologic responses to infection are often nonspecific. Strains of yellow fever virus from Africa and South America are distinguishable by special serologic tests. Strain variation in virulence for laboratory animals also occurs. No geographic differences have been shown in the clinical features of the human disease. Yellow fever virus is pathogenic for a variety of cell cultures, newborn mice, adult mice (when injected intracerebrally), and some monkey species.

DISTRIBUTION AND INCIDENCE. Yellow fever is distributed throughout much of tropical South America and subSaharan Africa. Between 50 and 300 cases of jungle yellow fever are recognized each year in South America. The virus is active in Brazil, Peru, Bolivia, Ecuador, Venezuela, and Colombia in forested and sparsely populated areas that are under limited cultivation and are drained by tributaries of the Amazon, Orinoco, and Magdalena rivers. Human cases reach a peak during the rainy months. Human cases are usually sporadic, but small epidemics (involving 20 to 50 persons) are not uncommon. Outbreaks are associated with monkey epizootics that appear at intervals and spread through natural corridors in forested areas. Central America, as well as parts of Paraguay and Argentina normally outside the enzootic zone, may be involved in waves of epizootic infection. The exact location of virus activity in the vast tropical forests of South America is difficult or impossible to ascertain at any given time, and indeed the virus is constantly moving, thus assuring a supply of susceptible hosts adequate for maintenance of the cycle.

In the Americas, urban yellow fever has not occurred in epidemic form since 1942 (in Brazil) largely because of the eradication of *Aedes aegypti* mosquitoes from population centers of South America. Nonetheless, *Ae. aegypti*-infested areas are increasing in juxtaposition to the jungle cycle. In the 1980s, moreover, *Ae. aegypti* has reinvaded many areas from which it had been eradicated, including coastal Brazil, Paraguay, Bolivia, Peru, and Ecuador, with the result that large outbreaks of dengue fever have occurred. The inescapable conclusion is that urban yellow fever will reappear.

In Africa, few sporadic cases are recognized annually; however, this reflects inadequate surveillance and diagnostic facilities. Large epidemics, which occur at irregular intervals in areas of West, Central, and East Africa between 0 and 15 degrees North, have involved as many as 100,000 cases, with 30,000 deaths. The vectors responsible for these epidemics are complex and involve both *Ae. aegypti* and sylvatic mosquito species. The most recent epidemic period began in 1986 and continued through 1988, with outbreaks in Nigeria and Mali involving many thousands of cases. The Nigerian epidemic in 1987 involved urban populations and was transmitted by *Ae. aegypti*.

TRANSMISSION AND EPIDEMIOLOGY. Two forms of yellow fever are classically distinguished on the basis of different mosquito vectors and vertebrate hosts involved in the cycle of virus transmission. These forms are clinically and pathoanatomically identical. In the urban form, yellow fever virus is passed from a viremic to a susceptible individual by *Ae. aegypti*, which breeds and bites in and around houses. A period of extrinsic incubation in the vector (9 to 12 days, temperature-dependent) is required before the virus can be transmitted. Jungle (or sylvan) yellow fever is a zoonotic infection acquired through the bite of forest mosquito vector species, which maintain the virus in a monkey-mosquito-monkey cycle (Fig. 110–2). The epidemiology of the disease in the Americas and in Africa differs and must be considered separately.

In the Americas, the virus is maintained as a wandering monkey epizootic in tropical forests, with *Haemagogus* species as the principal vector. Presence of the virus is sometimes evident on the basis of monkey deaths because some New World species, e.g., *Alouatta* (howler) monkeys, succumb to the infection. Humans acquire the disease during activities such as woodcutting, which bring them into contact with *Haemagogus* mosquitoes. Dramatic outbreaks have occurred when groups of unvaccinated laborers have penetrated jungle areas. *Haemagogus* mosquitoes may also bite in and around houses in cleared forest areas. The drought-resistant species *Sabethes chloropterus* plays a secondary role in the yellow fever cycle but may be important in maintaining transmission during the dry season.

In Africa, epidemics sustained by the peridomestic *Ae. aegypti* vector have occurred in both urban and rural environments of West Africa. In savannah and forest-savannah transition areas of West Africa, epidemic yellow fever has been transmitted by treehole-breeding *Aedes*, including *Ae. furcifer, africanus*, and *luteocephalus*, with both monkeys and humans as intermediate hosts (Fig. 110–2). Adult mosquitoes disappear during the long dry season, and the virus may survive in transovarially infected eggs of *Aedes* vectors. The virus has also been recovered from *Amblyomma* ticks, adding a new dimension to its natural history that requires further study.

In the extensive forests of Central and East Africa, a jungle cycle exists analogous to that in the Americas, with *Ae. africanus* as the major vector. Sporadic cases and epidemics in persons entering the forest or living at the forest fringe result from exposure to this mosquito, which bites near the forest floor during the daytime. In some areas, mosquitoes belonging to the *Ae. simpsoni* complex, link the jungle cycle with human populations and have been responsible for intensive interhuman transmission (Fig. 110–2).

Susceptibility. All races are equally susceptible to yellow fever infection. The disease is thought to be milder in native populations of Africa than in whites. However, this is probably a reflection of background immunity and cross-protection by related endemic flaviviruses, as some outbreaks of yellow fever involving Africans have been severe, with high death rates. In an epidemic in Gambia, the ratio of inapparent to apparent infection was estimated to be 2:1 in those with primary yellow fever infection and 22:1 in persons with prior exposures to heterologous flaviviruses. Nonimmune persons of all ages and both sexes are equally susceptible. The age and sex distribution is, however, determined by natural immunization and vaccination and by occupational exposures. In tropical America, adult males employed in woodcutting or agricultural pursuits are primarily affected by jungle yellow fever. In endemic areas of West Africa, disease has been most frequent in children, as a result of cumulative natural and vaccine immunity.

PATHOLOGY AND PATHOGENESIS
Pathology. Gross pathologic findings include icterus; cardiac enlargement; swelling and congestion of the kidneys; hemorrhages or petechiae of the mucous mem-

branes, stomach, duodenum, renal capsule, and urinary bladder; and small, bloody pleural and peritoneal effusions. The liver is usually normal in size, is red or yellow, and shows obliteration of the normal lobular pattern and a greasy consistency. Histopathologic changes of the liver may be characteristic, but atypical findings are common. Conditions with which yellow fever may be confused on the basis of histopathologic findings include Congo-Crimean hemorrhagic fever, Lassa fever, African (Marburg-Ebola virus) hemorrhagic fever, viral hepatitis, and leptospirosis. The typical yellow fever lesion is marked by cloudy swelling and then by coagulative necrosis of hepatocytes in the midzone of the liver lobule, sparing cells bordering the central vein (Fig. 22–1A). Eosinophilic degeneration of hepatocytes results in the formation of Councilman bodies and intranuclear eosinophilic granular inclusions (Torres bodies) (Fig. 22–1B and C). Multi- and microvacuolar fatty changes are nearly always present (Fig. 22–1D), especially after the eighth day of illness. An inflammatory response is absent or mild. The reticulin framework is preserved. Typical changes have been seen in biopsy specimens taken as early as the third day of illness; interpretation of biopsy or necropsy material obtained after the tenth day is often difficult. *Biopsy is, however, contraindicated as a diagnostic procedure owing to the high risk of hemorrhage.* Renal glomerular changes are relatively insignificant compared with acute tubular necrosis and fatty metamorphosis, which may be marked. The myocardial fibers show cloudy swelling, degeneration, and fatty infiltration. Lymphocytic elements in the spleen and nodes are depleted, and large mononuclear or histiocytic cells accumulate in the splenic follicles. The brain may show edema and petechial hemorrhages.

Pathophysiology. The pathophysiology of yellow fever is incompletely understood. Direct viral injury to the cells of major target organs, such as the liver, underlies the pathogenic process. Fatal cases usually present as fulminating hepatitis, with hemorrhage, toxemia, and shock. Some patients have prominent signs of acute renal failure, and deaths have been attributed to uremia. Acute tubular necrosis is probably secondary to hemodynamic causes or hepatocellular necrosis. Deaths, especially late in the disease, have occurred because of cardiac failure or arrhythmia, but are rare. Hemorrhage undoubtedly exacerbates hypotension and oliguria and may precipitate vascular collapse and death. Evidence for disseminated intravascular coagulation as the basis for the hemorrhagic diathesis has been obtained in a few cases, but its incidence is uncertain. Acidosis and hyperkalemia are terminal events. At present, the complex pathophysiologic interrelationships of yellow fever cannot be specified, and directions for specific therapeutic interventions are consequently undetermined.

CLINICAL MANIFESTATIONS AND COMPLICATIONS. The incubation period (interval between the bite of an infected mosquito and the onset of symptoms) is generally 3 to 6 days. Yellow fever infection produces a spectrum from mild, nonspecific, febrile illness to a fulminating, sometimes fatal disease with pathognomonic features. The precise frequency with which the

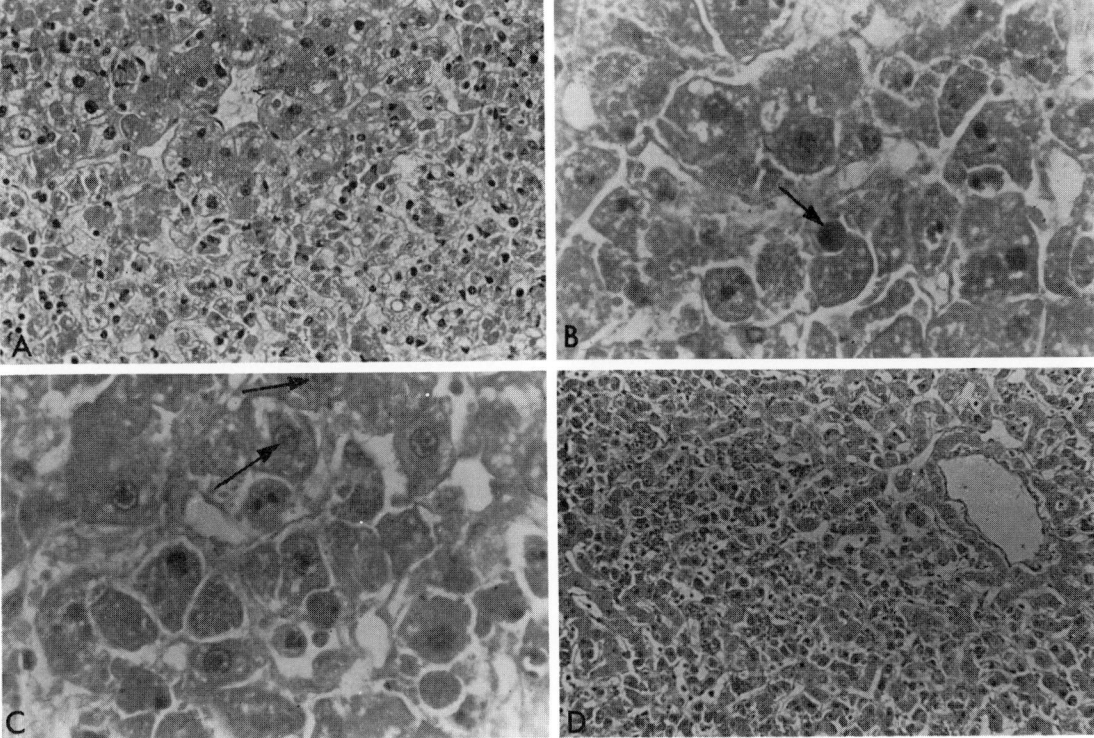

FIGURE 22–1. Fatal yellow fever: histopathologic changes in the liver. *A,* Central zone of a liver lobule, showing cytoplasmic degeneration, sinusoidal Councilman bodies, and sparing of hepatocytes around central vein. *B,* Acidophilic cytoplasmic degeneration of hepatocytes with Councilman body formation (arrow). *C,* Amorphous amphophilic mass in nucleus (Torres body, arrows): these are not viral inclusions, but are derived from host cell nuclear proteins. *D,* Midzonal necrosis of liver lobule. (*A* and *D,* courtesy of Armed Forces Institute of Pathology.)

various clinical forms occur is uncertain; however, abortive infections are the rule, and the classic symptoms of severe yellow fever are found in only 10 to 20% of cases.

Acute Febrile Illness. The mild case will not be suspected except in the setting of an epidemic. In its mildest form, yellow fever is characterized by sudden onset of fever and headache, without other symptoms, lasting 48 hours or less. In other patients, the fever is higher, the headache is more severe and accompanied by myalgia, there is slight albuminuria, and bradycardia occurs in relation to the presence of fever (Faget's sign). The illness lasts several days, with uneventful recovery.

Hemorrhagic Illness. Severe yellow fever begins abruptly with fever to 40C, chills, severe headache, lumbosacral pain, and generalized myalgia. The patient appears distressed and anxious, the conjunctivae are congested, the face and neck are flushed, the tongue is reddened at the tip and edges, and the breath is foul smelling. Anorexia, nausea, vomiting, and minor gingival hemorrhages or epistaxis may occur. Despite a persistent or rising temperature, the pulse may decrease. This syndrome, lasting approximately 3 days, corresponds to the *period of infection,* during which yellow fever virus is present in the blood. It may be followed by a *period of remission,* with defervescence and mitigation of symptoms, usually lasting several hours to 1 day. Fever and symptoms then reappear, with more frequent vomiting, epigastric pain, prostration, and the development of jaundice *(period of intoxication).* Viremia is generally absent, and antibodies appear during this phase. Hematemesis (coffee-ground material or black vomit, i.e., vomito negro), melena, metrorrhagia, petechiae, ecchymoses, and diffuse oozing from the mucous membranes may occur. Dehydration resulting from vomiting and increased insensible fluid losses is frequent. Renal dysfunction is marked by the sudden appearance of albuminuria, which may rapidly increase, and by diminishing urine output. The pulse remains unrelated to the fever, but may weaken as the blood and pulse pressures decrease. The patient recovers, either rapidly after a period of intoxication of 3 to 4 days or over a protracted course of up to 2 weeks. Yellow fever is fatal in 20 to 50% of severe cases. Deaths generally occur on the seventh to tenth day of illness and are preceded by increasing albuminuria, hemorrhages, rising pulse, hypotension, oliguria, and azotemia. Hypothermia, a severe agitated delirium, intractable hiccup, stupor, and coma are terminal signs.

Hepatic, renal, or myocardial involvement predominates in individual cases with clinical signs of relatively pure hepatitis, acute renal failure, or hypotension and hypokinetic heart failure. Pre-eminent central nervous system involvement, producing meningoencephalitic signs, has been described rarely. Atypical fulminant cases have been described, with death on the second or third day in the absence of hepatic or renal signs but are without virologic confirmation.

Physical findings during the period of intoxication include scleral and dermal icterus, hemorrhagic manifestations, epigastric (rarely hepatic) tenderness without enlargement, and abnormal vital signs.

The convalescent stage is sometimes prolonged, with profound weakness lasting 1 to 2 weeks. Late death, occurring at the end of convalescence or even weeks after recovery from the acute illness, is a rare phenomenon attributed to myocardial damage, cardiac arrhythmia, or cardiac failure. Suppurative parotitis (resulting from dehydration) and secondary bacterial pneumonia may complicate the disease.

Clinical Laboratory Findings. Leukopenia (neutropenia) occurs during the early phase of illness. Prolongation of the clotting, prothrombin, and partial thromboplastin times is marked in patients with jaundice. The platelet count may be decreased, and fibrin split products may be present in serum. The total and conjugated serum bilirubin may reach levels of 15 to 20 mg/dl. Serum alanine and aspartate aminotransferase levels are markedly elevated in all icteric patients (but inconstantly and to lower levels in anicteric patients), with peak values between days 5 and 10 of the illness, and return to normal by days 10 to 20. The alkaline phosphatase level is generally normal. Hypoglycemia has been noted in patients with severe hepatic damage.

During the period of infection, the urine may contain a small amount of albumin, which then increases on the fourth or fifth day, reaching levels of 3 to 5 (rarely as high as 40) gm/L. The urine contains bile; the cell sediment may be abnormal but is not diagnostically helpful. The cerebrospinal fluid is clear and without cells, but may be under increased pressure and may contain a mildly elevated protein concentration. Electrocardiographic (ST-T wave) abnormalities have been described.

PROGNOSIS AND TREATMENT. Up to 50% of patients with severe forms of yellow fever die. Patients have generally been cared for under primitive conditions, and the prognosis may improve with advanced intensive hospital care facilities. The prognosis is guarded for the patient who, after a brief remission, enters a period of intoxication with rising fever, jaundice, and albuminuria. Features that correlate with a poor prognosis include early onset of bilirubinemia and albuminuria, rising to high levels; marked prolongation of the prothrombin time (<25% of normal); severe hemorrhage; and the appearance of shock, coma, hypothermia, and intractable hiccup. Relapses have not been described. The possibility of late death from myocardial or renal injury must be considered.

Complete bed rest, supportive care, and close monitoring of vital functions are essential. During the period of infection, mild sedatives, nonsalicylate analgesics, and antiemetics may be indicated, and attention should be given to fluid and electrolyte balance. Supportive measures are of critical importance during the period of intoxication if vomiting is severe, if hemorrhage appears, or if hypertension, hypokinetic heart failure, oliguria, azotemia, and electrolyte and acid-base imbalance become evident. Dialysis may be indicated in patients with evidence of acute tubular necrosis. Cautious consideration may be given to early heparin treatment of disseminated intravascular coagulation if laboratory tests indicate its occurrence. Secondary bacterial infections or concurrent infections, malaria in particular, should be treated by the usual appropriate means. The benefits of antiviral chemotherapeutic agents or human interferon remain unknown, but animal experiments suggest that these measures are unlikely to be of use once clinical illness is well established.

DIAGNOSIS. Because the incubation period is sufficient to permit an infected person to travel a long distance, the diagnosis should be suspected in all patients with fever and jaundice who have recently been to tropical America or Africa. Specific diagnosis depends on histopathologic study, isolation of the virus, or demonstration of a specific antibody response. The virus is most readily isolated from serum obtained during the first 3 or 4 days of illness (period of infection), but it may be recovered from serum up to the twelfth day and occasionally from the liver at death. Viral antigen may be demonstrated in serum or liver tissue by enzyme immunoassay employing monoclonal antibodies. A retrospective definitive diagnosis is also possible by examining formalin-fixed liver for antigen by immunocytochemical techniques or for viral nucleic acid by hybridization.

Serology. Serologic methods useful in the diagnosis of yellow fever include hemagglutination-inhibition (HI), complement-fixation (CF), IgM enzyme-linked immunosorbent assay (ELISA), neutralization (N), fluorescence, and radioimmuno-assay tests. The HI, IgM and N antibodies appear within 1 week of onset; the CF antibodies appear later. Paired acute and convalescent phase specimens are required to establish the diagnosis based on a rise in antibody titer. Cross-reactions with other flaviviruses and the high prevalence of background immunity to flaviviruses in tropical populations render serodiagnosis difficult.

Differential Diagnosis. Mild yellow fever cannot be clinically distinguished from a wide array of other infections. In the presence of jaundice and the other signs of severe yellow fever, conditions that must be differentiated include viral hepatitis, Congo-Crimean hemorrhagic fever, Rift Valley fever, falciparum malaria, spirochetal infections (tick-borne relapsing fever and Weil's disease), typhoid, Q fever, typhus, and surgical, drug-induced, and toxic causes. Other diseases, usually without jaundice, that may be confused with yellow fever include Lassa, African (Marburg-Ebola virus), Bolivian, and Argentine hemorrhagic fevers.

PREVENTION AND CONTROL

Isolation. The patient with yellow fever should be isolated from contact with mosquitoes by being placed under netting or in a screened room.

Vaccination. Yellow fever 17D is a safe live attenuated vaccine providing long-lasting immunity in 95% or more of vaccines. For purposes of international certification, vaccination is considered valid for 10 years, but immunity has been documented to last more than 40 years and may be lifelong. Because yellow fever exists as a silent enzootic over wide areas of the tropics and appears in epidemic form with little warning and without early recognition, vaccination of travelers is imperative. As many countries with endemic yellow fever claim to be free of the disease (and so report to the World Health Organization), decisions regarding vaccination should *not* be based on official reports. A case in point is the unfortunate occurrence of 2 deaths from yellow fever in unvaccinated French tourists to Senegal, a country not officially requiring yellow fever vaccination. A general recommendation may be formulated as follows: Yellow fever is *potentially* active in the countries shaded in Figure 22–2; persons who plan to travel within these areas should be immunized unless visits are brief, e.g., several days, and confined to large urban centers. Immunity can be demonstrated within 10 days after vaccination. The vaccine is relatively unstable at ambient temperatures, and cold preservation, as directed by the manufacturer, is essential. Mild vaccine reactions rarely occur, and serious complications have been exceedingly uncommon. A total of 17 cases of encephalitis following 17D vaccination have been reported, of which one was fatal; nearly all cases have been in infants younger than 4 months of age. For this reason, the vaccine is not administered to infants 6 months of age or younger. In Africa, several outbreaks of severe and fatal bacterial infections following yellow fever vaccination have been reported; these were probably due to clostridial or streptococcal contamination of vaccine (after reconstitution) or syringe and needle.

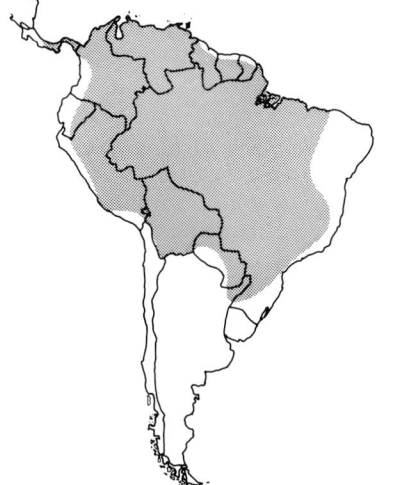
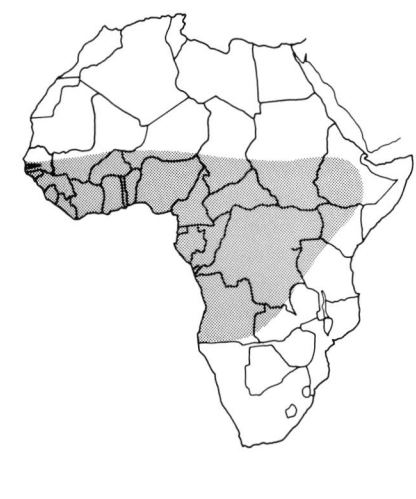

FIGURE 22–2. Regions of tropical America and Africa endemic for yellow fever or experiencing intermittent epidemics. Travelers to these areas should receive yellow fever immunization. Yellow fever does not occur in Asia, Australia, or the Pacific.

These unfortunate occurrences emphasize the need for scrupulous attention to handling and administration of the vaccine. No untoward consequences for the fetus have been recorded; but on theoretical grounds, pregnant women should not be vaccinated unless the risk of acquiring yellow fever is considered greater than the potential (undocumented) risk to the fetus. The vaccine is prepared in chicken embryos and should be used with caution in persons hypersensitive to egg proteins. The French neurotropic viral vaccine produced in mouse brain is no longer used; it caused allergic encephalomyelitis in children.

In the event of an epidemic, the disease may be controlled by mass vaccination and the use of insecticides to reduce infected vector populations.

BIBLIOGRAPHY

Germain M, Cornet M, Mouchet J, et al: La fièvre jaune selvatique en Afrique: Données récentes et conceptions actuelles. Med Trop (Marseilles) 41:31, 1981.
Monath, TP, Craven RB, Adjukiewicz A, et al: Yellow fever in the Gambia, 1978–1979: Epidemiologic aspects with observations on the occurrence of Orungo virus infection. Am J Trop Med Hyg 29:912, 1980.
Monath TP, Brinker KR, Chandler FW, et al: Pathophysiologic correlations in a rhesus monkey model of yellow fever. Am J Trop Med Hyg 30:431, 1981.
Strode GK (ed): Yellow Fever. New York, McGraw-Hill, 1951.

22.2.   LASSA FEVER

Susan P. Fisher-Hoch

DEFINITION. Lassa virus, the cause of Lassa fever (LF) is an arenavirus. Members of this family of viruses are natural parasites of rodents, in whom they establish chronic, but silent, lifelong infection. High-titer virus is excreted in the urine of the rodent, and humans may become infected as accidental hosts. Lassa virus, which causes hemorrhagic fever, is an important human pathogen. Although LF was first described in West Africa in the 1950s, the virus was not isolated from a patient with LF until 1969. LF occurs from Nigeria to Guinea, resulting in as many as 5000 deaths annually.

VIROLOGY. Lassa virus belongs to the arenaviruses, which are enveloped viruses with a mean diameter of 110 to 130 nm (range 50 to 300 nm). The virion density in sucrose is 1.17 gm/cm^3. The arenaviruses contain two segments of RNA encoding at least 3 gene products. The large segment (L) RNA encodes a protein of 180 to 200 kd believed to be the viral polymerase. The 3′ half of the small (S) RNA encodes a nucleoprotein in the viral-complementary sequence, and the 5′ half encodes the glycoprotein precursor in the viral sense sequence. The viral envelope is composed of two glycosylated proteins (GP1 and GP2), which are created by enzyme cleavage after translation. GP1 (MW 35 to 38) is the amino end and GP2 (MW 44 to 64) the carboxy end of the precursor. The single nucleocapsid protein of the arenaviridae range in molecular weight

from 54 to 68, and the viral polymerase is usually about 200.

EPIDEMIOLOGY AND ECOLOGY. The modes of transmission from rodent to human are not precisely known. Arenaviruses are stable, especially with low humidity, for several hours and they may be transmitted to rodents in the laboratory by aerosol. However, the sporadic pattern of human infection in the community does not support aerosol transmission. Direct contact of cuts and scratches on hands and feet with articles and surfaces contaminated by virus may be a more important and consistent mode of transmission.

Transmission

Rodent to Human. The only known reservoir of Lassa virus is *Mastomys natalensis*, one of the most common rodents in Africa. At least 2 species of *Mastomys* (diploid types with 32 and 38 chromosomes) inhabit West Africa, and both harbor Lassa virus. A third diploid type (with 36 chromosomes) in southern Africa, carries the closely related, Mopeia virus, which is not virulent for humans. These rodents, especially the species with 32 chromosomes, are highly commensal with humans. They are a common domestic rodent in West Africa. Their movement within a village is limited, usually near the house they occupy. Human infection rates are higher in households that have infected rodents and large household rodent populations. As all age groups and both sexes are affected, and antibody prevalence increases with age, it is assumed that most virus transmission to humans takes place in and around the homes. Rodent to human infection is highly associated with indiscriminate food storage and practices such as catching, cooking, and eating rodents.

Person to Person. Spread of Lassa virus in households is common although it is less frequent than rodent to human spread. Risk of infection is associated with direct contact with, nursing care of, or sexual contact with someone during the incubation or convalescent phases of illness.

Nosocomial Spread in Hospitals. This was prominent in the early epidemics. Experience shows that nosocomial transmission can be effectively prevented with simple isolation and barrier nursing techniques. However, the increasing use of intravenous therapy in West African hospitals with inadequate needle and syringe supplies has led to large-scale epidemics. Inadequate barrier nursing techniques, injuries with needles and other sharp instruments, surgery, and exposure to blood caused many infections in the past and could lead to nosocomial infections in the future.

Prevalence. Estimates of antibody prevalence range from 4 to 6% in Guinea to 15 to 20% in Nigeria, although in some villages in Sierra Leone as many as 60% of the population have evidence of past infection. In prospective studies, seroconversion to Lassa virus ranged from 5 to 20% of susceptible (seronegative) Sierra Leone villagers. Most of those infected were asymptomatic.

Disease: infection ratios ranged from 1:4 to 2:10, and the proportion of febrile illness associated with seroconversion ranged from 5 to 14%. Five to 8% of infected people were hospitalized, and, although overall fatality was as low as 2 or 3%, it rose to 15 to 20% in hospitalized cases and to 30% in women in the third trimester of pregnancy. Case-fatality in hospitalized children younger than age 15 was 12 to 15%. In 2 hospitals in Sierra Leone, LF accounted for 10 to 15% of all adult admissions and 30% of adult deaths, with a peak during the dryer months. LF is more common than previously suspected and probably results in more than 100,000 infections per year in West Africa. Furthermore, with so many living in poor-quality, rodent-infested housing and with the increasing indiscriminate use of needles in hospital practice, devastating epidemics could always occur.

PATHOPHYSIOLOGY

Pathology. Although the outcome in LF is directly associated with virus replication, tissue destruction is not a major component. The most frequent and consistent microscopic lesions in fatal human Lassa fever are variable hepatocyte necrosis with regeneration and focal necrosis of adrenal glands and spleen, with little, if any, lymphocytic inflammatory response. Although high virus titers occur in brain, ovary, pancreas, uterus, and placenta, no significant pathologic lesions have been observed in these organs.

Pathogenesis. The critical events in fatal disease are intractable hypovolemic shock, severe central nervous system (CNS) involvement, bleeding, and gross edema of the head and neck with pulmonary edema and respiratory distress. Some of these manifestations are due to disturbances in the intravascular compartment, particularly increased endothelial cell permeability. Platelet dysfunction correlates with severity of illness, and a marked decrease in prostacyclin production by endothelium has been measured in primates infected by Lassa virus. An inhibitor of platelet function has been identified in the serum of patients and nonhuman primates with severe LF. Disseminated intravascular coagulation is not a significant component of fatal LF; circulating platelet numbers are well maintained, and, in primates with severe Lassa infection, platelet and fibrinogen turnover have been normal, and there is no increase in fibrinogen breakdown products in humans. No clear evidence of virus replication in—and damage of—endothelium has been demonstrated; so, it must be concluded that shock and bleeding are due to disturbances in the functional hemostatic mechanisms of the intravascular compartment other than the coagulation cascade.

Immunity. The rapid development of antibodies is accompanied by lymphopenia and absence of tissue infiltration by lymphocytes, suggesting that some impairment may occur in the T-cell arm of the immune response. In primates the response to nonspecific antigens is markedly reduced during the acute phase of fatal infection. Lassa virus does not induce neutralizing antibodies in humans or primates during the acute or early convalescent phases of illness. In a minority of patients neutralizing activity may occasionally be detected several weeks or months into the illness. These antibodies do not appear to be associated with either virus clearance or immunity to reinfection. The cell-mediated immune response to Lassa virus appears to be critical to virus clearance and presumably protects against reinfection.

CLINICAL MANIFESTATIONS

Symptoms and Signs. Following an incubation period of 7 to 18 days, LF begins insidiously, with fever, weakness, and malaise. More than 50% of patients then experience joint and lumbar pain and 60% or more have a nonproductive cough. Most patients also have severe headache, usually frontal, and a painful sore throat. Many also develop a severe retrosternal chest pain, and about half have vomiting or diarrhea and abdominal pain. On physical examination, respiratory rate, temperature, and pulse rate are elevated and blood pressure may be low. About a third have conjunctivitis, and more than two thirds have pharyngitis, half of whom will have exudates, with diffusely inflamed and swollen posterior pharynx and tonsils, but with few if any petechiae.

Hospital Course. Up to a third of hospitalized patients progress to a prostrating illness 6 to 8 days after onset of fever. They are often dehydrated and the hematocrit is elevated. Bleeding occurs in only 15 to 20% of patients, limited primarily to the mucosal surfaces or occasionally conjunctival hemorrhages or gastrointestinal or vaginal bleeding. Also uncommon, but with poor prognosis, is edema of the face and neck. In the absence of peripheral edema, it indicates capillary leakage, rather than cardiac dysfunction or impaired venous return. About half have diffuse abdominal tenderness but there are no localizing signs and bowel sounds are usually active. Proteinuria occurs in two thirds of patients, and the blood urea nitrogen level may be moderately elevated.

Pulmonary and Cardiac. Pneumonitis and pleural and pericardial rubs develop in early convalescence in about 20% of patients, occasionally in association with congestive heart failure. Severe retrosternal or epigastric pain seen in many patients may be due to pleural or pericardial involvement. More than 70% of 32 patients had abnormal electrocardiograms. The changes included nonspecific ST-segment and T-wave abnormalities, ST-segment elevation, generalized low-voltage complexes, and changes reflecting electrolyte disturbance. None of the abnormalities correlated with clinical severity of infection, serum aminotransferase levels, or eventual outcome.

Neurologic. Signs are infrequent, but also carry a poor prognosis, progressing from fine tremors and confusion to severe encephalopathy with or without generalized seizures, but without focal signs. Cerebrospinal fluid (CSF) is usually normal; there may be a few lymphocytes/mm^3. Virus titers are lower in the CSF than in the serum.

Hematologic. The most significant hematologic changes are in platelet function. Although thrombocytopenia is moderate, even in severely ill patients, function is markedly depressed or even absent. This abnormality is usually maximal on admission to the hospital, and is characteristically present even when circulating platelet numbers remain normal. A circulating inhibitor of platelet function has been associated with severe disease; it specifically inhibits platelet-dense granule and adenosine triphosphate release, relatively sparing the thromboxane pathways.

Although the mean white blood cell count in LF on admission to hospital is 6000/mm³, there is characteristically early lymphopenia, relative thrombocytopenia, and sometimes a relative or absolute neutrophilia. Neutrophil counts as high as 30,000/mm³ have been recorded in severe cases. The inhibitor of platelet function also interferes with the generation of the chemotactic peptide formyl-methionylleucyl phenylalanine (FMLP)–induced superoxide generation in neutrophils.

Prognosis. Serum aminotransferase levels of greater than 150 are associated with a case-fatality rate of 50%. A second variable associated with outcome is the level of viremia; a blood virus level of greater than 1×10^3 is associated with an increasing case fatality. Both factors together carry a risk of death of 80%.

Complications

Maternal and Fetal Morbidity. LF may be a common cause of maternal mortality in many areas of West Africa. Two studies have shown that the case-fatality rate in pregnant women is about 20%. This is particularly the case in those infected during the third trimester of pregnancy, in whom high levels of virus replication have been found in placental tissue. A fourfold reduction in mortality was noted among women who spontaneously or were therapeutically aborted. Fetal loss was 87% and did not vary by trimester.

Deafness. Another important complication of LF is acute eighth nerve deafness. Nearly 30% of patients with LF infection have an acute loss of hearing in one or both ears. About half of the patients have a near or complete recovery, but in many the deafness is permanent.

Other less frequent complications are uveitis, pericarditis, orchitis, pleural effusion, and ascites. Renal and hepatic failure are not seen.

DIAGNOSIS

Clinical Diagnosis. All ages of children can be infected, and LF is difficult to diagnose because its manifestations are so general. In young babies, marked edema has been reported in severe infections. In older children, the disease may manifest as diarrhea or as pneumonia or simply as an unexplained prolonged fever.

Fever with pharyngitis, proteinuria, and retrosternal chest pain have a predictive value for LF of 81% and a specificity of 89%. Likewise, a triad of pharyngitis, retrosternal chest pain, and proteinuria in a febrile patient correctly predicted Lassa fever in an endemic area 80% of the time. However, these triads had sensitivities of only 50%. Bleeding and sore throat have a specificity for fatal outcome of 90%, however, these two criteria have a sensitivity of only 36%. On the other hand, vomiting and sore throat had a specificity of only 47% but a sensitivity of 89%.

Laboratory Diagnosis. Demonstration of a fourfold rise in antibody titer, isolation of virus, or demonstration of high-titer IgG antibody with virus-specific IgM antibody in association with compatible clinical disease all are means of establishing the diagnosis.

Antibodies. The most reliable and safe routine method for the laboratory is detection of virus-specific antibody by immunofluorescence (IFA). Slides of inactivated Lassa virus–infected tissue culture cells may be stored at −20C for 6 months or at −70C for several years. Generally, an IgG titer of at least 16 and IgM titer of 4 are considered specific for Lassa infection. Genetically engineered reagents should produce highly purified antigens, which in the future may avoid the false-positive reactions.

At least 50% of LF patients have measurable IgG or IgM antibodies by IFA by day 5 of illness, and virtually all have antibody by days 12 to 14. The IgG antibodies are directed against the glycoprotein and nucleocapsid of Lassa virus; they are often present simultaneously with high levels of viremia and during the most severe illness. Thus, antibody has little to do with recovery.

Virus Isolation. Virus may be isolated from serum specimens taken from acutely ill patients. Lassa virus requires laboratory biosafety level 4 facilities, so that any manipulation of live virus in tissue culture has to be performed in very specialized facilities. Lassa virus may easily be isolated in cell culture or suckling mice. Tissue culture should be harvested after 7 days, and tested by IFA for presence of virus. Mice are killed after 7 to 9 days and the brain harvested.

Specimens should be drawn into a vacuum tube system to minimize risk of spill, and the blood should be allowed to clot at room temperature. The serum is separated and placed in a sealable plastic vial for storage and/or transfer. Urine should be mixed with an equal amount of bovine serum albumin at pH 7.4 before freezing. Other fluids should be frozen undiluted. All of these specimens keep best if they are frozen at −70C or lower as soon as possible.

Viremia may be high and sustained (up to 4 weeks in some instances) in severe disease. Titers in milder cases are lower and of short duration. Lassa virus has been isolated from throat swabs during acute illness, but the titer is low and recovery variable. Virus has also been isolated from breast milk, spinal fluid, pleural and pericardial transudate, and autopsy material. Virus may be recovered for 1 to 2 months in urine, but its presence in urine during acute disease is sporadic.

Virus may be inactivated for safe laboratory manipulation for antibody studies by using heat, β-propriolactone, formalin, and ultraviolet radiation. Antigenic properties are best conserved by inactivation with gamma irradiation. Disinfection can be accomplished by washing with 0.5% phenol in detergent (for example, Lysol), 0.5% hypochlorite solution, formaldehyde, or peracetic acid.

Detection of Virus Protein or Nucleoproteins. Another reliable method of diagnosis is the detection of viral protein by monoclonal antibodies in tissue imprints (usually liver) on a microscope slide. This method has been used for postmortem diagnosis as well as for detecting lymphocytic choriomeningitis virus and Lassa virus antigens in rodent tissues using antinucleocapsid monoclonal antibodies. The nucleocapsid antigen is the most abundantly expressed antigen in infected cells during acute infection. Efforts to detect antigen in conjunctival scrapings, buffy coat preparations, cells from pharyngeal aspirates, and urinary sediment have not been successful. The use of cDNA probes is now allowing development of more sensitive methods of virus detection, and have now been adapted for diagnostic use, particularly using polymerase chain reaction (PCR) techniques on cells or tissue samples.

TREATMENT AND MANAGEMENT

Antiviral Therapy. Ribavirin, a guanosine analogue, is effective in treating acute Lassa fever. A 5- to 10-fold decrease in the case-fatality rate was demonstrated in patients treated with ribavirin compared with untreated patients when therapy was given within the first 6 days of illness. A smaller, but still significant, decrease in fatality was also demonstrated in patients treated later in illness. Patients with AST and viremia risk factors who were treated within the first 6 days of illness experienced a 5 to 9% case fatality. Those with the same risk factors receiving treatment more than 6 days after the onset of illness had a 26 to 47% fatality, compared with 52 to 78% mortality in those untreated. Furthermore, patients treated with ribavirin had a significant reduction in viremia regardless of outcome. The ribavirin was given as a 2-gm loading dose followed by 1 gm every 6 hours for 4 days, and then 0.5 gm every 8 hours for 6 more days.

Supportive Therapy. Since the pathogenesis is less reversible later in illness, patients treated after the first 5 or 6 days of illness require effective clinical management of their complications. Fluid, electrolyte, respiratory, and osmotic imbalances should be corrected to prevent clinical shock. However, even vigorous support of this kind may be insufficient to prevent fatal progression of advanced disease.

PREVENTION AND CONTROL

Rodent Control. The key to prevention and control would be to eliminate contact with rodents; this has been effective in trap-out studies in villages in Sierra Leone. However, the control of rodents as a broad approach to preventing LF is not realistic. Improvement of housing and food storage might reduce the domestic rodent population but such changes are not easily accomplished.

Efforts are currently being made in Sierra Leone to reduce transmission by education programs aimed at the population at risk. Emphasis on the known modes of transmission both from rodents and from other humans may help to reduce infections, but the effectiveness of these campaigns has yet to be evaluated.

Chemoprophylaxis. Because ribavirin is most effective when given early in disease it seems reasonable to assume that it would also be effective prophylaxis in the event of laboratory or hospital exposure to the disease. Although data on efficacy are lacking, it seems reasonable to recommend oral ribavirin as postexposure prophylaxis.

Vaccines. A candidate LF vaccine made by cloning and expressing the Lassa virus glycoprotein gene into vaccinia virus has proved highly successful in preventing severe disease and death in challenged monkeys. It is hoped that this vaccine will shortly be tested in humans for both safety and efficacy. At present, this is the most realistic and practical approach to control of this devastating public health problem.

Hospital Control. Although nosocomial transmission of Lassa virus occurred during the first outbreaks, basic barrier nursing methods (gloves, gowns, and masks) are highly effective in preventing secondary spread of the infection. Strict isolation with rigorous barrier nursing should be combined with full medical care, including surgery if indicated, to ensure the safety of the staff and survival of the patient.

Extensive nosocomial epidemics may result from reuse of inadequately sterilized equipment (needles, syringes, gloves, etc.) during surgery or midwifery. In this context, the importance of awareness by medical teams of the possibility of LF in patients with conditions such as abdominal pain or septic abortion cannot be overemphasized.

BIBLIOGRAPHY

Fisher-Hoch SP, McCormick JB, Auperin D, et al: Protection of rhesus monkeys from fatal Lassa fever by vaccination with a recombinant vaccinia virus containing the Lassa virus glycoprotein gene. Proc Natl Acad Sci USA 85:317, 1989.

Fisher-Hoch SP, McCormick JB, Sasso D, Craven RB: Hematologic dysfunction in Lassa fever. J Med Virol 26:127, 1988.

Fisher-Hoch SP, Mitchell SW, Sasso DR, et al: Physiological and immunological disturbances associated with shock in a primate model of Lassa fever. J Infect Dis 155:465, 1987.

Johnson KM, McCormick JB, King IJ, et al: Clinical virology of Lassa fever in hospitalized patients. J Infect Dis 155:456, 1987.

McCormick JB, King IJ, Webb PA, et al: Lassa fever. Effective therapy with ribavirin. N Engl J Med 314:20, 1986.

McCormick JB, King IJ, Webb PA, et al: A case-control study of the clinical diagnosis and course of Lassa fever. J Infect Dis 155:445, 1987.

McCormick JB, Webb PA, Krebs JW, et al: A prospective study of the epidemiology and ecology of Lassa fever. J Infect Dis 155:437, 1987.

Monath TP, Newhouse VF, Kemp GE, et al: Lassa virus isolation from *Mastomys natalensis* rodents during an epidemic in Sierra Leone. Science 185:263, 1974.

Price ME, Fisher-Hoch SP, Craven RB, McCormick JB: Prospective study of maternal and fetal outcome in acute Lassa fever during pregnancy. Br Med J 297:584, 1988.

Walker DH, McCormick JB, Johnson KM, et al: Pathologic and virologic study of fatal Lassa fever in man. Am J Pathol 107:349, 1982.

22.3. SOUTH AMERICAN HEMORRHAGIC FEVERS

Susan P. Fisher-Hoch

DEFINITION. The viruses causing South American hemorrhagic fevers are arenaviruses. As such they also cause persistent and, for the most part, silent infections of rodents. Humans, who are accidentally infected, develop a severe illness, sometimes with profuse hemorrhage.

Junin virus, the cause of Argentine hemorrhagic fever (AHF) and the first identified South American hemorrhagic fever virus, was isolated in 1958. Machupo virus, the cause of Bolivian hemorrhagic fever (BHF), was isolated in 1965. Both viruses were found to be related to Tacaribe virus isolated from Trinidad fruit bats. These viruses, together with numerous other nonpathogenic arenaviruses from South American rodents, have been assigned to the "Tacaribe complex," a group of antigenically related viruses that are distinct from the Old World arenaviruses, lymphocytic choriomeningitis virus, and Lassa viruses.

EPIDEMIOLOGY AND ECOLOGY. The viruses are transmitted from rodent to rodent both vertically and horizontally. Both of the South American viruses may cause illness and death in newborn mice or may induce persistence. Both induce a humoral immune response when transmitted to their suckling natural rodent hosts and may induce neutralizing antibody in the face of persistent infection. Machupo virus renders its major natural host *Calomys callosus* essentially sterile by causing the young to die in utero. Machupo virus also induces a hemolytic anemia in its rodent host with significant splenomegaly, often an important identifier of infected rodents in the field.

Argentine Hemorrhagic Fever. This was first recognized in the 1950s in the fertile farmland of northwestern Buenos Aires Province in Argentina. About 21,000 cases have been reported over 30 years. The disease is seasonal, with peaks each May. Although the average number of cases each year is about 360, wide annual fluctuations result in annual incidence ranging from 100 to 4000.

Reservoir Host and Transmission. The major rodent hosts for Junin virus are *Calomys musculinus* and *C. laucha*. Transmission from rodent to rodent is horizontal, not vertical, and is believed to occur through contaminated saliva and urine. The rodents are affected by the virus, with up to 50% fatality among infected suckling animals and stunted growth in many others. Unlike the peridomestic host of Lassa virus, these rodents occupy grain fields, and thus the group at risk is mainly field workers. The major routes of virus transmission to humans are probably through virus-infected dust and grain products in contact with cuts and abrasions on the skin, or possibly from dust generated by killing and scattering of infected rodents during mechanized farming.

Distribution. The disease has spread during the 30 years since its recognition from an area of 16,000 km² inhabited by a quarter of a million persons to an area greater than 120,000 km² with a population of more than 1 million. However, incidence in the earliest affected areas diminished after 5 to 10 years, possibly because the rodent population is adversely affected by the virus. Other possible explanations are changing farming practices and crops and human population fluctuations. Infection rates were high in operators of farm machinery, and a recent serosurvey in the endemic area showed an overall antibody prevalence of 12%, with a predominance in agriculture workers. One third of the seropositive individuals had no history of typical illness, suggesting that the case:infection ratio was about 2:3. The dynamics of Junin infection in human populations is clearly changing, but the basic reasons for these changes are unknown.

Bolivian Hemorrhagic Fever. Machupo virus is limited to a portion of the department of Beni in Bolivia. The only known reservoir for the virus is *C. callosus*, found in the highest density at the borders of tropical grassland and forest. This rodent apparently is distributed in the eastern Bolivian plains, as well as northern Paraguay and adjacent areas of western Brazil. By 1962, more than 1000 cases of BHF had been identified in a confined area of two provinces, with a 22% case fatality. The largest known epidemic of BHF involving several hundred cases followed a marked and unusual increase in the *Callomys* population in homes in the town of San Joaquin in 1963 and 1964. This seems to have been a unique event. There has been no increase in the geographic areas affected by BHF in the last decade, and virtually no cases have been reported.

PATHOPHYSIOLOGY

Pathology. Petechiae on the organ surfaces and ulcerations of the digestive tract have been described. Splenic hemorrhage is also common, and lymph nodes are enlarged from reticular cell hyperplasia. A major tendency to bleed is reflected in histologic observations of large areas of intra-alveolar or bronchial hemorrhage. Virus titers in serum are not as high as in Lassa fever, but the infection is also apparently pantropic.

Clinical observations lead to the conclusion that vascular endothelial dysfunction and subsequent circulatory failure are important causes of pathophysiologic changes in AHF and BHF. Persistent hypovolemic shock in the face of intravascular volume expanders suggest that this is caused by a loss of endothelial cell function and leakage of fluid into extravascular spaces. Microscopic examination shows a general alteration in endothelial cells and mild edema of the vascular walls, with capillary swelling and perivascular hemorrhage. As in Lassa fever, pulmonary edema is common in severely ill patients and intractable shock accounts for the majority of deaths from AHF and BHF. Observed cardiac involvement has been limited to hemorrhage and a lymphocytic infiltrate in the pericardium, and occasional interstitial myocarditis. It is likely, therefore, that there is a process similar to that in Lassa fever with failure of the intravascular compartment and leakage of fluids and macromolecules into the extravascular spaces, resulting in hemoconcentration and hypovolemic shock.

Immunity. The appearance of antibody, especially neutralizing antibody, in Junin infection coincides with disappearance of virus in the blood at the time the patient begins to recover from acute illness. This antibody may be effective in clearing virus during acute infection and may be sufficient to protect against future infections. This observation is supported by the fact that therapeutic efficacy of immune plasma in patients with Junin infection is directly associated with the titer of neutralizing antibody in the plasma given. Similar observations have been made in experiments with Machupo virus–infected monkeys. Furthermore, immediate reduction of viremia is associated with recovery from disease. Although elements of a cell-mediated immune response to Junin virus have been shown, its importance in virus clearance and subsequent protection are not known.

CLINICAL MANIFESTATIONS

Signs and Symptoms. AHF and BHF are clinically

similar diseases. Although in several respects they resemble the other hemorrhagic fever caused by an arenavirus, Lassa fever, there are important differences. Both AHF and BHF have insidious onset of a nonspecific illness consisting of malaise, high fever, general myalgia, lumbar pain, epigastric pain, conjunctivitis, retro-orbital pain, often with photophobia, and anorexia frequently progressing to nausea and vomiting. Although there may be a pharyngeal exanthem, there is no sore throat or cough. There is marked erythema of the face, neck, and thorax; lymph nodes are enlarged; and petechiae may be observed.

Complications. As in Lassa fever, organ function, other than the endothelial system, remains intact and histolopathologic lesions are minimal. Hepatitis is mild. Renal function is also well maintained although proteinuria and microscopic hematuria are common.

Hemorrhage and Shock. The critical period of shock is brief, lasting only 24 to 48 hours. A low white blood cell count is characteristic in acute disease. Nearly half of the patients with South American hemorrhagic fevers have hemorrhagic manifestation, most commonly epistaxis and/or hematemesis. Nevertheless, bleeding is not the cause of shock and death. Although platelet counts less than 100,000 mm^3 are invariable, alterations in clotting functions are minor, and disseminated intravascular coagulation is not a significant feature. The fluid loss and edema lead to irreversible shock and death in the most severely ill patients.

Neurological Findings. Fifty percent of AHF and BHF patients have neurologic symptoms such as tremors of the hands and tongue, progressing in some patients to delirium, oculogyrus, and strabismus. As in Lassa fever, the pathogenesis of central nervous system involvement is obscure, and there is no evidence for direct infection. A late neurologic syndrome has also been described, often associated with successful treatment with immune plasma and consisting mainly of cerebellar signs.

DIAGNOSIS

Antibodies. Neutralizing and complement-fixing antibody to Junin and Machupo viruses are usually detectable 3 to 4 weeks after the onset of illness. More recently, indirect fluorescent antibody (IFA) tests have detected antibodies by the end of the second week of illness. The IFA using inactivated infected cell monolayers (preferably by gamma irradiation) is the most commonly performed method for antibody detection. The slides may then be stored at −20C for 6 months or at −70C for several years. For determination of IgM antibodies the enzyme-linked immunosorbent assay (ELISA) may be superior to IFA.

Virus Isolation. The demonstration of effective therapy for AHF with immune plasma has increased the practical value of a rapid diagnostic test. Junin and Machupo viruses may be detected in serum by virus isolation using cell culture techniques or intracerebral inoculation of suckling mice. However, these reagents are classified as biosafety level 4 agents, and isolation should not be attempted without the protection of a high containment laboratory facility. Moreover, because virus isolation and identification require a few days to complete, it does not provide a rapid diagnosis. With

the emergence of genetically engineered antigens—obviating the need for production and inactivation of infectious reagents—antigen and nucleotide detection systems using ELISA or polymerase chain reaction (PCR) may simplify the diagnosis of acute clinical disease.

Disinfection of arenaviruses can be effectively accomplished by washing with 0.5% phenol in detergent (for example, Lysol), by 0.5% hypochlorite solution, or by formaldehyde or peracetic acid.

TREATMENT AND MANAGEMENT

Immune Plasma. In contrast to Lassa fever, convalescent-phase plasma has been shown to be highly successful in AHF, reducing the mortality from 16% to 1% in the patients treated in the first 8 days of illness. In treated patients, viremia is reduced within 24 hours, and clinical symptoms and hematologic alterations are less severe than in control cases receiving nonimmune plasma. Efficacy is directly related to the concentration of neutralizing antibodies.

Although immune plasma therapy is highly successful in patients treated early in disease, as with ribavirin-treated Lassa fever patients, those treated late in disease do not fare so well. Another problem has been the development of a late neurologic syndrome in about 10% of cases. It begins between 4 and 6 weeks after onset of acute illness and lasts less than a week. It is characterized by fever, headache, ataxia and intention tremors, and a mild cerebrospinal fluid pleocytosis with anti-Junin virus antibody in the cerebrospinal fluid. However, death from this syndrome is rare, and most patients recover within 3 months. Mild permanent damage to acoustic centers has been detected in a small group of patients. Furthermore, plasma therapy depends on collection, storage, and distribution of plasma from persons known to have had the disease, and screening to assess potency and freedom from adventitious agents such as those responsible for hepatitis, syphilis, and human immunodeficiency virus infection.

Chemotherapy. Ribavirin is the only drug shown to increase survival in experimentally infected primates, although a late neurologic syndrome has been described. Therapeutic use of ribavirin, particularly in the subgroup of patients presenting late in disease, is currently being explored.

PREVENTION AND CONTROL

Rodent Control. The ideal method of prevention is to prevent contact between rodents and humans. This principle was demonstrated in the outbreaks of BHF in the 1960s when rodent control programs in the villages were highly successful in eliminating the epidemic. The human-rodent encounter resulting in AHF occurs during the crop harvests, and with present technology it is difficult to imagine how control of noncommensal feral rodents could be accomplished. The best choice may be better protection of the agricultural worker from contact with rodent secretions and blood.

Vaccine. A live attenuated vaccine against AHF has been extensively evaluated in monkeys and is presently undergoing phase 2 testing in field trials in Argentina. This vaccine was derived from the XJ attenuated strain developed nearly 20 years ago. The initial strains of attenuated Junin virus were tested in volunteers, about one third of whom developed a fever with some constitutional symptoms. The current attenuated strain was developed in a cell line acceptable for human vaccine use and has been shown to have no adverse effects in primates, to prevent illness and death in vaccinated and subsequently challenged monkeys, and to be free of side effects in humans.

BIBLIOGRAPHY

Eddy GA, Wagner FS, Scott SK, Mahlaudt BJ: Protection of monkeys against Machupo virus by the passive administration of Bolivian hemorrhagic fever immunoglobulin (human origin). Bull WHO 52:723, 1975.

Elsner B, Schwarz E, Mando OG, et al: Pathology of 12 fatal cases of Argentine hemorrhagic fever. Am J Trop Med Hyg 22:229, 1973.

Enria DA, Franco SG, Ambrosio A, et al: Current status of the treatment of Argentine hemorrhagic fever. Med Microbiol Immunol 175:173, 1986.

Mackenzie RB, Beye HK, Valverde L, Garron H: Epidemic hemorrhagic fever in Bolivia. I. A preliminary report of the epidemiological and clinical findings in a new epidemic area in South America. Am J Trop Med Hyg 13:620, 1964.

Maiztegui JI, Fernandez NJ, de Damilano AJ: Efficacy of immune plasma in treatment of Argentine hemorrhagic fever and association between treatment and a late neurological syndrome. Lancet 2:1216, 1979.

Maiztegui JI, Feuillade M, Briggiler A: Progressive extension of the endemic area and changing incidence of Argentine hemorrhagic fever. Med Microbiol Immunol 175:142, 1986.

Melcon MO, Herskovits E: Complicaciones neurologicas tardias de la fiebre hemorragica argentina. Medicina (B Aires) 41:137, 1981.

Sabattini MS, de Rios LEG, Diaz G, Vega VR: Natural and experimental infection of rodents with Junin virus. Medicina (B Aires) 37:149, 1977.

Weissenbacher MC, Laguens RP, Coto CE: Argentine hemorrhagic fever. Curr Top Microbiol Immunol 134:79, 1987.

22.4. EBOLA AND MARBURG VIRUS INFECTIONS

Joseph B. McCormick

DEFINITION AND HISTORY. Marburg and Ebola viruses, members of the Filoviridae, burst from obscurity with spectacular outbreaks of severe, hemorrhagic fevers. Marburg virus appeared first and was isolated in 1967 in conjunction with 31 cases of fulminating febrile disease with hemorrhage in Europe (primarily in Marburg, Germany) among laboratory workers who were infected while preparing primary monkey kidney cell cultures from imported *Cercopithecus aethiops*. Nearly a decade later simultaneous outbreaks of another lethal hemorrhagic fever occurred in Zaire and Sudan. Ebola virus was associated with an outbreak of 318 cases and a case-fatality rate of 90% in Zaire and caused 150 deaths among 250 cases in Sudan. Numerous ecologic studies have failed to uncover the natural habitat of these viruses. Smaller outbreaks and single cases of each virus continue to occur periodically, particularly in East, Central, and southern Africa.

In late 1989, a hemorrhagic disease was recognized among cynomolgus macaques imported into the United States from the Phillippines. Strains of Ebola virus were isolated from these monkeys. Serologic studies in the Phillippines and elsewhere in Southeast Asia indicate that Ebola virus is a prevalent cause of infection among macaques. These observations raise serious concerns for transmission of Ebola viruses to humans exposed to wild-caught monkeys and extend the known geographic range of filoviruses to Asia.

ETIOLOGY. Detailed laboratory studies have placed these viruses into a newly designated family, the Filoviridae (*filo*, "threadlike"). The viruses are pleomorphic, with a highly variable length (up to 14,000 nm) apparently owing to concatamerization (Fig. 22–3). However, the average length of an infectious virion appears to be 790 nm for Marburg virus and 920 nm for Ebola virus. The virions are 80 nm in diameter with a helical nucleocapsid, a membrane made of 10-nm projections, and host cell membrane. The virions contain a unique single-stranded molecule of noninfectious (negative sense) RNA. The virus is composed of 7 polypeptides, a nucleoprotein, a glycoprotein, a polymerase, and 4 other undesignated proteins. Proteins are produced from polyadenylated monocistronic mRNA species transcribed from virus RNA. The replication in and destruction of the host cell is rapid and produces a large number of viruses budding from the cell membrane. The virus is destroyed by heating to 60C for 30 minutes as well as by exposure to ultraviolet light, gamma irradiation, lipid solvents, hypocholorite, and phenol-detergent disinfectants.

EPIDEMIOLOGY. Primary epidemics of Ebola and Marburg virus infections do not occur. All of the clusters or epidemics of infections by these viruses have resulted from person to person transmission, nosocomial spread, or laboratory infections. The mode of primary infection and the natural ecology of these viruses are unknown. Association with bats has been directly implicated in at least 2 episodes when individuals entered the same bat-laden cave in Eastern Kenya (one in 1980 and another in 1987). Both died of fulminant Marburg infections. The other episodes loosely implicating bats were the outbreaks of Ebola infections in Sudan in 1976 and 1979. In both instances, the primary infections were in workers of a cotton factory containing thousands of bats in the roof. In all instances, study of antibody in bats failed to detect evidence of infection, and no virus was isolated from bat tissue.

Marburg Virus Infection. The outbreak of Marburg virus in 1967 was caused by infection of individuals directly handling fresh monkey tissues in the laboratory. Several of the monkeys from which those tissues were taken also died of infection, but none of the animal handlers were infected. There were 31 human cases, 25 of which were primary infections and 6 of which were secondary cases. Five resulted from person to person contact at home or in the hospital and the sixth occurred as a result of sexual transmission of the virus several weeks after recovery. Virus was recovered from the semen of that patient's husband. The case-fatality rate in the 25 primary infections was 28%, but none of the 6 patients with secondary infections died. The source of infection to the monkeys was never determined, but it

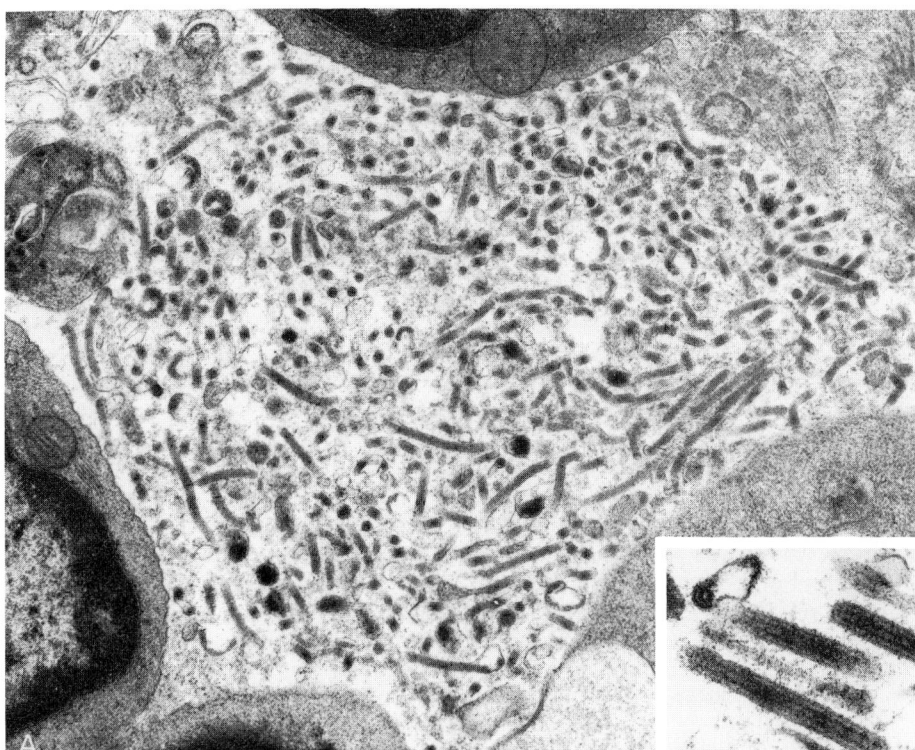

FIGURE 22–3. *A*, Thin-section electron micrograph of lymph node tissue (× 14,000). Ebola virions can be 10 μm in length and pleomorphic. *Inset*, Viral envelope around cylindric nucleocapsid at higher magnification (× 40,000). *B*, Ebola virus. Negative-stain electron micrograph (× 15,340) showing highly pleomorphic quality of extracellular viral particles, including elongated and branched forms. (*A* courtesy of Dr. John D. White; *B* courtesy of B. Geisbert.)

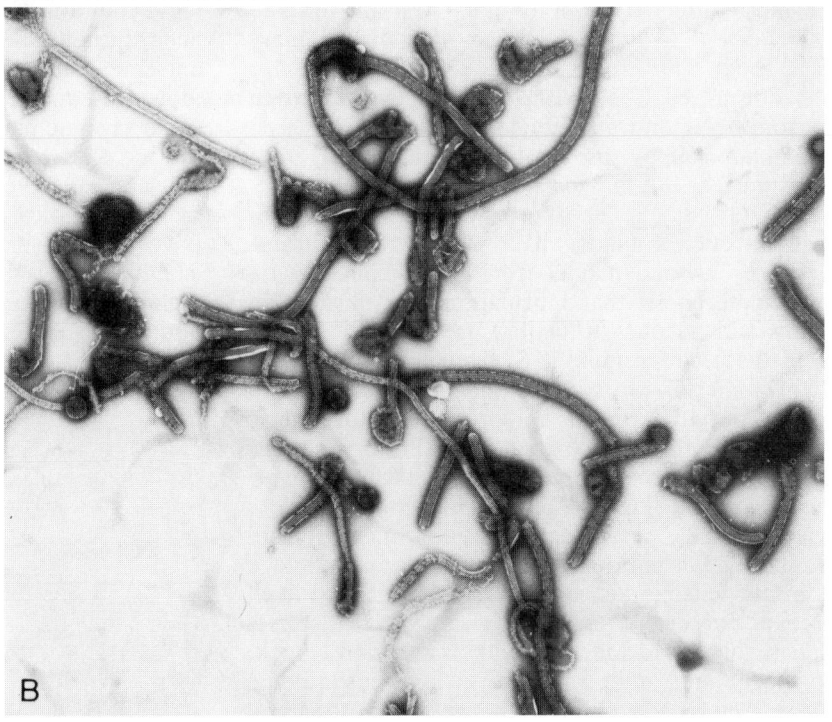

seemed clear that they were not the primary reservoir for the virus in view of the severity of disease and high fatality in these African Green monkeys. There have been several subsequent single cases or clusters of Marburg virus human infection in Kenya, Zimbabwe, and South Africa. A total of 4 index cases have resulted in 3 secondary infections. Three of 4 index cases died compared with none of the 3 secondary cases. A case fatality of 10 of 29 primary cases and none of 10 secondary cases is consistent with a reduction in viru-

lence following human to human transmission or possibly more intense and earlier medical care of secondary infections.

Ebola Virus Infection. There has been one large outbreak of Ebola virus infection in Zaire in 1976, and several single infections have been documented since that time. The index case in 1976 was never conclusively identified, but this large outbreak resulted in 280 deaths of 318 infections. The outbreak was primarily the result of person to person contact spread and transmission by contaminated needles in outpatient and inpatient departments of a hospital and subsequent person to person spread in surrounding villages. Risk factors for infection included injections at the hospital's outpatient department, nursing care of an ill patient, delivery of an abortus of a febrile woman, or preparation of a body at a funeral.

Further outbreaks of infections with an Ebola-related virus occurred in southern Sudan in 1976 and 1979. Both outbreaks were associated with an index case from the same nearby cotton-weaving factory. The outbreaks were caused by nosocomial and household person to person transmission. Two hundred eighty-four cases occurred in 1976 with a case-fatality rate of 53% (150 deaths), whereas 22 (65%) of 34 infections in 1979 were fatal. Investigations of risk factors for transmission in the 1976 and 1979 epidemics found physical contact with a patient to be the most important (Table 22–1). In this outbreak, there was a decreased case fatality following tertiary and quaternary transmission.

In serosurveys in Zaire, antibody prevalence to Ebola virus has been 3 to 7%. Serosurveys in noncontacts of patients in Sudan have had antibody prevalence of 1 to 4% to an Ebola-related virus. Because no formal surveillance for these viruses exists, the true incidence of disease is unknown.

The incubation period of primary Marburg disease appears to be 3 to 7 days, whereas that of secondary cases is about 5 to 8 days. The incubation period for needle-transmitted Ebola virus is 5 to 7 days and that for person to person transmitted disease is 6 to 12 days. The incubation period for the Ebola-related virus from Sudan is unclear but may be slightly longer.

PATHOGENESIS. The portal of entry in primary filovirus infection is unknown. Person to person transmission has resulted mainly from direct contact with infected material so that inoculation into minor skin abrasions and needle stick injury are of major importance in these circumstances. Such infections probably result in a shorter incubation period and more severe diseases. The virus appears to spread hematogenously and replicate in many organs. The histopathologic change is focal necrosis in many organs, including liver, lymphatic organs, kidney, testes, and ovaries. These lesions are usually not sufficient, even in the aggregate, to produce organ failure. The moderate organ damage seen in fatal infection is certainly not sufficient in itself to account for events associated with severe diseases and death, which include vascular dysfunction, shock, hemorrhage, and adult respiratory distress syndrome (ARDS). The most prominent changes are in the liver.

TABLE 22–1. Risk of Transmission of Ebola Virus by Degree of Person to Person Contact (Sudan, 1976 and 1979)

	1976			1979		
	Contacts	Cases	%	Contacts	Cases	%
Nursing care	48	39	81	60	24	40
Physical contact only	28	5	23	26	3	12
Entered room (no contact)	Not available			23	0	0

These are associated with elevated aspartate aminotransferase (AST) and alanine aminotransferase (ALT) with normal bilirubin and alkaline phosphatase levels. In addition the AST:ALT ratio is greater than 1, suggesting at least in part an extrahepatic source of AST. The central lesions appear to be those affecting the vascular endothelium and the platelets. The resulting manifestations are bleeding, especially in the mucosa, and extensive effusions in the pleura, abdomen, and pericardium. Animal studies have demonstrated a profound loss of in vitro platelet response to adenosine diphosphate and collagen, and a lack of endothelial cell production and prostacyclin. Capillary leakage appears to lead to loss of intravascular volume, bleeding, shock, and the ARDS seen in fatal infection. The exact mechanism of these events is unclear. A profound lymphopenia occurs initially, which is followed by marked neutrophilia in experimentally infected primates. However, there is little infiltration of inflammatory cells in areas of tissue damage. Laboratory evidence of only moderate disseminated intravascular coagulation (DIC) is present late in disease and probably is a consequence of the process rather than the underlying primary pathologic change.

CLINICAL MANIFESTATIONS

Symptoms and Signs. The diseases caused by all members of this family of viruses are similar in onset and evolution. Onset is abrupt, with fever, severe headache (usually periorbital and frontal), myalgia, and extreme malaise (Table 22–2). Conjunctivitis is common. A papular, eventually desquamating, rash may occur in some patients especially on the trunk and back. During the 3 or 4 days following onset, pharyngitis, nausea, and vomiting occur. Prostration and ghostlike facies are typical features (Fig. 22–4). Patients begin to have bleeding manifestations by 5 to 7 days of illness. The bleeding is primarily from the mucous membranes, including gastrointestinal tract, gingiva, nasopharynx, and vagina. Petechiae are not seen and ecchymoses are unusual. Patients die primarily of intractable shock associated with pulmonary insufficiency usually mani-

TABLE 22–2. Frequency of Symptoms and Signs in Fatal and Nonfatal Ebola Infections (Zaire, 1976)

	Fatal Infections			Nonfatal Infections		
	N	Frequency	%	N	Frequency	%
Symptoms						
Fever	231	226	98	34	20	59
Headache	210	202	96	34	20	59
Abdominal pain	201	163	81	34	17	50
Sore throat	207	164	79	34	11	32
Myalgia	206	163	79	34	16	47
Nausea	178	117	66	30	10	33
Arthritis	193	102	53	34	13	38
Signs						
Diarrhea	228	180	79	34	15	44
Bleeding	223	174	78	34	6	18
Oral/throat lesions	208	154	74	34	9	27
Vomiting	225	146	65	34	12	35
Conjunctivitis	208	121	58	34	12	35
Cough	208	75	36	34	6	18
Abortion	73	18	25	9	1	11
Jaundice	191	10	5	34	0	0

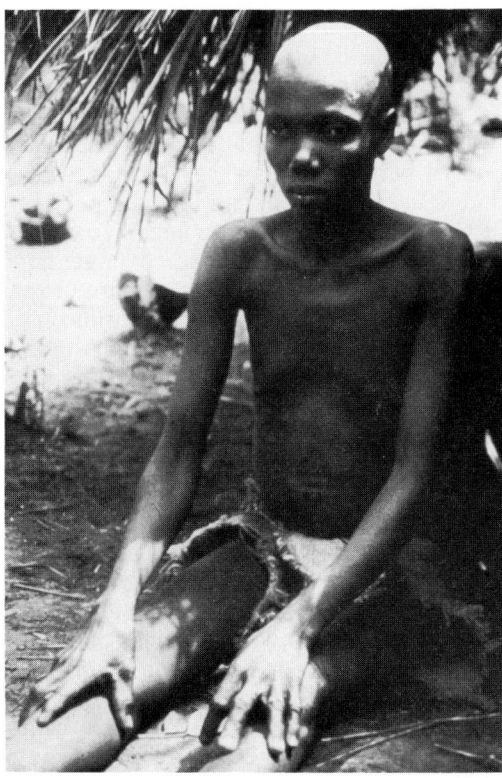

FIGURE 22–4. A case of Ebola virus disease in Zaire, 1976, showing the ghostlike facies typical of this highly lethal disease. The patient died 24 hours later.

fested as acute ARDS. Those with severe illness often have sustained high fevers and are delirious, combative, and difficult to control. Infection in pregnancy results in high maternal fatality and virtually 100% fetal death.

Laboratory Abnormalities. These include an early and often profound lymphopenia with a sudden shift to neutrophilia late in the infection. Thrombocytopenia is observed to levels not usually compatible with overt bleeding (50,000/mm³). However, studies in animals have shown that the platelets have profoundly abnormal in vitro aggregation. Levels of some enzymes are elevated, particularly AST and ALT (with AST > ALT). Specific liver-associated factors such as alkaline phosphatase and bilirubin levels are only mildly abnormal.

Differential Diagnosis. In the early stage of Ebola infection, any number of undifferentiated febrile illnesses that include malaria, influenza, arbovirus infection and bacterial infection, such as typhoid fever, would not be easily distinguished from Ebola virus disease. The appearance of a severe sore throat, chest and abdominal pain, and vomiting should make the clinician worry about this infection in the correct epidemiologic context. The persistence of vomiting and the onset of any signs of musocal bleeding are not only more specific clinical diagnostic signs but carry a high risk of fatal outcome.

LABORATORY DIAGNOSIS

Serology. The serologic method used in the discovery of Marburg and Ebola viruses was the indirect immunofluorescent assay, which remains the basic diagnostic serologic test for these viruses. The test is performed on a monolayer of infected and uninfected cells fixed on a microscropic slide. The cells are inactivated by gamma irradiation so that the assay may be performed in ordinary laboratory conditions, provided any acute serum specimen is also inactivated. Use of IgG- or IgM-specific conjugated antiserum permits a reasonably virus-specific immunoglobulin assay. Serologic tests may be confirmed by western blot or radioimmunoprecipitation. A rising antibody titer (fourfold) in paired serum or a high IgG titer (≥64) and presence of IgM antibody with a compatible clinical illness are also consistent with the diagnosis.

Virus Isolation. This is a highly useful diagnostic method and is performed on suitably preserved serum, blood, or tissue specimens stored at −70C or freshly collected. The virus may be isolated in Vero E-6 cells or SW-13 cells. The virus from Sudan is more fastidious and may require blind passage or use of animals such as suckling mice or guinea pigs.

In the event of a fulminant fatal infection, an impression preparation made from a postmortem liver biopsy may be probed with monoclonal antibodies for presence of virus antigen. This is particularly helpful when a rapid diagnosis is needed for subsequent clinical and epidemiologic decisions. Electron microscopy may also be used on tissue or blood specimens for a rapid diagnosis.

TREATMENT. No specific antiviral therapy presently exists for either Marburg or Ebola virus infections. Convalescent plasma has been used in a few instances, however, its value is doubtful. Convalescent plasma does not neutralize homologous virus in standard virus neutralization tests. In addition, it does not protect animals from simultaneous challenge with homologous virus. The danger of transmitting hepatitis and human immunodeficiency virus (HIV) reduce the attractiveness of its use, particular because its effectiveness is unknown. Human interferon has been used in 1 instance; however, in vitro studies have shown it to be without effect. Heparin has been advocated and used in some instances, but, because the filoviridae do not cause frank DIC, its use is without clear rationale, and it could prove detrimental. The most important aspect of the case is prevention of shock, ARDS, and accompanying complications.

Past recommendations for isolation of the patient in a plastic isolator have given way to the more moderate recommendation of strict barrier isolation with body fluid precautions. This presents no excess risk to hospital personnel and allows substantially better care to be given to the patient. The major factor in nosocomial transmission is the combination of the unawareness of the possibility of the disease by a worker who is also inattentive to the requirements of effective barrier nursing. After the diagnosis has been entertained and appropriate precautions used, the risk of nosocomial transmission is small.

PREVENTION AND CONTROL. The basic method of prevention and control is the interruption of person to person spread of the virus. The essential components of this task are the early identification of the clinical illness and appropriate precautions taken by family members and hospital workers. At present, the foundation of epidemic control of these diseases rests in early identification, case finding, and, most importantly, intervention in the spread of the disease within families. In rural areas, this may be difficult because families are often reluctant to admit members to the hospital because of limited resources and the culturally unacceptable separation of sick or dying patients from the care of their family. In rural clinics the careful decontamination of medical equipment after contact with blood or secretions, especially needles and syringes, is essential; these must never be used in a subsequent patient without sterilization. Finally, the observation of good nursing practices is paramount in preventing nosocomial spread.

Although a vaccine would have application in certain situations, e.g., for hospital personnel in endemic areas, in an outbreak situation, and for laboratory staff who work on these viruses, there is presently no vaccine available. Experience with human disease and primate infection suggests that a vaccine inducing a strong cell-mediated immune response will be necessary for virus clearance and adequate protection. Neutralizing antibodies are not observed in convalescent patients (within 6 to 10 weeks of recovery) nor do they occur in primates inoculated with killed vaccine. A vaccine expressing the glycoprotein in vaccinia is being prepared for laboratory evaluation.

BIBLIOGRAPHY

Baron RC, McCormick JB, Zubeir OA: Ebola virus disease in southern Sudan: Hospital dissemination and intrafamilial spread. Bull WHO 61:997, 1983.

Centers for Disease Control: Management of patients with suspected viral hemorrhagic fevers. MMWR 37(Suppl 3):1, 1988.

Fisher-Hoch SP, Platt GS, Neild GH, et al: Pathophysiology of shock and hemorrhage in a fulminating viral infection (Ebola). J Infect Dis 152:887, 1985.

Kiley MP, Cox NJ, Elliott LH, et al: Physicochemical properties of Marburg virus: Evidence for three distinct virus strains and their relationship to Ebola virus. J Gen Virol 69:1957, 1988.

Martini GA, Siegert R (eds): Marburg Virus Disease. New York, Springer, 1971.

Pattyn SR (ed): Ebola Virus Hemorrhagic Fever. Amsterdam, Elsevier/North Holland, 1978.

Report of an International Commission. Ebola hemorrhagic fever in Zaire, 1976. Bull WHO 56:271, 1978.

Report of a WHO International Study Team. Ebola hemorrhagic fever in Sudan, 1976. Bull WHO 56:247, 1978.

Sanchez AS, Kiley MP, Auperin DA, et al: The nucleoprotein gene of Ebola virus: Cloning, sequencing, and in vitro expression. Virology 170:81, 1989.

22.5. CRIMEAN-CONGO HEMORRHAGIC FEVER (CCHF)

Joseph B. McCormick

DEFINITION AND HISTORY. Crimean hemorrhagic fever is a tick-borne viral disease initially described in the Soviet Union in the 1930s. A virus was isolated in 1967 from an ill child in the Congo (now Zaire) and given the name of Congo virus. It was found in 1969 that the two viruses were closely related anti-

genically. The virus was renamed Crimean-Congo hemorrhagic fever (CCHF) virus. The disease is now known to occur from Eastern Europe through Asia, the Middle East, and all of Africa. Humans may be infected directly from the bite of a tick, by handling infected domestic animals, or by person to person spread via close contact with blood or secretions from an infected person.

ETIOLOGY. CCHF virus is a member of the *Nairovirus* genus of the Bunyaviridae, a large family of related viruses, most of which are transmitted to animals by insect or tick vectors. The spherical virions are 85 to 100 nm in diameter, with a unit membrane and regular surface projections. Because of the high biosafety level required for work with CCHF, most laboratory studies have been with closely related but less dangerous nairoviruses such as Hazara virus. Like all Bunyaviridae, the nairoviruses possess a tripartite negative sense (i.e., noninfectious) RNA genome. The nairoviruses differ from other genera in the molecular weights of the respective genomic segments, which are approximately 4.3, 1.5, and 0.6×10^6. The nucleocapsid core protein is about 50 kd, and the two glycosylated surface and membrane proteins 75 and 30 kd. In addition to recognized antigenic relationships, these properties are now used to distinguish the genus *Nairovirus* within the Bunyaviridae. The CCHF agent is the prototype of this taxon. Although coding strategies have not been resolved, on the basis of the familial coding strategy, it is assumed that the small RNA species encodes the nucleocapsid protein; that the middle RNA segment encodes the glycoprotein precursor, which is post-translationally cleaved to make the 2 virion glycoproteins; and that the large RNA segment encodes the virus-directed RNA polymerase.

ECOLOGY AND EPIDEMIOLOGY

Vectors and Reservoirs. CCHF virus is a parasite of ixodid (hard) ticks, which develop from eggs through 3 successive stages: larva, nymph, and adult. A blood meal is generally required at each postembryonic stage, and both sexes actively seek vertebrate hosts. Transovarial and/or trans-stadial transmission of CCHF virus occurs in several major tick vectors. It is therefore likely that ixodid ticks serve as both reservoir and vector of this agent. CCHF viruses have been isolated from at least 24 species and subspecies of ixodid ticks, belonging to 7 distinct genera. Among these are ticks of 1-, 2-, or 3-host types, and ticks with a wide mammalian host range.

The best-studied tick hosts and most important vectors to humans are *Hyalomma* spp., including *H. marginatum marginatum* of southeastern Europe and the Caspian region and *H. anatolicum anatolicum*, found in drier areas in southcentral Asia. Each is a 2-host species, the larva molting to nymph on the same animal, feeding then falling away to molt to an adult, which must find a new host animal. Adult *H. m. marginatum* prefer large domestic animals and avidly attack humans, whereas immature stages usually parasitize small ground-living or ground-feeding vertebrates, including birds. In contrast, all stages of *H. a. anatolicum* feed mostly on large domestic animals. Regardless, it is believed that the adult tick transmits infection to humans. Geographic variability of biologic behavior has important consequences for the epidemiology of CCHF.

Parasitization by ticks results in the infection of many domestic and wild animals and birds by CCHF virus. Certain birds such as rooks are not susceptible to infection from bites of ticks carrying CCHF virus and thus do not replicate virus; some data suggest, however, that ostriches may be effective viremic hosts. Nevertheless, transport of infectious ticks by birds may account for the wide geographic distribution of the virus. Mammals such as hares, cattle, sheep, and goats develop viremia, albeit low levels, when infected. The role, if any, of such viremias in amplification of virus infection in tick populations is unclear. The most important reservoirs as well as vectors of CCHF are infected ticks, which survive winter cold and which continue to support transovarial passage.

Human Epidemiology. The incubation period of CCHF is relatively brief, generally about 2 to 5 days, probably a consequence of direct hematogenous infection. The infectious dose of virus delivered by ticks is not known. Nosocomial infections may have an incubation of 5 to 9 days.

Seasonality. The seasonality of CCHF depends on the climate and the principal tick species. In the lower Volga and Don river basins of the Soviet Union where *H. m. marginatum* is the main vector, the disease occurs almost exclusively in the spring months of April to June when adult ticks become active. On the other hand, seasonality is much less pronounced in the Balkans, central Asia, and the Middle East, where the vector *H. a. anatolicum* and other ticks feed exclusively on domestic animals, although more cases are generally registered in the warmer months. Sheep shearing, particularly in autumn, may be a risk factor in infection. In Africa, mostly nonhemorrhagic human illness has been observed that is sporadic and without a clear seasonal pattern. More recently, however, CCHF has emerged as an important disease in the arid farming areas that have high tick populations, with peaks of disease in the spring and fall coinciding with maximal tick infestation.

Prevalence of Disease. Little is known about the illness:infection ratio of CCHF virus. In the southern Soviet Union, 1 in 5 infections resulted in clinical illness sufficient for individuals to seek medical attention. A recent study in an endemic region of South Africa suggests high illness:infection ratios in this area (70% of those with evidence of past infection were hospitalized with CCHF disease). These observations may be explained by poor identification of illness and or infections in some areas, or possibly differences in pathogenicity of viruses in different geographic areas. Furthermore, inapparent infection appears to be the rule for mammalian species, with the exception of humans.

The case-fatality rate, like the illness:infection ratio, appears to vary. This may be a consequence of the relative availability of medical and diagnostic services. There may be strain differences in virulence, but there are no studies to provide evidence for this or even for the existence of more than 1 CCHF virus able to infect humans. In the southern Soviet Union, where disease surveillance is more complete, milder disease forms are often noted and fatalities rarely exceed 5 to 10%. In South Africa from 1981 to 1986, the case-fatality rate was 35% with good medical facilities and surveillance. In central Asia and the Middle East, case-fatality rates of 35 to 50% are recorded, which may be higher in nosocomial outbreaks. These observations suggest that virus variation may be important in determining pathogenicity; however, in making comparisons, marked differences in the ability to diagnose and treat cases and existence of surveillance systems must be considered.

Occupational Exposure. CCHF in the Soviet Union is a disease of adults who handle and/or milk cattle, and any sex difference is a function of sex division in agricultural practice. Milkmaids in some areas and sheep handlers in others appear to be at greatest risk. CCHF equally infects males and females and persons of all age groups in central Asia and Iraq. This is explained by the "peridomestic" nature of the disease, which may occur even in urban areas, where people live in close daily proximity to sheep, goats, and camels and the associated infected ticks. The only case-control study of risk factors in human infections was in South Africa, and this did not show a positive association with tick infestation or animal slaughter. CCHF was, however, associated with handling of young sheep and with handling of goats (for vaccination, castration, ear notching, or tail docking). Antibody prevalence in domestic animals was high in this study (i.e., 15% of sheep, 39% of cattle, and 53% of goats); however, evidence of human infection was only 2.7%, and these were individuals with daily animal exposure.

Transmission. Accumulated experience suggests that transmission of CCHF virus occurs from bites of infected ticks or through contamination by blood or infected material from animals or other humans. The high prevalence in endemic areas of anti-CCHF antibodies in domestic animals and the relatively lower prevalence in humans shows transmission from animals to humans (whatever the route) to be infrequent. Animal infection may be associated with brief and low viremia and therefore would only occasionally result in human infection, depending on the type of human-animal interaction. In the recent study in South Africa, young animals (<6 months) were associated with disease transmission perhaps because of increased hazard due to higher and more prolonged viremia. Lacking are the correlation of animal infection, tick infestation, and population of ticks infected. It is clear that tick bites are frequent in persons living among domestic animals in CCHF endemic areas. The relatively low frequency of human CCHF infection therefore suggests that a minority of these bites result in infection, either because of low infection in ticks or inefficiency of virus transmission to humans.

PATHOPHYSIOLOGY AND PATHOLOGY. Viremia, thrombocytopenia, and lymphopenia are features of the acute disease process. Eosinophilic necrosis of the liver (Councilman bodies are present) without inflammatory reaction is a prominent pathologic observation. There is lymphoid depletion with significant necrosis of red and white pulp in the spleen. Hemorrhages are widely distributed in many organs, and death in this disease is often partially attributable to blood loss. The basic changes, however, most resemble those noted in Marburg and Ebola disease. Although it is highly possible that disseminated intravascular coagulation (DIC) is important in the pathogenesis of CCHF, definitive hematologic studies and pathologic evidence at autopsy are lacking.

CLINICAL MANIFESTATIONS

Symptoms and Signs. There is a rapid onset with severe headache, fever, chills, myalgia strongly localized to the lower back, joint pains, and epigastric pain. Conjunctivitis and a mild flushing of the face and chest, pharyngeal hyperemia, and petechiae on the palate are frequent. Bradycardia is typical. Diarrhea occurs occasionally. The fever may be high (40C). Patients are anorectic, irritable, or obtunded. Hemorrhage may begin as early as 3 to 5 days after onset. Epistaxis and gum bleeding are common. Hematuria, proteinuria, and azotemia are associated with severe disease and a poor prognosis. Bleeding may occur at any mucosal surface as well as from venipuncture sites, with development of large, huge, pressure-linked ecchymoses (Fig. 22–5). There is biochemical evidence of hepatocellular damage, which may be associated with severe hepatic impairment and uncontrolled bleeding. Pulmonary edema and hypovolemic shock, due to capillary leakage and blood loss, portend a fatal outcome. In severe cases, the combination of low platelet counts and hepatorenal failure may lead to DIC, but its relative importance to the hemorrhage is at present unclear. A variety of neurologic signs have been described, but these suggest encephalopathy rather than viral encephalitis, meningitis, or myelitis. Changes in affect and mood, including aggressive behavior, are described. Recovery may be

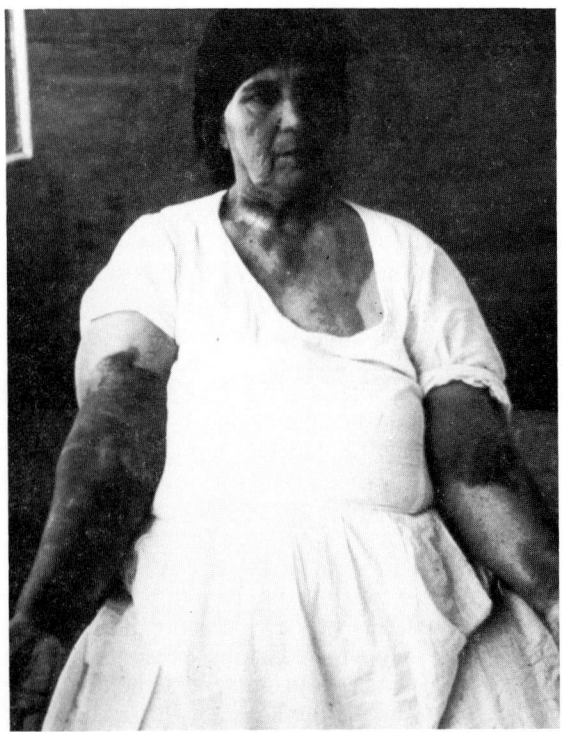

FIGURE 22–5. A patient with Crimean-Congo hemorrhagic fever, USSR. Of all the viral hemorrhagic fevers, CCHF is characterized by the most severe ecchymoses.

slow. Results of serosurveys suggest that subclinical or asymptomatic infections occur.

Laboratory Findings. The white blood cell count may be low ($<2000/mm^3$) in the early days of illness. Lymphopenia persists throughout the illness, while later in the disease (after 7 to 10 days), particularly in severe disease, a rise in neutrophils may be observed. Severe thrombocytopenia with counts below 20,000 per mm^3 is frequently encountered. Biochemical tests may show marked hepatocellular dysfunction and subsequent severe impairment of renal function.

DIAGNOSIS. Diagnosis of CCHF infection is made by isolation of the agent from blood of acutely ill patients or by immunologic methods. Suckling mice are highly susceptible to infection, and CCHF virus can be recovered from brain of these animals 3 to 6 days following inoculation and identified by a number of methods including hemagglutination-inhibition (HI), enzyme-linked immunosorbent assay (ELISA), neutralization, or immunofluorescence (IF) techniques. Several types of cultured cells may be used to isolate virus strains, but in most cases infection is not cytolytic. The virus is fairly stable in blood for up to 10 days at 4C, but transport at −50C or less is important for virus isolation.

Acute and convalescent paired sera are used to demonstrate an increase in virus-specific antibodies by ELISA or IF tests. These antibodies may be present 7 to 10 days after infection from CCHF virus, and neutralizing antibodies occur after day 14 to 16, but they persist for many years.

MANAGEMENT

Specific Measures. Treatment of acute CCHF with immune plasma had little success when attempted by Soviet workers, with no difference in duration of viremia or fever, or clinical outcome of 61 persons given 60 to 160 ml of plasma containing CCHF antibodies as compared with 88 subjects who received normal plasma. The virus is sensitive to ribavirin in vitro so intravenous chemotherapy early in disease is a potential approach, and preliminary clinical trials indicate efficacy.

Supportive. In addition to the careful management of fluid and electrolyte dynamics during the acute stages of disease, CCHF is the one viral hemorrhagic fever in which whole blood, platelets, and fresh plasma may be indicated. Such therapy needs to be accompanied by careful observations to determine if such therapy is truly beneficial.

Patient Isolation. Together with Lassa, Marburg, and Ebola viruses, CCHF, especially outside Africa, is an agent known for its propensity to produce nosocomial and intrafamilial secondary infection. Infectious blood and vomitus are the most likely vehicles of such transmission. Strict isolation, restriction of attendant personnel, and observance of enteric precautions are the minimum essentials to limit exposure of patient caregivers (Chapter 22.2).

PREVENTION AND CONTROL. Avoidance of tick bite or contact with blood from infected engorged ticks is the most effective strategy for prevention of infection. Repellents applied to skin, or better, soaked into clothing prior to its use, are the methods of choice. Slaughter of potentially viremic animals is also a hazard, and care should be taken to avoid contamination of cuts or mucous membranes by blood from viremic animals or from infected ticks damaged during such procedures as shearing, dehorning, or castration. Similarly, care of infected patients should avoid blood contact, and high-risk procedures such as mouth to mouth resuscitation are to be avoided.

A formalin-inactivated CCHF vaccine produced from brains of suckling mice has been reported and is currently used in Bulgaria in high-risk groups, such as farmers and border guards, but no efficacy data are available.

Reports from the Soviet Union have described the use of 2% hypochlorite to control virus-transmitting ticks. When used for dipping dairy cattle, it reduced tick infestation and CCHF infection rates among milkmaids. Reasonable control of adult ticks was achieved for about 6 weeks when it was applied at the rate of 50 to 100 L/ha to pastures. Longer lasting results were achieved with immature stages, which are the virus transmitters in subsequent years. There are also natural phenomena in nature which may also be effective. In the Rostov region of the Soviet Union, an exceptionally cold winter in 1968 to 1969 was followed by a fourfold reduction in disease in 1969 and the complete absence of human infection in 4 of the succeeding 5 years. *H. m. marginatum* virtually disappeared, but the cold-resistant *Rhipicephalus rossicus*, which rarely attacks humans, showed no such decline and continued to maintain CCHF. Since 1975, both *H. m. marginatum* and human disease have again increased.

BIBLIOGRAPHY

Burney MI, Ghafoor A, Saleen M, et al: Nosocomial outbreak of viral hemorrhagic fever caused by Crimean hemorrhagic fever–Congo virus in Pakistan, January 1976. Am J Trop Med Hyg 29:941, 1980.

Casals J: Antigenic similarity between the virus causing Crimean hemorrhagic fever and Congo virus. Proc Soc Exp Biol Med 131:233, 1969.

Casals J, Henderson BE, Hoogstraal H, et al: A review of Soviet viral hemorrhagic fevers, 1969. J Infect Dis 122:437, 1970.

Hoogstraal H: The epidemiology of tick-borne Crimean-Congo hemorrhagic fever in Asia, Europe, and Africa. J Med Entomol 15:304, 1979.

Simpson DIH, Knight EM, Courtois G, et al: Congo virus: A hitherto undescribed virus occurring in Africa. I. Human isolations—clinical notes. East Afr Med J 44:87, 1967.

Swanepoel R, Shephard AJ, Leman PA, et al: Epidemiologic and clinical features of Crimean-Congo hemorrhagic fever in southern Africa. Am J Trop Med Hyg 36:120, 1987.

Watts DM, Ksiazek TG, Linthicum KJ, Hoogstraal H: Crimean-Congo hemorrhagic fever. *In* Monath TP (ed): The Arboviruses: Epidemiology and Ecology, Vol II. Boca Raton, FL, CRC Press, 1988, pp 177–222.

Yu-Chen Y, Ling-Xiong K, Ling L, et al: Characteristics of Crimean-Congo hemorrhagic fever virus (Xinjiang strain) in China. Am J Trop Med Hyg 34:1179, 1985.

22.6. DISEASES CAUSED BY HANTAVIRUSES
(Hemorrhagic Fever with Renal Syndrome)

Joseph B. McCormick

DEFINITION AND HISTORY. Hemorrhagic fever with renal syndrome (HFRS) is the current appellation given to a disease first described in various parts of the world in the 1930s and now known to be caused by a collection of related viruses. These viruses persistently infect a variety of rodent species that occupy ecologic niches throughout the Far East and Eastern and Western Europe, and have been divided into 4 general serologic groups. These groups are determined primarily by the rodent host species; thus, Hantaan virus represents those viruses carried by *Apodemus* spp. rodents; the viruses carried by voles (*Clethrionomys* spp.) are represented by Puumala virus; and those carried by *Rattus* spp. are represented by Seoul virus. The group of viruses found in *Microtus* spp. have not yet been associated with human disease. More recently, a related virus has been isolated from *Mus musculus* in the United States, but its serologic relationship to the other viruses and to human disease is unknown.

The distribution of a particular virus is determined by the rodent it parasitizes. In rural areas field mice and/or voles often predominate and Hantaan or Puumala viruses prevail. In urban or semiurban settings, the virus type will be that carried by *Rattus* spp. Because different degrees of illness also depend on the infecting virus, severity is geographically distinct, with severe disease caused by Hantaan virus in the *Apodemus* habitats in the Far East and milder nephropathia epidemica in the vole habitats of Europe.

ETIOLOGY. The hantaviruses are members of the Bunyaviridae. The tripartite negative stranded genome consists of a large (L) RNA segment, which encodes the polymerase gene; a medium (M) RNA, which encodes the glycoprotein gene; and a small (S) RNA, which encodes the nucleoprotein gene. The nucleoprotein would appear to be the most conserved among the viruses, whereas the glycoprotein, the major component of the viral envelope is more antigenically variable. The two envelope glycoproteins result from post-translational processing of a glycoprotein precursor. These are also the sites of neutralizing epitopes now identified on both glycoproteins.

The viruses, particularly the vole-associated ones, are difficult to isolate and replicate to high titers. They replicate best in Vero E-6 or CV1 cells and maximal titers are achieved in 7 to 10 days. The viruses also replicate in suckling mice or gerbils.

EPIDEMIOLOGY AND ECOLOGY. Human disease depends on intimate contact with rodents, such as may occur in agricultural areas with high human and rodent population densities, during military campaigns or exercises, or in crowded urban housing.

Reservoirs. In the Soviet Far East, mainland China, and Korea, the best known rodent host is the Manchurian striped field mouse, *Apodemus agrarius*, but virus has now also been identified in *Clethrionomys* spp., especially in the Soviet Union, and *Rattus* spp. in China,

Korea, Japan, and Southeast Asia. A specific correlation was made in 1961 when 129 employees of a scientific institute in the Soviet Union became ill following the introduction into the institute of a large number of wild-caught rodents, including some *Apodemus sylvaticus*. In Korea, virus has been isolated from *A. sylvaticus* in forests and *A. agrarius* in secondary and wet forests and in fields, *Microtus* in grasslands, and *Clethrionomys* in settings such as forests, domestic gardens, and agricultural areas. In Scandinavia, the *Clethrionomys* spp. are the predominant hosts, which is probably true of most of the rest of Europe, with the exception of Greece, and possibly also other Balkan countries, where *Apodemus* spp. have been primarily implicated.

In the United States, viruses have been isolated from *Rattus* and *Microtus* spp.; although specific antibodies have been detected in human serum, evidence of overt human disease is still lacking. Human infections from infected laboratory rat colonies, however, have been reported in Japan, Korea, Belgium, and the United Kingdom.

Seasonality and Occupational Exposure. HFRS in the Soviet Union, China, and Korea may be epidemic or sporadic in agricultural, sylvatic, or urban settings. Rural epidemics occur in early summer and late fall. These are thought to be temporally related to harvests and migration of field rodents, particularly movement into houses at the onset of cold weather. Furthermore, the fall peak is apparently associated with *Apodemus* infections and the spring peak with *Rattus*. The disease was noted to be highly associated with dust production in a study of forest workers, and in France aerosol infection has also been implicated. During the numerous reports of epidemics during military campaigns, infections have been associated with trench warfare and bivouaks in the open.

Epidemics in the People's Republic of China have been increasing in size and can be large in some rural areas, creating an important public health problem. In Korea, much of the disease is sporadic, with fewer large clusters of cases. In Europe, especially Scandinavia, the disease is rural and associated with forestry or agricultural pursuits. The disease is sporadic, not epidemic, and most cases occur in winter.

Urban disease, such as reported originally from Japan and now from Korea and China, is sporadic and endemic, and is associated with crowded, rat-infested housing. Although the disease is apparently milder, it is possible that the scale of this problem is not yet appreciated, especially in some densely populated Asian urban centers.

Institutional epidemics associated with persistently infected colonized laboratory rats have also been recorded in several countries, including the Soviet Union, Japan, and Belgium. Some continuous rodent cell lines have been persistently infected and may also be a hazard to laboratory staff.

Transmission. There is no evidence for the spread of this virus from person to person, and no nosocomial transmission has been reported. The overwhelming evidence is that spread is from rodent to human through contact with infected rodent secretions or airborne transmission by infected dust particles.

It is clear that this group of viruses can be transmitted to persons of any age and depend only on the ecologic setting and opportunities for rodent-human contact. In rural areas, mostly adult males are affected, especially forestry and agricultural workers, but in urban and densely populated rural areas, both sexes and all age groups are involved, with increased risk associated with poor housing. In the Soviet Union, those tending peri-urban gardens are exposed; in Scandinavia, individuals with summer homes are at risk, with rodent contact occurring usually in sheds or barns.

Case-fatality rates vary widely, affected not only by the level of care given to the severely ill, but also by the particular infecting virus. However, the original distinctions are becoming less clear, and investigations are needed to focus on the details of association between the patient and the rodent reservoir. Trapping and identification of rodents from the patient's surroundings are essential elements in confirming the source of infection. Although the emergence of *Hantavirus* as a new genus of the Bunyaviridae might suggest vector transmission, there is now sufficient accumulated evidence to show that, although mite transmission in particular remains conceivable, vector transmission is not the most important source of human infection and is also unlikely to be of major importance in rodent to rodent spread.

PATHOGENESIS

Vascular Collapse. Virus may be isolated from serum or whole blood most often early in disease. The drop in viremia coincides with the appearance of antiviral antibody and with the onset of shock followed by renal disease, suggesting an immune-mediated origin. Extreme vascular instability with shock, oliguria or anuria, and bleeding are thus clinical hallmarks of severe HFRS. Substantial capillary leakage leads to extravasation of fluid and protein far in excess of the loss of erythrocytes. This results in periorbital and subscleral edema, and pulmonary edema, massive proteinuria, and finally the hypovolemic shock characteristic of severe HFRS. In certain severe cases, adult respiratory distress syndrome may also occur. An elevated hematocrit characterizes the hemoconcentration mainly during the shock/oliguric phase of the illness. Despite the clear physiologic failure of the endothelial cells, they do not appear histologically to be damaged.

Acute Renal Failure. A usually self-limited episode of acute renal failure following shock is a characteristic of HFRS and distinguishes it from most other viral hemorrhagic fevers. Kidney function rapidly deteriorates, sometimes to anuria, about 24 hours after the onset of shock, and dialysis may be required. Biochemical evidence of renal failure reflects the degree of oliguria or anuria. Postmortem examination has shown large and edematous kidneys, with medullary hemorrhage. There is commonly interstitial edema of the cortex with distention of Bowman's capsule and renal tubules by homogeneous, eosinophilic deposits. Antigen-antibody complexes have been reported in blood and tissues, including renal tissue. These observations support the notion that the renal tubular damage characteristic of HFRS may be caused by immune complex deposition.

Bleeding. Pathologic changes from the few fatal cases studied reflect the severe end of the spectrum. Vascular changes are prominent and are characterized by capillary dilation, erythrocyte diapedesis, focal hemorrhages, interstitial edema, and gross retroperitoneal edema. There is no evidence of direct invasion and lytic replication by the virus, though immunofluorescent studies in mice and humans show viral antigen on endothelium. It is possible that with or without immune complexes, virus may become adherent to endothelial cells or be able to establish a nonlytic infection.

Subendocardial hemorrhages, especially in the right atrium and atrial appendage, are described. Electrocardiographic changes may include arrythmias, heart block, and signs of pericarditis and myocarditis. Liver function test results may be mildly abnormal; in about 30% of patients examined postmortem, mild focal hepatic necrosis is seen in the outer zonal portion of lobules. There is no evidence of direct central nervous system involvement.

Although bleeding is rare, uncontrolled hemorrhage remains the most difficult problem for clinical management, with death occurring from intracranial bleeding. Other parynchemal neurologic involvement has not been observed. Severe thrombocytopenia is a uniform finding, with about half of the patients having less than 100,000 platelets/mm³. Consequently, petechiae are characteristic. Clinical and laboratory evidence do not suggest consumption coagulopathy or bleeding from hepatic failure. Disseminated intravascular coagulation (DIC) has been reported occasionally as a complicating terminal event, but not as a feature of the primary bleeding disorder. The genesis of the hemorrhagic diathesis in those patients who bleed is still obscure.

The white blood cell count may be elevated sometimes to between 10,000/mm³ and 20,000/mm³ and immature granulocytes are seen at the end of the first week. Lymphocytic cells become predominant during the second week of illness, but a marked neutrophilia may occur.

CLINICAL MANIFESTATIONS

Symptoms. The incubation period of HFRS ranges from 12 to 21 days, and mild or subclinical infections are common. Little is known about viral invasion, primary site of replication, and host response. There is evidence that infection can be acquired from airborne virus. Classically, the disease has been divided into febrile, hypotensive, oliguric, diuretic, and convalescent phases, but in practice these stages overlap. The prodromal stage is mild and nonspecific, but onset is usually abrupt with chills, high fever, lethargy, and dizziness. Frontal or retro-orbital headache may be accompanied by ocular pain and photophobia and blurring of vision. Mild myalgia and generalized aching, severe abdominal and back pain, anorexia, nausea, and vomiting are all common. There may also be an unproductive cough, but other than modest injection of the soft palate and tonsils, there is little evidence of respiratory tract involvement.

Signs. On examination, there is a typical erythematous facial flush, especially extending to the supraorbital ridges and spreading to the neck, shoulders, and upper thorax. There may be blanching on pressure and dermatographia. Petechiae on the soft palate and axillae are almost invariable, but may also be observed on the face, neck, upper thorax and axillary folds, hips, and thighs. The liver may occasionally be palpable, and the abdomen is soft, but most commonly there is abdominal and renal tenderness.

Clinical Course and Complications. Many patients make an uneventful though slow recovery after the febrile stage, but some deteriorate, entering the hypotensive phase, which usually begins as the temperature falls toward normal. If fever persists with hypotension, the prognosis is poor. Shock may occur by day 3, but usually not before day 5 or 6. This is mild and short lived in most patients, but in some it can be severe. Bleeding and increased number of petechiae may be seen and occasionally severe bleeding with convulsions and death, particularly when the infecting strain is transmitted by *Apodemus*. The oliguric phase follows within 24 hours of the onset of shock and may overlap with the hypotensive phase. Renal function deteriorates and the patient may become anuric and require dialysis. Recovery is then usually rapid, though hypertensive episodes may occur, and diuresis may be marked. Occasional deaths may still result from intracranial bleeding. Reports of case-fatality rates range from 1 to 10%, but overall about 4% can be expected in areas where *Apodemus* are found. Improvements in these rates usually result from physician experience in managing the particular problems associated with this disease.

Strain Variations in Severity. HFRS acquired from urban rats appears to be less severe, and the disease in Scandinavia acquired from voles has traditionally been described as a separate entity, *nephropathia epidemica,* which is considered to be milder still. Hemorrhage and shock are unusual, oliguria is rarely severe enough to warrant dialysis, and fatal outcome is virtually extraordinary. However, severe cases have been reported from France, Greece, Yugoslavia, and the Balkan countries where other *Apodemus* spp. have been implicated as hosts. The clinical distinction between diseases occurring in Asia and those in Europe has become less clear. In North America, viruses have been isolated, and serologic evidence of human infection observed, however, human disease has not been reported. It is possible that a mosaic of viruses with varying virulence exist, and prospective clinical studies are needed to understand the true illness associated with various virus strains and human disease.

DIAGNOSIS. Laboratory diagnosis of hantavirus infections can be made by demonstration of a rise in specific antibodies, demonstration of virus-specific IgM, and virus isolation.

Serology. A high proportion of patients with acute illness have IgM and IgG antibody at the time of hospital admission. Serologic assays include enzyme-linked immunoassays, including IgM capture, and immunofluorescence, which, although simple, may give false-positive results. Antibodies persist for up to 3 decades. Antibodies react to highest titer with homologous antigens, but in general, sera from patients infected by virus from *Clethrionomys* and *Rattus* react to higher titer against strains from *Apodemus* than *Apodemus*-derived strains to those transmitted by *Clethrionomys* or *Rattus*. Virus neutralization is strain specific; although laborious, it is the only method available for determining the probable infecting strain. Several of the *Hantavirus* epitopes appear to be conformationally dependent, so that radioimmunoprecipitation, rather than western blot, may be better in detecting antibody to individual viral proteins. Virus-specific DNA probes and peptides may eventually be helpful in determining strain differences both in serologic tests and in probing tissue specimens from wild-caught rodents.

Virus Isolation. Virus isolation requires careful handling and transport and storage of specimens at −70C and is labor intensive. It should only be attempted under biosafety level 3 or 4 conditions. The E-6 clone of Vero cells may be used, and, for greater sensitivity, isolation may be made by intracerebral inoculation of suckling mice or gerbils. A range of monoclonal antibodies is available for identification of isolates.

MANAGEMENT

Antiviral Therapy. Recent studies have shown that intravenous ribavirin may be useful in HFRS if given on or before the fourth day of disease. The dose of ribavirin and schedule have been similar to those described for Lassa fever (Chapter 22.2). Treatment with immune plasma would be inappropriate; it could have deleterious immunologic effects as well as being ineffective, because many patients already have neutralizing antibody on admission.

Supportive Therapy. Management of the patient should focus on fluid balance. Intravenous fluids during the febrile and shock phases may leak into the extravascular space, aggravating edema, particularly during the period of oliguria. Severe pulmonary edema may result in death. Patients may respond temporarily to vasopressors, but their use seems limited. In China, cyclophosphamide, which presumably inhibits immune-mediated damage, has been used, and, although reports are favorable, no rigorous controlled clinical trials have been done. Diuretics are relatively ineffective, and peritoneal dialysis or hemodialysis may be lifesaving in certain cases. With careful fluid management, most patients make a spontaneous and complete recovery. The occurrence of long-term renal damage, if any, is unknown. Uncontrolled hemorrhage remains the most intractable cause of death, but therapy such as heparin is contraindicated because there is no evidence for DIC as a major component of the bleeding disorder.

PREVENTION AND CONTROL. The variety of rodents and their ubiquity and success in many ecologic settings make the control of hantaviral infections by rodent control virtually impossible. Clearly, improvement of housing, and particularly food storage, will help prevent those cases caused by rodent invasion of houses. However, a large number of infections occur in rural settings associated with agricultural and forestry activities, which are not so amenable to rodent exclusion. Education of populations to avoid direct contact with rodents in these circumstances may only have marginal effect because the virus may be airborne.

Vaccination of selected populations appears to be the best prospect for control. Recently, formalin-inactivated vaccines have been prepared from infected suckling rat or mouse brain tissue. These vaccines have undergone preliminary trials in North and South Korea with encouraging results. Genetic engineering techniques are also being used to produce candidate recombinant vaccinia viruses or to produce high titers of viral proteins. However, studies on the strain variation likely to be encountered in a target population and on the epitope recognition involved in protection are needed to design an effective, safe vaccine with broad enough specificity to protect against a variety of strains.

BIBLIOGRAPHY

Fisher-Hoch SP, McCormick JB: Hemorrhagic fever with renal syndrome: A review. Abstracts on Hygiene and Communicable Diseases 60:R1, 1985.

Kulagin SM, Fedorova NI, Ketiladze ES: A laboratory outbreak of haemorrhagic fever with renal syndrome (clinical-epidemiological functions). Zh Mikrobiol Epidemiol Immunobiol 33:121, 1962.

Lahdevirta J: Nephropathia epidemica in Finland. A clinical, histological and epidemiological study. Ann Clin Res 3(Suppl 8):1, 1971.

Lee HW, Baek LJ, Johnson KM: Isolation of Hantaan virus, the etiologic agent of Korean hemorrhagic fever, from wild urban rats. J Infect Dis 146:638, 1982.

Lee HW, Lee PW, Johnson KM: Isolation of the etiologic agent of Korean hemorrhagic fever. J Infect Dis 137:298, 1978.

McCormick JB, Sasso DR, Palmer EL, et al: Morphological identification of the agent of Korean hemorrhagic fever (Hantaan virus), as a member of the Bunyaviridae. Lancet 1:765, 1982.

Schmaljohn CS, Hasty SE, Dalrymple JM, et al: Antigenic and genetic properties place viruses linked to hemorrhagic fever with renal syndrome into a newly-defined genus of Bunyaviridae. Science 227:1041, 1985.

Yanagihara R, Gajdusek DC: Hemorrhagic fever with renal syndrome: A historical perspective and review of recent advances. *In* Gear JHS (ed): CRC Handbook of Viral and Rickettsial Hemorrhagic Fevers. Boca Raton, FL, CRC Press, 1988, pp 151–188.

22.7.   KYASANUR FOREST DISEASE

Thomas P. Monath

DEFINITION. Kyasanur Forest disease (KFD) is a severe infection characterized by fever, hemorrhage, rash, and, frequently, neurologic signs.

ETIOLOGY AND HISTORY. The etiologic agent, KFD virus, is antigenically related to the virus causing tick-borne encephalitis and is a member of the tick-borne flavivirus complex. The first indication of the presence of the disease was in March 1957, when several deaths were noted among langur and macaca monkeys in the forest areas of the Shimoga District of Karnataka (then Mysore) State, southern India. Not only were monkeys dying in large numbers, but cases of febrile illness were also occurring among human beings. Studies initiated by the Virus Research Centre, Poona, India, led to the isolation of several strains of virus from humans, monkeys, and ticks; the viruses were antigenically very closely related, if not identical. The etiologic agent was named Kyasanur Forest disease virus after the locality from which it was first isolated, and the disease in humans was called Kyasanur Forest disease.

DISTRIBUTION AND INCIDENCE. The disease in humans appears to be restricted to Karnataka State, India. The disease is focal in nature, appearing in new districts coincident with deforestation and agricultural projects. Approximately 400 to 500 cases occur annually. Human cases occur mainly in the premonsoon season between mid-November and mid-April, with maximum incidence from February to mid-April. With the onset of the monsoon the number of cases tends to diminish, but sporadic cases occur throughout the year. Antibodies to KFD or a closely related virus have been found in Kutch and Saurashtra, far to the north of the affected area.

TRANSMISSION AND EPIDEMIOLOGY. The virus is transmitted to humans by nymphal *Haemaphysalis* ticks, especially *H. spinigera*. However, virus isolation has also been made from *Ixodes* species, *Dermacentor* species, and *Rhipicephalus* species. Strong evidence suggests that small mammals (rats, mice, squirrels, shrews, and probably bats) are involved in the maintenance and dispersal of KFD, with monkeys acting as amplifiers of the virus. Cattle play an important role as a source for blood meals of adult ticks, thereby assuring tick reproduction and population density, but they do not serve as effective viremic hosts. The virus is transmitted transstadially (but apparently not transovarially) in *Haemaphysalis* ticks.

Human infections are usually preceded by illness and death in the forest-dwelling langur and macaca monkeys. Infection of humans is an occupational disease, being mainly contracted by adult males who enter the forest. However, all ages and sexes are susceptible. The disease is not transmitted from person to person.

PATHOGENESIS AND PATHOLOGY. Viremia studies of human patients have shown that the virus is detected in the blood between the second and twelfth day of illness, with peak virus titers of 3 to 5 dex being obtained between the fourth and seventh day of illness.

Gross necropsy findings are those of generalized hemorrhage occurring as petechiae in the skin and in the lungs (causing signs of consolidation), body cavities, viscera, and gastrointestinal tract. The main pathologic features are parenchymal degeneration in the liver and kidneys, massive or patchy hemorrhagic pneumonitis, and increased prominence of reticuloendothelial tissue in the liver and spleen with marked erythrophagocytosis. The virus has been isolated from blood, liver, spleen, kidneys, lungs, heart, and skeletal muscle.

CLINICAL MANIFESTATIONS AND COMPLICATIONS. After an infective tick bite, there is an incubation period of 3 to 8 days before the sudden onset of fever and severe headache. This is followed by back pain, severe pain in the upper and lower extremities, and prostration. Relative bradycardia is frequently present. Inflammation of the conjunctivae is common and usually occurs early in the disease. The palate is suffused and often covered with maculopapular spots. A generalized lymphadenopathy has been noted, and many patients have bronchiolar involvement. The fever generally lasts 5 to 12 days and sometimes follows a biphasic course; a mild meningoencephalitis frequently occurs during the second phase. Albuminuria, leukopenia, and thrombocytopenia are usual findings. Hemorrhagic complications include epistaxis, hematemesis, hemoptysis, melena, and bleeding gums; uterine bleeding may sometimes occur. Serum alanine and aspartate aminotransferase levels are often raised. A small proportion of patients may die, usually 8 to 12 days after onset of illness. These patients develop coma or bronchopneumonia prior to death. The majority of patients, however, make an uneventful and complete recovery.

DIAGNOSIS. A detailed travel history will help differentiate between KFD and other hemorrhagic fevers. Specific diagnosis will require isolation and identification of the virus or evidence of antibody development between acute and convalescent sera. The virus is readily isolated from acute phase blood in suckling mice or tissue culture. An antigen can be prepared from mouse brain material, and this can be tested by the complement-fixation, hemagglutination-inhibition, or neutralization test using specific immune reference serum.

TREATMENT AND PROGNOSIS. The case-fatality rate is 8 to 10%. Patients have a prolonged convalescence with aesthenia and neuromuscular complaints. The treatment of KFD, like that of other hemorrhagic fevers, is mainly symptomatic and supportive. The control of dehydration and hemorrhage is critically important and will require close laboratory monitoring.

CONTROL AND PREVENTION. The disease is transmitted by ticks; however, methods designed to reduce tick populations are generally difficult. It is important, therefore, to educate the public about the mode of transmission by ticks and the means for personal protection. Persons working or playing in infected areas should examine their body for ticks at frequent intervals. The use of tick repellents may be of value. A formalinized tissue culture vaccine developed in India has been tested and appears safe and effective.

BIBLIOGRAPHY

Banerjee K: Kyasanur Forest disease. *In* Monath TP (ed): The Arboviruses: Epidemiology and Ecology, Vol III. Boca Raton, FL, CRC Press, 1988, pp 93–116.

Iyer CGS, et al: Kyasanur Forest disease. VI. Pathological findings in three fatal human cases of KFD. Indian J Med Sci 13:1011, 1959.

Lakshmana RR: Clinical observation on Kyasanur Forest disease cases. J Indian Med Ass 31:113, 1958.

Theiler M, Downs WG: The Arthropod-Borne Viruses of Vertebrates. An Account of The Rockefeller Foundation Virus Program, 1951–1970. New Haven, CN, Yale University Press, 1973.

PART III

BACTERIAL INFECTIONS
SECTION A
RICKETTSIAL INFECTIONS

GENERAL PRINCIPLES

Charles L. Wisseman, Jr.

The rickettsial diseases of man are variously distributed over the earth's tropical and temperate zones, some more or less worldwide and others with more restricted distributions (Table III A–1). Evidence is accumulating to indicate that some of these diseases constitute substantial, largely unrecognized health problems, especially in developing countries where laboratory diagnostic support is not yet readily available. The diseases consist of several clinical entities, usually acute, self-limited fevers, caused by bacteria of the family Rickettsiaceae. They fall naturally into the categories of typhus-like disease (typhus group, spotted fever group, and scrub typhus groups), Q fever, and trench fever (Tables III A–2 and III A–3). In addition, intraleukocytic organisms of the genus *Ehrlichia,* best known as pathogens of domestic animals, are being recognized as occasional causes of human disease (Chapter 27.2). Finally, *Bartonella bacilliformis,* a member of the family Bartonellaceae under the order Rickettsiales, causes human disease restricted to certain Andean regions of South America (Chapter 51).

DESCRIPTION. Although very different in many respects, organisms of the genera *Rickettsia, Coxiella,* and *Rochalimaea* are very small bacteria (the concept of their being intermediate organisms between bacteria and viruses is no longer tenable) with a gram-negative bacterium-like cell wall, bacterial-type internal structure (typical prokaryotic DNA arrangement with a genome size roughly equivalent to that of *Neisseria* and ribosomes), often a slime layer or microcapsule (Fig. III A–1), and a substantial independent metabolic activity. Organisms of the genus *Rickettsia* as well as *Coxiella burnetti* are obligate intracellular parasites, i.e., they grow only within eukaryotic host cells. *Rochalimaea quintana* grows on cell-free medium and extracellularly in the louse gut. Multiplication is by transverse binary fission. In addition, *C. burnetti* produces minute endospore-like structures that are quite resistant to adverse environmental factors (e.g., heat and desiccation) (Fig. III A–2). Members of the genus *Rickettsia* that have been studied and *C. burnetti* have endotoxins similar in physiologic action to those of gram-negative bacilli.

INTERACTIONS WITH HOST CELLS. All organisms of the genus *Rickettsia* have the capacity to pene-

trate through the host-cell plasma membrane into the cytoplasm, where they multiply free in the cytoplasm (Fig. III A–3). Spotted fever group rickettsiae can penetrate the host-cell nucleus. These as well as *R. mooseri,* unlike *R. prowazekii,* can escape through the plasma membrane without requiring complete host-cell destruction. *Coxiella burnetii* is probably taken in by endocytosis and grows within a membrane-bound vacuole. These differences in action on host-cell membranes are probably related to differences in disease patterns (host response) and immune mechanisms (Table III A–2). Active penetration of host cells correlates with mouse lethal toxic action and hemolytic properties. Although obligate intracellular-parasitic rickettsiae will grow in a wide variety of invertebrate and vertebrate host cells in cell cultures, in the intact mammalian host their growth is largely restricted to a very few cell types, i.e., endothelial cells (Fig. III A–4) and macrophages (Table III A–2).

NATURAL HISTORY
Transmission. All rickettsioses, except louse-borne typhus and trench fever, are zoonoses, i.e., they are maintained in nature in an enzootic cycle that involves vertebrate (usually mammalian) hosts and arthropod vectors (flea, tick, mite) (Fig. III A–5). Man becomes infected, usually from the vector, when he intrudes into the enzootic cycle. The rickettsiae of these zoonoses are not transmitted naturally from an infected human being to another or to mammals of the enzootic cycle. Man is only a "dead-end host" in these instances. The vectors responsible for transmission of rickettsiae from the enzootic cycle to man may be only a subset of those involved in the enzootic cycle. For example, rat lice, mites, and fleas have been implicated in the enzootic cycle of murine typhus, but only some of the fleas that feed on man are considered vectors of the human disease. Likewise, certain ticks, e.g., the rabbit tick *Haemaphysalis leporis-palustris,* may be vectors of Rocky Mountain spotted fever in the enzootic cycle, but they do not feed on or serve as vectors to man. In the case of murine typhus and spotted fever group infections, the mammalian component of the enzootic cycle serves not only as a host to the hematophagous vector but also as an amplifying host for the rickettsiae. Uninfected vectors feeding on a rickettsemic mammal can become infected. However, in scrub typhus, it has not been possible to demonstrate that chiggers become persistently infected by feeding on rickettsemic rodents.

The dominant cycles for louse-borne epidemic typhus

TABLE III A–1. Summary of Some Epidemiologic Features of Selected Rickettsial Diseases of Man

Disease	Organism	Natural Cycle		Usual Mode of Transmission to Man	Common Occupational or Environmental Association	Geographic Distribution
		Arthropod Vector	*Mammalian Host*			
Typhus Group						
Murine typhus	*Rickettsia mooseri (R. typhi)*	Flea	Rodents	Infected flea feces into broken skin or aerosol to mucous membranes	Rat-infested premises (shops, warehouses, grain elevators)	Scattered foci, worldwide
Epidemic typhus	*R. prowazekii*	Body louse	Man*†	Infected crushed louse or feces into broken skin or aerosol to mucous membranes	Lousy human population with louse transfer	Worldwide
Brill-Zinsser disease	*R. prowazekii*	Recrudescence months to years after primary attack of louse-bourne typhus			Unknown; ?stress	Worldwide
Spotted Fever Group (selected examples)						
Rocky Mountain spotted fever	*R. rickettsii*	Ixodid ticks*	Small mammals	Tick bite, mechanical transfer to mucous membranes	Tick-infested terrain, houses, dogs, ?airborne	Western Hemisphere
Boutonneuse fever	*R. conorii*	Ixodid ticks*	Rodents, dogs	Tick bite	Tick-infested terrains, houses, dogs	Mediterranean littoral, Africa, ?Indian subcontinent
Rickettsialpox	*R. akari*	Mouse mite*	Mice	Mouse mite bite	Unique mouse- and mite-infested premises (incinerators)	United States, USSR, Korea, ?Central Africa
Scrub Typhus (tsutsugamushi disease)	*R. tsutsugamushi* (multiple serotypes)	Chigger*	Rodents	Chigger bite	Chigger-infested terrain; secondary scrub, grass, airfield, golf courses	Asia, Australia, New Guinea, Pacific Islands
Q fever‡	*Coxiella burnetii*	?Ticks	Mammals*	Inhalation of dried airborne infective material; ?tick bite	Domestic animals or products, dairies, lambing pens, slaughterhouses	Worldwide
Trench fever‡	*Rochalimaea quintana*	Body louse	Man*	Infected crushed louse or feces into broken skin; ?aerosol to mucous membranes	Lousy human population with louse transfer	Africa, Mexico, ?South America, ?Eastern Europe

*Reservoir.

†Recent isolations of putative *R. prowazekii* from flying squirrels in the eastern United States have been implicated in human infection. Previous claims of involvement of domestic animals are now largely discounted.

‡Although *C. burnetii* and *R. quintana* differ from members of the genus *Rickettsia* and Q fever and trench fever differ clinically from the others, they are conventionally considered with the rickettsiae.

and trench fever involve only man and the human body louse, *Pediculus humanus humanus*. Man is host for the vector as well as amplifying host and reservoir for the rickettsiae. Lice infected with *R. prowazekii* by feeding on a rickettsemic typhus fever patient regularly die in 1 to 2 weeks, owing to massive destruction of midgut epithelial cells. In recent years, an enzootic cycle of an organism indistinguishable from *R. prowazekii* has been identified among flying squirrels (*Glaucomys volans*) in the eastern United States. Sporadic cases of typhus fever occur in people associated with flying squirrels (e.g.,

those squirrels nesting in attics). It is unknown if flying squirrels originally acquired *R. prowazekii* from man or if this is a relict of an archetypic prehuman enzootic cycle.

Although *Coxiella burnetii* may be readily isolated from ticks, the usual mechanism of transmission to man does not involve a vector. Sheep, cattle, and goats are the most common sources of *C. burnetii* infection. Convalescence from primary acute infection in these animals is accompanied by persistence of the organism. During subsequent pregnancies and lactation, the organ-

TABLE III A–2. Diversity in Human Rickettsioses Among Target-Cell Relationships, Basic Pathologic Lesions, and Type of Clinical Disease

Disease	Target Cell	Host-Cell Association	Basic Lesion	Clinical Manifestations
Typhus-like fevers				
Typhus group	Endothelial	Free intracytoplasmic	Vasculitis	Acute, self-limited fever
Scrub typhus	Endothelial	Free intracytoplasmic	Vasculitis	Acute, self-limited fever
Spotted fever group	Endothelial, smooth muscle	Free intracytoplasmic and intranuclear	Vasculitis	Acute, self-limited fever
Q fever	Reticuloendothelial	Intracytoplasmic vacuole	Granulomas	Acute, self-limited fever, "atypical pneumonia," subacute hepatitis, endocarditis
Trench fever	Unknown	Pericellular (in louse and cell culture)	Unknown	Recurring febrile episodes

isms multiply to large numbers in the placenta ($\sim10^8$/ gm of sheep placenta) and mammary glands. They are shed at birth, grossly contaminating the environment, and appear in the milk. Other animals, as well as the newborn, and man are readily infected from the contaminated environment—dust, milk, tissues, and excreta.

The mechanisms of transmission vary with the rickettsia and vector. In the tick-, mite-, and chigger-borne rickettsioses (spotted fever and scrub typhus groups), the organisms colonize the salivary glands of the vector and are transmitted by bite. In louse- and flea-borne rickettsioses (louse-borne typhus, murine typhus, trench fever), the organisms are confined to the gut, multiply in or on midgut epithelial cells, and are excreted in the feces. The inefficient mechanism of accidental contamination of the bite wound or breaks in the skin with infective feces or crushed lice or fleas is thought to be the usual method of transmission. The possibility of transmission by bite of the flea is being reinvestigated. The rickettsiae may remain infectious for some time in dried feces of lice and fleas. Abundant feces accumulate on the fur of animals (flea-borne murine typhus) or in the clothing of lice-infested people, contaminating the environment and possibly becoming airborne. As in the case of *C. burnetii,* man is highly susceptible to infection through the respiratory tract, conjunctivae, and mucous membranes.

The inefficiency of these transmission modes is offset by the abundant growth of the organisms in the louse or flea gut (10^7 to 10^8 organisms per individual) and their extremely high degree of infectivity. Only 1 or 2 viable *R. mooseri* (*R. typhi*) constitute a percutaneous ID_{50} for rats and mice. It is estimated that very few (probably <10) viable typhus, scrub typhus, spotted fever, and Q fever organisms constitute the infectious dose for man.

Reservoirs. The vector is also the main reservoir in tick-, mite-, and chigger-borne rickettsioses; the efficient transovarial passage from one generation to the next is adequate to ensure survival of the organisms. In contrast, transovarial transmission of rickettsiae does not occur in lice but may occur at low frequency in certain fleas. Persistent infection of man is the main reservoir mechanism for louse-borne typhus and trench fever. In

TABLE III A–3. Some Clinical Features of Selected Rickettsial Diseases

Disease	Usual Incubation Period (Days)	Eschar	Rash Onset (Day of Disease)	Rash Distribution	Rash Type	Usual Duration of Disease* (Days)	Usual Severity†	Duration of Fever after Chemotherapy (Hours)
Typhus Group								
Murine typhus	12 (range: 8–16)	None	5–7	Trunk, extremities	Macular, maculopapular	12 (range: 8–16)	Moderate	48–72
Epidemic typhus	12 (range: 10–14)	None	5–7	Trunk, extremities	Macular, maculopapular, petechial	14 (range: 10–18)	Severe	48–72
Brill-Zinsser disease		None		Trunk, extremities	Macular	7–11	Relatively mild	48–72
Spotted Fever Group								
Rocky Mountain spotted fever	7 (range: 3–12)	None	3–5	Extremities, trunk, face	Macular, maculopapular, petechial	16 (range: 10–20)	Severe	<48–72
Boutonneuse fever	5–7	Often present	3–4	Trunk, extremities, face, palms, soles	Macular, maculopapular, petechial	10 (range: 7–14)	Moderate	—
Rickettsialpox	9–17	Often present	1–3	Trunk, face, buccal mucosa	Papulovesicular	7	Relatively mild	—
Scrub typhus (tsutsugamushi disease)	12 (range: 9–18)	Often present	4–6	Trunk, extremities	Macular, maculopapular	14 (range: 10–20)	Mild to severe	24–36
Q fever	19 (range: 10–26)	None		None		6‡ (range: 2–21)	Relatively mild	48 (occasionally slow)

*Untreated disease.
†Severity can vary greatly.
‡Occasional chronic infections occur (e.g., hepatitis, endocarditis).

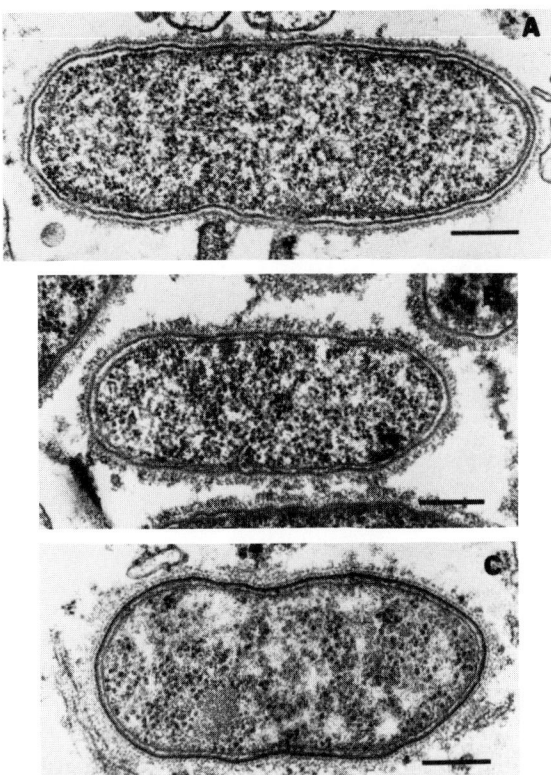

FIGURE III A–1. Comparison of ultrastructure as revealed by transmission electron microscopy of *R. prowazekii (A)*, *R. rickettsii (B)*, and *R. tsutsugamushi (C)*. Note the small residual slime layer stabilized by antibody, the inner and outer membranes, and the internal ribosomal structures. This outer envelope of *R. tsutsugamushi* differs from the others in thickness of the outer leaflet of the outer membrane. (Bar = 0.25 μm.) (From Silverman DS, Wisseman CL Jr: Infect Immunol 21:1020, 1978. Reprinted by permission.)

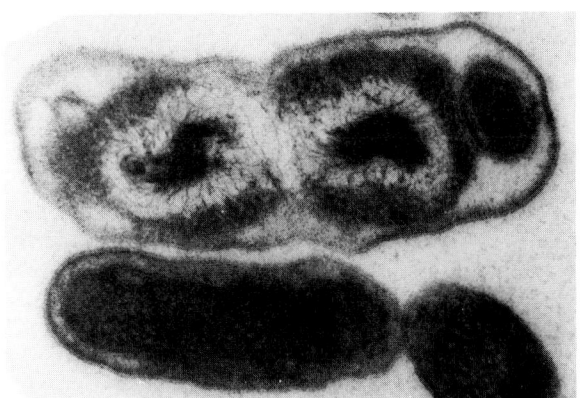

FIGURE III A–2. Transmission electron micrograph of *C. burnetii* showing small, dense, endospore-like structure. The small, dense forms are thought to account for the unusual stability of *C. burnetii*. (From McCaul TF, Williams JC: J Bacteriol 147:1063, 1981. Reprinted by permission.)

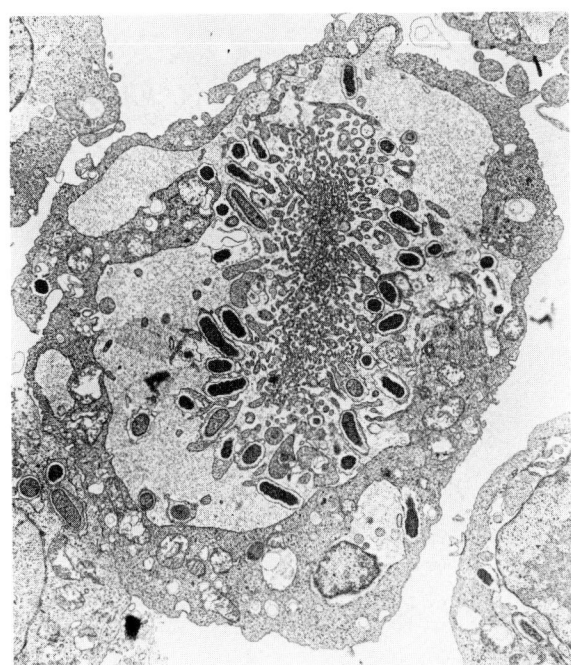

FIGURE III A–3. Transmission electron micrograph of chicken embryo fibroblast late in the infection cycle of *R. rickettsii*. Note the enormous swelling of the endoplasmic reticulum with entrapped organisms. Similar changes in the endoplasmic reticulum have been described in endothelial cells in a fatal case of RMSF. (From Silverman DS, Wisseman CL Jr: Infect Immunol 26:714, 1979. Reprinted by permission.)

louse-borne typhus, rickettsemia disappears with convalescence from acute primary disease. A nonsterile immunity develops, with *R. prowazekii* persisting in an ill-defined state, and recrudescence of infection and disease (Brill-Zinsser disease) with rickettsemia may occur months to many years later. The importance of the established flying squirrel enzootic cycle as a reservoir mechanism is unknown. In contrast, earlier reports of domestic livestock as possible typhus reservoirs were probably based on serologic artifacts and are not considered seriously now. With trench fever, *Rochalimaea quintana* is recoverable from the blood for months to years, even without relapses of clinical disease. The persistence of *C. burnetii* in domestic animals with pregnancy-associated recrudescences constitutes an effective reservoir mechanism, although perhaps not the only one. The reservoir mechanism of murine typhus is unknown.

PATHOGENESIS. Although there are sufficient differences to yield distinct clinical entities, the human diseases caused by members of the genus *Rickettsia* share many common features. Therefore, it is convenient to consider pathogenesis and immunity in a generalized framework. Q fever and trench fever are treated separately.

Pathology. Some local proliferation undoubtedly occurs at the inoculation site with all *Rickettsia* species. In some (e.g., scrub typhus, rickettsialpox, and boutonneuse fever), a visible lesion (the eschar) (see Fig. 25–1) develops at the inoculation site during the incubation period. The route(s) of dissemination of the infection from the inoculation site is not known. Regional lymphadenopathy (e.g., in scrub typhus) suggests lymphatic spread; however, the demonstration of rickettsiae in endothelial cells (Fig. III A–4) of small blood vessels at the inoculation site opens the possibility of direct hematogenous dissemination. Some dissemination to and proliferation in distant sites must take place during the incubation period, but the organs or tissues involved

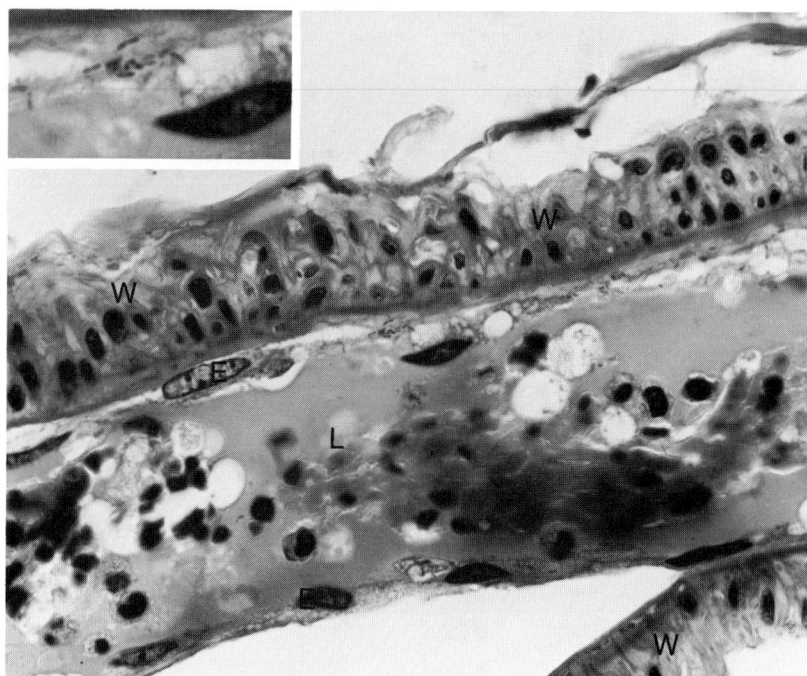

FIGURE III A–4. *R. rickettsii* within a vascular endothelial cell (*inset*) from a fatal case of human Rocky Mountain spotted fever (W = wall; E = endothelium; L = lumen). (Courtesy of Drs. Douglas Wear and Daniel Connor and the Armed Forces Institute of Pathology, Photograph Negative No. 79–15424.)

have not been identified in man. Patent rickettsemia probably appears only late in the incubation period, e.g., only a few hours prior to the onset of clinical disease in volunteers infected with *R. tsutsugamushi.* It is regularly present at the onset of symptoms and persists throughout the febrile period of disease, despite the appearance of humoral antibodies.

Vasculitis. Disseminated focal infection occurs in the endothelium of small blood vessels (capillaries, arterioles, and venules) of the skin, brain (Fig. III A–4), lungs, heart, liver, kidneys, and other organs. This multifocal, multiorgan vasculitis is the single most important known pathophysiologic feature of these diseases. Rickettsiae infect, multiply in, and damage endothelial cells, causing cell necrosis, hypertrophy, and proliferation. Loss of protein-rich fluid from the intravascular compartment into the tissues across damaged endothelium plays a prominent role in the pathophysiology of these disorders. Infection is limited to the endothelial cells in typhus and scrub typhus infections but may extend to all layers in Rocky Mountain spotted fever, causing necrosis of the media (Fig. III A–6). At the sites of endothelial damage, platelet-fibrin thrombi tend to form, which, along with endothelial hypertrophy and proliferation, partially or completely occlude the vascular lumen. The typical perivascular inflammatory response develops at infection sites, with polymorphonuclear and monocytic cells early and macrophages, lymphocytes, and occasional plasma cells later, coinciding approximately temporally with antibody response (Figs. III A–6 and III A–7). This sequence suggests that perhaps typically, the infection evolves through an early phase, with vascular damage being primarily the direct result of rickettsial infection, and a late phase, with additional vascular damage produced by immunologic mechanisms. The immunopathologic component is unproved but is consistent with the facts that in typhus and scrub typhus infections, patients appear more

"toxic" in this late phase and show greater vascular instability and that most deaths occur in the period after antibodies are demonstrable. However, the greater severity of vascular lesions with little perivascular cellular response, no antibody response, and unresponsiveness to antirickettsial therapy in rapidly fatal or fulminant cases of Rocky Mountain spotted fever suggests that in this disease direct rickettsiae-induced damage alone can initiate irreversible pathophysiologic changes. The significance of the leukocytoclastic vasculitis with IgA deposition on the basement membrane recently described in some severe Mediterranean spotted fever remains to be determined.

Complications. The disseminated vascular lesions can account for the multiorgan involvement and many of the clinical and pathophysiologic abnormalities seen in these infections, e.g., rash, edema and increased extravascular fluid space, hypovolemia, hypotension, and gangrene (in louse-borne typhus and Rocky Mountain spotted fever). These lesions can also account for the clotting abnormalities that have been recognized in several rickettsial diseases but that occur more regularly in severe form in Rocky Mountain spotted fever and may be a major factor contributing to death. The classic typhus nodules in the brain (Fig. III A–7), occurring most commonly in the midbrain and nuclear areas, are of the same vascular origin and, along with edema, help to explain the mental changes and cranial nerve deficits. In Rocky Mountain spotted fever, discrete microinfarcts may occur in the white matter of the brain (Fig. III A–8), with persisting electroencephalographic changes.

In addition to the typical perivascular lesions, the heart often shows some edema, a diffuse mononuclear infiltrate, and a minor amount of muscle necrosis. Nonspecific electrocardiographic changes are common. Despite this dramatic change in the appearance of the heart, limited studies during World War II suggested that cardiac function was not impaired. Congestive heart

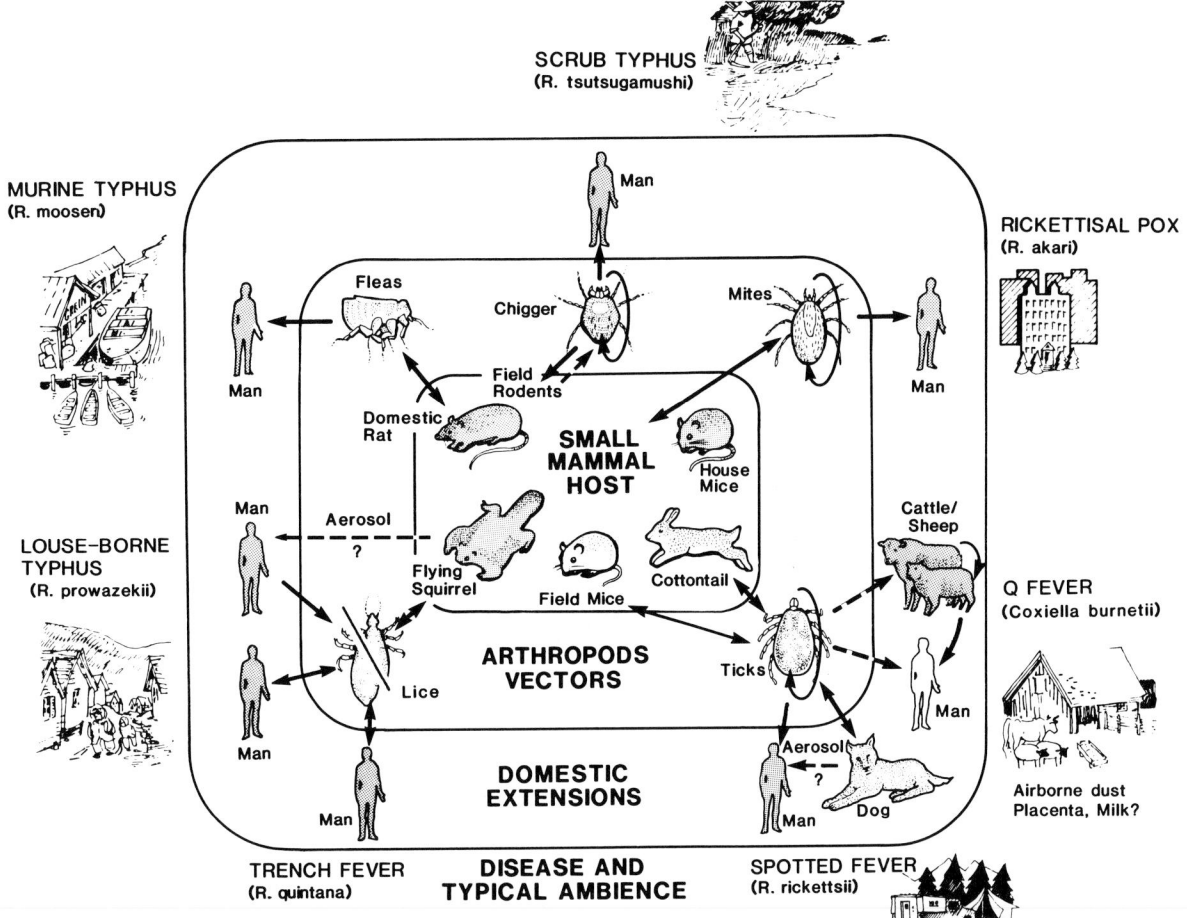

FIGURE III A–5. Schematic summary of some major interactions between rickettsial organisms, their small animal hosts and arthropod vectors, the participation of domestic animals, and examples of the typical ambience under which each rickettsial infection is contracted by man. Scrub typhus is transmitted in grassy, scrub, or transitional vegetation; by rickettsialpox in the incinerator areas of large apartment houses; by spotted fever through occupational or recreational activities in tick-infested terrain; by Q fever in the husbandry or use of sheep and cattle; by louse-borne typhus and trench fever where human body lice are prevalent, now largely confined to poverty-stricken mountain villages in some developing countries; and by murine typhus in rat-infested grain/food storage structures and warehouses. (Courtesy of Dr. J.K. Frenkel, University of Kansas Medical Center, Kansas City, KS.)

failure, with increased venous pressure, is uncommon. Nevertheless, the clinical significance of myocarditis has again come under scrutiny.

Typical perivascular lesions occur in the portal areas of the liver, along with nonspecific focal areas of fatty degeneration in hepatocytes. Blood levels of aminotransferases are elevated, even early in the disease. The kidneys show focal interstitial vascular lesions involving only a few nephrons. The characteristic oliguria and azotemia of typhus are attributable to prerenal causes, e.g., hypotension, hypovolemia, and tissue catabolism. Renal tubular necrosis has been observed in severe Rocky Mountain spotted fever. The lungs show a variable degree of interstitial-type pneumonitis on histologic examination and on radiography, regardless of the route of infection. Cough is a common early clinical manifestation, but physical signs are scant. Rarely, pulmonary symptoms and signs may be prominent at the onset. Pulmonary edema later is due to increased vascular permeability and not to congestive heart failure.

Immune Response. Immunity to the infecting rickettsial strain following recovery tends to be solid and long-lasting but of a nonsterile type, i.e., the rickettsiae are not entirely eradicated and may remain "latent" for months to years. The bases for immunity are not yet completely understood, although rapid advances are now being made. Antibodies, detectable after about 1 week of disease, are not rickettsiacidal, do not control intracellular rickettsial growth, and do not immediately control rickettsemia or disease, even though they may opsonize extracellular rickettsiae and facilitate their intraphagosomal destruction by macrophages. Cell-mediated immunity also develops. Immune T lymphocytes confer on nonimmune animals the capacity to control intracellular rickettsial growth. Immune T lymphocyte subsets (human CD 4+ and CD 8+) lyse rickettsia-infected target cells. Immune interferon (IFN-γ) kills intracellular rickettsiae and lyses infected cells. The role of suppressor cells, demonstrable under certain circumstances, remains unclear. The current consensus is that both antibody-mediated and cell-mediated mechanisms contribute to immunity but that cell-mediated mechanisms are more important in controlling intracellular parasitism.

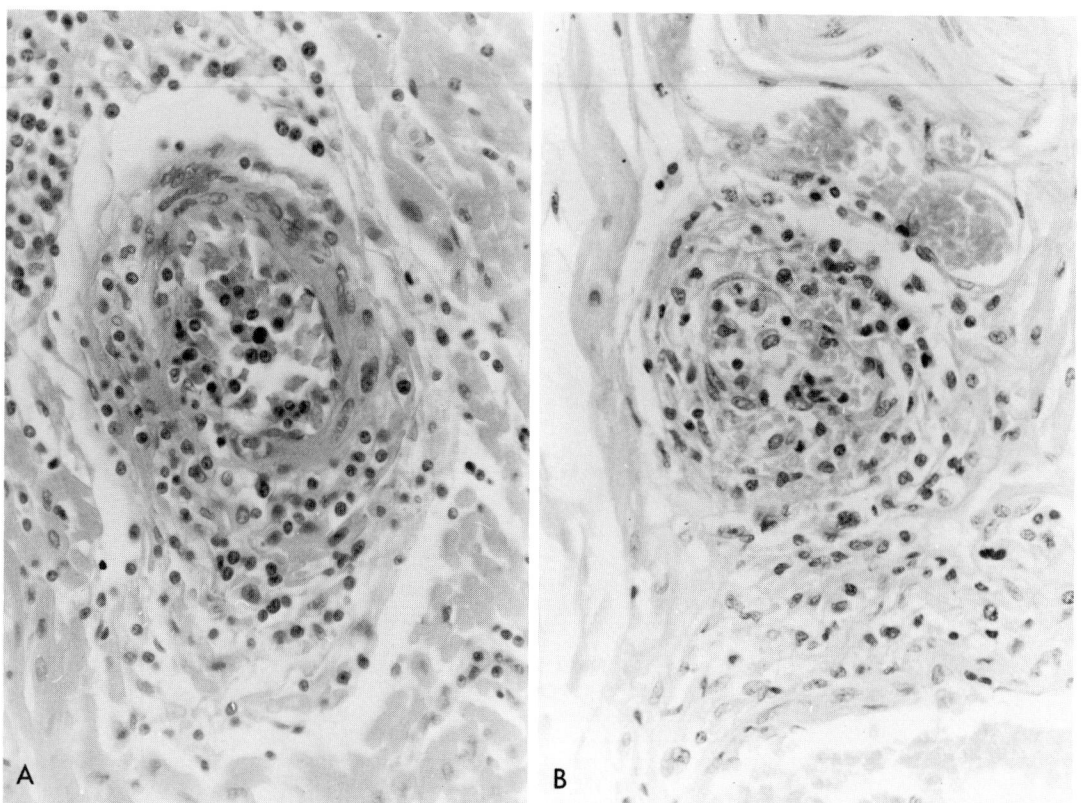

FIGURE III A–6. Comparison of vascular lesions in human louse-borne typhus fever *(A)* and Rocky Mountain spotted fever *(B)*.

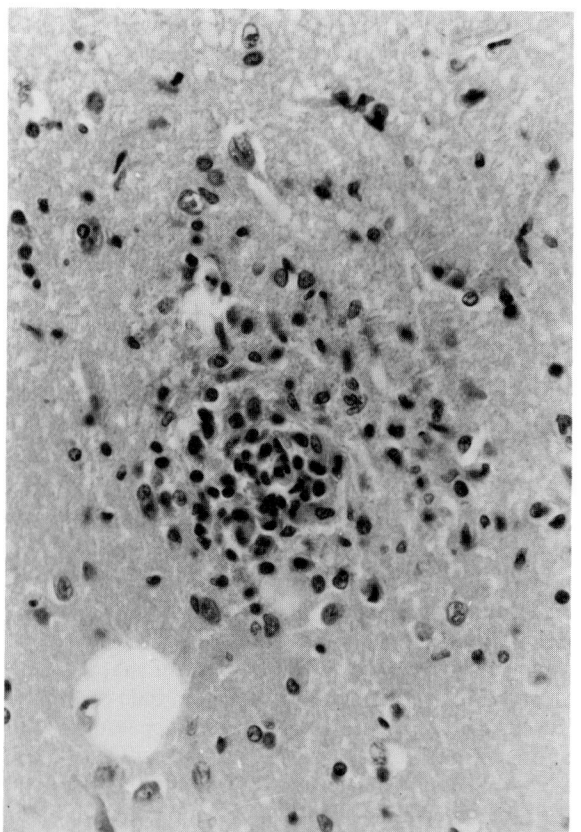

FIGURE III A–7. "Typhus nodule" in the brain of a patient with louse-borne typhus. Similar lesions are found in scrub typhus and, more rarely, in Rocky Mountain spotted fever.

GENERAL CLINICAL CONSIDERATIONS. In the classic forms, the typhus-like rickettsial diseases display many common clinical features that may vary in degree and in detail, e.g., fever, headache (Fig. 23–1), cough, prostration, rash (Figs. 23–2 and 24–1), altered mental state (Figs. 23–3 and 23–4), hypotension, and initial normal to low white blood cell count. However, one or more of the classic features may be absent in many patients, and, in some, unusual dominant presentations, e.g., acute abdomen or pneumonitis, may be misleading.

Differential Diagnosis. The signs and symptoms, especially at the onset, are those common to many acute infectious diseases; differential clinical diagnosis is difficult; and specific laboratory diagnostic methods are limited. Sometimes, an early sign such as an eschar can be helpful. However, an eschar (see Fig. 25–1) is variable even in the rickettsioses in which it occurs. Later clues may be rash (Figs. 23–2 and 24–1), hypotension, and/or changes in mental state (Figs. 23–3 and 23–4), but rickettsioses vary in severity, and not all cases are classic. Moreover, in many areas, other infectious diseases coexist that are confusing clinically, especially in the early period, when the correct choice of chemotherapy may be lifesaving (as with Rocky Mountain spotted fever, meningococcemia, or cerebral malaria). Therefore, a practitioner must be acutely sensitive to the different possibilities in areas of practice and must devise a strategy for the diagnosis and management, sometimes empirically on the basis of probabilities, of a rickettsiosis-like disease, using all available epidemiologic, clinical, and laboratory information. Simple observation of the patient for the development of diagnostic clinical

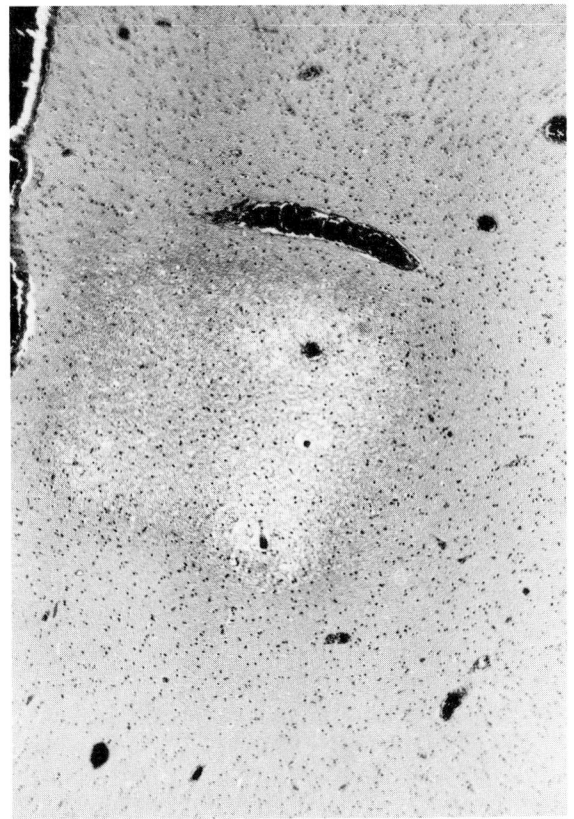

FIGURE III A–8. Microinfarct in white matter of the brain of a patient with Rocky Mountain spotted fever.

or laboratory features is a hazardous practice. In the United States, the single major factor contributing to the continuing 5% to 10% mortality rate of Rocky Mountain spotted fever is delay in the institution of specific chemotherapy.

Exposure. The history of potential exposure (e.g., by occupation, travel, or recreational activities in wilderness areas) or of tick or flea bite or the finding of an eschar or the presence of body lice is extremely important in alerting the physician to the possibility of a rickettsial disease. Modern air travel makes it possible for a person to return from any part of the world within the incubation period of a rickettsial disease, e.g., scrub typhus and Kenya tick typhus in travelers returning to the United States.

In a given area, certain diseases commonly cause difficult clinical differential diagnostic problems. For example, in the United States, diseases commonly confused with Rocky Mountain spotted fever are measles, meningococcemia, and enterovirus infection. In Central and East Africa, diseases that cause major differential diagnostic problems with louse-borne typhus are cerebral falciparum malaria, typhoid fever, and relapsing fever. Milder cases of typhus may be indistinguishable clinically from influenza. Treatment for one generally is not optimal or even effective for the other. Errors in both directions are not uncommon, resulting in the loss of critical time. In addition, in patients outside the United States or those newly arrived in the United States, rickettsial disease may be complicated by some other concurrent infection, such as malaria.

Therapeutic Trial. Outside the United States and Europe, laboratory facilities may be unavailable, and an empirical therapeutic approach is often successful. For example, when it is not possible to distinguish among malaria, typhus, and typhoid, a combination of chloramphenicol and chloroquine or another antimalarial agent appropriate for the resistance patterns of the area often gives a satisfactory clinical response; a patient suspected of having typhus who does not respond in 48 hours to a tetracycline drug can often be treated successfully with chloramphenicol.

It is important to remember that the antimicrobials commonly used in the practice of "covering" an acute febrile disease while awaiting return of laboratory results, e.g., beta-lactam and aminoglycoside antibiotics, have no antirickettsial action at the usual clinically attainable concentrations. The time lost in relying on this practice has contributed to fatalities in Rocky Mountain spotted fever.

LABORATORY DIAGNOSIS. Methods for retrospective diagnoses of rickettsial infections (isolation of the organism and serologic response) are reasonably well developed, although not universally available; methods for diagnosis in the acute phase of disease, when crucial decisions about specific chemotherapy must be made, are generally unsatisfactory but are improving.

Exclusion of Differential Diagnostic Problems. Examples include malaria smear, skin lesion smear for meningococci, demonstration of measles antigen in respiratory epithelial cells by fluorescence microscopy, and cultures for typhoid and other enteric fevers.

Direct Demonstration of Rickettsiae or Rickettsial Antigens. When positive, microscopic demonstration of rickettsiae in endothelial cells in skin biopsy specimens, especially of rash, by means of fluorescein-labeled antibodies permits a specific diagnosis within hours in the early critical stages of the disease. This has been especially useful in Rocky Mountain spotted fever but should be applicable to the typhus and scrub typhus groups as well.

Although theoretically feasible, demonstrable in certain experimental infections in animals, and sporadically reported in human disease, detection of rickettsial antigens in acute phase urine has been fraught with difficulty. Application of modern immunologic methods (e.g., immunodiffusion, counterimmunoelectrophoresis, radioimmunoassay, enzyme-linked immunosorbent assay [ELISA]) may improve sensitivity, specificity, and reliability and deserves concerted effort.

Isolation of Rickettsiae. The isolation of rickettsiae from the blood or tissues of a patient is hazardous, requires special laboratory facilities and trained personnel, usually does not yield results in time to influence patient management, and, therefore, was not encouraged as a routine procedure in the past. However, it is urgent to change this position, because methods are improving and because serologic retrospective diagnoses are ill equipped to identify new species or variants of rickettsiae. A growing diversity of rickettsial agents (e.g., the flying squirrel agent, *R. canada,* and new members of the spotted fever group) is being recognized in the United States and elsewhere, but their importance as causes of human disease remains unknown. Conventional serologic tests for retrospective diagnosis are largely group-specific, might not recognize variants at the species level, and would not detect infections with totally new agents. Isolation and characterization of the agent are the keystones of identification of new diseases.

A hospital laboratory equipped to isolate viruses and chlamydiae (e.g., laminar flow biosafety hood) can isolate rickettsiae safely. Isolations are usually made in guinea pigs (typhus, spotted fever group, Q fever), mice (scrub typhus), yolk sac of embryonated eggs or tissue culture. Especially promising for hospital laboratories is the recent adaptation of the shell vial method in which diluted whole blood is centrifuged onto a cell monolayer on a coverslip in shell vials. After washing, adding fresh medium, and incubating at 35°C in 5% CO_2:95% air for 4 to 5 days, coverslips are stained with Giménez stain or specific fluorescein-labeled antibody. This method has been applied successfully for the isolation of *Rickettsia conorii* from patients with Mediterranean spotted fever and should be applicable to other rickettsial diseases.

Rochalimaea quintana can be grown from blood on blood agar incubated for 10 to 14 days at 33°C in an atmosphere of 10% CO_2 in air. Colonies are minute and are best seen under a dissecting microscope. Smears stained with Giménez or Giemsa stain reveal minute bacillary or coccobacillary organisms.

Although isolation and identification of rickettsial agents are usually beyond the competence of the ordinary hospital laboratory, mechanisms do exist for accomplishing this. In the United States, properly collected and preserved specimens (frozen at −70°C or lower) can be sent through state health departments to the Centers for Disease Control in Atlanta, Georgia, where specially trained personnel and special facilities exist to handle and characterize such agents. Moreover, in the United States and elsewhere, the World Health Organization has established a series of reference laboratories capable of handling such agents.

Serologic Diagnosis. Serologic methods remain the mainstay of routine laboratory diagnosis of rickettsial infections and are also used for epidemiologic purposes. However, because an antibody response rarely occurs with any of the rickettsioses before the end of the first week of disease and because a rise in antibody titer is more or less essential to a solid diagnosis, convincing serologic diagnosis may become available only after the critical stage with respect to lifesaving decisions about chemotherapy. At present, serologic tests consist of (1) nonspecific tests (Weil-Felix reaction), generally available to hospital laboratories through commercially produced antigens (a part of the "febrile agglutinin" package) and (2) more specific tests, generally available at state health departments, the CDC, and the WHO reference laboratories. Rickettsial antigens for the diagnosis of Q fever and infections of the spotted fever group are becoming commercially available.

Weil-Felix Reaction. Based on unique sharing of polysaccharide antigens between certain *Proteus* strains and some rickettsiae, this agglutination test performed with suspensions of rough *Proteus* OX–2, OX–19, and OX-K strains has an historical aura and the advantages of simplicity, ready availability of antigens, and sensitivity to early antibody response. Some typical responses are recorded in Table III A–4. This test has serious limitations. It will not reliably discriminate between typhus and spotted fever group infections. It is not positive in Q fever or rickettsialpox. It is variably positive in Brill-Zinsser disease and in scrub typhus reinfections. False-positive reactions may occur in *Proteus* infections and with *Proteus* OX-K, relapsing fever, leptospirosis, and *Vibrio* infections. Despite these limitations and efforts to discourage its use in favor of more specific tests, the Weil-Felix test is likely to remain in use until the specific tests become readily available at the local hospital level. Properly used, it can help differentiate, for example, between typhoid and typhus on or soon after the patient's admission to the hospital, when decisions about treatment must be made. Confirmation can be obtained with specific tests at a later date from a reference laboratory.

Indirect Fluorescent Antibody (IFA) Test. The IFA test is currently the most widely used test for diagnostic and epidemiologic purposes. It can be applied to all rickettsial infections. It can be made group-specific or reasonably species-specific. IgG, IgM, and IgA antibody titers can be determined directly. Currently, the IFA test is the most reliable and sensitive test available for the serodiagnosis of scrub typhus. An immunoperoxidase test, which can be read under an ordinary light microscope, is widely used in Asia, especially for scrub typhus.

Agglutination Tests. Microagglutination tests with highly purified rickettsial suspensions still receive attention because they are simple to perform and highly sensitive and usually detect antibodies somewhat earlier in disease than does the complement fixation test. Persistence of antibodies has not yet been thoroughly documented. Group specificity is good. Species specificity appears to be fair among the spotted fever group, but some problems have been encountered in distinguishing between murine and epidemic typhus infections of man (as opposed to high specificity in rodents). This test requires large amounts of antigen compared with other tests. (*Note:* The agglutination test referred to here is not to be confused with the Giroud type of microscopic agglutination test, which is performed with relatively crude antigens and is often unreliable.)

Complement Fixation (CF) Test. For most of the

TABLE III A–4. Some Typical Reactions Obtained with the Weil-Felix Agglutination Test

Rickettsial Infection	Agglutination with *Proteus* Strain		
	OX-19	**OX-2**	**OX-K**
Typhus group	+ + +	+	0
Brill-Zinsser disease	Variable, often negative		
Spotted fever group	+ + +	+	0
	+	+ + +	
Rickettsialpox	0	0	0
Scrub typhus group	0	0	0/+ + +*
Q fever	0	0	0

*Not likely to be reliably positive in second and subsequent reinfections with different serotypes.

rickettsioses, except the scrub typhus group, the CF test was the standard of serodiagnosis and seroepidemiology for many years. With group ("soluble") antigens, sera can be screened for evidence of infection with any member of the typhus or spotted fever group, and with the "specific" rickettsial body antigens, the offending organism often can be identified by titer differences, depending in part on the time of specimen collection, previous exposure to related organisms, and other similar factors. In the case of Q fever, persisting high titers with phase I antigen suggest chronic infection (e.g., hepatitis and endocarditis).

Other Tests. Toxin neutralization tests, passive hemagglutination tests, and latex agglutination tests have special uses. New tests, e.g., the ELISA and dot-blot, are under development and evaluation. Western blot tests have special applications.

TREATMENT OF RICKETTSIAL DISEASES. The general principles of therapy are similar for all the common rickettsial diseases. Optimal management includes (1) specific antimicrobial therapy directed against the offending rickettsial agent; (2) supportive measures to correct physiologic abnormalities; (3) good nursing care to prevent serious complications; and (4) prompt, appropriate treatment of complications. In mild cases, patients treated early may require little more than the specific antimicrobial therapy. Vigorous supportive measures and good nursing may be lifesaving in severe cases. The treatment of acute Q fever is similar to that which will be described in the following section, but chronic infections pose different problems (see Chapter 26).

Antirickettsial Therapy. *Prompt, adequate antirickettsial therapy is the single most important factor in shortening the disease, reducing mortality, and speeding convalescence.* In uncomplicated cases, this may be the only medication required.

Antimicrobial agents of the tetracycline series are the drugs of choice for the treatment of all acute rickettsial diseases. Although also highly effective, chloramphenicol is not routinely recommended, unless tetracyclines cannot be used, because of the rare complication of aplastic anemia. The new quinolone drug, ciprofloxacin, inhibits the growth of typhus and spotted fever group rickettsiae and *Coxiella burnetii* in vitro. Preliminary reports indicate clinical efficacy in the treatment of Mediterranean spotted fever. These drugs shorten the course of disease dramatically and reduce fatality rates virtually to zero, except in neglected, complicated, or fulminating cases. The patient often begins to respond by 24 hours and is afebrile in 1 to 4 days, usually 2 to 3 days, depending on the specific rickettsia and the stage of disease at the time therapy is begun.

Penicillin, streptomycin, and sulfonamides are clinically ineffective. Practical concentrations of a wide range of aminoglycosides, semisynthetic penicillins, and cephalosporins do not inhibit the growth of *R. prowazekii* in vitro in cell cultures. *Except for chloramphenicol,* none of the drugs (ampicillin, amoxicillin, co-trimoxazole) used for the treatment of typhoid fever, a serious differential diagnostic problem in some areas, gives clinical and/or in vitro evidence of effectiveness in rickettsial diseases.

Tetracycline HCl is given orally in a total daily dose of 25 to 50 mg/kg of body weight. Two grams per day in divided doses at 4- to 6- or even 12-hour intervals usually suffice for adult patients. Chloramphenicol is given orally in amounts of 50 or 75 mg/kg of body weight per day for children and adults, respectively, usually in divided doses at 4- to 6- or even 12-hour intervals. *Doses larger than 25 mg/kg of body weight may be severely toxic for newborn infants.* Intravenous tetracycline is given in a dosage of 0.5 gm every 6 to 12 hours, to a maximum of 2 gm per day for adults. Chloramphenicol succinate, appropriately diluted, is given intravenously to adults in a dose of 1 gm every 8 to 12 hours. Parenteral therapy should be replaced with oral therapy as soon as the patient can swallow. When parenteral preparations are unavailable or intravenous drip therapy is impractical, oral preparations suspended in fluid may be administered by stomach tube.

Long-Acting Tetracyclines. The introduction of new lipotropic tetracycline derivatives that produce prolonged high blood and tissue levels after a single dose (i.e., doxycycline and minocycline) has literally revolutionized the management of *louse-borne typhus.* A single 100-mg dose of doxycycline will cure most adults, and a single 50-mg dose will cure most children, with only an occasional transient relapse that does not require additional therapy. A single 200-mg dose is rarely followed by relapse. Under extreme circumstances, single-dose doxycycline therapy, requiring only a single contact between patient and medical personnel, has been applied successfully on an outpatient basis. Unless in extremis from typhus or suffering from some unrelated disease, almost all patients will survive whether hospitalized, at home, or transiently disoriented in the bush. Single-dose doxycycline is currently the treatment of choice for louse-borne typhus. Comparable results have been obtained with minocycline, but because of its tendency to cause otitic complications, it is not recommended as a first-choice drug.

Experience with single-dose doxycycline treatment of other rickettsioses is limited. However, evidence indicates that a single 200-mg dose of doxycycline will cure scrub typhus, with some transient recrudescences (see Chapter 25). In contrast, limited observations in the United States suggest that a single dose will *not* suffice for the treatment of murine typhus or Rocky Mountain spotted fever, although a daily dose of 100 to 200 mg on a schedule described for tetracycline HCl is effective. However, reports from China indicate successful treatment of murine typhus with a single dose of doxycycline.

Precautions. The usual precautions are observed for administering antimicrobials, e.g., adjustment of dosage to compensate for problems of immaturity in infants and of renal or hepatic dysfunction of rickettsial or other origin, staining of developing teeth, changes in microbial flora and superinfection, pregnancy, drug sensitivities, or blood dyscrasias. These must be balanced against the risks of not treating the disease, i.e., mortality and complications. Abortion is common in untreated rickettsial disease. The short duration of required therapy with tetracyclines is considered by many physicians to pose no serious problem to young children and pregnant women and fetuses with regard to staining of teeth and bones.

Relapses. Because neither tetracycline HCl nor chloramphenicol is rickettsicidal under ordinary circumstances and because neither eradicates the organism from the body, ultimate freedom from clinical relapse (i.e., "cure") is probably dependent on an adequate immune response by the patient. The duration of therapy depends on the pharmacology of the particular drug employed; the susceptibility of the organism to and rate of recovery from the inhibitory effects of the drug; and the stage of the disease at the time therapy is begun. Although not necessarily the minimal effective regimen, a practical, conservative guide to duration of tetracycline or chloramphenicol therapy is to administer the drug until the patient has been afebrile for 48 hours and for an additional period until the total time elapsed from onset of disease is 12 to 14 days. Relapses respond to retreatment with the same drug. In fact, in many instances, "relapses" or recrudescences of fever are self-limited and resolve spontaneously about as rapidly as they do with additional chemotherapy.

Antimicrobial Resistance. Antimicrobial resistance has not been encountered in naturally occurring infections by members of the genus Rickettsia, although strains of *R. prowazekii* resistant to several antibiotics have been selected in the laboratory. In the case of *R. prowazekii, Rochalimaea quintana,* and *Coxiella burnetii,* conditions of infection and transmission provide a reasonably plausible opportunity for potential selection of antibiotic-resistant strains and their entry into the transmission cycle. Indeed, naturally occurring tetracycline-resistant strains of *C. burnetii* have been isolated in Cyprus. Moreover, the possibility exists that tetracycline- or chloramphenicol-resistant *R. prowazekii* is already latent somewhere in the world and that an outbreak or epidemic of infection with this antibiotic-resistant organism could emerge.

Supportive Therapy

Steroids. Although not rigorously controlled, studies have shown that corticosteroids given in conjunction with antimicrobial drugs may cause rapid defervescence, dramatic reversal of neurologic impairment (e.g., coma and difficulty in swallowing), and an apparent improvement in the general well-being of the patient without adversely affecting the infectious process in typhus. More limited observations with scrub typhus and Rocky Mountain spotted fever have shown similar apparently beneficial effects, although corticosteroids do not reverse clotting abnormalities in Rocky Mountain spotted fever. Clinical improvement in other parameters follows the administration of 100 mg of hydrocortisone intravenously and 200 to 300 mg of cortisone acetate intramuscularly in addition to 500 mg of tetracycline given parenterally upon admission. *(Falciparum malaria must be excluded by blood smear in patients at risk for both diseases.)* Often, within 24 hours, a patient with typhus is able to swallow the final dose of antibiotic (100 mg of doxycycline), to take oral fluids, to attend to elimination, and to move spontaneously to reduce the chances of developing pressure necrosis or thrombophlebitis. This therapy is reserved for seriously ill patients.

Fluid and Electrolyte Balance. Oral fluids sufficient to ensure a daily urine output of at least 1500 ml suffice for the conscious, cooperative patient without renal impairment. The comatose patient will require parenteral fluids to maintain an adequate urine output. Indeed, correction of dehydration and hypovolemia may improve renal function. However, excess salt and fluids contribute to the generalized edema, including pulmonary edema.

Cardiovascular Complications. The most prominent manifestations of the typhus, scrub typhus, and spotted fever groups of rickettsial diseases can be attributed to abnormalities of the cardiovascular system. Some degree of hypotension is common, and frequently in the second week of disease, severe hypotension is difficult to manage and is a leading cause of death. Its cause is only incompletely understood. However, it is assumed that the widespread focal lesions of the small vessels contribute to increased vascular permeability, hypovolemia, and collapse and may also account for some of the clotting abnormalities. This in turn would help explain certain complications—hemorrhage, vascular occlusion (e.g., gangrene [Fig. 23–6] and hemiplegia), and thrombophlebitis—and would suggest more rational approaches to their prevention and management, especially when specifically identified by laboratory tests.

Albumin may be used to combat hypoproteinemia. A transfusion of packed red blood cells can correct anemia. Heparin has been described by some as treatment for rickettsia-associated intravascular clotting, but others have failed to detect benefit from heparin in the clotting abnormalities accompanying Rocky Mountain spotted fever.

The management of peripheral vascular collapse with the following is empirical and largely of unproven benefit: (1) oxygen; (2) salt-poor concentrated albumin used judiciously as a plasma expander and to reduce edema; (3) vasopressor drugs, e.g., levarterenol bitartrate (Levophed); and (4) corticosteroids such as hydrocortisone.

Pulmonary edema is usually due to increased vascular permeability, not to congestive heart failure. and is exacerbated by excessive electrolytes and water. No guidelines are available for the use of diuretics, but if their use is contemplated, consideration should be given to the state of renal function.

Massive intravascular hemolysis, described in glucose–6-phosphate dehydrogenase-deficient subjects with murine or scrub typhus, has been managed successfully with dialysis.

Other Complications. Bacterial pneumonia, which is still common in epidemic typhus, or other bacterial infections are treated with antimicrobial agents according to the causative organisms and their sensitivity patterns. Gangrene, decubitus ulcers, and thrombophlebitis are treated by appropriate surgical and medical methods. Unless caused by a large destructive process (hemorrhage or thrombosis of a large vessel), neurologic abnormalities usually resolve with convalescence, although personality changes, electroencephalographic abnormalities, and deafness have been known to persist in some patients for months.

Nursing Care. Patients may be irrational, delirious

(Fig. 23–4), or agitated and may injure themselves or even attempt self-destruction. Close observation and restraint may be required. Comatose patients should be turned frequently to prevent pressure necrosis, thrombophlebitis, and hypostatic pneumonia. Special skin care and protection of bony prominences may be desirable in view of the vascular damage associated with the disease. Good oral hygiene reduces the chances of suppurative parotitis.

BIBLIOGRAPHY

General

Baca OG, Paretsky D: Q fever and *Coxiella burnetii:* a model for host-parasite interactions. Microbiol Rev 47:127, 1983.

Burgdorfer W, Anacker RL: Rickettsiae and Rickettsial Diseases. New York, Academic Press, 1981, pp 1–650.

Moulder JW: Comparative biology of intracellular parasites. Microbiol Rev 49:298, 1985.

Weiss E: The biology of rickettsiae. Annu Rev Microbiol 36:345, 1982.

WHO Working Group on Rickettsial Diseases: Rickettsioses: A continuing disease problem. Bull WHO 60:157, 1982.

Wisseman CL Jr: Selected observations on rickettsiae and their host cells. Acta Virol 30:81, 1986.

Laboratory Diagnosis

Brown GW, Shirai A, Rogers C, Groves MG: Diagnostic criteria for scrub typhus: probability values for immunofluorescent antibody and Proteus OXK agglutinin titers. Am J Trop Med Hyg 32:1101, 1983.

Clements ML, Dumler JS, Fiset P, et al: Serodiagnosis of Rocky Mountain spotted fever: comparison of IgM and IgG enzyme-linked immunosorbent assays and indirect fluorescent antibody test. J Infect Dis 148:876, 1983.

Dasch GA, Halle S, Bourgeois AL: Sensitive microplate enzyme-linked immunosorbent assay for detection of antibodies against the scrub typhus rickettsia, *Rickettsia tsutsugamushi.* J Clin Microbiol 9:38, 1979.

Doeller G, Doeller PC, Gerth H-J: Early diagnosis of Q fever: detection of immunoglobulin M by radioimmunoassay and enzyme immunoassay. Eur J Clin Microbiol 3:550, 1984.

Field PR, Hunt JG, Murphy AM: Detection and persistence of specific IgM antibody to *Coxiella burnetii* by enzyme-linked immunosorbent assay: a comparison with immunofluorescence and complement fixation tests. J Infect Dis 148:477, 1983.

Goldwasser RA, Shepard CC: Fluorescent antibody methods in the differentiation of murine and epidemic typhus sera: specific changes resulting from previous immunization. J Immunol 82:373, 1959.

Hays PL: Rocky Mountain spotted fever in children in Kansas: the diagnostic value of an IgM-specific immunofluorescence assay. J Infect Dis 151:369, 1985.

Hechemy KE, Anacker RL, Phillip RN, et al: Detection of Rocky Mountain spotted fever antibodies by a latex agglutination test. J Clin Microbiol 12:144, 1980.

Hechemy KE, Osterman JV, Eisemann CS, et al: Detection of typhus antibodies by latex agglutination. J Clin Microbiol 13:214, 1980.

Hechemy KE, Stevens RW, Saskowski S, et al: Discrepancies in Weil-Felix and microimmunofluorescence test results for Rocky Mountain spotted fever. J Clin Microbiol 9:292, 1979.

Kelley DJ, Wong PW, Gan E, Lewis GE Jr: Comparative evaluation of the indirect immunoperoxidase test for the serodiagnosis of rickettsial disease. Am J Trop Med Hyg 38:400, 1988.

Marrero M, Raoult D: Centrifugation–shell vial technique for rapid detection of Mediterranean spotted fever rickettsiae in blood cultures. Am J Trop Med Hyg 40:197, 1989.

Newhouse VF, Shepard CC, Redus MD, et al: A comparison of the complement fixation, indirect fluorescent antibody, and microagglu-

tination tests for the serological diagnosis of rickettsial diseases. Am J Trop Med Hyg 28:387, 1979.

Ormsbee R, Peacock M, Philip R, et al: Serologic diagnosis of epidemic typhus fever. Am J Hyg 105:261, 1977.

Philip RN, Casper LA, MacCormack JN, et al: A comparison of serological methods for diagnosis of Rocky Mountain spotted fever. Am J Epidemiol 105:56, 1977.

Philip RN, Casper EA, Ormsbee RA, et al: Microimmunofluorescence test for the serological study of Rocky Mountain spotted fever and typhus. J Clin Microbiol 3:51, 1976.

Rawlings JA, Elliott LB, Little LM: Comparison of a latex agglutination procedure with the microimmunofluorescence test for *Rickettsia typhi.* J Clin Microbiol 21:470, 1985.

Woodward TE, Pederson CE Jr, Oster CN, et al: Prompt confirmation of Rocky Mountain spotted fever: Identification of rickettsiae in skin tissues. J Infect Dis 134:297, 1976.

Worswick D, Marmion BP: Antibody response in acute and chronic Q fever and in subjects vaccinated against Q fever. J Med Microbiol 19:281, 1985.

Pathology

Pinkerton H, Strano AJ: Diseases caused by rickettsiae. *In* Binford CH, Connor DH (eds): Pathology of Tropical and Extraordinary Diseases, Vol 1. Washington, DC., Armed Forces Institute of Pathology, 1976, pp 87–100.

Chemotherapy

Kimbrough RC III, Ormsbee RA, Peacock MG: Q fever endocarditis: a three and one-half year follow-up. *In* Burgdorfer W, Anacker RL (eds): Rickettsiae and Rickettsial Diseases. New York, Academic Press, 1981, p 125.

Olson JG, Bourgeois AL, Fang RCY, Dennis DT: Risk of relapse associated with doxycycline therapy for scrub typhus. *In* Burgdorfer W, Anacker RL (eds): Rickettsiae and Rickettsial Diseases. New York, Academic Press, 1981, p 201.

Raoult D, Gallais H, De Micco P, Casanova P: Ciprofloxacin therapy for Mediterranean spotted fever. Antimicrob Agents Chemother 30:606, 1986.

Spicer AJ, Peacock MG, Williams JC: Effectiveness of several antibiotics in suppressing chick embryo lethality during experimental infections by *Coxiella burnetii, Rickettsia typhi* and *R. rickettsii. In* Burgdorfer W, Anacker RL (eds): Rickettsiae and Rickettsial Diseases, New York, Academic Press, 1981, p 375.

Wisseman CL Jr, Silverman DJ, Waddell A, et al: Penicillin-induced unstable intracellular spheroplast formation by rickettsiae. J Infect Dis 146:147, 1982.

Wisseman CL Jr, Waddell A: *In vitro* sensitivity of *Rickettsia rickettsii* to doxycycline. J Infect Dis 145:584, 1982.

Wisseman CL Jr, Waddell AD, Walsh WT: *In vitro* studies of the action of antibiotics on *Rickettsia prowazeki* by two basic methods of cell culture. J Infect Dis 130:564, 1974.

Yeaman MR, Mitscher LA, Baca OG: In vitro susceptibility of *Coxiella burnetii* to antibiotics, including several quinolones. Antimicrob Agents Chemother 31:1079, 1987.

23. THE TYPHUS GROUP

Charles L. Wisseman, Jr.

Three clinical and epidemiologic entities constitute the established diseases of the typhus group: (1) primary louse-borne epidemic typhus *(Rickettsia prowazekii),* (2) its recrudescent form, Brill-Zinsser disease *(R. prowazekii),* and (3) flea-borne murine typhus *(R. mooseri [R. typhi]).* These diseases are similar clinically and pathologically but differ in intensity of certain symptoms and signs, severity, and case-fatality rate. (See Tables III A–1 to III A–3 for summaries of selected features of the organisms, the diseases, and their epidemiologies.) This conventional listing of typhus group diseases has been complicated in the United States by (1) the isolation of a new species, *R. canada,* from ticks in Canada and California and its implication, on serologic grounds, as the possible cause of a Rocky Mountain spotted fever–like disease in Georgia; (2) the isolation of a rickettsia indistinguishable from *R. prowazekii* from flying squirrels in the eastern United States, and the recognition of sporadic human cases serologically identified as *R. prowazekii* infection in houses harboring flying squirrels; and (3) the strong 1-way serologic cross-reactions between *R. canada* and *R. prowazekii.* Much more information, especially isolation and characterization of the agents from human cases, is needed for clarification.

23.1.   EPIDEMIC LOUSE-BORNE TYPHUS FEVER

DEFINITION. Classic typhus fever is an acute infectious disease transmitted by the human body louse *(Pediculus humanus humanus)* and characterized clinically by sudden onset, sustained high fever of about 2 weeks' duration, a maculopapular rash, and altered mental state. Brill-Zinsser disease is a recrudescence of typhus that occurs months to years after primary infection, is caused by organisms persisting in tissues since the primary infection, and clinically resembles a mild form of classic typhus.

ETIOLOGY (III A, General Principles). *Rickettsia prowazekii* is the etiologic agent of both classic typhus fever and Brill-Zinsser disease (see Fig. III A–1). No evidence has been obtained for significant variations in antigenic composition or virulence for humans in strains from different areas, but attenuation has been observed as a laboratory phenomenon.

TRANSMISSION AND EPIDEMIOLOGY
(III A; General Principles)
Transmission
Epidemic Louse-Borne Typhus. The "classic" infection cycle is restricted to humans and the human body louse *(Pediculus humanus humanus),* although the organism can also grow in the head louse *(P. humanus capitis)* (Table III A–1). The louse acquires the rickettsiae by feeding on the blood of a typhus patient during the rickettsemic phase; large numbers of rickettsiae are excreted in the feces. The organisms are not transmitted by bite. Instead, crushed infective lice or louse feces contaminate bite sites or other breaks in the skin, or airborne infective louse feces gain access through the respiratory tract.

Brill-Zinsser Disease. In most areas, humans, through the phenomenon of persisting infection and subsequent recrudescence (Brill-Zinsser disease), are the only known interepidemic reservoir and the mechanism by which the rickettsiae are made available again to lice. Neither the factors that precipitate recrudescence nor the precise rate of recrudescence is known, although one estimate suggests a rate of less than 10 per 100,000 cases of primary infection. The efficiency with which

lice become infected with *R. prowazekii* is apparently less during feeding on patients with Brill-Zinsser disease than on patients with primary typhus. Nevertheless, this phenomenon is known to have initiated typhus outbreaks and probably also contributes to sustaining endemicity.

Distribution. One major key to epidemic typhus is the body louse vector. Typhus can occur anywhere when political, socioeconomic, environmental, and cultural factors predispose to lousiness and the transfer of lice among people. These factors are currently present in some mountainous areas of both hemispheres as well as in equatorial regions, in deserts (Sahara and Arabian Deserts) where heavy clothing is worn continuously, and in tropical regions among nearly naked populations whose waistbands or arm and leg ornaments provide harborage for lice. At present, the known distribution of louse-borne typhus fever includes mountainous regions of Mexico and Guatemala, the Andean highlands of South America, the Himalayan regions (including Afghanistan and Pakistan), mountainous or highland regions of Africa (i.e., Ethiopia, Burundi, Rwanda, and Lesotho), and northern China. Reservoirs in the form of typhus convalescents occur on all continents, but those derived from typhus contracted during and after World War II are diminishing in number.

Depending on many factors, louse-borne typhus can occur as a truly epidemic disease, as a prolonged endemic-epidemic disease (as in Ethiopia today), or as a highly endemic infection with sporadic, often unrecognized infections, especially in young age groups, but with sharp, sporadic village outbreaks involving all age groups (as in Andean countries today).

IMMUNITY (III A, General Principles). Susceptibility to louse-borne typhus is universal. Convalescence from infection is accompanied by a solid, long-lasting immunity against disease, although second infections have been described. The immune response consists of both humoral and cellular components that are demonstrable for many years. The immunologic defect that permits the occasional recrudescence (Brill-Zinsser disease) to occur is unknown. Cross-immunity is strong against murine typhus but not against Rocky Mountain spotted fever, with which there may be some serologic cross-reactions.

PATHOLOGY. The general pathologic and pathophysiologic features are described in III A, General Principles.

CLINICAL MANIFESTATIONS AND COURSE. The following description applies to untreated full-blown classic typhus fever in adults. The incubation period usually is from 8 to 12 days but may be as short as 6 days or as long as 15 days (Table III A–3). The disease may be divided into the prodromal, early, and late phases (Pathogenesis in III A, General Principles).

Prodromal and Early Phases. Prodromes of vague malaise and headache are not uncommon. The early phase is usually ushered in by the abrupt onset of fever, severe headache (Fig. 23–1), myalgia of the back and legs, and chills or chilly sensations. The headache is intense and intractable and persists day and night. Over the first 2 or 3 days, the temperature attains a level of about 39 to 41C, where it remains, with only slight fluctuations, until death or recovery. The skin is usually hot and dry. The face is flushed or dusky; the conjunctivas are suffused; photophobia is frequent. The mental state is dull. Weakness and prostration may be mild early after onset, but may become profound after 2 or 3 days. Unproductive cough with sparse physical findings occurs in about two thirds of the patients. Nausea, vomiting, and diarrhea occur but are uncommon. Constipation is usually present.

Late Phase

Rash. The characteristic rash appears between the fourth and seventh days and ushers in the late phase of disease. In some instances, it is preceded by a diffuse, transient erythema. The lesions first appear on the trunk and axillary folds and spread to the extremities, sparing the face, palms, and soles, except in severely ill patients. At first, the lesions are pinkish-red macules that blanch on pressure. The evolution of the rash depends on the severity of the illness. In mild cases, it may fade completely in 1 or 2 days; in cases of moderate severity, it may become maculopapular, possibly hemorrhagic, changing to a reddish-brown color and lasting for 1 to 2 weeks before fading; in severe cases, the lesions may be exceedingly numerous, almost confluent, quickly becoming hemorrhagic or purpuric. The rash may be absent in 5 to 10% of patients. With experience and proper lighting, the papular component may be seen without too much difficulty in dark-skinned persons (Fig. 23–2).

Cardiopulmonary Findings. At first, the pulse rate is slow in relation to the temperature, but by the end of the first week, it becomes rapid (110 to 140), weak, and frequently undulating or irregular. The blood pressure

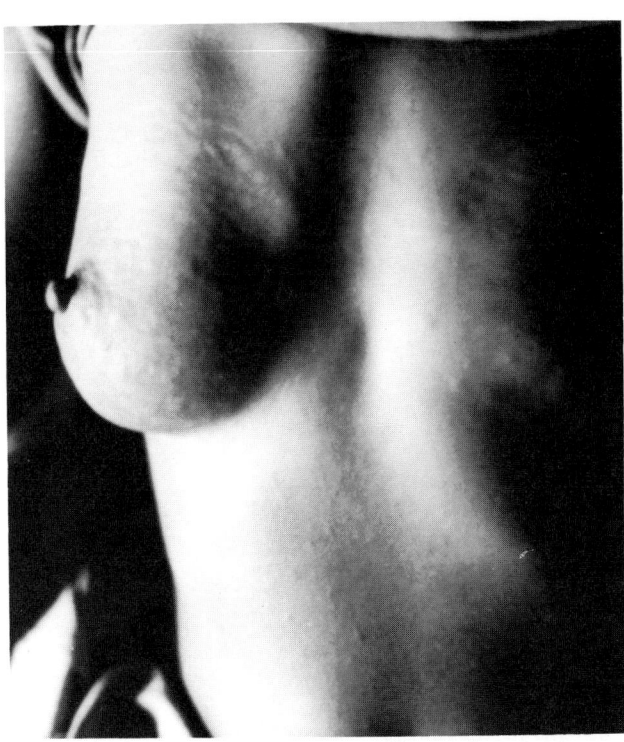

FIGURE 23–2. Louse-borne typhus fever. The rash in typhus is macular to maculopapular, pink and blanching under pressure early, and fixed and petechial late. The papular component may be seen under appropriate lighting conditions even when the erythema is masked in deeply pigmented skin.

is usually low, sometimes with a systolic pressure below 80 mm Hg, and there may be brief episodes of severe hypotension. Cyanosis may be present.

Neurologic Findings. The mental state progresses from dullness to stupor or, occasionally, coma (Fig. 23–3). The stupor may be interrupted by periods of delirium, excitement, or vigorous activity, during which the patient may exhibit self-destructive action or wander off into the bush (Fig. 23–4). Cranial nerves are selectively and variably involved (e.g., tinnitus, deafness, dysphagia, and dysphonia). Coarse tremors may appear.

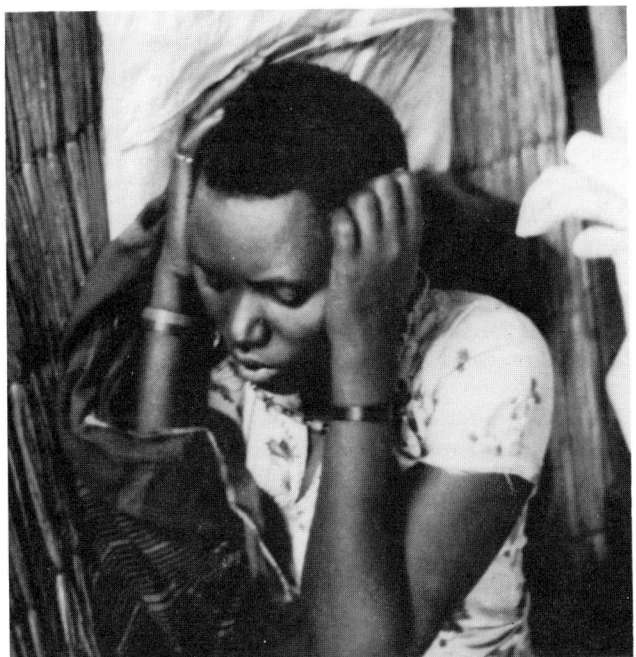

FIGURE 23–1. Louse-borne typhus fever. Headache, although not invariably a prominent feature, is commonly severe, constant, relentless, and incapacitating. Patients often describe it as the worst headache that they have ever had. Similar headache may be present in murine typhus, scrub typhus, spotted fever group infections, and Q fever.

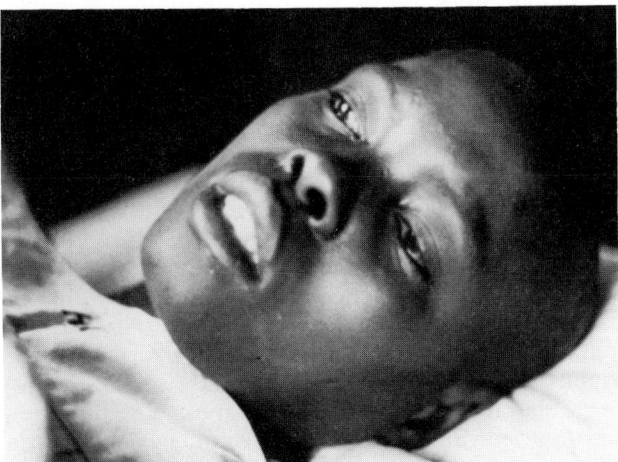

FIGURE 23–3. Louse-borne typhus fever. After a few days of untreated typhus fever, patients may sink into a semistuporous state with characteristic facies, lying immobile, staring unseeing, and responding only to strong external stimuli.

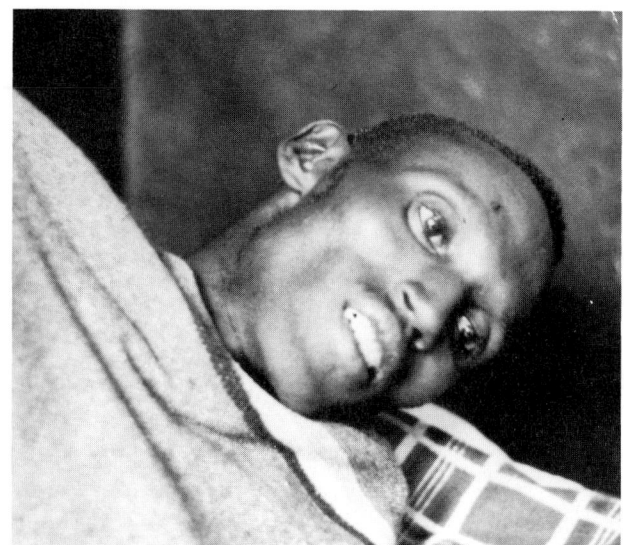

FIGURE 23–4. Louse-borne typhus fever. Delirium is a troublesome complication.

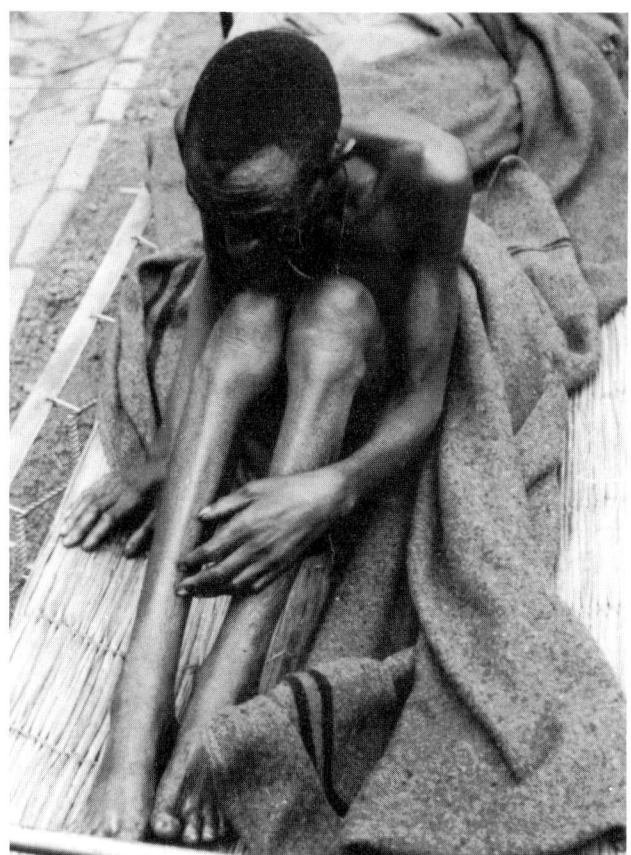

FIGURE 23–5. Louse-borne typhus fever. Three weeks after onset of disease, this formerly robust and well-developed young adult male shows the wasting, extensive loss of tissue mass, and debilitation typical of severe untreated typhus. Prompt early specific antirickettsial chemotherapy prevents this troublesome complication that needlessly prolongs convalescence.

Urinary and fecal incontinence is encountered in moderately or severely ill patients.

Laboratory Findings. Oliguria, proteinuria, and azotemia are common. Jaundice is rare, but elevations in serum aminotransferases may appear early. The white blood cell count may show leukopenia early; in the second and third weeks of the disease, it is normal or only slightly elevated, unless complications ensue. Eosinophils are absent or rare in the early stages of typhus. Anemia may develop in the second or third week.

Outcome. Death from untreated typhus usually occurs between the ninth and eighteenth days of illness. The terminal period is usually characterized by a profound stupor, peripheral vascular collapse, and severe renal failure. When recovery is the outcome, the temperature begins to decline after 14 to 18 days and reaches a normal level by rapid lysis in 2 or 4 days. The mental and physical states of the patient improve strikingly as the temperature falls, but strength returns more slowly (2 to 3 months) (Fig. 23–5).

Complications. Secondary bacterial bronchopneumonia, otitis media, and parotitis are common in untreated patients. Thrombosis may affect the large arteries, with serious results, e.g., hemiplegia. Thrombosis of small vessels in the skin may lead to gangrene, particularly of the toes, fingers, or ear lobes (Fig. 23–6). Necrosis of the skin may occur over the bony prominences, especially over the sacrum or greater trochanter.

Modified Disease. The severity of disease and the case-fatality rate increase with age, being less severe and often uncharacteristic in younger children, but increasing rapidly in those over the age of 40 years. In persons who contract typhus after having received killed typhus vaccine, the disease is greatly modified, with headache, fever of a few days' duration, and a transient rash but with rare complications and negligible mortality.

Brill-Zinsser Disease. Recrudescent typhus is similar to primary typhus except that it is milder. On the average, the fever is lower and of shorter duration, the rash is less intense and often absent, and the case-fatality rate is low.

LABORATORY DIAGNOSIS (III A, General Principles). *R. prowazekii* can be isolated from blood or tissues by inoculation of guinea pigs or directly in tissue culture. Diagnosis is usually made by demonstrating a rise in antibody titer by any one or combination of tests. The indirect fluorescent antibody (IFA) test is most useful in distinguishing among current primary typhus (early IgM response), recrudescent typhus or Brill-Zinsser disease (accelerated dominant IgG response), and past typhus infection (unchanging dominantly IgG titers). Differentiation between louse-borne and murine typhus can be made with species-specific complement fixation (CF) tests, absorption-type IFA tests, or toxin neutralization tests. The microagglutination test is convenient for field use but will not reliably differentiate between louse-borne and murine typhus infections in humans, as opposed to rodents and guinea pigs. Antibodies persist for many years.

PROGNOSIS. Depending on host factors, such as age, stress, nutritional state, other concurrent diseases, and perhaps the past typhus history of the population, the case-fatality rate in untreated typhus may range from 10% or less to 60%. Deep coma, severe hypotension, and tachycardia associated with falling body tem-

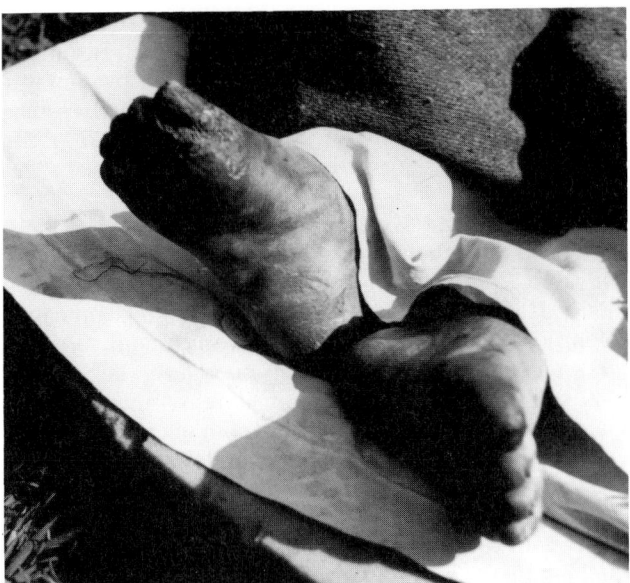

FIGURE 23–6. Louse-borne typhus fever. A small proportion of patients may develop some degree of dry gangrene, most commonly of the extremities. It may be limited to the tips of the fingers and toes but on occasion may involve all or part of the foot or even the entire lower leg. This patient shows gangrene of the distal part of the right foot and beginning necrosis of the left hallux. Partial débridement of the insensitive necrotic right hallux and foot was occurring during nightly visits of rats.

perature are signs of poor prognosis. However, even patients with these signs often respond dramatically to appropriate chemotherapy and supportive measures. Appropriate treatment reduces the mortality rate in ordinary severe typhus fever virtually to zero.

TREATMENT. Treatment is described in detail in III A, General Principles. A single 100- to 200-mg oral dose of the long-acting tetracycline doxycycline is the treatment of choice under ordinary circumstances. The response of uncomplicated typhus to specific antirickettsial chemotherapy, whether begun early or late, is highly predictable. The temperature returns to normal within 48 to 72 hours, averaging about 60 hours, accompanied by progressive lessening of headache and improvement of mental status. Occasionally manifestations such as deafness may appear during response to early therapy but subsequently subside. The occasional recrudescence of fever is usually mild and self-limited, but more severe recrudescences respond to retreatment with the same drug and dose. Other concurrent or intercurrent infections are treated by appropriate methods; gangrene may require surgical intervention.

Brill-Zinsser disease is managed in an identical manner. Because louse-borne typhus, especially in epidemic form, tends to occur under circumstances under which even the most elemental components of conventional medical care may not be available, it is heartening to know that the simple expedient of administering a single 100- to 200-mg dose of doxycycline will cure almost all patients.

PREVENTION AND CONTROL

Decontamination. Infected lice and louse feces on a patient with typhus present a special hazard to all nonimmune contacts, including physicians and atten-

dants, among whom infection is a common occupational hazard. Decontamination and delousing of the patient with typhus (including the head) and his or her clothing (including blankets and hats) are performed immediately on hospitalization. Clothing and bedding are best decontaminated by heat, because this will kill the lice as well as the rickettsiae. After the patient is decontaminated and deloused, isolation and quarantine are not necessary. Depending on the circumstances, it may be necessary to apply insecticides at appropriate intervals to prevent reinfestation with lice.

Louse Control. Control of louse-borne typhus currently depends heavily on control of the louse vector. When simple hygienic measures, e.g., bathing and laundering of clothes in hot water with detergent, cannot be followed, the application of insecticide dusts (10% DDT, 1% malathion, 1% lindane, or newer carbamates, depending on local louse resistance patterns) to fully clothed persons is effective for reducing louse populations and controlling disease in acute outbreaks. Insecticide resistance among body lice is a widespread and growing problem. Kits for testing insecticide susceptibility are available from the World Health Organization. The older methods of subjecting clothes and bedding to heat or fumigants, e.g., methyl bromide, are effective but cumbersome. It is possible but unproved that repellent-treated (e.g., with M-1960, permethrin, or diethyltoluamide) clothing would reduce the chances of louse acquisition. Insecticides alone are less effective for long-term louse control in areas where conditions conducive to lousiness persist and where louse strains resistant to insecticides can be, and are, selected. Long-term louse control or eradication depends on correcting the complex environmental, economic, cultural, educational, and political factors that contribute to lousiness.

Vaccine. Conventional typhus vaccines composed of killed organisms are no longer available in the United States, pending development of improved vaccines of proven protective potency. The attenuated E strain of *R. prowazekii*, when used as a living vaccine, is protective but may produce a mildly symptomatic, self-limited infection in 10 to 15% of recipients. It is not generally available in the United States.

Reduction of Exposure. Under current circumstances, the ordinary tourist is not likely to be exposed to louse-borne typhus, in contrast to murine typhus, even in endemic areas; nor are business persons, government representatives, archeologists, or engineering or construction workers likely to be exposed on assignment to most endemic zones if they maintain the usual separate households, pay attention to personal hygiene, and do not mix intimately with the affected local population. At high risk, however, are medical personnel and others who must treat or otherwise come into close contact with members of the affected populations. Depending on the circumstances, the wearing of insecticide- or repellent-treated clothing and the overnight exposure of clothing to a dichlorvos strip (No-Pest Strip) in an airtight bag may reduce exposure to lice.

Chemoprophylaxis. Under special short-term circumstances, when it is necessary to keep personnel disease free for a limited time, chemoprophylaxis with 100 mg of doxycycline once or twice a week might be effective. However, this has not been formally tested with louse-borne typhus to determine the optimal spacing of doses and duration of administration to permit subclinical immunizing infection. The disease might develop after the drug is discontinued. Close medical surveillance and prompt chemotherapy on the first or second day of illness reduce typhus to a relatively minor inconvenience, with possible return after a few days to sedentary or light physical activity for the otherwise healthy young adult. The practice of administering a single dose of doxycycline to healthy contacts of patients with typhus with the mistaken notion that it will prevent typhus reveals an ignorance of the interplay between a rickettsiostatic antibiotic and the developing immunity that is essential to control the infection; it can only be condemned. Delay of onset of disease is the likely outcome.

It is presumed that chemotherapy shortens the period of rickettsemia in typhus as it does in scrub typhus. Under primitive or overwhelming conditions, when louse control may not be possible, this would be expected to limit the time a patient is infectious for lice. However, the growth of rickettsiae in infected lice feeding on blood containing therapeutic levels of doxycycline is inhibited and the lice survive longer.

23.2. MURINE OR FLEA-BORNE TYPHUS FEVER

DEFINITION. Murine typhus fever is an acute infectious disease communicable from rodent hosts to humans sporadically, often by means of the rat flea (*Xenopsylla cheopis*). The disease is similar clinically to classic epidemic typhus except that it is milder.

ETIOLOGY (III A, General Principles). *Rickettsia mooseri (R. typhi)* shares some common antigenic determinants (epitopes) with *R. prowazekii* and *R. canada* but differs in specific epitopes, host range, and certain other biologic properties. Significant cross-immunity between *R. mooseri* and *R. prowazekii* is produced by infection but not by killed vaccines. DNA homology studies show a reasonably close relationship between *R. mooseri* and *R. prowazekii*, but the difference is sufficiently large to preclude easy transition from one to the other by simple variation or mutation, except on an evolutionary scale. Thus, *R. mooseri* is an unlikely source of some contemporary outbreaks of classic louse-borne epidemic typhus, as has been suggested, although limited outbreaks of louse-borne *R. mooseri* infection may have occurred.

TRANSMISSION AND EPIDEMIOLOGY (III A, General Principles)

Transmission. Murine typhus is not communicable from person to person. It is a zoonosis maintained in nature in a cycle involving rats and certain other small mammals as amplifying hosts and fleas and rat lice as vectors (Table III A–1). The rat flea (*Xenopsylla cheopis*) and other fleas are infected by feeding on rickettsemic rats and other small mammals, and the rickettsiae are excreted in the feces during the life of the flea.

Ecologic details are complex and may vary significantly from place to place. *R. mooseri* is usually not transmitted to humans by the bite of the flea, but rather by contamination of broken skin with infective feces or by inhalation of dried infective feces. Cases tend to occur sporadically, but sharp local outbreaks have been described.

Distribution and Exposure. Murine typhus is widely distributed over the world in areas penetrated by *Rattus rattus* and *Rattus norvegicus* and where the vector fleas coexist. It is grossly underestimated as a significant cause of febrile human disease in many tropical and subtropical areas where, untreated, it may have substantial economic consequences. In some areas, under appropriate conditions, *R. mooseri* may spill over from *Rattus* to other spatially closely associated small mammals (e.g., other rodents, shrews, and opossum) and to humans. Seasonal incidence of human infections appears to correlate with the period of abundance of vector fleas, which is in the summer months in the United States. Rats are commensal animals closely associated with buildings or structures containing food (such as warehouses, markets, grain elevators, and godowns). Hence, in some areas, acquisition of murine typhus by humans is often associated with certain places and occupations; in others, as in some tropical areas where heavy rodent infestation of dwellings is universal, infection is acquired in dwellings.

PATHOLOGY. Because of the low death rate in murine typhus, few postmortem studies have been done. It is assumed, however, that the lesions in humans, as is the case in experimental infection of laboratory animals, are similar to those in louse-borne typhus.

CLINICAL MANIFESTATIONS AND COURSE. The incubation period of murine typhus lasts from about 6 to 14 days. The symptoms are similar to those of louse-borne typhus, the principal differences being that murine typhus is, on the average, a milder and shorter-lasting disease, the rash is less extensive and persists for shorter periods, there are fewer complications, and the case-fatality rate is lower (Table III A–3).

Although murine typhus is often referred to as mild, and truly mild cases do occur, on the average the degree of mildness is only relative to louse-borne typhus. On an absolute scale, it can be severe and debilitating, and untreated patients may require 2 to 3 months to regain strength and weight. High fever (40 to 41C), prostration, delirium, and stupor or coma may occur. Other patients may have a low-grade fever (38 to 39C) and remain provisionally ambulatory.

DIAGNOSIS

Clinical Diagnosis. The diagnosis of murine typhus may be suspected when a patient has sustained fever of several days' duration accompanied by headache, generalized aches and pains, and a macular or maculopapular rash appearing on the trunk on the fifth or sixth day after onset of fever. The patient with murine typhus may give a history of activities that have brought her or him in contact with places where rats are numerous. However, there is often no definite recollection of a flea bite, and the clinical picture is nondescript. It is impossible on clinical evidence alone to distinguish an ordinary case of murine typhus from a case of Brill-Zinsser disease or a mild case of louse-borne typhus—or from a variety of other infectious diseases.

In many areas of the world where typhoid or other enteric fevers are common, where specific laboratory diagnostic tests are not readily available, and where chloramphenicol is routinely employed to treat enteric fevers, significant occurrence of murine typhus and sporadic louse-borne typhus may be unsuspected or unrecognized, being hidden among the enteric fevers by virtue of some clinical similarity and response to chloramphenicol. However, when ampicillin or trimethoprim-sulfamethoxazole is used for the treatment of suspected typhoid fevers, the typhus fevers do not respond, and their presence may then be unveiled.

Laboratory Diagnosis. Diagnosis can be made by specific rickettsial serologic tests or by isolation of the agent (III A, General Principles and Chapter 23.1). Prior immunization with louse-borne typhus vaccine may result in a dominant antibody response to *R. prowazekii* antigens in a subsequent *R. mooseri* infection.

IMMUNITY (III A, General Principles). Immunity is as described in louse-borne typhus, except that recrudescence (the equivalent of Brill-Zinsser disease) has not been recognized.

PROGNOSIS. The case-fatality rate is usually less than 5% in untreated patients and is virtually zero with rapid convalescence in patients with uncomplicated murine typhus treated with appropriate antirickettsial drugs.

TREATMENT. Treatment follows the guidelines presented in III A, General Principles with respect to the *multiple-dose* antimicrobial regimen. A single dose of doxycycline may not effect a cure.

PREVENTION AND CONTROL. Individual preventive measures include avoiding endemic foci where rats and their fleas abound (e.g., warehouses, storage areas, and grain elevators) and wearing repellent-treated clothing to prevent acquisition of fleas. A killed vaccine has been produced, but it has not been evaluated and is not available at present.

Rodent and Flea Control. General control measures are directed at reducing rat and flea populations. These include, among others, rat-proof construction and prevention of access of rats to food materials; reduction of rat populations by poison baits (e.g., warfarin and α-naphthylthiourea), trapping, or the introduction of poison gases into burrows; and reduction of the flea population through application of appropriate insecticides to rat runs or at bait stations. When contemplating a rodent control program, it is important to plan insecticide application for flea control prior to or simultaneously with the rodent control measures. This prevents the increased exposure of humans to fleas seeking alternative hosts. Resistance of fleas to insecticides is a growing problem.

BIBLIOGRAPHY

Al-Awadi AR, Al-Kazemi N, Ezzat G, et al: Murine typhus in Kuwait in 1978. Bull WHO 60:283, 1982.

Gaon JA, Murray ES: The natural history of recrudescent typhus (Brill-Zinsser disease) in Bosnia. Bull WHO 35:133, 1966.
Miller ES, Beeson PB: Murine typhus fever. Medicine 25:1, 1946.
Proceedings of the International Symposium of the Control of Lice and Louse-Borne Diseases. Washington, DC, December 4–6, 1972. Pan-American Health Organization Scientific Publication No. 263. Washington, DC, 1973.
Stuart BM, Pullen RL: Endemic (murine) typhus fever: Clinical observations of 180 cases. Ann Intern Med 23:520, 1945.
Traub R, Wisseman CL Jr, Farhang-Azad A: The ecology of murine typhus—a critical review. Trop Dis Bull 75:237, 1978.
Wisseman CL Jr: Concepts of louse-borne typhus control in developing countries: The use of the living attenuated E strain typhus vaccine in epidemic and endemic situations. *In* Kohn A, Klingberg MA (eds): Immunity in Viral and Rickettsial Diseases. New York, Plenum Publishing, 1972, pp 97–130.
Wisseman CL Jr, Wood WH Jr, Noriega AR, et al: Antibodies and clinical relapse of murine typhus following early chemotherapy. Ann Intern Med 57:743, 1962.
Wohlbach SB, Todd JL, Palfrey FW: The Etiology and Pathology of Typhus. Cambridge, MA, Harvard University Press, 1922.
Zarafonetis CJD: The typhus fevers. *In* Coates JB, Havens WP (eds): Internal Medicine in World War I. Vol II: Infectious Diseases. Washington, DC, Office of the Surgeon General, Department of the Army, 1963, pp 143–223.

24. THE SPOTTED FEVER GROUP

Charles L. Wisseman, Jr.

The spotted fever (SF) group is large and complex. Its members are widely distributed over the world and, except for *Rickettsia akari,* which is transmitted by mouse mites, are associated primarily with ixodid ticks, which serve as both vector and reservoir (Table III A–1; III A, General Principles). Laboratory methods have recently been developed for reliable differentiation of organisms. New information is evolving so rapidly that any summary should be viewed as tentative and subject to frequent revision.

Current information suggests that each major land mass has at least 1 tick-borne species that causes disease in humans, with some apparent overlap where major land masses join: *R. rickettsii* (Rocky Mountain spotted fever [RMSF], São Paulo tick typhus) in North, Central, and South America; *R. australis* (Queensland tick typhus) in northern Australia; *R. sibirica* (North Asian tick typhus) in the North Asian region of the Soviet Union and China, to the southern slopes of the Himalaya mountains in Pakistan, and to central Europe; and a putative new species causing the recently recognized spotted fever in Japan.

Diseases attributed to *R. conorii* are widely distributed: (1) the Mediterranean littoral from North Africa through southern Europe to Spain and the islands of Sicily and Corsica (fièvre boutonneuse, Marseille fever, Mediterranean spotted fever, fiebre botonosa); (2) subSaharan Africa (Kenya tick typhus and South African tick typhus diseases); (3) east to the Indian subcontinent (Indian tick typhus disease). However, the rickettsial strains causing human disease over this large area may not all be identical. South African strains are said to differ somewhat from classic North African *R. conorii.* Some spotted fever infections in Israel are caused by a strain sufficiently different to be proposed as a new species, *R. israeli.* Systematic study by more specific modern methods may show significant geographic strain variation.

Evidence for the occurrence of tick typhus in Southeast Asia is still fragmentary but suggestive. In Malaysia, patients with eschar, rash, and SF group antibodies have been recognized and the occurrence of SF group antibodies among small mammals suggests an enzootic cycle, but no SF group agent has yet been isolated. Early reports from French Indochina suggested the occurrence of tick typhus, but the implication of *R. conorii* was beyond the capacity of the serologic methods of the time. The so-called Thai tick typhus rickettsial strain was isolated from ticks and has not yet been associated with human disease.

Systematic study of ticks in the United States has revealed the presence of multiple new species of spotted fever group rickettsiae of no known pathogenicity for humans. Their prevalence in ticks may far exceed that of virulent *R. rickettsii*, even in areas highly endemic for RMSF. The tick isolate representing a new species from Switzerland has not yet been associated with human disease.

24.1. ROCKY MOUNTAIN SPOTTED FEVER

DEFINITION. Rocky Mountain spotted fever (RMSF) is also known as fiebre manchada (Mexico), fiebre petequial (Colombia), and fiebre maculosa or São Paulo typhus (Brazil). It is a mild to severe, frequently fatal, acute infectious disease of the Western Hemisphere caused by *Rickettsia rickettsii* and transmitted to humans by several species of ticks. The disease is characterized by sudden onset with chills and headache, fever of about 2 to 3 weeks' duration, and a rash on the extremities and trunk beginning about the fourth day of illness (Table III A–3).

ETIOLOGY. As noted, the disease is caused by *R. rickettsii*, the prototype species of the SF group of rickettsiae, the members of which share group antigens but can be differentiated by more specific tests. *R. rickettsii* share a minor antigenic component with typhus group rickettsiae, which might cause some confusion in serodiagnosis unless antigens of both groups are included in the tests. Although several other species of the SF group of rickettsiae have been isolated from ticks in the United States, to date only typical *R. rickettsii* have been isolated from infections of humans. Intensive efforts to isolate and characterize rickettsiae from patients are needed to clarify the role of other SF group agents as possible causes of human disease.

DISTRIBUTION AND INCIDENCE. Although originally encountered in Rocky Mountain states (Montana and Idaho), RMSF has been recognized in at least 46 states and now is actually more prevalent in the southern Atlantic states than in the West. In the eastern United States, it extends from Cape Cod, Massachusetts, and some adjacent islands, through a focus on Long Island, to Florida. Almost half of the cases in the United States occur in Maryland, Virginia, North Carolina, and Georgia and about 20% in the West South

Central region, with Oklahoma having the highest incidence (2.7/100,000) in 1987. The total number of reported cases per year in the United States rose steadily through the 1970s to more than 1000 about 1980, after which it slowly declined to 592 in 1987. The reasons for the waxing and waning of RMSF cases are not fully understood but may include abundance of ticks, extension of suburbs into tick-infested rural areas, increased recreational activities in wilderness areas, and better diagnosis and reporting. RMSF has also been recognized in several provinces of Canada, Mexico, Central America (Panama and Costa Rica), and South America (Colombia and Brazil).

TRANSMISSION AND EPIDEMIOLOGY. RMSF is a zoonosis maintained in a natural cycle between certain tick species and small rodents, rabbits, and larger mammals. Humans, a dead-end host for *R. rickettsii*, become infected when they intrude into this enzootic cycle, e.g., for recreational or occupational reasons, and are bitten by an infected tick.

Although multiple tick species (both hard and soft varieties) become naturally infected and may play a role in transmission among animals, the main tick vectors for man are hard (ixodid) ticks—the wood tick, *Dermacentor andersoni*, in the western United States; the dog tick, *Dermacentor variabilis*, in the eastern United States; *Amblyomma americanum* in Texas and Oklahoma; the brown dog tick, *Rhipicephalus sanguineus*, in northern Mexico (and introduced into the United States); and *Amblyomma cajennense* in Brazil and Colombia.

In some areas, RMSF tends to be sylvan or campestral, and certain occupational and recreational groups are at highest risk (e.g., ranchers, forestry workers, highway and railway workers, telephone lineworkers, hikers, and campers). In other areas, such as the eastern United States, rural and suburban populations of all age groups, including children, are at risk. Focal areas of high endemicity may exist within broad endemic regions as well as within urban settings. For example, in 1987 cases of RMSF were traced to a park within New York City where *R. rickettsii*–infected *Dermacentor variabilis* ticks were found. Dogs may bring infected ticks into households; removing the ticks from dogs may pose a hazard. RMSF is largely seasonal, paralleling the abundance and activity of the tick vectors. This is usually maximum in late spring and early summer, but transmission continues at a diminished rate into the fall, and a few cases are reported in the winter months. If *R. rickettsii* becomes established in the United States in the introduced dog tick *Rhipicephalus sanguineus*, which may colonize houses and kennels, the possibility exists for urban spotted fever in any season.

PATHOLOGY. The pathology of RMSF conforms to the description in III A, General Principles. Of special note is the fact that vasculitis in RMSF is not limited to the endothelium and is more severe than in typhus or scrub typhus, causing more pronounced thrombotic occlusions and necrosis of the muscular layers (Fig. III A–6). Microinfarcts occur with some frequency in the central nervous system (Fig. III A–7).

CLINICAL MANIFESTATIONS (Table 24–1). A

TABLE 24–1. Common Signs, Symptoms, and Laboratory Findings in Rocky Mountain Spotted Fever and Mediterranean Spotted Fever

Signs/Symptoms/Findings	RMSF* %	MSF† %
(Number of cases)	(262)	(199)
Fever	99	100
Fever >102F/39C	90	80
Headache	91	56
Conjunctivitis	30	9
Rash, maculopapular	82	96
Rash, petechial	49	10
Rash, palms/soles	74	79
Myalgia	47	36
Abdominal pain	52	
Stupor	26	10
Coma	9	
Meningismus	18	10
Lymphadenopathy	27	
Splenomegaly	16	6
Hepatomegaly	12	13
Jaundice	9	2
Myocarditis	5	11
Edema	18	
Renal insufficiency		6
Shock	7	
Death	4	2.5
Platelets <150,000/mm³	32	35
Blood urea nitrogen >25 mg/dl	12	6
Serum sodium <130 mEq/L	19	25
Elevated serum enzymes:		
Glutamic oxaloacetic transaminase	37	39
Alkaline phosphatase	10	21

*Rocky Mountain spotted fever. Adapted from Helmick CJ, et al: J Infect Dis 150:480, 1984.

†Mediterranean spotted fever. Adapted from Raoult D, et al: Am J Trop Med Hyg 35:845, 1986.

history of tick bite can be elicited in many, but not all, patients. In one study the triad of fever, rash, and history of exposure to ticks was present in only 67% of 262 cases during the illness. Variations in the incubation period (2 to 14 days, with an average of 7 days) and severity of disease occur in RMSF, with a tendency for an inverse relationship between the two. Severe disease often is preceded by a short incubation period (2 to 5 days).

Symptoms. When present, prodromes consist of anorexia, irritability, malaise, feverishness, and chilly sensations. Attacks may be so mild that the patient remains ambulatory or so severe that death may occur within 3 to 6 days of onset. The more typical infections are sudden in onset, with severe headache, chills, fever, prostration, myalgia (especially of the back and legs), nausea with occasional vomiting, conjunctival injection, and photophobia. There may be abdominal muscular pain, tenderness of muscles on palpation, and arthralgia.

Signs. Body temperature reaches to 39 to 40C in the first 2 days, is sustained at elevated levels for about 2 weeks, and declines by slow lysis over 3 or 4 days. Hyperthemia in the range of 41C is a serious sign. Body temperature falling to near or below normal levels in the face of severe hypotension and tachycardia carries a grave prognosis.

Rash. The characteristic rash appears about the fourth day (2 to 6 days after the onset of illness); it appears first about the wrists and ankles and then extends rapidly over all or most of the body (Fig. 24–1), including the palms, soles, face, and, occasionally, the mucous membranes of the mouth and throat. At first, the lesions are pink macules measuring 2 to 5 mm in diameter that blanch on pressure. In 2 or 3 days, they become fixed, darker red or purplish, and maculopapular, and around the fourth day, they become petechial. Hemorrhagic lesions may coalesce. The rash begins to disappear as the fever subsides but often remains as pigmented spots for weeks.

Cardiovascular Findings. Early in RMSF, the pulse is full, regular, and elevated in proportion to the fever. Later, it becomes more rapid and feeble, and some degree of hypotension develops. Increased vascular permeability results in increased extravascular fluid, hypovolemia, generalized edema, and episodes of pulmonary edema. The electrocardiogram may show minor ST deflections and prolonged PR intervals. In some cases, hypotension may attain shock levels, and gangrene of fingers, toes, ears, nose, or genitalia may develop. Thrombosis of larger vessels may lead to loss of a portion of a limb or to hemiplegia. The skin may become necrotic over bony prominences. Hemorrhage from the nose, gastrointestinal tract, or kidney may occur. Disturbances in hemostatic mechanisms have been recognized. Thrombocytopenia; activation of platelets, coagulation pathways, and the fibrinolytic system; and depletion of complement have been described, some evident even early in the disease.

Central Nervous System (CNS) Involvement. CNS involvement is manifested by restlessness, insomnia, delirium, stupor, and, in severe cases, coma. Convulsions, muscular rigidity, tremors, and athetoid movements may occur. Cranial nerve involvement is variable. Transient deafness is common, but peripheral neuritis is uncommon. Electroencephalographic changes may persist for many months. Urinary and fecal incontinence may be present in severe cases.

Involvement of Other Systems. The white blood cell count may be below 5000 cells/mm³ early in the disease and may exceed 10,000 cells/mm³ later in some patients. The liver may be enlarged, serum albumin depressed, prothrombin time prolonged, and bilirubin elevated, sometimes with jaundice. Various serum enzyme levels may be increased, indicating liver, lung, myocardial, and skeletal muscle damage. Oliguria and some azotemia are common in severe cases of RMSF. Anuria and marked azotemia occur in critically ill patients. Acute tubular necrosis may develop after prolonged hypotension. Complicating secondary bacterial infections (e.g., bronchopneumonia, otitis media, and parotitis) occur but are uncommon.

Convalescence may take weeks to months. When death occurs in nonfulminant RMSF, it usually does so late in the second week of disease (about 9 to 18 days after onset).

DIAGNOSIS. An acute febrile illness, with or without rash, in a person with a history of tick bite or exposure or possible exposure to ticks should alert the physician to the possibility of RMSF. Although other diseases, especially those with rash, may present tran-

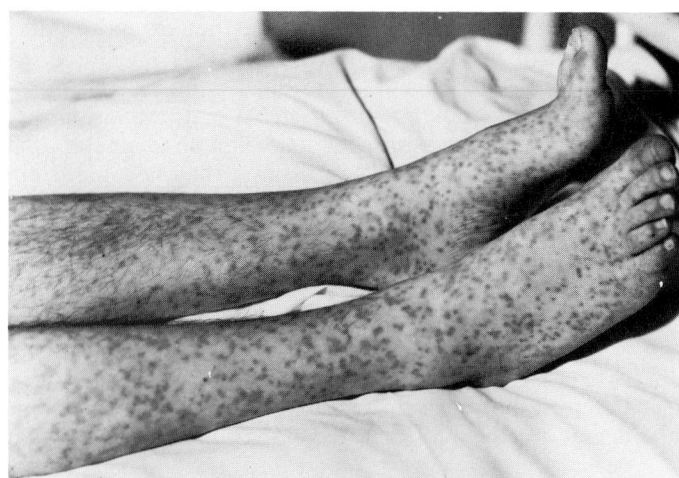

FIGURE 24–1. Rash in Rocky Mountain spotted fever. Note also the discoloration of the right hallux suggestive of incipient gangrene. (Courtesy of the Armed Forces Institute of Pathology, Photograph Neg. No. 67987-3.)

sient early differential diagnostic problems, the 2 diseases that have consistently caused the greatest confusion are measles and meningococcemia. The most promising laboratory method for providing a specific diagnosis early enough in the disease to permit effective therapeutic intervention is the demonstration by the fluorescent antibody technique of spotted fever group rickettsiae in skin biopsy specimens. Isolation attempts are encouraged, and serologic diagnostic methods (III A, General Principles) are useful and important but rarely yield results in time for most efficient management. Indeed, antibody response may not be detectable until about 6 weeks after onset.

PROGNOSIS. Mild cases occur, but the rapid, severe course in some patients makes it imperative to regard any suspected case of RMSF as a medical emergency. In untreated cases, the overall case-fatality rate is about 20%; the low (<10%) and high (>60%) rates in some areas are partly dependent on the age profile of the affected population. Prognosis depends on the severity of infection, host factors (e.g., age and the presence of other disease), and the time after onset when specific antirickettsial chemotherapy is started. Even with effective antirickettsial drugs available, the case-fatality rate has remained at about 5%. Analysis of fatal cases has shown that the single most important factor was delay in the institution of antirickettsial therapy. With the time between onset and death being as little as 3 to 6 days, the critical period when antimicrobial therapy can influence the outcome may be short.

TREATMENT. *Prompt administration of a tetracycline antibiotic, including doxycycline, or chloramphenicol, daily for about 6 days is the single most important specific therapeutic measure* (III A, General Principles). Because specific etiologic diagnosis may be impossible in the first few days of disease, any patient seriously considered (on the basis of history of potential exposure) to have RMSF should be treated as such while other diagnostic procedures continue.

Specific treatment of uncomplicated RMSF on the first or second day of disease usually results in rapid defervescence, sometimes by 24 to 48 hours, with few residua. In sharp contrast, in untreated severe cases, tissue damage caused by progressive infection may be accompanied by increasingly serious physiologic derangements, such as in the cardiovascular and blood clotting systems, which do not respond directly to antimicrobial therapy and which often are poorly responsive to specific therapeutic measures. A patient may progress to this dangerous state in 5 to 7 (or even fewer) days after the onset of disease. It is not uncommon for a patient with an unsuspected case of RMSF to enter the hospital after 2 to 4 days of fever and to become critically ill, perhaps even under the misguided security of some ineffective combination of β-lactam and aminoglycoside antibiotics, while routine diagnostic tests are still in progress.

PREVENTION AND CONTROL

Reduction of Exposure to Ticks. Individual preventive measures are directed primarily at prevention of tick bite. The chances of ticks attaching should be minimized by (1) avoiding places especially likely to harbor ticks; (2) wearing boots and protective clothing designed to exclude ticks (preferably impregnated with a tick repellent, such as N-N-butylacetanilide or permethrin); and (3) carefully inspecting the entire body once or twice daily to remove all ticks. Ticks usually crawl on the body or in the clothing for some time prior to attaching. Because the chance of transmission of RMSF is a function of the duration of attachment, early removal of an attached tick probably reduces the chances of infection. Ticks should be removed (from humans or dogs) with forceps, exerting gentle, steady traction so that the mouth parts are released intact from the skin. Contact between the tick and the fingers should be avoided, because rickettsiae in tick feces or body fluids may enter a break in the skin or be transferred to mucous membranes and thus initiate infection.

For families living in tick-infested areas, an especially effective preventive measure is for parents to establish the routine of examining themselves and their children for ticks every evening at bath time during the tick season.

Dogs frequently bring ticks into houses. Ticks should be removed from dogs with the same care as from humans. Acquisition of RMSF by inhalation of airborne dried infected tick feces from the dog's coat is suspected. Commercial repellent-impregnated plastic collars may reduce, but not necessarily eliminate, ticks on dogs. *Rhipicephalus sanguineus* may become established indoors.

Area control of ticks is still difficult and is usually considered impractical. Ticks are resistant to many insecticides. However, some measure of control may be achieved in small plots of ground, such as suburban lots, by intensive acaricidal treatment, the clearing of underbrush, intensive gardening or cultivation, and a reduction of the wild animal population. Changes in land use may affect tick populations. Some progress is being made toward identifying the specific habitat alterations that affect tick populations.

Chemoprophylaxis and Vaccine. If an attached tick is found it is best to place the person from whom such a tick has been removed under close observation, recording morning and evening temperatures for 2 weeks and instituting full antirickettsial chemotherapy immediately on documentation of a fever. Attempts at chemoprophylaxis, for which no effective regimen has been established, would most likely delay onset of disease, not prevent it, because of the primary rickettsiastatic action of available antirickettsial antimicrobials.

R. rickettsii vaccines have been removed from the market because of limited effectiveness.

BIBLIOGRAPHY

Bradford, WD, Hackel DB: Myocardial involvement in Rocky Mountain spotted fever. Arch Pathol Lab Med 102:357, 1978.

Bradford WD, Croker BP, Tisher CC: Kidney lesions in Rocky Mountain spotted fever. A light-, immunofluorescence-, and electron-microscopic study. Am J Pathol 97:381, 1979.

Fine D, Mosher D, Yamada T, et al: Coagulation and complement studies in Rocky Mountain spotted fever. Arch Intern Med 138:735, 1978.

Harrell GT: Rocky Mountain spotted fever. Medicine 28:333, 1949.

Hatwick MAW, O'Brien RJ, Hanson BF: Rocky Mountain spotted fever: Epidemiology of an increasing problem. Ann Intern Med 84:732, 1976.

Helmick CG, Bernard KW, D'Angelo LJ: Rocky Mountain spotted fever: Clinical, laboratory, and epidemiological features of 262 cases. J Infect Dis 150:480, 1984.

Linnemann CC Jr, Janson PF: The clinical presentations of Rocky Mountain spotted fever. Clin Pediatr 17:673, 1978.

McDade JE, Newhouse VF: Natural history of *Rickettsia rickettsii*. Annu Rev Microbiol 40:287, 1986.

Rao AK, Schapira M, Clements ML, et al: A prospective study of platelets and plasma proteolytic systems during the early stages of Rocky Mountain spotted fever. N Engl J Med 318:1021, 1988.

Salgo MP, Telzak EE, Currie B, et al: A focus of Rocky Mountain spotted fever within New York City. N Engl J Med 318:1345, 1988.

Walker DH, Mattern WD: Rickettsial vasculitis. Am Heart J 100:896, 1980.

Walker DH, Crawford CG, Cain BG: Rickettsial infection of the pulmonary microcirculation: The basis for interstitial pneumonitis in Rocky Mountain spotted fever. Hum Pathol 11:263, 1980.

24.2. TICK-BORNE RICKETTSIOSES OF THE EASTERN HEMISPHERE

DEFINITION AND ETIOLOGY. Three diseases, caused by 3 different members of the spotted fever (SF) group of rickettsiae, are currently the best recognized tick-borne rickettsioses of the Eastern Hemisphere and occur over distinct broad geographic areas: (1) Mediterranean spotted fever *(R. conorii)*, (2) North Asian tick-borne rickettsiosis *(R. siberica)*, and (3) Queensland tick typhus *(R. australis)*. Each is a zoonosis, with humans as accidental dead-end hosts, and is transmitted by the bite of one or more species of ixodid ticks (Table III A–1). The 3 diseases, mild to moderate in severity, closely resemble one another, with a short incubation period (averaging 5 to 7 days), a primary lesion (eschar, tache noire), a fever of a few days' to 2 weeks' duration, and a maculopapular to almost nodular rash that appears 3 to 5 days after onset (Table III A–3).

EPIDEMIOLOGY

Mediterranean and SubSaharan Spotted Fevers. (See III A, General Principles and the introduction to Chapter 24.) The brown dog tick, *Rhipicephalus sanguineus*, is the main vector for *R. conorii* and *R. israeli* in the Mediterranean littoral where disease is often acquired in and around human habitations. In subSaharan Africa the causative agent of the local disease (Kenya tick typhus, South African tick typhus) is transmitted by ticks that are parasitic on wild animals and, hence, the disease is acquired in rural areas, e.g., certain stretches of the South African veldt.

North Asian Tick-borne Rickettsiosis. Siberian tick typhus, now known to be caused by *R. siberica*, was first recognized as a clinical entity distinct from the other rickettsioses of the Soviet Union in the mid- to late-1930s. It has since been found distributed from European Russia through Siberia to the Soviet Far East, China, and possibly to the IndoPakistan subcontinent. Several species of ixodid ticks have been implicated as vectors in different geographic regions. Its acquisition is characteristically in a sylvan or rural setting.

Queensland Tick Typhus. This is usually acquired in rural areas heavily infested with the tick *Ixodes holocyclus;* a history of tick bite and an eschar are common. The agent *R. australis*, however, has been isolated only from the blood of patients. Antibodies have been detected in the blood of some small marsupials and a rat, suggesting a natural sylvan small animal–tick cycle.

PATHOLOGY. In fatal cases, which are few and usually limited to the aged and debilitated, the findings are similar to those in RMSF, except for the presence of the tache noire, the black, button-like, necrotic primary lesion that is generally found on the surface areas of the body ordinarily covered by clothing. Pathologic changes are found in the small blood vessels (III A, General Principles).

CLINICAL MANIFESTATIONS. The tick-borne rickettsioses that occur in different parts of the Eastern Hemisphere resemble one another closely.

Symptoms and Signs. After an incubation period of about 5 to 7 days, the disease begins with fever, headache, malaise, myalgia, and conjunctival injection. The primary lesion, which is present in most patients at the onset of fever, consists of a small ulcer 2 to 5 mm in diameter with a black center and a red areola; the regional lymph nodes are enlarged. The generalized erythematous maculopapular rash appears about the fourth day and quickly involves most of the body, including the palms and soles and often the face. In severe cases, the rash becomes hemorrhagic. Fever abates during the second week. The prognosis is good, except in the aged and debilitated. Complications and sequelae are unusual.

The Mediterranean spotted fever of southern Europe has received considerable attention in recent years by Italian, French, and Spanish investigators. Clinical features are remarkably similar to those of Rocky Mountain spotted fever (Table 24–1). Severe or malignant forms occur but the case-fatality rate in treated patients is low. Myocarditis, renal insufficiency, altered liver function, myositis, and thrombocytopenia are recognized. Cases with complicating acute leukocytoplastic vasculitis and with depressed serum complement levels have been described.

North Asian tick-borne rickettsiosis has been the subject of considerable laboratory and clinical observation by Soviet investigators. Mild hypotension, electrocardiographic changes, a reversal of the albumin: globulin (A:G) ratio in serum (depressed albumin and early increased alpha globulins, followed by increase in gamma globulins), and abnormal liver function tests are noteworthy.

DIAGNOSIS (III A, General Principles). The serologic test most commonly used at this time to detect antibody response in acute cases and for epidemiologic studies is the indirect fluorescent antibody test. As usually performed, even with *R. conorii* antigen, it is only SF group specific. Special modifications using a battery of SF group antigens are required to identify specifically the infecting species. Early diagnosis is possible by identifying the organism in biopsy specimens of rash or primary lesion with specific fluorescein- or peroxidase-labeled antibody. A shell vial tissue culture method simplifies the isolation of the organism from blood. In differential diagnosis, the typhus fevers, especially scrub typhus with its primary lesion, meningococcemia, and measles must be considered.

TREATMENT. The tetracycline drugs and chloramphenicol are as effective in patients with Mediterranean spotted fever and North Asian tick-borne rickettsiosis as in those with other rickettsioses (III A, General Principles). Mediterranean spotted fever responds to ciprofloxacin, a welcome alternative. Presumably, these antimicrobial agents are also applicable to the other tick-borne rickettsioses of the Eastern Hemisphere. All of the classically recognized SF group species and the newly recognized strains from Pakistan, Czechoslovakia, and Israel display susceptibility in vitro to doxycycline of the same order as *R. rickettsii* and presumably would respond to similar therapeutic regimens.

PROPHYLAXIS. Prevention of human disease is based on avoiding the bites of infected ticks. In Chapter 24.1, details are set forth regarding personal prophy-laxis, including the use of protective clothing, chemical repellents, and reduction of tick populations by measures involving terrain control. Experimental vaccines prepared from formalin-treated yolk-sac tissue infected with some of the 3 established Eastern Hemisphere rickettsiae under discussion are effective in animals, but commercial vaccines for human use are unproved and unavailable.

BIBLIOGRAPHY

Campbell RW, Abeywickrema P, Fenton C: Queensland tick typhus in Sydney: A new endemic focus. Med J Aust 1:350, 1979.

De Micco C, Raoult D, Benderitter T, et al: Immune complex vasculitis associated with Mediterranean spotted fever. J Infect 14:163, 1987.

Fan M-Y, Walker DH, Yu S-R, Liu QH: Epidemiology and ecology of rickettsial diseases in the People's Republic of China. Rev Infect Dis 9:823, 1987.

Fan M-Y, Yu X-J, Walker DH: Antigenic analysis of Chinese strains of spotted fever group rickettsiae by protein immunoblotting. Am J Trop Med Hyg 39:497, 1988.

Farfan AM, Fernandez CJ, Torrecillas FC, et al: Estudio clinico-epidemiologico de 164 casos de fiebre botonosa. Rev Clin Esp 176:333, 1985.

Grilo-Reina A, Perez-Jimenez F, Escauriaza J, et al: Fiebre botonosa. Estudio de los factores prognosticos. Rev Clin Esp 164:387, 1982.

Guardia J, Martinez-Vazquez JM, Moragas A, et al: The liver in boutonneuse fever. Gut 15:549, 1974.

Herrero-Herrero JI, Ruiz-Beltran R, Battle-Forondona J: The complement system in Mediterranean spotted fever. J Infect Dis 157:1093, 1988.

Hoogstraal, H: Ticks in relation to human disease caused by *Rickettsia* species. Ann Rev Entomol 12:377, 1967.

Kawamura A, Tanaka H: Rickettsiosis in Japan. Jpn J Exp Med 58:169, 1988.

Pennell DJ, Grundy HC, Joy MD: Mediterranean spotted fever presenting as acute leucocytoclastic vasculitis. Lancet 1:1393, 1988.

Raoult D, Gallais H, De Micco P, Casanova P: Ciprofloxacin therapy for Mediterranean spotted fever. Antimicrob Agents Chemother 30:606, 1986.

Raoult D, Gallais H, Ottomani A, et al: La forme maligne de la fièvre boutonneuse méditerranéenne. Presse Med 12:2375, 1983.

Raoult D, Weiller PJ, Chagnon A, et al: Mediterranean spotted fever: Clinical, laboratory and epidemiological features of 199 cases. Am J Trop Med Hyg 35:845, 1986.

San Jose A, Bosch JA, Arderiu A, et al: Myositis due to *Rickettsia conorii* infection. Trans R Soc Trop Med Hyg 82:346, 1988.

Uchida T, Uchiyama T, Koyama AH: Isolation of spotted fever group rickettsiae from humans in Japan. J Infect Dis 158:664, 1988.

24.3. RICKETTSIALPOX

DEFINITION. Rickettsialpox is a mite-borne rickettsial disease, mild and self-limited, characterized by an initial eschar-like lesion and a fever of a week's duration accompanied by headache, backache, and a generalized papulovesicular rash (Table III A–3).

ETIOLOGY. Rickettsialpox is caused by *Rickettsia akari,* a member of the SF group of rickettsiae, on the basis of shared group antigens, but with unique specific antigens and biologic properties.

DISTRIBUTION AND INCIDENCE. The disease has been reported from cities in the United States (e.g., New York, Boston, West Haven, Philadelphia, Pittsburgh, and Cleveland) and from the Soviet Union. In the first 3 years after the disease was described in 1946, about 500 cases were reported in the United States, mostly from New York. Since then, the number reported has declined markedly, possibly owing to underreporting or to control measures (Table III A–4).

TRANSMISSION AND EPIDEMIOLOGY. Although detailed information is sparse, it it is clear that rickettsialpox is a zoonosis that can involve house mice *(Mus musculus)* and mouse mites *(Allodermanyssus sanguineus)*. *R. akari* has also been isolated from rats in the Soviet Union and from voles (small field "mice") in Korea. It is unknown whether the basic natural cycle involves field rodents and their ectoparasites with occasional spillover into the mouse-mite cycle, or whether the latter is in fact the basic sustaining cycle. In the United States, the mouse-mite cycle, greatly amplified and concentrated in discrete foci artificially created and frequented by humans (e.g., improperly fired apartment house incinerators), was responsible for bringing *R. akari* and humans into effective contact. The unusually large mite population that infested the walls and floors of the incinerator rooms had access to people frequently entering the foci. Transmission is presumably by bite of the mite. Simple control measures directed at the mice and mites have virtually eliminated the human disease.

PATHOLOGY. As no fatal cases have been encountered, studies of the pathology of rickettsialpox have been limited to an examination of skin biopsy specimens. Histologically, the eschar of rickettsialpox resembles the eschars of scrub typhus and boutonneuse fever. The skin lesions composing the rash show a typical perivascular infiltration by mononuclear cells. Later, necrosis of the superficial epithelium leads to intraepidermal vesicle formation.

CLINICAL MANIFESTATIONS. The incubation period varies from about 10 days to 3 weeks. An initial lesion (the eschar) appears at the site of the mite bite about a week before the onset of fever in about 90% of the patients, gradually enlarging and progressing from a papular lesion through vesicle formation to form finally a dark encrusted lesion measuring 0.5 to 1.5 cm in diameter. The onset of an intermittent fever is sudden and is accompanied by chills or chilly sensations, drenching sweats, headache, anorexia, and photophobia. The fever ranges from about 38 to 40C, lasts for about a week, is accompanied by headache, lassitude, and myalgia, and then gradually subsides. A sparse eruption appears on the trunk, extremities, and mucous membranes between the first and fourth days of fever, beginning as discrete maculopapular lesions and evolving into a vesiculopapular rash. The vesicles are firm, are sometimes surrounded by erythema, and, on drying, form a dark crust that falls off without leaving a scar.

DIAGNOSIS. The clinical characteristics of rickettsialpox are so distinctive that, in most patients, a presumptive diagnosis may be made on clinical grounds. Chickenpox in adults poses the most difficult differential diagnostic problem. Important points in differentiation are the following: (1) The vesicles in rickettsialpox arise from the center of discrete papules. (2) The lesions tend to appear at the same time instead of in crops. (3) The average number of lesions is generally fewer than in chickenpox. (4) There is often an initial lesion (eschar) at the site of the mite bite. (5) Laboratory diagnosis depends on isolation of the agent and on serologic response measured by rickettsial group and specific antigens. (6) The result of the Weil-Felix test is negative (Table III A–4).

PROGNOSIS. Even without specific therapy, the course of the disease is benign, and the prognosis is excellent.

TREATMENT. Response to tetracycline drugs, given in multiple doses as outlined in III A, General Principles, is rapid and there is no relapse.

PREVENTION AND CONTROL. The transient evolution of rickettsialpox from a silent enzootic infection to a human disease problem was an artifact of urban living, and its apparent disappearance is probably a result of minor changes in human behavior. The prevention and control of rickettsialpox depend on rodent and mite control by (1) the elimination of mice and mouse harborages, which should include proper care and firing of incinerators in dwellings, and (2) the application of residual acaricides to walls and other mite-infested areas. No vaccines have been developed.

BIBLIOGRAPHY

Greenberg M, Pelliteri O, Klein IF, et al: Rickettsialpox—a newly recognized rickettsial disease. II. Clinical observations. JAMA 133:901, 1947.
Lackman DH: A review of information on rickettsialpox in the United States. Clin Pediatr 2:296, 1963.

25. SCRUB TYPHUS

Charles L. Wisseman, Jr.

DEFINITION. Scrub typhus, chigger-borne rickettsiosis, or tsutsugamushi disease is an acute, febrile, typhus-like disease of rural Asia transmitted by the bite of larval trombiculid mites (chiggers) (Table III A–1). The site of infection is often marked by an eschar accompanied by regional lymphadenitis.

ETIOLOGY. The disease is caused by infection with *Rickettsia tsutsugamushi (R. orientalis)* (Fig. III A–1). The organism differs somewhat from other members of the genus *Rickettsia*. It shares an antigen with Proteus OX-K. Multiple serotypes exist, often in the same endemic foci, which produce substantial homologous immunity but only transient cross-immunity in humans. Evidence exists for the occasional participation of more than 1 serotype in a single attack of scrub typhus. Virulence of strains for mice and humans varies from low to very high.

DISTRIBUTION. Scrub typhus is widely distributed in eastern and southern Asia and the islands of the western and southern Pacific. It is known as far north as the island of Hokkaido in Japan and the Primorye region of Asiatic USSR, as far south as the northern tip of Australia, and as far west as Pakistan and Tadzhikistan. Endemic infection is unknown in the Americas,

Europe, and Africa, but cases imported during the incubation period following infection in an endemic area have been recognized in the United States.

TRANSMISSION AND EPIDEMIOLOGY (III A, General Principles). Scrub typhus is acquired from the bite of infected larval trombiculid mites (chiggers). It is a zoonosis. Humans acquire the infection when they intrude into an enzootic focus. Four main elements are constant features of such foci: (1) *R. tsutsugamushi*; (2) chiggers of the *Leptotrombidium deliense* group (e.g., *L. deliense, L. akamushi, L. fletcheri, L. arenicola, L. pallidum,* and *L. pavlovskyi*); (3) wild rats, especially of the subgenus *Rattus*; and (4) transitional vegetation. The mites, whose larval "chiggers" are the only stage to feed on humans and rats, efficiently transmit the rickettsia from one generation to the next through the egg (transovarial passage) and probably constitute the main reservoir of *R. tsutsugamushi* as well as serving as vectors. Rats, especially wild rats of the subgenus *Rattus,* and other small mammals, e.g., field mice, voles, and shrews, serve as hosts for the parasitic larval mites. Some kind of transitional or secondary vegetation, e.g., cleared forest areas, the fringe vegetation along roads, forest trails, or streams, and abandoned agricultural areas, provides the habitat for the chigger-mammal association. Within such habitats, infected chiggers may occur in very circumscribed foci, or "mite islands," accounting for the marked focal distribution of scrub typhus cases and sudden outbreaks among field personnel. Suitable habitats are widely distributed from tropical to temperate zones and occur in such extreme settings as semideserts, alpine meadow and subarctic scree in the Himalayas, disturbed rain forests, and seashores. In temperate zones, the chiggers are usually active at some time during the warm months, although *L. scutellare*—transmitted *winter* scrub typhus occurs in the Izu Islands of Japan. In tropical or subtropical regions, the disease may be more prevalent at one time of the year than another, depending on rainfall, flooding, and other factors.

Scrub typhus is best known from outbreaks occurring among groups of nonimmune people entering into endemic areas, e.g., military personnel, road builders, agricultural land clearers, and other transmigrants. Systematic laboratory-supported studies of populations indigenous to endemic areas, as in Malaysia and the Pescadores Islands, have revealed infection rates as high as 3 to 4% per month and clinical scrub typhus as a leading cause of febrile disease requiring hospitalization. In such areas, there may be multiple sequential infections due to different serotypes of *R. tsutsugamushi,* with attendant modification of disease severity and loss of classic diagnostic features (e.g., no eschar, rash, or lymphadenopathy, and no Proteus OX-K agglutinin response). In other areas, changing socioeconomic conditions and political factors are modifying infection patterns. For example, urbanization and universal school attendance are decreasing infection rate in some areas, whereas in others, migration of populations from urban centers to rural or forested areas to increase agriculture is resulting in a substantial increase in disease.

IMMUNITY. Multiple serotypes of *R. tsutsugamushi* exist. Homologous immunity to the infecting strain persists at least up to a year, and perhaps longer, following an attack of scrub typhus, but cross-immunity to other serotypes is transient (about 1 to 2 months). Thus, it is possible for an individual to have multiple scrub typhus infections during his or her lifetime. There are conflicting reports on the duration of serum antibodies after infection, with decay of indirect fluorescent antibodies (IFA) within a year or two on the one hand and the persistence of complement-fixing antibodies and IFA for several years on the other. Reasons for these discrepancies are unknown. In mice, protective immunity appears to be dominantly cell mediated.

PATHOLOGY. The pathologic features of scrub typhus conform generally to those described in III A, General Principles. Of special note in scrub typhus is the primary local ulcer with regional and, later, generalized lymphadenopathy. Vascular thrombosis is less frequent than in epidemic typhus and Rocky Mountain spotted fever, but inflammatory lesions of larger arteries are more common.

CLINICAL MANIFESTATIONS AND COURSE. The spectrum of clinical severity of untreated scrub typhus ranges from inapparent or mild to severe or fatal, with mortality rates varying from 0 to more than 30% in different places and outbreaks (Table III A–3). The following description pertains to a classic, relatively severe, untreated case of primary scrub typhus.

Acute Illness. The bite of the infecting chigger, which may be on any part of the body, is usually unnoticed, but in roughly 60 to 70% of the primary infections and in substantially fewer second infections, a small, painless papule develops during the 6- to 18-day (usually 9- to 12-day) incubation period. It enlarges, undergoes central necrosis, and crusts to form the eschar or primary lesion (Fig. 25–1), which is well developed and healing at the onset of disease. The regional lymph nodes are enlarged and tender. Prodromes of headache, malaise, anorexia, and weakness may occur. The onset is usually acute. The fever rises progressively during the first few days to

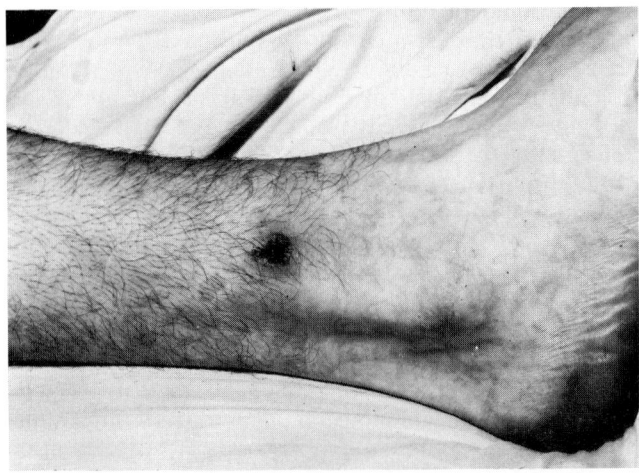

FIGURE 25–1. Eschar in scrub typhus. These may also be located on the trunk, neck, and arms and may be single or multiple. (Courtesy of the Armed Forces Institute of Pathology, Photograph Neg. No. D-4451.)

39.5 to 40.5C, sometimes accompanied by chills after about the third day and also accompanied by severe headache, ocular pain, conjunctival injection, anorexia, generalized aches, malaise, apathy, and cough. Interstitial pneumonitis is common. The pulse remains relatively slow. Toward the end of the first week, a macular rash (later sometimes papular) often appears, first on the trunk and then on the extremities. About this time, there is generalized lymphadenopathy, soft splenic enlargement, and sometimes hepatomegaly.

Episodes of scrub typhus fever after the primary infection, whether mild or severe, may exhibit no eschar, rash, or lymphadenopathy.

Convalescence and Complications. During the second week of disease, the temperature remains elevated, and signs of complex multiple organ system involvement appear. Apathy may give way to more pronounced signs of meningoencephalitis, i.e., delirium and restlessness, stupor, coma, convulsions, muscular weakness, hyperesthesias, and coarse intention tremors. Cranial nerves are selectively involved, with varying degrees of nerve deafness and papilledema and congestion of retinal vessels being common and dysarthria and dysphagia occurring less frequently. Signs of diffuse and focal myocarditis may appear—soft first heart sound, systolic murmurs, ectopic beats, occasional cardiac enlargement, transient gallop rhythm, and minor abnormalities of the electrocardiogram (i.e., prolonged PR interval and inverted T waves). Classic congestive failure is rare, but varying degrees of circulatory failure may appear, i.e., increasing pulse rate, falling blood pressure (commonly below 100 mm Hg systolic), rapid, shallow respirations, cyanosis, sweating, and cold, clammy skin. Gangrene is rare, but edema may be overt in severe cases. Clinical evidence of renal insufficiency is often absent, but oliguria or anuria occurs in some patients. Spontaneous diuresis is fairly common late in the febrile course or in early convalescence.

In untreated cases, defervescence is by lysis, usually after about 10 to 14 days (21 or more days in severe cases). In nonfatal cases, all abnormalities appear to be completely reversible, although convalescence is prolonged. Some conditions, e.g., cardiovascular instability, personality changes, and deafness, may persist for weeks to months. Long-term (10 years or more) follow-up of combat forces in the Far East and Southwest Pacific who survived scrub typhus in World War II failed to reveal any significant residua.

Laboratory Findings. An early leukopenia (1000 to 5000 white blood cells/mm³) gives way to slightly depressed or normal total white blood cell counts, which may become somewhat elevated late in the disease. Total serum proteins are usually normal or low, but the gamma globulin levels may be greater than the albumin level. Occasional clotting disturbances have been reported, including the disseminated intravascular coagulation syndrome. Jaundice is rare, but serum aminotransferase levels may be elevated. Albuminuria is common. Isosthenuria, oliguria, and azotemia may occur.

DIAGNOSIS. A typhus-like illness in a patient with a history of possible exposure in endemic areas and an eschar with regional lymphadenitis should alert the physician to the possibility of scrub typhus. Differential diagnosis may be difficult in some endemic regions where the clinical picture may suggest other rickettsial infections (especially tick-borne typhus, which may also cause an eschar) and other nonrickettsial infections (III A, General Principles). Furthermore, lack of eschar, lymphadenopathy, or rash in attacks after the primary infection makes it difficult to differentiate second and subsequent attacks from other acute febrile diseases on clinical grounds alone. The Weil-Felix test with Proteus OX-K is useful in primary infections because of general availability (Table III A–4). However, it is often negative in second and subsequent infections. The IFA and immunoperoxidase tests are currently the serodiagnostic methods of choice (III A, General Principles). The IgM response is good in primary infections and is suppressed in reinfections. Isolation can be accomplished by inoculating blood or tissue homogenates intraperitoneally into white mice.

TREATMENT. Tetracycline drugs, given as recommended in III A, General Principles, along with appropriate supportive measures, are the recommended treatment. A single 200-mg dose of doxycycline may be adequate treatment for cases of several days' duration, but relapses occur, especially in patients treated on or before the third day of disease. A second dose given 4 to 5 days after the first should eliminate relapses. Concurrent malaria should not be overlooked.

PROGNOSIS. In untreated scrub typhus, the mortality rate ranges from essentially zero to over 30% in different foci. Prompt antibiotic therapy reduces mortality virtually to zero.

PREVENTION AND CONTROL. Effective killed vaccines have not yet been developed to prevent scrub typhus. Transient cross-immunity among serotypes and more persistent homologous immunity can be induced by intentional infection with a virulent strain, followed by carefully timed chemoprophylaxis, which permits subclinical immunizing infection, but this procedure is not practical. Chemoprophylaxis with a long-acting tetracycline (doxycycline) is feasible. Weekly 200-mg doses of doxycycline, continuing for 6 weeks after the last exposure, prevent most clinical breakthroughs of infection.

Preventive measures against scrub typhus are directed primarily against the chigger vector. Mite-infected terrain should be avoided whenever possible. Individual prophylaxis against attack by larval mites consists of wearing protective clothing impregnated with a mite repellent, e.g., benzyl benzoate or M-1960, and applying diethyltoluamide to exposed skin. The vector population in and around campsites in endemic zones can be reduced by the following means: (1) by treating the area intensively with acaricides; (2) by reducing the rodent population through intensive poison-bait campaigns, and (3) by destroying vegetation (with bulldozers, power oil burners, and herbicides). Appropriate and relevant environmental, medical, and ecologic considerations must temper decisions on the use of persisting acaricides and herbicides, however.

BIBLIOGRAPHY

Bourgeois AL, Olson JG, Fang RCY, et al: Humoral and cellular responses in scrub typhus patients reflecting primary infection and reinfection with *Rickettsia tsutsugamushi.* Am J Trop Med Hyg 31:532, 1982.

Bourgeois AL, Olson JG, Ho CM, et al: Epidemiological and serological study of scrub typhus among Chinese military in the Pescadores Islands of Taiwan. Trans R Soc Trop Med Hyg 71:338, 1977.

Brown GW, Robinson DM, Huxsoll DL: Scrub typhus: A common cause of illness in indigenous populations. Trans R Soc Trop Med Hyg 70:444, 1976.

Brown GW, Robinson DM, Huxsoll DL: Serological evidence for a high incidence of transmission of *Rickettsia tsutsugamushi* in two Orang Asli settlements in peninsular Malaysia. Am J Trop Med Hyg 27:121, 1978.

Brown GW, Saunders JP, Singh S, et al: Single dose doxycycline therapy for scrub typhus. Trans R Soc Trop Med Hyg 72:412, 1978.

Deller JJ Jr, Russell PK: An analysis of fevers of unknown origin in American soldiers in Vietnam. Ann Intern Med 66:1129, 1967.

Kawamura A, Tanaka H: Rickettsiosis in Japan. Jpn J Exp Med 58:169, 1988.

Olson JG, Bourgeois AL: Changing risk of scrub typhus in relation to socioeconomic development in the Pescadores Islands of Taiwan. Am J Epidemiol 109:236, 1979.

Olson JG, Bourgeois AL, Fang RCY, et al: Prevention of scrub typhus: Prophylactic administration of doxycycline in a randomized double blind trial. Am J Trop Med Hyg 29:989, 1980.

Saunders JP, Brown GW, Shirai A, et al: The longevity of antibody to *Rickettsia tsutsugamushi* in patients with confirmed scrub typhus. Trans R Soc Trop Med Hyg 74:253, 1980.

Traub R, Wisseman CL Jr: The ecology of chigger-borne rickettsiosis (scrub typhus) (review article). J Med Entomol 11:237, 1974.

Twartz JC, Shirai A, Selvaraju G, et al: Doxycycline prophylaxis for human scrub typhus. J Infect Dis 146:811, 1982.

26. Q FEVER

Charles L. Wisseman, Jr.

DEFINITION. Q fever is an acute, usually self-limited rickettsial infection characterized by fever, headache, chills, myalgia, malaise, and, only rarely, rash. A variable proportion of patients show radiologic evidence of pneumonitis. Chronic forms with hepatitis or endocarditis occur. Infection is usually by inhalation of airborne organisms; an arthropod vector is not required.

ETIOLOGY (III A, General Principles). Q fever is caused by *Coxiella burnetii* infection. The organism, possibly the minute (0.2 μm) endospore-like form (Fig. III A–2), is resistant to heat (60C for 30 to 60 minutes, or weeks in blood clots at ambient temperature), desiccation, and disinfectants (0.5% formalin for 4 days). Strains from various parts of the world show no serologic variations. The organism undergoes variation from phase I to phase II, akin to smooth to rough variation, on passage in embryonated eggs but not in animals. Phase I, the only form seen in nature, possesses a surface antigenic material that has antiphagocytic properties.

DISTRIBUTION. *C. burnetii* infection is widely distributed throughout the world, but the clinical disease is not uniformly recognized. Infection may be more prevalent in dry climates than in wet ones.

EPIDEMIOLOGY AND TRANSMISSION. *C. burnetii* infection is a zoonosis. The natural history of its infection cycle is complex and not well understood in its entirety (Table III A–1). It has been isolated from a wide variety of arthropods (e.g., ticks, chiggers, lice, and flies) and wild and domestic animals. Humans are rarely, if ever, infected from arthropods, but rather from infected domestic animals, notably cattle, sheep, and goats, usually by inhalation of airborne organisms. This is probably just a "special case" within the total spectrum of transmission cycles, but in view of the universal dependency of humans on domesticated animals, it has assumed a dominant role in the case of the human disease.

Infection in Domestic Animals. *C. burnetii* infection of cattle, sheep, and goats causes no recognizable disease, although instances of late abortion have been attributed to it. In subsequent pregnancy, however, persisting organisms may grow to high titer ($\sim10^8$/gm) in the placenta and are shed at parturition with the placenta and fluids, heavily contaminating the environment with the resistant infectious organisms, which readily become airborne in dust. The organisms are also shed in the milk ($\sim10^5$/gm) and probably in urine and feces as well.

Infection in Humans. The most common mode of transmission to humans is by the respiratory route from infectious airborne dust or aerosols derived from infected domestic animals. The variations in the epidemiologic details are manifold. The acquisition of Q fever by people who consume infected raw milk is controversial, but such populations have a significantly higher seroconversion rate than those who do not consume raw milk.

Infection is most common in people who are associated with infected domestic animals (e.g., abattoir workers, ranchers, dairy farmers, and people who live in close association with their animals) or who live near domestic animals. People living miles downwind from an infected dairy have shown serologic evidence of infection. Outbreaks of Q fever have been described in villages following the passage of a flock of sheep, with the attendant dust, through the village. Human occupation of barns where infected animals had been kept has led to outbreaks (as in US Army personnel in Italy during World War II). Straw from barns and hides from infected animals may be the sources of infection, even when transported far from where the animals are quartered. Recently, cases of Q fever were traced to a parturient cat.

Laboratory outbreaks have been common. In one instance, a laboratory worker carried organisms home on his shoes and infected his landlord. Outbreaks in medical centers, involving both personnel and patients, have been traced to sheep brought into the centers for research purposes. Seroepidemiologic studies have shown evidence of human infection in areas where Q fever has rarely, if ever, been reported.

PATHOLOGY. Few autopsies have been performed on patients who have died from acute infection. In contrast to members of the genus *Rickettsia, Coxiella burnetii* appears to infect primarily cells of the reticuloendothelial system (Table III A–2). Instead of a vasculitis, the basic lesion in *C. burnetii* infection is a granuloma (Fig. 26–1). It may contain macrophages, monocytes, lymphocytes, plasma cells, and multinu-

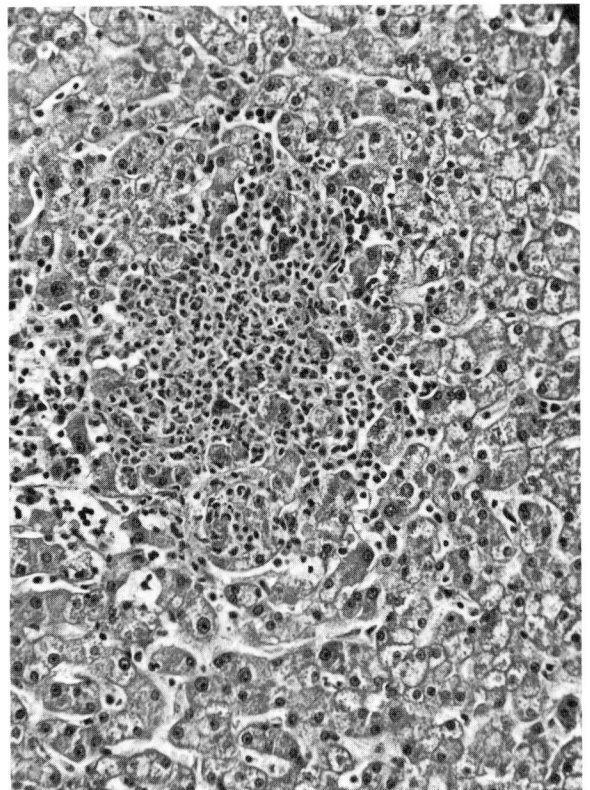

FIGURE 26–1. Focal granulomatous lesions in the liver of a patient with Q fever. (From Dupont HL, et al: Ann Intern Med 74:198, 1971.)

cleate giant cells. Some granulomatous lesions have a central clear area, the "doughnut" granuloma. Best described are those in the liver, lungs, and bone marrow. *C. burnetii* is often demonstrable by fluorescent antibody methods. Damage to parenchymal liver cells is not clear, although some unexplained amorphous material may be in sinusoids. However, the livers of guinea pigs infected heavily by the intraperitoneal route show multiple biochemical alterations.

IMMUNITY. Susceptibility is universal. Immunity following recovery from infection is solid and long-lasting, but nonsterile. The organisms are adapted to live and grow within phagocytic vacuoles of macrophages. In contrast to infection with members of the genus *Rickettsia,* immune serum, although it opsonizes for enhanced phagocytosis, does not initiate destruction within macrophage phagolysosomes. Antibodies detectable by complement fixation and microagglutination tests may fall below detectable or interpretable levels within 2 to 3 years after infection. Protective immunity is primarily cell mediated. Strong delayed-type hypersensitivity develops as a result of infection or vaccination with killed organisms. Skin tests for delayed-type hypersensitivity are the best correlates of prior infection and immunity. A chloroform-methanol–soluble fraction of the organisms has intrinsic toxic action and stimulates suppressor cells. It is thought to contribute to the persistence of the organisms in tissues, to an adjuvant action, to granuloma formation, and to the occasional "sterile abscesses" encountered at vaccination sites. Persistence of organisms after recovery from acute in-

fection is indicated by the later occurrence of *C. burnetii* endocarditis and of organisms in human placentas and milk.

CLINICAL MANIFESTATIONS AND COURSE. Most *C. burnetii* infections of humans are either inapparent or unrecognized. When clinical disease results from exposure, it begins after an incubation period of about 14 to 26 days (with an average of 19 days) with headache, chilly sensations, fever, myalgia, malaise, and anorexia. The acute, uncomplicated disease usually lasts between 3 and 6 days but occasionally exceeds 2 weeks, with fever fluctuating between 38 and 40C. Rash, although unusual, has been described (Table III A–3).

Pneumonitis. Pulmonary involvement is variable from outbreak to outbreak, occurring frequently (~60%) in some and rarely in others. It is usually benign and self-limited. When present, pulmonary involvement is usually manifested by a dry cough a few days after onset, productive of scant mucoid sputum and sometimes accompanied by chest pain. Fine crepitant rales may be heard on deep inspiration. Radiologic features are most often single or multiple, rounded, homogeneous segmental densities, usually in the lower lobes, visible after the third or fourth day (Fig. 26–2). The lesions may persist after the patient becomes afebrile, in rare cases for as long as 70 days. Pleural (and pericardial) effusion, as well as a persisting inflammatory pseudotumor containing *C. burnetii,* has been described.

Hepatitis. A common complication, causing chronic Q fever of variable duration, is hepatic involvement, which occurs in about one third of patients in some series. The liver may be enlarged and tender; fever persists; and biopsy reveals the presence of granulomas (Fig. 26–1). Some patients show relatively little bio-

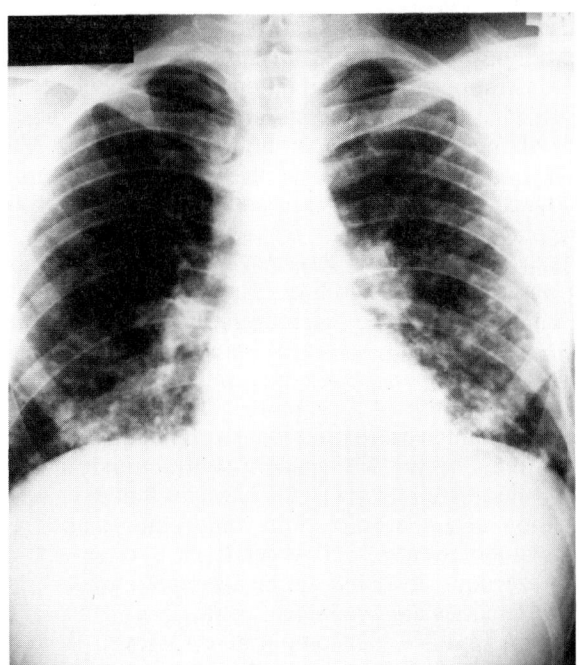

FIGURE 26–2. Chest radiograph of a patient with Q fever showing patchy densities predominantly in the lower lung fields 13 days after aerogenic exposure to *C. burnetii.* (From Dupont HL, et al: Ann Intern Med 74:198, 1971.)

chemical evidence of liver damage; others have been described with jaundice, abnormal liver function tests, and a clinical picture resembling viral hepatitis.

Endocarditis. A more serious complication is *C. burnetii* subacute endocarditis. Originally thought to be rare, it is now diagnosed with increasing frequency. The onset may be 2 to 20 years after the known or presumed acute infection. Predisposing conditions are abnormal valves (e.g., congenital bicuspid aortic valve and rheumatic mitral valve damage) and valvular prostheses. A significant number of patients have no evidence of preexisting valvular disease. Vegetations containing *C. burnetii* are formed. The disease resembles subacute bacterial endocarditis, except that ordinary blood cultures are negative. Findings include fever, anemia, elevated erythrocyte sedimentation rate, clubbing of the fingers, splenomegaly, and/or embolic phenomena. Associated hepatitis and glomerulonephritis with granular deposits containing immunoglobulins and complement have been described. The untreated disease is fatal in about 3 years.

DIAGNOSIS

Differential Diagnosis. Without some clue as to possible exposure, the clinical diagnosis of Q fever is difficult, because there are no pathognomonic signs. The uncomplicated disease may be confused with influenza or grippe (e.g., "Balkan grippe"). Pulmonary findings may suggest "atypical pneumonia" (Fig. 26–2); liver involvement may mimic viral hepatitis, and cardiovascular findings may suggest subacute bacterial endocarditis (blood culture negative). Granulomas in biopsy specimens must be differentiated from the lesions in other granulomatous diseases (e.g., tuberculosis, brucellosis, tularemia, syphilis, histoplasmosis, and sarcoidosis). It is essential to have adequate historical and epidemiologic information. A high index of suspicion and ready use of the laboratory are essential.

Antibody Detection. Diagnosis is usually made by demonstration of a rise in antibodies. In uncomplicated cases, Phase II complement-fixing (CF) antibodies appear about a week after onset, reach a peak in 3 to 4 weeks, and then decay over the next 24 to 36 months to low titers that usually are not considered significant. The phase I CF antibody response is either not significant or relatively low. Persisting high levels of phase I CF antibodies suggest chronic infection, e.g., hepatitis or endocarditis. The microagglutination and indirect fluorescent antibody tests are also useful, but the kinetics of antibody response are not so well defined.

Demonstration of Organisms. Organisms can sometimes be demonstrated in tissues (granulomas) or valve vegetations by the direct fluorescent antibody method, using fluorescein-labeled *C. burnetii* immune serum. Isolation in guinea pigs, mice, and embryonated eggs from blood, tissues, and vegetations is relatively easy but hazardous; it should not be attempted unless appropriate facilities are available.

TREATMENT. Uncomplicated Q fever is a self-limited disease. Treatment by the multiple-dose regimen (III A, General Principles) with tetracycline, doxycycline, or chloramphenicol causes defervescence in 36 to 48 hours. Pulmonary lesions and chronic Q fever with hepatitis respond to antimicrobial therapy but do so more slowly.

Antibiotic Resistance. During outbreaks of Q fever in Cyprus, patients did not respond well to tetracycline therapy, and *C. burnetii* strains from Cyprus showed increased resistance to tetracyclines. Therefore, the physician should be alert to the possibility of antibiotic resistance in Q fever and chronic *C. burnetii* infections.

Endocarditis. Endocarditis poses a life-threatening problem in Q fever. Because the drugs effective against *C. burnetii* are primarily rickettsiostatic, antibiotic therapy must be prolonged (for months) and may not be successful. Some combination of doxycycline and trimethoprim or rifampin or lincomycin has been used. (Trimethoprim is inhibitory for *C. burnetii* in the laboratory but is neither inhibitory nor clinically effective against *Rickettsia* species.) Valvular replacement is indicated for mechanical reasons but is controversial as therapy for the endocarditis because of the tendency for recurrence of endocarditis on the prosthetic valve.

PROGNOSIS. Death is rare in uncomplicated Q fever, with or without antibiotic therapy. The course of chronic Q fever is substantially shortened by therapy. However, mortality from Q fever endocarditis remains high.

PREVENTION AND CONTROL. Domestic animals are the source of most human infections with *C. burnetii,* but because the infection in animals produces no apparent illness or significant economic loss, there has been no incentive to prevent infection in domestic animals. However, outbreaks of Q fever in medical centers where sheep were used for research purposes led to vigorous attempts to exclude *C. burnetii* infection from animals destined for research use by several methods. These include attempts to establish infection-free flocks, sometimes aided by the use of killed vaccines, screening of sheep for *C. burnetii* antibodies (unreliable because not all animals excreting organisms are seropositive), housing and conducting research on sheep only in high-containment facilities, and simply conducting research requiring sheep in isolated or remote facilities.

Vaccine. An effective killed phase I *C. burnetii* vaccine for use in humans exists but is not commercially available. When given to persons who have had inapparent or clinically overt Q fever, the vaccine tends to produce systemic and local reactions, sometimes with the development of a chronic "sterile abscess" (granuloma) at the site of inoculation. Exclusion from vaccination of persons sensitive to *C. burnetii,* determined by means of a skin test, markedly reduces the incidence of reactions and appears to be a practical procedure for persons at special risk, e.g., laboratory workers, ranchers, veterinarians, and dairy farmers.

BIBLIOGRAPHY

Aitken ID, Boegel K, Cracea E, et al: Q fever in Europe: Current aspects of aetiology, epidemiology, human infection, diagnosis and therapy. Infection 15:323, 1987.

Anonymous: Q fever at a university research center. MMWR 28:333, 1979.

Babudieri B: Q fever: A zoonosis. Adv Vet Sci 5:81, 1959.

Dupont HL, Hornick RB, Levin HS, et al: Q fever hepatitis. Ann Intern Med 74:198, 1971.

Fiset P, Woodward TE: Q fever. *In* Evans AS, Feldman HA (eds): Bacterial Infections of Humans. Epidemiology and Control. New York, Plenum Publishing, 1983, pp 435–448.

Langley JM, Marrie TJ, Covert A, et al: Poker players' pneumonia. An urban outbreak of Q fever following exposure to a parturient cat. N Engl J Med 319:354, 1988.

Marmion BP, Higgins FE, Bridges JB, Edwards AT: A case of acute rickettsial endocarditis with a survey of cardiac patients with this infection. Br Med J 2:1264, 1960.

Marmion BP, Kyrkou M, Worswick D, et al: Vaccine prophylaxis of abattoir-associated Q fever. Lancet 2:1411, 1984.

Palmer SR, Young SEJ: Q-fever endocarditis in England and Wales, 1975–81. Lancet 2:1448, 1982.

Ruppanner R, Brooks D, Morrish D, et al: Q fever hazards from sheep and goats used in research. Arch Environ Health 37:103, 1982.

Sawyer LA, Fishbein DB, McDade JE: Q fever: Current concepts. Rev Infect Dis 9:935, 1987.

Sawyer LA, Fishbein DB, McDade JE: [Q fever in patients with hepatitis and pneumonia: Results of laboratory-based surveillance in the United States.] J Infect Dis 158:497, 1988.

Spelman DW: Q fever. A study of 111 consecutive cases. Med J Aust 1:547, 1982.

Spicer AJ: Investigation of *Coxiella burnetii* infection as a possible cause of chronic liver disease in man. Trans R Soc Trop Med Hyg 73:415, 1979.

Spicer AJ, Peacock MG, Williams J: Effectiveness of several antibiotics in suppressing chick embryo lethality during experimental infections by *Coxiella burnetii, Rickettsia typhi* and *R. rickettsii. In* Burgdorfer W, Anacker RL (eds): Rickettsiae and Rickettsial Diseases. New York, Academic Press, 1981, pp 375–383.

Srigley JR, Vellend H, Palmer N, et al: Q fever. The liver and bone marrow pathology. Am J Surg Pathol 9:752, 1985.

Stoker MGP, Marmion BP: The spread of Q fever from animals to man: The natural history of a rickettsial disease. Bull WHO 13:781, 1955.

Tigertt WD, Benenson AS, Gochenour WS: Airborne Q fever. Bacteriol Rev 25:285, 1961.

Turck WP, Howitt G, Turnberg LA, et al: Chronic Q fever. Q J Med 178:193, 1976.

Varma MPS, Adgey AAJ, Connolly JH: Chronic Q fever endocarditis. Br Heart J 43:695, 1980.

27. MISCELLANEOUS RICKETTSIAL INFECTIONS

Charles L. Wisseman, Jr.

27.1. TRENCH FEVER

DEFINITION. Trench fever (5-day fever, Wolhynia fever) is an acute louse-borne febrile disease caused by infection with *Rochalimaea quintana* and characterized by fever, headache, and muscle and joint pains of a few days' duration, with a tendency for relapse.

ETIOLOGY. (III A, General Principles). *R. quintana* is a small, rickettsia-like, gram-negative bacillus that grows in cell-free artificial medium in vitro, in an extracellular but cell-associated pericellular localization in the louse midgut, in cell culture, and in an undefined blood element-associated state in humans. It is related but not identical to the vole agent for which the separate taxon *R. vinsonii* has been proposed.

EPIDEMIOLOGY, TRANSMISSION, AND DISTRIBUTION. Trench fever was first recognized in World War I and again in World War II. It is transmitted by the human body louse, *Pediculus humanus humanus,* in which it grows extracellularly in the midgut and is excreted in the feces (Table III A–1). The louse acquires the organism from the blood of an infected person, in whose blood the organisms persist for months to years whether or not relapses of clinical disease occur. Under epidemic circumstances, infected lice may be collected from a high proportion (15% to 40%) of apparently healthy persons in the affected population. The louse does not die from *R. quintana* infection. The epidemiology of trench fever is similar to that of louse-borne typhus; trench fever occurs under similar circumstances and sometimes concurrently (Chapter 23). The clinical disease is seldom recognized outside of epidemics. Nevertheless, studies have shown its presence in Mexico, North Africa, and Eastern Europe, and it is likely to be present in other louse-ridden populations.

PATHOLOGY. Because the disease is not fatal, little is known of the pathology.

IMMUNITY. Little is known about immunity in trench fever, except that it is unusual. The organisms are present in the blood from the primary attack through the closely associated relapses and, often, for at least 1 to 3 months afterward. Following this, the presence of organisms in the blood is highly variable—almost continuously for months up to at least a year; intermittently present for months to several years with or without late clinical relapses; or recrudescence after as long as 8 years. Late relapses may be precipitated by other intercurrent infections, typhoid vaccine, or malignancy. Some people constantly exposed to reinfection have no subsequent episodes of disease. Others with the same exposure have 1 or more clinical episodes; however, it is difficult to learn whether these are relapses or new infections. Antibodies, measurable by several serologic methods, appear during the initial episode, usually in low titer, and persist in some but are transient in others. Immune serum, containing detectable antibodies, plus complement fails to kill the organisms. Nothing is known about cell-mediated immunity.

CLINICAL MANIFESTATIONS AND COURSE. In some volunteer studies, the incubation period has been as short as 4 to 7 days; in others and in natural infection, the incubation period has varied between 14 and 35 days (with an average of 22 days). The clinical disease is highly variable: (1) it is negligible or abortive; (2) there is a single acute febrile attack of 3 to 4 days' duration; (3) there is a "typhoidal" type with sustained fever; and (4) sometimes, there are single or multiple relapses over a short (1- to 2-month) period to several years. The classic quintana form of multiple relapses at intervals of 4 to 6 days between onset of each episode is not typical.

A more or less "typical" episode is characterized by sudden onset of fever with chills, headache, ocular pain, pain in bones, joints, and muscles, especially those of the shins, thighs, and back, profuse sweating, and malaise. These features peak in 2 to 3 days and subside in about the same length of time. Some patients exhibit a macular rash. Relapses may simulate the primary episode or may simply be a febrile episode of a few hours' duration accompanied by some symptoms of the primary episode.

DIAGNOSIS. Unless trench fever occurs in a louse-ridden population in numbers sufficient to attract notice to the relapsing nature of the disease, clinical diagnosis is difficult, and sporadic cases are not likely to be recognized as distinct from many other short, acute febrile diseases. The relapsing form should be differentiated from the far more serious relapsing fever, which, along with louse-borne typhus, may occur under the same circumstances.

The organisms can be isolated readily from the blood by cultivation on blood agar in a carbon dioxide–enriched atmosphere (III A, General Principles) or by xenodiagnosis with clean lice. Complement fixation, microagglutination, indirect fluorescent antibody, and enzyme-linked immunosorbent assay (ELISA) tests have been described for the detection of antibodies. All present special problems. The kinetics of antibody response are not established.

TREATMENT. The organism is sensitive in vitro (on artificial medium) to tetracycline antibiotics and chloramphenicol. Limited experience suggests that the clinical disease will respond to tetracycline therapy, but nothing is known of the effect of such treatment on the long-term persistence of the organism.

PROGNOSIS. Deaths are rare in untreated disease, but the relapsing nature of the disease may produce some disability.

PREVENTION AND CONTROL. Control of body lice, as described for louse-borne typhus (Chapter 23.1), is the only known practical means of control and prevention.

BIBLIOGRAPHY

Byam W, Carrol JH, Churchill JH, et al: Trench Fever. A Louse-borne Disease. London, Oxford University Press, 1919, pp 1–196.
Kostrzewski J: The epidemiology of trench fever. Med Dosw Microbiol 11:1, 1950.
Myers WF, Wisseman CL Jr, Fiset P, et al: The taxonomic relationship of vole agent to *Rochalimaea quintana*. Infect Immunol 26:976, 1979.
Strong RP, Swift HF, Opie EL, et al: Trench Fever. London, The American Red Cross Society and Oxford University Press, 1918, pp 1–446.
Vinson JW: *In vitro* cultivation of the rickettsial agent of trench fever. Bull WHO 35:155, 1966.

27.2. EHRLICHIOSIS

Organisms of the genus *Ehrlichia* are best known as the etiologic agents of diseases of domestic animals, e.g., canine ehrlichiosis *Ehrlichia canis*). They grow in vacuoles within circulating leukocytes, monocytes, lymphocytes, and/or granulocytes depending on the species. Where known, the vectors are ticks (e.g., *Rhipicephalus* spp., *Ixodes* spp., and *Hyalomma* spp.). Recognition of *Ehrlichia* spp. as human pathogens is a recent and evolving phenomenon.

Sennetsu fever (glandular fever), known under various local names, is an infectious mononucleosis-like disease restricted to localities in western Japan. It may vary from a mild form with headache, slight back pain, and low fever to a severe febrile disease with lymphadenopathy and an increase in peripheral blood lymphocytes, many atypical. The disease responds to tetracycline therapy. The organism isolated from patients, which will grow in dog or human monocyte cultures, was originally named *Rickettsia sennetsu* but recently has been reclassified as *Ehrlichia sennetsu* on the basis of shared antigenic determinants with *E. canis*. Its reservoir and mode of transmission remain unknown.

Human ehrlichiosis in the United States was first recognized as a severe febrile disease in 1987 on serologic grounds, i.e., appearance of antibodies reactive with *E. canis* antigen. Cytoplasmic inclusions were seen in blood neutrophils, lymphocytes, and monocytes. Serologic evidence for human ehrlichiosis in the United States is now accumulating rapidly, from Texas and Oklahoma to New Jersey. Many of the cases have been detected by tests for anti-*Ehrlichia* antibodies when sera submitted from patients with suspected Rocky Mountain spotted fever were found to be negative for antibodies against *R. rickettsii* and *Borrelia burgdorferi*. At the time of this writing, a tentative pattern seems to be emerging of a tick-associated, mild to moderately severe, acute infection exhibiting many nonspecific signs and symptoms similar to those of Rocky Mountain spotted fever, e.g., fever, chills, headache, myalgia, and anorexia/nausea/vomiting. Rash occurs, but in a minority of cases. Leukopenia, thrombocytopenia, and elevated liver function test results have been common. Tetracycline appears to be effective therapy. The agent causing human ehrlichiosis has not yet been isolated and identified, nor has the vector been identified. The epidemiologic features are not typical of *Rhipicephalus sanguineus*–transmitted *E. canis* infection of dogs. Recently, serologic evidence has been obtained for the occurrence of human ehrlichiosis in the Soviet Union. Human ehrlichiosis may prove to be a widespread but previously unrecognized problem.

BIBLIOGRAPHY

Anonymous: Human ehrlichiosis—United States. MMWR 37:270, 1988.
Harkess JR, Ewing SA, Crutcher JM, et al: Ehrlichiosis in Oklahoma. J Infect Dis 159:576, 1989.
Kelly DJ, Labarre DD, Lewis GE Jr: Effect of tetracycline therapy on host defense in mice infected with *Ehrlichia sennetsu*. *In* Lieve L (ed): Microbiology—1986. American Society for Microbiology, Washington, DC, 1986, pp 209–212.
Maeda K, Markowitz N, Hawley RC, et al: Human infection with *Ehrlichia canis*, a leukocytic rickettsia. N Engl J Med 316:853, 1987.
Petersen LR, Sawyer LA, Fishbein DB, et al: An outbreak of ehrlichiosis in members of an army reserve unit exposed to ticks. J Infect Dis 159:562, 1989.
Rapmund G: Rickettsial diseases of the Far East: New perspectives. J Infect Dis 149:330, 1984.
Ristic M, Huxsoll DL: Genus IV. Ehrlichieae Moshkovski 1945, 18AL. *In* Krieg NR, Holt JG (eds): Bergey's Manual of Systematic Bacteriology. Baltimore, Williams & Wilkins, 1984, pp 704–709.
Tachibana N: Sennetsu fever: The disease, diagnosis, and treatment. *In* Lieve L (ed): Microbiology—1986. Washington, DC, American Society for Microbiology, 1986, pp 205–208.
Taylor JP, Betz TG, Fishbein DB, et al: Serological evidence of possible human infection with *Ehrlichia* in Texas. J Infect Dis 158:217, 1988.

SECTION B

CHLAMYDIAL INFECTIONS

GENERAL PRINCIPLES

Hugh R. Taylor
and Thomas A. Bell

ETIOLOGY AND HISTORY. Trachoma is the prototypic chlamydial infection and was recognized in ancient times. Chlamydiae were detected with cytologic stains in the early twentieth century in specimens from persons with trachoma and, soon thereafter, in infants with conjunctivitis and their parents. Chlamydiae were first cultivated in the 1950s. The widespread importance and frequency of genital and infant chlamydial infections were first appreciated in the 1960s.

Chlamydiae were once thought to be viruses but are actually gram-negative bacteria that lack muramic acid in their cell walls and their own respiratory systems and are thus obligate intracellular parasites. Taxonomically, chlamydiae are in 1 order, Chlamydiales, which has 1 family, Chlamydiaceae, which contains 1 genus, *Chlamydia*. The genus contains 3 accepted species, *C. trachomatis* and *C. psittaci,* and a new species, *C. pneumoniae*, formally called TWAR. *C. trachomatis* is composed of two main biovars—the lymphogranuloma venereum agents and the oculogenital serovars, which may be distinguished by several well-described serovars with distinctive antigens in the outer membrane protein. *C. psittaci* is a diverse species that has been poorly characterized. Strains that infect psittacine birds seem to differ from those that infect poultry. Several mammals and marsupials have species-specific strains. Chlamydiae are susceptible to erythromycins, tetracyclines, and rifampin. *C. psittaci* and *C. pneumoniae* strains are resistant to sulfonamides, whereas *C. trachomatis* is susceptible.

LIFE CYCLE. Chlamydiae have a complex and unique life cycle. The infectious form, the 350-nm elementary body, induces its own phagocytosis by the host cell at a specific receptor site. It develops within the cell's phagosome, which is prevented from fusing with intracellular lysosomes. Within 6 to 8 hours, the elementary body enlarges and becomes a metabolically active initial or reticulate body, which multiplies by binary fission for an additional 10 to 15 hours. The reticulate body then reorganizes and consolidates into new elementary bodies, which are released to infect other cells. The reticulate body and accumulated elementary bodies compose the characteristic intracytoplasmic inclusions (Fig. III B–1).

The inclusions stain with Giemsa stain. *C. trachomatis* also stains with iodine because its cell wall and matrix are rich in glycogen. All species stain with labeled genus-specific monoclonal antibodies. Individual serovars of *C. trachomatis* may be stained with specific monoclonal antibodies.

INFECTION

***Chlamydia psittaci* Infection.** *C. psittaci* strains are found among many mammals, marsupials, and birds. Generally, humans are not susceptible to infection with most mammalian strains of *C. psittaci;* a notable exception is the ovine abortion agent, which may cause miscarriage in women. Avian strains, however, can cause infection in humans—psittacosis or ornithosis (Chapter 31). Such infections are most common in those slaughtering and dressing poultry and in owners of pet psittacine birds, especially parrots and parakeets. Manifestations of psittacosis include fever that may be low or high, and sometimes severe pneumonia, fever, malaise, anorexia, myalgia, headache, and, occasionally, splenitis, hepatitis, and myocarditis. The differential diagnosis includes influenza, typhoid fever, Q fever, legionellosis, and *Mycoplasma pneumoniae* infection.

The treatment of choice for psittacosis is tetracycline, 500 mg by mouth or 250 mg intravenously 4 times a day for 14 to 21 days. Children less than 8 years old may be treated with erythromycin 12.5 mg/kg 4 times a day by mouth or, if necessary, intravenously.

***Chlamydia trachomatis* Infections.** Humans are the only natural host of *C. trachomatis*. Other primates are susceptible to experimental infection. Endemic trachoma is usually caused by serovars A, B, Ba, and C (Chapter 28); genital infections, by B, D, E, F, G, H, I, J, and K; and lymphogranuloma venereum by L_1, L_2, and L_3 (Chapter 29).

Genital Infections. In developed countries, genital infection with *C. trachomatis* is more common than with

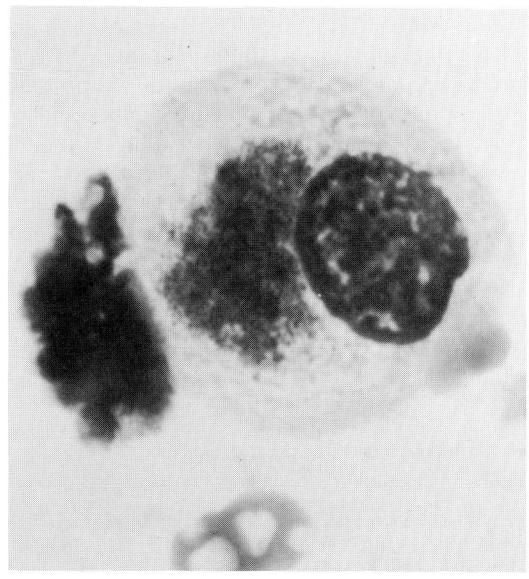

FIGURE III B–1. An epithelial cell with a prominent intracytoplasmic inclusion: superior tarsal conjunctival scraping from a patient with inclusion conjunctivitis (Giemsa stain).

Neisseria gonorrhoeae. Information about the relative frequencies of these 2 infections in developing nations is sparse. *C. trachomatis* causes about 40% of nongonococcal urethritis in men and occurs concurrently with *N. gonorrhoeae* in as many as 50% of cases of the latter. In women, *C. trachomatis* causes mucopurulent cervicitis, urethritis, endometritis, salpingitis, perihepatitis (Fitz-Hugh–Curtis syndrome), and late postpartum endometritis. At least one third of infected males and half of infected females have no symptoms (Chapter 30).

Perinatal Infections. *C. trachomatis* infections of pregnant women are common in developed and in developing countries. The prevalence varies inversely with maternal age. Approximately three fourths of infants born vaginally to infected women become infected. These infections may remain latent for several months after birth. Less commonly, infants born by cesarean section may also be infected. The anatomic sites most commonly infected in infants are the conjunctiva, often manifested as a purulent conjunctivitis, and the nasopharynx, often manifested as chronic nasal congestion. The most serious manifestation of perinatal chlamydial infection is pneumonia, which may range in severity from mild to fatal if untreated. In many areas, *C. trachomatis* is the most common cause of purulent conjunctivitis in the first month of life and of afebrile pneumonia in the first 3 months. Infants infected with *C. trachomatis* at birth may harbor the organism for months or years. The relation of such infections to trachoma is unknown. Empiric therapy of conjunctivitis in children of the appropriate age should include antichlamydial drugs. They may be treated with erythromycin in a dosage of 12.5 mg/kg 4 times a day for 14 days, or with a sulfonamide in an appropriate dosage if the infant is no longer jaundiced. Topical treatment is neither effective nor necessary (Chapter 28).

Chlamydia pneumoniae Infections. *C. pneumoniae* is a newly identified species. It is unique to humans, although experimentally induced infections can occur in animals. It causes upper and lower respiratory tract infections and conjunctivitis. The prevalence of antibodies to *C. pneumoniae* in children is low, increases in adolescence, and reaches a maximum of approximately 50% in middle adulthood. Infections may occur sporadically or in small and slowly spreading epidemics. *C. pneumoniae* pneumonia, which constitutes approximately 10% of "atypical" pneumonias in temperate climates and an unknown proportion in the tropics, is not clinically distinguishable from that caused by *Mycoplasma pneumoniae*. Diagnosis is technically difficult. Tetracycline and erythromycin are the drugs of choice, but the optimal dosage and duration have not been determined.

BIBLIOGRAPHY

Becker Y: The chlamydia: Molecular biology of procaryotic obligate parasites of eucaryocytes. Microbiol Rev 42:274, 1978.
Beer RJS, Bradford WP, Hart RJC: Pregnancy complicated by psittacosis acquired from sheep. Br Med J 284:1156, 1982.
Grayston JT, Wang S-P: New knowledge of chlamydiae and the disease they cause. J Infect Dis 132:87, 1975.
Grayston JT, Kuo C-C, Wang S-P, Altman J: A new *Chlamydia psittaci* strain, TWAR, isolated in acute respiratory tract infections. N Engl J Med 315:161, 1986.
Schachter J: Chlamydial infections. N Engl J Med 298:428, 490, 540, 1978.
Schachter J, Grossman M, Sweet RL, et al: Prospective study of perinatal transmission of *Chlamydia trachomatis*. JAMA 255:3374, 1986.
Stagno S, Brasfield DM, Brown MB, et al: Infant pneumonitis associated with cytomegalovirus, *Chlamydia, Pneumocystis,* and *Ureaplasma*: A prospective study. Pediatrics 68:322, 1981.
WHO Working Group: Extra-ocular chlamydial infection. Bull WHO 64:481, 1986.

28.   TRACHOMA AND INCLUSION CONJUNCTIVITIS

Hugh R. Taylor

TRACHOMA

DEFINITION. Trachoma is a chronic follicular conjunctivitis endemic in many "developing" areas. The infection is usually initially acquired in early childhood. Subsequent blindness usually occurs in middle age. The final stage, corneal scarring, results from progressive scarring and distortion of the upper eyelid.

ETIOLOGY. Trachoma results from infection with *Chlamydia trachomatis,* usually serotypes A, B, Ba, or C. A single infection with *C. trachomatis* usually produces an acute or subacute self-limited follicular conjunctivitis, i.e., inclusion conjunctivitis. Repeated episodes of reinfection seem necessary for sustained inflammation and the characteristic scarring. Trachoma may be a chronic delayed hypersensitivity response to the persistent chlamydial infection of the epithelium, which is maintained by repeated reinfection.

DISTRIBUTION AND INCIDENCE. Trachoma is one of the most common infectious diseases, affecting an estimated 500 million people. It is the leading infectious cause of blindness in the world; 7 to 10 million people are blind as a result of trachoma. In some endemic areas, everyone over the age of 1 year has some signs of trachoma, and 25% of those over 60 years old are blind from it.

Trachoma occurs in areas of poor personal and community hygiene. It was common in Europe and much of North America in the 1800s but disappeared as hygiene improved. Trachoma is most common in North and sub-Saharan Africa, the Middle East, and the Indian subcontinent. It also occurs in areas of Central and South America, Australia, and the Pacific. It tends to be more common in hot, dry areas, which also often have the poorest hygiene.

EPIDEMIOLOGY. Chlamydiae are moderately contagious, and relative "immunity" develops to subsequent reinfection. Repeated episodes of reinfection are necessary for the development of trachoma. Chlamydial infections, including trachoma, are not necessarily confined to the eye but can infect other epithelial surfaces. Chlamydia can be cultured from the nasopharynx and rectum of children in endemic areas.

It appears that most of the transmission of trachoma

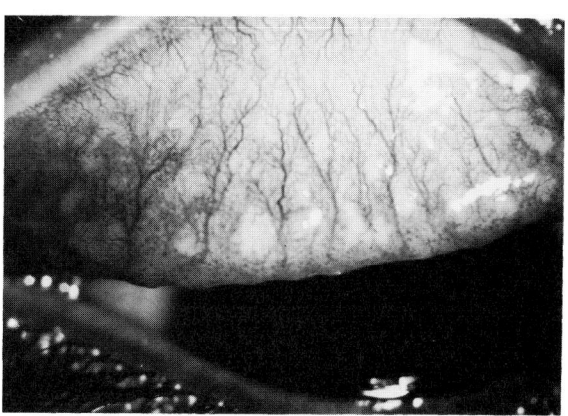

FIGURE 28–1. Superior tarsal conjunctiva of a child with trachoma. The upper lid has been everted, showing several large white follicles, especially along the upper border of the tarsal plate. The tiny dark dots are papillae.

occurs within the family, especially between young children and their mothers or caretakers. In this regard, trachoma can be regarded as a disease of the crèche. Transmission is favored by poor hygiene. Recent epidemiologic studies have singled out the lack of facial cleanliness in children as being of key importance in facilitating transmission, at least in some areas. Lack of adequate water for personal washing and for washing clothes leads to collection and persistence of infected secretions on the face, hands, and clothes. Inadequate sleeping space and poor ventilation may also permit spread by direct contact or by transmission through bedding. Inadequate food storage and poor rubbish or sewage disposal support flies, which can transmit infected ocular secretions.

The chronically inflamed conjunctiva is susceptible to secondary bacterial infection. The chlamydial and bacterial infections have a synergistic effect and produce more severe disease, leading to accelerated development of conjunctival scars and corneal ulceration with subsequent scarring. Bacterial superinfection also produces a more copious mucopurulent discharge, which enhances transmission of chlamydiae.

PATHOGENESIS AND PATHOLOGY. Intracyto-plasmic inclusions in epithelial cells, which stain blue with Giemsa stain (Halberstaedter-Prowazek bodies), are characteristic of chlamydial infection. Inclusions are most common in conjunctival scrapings taken from patients with acute infection. Early in the disease, the conjunctiva shows an acute inflammatory response, but soon mononuclear cells and plasma cells are also present. The most characteristic histologic finding in trachoma is the presence of follicles in the superior tarsal conjunctiva. These are germinal centers surrounded by small lymphocytes. They are believed to be part of a delayed-type hypersensitivity reaction to chlamydial antigens, and the continuing cell-mediated immune response leads to fibrosis and conjunctival scarring. Often, the conjunctival epithelium is invaded by polymorphs and mononuclear cells, and it may thin to a single layer over the surface of a follicle. Later, necrosis in the follicles leads to subconjunctival scarring. Contraction of this scar tissue leads to distortion of the tarsal plate, producing entropion and trichiasis, which in turn lead to corneal opacification and blindness. Pannus is initially an inflammatory infiltrate, which is replaced by fibrous tissue and new blood vessels.

CLINICAL MANIFESTATIONS AND COMPLICATIONS. Trachoma usually produces few symptoms until its final stages when trichiasis (inturning of the eyelashes) develops. A superimposed bacterial conjunctivitis causes a mucopurulent discharge. In the absence of secondary conjunctivitis, the symptoms may be mild and ignored (even if medical care is available) as are a purulent nasal discharge, chronic serous otitis media, and a productive cough, which also may be due to an initial chlamydial infection followed by secondary bacterial infection.

The most obvious sign of trachoma during the stage of active inflammation is the follicle, either in the superior tarsal conjunctiva or at the corneal limbus (Figs. 28–1 and 28–2). Follicles are large, pale yellow or white spots which may be slightly elevated and are 0.25 to 2 mm in diameter. Those on the limbus are often a dirty gray and may be semitranslucent (Fig. 28–3).

Active inflammation is also accompanied by marked thickening of the conjunctiva. This can be recognized

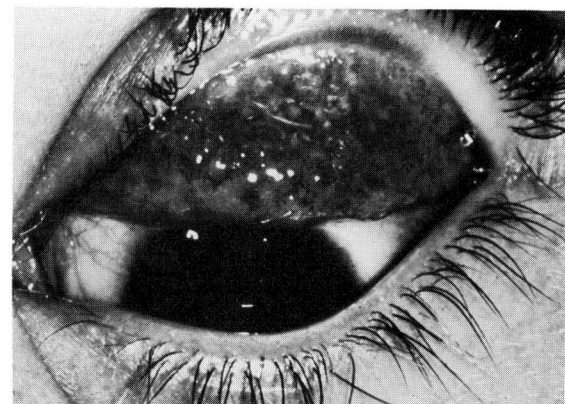

FIGURE 28–2. An intense inflammatory response to trachoma. Follicles extend over most of the superior tarsal conjunctiva; some are confluent. The inflammation and hyperemia have caused spontaneous hemorrhages.

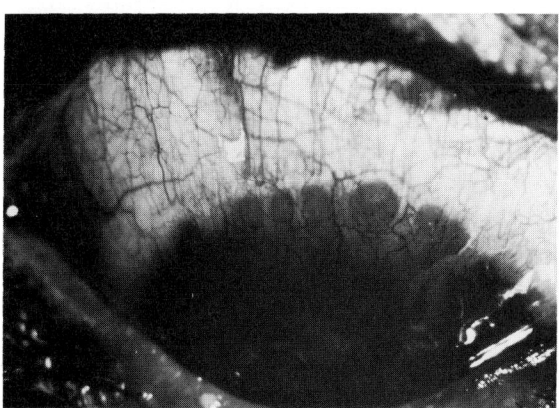

FIGURE 28–3. Superior cornea of a child with active trachoma showing large, gray, fleshy limbal follicles. Corneal pannus extends several millimeters into the cornea.

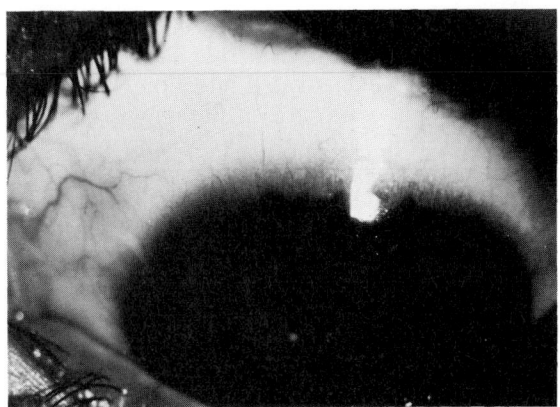

FIGURE 28–4. Superior limbus of a child with trachoma showing many Herbert's pits and about 1 mm of corneal pannus.

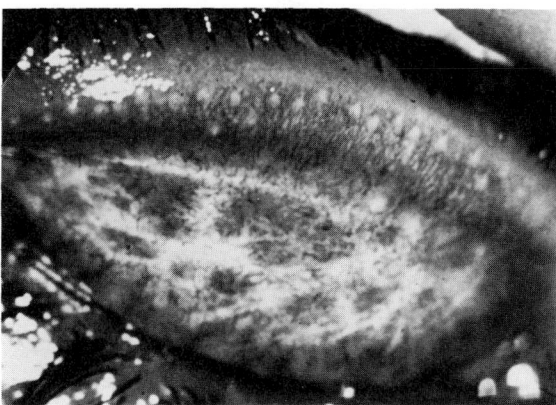

FIGURE 28–6. Strong, organized bands of scarring of the superior tarsal conjunctiva in an adult, with distortion of the line of openings of the meibomian glands as they are dragged onto the tarsal surface by scarring. (Courtesy of Professor F. C. Hollows.)

by the obscuration of tarsal blood vessels or the presence of conjunctival papillae. Papillae appear as small, pinpoint red dots (Fig. 28–4). They are not specific for trachoma. Papillae appear before trachomatous follicles and also may be the only sign of ongoing active inflammation in eyes of young children or older persons, who usually have no follicular response. The papillary response increases dramatically with bacterial secondary infection. The intensity of the papillary response in the presence of follicles is a good index of the severity of the inflammation and infection.

Fine conjunctival scars gradually appear. Occurring first as small stellate figures, they gradually accumulate to form a basketweave network (Fig. 28–5). With time, this consolidates to form strong bands of scar tissue (Fig. 28–6). Sometimes, an especially prominent band, Arlt's line, develops a few millimeters above and parallel to the lid margin. Follicles seem to blend into the scars and may be difficult to distinguish.

Scarring of the conjunctiva impedes the normal protective role of this mucous membrane and leads to distortion and buckling of the tarsal plate. The scar tissue contracts like the string of an archer's bow, causing the lid margin to rotate inward, leading to entropion. The earliest sign of this is the irregular migration of the openings of the meibomian glands onto

the inner surface of the lid (Fig. 28–6). This is followed by turning in of the lashes, which rub on the cornea, causing trichiasis (Fig. 28–7). The continual abrasion of the cornea rapidly leads to corneal edema, ulceration, and scarring—the main route by which trachoma leads to blindness.

Inflammatory infiltrate and punctate keratitis may occur in the superior cornea during active inflammation; corneal stromal opacification and new vessels later develop to produce the superior corneal pannus characteristic of trachoma (Figs. 28–3 and 28–4). The pannus may extend several millimeters across the cornea and, in rare cases, may reach the central cornea and affect vision. More often, however, blood vessels will extend from the pannus to an area of corneal ulceration and lead to a vascularized leukoma. As the pannus advances across the cornea, it bypasses the sites of limbal follicles. After the follicles resolve, clear depressions are left, surrounded on 3 sides by pannus. These depressions are known as "Herbert's pits" (Fig. 28–4).

Some investigators have described a decrease in the tears in those with cicatrizing trachoma, but no specific abnormality in tear function has been shown. The eyes are often more moist (watery) than usual, and there may even be maceration from chronic conjunctivitis.

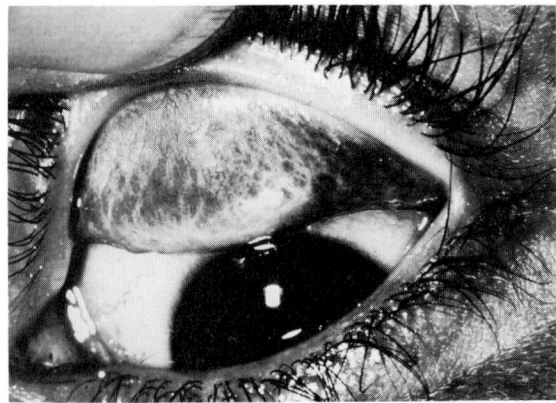

FIGURE 28–5. The superior tarsal conjunctiva of a child with trachoma, showing an extensive "basketweave" network of conjunctival scarring. Although no follicles are obvious, active inflammation is indicated by the numerous papillae.

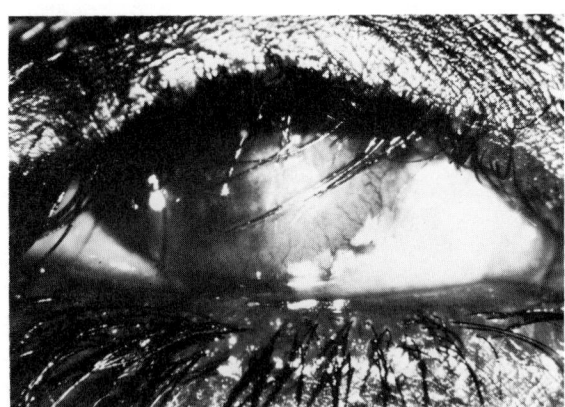

FIGURE 28–7. Early trichiasis in an adult with advanced cicatricial trachoma. The medial lashes of the upper lid rub on the cornea, which has become opaque and vascularized.

The presence of signs of cicatrization, i.e., tarsal scarring, entropion and trichiasis, pannus, and Herbert's pits, indicates that that eye has had active inflammatory trachoma in the past. Follicles (either tarsal or limbal) and inflammatory thickening indicate an active inflammatory response at time of examination.

Trachoma and inclusion conjunctivitis present a spectrum of chronicity. Inclusion conjunctivitis develops following an isolated episode of infection, whereas repeated infection is needed to maintain trachoma. Putative relapses of trachoma are almost certainly due to episodes of reinfection.

DIAGNOSIS

Clinical Diagnosis. Trachoma is usually diagnosed on clinical grounds. The old 4-stage classification introduced by MacCallan in 1930 has been superseded and is now seen as no longer useful. A new simplified grading scheme has been developed by WHO (Table 28–1).

Laboratory Diagnosis. Several tests can be used to make a laboratory diagnosis of trachoma. Previously, the most common was a Giemsa stain of a conjunctival scraping; the characteristic inclusions were sought in the epithelial cells (see Fig. III B–1). The organism may be cultured in either embryonated hens' eggs or one of several tissue culture systems, the best of which is McCoy cells treated with cycloheximide. Antigen detection methods using commercially available kits or reagents have been improved so that they are suitable for field use. Direct fluorescent antibody (DFA) cytology uses fluorescein-labeled monoclonal antibodies to identify chlamydial elementary bodies in conjunctival smears (Fig. 28–8). Enzyme immunoassay (EIA) methods use enzymes linked to antibodies to detect antigen in conjunctival swabs. In general, these tests give similar results, although each has its own advantages and disadvantages, but both are much more sensitive than Giemsa cytology and much cheaper than culture. Methods that detect chlamydial nucleic acids are still in the developmental phase.

The finding of antichlamydial antibodies in serum or tears indicates the occurrence of past infection but is not diagnostic for current infection. However, in infants, it is diagnostic if IgM antibodies are present and the presence of IgA antibodies in tears is suggestive of infection.

Differential Diagnosis. Conditions producing a follicular conjunctivitis and causing conjunctival scarring can be confused with trachoma. Viral infection is the most common nonchlamydial cause of follicular conjunctivitis; it is an acute and self-limiting infection that usually shows significant resolution within 2 weeks. A toxic follicular conjunctivitis may occur with molluscum contagiosum, prolonged use of topical drugs, and allergy to eye cosmetics. The large papillae of vernal catarrh may be confused at times with follicles. In otherwise healthy eyes, follicles may be found in the fornix conjunctivae, especially in the inferior fornix. This occurs most commonly in young children and is called "folliculosis." There is no other sign of inflammation, and the follicles do not involve the superior tarsus. The other differential diagnoses are different presentations of chlamydial infection and include inclusion conjunctivitis and the pre-

TABLE 28–1. World Health Organization Simplified Trachoma Grading Scheme

TF:	Trachomatous inflammation—follicular; 5 or more follicles (≥0.5 mm) in the upper tarsal conjunctiva
TI:	Trachomatous inflammation—intense; inflammatory thickening of tarsal conjunctiva obscuring more than half of the normal deep tarsal vessels
TS:	Trachomatous conjunctival scarring; easily visible scarring in the tarsal conjunctiva
TT:	Trachomatous trichiasis; at least 1 eyelash rubbing on the eyeball
CO:	Corneal opacity; easily visible opacity over the pupil obscuring at least part of the pupil margin

sumed chlamydial infections of Axenfeld's chronic follicular conjunctivitis and Thygeson's chronic follicular keratoconjunctivitis.

Conditions that produce tarsal scarring and are likely to be confused with trachoma include trauma, previous chalazion, and severe bacterial conjunctivitis.

TREATMENT AND PROGNOSIS. Chlamydiae are susceptible to many antimicrobials, including sulfonamides, tetracycline, erythromycin, and rifampin. Previously, standard treatment of trachoma was 1.0% tetracycline ointment or 1.0% oily tetracycline drops used 2 to 4 times a day for 1 to 3 weeks and possibly repeated up to 6 times at monthly intervals. Systemic treatment may provide an alternative, although topical tetracycline should continue to be used for mass treatment until the risks and benefits of mass systemic treatment are more clearly defined. Tetracycline, which is inexpensive, safe, and effective, should not be given to pregnant women or to children under 8 years of age. Sulfonamides, especially sulfamethoxazole combined with trimethoprim, are usually well tolerated but have rare serious side effects, e.g., the Stevens-Johnson syndrome. Erythromycin also is safe and effective but must be given 4 times a day. Systemic chemotherapy should be given for 3 weeks. If significant bacterial conjunctivitis coexists, it should be treated with topical antibiotics. This strategy is effective for treating sporadic cases, but without some community-based intervention patients in endemic areas

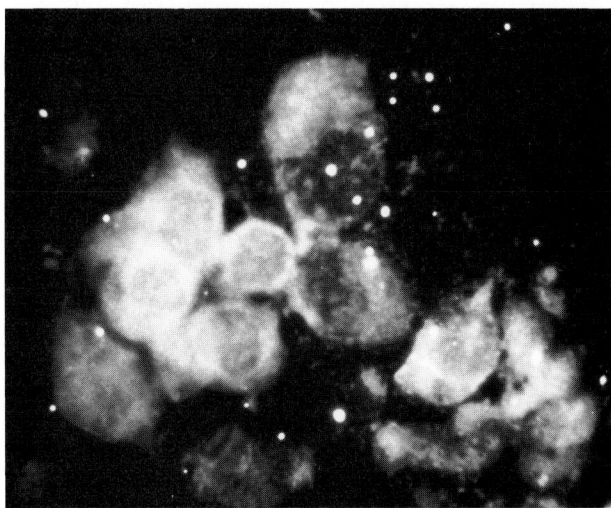

FIGURE 28–8. Direct fluorescent antibody (DFA) cytology preparation. The free chlamydial elementary bodies are stained brightly with a fluorescent-labeled monoclonal antibody.

will rapidly become reinfected. Copper sulfate and the expression of follicles may be harmful and are no longer advocated, as they are likely to cause even more conjunctival scarring.

Trichiasis should be treated. Single lashes may be epilated, and epilation by the patient or relatives should be encouraged. However, it is only of temporary benefit because the lashes will promptly regrow. Lid surgery is needed to evert the lashes; some procedures have a high failure rate and may lead to further problems caused by poor lid closure if not carefully performed. Trichiasis surgery is most important, however, because it can often greatly improve vision or prevent the development of blindness.

PREVENTION AND CONTROL. The aim of prevention is to break the transmission of infection and thereby reduce the frequency of exposure to the extent that episodes of reinfection do not occur often enough to cause blinding trachoma. In many areas, chlamydiae cannot be eliminated from the environment. The key to reducing transmission is good personal and community hygiene; any measures that improve hygiene are likely to lessen trachoma. These may include the provision and proper use of adequate water supplies, housing, food storage, fly control, and rubbish and sewage disposal, although recent studies suggest that improved facial cleanliness in children may be of prime importance.

For the short term, antibiotics can be used in 2 ways, either directly to attack the infectious pool itself or indirectly by reducing the transmission of chlamydiae. The intermittent use of topical antibiotics, e.g., tetracycline, can reduce transmission indirectly. Antibiotics mainly reduce bacterial secondary infection, which in turn reduces the intensity of inflammation and the amount of ocular discharge, thereby reducing transmission. Topical antibiotics can also temporarily clear the conjunctiva of chlamydiae, but, once discontinued, the eye is likely to be reinfected either endogenously from other epithelial surfaces or exogenously.

When using antibiotics to reduce the infectious pool, one must treat all components of the pool. Antibiotics must be given systemically to reach all infected surfaces. To reach all those infected or potentially infected, the entire "living unit" should be treated. In some cases, this may be a family or household; at other times, a segment of the community or the entire community may need to be treated. Therefore, antibiotic treatment aimed at reducing the infectious pool must be given systemically as mass treatment.

INCLUSION CONJUNCTIVITIS

DEFINITION. Inclusion conjunctivitis is an acute conjunctivitis caused by *C. trachomatis*. In neonates, it is usually purulent and severe and is associated with extraocular infection. In adults, it is often a more chronic, follicular conjunctivitis and is usually associated with urogenital infection.

DISTRIBUTION AND INCIDENCE. Inclusion conjunctivitis has a worldwide distribution, although its prevalence tends to vary inversely with the prevalence of trachoma. In areas with poor hygiene and hence more frequent episodes of reinfection often with eye to eye transmission, trachoma predominates. In areas with better hygiene and therefore less frequent episodes of reinfection, inclusion conjunctivitis is more common and is usually the result of sexual transmission.

ETIOLOGY. Inclusion conjunctivitis is caused by *C. trachomatis,* usually of the "genital" immunotypes—D through K. Trachoma strains have been isolated from cases clinically indistinguishable from inclusion conjunctivitis, and the disease caused by genital strains may be indistinguishable from trachoma. Animal experiments indicate that the serotype is less important than the frequency of reinfection.

EPIDEMIOLOGY. Inclusion conjunctivitis usually results from the inoculation of the eye with infected genital secretions. Although inclusion conjunctivitis can be transmitted by eye-finger-eye contact and there have been classic outbreaks associated with communal bathing, most transmission is sexually related. About one half of the infants delivered vaginally by mothers with chlamydial cervicitis will develop inclusion conjunctivitis, and some studies have shown that 5 to 30% of pregnant women have chlamydial cervicitis. Neonatal inclusion conjunctivitis usually appears 4 to 12 days after birth.

In adults, inclusion conjunctivitis is often associated with genital infection. The incubation period in adults is usually 7 to 14 days.

CLINICAL MANIFESTATIONS AND COMPLICATIONS. In neonates, inclusion conjunctivitis is a mucopurulent conjunctivitis. It causes lid swelling and hyperemia and edema of the conjunctiva. Rarely, untreated cases develop some conjunctival scarring and corneal pannus.

In adults, inclusion conjunctivitis causes an acute follicular conjunctivitis, often with preauricular lymphadenopathy. There is usually a mild to moderate watery or mucopurulent discharge, which is less severe than that of herpetic or adenoviral keratoconjunctivitis. Diffuse superficial punctate keratitis or, less often, subepithelial infiltrates may occur. Often, other evidence of chlamydial infection exists, such as genital infection or otitis media. Anterior uveitis is a rare manifestation.

DIAGNOSIS. Inclusion conjunctivitis is usually diagnosed clinically and confirmed by cytologic examination. Conjunctival smears may show epithelial cells that contain the intracytoplasmic inclusions, best seen with Giemsa stain (Fig. III B–1). A mixed inflammatory cell response containing both polymorphs and lymphocytes is characteristic. However, the diagnosis is better made with a DFA cytology test using a monoclonal antibody directed against the surface of the elementary body (Fig. 28–8). DFA cytology can detect free elementary bodies and is highly sensitive and specific.

The most important differentiation in neonates is gonococcal ophthalmia neonatorum, which is usually more severe, appearing within the first 8 days of life. The typical gram-negative intracellular diplococci are usually seen in smears and can be grown on chocolate agar in 5% carbon dioxide. Inclusion conjunctivitis should be differentiated also from adenovirus and herpes simplex keratoconjunctivitis.

TREATMENT AND PROGNOSIS. Chlamydial infection in neonates is potentially serious. These infants should be treated with systemic antibiotics. Erythromycin given as a weight-adjusted dose (50 mg/kg/day in 4 divided doses) is the preferred treatment and should be used for 3 weeks. Topical antibiotics—either erythromycin, tetracycline, or sulfonamides—can also be used 4 times a day if there is a marked discharge to reduce more rapidly the risk of spreading infection.

Adults should receive systemic tetracycline, erythromycin, or sulfonamides for 3 weeks. Again, topical antibiotics can also be used if there is a marked mucopurulent discharge. Sexual partners should be examined and treated. Although persistent infection may occur, recurrences are usually the result of reinfection.

PREVENTION AND CONTROL. The prevention of inclusion conjunctivitis is difficult. Treatment of patients and consorts is important, as are the identification and treatment of infected pregnant women. Credé's prophylaxis with silver nitrate drops in the eyes of infants is ineffective in preventing chlamydial infection. A single conjunctival application of erythromycin ointment at birth reduces the incidence of ocular infection but not that of nasopharyngeal or respiratory chlamydial infection. It seems that to be effective antibiotic prophylaxis must be given at the time of delivery and not delayed for several hours.

BIBLIOGRAPHY

Dawson CR, Jones BR, Tarizzo ML: Guide to Trachoma Control. Geneva, WHO, 1981.

Dawson CR, Schachter J: Strategies for treatment and control of blinding trachoma: Cost effectiveness of topical or systemic antibiotics. Rev Infect Dis 7:768, 1985.

Grayston JT, Wang S-P, Yeh L-J, et al: Importance of reinfection in the pathogenesis of trachoma. Rev Infect Dis 7:717, 1985.

Hammerschlag MR, Chandler JW, Alexander ER, et al: Erythromycin ointment for ocular prophylaxis of neonatal chlamydial infection. JAMA 244:2291, 1980.

Hollows FC: Community-based action for the control of trachoma. Rev Infect Dis 7:777, 1985.

Jones BR: The prevention of blindness from trachoma. Trans Ophthalmol Soc UK 95:16, 1975.

Jones BR, Darougar S, Mohsenine H, et al: Communicable ophthalmia: The blinding scourge of the Middle East. Yesterday, today and ? tomorrow. Br J Ophthalmol 60:492, 1976.

Rapoza PA, Quinn TC, Kiessling LA, et al: Assessment of neonatal conjunctivitis with a direct immunofluorescent monoclonal antibody stain for *Chlamydia*. JAMA 255:3369, 1986.

Schachter J, Dawson CR: Human Chlamydial Infection. Littleton, MA, PSG Publishing, 1978.

Taylor HR, Millan-Velasco F, Sommer A: The ecology of trachoma: An epidemiological study of trachoma in Southern Mexico. Bull WHO 63:559, 1985.

Taylor HR, Sommer A: Risk-factor studies as an epidemiologic tool. Rev Infect Dis 7:765, 1985.

Thylefors B, Dawson CR, Jones BR, et al: A simple system for the assessment of trachoma and its complications. Bull WHO 65:485, 1987.

Wilson MC, Millan-Velasco F, Tielsch JM, et al: Direct-smear fluorescent antibody cytology as a field diagnostic tool for trachoma. Arch Ophthalmol 104:688, 1986.

29. LYMPHOGRANULOMA VENEREUM

Peter L. Perine

DEFINITION. Lymphogranuloma venereum (LGV) is a sexually transmitted disease caused by *Chlamydia trachomatis*. Known variously as tropical or climatic bubo, strumous bubo, lymphopathia venereum, Nicolas-Favre disease, and lymphogranuloma inguinale, it is primarily a disease of lymphatic and anogenital tissue.

The clinical course of LGV is conventionally separated into 3 more or less distinct stages—primary, secondary, and late or tertiary. The infrequently seen initial or primary lesion appears at the site of infection. The first manifestations of disease usually occur during the secondary stage, some 3 to 6 weeks after infection, and are of 2 types: acute inguinal lymphadenitis, often leading to bubo formation (the inguinal syndrome), or a hemorrhagic proctocolitis (the anogenitorectal syndrome). Tertiary lesions evolve over a period of several years and take the form of locally destructive chronic ulcerations, fistulas, abscesses, genital elephantiasis, and stricture. Late complications are prevented by adequate antibiotic treatment during the early stage of infection.

ETIOLOGY. Only 3 of the 15 recognized immunotypes of *C. trachomatis,* designated L1, L2, and L3, cause the bubonic lymphadenitis and systemic symptoms characteristic of LGV. This reflects the greater invasive potential of LGV immunotypes compared with the other immunotypes of *C. trachomatis* (Chapter 28). For example, LGV chlamydiae are more cytopathogenic and usually cause a fatal meningoencephalitis when inoculated intracerebrally into mice, whereas other *C. trachomatis* immunotypes do not. These distinctions have little clinical significance except that non-LGV serotypes can cause a milder form of proctitis in homosexual men.

HISTORY. The different manifestations of LGV were considered to be variations of syphilis until Wassermann introduced his test for the detection of syphilis antibody in 1906. Together with the darkfield microscopic technique for identification of *Treponema pallidum,* the Wassermann test differentiated the primary lesion and the inguinal lymphadenitis accompanying primary syphilis as well as the inguinal buboes caused by chancroid from those caused by LGV. The first definitive description of acute LGV, including hemorrhagic proctitis, was written by Durand, Nicolas, and Favre in 1913.

Climatic or tropical bubo was not associated with LGV until the mid 1920s. This disease was particularly common in soldiers and sailors serving in the tropics who consorted with local prostitutes. Attempts to isolate bacteria on usual culture media were unsuccessful. Based on its epidemiology, tropical bubo was regarded as a sexually transmitted disease of unknown etiology until 1925, when Frei introduced a specific LGV skin test. This test established the common etiology of tropical bubo and LGV.

The original Frei skin-test antigen was prepared from heat-inactivated pus aspirated from unruptured LGV inguinal buboes. This antigen produced a tuberculin-like reaction when inoculated into the skin of an LGV patient with an infection of at least 2 to 6 weeks' duration. Once established, this skin hypersensitivity was usually lifelong. However, other chlamydial infections such as nonspecific urethritis, trachoma, and psittacosis also produced positive Frei tests. The Frei test was also negative in many patients with early LGV. Despite these deficiencies, the Frei test led to the recognition that rectal stricture, genital elephantiasis, and various rectal fistulas were complications of LGV.

LGV chlamydiae were first isolated in the 1930s from infected human tissue by intracerebral inoculation of mice and later by inoculation of the yolk sac of embryonated eggs. Egg culture provided a less hazardous and a more plentiful source of Frei antigen both for the Frei test and for serologic tests to detect complement-fixing (CF) chlamydial antibodies. More specific serodiagnostic tests for LGV and for isolation of LGV chlamydiae in tissue culture were introduced in the 1960s.

EPIDEMIOLOGY. LGV is sporadic in North America and Europe, although focal areas of endemicity, usually seaports, are recognized. The disease is endemic in several areas of East and West Africa, India, Southeast Asia, the Caribbean, and Brazil. The highest prevalence may be in Addis Ababa, Ethiopia, where several thousand cases are reported annually.

Prevalence studies of LGV based on the results of Frei skin tests or CF serologic tests should be interpreted with caution. Neither of these diagnostic tests is specific for LGV because they both employ an antigen present in all chlamydiae. In almost every instance in which the prevalence of LGV was based on positive skin tests or CF serologic tests, it was grossly overestimated.

The relatively infrequent occurrence of the acute inguinal syndrome or anogenitorectal syndrome in women who are named as sexual contacts of males with proven cases of LGV suggests that women may be carriers of LGV chlamydiae and serve as the reservoir of infection. Women can develop asymptomatic LGV endocervicitis. The duration of contagiousness in women can be several weeks or months, which argues strongly for the prophylactic treatment of sexual partners of LGV patients to prevent reinfection.

The risk of acquiring LGV following exposure is not known. LGV often coexists with gonorrhea or syphilis, both of which are transmitted with greater frequency than LGV.

Extragenital transmission of LGV is rare, but open, draining buboes pose a risk for nursing personnel. Laboratory-acquired infections have also been reported.

PATHOPHYSIOLOGY. The complex reproductive cycle of chlamydiae terminates with the death of infected host cells and the discharge of infectious elementary bodies into the extracellular tissues and secretions. These small bodies measuring 350 nm in diameter contain immunotype-specific antigens on their surface. In a process not yet defined, the elementary body attaches to the surface of another cell, enters the cell by phagocytosis, and begins another reproductive cycle.

LGV chlamydiae have an inherent preference for the cells and tissues they parasitize. They usually invade mucosal epithelial cells of the urogenital tract or the columnar epithelium lining the urethra, rectum, or endocervix. Unlike other chlamydiae, LGV immunotypes invade submucosal tissue and enter lymphatic vessels, which carry the organisms to the lymph nodes draining the site of infection, and from there they spread systemically. Systemic spread causes the constitutional symptoms that are characteristic of the acute stages of infection. Rarely, a meningoencephalitis occurs. Systemic spread is ultimately limited by the humoral and cell-mediated immune response, although the organisms may persist in anogenital tissue in the absence of antibiotic treatment. Persistence of LGV within host cells probably protects them from immune-mediated destruction.

Although multiplication of LGV chlamydiae destroys host cells, as in the case of trachoma, further tissue injury is caused by bacterial superinfection of LGV ulcerations and fistulas. Tissue damage during acute LGV may be caused by hypersensitivity to chlamydial antigens with the formation of necrotic, granulomatous lesions found both within the mucosa and within lymph nodes. Repeated exposure to LGV chlamydia may be important in developing symptomatic disease. Late sequelae of LGV are rare today because of the use of antibiotics.

CLINICAL MANIFESTATIONS. Inguinal buboes are the most common manifestation of LGV. They are predominant in men, with male:female ratios often exceeding 4:1. Women and homosexual men usually present with hemorrhagic proctocolitis and the overwhelming majority of late LGV complications such as rectal stricture, rectovaginal fistulas, and genital elephantiasis occur in women.

Primary LGV. The initial or primary lesion of LGV appears at the site of infection after an incubation period of 7 to 21 days. It can be a papule, a herpetiform lesion, an erosion or ulceration, or a nongonococcal urethritis or endocervicitis. A primary lesion is found in only 10 to 30% of men and in fewer women. In men, the most common sites of the papule, ulcer, or herpetiform lesion are on the prepuce, glans, and shaft of the penis. In women, they usually appear on the posterior vaginal wall or on the labia. Most primary lesions on the skin or mucous membrane are asymptomatic and inconspicuous and heal within a few days. LGV urethritis and cervicitis may be indistinguishable from those caused by other immunotypes of *C. trachomatis*. The primary lesion in the case of urethritis may be intraurethral.

Extragenital primary LGV lesions are usually painful, ulcerated, and accompanied by tender enlargement of the lymph nodes draining the lesion. Conjunctivitis can develop by direct inoculation or autoinoculation of LGV into the eye and may be accompanied by a preauricular lymphadenopathy and lymphedema of the eyelids, a form of "Perinaud's oculoglandular syndrome."

Secondary LGV. The symptoms and signs of secondary LGV appear 2 to 6 weeks after infection and are usually the first manifestations of infection. A variety of lesions can present (Table 29–1) because of local and systemic spread of chlamydiae. Constitutional symptoms, including hectic fever, headache, myalgia, and anorexia, are especially common during this stage and resemble influenza. The majority of patients, however,

TABLE 29–1. Manifestations of Lymphogranuloma Venereum

Manifestation	Early and Late Complications
Primary herpetiform lesion, papule, or ulcer (genital and remote)	Meningitis (rare) Regional lymphadenitis
Primary nongonococcal urethritis, endocervicitis	Urethral stricture; fistula; salpingitis; parametritis
Secondary inguinal syndrome, lymphangitis/lymphadenitis, bubo formation	Bubonulus or local abscess; sinus tracts; genital elephantiasis; fistulas; chronic ulceration
Secondary anorectal syndrome, proctocolitis	Rectal stricture; rectovaginal and perirectal abscesses; fistulas in ano; lymphorrhoids; chronic ulceration; genital elephantiasis (esthiomene)
Other	Generalized lymphadenitis; hepatosplenomegaly; erythema nodosum; erythema multiforme; polyarthritis; extragenital ulcerations

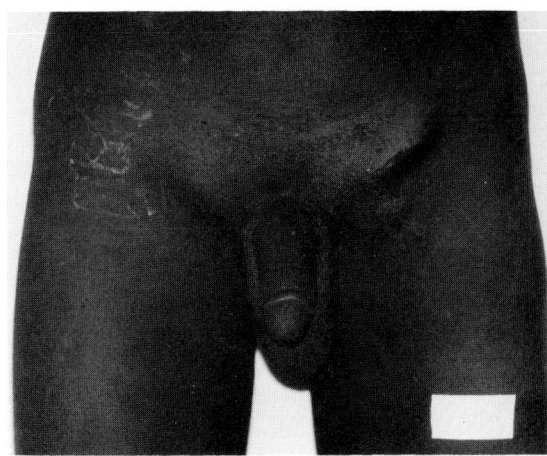

FIGURE 29–1. Lymphogranuloma venereum. Bilateral inguinal buboes with separation of the matted left inguinal and femoral lymph nodes by the inguinal ligament, creating the pathognomonic sign of the "groove."

develop either the *inguinal syndrome* or the *anogenitorectal syndrome,* depending on the site of the initial infection or primary lesion.

Inguinal Syndrome. This is the most common manifestation of secondary LGV. It occurs predominantly in men because of the location of the primary lesion; the lymphatics of the penis and scrotum drain into the superficial and deep inguinal glands. The syndrome begins with rapid, painful enlargement of the inguinal lymph nodes. The femoral lymph nodes may enlarge as well, and the inelastic inguinal ligament may separate or cleave the enlarged inguinal and femoral nodes, thereby creating a "groove," which is considered to be virtually diagnostic of LGV lymphadenitis (Fig. 29–1). The nodes are matted together as they enlarge by a plastic periadenitis. Within 1 or 2 weeks, a glandular inguinal mass forms and attaches to skin and subcutaneous tissue. The overlying skin often has a characteristic livid discoloration ("blue balls"). Two thirds of the inguinal buboes are unilateral, and about three fourths suppurate and rupture within 2 weeks of their appearance. Multiple sinuses form and drain thick, yellowish pus, giving the inguinal region the appearance of the mouthpiece of a watering pot, a condition termed "poradenitis."

Rupture of the bubo usually relieves the pain and fever, but sinus drainage may continue for several weeks. Healing produces characteristic calluses and contracted scars in the inguinal region. Scarring may obstruct lymphatic drainage of the penis and scrotum and produce genital elephantiasis. The majority of patients, however, experience no serious sequelae.

Dorsal penile lymphangitis may also precede or accompany the inguinal bubo. The lymphatic vessels are visibly swollen and tender. A large, tender nodule or "bubonulus" may form along the course of the dorsal penile lymphatics. Occasionally, the bubonulus ruptures and forms sinus tracts, fistulas extending to the urethra, or chronic ulcerations, which can result in fibrotic, deforming scars at the base of the penis and scrotum.

Anogenitorectal Syndrome. This occurs predominantly in women, because the lymphatics of the posterior vagina and cervix, the areas that are the most common sites of the primary infection in women, drain to the deep iliac, anorectal, and presacral lymph nodes. The rectovaginal septum is particularly rich in lymphatics, which carry LGV chlamydiae to the rectal mucosa and surrounding tissue. LGV may also be directly inoculated into the rectum by anal intercourse.

The early symptoms of rectal LGV are anal pruritus, anorectal pain, and a bloody, mucous rectal discharge. The rectal mucosa becomes diffusely hyperemic and friable after several weeks. Multiple small, superficial ulcerations with irregular borders are gradually replaced by granulation tissue. This inflammatory process involves the entire bowel wall, and bacterial superinfection causes a bloody, mucopurulent rectal discharge. The inflammation is usually limited to the rectosigmoid colon below the level of the peritoneal reflection and cannot be easily differentiated from other causes of inflammatory bowel disease.

Fever, rectal pain, and tenesmus are common during the early stages of the anogenitorectal syndrome. The left lower quadrant of the abdomen is tender, and the pelvic colon may be palpably thickened. The rectal mucosa feels granular on digital examination, and enlarged lymph nodes may be palpated beneath the bowel wall.

Tertiary Lesions. If untreated, the granulation tissue can erode the rectovaginal septum and form a fistula, or it may contract slowly, causing a rectal stricture with partial or complete bowel obstruction. Symptoms at this stage include various degrees of constipation, abdominal distention, colic, and passage of "pencil" stools. The stricture is usually located between 2 and 5 cm from the anocutaneous margin, where the perirectal lymphatics are the richest. The rectal mucosa below the stricture and the skin around the anus are also frequent sites for formation of perirectal abscesses, anal fissures, fistulas in-ano, and ischiorectal fistulas. Obstruction of the lymphatic drainage of the distal rectum may cause outgrowths of perianal lymphatics (lymphorrhoids), which grossly resemble hemorrhoids. Perianal lymphatic obstruction in women may also cause lymphedema and chronic ulceration of the external genitalia with formation of fistulas and extremely painful destructive lesions, collectively referred to as "esthiomene." This process may destroy the anus and perineum as well as the rectovaginal septum.

Miscellaneous Manifestations. A variety of rashes, e.g., erythema nodosum and erythema multiforme, are common in both early and late LGV. Constitutional symptoms always accompany extragenital primary LGV ulceration. Follicular conjunctivitis may occur at any time during the course of untreated LGV by autoinoculation of infected secretions into one or both conjunctivae.

DIAGNOSIS. The laboratory diagnosis of LGV is best made by isolating LGV chlamydiae from infected tissue or secretions in tissue culture, in ovo, or by mouse-brain inoculation. However, because chlamydia culture is available only in specialized laboratories, the diagnosis of LGV is usually based on the clinical findings together with a positive serologic test for chlamydial antibody.

In areas where LGV is prevalent, clinical diagnosis together with an LGV-positive CF test is usually sufficient to establish the diagnosis. In acute LGV infections, the higher the CF titer, the more secure the diagnosis. A fourfold or greater increase in CF titer between acute and convalescent serum specimens is also diagnostic.

Serologic Tests. The two most common types of LGV serologic tests are distinguished by the type of antigen used. The LGV CF assay uses a heat-stable antigen made from any strain of *Chlamydia* grown in egg or tissue culture, usually a strain of LGV or *C. psittaci*. This genus antigen is present in all *Chlamydia* and reacts with antibody produced in any chlamydial infection. This lack of specificity does not detract from the usefulness of the CF assay, however. It is almost always positive in high titer during the acute stages of LGV. The titer falls rapidly after antibiotic treatment.

The second category of serologic tests uses an indirect fluorescent antibody technique to detect antibody specific for *C. trachomatis*. This microimmunofluorescent (micro-IF) assay is more sensitive and specific for detecting LGV antibody, but like the CF test, a positive result indicates only that the patient has at some time been infected with *C. trachomatis*. Although the micro-IF titer to LGV antigens is high in most acute infections, the complexity of the test is such that the test is performed routinely only in reference laboratories.

Skin Test. The once popular Frei skin test is rarely used today because of its lack of sensitivity and specificity. The standardized antigen used in the test is no longer produced commercially.

Biopsy and Smears. Biopsy of infected lymphatic tissue may show characteristic "stellate microabscesses" during the early stages of LGV, but these lesions are also found in other diseases. Cytologic examination of smears made from infected secretions or tissue may reveal intracytoplasmic inclusion or elementary bodies if the preparation is stained with fluorescein-labeled chlamydial commercially available antibody (Fig. 28–8). This technique requires the use of a fluorescent microscope and cannot distinguish between serovars of *C. trachomatis*.

Differential Diagnosis. In areas where LGV is sporadic or of low incidence, the diagnosis should be made with caution. Other diseases that are frequently mistaken for bubonic LGV are genital herpesvirus infections, Hodgkin's disease, and primary syphilis. Occasionally, a surgeon mistakes the acute inguinal LGV bubo for an incarcerated inguinal hernia. The LGV anogenitorectal syndrome is clinically indistinguishable from acute amebic dysentery, idiopathic ulcerative proctocolitis, and Crohn's disease.

TREATMENT. The highly variable clinical course of LGV makes evaluation of therapy difficult, if not impossible. Most LGV lesions heal spontaneously, and only a rare patient suffers serious sequelae.

Antibiotics. A variety of different antimicrobial agents have been used to treat the acute manifestations of LGV, including tetracyclines, sulfonamides, chloramphenicol, rifampin, and erythromycin. None appears to be singularly effective. In the inguinal syndrome, drug treatment is only marginally better than symptomatic treatment alone. Nevertheless, these drugs limit or prevent secondary bacterial infection of LGV lesions and usually provide some measure of symptomatic improvement. There is, however, debate as to what constitutes adequate dosage and duration of therapy.

Tetracycline hydrochloride, 500 mg 4 times daily by mouth for 2 to 4 weeks, is recommended for treatment of the acute inguinal and anogenitorectal syndromes. Patients unable to tolerate tetracycline may be given erythromycin, 500 mg 4 times daily for 2 to 4 weeks, or co-trimoxazole, 2 tablets containing 80 mg of trimethoprim and 400 mg of sulfamethoxazole given orally twice a day for 14 days. Unruptured fluctuant buboes should be aspirated with a large-bore needle and a syringe, as needed, to prevent sinus tract formation. Open lesions should be covered with a nonadherent dressing soaked in an antiseptic solution to prevent autoinoculation or nosocomial infection.

Surgery. The late complications of LGV such as esthiomene, rectal stricture, and fistulas may require surgery. Because much of the inflammation accompanying late LGV lesions is caused by bacterial superinfection, it should be preceded by a prolonged course of antibiotic treatment. This may cause small fistulas to close spontaneously and limit the extent and complexity of the surgery required to restore normal function.

PREVENTION AND CONTROL. The methods used to prevent and to control LGV are similar to those used in all sexually transmitted diseases. Every effort should be made to identify, locate, and treat concurrently the sexual partners of patients with acute LGV. If this is not possible, sufficient medication should be given to the patient for his or her sexual partner to take to prevent "ping-pong" reinfections.

BIBLIOGRAPHY

Greaves AB, Hilleman MR, Taggart SR, et al: Chemotherapy in bubonic lymphogranuloma venereum. Bull WHO 16:277, 1957.
Klotz SA, Drutz DJ, Tam MR, et al: Hemorrhagic proctitis due to lymphogranuloma venereum serogroup L2. N Engl J Med 308:1563, 1983.

Koteen H: Lymphogranuloma venereum. Medicine 24:1, 1945.

Quinn TC, Goodell SE, Mkrtichian E, et al: *Chlamydia trachomatis* proctitis. N Engl J Med 305:195, 1981.

Schachter J, Osoba AO: Lymphogranuloma venereum. Br Med Bull 39:151, 1983.

30. NONGONOCOCCAL URETHRITIS AND CERVICITIS

Thomas A. Bell and Peter L. Perine

DEFINITION. Nongonococcal urethritis (NGU) is a symptom complex occurring in men who have a nongonococcal urethral discharge with or without dysuria. The equivalents of NGU in women are the acute urethral syndrome and nongonococcal mucopurulent cervicitis. The acute urethral syndrome consists of urinary frequency or urgency and dysuria in the absence of urethral discharge. It differs from acute cystitis and other types of urinary tract infection by affecting principally the urethra, and by the quantity of pus cells and bacteria present in voided urine. Nongonococcal cervicitis is usually asymptomatic or is associated with a mild to moderate vaginal discharge.

ETIOLOGY. The known infectious causes of NGU are listed in Table 30–1. Immunotypes (serovars) band D through K of *Chlamydia trachomatis* are the principal causes of NGU. The role of *Ureaplasma urealyticum* (formerly called T-strain mycoplasma) is controversial because it is often isolated with the same frequency in normal men who are as sexually active as men with NGU. Organisms that do not cause NGU are *Gardnerella (Hemophilus) vaginalis,* commensal bacteria of the urethra and vagina, cell wall–deficient ("L-form") *Neisseria gonorrhoeae, Corynebacterium genitalium,* and *Corynebacterium pseudogenitalium.* Noninfectious causes of NGU have been proposed but never proven.

EPIDEMIOLOGY

Nongonococcal Urethritis. This is a sexually transmitted disease of men. In Europe and North America, it is more common than gonococcal urethritis. The prevalence of NGU in the tropics is largely unknown because the specialized laboratory techniques needed to identify *C. trachomatis* and other causes of NGU are not routinely available in developing countries. The incidence of NGU is much less than that of gonococcal urethritis. The urethral discharge and dysuria of NGU may not be severe enough to cause men to seek treatment. In areas where trachoma is endemic, the incidence of NGU may also be affected by cross-immunity between trachoma and NGU serovars.

TABLE 30–1. Causes of Nongonococcal Urethritis

Organisms	Percentage of Cases
Chlamydia trachomatis	40–50
Ureaplasma urealyticum	20–25
Herpes simplex virus	<5
Trichomonas vaginalis	<5
Candida	<5
Unknown	20–30

Postgonococcal Urethritis. This syndrome consists of dual infection of the urethra by *N. gonorrhoeae* and the agents causing NGU. *C. trachomatis* can be isolated from 20 to 35% of heterosexual men with gonorrhea in North America and in Southeast Asia.

Nongonococcal Cervicitis. The prevalence of nongonococcal cervicitis is probably equal to that of NGU in most parts of the world. *C. trachomatis* has been isolated from 30 to 50% of female sexual partners of men with chlamydia-positive NGU. Infected women are at risk for developing complications such as salpingitis.

CLINICAL MANIFESTATIONS

Urethritis. The urethral discharge of NGU begins after an incubation period of 7 to 21 days. The first symptom is a slight mucoid or mucopurulent discharge with or without dysuria. In contrast to the urethral discharge of gonorrhea (Table 30–2), the discharge of NGU often is not spontaneous and may be detectable only after the urine has been held for several hours or overnight in the bladder. Symptoms are often ignored by the patient and may persist for several weeks before resolving spontaneously. The discharge occasionally increases in volume and consistency to become indistinguishable from that of gonorrhea. Complications are rare.

Testicular Infection. Ascending infection of the urogenital tract can produce prostatitis, epididymitis, and orchitis. Acute epididymitis occurs in about 2% of cases, particularly in NGU caused by *C. trachomatis.* This type of epididymitis is especially common in men under 35 years of age. The onset is usually gradual, with increasing swelling and tenderness of one or both epididymides. Inguinal and testicular pain causes the patient to seek medical care. Untreated, the condition progresses and the testicle becomes inflamed, making differentiation from torsion of the spermatic cord or testicular appendages, hernia, and hydrocele virtually impossible. This induration may take several months to resolve and may leave the patient sterile or with a urethral stricture.

Infection in Other Sites. The chlamydiae of NGU can also cause inclusion conjunctivitis by autoinoculation, and proctocolitis following inoculation of the rectal mucosa during anal intercourse. Proctocolitis is rare in heterosexual men.

DIAGNOSIS. In the early stages of urethritis, infected epithelial cells of the urethra appear in the urine, as do increased numbers of polymorphonuclear leukocytes. The 2-glass urine test, in which 20 to 40 ml of the

TABLE 30–2. Comparison of Nongonococcal and Gonococcal Urethritis

	Nongonococcal	Gonococcal
Incubation (days)	7–21	2–7
Onset	Gradual	Abrupt
Dysuria	Variable; mild or absent	Frequent; moderate to severe
Urethral discharge		
Clear	20%	Rare
Mucopurulent	60%	25%
Purulent	20%	75%
Complications	Rare	Common

first voided urine is collected into 2 cylindrical glass containers, is a useful clinical diagnostic guide. In acute urethritis, small round or comma-shaped "flakes" composed of desquamated epithelial cells and leukocytes are visible in the first urine container when it is viewed through transmitted light. In severe inflammation, chunks of cellular debris may be seen sinking to the bottom of the glass. The presence of small "threads" in the urine indicates inflammation of the seminal vesicles or the prostate; "flakes" or "threads" in both urine containers indicate posterior urethral inflammation, cystitis, or upper urinary tract infection.

The diagnosis of NGU is one of exclusion. A presumptive diagnosis of NGU can be made by microscopic examination of a Gram-stained smear of urethral exudate. There must be at least 5 polymorphonuclear leukocytes in a × 1000 power field and no gram-negative intracellular diplococci. The diagnosis of NGU should be confirmed by a negative culture for *N. gonorrhoeae*. It is not feasible to establish the etiology of NGU unless tests for *C. trachomatis* are available, which is rare in the tropics.

TREATMENT

Acute Infections. The tetracyclines are the drugs of choice for treatment of NGU. Tetracycline hydrochloride in a dose of 500 mg by mouth 4 times daily for 7 days is highly effective and inexpensive. Doxycycline, 100 mg by mouth twice daily for 7 days, is more convenient but is no more effective than generic tetracycline. It is more expensive and has side effects such as vomiting or ataxia, which may cause the patient to discontinue therapy.

Patients allergic to tetracyclines can be treated with erythromycin, 250 to 500 mg 4 times a day for 7 days. The penicillins, spectinomycin, and metronidazole (except for the few patients infected with *T. vaginalis*) are ineffective and should not be prescribed.

Treatment with tetracycline or erythromycin will cure about 80% of patients with NGU. The remainder will have persistent symptoms or will relapse within 6 weeks of treatment.

Persistent or Recurrent Infection. Persistent NGU should alert the physician to the possibility of infection by *T. vaginalis*, yeast, or herpes simplex virus or failure by the patient to take the prescribed drug correctly. Relapse is more likely than reinfection, although the physician should always be alert to the possibility of the latter.

The treatment of persistent or recurrent NGU is controversial. Most experts recommend a 7-day trial of erythromycin if tetracycline was given first, or vice versa. Others recommend a 2- or 3-week course of erythromycin or tetracycline. Doxycycline may be indicated if the patient has prostatitis, because this drug reaches relatively high concentrations in prostatic tissue. A small proportion of patients with NGU will have persistent or intermittent symptoms for several months and deny sexual re-exposure. Such patients should be carefully evaluated for chronic prostatitis, urethral stricture, self-induced penile trauma, or other urologic disease. Many chronic NGU patients have a psychogenic component to their illness that may require psychiatric evaluation.

There is no evidence that moderate alcohol consumption interferes with treatment.

PREVENTION AND CONTROL. Prevention of NGU and the serious complications of chlamydial infection in women and neonates requires identification and treatment of both regular and casual female sexual partners. Ideally, both the patient and his sexual partner(s) should be treated simultaneously and abstain from sexual intercourse until therapy has been completed to prevent reinfection.

BIBLIOGRAPHY

Berger RE, Alexander ER, Monda GD, et al: *Chlamydia trachomatis* as a cause of acute "idiopathic" epididymitis. N Engl J Med 298:301, 1978.

Bowie WR: Etiology and treatment of nongonococcal urethritis. Sex Transm Dis 5:27, 1978.

Brunham RC, Paavonen J, Stevens CE, et al: Mucopurulent cervicitis–the ignored counterpart in women of urethritis in men. N Engl J Med 311:1, 1984.

Forsey T, Darougar S: Chlamydial infections. Baillère's Clin Trop Med Comm Dis 2:59, 1987.

Judson FN: Epidemiology and control of nongonococcal urethritis and genital chlamydial infections: A review. Sex Transm Dis 8:117, 1981.

Stamm WE, Guinan ME, Johnson C, et al: Effect of treatment regimens for *Neisseria gonorrhoeae* on simultaneous infection with *Chlamydia trachomatis*. N Engl J Med 310:545, 1984.

Woodland RM, Darougar S: Non-specific genital infections. Baillère's Clin Trop Med Comm Dis 2:33, 1987.

31. PSITTACOSIS

Fred P. Paleologo

DEFINITION. Psittacosis, also known as ornithosis, is a bird-associated zoonosis caused by *Chlamydia psittaci*. This disease usually manifests acutely with fever, influenza-like symptoms, and a dry cough often indicative of pneumonia. Another rarer but more serious presentation of this infection is endocarditis, possibly with arterial embolization. In addition to causing human disease, this pathogen is also of economic importance to the poultry, sheep, and cattle industries.

HISTORY. The first description of psittacosis was in 1879 by Ritter, a Swiss physician who described an outbreak of what he called "pneumotyphus" in 7 cases, including 3 fatalities. Although he suspected caged pet parrots and finches as the source of infection, transmission by birds was not proved until after the study of several outbreaks in Europe over the next 15 years. The name "psittacosis"—taken from *psittakos*, the Greek word for parrot—was first given to this disease after an outbreak in Paris in 1892. Because it is now known that many nonpsittacine birds can transmit the disease, some recommend using the more general name "ornithosis" (from *ornis*, the Greek word for bird).

From 1929 to 1930, a pandemic of the disease with over 700 cases in 12 different countries was caused by widespread importation of large numbers of infected birds from South America. More recently, recognition of epidemics associated with the turkey-processing industry and human to human transmission (likely due to *C. pneumoniae*) led to increased research interest.

ETIOLOGY. When the etiologic agent of psittacosis was discovered by Bedson in 1930, it was initially thought to be a large virus. Later, it was shown to be an obligate intracellular bacteria with a cell wall and a genome that contains both DNA and RNA. *C. psittaci* can be seen as a 0.3- to 1.0-μm cytoplasmic inclusion in host cells.

The other species of *Chlamydia* pathogenic for humans are *C. trachomatis* and the newly described *C. pneumoniae*.

Distribution and Transmission. Psittacosis is worldwide in distribution. The disease has no seasonal pattern and is usually sporadic; however, epidemics do occur. Outbreaks are most often associated with exposure to caged pet birds (e.g., at pet shops), domestic and wild pigeons, and fowl (i.e., turkeys, chickens, and ducks), especially at commercial processing plants. Many species of birds may be healthy carriers of *C. psittaci* and not excrete the organism under normal conditions. At times of stress and during breeding, their resistance is lowered and they may excrete the organism. When young birds are infected, they may either die or become carriers. In as many as 20% of cases, no exposure to birds can be determined. Here, the disease is probably the result of a brief, unremembered yet infectious contact. Sporadic secondary human to human spread in disease acquired from birds is also possible. In fatal human cases, patients are highly infectious shortly before death.

The infectious agents, called elementary bodies, are found in dried urine and feces and in tissues from infected birds. They are dense, spherical bodies measuring 0.2 to 0.4 μm in diameter. Elementary bodies have a rigid cell wall similar to that of gram-negative bacteria and contain both DNA and RNA, but they have little metabolic activity. These infectious agents are inhaled by the host, whereupon they induce phagocytosis by the host cell. The elementary body cell wall inhibits phagolysosome fusion, and the invaginated host cell membrane containing the elementary body forms the "inclusion body." Later in the course of the infection, the host cell membrane incorporates elementary body antigen into its surface.

Infected cells are carried from the lung to the reticuloendothelial system where they replicate in the liver and spleen. The organism then invades the lung and other organs by hematogenous spread. Another source of infection may be aerosols from infected tissues, such as in poultry-processing plants.

After phagocytosis, the developing inclusion body enlarges over the first 12 postinfection hours to form a "reticulate body" measuring 0.7 to 1.0 μm in diameter. This form is not infectious and is incapable of surviving outside the host cell. It is metabolically active, but is unable to synthesize high-energy compounds such as adenosine triphosphate and guanosine triphosphate. It utilizes nutrients, nucleotide precursors, and energy compounds made by the host cell to replicate itself by binary fission. Because of this, *Chlamydia* are sometimes referred to as "energy parasites." At 20 hours, the host cell nucleus is displaced by the large developing reticu-

late bodies. By 30 hours, cell wall synthesis has led to the formation of progeny elementary bodies. At this stage, the intracytoplasmic inclusion bodies contain both developing reticulate and formed elementary bodies. These are intracellular bacterial microcolonies within the phagosome. After cell lysis, elementary bodies are released into the extracellular environment for subsequent infection of other susceptible cells.

CLINICAL MANIFESTATIONS AND PATHOLOGY

Initial Symptoms. The incubation period for psittacosis ranges from 7 to 15 days (usually 10 days), but may be as long as 21 days. Clinical disease usually has a rapid onset with sudden chills and high fever (up to 40C). Alternatively, it may develop slowly over several days with increasing fever and malaise. As with other intracellular infections (e.g., typhoid fever and brucellosis), there may be a relative bradycardia for the degree of fever. Diffuse headache is a prominent symptom, and myalgias, diaphoresis, arthralgias, weakness, and anorexia are common.

Pneumonia. Pneumonia, with disproportionately few signs of consolidation on examination, is a common finding that may either be noted on presentation or develop later in the course of the disease. The typical dry cough, occasionally with small amounts of mucopurulent or blood-tinged sputum, and fine crepitant rales often underestimate the pulmonary involvement demonstrated on chest x-ray film. There is no characteristic x-ray infiltrate pattern that can be used to make this diagnosis. More than one lobe is involved in approximately 40% of cases, and radiologic resolution of abnormalities is slow. Half will resolve within 4 weeks; however, 30% may still have abnormalities on x-ray film at 12 weeks. Hyperpnea and dyspnea are relative to the amount of pulmonary involvement. Hypoxia is sometimes severe and may lead to cyanosis and decreased mental status. Pleural and pericardial rubs and pleural effusions may be noted. On histologic examination of the lung, mononuclear cells predominate in the thickened alveolar walls, and a gelatinous exudate with few mononuclear cells is found in the alveoli.

Generalized Findings. Hepatomegaly is common, and splenomegaly may be present in up to 70% of cases. On histologic examination, focal areas of necrosis with a predominance of mononuclear cells can be seen in both organs. Hepatitis occurs, occasionally with hepatic granuloma formation; however, marked abnormality of liver function is unusual. Splenomegaly with atypical pneumonia is suggestive of the diagnosis. The white blood cell count is often normal, but may be mildly elevated or decreased.

A Horder's spot rash, described as a reddish-brown, slightly raised, blanching maculopapular rash slightly darker than the "rose spots" of typhoid fever, may be seen. Other cutaneous manifestations such as acrocyanosis, superficial venous thromboses, splinter hemorrhages under the fingernails in the absence of endocarditis, erythema nodosum, and Stevens-Johnson syndrome have also been reported.

Complications. There have been a few case reports of Reiter's syndrome, a triad of asymmetrical polyarthritis, conjunctivitis, and the presence of HLA-B27 antigen, associated with psittacosis. In these cases, the joint involvement is a reactive arthritis, which responds to treatment with corticosteroids. Infectious arthritis in which *C. psittaci* was isolated from synovial fluid has also been reported.

Meningoencephalitis, disseminated intravascular coagulation, Guillain-Barré syndrome, a rheumatic fever–like syndrome, pharyngitis, laryngitis, epistaxis, follicular keratoconjunctivitis, thrombophlebitis, and nonspecific gastrointestinal symptoms (e.g., nausea, vomiting, and diarrhea) have been reported.

Endocarditis, myocarditis, and pericarditis may occur. Onset may be rapid or insidious. Evidence of prior abnormality of the aortic or mitral valves (e.g., bicuspid aortic valve or history of rheumatic fever) is common. Culture-negative endocarditis should cause the physician to suspect the diagnosis. Embolism with arterial occlusion may be a rare presenting sign.

DIAGNOSIS. Difficulty in diagnosing this disease has undoubtedly resulted in underestimates of its incidence. Serology or isolation of the organism are the primary methods of confirming the diagnosis.

Serology. The complement-fixation (CF) test detects a common heat-stable, group-specific cell wall antigen. This test is genus specific and cannot differentiate between antibody to *C. psittaci*, *C. pneumoniae*, and *C. trachomatis*. The microimmunofluorescence (micro-IF) test is both sensitive and specific and can differentiate between species.

Culture. Culture of the organism from sputum, blood, or infected tissue specimens can be done in mice, embryonated eggs, or tissue culture using irradiated McCoy or HeLa cell lines. Tissue culture is more effective than egg yolk sac inoculation in recovering *Chlamydia* from clinical specimens. Cultures are highly infectious and this procedure should be done only at specialized laboratories with adequate safety facilities.

Fluorescent Antibody Stains. Monoclonal antibodies are proving to be increasingly important in the diagnosis of this infection. Immunofluorescent antibody staining of elementary bodies or inclusions can make species-specific diagnosis (Fig. 28–8).

PROGNOSIS AND TREATMENT. Psittacosis is usually a mild to moderately severe illness. The 20 to 40% mortality of the preantibiotic era has declined to less than 1% with current treatment. Patients with mild infections usually recover within a week; however, recovery from more severe infections may require 3 weeks or longer. Elderly persons, especially those with a serious pre-existing illness, may tend to have a more severe clinical course.

Tetracycline (2 to 3 gm/day in divided doses) is effective in treatment of psittacosis infection in non-pregnant adults. Clinical response may take 2 to 3 days or longer. Therapy continuing for 10 to 14 days beyond defervescence will decrease the rate of relapse. Chloramphenicol has been used in the past but is less effective than tetracycline. Similarly, penicillin will inhibit cell wall synthesis in the reticulate body, but it is not a drug of choice. Doxycycline (100 mg/day orally for 10 days) has been reported to be an effective prophylaxis for nonpregnant adults exposed to an infectious contact. Erythromycin is useful when tetracycline is contraindicated (e.g., pregnant women, young children, and those with drug allergy).

In cases of chlamydial endocarditis, replacement of the diseased valve is usually necessary; however, there have been reports of cure with prolonged courses of antibiotic treatment alone using erythromycin and rifampin. These drugs are also useful in patients who are not cured with a course of treatment with tetracycline.

PREVENTION AND CONTROL. Many countries require that cases of psittacosis be reported to local health authorities to facilitate early detection and investigation of epidemics and to enforce quarantine and antibiotic treatment of potentially infected birds. Control programs have not been as successful as desired owing to failure both to adhere to regulations and to ensure that treated birds receive an effective dose of tetracycline. Infected birds should be carefully treated or destroyed because, in avian epizootics, large doses of tetracycline may only suppress the infection. Contaminated areas should be thoroughly cleaned with a phenolic disinfectant compound to destroy infectious agents.

BIBLIOGRAPHY

Anderson DC, Stoesz PA, Kaufman AF: Psittacosis outbreak in employees of a turkey-processing plant. Am J Epidemiol 107:140, 1978.

Bedson SP, Western GT, Simpson SL: Observations on the aetiology of psittacosis. Lancet 1:235, 1930.

Bromage DJ, Jeffries DJ, Philip G: Embolic phenomena in chlamydial infection. J Infect 2:151, 1980.

Darougar S, Forsey T, Brewerton DL, et al: Prevalence of antichlamydial antibody in London blood donors. Br J Vener Dis 56:404, 1980.

Dimmit SB, Pearman JW, Woollard KV: Chlamydial endocarditis. Aust NZ J Med 15:340, 1985.

Jones RB, Priest JB, Kuo CC: Subacute chlamydial endocarditis. JAMA 247:655, 1982.

MacFarlane JT, MacRae AD: Psittacosis. Br Med Bull 39:163, 1983.

MacFarlane JT, Miller AC, Roderick Smith WH, et al: Comparative radiographic features of community acquired Legionnaires' disease, pneumococcal pneumonia, mycoplasma pneumonia, and psittacosis. Thorax 39:28, 1984.

Schachter J: Chlamydial infections. N Engl J Med 298:428, 490, 540, 1978.

Schachter J, Sugg N, Sung M: Psittacosis: The reservoir persists. J Infect Dis 137:44, 1978.

SECTION C

SPIROCHETAL INFECTIONS

GENERAL PRINCIPLES

Thomas Butler

DEFINITION AND ETIOLOGY. The spirochetes are an important group of bacteria that are capable of causing many diverse diseases of humans and animals. The 3 genera of pathogenic spirochetes are *Borrelia*, *Leptospira*, and *Treponema*. Spirochetes are classified as bacteria because they share the typical features of other bacteria. For example, they are single celled and have an outer membrane or cell wall. They are prokaryotes, i.e., the nuclear material is not organized into chromosomes or bounded by a nuclear membrane, and multiplication occurs by binary fission. The spirochetes contain both DNA and RNA and are capable of cellular metabolism and protein synthesis. Furthermore, they are susceptible to the action of antibiotics. On the other hand, they differ from other bacteria by their unique helical structure, spiraling motility, and growth requirements. They range in length from about 5 to 40 μm. Their motility appears to be a rotational corkscrew-like motion but actually consists of complex patterns of contrarotation of opposite ends, helical waves, and flexing motions. The organelles of motility are flagella, which vary in number from 1 to 20 in the pathogenic spirochetes and are unique by their location between the outer membrane and inner cytoplasmic membrane. In general, the spirochetes are fastidious in their growth and require long-chain fatty acids. They will not form colonies on agar medium, but the *Leptospira* and *Borrelia* can be cultivated in media supplemented with bovine serum albumin and rabbit serum. Certain treponemes are even more fastidious because of extreme sensitivity to oxygen (i.e., it is toxic in greater than minute amounts) outside of mammalian tissues and have defied all attempts at in vitro cultivation.

EPIDEMIOLOGY AND DISTRIBUTION. Spirochetes are ubiquitous in nature. In addition to the pathogenic genera, there are free-living spirochetes that inhabit bodies of water, marshes, and sewage. Animals such as the mollusks have their digestive tracts colonized by spirochetes. Spirochetes colonize the oral cavities and intestinal tracts of humans and other animals, in which they constitute part of the normal endogenous bacterial flora. Only rarely are these spirochetes associated with disease, and the pathogenic roles of these endogenous spirochetes in initiating certain diseases are unclear. One such disease is periodontitis, in which the oral treponemes on the subgingival plaque proliferate to much greater than usual numbers when there is inflammation, tissue destruction, and bone loss. Acute necrotizing ulcerative gingivitis, or trench mouth, is another sort of oral inflammation in which oral spirochetes appear to play a pathogenic role. Another ex-

ample of oral inflammation is Vincent's angina, a form of tonsillitis in which *Borrelia vincentii* spirochetes exist in large numbers. In the swine intestine, *Treponema hyodysenteriae* is capable of invading the epithelial cells and producing dysentery.

Some of the human pathogenic spirochetes, particularly the leptospires and the tick-bone *Borrelia*, are adapted to animal hosts in nature. Rodents, as well as dogs and farm animals, are the largest reservoirs for these zoonotic infections, and humans are only accidental hosts. On the other hand, the pathogenic *Treponema* species and the louse-borne *Borrelia* are adapted to humans, the major reservoir for infection.

In the following chapters, several of the important spirochetal diseases will be considered. These are all caused by the introduction of exogenous spirochetes into the body of the infected person. The relapsing fevers and Lyme disease are caused by *Borrelia* species, which circulate in the blood in large numbers (Chapters 34 and 36). Leptospirosis is a common infection of humans caused by *Leptospira interrogans* (Chapter 35). *Treponema pallidum* is the cause of syphilis, a frequently transmitted venereal infection. Important nonvenereal treponemal infections that produce skin diseases are yaws caused by *T.P. pertenue* and pinta caused by *T.p. carateum* (Chapter 32).

BIBLIOGRAPHY

Harwood CS, Canale-Parola E: Ecology of spirochetes. Annu Rev Microbiol 38:161, 1984.
Holt SC: Anatomy and chemistry of spirochetes. Microbiol Rev 42:114, 1978.
Johnson RC: The spirochetes. Annu Rev Microbiol 31:89, 1977.

32. SYPHILIS AND THE ENDEMIC TREPONEMATOSES

Peter L. Perine

DEFINITION. Syphilis and the endemic treponematoses—yaws, endemic syphilis, and pinta—are a group of chronic diseases caused by spirochetes belonging to the genus *Treponema*. The cause of venereal and nonvenereal syphilis is *Treponema pallidum* subsp. *pallidum* and subsp. *endemicum*, respectively; the cause of yaws is *T. pallidum* subsp. *pertenue;* and the cause of pinta is *T. carateum*. These closely related, morphologically identical treponemes cause production of antitreponemal antibodies during infection that cannot be differentiated by conventionally used serologic tests. The only means of distinguishing these organisms is by the pattern of infection they produce in humans and in experimentally infected animals and by certain epidemiologic differences (Table 32–1). The most notable feature of the treponemal diseases, particularly venereal syphilis, is the progression of disease by stages, designated primary, secondary, and tertiary. Each stage is separated by a period of latency and has different manifestations and lesion morphology.

ETIOLOGY. The spirochetes of yaws, pinta, and venereal and nonvenereal syphilis—collectively called the pathogenic treponemes—are thin, corkscrew-shaped organisms measuring 0.3 μm in diameter and 7 to 20 μm in length. They tolerate only minute concentrations of oxygen and are readily killed by exposure to atmospheric oxygen, soaps, detergents, and mild antiseptic solutions. None of the pathogenic treponemes grow in artificial culture. The only means of isolating pathogenic treponemes from infected tissue or growing these organisms for use in diagnostic tests is by animal inoculation. The laboratory animal commonly used is the male rabbit, which, when inoculated intratesticularly with *T. pallidum* subsp. *pallidum* or subsp. *pertenue,* regularly develops an acute orchitis. The only animals susceptible to *T. carateum* infection besides humans are apes.

Because of their susceptibility to drying and oxygen, the pathogenic treponemes have limited survival on exposed body surfaces and in infected secretions. Transmission of infection takes place by close person to person contact, which is almost always sexual in the case of venereal syphilis. Both *T. pallidum* subsp. *pallidum* and subsp. *pertenue* are able to penetrate mucous membranes, but intact skin is a formidable barrier to infection. In yaws and possibly pinta, most infections occur by contamination of small cutaneous lacerations, abrasions, or insect bites with infectious exudate from a person with primary or secondary lesions.

PATHOPHYSIOLOGY. The pathogenic mechanisms in treponemal infections are poorly understood. The treponemes produce no known toxic substances and do not directly cause cell death. Much of the pathology is attributed to the immune response of the host to the treponeme. Because the favorite tissue location of treponemes is in the perivascular lymph spaces, much of the pathology results from obliterative endarteritis and periarteritis initiated by immune lymphocytes. Evidence for immune-mediated pathology is the observation that infection by *T. pallidum* subsp. *pallidum* before the fifth month of gestation, which is the age of fetal immunocompetence, does not produce histopathologic signs of infection.

The extent of immunopathology depends to a large degree on the particular treponeme. *T. pallidum* subsp. *pallidum* can damage any organ or tissue of the host; *T. pallidum* subsp. *pertenue* damages only skin and osseous tissue; and *T. carateum* damages only the superficial layers of the skin. This phenomenon probably represents an inherent property of the individual treponeme, because all are capable of systemic invasion.

32.1. SYPHILIS

EPIDEMIOLOGY. Syphilis *(lues venerea)* first appeared in Europe in the late fifteenth century, shortly after Columbus returned from America. Whether the disease was carried back to Europe by the explorers or arose by mutation of an indigenous European treponeme remains a matter of historical controversy. Nevertheless, syphilis was recognized as a new disease and spread with amazing rapidity as the "great pox."

The early descriptions of syphilis indicate that destructive skin lesions were the predominant manifestations and that death was common in the early stages of infection. Over the next 5 centuries, syphilis evolved to become a less virulent and more chronic infection. Death and disability occurred in the tertiary stage after a quiescent or latent period of several years or decades.

The incidence of syphilis throughout the world has declined steadily since 1860, except for temporary increases during wars. In North America and Europe, the number of reported cases of all types of venereal syphilis has decreased more than 90% since the introduction of penicillin therapy in 1945. However, infectious syphilis is increasing in prevalence in many urban areas of Africa and Asia that were formerly relatively free of syphilis. As with other sexually transmitted diseases, the increase in venereal syphilis is directly related to the increasing urbanization and industrialization of many parts of the tropical world and, possibly, to changes in social mores leading to increased sexual permissiveness and promiscuity.

Most cases of syphilis are contracted during sexual intercourse. Otherwise, intimate contact with infected tissue or contaminated fomites is required. The risk of infection after exposure as revealed by contact tracing is highly variable but averages 12% in the United States.

CLINICAL MANIFESTATIONS
Primary Syphilis. *T. pallidum* subsp. *pallidum* penetrate intact mucous membranes or abraded skin. Systemic invasion occurs almost immediately; spirochetes

TABLE 32–1. Epidemiologic Features of Syphilis and the Endemic Treponematoses

	Venereal Syphilis	Endemic Syphilis	Yaws	Pinta
Geographic area	Urban, worldwide	Rural, arid Africa, Asia	Rural, humid tropics	Rural, semiarid Central and South America
Seasonal variations	None	Increases rainy season	Increases rainy season	?
Peak incidence (age)	20–30	2–10	4–15	18–30
Transmission				
Congenital	Frequent	Rare, if ever	Never	Never
Venereal	Usual	Rare	Never	Never
Direct (skin)	Occasional	Common	Usual	Probable
Fomite (utensils)	Rare	Usual	?	Never

enter the subcutaneous blood vessels and lymphatics at the site of infection and disseminate to most organs and tissues within hours.

The characteristic primary lesion, the *chancre,* develops at the site of infection after an incubation period of 9 to 90 days, with an average of 3 weeks. The chancre first appears as a small papule, which rapidly erodes to form a shallow, painless, punched-out ulcer with indurated margins, measuring up to 3 cm in diameter. It usually is covered by a thin crust, which is easily removed, and the serous exudate from the hard, granular base of the chancre contains many spirochetes. The lymph nodes draining the lesion are often discretely enlarged, firm, and painless. More than 90% of the chancres in heterosexual men are on the prepuce, coronal sulcus, glans, or shaft of the penis. Chancres in women may be seen on the labia or perineum, but most are hidden on the cervix, vaginal wall, or posterior fourchette and are often so inconspicuous that they escape notice. Multiple chancres occur infrequently and are usually situated close together; these represent either multiple sites of infection or autoinoculation.

Extragenital chancres are rare and, in contrast to genital chancres, are usually painful. Occurring anywhere on the body, they are usually seen on the lips, nipples, and oral and rectal mucosa as the result of extragenital sexual behavior. Lymphadenopathy, which usually accompanies extragenital chancres, is a valuable diagnostic finding. Whatever their location, most chancres heal without scar formation in 3 to 6 weeks. After the chancre heals, the patient is immune to reinfection ("chancre immunity").

Secondary Syphilis. The secondary stage of syphilis begins within 3 weeks to 6 months (average, 6 weeks) after the chancre heals. In some cases, the chancre may still be present. The clinical manifestations of secondary syphilis are protean because any organ or tissue may be involved. Most frequent are a variety of rashes that have little in common, except that they are usually painless, nonpruritic, and almost never vesicular or bullous. The rash may be macular, papular, follicular, papulosquamous, or pustular and may involve both the skin and mucous membranes. If generalized, it tends to be a bilateral, symmetrical eruption, more prominent on the face and thorax and often involving the palms and soles.

Certain types of cutaneous lesions have a close association with secondary syphilis. These include *condylomata lata*—broad, moist, grayish-white, exudative lesions that appear in the intertriginous areas of the perineum, scrotum, vulva (Fig. 32–1), and axilla; *mucous patches*—oval, shallow ulcers often covered by a grayish-white membrane that are found in the mouth and on the moist surfaces of the genitalia; *follicular syphilids*—small papular lesions involving hair follicles, which cause temporary, patchy hair loss (alopecia areata) of the eyebrows, beard, and scalp hair; *papulosquamous syphilids*—indurated papules with peripheral scales, usually found on the palms and soles; and *nummular syphilids*—coinlike lesions with sharply defined borders, usually seen on the face or perineum, especially in dark-skinned people (Fig. 32–2).

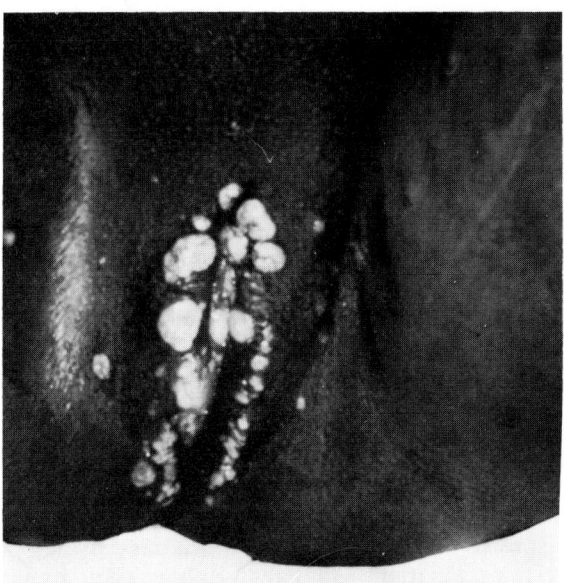

FIGURE 32–1. Venereal syphilis. Raised condylomata lata of secondary syphilis, which are usually found in the warm, moist areas of the body such as the perineum, anal cleft, and axilla.

Although most of the rashes of secondary syphilis heal within a few weeks without scar formation, some may persist for several months. Moreover, as many as 25% of untreated patients will experience one or more mucocutaneous relapses within 2 years of infection. Relapse lesions tend to be asymmetrically distributed and of a more exudative nature, such as condyloma latum or mucous patches.

Constitutional symptoms, including mild fever, malaise, headache, and anorexia, may accompany secondary syphilis, with or without cutaneous lesions. Generalized, discrete, nontender lymphadenopathy is common, and occasionally the spleen is palpable. Acute meningitis, hepatitis, nephrosis, arthritis, periostitis, ir-

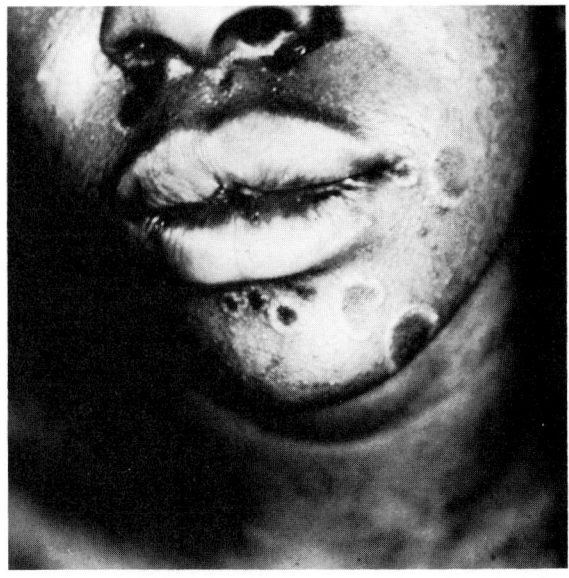

FIGURE 32–2. Coinlike, or nummular, secondary syphilis lesions on the face. These lesions characteristically occur in dark-skinned people.

idocyclitis, and anterior uveitis are uncommon but well-documented manifestations of secondary syphilis.

Latent Syphilis. The disappearance of the lesions of secondary syphilis is followed by another period of quiescence or *latency,* which may last for 20 years or longer. The latent period is arbitrarily divided into early and late latent syphilis, the early latent period being the first 2 years during which secondary lesions may recur. The only evidence of infection in latent syphilis is a reactive serologic test for syphilis. In the preantibiotic era, only one third of patients with latent syphilis progressed to develop lesions of tertiary syphilis.

Tertiary Syphilis. The three types of tertiary syphilis in decreasing order of frequency are cardiovascular syphilis (80%), gummatous syphilis (10%), and meningovascular or parenchymatous neurosyphilis (10%). All forms of tertiary syphilis are rarely diagnosed anywhere in the world today. This is often attributed to the widespread use of antibiotics, which may by happenstance cure a patient with latent syphilis when given for other reasons (e.g., respiratory tract infections, other venereal diseases).

Cardiovascular Syphilis. The cardiovascular lesions are caused by destruction of the wall of the thoracic aorta by immune-mediated thrombosis (obliteration) of the vasa vasorum, which supplies blood to this structure. The elastic fibers are weakened, and the aorta dilates, forming an *aneurysm.* If the dilatation occurs near the aortic valve, the valve cusps are separated and *aortic insufficiency* results. This leads to left ventricular enlargement and may terminate in a refractory type of congestive heart failure. Frequently, the changes in the aortic wall cause narrowing of the coronary ostia, impairing coronary flow, as manifested by angina pectoris.

Gummatous Syphilis. Gummatous syphilitic lesions histologically resemble tuberculomas, an area of coagulation necrosis surrounded by epithelioid cells and fibrous tissue. Varying greatly in size, gummas may be found in any tissue of the body. Although they may impair normal function as a result of the fibrous tissue reaction, they are usually "benign" because they seldom cause physical incapacity or death. Gummas are most frequently found in the liver, where they form irregular lobules separated by fibrous bands. On the skin, they form round ulcerative lesions that resemble the lesions of yaws. Gummas of bone and cartilage are destructive and may perforate the hard palate and nasal septum. In the heart, they may interrupt the conduction system and cause a variety of cardiac arrhythmias. Gummas have become rare since the advent of penicillin, probably because they are cured by low doses of penicillin and other antibiotics.

Meningovascular Neurosyphilis. This is caused by an obliterative endarteritis in the central nervous system. Symptoms are extremely varied because lesions may involve any part of the nervous system and may be sharply focal or diffuse. Focal cerebral lesions commonly produce hemiplegia or a selective neuropathy, especially of the third cranial nerve. Diffuse cerebral lesions cause severe headache, mental changes, and convulsions.

Parenchymatous Neurosyphilis. This includes the tabetic and paretic forms and differs from meningovascular neurosyphilis in that there is a comparative absence of vascular lesions and a tendency for the lesions to be selective in their distribution. Involvement of the spinal cord is common and usually affects the dorsal roots, causing pain, weakness of the lower limbs, flaccid paraplegia, and loss of sensation below the level of the lesion. *Tabes dorsalis* is characterized by attacks of "lightning" pains, paresthesias of the lower extremities, and ataxia. Appreciation of painful stimuli is lost, and painless arthropathies, i.e., Charcot's joints, result from unrecognized hyperextension and trauma to the joint. More common are painless, trophic ulcers of the feet that resemble those of diabetes mellitus. *Tabetic crises* are rare, paroxysmal, painful disorders of function of abdominal viscera that may simulate an acute surgical emergency. The symptoms of *general paresis* are those of a progressive dementia accompanied by generalized or focal seizures with or without manifestations of tabes dorsalis.

The *Argyll Robertson* pupil, one of the most common abnormalities seen in neurosyphilis today, consists of small, irregular, fixed pupils, with synechiae at the inner edge of the irides, which accommodate but do not react to light. A fulminating arachnoiditis-producing degeneration of the optic nerve and blindness (primary optic atrophy) occurs in both meningovascular and parenchymatous neurosyphilis but are associated more often with tabes dorsalis.

Congenital Syphilis. Transplacental passage of *T. pallidum* subsp. *pallidum* to the fetus may occur at any time during gestation, but the probability of congenital infection decreases with the duration of untreated infection in the mother. The infant may be stillborn but more often is born alive without any of the signs of congenital syphilis. These include a mucopurulent nasal discharge ("snuffles"), any of the skin rashes of secondary syphilis, including bullous lesions, generalized desquamation of the skin, hepatosplenomegaly, ascites, pneumonia, osteoperiostitis of the long bones, and failure to thrive. Most infants who develop early congenital syphilis do so between 3 weeks and 6 months of age. Late congenital syphilis is defined as congenital syphilis that has persisted beyond 2 years of age. In two thirds of patients with latent congenital syphilis, the only evidence of infection is a reactive serologic test for syphilis. The signs and symptoms of this stage may represent previous damage in utero or in early life or may result from continued disease activity. The stigmata of late congenital syphilis include interstitial keratitis, dental abnormalities of permanent teeth, and eighth nerve deafness (Hutchinson's triad), and any of the lesions of tertiary syphilis.

DIAGNOSIS. Syphilis is known as the "great imitator" because it may mimic any disease manifesting local or generalized symptoms and lesions. Syphilis frequently accompanies other venereal infections, which should be excluded by clinical and laboratory examination.

Darkfield Microscopy. The most specific diagnostic test for infectious syphilis (primary, secondary, and early congenital) is a darkfield microscopic examination of exudate obtained from a suspicious lesion. *T. pallidum* spirochetes are between 1 and 3 red blood cell diameters in length and appear as thin, coiled silver threads on a dark background. They have a rapid spinning movement along their longitudinal axis. They often flex in the middle, or "whiplash," while keeping their corkscrew appearance. Darkfield examination of lesions in the oropharynx, rectum, cervix, and vagina should be interpreted with caution because the specimen may contain saprophytic *Borrelia* or nonpathogenic treponemes, which are difficult to distinguish morphologically from *T. pallidum.*

Serologic Tests. In all stages of acquired and congenital syphilis, the diagnosis is supported but not established by a reactive serologic test for syphilis. These tests are of 2 general types. The first and oldest are the *nontreponemal antigen tests* which use cardiolipin, an alcoholic extract of beef heart and a normal constituent of mammalian cells, as antigen. The second type of serologic test uses *T. pallidum* or closely related treponemal antigens. Examples of the nontreponemal antigen tests are the Venereal Disease Research Laboratory (VDRL), Kolmer, and rapid plasma reagin (RPR) tests, which detect antibodies by flocculation, complement fixation, and agglutination, respectively. The nontreponemal antigen tests do not vary significantly in their sensitivity or specificity for syphilis. They are excellent screening tests for most stages of syphilis, and their titer is a good measure of disease activity. Many diseases induce antibodies to cardiolipin and cause a biologic false-positive (BFP) reaction. A BFP reaction is most frequently encountered in autoimmune diseases and viral, chronic bacterial, and parasitic infections. A positive nontreponemal antigen test result should always be confirmed by a more specific treponemal antigen test in the absence of a darkfield-positive lesion.

The treponemal antigen tests include the *Treponema pallidum* immobilization (TPI) test, in which motile *T. pallidum* are immobilized in vitro by antibody; the *T. pallidum* hemagglutination assay (TPHA) test that uses as antigen *T. pallidum* adsorbed to erythrocytes; and the fluorescent treponemal antibody (FTA) test, which uses lyophilized *T. pallidum* as antigen in an indirect fluorescent antibody technique. To increase FTA specificity, the test serum may be diluted in a "sorbent" prepared from the nonpathogenic treponemes. This procedure removes antibodies produced in response to the presence of nonpathogenic treponemes in the gastrointestinal flora and is known as the FTA-ABS test. Although these tests vary in their sensitivity, BFP reactions are rarely seen in the FTA and TPHA tests. Because of its complexity, the TPI test is rarely performed today.

Laboratory Abnormalities. A mild polymorphonuclear leukocytosis, elevated sedimentation rate, hypergammaglobulinemia, rheumatoid factor activity, and cryoglobulinemia may occur in late primary, secondary, congenital, and tertiary syphilis. Liver enzymes are elevated in syphilitic hepatitis. Anemia is common in early congenital syphilis.

Cerebrospinal fluid abnormalities may occur during any stage of syphilis, particularly in patients with meningovascular or parenchymatous neurosyphilis. These abnormalities include a mild mononuclear cell pleocytosis (to 100 cells/mm^3), a reactive serologic test for syphilis, and increased protein.

Histopathology. The histopathology of syphilitic lesions may show pathognomonic changes supporting the diagnosis, particularly if spirochetes can be demonstrated by special stains.

TREATMENT. The recommended treatment for syphilis is outlined in Table 32–2. Antibiotic treatment of syphilis should include pretreatment and post-treatment quantitative VDRL tests, which are the only means of detecting persisting infection or reinfection after cutaneous syphilitic lesions have healed. Antibiotics other than penicillin should not be used unless penicillin allergy is well documented by history or by skin testing (Table 32–3). Because it is necessary to maintain a treponemicidal blood level for 7 to 10 days to be certain of a cure, the longer-acting penicillin preparations are recommended.

Post-treatment Observations. The initial dose of any treponemicidal medication may provoke a *Jarisch-Herxheimer reaction,* and the patient should be told to anticipate this possibility. Beginning 6 to 12 hours after penicillin injection, the reaction consists of chills, fever, and headache accompanied by a leukocytosis and aggravation of local syphilitic lesions. The reaction is attributed to the release of endotoxin-like substances from treponemes. It is not a drug allergy and requires no specific treatment.

TABLE 32–2. Treatment of Venereal Syphilis with Penicillin*

	Benzathine Penicillin G		Aqueous Procaine Penicillin G		
	Dose (million units)	*Number of Injections (one a week)*	*Dose (million units)*	*Number of Injections (one a day)*	**Post-treatment Serology**
Early syphilis (primary, secondary, early latent)	2.4	1	6.0	10	Third, sixth, and twelfth months
Late latent syphilis and late benign syphilis	7.2	3	9.0	15	Every 3 months for first year, and every 6 months for second year
Cardiovascular syphilis and neurosyphilis	—	—	12.0	20	As above
Early syphilis in pregnancy	2.4	1	6.0	10	Monthly during pregnancy, then as above, depending on stage
Congenital syphilis†	50,000 units/kg	1	50,000 units/kg	10	Same as for primary syphilis

*Adapted from Treponemal Infections. WHO Technical Report Series 674, 1982.

†In late congenital syphilis, the total dose of penicillin, erythromycin, or tetracycline should not exceed dosage used for comparable stage of acquired syphilis.

TABLE 32–3. Treatment of Venereal Syphilis in Penicillin-Allergic* Patients

	Tetracycline Hydrochloride† (500 mg by mouth 4 times daily)		Erythromycin‡ (500 mg by mouth 4 times daily)	
	Total Dose	*Days*	*Total Dose*	*Days*
Syphilis of not more than 2 years' duration	30 gm	15	30 gm	15
Syphilis of more than 2 years' duration	60 gm	30	60 gm	30

*Not indicated unless penicillin allergy is carefully documented.
†*Not* in pregnancy or in children under 8 years of age.
‡*Not* the estolate.

Spirochetes disappear from cutaneous syphilitic lesions within 48 hours after penicillin treatment, and the lesions heal rapidly. In rare cases of neurovascular and congenital syphilis, and more commonly in HIV-infected persons, viable treponemes have persisted in the central nervous system (CNS) despite recommended doses of parenteral penicillin. In these patients, prolonged or repeated courses of aqueous procaine penicillin may be indicated.

Most patients with seropositive primary and secondary syphilis become seronegative 6 to 12 months after treatment. Those who continue to be seropositive 18 to 24 months after treatment should undergo spinal fluid examination to rule out CNS involvement. Retreatment should be given if clinical signs or symptoms of syphilis persist or recur, if an initial high-titer nontreponemal antigen test fails to decrease fourfold within a year, or if the titer increases fourfold. A titer increase usually indicates reinfection rather than treatment failure. For patients with primary and secondary syphilis, the failure rates for penicillin treatment range from 0 to 4% after 1 year of observation to as high as 11% after 2 years of observation. Failure rates are higher in HIV-infected patients.

Patients with latent and tertiary syphilis may continue to be seropositive ("serofast") with stable, low VDRL titers after 2 years of observation. This persistent seropositivity does not indicate treatment failure or reinfection, and these patients are likely to remain seropositive for their lifetimes even if retreated. Unfortunately, much of the tissue damage in late congenital, neurovascular, and cardiovascular syphilis is irreversible; treatment is given in hope of preventing further damage and deterioration of function.

Concomitant Gonorrhea. Dual infections of early syphilis and gonorrhea should be treated as if each disease were a separate entity, because the penicillin schedules recommended for the treatment of syphilis do not produce high enough blood levels to cure gonorrhea. However, incubating syphilis is cured by the recommended dosages of aqueous procaine penicillin G given for treatment of uncomplicated gonorrhea.

PREVENTION AND CONTROL. Every case of infectious syphilis should be regarded as a potential source of an epidemic. Every effort should be made to find recent sexual contacts of patients with infectious syphilis. These contacts should be treated with penicillin even if they are asymptomatic and seronegative to prevent both the spread of infection and reinfection of the treated partner. This is often referred to as "epidemiologic" treatment.

BIBLIOGRAPHY

Clark EG, Danbolt NN: The Oslo study of the natural course of untreated syphilis. Med Clin North Am 58:613, 1964.
Hart G: Syphilis tests in diagnostic and therapeutic decision making. Ann Intern Med 104:368, 1986.
Jaffee HW: The laboratory diagnosis of syphilis: New concepts. Ann Intern Med 83:846, 1976.
Sparling PF: Diagnosis and treatment of syphilis. N Engl J Med 284:642, 1971.

32.2. YAWS

EPIDEMIOLOGY. Yaws (*framboesia tropica, pian*) occurs in warm, humid tropical regions of Africa, Asia, South America, and Oceania where little clothing is worn and hygiene is poor. It is spread by direct contact with skin lesions or contaminated fingers and fomites. More than 90% of cases begin before the age of 15 years, and a high percentage of the population is infected in endemic areas. Yaws was one of the world's most prevalent diseases before the initiation of mass treatment campaigns with penicillin by the WHO in 1949.

Yaws differs from pinta in being more contagious and invasive, involving the osseous system as well as the skin. Unlike the case with venereal syphilis, congenital transmission does not occur.

CLINICAL MANIFESTATIONS. *Treponema pallidum* subspecies *pertenue* cannot penetrate unbroken skin, and the initial lesion, the "mother yaw," appears after 2 to 8 weeks' incubation as a papule at the site of a recent skin abrasion or laceration, usually on the legs or buttocks. The papule increases in diameter (3 to 5 cm) to become a raised, raspberry-like lesion known as a papilloma. The papilloma persists for 1 to 3 months and is often accompanied by regional lymphadenopathy (Fig. 32–3). Secondary papillomas erupt locally or elsewhere on the body before or several weeks after the mother yaw heals (Fig. 32–4). These lesions usually occur in crops, have a moist appearance around the nose and mouth (Fig. 32–5), and are hard, fissured, and painful on the palms and soles. Palmar and plantar yaws prevent normal gait and use of the hands; the patient may be able to walk only by placing his or her weight on the sides of the feet, so that the gait resembles that of a crab ("crab" yaws) (Fig. 32–6). Bone involvement produces painful swelling of the fingers (dactylitis), nose, and tibia (osteoperiostitis). Secondary lesions may relapse repeatedly over a period of 5 years. They may leave "tissue paper" scars, especially if they are secondarily infected by other types of bacteria.

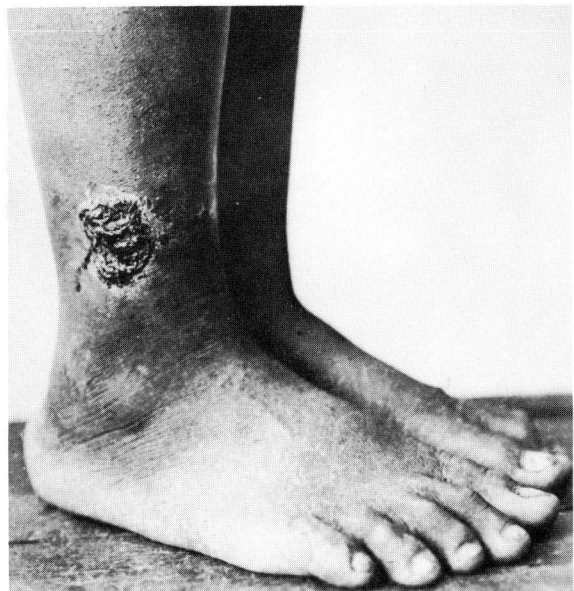

FIGURE 32–3. Yaws. The mother yaw, most frequent on the extremities, begins as a hyperkeratotic papilloma that later undergoes shallow ulceration. (Courtesy of the Armed Forces Institute of Pathology. Photograph Neg. No. 39207.)

Tertiary lesions develop 5 to 10 years after infection in about 10% of patients, with or without an intervening latent period. The most common lesions are chronic ulcerations of the extremities (Fig. 32–7) and face (Fig. 32–8), which mutilate and disfigure. Another late lesion is hyperkeratosis with fissuring of the soles, known as

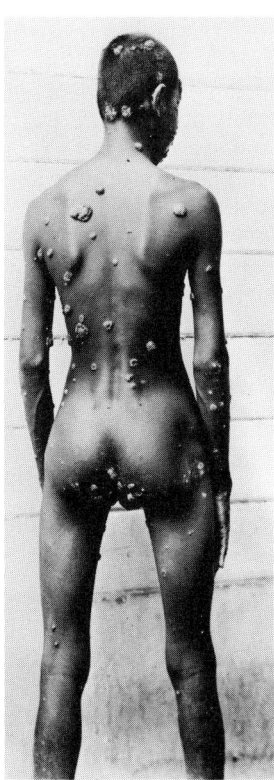

FIGURE 32–4. The elevated papillomatous nodules characteristic of early yaws are widely distributed and painless. (Courtesy of the Armed Forces Institute of Pathology. Photograph Neg. No. 39205.)

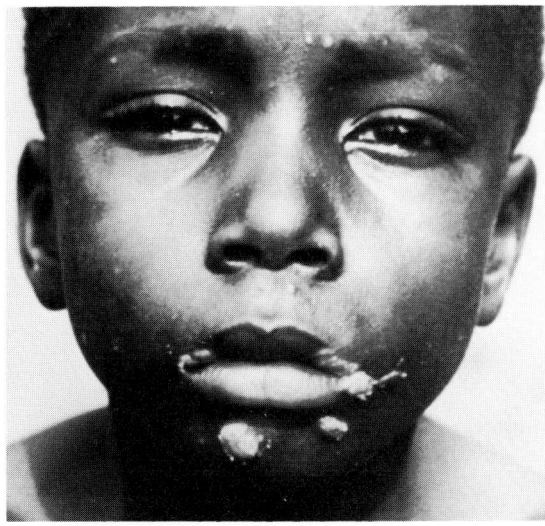

FIGURE 32–5. Early mucocutaneous yaws with papillomas on the chin and scattered papules elsewhere on the face. Identical mucocutaneous lesions are found in endemic syphilis. These lesions are highly infectious.

"dry crab yaws." There are no visceral, cardiac, or nervous system lesions.

DIAGNOSIS. Demonstration of *T. pertenue* by darkfield microscopic examination of exudate from a suspected lesion and seroreactivity in both nontreponemal and treponemal antigen tests serve to distinguish yaws

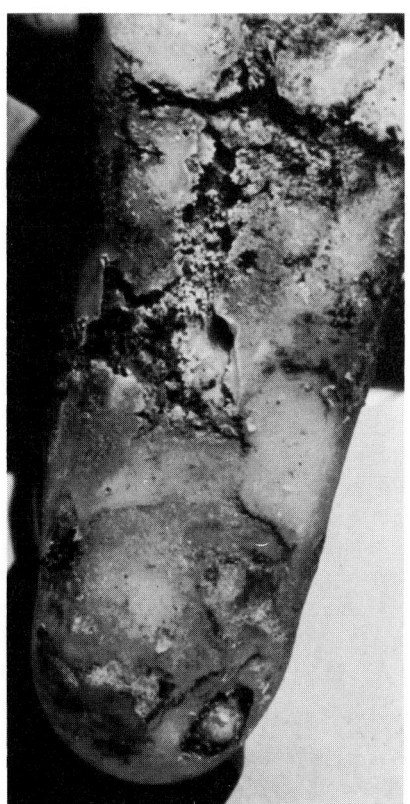

FIGURE 32–6. Early plantar or "crab" yaws. Yaws papillomas and hyperkeratoses are exquisitely painful and cause the patient to walk on the sides of the feet, which produces a gait resembling that of a crab.

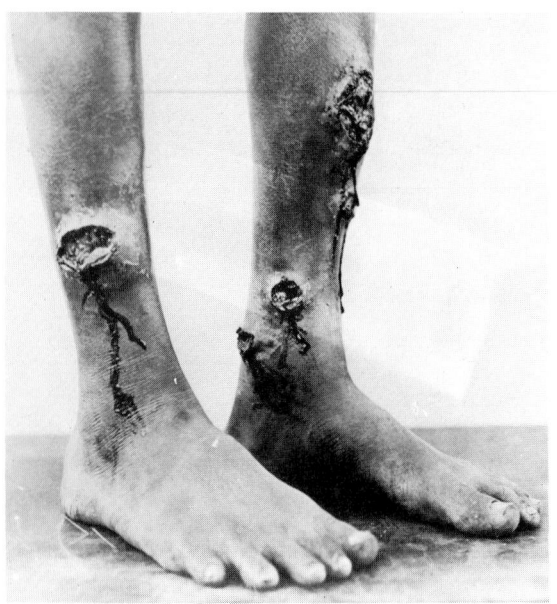

FIGURE 32–7. Two of the late complications of both yaws and nonvenereal syphilis are illustrated. The bowing deformity of the left leg is probably caused by hypertrophic periostitis. The deeply ulcerated draining lesions are gummas. (Courtesy of the Armed Forces Institute of Pathology. Photograph Neg. No. 40815.)

from other conditions, except venereal and endemic syphilis.

TREATMENT AND CONTROL. Benzathine penicillin G, 2.4 million units intramuscularly in adults and half doses in children under 10 years old, rapidly cures early lesions and prevents relapses. When the prevalence

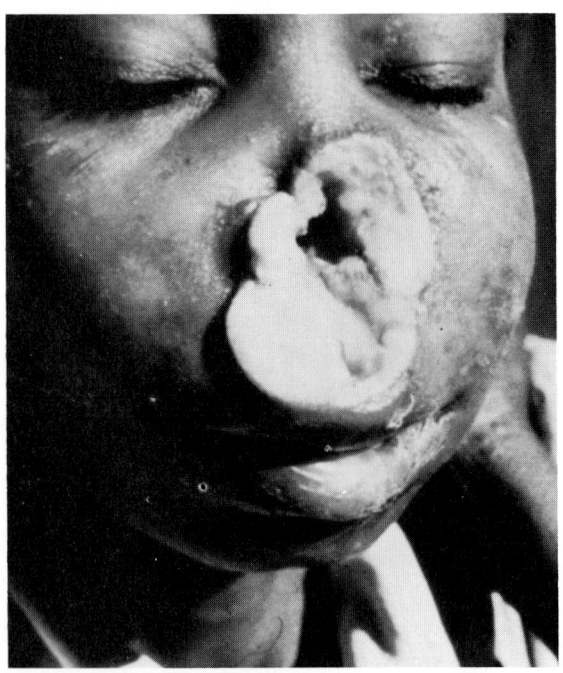

FIGURE 32–8. Gangosa of yaws and endemic syphilis. This begins as mucocutaneous lesions of the nares during the early stages of infection. Although a characteristic lesion of late yaws and endemic syphilis, it may also occur in children who are infected for relatively short periods of time.

of active clinical yaws is 10% or higher, all members of the community should be treated; with less than 5% prevalence, only afflicted individuals and close contacts are treated. Patients allergic to penicillin are given tetracycline (erythromycin if less than 8 years old) in a dose similar to that used for venereal syphilis.

Control of yaws by conducting a mass penicillin treatment campaign requires careful coordination and planning; the aim is to create an ever-enlarging yaws-free area. Ongoing surveillance to detect new or relapsed cases in treated populations is critical to prevent recrudescence of the disease. Failure to maintain active surveillance for yaws is one of the reasons why the disease dramatically increased in prevalence in parts of West Africa in the 1970s.

BIBLIOGRAPHY

Burke JP, Hopkins DR, Hume JC, et al: International symposium on yaws and other endemic treponematoses, Washington, D.C., 1984. Rev Infect Dis 7(Suppl 2):S217, 1985.
Hackett CJ, Guthe T: Some important aspects of yaws eradication. Bull WHO 15:869, 1956.

32.3. ENDEMIC SYPHILIS

Endemic, nonvenereal syphilis *(bejel, njovera)* occurs in arid, dry regions among the nomadic and seminomadic people of the Middle East, North Africa, and the Eastern Mediterranean. Unlike yaws, the initial lesions are "mucous patches" of the secondary type localized to the oral mucosa. These are soon followed by the appearance of moist papules in the axilla and skin folds. Other early lesions are macular or resemble those of secondary venereal syphilis. Palmar and plantar hyperkeratoses occur frequently and are indistinguishable from yaws (Fig. 32–6). Late destructive lesions of the nasopharynx ("gangosa") (Fig. 32–8) and long bones (Fig. 32–7) occur more frequently than in yaws. Isolated cases of cardiovascular syphilis and neurosyphilis have been reported. The diagnosis, treatment, and control of endemic syphilis are similar in all respects to those of yaws.

BIBLIOGRAPHY

Csonka G, Pace J: Endemic nonvenereal treponematoses (Bejel) in Saudia Arabia. Br J Vener Dis 60:293, 1984.
Guthe T, Luger A: The control of endemic syphilis of childhood. Dermatol Internationalis 5:179, 1966.
Perine PL, Hopkins DR, Niemal PLA, et al: Handbook of Endemic Treponematoses. Geneva, World Health Organization, 1984, 59 pp.
Proceedings of the intra-regional meeting on yaws and other endemic treponematoses, Cipanas, Indonesia. Southeast Asian J Trop Med Public Health 17(Suppl):1, 1986.

32.4. PINTA

EPIDEMIOLOGY. Pinta *(mal del pinto)*, a nonvenereal skin infection caused by *Treponema carateum,* is found today only among isolated, rural populations of

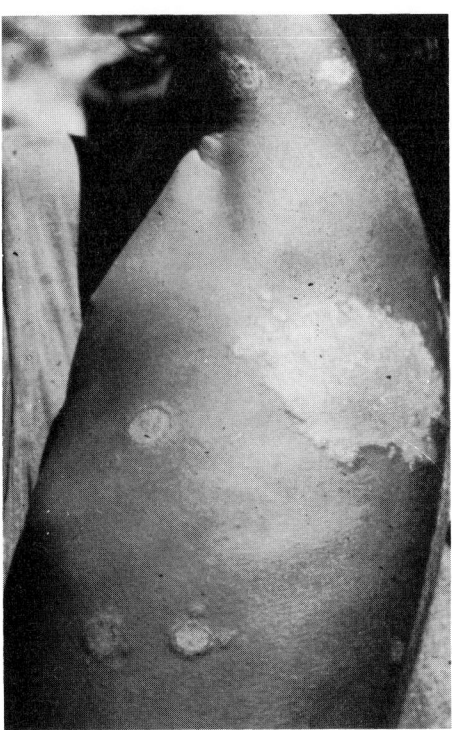

FIGURE 32–9. Pinta. Large primary and secondary lesions in a young child from Venezuela. (Courtesy of the Armed Forces Institute of Pathology. Photograph Neg. No. 75–5536–2.)

South and Central America and Mexico. The exact mode of transmission is unknown, but prolonged close personal contact is required. Because of its infrequent transmission and the improving standards of living and medical care in areas where pinta is endemic, the disease is rare today.

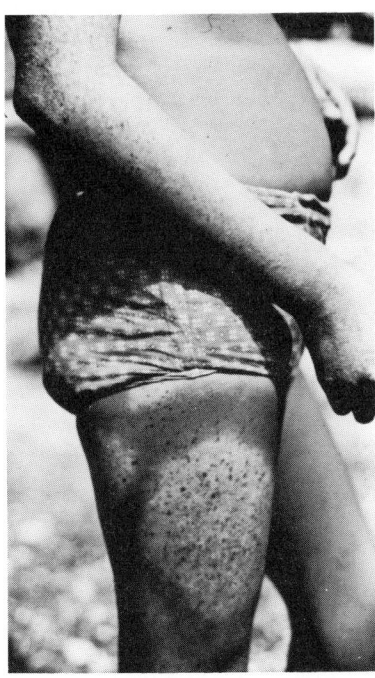

FIGURE 32–10. Late pinta. Hypopigmentation and hyperpigmentation of the right arm, forearm, and thigh. (Courtesy of the Armed Forces Institute of Pathology. Photograph Neg. No. 75–5536–3.)

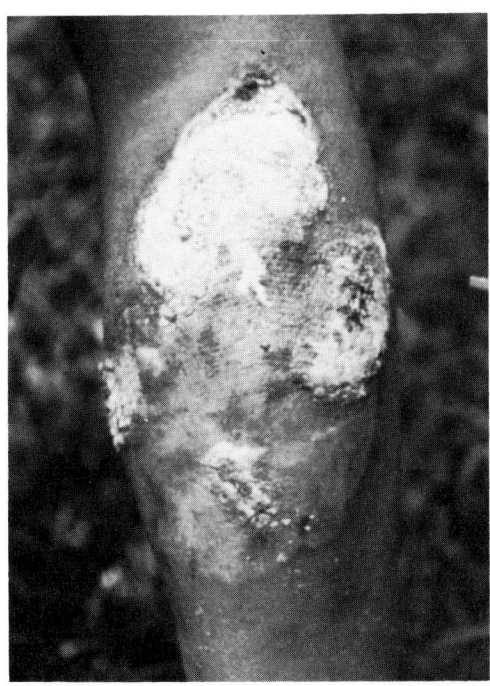

FIGURE 32–11. Pinta. Dyschromic lesion on the calf in various stages of healing. Only the dermis is involved, and the complications of pinta are cosmetic.

CLINICAL MANIFESTATIONS. The initial (primary) lesion is a small, erythematous papule at the site of infection; it appears within 10 days after inoculation, usually on the legs or face. The papule grows over the next 2 to 3 months to become a flattened, scaly plaque up to 10 cm in diameter with irregular margins. This is followed, in 5 to 18 months, by secondary lesions called *pintids,* which are flat, bluish-brown, hyperpigmented macules on the exposed surfaces, including the face (Fig. 32–9). The primary lesion merges with adjacent secondary pintids, and as the lesions progress toward the tertiary stage, they become hyperkeratotic and achromic. The epidermis is atrophic, and permanent cosmetic disfigurement results (Fig. 32–10). The disease is limited to the skin (Fig. 32–11). General clinical symptoms and signs, except for occasional enlargement of regional lymph nodes, are absent during all stages of infection.

DIAGNOSIS. Pintids may resemble psoriasis, lichen planus, leprosy, and other skin diseases. In pinta, treponemes are easily demonstrated by darkfield examination of scrapings taken from the periphery of primary and early secondary lesions. The VDRL serologic test is positive in approximately 60 to 75% of cases during the secondary stage and in most cases of tertiary pinta.

TREATMENT AND CONTROL. Benzathine penicillin G, 2.4 million units intramuscularly at 1 treatment session, is recommended. Children less than 10 years of age are given half doses. Only family contacts require prophylactic penicillin treatment.

BIBLIOGRAPHY

Fohn MJ, Wignall FS, Baker-Zandor SA, et al: Specificity of antibodies from patients with pinta for antigens of *Treponema pallidum* ssp. *pallidum.* J Infect Dis 157:32, 1988.

Sosa-Martinéz J, Peralta S: An epidemiologic study of pinta in Mexico. Am J Trop Med Hyg 10:556, 1961.

33. TROPICAL PHAGEDENIC ULCER

Wayne M. Meyers and Ronald C. Neafie

DEFINITION. Tropical phagedenic ulcer (TPU) is a painful, foul-smelling, necrotizing ulcer of the skin and subcutaneous tissue. Most ulcers are on the foot or leg.

ETIOLOGY AND HISTORY. Le Dante may have been the first to comment on the bacterial flora of lesions that were probably TPU. In 1884 he reported fusiform bacilli in ulcers in patients in Guiana but credited other observers with earlier clinical descriptions. The fusospirochetal etiology of TPU has long been suspected, and recent detailed microbiologic studies support this concept. There is, however, growing evidence that TPU is not caused by one or even two species of organisms but may be a remarkable example of the interaction of a variety of microbes: fusobacteria (? *Fusobacterium nucleatum*), a spirochete (? *Treponema vincenti*), and other unidentified aerobic and anaerobic organisms.

EPIDEMIOLOGY AND DISTRIBUTION. TPU is virtually limited to the tropics and subtropics. The disease is more common in males, in rural environments, and in the rainy season. The major endemic areas are the tropical countries of Africa, Asia, and South America as well as New Guinea, the Pacific Islands, Central America, and the West Indies. Thus, most endemic areas are between 35° North and 10° South latitudes. Malnutrition and poor hygienic conditions are common in the endemic areas and may play a role in transmission and susceptibility; however, otherwise healthy individuals are often afflicted. The source of the infectious agent is unknown, but the fusospirochetal organisms found in the ulcers are similar to organisms that commonly inhabit the oral cavities of humans and some domesticated animals. Some authorities have speculated that there is a relationship between poor oral hygiene and TPU. Other investigators believe that the infectious agents are saprophytes in soil and mud. Patient-to-patient transmission is uncommon, but experimental inoculation of exudates from lesions of patients to healthy volunteers produces typical TPU.

PATHOGENESIS AND PATHOLOGY. A history of trauma or insect bite at the ulcer site can often be elicited. Perhaps contamination of this site by saliva or other materials introduces the infectious microorganism(s). The predominant, even nearly exclusive, location of advanced ulcers on the lower leg and foot may be related to exposure to contamination, dependency of the lower limb, and poor blood supply to the lower leg. Neglect of early lesions contributes to advanced ulceration and scarring. Once the microorganisms are sufficiently established in lesions, they may produce toxins that cause the typical excruciating pain and tissue necrosis of TPU. Butyrates elaborated by fusiform bacilli have been suggested as candidate toxins.

The histopathologic changes in early preulcerated lesions have not been reported, but sections through the margin and crater of the ulcerated area of a TPU reveal a necrotic coagulum of cellular debris and fibrin on the surface. This coagulum contains numerous fusiform and spirochetal organisms. Below this coagulum there is granulation tissue infiltrated by acute and chronic inflammatory cells. Many small blood vessels in the base of the ulcer are thrombosed, and others are narrowed by proliferating endothelial cells; however, the vasculitis does not appear to be primary. The margin of the ulcer is acanthotic or pseudoepitheliomatous, and dense fibrosis surrounds the lesion.

CLINICAL MANIFESTATIONS. Lesions are nearly always single and begin as a small, painful, tender, erythematous, edematous area, which over 3 to 7 days becomes a pustule 1 or 2 cm in diameter that ulcerates and discharges sanguineous pus. The lesion is malodorous, and the base is covered by a necrotic slough. If untreated, tissue necrosis advances, forming an enlarging rounded ulcer, and may penetrate to underlying structures including fascia, muscle, tendons, and ultimately bone (Fig. 33–1). Regional lymphadenopathy and mild to moderate systemic symptoms may be present in the early stages. As the ulcer enters the chronic phase the epithelium piles up at the margin and the base of the ulcer and surrounding tissues are scarred, frequently breaking down and becoming secondarily infected (Fig. 33–2). Without treatment the average duration is several months, but ulcers may persist for up to several decades.

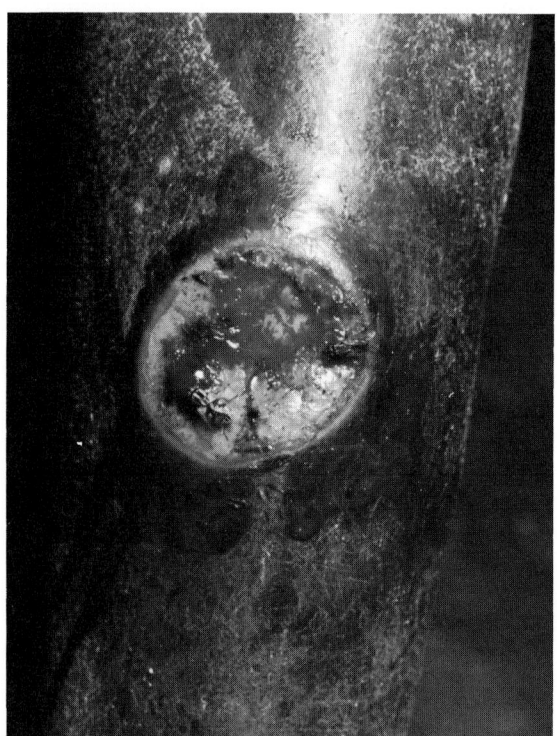

FIGURE 33–1. Typical early active tropical phagedenic ulcer over the lower one third of the pretibial area of an African patient. Note that the malodorous necrotic ulcer crater and the draining serous fluid have attracted flies. The ulcer margin is elevated by a hypertrophic epidermis. (Photograph by Dr. D.H. Connor. Courtesy of the Armed Forces Institute of Pathology. Photograph Neg. No. 68-658.)

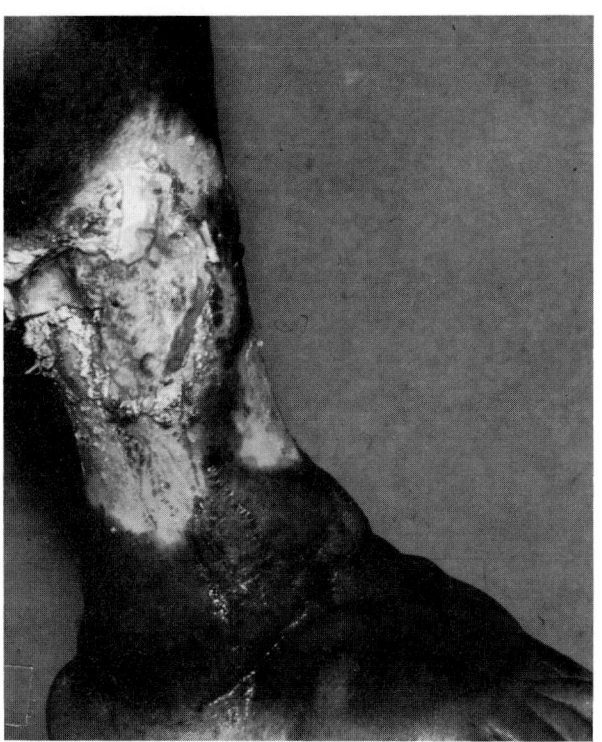

FIGURE 33–2. Old tropical phagedenic ulcer showing frayed scarring. The circumferential scar has caused lymphedema of the foot. (Photograph by Dr. D.H. Connor. Courtesy of the Armed Forces Institute of Pathology. Photograph Neg. No. 74-5309.)

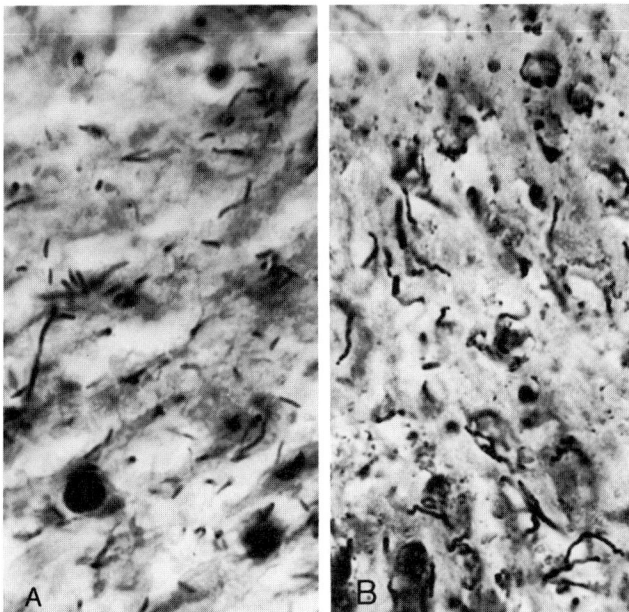

FIGURE 33–3. Exudates from the ulcer crater of active tropical phagedenic ulcers contain fusiform bacilli and spirochetes. *A,* Tissue Gram stain demonstrates the fusiform bacilli. Humberstone stain, × 1200. (Photograph Neg. No. 68-1876.) *B,* Warthin-Starry stain showing the spirochetal organisms. (Courtesy of the Armed Forces Institute of Pathology. Photograph Neg. No. 74-11309.)

Most ulcers are 2 to 5 cm in diameter and rarely exceed 10 cm in diameter. Ordinarily there is a gradual nonpigmented re-epithelialization over the scarred base of the ulcer. If the ulcer is large, there may be contractures. Squamous cell carcinoma sometimes develops at the ulcer site. This may be related to the chronic inflammation, or to actinic stimulation of the nonpigmented epithelium at the healing or healed ulcer site.

DIAGNOSIS. "Once seen, once smelled, never forgotten" is a well-known maxim concerning TPU among physicians experienced in clinical tropical medicine. The demonstration of fusiform bacilli and spirochetes in ulcer exudates, or in histologic sections of an ulcer from the lower leg or foot, is strong evidence for TPU (Fig. 33–3). The differential diagnosis is not usually a problem. TPU are most frequently confused with Buruli ulcers, diphtheritic ulcers, and yaws; however, ulcers of *Mycobacterium ulcerans* are undermined and smears often reveal acid-fast bacilli; diphtheritic ulcers are "punched out," have a diphtheritic membrane, and contain diphtheroids; and ulcers caused by yaws have irregular contours. The histopathologic changes in all these lesions are often diagnostic.

TREATMENT AND PROGNOSIS. Early recognition followed by treatment is ideal but rarely possible. There have been no published reports of the therapy of early lesions, but one of the authors (WMM) treated several lesions in the preulcerative or very early ulcerative stage with penicillin intramuscularly. There was rapid resolution of the lesion.

Unfortunately, most patients present with advanced painful ulceration that has severely limited their activity and productivity. Much has been written describing various topical treatments and dressings, but it is sufficient to clean the ulcer by routine methods (e.g., hydrogen peroxide), apply bland dry dressings, and give systemic antibiotics. Penicillin is usually employed at 500,000 to 1 million units IM daily for 7 to 20 days. Long-acting penicillin may be used as outpatient therapy. Metronidazole (800 mg twice daily for 1 or 2 weeks) is effective against fusobacteria and may accelerate healing.

Large ulcers should be skin-grafted following successful systemic therapy and the development of healthy granulation tissue.

If carcinomatous changes are suspected, a biopsy specimen should be taken to establish the diagnosis. Squamous cell carcinomas developing in TPU lesions are locally invasive and eventually destroy soft tissue and bone, but metastases are rare. Local wide excision is the preferred treatment. Amputation is sometimes necessary with massive lesions, or when bone is destroyed.

BIBLIOGRAPHY

Adriaans RB: Tropical ulcer—a reappraisal based on recent work. Trans Soc Trop Med Hyg 82:185–189, 1988.

Connor DH, Neafie RC: Tropical phagedenic ulcer. *In* Binford CH, Connor DH (eds.): Pathology of Tropical and Extraordinary Diseases. An Atlas. Washington DC, Armed Forces Institute of Pathology, 1976, pp 199–201.

34. RELAPSING FEVER

Thomas Butler

DEFINITION. Relapsing fever is an acute febrile illness of humans caused by blood spirochetes belonging to *Borrelia* species. The two major kinds are louse-borne relapsing fever, for which the human is the reservoir and the body louse is the vector, and tick-borne relapsing fever, for which rodents and other animals are the predominant reservoirs and ticks are the vectors. The relapsing fevers are distributed worldwide in both tropical and temperate climates. The natural course of relapsing fever consists of one or more phases of fever and spirochetemia, which last for several days and are separated by afebrile intervals of several days without spirochetemia. Relapsing fever is usually a self-limited disease, but high mortality rates have been recorded during epidemics of louse-borne relapsing fever.

ETIOLOGY. Relapsing fevers are caused by blood spirochetes of *Borrelia* species, which belong to the order of bacteria called Spirochaetales. *Borrelia* species differ from the other two genera of pathogenic spirochetes, *Leptospira* and *Treponema,* by structure, biochemical characteristics, and antigenic determinants.

Borrelia spirochetes are spiral organisms that measure 5 to 40 μm in length and about 0.5 μm in diameter. They are too thin to be seen reliably by light microscopy of wet preparations, but they are easily visible when viewed by darkfield or phase contrast microscopy. They are stainable with aniline dyes, such as Wright's and Giemsa stains, and can be visualized well in tissue by the application of silver stains, such as the Dieterle and Warthin-Starry stains. Like other bacteria, these spirochetes possess an outer cell wall (outer envelope) and an inner cytoplasmic membrane that contains muramic acid. Between the cell wall and cytoplasmic membrane, there are 15 to 20 flagella, the organelles of motility. They are anchored to the ends of the spirochete and wrap around its body until they meet at the middle region. In 3 dimensions, the spirochetes have a helical configuration consisting of about 5 to 10 coils with amplitudes of about 1 to 4 μm. Under darkfield or phase contrast microscopy, *Borrelia* spirochetes display an active corkscrew-like motility, which consists of rotation and helical waves, giving translational movement to the organisms. Inside the cytoplasmic membrane are ribosomes, DNA, and RNA. These prokaryotic organisms divide by transverse binary fission.

Borrelia organisms are microaerophilic and fermentative in their growth characteristics. Like other pathogenic spirochetes, they require long-chain fatty acids for growth. They can be cultivated in Kelly's medium, which is a complex broth containing proteose peptone, tryptone, bovine serum albumin, rabbit serum, *N*-acetylglucosamine, citric acid, and pyruvate in addition to glucose and salts. *B. recurrentis*, the agent of louse-borne relapsing fever, is more fastidious than the tick-borne *Borrelia* species and requires the further addition of asparagine and choline to Kelly's medium. The *Borrelia* organisms grow slowly in Kelly's medium, with doubling times of 18 to 26 hours.

The species names of the tick-borne *Borrelia* are derived from the species names of *Ornithodoros* tick vectors that carry them. The more common ones in North America are *B. turicatae, B. hermsii,* and *B. parkeri,* and, in Africa, *B. duttonii.* The classification of Borrelia is not based on biochemical or antigenic characteristics that could be standardized for laboratory diagnosis.

Borrelia spirochetes do not possess or produce any known toxins. They produce fever when injected into rabbits but do not possess endotoxin. In general, *Borrelia* spirochetes do not elicit acute inflammation, do not produce abscesses, and are confined predominantly to the plasma space of their mammalian hosts.

The relapsing feature of *Borrelia* infection has been attributed to antigenic variation in the infecting population of spirochetes. In experimental infections of rats with *B. hermsii,* separate serotypes emerged sequentially during relapses and specific antibody appeared in response to each of the antigenic variants. Each of 25 serotypes of *B. hermsii* expresses different variable major proteins that are encoded by genes located on linear plasmids of the spirochete.

HISTORY. The name *relapsing fever* was coined by Craigie in 1843 in Edinburgh. A year later in the same city, Henderson differentiated this disease from typhus fever. The etiologic agent of relapsing fever, however, was first established in Berlin in 1873 by Obermeier, who used a microscope to observe spirochetes in the blood of patients. The transmission of *Borrelia* spirochetes by arthropod vectors was suggested in 1891 by Flugge, who postulated the body louse as a vector, and in 1905 by Dutton and Todd, who demonstrated the infection in the *Ornithodoros* ticks of Africa. The genus name *Borrelia* was proposed in 1907 in honor of the French bacteriologist Amédée Borrel.

Relapsing fever is certainly a disease of antiquity, and its known epidemic potential—particularly in times of war, migrations, and other conditions that favor human crowding and poor hygiene—suggests that relapsing fever has had a major impact on human history. Before the advent of microscopic diagnosis, however, it was not possible to distinguish relapsing fever reliably from similar scourges of humanity such as malaria, typhoid fever, and typhus fever. Therefore, the history of relapsing fever before 1873 is only speculative. In the twentieth century, Bryceson has described evidence for 7 major epidemics of louse-borne relapsing fever. These outbreaks occurred between 1910 and 1945 in North Africa, Sudan, Ethiopia, West Africa, Central Africa, Eastern Europe, and Russia. There were an estimated 15 million cases, with over 5 million deaths and case-fatality rates as high as 73%.

DISTRIBUTION AND INCIDENCE. The geographic distribution of the relapsing fevers is widespread, with occurrence in most continents of the world, including the Americas, Europe, Africa, and Asia. The only areas believed to be entirely free of the relapsing fevers are Australia, New Zealand, and Oceania. Epidemic relapsing fever refers to the louse-borne kind and endemic or sporadic relapsing fever to the tick-borne variety.

Epidemic Relapsing Fever. Louse-borne relapsing fever has disappeared from the United States but still occurs in parts of South America, Europe, Africa, and Asia. From 1960 to 1979, louse-borne relapsing fever was documented in Ethiopia and Sudan. Although accurate statistics on the incidence of this disease are not available, Ethiopia appears to be the country with the highest prevalence, estimated to be 10,000 or more cases per year.

Endemic Relapsing Fever. Tick-borne relapsing fever occurs in endemic foci in southern British Columbia, in the western United States, in the plateau regions of Mexico, and in Central and South America. This disease is present in all areas of Africa except the Sahara Desert and the rain-forest belt. It occurs also in Spain and Portugal. In Asia, tick-borne relapsing fever has been reported in Cyprus, Israel, Syria, Turkey, Iraq, Iran, southern Russia, China, Afghanistan, and India. Accurate statistics on tick-borne relapsing fever are not available, but the sporadic nature of human contact with rodent ticks and the small numbers of established diagnoses suggest that this form of relapsing fever occurs less frequently in humans than louse-borne relapsing fever.

EPIDEMIOLOGY AND TRANSMISSION. The two types of relapsing fever, louse-borne and tick-borne, differ so much in their epidemiology that they must be considered separately.

Epidemic Relapsing Fever. The only species of *Borrelia* that causes louse-borne relapsing fever is *B. recurrentis*. Its vector is the human body louse, *Pediculus humanus humanus* (Fig. 114–1), and the only known natural reservoir is humans. Thus, the cycle of infection is simply from person to person by means of the louse. Body lice acquire the infection by feeding on a spirochetemic person, and they remain infected for their entire life span, which is 10 to 61 days under laboratory conditions. The ingested spirochetes pass through the esophagus to the midgut, where they penetrate the gut epithelium to reach the hemolymph in which they multiply. Spirochetes do not reach the salivary glands or ovaries of the lice. Therefore, infection is not transmitted to people by bites of lice, and infection cannot be transmitted transovarially to offspring of infected lice. Infection is believed to be transmitted after the crushing of lice on the skin, which allows liberated spirochetes to penetrate through a bite site or through intact skin. Body lice prefer the normal human body temperature of 37°C to higher temperatures; thus, lice are likely to leave the skin of a febrile patient to go to another person. This may explain, in part, the rapid transmission of infection during epidemics.

The persons at greatest risk for acquiring louse-borne relapsing fever are those living under crowded, unhygienic conditions that favor infestation with body lice. Migrant workers and soldiers in war are particularly prone to develop this infection. Males are at much greater risk than females, presumably because their lives more commonly expose them to infected lice. A strain-specific and short-lived acquired immunity develops after the infection. This immunity helps to explain why migrant workers coming into an endemic area are more susceptible to infection than are the permanent inhabitants. In some endemic areas, such as Addis Ababa, Ethiopia, there is an increase in incidence during the cool winter season when people wear heavier clothing that becomes louse-infested. In lowland regions of tropical equatorial Africa, where people wear scantier clothing, this infection has been reported but seems to occur less frequently than at higher altitudes.

Endemic Relapsing Fever. The species of *Borrelia* that cause tick-borne relapsing fever are numerous and include *B. duttonii* in East Africa, *B. hispanica* in Spain, *B. persica* in Asia, and *B. hermsii* and *B. turicatae* in North America. These various species cannot be reliably differentiated in the laboratory but usually are determined by the species of tick (which often have the same species names) or by the geographic region in which the infection occurred. The vectors of these organisms are argasid ticks of the genus *Ornithodoros* (Figs. 112–4 and 114–17). The major reservoirs of the tick-borne relapsing fevers are wild rodents, including squirrels, deer mice, rats, chipmunks, and rabbits, and, occasionally, lizards, toads, turtles, and owls. The infection is passed between the reservoir animals by tick bites, and humans become accidental hosts when they come into contact with infected animal ticks. The exception to the animal reservoirs may be *B. duttonii* in East Africa, which is carried by the domestic tick *Ornithodoros moubata* and for which humans appear to be the reservoir.

Ticks acquire the infection by biting and sucking blood from a spirochetemic animal. The spirochetes, after entering the hemocoelom, invade other tissues of the tick, including the salivary glands, the coxal glands on the legs, and the ovaries. Transmission of the infection to animals or humans follows either injection of infected saliva through the bite site or secretion of infected coxal fluid that enters through the bite site or intact skin. Ticks are more durable vectors than body lice, being able to survive as long as 15 years between blood meals and to harbor viable spirochetes for years. In addition, female ticks can pass *Borrelia* spirochetes transovarially to their offspring, thus permitting ticks to be infective without having previously bitten an infected host.

Persons at greatest risk of infection are those who come into contact with infected ticks from wild rodents. In the United States, the largest outbreak of tick-borne relapsing fever occurred in 62 campers and employees in the National Park at the northern rim of the Grand Canyon, Arizona, in 1973. They had all slept in log cabins that were inhabited by wild rodents. Another outbreak in the state of Washington affected 42 Boy Scouts, who also camped out in a log cabin. In tropical countries, people who live in dwellings that are not rodent-proof are prone to infection. In East Africa, where ticks have become domesticated and humans have become a reservoir of tick-borne relapsing fever, people living in the endemic areas develop immunity to the disease. In fact, some village people are known to plant ticks in their houses and to allow themselves deliberately to be bitten by ticks to ensure continuous immunity. Neonates have acquired infection from their mothers' blood. Transmission of spirochetes in these cases occurred presumably by the transplacental route before birth or by exchange of blood at the time of birth.

PATHOGENESIS AND PATHOLOGY

Pathogenesis. After exposure to an infected louse or tick, spirochetes enter the body through the skin and into the subcutaneous tissue, where they have access to the systemic and lymphatic circulations. There are no symptoms during the incubation period, estimated to last from 4 to 18 days, while the spirochetes are dividing in the blood plasma. No local lesions develop at the skin site of entry, and there is no evidence for an intracellular phase of multiplication or for sites of attachment of spirochetes to host cells. After the spirochetes have built up to a concentration of 10^6 to 10^8/mL of blood, symptoms begin suddenly. At this early stage of illness large numbers of spirochetes are regularly present in the plasma space. A small proportion of the spirochetes are within circulating polymorphonuclear phagocytes, and some spirochetes have been phagocytosed by fixed macrophages of the reticuloendothelial system of the spleen, liver, and bone marrow. Although occasionally found in other tissues (e.g., the brain, hepatic cells, kidney, and subcutaneous tissues), spirochetes do not appear to proliferate in these extravascular sites or to elicit inflammatory reactions.

The pathogenesis occurs in the presence of massive numbers of circulating spirochetes. Although *Borrelia* spirochetes do not possess endotoxin or any identified exotoxins, the spirochetes themselves are pyrogenic. The pyrogenic principle resides in the body or outer envelope of the spirochete, is heat-stable, and acts by stimulating mononuclear phagocytic cells to elaborate leukocytic pyrogen (interleukin-1). Because platelet production by the bone marrow is normal, the thrombocytopenia of relapsing fever, which causes petechiae and sometimes other hemorrhagic phenomena, results from sequestration of platelets. In addition, there is disseminated intravascular coagulation. During acute relapsing fever, levels of serum complement, Hageman factor, and prekalikrein are decreased, suggesting that activation of certain plasma proteins contributes to the pathogenesis of features such as hypotension and disseminated intravascular coagulation.

Most patients with relapsing fever recover from their illness either with or without antibiotic treatment. Patients develop antiborrelial antibodies, which can agglutinate, kill, or opsonize spirochetes. In the presence of opsonizing antibody, spirochetes are rapidly phagocytosed and digested by polymorphonuclear leukocytes. These antibodies also participate in rendering patients immune to future infection with the same serotype of *Borrelia.*

Pathology. Autopsies performed in Ethiopia and Sudan in fatal cases of louse-borne relapsing fever showed characteristic lesions in the spleen, liver, heart, and brain. The spleen is enlarged to as much as 900 gm, and the cut surface shows white microabscesses, which consist of necrosis and hemorrhage in the white pulp. Occasionally, there are splenic infarcts and splenic rupture. The liver is also enlarged, often to over 2000 gm. The midzonal regions show scattered necrosis and hemorrhage, and Kupffer cells are enlarged and numerous.

The heart is normal in size but frequently shows myocarditis, with interstitial edema and a cellular infiltrate of lymphocytes and plasma cells. The brain usually shows cerebral edema, and in some cases, there is hemorrhage into the subarachnoid space or cerebrum. Thus, the immediate causes of death in relapsing fever are varied and, in any particular case, may be liver failure, cerebral hemorrhage, or acute cardiac arrhythmia due to myocarditis.

CLINICAL MANIFESTATIONS. The illness begins abruptly with shaking chills, fever, headache, and fatigue. Most patients have these symptoms almost continuously throughout the day, whereas some patients report the intermittent appearance of these symptoms several times a day. Patients complain frequently of myalgias, arthralgias, anorexia, dry cough, and abdominal pains. These symptoms are usually mild on the first day of illness and increase in intensity over a few days, leading to prostration and a visit to a physician. The nonspecific nature of this symptomatology leads patients or their physicians to believe they have a flulike illness.

The temperature is elevated in the range of 38.5° to 40° C, and the pulse rate is increased to about 115 beats/min. The blood pressure is lowered to about 105/70 mm Hg. Patients appear lethargic. Physical signs that are common but not regularly present are conjunctival injection, petechial skin rash that is more apparent on the trunk than on the extremities, and palpable liver and spleen. Jaundice is present occasionally. Generalized muscle weakness is common. Some patients display mental confusion or delirium, and some have nuchal rigidity.

The laboratory results show a positive blood smear for spirochetes. The white blood cell count is usually normal, with increased band forms and decreased eosinophils. The platelet counts are often less than 50,000/mm³, and there may be prolongations of the prothrombin time and partial thromboplastin time and increased titers of fibrinogen–fibrin degradation products. Liver function tests are frequently abnormal, with serum alanine aminotransferase elevations and bilirubin elevations that are evenly divided between the conjugated and unconjugated fractions. Renal function tests often show mild abnormalities of the serum urea nitrogen and creatinine values, and patients may have proteinuria and microscopic hematuria.

DIAGNOSIS

Visualization in Peripheral Blood. The diagnosis of relapsing fever depends on the demonstration of spirochetemia. In most patients, this is readily accomplished by obtaining peripheral blood by either finger-stick or venipuncture and preparing a thin film on a microscope slide. *Borrelia* spirochetes are stained blue by aniline dyes. Thus, a routine blood smear stained with Wright's or Giemsa stain is adequate. Blood smears, thin and thick, prepared for examination for malaria parasites are also satisfactory for spirochete examination. The spirochetes are 5 to 20 μm in length and lie in the plasma spaces between blood cells or may overlie the blood cells (Fig. 34–1). Febrile patients with relapsing fever typically have large numbers of spirochetes in the blood, about 10^6 to 10^8/mL, or several per high-power

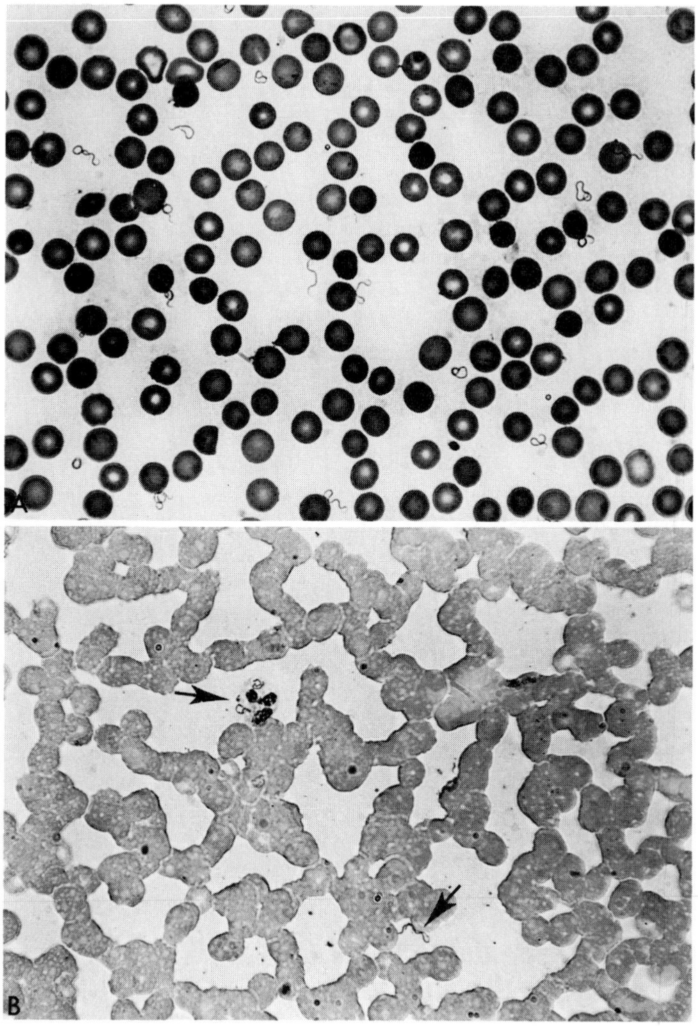

FIGURE 34–1. *A,* Blood smear from a patient with louse-borne relapsing fever stained with Wright's stain showing *Borrelia* spirochetes. *B,* Blood smear stained with Warthin-Starry stain after antibiotic treatment showing intracellular spirochetes in a polymorphonuclear leukocyte (*top arrow*) and a single extracellular spirochete (*bottom arrow*).

field. Patients who are afebrile in the interval between relapses have negative smears and should be re-examined when the fever reappears.

Spirochetemia may be detected alternatively by dark-field or phase contrast microscopy. A drop of fresh blood is diluted with another drop of 0.9% NaCl and covered with a coverslip. Spirochetes are readily identified by their characteristic rotational motility.

Culture or Animal Isolation. For purposes of special investigation or research, additional diagnostic tests of culture and animal inoculations can be used. *Borrelia* organisms are fastidious and slow-growing but can be cultivated in Kelly's broth medium. Infected blood is inoculated into broth and allowed to incubate for about a week. Likewise, infected blood can be inoculated intraperitoneally into laboratory mice or rats and the blood of these animals examined daily for 14 days for spirochetemia. Tick-borne *Borrelia* species are more readily cultivated in Kelly's medium and recoverable from laboratory animals than are the louse-borne *B. recurrentis.*

Epidemiology and Vector Examination. The distinction between louse-borne and tick-borne relapsing fever is made by knowing the geographic distribution of the types of relapsing fever and obtaining information about

contact with lice or ticks. If the vectors can be collected from the patient or the household, they can be dissected and the hemolymph or coxal fluid examined microscopically for the presence of spirochetes.

Serology. Serologic testing has been employed in endemic areas for purposes of seroepidemiology and examination of convalescent patients. Serum of convalescent patients contains antibodies that produce agglutination and immobilization of living spirochetes and fix complement during reaction with spirochetal antigens. None of these tests, however, is standardized or commercially available for general use.

TREATMENT AND PROGNOSIS

Antibiotics. The relapsing fevers are effectively treated with tetracycline and erythromycin. Tetracycline is the treatment of choice except in children less than 7 years old and in pregnant women, in which cases tetracycline may stain developing teeth. Studies in Ethiopia indicate that a single 500-mg oral dose of tetracycline is as effective in clearing spirochetemia and preventing relapse as a longer course of treatment. Erythromycin, 500 mg given orally as a single dose, is equally effective and is a satisfactory alternative to tetracycline. For patients unable to take oral medication, intravenous injections of 250 mg of tetracycline or erythromycin are curative. For children who weigh less than 30 kg, the dosage of tetracycline or erythromycin should be reduced to approximately 10 mg/kg. Penicillin G has been used to treat relapsing fever, but its use has been associated with slow clearance of spirochetes and relapses following treatment.

Jarisch-Herxheimer Reaction. In most patients with louse-borne relapsing fever and in some with tick-borne relapsing fever, antibiotic treatment provokes a distressing Jarisch-Herxheimer reaction. As depicted in Figure 34–2, which shows the mean values of 32 Ethiopian patients with louse-borne relapsing fever treated with erythromycin, a rigor occurred 2 or 3 hours after treatment in 28 patients. Subsequently, temperature rose sharply and blood pressure declined while spirochetes were cleared from the blood. Patients are extremely uncomfortable during the reaction, feeling very cold with severe headache and myalgia. Often they express a sense of impending doom: "This is much worse than my illness was before treatment." During the Jarisch-Herxheimer reaction, blood leukocyte and platelet counts sharply decrease and spirochetes disappear from the plasma. Patients may require intravenous infusions of 0.9% NaCl to maintain adequate blood pressure. Deaths rarely occur during the reaction. Over several hours, temperature declines and patients feel better. Attempts to ameliorate the severity of the reaction by giving antipyretic or anti-inflammatory drugs have not been entirely successful. The best approach is to anticipate the reaction and to provide intensive nursing care and intravenous fluid support during the first day of treatment.

Prognosis and Relapses. The prognosis is favorable for complete recovery in 95% or more of treated cases

of relapsing fever. Bad prognostic signs are the presence of jaundice, high spirochete counts in the blood, and hypotension. More than half of neonatal patients with relapsing fever die. The prognosis for untreated disease is grave in the case of louse-borne relapsing fever, for which mortality rates of 40% have been reported during epidemics. Untreated cases also experience relapses. In louse-borne relapsing fever, the first attack lasts about 6 days and is followed by an afebrile period of about 9 days. There usually is 1 relapse, which lasts only about 2 days. In tick-borne relapsing fever, the first attack lasts about 3 days and is followed by an interval of about 7 days, after which an average of 3 relapses occur, each lasting about 2 days. Relapses are usually milder in intensity than the first attacks.

PREVENTION AND CONTROL. Available approaches for the control of the relapsing fevers include the detection and treatment of human cases, vector control, rodent control, and public health education. Vaccines are not available for the prevention of relapsing fever.

Epidemic Relapsing Fever. For louse-borne relapsing fever, the detection and treatment of cases have the effect of reducing the reservoir of infection and, consequently, reducing transmission. More important is the control of louse infestation. Instructing people to bathe and wash their clothes is the rational approach, but compliance is likely to be low. Delousing of clothing and bodies with insecticides (e.g., DDT) can be employed, as can the application of insect repellants. In known epidemic situations, prophylactic antibiotics are a temporary measure to contain spread of infection to persons at high risk. The eventual control of this disease requires improvements in personal hygiene and housing conditions.

Endemic Relapsing Fever. For tick-borne relapsing fever, the treatment of human cases has no impact on the animal reservoirs. It is not possible to control this infection in wild rodents. Campers and hikers going into endemic areas should be advised to avoid staying in cabins that are inhabited by rodents and their ticks and to apply topical tick repellants to their skin. In endemic areas of Africa, people need to be assisted in building rodent-proof houses.

BIBLIOGRAPHY

Ahmed MAM, Abdel-Wahab SM, Abdel-Malik MD, et al.: Louse-borne relapsing fever in the Sudan: A historical review and a clinicopathological study. Trop Geogr Med 32:106, 1980.

Barbour AG, Hayes SF: Biology of *Borrelia* species. Microbiol Rev 50:381, 1986.

Bryceson ADM, Parry EHO, Perine PL, et al.: Louse-borne relapsing fever: A clinical and laboratory study of 62 cases in Ethiopia and a reconsideration of the literature. Q J Med 39:129, 1970.

Burgdorfer W: The epidemiology of the relapsing fevers. *In* Johnson RC (ed.): The Biology of Parasitic Spirochetes. New York, Academic Press, 1976, pp 191–200.

Butler T, Jones PK, Wallace CK: *Borrelia recurrentis* infection: Single dose antibiotic regimens and management of Jarisch-Herxheimer reaction. J Infect Dis 137:573, 1978.

Butler T, Hazen P, Wallace CK, et al.: *Borrelia recurrentis* infection: Pathogenesis of fever and petechiae. J Infect Dis 140:665, 1979.

Butler T, Aikawa M, Habte-Michael A, et al.: Phagocytosis of *Borrelia*

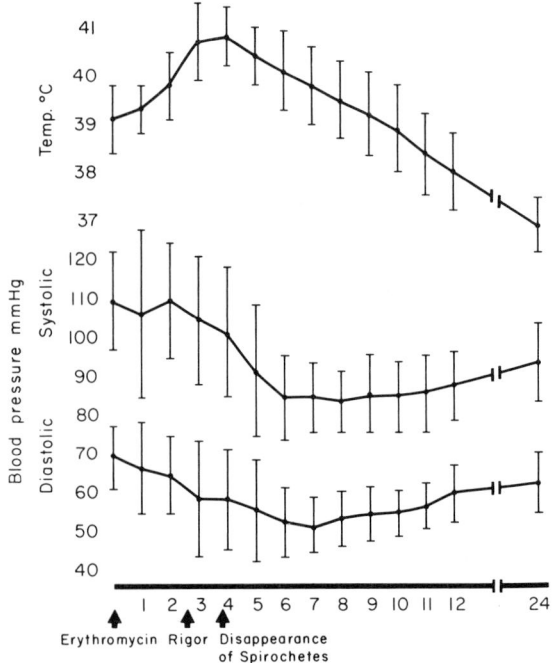

FIGURE 34–2. Changes in temperature and blood pressure during Jarisch-Herxheimer–like reaction. Thirty-two patients with louse-borne relapsing fever were treated with erythromycin, 500 mg orally.

recurrentis by polymorphonuclear leukocytes is enhanced by antibiotic treatment. Infect Immun 28:1009, 1980.

Horton JM, Blaser MJ: The spectrum of relapsing fever in the Rocky Mountains. Arch Intern Med 145:871, 1985.

Judge DM, Samuel I, Perine PL, et al.: Louse-borne relapsing fever in man. Arch Pathol 97:136, 1974.

Warrell DA, Perine PL, Krause DW, et al.: Pathophysiology and immunology of the Jarisch-Herxheimer-like reaction in louse-borne relapsing fever: Comparison of tetracycline and slow-release penicillin. J Infect Dis 147:898, 1983.

Yagupsky P, Moses S: Neonatal *Borrelia* species infection. Am J Dis Child 139:74, 1985.

35. LEPTOSPIROSIS

George Watt

DEFINITION. Leptospirosis is a worldwide zoonosis with diverse clinical findings ranging from asymptomatic infection to renal failure and death. Severe, icteric infection is commonly referred to as Weil's disease. The causative agent, *Leptospira interrogans,* is a single species of spirochete with multiple serotypes arranged in antigenically related groups. Old terms such as peapicker's disease, swineherd's disease, and canicola fever, which linked specific serotypes with distinct disease manifestations, are inaccurate and confusing and should no longer be used.

ETIOLOGY. The responsible organism is a tightly coiled, motile spirochete with one axial filament and hooked ends (Fig. 35–1). Leptospires are aerobic and approximately 0.1 μm in diameter and from 6 to 20 μm in length. Unstained organisms can be seen only by darkfield or phase-contrast microscopy. Silver staining is the method of choice for demonstrating leptospires in tissue specimens.

The taxonomy of leptospires is evolving. At present, the genus *Leptospira* is said to contain two species: *interrogans,* which is pathogenic, and *biflexa,* which is saprophytic. Stable antigenic differences allow subclassification into serotypes, referred to in the literature as serovars (serovarieties). Antigens common to several serovars permit arrangement into broader serogroups. Over 170 serovars and 18 serogroups have been identified for *L. interrogans.*

HISTORY. In 1886 Weil described the first cases of a severe icteric illness that he recognized as a new clinical entity. The causative organism was first seen in 1907 in sections of kidney tissue from a patient dying during a yellow fever epidemic. However, it took until 1915 for Inada to successfully culture the spirochete and prove its association with Weil's disease. Leptospires were recovered from a Norway rat in 1917, and the first human case connected with rat exposure was reported in 1922.

EPIDEMIOLOGY

Distribution and Prevalence. *L. interrogans* infection has its greatest impact in the tropics, though its distribution is worldwide. Most infections go unrecognized and unreported partly because leptospirosis is often confused with other entities and partly because a conclusive diagnosis is often difficult to make. Indirect evidence suggests that leptospirosis is of greatest public health importance in Southeast Asia and Latin America. It was shown to be a major cause of fever of unknown origin in both Malaysia and Vietnam, and antibody positivity rates were 27% in Thailand, 23% in Vietnam, and 37% in rural Belize. Leptospirosis also remains an important public health problem in other parts of Asia, eastern and southern Europe, Australia, and New Zealand. It is primarily of veterinary importance in the United States, where only 50 to 150 human cases are reported annually.

Animal Reservoirs. Leptospires nest in the renal tubules of mammalian hosts and are shed with the urine. They can survive for several months in the environment under moist conditions, particularly in the presence of warmth (above 22C) and a relatively neutral pH (pH 6.2 to 8). These conditions are found year round in the tropics but only during the summer and autumn months in temperate climates. Survival is inhibited by contaminated water and by salinity.

Among the roughly 160 mammalian species harboring organisms, rodents are the most important reservoir. Carrier rates of over 50% have been measured in Norway rats, which shed massive numbers of organisms for life without showing clinical illness. Some serovars appear to be preferentially adapted to select mammalian hosts. For example, serovar *icterohaemorrhagiae* is primarily associated with the Norway rat, *canicola* with dogs, and *pomona* with swine and cattle. However, a particular host species may serve as a reservoir for one or more serovar and a particular serovar may be hosted by many different animal species.

Transmission to Man. The transmission of infection from animal to man usually occurs through contact with contaminated water or moist soil. The streets of some crowded Asian cities that become submerged during the rainy season and have large rat populations provide

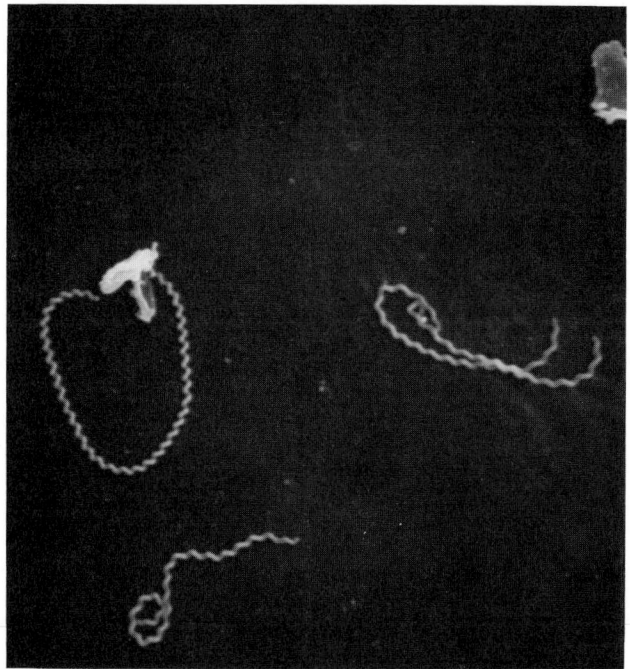

FIGURE 35–1. Typical leptospires viewed under electron microscopy at a magnification of 4000 ×. (Courtesy of J. Bruce McClain.)

ideal conditions for the transmission of disease. Jungle swamps and mud are rich sources of pathogenic organisms. Less frequently, leptospirosis is acquired by direct contact with the blood, urine, or tissues of infected animals. Transmission via laboratory accidents or breast milk has been reported but is rare. Organisms enter man through abrasions of the skin or through the mucosal surface of the eye, mouth, nasopharynx, or esophagus.

Occupational Risk. People working in a milieu that associates rats or infected livestock with water are especially prone to infection. Certain agricultural laborers are at high risk, and intense exposure to leptospires has been documented in rice, sugar cane, and rubber plantation workers. Others with hazardous occupations include abattoir workers, fish and poultry processors, butchers, ditch diggers, and sewer workers. Many residents of the tropics are infected by wading through streets flooded by leptospire-contaminated water. Epidemiologic patterns in the United States and United Kingdom have changed. Recreational exposure and animal contact at home have replaced occupational exposure as the chief source of disease.

PATHOGENESIS AND PATHOLOGY. Much of the pathogenesis of leptospirosis remains unexplained. The most striking finding in severe disease is the paucity of histopathologic lesions in the kidneys and livers of patients with marked functional impairment of these organs. This disparity indicates damage at the subcellular level—perhaps caused by a toxin. Fatally infected animals and some human patients exhibit changes similar to those produced by the endotoxemia of gram-negative bacteremia. An endotoxin-like substance is present in the cell wall of leptospires but lacks the ketodeoxyoctanoate of true endotoxin. Additional evidence for toxic effect is that patients with icteric disease typically have marked leukocytosis, but there is an absence of leukocytic infiltrates in organs. Patients who survive severe leptospirosis have complete recovery of hepatic and renal function, a finding consistent with the lack of structural damage to these organs.

Kidneys. Renal failure is the most important cause of death in leptospirosis. It is due primarily to acute tubular necrosis; impaired renal perfusion constitutes the fundamental nephropathic change. Oliguria is rapidly reversed by intravenous fluid administration in many patients, suggesting that volume depletion is frequent. Hypovolemia in leptospirosis is multifactorial: insensible water loss due to high fever, diminished intake of fluid, vomiting, diarrhea and, infrequently, gastrointestinal hemorrhage. A defect in the kidney's ability to concentrate urine is common and increases fluid loss. In some patients, widespread endothelial injury causes a shift of fluid from the intravascular to the extracellular space; hypotension of cardiac origin occurs rarely. The majority of cases of renal dysfunction are reversible with correction of hypovolemia and the resultant improvement in renal perfusion.

Leptospires are frequently found in human renal tissue (Fig. 35–2), but their role in mediating kidney damage is unknown. Interstitial nephritis is found primarily in individuals who have survived until inflam-

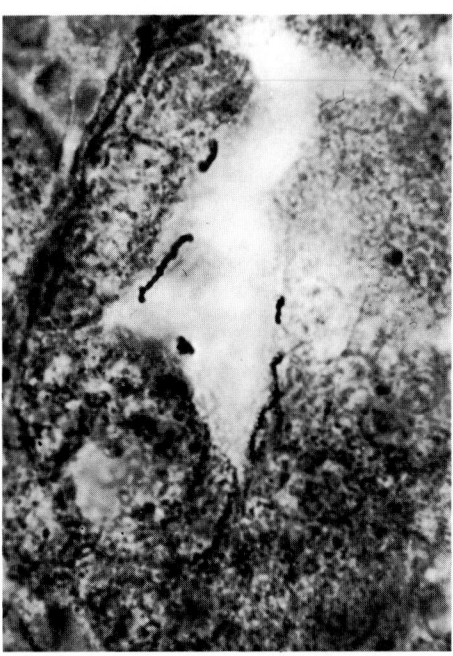

FIGURE 35–2. Leptospires in a renal tubule (Warthin-Starry stain, × 1320). (Courtesy of the Armed Forces Institute of Pathology, Photograph Neg. No. 60-1525.)

mation has had an opportunity to develop, but is frequently absent in patients whose disease is characterized by a fulminant course.

Hemorrhage. A prominent feature of experimental leptospirosis is a progressively severe hemorrhagic diathesis. In humans, bleeding is generally restricted to the skin or mucosal surfaces, but occasionally massive gastrointestinal hemorrhage or bleeding into a vital organ occurs. Coagulopathy and thrombocytopenia are present either together or separately in many patients with leptospirosis but do not adequately explain bleeding. By exclusion, capillary damage is the postulated mechanism, and toxins have been suggested as the mediators of endothelial injury.

Liver. Jaundice is the most noticeable clinical finding in cases of hepatic dysfunction, but its pathogenesis remains unexplained. Neither hemolytic anemia nor hepatocellular necrosis is a prominent feature of leptospirosis. The most severe hepatic pathologic changes are seen when organisms are difficult to demonstrate in tissue, again suggesting subcellular toxic or metabolic effects.

Meningitis. Organisms easily enter the cerebrospinal fluid during leptospiremia, and this is thought to explain the high incidence of meningitis. However, signs of meningeal irritation are not due to the invasion of the meninges by leptospires, a process that elicits little reaction. Organisms are isolated frequently from cerebrospinal fluid that is otherwise normal and from individuals without clinically detectable nervous system involvement. Symptoms of meningitis coincide with the development of antibody and disappearance of leptospires from the blood and cerebrospinal fluid, suggesting an immunologic mechanism. Pathologic changes are minimal or absent, and the prognosis is excellent.

Cardiopulmonary System. Pulmonary involvement in leptospirosis is generally the result of hemorrhage rather than of inflammation. Localized or confluent hemorrhagic pneumonitis is the usual finding, with petechial and ecchymotic hemorrhages noted throughout the lungs, pleura, and tracheobronchial tree. Pulmonary capillary damage could be the result of a toxin, since leptospires have not been demonstrated in pulmonary tissue. Focal hemorrhagic myocarditis has been reported, but hypovolemia, electrolyte imbalance, and uremia are more frequent causes of cardiac dysfunction.

Skeletal Muscle. The myalgias typical of early disease appear to be due to active invasion of skeletal muscle by leptospires. Muscle pain ends as antibody titers develop and organisms are cleared from the blood. Muscle biopsies in patients with early illness demonstrate vacuolation of the myofibrillar cytoplasm, loss of cellular detail, and fragmentation. Leptospiral antigen can be demonstrated by fluorescent antibody techniques. Pathologic changes are usually absent in the muscles of patients dying during the second week of disease.

Eye. The aqueous humor provides a protective environment for leptospires, which readily enter the anterior chamber of the eye during the leptospiremic phase of disease. There they can remain viable for months, despite the development of serum antibodies. Uveitis is frequent, appearing weeks or months after the onset of disease and has been attributed to the persistence of organisms in the anterior chamber.

CLINICAL AND LABORATORY FINDINGS

General Features. Serologic surveys of workers at high risk confirm that subclinical infection is common. Among individuals unaware of illness due to leptospirosis, 16% of abattoir workers and 40% of rice farmers were found to have antibodies. Less than 10% of symptomatic infections result in severe, icteric illness. Even relatively virulent serovars such as *icterohaemorrhagiae* lead more often to anicteric than to icteric disease. A higher percentage of patients with severe infections is seen in hospitals in the tropics because patients with mild cases are often not admitted.

After accidental laboratory exposure or immersion in contaminated water, the incubation period has shown extremes of 2 and 26 days. The standard interval is 1 to 2 weeks; the average is 10 days. The duration of the incubation period has no prognostic significance. Once symptoms develop, they are said to follow a biphasic course: After an initial febrile illness, there is defervescence of fever and symptomatic improvement, followed by a second period of disease. However, a clear demarcation between the first and second stages is atypical of icteric leptospirosis; in mild cases the distinction can be unclear, or the second stage may never occur. Thus a history of a biphasic illness supports the diagnosis of leptospirosis, but its absence does not rule it out.

Anicteric Leptospirosis

Symptoms and Signs. The onset of symptoms is typically abrupt: Patients can time the beginning of their illness to within 1 or 2 hours. Headache, fever, chills, and myalgias are the most frequently reported initial symptoms. Headache is usually frontal, less often retro-orbital, and occasionally bitemporal or occipital. It is generally intense, persistent, and poorly controlled with nonprescription analgesics. Fever is high, with one or more daily peaks that often exceed 40C (103F) and are preceded by rigors. Muscle pain can be excruciating and occurs most commonly in the thighs, calves, lumbosacral region, and abdomen. Some patients with leptospirosis have intense abdominal wall pain with tenderness and fever mimicking an acute surgical abdomen. There are numerous reports of inappropriate surgical interventions, particularly appendectomies. Myalgias adjacent to the cervical spine can cause nuchal rigidity and suggest meningitis in a patient with headache and fever. Lumbar puncture is often performed, but cerebrospinal fluid obtained during the first week of illness is acellular with normal protein and glucose content.

Leptospires can be isolated from the blood for 4 to 9 days after the onset of illness. Many other symptoms can occur during this "leptospiremic" phase (Table 35–1). Nausea, vomiting, diarrhea, and sore throat are especially frequent. Cough and chest pain figure prominently in reports of patients from Korea and China. Up to a quarter of Korean patients present with pneumonia.

Conjunctival suffusion is the most characteristic and diagnostically helpful physical sign in the leptospiremic phase. It usually appears 2 or 3 days after the onset of fever and involves the bulbar conjunctiva. Redness decreases in intensity toward the cornea. It is not a conjunctivitis—pus and serous secretions are absent, and there is no matting of the eyelashes and eyelids. Suffusion gradually fades over a period of 3 days to 3 weeks. The marked variation in the reported incidence of this finding is due more to the diligence with which suffusion is sought than to true differences in the frequency with which it occurs. Unless specifically looked for, mild suffusion can easily be overlooked. Less common and less distinctive signs include pharyngeal injection, splenomegaly, hepatomegaly, lymphadenopathy,

TABLE 35–1. The Most Common Clinical Manifestations of 208 Leptospirosis Patients in Puerto Rico*

	Anicteric (106 Cases)	Icteric (102 Cases)
Symptoms (% of cases)		
Fever	100	99
Myalgia	97	97
Headache	82	95
Chills	84	90
Sore throat	72	87
Nausea	71	81
Vomiting	65	75
Eye pain	54	38
Diarrhea	23	30
Decreased urine	20	30
Cough	15	32
Hemoptysis	5	14
Signs (% of cases)		
Conjunctival injection	100	98
Muscle tenderness	70	79
Hepatomegaly	60	60
Pulmonary findings	11	36
Lymphadenopathy	35	12
Petechiae and ecchymoses	4	29

*Adapted from Diaz-Rivera RS, et al: Zoonosis Res 2:159, 1963.

and skin lesions. These may be macular, papular, erythematous, urticarial, or hemorrhagic.

Within a week most patients become asymptomatic, although occasionally disease persists for more than a month. After several days of apparent recovery, the illness resumes in some individuals. Manifestations of the second stage are more variable than those of the initial illness. Symptoms last from 2 to 4 days in most patients, fever is not so high, and myalgias and gastrointestinal disturbances are less severe. Leptospires disappear from the blood, cerebrospinal fluid, and tissues but appear in the urine. Serum antibody titers rise—hence the term "immune" phase.

Meningitis is the hallmark of this stage of leptospirosis. Cerebrospinal fluid pleocytosis can be demonstrated in 80 to 90% of all patients during the second week of illness, although only about 50% will have clinical signs and symptoms of meningitis. Pleocytosis usually lasts 1 to 3 weeks but occasionally may persist for 60 to 80 days. Meningeal signs can last several weeks but usually resolve within a day or two. Neurologic manifestations other than meningoencephalitis occur occasionally.

Uveitis is a late manifestation of leptospirosis. Although it is seen as early as the third week of illness, the average is 4 to 8 months, and intervals of up to 1 year have been reported. The anterior uveal tract is most frequently affected, and pain, photophobia, and blurring of vision are the usual symptoms. Iridocyclitis can be unilateral or bilateral; the prognosis is generally good.

Laboratory Findings. The white blood cell count may be low, normal, or elevated, but neutrophilia is usually found, whatever the total count. The erythrocyte sedimentation rate is consistently elevated. Urinalysis may show proteinuria, pyuria, and microscopic hematuria. Enzyme markers of skeletal muscle damage, such as creatinine phosphokinase and aldolase, are elevated in the sera of 50% of patients during the first week of illness.

Chest radiographs in patients with pulmonary manifestations show a variety of abnormalities, but none is pathognomonic of leptospirosis. The most common finding is small, patchy, snowflake-like lesions in the periphery of the lung fields—either restricted to a few intercostal spaces or disseminated widely. Other patterns include confluent infiltrates or massive consolidation, which represent hemorrhage, and solitary, patchy lesions with ill-defined margins.

Lumbar puncture during the second week of illness reveals changes characteristic of aseptic meningitis. Cerebrospinal fluid pressures and cell counts are generally less than 200 mm H_2O and 500/mm^3, respectively. There is an early, transient predominance of polymorphonuclear leukocytes, after which lymphocytes are the dominant cell type. Protein concentrations range from normal to 300 mg/dl, and glucose values are normal.

Icteric Leptospirosis (Weil's Disease). This dramatic, life-threatening illness is characterized by jaundice, renal dysfunction, hemorrhagic manifestations, and a high mortality rate; a clear-cut biphasic disease pattern is atypical. The key differences between icteric and anicteric leptospirosis are summarized in Table 35–2. The

TABLE 35–2. Salient Differences Between Icteric and Anicteric Leptospirosis*

	Icteric (Weil's Disease)	Anicteric
Jaundice	+ + +	+
Leukocytosis	+ + +	−
Hemorrhage	+	−
Renal failure	+	−
Death	+	−
Aseptic meningitis	−	+
Disturbances of consciousness†	+	+

*(−) = rare or absent; (+) = can occur; (+ + +) = characteristic.

†Due primarily to uremia in severe disease and to encephalitis in anicteric cases.

clinical picture is variable and may be dominated by symptoms of renal, hepatic, or vascular dysfunction. With adequate supportive care the case fatality rate is less than 10 per cent, but is generally much higher in the tropics because facilities are lacking and patients present late in the course of illness.

Though jaundice is the hallmark of severe leptospirosis, fatalities do not occur because of liver failure. The degree of jaundice has no prognostic significance, but its presence or absence does—virtually all leptospirosis deaths occur in icteric patients. Icterus first appears between the fifth and ninth days of illness, reaches maximum intensity 4 or 5 days later, and continues for an average of 1 month. Hyperbilirubinemia results from increases in both conjugated (direct) and unconjugated (indirect) bilirubin, but elevations of the direct fraction predominate.

Other signs of hepatic dysfunction usually accompany jaundice. Prolongations of the prothrombin time occur commonly and are easily corrected by the administration of vitamin K; modest elevations of serum alkaline phosphatase are typical. Jaundice is not associated with marked hepatocellular necrosis—greater than fivefold increases of transaminase (aminotransferase) levels are exceptional. Hepatomegaly is found in the majority of patients (Table 35–1), and hepatic percussion tenderness is a reliable clinical marker of continuing disease activity. There is no residual liver dysfunction in survivors of Weil's disease, consistent with the absence of structural damage seen on pathologic examination of this organ.

Bleeding is occasionally seen in anicteric cases but is most prevalent in severe disease (Tables 35–1 and 35–2). Purpura, petechiae, epistaxis, bleeding of the gums, and minor hemoptysis are the most common hemorrhagic manifestations, but deaths due to subarachnoid hemorrhage and exsanguination from gastrointestinal bleeding occur. Adrenal hemorrhage has been reported but is rare. Conjunctival hemorrhage is an extremely useful diagnostic finding, and when combined with scleral icterus and conjunctival suffusion, produces eye findings pathognomonic of leptospirosis.

Laboratory findings in severe disease are nonspecific but helpful in the differential diagnosis. Jaundiced patients usually have leukocytosis in the range of 15,000 to 30,000/mm^3. Extremely high counts have been reported, but whatever the absolute number of white cells, neutrophilia is constant. Anemia is common and multifactorial; blood loss and azotemia contribute frequently, intravascular hemolysis less often. Mild thrombocytopenia occurs often, but decreases in platelet count sufficient to be associated with bleeding are exceptional.

Life-threatening renal failure is a complication of icteric disease, though all forms of leptospirosis may be associated with mild kidney involvement. Prompt recognition and appropriate management of renal dysfunction in severe leptospirosis is the key to patient survival. Oliguria or anuria usually develops during the second week of illness, although it may appear as early as the third or fourth day. Despite extremely elevated serum creatinine levels, renal recovery can be achieved in most patients without dialysis provided that some urine output is present. Complete anuria is a grave prognostic sign, often seen in patients who present late in the course of illness with frank uremia and irreversible disease.

Most oliguric patients have decreased renal perfusion and respond to fluid challenge with increased urine output, but there is rapid progression to acute tubular necrosis and anuria if hypovolemia is not corrected. Signs of hypovolemia include flat neck veins, reduced ocular tension, poor skin turgor, and postural hypotension; urine specific gravity is high. Occasional individuals have renal deterioration despite vigorous fluid therapy. Because renal failure develops very quickly in leptospirosis, symptoms and signs of uremia are frequently encountered. Anorexia, vomiting, drowsiness, disorientation, and confusion are seen early and progress to convulsions, stupor, and coma in severe cases. Disturbances of consciousness in a patient with severe leptospirosis are usually due to uremic encephalopathy, whereas in anicteric cases aseptic encephalitis is the usual cause (Table 35–2). Renal function eventually returns to normal in survivors of Weil's disease, though detectable abnormalities may persist for several months.

Childhood Disease. Pediatric leptospirosis shares many features with adult disease but has several distinct clinical features. Hypertension, acalculous cholecystitis, pancreatitis, abdominal causalgia, and skin lesions that may desquamate or become gangrenous have been reported. Cardiopulmonary arrest sometimes occurs.

DIFFERENTIAL DIAGNOSIS

Anicteric Leptospirosis. The typical leptospirosis patient has a history of contact with animals or contaminated water, severe myalgias, and conjunctival suffusion. Atypical or mild cases are often confused with other entities, but because of a low index of suspicion and the disease's protean manifestations, the diagnosis is often missed even in typical cases. *L. interrogans* infection was included in the admitting differential diagnosis in less than 25% of over 1000 confirmed cases reported by the Centers for Disease Control since 1949, and in another series of 483 proven cases, only 17% of patients were initially thought to have leptospirosis. Aseptic meningitis is the most common clinical impression in leptospirosis patients; fever of unknown origin, influenza, appendicitis, and gastroenteritis are other frequent diagnoses.

Weil's Disease. Viral hepatitis is a common misdiagnosis in patients with Weil's disease. Conjunctival suffusion, severe myalgias, and a history of water or animal contact are very helpful diagnostic clues in jaundiced patients, as they are in anicteric individuals. Leukocytosis, elevated serum bilirubin levels without marked transaminase elevations, and renal dysfunction are typical of leptospirosis but unusual in hepatitis. Malaria, typhoid fever, scrub typhus, and Hantaan virus infection (hemorrhagic fever with renal syndrome) are important differential diagnoses in the tropics. Marked leukocytosis and a negative malaria smear argue against *Plasmodium falciparum* infection; jaundice, severe renal dysfunction, and leukocytosis militate against typhoid fever. Differentiating leptospirosis from scrub typhus and Korean hemorrhagic fever in areas where these diseases coexist is more difficult. Both are associated with animals, and both can cause conjunctival suffusion. Splenomegaly and generalized lymphadenopathy are characteristic of scrub typhus but not leptospirosis, whereas jaundice and leukocytosis are unusual in *Rickettsia tsutsugamushi* infections. Korean hemorrhagic fever is transmitted by infected rodent urine, and mixed infections with *L. interrogans* and Hantaan virus have been reported. Liver disease is not usually a prominent manifestation of Korean hemorrhagic fever.

Childhood Disease. Some features of pediatric leptospirosis, such as desquamation, myocardial involvement, and hydrops of the gallbladder, suggest Kawasaki's disease (mucocutaneous lymph node syndrome).

DIAGNOSIS

General Considerations. The diagnosis of leptospirosis is usually based on serology. Culturing *L. interrogans* is not difficult, though this organism grows so slowly that isolation results may be delayed for up to 8 weeks—too late to benefit acutely ill patients. Animal inoculation offers no greater chance than culture for recovery of leptospires. Direct examination of blood or urine by darkfield microscopy is not only insensitive but often erroneous; it should not be performed except by highly skilled specialists.

Serology. The macroscopic slide agglutination test is the only serologic method that is commercially available. Killed or formalinized organisms, usually those prevalent in North America, are combined into several antigenic pools. Unfortunately, serovars present in the tropics are sometimes not well represented in these pools, so that sera from leptospirosis patients in tropical areas may test negative. In addition to problems with sensitivity, the specificity of this test has been questioned.

The microscopic agglutination test is considered the serodiagnostic method of choice for leptospirosis, but its complexity limits its use to reference laboratories. Dilutions of patient sera are applied to live, pathogenic leptospires. The results are viewed under dark-field microscopy and expressed as the percentage of organisms cleared from the field by agglutination. To ensure detection of antibodies that may be provoked by any of the large number of different serovars, it is necessary to use a battery of antigens—usually 24. This test does not reliably identify the infecting serovar because of frequent cross-reactivity.

A group of tests that have shown great promise rely on detecting genus-specific antibody by using a serovar of *L. biflexa* as antigen. This test has the advantage of being simple (only one antigen is needed) and safe (nonpathogenic organisms are employed). Both the IgM-specific dot-ELISA (enzyme-linked immunosorbent assay) and the genus-specific microagglutination test were shown to be effective at diagnosing leptospirosis in an endemic area.

Agglutinating antibodies generally do not reach detectable levels until the sixth to twelfth day of illness and rise to maximum levels by the third or fourth week. It is usually necessary, therefore, to obtain acute and convalescent sera; a fourfold rise in antibody titer or greater after the onset of a disease compatible with leptospirosis is considered confirmation. Genus-specific tests detect antibodies slightly earlier but may not detect antibodies late in convalescence. Single high titers (e.g., >1:400) or a positive dot-ELISA are diagnostic. Genus-specific tests are not appropriate for epidemiologic studies because of the short duration of the antibodies that they detect.

Isolation Procedures. Isolation of leptospires from blood or cerebrospinal fluid is possible during the first 10 days of clinical illness. Organisms usually appear in the urine during the second week and may persist for several months, thus permitting diagnosis by urine culture in untreated patients even after clinical illness is over. Leptospires are not difficult to isolate, provided that specialized media are used—organisms will not grow in the standard media used for isolation of pathogens from blood or urine. If specialized media are not immediately available, leptospires will remain viable for up to 11 days in blood anticoagulated with sodium oxalate. Repeated attempts at isolation will increase the diagnostic yield.

Isolations are usually made from urine, but too much urine inhibits growth. Best results are obtained by diluting 0.1 ml of urine, obtained as sterilely as possible, with 0.9 ml of buffered saline and then making 4 additional dilutions. These different concentrations are then inoculated into 5 ml of Fletcher's or EMJH semisolid medium and incubated at 28C to 30C in the dark for at least 5 to 6 weeks. For either blood or cerebrospinal fluid, the same procedures are followed beginning with from 1 to 4 drops of sample liquid. Isolates can be sent to reference centers for identification of the responsible serovar.

THERAPY

Supportive Therapy. Proper symptomatic treatment and supportive care are essential for a good outcome in cases of severe leptospirosis. Meticulous attention must be paid to fluid and electrolyte balance and patients aggressively rehydrated when necessary. Ensuring adequate renal perfusion prevents renal failure in the vast majority of oliguric individuals. Rarely, patients present late in the course of disease with symptomatic uremia and anuria. Such individuals rarely respond to conservative measures and have a high mortality rate.

Peritoneal dialysis is preferred to hemodialysis in patients who require it. Renal failure in leptospirosis is hypercatabolic, so frequent dialysis may be necessary.

Massive hemorrhage is uncommon in leptospirosis, but lesser amounts of bleeding occur frequently and decrease renal perfusion by worsening hypovolemia. A careful search should be made for sources of occult blood loss; blood should be transfused as necessary; and parenteral vitamin K should be administered in the event of a prolonged prothrombin time. Meningoencephalitis is a nonfatal but extremely unpleasant complication of *L. interrogans* infection and is thought to be of immune origin. The possible role of corticosteroids as adjunctive therapy for meningitis should be evaluated by controlled trials.

Antibiotic Treatment. A wide range of antibiotics are active against *L. interrogans* both in vitro and in experimental infections in animals. The list includes penicillin, ampicillin, the tetracyclines, some third-generation cephalosporins, and some quinolones. Whether or not antibiotics are effective in the treatment of human disease has been debated for over 40 years because of conflicting data from uncontrolled trials. However, in recent double-blind, placebo-controlled studies, doxycycline shortened the course of early leptospirosis, and intravenous penicillin decreased the duration of both symptoms and renal dysfunction in severe, late disease (Figs. 35–3 and 35–4). In these studies, antibiotics eliminated leptospiruria (Fig. 35–5). Antimicrobials may prevent the development of renal failure if the presence of leptospires in the kidney and their passage in the urine mediates the development of renal damage. Antibiotics should therefore be given to all patients with leptospirosis, regardless of when in their disease course they are seen. Doxycycline is given at doses of 100 mg orally twice a day for 1 week. Patients who are vomiting or are seriously ill require parenteral therapy. Intravenous penicillin G is administered as 1.5 million units every 6 hours for 1 week. Early reports that a Jarisch-Herxheimer reaction occurs within 4 to 6 hours after initiation of penicillin treatment have not been confirmed.

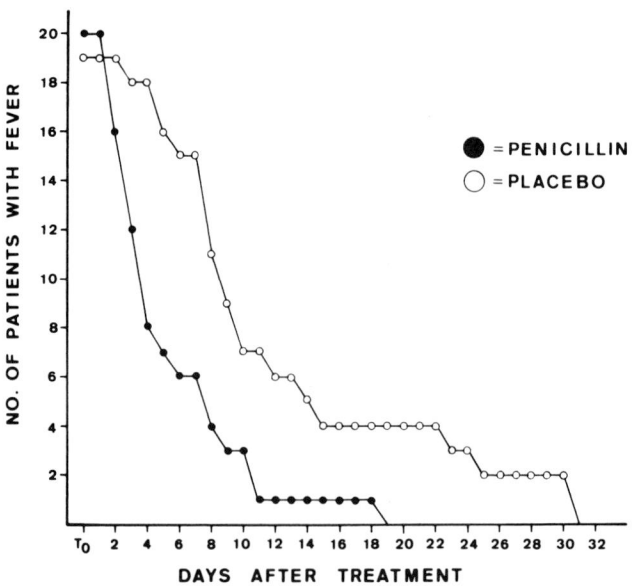

FIGURE 35–3. The effect of penicillin on the duration of fever in patients with Weil's disease. By day 4 more than half the penicillin-treated patients *(closed circles)* were afebrile, compared with only 1 of 19 patients in the placebo group *(open circles)*. (From Watt G, et al: Lancet 1:433, 1988. Reprinted by permission.)

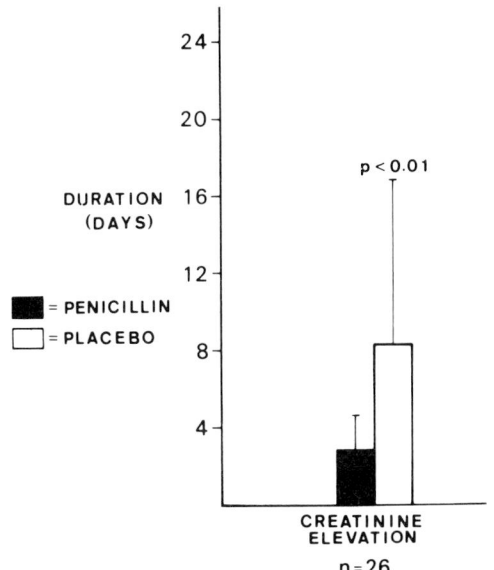

FIGURE 35–4. The duration of creatinine elevation in 26 patients with Weil's disease. Note that abnormal values persisted more than three times as long in patients who received placebo than in those who were treated with penicillin (p < 0.01).

PREVENTION. Doxycycline, 200 mg taken once a week, prevents infection by *L. interrogans*. Widespread use of doxycycline prophylaxis is not indicated, but it can benefit those who are at high risk for a short time, such as military personnel and certain agricultural workers.

Infection by leptospires confers only serovar-specific immunity—second attacks due to different serovars can occur. Vaccines directed against regionally prevalent serovars are currently used in domestic animals and serve as a useful control measure. Immunization of groups of workers with high morbidity rates has successfully protected miners in Japan and Poland as well as rice field laborers in Italy and Spain. However, the efficacy and safety of human leptospiral vaccines have yet to be conclusively demonstrated. Surface decontamination, wearing protective clothing, and rodent control are preventive methods applicable to some work environments.

Prevention of leptospirosis in the tropics is particularly difficult. The large animal reservoir of infection is impossible to eliminate, the occurrence of numerous serovars limits the usefulness of a serovar-specific vaccine, and the wearing of protective clothing (e.g., rubber boots in rice fields) is both prohibitively expensive and impractical. Improved control will result only from a rise in the standard of living and betterment in general hygiene and sanitation.

BIBLIOGRAPHY

Berman SJ, Tsai CC, Holmes KK, et al: Sporadic anicteric leptospirosis in South Vietnam. Ann Intern Med 79:167, 1973.

Deller JW, Russell PK: Fevers of unknown origin in American soldiers in Vietnam. Ann Intern Med 66:1129, 1967.

Diaz-Rivera RS, Hall HE, Ramos-Morales KY, et al: Leptospirosis in Puerto Rico. Clinical aspects of human infection. Zoonosis Res 2:159, 1963.

Edwards GA, Domm BM: Human leptospirosis. Medicine 39:117, 1960.

Faine S (ed): Guidelines for the Control of Leptospirosis. Geneva, World Health Association, 1982.

Feigin RD, Anderson DC: Human leptospirosis. CRC Crit Rev Clin Lab Sci 5:413, 1975.

Heath CW Jr, Alexander AD, Galton MM: Leptospirosis in the United States: Analysis of 483 cases in man, 1949–1961. N Engl J Med 273:857, 915, 1965.

Johnson RC: The Biology of Parasitic Spirochetes. New York, Academic Press, 1976.

McClain JBL, Ballou WR, Harrison SH, et al: Doxycycline therapy of leptospirosis. Ann Intern Med 100:696, 1984.

Pappas MG, Ballou WR, Gray MR, et al: Rapid serodiagnosis of leptospirosis using the IgM-specific dot-ELISA: comparison with the microscopic agglutination test. Am J Trop Med Hyg 34:346, 1985.

Sitprija V, Pipatanagul V, Mertowidjojo K, et al: Pathogenesis of renal disease in leptospirosis: clinical and experimental studies. Kidney Int 17:827, 1980.

Takafuji ET, Kirkpatrick JW, Miller RN, et al: An efficacy trial of doxycycline chemoprophylaxis against leptospirosis. N Engl J Med 310:497, 1984.

Watt G, Padre LP, Tuazon L, et al: Placebo-controlled trial of intravenous penicillin for severe and late leptospirosis. Lancet 1:433, 1988.

Watt G, Alquiza LM, Padre LP, et al: The rapid diagnosis of leptospirosis: a prospective comparison of the dot-ELISA and the genus-specific microscopic agglutination test at different stages of illness. J Infect Dis 157:840, 1988.

Welsh JD, Sulzer CR, Douglas HL: Leptospiral seroreactors in the Mekong delta of South Vietnam. Southeast Asian J Trop Med Public Health 3:205, 1972.

Wong ML, et al: Leptospirosis: A childhood disease. J Pediatr 90:532, 1977.

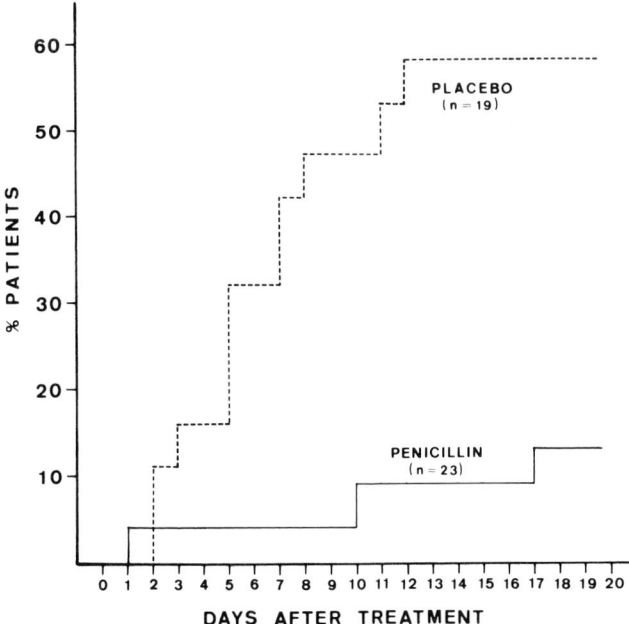

FIGURE 35–5. The cumulative percentage of patients in the same study from whom leptospires were isolated by urine culture after treatment began. Note that isolations continued to be made from the placebo group *(dotted line)*, whereas penicillin *(solid line)* prevented leptospiruria. (From Watt G, et al.: Lancet 1:433, 1988. Reprinted by permission.)

36. LYME DISEASE

Fred P. Paleologo

DEFINITION. Lyme disease is a tick-borne zoonosis caused by infection with the spirochete *Borrelia burgdorferi*. It is most commonly spread to humans by the bite of the infected nymphal stage of hard ticks (genus *Ixodes*). Major disease manifestations have been grouped into three stages: stage 1 (localized)—generalized flulike symptoms and a characteristic skin rash, erythema chronicum migrans (ECM); stage 2 (disseminated—neurologic or cardiac abnormalities, or both; and stage 3 (persistent)—arthritic manifestations that can lead to destructive joint disease in severe cases. Disease activity generally follows a fluctuating course of exacerbations and remissions.

In Europe, where disease caused by this spirochete is often called "Lyme borreliosis," additional findings of *acrodermatitis chronica atrophicans, lymphadenosis benigna cutis, and Bannwarth's syndrome (tick-borne meningopolyneuritis, also called lymphocytic meningoradiculitis)* are frequently noted.

Lyme disease, with its increasing incidence, distribution, and myriad clinical expressions, is surpassed in importance only by the acquired immunodeficiency syndrome (AIDS) as one of the most significant newly recognized diseases.

HISTORY. Lyme disease, initially described as "Lyme arthritis," was first recognized in 1975 because of an unusual incidence of arthritis in two neighboring communities. A high degree of correlation was found between recurrent bouts of arthritis and prior or concurrent presence of ECM, a rash first described in Sweden in 1909 and later thought to be secondary to spirochetal infection. Further investigations were undertaken in the index area, several communities near the town of Lyme, Connecticut, where patient histories suggested an association between ECM and tick bites.

Early detailed epidemiologic and entomologic investigations demonstrated a peak seasonal onset of disease in summer and early fall and implicated the white-tailed deer tick *Ixodes dammini* (also the vector for *Babesia microti*) and possibly other closely related tick species as vectors. Study of *I. dammini* led to the 1982 discovery of a new spirochete by Burgdorfer and Barbour. This spirochete, found in the midgut, hindgut, and rectal ampulla of the infected tick, was initially called the "*I. dammini* spirochete.*" In experimental animals, bites by infected ticks could produce a rash similar to ECM, but early investigations failed to show the spirochete in unfed tick larvae. This suggested a possible animal reservoir in the transmission cycle. The spirochete was subsequently determined to belong to the genus *Borrelia* and is now called *Borrelia burgdorferi*.

GEOGRAPHIC DISTRIBUTION. Lyme disease has been reported from 20 countries on 4 continents (North America, Europe, Australia, and Asia [Japan]), with most reported cases coming from the United States and Europe. There is also one preliminary report, based on serologic evidence, that suggests the presence of Lyme

disease in Egypt; however, the possibility of cross reactivity to other *Borrelia* species cannot be ruled out.

In the United States, indigenous cases of the disease have been reported from 43 states, and both its incidence and distribution are increasing. Three main regions are endemic for Lyme disease: the Northeast (Connecticut, Delaware, Maryland, Massachusetts, New York, New Jersey, Pennsylvania, and Rhode Island); the Midwest (Wisconsin and Minnesota); and the West (California, Oregon, Nevada, and Utah); with approximately 80% of cases being reported from the Northeast. This distribution of disease correlates with the distribution of tick vectors. Although Lyme disease is the most commonly reported vector-borne disease in the United States, Rocky Mountain spotted fever persists as the most commonly reported vector-borne disease in the southern and mountain regions (Fig. 36–1). Lyme disease is the most common arthropod-borne infection in Europe, having been reported from most countries and is a frequent zoonotic disease in much of the Soviet Union. Both wild and domestic animals are susceptible to infection, but detectable illness has been reported to occur only in domestic animals (e.g., cattle, dogs, and horses).

INCIDENCE. In a study of 1149 cases reported to the Connecticut health authorities during 1984–1986, it was determined that the overall incidence of Lyme disease among residents was 22/100,000 population with a range of 0 to 1156/100,000 in specific communities. The 5-year age-specific incidence ranged from a high of 39/100,000 population in 5- to 9-year olds to 11/100,000 in 20- to 24-year olds. Based on national data reported in 1987, the regional incidence per 100,000 population in the United States varied from a low of less than 0.1 in the mountain region to a high of 6.1 in the mid-Atlantic region. Age-specific incidence remained highest in children under 15 years of age and for those 25 to 44 years old.

In a study of Lyme disease in the United States during 1983–1984, 80% of reported cases occurred in a 4-month period between May and August, with the peak inci-

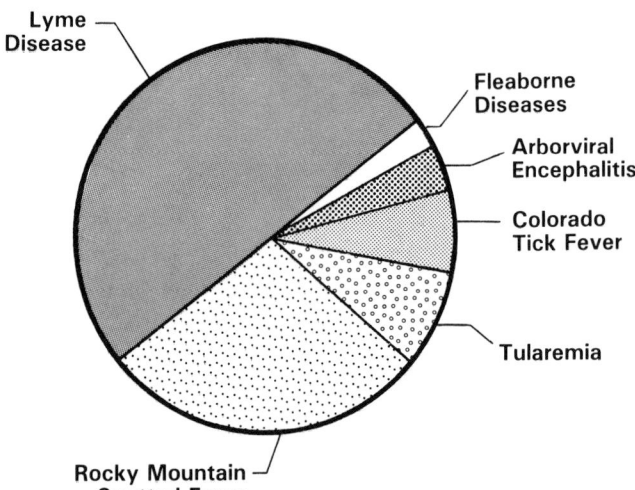

FIGURE 36–1. Reported cases of vector-borne diseases in the United States, 1983–1987. (From Morbidity and Mortality Weekly Reports. MMWR 38:670, 1989.)

dence in July. This correlated with the period of highest human exposure to the vector. In 1987–1988, it was noted that 64% of patients from the Northeast and North Central regions had onset of illness during the same period. Although 33% of patients from the Pacific region also had onset during these months, more cases occurred in this region from January through May.

ETIOLOGY. The *"I. dammini* spirochete*" (B. burgdorferi)* is the longest and narrowest of the *Borrelia* species, measuring 20 to 30 μm in length and 0.2 to 0.3 μm in transverse diameter. It has an outer membrane and 7 to 11 flagella. Data suggest that the outer membrane can undergo antigenic variation and that plasmids play a role in pathogenicity. The organism is microaerophilic and can be grown in vitro, with prolonged incubation at 33°C on a modification of Kelly's medium, a medium used to culture other *Borrelia* species. Initial clinical isolates of the spirochete came from three very different types of specimens: the blood of a patient who had been ill for 2 days with ECM and systemic symptoms; a skin biopsy of the periphery of an ECM rash present for 3½ weeks; and the cerebrospinal fluid of a patient ill for 2½ months with ECM, arthritis, and chronic meningoencephalitis. These successful isolations represented only a small percentage of the isolations attempted using patient specimens. In contrast, recovery of the organism from infected ticks was considerably easier.

TRANSMISSION

Vectors. The primary tick vector species are from the *I. ricinus* complex: *I. dammini* (white-tailed deer or northern deer tick) in the northeastern and midwestern United States (Figs. 36–2 and 112–5); *I. pacificus* (western black-legged tick) in the western United States; and *I. scapularis* (common black-legged tick), a possible vector in the southern United States. *I. ricinus* (European castor bean tick) is the primary vector in Europe, and one report of Lyme disease from Japan implicates *I. persulcatus* (taiga tick) as the probable vector. Addi-

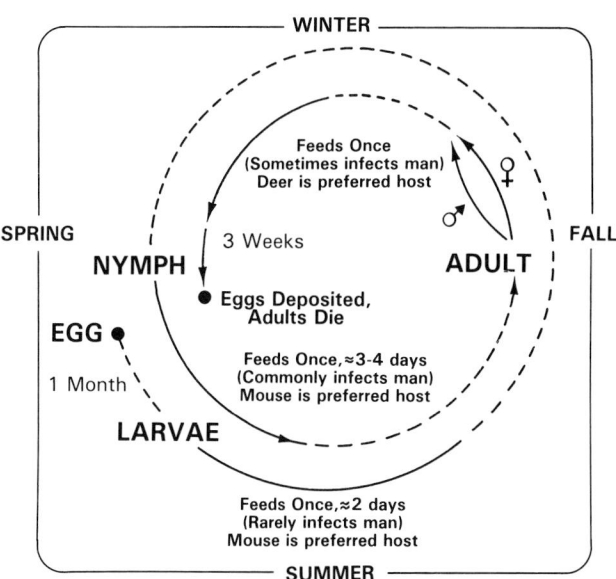

FIGURE 36–3. Schematic representation of the 2-year life cycle of *Ixodes dammini.* (Adapted from Spielman A, et al: Ann Rev Entomol 30:439, 1985. Reprinted by permission.)

tionally, *Amblyomma americanum* (Lone Star dog tick) and *Dermacentor variabilis* (wood or American dog tick) have been found to be infected with *B. burgdorferi* and may be occasional vectors in certain areas. The spirochete has been isolated from horseflies, deer flies, and mosquitoes, but the importance of these insects in the transmission cycle is unknown.

Life Cycle. Ixodids tend to be three-host ticks, with immature (larval and nymphal) and adult stages feeding on very different sizes and types of hosts. *I. dammini* was recognized as a separate species in 1979. It is a nearly uniform, brownish red tick, the adult being about the size of a sesame seed (Figs. 36–2 and 112–5). It has a 2-year developmental cycle, in which most adults both feed and mate on the deer host in October and November of the second year (Fig. 36–3). After mating, the adult females leave their host, lay their eggs, and die. The eggs produced will later hatch and develop into pinhead-sized 6-legged larvae that attach and feed during the following August through October. The 8-legged nymphs of this generation attach and feed during the following May through July. Based on data from experimental infection of rabbits, it is believed that the spirochete is most likely carried over from the nymphal stage to the adult stage in the midgut diverticula of the tick.

Tick population density decreases significantly with each successive stage, probably owing to difficulties in surviving winters and finding and feeding on a suitable host. The tick locates its host by "questing." In this behavior pattern, the tick will climb to the tip of vegetation (e.g., grass or brush), especially in areas near woods and along animal trails or paths. When a potential host comes in contact with this vegetation, the waiting tick transfers to the host and attempts to feed. Adult ticks often feed for several days. The bite is usually painless, and because of the tick's small size and coloration, it can easily go unnoticed. There are two hy-

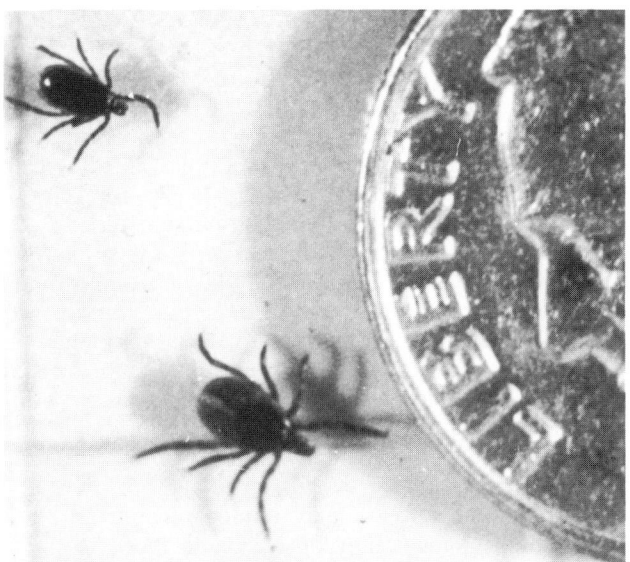

FIGURE 36–2. Adult male (upper) and female (lower) *Ixodes dammini.* (Courtesy of Dr. A. Main.)

potheses to suggest how the spirochete is inoculated into the host. The first is that in a systemically infected tick, the spirochete passes through the salivary gland into the feeding cavity to infect the host. The second is that, during feeding, the tick regurgitates into the feeding cavity, thus carrying forward spirochetes from the midgut diverticula to infect the host. Since a prolonged feeding time is required for the adult tick to infect its host, this limits its vectorial capacity and highlights the importance of early tick removal in prevention of infection.

Reservoir Hosts. Although all stages of the infected tick can spread the disease to humans, the infected nymph is most commonly associated with human infection (Fig. 36–3). While it is possible for *I. dammini* larvae to become infected transovarially, this is a rare occurrence. Instead, these ticks usually acquire *B. burgdorferi* when feeding on the infected white-footed mouse *(Peromyscus leucopus)* in its burrow. Generally, the mouse acquires the spirochete from the bite of an infected nymph. Infected mice, which have no inflammatory response to spirochetemia, then serve as the infectious reservoir for the next generation of uninfected larval ticks. This mouse species is a very competent reservoir host and the preferred host for both immature forms (larvae and nymph) of *I. dammini*. It is also the primary reservoir of *Borrelia burgdorferi* in the United States. Other reservoir hosts include many small feral mammals (e.g., squirrels, chipmunks), some birds, and possibly horses. The present list of known and potential vector and reservoir species will probably increase.

In the United States, white-tailed deer *(Odocoileus virginianus)* are the primary host for *I. dammini* adults. Infestation of white-tailed deer serves as a necessary amplification phase for the growth of the tick population. *Ixodes pacificus* is commonly found on deer in California; it also infests cattle and readily bites humans. Many believe that an increase in the number of deer in the United States during the last 50 years is the cause of the marked increase in this tick population and, consequently, the increasing incidence, prevalence, and distribution of Lyme disease. Successful feeding on this final host allows the tick to reproduce, and the mobility of the deer serves to disseminate the tick (Fig. 36–3). In a study wherein deer were eliminated from an island, a significant decrease in the tick population was noted. It took several years for all stages of the tick population to decrease, however, owing to the 2-year life cycle. Larval infestation of passerine birds can greatly disperse the tick, especially in the case of migrating birds. The unique ability of *B. burgdorferi* to infect both mammals and birds is also a factor in dissemination of this pathogen.

CLINICAL MANIFESTATIONS AND PATHOLOGY.

The clinical spectrum of Lyme disease is variable and may depend upon specific characteristics of the host and pathogen. Systemic complications are intermittent and fluctuate in severity. The disease often occurs in three stages (Table 36–1), but symptoms may not be present until late in the course of infection. It has been estimated that in the United States as many as 10% of those persons infected may be asymptomatic, whereas

TABLE 36–1. Clinical Manifestations of Lyme Disease

Stage 1	**Localized (1–3 weeks after infectious bite)**
	Flulike symptoms, fever
	Erythema chronicum migrans (ECM)
	Often undetected
Stage 2	**Disseminated (usually weeks to months later)**
	May be initial presentation
	Neurologic dysfunction
	Meningoencephalitis (chronic)
	Cranial neuropathy (Bell's palsy)
	Peripheral radiculopathy
	May have residual deficit
	Cardiac abnormalities
	Conduction defects
	Atrioventricular block
	May require pacemaker
	Myocarditis
Stage 3	**Persistent (weeks to years after onset)**
	Arthritis
	Recurrent oligoarthritis (usually large joints)
	Migratory polyarthritis
	May resolve or progress to destructive joint disease

in Europe the percentage is probably greater. Some suggest that the ratio of apparent to inapparent infection may be as high as 1:1.

Stage 1 (Localized)—Generalized Symptoms and Rash. This stage is usually the initial clinical presentation of Lyme disease and generally follows an infectious tick bite by 1 to 3 weeks. It is manifested as a flulike syndrome, with some combination of fever, headache, stiff neck, backache, sore throat, myalgias, arthralgias, regional lymphadenopathy, nausea, vomiting, malaise, or fatigue lasting 2 days to 10 weeks (median, 4 weeks) as well as development of the characteristic rash, erythema chronicum migrans.

Erythema Chronicum Migrans. ECM, also known as erythema migrans, is a macular, sometimes papular, skin lesion manifested as enlarging erythema with a paler center, less frequently with confluent erythema or a bluish center (Fig. 36–4). The lesion may be somewhat indurated and warm to the touch, but it is not painful. These lesions are often multiple and are at the sites of tick bites (Fig. 36–5). Common sites for ECM are the thigh, groin, and axilla. Later, satellite lesions may develop. The primary lesion of ECM averages 16 cm varying from 6 to 52 cm and persists for up to 10 weeks (average, 3 weeks) before fading spontaneously. The rash can persist as long as 14 months. Histologically, the skin shows edema and mononuclear cell infiltration, and spirochetes may be demonstrated on biopsy. This skin lesion represents a local reaction at the site of early replication of *B. burgdorferi*. Studies have shown that ECM in the United States is more common after infectious bites by adult as compared with larval ticks.

Laboratory Findings. The differential leukocyte count may reveal a mild lymphocytosis. An elevated erythrocyte sedimentation rate (ESR) of > 20 mm/hr is often present. Mild abnormalities in tests of liver function may also be present.

Often, Lyme disease may not be recognized at this stage. Skin changes may be absent in more than 25% of patients, and systemic symptoms may either be absent or be so subtle as to go unnoticed. Clinical findings may

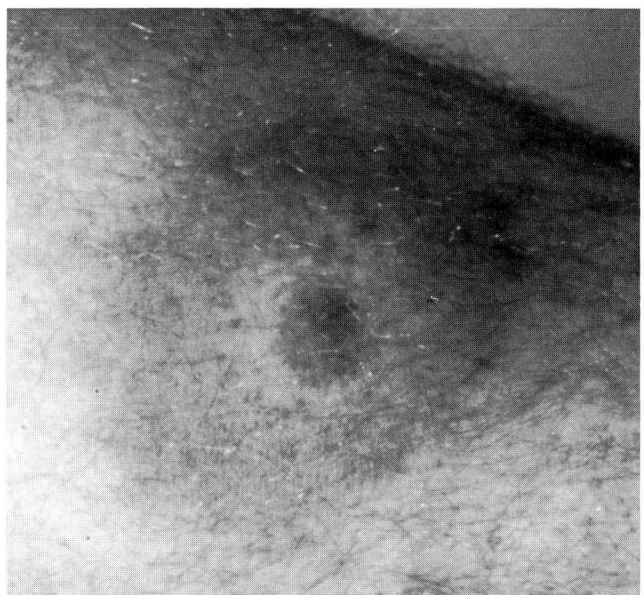

FIGURE 36–4. Erythema chronicum migrans (ECM) on the lower extremity, showing an annular erythematous lesion with central punctum, surrounded by zone of clearing and peripheral erythema. (Courtesy of the Department of Dermatology, National Naval Medical Center, Bethesda, MD.)

be attributed to another disease, especially in the absence of either a high index of suspicion or a history of tick bites or exposure to ticks.

Stage 2 (Disseminated)—Neurologic and Cardiac Manifestations. This stage tends to follow the onset of disease by weeks to months; however, patients may present with neurologic or cardiac abnormalities as the initial manifestation of their disease. Severe fatigue and malaise are common.

Neurologic Disease. Neurologic dysfunction has been associated with tick bites, both with and without ECM.

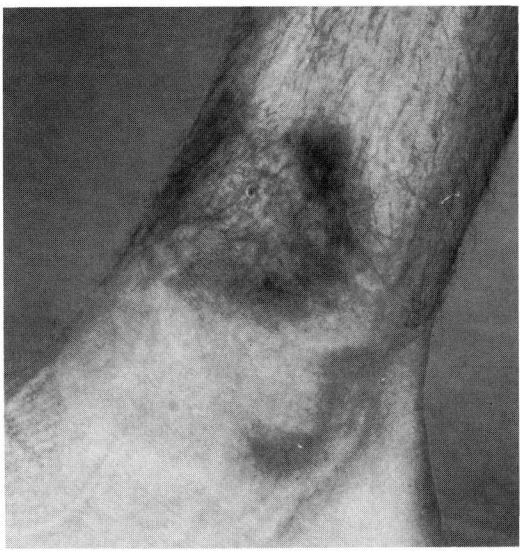

FIGURE 36–5. Erythema chronicum migrans (ECM) lesion on the ankle, showing a central punctum at the site of a tick bite, with a surrounding clear zone and peripheral erythema. (Courtesy of the Department of Dermatology, National Naval Medical Center, Bethesda, MD.)

In this stage, symptoms often begin with headache and stiff neck. Headache is often episodic but can be quite severe. When ECM occurs in the initial presentation of disease, it is often still present when symptoms of advanced disease occur. The most common neurologic finding is fluctuating meningoencephalitis, ranging in duration from 1 to 9 months, with superimposed cranial neuropathy (e.g., unilateral or bilateral facial palsies) and radiculoneuropathy. The spectrum of abnormalities may include fluctuating aseptic meningitis and encephalitis or chorea, cerebellar ataxia, cranial neuritis, motor and sensory radiculoneuritis, mononeuritis multiplex, and myelitis, either as isolated findings or in various combinations. Neurologic abnormalities may recur or become chronic.

Cardiac Disease. Cardiac findings are seen in 4 to 10% of cases and can be subtle or pronounced. Abnormalities primarily consist of conduction defects, ranging in severity from mild aberrations in conduction to fluctuating atrioventricular block or complete heart block. Myocarditis or pericarditis also may occur. Cardiac symptoms ensue at an average of 5 weeks (range, 4 days to 7 months) after the onset of disease. ECM is noted in 85% of patients who are diagnosed as having Lyme carditis. Syncope, shortness of breath, dizziness, and palpitations are common presenting signs and symptoms. Cardiac symptoms may resemble those of rheumatic fever, but in the carditis of Lyme disease, complete heart block occurs more frequently (usually in otherwise healthy young men), myopericardial involvement is usually milder, and the heart valves are not affected. The duration of cardiac involvement may be 3 to 6 weeks. Symptoms usually resolve with treatment.

Stage 3 (Persistent)—Arthritis. The arthritis of Lyme disease tends to be characterized by brief episodes of recurrent oligoarthritis of the larger joints, especially the knee, or migratory polyarthritis beginning days to months after the onset of ECM. Unlike those with rheumatoid arthritis, patients with Lyme arthritis do not have rheumatoid factor and serum antinuclear antibodies. In addition, asymmetric polyarthritis, morning stiffness, and subcutaneous nodules are rarely present in Lyme disease. Joint involvement has been mistaken for juvenile rheumatoid arthritis and suppurative arthritis. Lyme arthritis may resolve completely or progress to chronic arthritis with pannus formation and cartilage erosion. *Borrelia burgdorferi* spirochetes can be demonstrated in the tissues and joint fluid, supporting the theory that the arthritis is due, at least in part, to the persistent presence of organisms in chronic infection. The number of patients with joint involvement has been reported to decrease at a rate of 10 to 20% per year, and arthritis rarely persists for more than several years.

In the study of 1149 patients from Connecticut, 83% had ECM, 24% had arthritis, 8% had neurologic manifestations, and 2% had cardiac involvement. Among those with arthritis, the affected joint was the knee in 89%, the shoulder in 9%, the ankle in 7%, and the elbow in 2%. Arthritis was more likely to develop in patients under 20 years of age. An important finding was that the majority of patients with arthritis did not report a prior ECM rash.

GEOGRAPHIC VARIATIONS IN SYMPTOM COMPLEXES.

Like syphilis, the Lyme disease complex encompasses a broad spectrum of signs and symptoms. Basic patterns of recognized disease are similar, and, with increasing awareness, manifestations once thought unique to a specific area are being recognized in other areas.

Clinical Variation. The pattern of disease differs between Europe and the United States. ECM and neuritis are prominent features of the disease in both areas, but neurologic complications are more common in Europe. Bannwarth syndrome, a triad of meningoencephalitis, cranial neuritis, and radiculoneuritis, is often seen in Europe but not in the United States. Further, the skin manifestations of acrodermatitis chronica atrophicans (ACA), a bluish red induration that usually occurs on the skin of an extremity and progresses to atrophy, and lymphadenosis benigna cutis (LBC), a red to violaceous skin nodule thought to be associated with tick bites, are often seen in Europe but are rare in the United States and the United Kingdom. Arthritis and carditis, however, are more common in the United States. It has been suggested that the lower incidence of arthritis in Europe is due to the more frequent use of antibiotics in treating ECM in Europe. This treatment became widely practiced in the United States only in the early 1980s. Lymphocytoma has been reported from Europe as a rare finding.

Antigenic Variation. Antigenic variation between strains of *B. burgdorferi* isolated from the United States and Europe has been noted in several studies. One study noted great diversity in expression of a major spirochete protein called the outer surface protein A (OspA). Isolates from the United States and from Europe were obtained from human, animal, and tick specimens. With the use of polyacrylamide gel electrophoresis and monoclonal antibodies, 25 United States isolates, with only one exception, were found to be homogeneous in the type of OspA that they produced. This protein differed from the OspA proteins produced by 21 European isolates, a reflection of differences in genome of the isolates. Variability among isolates from the United States is increasing.

OTHER COMPLICATIONS.

A variety of other clinical problems have been attributed to infection with this spirochete. Among these are the adult respiratory distress syndrome, granulomatous hepatitis, panophthalmitis, ischemic optic neuropathy, pseudotumor cerebri, memory loss, dementia, and irreversible myelopathy. Demyelinating processes or an acute transverse myelitis, sometimes confused with multiple sclerosis, have also been reported.

A syndrome noted late in the disease, described as progressive encephalomyelitis, has been reported from Europe. Patients have spastic paraparesis, bladder dysfunction, ataxia, seventh or eighth cranial nerve deficits, dementia, or cognitive impairment.

Patients may report nonspecific complaints, especially fatigue, as lingering manifestations of infection with *B. burgdorferi*. These symptoms can be particularly frustrating and debilitating to the patient as well as posing a diagnostic and therapeutic challenge to the physician.

LYME DISEASE IN PREGNANCY.

Information regarding the effects of infection with *B. burgdorferi* during pregnancy is limited. Transplacental infection of the fetus has been demonstrated. There have been reports of intrauterine fetal demise, prematurity, birth defects (syndactyly, cortical blindness), and rash in the newborn in cases in which women developed Lyme disease during pregnancy. A causal association for these abnormalities, however, has not yet been demonstrated. There has also been one report demonstrating *B. burgdorferi* in the brain and liver of a full-term newborn who died shortly after birth. The mother had developed ECM during the second month of pregnancy and had been treated with oral penicillin. This association may be a significant consideration in evaluating the adequacy of oral therapy alone for pregnant women who develop Lyme disease. The actual incidence of complications due to infection with *B. burgdorferi* during pregnancy is not yet established.

IMMUNE RESPONSE.

Lyme disease has characteristics of both autoimmune and infectious diseases. There is a higher frequency of the histocompatibility antigen HLA-DR2 among patients with ECM who later develop arthritis. This antigen is also associated with ACA but not with Bannwarth syndrome. A significantly greater frequency of HLA-DR4, often associated with HLA-DR3 or HLA-DR2, has been demonstrated in a group of patients with arthritis who were refractory to multiple courses of antibiotic therapy. Both genetic predisposition on the part of the host and genetic variation on the part of the pathogen probably play a role in determining exact disease manifestations.

Antibody Responses. *Borrelia burgdorferi*–specific immunoglobulin M (IgM) antibody titers tend to peak in the third to sixth week of illness, but elevated titers may not be detected in early infection. Antispirochete IgG is often detected 6 weeks or more after the onset of ECM, and titers usually peak months later, often during bouts of arthritis. In one study, 94% of patients with involvement of the central nervous system, heart, or joints had IgG titers of 1:128 or greater. Similar results have been reported in patients from Europe with later manifestations of the disease (neurologic disorders and ACA). Patients with infectious mononucleosis occasionally have elevated IgG antibody titers to *B. burgdorferi*.

In studies of the immune response to this disease, it has been shown that high total IgM levels correlate with disease activity and that titers of *B. burgdorferi*–specific IgM correlate directly with total IgM levels. When ECM is present, elevated IgM levels tend to predict subsequent neurologic, cardiac, or joint involvement. During disease, elevated IgM levels are associated with a decreased number of T cells, a heightened cellular immune response, and decreased suppressor cell activity. Studies have shown serial IgM levels to be the best serologic indicator of disease activity. Generally, increased serum IgM and decreased serum IgG and IgA levels were noted with a flare of the disease, and a reverse pattern occurred during quiescent periods and resolution. Some patients treated with antibiotics may have a later flare of the disease with an associated heightened lymphoproliferative response to *B. burgdorferi* antigens without a serologic response. This may not be a specific finding, however. Antibiotic treatment early in the disease is also associated with disappearance of the specific antibody response within months of therapy, thereby making patients more susceptible to reinfection at a later time.

Complement Activity. Studies have shown abnormal serum C1q binding activity at the onset of ECM. This persisted among patients who subsequently developed arthritis and either neurologic or cardiac complications. In those patients who developed only arthritis, abnormal serum C1q binding activity tended to disappear, but abnormal binding was always present in the synovial fluid of affected joints and at higher levels than in serum. This synovial activity correlated with the concentration of synovial fluid granulocytes but not with intra-articular levels of CH_{50}, C3, or C4. The physical properties of the C1q reactive material were consistent with antigen-antibody complexes of high affinity. This supports the belief that ECM is the initial manifestation of an immune-mediated inflammatory reaction associated with immune complexes. Serum complement levels and activity are decreased with systemic involvement.

DIAGNOSIS
Clinical Findings. The history of a tick bite or the occurrence of ECM is a very helpful clue to the diagnosis, but the tick bite often goes unnoticed and ECM may be unnoticed, misdiagnosed, or absent. This highlights the importance of epidemiologic association and clinical suspicion in diagnosing this potentially serious but treatable infectious disease.

Histopathology and Culture. Direct demonstration of the organism by special staining of human biopsy specimens or by culture is possible but difficult. Skin biopsies taken from the outer edge of the ECM lesion and stained with the Warthin-Starry or Dieterle silver impregnation method may reveal organisms in more than half the cases. Isolation of the organism by blood culture is successful in less than 10% of cases.

In patients with myocarditis, Dieterle silver impregnation stains of endomyocardial biopsy specimens may detect sparse spirochetes in the myocardium and cardiac blood vessels. Histopathology studies reveal a lymphocytic infiltrate. Active myocarditis can be demonstrated by gallium-67 citrate (Ga-67) radioisotope scanning in both children and adults.

Serology. Serologic tests are the most important means of confirming the diagnosis of Lyme disease. The indirect fluorescent antibody test (IFA), an enzyme-linked immunosorbent assay (ELISA), and the microscopic agglutination (MA) test all have a high degree of cross-reactivity with sera from patients with Lyme disease, louse-borne or tick-borne relapsing fevers (Chapter 34). This is probably due to the presence of shared antigens. *Borrelia burgdorferi* organisms also share common flagellar polypeptide antigens with treponemes. Sera from patients with Lyme disease can give a false positive reaction in the fluorescent treponemal antibody absorption test (FTA-ABS) for syphilis; however, the Venereal Disease Research Laboratories (VDRL) test usually remains negative. The VDRL test, as well as

the rapid plasma reagin (RPR) test for syphilis, can be helpful in distinguishing between these two spirochetal infections (Chapter 32.1).

There is also serologic evidence that in areas endemic for both Lyme disease and babesiosis, patients are concurrently exposed to both organisms and may be doubly infected by the common vector, *I. dammini* (Chapter 77). Some have recommended testing for both diseases when either is diagnosed.

In a study of patients with ECM, the sensitivity of serology was 30% by IFA and 24% by ELISA. When serum was obtained 21 or more days after onset of symptoms, the sensitivity of tests increased to 45% (IFA) and 32% (ELISA). Serologic diagnosis early in the disease is difficult at best, and caution in interpreting results is necessary. Diagnostic sensitivity and specificity in early disease is improving with use of newer IgM antibody-capture enzyme immunoassays and confirmatory Western blot analysis.

The problems with sensitivity of serologic tests, cross-reactivity, lack of standardization between tests and among different laboratories performing the same test, and the wide clinical spectrum of Lyme disease highlight the importance of epidemiologic history and clinical correlation. New sensitive and specific diagnostic methods, such as the DNA polymerase chain reaction (PCR) to detect *B. burgdorferi* DNA, hold promise for the future.

TREATMENT. In an early study, it was found that treatment with oral penicillin or tetracycline significantly decreased the time required for resolution of ECM, but treatment with erythromycin did not. Penicillin also appeared to prevent or attenuate subsequent arthritis. Later studies showed that patients treated with tetracycline were less likely to develop neurologic, cardiac, or joint manifestations. Jarisch-Herxheimer reactions can complicate the antibiotic therapy of Lyme disease. In one study, this occurred in 4 of 66 cases (6%). Milder forms of this reaction may occur much more commonly, but this is not usually a significant clinical problem.

The duration of therapy for all stages of Lyme disease should be guided by clinical response. Antibiotic therapy to prevent or cure the later stages is not always successful, and treatment failures may occur with any of the present regimens. Since treatment regimens continue to be improved, clinicians should keep abreast of current recommendations.

Stage 1 Disease
Antibiotic Therapy. The recommended treatment for men, nonpregnant women, and children more than 8 years old with stage 1 Lyme disease is 250 to 500 mg oral tetracycline four times a day for 10 to 30 days, with duration of therapy depending on clinical response. Oral doxycycline in a dose of 100 mg twice daily for adults is also effective. For younger children, therapy with amoxicillin (40 mg/kg/day) in divided doses for the same duration has been recommended. Phenoxymethyl penicillin (50 mg/kg/day) is an alternative. Depending on the severity and duration of symptoms and the response to therapy, a higher dosage and longer duration of therapy may be appropriate. In the case of penicillin allergy or contraindication to treatment with tetracycline

compounds, erythromycin 30 mg/kg/day for 15 to 30 days has been recommended to prevent later stages of the disease, but this regimen may be less effective.

Pregnant or lactating women may be given amoxicillin. It is not clear whether oral antibiotic therapy alone is sufficient to prevent problems consequent to fetal infection. Many authors recommend parenteral antibiotic therapy if Lyme disease develops during pregnancy.

Stage 2 Disease

Antibiotic Therapy. High-dose intravenous penicillin G was the first therapy shown to have a highly beneficial effect in treatment of severe complications of Lyme disease. Recently, parenteral ceftriaxone in a dose of 1 to 2 gm twice daily for 14 days was reported to be effective in patients with chronic sequelae of Lyme disease whose fatigue, arthritis, or peripheral nervous system manifestations had proved refractory to treatment with high-dose penicillin. The very long half-life of ceftriaxone and its ability to penetrate both normal and inflamed meninges are believed to be important factors in its high rate of success. For treatment of mild neurologic symptoms, oral doxycycline, tetracycline, or amoxicillin may be used at the same dosage as for stage 1 disease, with a treatment duration of at least 1 month. High-dose intravenous penicillin (20 million units penicillin G/day in divided doses for 10 days) decreased the time required for resolution of meningeal symptoms to 1 week, compared with an average of 29 weeks in a group of patients treated with prednisone alone. In both groups an average of 7 to 8 weeks was required for complete recovery from motor deficits.

Current recommendations for treatment of serious neurologic disease are for intravenous penicillin G, 20 to 24 million units/day in divided doses for 10 to 14 days. Intravenous ceftriaxone in a dose of 2 gm/day for 14 days also may be effective. For isolated facial palsy or ACA, oral regimens may be used.

Anti-inflammatory Therapy. Studies have shown that corticosteroids rapidly suppress meningeal symptoms but do not affect established parenchymal lesions that may leave patients with residual muscle weakness. Therapy with prednisone appears to hasten resolution of carditis and may decrease conduction defects; however, use of nonsteroidal anti-inflammatory agents or aspirin is the preferred therapy in the absence of meningoencephalitis, complete atrioventricular block for longer than 1 week, or deterioration of cardiac function with cardiomegaly.

Therapy of Cardiac Complications. Complete heart block usually resolves in 7 to 10 days with antibiotic therapy, but some less life-threatening conduction defects may persist. In patients with high-degree atrioventricular block, hospitalization with continuous cardiac monitoring and aggressive antibiotic therapy is recommended. Temporary cardiac pacemaker insertion is often necessary. Antibiotic therapy with 2 gm/day of intravenous ceftriaxone (80 mg/kg/day in children) or 20 to 24 million units intravenous penicillin G/day (250,000 units/kg/day in children) should be given for 10 to 21 days, depending on clinical response. The oral antibiotic regimens for early disease may be used in patients who

have only first-degree atrioventricular block with a PR interval less than 0.30 seconds and who have no other symptoms. Close clinical follow-up is appropriate.

Stage 3 Disease

Antibiotic Therapy. Treatment of established arthritis with penicillin produces clinical improvement. However, studies showed that only 7 of 20 patients given 2.4 million units of benzathine penicillin/week, for 3 weeks were cured, and only 11 of 20 treated with high-dose intravenous penicillin G were cured. Those patients who had previous antibiotic treatment for ECM as well as those who had never received intra-articular corticosteroids showed a better response. Treatment of Lyme arthritis with intravenous ceftriaxone or penicillin G, in the same regimens as used for severe cardiac abnormalities, has been recommended. Patients with less severe disease may benefit from a 1-month course of oral doxycycline or amoxicillin, but the clinical response may be delayed.

PREVENTION AND CONTROL

Tick Control. Foremost in the prevention of Lyme disease is avoidance of potentially infectious tick bites (Chapter 112). In tick-infested areas, margins of trails, brush, and grassy areas should be avoided. Grass should be kept mown, and the brush along trails, near buildings, and in other areas that people frequent should be removed. Clothing can be an effective barrier. Wearing long pants and long-sleeved shirts and tucking shirt tails into pants and pant legs into boots or socks will decrease the access of ticks to sites where they can feed. Wearing light-colored clothes facilitates detection and removal of ticks, since they are easier to see. Tick repellents applied to pants, socks, and shoes may also be helpful.

Frequent inspection of the skin for ticks is important. Prompt removal of an infected tick may prevent disease transmission. Ticks should not be grasped or removed with the fingers. Instead, they should be gently removed with forceps or tweezers by grasping as close as possible to the skin surface. The mouth parts should be gently and steadily pulled straight away from the skin, taking care not to twist or jerk the tick. If the tick body ruptures or parts of the tick remain embedded in the skin, a physician should be consulted. The tick should not be crushed but rather placed in alcohol or other disinfectant for disposal. The bite should be cleaned with soap and water and the hands of the person removing the tick thoroughly washed. An antiseptic should be applied to the site of the tick bite and any contaminated surfaces. The same procedure should be used when removing ticks from animals.

Reservoir Control. White-tailed deer are the primary host of the adult tick and are believed to be essential for the development of large populations of *I. dammini.* Elimination of deer from an infested area has been shown to greatly reduce the tick population and may provide an effective means of control.

Widespread application of insecticides has not proved an effective means of controlling ticks. Recently, a simple device, consisting of a small cardboard tube filled with cotton impregnated with the acaricide permethrin, has been used in areas where the agents of Lyme disease and babesiosis are enzootic. The white-footed mouse, the primary host for immature stages of *I. dammini*, actively accumulates the impregnated cotton as nesting material for its burrow, where immature (larval) ticks are concentrated. Larval ticks are killed by contact with the acaricide-impregnated cotton during feeding or when they drop from the mouse onto the treated cotton. Laboratory-reared *I. dammini* failed to attach to wild caught mice from treated areas, and most of these experimentally exposed ticks died. In field tests, this method has decreased the overall prevalence of infected ticks by 72%. In contrast, this treatment had no effect on the rate of infestation of voles *(Microtus pennsylvanicus)*, which do not use the cotton as a nesting material.

Permethrin, when applied to clothing, will not repel questing adult ticks; however, brief exposures to treated clothing can make all stages of the tick moribund.

BIBLIOGRAPHY

Barbour AG: The diagnosis of Lyme disease: Rewards and perils. Ann Intern Med 110:501–502, 1989.

Benach JL, Coleman JL, Skinner RA, et al: Adult *Ixodes dammini* on rabbits: A hypothesis for the development and transmission of *Borrelia burgdorferi*. J Infect Dis 155:1300–1306, 1987.

Burgdorfer W, Barbour AG, Hayes SF, et al: Lyme disease—A tick-borne spirochetosis? Science 216:1317–1319, 1982.

Craft JE, Grodzicki RL, Steere AC: Antibody response in Lyme disease: Evaluation of diagnostic tests. J Infect Dis 149:789–795, 1984.

Dattwyler RJ, Halperin JJ, Pass H, et al: Ceftriaxone as effective therapy in refractory Lyme disease. J Infect Dis 155:1322–1325, 1987.

Dattwyler RJ, Volkman DJ, Luft BJ, et al: Seronegative Lyme disease: Dissociation of specific T- and B-lymphocyte responses to *B. burgdorferi*. N Engl J Med 319:1441–1446, 1988.

Donahue JG, Piesman J, Spielman A: Reservoir competence of white-footed mice for Lyme disease spirochetes. Am J Trop Med Hyg 36:92–96, 1987.

Duffy J, Mertz LE: Serologic testing for Lyme disease. Ann Intern Med 103:458, 1985.

Duray PH: Clinical pathologic correlations of Lyme disease. Rev Infect Dis (Suppl) 6:S1487–S1493, 1989.

Lastavica CC, Wilson ML, Berardi VP, et al: Rapid emergence of a focal epidemic of Lyme disease in coastal Massachusetts. N Engl J Med 320:133–137, 1989.

Lyme Disease—United States, 1987 and 1988. MMWR 38:668–672, 1989.

Magnarelli LA, Anderson JF, Johnson RC: Cross-reactivity in serological tests for Lyme disease and other spirochetal infections. J Infect Dis 156:183–188, 1987.

Markowitz LE, Steere AC, Benach JL, et al: Lyme disease during pregnancy. JAMA 255:3394–3396, 1986.

McAlister HF, Klementowicz PT, Andrews B, et al: Lyme carditis: An important cause of reversible heart block. Ann Intern Med 110:339–345, 1989.

Moffat CM, Sigal LH, Steere AC, et al: Cellular immune findings in Lyme disease. Am J Med 77:625–632, 1984.

Muhlemann MF, Wright DJM: Emerging pattern of Lyme disease in the United Kingdom and Irish Republic. Lancet 1:260–262, 1987.

Reik L, Burgdorfer W, Donaldson JO: Neurologic abnormalities in Lyme disease without erythema chronicum migrans. Am J Med 81:73–78, 1986.

Ryberg B: Bannwarth's syndrome (lymphocytic meningoradiculitis) in Sweden. Yale J Biol Med 57:499–503, 1984.

Schmid GP: The global distribution of Lyme disease. Rev Infect Dis 7:41–50, 1985.

Spielman A, Clifford CM, Piesman J, et al: Human babesiosis on Nantucket Island, USA: Description of the vector, *Ixodes* (Ixodes *dammini*, n. sp. (Acarina: *Ixodidae*). J Med Entomol 15:218–234, 1979.

Steere AC: Lyme disease. N Engl J Med 321:586–596, 1989.

Steere AC, Bartenhagen NH, Craft JE, et al: The early clinical manifestations of Lyme disease. Ann Intern Med 99:76–82, 1983.

Steere AC, Grodzicki RL, Kornblatt AN, et al: The spirochetal etiology of Lyme disease. N Engl J Med 308:733–740, 1983.

Steere AC, Schoen RT, Taylor E: The clinical evolution of Lyme arthritis. Ann Intern Med 107:725–731, 1987.

Steere AC, Taylor E, Wilson ML: Longitudinal assessment of the clinical and epidemiological features of Lyme disease in a defined population. J Infect Dis 154:295–300, 1986.

Treatment of Lyme disease: Med Lett Drugs Ther 31:57–60, 1989.

Weber K, Bratzke H-J, Neubert U, et al: *Borrelia burgdorferi* in a newborn despite oral penicillin for Lyme borreliosis during pregnancy. Pediatr Infect Dis J 7:286–289, 1988.

Wilson ML, Telford SL, Piesman J, et al: Reduced abundance of immature *Ixodes dammini* (Acari: *Ixodidae)* following elimination of deer. J Med Entomol 24:224–228, 1988.

SECTION D

ENTERIC BACTERIAL INFECTIONS

GENERAL PRINCIPLES

Karen L. Kotloff and David R. Nalin

Bacterial diarrhea is a leading cause of death in children. The burden of disease occurs in developing countries, where there are insufficient food supplies, poor sanitation and hygiene, undereducation, and lack of access to health services. Under such conditions, diarrhea and malnutrition interact synergistically and lead to high childhood mortality rates (Chapter 109.1).

EPIDEMIOLOGY

Global Impact of Diarrhea. In the developing world, it has been estimated that more than 1 billion episodes of diarrhea occur each year and result in 4 million to 5 million deaths in children less than 5 years old. An infant or toddler living in Africa, Asia, or Latin America may experience up to 10 episodes of diarrhea per year (median 3.3). Although most illnesses are mild, nearly 5% require hospitalization, and 0.4 to 0.8% are fatal. Death occurs chiefly from dehydration, but underlying malnutrition markedly reduces the child's ability to survive a diarrheal illness.

Age Incidence. The overall incidence of diarrhea peaks in the 6- to 24-month age group and declines slowly thereafter. Similarly, mortality is highest under the age of 2 years; about 20 deaths per 1000 children younger than 2 years occur each year in the developing world. Factors that influence the age-related incidence of diarrhea are the duration of breast feeding, introduction of foods that may be contaminated with pathogens, presence or absence of maternal transplacental antibodies, and immunity related to previous exposure.

The likelihood of infection with specific pathogens may vary according to age. Whereas the peak incidence of *Escherichia coli* diarrhea occurs in the first year of life, shigellosis and cholera are more likely to occur in 2- to 4-year-olds. The peak incidence of typhoid fever is in the school-age and adolescent years. Factors specific to each pathogen, such as reservoir and infectious dose, may also influence age-specific attack rates. In some instances, the presence of pathogen-specific intestinal receptors may be developmentally regulated. For example, in animal models the appearance of intestinal binding sites, such as the glycolipid receptors for Shiga toxin and the carbohydrate binding moiety for *Clostridium difficile* toxin, is age-related and coincides with the time at which the species first becomes susceptible to the effects of the toxin.

Reservoirs and Sources of Contamination. *Salmonella, Yersinia,* and *Campylobacter* have animal reservoirs and may be transmitted to humans by contact with the feces of fowl or other domestic animals or by ingestion of undercooked foods of animal origin. Vibrios naturally exist in estuarine environments, while man is the only known reservoir for shigellosis. Largely because of its low infectious dose, *Shigella* is most often spread by direct person-to-person contact, especially in settings of limited available water and poor personal hygiene. Perhaps the single most important mode of transmission of enteric organisms to young children is contamination of weaning foods; this can result from inadequate heating of contaminated food and water or delayed consumption of foods after boiling, as well as the use of contaminated bottles and utensils. Houseflies may also disseminate enteric pathogens in warm climates.

CLINICAL FEATURES OF DIARRHEA. The prevailing symptom resulting from enteric bacterial infection is diarrhea, which is generally defined as an increase in the fluidity and frequency of stools. Passage of 3 or more loose or watery stools in a 24-hour period is a commonly accepted definition. However, because healthy infants may produce stools that are unformed and of variable frequency, it is important to consider the mother's impression of what constitutes diarrhea for her child. Two forms of diarrhea are commonly described: *acute watery diarrhea (AWD),* defined as stools of grade III or greater consistency (Table III D–1), possibly leading to dehydration if loss of fluid and electrolytes exceeds replacement; and *dysentery,* which refers to the presence of blood and mucus in the stools, often accompanied by high fever, chills, convulsions, or tenesmus in severe cases. *Persistent* or *prolonged diarrhea* has been operationally defined as an episode lasting at least 14 days, although it must be kept in mind that the duration of acute diarrhea represents a continuum, with most episodes ending within 7 days.

The stool-grading system shown in Table III D–1 has proved clinically useful for guiding therapy and for determining prognosis in AWD. Volunteer studies have revealed that stool consistency proceeds from grade I to grade V as AWD progresses and gradually reverses as diarrhea wanes. Grade V (rice-water) stools are totally watery and translucent, as is seen with cholera gravis.

DEHYDRATION. The loss of body water and electrolytes in excess of replacement leads to dehydration. If losses continue, acidosis, cardiovascular collapse, and death may ensue. For several reasons, young infants are particularly susceptible to dehydration. First, they have a greater surface area per kilogram, which results in increased relative losses of water through transpiration and diarrhea. Second, the concentrating mechanism of the young infant's kidneys may be immature and less able to conserve water. Last, the thirsty infant must depend on others to provide adequate fluid replacement.

Correlation between clinical signs and the degree of dehydration (Table III D–2) can be variable, but clinical experience suggests that once the child has signs of dehydration, at least 5% of body weight has been lost. Clinical estimation of the degree of dehydration is helpful in determining fluid deficit for replacement therapy if previous weight measurements are not available for calculating the percentage of weight lost (Table III D–2). The amount of fluid in milliliters to be replaced should equal the estimated weight deficit in grams.

Concurrent conditions that may aggravate net fluid losses include fever, vomiting, high ambient temperature, and voluntary withholding of fluids as an ill-advised therapeutic measure. Stool electrolyte composition is more closely related to the rate of purging than to specific etiology (Table III D–3). Hypernatremia may result from excess free water loss and/or replacement of losses with hypertonic solutions, most notably hypertonic solutions of nonabsorbable composition. Conversely, excess intake of free water may lead to hyponatremia. Ingestion of potassium-free liquids during diarrhea can cause hypokalemia. A sometimes fatal manifestation seen occasionally in children with AWD is hypoglycemia, which may be related to starvation.

MALNUTRITION AND POSTINFECTIOUS MALABSORPTION. Infectious diarrhea has a marked adverse effect on the growth of children (Chapter 109.1). Events occurring during diarrhea that may lead to a decreased availability of nutrients include catabolism, reduced dietary intake, vomiting, accelerated intestinal transit time, loss of endogenous nutrients through the injured gut epithelium, decreased levels of digestive enzymes, and malabsorption. These energy losses may be further accentuated by increased caloric requirements imposed by fever and other metabolic responses to infection. The annual weight loss attributable to diarrhea has been estimated at 25 to 75% of expected annual

TABLE III D–1. Stool Grading System

I. Normal formed
II. Soft formed
III. Semiliquid, takes shape of container
IV. Totally watery, few particles, opaque
V. Totally watery, translucent ("rice-water")

weight gain, and nutritional supplementation must be provided to replenish the deficit and permit catch-up growth. Given the added problem of insufficient food supplies in areas where weanling diarrhea rates are high, it is not surprising that malnutrition is prevalent. The ill-advised practice of withholding food during diarrheal illnesses can exacerbate this condition.

The child with malnutrition, in turn, may experience more severe and more prolonged episodes of diarrhea compared with the well-nourished child and is 2 to 8 times more likely to die from one of these illnesses. Decreased gastric acidity, lowered gut motility, reduced mitotic index of mucosal cells, and defects in cell-mediated immune function and IgA secretion may contribute to the increased risk and severity of intestinal infection in the malnourished state.

Mucosal injury seen especially with invasive enteropathogens is associated with malabsorption. Diminished lactose, D-xylose, folate, and vitamin B_{12} absorption may persist after each attack. However, recent studies suggest that milk and cereal mixtures, lactose-free diets, and human milk are well tolerated during episodes of diarrhea and may, in fact, hasten intestinal healing, shorten the duration of illness, and improve nutritional outcome. On the other hand, feeding undiluted lactose-containing nonhuman milk as the sole nutrient to children with persistent diarrhea has resulted in greater purging and risk of dehydration in some individuals. Determining optimal refeeding regimens for acute and persistent diarrhea is thus an important area for future research.

ETIOLOGY. The development of new laboratory techniques has made it possible to identify an enteropathogen in most clinically significant diarrheal illnesses.

TABLE III D–2. Clinical Features of Dehydration

Mild Dehydration
≤5% body weight loss
Alert
Thirsty, mucosa may be slightly dry

Moderate Dehydration
6–10% body weight loss
Sleepy or irritable
Tachypnea and tachycardia
Thirsty, dry mouth, decreased urine output
Sunken eyes and fontanelle
Absent tears
Diminished skin turgor

Severe Dehydration
>10% dehydration
Very weak, sleepy, or obtunded
Tachypnea, hyperpnea, tachycardia with weak or absent pulse, hypotension
Very dry mouth, anuria
Eyes dry and sunken, very depressed fontanelle
Absent tears
Markedly diminished skin turgor

TABLE III D–3. Electrolyte Composition in Diarrhea of Various Etiologies

	Concentrations (mmol/L) in Stool			
Etiology	Na^+	K^+	Cl^-	HCO_3^-
Rotavirus	37	38	22	6
ETEC	53	37	24	18
Pediatric cholera	88	30	86	32
Adult cholera	135	15	100	44

Many bacterial agents have been reported to have possible associations with diarrheal disease (Table III D–4), but 6 genera are of major public health importance: *Salmonella* (Chapter 39), *Shigella* (Chapter 37), *Campylobacter* (Chapter 41.2), *Yersinia* (Chapter 41.3), *Vibrio* (Chapter 40), and the diarrheagenic classes of *E. coli* (enterotoxigenic *E. coli* [ETEC], enteropathogenic *E. coli* [EPEC], enteroinvasive *E. coli* [EIEC], enterohemorrhagic *E. coli* [EHEC], and a recently described but less well characterized class of enteroaggravative *E. coli* [EAggEC]) (Chapter 41.1). Two other putative enteropathogens, *Aeromonas hydrophila* and *Pleisiomonas shigelloides*, have been the object of much interest, but their role as human enteropathogens remains controversial. The epidemiologic importance of each pathogen varies with the age of the host, season, geographic locale, and clinical presentation.

Endemic Diarrhea in Infants and Children. The etiology and epidemiology of diarrheal illness can best be determined by conducting prospective community-based surveillance. Such studies have shown that worldwide ETEC is the single most common cause of diarrhea among children less than 5 years of age. In Bangladesh and Brazil ETEC was demonstrated in 20 to 30% of all diarrheal episodes and caused 2 to 3 episodes per child during the first year of life. Other bacterial agents of

TABLE III D–4. Etiologic Agents of Bacterial Enteritis in Man

Established Pathogens
Bacillus cereus
Campylobacter species
Clostridium difficile
Clostridium perfringes
Enterohemorrhagic *Escherichia coli*
Enteroinvasive *Escherichia coli*
Enteropathogenic *Escherichia coli*
Enterotoxigenic *Escherichia coli*
Salmonella species
Shigella species
Staphylococcus aureus
Vibrio cholerae
Vibrio parahaemolyticus
Yersinia enterocoliticia

Newly Recognized and Possible Pathogens
Aeromonas hydrophilia
Bacteroides fragilis
Citrobacter freundii
Edwardsiella tarda
Enteroaggregative *Escherichia coli*
Escherichia coli with diffuse adherence to HEp-2 cells
Klebsiella species
Kluyvera species
Plesiomonas shigelloides
Other *Vibrio* species

importance in the community, namely *Shigella, Campylobacter,* and EPEC, each account for 5 to 15% of episodes in countries such as Bangladesh, Brazil, and Peru.

Acute Dehydrating Diarrhea in Infants and Children. When episodes of acute dehydrating diarrhea have been examined, ETEC has been a leading cause of illness, surpassed only by rotavirus. Together these two agents were found in more than 70% of life-threatening dehydrating illnesses in Bangladesh. While many other bacterial agents can produce dehydration, EPEC, *Campylobacter* spp., and *Shigella* spp. are most frequently encountered.

Persistent Diarrhea and Malnutrition. Most of the bacterial agents capable of causing acute diarrhea have also been found in patients with persistent diarrhea. Two groups of organisms have been identified in children with persistent diarrhea: (1) those that are isolated with similar frequency from episodes of acute and prolonged diarrhea, suggesting that they are not especially able to induce prolonged illness. These include *Shigella,* ETEC, nontyphoidal *Salmonella, Campylobacter,* and *Aeromonas;* and (2) those that are isolated with greater frequency from episodes of prolonged diarrhea, suggesting a propensity to induce prolonged illness; these include EPEC, EAggEC, and the protozoan *Cryptosporidium* (Chapter 70). Another possible etiology of persistent diarrhea is colonization of the upper bowel with flora normally found in the distal intestine, thus interfering with the secreting and absorbing areas of the jejunum and ileum. The negative impact of persistent diarrhea on nutritional status has been established in many studies, but whether particular pathogens cause malnutrition independent of their association with persistent diarrhea is unknown.

Diarrhea-Associated Mortality. Pathogen-specific diarrheal mortality rates were estimated by the Institute of Medicine in 1984 for children less than 5 years of age in Africa, Asia, Latin America, and Oceania. The fatality rate per 1000 treated cases was estimated to be 1.8 for ETEC diarrhea, 4.0 for shigellosis, and 15.7 for endemic and pandemic cholera in Asia and Africa. Substantial reductions in mortality due to ETEC and cholera are expected with proper use of oral rehydration therapy.

Pandemic Diarrhea. The toll of endemic diarrhea on public health is further increased by the scourge of severe illness associated with pandemics of *Vibrio cholerae* 01 (Chapter 40.1) and *Shigella dysenteriae* type 1 (Chapter 37). These pandemics have been spreading across Africa, Asia, and Oceania since recrudescing in the 1960s. High attack rates of severe illness are seen in all age groups when previously unexposed populations are affected.

Traveler's Diarrhea. While regional differences exist in the relative importance of various agents, most cases of diarrhea in travelers and foreign residents in developing countries are attributable to bacterial enteropathogens (Chapters 3 and 117). Overall, ETEC is the predominant agent seen, but other important pathogens include *Shigella, Campylobacter, Salmonella,* EPEC, EIEC, and in some settings nonbacterial agents such as

rotavirus (Chapter 18.2), *Giardia* (Chapter 69), and *Cryptosporidium.*

Diarrhea in AIDS. Diarrhea is a common complication of AIDS both in Africa and in Western countries (Chapter 15.1). In Africa, chronic diarrhea associated with wasting is a common presenting feature of AIDS and has been termed "slim disease." The principal agents responsible for this illness are *Cryptosporidium, Isospora* (Chapter 71.2), atypical mycobacteria (Chapter 61.2), *Salmonella,* and cytomegalovirus, but other bacterial enteropathogens such as *Campylobacter* and *Shigella* have been found. Complications associated with bacterial enteritis, including bacteremia, persistent infection, and relapse, occur with increased frequency in persons with AIDS.

PATHOGENESIS. Following ingestion, the organism must reach the intestinal lumen and proliferate, thus overcoming natural host defenses which include gastric acidity, intestinal motility, competing intestinal flora, local mucin production, bile salts, and systemic and local secretory antibody. The competence of host defenses may be modulated by numerous factors, including age, state of nutrition, concurrent infections, immunologic history, and genetic susceptibilities. Normal gastric acidity is a potent barrier against gut colonization by acid-sensitive organisms, which require large infective inocula when water is the vehicle, e.g., 10^{11} *V. cholerae* or 10^5 *Salmonella typhi,* doses far exceeding surface water counts. However, in the presence of conditions associated with hypochlorhydria, such as malnutrition, or when ingested with certain alkaline foods or acid-inhibiting diets, the infective inoculum of acid-sensitive organisms such as *V. cholerae, E. coli,* and *Salmonella* is reduced and the risk of infection increased.

Pathogenic bacteria possess multiple virulence factors (Table III D–5). These factors permit gut colonization, alteration of intestinal ion-transport processes, destruction of intestinal cells either by direct invasion or by elaboration of toxins, and, as occurs with *S. typhi* and *Salmonella paratyphi,* mucosal penetration, without destruction, to produce systemic illness. In the sections that follow, general concepts regarding pathogenesis of bacterial enteric infection will be presented.

Pathologic Site. The enteric bacterial infections can be classified by the anatomic region of the intestinal tract that is their chief target (Table III D–6). In general, noninvasive enterotoxigenic pathogens, e.g., *V. chol-*

TABLE III D–5. Some Virulence Factors of Enteric Bacteria

Adhesins and fimbrial colonization factors
Acid resistance
Motility
Ability to utilize nutrients
Immunosuppression (cholera toxin)
Gut flora suppressor substances (colicins)
Mucinase
Factors making binding sites available (neuraminidase)
Enterotoxin, endotoxin, and cytotoxin
Invasiveness
Pyrogenicity
Emetogenic substances
Immunolytic enzymes (IgA protease)
Modulators of gut motility

TABLE III D–6. Small Bowel Versus Large Bowel Diarrhea

	Proximal Bowel Diarrhea (Small Intestine)	Distal Bowel Diarrhea (Ileocolonic)
Etiologic Agents (partial list)		
Bacteria	*Vibrio cholerae* *Vibrio parahaemolyticus* *Escherichia coli*	*Shigella* species *Salmonella* species *Escherichia coli* *Yersinia enterocolitica* *Campylobacter jejuni*
Protozoa	*Giardia lamblia*	*Entamoeba histolytica*
Viruses	Rotavirus 27 nm viruses	Unknown
Mechanism	Chiefly enterotoxic, noninvasive, affects epithelium only	Chiefly invasive, ulcerogenic Cytotoxicity
Symptoms	Upper and midabdominal pain and borborygmi Anorexia, nausea, and vomiting High-volume watery diarrhea	Right and left lower quadrant pain, occasional tenesmus Foul, low-volume bloody mucoid diarrhea
Complications	Dehydration, shock, and renal failure Electrolyte abnormalities	Toxic megacolon, rectal prolapse, septicemia Hemolytic-uremic syndrome Reactive arthritis, Reiter's syndrome

erae, ETEC, and EPEC, affect the proximal and mid–small bowel, whereas invasive organisms, e.g. *Shigella, Campylobacter, Salmonella, Yersinia,* and EIEC, predominantly affect the terminal ileum and colon. Thus, small bowel bacterial diarrhea is associated with few anatomic mucosal changes, whereas large bowel diarrhea is characterized by ulceration, pyogenic and inflammatory reactions, and bleeding (Fig. 73–5*N*). A possible exception is the noninvasive organism EHEC, which elaborates cytotoxins known as Shiga-like toxins that act locally on the colonic mucosa to produce bloody diarrhea.

Colonization. Noninvasive pathogens must adhere to specific receptors on the enterocytes to resist intestinal peristalsis and deliver enterotoxin to the mucosa surface. ETEC fimbrial adherence factors, designated as colonization factor antigens (CFA)/I, CFA/II complex, CFA/IV complex (PCF 8775), and less importantly, CFA/III and PCF 0159, are well characterized and consist of either rigid or wiry and flexible structures composed of protein subunits on the surface of the organism. A fimbrial adhesin, tcp, has also been identified for *V. cholerae.* Although a requirement for attachment is known for other noninvasive pathogens, the nature of these specific adhesins is not clear. For EPEC, and possibly EHEC, the process of attachment produces a unique histopathologic lesion in the intestine characterized by effacement of the enterocyte membrane with destruction of the brush border microvilli and disruption of the underlying cytoskeleton. This lesion appears to play an important role in the pathogenesis of EPEC (and possibly EHEC) diarrhea.

Toxin Production. Enterotoxins, such as cholera toxin (CT), heat-labile toxin (LT), heat-stable toxin (ST), and their variants, are responsible for the derangements in fluid and electrolyte balance seen with secretory diarrhea, of which cholera (Chapter 40) and ETEC (Chapter 41.1) are the prototypes. Cellular injury resulting from the potent Shiga cytotoxin contributes to the pathogenesis of bloody diarrhea and hemolytic-uremic syndrome seen in *S. dysenteriae* type 1 and EHEC infection. *C. difficile* elaborates a cytotoxin that injures the colonic epithelium and increases vascular permeability (Chapter

55.4). This results in leakage of fluid into the colon, and in severe cases pseudomembranous colitis may occur. Toxin-producing bacteria, such as *Staphylococcus* and *Bacillus cereus,* are important in the etiology of food poisoning. Several bacterial enteropathogens elaborate various other enterotoxins, cytotoxins, and exotoxins whose role in the pathogenesis of diarrhea remains unclear.

Epithelial Cell Invasiveness. Invasion and proliferation within colonic epithelial cells is the fundamental virulence factor of *Shigella* and EIEC. These cytotoxic organisms multiply and spread within the intestinal mucosa and incite an intense polymorphonuclear inflammatory response, creating microabscesses and ulcers that leak blood and exudate into the stool. Although epithelial cell invasion also occurs after *Salmonella* infection, in contrast to shigellae, salmonellae do not multiply within and destroy epithelial cells. Instead, they pass into the lamina propria, where they elicit a specific inflammatory reaction. Other bacterial enteropathogens such as *Campylobacter* and *Yersinia* have invasive properties, but these are less well understood. Many invasive diarrheas have a secretory component that may be attributable to impaired reabsorption of fluid by the damaged colon, active secretion of fluid and electrolytes mediated by enterotoxins, or release of cell-associated substances that stimulate an inflammatory reaction, thereby inducing intestinal secretion.

INFECTION-DERIVED IMMUNITY. The correlates of protective immunity against bacterial diarrhea are not well understood. Epidemiologic data suggest that prior infection with ETEC, *Shigella, S. typhi,* and *V. cholerae* O1 confers protection against subsequent infections. Support for this view comes from the observation that incidence declines with age in endemic populations, whereas previously unexposed adults, such as foreign travelers to endemic areas, remain susceptible. Furthermore, volunteers experimentally infected with cholera, ETEC, *Shigella,* and *Campylobacter jejuni* were protected against subsequent challenge with homologous strains. The importance of secretory immunity has been inferred from observations that orally administered secretory antibody in human breast milk and in experimentally administered hyperimmune cow's milk can confer protection against cholera and ETEC diarrhea.

GENERAL PRINCIPLES OF THERAPY. The specific aims of therapy are (1) restoration of water and electrolytes lost in stools, vomitus, sweat, and expired air, using replacement solutions approximating the composition of the fluids lost; (2) early nutritional support; (3) antibiotic therapy in selected cases of severe bacterial illness; (4) replacement of significant blood and albumin deficits as can be seen in malnourished patients who develop epidemic *S. dysenteriae* I dysentery; and (5) specific therapy for renal, hematologic, vascular, infectious, metabolic, and arthritic complications.

Water and Electrolyte Replacement. Evidence that glucose-coupled sodium and water transport remains intact during infectious diarrhea caused a revolution in rehydration and maintenance therapy. These seminal observations in the 1960s led to the discovery that incorporation of glucose into an oral polyelectrolyte solution replaces intestinal fluid losses during AWD. Oral rehydration solution (ORS) was taken to the field to treat cholera in Bangladesh in 1968 and has repeatedly been shown to be a practical method for preventing and treating dehydration in patients with diarrhea, regardless of etiology. ORS has proved to be safe and effective in all age groups, including neonates, and in diarrhea patients with numerous underlying conditions, including malnutrition. Subsequent mass implementation efforts have made ORS available to nearly 60% of children in developing countries. The target of the World Health Organization (WHO) is the use of ORS in 50% of cases of diarrhea by 1990 and the prevention of 1.5 million child deaths.

Oral rehydration therapy (ORT) works only when an electrolyte solution containing one or more substrates that enhance salt and water absorption, e.g., glucose or amino acids, is used. The normal mechanism for salt and water absorption is impaired during an episode of diarrhea; thus administration of substrate-free electrolyte solutions may exacerbate fluid losses. ORS ingredients are far cheaper and easier to administer than intravenous solutions and are widely available. Preparation requires only clean water and a 1-liter container in which to mix the salt and substrate.

Universal implementation of ORT requires educational programs that integrate ORT into culturally accepted patterns of child care in homes and health facilities. In some countries, village mothers, midwives, and healers have been trained as local ORT dispensers and teachers. At centers treating many infants, health education needs are best met by posting a trained paramedical worker in the emergency room or outpatient clinic. In either case, having a health worker effectively communicate the few essential points to the mother (Fig. III D–1) should improve home therapy skills, reduce dehydration, and lower the need for hospital admission during subsequent attacks.

Composition of ORS

Sodium and Water Content. ORS should be prepared daily by mixing 1 packet with 1 liter of potable water (or the correct amount for the particular preparation)

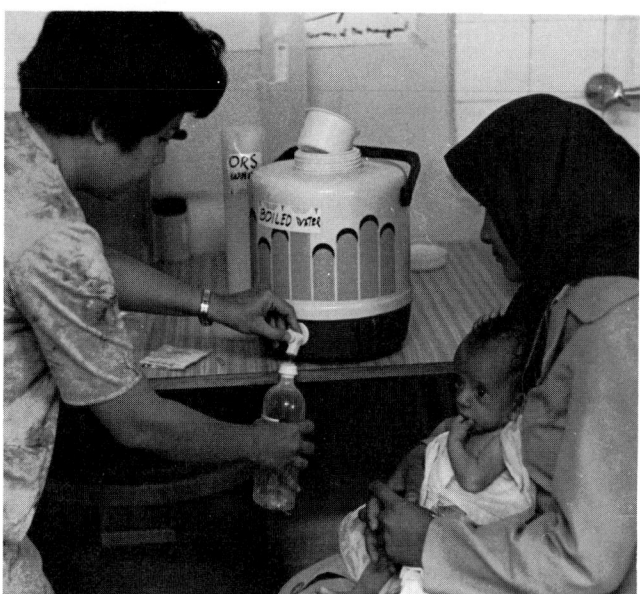

FIGURE III D–1. An aide in a primary health care facility is explaining to a Jordanian mother how to make up ORS to treat her moderately dehydrated infant.

using clean utensils. While lower sodium concentrations are useful to treat mild dehydration in developed countries, experience suggests that standard therapy with ORS containing 90 mmol/L of sodium (WHO-ORS) is necessary to treat the moderate to severe dehydration seen in developing countries (Table III D–7). Whereas one extensively used regimen calls for replacement of one third of the deficit with free water (the 2:1 method), WHO currently recommends replacement of the total fluid deficit with ORS alone. Nevertheless, to avoid such complications as hypernatremia and edema, it is recommended that plain water be offered after the initial phase of rehydration.

Base and Base Precursors. Bicarbonate and base precursors (citrate, acetate, and lactate) have been added to ORS to correct acidosis. All but lactate offer the additional advantage of promoting absorption of sodium and water in the intestine. Because bicarbonate-containing formulations lack stability owing to bicarbonate-glucose interactions during prolonged storage, WHO currently recommends the use of citrate in ORS.

Substrate. Based on intestinal perfusion studies show-

TABLE III D–7. Ingredients of WHO Oral Rehydration Solution (ORS)

Ingredient	Amount
In gm/L	
Glucose (% anhydrous glucose)	20 (2)
NaCl	3.5
KCl	1.5
Trisodium citrate, dihydrate*	2.9
In mmol/L	
Glucose (% anydrous glucose)	111
Na⁺	90
Cl⁻	80
K⁺	20
Citrate*	10

*Can substitute $NaHCO_3^-$ 2.5 gm/L (HCO_{3-} 30 mmol/L)

ing that maximal absorption of salt and water together occurs with glucose concentrations of 80 to 140 mmol/L at glucose: sodium ratios of approximately 1:1, standard ORS contains 111 mmol/L of glucose and 90 mmol/L of sodium. Although this formulation reduces net stool losses and can prevent and correct dehydration, it does not reduce gross stool output. Efforts are thus under way to develop improved substrates. Sucrose-containing ORS offers the advantage of being cheap and available in many households; however, electrolyte corrections may be slower in comparison with glucose ORS. Evidence that sodium-coupled intestinal transport of amino acids and dipeptides is preserved during diarrhea and may be additive to that of glucose prompted trials of other solutes, either singly or in combination, but none has proved to be consistently superior to standard WHO-ORS. In recent years, impressive results have been obtained with the use of food-based ORS formulations made from gruel mixtures commonly used in weaning diets around the world, such as rice, maize, millet, wheat, sorghum, and potato. Compared with standard ORS, cereal-based solutions have been shown to decrease both gross stool output and the need for ORS during acute diarrhea. The observed benefits may be due to several factors. It has been hypothesized that by using polymers that are hydrolyzed slowly, greater concentrations of glucose and amino acids might be delivered to the intestine with less osmotic penalty in comparison with monomeric substrates. Furthermore, amino acids and glucose in combination may surpass the amount of intestinal fluid absorption achievable with a single substrate. Finally, food-based ORT is nutritious and thus may contribute to more rapid intestinal healing and diminished malnutrition. If these advantages, particularly the observable impact on stool output combined with the use of locally available formulations, are appreciated by local ORS dispensers and users, compliance with therapy may increase. However, it must be emphasized that only formulations with proven efficacy should be used.

Therapeutic Management of Dehydration. Therapy has been classified by WHO according to disease severity, as follows.

Plan A for Home Treatment of Diarrhea. Infants with diarrhea who have no signs of dehydration and have lost less than 2.5% of their body weight can be treated at home, as can children who have already been treated for dehydration and have improved. Parents must learn 3 vital principles for treating diarrhea in the home: (1) Give the child more fluids than usual, using the recommended home fluid or food-based fluids such as gruel, soup, or rice water. Offer breast milk or half strength milk feeds frequently. (2) If the child is already weaned, give small amounts of nutritious, easily digestible food at frequent intervals. Recommended menu items include freshly prepared mixes of cereal and beans, meat, or fish with added oil for extra calories, eggs, dairy products, and fresh fruit juices. Following recovery, offer one extra meal each day for 1 week or until weight has returned to normal. (3) Take the child to a health worker if he or she is not getting better, if signs of dehydration develop, or if the child passes many stools, has diminished intake, or develops a fever. Parents must be taught to look for easily recognizable signs of dehydration, e.g., sunken eyes (Fig. 40–2), and excessive thirst, and to pinch the dorsum of the hand or the belly skin to determine skin elasticity or turgor (Fig. III D–2).

It may be necessary to teach the mother to use ORS at home to replace ongoing diarrheal losses in the nondehydrated child, or even to treat dehydration if access to health care is limited. The parent should be told to give 50 to 100 ml (1/4 to 1/2 large cup) of ORS solution after each stool for a child under 2 years of age, or 100 to 200 ml (1/2 to 1 large cup) for older children. (Adults should drink ad libitum.) If the child vomits, ORS should be withheld for 10 minutes then given more slowly, e.g., a spoonful every 2 to 3 minutes.

Plan B for Treatment of Mild to Moderate Dehydration. The provider (preferably the parent) should give as much ORS as the child will accept in 4 to 6 hours, by spoon-feeding if the child is weak, until he or she can tolerate drinking (Fig. III D–3). A minimum of 50 ml/kg body weight should be given to the mildly (≤5%) dehydrated and 100 ml/kg to the moderately (6 to 10%) dehydrated patient. Hydration status should be reassessed after 4 to 6 hours and the decision made either to proceed to Plan A or to continue on Plan B. A simple bedside record sheet is helpful for assessing fluid balance in clinics (Fig. III D–4). If the child is to continue on Plan B, begin milk feeds and solid foods. If the child is not breast-fed, give 100 to 200 ml of clean water before continuing ORS. About 95% of infants with mild to moderate dehydration can be managed with ORS alone and no intravenous fluids, and most are successfully treated within 6 hours.

Adults with dehydration should drink 250 ml of ORS

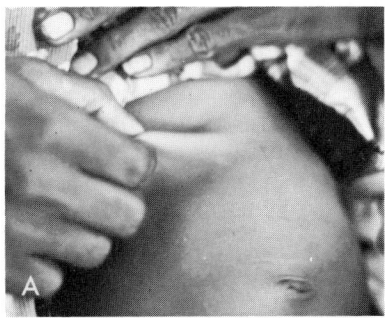
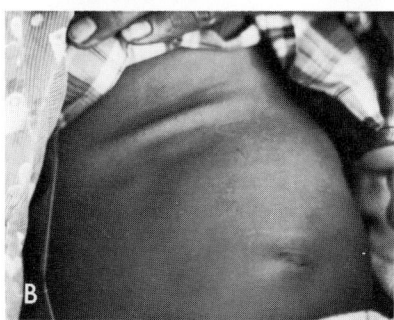

FIGURE III D–2. Parents should be taught the significance of examining skin elasticity as a bedside guide to oral rehydration fluid requirements. *A,* Skin is pinched. *B,* If dehydration is present, a fold remains.

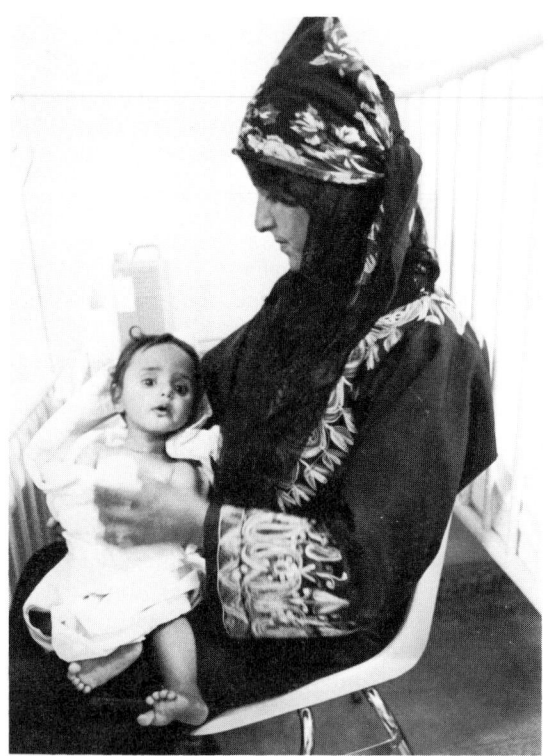

FIGURE III D–3. A Jordanian mother administers ORS to her moderately dehydrated infant during rehydration. (Courtesy of Al Bashir Hospital, Amman.)

each hour until rehydrated. Additional plain water is permitted ad libitum.

Plan C for Treatment of Severe Diarrhea. Patients in shock from more than 10% dehydration may be anuric with depressed mental status and a rapid, thready, or undetectable radial pulse. They require immediate intravenous rehydration with Ringer's lactate or other, less suitable solutions such as normal saline and 5% dextrose in half-normal saline (Table III D–8); blood and plain 5% dextrose have no role in rehydration. Adequate access for intravenous infusion can usually be established via the arm veins. For patients arriving in terminal condition, femoral vein infusion can be lifesaving; when the patient stabilizes, however, peripheral access should be sought.

The rate of infusion must be tailored to the clinical picture. In general, infants are given 30 ml/kg body weight over 1 hour followed by 40 ml/kg over the next

2 hours. If adequate progress has been made, oral therapy with ORS can be instituted at a rate of 40 ml/kg body weight over the next 3 hours. Thereafter, Plan A or B may be followed as indicated; however, 100 to 200 ml of plain water should be given before continuing with ORS. As soon as the infant is able to suck, breast feeding may begin.

For older children and adults, intravenous therapy is begun at a rate of 100 ml/kg body weight over 3 hours (initially as fast as possible until the radial pulse is easily palpable), followed by ORS supplemented with plain water as desired.

Oral rehydration using a nasogastric tube is an alternative for infants who cannot drink. It can also be used for those in shock in whom intravenous access cannot be obtained or when supplies are unavailable. The recommended rate is 20 ml/kg per hour or higher if clinically indicated. Treatment must be reevaluated if the abdomen becomes distended. Adult cholera patients in shock due to dehydration have been successfully rehydrated without any IV fluids, using ORS at rates of 1 L/hour.

Correction of Serum Electrolyte Derangements. Recent studies have demonstrated that, compared with intravenous therapy, correction of electrolyte abnormalities is more gradual when ORT is used and that this may result in fewer central nervous system complications during rehydration. The occurrence of convulsions may be further diminished with "slow" (12 hour) replacement of fluid deficit in hypernatremic dehydration. Standard ORS contains 20 mmol/L of potassium (Table III D–7), compared with 30 to 40 mmol/L in some infant diarrheal stools (Table III D–3). Thus, to avoid complications related to hypokalemia in actively purging children, some centers have adopted a modified ORS containing 25 to 30 mmol/L of potassium. In addition, ongoing potassium supplementation via foods (banana, fruit juices, coconut water) is advised. In most instances, acidosis can be corrected with ORS alone, a benefit attributed to the addition of base or base precursors plus the effect of restoring vascular volume and renal perfusion.

Correction of Hypoglycemia. This potentially devastating complication is best prevented by adding glucose to IV electrolyte solutions (Table III D–8). ORT and early diet help avoid it, but signs of lethargy, hypothermia, or convulsions linked to hypoglycemia demand IV glucose.

SIMPLE BEDSIDE INTAKE AND OUTPUT FORM FOR INFANTILE DIARRHEA

DATE	BOTTLE NUMBER	AMOUNT (CC)	TYPE OF FLUID (ORS, WATER, MILK)	TIME STARTED	TIME ENDED	VOMIT YES/NO	SKIN ELASTICITY (decreased/normal)	STOOL GRADE

FIGURE III D–4. This record sheet is useful for lower-grade infantile diarrheas for which clinical monitoring of improvements in signs of dehydration is a sufficient guide to progress of therapy.

TABLE III D–8. Intravenous Rehydration Solution Ingredients

Name of Solution	Concentrations (in gm/L or ml/L)*					Resulting Electrolyte Concentrations (in mEq/L)			
	NaCl	KCl	NaHCO₃	Na Acetate	Glucose	Na⁺	K⁺	HCO₃⁻†	Cl⁻
Dacca solution	5	1	4	—	Add: 2 ml of 50% glucose per liter	133	13	48	98
Acetate solution	5	1	—	6.5	"	134	13	48	98
Lactate Ringer's solution	6.2	0.4	2.3 (as lactate)	—	"	130	4	28	109
Normal saline (NS)	9	—	—	—	—	154	—	—	154
Diarrhea solution "A" (Adults, older children) To make up 1 liter:	500 ml NS	+ 15 ml KCl‡	+ 50 ml 7.5% NaHCO₃	—	Add to 435 ml of 5% glucose	122	15	45	92
Diarrhea solution "B" (Infants) To make up 1 liter:	333 ml NS	+ 15 ml KCl‡	+ 33 ml 7.5% NaHCO₃	—	Add to 619 ml of 5% glucose	81	15	30	66

*gm/L for first four solutions; ml/L for last two solutions.
†Or equivalent from base precursors (acetate, lactate).
‡Containing 1 mEq K⁺/ml.

Antibiotics and Other Adjuvant Therapy

Antibiotics. These are ineffective in most episodes of diarrhea and in some cases may prolong illness. Indiscriminate use fosters development of multiresistant organisms in many areas of the world, which interferes with effective therapy when it is indicated to treat severe or complicated illness. The primary indications for antibiotics are (1) as an adjunct to ORT in moderate to severe cholera (Chapter 40.1), and (2) treatment of *Shigella* dysentery (Chapter 37). Dysentery is often caused by *Shigella,* and these patients should be given antibiotics whether or not stool cultures are available to identify the cause. Treatment of suspected *Campylobacter* dysentery may be of some benefit if instituted very early in the illness (Chapter 41.2). Although antibiotics are not useful for treating uncomplicated *Salmonella* gastroenteritis, they are indicated when there is increased risk of bacteremic complications, such as in infants younger than 3 months, in patients with malignancies or other immunosuppressive conditions, and when typhoid fever is suspected (Chapters 38 and 39). In areas where ETEC is prevalent, antibiotics are useful in the treatment of traveler's diarrhea (Chapters 41.1 and 117) but are not recommended to treat endemic ETEC diarrhea, which is generally self-limited and amenable to ORT alone. In young infants, especially those with malnutrition, diarrhea may be accompanied by septicemia, which must be promptly treated with antibiotics directed against the likely etiologic agent.

Antisecretory Agents. The use of available antisecretory agents, such as aspirin, indomethacin, chlorpromazine, somatostatin, and loperamide, is not recommended; overall, none exceeds ORS in safety and efficacy. Opiates and their derivatives, such as loperamide and diphenoxylate, are widely used as antiperistaltic agents. However, these drugs may actually prolong pathogen excretion and exacerbate illness due to invasive pathogens; thus they are not recommended to treat diarrhea in developing countries. Bulk-forming agents, such as kaolin and pectin, increase stool consistency but do not retard fluid losses and are thus of no benefit. Bacteriotherapy, or enteric administration of nonpathogenic organisms such as lactobacilli, *Streptococcus faecalis,* or multiorganism cocktails, is thought to prevent or treat diarrhea by inhibiting growth of pathogens, but the efficacy of this approach has not been established in controlled studies.

Bismuth subsalicylate, which has both antisecretory and antimicrobial properties, may have a role in the prevention of traveler's diarrhea but should be used with caution in persons with aspirin hypersensitivity or bleeding diathesis and is not recommended for young children.

MORTALITY RELATED TO DIARRHEA AND ITS COMPLICATIONS. The most common cause of diarrhea-related mortality is dehydration, a potentially avoidable outcome with the advent of ORS. Nevertheless, some children die from diarrhea even after rehydration therapy. In a study performed in Bangladesh, the most common terminal events following rehydration therapy were sepsis, hypoglycemia, and hypokalemia. Generally speaking, mortality was greatest in patients with underlying malnutrition and in those with severe colitis. Aspiration pneumonia after vomiting was a cause of serious morbidity and even death.

Improper use of ORS can have severe sequelae. Delay or inadequate rehydration with ORS can result in irreversible shock and renal failure, leading to death. Homemade or improperly mixed ORS solutions may contain erroneous quantities of salt and sugar and result in serious electrolyte disturbances. Inadequate replacement of deficits in potassium and glucose can be fatal.

PREVENTION OF DIARRHEA. While many deaths from acute dehydration can be prevented with ORT, there is a need to institute long-term measures that prevent diarrheal morbidity. The protection against diarrhea conferred by breast-feeding is well recognized and has been attributed both to the immunologic properties of breast milk and to diminished exposure to environmental contamination in the breast-fed infant. Mothers should be encouraged to breast-feed exclusively for 4 to 6 months and to continue breast-feeding for at least the first year.

Educational programs that lead to culturally accepted

changes in hygienic practices and health behaviors are needed. Interventions that have proved efficacious include introduction of soap, handwashing after defecation and before eating or preparing food, and proper disposal of feces. Practices that decrease contamination of weaning foods should also be taught. Ongoing efforts to improve water supply, sanitation, and housing are expected to diminish diarrheal morbidity and improve infant survival, as are effective nutritional interventions.

Of great importance is the development of vaccines to prevent enteric infection and effective delivery of those vaccines with proven indirect benefit against diarrheal mortality, such as measles vaccine. The focus of recent research has been to develop oral vaccines that elicit local immunity in the intestine and prevent initial attachment, penetration, and local toxinogenicity. Efforts to develop safe and effective oral vaccines against rotavirus diarrhea, cholera, ETEC diarrhea, typhoid fever, and shigellosis are in progress.

BIBLIOGRAPHY

DiJohn D, Levine MM: Treatment of diarrhea. Infect Dis Clin North Am 2:719–745, 1988.

Finlay BB, Falkow S: Common themes in microbial pathogenicity. Microbiol Rev 53:210–230, 1989.

Guzman C, Pizarro D, Castillo B, Posada G: Hypernatremic diarrheal dehydration treated with oral glucose-electrolyte solution containing 90 or 75 mEq/l of sodium. J Pediatr Gastroenterol Nutr 7:694–698, 1988.

Levine MM, Losonsky G, Herrington D, et al: Pediatric diarrhea: the challenge of prevention. Pediatr Infect Dis 5:S29–S43, 1986.

Molla AM, Molla A, Nath SK, Khatun M: Food-based oral rehydration salt solution for acute childhood diarrhoea. Lancet 2:429–431, 1989.

Molla AM, Molla A, Rohde J, Greenough WB III: Turning off the diarrhea: The role of food and ORS. J Pediatr Gastroenterol Nutr 8:81–84, 1989.

Nalin DR, Cash RA, Islam R, et al: Oral maintenance therapy for cholera in adults. Lancet 2:370, 1968.

Nalin DR, Harland E, Ramlal A, et al: Comparison of low and high sodium and potassium content in oral rehydration solutions. Pediatrics 97:848, 1980.

Rennels MB, Levine MM: Classical bacterial diarrhea: perspectives and update—Salmonella, Shigella, Escherichia coli, Aeromonas and Plesiomonas. Pediatr Infect Dis 5:S91–S100, 1986.

Taylor CE, Greenough WB: Control of diarrheal diseases. Annu Rev Public Health 10:221–244, 1989.

World Health Organization: The treatment and prevention of acute diarrhoea: Practical guidelines. Geneva, WHO, 1989.

37. SHIGELLOSIS

Myron M. Levine

DEFINITION. Shigellosis is an acute bacterial infection of the intestinal tract, predominantly involving the terminal ileum, colon, and rectum, caused by organisms of the genus *Shigella*. The spectrum of illness is broad, extending from subclinical infections and mild watery diarrhea to fulminating dysentery manifested by high fever, chills, toxemia, tenesmus, and the passage of multiple scanty stools of blood and mucus. Strictly speaking, dysentery implies the presence of blood and mucus in stools, of which *Shigella* is the most common

cause. However, bacillary dysentery has become synonomous with all clinical presentations of shigellosis.

ETIOLOGY. Shigellae are nonmotile, gram-negative, rod-shaped bacteria within the family Enterobacteriaceae. Four species or groups of *Shigella* are recognized based on biochemical and serologic differentiation: *S. dysenteriae* (group A); *S. flexneri* (group B); *S. boydii* (group C); and *S. sonnei* (group D). Groups A, B, and C have multiple serotypes and subtypes, whereas only a single serotype of group D is recognized. *S. dysenteriae* 1, so-called Shiga's bacillus, is a unique serotype that causes the most severe clinical illness, manifests pandemic behavior, and is particularly difficult to cultivate. *S. flexneri* and *S. dysenteriae* serotypes predominate in the less developed world, while *S. sonnei* is the most frequent isolate in industrialized countries.

HISTORY. Bloody diarrhea accompanied by tenesmus and abdominal cramps was described by Hippocrates, who also recognized the seasonality of this disease, which peaked in summer. Throughout recorded history, bacillary dysentery has afflicted military units and played a decisive role in military campaigns. The outcome of many a battle has been influenced by a dysentery epidemic in one of the opposing armies, thereby altering the course of history. *Shigella* was first identified by Kiyoshi Shiga at the end of the nineteenth century, at a time when extensive epidemics were sweeping the islands of Japan accompanied by high case fatality.

DISTRIBUTION AND INCIDENCE. *Shigella* infections occur throughout the world, from the tropics to the Arctic wherever personal hygiene is compromised. Thus, shigellosis is endemic among toddlers and preschool children in less developed countries, while in industrialized countries it occurs in custodial institutions for the mentally retarded and the insane and in some day care centers for preschool children.

Prospective household surveillance of cohorts of children for diarrheal disease in less developed countries has shown that the peak incidence of *Shigella* infections occurs in the second and third years of life. During this early age, approximately 3 to 6 episodes of diarrhea per child per year occur, and about 10% of the episodes are due to *Shigella*. Worldwide, shigellosis is a formidable public health problem. A study by the Institute of Medicine estimates that annually *Shigella* causes 250 million cases of diarrheal illness and 654,000 deaths throughout the world.

Shiga dysentery due to *S. dysenteriae* 1 can occur in pandemics. Pandemics have been observed in Central America in the late 1960s, Bangladesh in the early 1970s, Central Africa in the late 1970s and early 1980s, and south Asia in the mid-1980s (Table 37-1). These pandemics have all involved *S. dysenteriae* 1 strains that exhibited multiple antibiotic resistances and were often accompanied by severe clinical illness and high case fatality in all age groups.

TRANSMISSION AND EPIDEMIOLOGY. Other than primates in captivity, man serves as the only reservoir and natural host for *Shigella*. As few as 10 *Shigella* organisms can cause overt clinical illness in volunteers. This finding corroborates the epidemiologic

TABLE 37–1. Epidemics of Shiga (*Shigella dysenteriae* 1) Dysentery Throughout the World Since the Late 1960s

Years	Countries Affected	Resistance to Clinically Relevant Antibiotics
1968–1970	Guatemala, El Salvador, Nicaragua, Honduras, Costa Rica, southern Mexico	Tetracycline, sulfas, chloramphenicol
1972	Mexico	Tetracycline, sulfas, chloramphenicol, ampicillin
1972–1977	Bangladesh	Tetracycline, sulfas, chloramphenicol, ampicillin (some strains)
1974–1978	Southern India	Tetracycline, sulfas, chloramphenicol, ampicillin
1979–1986	Zaire, Rwanda, Burundi	Tetracycline, sulfas, chloramphenicol, ampicillin
1984–present	India, Burma, Bangladesh, southern China, Thailand, Nepal	Tetracycline, sulfas, ampicillin, trimethoprim-sulfamethoxazole

observations that indicate the ready transmission of *Shigella* by direct fecal-hand-oral contact in propagated epidemics. The low inoculum required for transmission also explains why spread of *Shigella* easily ocurs wherever crowding, poor sanitation, and primitive personal hygiene coexist. Less commonly, *Shigella* is transmitted by contaminated food or water vehicles. Other epidemiologic data suggest that under certain conditions, as found seasonally in many less developed areas, *Shigella* may be transmitted by house flies. Shigellosis has also been recognized to occur with increased frequency in male homosexuals, in whom the infection is transmitted by oral-anal contact.

PATHOGENESIS AND PATHOLOGY. The cardinal feature of the pathogenesis of *Shigella* infection is the capacity of the bacilli to invade enterocytes, multiply therein, and cause cell death. Shigellae that lose their invasive potential are no longer pathogenic. The ability to invade epithelial cells involves both chromosomal genes and a large (120 to 140 MD) enteroinvasiveness plasmid; the latter is necessary for the expression of several outer membrane proteins required for shigellae to gain entry into the enterocyte.

Intraepithelial proliferation of shigellae followed by death of the enterocytes results in discharge of the bacteria into the lamina propria. This is accompanied by a striking influx of polymorphonuclear leukocytes into the lamina propria. With progression of the mucosal infection, death of enterocytes leads to small ulcers, hemorrhage, microabscesses, and the presence of many leukocytes in the fecal material.

One serotype, *S. dysenteriae* 1, produces relatively large amounts of a highly potent exotoxin, so-called Shiga toxin. This toxin exhibits several biologic activities: It is cytotoxic for HeLa and Vero cells in nanogram quantities; following inoculation of guinea pigs, mice, or rabbits, hindlimb paralysis becomes evident, so Shiga toxin has been called a neurotoxin; inoculated into an ileal loop, it acts as an enterotoxin and induces intestinal secretion. Shiga toxin is a powerful inhibitor of protein synthesis. With perhaps rare exceptions, only *S. dysenteriae* 1 elaborates true Shiga toxin. Other *Shigella* serotypes elaborate small quantities of other cytotoxins. While some of these other cytotoxins may be partially or even completely neutralized by Shiga antitoxin, demonstrating antigenic cross-reactivity, these strains of other serotypes do not hybridize with DNA probes specific for the genes of true Shiga toxin. Thus, these other toxins, even if immunologically related, are genetically distinct from true Shiga toxin.

The exact role of Shiga toxin in the pathogenesis of Shiga dysentery is not known. Both animal experiments and volunteer studies show that mutants of *S. dysenteriae* 1 that retain invasive potential while lacking the ability to elaborate true Shiga toxin are capable of causing diarrhea and dysentery virtually indistinguishable from that caused by strains that produce Shiga toxin. In neither man nor monkeys was the amount of watery diarrhea diminished in infection with the strain lacking Shiga toxin, although in monkeys less blood in stools was seen. The most prominent effect of Shiga toxin in monkeys appeared to be the occurrence of vascular damage. One report in humans suggests that among *Shigella* strains that elaborate cytotoxins other than Shiga toxin, those that show increased cytotoxin expression are associated with more severe clinical illness as measured by higher fever and more blood in stools.

One much-feared complication of shigellosis, the hemolytic-uremic syndrome, is attributed to the effects of Shiga toxin. This syndrome is an uncommon but often fatal complication seen with *S. dysenteriae* 1 (Shiga bacillus) infection. Notably in industrialized countries, enterohemorrhagic *Escherichia coli* (most commonly of serotypes 0157:H7 and 026:H11) that elaborate Shiga toxin have also been incriminated as etiologic agents of the hemolytic-uremic syndrome (Chapter 41.1).

Bacteremia is generally uncommon in shigellosis. An exception is *S. dysenteriae* 1 infection in malnourished children.

The major sites of pathology include the mucosa of the terminal ileum and the colon. When visualized by proctoscopy, the mucosa is edematous and covered with mucus and shows interspersed hemorrhages (Fig. 73–5*N*). Biopsy of a typical affected area reveals a striking polymorphonuclear leukocyte infiltration, congestion of blood vessels, edema, and ulceration of the overlying mucosa (Fig. 37–1).

CLINICAL MANIFESTATIONS. The spectrum of clinical illness due to *Shigella* includes asymptomatic infection; mild diarrheal illness indistinguishable from that caused by many other bacterial, viral, or protozoal agents; and severe dysentery. The incubation period is usually 1 to 4 days but may be as long as 6 to 8 days with *S. dysenteriae* 1 infection. While any serotype can cause either mild diarrhea or fulminating dysentery, *S. sonnei* tends to be more frequently associated with mild ("catarrhal") enteritis, and *S. flexneri* and *S. dysenteriae* serotypes with more severe clinical illness. *S. dysenteriae* 1 is particularly feared because of the severity of the clinical illness and the frequency of major complications.

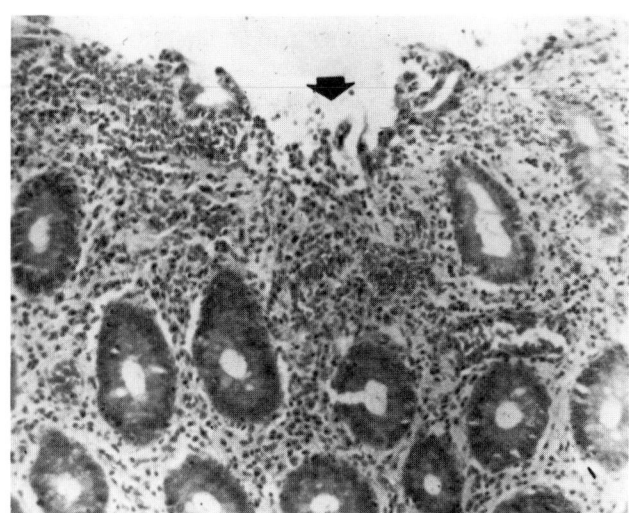

FIGURE 37–1. A rectal biopsy from the patient with Shiga dysentery whose proctoscopic examination results are shown in Figure 73–5N. The biopsy demonstrates hemorrhage, vascular congestion, intense infiltration of the lamina propria with polymorphonuclear leukocytes, and a mucosal ulceration (arrow).

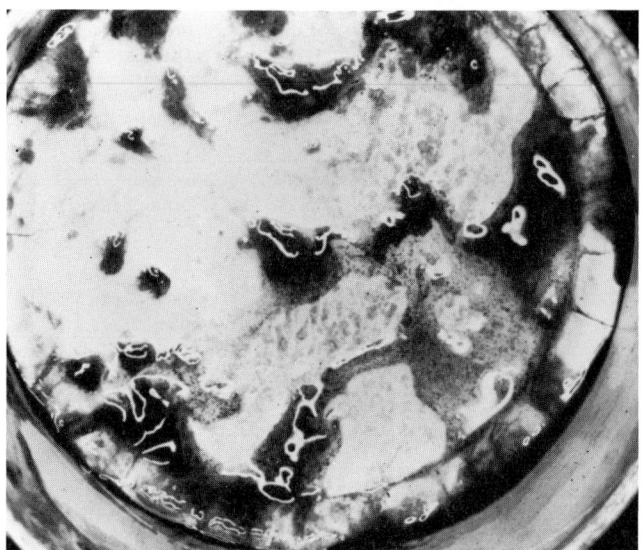

FIGURE 37–2. A typical dysenteric stool. Note the scanty discharge consisting virtually entirely of blood and mucus. At the height of the dysenteric illness, such stools can be passed with great frequency (e.g., every 1 or 2 hours) accompanied by severe tenesmus.

Shiga dysentery is often characterized by high fever, toxemia, disabling abdominal cramps, tenesmus, frequent bloody mucoid stools (Fig. 37–2), vomiting, and convulsions (in pediatric patients).

In shigellosis there is often a progression of disease through several fairly distinct phases. Toxemia, malaise, and high fever are often present at the onset of clinical illness followed by some hours of watery diarrhea. When convulsions occur as part of shigellosis in children, they accompany the early phase of illness. Lastly, the dysenteric phase begins manifested by lower abdominal cramps, tenesmus, and the passage of scanty stools of blood and mucus (Fig. 37–2).

Complications. Diarrheal dehydration may accompany *Shigella* infection in infants and young children but is less common in groups. Convulsions may be considered an uncommon presentation of acute disease in children rather than as a complication per se.

The hemolytic-uremic syndrome, leukemoid reactions, and severe hypoproteinemia are recognized complications of Shiga dysentery. In hemolytic-uremic syndrome a disseminated intravascular coagulopathy occurs with massive hemolytic anemia, the presence of fragmented erythrocytes (schistocytes) in the peripheral blood smear, severe thrombocytopenia, and acute renal failure. Electron microscopic examination of the kidney in such patients reveals immune complexes, fibrin-platelet deposits, endocapillary cell lysis, and necrosis of glomerular and tubular epithelial cells. In the leukemoid reactions of Shiga dysentery, polymorphonuclear leukocyte counts exceeding 100,000 per mm³ have been recorded. The exudation of proteins through the extensive mucosal damage in the intestine of young children with Shiga dysentery can lead to a precipitous drop in plasma protein levels, resulting in an acute kwashiorkor syndrome characterized by edematous extremities (Fig. 37–3).

Rarely, Reiter's syndrome can follow shigellosis, par-

ticularly that due to *S. flexneri* or *S. dysenteriae* serotypes. This hypersensitivity reaction, manifestd by reactive arthritis (joint fluid cultures are sterile) and conjunctivitis or uveitis, is most frequent in patients having histocompatibility antigen HLA-B27.

In infants or young children with severe shigellosis, rectal prolapse can occur. *Shigella* also occasionally causes vaginitis in young girls.

DIAGNOSIS

Clinical and Laboratory. There are no characteristic features of shigellosis detectable on physical examina-

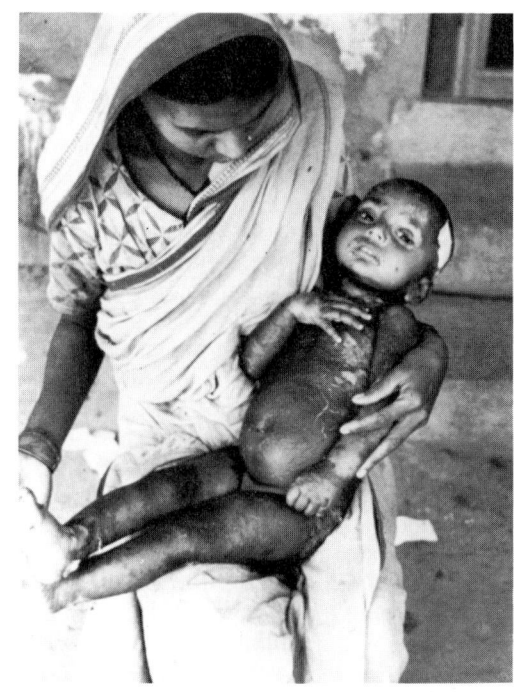

FIGURE 37–3. A Bangladeshi child with severe hypoproteinemia and acute onset of nutritional edema following Shiga dysentery. (Courtesy of Dr. M. Mujibur Rahaman.)

tion. Consequently, considerable emphasis is placed on the medical history. The white blood count is variable but often is elevated with a shift to the left.

Stool Culture. A specific diagnosis can usually be made within 48 hours by means of bacteriologic culture; however, special attention must be paid if *S. dysenteriae* 1 is suspected, since this serotype is notoriously difficult to cultivate. Culture of a fresh stool is optimal. If this is not possible, buffered glycerol saline makes the best transport medium for rectal swabs if *Shigella* is suspected. The combination of a selective medium such as xylose-lysine-deoxycholate (XLD) agar and a differential (noninhibitory) medium such as MacConkey's agar should be used. Culture of 2 or more specimens from the patient increases the likelihood of isolating *Shigella*. If an outbreak of *S. dysenteriae* 1 is suspected, Tergitol-7 agar is particularly useful in detecting this serotype, although XLD agar also functions quite well.

Serology. In investigation of outbreaks where the serotype is known but coprocultures may not be readily obtainable, measurement of serum antibodies to the O antigen of the specific *Shigella* serotype by passive hemagglutination of ELISA techniques is very useful for serodiagnosis.

Stool Microscopy. Patients with a clinical syndrome suspicious for *Shigella* infection should have a drop of stool mucus mixed with a drop of saline, smeared and dried on a slide, lightly heat-fixed, stained with methylene blue or Gram stain, and examined by light microscopy for the presence of fecal leukocytes. Virtually all patients with shigellosis have polymorphonuclear leukocytes in abundance in such smears (Fig. 37–4). Although a nonspecific test, this provides evidence that a bacterial pathogen has invaded the intestinal mucosa. Other bacterial enteropathogens that cause a dysenteric syndrome and are associated with abundant fecal leukocytes are *Campylobacter jejuni*, enteroinvasive *E. coli*, *Yersinia enterocolitica*, and *Salmonella* causing nontyphoidal infections. The presence of fecal leukocytes in

an acutely ill patient with clinical features of shigellosis provides sufficient indication to initiate therapy for shigellosis while awaiting the results of coprocultures. Stool microscopy in a patient with dysenteric stools will also differentiate amebic dysentery from enteroinvasive bacterial infection. The former does not have abundant fecal leukocytes, but amebic trophozoites are visible.

Differential Diagnosis. Mild forms of shigellosis not accompanied by overt dysentery are indistinguishable from acute watery diarrhea due to any infectious etiology and should be treated, as any diarrhea, with oral rehydration. Bacillary dysentery due to *Shigella* is clinically very similar to dysentery caused by *C. jejuni, Y. enterocolitica, Salmonella,* or enteroinvasive *E. coli*. Amebic dysentery does not manifest the high fever and constitutional symptoms of shigellosis. Furthermore, amebic infection can be differentiated by direct stool microscopy (Chapter 68). Bacillary and amebic dysentery can also be distinguished by sigmoidoscopic examination. In shigellosis the observed mucosal ulcerations appear punched-out and are not undermined, as they often are in amebic infection.

TREATMENT AND PROGNOSIS. The therapy of shigellosis can be divided into four phases: emergency treatment of life-endangering complications, supportive measures, specific antimicrobial drugs, and health education.

Potentially Life-Endangering Emergencies. Shock accompanying severe diarrheal dehydration can occur in acute shigellosis, especially in infants. It must be vigorously combated with a rapid intravenous infusion of Ringer's lactate, isotonic saline, or a similar solution given as rapidly as possible. This bolus of fluid quickly expands the intravascular volume and begins to correct the signs of shock. Continuing rehydration in such patients must then proceed with either intravenous hypotonic electrolyte solutions or, preferably, oral glucose-electrolyte solutions. Acidosis is corrected in the course of rehydration (III D, General Principles).

Convulsions are a well-recognized complication of shigellosis in infants and children. As with convulsions of any cause, aspiration, airway obstruction, and head trauma can occur during loss of consciousness and become more life-threatening than the underlying infection. Convulsions should be treated with intravenously administered diazepam (up to 10 mg) or phenobarbital (5 mg/kg body weight). The high fever usually associated with *Shigella* convulsions in children should be lowered with oral acetaminophen and by sponging the child in a tepid water bath.

Supportive Measures. Significant dehydration should be treated mainly with oral rehydration as described in III D, General Principles.

Agents that suppress intestinal motility, such as diphenoxylate, loperamide, and tincture of opium, are to be avoided in known or suspected shigellosis. Such agents may prolong the duration of fever and excretion of shigellae. Guinea pigs ordinarily are naturally resistant to *Shigella* infection. However, administration of antimotility agents renders them quite susceptible.

There is no evidence that common antidiarrheal preparations such as kaolin-pectin formulas, lactobacilli, or

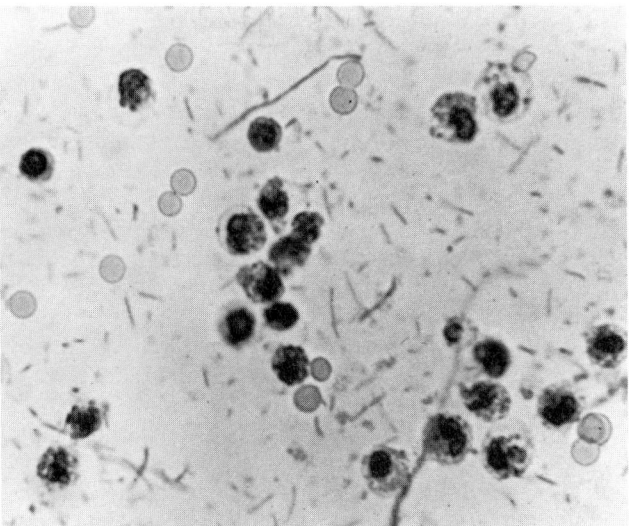

FIGURE 37–4. Demonstration of abundant fecal leukocytes and some red blood cells in stool mucus of a patient with dysentery due to *Shigella flexneri* type 2a. Stained with methylene blue and examined under high dry lens (450 ×).

bismuth salicylate have a significantly beneficial effect on the clinical or bacteriologic course of shigellosis. Nor is there evidence to suggest that these agents are deleterious and therefore contraindicated.

Specific Antimicrobial Therapy. Results of many controlled clinical trials have shown that appropriate antibiotics significantly decrease the duration of fever, diarrheal illness, and excretion of the pathogen in *Shigella* infections. This cumulative experience in conjunction with the fact that man is the natural reservoir and host of this infection, which is transmitted by contact, provides a compelling rationale for treating all persons with shigellosis with antibiotics. This must be reconciled with the reality that only a few antibiotics have proven clinical efficacy in patients (even though many more show good activity in vitro against *Shigella*) and that widespread use of these effective antibiotics eventually leads to the emergence of resistant *Shigella* strains. Sulfonamides, the drugs of choice in the 1940s, were of little practical use by the mid-1950s because of resistance and were replaced by tetracycline. Widespread resistance to tetracycline resulted in ampicillin's becoming the drug of choice in the 1960s.

Trimethoprim-sulfamethoxazole replaced ampicillin as the most important antibiotic in the late 1970s and early 1980s because of widespread resistance to ampicillin. Treatment with trimethoprim-sulfamethoxazole is given for 5 days. The adult dosage is 160 mg of trimethoprim and 400 mg of sulfamethoxazole every 12 hours. Children should receive 10 mg/kg trimethoprim and 50 mg/kg sulfamethoxazole daily in two divided doses given every 12 hours.

In the late 1980s, members of the quinolone family of antimicrobials, such as nalidixic acid, ciprofloxacin, and norfloxacin, became increasingly important in the treatment of *Shigella* infections that manifest resistance to other previously useful antibiotics. Particularly in dysentery due to *S. dysenteriae* 1, the quinolones have proved helpful. Ciprofloxacin has been used only in adults, while nalidixic acid has been used in all age groups, including infants and young children.

Health Education. Because *Shigella* is so readily transmitted from person to person and is spread with minute numbers of organisms, it is important to emphasize the importance of handwashing with soap after each defecation. Intervention studies have demonstrated the effectiveness of handwashing with soap and water in interrupting transmission of *Shigella*. Other studies have shown that the incidence of *Shigella* disease diminishes with increasing availability of water, even if the water is not potable.

PREVENTION AND CONTROL. Provision of adequate sanitation and proper hygiene practices make the chance of acquiring *Shigella* minimal. In high-risk situations where local conditions favor transmission, attempts must be made to initiate a high standard of personal and food hygiene. This includes compulsive handwashing with soap and water after defecation and before food preparation. Food preparation and eating areas should be kept free of flies.

Mass antibiotic therapy has been used with varying results in closed populations, such as in custodial institutions. While occasional successes have been reported, the general experience is that it usually fails.

For decades there have been attempts to prepare oral vaccines to prevent shigellosis. In the 1960s, streptomycin-dependent *Shigella* vaccines and the T₃₂ colonial mutant (*S. flexneri* 2a) strain were shown to be safe and protective when used as live oral vaccines. These vaccines suffered drawbacks, however, and never gained widespread usage. Research is continuing to develop improved live oral *Shigella* vaccines that will be safe and will provide a high level of broad-spectrum, long-lived immunity following 1 or 2 oral doses.

BIBLIOGRAPHY

Butler T, Islam MR, Bardhan PK: The leukemoid reaction in shigellosis. Am J Dis Child 138:162, 1984.
DiJohn D, Levine MM: Treatment of diarrhea. Infect Dis Clin North Am 2:719, 1988.
Gangarosa EJ, Perera DR, Mata LJ, et al: Epidemic Shiga bacillus dysentery in Central America. II. Epidemiologic studies in 1969. J Infect Dis 122:181, 1970.
Harris JC, DuPont HL: Fecal leukocytes in diarrheal illness. Ann Intern Med 76:697, 1972.
Khan MU, Shahidullah M: Interruption of shigellosis by handwashing. Trans R Soc Trop Med Hyg 76:164, 1982.
Levine MM: Bacillary dysentery. Mechanisms and treatment. Med Clin North Am 66:623, 1982.
Levine MM, DuPont HL, Formal SB, et al: Pathogenesis of *Shigella dysenteriae* 1 (Shiga) dysentery. J Infect Dis 127:261, 1973.
Raghupathy P, Date A, Shastry JCM, et al: Haemolytic uremic syndrome complicating *Shigella* dysentery in South Indian children. Br Med J 1:1518, 1978.
Rahaman MM, Khan MM, Aziz KMS, et al: An outbreak of dysentery caused by *Shigella dysenteriae* type 1 on a coral island in the Bay of Bengal. J Infect Dis 132:15, 1975.
Shiga K: The trend of prevention, therapy and epidemiology of dysentery since the discovery of its causative organism. N Engl J Med 215:1205, 1936.

38.   TYPHOID FEVER

Stephen L. Hoffman*

DEFINITION. Typhoid fever is an acute systemic illness caused by infection with *Salmonella typhi*. It is characterized by (1) prolonged fever, (2) sustained bacteremia without endothelial or endocardial involvement, and (3) bacterial invasion of and multiplication within the mononuclear phagocytic cells of the liver, spleen, lymph nodes, and Peyer's patches. Paratyphoid fever is a pathologically and clinically similar, but generally milder, illness that is caused by many species of salmonellae but most commonly by *S. paratyphi* A, *S. schottmuelleri*, and *S. hirschfeldii*. Enteric fever refers to either typhoid or paratyphoid fever. Unless otherwise stated, the term typhoid fever will be used in this chapter to refer to either typhoid or paratyphoid fever.

HISTORY. Although Hippocrates may have written about typhoid fever, it was not until the early nineteenth

---

*The opinions or assertions herein are those of the author and are not to be construed as official or as reflecting the views of the U.S. Navy or the naval service at large.

century that French workers described the clinical and pathologic features of the "dothoienenterite" (boil of the intestine) that was endemic in Paris. In 1829 Pierre Louis first called it typhoid, meaning "typhus-like," but he did not distinguish between the typhoid of Paris and typhus that was then common in Great Britain. Thus both typhoid and typhus take their names from the Greek "typhos," which means smoke and refers to the apathy and confusion associated with fever that are such prominent features of the fully developed clinical syndromes and also to the belief that the diseases had their origin in miasmic vapors. In 1837 William Wood Gerhard, a former student of Louis's working in Philadelphia, clearly differentiated typhoid from typhus fever, both clinically and pathologically. He wrote:

The anatomical characters of these varieties of fevers are peculiar to themselves and it is (as) impossible to substitute the lesion of the follicles of the small intestine observed in typhoid fever from (for) the pathological phenomena of typhus as it is by other treatment or means to transform the eruption of measles into the pustules of smallpox.

In 1880 Eberth described *Bacillus typhosus* in histologic sections of mesenteric lymph nodes and the spleen. Four years later Gaffky successfully cultured *S. typhi* and stressed that the infection was waterborne and not airborne. In 1896 Achard and Bensaude isolated *S. paratyphi* B and first used the term paratyphoid fever. In the same year Widal described the Widal reaction, and Wright from England and Pfeiffer from Germany introduced the first vaccination against typhoid.

Until 1948 there were no other major advances in typhoid research. Modifications of the first inactivated whole-cell vaccines were used for prevention, the Widal test and culture were used for diagnosis, and patient management was supportive, the outcome being highly dependent on the quality of nursing care. In 1948 Woodward and colleagues, who were working in Malaysia to determine whether chloramphenicol was effective for treating typhus, found that one of their suspected typhus patients had typhoid fever and that chloramphenicol rapidly cleared the bacteremia and markedly shortened the duration of the illness. Since then, chloramphenicol has been the antimicrobial agent of choice for treating both typhoid and paratyphoid fever. In the 1970s and 1980s, live oral attenuated, and Vi capsular polysaccharide *S. typhi* vaccines were developed and shown to be effective in large field trials. These vaccines are likely to soon replace whole-cell vaccines.

ETIOLOGY

Salmonella typhi. *S. typhi* is similar to other salmonellae in that it is a gram-negative, flagellated, nonencapsulated, nonsporulating, facultative anaerobic bacillus. It ferments glucose; reduces nitrate to nitrite; synthesizes peritrichous flagella when motile; has a somatic (O) antigen (oligosaccharide), a flagellar (H) antigen (protein), and an envelope (K) antigen (polysaccharide); and has a lipopolysaccharide macromolecular complex called endotoxin that forms the outer portion of the cell wall (Fig. 38–1). The endotoxin is composed of three layers: outer (O-oligosaccharide), middle (R-core), and basal (lipid A). *S. typhi* is also

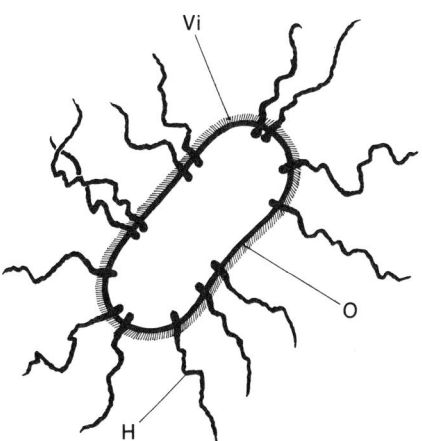

FIGURE 38–1. A schematic diagram of a single *Salmonella typhi* cell showing the locations of the H (flagellar), O (somatic), and Vi (K-envelope) antigens. (From Thomason BM, Cherry WB, Moody MD: J Bacteriol 74:525, 1957. Reprinted by permission.)

capable of developing R-plasmid–transmitted antimicrobial resistance.

Salmonella enteritidis. Paratyphoid fever is caused by organisms of the species *S. enteritidis.* The bacteria that most frequently cause paratyphoid fever are formally named *S. enteritidis* bioserotype paratyphi A, *S. enteritidis* bioserotype paratyphi B, and *S. enteritidis* bioserotype paratyphi C, but they are commonly referred to as *S. paratyphi* A, *S. schottmuelleri,* and *S. hirschfeldii,* respectively.

Characteristics and Classifications. All salmonellae grow on simple media; however, specimens are usually cultured on a selective medium, such as *Salmonella-Shigella* agar, to avoid the overgrowth of salmonellae by other enteric bacteria. The various salmonellae are differentiated on the basis of biochemical reactions and by serologic reaction, i.e., agglutination patterns with O, H, and Vi homologous antisera. The biochemical differences between *S. typhi, S. paratyphi* A, and *S. schottmuelleri* (paratyphi B) are summarized in Table 38–1. Serologic classification using the Kauffman-White agglutination scheme of antigenic analysis is summarized in Table 38–2. Among the salmonellae, only *S. typhi* and *S. hirschfeldii* (paratyphi C) have the important K antigen called the Vi antigen. Vi stands for virulence, and *S. typhi* microorganisms with this antigen are thought to be more virulent than those without, possibly because the envelope protects the somatic O antigen from bactericidal antibody (Fig. 38–1).

DISTRIBUTION AND INCIDENCE. Patients with typhoid and paratyphoid fever are encountered in all parts of the world but are now primarily found in those countries of the developing world where sanitary conditions are poor. In the Spanish-American War, one fifth of the United States troops had typhoid fever, and over 1500 died of typhoid. In the South African Boer Wars, the British Army lost more men to typhoid (8225 deaths) than it did to wounds (7582 deaths). When Sir William Osler published his first textbook of medicine in 1892, the first chapter was on typhoid, and in 1909 Osler estimated that there were 500,000 cases per year in the United States, with 35,000 to 40,000 deaths caused

TABLE 38–1. Biochemical Differences Between *S. typhi*, *S. paratyphi* A, and *S. schottmuelleri*

	S. typhi	*S. paratyphi* A	*S. schottmuelleri*
Acid from glucose	+	+	+
Gas from glucose	−	+ (trace)	+
Hydrogen sulfide production	+ (trace −5%)	− (10% late +)	+
Citrate utilization	+	− (25% late +)	+
Lysine decarboxylase	+	−	+
Ornithine decarboxylase	−	+	+

by typhoid. In 1988 there were 436 cases of typhoid fever in the United States, the majority of which were acquired outside the country. There has been an equally dramatic decrease in the annual incidence of reported typhoid in most European countries. In most areas of the world, typhoid fever is much more common than paratyphoid fever.

Although not a major problem in the developed world, typhoid is considered by many to be one of the most important and underreported diseases in the developing world. The underreporting is due to the fact that a positive blood culture is often required for diagnosis, and many patients with typhoid are treated where there are no bacteriology facilities. However, recent studies in Chile, Nepal, South Africa, and Indonesia have documented annual blood culture–positive attack rates ranging from approximately 100/100,000/year (Chile) to over 1000/100,000 population/year (Indonesia). It has been estimated that the worldwide incidence (excluding China) of typhoid fever is approximately 12,500,000 cases per year, with greater than 62% of cases occurring in Asia and 35% in Africa. In some areas it has been estimated that typhoid fever is responsible for 2 to 5% of all deaths.

Hospital case-fatality rates for typhoid fever are still high (1 to 30%) in many parts of the developing world. Since typhoid frequently kills young adults, many of whom have recently finished school, entered the work force, and become parents, the economic and social impact of typhoid on the family and society is often dramatic.

EPIDEMIOLOGY

Source of Infection. *S. typhi*, *S. paratyphi* A, and *S. schottmuelleri* infect only humans. Thus, all cases of typhoid fever and most cases of paratyphoid fever could theoretically be traced back to another infected human. The stool and, less commonly, the urine of carriers and those with or recovering from acute infections are the source of the organism. It is generally believed that 3% of patients with acute typhoid fever become carriers, but this rate is a function of the age and health of the patient. The carrier rate increases with increasing age and prevalence of gallbladder disease. Fecal carriers usually outnumber urinary carriers 10 to 1, but in areas

endemic for *Schistosoma haematobium* urinary carriers are often more common. The carrier rate within communities varies considerably.

Method of Transmission. The infection is most commonly acquired by ingestion of contaminated food or water but may rarely be transmitted by direct finger-to-mouth contact with the feces, urine, respiratory secretions, vomitus, or pus from an infected individual. The stools of chronic carriers usually contain from 10^6 to 10^9 organisms per gram. *S. typhi* can survive for several weeks in water, ice, dust, or dried sewage and on clothing but survives in raw sewage for less than a week. It can also survive and multiply in milk or milk products without altering the appearance of the milk.

Food can be infected directly by water used to wash it or prepare it, by carriers, by fomites and dust, and probably by flies. In many cases the initial concentration of organisms is too low to cause human disease, but under optimal environmental conditions the organisms can multiply in food. In the case of shellfish such as oysters and mussels, the polluted water in which they live may not have a high enough concentration of organisms to cause disease in a swimmer who ingests small amounts of water. However, since the shellfish filters up to 50 gallons of water per day and concentrates the microbial content, the aficionado of raw shellfish from polluted water may be presented with an enormous dose of *S. typhi*.

Factors that Influence Infectivity. Studies done in human volunteers using the Quailes strain of *S. typhi* showed that in healthy, previously unvaccinated male adults, ingestion of 10^5 organisms led to clinical disease in 25% of volunteers (ID_{25}); ingestion of 10^7 organisms caused disease in 50% (ID_{50}); and 10^9 organisms caused disease in 95% (ID_{95}). As the number of organisms increased, the incubation period decreased, but the clinical syndrome was unchanged. Nothing is known about the relationship between differences in strains of *S. typhi* and infectivity except that strains that do not have Vi antigen are less infective and less virulent. A gastric pH of < 2 will kill most of the organisms; those patients who chronically ingest antacids, have had a gastrectomy, or have low gastric acidity for other reasons require lower numbers of organisms to produce clinical

TABLE 38–2. Antigenic Analysis by the Kauffman-White Scheme of the Organisms Causing Typhoid and Paratyphoid Fever

	O Antigen Group	O Antigens	H Antigens		K Antigens
			Phase 1	*Phase 2*	
S. paratyphi A	A	1, 2, 12	a	—	—
S. schottmuelleri	B	1, 4, 5, 12	b	1, 2	—
S. hirschfeldii	C	6. 7	c	1, 5	Vi
S. typhi	D	9, 12	d		Vi

disease. Parenteral vaccination confers a fairly strong immunity, which may be overcome by increasing the infecting dose.

Patterns of Disease in the Community

Developed Countries. In industrialized nations with good sewage and water supply systems, most cases of typhoid fever are sporadic and either are imported or can be traced to contact with a chronic carrier. There are intermittent epidemics that are generally attributed to a common source exposure. In 1964, in Aberdeen, Scotland, 507 cases of typhoid fever occurred that were traced to ingestion of canned corned beef from Argentina. The leaky cans had been cooled in sewage-contaminated river water after canning. In 1973, there were 225 cases of typhoid fever in a migrant farm labor camp in Dade County, Florida. The laborers were infected by drinking from the camp water supply system, which had a defective chlorinator and probably had been contaminated by a mentally retarded girl who acquired the infection from a chronic carrier who lived next door to her. In 1981, 76 cases of typhoid fever occurred in San Antonio, Texas. They were traced to a tortilla shop where one employee had *S. typhi* in his stool. In 1986, 10 cases of typhoid fever were acquired in a fast food restaurant in Silver Spring, Maryland. They were traced to a shrimp salad prepared by an 18-year-old asymptomatic carrier who worked in the restaurant.

Developing World. Epidemics also occur in the tropics and subtropics, but the majority of cases are reported in areas where typhoid fever is endemic. In these locations there are so many sick or recovering individuals that chronic carriers may be less important in transmission than they are in the industrialized world. The incidence is frequently seasonal, with a peak in the hot, dry months of the year when the concentration of organisms in water is increased—not diluted by rains. In some areas the incidence is reported to peak during the rainy season, when flooding apparently breaks down the systems that separate sewage from drinking water.

In areas where typhoid fever is endemic, it is likely that more than 95% of patients are treated as outpatients by local physicians. Thus, hospital-based incidence figures may underestimate actual incidence by 15 to 25 times. In most areas of the developing world, the reported incidence of typhoid fever is at least 2 to 3 times that of paratyphoid fever, except during epidemics and in infants.

Age. The age-specific attack rates of typhoid fever must reflect exposure to the organism and the development of a protective immune response. Osler observed that typhoid fever was primarily a disease of late adolescence and early adulthood, and most current data derived from studies of hospitalized patients in the developing world support this observation. However, in recent years prospective studies of outpatients in endemic areas have shown that even where the incidence in inpatients is highest in adolescents and young adults, the overall incidence of blood culture–confirmed disease is generally highest in children aged 3 to 9 years, declining significantly in late adolescence. The difference between hospital-based and outpatient studies may reflect the fact that older adolescents and young adults become more ill with *S. typhi* infection and require hospitalization more often than do children. Infants and children can certainly develop life-threatening typhoid fever, although the case-fatality rates for hospitalized children are generally lower than for adults.

Antibiotic Resistance. In the 1970s there were large epidemics of typhoid fever in Mexico (> 10,000 cases) and Southeast Asia caused by strains of *S. typhi* that exhibited R-plasmid–mediated resistance to chloramphenicol. The Mexican outbreak was caused by a single Vi phage type that was later found to have been responsible for cases of typhoid fever reported from Switzerland, the United Kingdom, and the United States (especially Los Angeles). Subsequent to this epidemic, resistance has not been a major problem in this part of the world. The cases in Southeast Asia were caused by at least 11 different phage types of *S. typhi,* making the continued spread of resistance much more likely than in Mexico. Fortunately, in most areas of Southeast Asia, few isolates of *S. typhi* are now resistant to chloramphenicol. In recent series from India, Singapore, and Indonesia, less than 3% of *S. typhi* isolates were resistant to chloramphenicol. In a study of isolates from 100 patients in Bangkok, Thailand, 45% were found to be resistant. However, in recent years the incidence of resistance has diminished considerably in Thailand.

PATHOGENESIS AND PATHOLOGY. The hallmark of the syndrome is bacterial invasion of and multiplication within the mononuclear phagocytic cells in the liver, spleen, lymph nodes, and Peyer's patches of the ileum. Our knowledge of the sequence of events following ingestion of an infective dose of *S. typhi* is derived from studies of human volunteers and chimpanzees experimentally infected with *S. typhi* and of mice infected with *S. enteritidis* serotypes enteritidis and typhimurium. However, this information is incomplete, and the theories of pathogenesis are not well substantiated. For example, there is still no well-documented explanation for the pathogenesis of the mental confusion and other central nervous system manifestations that led to the disease's being called typhoid.

Proposed Sequence of Events

Mucosal Penetration. After ingestion the organisms pass through the upper gastrointestinal tract to the small intestine, where they attach preferentially to the tips of the villi and either invade directly or multiply for several days before invading. Since less than 5% of the villi are involved, it is hypothesized that there are specific receptor sites on the villi, but these receptors have not been identified. Stool cultures are positive for several days after *S. typhi* ingestion and then become negative until after the onset of clinical illness. Human volunteer studies have shown that invasion can take place in the jejunum, and animal studies suggest that it occurs in the ileum. After penetration (mechanism unknown), the organisms pass to the intestinal lymphoid follicles and the draining mesenteric lymph nodes; some also pass into the systemic circulation, where they are filtered out by the reticuloendothelial cells of the liver and spleen. The salmonellae then multiply within the mononuclear phagocytic cells of the lymphoid follicles, lymph nodes, liver, and spleen. At this stage there are subtle degenerative, proliferative, and granulomatous changes in the villi, crypt glands, and lamina propria of the small bowel and in the mesenteric lymph glands. These changes are reversible and unassociated with clinical symptoms.

Dissemination and Organ Invasion. At a critical point (which is probably a function of numbers of bacteria, bacterial virulence, and the host's immune response), a sufficient number of organisms and possibly other mediators that induce clinical symptoms are released from this sequestered intracellular habitat in the intestinal and mesenteric lymph system and pass through the thoracic duct and into the general circulation. This marks the end of the incubation period, which may last from 3 to 60 days but is usually 7 to 14 days.

During this bacteremic phase the organisms may invade any organ but are most commonly found in the liver, spleen, bone marrow, gallbladder, and Peyer's patches in the terminal ileum. They invade the gallbladder either directly from the blood stream or from the bile and then reappear in the intestine, where they are excreted in the stool and reinvade through the intestinal wall. At most tissue sites the organisms are again taken up by, and multiply within, the mononuclear phagocytic cells.

Pathology. The basic histologic finding in typhoid fever is infiltration of tissues by macrophages (typhoid cells) containing bacteria, erythrocytes, and degenerated lymphocytes. Aggregates of these macrophages are called typhoid nodules (Fig. 38–2). They are most commonly found in the intestine, mesenteric lymph nodes, spleen, liver, and bone marrow but may be found in the kidneys, testes, and parotid glands.

Intestine. In the intestine there are four classic pathologic stages. *Hyperplastic* changes begin during the first week of illness and primarily involve Peyer's patches of the ileum and solitary lymphoid follicles of the cecum but may involve any lymphoid tissue in the intestine. Almost all infiltrative cells are mononuclear; typhoid

nodules are common. If the hyperplasia does not resolve, *necrosis* of the intestinal mucosa develops, usually after 7 to 10 days of clinical illness (Fig. 38–3). Sloughing of the mucosa follows and results in the development of an *ulcer* that may bleed (Fig. 38–3). The ulcers conform in shape and distribution to the location of the lymphoid follicles, are largest in the ileum, and are almost always found on the antimesenteric border of the intestines. These ulcers may perforate into the peritoneal cavity. Perforations are single and measure less than 1 cm in 80% of cases; 90% are found within 60 cm of the ileocecal valve. When healing takes place, it is usually complete, without scarring.

Mesenteric Lymph Nodes, Spleen, and Liver. In the mesenteric lymph nodes, the sinusoids are enlarged and distended by large collections of macrophages and reticuloendothelial cells. The nodes become soft and swollen and often contain areas of focal necrosis. The spleen is enlarged, red, soft, and congested. Its serosal surface may have a fibrinous exudate. Microscopically the red pulp is congested and contains typhoid nodules. The liver is usually enlarged. Hypertrophy and hyperplasia of the Kupffer cells produce the typhoid nodules. There is frequently focal hepatic necrosis and cloudy swelling of hepatocytes. The gallbladder is usually slightly hyperemic and may, in rare instances, show evidence of cholecystitis.

Other Organs. These are less frequently involved during typhoid fever and usually have lesions attributed to toxic factors. The heart may be flabby with dilated ventricles, and microscopically there is often a nonspecific pattern of necrosis with degeneration and fatty infiltration of the myocardial cells. The lungs show interstitial pneumonitis and bronchitis, and skeletal muscles may show Zenker's degeneration. The most common lesion found in the kidneys is swelling and albuminous degeneration of the proximal tubular epithelium, but interstitial nephritis, glomerulonephritis, and pye-

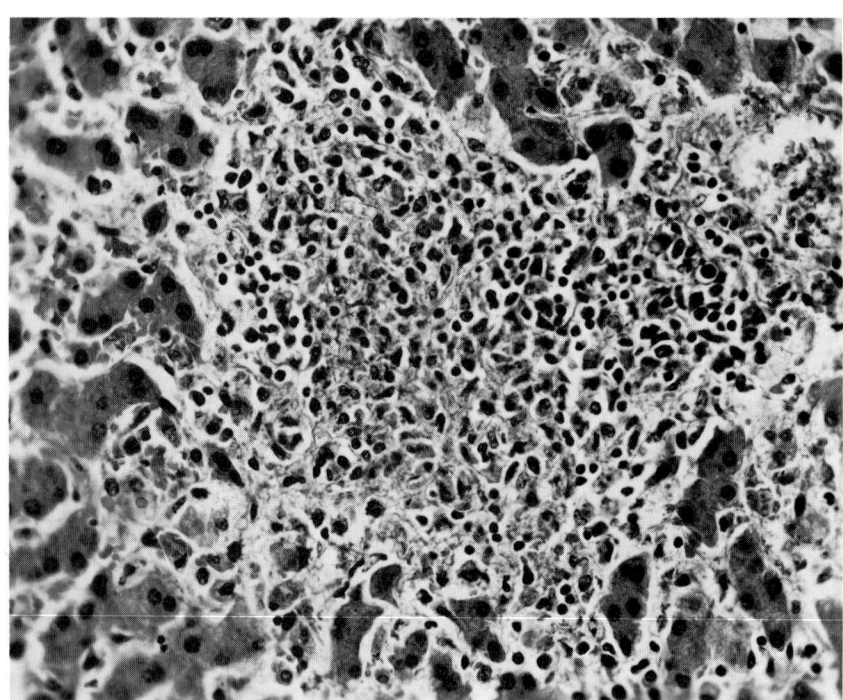

FIGURE 38–2. A typhoid nodule in the liver during the stage of active invasion. This lesion is principally composed of macrophages (center) with variable numbers of lymphocytes and plasma cells (periphery). (× 305.) (Courtesy of the Armed Forces Institute of Pathology. Photograph Neg. No. 72–4603.)

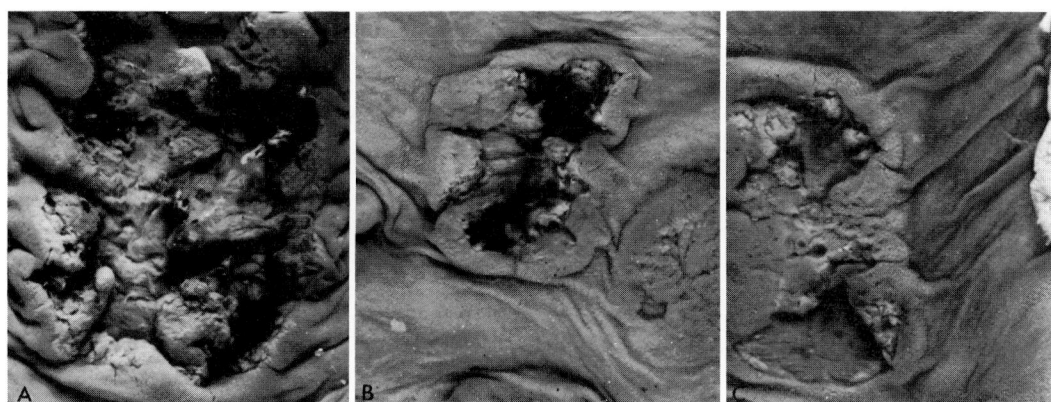

FIGURE 38–3. Peyer's patches in the ileum showing several stages in a single specimen. *A.* Active ulceration. *B,* Necrosis. *C,* The sloughing of necrotic tissue has left the muscularis bare. (Courtesy of the Armed Forces Institute of Pathology, Photograph Neg. No. 64–3208–2.)

lonephritis have been noted. Central nervous system changes have been poorly described, but ring hemorrhages, capillary thrombi, perivenous demyelinating leukoencephalitis, and meningitis have been reported. Occasionally, focal lesions such as osteomyelitis, brain abscess, and spleen and liver abscesses have been reported. These lesions are almost always characterized by polymorphonuclear instead of mononuclear response.

Pathogenesis of Organ Dysfunction and Toxemia. A hypothesis for the pathogenesis of typhoid fever must explain (1) the inflammatory and necrotic changes at the sites of multiplication of the organism in the intestine, liver, spleen, and lymph nodes; (2) the prolonged pyrexia and toxemia; and (3) the pathologic changes and functional derangements in organs such as the heart, lungs, brain, and kidneys, where typhoid nodules and *S. typhi* are generally not found.

Until the past decade most authorities thought that the necrotic changes in the intestine, liver, spleen, and lymph nodes were the result of tissue hypoxia secondary to small vessel occlusion by typhoid nodules, and that the systemic manifestations and dysfunction of other organs were caused by circulating endotoxin. There is now evidence that neither small vessel occlusion nor circulating endoxin plays a major role in the pathogenesis of typhoid fever.

Endotoxin. The role of endotoxin in the pathogenesis of typhoid fever is unclear. Investigators at the University of Maryland showed that when *S. typhi* endotoxin was initially injected into human volunteers, it produced chills, fever, headaches, myalgias, anorexia, nausea, thrombocytopenia, and leukopenia, as in typhoid fever. After these volunteers had received repeated injections of endotoxin, they became unresponsive (tolerant) to it, but when the tolerant individuals were challenged with *S. typhi,* they developed classic typhoid fever. Since typhoid fever is an unrelenting, sustained illness when not treated with antibiotics, the fact that the volunteers developed tolerance to endotoxin suggests that circulating endotoxin does not cause the symptoms and signs of naturally acquired typhoid fever. Furthermore, the facts that endotoxin-tolerant volunteers developed typhoid fever after rechallenge and that circulating endotoxin as detected by limulus assay is not present in many

patients with typhoid make it even less likely that circulating endotoxin plays a major role in the pathogenesis of the disease.

Immune Complexes and Other Immunologic Reactions. Several investigators have found circulating immune complexes in patients with typhoid fever, and others have noted immune complexes in renal biopsy specimens taken from typhoid patients with glomerulonephritis and nephrotic syndrome. The significance of these complexes is unknown. Other investigators have hypothesized that some of the less common central nervous system manifestations of typhoid fever, such as Guillain-Barré syndrome, perivenous leukoencephalitis, and transverse myelitis, are due to an immune reaction, but there is no good evidence to support these hypotheses.

Disseminated Intravascular Coagulation. Although there have been several reports of clinically classic disseminated intravascular coagulation (DIC) in typhoid patients, this is a rare complication. On the other hand, recent work indicates that many patients with *S. typhi* infections have laboratory evidence of DIC without bleeding and may have localized DIC within organs.

Metabolic and Nutritional Factors. Various authors have suggested that anemia, vitamin deficiencies, zinc and other trace metal deficiencies, thyroid dysfunction, tryptophan metabolites, other amino acids, and the time of the day that infection occurs or treatment is initiated are all important in the pathogenesis of the disease and the host's ability to mobilize adequate defenses. Although it is likely that many of these factors may be important in determining the ultimate expression of the disease, it is unlikely that any of them is the major determinant of how the disease is expressed or how the host defends against the infection.

Proposed Pathogenesis. The unique feature of typhoid fever is the relationship between *S. typhi* and macrophages in the liver, spleen, intestinal lymphoid follicles, and mesenteric lymph nodes. Macrophages can produce an array of functionally active cytokines. These include tumor necrosis factor (cachectin), IL–1, and interferons. Macrophages are also an important source of arachidonate metabolites and reactive oxygen intermediates. These macrophage products can cause cellular necrosis, stimulation of the immune system, vascular instability, initiation of the clotting mechanism, bone marrow depression, fever, and other abnormalities associated with typhoid fever. It is likely that *S. typhi* endotoxin stimulates the macrophages to release these substances, which locally mediate the intestinal and hepatocellular necrosis found in the disease and which, when released systemically, cause most of the other manifestations of the disease.

Although immune complexes, other immune reactions, and metabolic disturbances probably cause some of the less common manifestations of the disease, it is doubtful that they play a significant role in the pathogenesis.

IMMUNOLOGIC RESPONSE. Typhoid fever induces both systemic and local humoral and cellular immune responses. Although there have been many descriptive studies of the immune responses associated with *S. typhi* infection and with immunization with typhoid vaccines, the roles of specific immune mechanisms in the development of resistance to reinfection with *S. typhi*, pathogenesis of typhoid, and complete elimination of bacteria from infected individuals have not been clearly established. Some have suggested that infection with typhoid confers long-lasting immunity to reinfection, but the high incidence of typhoid fever in young adults in endemic areas and the results of volunteer studies indicate that this is not the case. Fifteen volunteers who had ingested 10^5 organisms and developed acute typhoid fever were rechallenged with 10^5 organisms (expected to cause infection in 25% of individuals) a mean of 20 months after the first infection. Five (33%) developed acute typhoid fever again. The fact that hospital-based studies indicate that the incidence of severe typhoid fever is higher in older adolescents and young adults than in young children suggests that an acquired immune response may play a role in the pathogenesis of severe disease. Relapse may reflect the inadequate development of an appropriate anti–*S. typhi* immune response.

Antibodies. *S. typhi* specific secretory IgA in the small intestine may be important in determining whether mucosal penetration takes place. A study from India has reported that patients with typhoid fever have lower levels of IgA in intestinal secretions than do control subjects. *S. typhi*–specific IgA has been demonstrated in the feces and intestinal fluid of volunteers immunized with the oral typhoid vaccne Ty21a.

Development of specific antibodies during typhoid fever has been well documented. Circulating IgG, IgM, and in some cases IgA antibodies to *S. typhi* O, H, Vi, and porin antigens have been identified. Not all individuals with typhoid fever develop antibodies to these antigens. Fourfold titer rises to O, H, and Vi antigens were documented in 75%, 75%, and 40%, respectively, of volunteers experimentally infected with *S. typhi.* Immunization with the Vi antigen vaccine and the oral vaccine Ty21a (see section on vaccines) induce antibodies to Vi antigen and O antigen (IgG and IgA), respectively; immunization with the killed typhoid vaccines can induce antibodies to O, H, and Vi antigens. It has not been proved that these antibodies are responsible for the protective immunity found after administration

of these vaccines. However, the developers of the Vi vaccine attribute the vaccine-induced protection to antibodies against Vi antigen. Interestingly, a study in Sweden showed that an O, H, and Vi antigen-free fraction of *S. typhi* induced serum antibodies in rabbits and that this serum protected chicken embryos against lethal doses of *S. typhi*. Work has begun only recently to determine the fine specificity of antigen-specific antibody responses.

Cellular Immune Responses. A major characteristic of typhoid fever is the activation of macrophages. Phagocytosis is a major host defense mechanism, and substances released from macrophages, including cytokines, reactive oxygen intermediates, and arachidonic acid metabolites, probably play a significant role in the pathogenesis of the disease. Several small studies from India have suggested that patients who do not develop cell-mediated immunity as measured by the leukocyte migration inhibition test have an increased incidence of complications and relapse, but investigators in Sri Lanka using similar techniques did not find this relationship. Immune cells may also play an important role in the protective immunity induced by immunization, but this response has not been adequately characterized. It has been proposed that the protective immunity induced by immunization with the oral typhoid vaccine Ty21a may be mediated by antibody–dependent cellular cytotoxicity involving IgA antibodies against *S. typhi* and CD4+ T cells, since volunteers immunized with Ty21a have been shown to develop this immune response.

CLINICAL MANIFESTATIONS. The clinical presentation of typhoid fever is variable, but nearly all patients have fever, and most have a headache. The range of clinical manifestations and severity of the illness varies, depending upon the patient population. Clinicians who see outpatients in an endemic area of the developing world will find that their typhoid patients are moderately ill, that less than 10% will require hospitalization, that complications are rare, and that the case-fatality rate will be less than 1%. Hospital-based physicians in the same area will see typhoid patients who are much sicker and have a greater range of symptoms, signs, and complications; the case-fatality rate may range up to 30%. If one sees typhoid patients in the developed world, nearly all patients will be hospitalized, but the clinical severity, complications, and case-fatality rates will be comparable to those in outpatients in the developing world. In many cases, the most severely ill patients will have been sicker for longer periods than those who are moderately ill, but this is not always so. The strain of *S. typhi,* the number of organisms ingested, the general and nutritional condition and immunologic status of the patient, and, possibly, the genetic makeup of the host may influence the clinical presentation.

Untreated Typhoid Fever. After ingestion of the organisms, 10 to 20% of patients will have transient diarrhea. These patients, as well as all others, remain asymptomatic during the incubation period, which usually lasts 7 to 14 days but can be as short as 3 days and as long as 60 days, depending on the number of organisms ingested. As the stage of sustained bacteremia

TABLE 38–3. Symptoms Expected on Admission in Hospitalized Typhoid Patients in Endemic Areas of the Developing World

Symptom	%	Symptom	%
Fever	99	Cough or chest discomfort	35
Weakness	99	Vomiting	35
Anorexia	85	Myalgia, arthralgia	35
Headache	85	Confusion	25
Dizziness	80	Sore throat	20
Abdominal pain	50	Decreased hearing	15
Nausea	50	Blood in stool or melena	12
Chills	50	Epistaxis	10
Diarrhea	45	Dysuria	2
Constipation	40	Seizures	2

develops, the incubation period ends and the patient notices the onset of fever, which classically increases daily in a stepwise fashion but may be remittent or sustained. At this point the patient will usually have a flulike syndrome with headache and malaise, will frequently have a sore throat, anorexia, nausea, abdominal pain, and myalgias, but may have any of the symptoms listed in Table 38–3. By the end of the first week after the onset of symptoms the fever is sustained, and the patient is often toxic and may have any of the symptoms and signs listed in Tables 38–3 and 38–4.

The fever remains sustained during the second week and by the third week begins to come down spontaneously by lysis. Intestinal perforation and/or hemorrhage can occur at any stage of the illness, but these findings classically occur during the third week. The illness can go on for several months, although by the end of the fourth week the temperature usually returns to normal, and except for individuals with metastatic foci in whom cholecystitis, osteomyelitis, and soft tissue abscesses may develop, most patients have recovered. It is at this stage that most relapses occur.

Clinical Course and Manifestations in Patients Who Receive Antimicrobials. Antimicrobials shorten the course, reduce the rate of complications if begun early, and reduce the case-fatality rate; some may increase the relapse rate. During volunteer studies in Maryland more than 400 patients with typhoid fever were treated within 3 days of the onset of fever, and the complication and case-fatality rates were 0.

Symptoms. The approximate frequencies of symptoms expected in hospitalized patients in endemic areas are summarized in Table 38–3. Before hospitalization, most

TABLE 38–4. Physical Signs Expected on Admission in Hospitalized Typhoid Patients in Endemic Areas of the Developing World

Common		Less Common	
Sign	*%*	*Sign*	*%*
Fever	98	Disorientation	25
Coated tongue	95	Relative bradycardia	15
Apathy	70	Rales or rhonchi	15
Hepatomegaly	50	Delirium	15
Abdominal pain	45	Severely toxic	10
Rose spots	0–50	Decreased hearing	10
Moderately sick	45	Stiff neck	10
Toxic	45	Stupor	2
Splenomegaly	35	Focal neurologic findings	1

of these patients will have been ill for 6 to 12 days, most will have seen a health care provider at some point, and most will have received short courses of antibiotics, often with chloramphenicol. Fever is universal and, although present daily, is usually higher in the late afternoon and evening. Chills and dull frontal or diffuse headaches are common. The headaches often prevent patients from sleeping comfortably. Most patients are anorexic. They complain of abdominal pain but cannot localize it well. Both diarrhea and constipation are common; normal bowel function is unusual. Children frequently have diarrhea. Bloody dysentery is occasionally encountered. The incidence of cough and chest discomfort varies considerably. Sore throats are common during the first week of illness but less common later. Dysuria is more commonly encountered in parts of the world where *Schistosoma haematobium* is endemic. Epistaxis, which was a common finding in the preantibiotic era, is much less common now. Seizures are occasionally reported, being more common in children below 5 years of age. If the family is interviewed, a history of intermittent confusion is frequently reported.

Signs. On physical examination the patient is generally moderately ill to toxic; however, 10 to 15% of patients will be severely toxic and may be hyperpyrexic (Table 38–4). He or she will be lying apathetically immobile in bed, often staring blankly, but will be arousable. About 10% of patients are severely agitated and 5% obtunded. Disorientation is common, as is frank delirium. Stupor and coma are infrequent. If the patient is hypovolemic from blood loss or dehydration, hypotension or shock may be present. Characteristic gram-negative septic shock is uncommon on admission but does occur after intestinal perforation, in patients with severe typhoid fever without obvious perforation, and as a preterminal event. Relative bradycardia, once considered to be a classic finding in typhoid fever, is now encountered in less than 25% of patients. Rose spots, which are blanching, red, maculopapular lesions measuring 2 to 4 mm, are most frequently found on the abdomen and chest but can be seen on the extremities and back. Rose spots are less frequently found in dark-skinned patients. The tongue is covered with a thick, "furry," white-to-brown coating that spares the bright red tips and edges. The incidence of respiratory findings varies, but signs consistent with bronchitis (15%) are more common than those of lobar consolidation (1 to 8%).

The abdominal examination is frequently difficult to interpret. In classic descriptions, the abdomen is said to be "doughy," and the examiner easily palpates loops of bowel filled with air and fluid and finds diffuse lower quandrant tenderness. In recent reports, diffuse abdominal pain with moderate guarding has often been described. Frequently, it is difficult for the examiner to be certain that perforation has not occurred. The spleen or liver is enlarged in 30 to 50% of patients, and although both organs can become quite large, more commonly they are moderately enlarged, with the liver palpable 2 or 3 cm below the right costal margin and the spleen palpable on deep inspiration or 1 or 2 cm below the left costal margin. Both organs are usually soft and moderately tender. Occult blood is found in the stool of 20 to 30% of patients.

Complications and Unusual Manifestations

Intestinal Perforation. Intestinal perforation occurs in about 3% of hospitalized patients. It usually occurs during the third week of illness but can happen during the first week. The patient with perforation has the usual symptoms of typhoid fever and complains of severe abdominal pain that often is localized to the right lower quandrant but may be diffuse. Bowel sounds are absent in 50% of cases. About 75% of patients will have guarding, rebound tenderness, and rigidity, particularly in the right lower quadrant. Some patients will have an absence of hepatic dullness because of free air in the abdomen, but a pneumoperitoneum is present on x-ray in only 50 to 70% of patients. Perforation causes a marked sudden rise in pulse, fall in blood pressure, and onset of severe pain. In most patients the diagnosis is not difficult. However, as noted above, approximately 25% of patients will not have classic findings of peritonitis and perforation, and in these individuals the diagnosis is difficult. It is sometimes quite difficult to decide whether a patient has perforation, impending perforation, or just severe typhoid abdominal pain. In the appropriate clinical setting, a rising white blood cell count with a shift to the left is suggestive of perforation but probably occurs in less than half of patients with perforation.

Intestinal Hemorrhage. Intestinal hemorrhage occurs in up to 15% of cases. Patients may or may not be toxic. The bowel usually does not perforate, and bleeding is sometimes heavy enough to cause shock. If blood replacement can keep up with losses, the hemorrhaging is usually a self-limiting process, not requiring surgery. About 25% of patients with typhoid fever have minor bleeding that does not require transfusion.

Neuropsychiatric Manifestations. In recent years, reports from India, Indonesia, and Africa (particularly Nigeria) have documented a wide spectrum of neuropsychiatric manifestations of typhoid fever. In some series, half the patients have had disorders of mental status. The most common findings are disturbances of the level of consciousness that range from disorientation to delirium, obtundation, stupor, and coma. Delirium, stupor, and coma are grave prognostic signs associated with case-fatality rates that have exceeded 40%. Delirium often persists after the temperature and metabolic function have returned to normal, and there is no good explanation for its pathogenesis.

Other less commonly encountered central nervous system findings are seizures, typhoid meningitis, encephalomyelitis, transverse myelitis with spastic paraplegia, peripheral or cranial neuritis, and Guillain-Barré syndrome. Psychotic syndromes, including schizophrenia-like illnesses, mania, depression, and catatonia, have been described, especially in Africa.

Cardiovascular Manifestations. Myocarditis occurs in 1 to 5% of typhoid patients, whereas nonspecific electrocardiographic changes occur in 10 to 15% of patients. Patients with myocarditis may have no cardiovascular symptoms or may have chest pains, congestive heart failure, arrhythmias, or cardiogenic shock. When myocarditis occurs in young children, it is frequently a serious complication. Electrocardiographic findings are the same as in any myocarditis. Pericarditis rarely occurs, but "peripheral vascular collapse" without other cardiac findings is being described increasingly. Deep venous and arterial thromboses are uncommon.

Hepatobiliary Manifestations. Asymptomatic typhoid hepatitis is a common finding; in fact, most patients have minor elevations of the serum enzymes, e.g., AST and ALT. Jaundice with or without major elevations of hepatic enzymes occurs in 1 to 2% of patients, as does acute cholecystitis. Acute or chronic cholecystitis may occur months to years after an episode of typhoid fever. Culture of stones and/or bile yields *S. typhi* in these cases.

Genitourinary Manifestations. About 25% of patients excrete *S. typhi* in the urine at some point during their illness. Transient proteinuria is the most common urinary abnormality and in some cases is due to an immune complex–mediated glomerulonephritis. On occasion the glomerulonephritis may present as renal failure or nephrotic syndrome, and in these cases the prognosis is poor. In severely ill patients, acute tubular necrosis may develop, and in patients with severe intravascular hemolysis, which may or may not be associated with glucose–6-phosphate dehydrogenase (G–6-PD) deficiency, renal failure can occur. Both pyelonephritis and cystitis occur in typhoid patients.

Other Complications. Disseminated intravascular coagulation is rarely of clinical importance, but thrombocytopenia, hypofibrinogenemia, elevated prothrombin time (PT) and partial thromboplastin time (PTT), and elevated levels of fibrin degradation products can be found in most patients. The hemolytic-uremic syndrome and severe intravascular hemolysis have been reported. Because of the sustained bacteremia, focal infections can develop at any site of the body, but these occur rarely. The most common sites of infection are in the bones (extremities, spine, ribs), but infections have been reported in the brain, liver, spleen, muscles, breast, thyroid, salivary glands, and cervical lymph nodes. In the past, thrombophlebitis, parotitis, and decubitus ulcers were common complications, but they are now rare.

Relapse. Relapse occurred in 5 to 10% of patients in the preantibiotic era, and although initial reports in the 1950s and 1960s suggested that relapse increased to 10 to 20% in antibiotic-treated patients, most recent series have not reported increased relapse rates in treated patients. Fever generally returns about 2 weeks after the cessation of antibiotic therapy or in untreated patients about 2 weeks after defervescence. However, relapse can occur during convalescence when the patient is afebrile but is still symptomatic and on antibiotics, and it has been reported several months after the initial illness. The relapse syndrome is usually, but not always, milder than the initial syndrome.

Typhoid in Children Less Than 5 Years of Age. *S. typhi* infections have been acquired congenitally, and there have been many case reports in neonates. The clinical presentation in children less than 5 years of age, and especially less than 1 year of age, is less predictable than in adults. It ranges from an extremely mild illness, often diagnosed as a viral infection but treated with antimicrobials, to severe typhoid fever with hospital mortality rates reaching 30%. Children with typhoid fever frequently have diarrhea and vomiting, and up to 20% may have convulsions. Typhoid meningitis, although reported in adults and older children, is found almost exclusively in children less than 5 years of age. Paratyphoid fever, particularly in infants, may also cause severe disease with high case-fatality and complication rates. In Indonesia, paratyphoid in children is often caused by the multiple antimicrobial–resistant *S. oranienburg* (C_1).

Geographic Variations. Reports from Indonesia, India, Nepal, and some areas of Africa have described patients with abnormal levels of consciousness or shock who have a much higher case-fatality rate than do those with normal mental status. These cases of severe typhoid fever with high mortality have rarely been reported from the Americas. It is not clear whether the difference in severity is a function of the host, bacteria, or epidemiologic factors. In areas of endemic schistosomiasis, a syndrome of prolonged, intermittent fever and *Salmonella* sp. bacteremia associated with mild active chronic schistosomiasis has been documented (Chapter 96). The pathogenesis of this syndrome is unknown; however, it may be linked to the abnormal immune response seen in chronic schistosomiasis and/or the tegmental attachment of bacteria to the adult schistosome worm. Chronic *Salmonella* sp. urinary carriage is common in areas with endemic *Schistosoma haematobium* and is undoubtedly related to the obstructive uropathy of urinary schistosomiasis. These patients may experience intermittent fever and bacteremia secondary to the resultant pyelonephritis. Patients with opisthorchiasis (liver fluke infection) may have intrahepatic as opposed to gallbladder carriage, and these individuals may have asymptomatic carriage or recurrent cholangitis. (Chapter 98.1).

Chronic Carriers. A person who excretes the organism in the stool 1 year after the initial illness is considered to be a carrier. Although 20% of typhoid patients will excrete the organism for 2 months after the onset of illness, and 10% for 3 months, only 3% of patients go on to become carriers. The prevalence is higher in females and in the elderly and is probably correlated with the prevalence of cholelithiasis. Most carriers are asymptomatic, and in some series up to 25% could not give a history compatible with acute typhoid fever. Individuals with abnormalities of the genitourinary system, including schistosomiasis, have a much higher prevalence of urinary carriage than do those with a normal system.

Laboratory Findings. At the time of hospital admission most patients will be moderately anemic, have an elevated erythrocyte sedimentation rate, and a platelet count reduced to about 150,000. The white blood cell count will often be about 5000 to 6000/μm but may range from 1200 to over 20,000/μm. The differential count is usually normal or shifted slightly to the left, but there may be a relative lymphocytosis, especially later in the disease. Most patients will have slightly elevated prothrombin and partial thromboplastin times,

decreased fibrinogen levels, and circulating fibrin degradation products. Serum enzymes, e.g., AST and ALT, are usually elevated to values that are twice normal, as is the serum bilirubin. Hyponatremia and hypokalemia are commonly encountered but are usually not severe. Renal function is usually normal. The urine often has low levels of protein and a few white blood cells.

DIAGNOSIS. The diagnosis of typhoid fever is suspected by the clinician; is suggested by assays that identify *Salmonella* sp. antibodies, antigens, or DNA; and is confirmed by isolation of the organism. The Widal reaction is indicative of typhoid fever in only 40 to 60% of patients at the time of admission, and although the organism can be isolated from 95% of patients, identification takes at least 18 hours and often 4 days. Thus, investigations are under way to develop more sensitive laboratory methods for making the rapid, presumptive diagnosis of typhoid fever.

Isolation of the Organism

Bone Marrow Aspirates. Culturing bone marrow aspirates is the single most sensitive method of isolating *S. typhi* from patients with typhoid fever. The diagnosis of typhoid cannot be excluded, and the sensitivity of other diagnostic techniques cannot be established without a bone marrow aspirate (BMA) culture. BMA cultures are positive in 80% to 95% of patients, even in those who have been taking antibiotics for several days, and regardless of how long they have been ill.

Blood Cultures. The blood culture is positive in 40% to 80% of patients. When experimentally infected human volunteers had daily cultures prior to antibiotic therapy (mean number of cultures was 5.8), only 75% had positive blood cultures. In the Dade County, Florida, epidemic (see under Epidemiology), only 55% of hospitalized patients with typhoid fever had positive blood cultures. The sensitivity of blood cultures is greatest during the first week of illness, is reduced by prior ingestion of antibiotics, and is directly related to the quantity of blood cultured and the ratio of culture broth to blood. Repeating blood cultures may improve the yield. Reports from South Africa indicated that culturing blood clots in the presence of streptokinase was 50% more sensitive than culturing whole blood. This finding was not confirmed in studies in Indonesia. A major limitation of conventional culture techniques is that it takes a minimum of 48 hours, and often 72 hours, from specimen acquisition, until identification of the organism in culture. Recent work carried out in Indonesia indicates that when the mononuclear cell fraction of blood is cultured, a procedure that concentrates organisms and presumably removes inhibitory serum factors, or when organisms are concentrated by lysis-centrifugation, 100% of cultured organisms can be identified within 18 hours of specimen acquisition.

Intestinal Fluid and Fecal Cultures. Culturing intestinal secretions collected on duodenal string capsule has a sensitivity of 60% to 80%. The sensitivity can be improved by culturing two specimens and leaving the string capsule in place overnight; sensitivity may increase during the third week of illness. A 1-gm stool culture is reportedly more sensitive than a *rectal swab culture* but is much more difficult to obtain. A single admission rectal swab culture can be expected to detect *S. typhi* in 30% to 40% of patients; the sensitivity increases with length of illness. Because of irregular shedding, several stool cultures may be necessary to identify carriers.

Cultures of Other Biologic Samples. Urine cultures are reported to be positive in 5 to 10% of patients, except in areas endemic for *Schistosoma haematobium,* where the positivity rate increases markedly. *S. typhi* has been isolated from the cerebrospinal fluid, peritoneal fluid, mesenteric lymph nodes, resected intestine, pharynx, tonsils, abscesses, bone, and other sites. In a single study, culturing skin snips of rose spots had a sensitivity of 63%.

Culture Techniques. Bone marrow aspirates and blood are cultured in a selective medium such as 10% aqueous oxgall or a nutritious medium such as tryptic soy broth, containing a complement and phagocytic inhibitor, e.g., sodium polyanetholesulfonate. One-half to one ml of BMA and 8 to 15 ml of blood are cultured at a 1:10 ratio in broth (e.g., 1.0 ml of BMA or 10 ml of blood in 9 ml or 90 ml of 10% oxgall, respectively). The cultures are incubated at 37°C for at least 7 days, and subcultures are made every day to one selective medium such as MacConkey's and one inhibitory medium such as Salmonella-Shigella agar. Suspected colonies are identified by standard biochemical reactions and by incubation with specific antisera. Rockhill and Lesmana have shown that a staphylococcal protein A coagglutination technique can be used to identify colonies as soon as they appear on culture plates.

After isolation, the organism should be tested for antimicrobial sensitivity. If it is resistant to chloramphenicol, it should be checked for the presence of R-plasmids.

Serologic and Other Tests

Widal Test. The standard serologic test in use for the diagnosis of typhoid fever is the Widal reaction, which measures agglutinating antibodies to the O and H antigens of *S. typhi.* Numerous studies have now shown that the sensitivity, specificity, and predictive values of this test vary dramatically among laboratories. This wide variation is caused by differences in patient populations, antigens, and techniques. Thus, if physicians do not know the sensitivity, specificity, and predictive values for the test in their laboratory and in their patient population, the results are almost uninterpretable. On the other hand, if these values are known, the Widal test can be useful.

The Widal test is inherently nonspecific because (1) all group D salmonellae have the same O antigens (9, 12) as *S. typhi* and all groups A and B salmonellae have the O antigen (12) (Table 38–2); (2) all group D salmonellae have the same d phase 1 H antigen as *S. typhi;* and (3) H antibody titers remain elevated for long periods after infection or immunization. The Widal test has a low sensitivity because (1) a significant number of culture-positive patients never develop detectable antibody as measured by this test, and (2) in those who do develop an antibody titer, the titer frequently begins to rise before the onset of clinical disease, making it difficult to demonstrate a fourfold rise in titer.

Studies in endemic areas have shown the sensitivity

of a single elevated O antibody titer ($\geq$ 1:40 in Mexico and Indonesia, $\geq$ 1:480 in Rhodesia) to vary from 50 to 90% and the specificity of the same titer to vary from 70 to 99%. In Indonesia an O antibody titer of $\geq$ 1:40 measured by the rapid, Widal slide agglutination test (results available to the physician within 45 minutes of specimen acquisition) was shown to have a positive predictive value of 96%. Although not useful when negative, when the test was positive the health care provider could be 96% certain that the patient had typhoid fever. The sensitivity of a single H titer is similar, but the specificity is much lower. In endemic areas a fourfold rise in O and/or H antibody titer is generally found in less than 40% of culture-positive patients. In nonendemic areas the sensitivity is usually the same as in endemic areas, whereas the specificity is generally higher.

An agglutination reaction using O and/or H antigens from *S. paratyphi* A and *S. schottmuelleri* to diagnose paratyphoid fever has similar deficiencies. A Vi agglutination reaction has been used in screening for *S. typhi* carriers. The reported sensitivity and specificity are 70 to 80% and 80 to 95%, respectively.

Other Tests. In recent years a number of techniques have been developed for detecting *S. typhi* antibodies in serum; *S. typhi* antigen in blood, serum, and urine; and *S. typhi* DNA in blood and stool. Preliminary results have been excellent for a number of assays, but none of the assays is currently in widespread use.

Differential Diagnosis

Endemic Areas. During the first week of illness, it is difficult to clinically distinguish typhoid fever from many other febrile illnesses. Thus the physician must suspect typhoid fever, order appropriate cultures, and consider treatment prior to obtaining bacteriologic confirmation. During the second week of febrile illness, the range of possibilities is narrowed, particularly if the other locally prevalent diseases that can cause prolonged fever are known. These include other bacterial diseases such as endocarditis, brucellosis, tularemia, tuberculosis, and abscesses; rickettsial infections such as typhus; protozoan infections such as malaria, visceral leishmaniasis, amebic liver abscess, and toxoplasmosis; and noninfectious diseases such as connective tissue diseases and lymphoproliferative disorders.

Physicians practicing in the tropics frequently see patients with fevers lasting for 7 to 10 days who have nonspecific clinical findings compatible with typhoid and negative bacteriologic tests and who recover either without antimicrobial treatment or after empirical treatment with a broad-spectrum antibiotic. It is likely that many of these patients have viral infections. It should be noted that the spleen in typhoid fever is generally smaller and softer than the spleen in malaria.

Developed Countries. Unless there is an epidemic, most cases will be imported. The physician must remember to take a travel history, suspect typhoid fever in febrile patients returning from endemic areas, and order appropriate cultures. The differential diagnosis will include those diseases prevalent in the areas visited as outlined above and all other causes of prolonged fever (Chapter 105). Typhoid should also be suspected in patients who have not traveled and who have prolonged fever.

If the diagnosis of typhoid fever is considered, and particularly if the patient is toxic and/or has had previous antibiotics, a bone marrow aspirate culture should be used as a primary diagnostic tool.

TREATMENT. In most cases of typhoid fever successful treatment requires prompt diagnosis, use of an appropriate antibiotic, and bed rest at home. In many endemic areas more than 90% of patients are managed in this way, and case-fatality rates for such patients are less than 1%. In some areas of Indonesia, India, Nepal, and a number of countries in Africa, 20 to 30% of patients with typhoid who are admitted to hospital are severely ill, and unless they receive intensive care, appropriate doses of corticosteroids, and surgery when indicated, may have case-fatality rates of 10 to 20%. Management of hospitalized patients requires (1) proper use of antibiotics; (2) good nursing care; (3) adequate nutrition; (4) careful attention to fluid and electrolyte balance; (5) prompt diagnosis and treatment of intestinal perforation, intestinal bleeding, and other complications; and (6) the use of high-dose corticosteroids in severely ill patients.

Antibiotics. Chloramphenicol is still the most widely used antibiotic for treating typhoid fever patients and is the standard for judging other antibiotics. It produces defervescence and relief of symptoms in most patients within 3 to 4 days, has reduced the preantibiotic era case-fatality rates of 10 to 15% to 1 to 4%, and cures approximately 90% of patients. Its major disadvantages are (1) it does not reduce the relapse rate; (2) it has no effect on the convalescent excretor or chronic carrier; (3) it causes aplastic anemia in 1 in every 10,000 to 50,000 patients; and (4) it is not useful for treating R-plasmid–mediated, chloramphenicol-resistant strains of *S. typhi.* Chloramphenicol's advantages are that it is inexpensive, widely available, and rarely associated with any short-term side effects noticeable to the patient.

Although effective in vitro against *S. typhi,* sulfonamides, tetracyclines, and aminoglycosides are not useful therapy, probably because they are ineffective at the low pH of the phagolysomes containing *S. typhi* within reticuloendothelial cells. Ampicillin, amoxicillin, and trimethoprim-sulfamethoxazole have been used successfully by a number of investigators in large series of patients. Trimethoprim alone has been effective in small groups of patients. In the past decade, third-generation cephalosporins, particularly ceftriaxone and cefoperazone, and fluoroquinolones including norfloxacin, ciprofloxacin, ofloxacin, and pefloxacin have all been shown in a number of small studies to be at least as effective as chloramphenicol in treating typhoid fever. Studies in animals indicate that the third-generation cephalosporins are quite effective in the acid environment of reticuloendothelial cells and that cefoperazone in particular, but also ceftriaxone, is excreted in high concentration into the biliary tract. Fluoroquinolones also have intracellular antibacterial activity. The in vivo activity of these compounds against *S. typhi* has been attributed to these characteristics.

Most studies have shown that in acute chloramphenicol-sensitive *S. typhi* infections, chloramphenicol produces more rapid defervescence than do ampicillin, amoxicillin, and trimethoprim-sulfamethoxazole, and a higher rate of clinical cure than does ampicillin. The use of amoxicillin or trimethoprim-sulfamethoxazole has generally been associated with clinical cure rates comparable to those of chloramphenicol as well as lower relapse and convalescent excretor rates. Reports thus far suggest that the rate of clinical cure is excellent, and relapse rates are quite low with fluorinated quinolones and cefoperazone.

Ampicillin, amoxicillin, and trimethoprim-sulfamethoxazole are all effective against *S. typhi* with R-factor–mediated resistance to chloramphenicol, but R-factor resistance to ampicillin has been reported. Presumably, these strains would also be resistant to amoxicillin, making trimethoprim-sulfamethoxazole the drug of choice for resistant infections.

The dosage regimens listed in Table 38–5, if given for 7 to 10 days after defervescence, will provide the best available cure rates and the lowest relapse rates. None of the available antibiotics can be considered ideal, since deaths and relapses still occur. An antibiotic is needed that is effective against multiresistant strains of *S. typhi,* can penetrate to the intracellular locations where the bacteria multiply, and can effect a cure without relapse or chronic carriage. A number of reports suggest that as more experience is gained with third-generation cephalosporins and quinolones, they may prove superior to chloramphenicol in fulfilling these requirements. Intravenous cefoperazone, 100 mg/kg/day in two doses until defervescence, and then 50 mg/kg/day for a total of 14 days, and intravenous or intramuscular ceftriaxone, 50 to 60 mg/kg/day in two doses for a total of 7 to 10 days, can be expected to cure more than 90% of patients. In several studies, higher doses of ceftriaxone and cefoperazone have been shown to cure typhoid fever when given in short (3- to 5-day) courses. Ciprofloxacin (500 mg BID for 14 days), norfloxacin and ofloxacin (400 mg BID for 10 days), and pefloxacin (400 mg TID for 15 days) have also been highly efficacious in a number of small series. Quinolones can be used only in adults.

Supportive, Nutritional, and Nursing Care. Toxic patients with typhoid fever are frequently immobile or agitated, anorexic or incapable of eating, and highly febrile. They must be turned and bathed frequently, fed intravenously or carefully by mouth, and cooled with a cooling blanket or by using tepid sponge baths supplemented by a fan to enhance evaporation. They must be protected against aspiration and observed for signs of intestinal perforation or hemorrhage and shock. Many authorities recommend avoidance of antipyretics, since they are reported to cause precipitous drops in temperature as well as hypotension; however, they may be used if the temperature remains over 39.5°C after other measures have been tried. Patients who do not have a paralytic ileus, suspected perforation, or severe abdominal pain should be encouraged to eat whatever they like, since maintenance of good nutritional status is more important than an unsubstantiated concern about some foods precipitating intestinal perforation or hemorrhage. Vitamin supplementation is recommended.

TABLE 38–5. Antimicrobial Treatment of Typhoid and Paratyphoid Fever

Antibiotic	Preferred Route of Administration	Daily Dosage	Doses per Day	Duration*
Chloramphenicol	PO/IV†	50 mg/kg	4	7–10 days After defervescence
Trimethoprim-sulfamethoxazole	PO/IV	6.5–10 mg/kg‡§	2–3	" "
Amoxicillin	PO	75–100 mg/kg	3	" "
Ampicillin	PO/IV/IM	100–150 mg/kg	4	" "
Third-generation cephalosporins		See text		
Quinolones		See text		

*Many authorities recommended halving the daily dosage after the patient has been afebrile for 2 days.
†Absorption is poor and erratic if given intramuscularly.
‡The mg/kg dosage refers to the trimethoprim component.
§There are a variety of recommendations in the literature; most investigators have used the twice daily lower dosage regimen.

Some patients may require total parenteral nutrition, but this is infrequent.

Fluid and Electrolyte Balance. Most patients can be managed without intravenous therapy. Patients with severe typhoid fever have poor oral intake, have high insensible water losses, and tend to become dehydrated with hyponatremia and hypokalemia. Vomiting or diarrhea exacerbates the situation. Initial fluid replacement therapy should provide for maintenance needs, insensible losses, and replacement for dehydration. A typical 50 kg patient who is not in shock will require 3 to 4 liters of fluid the first day. Thereafter, records of input and output should be kept and used in managing the patient. If possible, electrolyte determinations should be performed frequently. If not possible, the patient should receive liberal quantities of sodium, chloride, and potassium unless renal failure is suspected.

Corticosteroids. Since Woodward and Smadel's observations in 1951, the use of corticosteroids in severe typhoid fever has been controversial. Corticosteroids dramatically shorten the toxic febrile stage in typhoid fever, but until 1982 there was no proof that they reduced mortality. Studies in Indonesia by Hoffman, Punjabi, and colleagues have shown that prompt administration of high-dose dexamethasone unequivocally reduces mortality in patients with severe typhoid fever without increasing the incidence of complications, carriers, or relapse among survivors. Patients with suspected typhoid fever who are delirious, obtunded, stuporous, comatose, or in shock (severe typhoid fever) should immediately receive dexamethasone or an equivalent corticosteroid. After antimicrobial therapy is started, an initial dose of 3 mg/kg of dexamethasone should be administered by slow intravenous infusion over 30 minutes. This is followed by 1 mg/kg of dexamethasone given at the same rate every 6 hours for 8 additional doses, the total duration of corticosteroid therapy being 48 hours. Patients with normal mental and circulatory status do not require corticosteroids, but those with borderline mental and/or circulatory status should be monitored every 15 minutes in an intensive care unit. If their condition deteriorates, they should receive dexamethasone or an equivalent corticosteroid immediately, since a delay in institution of this therapy has been shown to significantly increase mortality.

Complications

Intestinal Perforation. Generalized peritonitis and large quantities of pus are often found in patients with intestinal perforation, while walling-off of the perforation is infrequent. If a well-trained surgeon, anesthesiologist, and operating room staff and the necessary equipment are available, operative management of typhoid perforation is indicated (Chapter 12). If these are not available, the choice between operative and nonoperative management is controversial and must be individualized. There have been no controlled trials comparing operative and medical management, but patients with clinical evidence of perforation have been successfully managed without surgery. Advocates of medical management point out that the intestinal lesions are friable, are sometimes larger than they appear, and tend to slough and that patients with perforation are usually very ill and withstand surgery poorly regardless of the sophistication of the surgeon and facilities.

In all cases the patient should be started on chloramphenicol; placed on nasogastric suction; resuscitated with fluids, blood, and oxygen as needed; and given corticosteroids if severely toxic. Most authorities would recommend at least one more antibiotic to cover enteric organisms not sensitive to chloramphenicol.

It is preferable to stabilize the patient before surgery, but the operation should not be delayed for more than several hours after diagnosis. At operation, the ileum as well as the cecum and proximal large bowel should be examined for perforations, and one of several procedures should be performed, e.g., intestinal resection and primary anastomosis, or wedge excision or debridement of the ulcer with primary closure of the perforation (both single- and double-layer closures have been advocated). Most surgeons will suture sites of impending perforation with serosal-to-serosal approximation. The peritoneal cavity is then lavaged, and the abdomen is closed, with or without drainage. Standard postoperative care is practiced. As the interval between perforation and surgery increases and the preoperative status of the patient worsens, the case-fatality rate increases. Mortality rates of 10 to 32% have been reported in recent series.

Intestinal Hemorrhage. In most cases, intestinal hemorrhage, even when massive, can be managed with general supportive care and vigorous replacement of blood. Occasionally the use of platelets, fresh frozen plasma to replace clotting factors, or intestinal resection will be necessary, but this is uncommon. If the patient does not have an abnormal level of consciousness or shock, the case-fatality rate will be less than 1%.

Other Complications. Renal failure, pneumonia, respiratory failure, myocarditis, arrhythmias, cardiac failure, shock, meningitis, localized abcesses, arthritis, osteomyelitis, hemolytic anemia, and cholecystitis are all occasionally encountered and should be managed with antimicrobials and standard medical and/or surgical practices. Disseminated intravascular coagulation may sometimes be clinically significant, in which case platelet, blood, and clotting factor transfusions may be necessary. There is no evidence that heparin therapy is useful in typhoid.

Relapse. Relapse should be treated in the same way as the first attack.

Carriers. In the absence of cholelithiasis, the majority of carriers can be cured by a course of oral ampicillin or amoxicillin, 100 mg/kg/day, plus probenecid, 30 mg/kg/day, or trimethoprim-sulfamethoxazole, two tablets twice daily, for 3 months. In the presence of cholelithiasis the foregoing regimen should be tried before surgical intervention is considered; in most cases, however, antimicrobial treatment alone will not be successful and cholecystectomy as well as the same antimicrobial regimen will be required. A cure rate of 80 to 90% can be effected by combined surgical and antimicrobial treatment. Cure rates of approximately 80% have been reported with 28 days of ciprofloxacin, 750 mg BID, and with norfloxacin, 400 mg BID. Some chronic urinary carriers of *S. typhi* are infected with *Schistosoma haematobium*. The schistosomiasis should be treated first, and then the patient should receive an antibiotic.

Prognosis. The prognosis is dependent upon the patient population and the geographic area. In an epidemic in developed countries, patients will generally be seen and treated promptly, have a case-fatality rate of less than 1%, and have a low incidence of complications. The majority of patients in endemic areas will be treated as outpatients and have case-fatality and complication rates comparable to those expected in an epidemic in developed countries.

In Central and South America, hospitalized patients are reported to have mortality rates of less than 1%. In some endemic areas, including Indonesia, Nigeria, India, and Nepal, severe typhoid fever (abnormal level of consciousness or shock) is common among hospitalized patients. These patients with severe typhoid fever may have a mortality rate as high as 50% if they are not treated with high-dose dexamethasone therapy.

Nearly all studies report much lower complication, case-fatality, relapse, and carrier rates with paratyphoid fever. There have been a number of reports of particularly severe paratyphoid fever in young children and infants, in whom complication and case-fatality rates have been similar to those in patients with typhoid fever. (Chapter 39).

PREVENTION AND CONTROL

Nonendemic Areas. In developed countries, prevention is now the responsibility of sanitation, water supply, and public health officials. Individuals need not take any special precautions. Chronic carriers should be identified and treated. In the past, considerable time and money have been devoted to screening food handlers, but in many countries this is no longer considered

necessary. In the event of an epidemic, the source of the infection must be identified and eliminated, and any breakdown in the water delivery and sewage systems must be repaired. The general populace must be informed of the need to adhere to standard hygiene practices.

Endemic Areas. Individuals can minimize their chances of developing enteric fever by paying careful attention to the quality of the food and water that they ingest and by receiving immunizations. *S. typhi* in water is killed by heating to 57°C, iodination, and chlorination. *S. typhi* in food is killed at the same temperature, but the food must be heated uniformly for several minutes. Travelers to or residents of endemic areas should drink only boiled or bottled water; avoid eating fresh, uncooked vegetables, or unpeeled fruit that have not been thoroughly washed in iodinated or chlorinated water; and use discretion when eating in restaurants or food stalls. Reduction of endemicity will depend on improvements in water supply and sewage systems and education of the populace as to proper hygiene and food and water preparation practices. Mass immunization can be extremely useful.

Vaccines

S. typhi Vaccines. The first parenteral killed typhoid vaccine was introduced in 1896. By 1912, all United States military personnel were required to receive it, but it was not until the 1960s that the vaccine's efficacy was established in field trials. The World Health Organization sponsored trials in typhoid-endemic areas of Poland, Yugoslavia, Guyana, and the Soviet Union and demonstrated that both phenol- and acetone-inactivated vaccines offered 51% to 88% protection to children and young adults. The acetone-inactivated vaccine, which preserves Vi antigen, was moderately more effective than the phenol-inactivated vaccine. In Poland and Guyana, one dose of the vaccine was as effective as two doses. This was probably due to vaccine stimulation of an immune system that had already experienced *S. typhi* infection.

Studies at the University of Maryland showed that the same vaccines used in the WHO studies gave 67% protection to volunteers who ingested an ID_{25} (10^5 organisms) of *S. typhi* but did not offer any protection to those who ingested an ID_{50} (10^7 organisms). At the ID_{25}, those who became infected had a longer incubation period, a milder illness, and a lower incidence of relapse than those who did not receive the vaccine. These volunteer studies also suggested that some efficacy may last up to 12 years.

Thus, the standard typhoid vaccine is effective in individuals from endemic and nonendemic areas but offers only partial protection, is associated with local and systemic side effects in 25 to 50% of recipients, and must be given parenterally. Because of these drawbacks, other vaccines have been developed. A galactose epimerase (gal E) mutant of *S. typhi* (Ty 21a) developed by Germanier is now being used as an oral vaccine. In volunteers in Maryland, 5 to 8 doses conferred 87% protection against an ID_{50}. Field studies suggest an inverse relation between the level of transmission of typhoid in an area and protective efficacy. In 6- to 7-

year-old Egyptians (incidence in controls, 46 cases/100,000/year) the protective efficacy was 96% after 3 years. In 6- to 21-year-old Chileans (incidence in controls, 103 cases/100,000/year) efficacy was 67% after 3 years; and in 3- to 19-year-old Indonesians (incidence in controls, 1206 cases/100,000/year) efficacy was 53% after 2.5 years. In Chile the protective efficacy has remained stable for 5 years. The vaccine does not contain Vi antigen and is thought to induce a protective cellular immune response.

A parenteral vaccine that includes the Vi antigen has been developed and studied by Robbins and coworkers. In 5- to 44-year-old Nepalese (incidence in controls, 654 cases/100,000/year), a single injection of the vaccine was not associated with significant side effects and conferred a protective efficacy of 72% after 17 months. In South African schoolchildren (approximate incidence in controls, 470 cases/100,000/year), the Vi vaccine had a protective efficacy of approximately 64% during 21 months of surveillance. It is thought that antibodies to Vi antigen are responsible for the protective immunity.

The TAB vaccine, which contains killed *S. typhi* (T), *S. paratyphi A* (A), and *S. paratyphi B* (B), is associated with more side effects than is the *S. typhi* vaccine and has never been shown to be of value in preventing paratyphoid fever. It is no longer recommended.

Vaccine Recommendations. Although there have been no comparative studies, current data indicate that both Ty 21a and the Vi antigen vaccine are as effective, if not more effective, than the standard parenteral typhoid vaccine and are not associated with the side effects found after immunization with the latter. Ty 21a is now available in the United States, but the Vi antigen vaccine is not. Where available, use of either of these vaccines alone would be preferable to the standard vaccine. Since the vaccines work through different mechanisms, some have advocated use of both in the same individual. Where these new vaccines are unavailable, the standard vaccine should be administered. Routine typhoid vaccination should be given to those traveling to or living in areas where typhoid is endemic. This includes most countries of the developing world. Routine vaccination is not recommended in those countries where incidence is low, as in the United States and Europe, not even during disasters or for family contacts. During disasters or in refugee camps in endemic areas, mass immunization should be considered, recognizing that provision of safe food and water is of primary importance.

Immunization.

Standard Parenteral Vaccine. Adults and children 10 years and older are given 0.5 ml subcutaneously on two occasions 4 or more weeks apart. Children less than 10 years of age receive half the dose on the same schedule. If there is insufficient time for two doses at the interval specified, one dose a week for 3 weeks may be given. A booster dose every 3 years is recommended. Repeat primary immunization is never necessary.

Ty 21a. As of late 1990 the only commercially available product is an enteric-coated formulation (Vivotif Berna, Berna Products Corp.). Four capsules should be given at intervals ranging from 2 days to several weeks.

Field studies now suggest that a lyophilized preparation that is reconstituted in liquid just prior to ingestion and administered with sodium bicarbonate is more effective than the enteric-coated capsule. This preparation should become commercially available soon. Current data indicate that vaccine efficacy lasts for at least 3 and perhaps 5 years.

Vi Antigen Vaccine. A single 25 μm dose is administered intramuscularly. Long-term efficacy data are not available.

BIBLIOGRAPHY

Acharya IL, Lowe CU, Thapa R, et al: Prevention of typhoid fever in Nepal with the Vi capsular polysaccharide of *Salmonella typhi*. N Engl J Med 317:1101–1104, 1987.

Bitar R, Tarpley J. Intestinal perforation in typhoid fever: A historical and state-of-the-art review. Rev Infect Dis 7:257–271, 1985.

Butler T, Bell WR, Levin J, et al: Typhoid fever: Studies of blood coagulation, bacteremia, and endotoxemia. Arch Intern Med 138:407–410, 1978.

Butler T, Rumans L, Arnold K: Response of typhoid fever caused by chloramphenicol-susceptible and chloramphenicol-resistant strains of *Salmonella typhi* to treatment with trimethoprim-sulfamethoxazole. Rev Infect Dis 1 4:551–561, 1982.

Duggan MB, Beyer L: Enteric fever in young Yoruba children. Arch Dis Child 50:67–71, 1975.

Edelman R, Levine MM: Summary of an international workshop on typhoid fever. Rev Infect Dis 8:329–349, 1986.

Gilman RH, Terminel M, Levine MM, et al: Relative efficacy of blood, urine, rectal swab, bone-marrow and rose-spot cultures for recovery of *Salmonella typhi* in typhoid fever. Lancet 1:1211–1213, 1975.

Gulati PD, Saxena SN, Gupta PS, Chuttani HK: Changing pattern of typhoid fever. Am J Med 45:544–548, 1968.

Hoffman SL, Flanigan TP, Klaucke D, et al: The Widal slide agglutination test, a valuable rapid diagnostic test in typhoid fever patients at the Infectious Diseases Hospital of Jakarta. Am J Epidemiol 123:869–875, 1986.

Hoffman SL, Punjabi NH, Rockhill RC, et al: Duodenal string-capsule culture compared with bone-marrow, blood, and rectal-swab cultures for diagnosing typhoid and paratyphoid fever. J Infect Dis 149:157–161, 1984.

Hoffman SL, Edman DC, Punjabi NH, et al: Bone marrow aspirate culture superior to streptokinase clot culture and 8 ml 1:10 blood-to-broth ratio blood culture for diagnosis of typhoid fever. Am J Trop Med Hyg 35:836–839, 1986.

Hoffman SL, Punjabi NH, Kumala S: Reduction of mortality in chloramphenicol-treated severe typhoid fever by high-dose dexamethasone. N Engl J Med 310:82–88, 1984.

Hoffman TA, Ruiz CJ, Counts GW, et al: Waterborne typhoid fever in Dade County, Florida: Clinical and therapeutic evaluations of 105 bacteremic patients. Am J Med 59:481–487, 1975.

Hornick RB, Greisman S: On the pathogenesis of typhoid fever. Arch Intern Med 138:357–359, 1978.

Klotz SA, Jorgensen JH, Buckwold FJ, Craven PC: Typhoid fever. An epidemic with remarkably few clinical signs and symptoms. Arch Intern Med 144:533–537, 1984.

Klugman KP, Koornhof HJ, Schneerson R, et al: Protective activity of Vi capsular polysaccharide vaccine against typhoid fever. Lancet 2:1165–1169, 1987.

Levine MM, Black RE, Ferreccio C, et al: Large-scale field trial of TY21A live oral typhoid vaccine in enteric-coated capsule formulation. Lancet 2:1049–1052, 1987.

Meier DE, Imediegwu OO, Tarpley JL: Perforated typhoid enteritis: operative experience with 108 cases. Am J Surg 157:423–427, 1989.

Murphy JR, Wasserman SS, Baqar S, et al: Immunity to *Salmonella typhi*: considerations relevant to measurement of cellular immunity in typhoid-endemic regions. Clin Exp Immunol 75:228–233, 1989.

Osuntokun BO, Bademosi O, Ogunremi K, et al: Neuropsychiatric manifestations of typhoid fever in 959 patients. Arch Neurol 27:7–13, 1972.

Punjabi NH, Hoffman SL, Edman DC, et al: Treatment of severe typhoid fever in children with high dose dexamethasone. Pediatr Infect Dis J 7:598–600, 1988.

Rajagopalan P, Kumar R, Malaviya AN: Immunological studies in typhoid fever. I. Immunoglobulins, C3, antibodies, rheumatoid factor and circulation immune complexes in patients with typhoid fever. Clin Exp Immunol 44:68–73, 1981.

Rubin FA, McWhirter PD, Burr D, et al: Rapid diagnosis of typhoid fever through identification of *Salmonella typhi* within 18 hours of specimen acquisition by culture of the mononuclear cell/platelet fraction of blood. J Clin Microbiol 28:825–827, 1990.

Rubin FA, McWhirter PD, Punjabi NH, et al: Use of a DNA probe to detect *Salmonella typhi* in the blood of patients with typhoid fever. J Clin Microbiol 27:1112–1114, 1989.

Soe GB, Overturf GD: Treatment of typhoid fever and other systemic salmonelloses with cefotaxime, ceftriaxone, cefoperazone, and other newer cephalosporins. Rev Infect Dis 9:719–736, 1987.

Stanley PJ, Flegg PJ, Mandal BK, Geddes AM: Open study of ciprofloxacin in enteric fever. J Anitmicrob Chemother 23:789–791, 1989.

Stuart BM, Pullen RL: Typhoid: Clinical analysis of three hundred and sixty cases. Arch Intern Med 1946; 78:629–661, 1946.

Tagliabue A, Villa L, De Magistris MT, et al: IgA-driven T cell–mediated anti-bacterial immunity in man after live oral Ty 21a vaccine. J Immunol 137:1504–1510, 1986.

Wahdan MH, Serie C, Cerisier Y, et al: A controlled field trial of live *Salmonella typhi* strain Ty 21a oral vaccine against typhoid. Three-year results. J Infect Dis 145:292–295, 1982.

Woodward TE, Smadel JE: Management of typhoid fever and its complications. Ann Intern Med 60:144–157, 1964.

39. NONTYPHOIDAL *SALMONELLA* INFECTIONS

Robert Longfield

DEFINITION. Salmonellosis is usually a self-limited acute infection of the intestine and rarely other anatomic sites that occurs worldwide in many animal species and in humans. Infection is readily transmitted to humans by contaminated food or under conditions of poor personal hygiene. Clinical *Salmonella* syndromes include acute enterocolitis, enteric (paratyphoid) fever, and bacteremia with or without focal infection. These syndromes tend readily to overlap or to evolve. Transient asymptomatic intestinal infection is common; however, chronic intestinal, biliary, or urinary tract carriage occurs less frequently than with *Salmonella typhi*.

ETIOLOGY. Salmonellae are nonsporulating, nonencapsulated, aerobic, gram-negative bacilli that comprise three species: *S. typhi* (1 serotype) (Chapter 38), *S. choleraesuis* (1 serotype), and *S. enteritidis* (over 1700 serotypes). For convenience, *Salmonella* serotypes are abbreviated as in the following example: *S. enteritidis* serotype *agona* is abbreviated *S. agona*. The "Arizona group" was designated formerly a separate genus, but these isolates are presently considered closely related to *Salmonella* strains. Although salmonellae do not form spores, they readily remain dormant in a desiccated state, within living cells, or in necrotic tissue.

Cultural Characteristics. Most salmonellae ferment maltose, mannitol, and glucose, producing acid and gas, but do not ferment sucrose or lactose. However, in the 1970s, a strain of lactose-fermenting *S. typhimurium* was readily confused with *Escherichia coli* during an epidemic in Brazil. Except for *S. gallinarum/pullorum*, all salmonellae exhibit motility by peritrichous flagella.

Classification. Salmonellae, like other enteric gram-negative bacilli, possess lipopolysaccharide somatic (O) antigens, which have been grouped A to Z, with additional numbered categories; however, more than 90% of human isolates are included in groups A through E (Table 39–1). Rough strains lacking O antigens are often nonpathogenic. Protein flagellar H antigens exhibit phase variation under different culture conditions. A given phase 1 antigen is generally shared by only a few *Salmonella* serotypes, whereas a phase 2 antigen is more widely distributed and less serotype-specific. The heat-labile Vi (virulence) antigen found in *S. typhi* is also carried by *S. hirschfeldii* (*S. paratyphi* C). In most microbiology laboratories, clinical *Salmonella* isolates are identified as to species on the basis of fermentation reactions and group-specific O agglutinations. Using serologic methods developed by Kauffmann and White, large *Salmonella* typing centers (Atlanta, Copenhagen, London) can provide the identification of isolates necessary for an epidemiologic investigation. Bacteriophage typing may be feasible also for isolates of certain relatively common serotypes. In any given year, fewer than 200 *Salmonella* serotypes are responsible for human disease. In the United States in 1986, 10 serotypes represented 73% of identified human isolates: *S. typhimurium*, *S. enteritidis*, *S. heidelberg*, *S. newport*, *S. hadar*, *S. infantis*, *S. agona*, *S. montevideo*, *S. muenchen*, and *S. braenderup*. *S. typhimurium* is the most common serotype both in the United States and worldwide.

EPIDEMIOLOGY

Incidence and Distribution. Widespread among members of the animal kingdom, salmonellae are responsible for human disease on a global basis. Although the incidence of typhoid fever has declined in many developed nations, the incidence of nontyphoidal salmonellosis may actually be rising. Despite identical mecha-

TABLE 39–1. Kauffmann-White Classification of Common *Salmonella* Serotypes†

Serotype	Group	O Antigens	H Antigens Phase 1	H Antigens Phase 2
S. paratyphi A	A	(1),* 2,**, 12	a	—
S. schottmuelleri	B	1, *4*, (5), 12	b	1, 2
S. typhimurium	B	1, *4*, (5), 12	(i)	1, 2
S. heidelberg	B	1, *4*, 5, 12	r	1, 2
S. canada	B	*4*, 12	b	1, 6
S. saint-paul	B	1, *4*, 5, 12	e, h	1, 2
S. hirschfeldii	C₁	6, *7*	c	1, 5
S. bareilly	C₁	6, *7*	y	1, 5
S. choleraesuis	C₁	6, *7*	c	1, 5
S. montevideo	C₁	6, *7*	g, m, s	—
S. oranienburg	C₁	6, *7*	m, t	—
S. newport	C₂	6, *8*	(e, h)	1, 2
S. typhi	D	*9*, 12	d	—
S. enteritidis	D	1, *9*, 12	g, m	—
S. pullorum/gallinarum	D	(1), *9*, 12	—	—
S. anatum	E	*3*, 10	e, h	1, 6
S. vancouver	I	*16*	c	1, 5

*Parentheses indicate that antigenic determinant may be absent or difficult to detect.

**Italicized* number signifies major determinant of group.

†Modified from Rubin RH, Weinstein L: Salmonellosis: Microbiologic, Pathologic, and Clinical Features. New York, Stratton Intercontinental Medical Book Corp., 1977.

nisms for reporting *Shigella* isolates to the Centers for Disease Control (CDC), the number of human isolates of *Salmonella* has continued to rise disproportionately over the past 30 years (Fig. 39–1). In the United States, over 42,000 human *Salmonella* isolations were reported in 1986. This figure probably underestimates the actual incidence of salmonellosis by 100-fold. The estimated occurrence of several million annual cases of salmonellosis in the United States assumes substantial medical and economic significance when extrapolated to the world population. Coinciding with seasonal outbreaks of food poisoning, most human isolates in the temperate zones are obtained during the summer and fall. Although there is no preponderance by sex, children and the elderly are disproportionately represented among reported cases (Fig. 39–2).

Outbreaks. Fifty-five percent of *Salmonella* isolations occur in small sporadic epidemics, usually within households. Among household contacts, 20 to 35% will be infected also. Institutional outbreaks have occurred in acute care hospitals, pediatric wards, nurseries, and nursing homes. Communal banquet-, school-, restaurant-, and foodstore-related epidemics are common also.

Occurrence in the Tropics. In 1980, among children in an indigenous community of South Africa, *Salmonella* was the second most common (17%) cause of acute summer diarrhea behind *E. coli* (43%). In Kenya, *Salmonella* caused 4% of acute adult diarrhea. Good surveillance studies are lacking, but *Salmonella* appears to cause diarrhea to a similar extent in other developing nations, although the prevalence of individual serotypes varies widely over time and from region to region.

Reservoir Hosts. *S. typhi* and *S. paratyphi* infect humans exclusively. *S. schottmuelleri* (*S. paratyphi* B), *S. hirschfeldii* (*S. paratyphi* C), and *S. sendai* infect humans principally but may incidentally infect animals. Almost all other serotypes infect either humans or animals, and virtually any animal species may harbor these organisms. Surveys in the United States reveal

Salmonella infection in chickens (50%), turkeys (41%), eggs (21%), swine (7 to 50%), and cattle (24%). Animals become infected from their environment or from contaminated feed. Infected animals may transmit salmonellosis among themselves during transport, holding, or butchering. Abattoir workers and food handlers may become infected readily and transmit *Salmonella*.

Conditions with Increased Incidence of *Salmonella* Infection

Hemolytic Disorders. Sickle cell anemia and other hemoglobinopathies (Chapter 5), acute bartonellosis (Chapter 52), and possibly malaria dramatically enhance susceptibility to *Salmonella* bacteremia. In patients with these disorders, macrophages are laden often with hemoglobin, impairing their ability to clear blood-borne salmonellae. In one study in Africa, 44% of patients with *Salmonella* bacteremia or meningitis were found to have sickle cell anemia (SS), whereas the incidence of SS in the general population was only 2%. *Salmonella* accounts for less than 1% of hematogenous osteomyelitis in normal hosts but is a frequent cause of such infections in patients with SS.

Schistosomiasis. Chronic or recurrent *Salmonella* bacteremia has been reported among patients with schistosomiasis in Egypt and Brazil (Chapter 96). In the urinary tract, fibrosis, scarring, and stone formation induced by *Schistosoma haematobia* promote chronic urinary carriage of salmonellae.

Other Chronic Conditions. Salmonella sepsis occurs more frequently in patients with serious underlying diseases, e.g., alcoholism, hepatic cirrhosis, inflammatory bowel disease, systemic lupus erythematosus, leukemia, lymphoma, other neoplasms, and chronic granulomatous disease. Patients with the acquired immunodeficiency syndrome (AIDS) (Chapter 15.1) and renal transplant recipients have an increased incidence of nontyphoidal *Salmonella* bacteremia and local suppuration. Salmonellae have not been implicated frequently as causing the gay bowel syndrome, rather AIDS-associated salmonellosis has been reported from all groups at increased risk for AIDS. The presence of scarred, necrotic, or recently traumatized tissue, e.g., tumors, cysts, bone infarcts, hematomas, effusions, and arterial aneurysms, favors the localization of blood-borne salmonellae.

Transmission

Food. Contaminated food is understandably the most frequent vehicle for transmission of salmonellosis (Table 39–2). Outbreaks are often traced to commercially processed meat and meat products, inadequately cooked poultry, eggs, and unpasteurized milk or dairy products. Food may become tainted during preparation on working surfaces or with utensils contaminated previously with salmonellae. Poultry products are responsible for over half of the common source epidemics. Salmonellae may be found on the shells of fecally contaminated eggs, between the shell and shell membrane, or in yolks of intact eggs from hens with ovarian infection. Pooling of eggs for freezing or drying increases the risk of contamination. Pork, beef, and lamb are implicated in 13% of salmonellosis epidemics.

Animals. Pets, e.g., dogs, cats, birds, and turtles, are

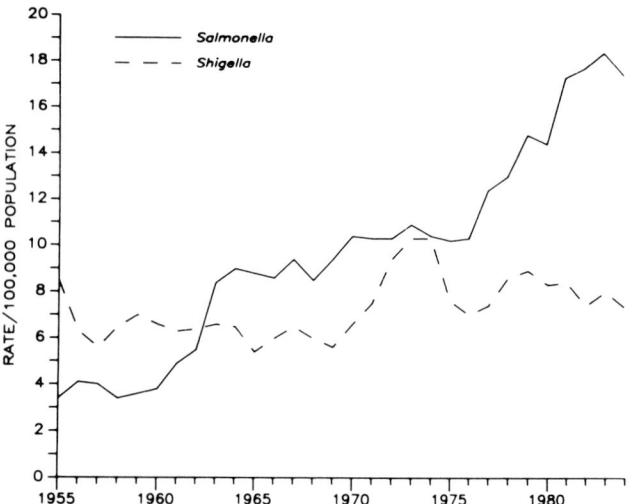

FIGURE 39–1. *Salmonella*(—) and *Shigella*(– –) infections reported to the Centers for Disease Control, 1955–1984. Rates are per 100,000 population in the United States. *Salmonella* rate excludes infections due to *S. typhi*. (From Chalker RB, Blaser MJ: Rev Infect Dis 10:111, 1988. Reprinted by permission.)

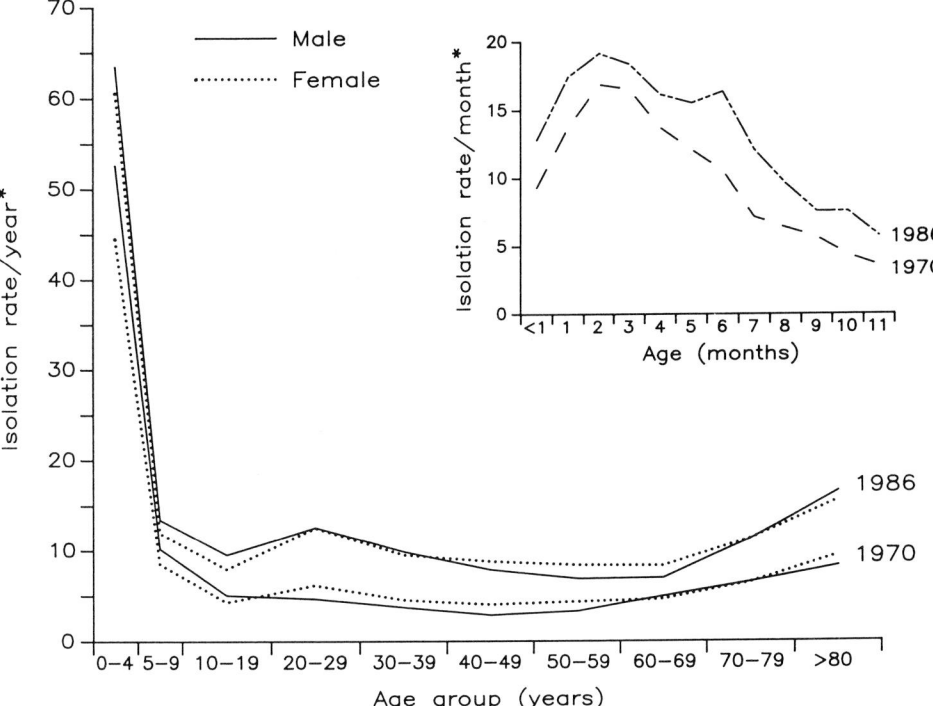

FIGURE 39–2. Rate of reported isolates of *Salmonella* by age in the United States, 1970 and 1986. (Courtesy of the Centers for Disease Control, Atlanta, Georgia.)

*Per 100,000 population

implicated in 3% of outbreaks of salmonellosis. Turtle-related salmonellosis has been virtually eliminated in the United States and Canada by legislation banning the distribution and sale of pet turtles less than 4 inches in carapace diameter.

Other Causes. Flies and other insects, gastrointestinal endoscopes, and even human breast milk have been reported to transmit *Salmonella*. Pharmacologic products implicated in transmission include carmine dye, bile salts, pepsin, gelatin, vitamins, and extracts of liver, pancreas, thyroid, pituitary, and adrenal cortex. Contaminated marijuana and, most recently, the ingestion of capsules of dried, ground rattlesnake meat have been responsible for scattered cases of enterocolitis in the United States. However, contaminated water is rarely implicated in *Salmonella* transmission except in developing nations.

Fecal-Oral Route. Direct human-to-human transmission of salmonellosis via the fecal-oral route, although less common than with shigellosis, has been underesti-

TABLE 39–2. Mode of Transmission in 500 Outbreaks of Human Salmonellosis in the United States (1966–1975)*

Source	% Total
Poultry	17
Meat	13
Person to Person	10
Eggs	6
Dairy products	4
Pets	3
Miscellaneous	19
Unknown	28
Total	100

*Prepared from data from the Centers for Disease Control, Atlanta, Georgia, 1977.

mated and may play a significant role in the amplification of infection under crowded, unhygienic conditions. Nursery and pediatric ward outbreaks have occurred in which direct cross-infection between neonates was the likely mode of spread. Neonates may become infected also by fecal-oral spread during labor or delivery, by direct contact with contaminated persons, by fomites such as feeding tubes, by food, and, possibly, by aerosol transmission. Neonates convalescing from salmonellosis are a hazard to other family members: 50% are culture-positive at 3 months, and 10% may be positive for 1 to 2 years.

Nosocomial Salmonellosis. Nosocomial epidemics accounted for 28% of all salmonellosis epidemics in the United States between 1963 and 1972. Often due to contaminated food or medicine with subsequent person-to-person spread, hospital-associated salmonellosis outbreaks carry a high mortality rate (7 to 9%).

International Spread. The mass production of food and animal feeds and their global distribution have contributed to the spread of *Salmonella* serotypes, some with disturbing antimicrobial resistance. *S. agona*, a rare isolate prior to 1970, was recovered from human cases in Peru in 1971 and subsequently produced epidemics of enterocolitis in Europe and the United States. Contaminated Peruvian fishmeal, used as poultry feed, proved to be the source. *S. eastbourne*, also an uncommon serotype, was introduced into the United States and Canada in 1974 in chocolate from contaminated African cocoa.

Infected travelers may spread *Salmonella* serotypes also. In 1969, antibiotic-resistant *S. wien* was first encountered among patients in a large Algerian pediatric hospital. Extensive outbreaks of gastroenteritis occurred around the Mediterranean, and 2 small outbreaks in the

United States were associated subsequently with persons arriving from Europe. Nontyphoidal *Salmonella* cause a small but significant proportion of diarrhea among travelers to developing nations.

Antibiotic-Resistant Strains. In the 1960s, 1970s and 1980s, a number of species of *Salmonella* causing clinical infection have acquired persistent, high-level resistance to ampicillin, chloramphenicol, and TMP-SMZ. Antibiotics added to animal feed as growth enhancers are thought to contribute to the emergence of some antibiotic-resistant *Salmonella* strains. In the United States, recent studies using restriction endonuclease "fingerprinting" of the DNA from antibiotic-resistant (R) plasmids from *Salmonella* isolates helped to clarify the relationship between resistant strains encountered in animals and those causing human disease. Identical or nearly identical R plasmids were found in salmonellae isolated from animals and persons in widely separated regions. Geographically dispersed human cases appeared to cluster in time, suggesting dissemination of a common source item by the food distribution system. The effect on human salmonellosis of antimicrobial use in domestic animals may be estimated more accurately using this sensitive method.

The presence or subsequent acquisition of antimicrobial resistance has characterized a number of salmonellosis outbreaks in both developed and developing nations. The emergence of resistance, such as that seen to TMP-SMZ among 76% of *Salmonella* in Brazil in the early 1980s, is highly variable but constitutes an area of concern. Unlike the common source contamination associated often with *Salmonella* outbreaks, most of the epidemics due to these clinically resistant strains seem to occur among hospitalized neonates or children via person-to-person spread. Prior use of antimicrobials for the empirical treatment of febrile syndromes including enterocolitis appears to be a significant risk factor for the acquisition of antimicrobial-resistant *Salmonella* infections.

Chronic Carriers. *S. typhi*, *S. paratyphi*, and *S. schottmuelleri* induce chronic biliary or urinary tract carriage in 1 to 3% of infected patients. Women are 3 times as likely as men to become chronic carriers. Infection with other serotypes rarely results in true chronic carriage (excretion of the organism for 12 months or more). Carefully performed surveys have estimated the prevalence of asymptomatic human carriage of these serotypes to be approximately 0.2%; however, 5.4% of children under 2 years of age continue to excrete nontyphoidal salmonellae 12 months after infection. Hepatic infection with the fluke *Opisthorchis sinensis* has been associated also with chronic carriage of *Salmonella*. The majority of *Salmonella* stool isolates from asymptomatic persons represent quiescent infection or transient convalescent carriage.

PATHOLOGY. *Salmonella* enterocolitis contributes to mortality primarily in infants, the aged, and persons with underlying disease. At autopsy, the mucosa of the ileum and colon is red and swollen with petechial hemorrhages. Ulceration of Peyer's patches occurs less frequently than in typhoid fever. In neonates, the stomach and small bowel may be involved also, with extensive inflammation, ulceration, hemorrhage, and edema. Intestinal lesions are absent often in patients succumbing to primary *Salmonella* bacteremia. Localized metastatic infections manifest the characteristic histopathology of abscess, osteomyelitis, endarteritis, and meningitis.

In experimental primate infection, hyperemia of the colon with abundant mucus and microscopic acute colitis are present 24 hours after initial *Salmonella* infection. Blood, lymph node, liver, and other organ cultures may be positive at this time. With overwhelming infection, death results from septic shock, and acute colitis may be the only histologic lesion. Pancreatitis and renal tubular necrosis may develop with protracted shock.

PATHOGENESIS. *Salmonella* may proliferate rapidly in contaminated food that is either improperly heated or inadequately refrigerated. Exposure to such food appears quite common, and the presence or absence of clinical infection depends on the inoculum ingested, the virulence of the *Salmonella* strain, and the status of the human host. Infection may be asymptomatic or may present as acute enterocolitis, enteric fever, or bacteremia with or without local suppuration.

Inoculum. The dose of *Salmonella* required to produce enterocolitis in normal adults has been estimated to be 10^5 to 10^6 bacilli. In general, the ingestion of 10^3 to 10^4 bacilli causes transient asymptomatic carriage; however, common source epidemics have occurred in which 10^2 to 10^3 bacilli produced symptomatic illness. The infective dose varies widely for different *Salmonella* serotypes, e.g., *S. newport*—10^5, *S. anatum*—5×10^6, *S. melagridis*—5×10^7, *S. pullorum*—10^9.

Virulence. Considerable differences in virulence exist among serotypes, e.g., *S. anatum* commonly causes inapparent infection or enterocolitis, whereas *S. choleraesuis* commonly causes bacteremia or local suppuration. Within a given *Salmonella* serotype, dramatic differences in virulence by strain may be evident. In one outbreak of *S. typhimurium*, 60% of patients were noted to have dysentery and unusually prolonged symptoms (mean 10.8 days). A single *Salmonella* strain may produce either asymptomatic or rapidly fatal illness, depending on the host status.

Protective Factors. Host gastric acidity appears to be an important defense mechanism, as salmonellae are rapidly killed at a pH of 2.0 (III D, General Principles). Since salmonellosis occurs in patients with normal gastric function, a large inoculum and the buffering of gastric acid or the physical protection of bacilli by food may nullify the gastric acid barrier. Oral antacids and gastrectomy or an increased rate of gastric emptying will reduce the infective dose. Water-containing low inocula of salmonellae (10^2 to 10^3) may pass rapidly through the stomach and induce infection.

In Infants. The inoculum of *Salmonella* required to infect neonates is lower than that for adults. During the newborn period, infection is promoted by a high average gastric pH, frequent milk feedings, which buffer gastric acid, and relatively rapid gastric emptying. The incidence of *Salmonella* enterocolitis is generally reduced in breast-fed infants, perhaps because they are not exposed to contaminated bottles. Mothers who have been naturally infected with or immunized against *Salmonella* secrete species-specific O and H agglutinins in colostrum and breast milk. Although agglutinins appear to retain their specific activity in the gut, they are neither bactericidal nor bacteriostatic in vitro. Maternal IgG antibodies transmitted to the fetus in late pregnancy may actually suppress the development of active humoral immunity in those neonates who subsequently develop *Salmonella* enterocolitis; however, no adverse consequences have been demonstrated.

Mucosal Attachment and Invasion. Salmonellae that survive the transit through the stomach and upper intestine may localize and multiply in the ileum and colon. The normal bacterial flora are thought to exert anti-*Salmonella* activity by the elaboration of short-chain fatty acids and perhaps other substances. Antimicrobials that inhibit colonic flora substantially reduce the inoculum of *Salmonella* required to cause infection. The preferential attachment of bacilli to the villous tips of the ileal and colonic mucosa suggests a specific receptor. Upon attachment, salmonellae induce local degeneration of mucosal cell microvilli, advance into a vacuole that migrates through the cell to the basal membrane, and are discharged directly into the lamina propria. Polymorphonuclear leukocytes attracted to the lamina propria may damage the colon secondarily by the release of lysosomal enzymes. Inflammation of the lamina propria and resultant smooth muscle spasm are thought to be responsible for the cramping abdominal pain and tenesmus. Mucosal damage is rarely sufficient to produce dysentery.

Immunity. The nature of the immune response elicited in the lamina propria determines whether *Salmonella* infection remains localized or becomes disseminated. Unlike *S. typhi*, which induces a mononuclear response with early invasion of lymphatics, regional lymph nodes, and the blood stream, nontyphoidal *Salmonella* elicit a polymorphonuclear response and generally remain confined to the lamina propria in healthy adults. Infants experience bacteremia more frequently than adults, ostensibly because their bacteria-localizing immune defenses are immature.

Mechanism of Diarrhea. Invasion of the lamina propria appears to be a prerequisite for diarrhea in nontyphoidal *Salmonella* infections, because large inocula of killed salmonellae fail to evoke diarrhea. Using the infant mouse and rabbit ileal assays for the heat-stable enterotoxin of *Escherichia coli*, a delayed-acting (18 to 24 hours), heat-labile enterotoxin has been isolated from nontyphoidal *Salmonella*. The toxin is active in vitro against Chinese hamster ovary cells and is neutralized by cholera antitoxin, indicating that its mechanism of action probably involves the adenyl cyclase system (Chapter 40). In experimental animals, pretreatment with the prostaglandin synthesis inhibitor indomethacin abolishes both fluid secretion and the adenyl cyclase activation induced by *Salmonella*. In similar experiments with *Vibrio cholerae*, indomethacin pretreatment partially reduces fluid secretion but has no effect on adenyl cyclase activation. The toxins of *Salmonella* and *V. cholerae* are thereby thought to modulate the mucosal cell adenyl cyclase system by different mechanisms. Polymorphonuclear leukocytes in the lamina propria may synthesize and release prostaglandins, resulting in adenyl cyclase activation and secretory diarrhea. There is no evidence in salmonellosis that any portion of the intestine leaks fluid passively, nor is there any discernible defect in fluid absorption.

Local Suppuration. Localized *Salmonella* infection generally involves typical abscess formation with a polymorphonuclear leukocytic response, even in abscesses due to *S. typhi*. Any organ or tissue may be involved.

Sickle Cell Anemia (SS). *Salmonella* is more common than *Staphylococcus aureus* as an etiologic agent of osteomyelitis in patients with SS who characteristically incur bony infarction. These individuals frequently acquire infarction-related autosplenectomy during childhood. In one study, heat-labile serum factors (principally components of the alternative pathway for complement activation) that are necessary for the opsonization of *S. typhimurium* were found to be deficient in 12 of 28 patients with SS.

Acquired Immunodeficiency Syndrome (AIDS). Recurrent *Salmonella* bacteremia despite antimicrobial treatment may be the initial manifestation of AIDS or complicate the course of established AIDS. Impaired cell mediated immunity, ongoing hemolysis, prior use of antimicrobials, or increased exposure to the pathogen may account for the increased frequency of salmonellosis in AIDS.

Relapse and Chronic Carriage. Relapse in typhoid fever is thought to be due to the intracellular persistence of organisms in macrophages. Except in the setting of AIDS, relapse tends to occur less commonly with nontyphoidal *Salmonella* that produce clinical enteric fever. Hematogenous seeding of an abnormal or calculous gallbladder is the likely cause of chronic carriage.

CLINICAL MANIFESTATIONS. Following the ingestion of contaminated food, an incubation period of 8 to 48 hours is required for *Salmonella* multiplication and mucosal invasion.

Enterocolitis. Transient nausea and vomiting are common early symptoms. An initial chill occurs in 30% of patients, and a fever of 38 to 39C is a common, if not invariable, finding. Most patients experience colicky periumbilical and lower quadrant abdominal pain, with a few to as many as 40 stools per day. Abdominal pain is severe occasionally and, when associated with hyperactive bowel sounds and local rebound tenderness, may suggest appendicitis. Surgery in this setting often yields a normal appendix; however, ileitis or appendicitis, with or without perforation, may be encountered. Frequently, stools test positive for occult blood but rarely demonstrate the gross blood or mucus of *Shigella* dysentery. Acute proctitis and colitis, heralded by tenesmus and small-volume blood stools, may be confirmed by sigmoidoscopy in a minority of patients. Intestinal perforation and toxic megacolon are rare. Patients exhibiting "cholera-like," watery diarrhea are exceptional; however, fluid and electrolyte depletion may be profound and may lead to hypovolemic shock. The symptoms of enterocolitis subside usually in 2 to 5 days; therefore, fever and diarrhea persisting beyond 7 days should suggest a suppurative complication of salmonellosis or an alternative diagnosis. Bacteremia follows enterocolitis in 1 to 4% of adults.

Routinely, children experience symptoms for a longer duration (mean of 8.7 days) and manifest dysentery and profound dehydration more frequently than adults. Among neonates, 15% exposed to *Salmonella* will remain uninfected, and 10 to 40% will have only asymptomatic infection. Enterocolitis develops in 25 to 50% and may be chronic and indolent or acutely necrotizing with high mortality. A recent study observed that 6 of 91 infants (6.5%) studied prospectively with *Salmonella* enteritis had a positive blood culture. Other studies place the bacteremia rate among such patients at 14 to 45%.

Paratyphoid Fever. The incubation period of enteric (paratyphoid) fever, usually 6 to 18 days, may be as long as 30 to 60 days and is inversely proportional to the number of organisms ingested. Although any serotype may do so, *S. paratyphi*, *S. schottmuelleri*, *S. hirschfeldii*, *S. heidelberg*, *S. typhimurium*, and *S. choleraesuis* characteristically produce human enteric fever. Often preceded by symptoms of enterocolitis, fever becomes sustained and increases in a stepwise fashion. Associated symptoms include malaise (90%), cough (90%), anorexia (80%), myalgias and arthralgias (up to 60%), headache (34%), and pharyngitis (20 to 40%). Rose spots occur less frequently than with *S. typhi*. Rare complications include hepatitis, hepatomegaly, seizures, and an illness similar to Guillain-Barré syndrome. Paratyphoid fever is generally of shorter duration and milder and causes less mortality than typhoid fever.

Primary Bacteremia. *Salmonella* bacteremia cannot be distinguished clinically from other causes of sepsis. Protracted, hectic fever, recurrent chills, anorexia, and weight loss are present; however, gastrointestinal symptoms, rose spots, and leukopenia are often absent, and stool cultures are negative. In the United States, *S. choleraesuis*, *S. paratyphi*, *S. dublin*, and *S. typhi* are the 4 serotypes most commonly associated with septicemia.

Endovascular Infection. When more than 50% of the blood cultures of a given patient are positive (high-grade bacteremia) or when *Salmonella* bacteremia recurs after apparently adequate treatment, an endovascular focus such as endocarditis or mycotic aneurysm should be suspected.

Mycotic Aneurysm. Persistent fever following enterocolitis and the presence of a known aortic aneurysm or the development of chest, back, or abdominal pain should suggest this diagnosis. Salmonellae occasionally seed atherosclerotic aneurysms of the thoracic or abdominal aorta or iliac vessels. Less commonly, infection may extend directly to the aorta from adjacent vertebral osteomyelitis or complicate prosthetic vascular grafts. *S. choleraesuis* is the most common isolate. Often fatal outcome is due to arterial rupture or a surgical complication. Iliac arteritis carries a better prognosis than aortic mycotic aneurysm. *Salmonella* infection has been reported with patient ductus arteriosus, coarctation of the aorta, arteriovenous fistula, idiopathic cystic medial necrosis, syphilitic aortitis, prosthetic valves, vascular grafts, and rarely with normal arteries.

Endocarditis. *Salmonella* endocarditis produces rapid and extensive valvular destruction and perforation. Myocardial abscesses, purulent pericarditis, and major emboli are common. Mural endocarditis occurs much more typically with *Salmonella* than with other organisms. *S. choleraesuis* and *S. typhimurium* are frequent isolates. Mortality is high despite combined surgical and antimicrobial therapy.

Pulmonary Infections. Pneumonia and empyema are most often present in the elderly and in patients with diabetes mellitus, malignancy, and cardiac or pulmonary disease.

Central Nervous System Infections. *Salmonella* meningitis often involves neonates and children under the age of 2 years (95% of cases). In a recent study from Brazil, *Salmonella* accounted for 2.3% of all cases of bacterial meningitis but 52% of all cases due to gram-negative enteric bacilli. Fever and meningismus may be absent in patients at both extremes of age. Prematurity, the presence of an immune deficiency, and obstetric trauma increase the risk of neonatal *Salmonella* meningitis. Subdural or epidural empyema, brain abscess, ventriculitis, and obstructive hydrocephalus are common complications. *S. choleraesuis*, *S. typhimurium*, *S. enteritidis*, and *S. schottmuelleri* are frequent cerebrospinal fluid isolates.

Osteomyelitis. Conditions predisposing to bone infection include sickle cell anemia and other congenital hemoglobinopathies, diabetes mellitus, systemic lupus erythematosus, and corticosteroid therapy. Any bone may be infected; however, the long bones, spine, and costosternal junctions are involved most frequently. Often infection involves both the diaphysis and epiphysis, with frequent erosion into an adjacent joint space. Vertebral osteomyelitis due to *Salmonella* is indistinguishable clinically and radiographically from that due to other agents. Disk spaces are involved early, bony lesions appear late, and mediastinal or paravertebral abscesses are common. *S. choleraesuis* and *S. typhimurium* are the prevalent organisms.

Arthritis. Pyogenic arthritis is a complication in 0.2 to 0.3% of patients hospitalized with salmonellosis. Many patients are under 12 months of age, and 55% are under 6 years old. Antecedent diarrhea is reported in only half of the patients. Commonly involved joints include knees, shoulders, hips, and sacroiliac joints. Hematogenous seeding occurs more frequently than does direct extension of *Salmonella* infection from adjacent osteomyelitis. Prosthetic joint implants may become infected occasionally following *Salmonella* bacteremia.

Male adults, predominantly with clinical enterocolitis due to *S. typhimurium*, may manifest Reiter's syndrome rarely. Urethritis has been inconspicuous in most reported cases, with many of these patients bearing histocompatibility antigen HLA-B27.

Genitourinary Tract Infections. Urinary tract infections with *Salmonella* are infrequent accompaniments of urolithiasis or underlying structural abnormalities. Testicular abscesses and epididymitis in males and ovarian abscesses and salpingitis in females comprise the most common genital sites of involvement.

Other Local Infections. Splenic abscesses are rare; however, *Salmonella* is implicated in 15% of reported cases. Soft-tissue abscesses afflict less than 1% of patients hospitalized with salmonellosis in the United States. Surgical wound infection due to *Salmonella* has been reported to follow cholecystectomy in chronic carriers.

DIAGNOSIS

Differential Diagnosis

Enterocolitis. On initial clinical and laboratory examination, it is often difficult to distinguish acute diarrheal disease due to *Salmonella* from that due to other infectious or noninfectious causes. The presence of fecal polymorphonuclear leukocytes also favors the diagnosis of shigellosis, invasive *Escherichia coli, Vibrio parahaemolyticus, Yersinia enterocolitica,* or *Campylobacter jejuni,* and pseudomembranous (antibiotic-associated) colitis. Fecal leukocytes are observed also in patients with acute inflammatory bowel disease. Salmonellosis should be included in the differential diagnosis of the acute abdomen and of acute colitis.

Paratyphoid Fever and Local Suppuration. As with diarrheal disease, bacteremia and local suppuration due to Salmonella are best differentiated from those due to other etiologic agents by cultural isolation of the organism. Postdysenteric, reactive arthritis has also been reported with Shigella, Yersinia, and most recently, *Campylobacter jejuni* infections. *Salmonella* osteomyelitis can clinically and radiographically mimic intraosseous sickling, and bone biopsy may be required for the diagnosis.

Culture. The diagnosis of *Salmonella* enterocolitis requires isolation of the organism from stool. Culture of 4 to 5 gm of stool yields more consistent recovery than does a rectal swab. Contaminated specimens (stool, urine, sputum) require inoculation on an assortment of differential and selective media. MacConkey's agar (MC) and either Hektoen enteric agar (HE) or xylose-lysinedeoxycholate agar (XLD) are appropriate solid media for initial isolation. Small numbers of salmonellae may be missed occasionally by direct plating of specimens. Prior to plating on selective media, inoculation of selenite or gram-negative enrichment broth enhances recovery. Enrichment broth should be employed routinely for serial stool specimens from suspected *Salmonella* carriers. Upon isolation, lactose-negative colonies (MC), which produce black pigment (H_2S:HE or XLD), are selected for confirmatory biochemical identification and O serogrouping.

Salmonellae may be isolated readily from normally sterile body sites using simple, nonselective media, e.g., blood agar, chocolate agar, and nutrient broth. Selective media might inhibit growth and prevent recovery of organisms from usually sterile sites. In enteric fever, stool cultures are positive during the prodromal and convalescent phases; positive blood and urine cultures coincide with the febrile phase; and rose spots, when present, may yield the causative organism on culture.

Fecal Smears. Direct fluorescent antibody examination of fecal smears may permit rapid, specific diagnosis of *Salmonella* enterocolitis; however, this test is currently investigational, and the requirement for a fluorescence microscope may ultimately limit its application in developing countries.

Blood Tests. Blood leukocyte counts are often normal in enterocolitis, reduced in enteric fever, and elevated in localized suppuration. Results of the O agglutination test are highly variable and are not helpful in the diagnosis of nontyphoidal salmonellosis. Critical studies are lacking to determine the specificity and clinical significance of positive or rising agglutinin serologic tests. A positive culture remains the cornerstone in the diagnosis of salmonellosis.

TREATMENT. Successful therapy of patients with nontyphoidal salmonellosis depends on diligent supportive care and prescription of specific antimicrobials for specific septic or suppurative complications.

Supportive Therapy. Central to the successful management of *Salmonella* enterocolitis is the correction of fluid and electrolyte imbalance and the prevention of circulatory collapse. Oral rehydration with isotonic glucose-electrolyte solutions is an economical and practical alternative to intravenous rehydration for most patients (General Principles, III D). Inhibitors of bowel motility may delay excretion of the organism, prolong symptoms, and enhance the likelihood of *Salmonella* bacteremia and are not recommended except in limited amounts for control of severe abdominal cramps. Opiates and atropine-like antimotility agents may mask serious extracellular fluid losses by causing sequestration of large volumes of fluid in the intestinal lumen. Oral or parenteral nutritional supplementation can be critical in children and in patients who are malnourished at the onset or who have prolonged salmonellosis.

Antimicrobial Therapy

Enterocolitis. Many antimicrobials have been employed to treat enterocolitis; none has proved to hasten recovery, and all prolong convalescent carriage, presumably by suppressing normal fecal flora. Consequently, antimicrobials are contraindicated for the majority of patients, including neonates, with *Salmonella* enterocolitis. Patients with enterocolitis and hemoglobinopathies, AIDS, other serious underlying diseases or suspected bacteremia should receive appropriate parenteral antimicrobials.

Paratyphoid Fever. Chloramphenicol is the antibiotic of choice for paratyphoid or enteric fever and is administered orally or intravenously every 6 hours in doses of 25 to 50 mg/kg/day for 14 days. For sensitive strains, a regimen of ampicillin or amoxicillin, 100 mg/kg/day for 14 days in 3 or 4 divided doses, often will be effective; however, ampicillin resistance is encountered frequently. Trimethoprim (10 mg/kg/day)-sulfamethoxazole (50 mg/kg/day) (TMP-SMZ), given orally in divided doses every 12 hours for 14 days, is an alternative regimen.

The relapse rate for paratyphoid fever in Singapore (1979) was 8.9%. As in typhoid fever, relapse occurs generally with organisms sensitive to the original antimicrobials.

Primary Bacteremia and Local Suppuration. Chloramphenicol is the initial agent of choice also for *Salmonella* bacteremia and local suppuration. The initial dose, 50 mg/kg/day may be reduced after several days to 25 mg/kg/day and continued for 2 to 6 weeks, depending on clinical response and the adequacy of surgical drainage. If the strain is sensitive, amoxicillin or ampicillin is preferred for long-term treatment in order to avoid bone marrow suppression. High-dose ampicillin is preferred also in the treatment of *Salmonella* endocarditis, as treatment failures have been reported with chloramphenicol. Prosthetic replacement of the involved valve is required often. Mycotic aneurysms of the thoracic or abdominal aorta require surgical resection and intensive antimicrobial therapy. Four to 6 weeks of parenteral therapy have been recommended for the initial management of *Salmonella* osteomyelitis. Unfortunately, relapse of infection and chronic osteomyelitis occurs in 40 to 50% of patients. TMP-SMZ, amoxicillin, and ciprofloxacin, a quinolone, are well absorbed after oral administration, and the prolonged administration of one of these agents may be useful in the treatment or suppression of localized *Salmonella* infections. Long-term suppression may become necessary in the setting of relapsing renal transplantation or AIDS-associated salmonellosis. Recently, third generation cephalosporins, including cefotaxime, ceftazidime, ceftriaxone, and moxalactam, have cured a number of patients with *Salmonella* meningitis or osteomyelitis. Although extensive comparative studies have not been done, these agents represent acceptable alternative antimicrobials for the treatment of multiresistant salmonellosis. Aminoglycosides, tetracyclines, cephalosporins, polymyxins, and paromomycin demonstrate in vitro activity against *Salmonella* but have been ineffective in treating patients. Although encouraging, clinical experience with the quinolones remains limited, and further studies are required before these agents can be recommended for routine use.

Chronic Carriers. Chronic biliary carriers of nontyphoidal *Salmonella* are managed as typhoid carriers. Cholecystectomy and therapy with a firstline antimicrobial has often resulted in the eradication of carriage. The benefits of eliminating asymptomatic carriage must be weighed against the risk and expense of surgery. The combination of rifampin and TMP-SMZ resulted in the cure of 35 of 40 chronic *S. typhi* carriers, 7 of 19 *S. schottmuelleri* carriers, and 6 of 28 *S. enteritidis* carriers. Cefoperazone and, particularly, ceftriaxone may prove to be useful for once-daily parenteral therapy to eradicate carriage. Both agents offer the advantages of sustained serum half-life, enhanced biliary concentrations, and potential penetration into gall stones. Failure to eradicate carriage may be due occasionally to sequestration of the organism outside the gallbladder.

PROGNOSIS. *Salmonella* enterocolitis is rarely fatal in healthy adults. Infants, the elderly, and patients with serious underlying disease incur a greater risk of mortality. The case-fatality rate approaches 20% in patients with *S. choleraesuis* bacteremia. However, patients who have bacteremia due to other nontyphoidal *Salmonella* have a lower fatality rate in general than patients with sepsis due to other Enterobacteriaceae. Salmonellosis causes unusually severe mortality in hospital-associated outbreaks, with the rates being 2.3% overall, 7.0% in newborn nurseries, and 8.7% in nursing homes. Neonatal meningitis results in an 85% mortality rate despite early specific therapy. Endocarditis and mycotic aneurysm due to *Salmonella* carry a poor prognosis also.

PREVENTION

Sanitation. The control of human-to-human spread of salmonellosis depends on good personal hygiene; a reliable, uncontaminated water supply; proper sewage disposal; the identification, treatment, and follow-up of chronic carriers; and the isolation of acute cases. Known chronic carriers should not be employed as food handlers or as health care or child care providers. Owing to the gravity of nosocomial outbreaks, particular attention should be paid to the application of enteric precautions for patients hospitalized with enterocolitis. Clinical data strongly support the role of breast-feeding in protection of neonates and infants against *Salmonella* infection.

Vaccines. No immunization is available currently to prevent nontyphoidal salmonellosis. Parenteral or oral immunization with killed nontyphoidal *Salmonella* vaccines has not proved effective in preventing disease in humans.

Zoonotic Spread. Detection and control of salmonellosis among animals and reduction in the contamination of food products from animals will not be easily accomplished. Heat treatment or pasteurization of animal feeds has curtailed the spread of *Salmonella* in some instances but may not be economical on a widespread basis. Improvement in the hygienic conditions encountered in the transport, holding, and slaughtering of animals and in food processing, distribution, and preparation remains a constant challenge.

BIBLIOGRAPHY

Black PH, Kunz LJ, Swartz MN: Salmonellosis—A review of some unusual aspects. N Engl J Med 262:811, 864, 921, 1960.
Centers for Disease Control: Salmonella Surveillance Annual Summary 1986, Atlanta, Georgia.
Chalker RB, Blaser MJ: A review of human salmonellosis: III. Magnitude of Salmonella infection in the United States. Rev Infect Dis 10:111, 1988.
Cohen JI, Bartlett JA, Corey GR: Extra-intestinal manifestations of Salmonella infections. Medicine 66:349, 1987.
Gunn RA, Loarte FB: Salmonella enterocolitis: Report of a large food-borne outbreak in Trujillo, Peru. Bull Pan Am Health Organ 13:162, 1979.
Kauffmann F: Serologic Diagnosis of Salmonella Species, Kauffmann-White Schema. Baltimore, Williams & Wilkins, 1972.
O'Brien TF, Hopkins JD, Gillece ES, et al.: Molecular epidemiology of antibiotic resistance in Salmonella from animals and human beings in the United States. N Engl J Med 307:1, 1982.
Turnbull PCB: Food poisoning with special reference to salmonella. Its epidemiology, pathogenesis and control. Clin Gastroenterol 8:663, 1979.

40.   CHOLERA AND OTHER VIBRIOSES

David R. Nalin and J. Glenn Morris, Jr.

DEFINITION. Cholera is a disease characterized by profuse, watery, typically rice-water diarrhea. It is caused by O group 1 strains of *Vibrio cholerae* that produce a protein enterotoxin known as cholera toxin. Dehydration is rapid and severe and, if untreated, may lead to death within 24 hours of onset of symptoms. *V.*

cholerae of other O groups (non-O1 *V. cholerae*), and other *Vibrio* species, may cause diarrhea of mild to moderate severity, and some *Vibrio* species have been implicated as a cause of wound infections and septicemia (Table 40–1).

40.1. *VIBRIO CHOLERAE* O GROUP 1 (CHOLERA)

ETIOLOGY. *V. cholerae* is a curved gram-negative bacterium with a characteristic rapid wobbly helical motility seen on darkfield or phase contrast microscopy. Two classification schemes are in common usage based on O antigens of *V. cholerae:* the Smith typing system (used by the Centers for Disease Control [CDC]) uses sera raised to live organisms and contains more than 70 O groups; the Sakazaki system, which uses heat-killed organisms, contains about 60 O groups. In both systems, strains responsible for cholera have been placed in O group 1 (*V. cholerae* O1).

V. cholerae O1 has two biotypes, the classic and the El Tor. These differ in biochemical and epidemiologic parameters and by reason of El Tor's hemolytic characteristic, polymyxin B resistance, milder spectrum of disease, choleraphage IV resistance, and greater hardiness in the environment. Each biotype has two distinct and one intermediate serotype (Ogawa, Inaba, and Hikojima, respectively). Immunity is serotype-specific, but cross-immunity occurs, chiefly when Inaba confers immunity against the Ogawa serotype.

HISTORY. The classic work of John Snow during the London cholera epidemics of the 1830s elucidated many of the salient characteristics of cholera epidemiology and illustrated the importance of providing hygienic water to prevent water-borne outbreaks. During this period, O'Shaughnessy pioneered chemical analyses of blood and stool in patients with cholera, and Thomas Latta of Leith was inspired by these analyses to conceive of replacing the water and salts lost in the copious cholera diarrhea by means of intravenous infusions.

These workers conceived of an infectious "principle," the nature of which awaited the later discovery of the vibrio by Pacini.

The disease has encompassed the globe in a series of pandemics. The seventh pandemic began in 1961 in the Celebes (Sulawesi) and has continued since, spreading westward across Asia through trade, tourism, and pilgrimage routes and affecting Europe and Africa. During its course, the classic biotype, for unknown reasons, has been almost entirely replaced by El Tor.

DISTRIBUTION AND INCIDENCE. Cholera has demonstrated its potential for worldwide distribution. In the last century, cases were common in North and South America as well as in Europe, Asia, and Africa. In recent years it has spread across Asia (the Philippines, Taiwan, Thailand, India, Pakistan, Bangladesh, Sri Lanka, the Soviet Union, and China) to Europe (Italy, Czechoslovakia, Spain), Africa (Tanzania, South Africa, Togo, Kenya, Zaire, and other countries) and to the South Pacific (Fig. 40–1). The current pandemic has not spread to South America, but cases have been reported along the Gulf Coast of the United States and Mexico. Cholera appears to have established endemic foci in many of these areas, with the number of countries reporting cases remaining relatively constant since the late 1960s (Fig. 40–2).

In 1986, 36 countries reported a total of 46,473 cholera cases to the World Health Organization. A number of countries known to have endemic cholera did not report cases, however, and, in some countries that did report, it is likely that the reported cases reflect only a small fraction of the actual number of cases that occurred. In endemic areas such as Bengal, clinical case-attack rates vary from 2 to 6 per 1000 population per year, but inapparent or asymptomatic infections are estimated to be 5 to 27 times more common. The fall and winter outbreaks in these areas may cause up to 500,000 deaths annually throughout India and Bangladesh in peak years. At one hospital serving Dhaka, Bangladesh, up to 400 patients with severe dehydration have been admitted daily during the late fall epidemic peaks.

EPIDEMIOLOGY. In endemic areas, cholera is rare under 1 year of age, because infants are protected by factors such as maternal antibodies acquired transplacentally or in breast milk. In nonendemic areas, however, infants may be affected, as in a Bahrein outbreak caused by contaminated infant formula. Weaning malnutrition (with associated hypochlorhydria) along with increasing contact with contaminated water leads to the peak incidence in the nonimmune 2- to 4-year age group. Up to 20% of cholera cases, however, occur in young adults in the child-rearing age group, and the nutritional and economic consequences of loss of a parent often prove fatal to surviving members of impoverished families. For unknown reasons, persons with blood group O are significantly more likely to have severe disease.

TRANSMISSION. Water is probably the primary vehicle of infection for cholera, but some outbreaks have been associated with a common food source. Foods, usually those in contact with contaminated water, have been the source of outbreaks in many newly infected areas: these foods have included mussels (Italy),

TABLE 40–1. *Vibrio* **Species Implicated as a Cause of Human Disease**

Species	Clinical Presentation		
	GI	*Wound/Ear*	*Septicemia*
V. cholerae			
O1	+ +	−	
Non-O1	+ +	+	−
V. parahaemolyticus	+ +	+	−
V. fluvialis	+ +		
V. mimicus	+ +	+	
V. hollisae	+ +		−
V. furnissii	+ +		
V. vulnificus	+	+ +	+ +
V. alginolyticus		+ +	
V. damsela		+ +	
V. albensis		+ +	
V. cincinnatiensis			+
V. carchariae			+
V. metschnikovii	?		?

GI = gastrointestinal; + + = most common presentation; + = other clinical presentations; − = rare presentation.

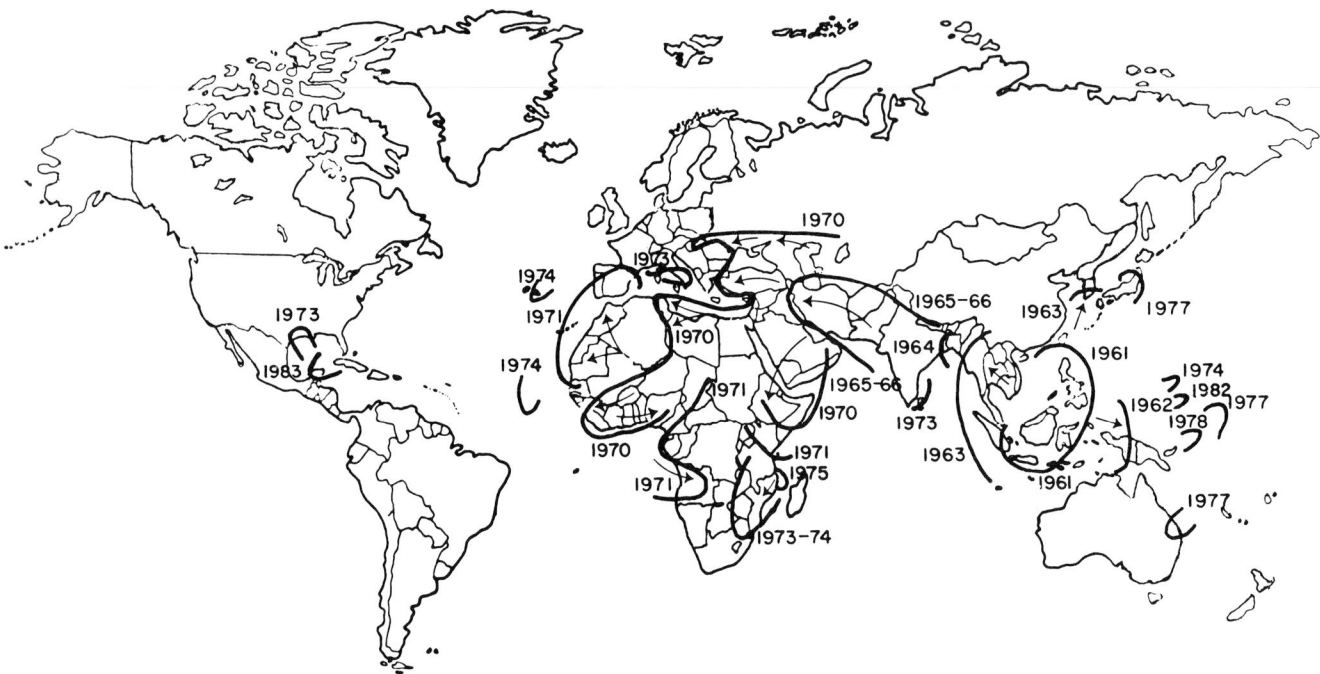

FIGURE 40–1. Extension of El Tor cholera 1961–1988.

salted fish (Guam), raw cockles and commercially bottled water (Portugal), crab (Louisiana), and possibly raw vegetables (Israel). Cholera is not easily spread by person-to-person contact. Nosocomial transmission has been documented, and care should be taken to ensure that water and food served to other patients within a hospital are not contaminated with the organism.

V. cholerae concentrations in surface water of endemic areas (under 10^2 organisms per liter) are usually far below doses (10^{11} organisms) needed to cause disease in most healthy normochlorhydric volunteers. Tropical hypochlorhydria is an important factor facilitating cholera spread. Gastrectomy and other causes of low acid production are also predisposing factors. In volunteer studies at the University of Maryland, the infective inoculum of the El Tor biotype was lowered when given with milk or with rice and fried fish, similar to the diet in Bengal. Alkaline dietary residues, inhibition of acid secretion by

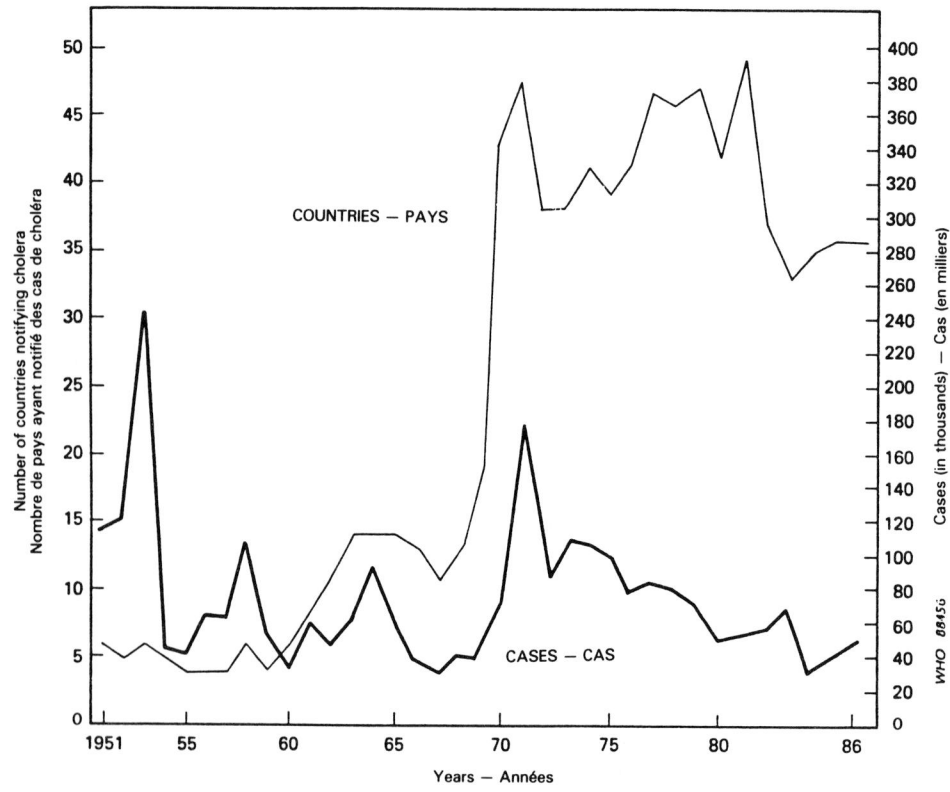

FIGURE 40–2. Incidence of cholera and number of countries notifying cases 1951–1986. (From Martinez CA, Barua D, Merson MH: World Health Stat Q 41:74, 1988. Reprinted by permission.)

dietary fats, or adsorption of vibrios to cells or to food particles may all protect them from gastric acid. In addition, vibrios adhere to and multiply readily on moist chitin of shrimp or crab shell particles and produce chitinase, which enables them to digest these particles. Adsorption to chitin protects *V. cholerae* from the lethal effects of hydrochloric acid.

In each endemic area, cholera has a sharply defined seasonal peak that occurs earlier in the year as one moves westward, possibly linked to variations in monsoon onset and local ecologic factors. In East Bengal (Bangladesh), epidemics start at the end of the monsoon (August to September) when floodwaters are high and peak during October to December as waters dry up. By January, cases have sharply diminished and few are seen until the smaller spring wave (April to June) begins. In West Bengal (Calcutta), in contrast, the spring wave is prominent and the winter wave, until recently, was absent.

By the time index cases are detected in each locality, the disease has typically already spread throughout the community. This occurs because the inapparent-to-apparent case ratio is high and initial cases are often misdiagnosed or not brought to official attention. Patients with inapparent infection typically cease excreting vibrios within 10 days, but vibrios excreted in feces during the subclinical infection serve to contaminate environmental water, facilitating infection of more susceptible individuals. Long-term gallbladder carriers are rare.

The fate of *V. cholerae* O1 in the environment needs further study. Outside of traditional endemic areas, increasing evidence suggests that pathogenic strains of *V. cholerae* O1 can persist in the environment adhering to chitinaceous fauna, certain algae, or higher aquatic plants, or as free-living organisms for extended periods. In the United States, a single strain (as identified by a unique *Hin*dIII site in the cholera toxin gene) appears to have been responsible for more than 50 cases of cholera since 1973. This strain has been isolated from the Gulf Coast environment, and appears, in many instances, to have been transmitted by inadequately cooked shellfish that carried the organism. Colonization of the gut of the Blue crab has been reported. Intriguing data also suggest that *V. cholerae* O1 can become "nonculturable," permitting it to persist undetected in the environment; further work is needed to define conditions that promote a shift to these dormant, nonculturable forms and to determine the role played by such forms in the epidemiology of the disease.

IMMUNE RESPONSES. Volunteer studies and a study of endemic cholera in rural Bangladesh suggest long-lasting antibacterial and possibly antitoxic immunity. Other studies in endemic areas, however, indicate that sequential infections with heterologous serotypes are not rare. In the latter studies, repeat infections, not always with accompanying clinical attacks, are as likely in individuals with prior attacks as in those not previously clinically ill. Coexisting malnutrition, hypochlorhydria, or parasite-related immunosuppression may influence the efficacy or duration of the immune response. The immunomodulatory effects of cholera toxin itself may play a role as well.

PATHOGENICITY AND PATHOPHYSIOLOGY. After ingestion and stomach transit, surviving vibrios must multiply and colonize the small bowel. Success of colonization depends on motility; pili; production of colicins, mucinase, and neuraminidase; and availability of intestinal mucosal binding sites for organisms and enterotoxin. Pathogenic *V. cholerae* strains can adhere to buccal epithelial cells and to gut cell surfaces. Adherence appears to be mediated primarily by the *tcp*A pilus; in volunteer studies, strains containing mutations in the *tcp*A gene were unable to colonize. Expression of *tcp*A is controlled by the *tox*R gene, a gene that regulates expression of a variety of virulence-associated factors, including cholera toxin.

Cholera Toxin. A protein enterotoxin, cholera toxin, is the primary factor responsible for the severe diarrhea seen in patients with clinical cholera. The cholera toxin gene (of which there may be multiple copies) is carried in the chromosome of toxigenic *V. cholerae* O1 strains. Cholera toxin consists of cyclase-activating (A) and 5 binding or light (B) subunits (choleragenoid) of 28,000- and 11,600-dalton molecular weight, respectively. The B subunit itself is nondiarrheagenic but binds the toxin molecule to GM_1 ganglioside in the cell membrane, permitting the active A moiety to enter the cell. Subsequently, adenyl cyclase activity inside the basolateral enterocyte border is enhanced by adenyl diphosphonucleotide (ADP) ribosylation of the enzyme. The site at which cholera toxin/NAD$^+$ activates by ADP ribosylation is the guanine nucleotide–binding activatory subunit of adenylate cyclase. The ADP-ribosyltransferase activity of the toxin leads to covalent modification of a 42,000-dalton guanyl nucleotide–binding protein and related proteins, which may increase adenyl cyclase activation by inhibiting the normal turn-off reaction of guanyl triphosphonucleotide hydrolysis. The resulting increase in cell cyclic adenosine monophosphate (cAMP) is associated with the net secretion of water and electrolytes into the gut lumen, but the final mechanism linking cyclic nucleotide–dependent protein phosphorylation and other biochemical alterations to electrolyte secretion remains unclear. Cholera toxin facilitates calcium transport in jejunal brush border vesicles, and calcium-calmodulin controls cAMP production, suggesting a possible role in intestinal secretion.

A protein cofactor may be required for ADP ribosylation by cholera toxin of the stimulatory guanine nucleotide–binding regulatory protein of the cyclase system. This cofactor is itself a GTP–binding protein. ADP ribosylation requires GTP and the endogenous guanine nucleotide–binding protein (a G protein) known as ARF (ADP ribosylating factor). The degree of ARF enhancement of cholera toxin ADP-ribosyltransferase activity can vary, and factors influencing it might account for variations in disease severity.

Although cholera toxin is the critical diarrheagenic factor in cholera, *V. cholerae* O1 strains that do not carry the cholera toxin gene, or from which the cholera toxin gene has been deleted by genetic techniques, have been associated with human disease. It has been postulated that these strains carry another toxin or toxins that can cause diarrhea; such toxins have yet to be characterized. An effect of supernatants of classic cholera toxin–negative strains on tight junctions has been shown, and Shiga-like toxin or other cytotoxins may play a role.

PATHOLOGY. Small bowel biopsy specimens from patients with cholera have virtually normal histologic appearance. Only slight villous crypt dilatation is present due to crypt cell secretion of cholera fluid. An increase in discharged goblet cells leads to increased mucus in cholera stools. Villous tip cells are morphologically intact, but their absorptive capacity for plain saline is reduced.

Changes in Electrolyte Metabolism. The chief effect of cholera toxin in humans and in dogs is a 70% reduction in unidirectional influx of water and ions from gut lumen into gut mucosal cells. A slight increase in outflux from cell to lumen may also occur. The net sum of these 2 movements (influx and outflux) yields the net secretion observed. In canine jejunum, cholera toxin reduces unidirectional influxes of many molecules, including tritiated water and ^{14}C-labeled urea; the water becomes totally nonabsorbable. In short-circuited tissue preparations, chiefly chloride absorption is inhibited. Cholera toxin thus causes a diffuse decrease in gut mucosal permeability to a wide range of molecules, leading, in turn, to a shift from primarily absorptive to primarily secretory osmoregulating mechanisms. Thus, net chloride and sodium absorption are absent and net secretion is present during cholera; glucose, potassium, and bicarbonate absorption, however, remain intact in cholera and allied diarrheas, as does glucose-linked enhancement of sodium and water absorption. Thus, although plain salt water is nonabsorbable during cholera and aggravates the diarrhea, the addition of glucose renders the solution absorbable and thereby provides the physiologic basis of oral rehydration and maintenance therapy. Galactose and certain amino acids (glycine, alanine) have an effect similar to that of glucose. Fructose is ineffective.

CLINICAL MANIFESTATIONS

Symptomatology. After an incubation period of about 45 hours, cholera diarrheal fluid accumulates, filling the small intestinal lumen to the point of causing gut distention, increased intestinal motility, decreased transit time, and diarrhea. All other clinical symptoms result entirely from the effects of loss of fluid and electrolytes in stool and vomitus. These changes lead to circulatory collapse, diminished total body water, and decreased plasma volume. These alterations, coupled with the acidosis that results from stool bicarbonate loss, lead to peripheral venospasm, pooling of remaining circulating blood volume in the heart and lungs, and ultimately circulatory failure and death. The cause and mechanism of vomiting in cholera and other intestinal infections are unknown; gut distention may be contributory. Septicemia and toxin absorption play no role in cholera pathogenesis.

Most cholera infections are, however, asymptomatic or cause only mild symptoms indistinguishable from other mild diarrheas; such patients rarely seek therapy. In most clinically apparent cases the first symptom is diarrhea that progresses over several hours from grade III to grade IV or V (Table III D–1). Typically, vomiting occurs early and abruptly; it occasionally begins before diarrhea and usually before dehydration or acidosis appears. Brief fever occurs in 25% of hospitalized cholera patients. Fever heralds clinical symptoms in volunteers infected with *V. cholerae* as well, particularly with the El Tor biotype. Early symptoms that are more prominent in adults with cholera than in adults with *E. coli* or rotavirus diarrhea include borborygmi and abdominal fullness, heralding emesis.

The diarrhea rate may quickly reach 500 to 1000 mL/hr, leading rapidly to tachycardia, hypotension, and vascular collapse due to dehydration. As dehydration progresses, the tongue becomes dry, urine production ceases, skin turgor and elasticity decrease, eyes become deeply sunken (Fig. 40–3), fingers become wrinkled, and the voice becomes raspy. Severe acidosis is associated with a Kussmaul breathing pattern. Although patients are prostrated and weak, they remain conscious, albeit sometimes obtunded. If coma occurs, further diagnostic workup is necessary to rule out complicating disorders.

Laboratory Abnormalities. Sodium and potassium loss from muscle accompanies electrolyte depletion and leads to cramps in the extremities and abdominal muscles. Water depletion is reflected by increased plasma protein concentrations and elevated hematocrit values; the plasma bicarbonate level falls with progressive loss of plasma bicarbonate into stool. The resulting acidosis elevates plasma potassium levels despite overall body potassium depletion. Plasma sodium and chloride concentrations remain in the normal range. Cumulative potassium loss may result in severe potassium depletion with or without hypokalemia in convalescence; ventricular dysrhythmias, muscle weakness, paralytic ileus, and nephropathy may result. Hypoglycemia occurs in patients, mostly children with cholera, and causes permanent brain damage. It appears to be primarily due to a failure of gluconeogenesis.

Complications. Complications consist chiefly of aspiration pneumonia after vomiting, and the chronic effects of improperly managed electrolyte deficits or hypoglycemia. Among properly treated patients deaths are rare (< 1%) and are associated chiefly with coexisting pulmonary disease and antecedent severe malnutrition. Infusion of large volumes of cold intravenous fluids into patients with cholera may cause skeletal muscle fasciculation.

DIAGNOSIS. The clinical diagnosis is based on the rapid onset of diarrhea and vomiting with dehydration and the profuse, translucent, fishy-smelling rice-water stool (Fig. 40–4). A presumptive bacteriologic diagnosis can be made by phase contrast or darkfield microscopy of a hanging-drop preparation of fresh liquid stool by detecting the characteristic helical vibrio motion. Stool spirochetes have a screwlike motion that experienced workers can easily distinguish from that of *V. cholerae*. The addition of a drop of group O1 antiserum to the slide stops and kills only vibrios.

Culture. A fresh rectal swab or stool specimen should be plated directly on suitable media such as thiosulfate-citrate-bile salt-sucrose (TCBS), Monsur's agar, MacConkey's agar, or blood agar. Suspected vibrio colonies

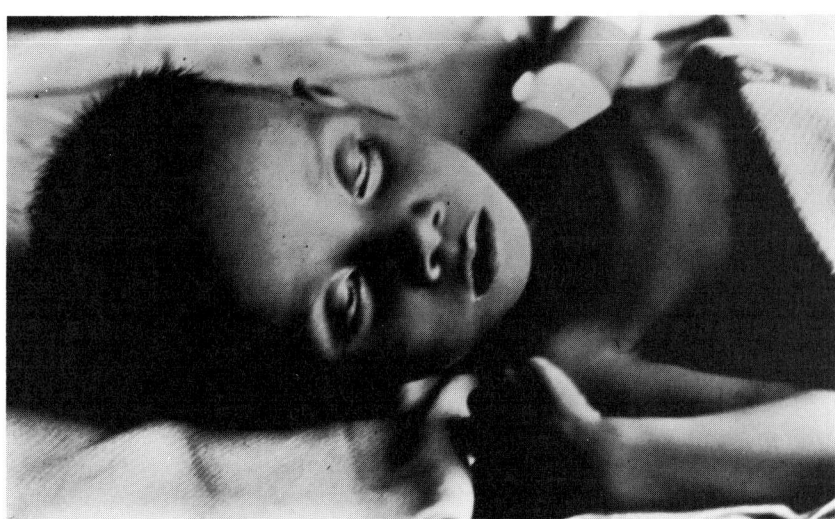

FIGURE 40–3. Filipino child with severe dehydration from cholera. Note sunken eyes.

are confirmed by seroagglutination with group O1 and Ogawa and Inaba antisera. Enrichment media (e.g., Monsur's fluid or alkaline peptone water with tellurite 1:200,000) also can be inoculated and subcultured after 6 and 18 hours of incubation. This is useful chiefly for processing stools from carriers, from patients treated late in the course of their disease, or only partially treated cases. Ordinary filter paper soaked with liquid stools and placed in a sealed plastic bag is suitable for sending to a laboratory from the field. *V. cholerae* in such specimens survive for 1 week. Vibrios in 1 gm of a patient's stool inoculated into plain sterile 1% sodium chloride solution survive for over 3 months at 37°C. Cultured cholera vibrios can be confirmed by seroagglutination with group O1 and type-specific antisera.

DNA Probes. Toxigenic *V. cholerae* O1 strains can be rapidly identified on colony blots using a DNA probe for the cholera toxin gene. Probes to detect sequences encoding hemolysin, lysogenic phage, and a toxin-regulating element also have been reported. DNA probes already are finding wide usage in epidemiologic studies. Because of the technical difficulties involved, they are not a substitute for standard microbiologic techniques in clinical situations. It is likely, however, that, with further refinements, these and other high-technology diagnostic systems will find increasingly wide application.

Serology. After an acute episode of cholera, almost all persons show a sharp rise in vibriocidal antibody titer. A rise in the titer of antibodies directed against cholera toxin also occurs; in contrast to the vibriocidal response, however, the antitoxic response may be blunted by early antibiotic therapy. Where acute and convalescent sera are available, the identification of a sharp rise in the titer of vibriocidal and antitoxic antibodies is virtually diagnostic for cholera; similarly, the presence of very high antibody titers in convalescent sera is strongly suggestive of the diagnosis. The significance of low levels of vibriocidal and antitoxic antibodies in population-based surveys is somewhat more problematic: related antigens, such as those of *Brucella, Citrobacter,* or *Yersinia,* can stimulate a vibriocidal response, whereas antitoxic antibodies directed against the heat labile (LT) toxin of enterotoxigenic *E. coli* are detected by assays for anti–cholera toxin antibodies.

DIFFERENTIAL DIAGNOSIS. In epidemic set-

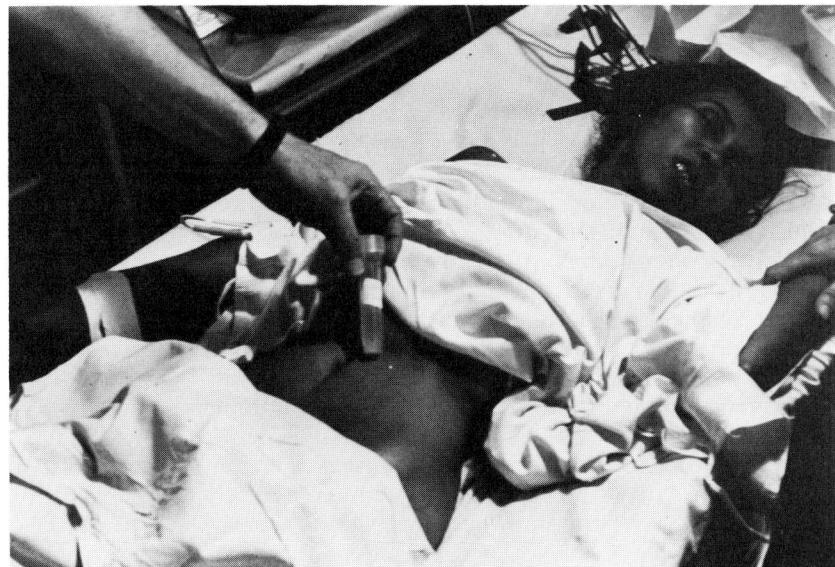

FIGURE 40–4. Filipino woman with severe dehydration from cholera being rehydrated intravenously while lying on a cholera cot. Test tube contains some of her rice-water stool.

tings, no other disease can consistently cause severe, life-threatening diarrhea and dehydration in adults. In individual cases, diarrhea that approaches the severity of cholera can be caused by other diarrheal pathogens, including enterotoxigenic *E. coli* and strains of non-O1 *V. cholerae*. Among children, rotavirus also can be a cause of severe, dehydrating diarrhea. These disorders respond to the same therapeutic fluid regimen as cholera.

Among noninfectious causes, acute arsenic poisoning is sometimes mistaken for cholera. Rare adenomas that produce vasoactive intestinal polypeptide (VIP) and related tumors may present with cholera-like diarrhea.

TREATMENT. The treatment of cholera consists of prompt replacement of the water and salts lost in the copious diarrhea and vomitus. In addition to rehydration and maintenance fluids, antibiotics such as tetracycline lessen the duration and volume of diarrhea, thereby reducing fluid therapy needs. A normal or light diet should be resumed on completion of rehydration a few hours after admission, early in the maintenance phase.

Water and salts can be replaced intravenously or orally (using oral glucose-electrolyte solutions, III D, General Principles). Because important details of cholera therapy differ from those of milder diarrheas, the salient points will be reviewed from the perspective of cholera.

Patients in Shock. Patients in shock as a result of the dehydration of cholera (i.e., no detectable radial pulse) should receive immediate intravenous (IV) fluid infusion equivalent to 10% (or proportionally less for obese subjects) of admission body weight (Fig. 40–4) administered over 2 to 3 hours. A scale is useful when placed at the ward door where the collapsed patient and a supporting attendant can be weighed together and then the attendant's weight deducted. Alternatively, weight can be estimated and measured after initial IV fluid therapy enables the patient to stand. Femoral vein infusion can be life-saving and avoids the high risk of death accompanying delay in initiating rehydration of patients in shock.

Optimal cholera therapy demands special intravenous and oral rehydration solution (ORS) compositions. The best IV solutions for cholera (or nonvibrio cholera) therapy are the acetate or the Dacca (now Dhaka) solutions (Table III D–8), which replace all the key electrolytes lost in the stool (Table III D–3); 1 or 2% glucose should be added to prevent hypoglycemia. Similar solutions can be made by using appropriate proportions of sterile intravenous dextrose, normal saline, and injectable KCl and $NaHCO_3$.

Early bicarbonate therapy greatly reduces the hazards of overhydration by correcting peripheral venospasm that accompanies acidosis. Prompt use of oral glucose-electrolyte maintenance solutions that contain bicarbonate and potassium makes it safer to correct shock rapidly by IV rehydration with normal saline or similar isotonic saline solutions. Prompt correction of volume deficit alone leads quickly to return of normal renal function, and the base or base precursor in the solution promptly corrects acidosis. Citrate can be used instead of bicarbonate to provide base, enhancing packet shelf-life. Oral

water should be available and permitted as wanted, in addition to calculated oral or IV fluids.

Oral Therapy. About 90% of cholera patients without shock are successfully rehydrated and maintained with ORS alone (Table III D–6). The remainder require initial IV rehydration equal to 5 or 10% of body weight before starting oral maintenance. In patients with circulatory collapse, the 10% rule is followed. Patients in shock receive initial rapid IV rehydration fluid volumes equivalent to 10% of their body weight (or, if obese, until vital signs are normal). Unlike low purging rate infantile noncholera diarrheas in which the 2:1 regimen is used, high purging rate cholera diarrhea is linked with higher stool sodium and lower stool potassium concentrations. These demand higher sodium and chloride concentrations and lower potassium concentrations in replacement solutions for cholera, compared with those for pediatric cholera or for noncholera diarrhea. Oral therapy for pediatric cholera is effective with several formulas such as UNICEF's Oralyte formula (Table III D–6). Measured losses are replaced volume for volume with ORS, or enough ORS is given hourly to maintain signs of normal hydration. In cholera, stool volumes are best monitored using a cholera cot (Figs. 40–4 and 40–5).

In cholera patients with very high diarrhea rates (rarely in noncholera patients), nasogastric infusion of Oralyte or of an adult cholera oral therapy formula (Table III D–7) is useful. This spares the patient frequent night awakenings to drink oral solutions by infusing the ORS through (used) clean IV tubing that connects a nasogastric tube to an inverted cleaned IV-type bottle filled with ORS. The oral solution need not be sterile; it can be prepared using boiled water made tepid, but it should not be boiled after mixing the ingredients.

It is easier and therapeutically more rational to use a special oral solution formula for adults with severe cholera. Such an adult solution is similar to Oralyte but has 4.2 g/L of NaCL, 4.0 g/L $NaHCO_3^-$, and 1.8 g/L KCl. The Oralyte formula (Table III D–6) does not match adult cholera stool composition, so net sodium, chloride, and potassium losses often develop during therapy with this formula, even when adult patients can drink hourly volumes equivalent to 1.5 times their stool volumes. Many such patients cannot drink that much; therefore, therapeutic failure rates increase when using that formula and regimen, especially in severe cases. Extensive field trials in patients with profuse cholera diarrhea whose shock was corrected with IV fluids before using the adult oral maintenance therapy formula have yielded the highest oral therapy success rates. Only 4.4% needed IV maintenance after initial rehydration, case-fatality rates were less than 0.5%, and electrolyte balance was positive. With the adult formula, patients need drink only enough ORS to match the volume of fluid lost. When extra oral water is permitted as desired, this formula also can be used for children with cholera. For mild cholera or for noncholera diarrhea, the Oralyte formula is equally effective in adults and children.

Oral Maintenance. When oral maintenance is used to treat cholera, total IV fluid requirements of patients

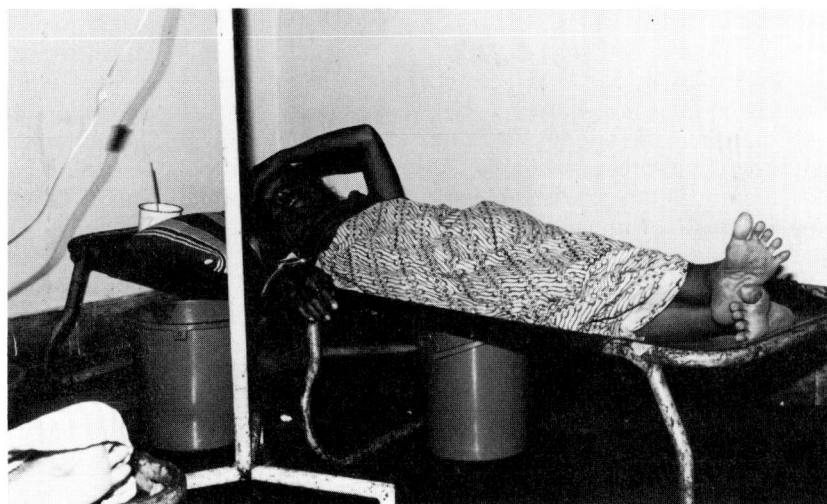

FIGURE 40–5. Bangladesh woman with acute cholera lying on cholera cot. Note plastic bucket under hole in cot to catch the stool.

with circulatory collapse are reduced by 80%, and most patients with a palpable radial pulse on admission need only oral rehydration and oral maintenance therapy with no IV fluids at all. In cholera epidemics, this oral regimen is crucial, because it stretches limited IV stocks.

Adults with profuse cholera diarrhea should initially drink 750 to 1000 mL of solution hourly for several hours. Oral therapy should begin as soon as shock is corrected with initial IV rehydration fluids, or earlier if no shock is present (or no IV fluid available).

Children with profuse watery diarrhea should drink 250 to 500 mL hourly, depending on weight, age, and diarrhea rate. The specific amounts can be adjusted to match initial rates of stool loss. During the first 4 to 6 hours of therapy, the individual rate of stool loss becomes apparent by checking clinical signs of hydration and the level of stool losses accumulating in the calibrated bucket under the cholera cot (Fig. 40–5). In subsequent 6-hour intake and output periods, the hourly amount of oral therapy given during each period should equal the mean hourly amount of fluid loss during the preceding intake and output period (Table 40–2) or the amount of fluid therapy needed to maintain clinical signs of normal hydration. Fluid therapy for cholera stops when profuse diarrhea stops, that is, when stool is grade III or less (Table III D–1).

Antibiotics. Antibiotics can be started 1 to 2 hours after initiating rehydration. Parenteral antibiotics offer no advantage. Tetracycline is the drug of choice. The optimal dose schedule is 250 mg for adults and 125 mg for children, given orally every 6 hours for 4 days.

Tetracycline prophylaxis is not advisable, since substantial benefits have not been demonstrated and such usage leads to resistant strains.

Although the incidence of dental staining after short-course tetracycline is less well documented than after long courses, young children and pregnant women can be treated alternatively with furazolidone. In practice, the efficacy, cost, availability, and therapeutic need for an antibiotic often outweigh the undefined dental risks in endemic cholera areas, in which dental staining due to pan chewing and other practices overshadows other dental problems. Furazolidone is given as tablets or syrup, 100 mg orally to adults or 50 mg to children, every 6 hours. Chloramphenicol and trimethoprim–sulfamethoxazole are slightly less effective but can be used if other drugs are not available. Newer quinolones such as norfloxacin and ciprofloxacin are effective in vitro, and a controlled comparative clinical trial of norfloxacin showed superiority to trimethoprim-sulfamethoxazole and placebo. Antibiotic resistance is becoming an increasingly severe problem, particularly in East Africa, and sensitivity of prevalent cholera strains to antibiotics should be checked periodically.

Antiemetics and Other Therapies. Complicating disorders such as aspiration pneumonia require additional antibiotics, usually a penicillin. Antiemetics have undergone no controlled trial, and, with few exceptions, vomiting disappears without any therapy other than rehydration a few hours after dehydration and acidosis are corrected. There is no role in cholera therapy per se for antidiarrheas, analeptics, adrenal corticosteroids,

TABLE 40–2. Cholera Oral Therapy Sheet

Admission body weight = 30kg								
				Volume (L)				
Time	IV	Oral Intake	Vomitus	Intake Minus Vomitus	Stool	GNB	Cumulative GNB	Urine
11 AM	3	Admission IV rehydration to correct shock.						
12 noon	0	Start oral solution maintenance with oral rehydration solution (ORS).						
6 PM	0	3	0.5	2.5	2	+0.5	+0.5	0.2
12 midnight	0	2	0	2	1.8	+0.2	+0.7	0.2
6 AM	0	2	0	2	1.5	+0.5	+1.2	0.2

GNB = gut net balance; ORS = oral rehydration solution.

aspirin, or other drugs. Chlorpromazine, believed to reduce cyclase activity, caused modest reduction in diarrhea rates in one study but not in another. Chlorpromazine does not, however, obviate the need for IV and oral fluid therapy and it causes stupor, interfering with these and other aspects of therapy. A reduction in oral therapy failure rates in pediatric patients with severe cholera treated with chlorpromazine has been reported; presumably, this may relate to chlorpromazine's antiemetic activity, but emesis data were not reported by the investigators. Lodoxamide, a calcium antagonist, inhibits the secretory response to cholera and *E. coli* enterotoxins, but no clinical trial of a calcium antagonist has been reported. No consistent clinical reduction of diarrhea duration or volume has been shown in clinical trials testing salicylates, indomethacin, or other potential toxin antagonists. Protease inhibitors can block activation of adenylate cyclase and may merit experimental therapeutic studies in cholera.

Management of Cholera Epidemics. Epidemics, during which hospitals may admit 200 patients in shock daily, demand special management. IV fluids and ORS ingredients or packets need to be stockpiled; UNICEF's Oralyte packet has a 2- to 3-year shelf-life, but plastic bags containing enough freshly bought and weighed glucose, salt, baking soda (*not* baking powder) or trisodium citrate and potassium chloride to provide 10 L of ORS can be made up daily and dissolved in 10 L of previously boiled tepid water in plastic carboys as needed (Fig. III D–1). Rice water or boiled rice gruel can substitute for glucose, as can sucrose, though the latter is slightly less effective than glucose; addition of 100 mM glycine to the glucose-ORS solution enhanced its efficiency in four studies of cholera. The ORS can be dispensed to patients' bedsides in plastic 1-L bottles with cups. In endemic areas, cholera cots and calibrated buckets (Fig. 40–5) should be kept available in storage until needed. Facilities for mass chemical or heat decontamination of stools before release into sewerage need to be devised to avoid hospital and perihospital spread of infections.

Therapy should be streamlined and a single available appropriate solution used for all patients. The accent is on rapid (1- to 2-hour) correction of shock with IV fluids followed by a prompt shift to oral maintenance therapy. Most patients with a palpable radial pulse should receive oral therapy alone.

If patients exceed available bed space, additional cholera cots can be quickly set up in tents. Use of the 10% rule for correction of shock is facilitated by placing a scale on the ward for measuring admission weight. Adequate oral and intravenous solutions, IV tubing, scalp-vein and conventional needles, and recording of intake and output data on a simple bedside form (Table 40–2) are essential.

PROGNOSIS. Prompt therapy according to the listed guidelines yields a cholera case-fatality rate of less than 1%; the few deaths are in the aged or very young with major complicating (chiefly pulmonary) diseases. The diarrhea rate is higher in pregnant patients and in those who arrive in shock.

PREVENTION AND CONTROL. Mass antibiotic prophylaxis is impractical and leads to antibiotic resistance, which has not become irreversible.

Vaccination. Cholera toxoid vaccine has been of no practical value. Cholera somatic antigen vaccine is of limited value and has not proved practical for cholera control; it gives a 50% reduction in case-attack rates for only a few months. A peanut-oil adjuvanated somatic antigen gave 2 years' protection from cholera in a Philippine trial but caused sterile abscesses. Mass vaccination with available vaccines is far more costly than treatment alone and saves fewer lives. Vaccinees who get cholera do not have an attenuated form of the disease.

A variety of oral and parenteral vaccines are undergoing experimental tests, but much work remains to be done. Results of the most recent trials indicate that 3 doses of an oral vaccine that consists of purified cholera toxin B subunit and killed vibrios provided about 60% protection during 12 months. Early results showed transient protection of children under six. Reductions in all diarrheas occurred, but the relation to vaccination versus annual background variations is questionable. Attenuated strains of *V. cholerae* O1 prepared by recombinant DNA techniques with deletion of genes encoding the A cholera toxin subunit (e.g., CVD 103-HgR) offer promise for new vaccine trials.

Organization of Therapy During Epidemics. Advanced planning is essential in areas in which cholera is endemic. This includes training in modern therapy for doctors, nurses, and paramedics and stockpiling of oral and IV therapy supplies and cholera cots at designated cholera treatment centers. Each city of 100,000 or more in endemic areas should have a designated treatment center with a coordinator and all needed supplies and equipment.

Provisions of sanitary stool disposal and potable germ-free water are essential public health control measures, but they fail without simultaneous public health legislation with enforcement and education to motivate change in the habits of exposed populations.

BIBLIOGRAPHY

Barua D, Burrows W: Cholera. Philadelphia, WB Saunders, 1974.

Cash RA, Lehman JS, Hare RS, et al.: Renal function in acute Asiatic cholera. Trans R Soc Trop Med Hyg 67:217, 1973.

Cash RA, Nalin DR, Rochat R, et al.: A clinical trial of oral therapy in a rural cholera-treatment center. Am J Trop Med Hyg 19:653, 1970.

Cash RA, Toha KMM, Nalin DR, et al.: Acetate in the correction of acidosis secondary to diarrhea. Lancet 2:302, 1969.

Clemens JD, Harris SR, Khan MR, et al.: Impact of B subunit killed whole cell and killed whole-cell–only oral vaccines against cholera upon treated diarrhoeal illness and mortality in an area endemic for cholera. Lancet 1:1375, 1988.

Glass RI, Becker S, Huq MI, et al.: Endemic cholera in rural Bangladesh, 1966–80. Am J Epidemiol 116:959, 1982.

Harvey RM, Enson Y, Lewis ML, et al.: Hemodynamic studies on cholera: Effects of hypovolemia and acidosis. Circulation 37:709, 1968.

Hirschhorn N, Kinzie JL, Sachar DB, et al.: Decrease in net stool output in cholera during intestinal perfusion with glucose-containing solutions. N Engl J Med 279:176, 1968.

Kaper JB, Morris JG Jr, Nishibuchi M: DNA probes for pathogenic

Vibrio species. *In* Tenover FC (ed.): DNA Probes for Infectious Diseases. Boca Raton, FL, CRC Press, 1989.

Levine MM, Kaper JB, Herrington D, et al.: Volunteer studies of deletion mutants of *Vibrio cholerae* O1 prepared by recombinant techniques. Infect Immun 56:161, 1988.

Levine MM, Nalin DR, Craig JP, et al.: Immunity of cholera in man: Relative role of antibacterial versus antitoxic immunity. Trans R Soc Trop Med Hyg 73:3, 1979.

Levine RJ, Khan MR, D'Souza S, et al.: Failure of sanitary wells to protect against cholera and other diarrheas in Bangladesh. Lancet 2:86, 1976.

Morris JG Jr, Black RE: Cholera and other vibrioses in the United States. N Engl J Med 312:343, 1985.

Mosley, WH, Bart KJ, Sommer A: An epidemiological assessment of cholera control programs in rural East Pakistan. Int J Epidemiol 1:5, 1972.

Nair GB, Sarkar BL, De SP, et al.: Ecology of *Vibrio cholerae* in the freshwater environs of Calcutta, India. Microbiol Ecol 15:203, 1988.

Nalin DR, Levine RJ, Levine MM, et al.: Cholera, non-vibrio cholera, and stomach acid. Lancet 2:856, 1978.

Peterson JW, Berg WD, Coppenhaver DH: Synthesis of protein in intestinal cells exposed to cholera toxin. Proc Soc Exp Biol Med 186:174, 1987.

Phillips RA: Water and electrolyte losses in cholera. Fed Proc 23:705, 1964.

Pollitzer R: Cholera. Geneva. WHO Monogr No. 43, 1959.

Siddique AK, Akdam K, Islam Q: Why cholera still takes lives in rural Bangladesh. Trop Doct 18:40, 1988.

Watten RH, Morgan FM, Songkhla, et al.: Water and electrolyte studies in cholera. J Clin Invest 38:1879, 1959.

40.2. NON-O1 *VIBRIO CHOLERAE*

During the past 2 decades, there has been increasing recognition that *V. cholerae* strains of O groups other than 1 (non-O1 *V. cholerae*) also are able to cause human disease. Non-O1 strains have been implicated in outbreaks of food-borne disease, isolated from as many as 13% of patients with cholera-like disease during cholera epidemics, and identified in stool samples from patients with gastroenteritis in Asia, Africa, Europe, Australia, and North and South America.

DISTRIBUTION AND EPIDEMIOLOGY. Non-O1 *V. cholerae* is part of the normal, free-living (autochthonous) bacterial flora in estuarine areas throughout the world; in areas such as the US Gulf Coast, non-O1 strains are several orders of magnitude more common than O1 strains in the environment. Isolation has been reported from fresh water, and infections have occurred after exposure to freshwater inland lakes. Non-O1 *V. cholerae* also has been isolated from a variety of wild and domestic animals, including 6% of seagulls sampled in England and 14% of dogs in Calcutta.

Non-O1 strains are a common isolate from shellfish in the United States, particularly from filter-feeders such as oysters. In a study conducted by the US Food and Drug Administration, non-O1 *V. cholerae* was isolated from 111 (14%) of 790 samples of freshly harvested oyster shellstock. Although non-O1 *V. cholerae* has been shown to be a frequent isolate in raw shellfish in other geographic areas, it is clear that the organism can be transmitted by a variety of routes. In a study in the Ban Vinai refugee camp in Thailand, non-O1 strains were isolated from 4% of vegetable samples, 39% of meat samples, and 16% of drinking water samples; in Cancun,

Mexico, 86% of untreated well water samples were culture-positive for non-O1 *V. cholerae*.

Despite the frequency with which they have been identified in the environment, non-O1 strains generally account for only a small proportion of cases of sporadic diarrheal disease in developing countries. In one study in Cancun, Mexico, non-O1 *V. cholerae* was isolated from 16% of persons with diarrhea; in most other studies, isolation rates have ranged from less than 1 to 3% of persons with diarrhea.

PATHOGENICITY AND PATHOPHYSIOLOGY. The relatively low rate of isolation of non-O1 *V. cholerae* from patients, as compared with the environment, may be a reflection of differences in virulence among strains: that is, it is possible that only a minority of non-O1 *V. cholerae* strains carry the necessary virulence factors to cause human disease. Some non-O1 strains are known to produce cholera toxin; studies of hospitalized patients in Bangladesh suggest that persons infected with cholera toxin–producing strains have more severe gastrointestinal symptoms than those infected with strains that do not produce cholera toxin. Other proposed virulence factors have included the El Tor and Kanagawa hemolysins, a Shiga-like toxin, various cell-associated hemagglutinins, and a 17–amino acid, heat-stable enterotoxin (designated NAG-ST) that closely resembles the heat-stable toxin produced by enterotoxigenic strains of *E. coli*. It also has been suggested that virulence depends on the ability of a non-O1 *V. cholerae* strain to colonize the intestine, as demonstrated in rabbits by using the removable intestinal tie–adult rabbit diarrhea (RITARD) model.

CLINICAL MANIFESTATIONS. Non-O1 *V. cholerae* has been associated with gastroenteritis, wound and ear infections, and septicemia. Gastroenteritis can occur in healthy persons. When a non-O1 *V. cholerae* strain that produced NAG-ST (but not cholera toxin) was administered to volunteers, 6 of 10 developed diarrhea. Although illness was generally mild, 1 volunteer had over 5 L of diarrhea, with typical rice-water stools. The median incubation period in these studies was 10 hours (range, 5.5 to 96 hours), with a median duration of illness of 21 hours (range, 3.5 to 48 hours). These results are in agreement with reports from non-O1 *V. cholerae* food-borne disease outbreaks, in which symptoms tended to be mild, with a short incubation period and a short duration of illness. Septicemia occurs primarily in persons who are immunocompromised or who have underlying liver disease; the mortality rate for persons with septicemia exceeds 50%.

DIAGNOSIS AND THERAPY. Techniques for isolation of non-O1 *V. cholerae* are identical to those used for *V. cholerae* O1, with non-O1 strains differentiated by their failure to agglutinate in O1 antisera. Persons with acute non-O1 *V. cholerae* gastroenteritis do not show a rise in titer of vibriocidal antibodies.

Treatment of persons with severe diarrhea is the same as that used in management of patients with cholera. No data on antibiotic efficacy are available, but use of tetracycline appears reasonable in severe cases.

BIBLIOGRAPHY

Kaper JB, Morris JG Jr, Nishibuchi M: DNA probes for pathogenic
   Vibrio species. *In* Tenover FC (ed.): DNA Probes for Infectious
   Diseases. Boca Raton, FL, CRC Press, 1989.
Morris JG Jr, Black RE: Cholera and other vibrioses in the United
   States. N Engl J Med 312:343, 1985.
Morris JG Jr, Takeda T, Tall BD, et al.: Experimental non-O group
   1 *Vibrio cholerae* gastroenteritis in humans. J Clin Invest 85:697,
   1990.

40.3. *VIBRIO PARAHAEMOLYTICUS*

V. parahaemolyticus is a well-recognized cause of diarrheal disease throughout the world. In Japan, it is the most common cause of food-borne illness. Illness tends to be mild, but cases of severe diarrhea and dysentery have been reported.

DISTRIBUTION AND EPIDEMIOLOGY. As with non-O1 *V. cholerae*, *V. parahaemolyticus* is part of the normal, free-living bacterial flora in estuarine areas throughout the world. The organisms are halophilic (salt loving) and are a common isolate from estuarine and marine water, sediment, suspended particulates, plankton, fish, and shellfish. In temperate climates, isolation is seasonal, *V. parahaemolyticus* apparently passing the winter in sediment and then proliferating as water temperatures rise.

In Japan, *V. parahaemolyticus* has been implicated as the etiologic agent in 24% of reported cases of food-borne disease. In the United States, it has been associated with a number of major food-borne disease outbreaks, often involving mishandling of seafood after cooking. Reported isolation rates from patients with diarrhea vary widely, ranging from 11% in Calcutta and 10.7% in Thailand to 2.6 to 3.7% in Indonesia and 1.5% in Korea. Illness is frequently, but not exclusively, associated with eating seafood.

PATHOGENICITY AND PATHOPHYSIOLOGY. Although the exact mechanisms by which *V. parahaemolyticus* causes human disease have yet to be determined, gastrointestinal pathogenicity is strongly correlated with hemolytic activity: more than 95% of *V. parahaemolyticus* strains associated with gastroenteritis are hemolytic on Wagatsuma agar (the Kanagawa phenomenon) compared with 1% or less of environmental isolates. At least four hemolytic constituents have been described for *V. parahaemolyticus,* including a heat-stable and heat-labile direct hemolysin. The heat-stable direct hemolysin (*tdh*) has been most extensively studied: it is a protein with a molecular weight of 42,000 daltons and an apparent subunit structure, is lethal for mice, is active in guinea pig skin–bluing assays, and has enterotoxic activity in suckling mice. The *tdh* gene has been cloned; nonhemolytic strains of *V. parahaemolyticus* lack the *tdh* gene sequences.

Although virulence is correlated with hemolytic activity, nonhemolytic strains have been isolated from patients with diarrheal disease. The clinical significance of these strains—and the possible virulence factors that they may carry—remain to be determined.

CLINICAL MANIFESTATIONS. In a summary of 8 culture-confirmed US outbreaks, symptoms included diarrhea (98% of patients), abdominal cramps (82%), nausea (71%), vomiting (52%), headache (42%), fever, rarely above 38.9°C (27%), and chills (24%). Incubation periods ranged from 4 to 96 hours. Illness was usually self-limited, with a median duration of 3 days. A dysentery-like syndrome has been reported in association with *V. parahaemolyticus* cases in India and Bangladesh; the incubation period for the dysentery-like form of the disease may be as short as 2.5 hours (range, 1 to 9 hours). Although apparently rare, cases of dysentery associated with *V. parahaemolyticus* have been reported in the United States. Septicemia due to *V. parahaemolyticus* can occur, but it appears to be limited to persons with underlying problems with host defenses.

DIAGNOSIS AND THERAPY. *V. parahaemolyticus* grows well on blood agar and other nonselective media. Isolation from stool generally requires use of a selective medium such as TCBS; *V. parahaemolyticus* does not ferment glucose; consequently, colonies on TCBS are blue-green. Species identification is based on standard biochemical tests. The organism does not grow in media containing 0% sodium chloride (as *V. cholerae* does), but it grows in relatively high-salt concentrations, including 6 and 8% NaCl. Potentially pathogenic strains can be identified based on hemolytic activity on Wagatsuma agar or hybridization with DNA probes for the *tdh* gene.

Patients with diarrhea should be managed as described for other diarrheal pathogens. No good data on antibiotic efficacy are available; in severe cases, use of tetracycline (or possibly one of the newer quinolones such as norfloxacin or ciprofloxacin) appears reasonable.

40.4. *VIBRIO VULNIFICUS*

V. vulnificus is a recently identified halophilic *Vibrio* species that has been implicated as a cause of severe wound infections, septicemia, and possibly gastroenteritis. It is similar biochemically to *V. parahaemolyticus,* and it is possible that some severe infections previously attributed to *V. parahaemolyticus* were actually due to *V. vulnificus.*

DISTRIBUTION AND EPIDEMIOLOGY. As with other *Vibrio* species, *V. vulnificus* is a free-living estuarine organism that is frequently isolated from water and shellfish, particularly oysters. In the United States, it is the most common cause of serious *Vibrio* infections. The incidence of *V. vulnificus* infections in coastal US states approximates 0.5 cases per 100,000 population per year, with primary septicemia accounting for two thirds of cases. Although it is likely that the organism is present in other parts of the world, few data are available on infections outside of the United States.

PATHOGENICITY AND CLINICAL MANIFESTATIONS. Occurrence of primary septicemia due to *V. vulnificus* (i.e., septicemia without an obvious focus of infection) is significantly associated with eating raw oysters. Susceptibility appears to be limited to certain high-risk groups of patients, however, particularly those with hemochromatosis, cirrhosis, and hematologic and other disorders associated with immunosuppression, renal failure, and diabetes. Wound infections are associated with contamination of wounds with sea water. Whereas wound infections can occur in otherwise healthy persons, deaths associated with wound infections have occurred almost exclusively among persons in these same high-risk groups.

One third of patients with primary septicemia present in shock or become hypotensive within 12 hours of hospital admission. Three fourths of patients have distinctive bullous skin lesions. Thrombocytopenia is common, and evidence often is seen of disseminated intravascular coagulation. Complications such as gastrointestinal bleeding are not infrequent. More than half of patients with primary septicemia die; the mortality rate exceeds 90% for those who become hypotensive. Persons with septicemia often have symptoms of gastroenteritis, and data suggest that the organism can cause gastroenteritis in the absence of septicemia.

DIAGNOSIS AND TREATMENT. *V. vulnificus* can be isolated on blood agar and other nonselective media, including media used in commercial blood culture systems. TCBS is the preferred medium for isolation from stool. Identification is based on standard biochemical tests; identity can be confirmed using DNA probes.

The fulminant nature of *V. vulnificus* septicemia and wound infections necessitates prompt, aggressive therapy. The diagnosis always should be considered in susceptible patients with a history of oyster consumption or seawater exposure, particularly if bullous skin lesions are present. Appropriate therapy should be initiated even before culture results are available. Some studies suggest that successful therapy depends on early administration of antibiotics. Although data are limited, tetracycline appears to be the drug of choice.

40.5. OTHER *VIBRIO* SPECIES

A number of other *Vibrio* species also have been associated with human disease (Table 40–1). *V. fluvialis* is a newly named species that includes strains previously designated as enteric group EF-6 or group F vibrios. *V. fluvialis* was associated with a large outbreak of diarrheal disease that occurred in Bangladesh in 1976–1977. Reported clinical features included diarrhea (100% of cases), vomiting (97%), abdominal pain (75%), moderate-to-severe dehydration (67%), and fever (35%); on microscopic examination, 75% of patients were found to have leukocytes and blood cells in their stools. There has been at least 1 reported death associated with the organism in the United States.

V. mimicus, *V. hollisae*, and *V. furnissii* also have been associated with diarrheal disease. *V. mimicus* is a newly named species that includes isolates previously classified as sucrose-negative *V. cholerae*. Strains previously identified as enteric group EF-13 are now included in the species *V. hollisae*. *V. furnissii* includes aerogenic strains (strains that produce gas from glucose) that were classified as biovar II of *V. fluvialis*. *V. alginolyticus* and

V. damsela have been implicated as the cause of infections in wounds exposed to sea water. There is a single report of isolation of *V. cincinnatiensis* from a patient with septicemia and meningitis. *V. carchariae* was isolated from a patient with an infected shark bite.

Diagnosis is based on isolation of the organism from stool, blood, or wound cultures. With the exception of *V. hollisae*, the medium of choice for isolation from stool is TCBS. Diarrheal disease is best managed with appropriate fluid therapy. Isolates are almost uniformly sensitive to tetracycline; norfloxacin and ciprofloxacin provide possible alternative therapies.

41. MISCELLANEOUS BACTERIAL ENTERITIDES

41.1. DIARRHEA CAUSED BY *ESCHERICHIA COLI*

Myron M. Levine

DEFINITION. In recent years it has become increasingly recognized that *Escherichia coli* cause a wide spectrum of diarrheal illnesses in different age groups, diverse geographic areas, and under varying epidemiologic conditions. *Escherichia coli* that cause diarrhea can be conveniently divided into 5 major categories: (1) enterotoxigenic *E. coli* (ETEC); (2) enteroinvasive *E. coli* (EIEC); (3) enteropathogenic *E. coli* (EPEC); (4) enterohemorrhagic *E. coli* (EHEC) and; (5) enteroaggregative *E. coli* (EAggEC). Each of these categories of diarrheagenic *E. coli* has a different pathogenesis, possesses distinct virulence properties, comprises a separate set of O:H serotypes, usually manifests a characteristic clinical syndrome, and exhibits a particular epidemiologic pattern.

HISTORY. EPEC were the first *E. coli* to be recognized as agents of diarrheal illness in humans. They were incriminated initially in the 1940s as an important cause of sporadic diarrhea in young infants in the community and as a cause of outbreaks of diarrhea in hospital nurseries in both industrialized and less-developed countries.

ETEC were first associated with cholera-like severe watery diarrhea in adults in the Indian subcontinent in the late 1960s. Later they were shown to be an important cause of diarrheal dehydration in infants in less-developed countries and to be the single most frequent etiologic agent of travelers' diarrhea.

EIEC have been known since 1970 to cause diarrhea and dysentery. EHEC have been recognized only since 1982 when they came to prominence as a cause of a multistate outbreak in the U.S.A.. Lastly, EAggEC, first described in 1987, were originally referred to by the cumbersome term enteroadherent-aggregative *E. coli;* this was subsequently shortened to enteroaggregative *E. coli.*

BACTERIOLOGY. *E. coli* can be defined serologically on the basis of their O (lipopolysaccharide antigen)

serogroup and H (flagellar) antigen type. More than 171 distinct O serogroups are currently recognized, and there are at least 70 H types. In addition, many *E. coli* also express polysaccharide capsular (K) antigens. Determination of the O:H serotype of *E. coli* has played an important role in understanding both the pathogenesis and the epidemiology of *E. coli* diarrhea. Each of the 5 categories of diarrheagenic *E. coli* falls into a relatively restricted set of O:H serotypes distinct for that category.

With diarrheagenic *E. coli*, critical virulence properties, peculiar to that category, are coded by genes located on plasmids. This phenomenon has been utilized to advantage in the preparation of diagnostic reagents. DNA sequences from the various virulence plasmids have been successfully employed as sensitive and specific gene probes to identify isolates as belonging to these categories of *E. coli*.

ETEC. ETEC elaborate a heat-labile (LT) and/or a heat-stable (ST) enterotoxin. The former closely resembles cholera toxin in amino acid sequence, structure, and pharmacological mode of action, whereas, the latter is a small polypeptide with a different mode of action. ETEC from diverse geographic areas fall within a limited number of O:H serotypes. Whereas many other serotypes can be toxigenic also, the recurrent O:H serotypes appear to be successful ETEC clones that have spread far and wide. Usually these serotypes elaborate both LT and ST and possess fimbrial colonization factors. The most common O serogroups of ETEC include 06, 08, 015, 020, 025, 027, 063, 078, 080, 085, 0114, 0115, 0128ac, 0148, 0153, 0159, and 0167.

EIEC. This category of diarrheagenic *E. coli* closely resembles *Shigella*: like *Shigella* they possess a 140 mD enteroinvasiveness plasmid that is necessary for the bacteria to invade epithelial cells; they cause clinical dysentery; the O antigens of EIEC show cross-reactions with *Shigella* O antigens. The main O serogroups in which EIEC fall include 028ac, 029, 0112, 0124, 0136, 0143, 0144, 0152, 0164, and 0167. Many EIEC also resemble *Shigella* by their inability to ferment lactose.

EPEC. The major EPEC O serogroups include 055, 086, 0111, 0119, 0125, 0126, 0127, 0128ab, and 0142. Virulence properties of EPEC are coded by both plasmid and chromosomal genes. The EPEC Adherence Factor (EAF) plasmid is necessary for EPEC to attach to epithelial cells. EPEC strains attach to HEp-2 cells in tissue culture by a characteristic pattern, so-called localized adherence, that gives the appearance of microcolonies; this attachment requires the presence of the EAF plasmid. Chromosomal genes code for the ability to cause effacement of microvilli of enterocytes, another characteristic of EPEC.

EHEC. In 1982 a multistate epidemic of hemorrhagic colitis that occurred in the U.S.A. was shown to be due to serotype 0157:H7. Whereas the main EHEC serotype is 0157:H7, other serotypes fall into this category also, e.g., 026:H11 and 0111:H8. EHEC strains can also cause the hemolytic-uremic syndrome. EHEC elaborate potent cytotoxins called Shiga-like toxins I and II (because of their close resemblance to Shiga toxin of *S. dysenteriae* 1); these are also called Vero toxins I and II.

Elaboration of these toxins is dependent upon the presence of certain phages carried by the bacteria. In addition, EHEC strains have a plasmid that codes for fimbriae involved in attachment of the bacteria to intestinal mucosa.

EAggEC. These *E. coli* manifest a characteristic aggregative pattern of adherence to HEp-2 cells in tissue culture. The presence of the characteristic plasmid of EAggEC is necessary for the aggregative phenomenon, the expression of novel fimbriae, and the elaboration (at least in some strains) of O antigen. The EAggEC O:H serotypes are being identified slowly. 03, 015, 073, 077, and 089 are common, and H33 and H2 are common H types encountered. Many EAggEC O antigens appear to be new and have not been given official O group numbers yet.

DISTRIBUTION AND INCIDENCE

ETEC. This is an infection of developing countries. During the first 3 years of life, young children in these areas experience multiple ETEC infections. ETEC infection in young children in less-developed countries, even when clinically mild, has been shown to be associated with adverse nutritional consequences. After rotavirus, ETEC is the second most common cause of diarrheal dehydration in infants in the Indian subcontinent. ETEC also readily infect travelers from industrialized countries who visit less-developed countries. In various studies of travelers' diarrhea, ETEC have accounted for 25 to 75% of cases.

EIEC. These infections are endemic in less-developed countries. However, studies of pediatric diarrhea in several developing countries have shown that EIEC are not common pathogens, usually accounting for less than 5% of diarrheal infections overall. Occasional infections and outbreaks of EIEC diarrhea in industrialized countries have been reported.

EPEC. Clinical infections due to EPEC are almost entirely limited to the first 6 months of life. Since the late 1960s, EPEC have largely disappeared as an important cause of infant diarrhea in North America and Europe. However, EPEC remains a major agent of infant diarrhea in many developing areas, including South America, Southern Africa, and Asia. Some studies of infant diarrhea in South America have shown EPEC to be the most common bacterial diarrheal pathogen. In less-developed countries, outbreaks of EPEC in infant nurseries and among hospitalized infants are still common.

EHEC. Since 1982, EHEC, in particular serotypes 0157:H7 and 026:H11, have emerged as enteric pathogens of public health importance in the United States, Canada, Europe, and the cone of South America, with multiple reports of outbreaks of hemorrhagic colitis, hemolytic-uremic syndrome, and diarrhea in nursing homes, day care centers, schools, and the community. Little is known of the epidemiology of EHEC in less-developed countries.

EAggEC. EAggEC appear to be an important cause of infant diarrhea in some parts of the world, including Latin America and India. In the Indian subcontinent they are the most common cause of persistent diarrhea in infants.

TRANSMISSION AND EPIDEMIOLOGY

ETEC. ETEC infections are largely species-specific. Thus, infected humans comprise the reservoir for ETEC strains that cause diarrhea. ETEC are transmitted by contaminated food and less often by contaminated water. Transmission via contaminated weaning foods may be particularly important in leading to infection in infants. Direct contact transmission by means of fecally-contaminated hands is believed to be rare.

EIEC. Infected persons are believed to comprise the reservoir for EIEC. Available evidence suggests that EIEC are transmitted by contaminated food.

EPEC. Infected individuals represent the reservoir for EPEC infection. Transmission of EPEC occurs by contaminated infant formula and weaning foods. Epidemiologic studies in infant nurseries in the 1950s showed that transmission by fomites and by contaminated hands can occur.

EHEC. Both calves and humans can develop hemorrhagic colitis due to EHEC. Cattle are believed to be the reservoir of EHEC. Infected persons may serve also as a reservoir for transmission within custodial institutions. Transmission occurs by means of contaminated food, most often poorly-cooked beef. Sustained outbreaks in custodial institutions have been observed suggesting that nosocomial transmission by direct contact may occur in high-risk populations.

EAggEC. The reservoir of these diarrheal pathogens has not been elucidated yet, nor is much known about the modes of transmission of this new category of diarrheagenic *E. coli.*

PATHOGENESIS AND PATHOLOGY

ETEC. For ETEC, the proximal small intestine is the critical site of host-parasite interaction. Here, they colonize by means of fimbrial colonization factors and elaborate LT or ST. LT, which closely resembles cholera toxin, activates the enzyme adenylate cyclase in enterocytes leading to an intracellular accumulation of cyclic adenosine monophosphate (cAMP). This results in diminished absorption by villus tip cells and overt secretion by crypt cells. ST is a small polypeptide that activates guanylate cyclase causing accumulation of cyclic guanosine monophosphate (cGMP); ST is not immunogenic in the course of natural infection.

ETEC possess attachment or colonization factors that allow them to overcome the peristaltic defense mechanism of the small intestine. Heretofore, all the characterized colonization factors have proven to be fimbriae, i.e., hair-like, filamentous protein organelles on the surface of the *E. coli* that are notably thinner than flagellae.

There is no morphological damage to the intestinal mucosa discernible by either light or electron microscope in ETEC infections. The sometimes copious diarrhea that occurs with ETEC infection in the absence of pathological changes to the intestine is due to the effects of LT and/or ST.

EIEC. EIEC have a predilection for colonic mucosa as the favored site of host parasite interaction. The large 140 mD plasmid found in EIEC codes for outer membrane proteins involved in the invasiveness process whereby EIEC gain entry to enterocytes. After invasion,

EIEC proliferate within colonocytes leading to cell death. EIEC infections are characterized by intense polymorphonuclear leukocyte infiltrations into the colonic mucosa. A simple stain of the fecal mucus reveals sheets of polymorphonuclear leukocytes.

EPEC. EPEC strains do not elaborate LT or ST nor do they exhibit the epithelial cell invasiveness of EIEC. Rather, they cause diarrhea by other mechanisms. EPEC have two major steps in their pathogenesis. The first involves a plasmid-mediated attachment to epithelial cells. This is followed by effacement of microvilli, a trait coded by chromosomal genes, which leads to a distinctive ultrastructural histopathological lesion in the intestine, typically without further invasion. Often bacteria are closely adherent to the membrane of the enterocyte with the membrane partially enveloping the bacterium.

The EAF plasmid is necessary for full expression of the pathogenicity of EPEC. The EAF plasmid is involved in the expression of a bacterial surface (outer membrane) protein that appears to be critical in the pathogenesis of EPEC diarrhea and perhaps in mediating protective immunity. This protein has been found in all the important EPEC serotypes, e.g., those in serogroups 055, 0111, 0119, 0127, and 0142, but not in ETEC, EIEC, and pyelonephritis-associated or meningitis-associated strains of *E. coli.*

EHEC. 0157:H7, 026:H11, and other EHEC strains from persons with hemorrhagic colitis and the hemolytic-uremic syndrome elaborate phage-encoded potent cytotoxins active on HeLa and Vero cells. One of these toxins, so-called Shiga-like toxin I (SLTI) or Verotoxin 1 (VT1), is identical apparently to the potent cytotoxin/neurotoxin/enterotoxin produced by *S. dysenteriae* 1 (Shiga toxin) and is neutralized by Shiga antitoxin. Many strains elaborate also a second potent cytotoxin (Shiga-like toxin II or Verotoxin 2) that is not neutralized by Shiga antitoxin. In addition, 0157:H7 and other EHEC strains possess a plasmid that plays a role in virulence by encoding the production of a newly-recognized variety of fimbriae that apparently mediates attachment to gut-derived epithelial cells in tissue culture.

Several animal models have been developed that demonstrate the pathologic features of EHEC infection. In electron photomicrographs, attached and effaced enterocytes are evident with effacement of the microvilli, a lesion resembling that due to classic serotype enteropathogenic *E. coli* (EPEC). Nevertheless, in gnotobiotic piglets, the two types of infection, EHEC versus EPEC, can be clearly differentiated by anatomic site of involvement, severity of lesions, and degree of polymorphonuclear cell infiltration. EPEC involve the entire intestine of piglets, EHEC only the cecum and colon. EPEC lesions are generally less severe; some infiltration by leukocytes is seen with EPEC (but not with EHEC) infection.

EAggEC. The newest category of diarrheagenic *E. coli* are strains that show a characteristic "aggregative" pattern of adherence to HEp-2 cells. In this pattern, the bacteria form aggregates that give a "stacked brick" appearance. Studies of EAggEC infection of piglets reveal the same stacked brick aggregative pattern of the bacteria in vivo as they attach to enterocytes. EAggEC do not elaborate LT or ST, do not manifest *Shigella*-like invasiveness, do not cause the histopathological lesion of EPEC, and are negative with the EHEC, EPEC, EIEC, and ETEC DNA probes. EAggEC cause a distinct histopathological lesion of the intestine discernible by light microscopy. In its most severe manifestation, this lesion is marked by damage to enterocytes on the tips and sides of the blunted villi leaving a hemorrhagic core.

CLINICAL MANIFESTATIONS AND COMPLICATIONS

ETEC. Incubations as short as 10 to 12 hours have been observed in outbreaks and in volunteer studies with certain LT-only and ST-only strains. The incubation of LT/ST diarrhea in volunteer studies has usually been 24 to 72 hours. The clinical features of ETEC infection are watery diarrhea, nausea, abdominal cramps, and low-grade fever. Occasionally, particularly with strains that are prevalent in the Indian subcontinent, severe cholera-like purging can occur.

EIEC. Incubations as short as 10 and 18 hours have been observed in volunteer studies and in outbreaks, respectively. Clinically, the illness is marked by fever, severe abdominal cramps, malaise, toxemia, and watery diarrhea followed by gross dysentery consisting of scanty stools of blood and mucus. More severe forms of clinical illness due to EIEC are clinically indistinguishable from bacillary dysentery due to *Shigella*.

EPEC. Often, incubation periods in volunteer studies have been as short as 9 to 12 hours. It is not known whether the same incubation applies to infants who acquire infection by natural transmission. Diarrheal disease due to this category is virtually confined to infants less than 6 months of age where it causes watery diarrhea with mucus, fever, and dehydration. EPEC diarrhea in infants can be quite severe and may be associated with high-case fatality.

EHEC. An outbreak of hemorrhagic colitis in the United States drew attention to an unusual clinical syndrome of diarrheal disease and a new bacterial enteric pathogen; the causative organism, *Escherichia coli* 0157:H7, was a serotype not recognized previously as a cause of diarrheal disease in humans. The clinical syndrome was notable because bloody but copious diarrhea, unaccompanied by fecal leukocytes, was seen in afebrile patients; these features distinguish it from classic dysentery due to *Shigella* or enteroinvasive *Escherichia coli* (EIEC), which is characterized by fever and scanty stools of blood and mucus containing many fecal leukocytes. The incubation period of EHEC illness is estimated to range from 12 to 60 hours with a median of 48 hours.

EAggEC. The incubation of diarrhea due to these pathogens is estimated to be 20 to 48 hours. The most common syndromes associated with EAggEC are acute and persistent diarrhea. Bloody stools occur in approximately 15% of EAggEC infections.

DIAGNOSIS

Laboratory Identification. Specialized bacteriological methods must be utilized to identify the different categories of diarrheagenic *E. coli*, because they will not be detected by routine stool cultures. ETEC can be identified by demonstrating toxin production of the strains by immunoassays or bioassays or by DNA probe techniques that identify LT and ST genes in colony blots. EIEC can be confirmed by an immunoassay that detects specific outer membrane proteins associated with epithelial cell invasiveness, a bioassay (the guinea pig keratoconjunctivitis test), or DNA probes that detect the enteroinvasiveness plasmid. EPEC can be identified by agglutination with antisera that detect EPEC O serogroups, by demonstrating localized adherence to HEp-2 cells, or by the EPEC adherence factor (EAF) DNA probe; there is a 99% correlation between the detection of localized adherence and EAF probe positivity. EHEC can be diagnosed by demonstrating the presence of Shiga-like toxins, by serotyping (e.g., identifying 0157:H7 or 026:H11), or by DNA probes that identify the toxin genes or the presence of the EHEC plasmid. The most available method to identify EAggEC is by the HEp-2 assay, wherein these strains cause a characteristic aggregative pattern as they attach to one another and to the HEp-2 cells. A DNA probe to identify EAggEC has also been described recently.

TREATMENT AND PROGNOSIS

Nonspecific Therapy. As with all forms of diarrheal illness, particularly in infants and young children, oral rehydration should be instituted promptly to prevent significant dehydration. Other nonspecific interventions, such as antimotility agents, are not indicated and with some forms of *E. coli* diarrhea (e.g., EIEC or EHEC) may possibly cause harm.

Specific Antibiotic Therapy. For travelers' diarrhea where ETEC infection is likely, it is recommended that prompt antimicrobial therapy be initiated with trimethoprim/sulfamethoxazole (twice daily for 5 days). For adult travelers, ciprofloxacin (750 mg twice daily for 5 days) serves as an alternative that is active against *Shigella* as well. In contrast, suspected ETEC infection in indigenous persons in endemic areas should not be treated routinely with antibiotics, because the background immunity tends to make most cases short-lived, prompt oral rehydration suffices in most cases, and unnecessary use of antibiotics drives up health care costs and encourages resistance.

Clinical bacillary dysentery, which may be caused by EIEC, *Shigella*, or *Campylobacter*, should be treated with the combination of trimethoprim/sulfamethoxazole and erythromycin. The new generation quinoline antibiotics, such as ciprofloxacin, also appear promising, at least for use in adults.

Known or suspected EPEC diarrheal infections in young infants that are clinically severe or persistent should be treated with a course of trimethoprim/sulfamethoxazole, which has been shown to significantly ameliorate the severity of clinical illness in controlled studies in Ethiopian infants.

There are no published results of controlled studies yet available to suggest whether antibiotic therapy favorably influences the course of EHEC or EAggEC infections. Controlled studies investigating the effect of antibiotics on persistent diarrhea due to EAggEC are in progress.

PREVENTION AND CONTROL

Period of Transmissibility. This is believed to be limited to the duration of excretion of the pathogenic *E. coli*. Excretion due to ETEC, EPEC, and EAggEC may be prolonged, whereas that due to EHEC is notably short.

Control Measures. Vaccines are not yet available against any of the categories of diarrheagenic *E. coli*, although much research is ongoing to develop a vaccine against ETEC; some candidate vaccines have already entered clinical trials.

For travelers, attention to food hygiene and sources of water represent important preventive measures. This includes care to avoid eating uncooked vegetables, salads, condiments that have sat for long periods at ambient temperatures, and other unheated foods. In the prevention of infant diarrhea due to diarrheagenic *E. coli*, it has been shown repeatedly that the longer weaning foods are stored without refrigeration, the greater the degree of coliform contamination.

When an individual in a family or other cohabiting unit has diarrhea, presumably or confirmed to be due to diarrheagenic *E. coli*, it is important that handwashing be practiced after defecation or after changing the infant's diapers.

BIBLIOGRAPHY

Bhan MK, Raj P, Levine MM, et al.: Enteroaggregative *Escherichia coli* associated with persistent diarrhea in a cohort of rural children in India. J Infect Dis 158:70, 1989.

Black RE, Merson MH, Huq I, et al.: Incidence and severity of rotavirus and *Escherichia coli* diarrhoea in rural Bangladesh. Lancet 1:141, 1981.

Cleary TG, Lopez EL: The Shiga-like toxin-producing *Escherichia coli* and hemolytic uremic syndrome. Pediatr Infect Dis 8:720, 1989.

DiJohn D, Levine MM: Treatment of diarrhea. Infect Dis Clin N Am 2:719, 1988.

DuPont HL, Reves RR, Galindo E, et al.: Treatment of travelers' diarrhea with trimethoprim/sulfamethoxazole and with trimethoprim alone. N Engl J Med 307:841, 1982.

Levine MM: *Escherichia coli* that cause diarrhea: Enterotoxigenic, enteropathogenic, enteroinvasive, enterohemorrhagic, and enteroadherent. J Infect Dis 155:377, 1987.

Levine MM, Edelman R: Enteropathogenic *Escherichia coli* of classical serotypes associated with infant diarrhea—epidemiology and pathogenesis. Epidemiol Rev 6:31, 1984.

Levine MM, Prado V, Robins-Browne RM, et al.: DNA probes and HEp-2 cell adherence assay to detect diarrheagenic *E. coli*. J Infect Dis 158:224, 1988.

Merson MH, Morris GK, Sack DA, et al.: Travelers' diarrhea in Mexico: A prospective study of physicians and family members attending a congress. N Engl J Med 294:1299, 1976.

Nataro JP, Kaper JB, Robins-Browne R, et al.: Patterns of adherence of diarrheagenic *Escherichia coli* to HEp-2 cells. Pediatr Infect Dis 6:829, 1987.

Riley LW, Remis RS, Helgerson SD, et al.: Hemorrhagic colitis associated with a rare *Escherichia coli* serotype. N Engl J Med 308:681, 1983.

Taylor DN, Echeverria P, Sethabutr O, et al.: Clinical and microbiologic features of *Shigella* and enteroinvasive *Escherichia coli* infections detected by DNA hybridization. J Clin Microbiol 26:1362, 1988.

Vial PA, Robins-Browne RM, Lior H: Characterization of enteroadherent-aggregative *Escherichia coli*, a putative agent of diarrheal disease. J Infect Dis 158:70, 1988.

41.2. CAMPYLOBACTER ENTERITIS

Thomas Butler

DEFINITION. *Campylobacter* enteritis is one of the most common causes of acute bacterial diarrhea throughout the world affecting mostly children in tropical countries, adult travelers to tropical countries, and adults and children in food-borne outbreaks in developed countries. It is caused by *Campylobacter jejuni* and less often by *C. coli*, thermophilic gram-negative bacilli that have their natural reservoirs in the intestinal tracts of chickens, cattle, and domestic animals. Transmission of the infection to humans occurs through ingestion of contaminated chicken, other meats, milk, or by direct contact with animal feces. The disease is characterized by acute watery diarrhea or dysentery, fever, and abdominal pain that is usually self-limited over a few days.

ETIOLOGY. Previously classified as *Vibrio fetus* and "related vibrios," *Campylobacter* came to be recognized as a separate bacterial genus in the 1960s. The 2 species of human enteric pathogens are *C. jejuni* and *C. coli*, whereas *C. fetus* (previously *V. fetus*) is an opportunistic pathogen of immunocompromised patients and can be cultured from the blood. The importance of *Campylobacter* as a human pathogen was missed until the 1970s, because it does not grow on routine bacteriological media for stool pathogens. The development of Butzler's and Skirrow's selective media took advantage of the natural antibiotic resistance and the microaerophilic and thermophilic (42C) characteristics of *Campylobacter* to obtain its growth among the multitude of normal enteric flora.

Campylobacter species are gram-negative rods about 1.5 to 3.5 μm in length and 0.2 to 0.4 μm in width that have varied morphologies on gram stain, including curved or comma-shaped rods, spirals, and "sea gull" forms. One or more flagella impart a darting rapid motility easily observable when liquid stool is viewed by phase contrast or dark field microscopy. The organisms grow selectively well on tryptic soy agar supplemented with sheep blood and containing bacitracin, novobiocin, cycloheximide, colistin, and cefazolin. The plates are incubated at 42C for 1 to 2 days under microaerophilic conditions, such as in a candle jar containing 5 to 10% oxygen and 3 to 10% carbon dioxide. Colonies are confirmed as *Campylobacter* by showing positive results in oxidase and catalase tests, sensitivity to nalidixic acid, and resistance to cephalothin. *C. jejuni* is distinguished from *C. coli* by its ability to hydrolyze hippurate. The more important enteric pathogen is *C. jejuni*, but many diagnostic laboratories do not distinguish between the species in routine work.

Two different serotyping schemes are used to distinguish among strains of *Campylobacter*. Twenty-one Lior serotypes based on the heat-labile flagellar proteins have been described, and a scheme based on heat-stable or Penner serotypes has identified 23 different serotypes.

EPIDEMIOLOGY. Among children less than 5 years old living in tropical and developing countries of Central and South America, Africa, and Asia, *Campylobacter* enteritis ranks with rotavirus, enterotoxigenic *E. coli*, and shigellosis as a leading cause of acute diarrhea. Recent surveys of childhood diarrhea in the tropics showed that *Campylobacter* was isolated from the stool cultures of 8 to 23% of cases with the highest rate of infection (25%) reported in infants with diarrhea in Bangladesh. Older children and adults are infected less frequently because of immunity acquired in early childhood. Children without diarrhea in tropical countries frequently show asymptomatic infection. Infections caused by *C. coli* are more likely to be asymptomatic than ones caused by *C. jejuni*. The ratio of cases of diarrhea to all persons infected with *Campylobacter* is highest in infancy and declines with increasing age. This case-to-infection ratio was 50% in Mexican children 1 to 6 months old and declined thereafter. The peak infection rate in Mexican children was 3.5 episodes per year in the age group 12 to 17 months. The reinfections are due to different serotypes of *Campylobacter*. These high rates of infection in infancy in developing countries result in acquisition of anti*Campylobacter* serum antibodies, which were shown in Thailand to reach a peak in children less than 2 years old. Symptomatic infections in Mexican children were shown to confer protective immunity, whereas asymptomatic infections did not result in protective immunity. The most prevalent Lior serotypes in Thai children are 4, 28, and 36.

In contrast to the hyperendemic situation in the tropics, *Campylobacter* infections in developed countries are less frequent, are rarely asymptomatic, and affect adults more often. Outbreaks are identified sometimes, affecting both children and adults, and may be traced to contaminated sources of chicken, raw milk, raw hamburger meat, or raw clams. *Campylobacter* is a common cause of diarrhea in travelers from developed countries who return from the tropics. Among American college students this is the most frequent form of diarrheal illness. Among homosexual men in the United States, including some with AIDS, *Campylobacter* was recovered from 20% of diarrheal cases. The most prevalent Lior serotypes in American students were 1,4,9, and 33, and the most prevalent Penner serotypes were 1,2,4, and 5.

Campylobacter enteritis occurs during all seasons without any variation by month in tropical countries. In developed countries, there may be an increased incidence of infection during summer months corresponding to the time of holiday travel, as was reported in Finland. Among college students in Georgia, the highest incidence of *Campylobacter* enteritis was in the spring.

The distribution of *C. jejuni* in nature indicates it is a zoonotic infection; humans are an accidental host. These bacteria inhabit the intestinal tracts of a variety of birds, including chickens, turkeys, and water fowl; farm animals, including pigs, cows, sheep, goats, and horses; domestic dogs and cats; and wild rodents and monkeys. These animals are infected frequently and do not usually show signs of illness. For example, in Peru, 61% of household chickens had infected feces.

Transmission of infection to humans occurs by ingestion of the organism. This occurs usually when food is contaminated, such as incompletely cooked chicken and other meats or unpasteurized milk. Direct contact with animal feces is probably important in tropical countries like Peru, where children are exposed to chicken droppings in and near their houses. Viable bacteria can survive in chicken droppings for about 4 days. Contact with cats and dogs is significant also, and water-borne outbreaks occur. Secondary spread of infection from person-to-person has not been documented, although household contacts of cases have higher rates of infection than persons living in houses without cases of infection. This increased rate of infection in household contacts is attributable to common sources of exposure to contaminated foods or animals. In developing countries, the highest rates of infection occur in homes of persons of low socioeconomic status living under unsanitary conditions, often with dirt floors and without running water. Food handlers who are asymptomatic excretors of *C. jejuni* are not a significant source of infection for the community.

PATHOGENESIS. To initiate infection, organisms must be ingested. The infective dose is estimated to vary from 500 to 10^6 bacteria. Volunteers who ingested inocula of these sizes became ill. *C. jejuni* is killed by acid at about pH 2.3, indicating that gastric acid is an effective barrier against infection and that ingestion of organisms with milk or other food that neutralizes acid may enhance infection by reducing the required inoculum. The incubation period varies from 1 to 7 days and is usually 2 to 4 days. During the incubation period, illness, and convalescence, *C. jejuni* multiplies in the intestine and is excreted in feces in quantities of 10^6-10^9 organisms/gm of stool. The duration of fecal excretion varies from about 8 days in children 1 to 5 years old to 14 days in infants and up to 3 months in adults not treated with antibiotics.

After *C. jejuni* have traversed the stomach, they adhere to the intestinal epithelial cells. Some of the bacteria invade epithelial cells leading to ulcerated mucosa and bloody diarrhea. The regions of the intestine most affected are the jejunum, terminal ileum, and colon. Biopsies of infected intestines show inflammatory infiltrates in the lamina propria, crypt abscesses, and mucosal ulceration. Bacteria gain access to the blood stream, but bacteremia is uncommon because most strains of *C. jejuni* are susceptible to the bacteriolytic action of serum complement. Watery diarrhea during infection may be attributed to the action of an enterotoxin, which is a heat-labile protein with a molecular weight of about 60,000 that is produced by some strains of *C. jejuni*. This enterotoxin resembles cholera toxin and the heat-labile enterotoxin of *E. coli* in its activation with the enzyme adenylate cyclase. *C. jejuni* produces a cytotoxin also, which might play a role in epithelial cell destruction in the ulcerated mucosa. Bloody diarrhea is more likely to be caused by *C. jejuni* than *C. coli*.

CLINICAL FEATURES. The 3 consistent clinical features of *Campylobacter* enteritis are fever, diarrhea, and abdominal pain. The diarrhea may be either watery or dysenteric with the presence of blood or mucus in liquid stool. In developing countries most children present with watery diarrhea rather than dysentery, whereas a larger portion of patients in developed countries report dysenteric disease. Fever, nausea, vomiting, and malaise may precede the onset of diarrhea by a day or more, and such nonspecific constitutional symptoms may be more severe than the diarrhea itself. The disease is usually self-limited and lasts 1 to 7 days. Severity of disease varies widely with stool frequency from once to more than 8 times a day. Most cases are mild, but about 20% of cases will have prolonged severe disease with high fever, grossly bloody stools, and relapses. The abdominal pain may be severe and, because it is sometimes localized to the right lower quadrant, patients with this infection have been subjected to laparotomy for suspected appendicitis. Cases of toxic megacolon, pseudomembranous colitis, and massive rectal bleeding have been reported. In homosexual males, *Campylobacter* infection is associated with diarrhea more often than with proctitis.

Although fatalities are rare from this illness, children in tropical countries with severe diarrheal syndromes commonly die. In Bangladesh, *Campylobacter* was the fourth most common cause of diarrhea in children who died, and most of these children showed severe colitis and the complicating conditions of pneumonia, septicemias with other organisms, and malnutrition. Less common complications reported in patients with *Campylobacter* enteritis include hypoglycemia, pancreatitis, peritonitis, and cholecystitis. A reactive arthritis may develop in patients who have the HLA-B27 haplotype.

Usually examination of stool reveals fecal leukocytes and sometimes red blood cells. Often, a Gram stain of stool shows bacterial forms, including spiral or "seagull" shapes, suggestive of *Campylobacter* morphology. The white blood cell count is normal or elevated slightly and may show an increased percentage of band forms. The erythrocyte sedimentation rate and C-reactive protein concentration are elevated as reflections of acute intestinal inflammation.

DIAGNOSIS. The diagnosis of *Campylobacter* enteritis requires isolation of the bacterium from stool cultures. This requires selective media, such as Campy-BAP, incubation at 42C, and a microaerophilic environment, such as a candle jar or Gas-pak. Identification follows standard bacteriological techniques. Fresh stool should be examined for the presence of leukocytes and to exclude the possible presence of trophozoites of *Entamoeba histolytica*. As the differential diagnosis includes other enteric pathogens, stool should be cultured also for species of *Salmonella, Shigella, Vibrio,* and *Yersinia* and, when diagnostic facilities are available, for enterotoxigenic *E. coli* and rotavirus. Examination of diarrheal stools for other pathogens in the tropics is important, because it was shown in Bangladesh that most patients with *Campylobacter* infections were infected with other diarrheal pathogens also.

Endoscopy is not advised routinely; however, when inflammatory bowel disease is considered in the differential diagnosis, colonoscopy with biopsy may be performed. The colonic mucosa will show erythema, superficial ulcerations, and friability, and the biopsy will reveal characteristically acute inflammation and crypt abscesses.

TREATMENT. As in other diarrheal diseases, the most important therapeutic approach is rehydration, which can be carried out with either isotonic intravenous fluids or oral rehydration solutions (Section III D, General Principles). Severe dehydration due to this disease is infrequent. Use of antibiotics in *Campylobacter* infection is controversial. Clinical trials comparing erythromycin with a placebo did not show significant differences in clinical responses in this self-limited disease. Stool cultures will be rendered negative for *Campylobacter* earlier in antibiotic-treated patients, but this does not prevent spread of infection to other persons. Therefore, the majority of patients should not be treated with antibiotics. In patients with severe bloody diarrhea, however, treatment with erythromycin should be considered. Most strains of *C. jejuni* are susceptible to erythromycin, tetracyclines, aminoglycosides, clindamycin, chloramphenicol, and quinolones, including nalidixic acid, norfloxacin, ciprofloxacin, and ofloxacin. Plasmids mediating resistance to tetracycline, kanamycin, and chloramphenicol in *C. jejuni* have been reported. Beta-lactamase production occurs in about 15% of strains, and ampicillin should not be used to treat patients. Erythromycin resistance, rare in *C. jejuni*, is more common in *C. coli* and is mediated chromosomally.

PREVENTION AND CONTROL. Reducing the hyperendemic transmission of *Campylobacter* infection in developing countries requires improvements in basic hygiene and living conditions of the people. Because children acquire infection in infancy and early childhood by ingesting contaminated food and by direct contact with animals, household methods of food preparation must be improved, and animals, especially chickens, must be kept away from people's homes. Handwashing before meals is a good preventive measure against most enteric infections.

In developed countries, transmission of *Campylobacter* infection could be reduced by cooking meats thoroughly and avoiding contamination of other foods by the juices of uncooked meats. Travelers to tropical countries should take the usual precautions to avoid most uncooked foods and to ensure that their cooked food is served fresh and thoroughly cooked.

BIBLIOGRAPHY

Abimiku AG, Dolby JM: Cross-protection of infant mice against intestinal colonisation by *Campylobacter jejuni*: Importance of heat-labile serotyping (Lior) antigens. J Med Microbiol 26:265, 1988.

Billingham JD: Campylobacter enteritis in the Gambia. Trans R Soc Trop Med Hyg 75:641, 1981.

Blaser MJ, Reller LB: Campylobacter enteritis. N Engl J Med 305:1444, 1981.

Butler T, Islam M, Azad AK, et al.: Causes of death in diarrhoeal diseases after rehydration therapy: An autopsy study of 140 patients in Bangladesh. Bull WHO 65:317, 1987.

Calva JJ, Ruiz-Palacios GM, Lopez-Vidal AB, et al.: Cohort study of intestinal infection with *Campylobacter* in Mexican children. Lancet 1:503, 1988.

Deming MS, Tauxe RV, Blake PA, et al.: *Campylobacter* enteritis at a university: Transmission from eating chicken and from cats. Am J Epidemiol 126:526, 1987.

Duffy MC, Benson JB, Rubin SJ: Mucosal invasion in *Campylobacter* enteritis. Am J Clin Pathol 73:706, 1980.

Glass RI, Stoll BJ, Huq MI, et al.: Epidemiologic and clinical features of endemic *Campylobacter jejuni* infection in Bangladesh. J Infect Dis 148:292, 1983.

Grados O, Bravo N, Black RE, et al.: Pediatric campylobacter diarrhoea from household exposure to live chickens in Lima, Peru. Bull WHO 66:369, 1988.

Ho DD, Ault MJ, Ault MA, et al.: *Campylobacter* enteritis. Early diagnosis with Gram's stain. Arch Intern Med 142:1858, 1982.

Laughon BE, Vernon AA, Druckman DA, et al.: Recovery of *Campylobacter* species from homosexual men. J Infect Dis 158:464, 1988.

Pitkanen T, Ponka A, Pettersson T, et al.: *Campylobacter* enteritis in 188 hospitalized patients. Arch Intern Med 143:215, 1983.

Taylor DE, Courvalin P: Mechanisms of antibiotic resistance in *Campylobacter* species. Antimicrob Agents Chemother 32:1107, 1988.

Taylor DN, Echeverria P, Pitarangsi C, et al.: Influence of strain characteristics and immunity on the epidemiology of *Campylobacter* infections in Thailand. J Clin Microbiol 26:863, 1988.

Walker RI, Caldwell MB, Lee EC, et al.: Pathophysiology of *Campylobacter* enteritis. Microbiol Rev 50:81, 1986.

41.3. *YERSINIA ENTEROCOLITICA* INFECTIONS

Thomas Butler

DEFINITION. *Yersinia enterocolitica* is a gram-negative rod bacterium that is a newly recognized enteric pathogen. It produces diarrhea and fever and can cause severe abdominal pain that mimics acute appendicits. Common pathologic lesions are acute enteritis and mesenteric lymphadenitis. *Y. enterocolitica* has its natural reservoir in the intestines of pigs, goats, dogs, and other animals. Humans become infected by ingesting contaminated particles, food, or water.

ETIOLOGY. *Y. enterocolitica* is a member of the bacterial order Enterobacteriaceae. Accordingly, it is a gram-negative rod, is oxidase negative, and grows on agars containing bile salts. It does not ferment lactose and grows faster at 25C than at 37C. Out of the 34 different O serotypes that have been identified, the only ones that are commonly associated with human disease are types 3 and 9 (in Canada and Europe) and type 8 (in the United States). Like other gram-negative bacteria, *Y. enterocolitica* contains a lipopolysaccharide endotoxin in its cell wall that may be responsible, in part, for the fever and inflammation in this disease. Virulence depends on a plasmid that encodes V and W antigens and makes the bacterium dependent on calcium for growth at 37C. This bacterium has been shown to elaborate an enterotoxin that is also plasmid-mediated, resembles the heat-stable enterotoxin of *E. coli*, and may cause the diarrhea associated with this infection.

EPIDEMIOLOGY. Infection caused by *Y. enterocolitica* is distributed worldwide. Large numbers of confirmed cases have been reported in Europe, Canada, the United States, and Japan. This infection has been reported also from Africa and Asia, but it appears to be an infrequent cause of tropical diarrhea. In the United States, infection with *Y. enterocolitica* appears to be rare when compared to infection with *Salmonella* and *Shigella* species, but in European countries, such as Finland, Sweden, and the Netherlands, the incidence of infection is higher. Adults and children are both susceptible to infection. Males acquire the infection more commonly than females. The natural reservoirs of infection are farm animals, especially pigs and goats, and other domestic animals, including dogs and cats. These animals harbor the bacteria in their intestines and excrete them in feces. Humans become infected by ingesting food or water contaminated by animal feces or directly by the ingestion of fomites. In Europe, ingestion of uncooked pork is associated with infection. Person-to-person transmission seems to be rare. Outbreaks in the United States have occurred in a family with a sick dog, in a school at which chocolate milk was discovered to be the source of infection, and following ingestion of milk that got contaminated at a dairy after pasteurization. There are no clear seasonal patterns of infection.

PATHOGENESIS OF CLINICAL SYNDROMES. An inoculum as high as 10^9 organisms may be required to produce infection. During the incubation period, estimated at 4 to 10 days, bacteria proliferate in the small bowel; invade the mucosa, especially that of the ileum; and elicit an acute inflammatory response. Ulcerations may occur and polymorphonuclear leukocytes appear in the stool. Some bacteria migrate via the lymphatics to the mesenteric lymph nodes, where inflammation occurs. The initial symptoms will include fever and either diarrhea or abdominal pain. In these instances, the corresponding pathologic finding is terminal ileitis and/or mesenteric lymphadenitis. The tissues are affected by acute inflammation, thrombosis of blood vessels, hemorrhage, and necrosis. The diarrhea results from either the mucosal invasion by bacteria or the action of an enterotoxin molecule. Diarrhea varies from being semisolid or watery to grossly bloody. In some patients the abdominal pain is severe and located in the right lower quadrant and may be mistaken for appendicitis; the appendix is usually normal. A few days later, some patients may develop extraintestinal complications of arthralgias, arthritis, and erythema nodosum. As the synovial and cutaneous tissues in these syndromes are sterile, an immunologic reaction has been postulated to explain their pathogenesis. Individuals with HLA-B27 haplotype are more susceptible to arthritis, Reiter's syndrome, and ankylosing spondylitis. Septicemia is a rarer complication that occurs in the setting of prior liver disease, malignancies, immunosuppressive therapy, hemolytic diseases such as thalassemias, and in hemochromotosis, especially when iron chelator therapy is given. Antibodies appear in the blood against the O antigen and other antigens of *Y. enterocolitica*, and nearly all infections are self-limited. Rare fatal cases have occurred, with extensive ulceration and necrosis of the intestine and septicemia.

DIAGNOSIS. The diagnosis requires the isolation of *Y. enterocolitica* from stool, blood, or surgical specimens. The number of bacteria in stool may be small, and a cold-enrichment technique may be required. A rectal swab or piece of stool is placed into 0.067 M phosphate-buffered saline at a pH of 7.6 and incubated at 4C for 4 weeks. Most other stool bacteria die, whereas *Y. enterocolitica* will grow. At weekly intervals, subcultures should be made onto MacConkey agar. Identification is made by finding nonlactose-fermenting colonies that on triple-sugar-iron agar give an acid/acid reaction without gas or hydrogen sulfide and are positive for urease. A serologic diagnosis can be made by showing a rise in agglutinin titer in paired serum specimens. The existence of cross-reacting antigens in the genera *Brucella, Vibrio,* and *Salmonella* indicates that false-positive serologic results sometimes occur.

TREATMENT AND PROGNOSIS. Infection with *Y. enterocolitica* is usually self-limited and so rarely diagnosed that it is impossible to assess the benefits of antibiotic treatment. Most isolates are susceptible to streptomycin, gentamicin, tetracycline, chloramphenicol, and trimethoprim-sulfamethoxazole and resistant to the penicillins and cephalosporin antibiotics. It is important to suspect the diagnosis in patients with severe abdominal pain to avoid unnecessary surgery for appendicitis. The recognition that early fever accompanies *Y. enterocolitica* infection may be helpful, as is epidemiologic information pertaining to outbreaks in the community.

PREVENTION AND CONTROL. The presumed origin of *Y. enterocolitica* infection in farm and domestic animals suggests that transmission may be similar to that of *Salmonella.* Meat products, dairy products, and other farm produce should periodically be examined for content of *Y. enterocolitica.* During outbreaks, public health authorities should identify sources of infection in food, water, or persons.

BIBLIOGRAPHY

Carniel E, Butler T, Hossain S, et al: Infrequent detection of *Yersinia enterocolitica* in childhood diarrhea in Bangladesh. Am J Trop Med Hyg 35:370, 1986.

Cornelis G, Laroche Y, Balligand G, et al: *Yersinia enterocolitica,* a primary model for bacterial invasiveness. Rev Infect Dis 9:64, 1987.

Marks MI, Pai CH, LaFleur L, et al.: *Yersinia enterocolitica* gastroenteritis: A prospective study of clinical, bacteriologic, and epidemiologic features. J Pediatr 96:26, 1980.

Prpic JK, Davey RB (eds.): The Genus *Yersinia*: Epidemiology, Molecular Biology and Pathogenesis. Karger, Basel, 1987.

Tauxe RV, Vandepitte J, Wauters G, et al.: *Yersinia enterocolitica* infections and pork: The missing link. Lancet 1:1129, 1987.

SECTION E

BACTERIAL MENINGITIS

42. MENINGOCOCCAL DISEASE

Brian M. Greenwood

DEFINITION. Meningococcal disease is the term used to describe the various clinical syndromes that may follow infection with *Neisseria meningitidis.* These include septicemia, meningitis, arthritis, pericarditis, conjunctivitis, pharyngitis, pneumonia, urethritis, and proctitis.

ETIOLOGY. Meningococcal disease is caused by a gram-negative, bean-shaped diplococcus. The meningococcus grows on standard blood agar plates but grows best on enriched media such as Mueller-Hinton agar. Growth is enhanced by an atmosphere of 5% CO_2, which can be achieved in a candle jar. The meningococcus does not ferment lactose, unlike the related organism *N. lactamica.* Meningococci are delicate organisms that are sensitive to freezing or overheating.

Differences in the antigenic structure of the meningococcal capsular polysaccharide define 8 major serogroups—groups A, B, C, X, Y, Z, 29e, and W135. Organisms that belong to group A, B, or C are responsible for most cases of clinical disease, but meningococcal pneumonia usually is caused by group Y meningococci. Group B and C meningococci cause most endemic cases of meningococcal disease in Europe and the United States, whereas most major epidemics of meningococcal infection, especially those that occur in tropical Africa, are caused by organisms belonging to serogroup A.

Meningococci also can be typed by their outer membrane proteins and lipopolysaccharides. Serotyping done in this way is useful in epidemiologic studies (e.g., in charting the spread of a new meningococcal strain). Meningococci can be differentiated further by electrophoresis of some of their enzymes or by electrophoresis of their DNA. Using a combination of outer membrane protein and isoenzyme typing, it has been shown that most epidemics of group A meningococcal disease are caused by bacteria that belong to a single clone. DNA fingerprinting is most useful in establishing that two meningococcal isolates, for example, those obtained from a patient and a family contact, are closely related bacteria.

Most meningococci are still sensitive to penicillin and chloramphenicol, but reports have been made from Europe, especially from Spain, of the isolation of meningococci from humans that have an increased resistance to penicillin. Many meningococci are resistant to sulfonamides, especially in tropical Africa, but there has been a fall in the level of sulfonamide resistance in recent years in some areas.

DISTRIBUTION AND INCIDENCE. The meningococcus is an ubiquitous organism that causes meningitis throughout the world. Outbreaks of meningococcal disease have been recorded in Alaska as well as in countries on the equator. In most tropical developing countries, the pneumococcus is a more important cause of meningitis than the meningococcus (Chapter 43). This situation is reversed in an area of sub-Saharan Africa—the African meningitis belt—where major epidemics of meningococcal disease have been recorded every 5 to 10 years since the beginning of the century. The meningitis belt, first defined by Lapeyssonnie, extends from

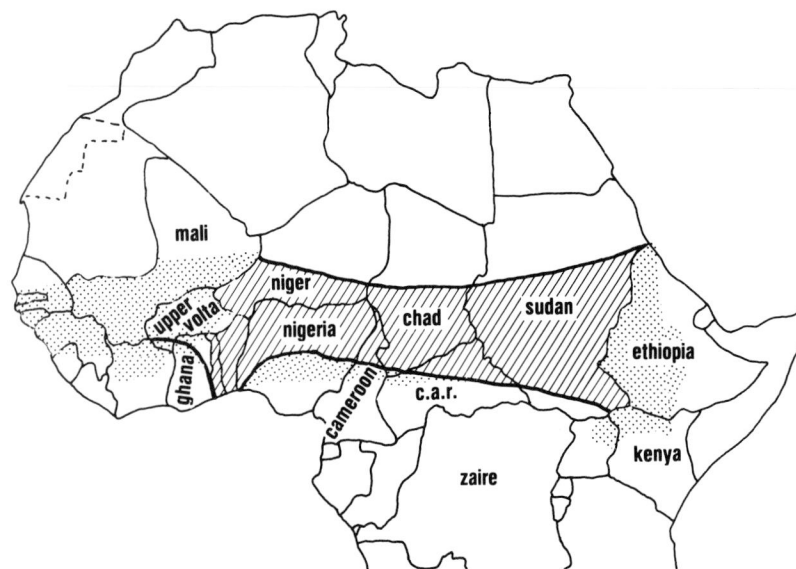

FIGURE 42–1. The African meningitis belt. The shaded area indicates the area of the belt as originally defined by Lapeyssonnie. Dotted areas indicate regions where outbreaks of meningococcal disease with epidemiologic features characteristic of the African meningitis belt have sometimes been recorded. (Adapted from Lapeyssonnie L: Bull WHO 28(Suppl 3):3, 1963.)

the Sudan in the east to Mali in the west (Fig. 42–1). To the north, it is bounded by the Sahara; it is limited to the south by the rain forests of West and Central Africa, where epidemics of meningococcal disease rarely occur. During major epidemics, outbreaks of meningococcal disease may extend as far west as Gambia, and seasonal outbreaks of meningococcal disease occur in Ethiopia. Outbreaks in Egypt and other parts of North Africa do not usually show the characteristic epidemiologic features of meningococcal disease in the northern African savanna. Major outbreaks of meningococcal infection have been recorded occasionally in many other parts of the tropics and subtropics (e.g., recent epidemics in Saudi Arabia and Nepal), but in no other area of the world have epidemics occurred with the frequency or the severity recorded in the northern savanna region of Africa.

Some 1 million cases of meningococcal disease have been reported to the health authorities of the countries of the African meningitis belt during the past 40 years; the true incidence of the infection is likely to be several times higher. During the 1950–1951 epidemic, 100,000 cases and 15,000 deaths were recorded in northern Nigeria alone. During a more recent outbreak in the same area, nearly 1000 cases of suspected meningococcal disease were seen at one general hospital during the course of a single day.

EPIDEMIOLOGY

Transmission. Meningococcal infection usually is transmitted from person to person by respiratory droplets, but occasional cases of sexual transmission have been recorded. Most infected subjects become asymptomatic nasopharyngeal carriers rather than cases of clinical disease. The ratio of clinical to subclinical infections varies from situation to situation; it is highest during epidemics, but it is rarely less than 1:100. Spread of meningococci is favored by overcrowding. The risk of infection is high in close contacts of a patient with clinical disease. In developed countries, most adults are immune to meningococcal infection as a result of immunization by an asymptomatic nasopharyngeal menin-

gococcal infection or as a result of infection with a related organism such as *N. lactamica.* In Europe and the United States, meningococcal infection is endemic. Cases occur sporadically over a wide area, sometimes with some local clustering, and there are only modest variations in the incidence of the infection from year to year. In such communities, most cases of meningococcal disease are seen in the young, although an increase has occurred in the incidence of meningococcal disease among teenagers in northern Europe.

African Meningitis Belt. Within the African meningitis belt, the epidemiology of meningococcal infection differs in a number of important respects from that observed in populations in which the infection is highly endemic (Table 42–1). Within the meningitis belt, epidemics of meningococcal infection occur every 5 to 10 years, each lasting for 2 or 3 dry seasons. Thus, in northern Nigeria, major outbreaks were recorded in 1949–1950, 1960–1962, 1970–1971, and 1977–1979. During these epidemics, most of the population probably was immunized by clinical or subclinical infection with the epidemic strain, and a further outbreak probably could not occur until a sufficiently large, new, nonimmune population redeveloped as a result of births and immigrations.

In the savanna region of Africa, outbreaks of meningococcal disease show a marked seasonal association, nearly always starting during the middle of the dry season, when it is hot, dry, and dusty, and ceasing

TABLE 42–1. Comparison of the Epidemiologic Features of Meningococcal Infection in the Northern Savanna of Africa and in Developed Countries

	Savanna of Africa	Developed Countries
Dominant serotype	Group A > group C	Group B and group C
Pattern of infection	Epidemic	Endemic
Seasonal prevalence	Dry season	Winter
Maximal age incidence	5–14 yr	<5 yr
Pattern of spread	Child to child	Adult to infant

abruptly with the onset of the rains (Fig. 42–2). Epidemics rarely spread into areas where the absolute humidity remains above 10 gm/m³ throughout the year. Studies in Upper Volta and in Nigeria showed that the rate of nasopharyngeal acquisition of meningococci is not affected by seasonal changes. Thus, it is likely that environmental factors associated with the dry season alter the ratio of clinical to subclinical infection rather than causing an overall increase in the incidence of meningococcal infection. A high temperature and a low absolute humidity may damage the local defenses of the nasopharynx, thus favoring systemic infection. In Egypt, however, the meningitis season occurs during the cool, damp months.

During African epidemics, most cases of meningococcal disease occur in children aged 5 to 14 years, in contrast to the much earlier onset of the infection in Europe and the United States. In Nigeria, the infection is uncommon in children under the age of 2 years, and carriage as well as clinical infection is found most frequently in older children, suggesting that within the African meningitis belt spread of meningococcal infection is usually from child to child.

During epidemics, the spread of meningococcal disease often appears to be haphazard, some communities being severely affected while neighboring communities are spared. This was observed during an epidemic of group A meningococcal disease in The Gambia, the first for many years. In some villages, attack rates as high as 1:20 were recorded whereas no cases were seen in neighboring villages. In affected villages, some households had several cases while neighboring households had none. No reasons could be found for this patchy distribution of cases, which has been observed in other epidemics.

PATHOLOGY AND PATHOGENESIS

Pathology. Postmortem examination of a patient who has died from acute meningococcemia may show only a few abnormalities. Petechiae usually are present, and there may be larger hemorrhages into organs such as the adrenals. Signs of encephalitis or pulmonary edema may be found. Microscopy may show extensive damage to small blood vessels. The pathologic features of meningococcal meningitis are characteristic of those of acute bacterial meningitis (Chapter 43).

Pathogenesis. Meningococci produce large amounts of endotoxin, which is probably important in the pathogenesis of the peripheral circulatory collapse characteristic of acute meningococcemia and in the pathogenesis of the acute meningeal inflammatory changes found in patients with meningococcal meningitis. Endotoxin can stimulate the release of tumor necrosis factor (TNF) by macrophages and other cells. TNF can produce many of the pathophysiologic changes seen in meningococcemia, and elevated plasma levels of TNF have been demonstrated in patients with meningococcemia. Thus, TNF is probably an important mediator of tissue damage in this infection.

Extensive hemorrhage may be present in the adrenal glands of patients who have died from shock, but this lesion is sometimes found in patients who have died from acute meningococcemia but who have maintained a normal blood pressure throughout their illness. Most patients with acute meningococcemia have elevated plasma cortisol levels and respond normally to stimulation with ACTH. Thus, it is likely that factors other

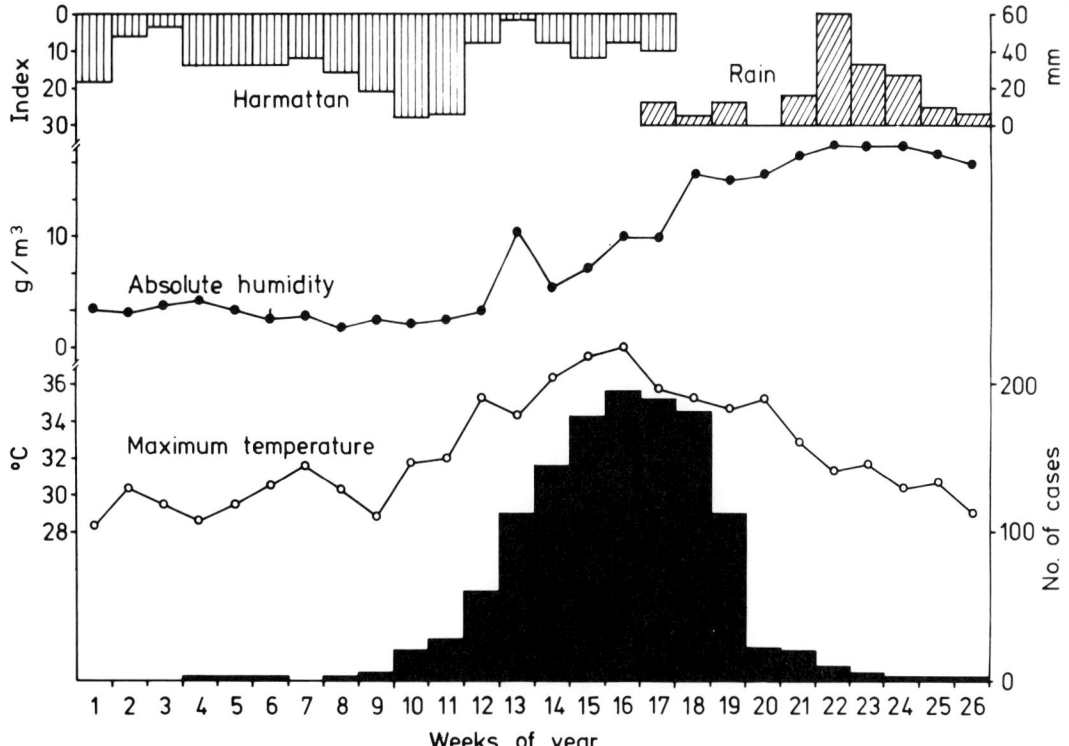

FIGURE 42–2. Relationship of an epidemic of meningococcal meningitis in northern Nigeria to seasonal climatic changes. The harmattan is a dry, dusty wind that blows from the Sahara. (From Greenwood BM, et al.: Trans R Soc Trop Med Hyg 73:557, 1979.)

than acute adrenocortical insufficiency are responsible for shock in most patients with this condition.

A patient with acute meningococcemia or meningococcal meningitis may have arthritis, cutaneous vasculitis, episcleritis, or pericarditis several days after the onset of illness, at a time when the early clinical features of the infection are lessening. Such lesions are usually sterile. Biopsy specimens of an affected area of skin or synovium show a vasculitis. Serologic studies indicate that these lesions occur most frequently in patients whose serum contains polysaccharide antigen and that they appear at a time when antigen disappears from the serum and circulating antibody can first be detected (Fig. 42–3), suggesting that the lesions are the result of the local formation of immune complexes at sites where meningococci have settled during the septicemic phase of the illness. This is supported by the fact that antigen, antibody, and complement can be demonstrated by immunofluorescence around affected small blood vessels.

CLINICAL MANIFESTATIONS

Pharyngitis. Although most meningococcal infections of the nasopharynx are asymptomatic, meningococci occasionally can produce a mild pharyngitis that is clinically indistinguishable from that caused by many other organisms.

Acute Meningococcemia

Symptoms. Acute meningococcemia can strike with frightening rapidity—a patient may be well at breakfast time but dead by the same afternoon. The early clinical features of the condition—fever, headache, and general malaise—are indistinguishable from those of many less serious infectious diseases. Diarrhea is sometimes an early feature of acute meningococcemia, and it may be severe enough to suggest a diagnosis of acute gastroenteritis.

Signs. Initial clinical examination may show no abnormalities apart from fever and tachycardia. The appearance of petechiae often is the first indication of the potentially serious nature of a patient's illness. Petechiae may be present in the conjunctivae and on the palate, a useful diagnostic sign in patients with dark skin (Fig. 42–4). Later, more extensive ecchymoses may appear. Cardiovascular signs may be present when a patient is first seen, but they frequently do not appear until a few hours after a patient has been admitted to the hospital. A third heart sound may be heard, and the electrocardiogram is often abnormal, showing features of myocarditis. The blood pressure may be low, and it may continue to fall despite treatment. Patients with acute meningococcemia frequently are confused, and their level of consciousness may deteriorate progressively.

Laboratory Findings. Examination of the blood usually shows a polymorphonuclear neutrophilic leukocytosis, but a severely ill patient may be leukopenic. Thrombocytopenia is usually present, and some patients are found to have other abnormalities, such as a raised level of fibrin degradation products, suggesting disseminated intravascular coagulation. Blood culture is frequently positive, and meningococcal capsular polysaccharide antigen usually can be detected in the serum. By definition, patients with acute meningococcemia have clear cerebrospinal fluid (CSF), but there may be a slight increase in the CSF white cell count.

Early Complications. Disseminated intravascular coagulation can occur as an early complication of acute meningococcemia, and it can lead to severe, and sometimes fatal, hemorrhage. Even when an episode of shock has been overcome successfully, survival of a patient with acute meningococcemia cannot be guaranteed. Severe pulmonary edema may occur during the first few days of illness, and some patients remain unconscious for a prolonged period, perhaps because of an associated encephalitis. Acute renal failure may develop in a patient who has been severely hypotensive.

Late Complications. At least 10% of patients who

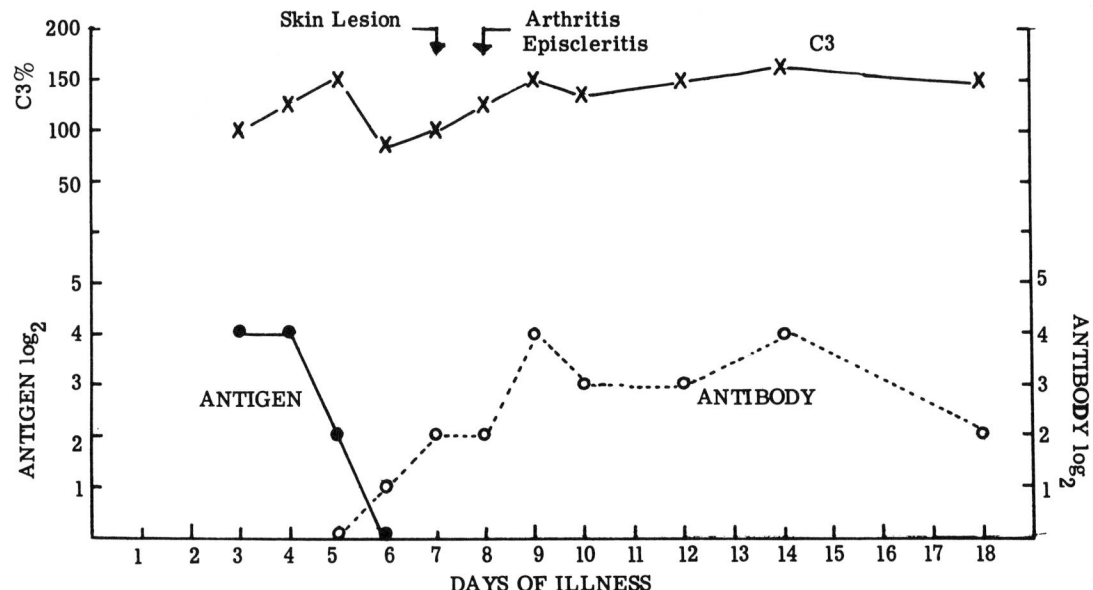

FIGURE 42–3. Serologic changes in a patient with meningococcal meningitis in relation to the development of late allergic complications. (From Greenwood BM, et al.: Br Med J 2:737, 1973.)

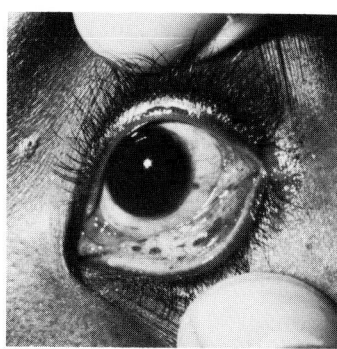

FIGURE 42–4. Conjunctival petechiae in a patient with meningococcal meningitis. (Photograph kindly provided by Professor D. A. Warrell.)

survive the early phase of acute meningococcemia develop late allergic complications. These include a monoarthritis or a polyarthritis, cutaneous vasculitis and ulceration, episcleritis, and pericarditis. These lesions probably result from the formation of immune complexes at these sites. Vasculitis can occasionally be severe, leading to extensive ulceration (Fig. 42–5) and even gangrene of distal extremities. Accumulation of pericardial fluid can give rise to tamponade.

Chronic Meningococcemia. This is a rare condition characterized by episodes of fever, rash, arthritis, and splenomegaly associated with intermittent meningococcemia.

Meningitis

Signs and Symptoms. Patients with meningococcal meningitis show the clinical features of acute bacterial meningitis (Chapter 43). The presence of petechiae is a helpful diagnostic sign, since petechiae are rarely seen in patients with other types of meningitis. A few patients with meningococcal meningitis show signs of acute meningococcemia, such as hypotension.

Laboratory Findings. Laboratory investigations show a peripheral blood polymorphonuclear neutrophilic leukocytosis. Blood culture is sometimes positive, and meningococcal antigen is demonstrable in the serum of about 10% of patients. Examination of CSF shows the characteristic changes of acute pyogenic meningitis (Chapter 43). Gram staining may show gram-negative diplococci both with and without leukocytes, and culture is usually positive, provided that no antibiotic treatment has been given. Meningococcal antigen is present in the CSF of about 80% of patients.

Complications. Patients with meningococcal meningitis only rarely have local complications such as an extradural empyema. However, activation of herpes simplex infection is observed frequently. About 10% of patients with meningococcal meningitis, especially older patients and those who are initially serum antigen–positive, have late allergic complications. Deafness is the most important long-term complication of meningococcal meningitis. A study done in The Gambia showed that 6 of 157 patients had severe sensorineural hearing loss 6 to 12 months after their illness.

Other Clinical Syndromes. Meningococci are an occasional cause of pneumonia, urethritis, cervicitis, proctitis, and conjunctivitis; these syndromes have no characteristic clinical features.

DIAGNOSIS

Pharyngitis. Meningococcal infection of the nasopharynx is established by a positive culture from a nasopharyngeal swab. The identification of meningococci is aided by the use of a selective medium, such as Thayer-Martin medium, which allows the growth of meningococci but inhibits the growth of many other nasopharyngeal bacteria.

Acute Meningococcemia. The early clinical features of acute meningococcemia are indistinguishable from those of many other acute infections. Thus, clinical diagnosis is often impossible unless it is known that the patient has been in close contact with a case of meningococcal disease. The detection of petechiae in a febrile patient should suggest a possible diagnosis of acute meningococcemia, but many other organisms can cause a febrile illness associated with petechiae and hemorrhages. A diagnosis of acute meningococcemia is confirmed by the detection of meningococcal antigen in the serum or by a positive blood culture. Provided that high-quality antisera are used, sera from most patients with acute meningococcemia give a positive result on counterimmunoelectrophoresis, thus rapidly establishing the diagnosis.

Chronic Meningococcemia. The diagnosis of chronic meningococcemia is established by blood culture.

Meningitis. The clinical and laboratory diagnosis of meningococcal meningitis is discussed in Chapter 43. CSF is sterile and negative for meningococcal antigen

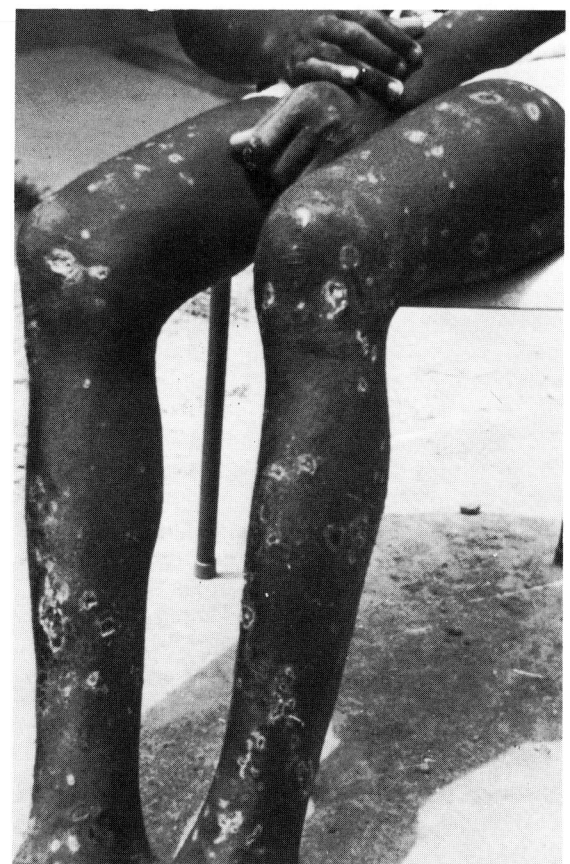

FIGURE 42–5. Cutaneous ulcerative skin lesions in a patient who had acute meningococcemia.

in about 10 to 20% of patients with meningococcal meningitis. A diagnosis can be made in these patients only by measurement of antibody levels in acute and convalescent phase sera. Culture- and antigen-negative patients have an excellent prognosis, perhaps because they had some pre-existing immunity at the time of infection.

TREATMENT

Acute Meningococcemia

Supportive Therapy. A patient with acute meningococcemia should be managed in an intensive care unit whenever possible. Fluid balance, acid-base status, and central venous pressure should be monitored whenever practicable. Two main approaches to the management of the peripheral circulatory collapse that kills many patients with acute meningococcemia have been used. Infusion of plasma or dextran increases the venous return to the heart and improves cardiac output, but such infusions can precipitate pulmonary edema. Alternatively, peripheral vascular resistance can be increased by an intravenous infusion of a sympathomimetic amine such as norepinephrine. The rate of infusion should be adjusted to maintain the systolic blood pressure at around 100 mm Hg. An average rate of infusion for an adult is 10 μg/min. Norepinephrine also increases myocardial contractility. The blood pressure of most patients with acute meningococcemia can be maintained by a combination of these two forms of treatment. Some patients who do not respond to dextran infusion and sympathomimetic amines are helped by an intravenous infusion of phentolamine in a dose for an adult of 20 to 80 μg/min. Phentolamine antagonizes the constricting effect of norepinephrine on small blood vessels, but it does not impair its action on the heart. An infusion of phentolamine may reduce the effective plasma volume, necessitating further fluid replacement.

The role of corticosteroids in the treatment of acute meningococcemia is uncertain. Because occasional patients with acute meningococcemia have low plasma cortisol levels, some physicians recommend that hydrocortisone or prednisone should be given in conventional therapeutic doses to hypotensive patients with acute meningococcemia unless normal plasma cortisol levels can be demonstrated. Studies in animals have shown that corticosteroids have some prophylactic action against endotoxin shock but only when they are given in massive doses. Massive doses of methylprednisone (e.g., 1 or 2 gm) have been given to patients with acute meningococcemia, but the value of this expensive form of therapy has not been clearly established.

Heparin is sometimes given to patients with acute meningococcemia in an attempt to control bleeding, but controlled trials have shown that heparin therapy is ineffective. Plasmapheresis has been tried with apparent success in a few patients with life-threatening acute meningococcemia, but no controlled trials have been done.

Antibiotics. Penicillin is the antibiotic of choice for the treatment of acute meningococcemia. It should be given by intravenous infusion in high doses (4 megaunits every 6 hours for an adult) during the critical phase of the illness. In survivors, this can be changed subse-

quently to intramuscular injections. Penicillin should be given for at least 7 days. Chloramphenicol is an effective alternative for patients who cannot be given penicillin for any reason.

Meningitis. The standard method of treatment of meningococcal meningitis with crystalline penicillin (Chapter 43) is unsuitable for the management of the many patients who require treatment during an epidemic. During an epidemic, it may be necessary to establish temporary treatment centers in schools and similar buildings and to recruit untrained staff to help with patient care. In these circumstances, a treatment schedule that relies on a limited number of injections is required. An oily suspension of chloramphenicol (Tifomycine), given in a single injection (3 gm for an adult), has been shown to be safe and effective. A single injection of ceftriaxone is a possible alternative, but this antibiotic is expensive.

PROGNOSIS. The outcome of acute meningococcemia is variable. Occasional patients have only a mild illness characterized by fever, petechiae, and a positive blood culture. In the savanna region of Africa, such cases are seen most frequently toward the end of an epidemic, when the mortality from the infection falls. Unfortunately, the outlook for most patients with acute meningococcemia is grave. During an outbreak of group A meningococcal disease in Nigeria, the overall mortality rate among 47 patients with meningococcemia was 43%; this is representative of the very high mortality from this condition that exists in many parts of the world. Mortality is especially high among patients who have neurologic signs or hypotension at the time of presentation. Death may occur from shock or hemorrhage during the early phase of the infection, or it may occur later as a result of pulmonary edema, renal failure, or residual neurologic damage. Survivors of the acute phase of the illness usually make a complete recovery.

In contrast to the poor prognosis of patients with acute meningococcemia, the outlook for patients with meningococcal meningitis is good. Most series indicate a mortality rate from this infection of less than 10%. Residual neurologic damage is unusual, with the exception of deafness; bacterial meningitis is a major cause of deafness in many developing countries. Deafness can prove to be a severe disability to a young child in a developing country where supportive facilities for the deaf are limited.

PREVENTION. Overcrowding and poor living conditions favor the spread of infections transmitted by respiratory droplets; a general improvement in living standards has helped to reduce the incidence of meningococcal disease in industrialized countries during the

TABLE 42–2. Recommended Dosage of Sulfonamides or Rifampicin for the Chemoprophylaxis of Meningococcal Disease*

	Sulfadiazine	Rifampicin
Adults	1 gm b.i.d.	600 mg b.i.d.
Children 1–12 yr	500 mg b.i.d.	10 mg/kg b.i.d.
Infants <1 yr	500 mg/day	5 mg/kg b.i.d.

*Treatment is given for 2 days.

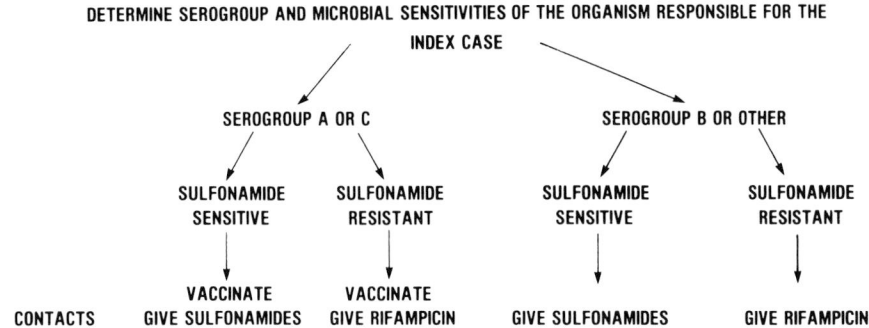

Note: If the organism responsible for the outbreak cannot be identified, contacts should be vaccinated with A + C vaccine and given rifampicin.

FIGURE 42–6. Scheme for the management of close contacts of a patient with meningococcal disease.

past 50 years. During epidemics of meningococcal disease, a high attack rate may occur in residential institutions (e.g., boarding schools and military barracks), and it may be wise to close such institutions until the epidemic is over. It is doubtful whether other measures that have been adopted in the past, such as closure of local markets and prevention of family gatherings, are of much value.

Chemoprophylaxis. Chemoprophylaxis has been used widely in the past to control outbreaks of meningococcal infection in schools and barracks and to protect close household contacts of a patient from the infection (Table 42–2). Sulfonamides, which are safe and inexpensive, eradicate sensitive strains of meningococci from the nasopharynx and thus interrupt transmission of the infection. Many strains of meningococci, however, especially those isolated in tropical Africa, are resistant to sulfonamides, and these drugs should no longer be used for prophylaxis unless it is known for certain that the epidemic strain is sensitive to sulfonamide. Rifampicin and minocycline are effective in eliminating sulfonamide-resistant meningococci from the nasopharynx. The tendency of minocycline to produce troublesome side effects has limited the use of this antibiotic for chemoprophylaxis. When used for prophylaxis, rifampicin rapidly induces the appearance of resistant strains of meningococci, and there is a theoretical risk that widespread use of rifampicin for meningococcal prophylaxis could encourage the emergence of rifampicin-resistant strains of *Mycobacterium tuberculosis* and *M. leprae* in areas in which infection with these two organisms is prevalent. Rifampicin is expensive, reducing further its usefulness as a prophylactic against meningococcal infection in tropical developing countries. Recently it has been shown that ceftriaxone given by injection and oral ciprofloxacin can eliminate carriage, but these drugs are expensive.

Vaccination. Vaccines comprising purified group A or C meningococcal polysaccharides are effective in preventing clinical infection with these two organisms. Group B meningococcal polysaccharide is poorly immunogenic and cannot be used as a vaccine. Progress has been made, however, toward the development of group B meningococcal outer-membrane protein vaccines. One such vaccine is being used extensively in Cuba, and trials of another have been started in Norway. Meningococcal polysaccharide vaccines are poorly immunogenic in the young, and they induce little immunologic memory.

Although there is clear evidence that meningococcal polysaccharide vaccines prevent meningococcal disease, there is still some uncertainty about how these vaccines can be used most effectively to control meningococcal infection. Because close contacts of a patient with group A or C meningococcal infection are at high risk, it is generally agreed that they should be vaccinated and given chemoprophylaxis (Fig. 42–6). Existing meningococcal vaccines offer an excellent means for controlling localized outbreaks and larger epidemics of meningococcal infection. Studies undertaken in various parts of the world have shown that mass immunization at the village, city, or nation level is highly effective in bringing outbreaks of group A or C meningococcal disease rapidly under control (Fig. 42–7). Vaccination of only those

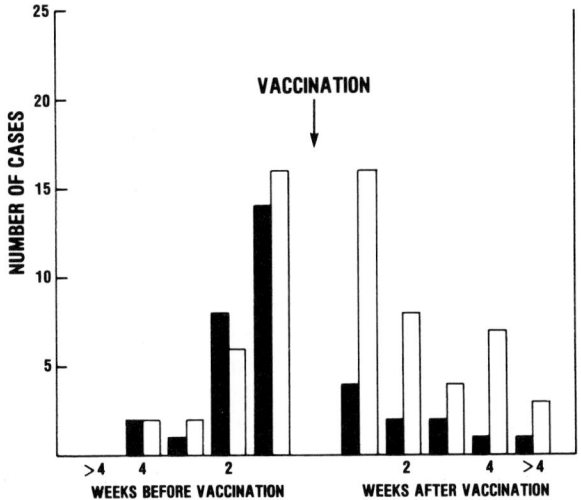

FIGURE 42–7. Influence of vaccination on an outbreak of group A meningococcal disease in a rural area in northern Nigeria. The number of cases of proven group A meningococcal meningitis in vaccinated villages (black bars) and in control villages (white bars) are shown. Only 2 of the 10 patients with meningitis from vaccinated villages after vaccination had been undertaken had been immunized. The remainder had been away from their village on the day that vaccination was performed. (From Greenwood BM, Wali SS: Lancet 1:729, 1980.)

subjects in the age group with a high risk of infection saves a great deal of vaccine and may be only marginally less effective than vaccination of the entire population. If vaccination is used to control an epidemic, immunization must be initiated as soon as possible after the outbreak has started.

Whether meningococcal capsular polysaccharide vaccines should be given routinely in areas in which epidemics are frequent is uncertain because of doubts over the duration of protection that they provide in children. In a trial in Burkina Faso, protection against meningitis was found to be only transitory in children immunized before the age of 4 years. It might be possible to introduce routine meningoccal vaccination on school entry, but routine immunization of children probably has to wait for the development of capsular polysaccharide protein conjugate vaccines that are immunogenic in young children and whose administration can be incorporated into existing infant immunization schedules. Several conjugate vaccines are being developed and will soon be entering clinical trials.

BIBLIOGRAPHY

Greenwood BM, Bradley AK, Cleland PG, et al.: An epidemic of meningococcal infection at Zaria, northern Nigeria. I: General epidemiological features. Trans R Soc Trop Med Hyg 73:557, 1979.

Greenwood BM, Greenwood AM, Bradley AK, et al.: Factors influencing susceptibility to meningococcal disease during an epidemic in The Gambia, West Africa. J Infect Dis 14:167, 1987.

Lapeyssonnie L: La meningite cerebrospinale en Afrique. Bull WHO 28(Suppl 3):3, 1963.

Olyhoek T, Crowe BA, Achtman M: The clonal population structure of *Neisseria meningitidis* serogroup A isolated from epidemics and pandemics between 1915 and 1983. Rev Infect Dis 9:665, 1987.

Reingold AL, Broome CV, Hightower AW, et al.: Age-specific differences in duration of clinical protection after vaccination with meningococcal polysaccharide A vaccine. Lancet 2:114, 1985.

Rey M: Treatment of purulent meningitis in developing countries. *In* Williams JD, Burnie J (eds.): Bacterial Meningitis. London, Academic Press, 1987, p 211.

Waage A, Halstensen A, Espevik T: Association between tumor necrosis factor in serum and fatal outcome in patients with meningococcal disease. Lancet 1:355, 1987.

Wali SS, Macfarlane JT, Weir WRC, et al.: Single injection treatment of meningococcal meningitis. 2: Long-acting chloramphenicol. Trans R Soc Trop Med Hyg 73:698, 1979.

Whittle HC, Abdullahi MT, Fakunle FA, et al.: Allergic complications of meningococcal disease. 1: Clinical aspects. Br Med J 2:733, 1973.

43.   ACUTE BACTERIAL MENINGITIS

Brian M. Greenwood

DEFINITION. Acute bacterial meningitis is the condition that results from invasion of the meninges by bacteria that induce an acute inflammatory response. This acute inflammatory reaction, which involves the arachnoid and the pia mater, is characterized by a polymorphonuclear neutrophil leukocyte exudate.

ETIOLOGY. Many species of bacteria can cause acute bacterial meningitis (Table 43–1), but surveys undertaken in various parts of the world have shown

TABLE 43–1. Organisms Identified Most Frequently as a Cause of Bacterial Meningitis

Acute Meningitis	Chronic Meningitis
Streptococcus pneumoniae	*Mycobacterium tuberculosis*
Haemophilus influenzae	*Treponema pallidum*
Neisseria meningitidis	*Borrelia burgdorferi*
Escherichia coli	
Other gram-negative bacilli	
Listeria monocytogenes	
Salmonella species	
Leptospira species	
Staphylococcus aureus	
Group B streptococci	

that 3 organisms—*Streptococcus pneumoniae, Haemophilus influenzae,* and *Neisseria meningitidis*—account for about three fourths of all cases. A study of 569 patients with proven acute bacterial meningitis admitted to hospital in Dakar, Senegal, during the period from 1974 to 1976 showed that 41% of cases were due to infection with a pneumococcus, 30% were due to infection with *H. influenzae,* and 7% were due to infection with a meningococcus. These findings reflect a pattern of acute bacterial meningitis that is typical of many tropical developing countries. In some parts of tropical Africa, however, the meningococcus is a more frequent cause of acute bacterial meningitis than the pneumococcus (Chapter 42). Most cases of *H. influenzae* meningitis are caused by bacteria belonging to type b. The suggestion has been made, however, that in some tropical countries such as Papua New Guinea, type a and nontypable *H. influenzae* may be more important causes of meningitis than in Europe or the United States.

INCIDENCE AND DISTRIBUTION. Hospital surveys undertaken in several developing countries have shown that meningitis accounts for 1 to 2% of all admissions. Few population data are available on the incidence of acute bacterial meningitis in tropical developing countries. Figures from Dakar, Senegal, suggest that the risk of a Senegalese child's being affected with acute bacterial meningitis before the age of 5 years is at least 1:500. This risk is probably higher in areas in which outbreaks of meningococcal infection frequently occur. Studies of deaths in children in a rural area of the Gambia suggest that as many as 1 in 100 die of acute bacterial meningitis before reaching age 5.

Infection with the pneumococcus or with *H. influenzae* occurs throughout both the wet and the dry tropics. Meningococcal infection is most prevalent in the northern savanna region of tropical Africa, where major outbreaks of this infection often occur (Chapter 42).

EPIDEMIOLOGY. The pneumococcus, the meningococcus, and *H. influenzae* are usually spread from person to person by respiratory droplets. There are no known animal reservoirs of these infections. Each of these 3 organisms can colonize the nasopharynx to produce an asymptomatic carrier. Asymptomatic carriers greatly outnumber cases of clinical disease and are the main source of infection. In some tropical countries, most infants are colonized with the pneumococcus and with *H. influenzae* in the first few months of life.

Predisposing Factors. A number of factors predisposing to acute bacterial meningitis have been identified, but it is uncertain what determines whether an individual infected with a pneumococcus, a meningococcus, or *H. influenzae* becomes an asymptomatic carrier or a patient with clinical disease. The presence or absence of circulating antibody at the time of infection is one important factor. It is possible that damage to the local defenses of the nasopharynx by a virus or by adverse climatic conditions predisposes to systemic infection. Patients with a primary or an acquired defect in humoral immunity show an increased susceptibility to pneumococcal and meningococcal infection. An anatomic defect resulting from trauma or surgery that allows access of bacteria in the nasopharynx to the inside of the skull also predisposes to these infections. Sickle cell disease is an important predisposing factor to pneumococcal meningitis in areas of the tropics in which this condition is prevalent. The incidence of pneumococcal infection is at least 10 times higher in people with the hemoglobin genotype SS than in those with a normal genotype. Malnutrition predisposes to infection of the meninges with organisms of low virulence, such as nontyphoidal salmonellae, that rarely cause meningitis in a healthy subject.

Age Distribution. Age has an important influence on susceptibility to different forms of acute bacterial meningitis (Fig. 43–1). Acute bacterial meningitis in the neonate is caused most frequently by gram-negative bacilli such as *Escherichia coli* or, more rarely, by group B streptococci. The pneumococcus and *H. influenzae* are the main causes of meningitis in children under the age of 1 year; meningitis due to *H. influenzae* is rare in subjects over age 5. In some tropical countries, meningitis attributable to *H. influenzae* occurs at an even earlier age than in Europe or the United States, with a peak incidence at about 6 months. The meningococcus is the most frequent cause of meningitis in older children, whereas the pneumococcus is the main cause of meningitis in the elderly.

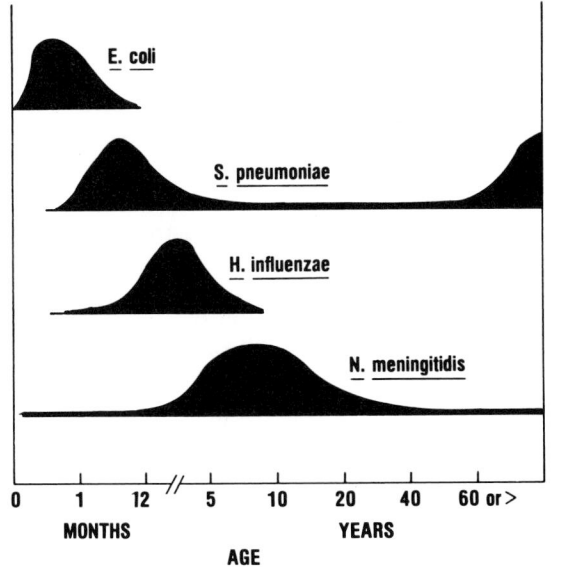

FIGURE 43–1. The age distribution of 4 important types of acute bacterial meningitis in a tropical African country where meningococcal meningitis is prevalent at a later age than in developed countries.

Transmission. Pneumococcal, meningococcal, and *H. influenzae* infections are endemic in most communities. Small outbreaks of pneumococcal or *H. influenzae* infection may occur among subjects living in crowded conditions, but epidemics of these infections are rare. In contrast, large epidemics of meningococcal disease occasionally occur in communities in which the infection is usually endemic.

Person-to-person spread of infection often can be observed during the course of outbreaks of meningococcal disease. The incidence of secondary cases is higher during an epidemic than during periods when transmission is endemic. During a large epidemic of group A meningococcal infection in northern Nigeria, 10% of hospital patients gave a history of close contact with a previous case of the infection. During this outbreak, the risk of secondary infection was high in close family contacts, especially among siblings of a patient, among whom the secondary attack rate was about 1:30. A similar pattern of intrafamily spread has been observed during other outbreaks of meningococcal disease. *H. influenzae* also can spread within households in a manner similar to that of the meningococcus. Studies in the United States have shown that the risk of infection in a sibling of a patient may be as high as 1 in 20 when the sibling is under the age of 1 year. In the United States, day-care centers are thought to play an important part in the spread of *H. influenzae* infections. In contrast, secondary spread of pneumococcal disease within households is rarely observed.

PATHOLOGY AND PATHOGENESIS

Pathology. The brain of a patient who has died from acute bacterial meningitis usually is covered with a thick exudate that extends inward along the perivascular spaces. An extradural effusion may be present, and medullary coning may be seen. When the brain is cross-sectioned, dilatation of the ventricles may be noted. On microscopy, the meninges show the characteristic features of an acute inflammatory response—a fibrinous exudate, hyperemia, and infiltration with polymorphonuclear neutrophilic leukocytes. Gram staining may show the causative organism within leukocytes or lying free in a fibrinous exudate. The lining of the ventricles may show acute inflammatory changes similar to those observed in the meninges. Inflammatory cells are sometimes seen in the brain substance of a patient who has died from meningococcal meningitis, indicating the presence of an associated encephalitis. Microscopy may show inflammatory changes in cerebral arteries and veins, especially if the patient has died from pneumococcal meningitis.

Postmortem examination of the rest of the body may show foci of infection at other sites. Thus, otitis media or pneumonia may be found in a patient who has died from pneumococcal meningitis, and bone or joint lesions are sometimes found in a young child who has died from a systemic *H. influenzae* infection. Some of the pathologic features of acute meningococcemia (Chapter 42) may be present in cases of meningococcal meningitis.

Pathogenesis. The pathogenesis of many of the clinical features of acute bacterial meningitis is incompletely understood. It is probable that most cases of pneumococcal, meningococcal, and *H. influenzae* meningitis follow spread of infection from the nasopharynx into the systemic circulation, with subsequent seeding of bacteria to the meninges. Some pneumococcal meningeal infections, however, probably follow invasion of the blood stream by bacteria present in a consolidated area of lung.

Once bacteria reach the meninges, they initiate an acute inflammatory response. In the case of meningococcal and *H. influenzae* type b infections, release of endotoxin may stimulate the production of mediators of inflammatory reactions such as tumor necrosis factor and interleukin-1. In the case of the pneumococcus, which does not possess an endotoxin, inflammatory changes are induced by cell wall components including peptidoglycans. Both endotoxin and some pneumococcal capsular polysaccharides can activate complement to produce chemotactic breakdown products such as C5a, which may attract further leukocytes to the inflamed meninges.

Acute bacterial meningitis may be accompanied by marked changes in cerebral metabolism. Transfer of glucose across the blood–brain barrier is defective, and there is a shift toward anaerobic carbohydrate metabolism in the brain.

IMMUNITY. Epidemiologic and laboratory studies suggest that protection against pneumococcal, meningococcal, and *H. influenzae* infection is mediated mainly by antibody. The possible protective role of cell-mediated immunity in these infections has undergone little investigation. The formation of antibody to the capsular polysaccharide antigens of the meningococcus, the pneumococcus, and *H. influenzae* can be stimulated by asymptomatic nasopharyngeal carriage as well as by clinical infection. Antibody to the capsular polysaccharides of these 3 organisms also can be formed as a result of infection with harmless bacteria that share antigens with them. Thus, asymptomatic infection with *Neisseria lactamica*, a frequent commensal of the nasopharynx of young children, can induce the formation of antibodies that are bactericidal for virulent strains of meningococci. Similarly, infection with the harmless strain of *E. coli* 075:K 100:H5 induces the formation of antibodies that cross-react with *H. influenzae* type b capsular antigens.

As a result of one or another of these immunizing mechanisms, most adults possess bactericidal antibodies to meningococci, *H. influenzae*, and some serogroups of pneumococci. Prospective studies in American military recruits have shown clearly that adults who lack bactericidal antibodies to the meningococcus are susceptible to subsequent clinical infection with this organism.

CLINICAL MANIFESTATIONS

Symptoms and Signs. The usual presenting symptoms of acute bacterial meningitis are headache, backache, fever, and general malaise. Other common symptoms are photophobia and vomiting. Convulsions may occur, especially in young children. The onset of acute bacterial meningitis is usually sudden, and, provided that transport is available, most patients reach the hospital within 2 or 3 days of the start of their illness. Several studies have shown that patients with a long history of this illness have a good prognosis, presumably because they have mild disease.

On initial examination, most patients with acute bacterial meningitis are febrile and have signs of acute meningeal inflammation. The neck is stiff, and Kernig's sign is positive (Fig. 43–2). Consciousness may be impaired to a degree that ranges from mild confusion to deep coma. Bradycardia and, in young infants, bulging of the anterior fontanelle may be present, indicating raised intracranial pressure, but papilledema is rarely seen. A sixth cranial nerve palsy is the most frequently encountered localized neurologic sign. Third, seventh, and eighth cranial nerve palsies are encountered less frequently. Neurologic abnormalities may be detected in the limbs but are unusual.

General examination may show signs outside the central nervous system. Many patients with meningococcal meningitis have petechiae. In dark-skinned subjects, these are seen best in the conjunctiva (Fig. 42–4) or on the soft palate. A patient with meningococcal meningitis often has signs of myocardial damage, such as a third heart sound or an arrhythmia. Patients with pneumococcal meningitis may have signs of the sinusitis, otitis media, or pneumonia from which their infection derived. Widespread dissemination of bacteria through the circulation may have produced pyogenic lesions at sites other than the meninges.

Blood Tests. A patient with acute bacterial meningitis usually has a polymorphonuclear neutrophilic leukocytosis. Thrombocytopenia may be present, especially when there is associated septicemia. Blood culture is positive in about two thirds of patients with *H. influenzae* meningitis, but a positive culture is obtained in a lower proportion of patients with pneumococcal or meningococcal meningitis. Polysaccharides derived from the capsule of the causative bacterium can be found in the serum or urine of some patients with pneumococcal, meningococcal, *H. influenzae*, or *E. coli* meningitis.

Cerebrospinal Fluid. The cerebrospinal fluid (CSF) of a patient with acute bacterial meningitis is usually turbid and under pressure. On laboratory examination, a high white cell count, mainly polymorphonuclear neutrophilic leukocytes, a high protein level, and a low glucose level are found. The CSF glucose is usually lower than the glucose content of a blood sample collected at the time that lumbar puncture was performed. Examination of a spun deposit of CSF may show the causative organism directly, and culture is usually positive. Bacterial polysaccharide capsular antigens are frequently present. Some of the other nonspecific changes that have been described in CSF samples obtained from patients with acute bacterial meningitis are presented in Table 43–2.

Complications. Local complications of acute bacterial meningitis include the formation of an extradural effusion or empyema and thrombosis of cerebral vessels; both of these complications may result in a deterioration of the patient's neurologic state. Occasionally, raised intracranial pressure causes medullary coning. Widespread dissemination of the causative bacterium may produce pyogenic lesions at distant sites such as the joints and eyes.

About 10% of patients with meningococcal meningitis have arthritis, cutaneous vasculitis, episcleritis, or pericarditis. These late complications probably have an allergic cause (Chapter 42).

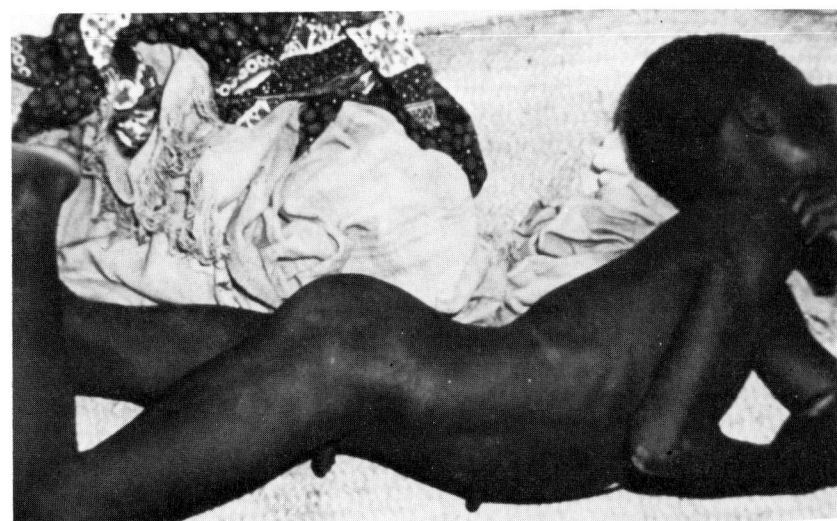

FIGURE 43–2. Acute bacterial meningitis in a 10-year-old Nigerian boy who had severe neck retraction.

Herpes simplex infection is a common complication of acute bacterial meningitis, especially when the infection is caused by a meningococcus. Usually, herpetic lesions appear around the mouth 2 or 3 days after a patient's admission to the hospital. Occasionally, the virus spreads extensively to involve the eyes or limbs. Activation of herpes infection in patients with acute pyogenic meningitis is probably a consequence of the generalized impairment of cellular immunity that is associated with this condition.

DIAGNOSIS

Clinical. A clinical diagnosis of acute bacterial meningitis usually can be made in adults and older children on the basis of a patient's characteristic symptoms and signs. The characteristic clinical features of acute meningitis may be absent, however, in the very young and in the old. Thus, meningitis must be considered as a possible diagnosis in any child with febrile convulsions and in any elderly patient who suddenly becomes confused. A malnourished child with meningitis may be afebrile, and meningitis must be considered as a possible cause for failure to thrive. Meningism associated with an upper respiratory tract or other infection may suggest a clinical diagnosis of meningitis; if there is any doubt, lumbar puncture must be performed. A cerebral abscess usually causes more marked localized neurologic signs and less marked signs of meningeal irritation than acute meningitis.

Acute bacterial meningitis usually can be differentiated clinically from tuberculous meningitis on the basis of a history of a sudden and shortlasting illness, but often it is not possible to differentiate acute bacterial

TABLE 43–2. Characteristic CSF Changes in Acute Bacterial Meningitis

↑ Cell count—mainly polymorphonuclear neutrophilic leukocytes
↑ Total protein
↑ IgG and IgM
↓ Glucose
↑ Lactic acid
↑ Lactic acid dehydrogenase
↑ Fibrin degradation products
↑ C-reactive protein

meningitis from acute viral meningitis on clinical grounds alone. Careful clinical examination may provide a clue to the cause of acute bacterial meningitis. The detection of petechiae suggests a diagnosis of meningococcal meningitis, since petechiae are found only rarely in patients with other forms of bacterial meningitis, whereas the presence of otitis media or pneumonia favors a diagnosis of pneumococcal disease.

General examination may show features of a predisposing factor to acute bacterial meningitis such as sickle cell disease. A detailed search for any possible mechanical or immunologic predisposing factor should be made in any patient who has had meningitis. A firm diagnosis of acute bacterial meningitis can be established only by lumbar puncture, which should be performed whenever this diagnosis is seriously considered. Opinion in developed countries is divided as to whether it is necessary to perform lumbar puncture in all children with febrile convulsions. In developing countries, where meningitis is common, it is probably wise to do so unless an obvious alternative cause for their convulsions can be found. Lumbar puncture should be performed in all patients thought to have cerebral malaria because detection of malaria parasitemia does not exclude coexisting meningitis.

Laboratory. A turbid CSF gives immediate confirmation of a clinical diagnosis of meningitis. A clear sample, however, does not exclude this diagnosis, because at least 200 cells/mm³ must be present before CSF appears turbid to the naked eye. Thus, a CSF cell count must be made before a diagnosis of meningitis can be confidently excluded. A spun deposit of CSF should be examined without staining for motile amebas, because organisms such as *Naegleria fowleri* can produce clinical and laboratory findings indistinguishable from those of acute bacterial meningitis (Chapter 80). Identification of *Naegleria* in a stained preparation is difficult. Examination of a Gram-stained deposit allows the characteristics of the leukocytes present in the CSF to be determined. Polymorphonuclear neutrophilic leukocytes predominate in CSF obtained from patients with acute bacterial meningitis, whereas most white cells present in the CSF of patients with viral meningitis are lymphocytes. CSF obtained from patients with tuberculous meningitis usually contains cells of both types (Chapter 61). Caution is needed in the interpretation of CSF cell findings in a patient with acute meningitis who has received antibiotic treatment before lumbar puncture was performed, since CSF of partially treated patients with acute bacterial meningitis may contain both polymorphonuclear neutrophils and lymphocytes. A low ratio of CSF glucose to blood glucose is found frequently in patients with acute bacterial meningitis and tuberculous meningitis but not in patients with acute viral meningitis. Elevation of CSF levels of lactic acid, lactic acid dehydrogenase, and immunoglobulins G and M favors a diagnosis of acute bacterial meningitis as opposed to a diagnosis of acute viral meningitis, but, in general, these investigations are of limited diagnostic value. A raised serum level of C-reactive protein also favors a diagnosis of bacterial as opposed to viral meningitis, but this test has a low specificity.

The cause of acute bacterial meningitis usually can be identified by Gram stain and by culture of a spun deposit of CSF, and the antibiotic sensitivities of the cultured organism can be determined. Staining with acridine orange rather than Gram stain can increase the sensitivity of bacterial detection by microscopy. Difficulties may be experienced with both of these routine bacteriologic techniques. Gram stains may be misinterpreted, especially when performed by inexperienced staff in a clinical sideroom, and culture is frequently negative in patients who have already received an antibiotic. Diagnostic tests that depend on the detection of bacterial products in CSF rather than on the detection of live bacteria are especially useful in partially treated patients. Endotoxin can be detected in CSF from nearly all patients with meningococcal, *H. influenzae*, or *E. coli* meningitis by the limulus lysate test, but this assay does not differentiate among these 3 organisms, which require different treatment. Demonstration of capsular polysaccharide antigens in the CSF has been used to diagnose acute bacteriologic meningitis for more than 50 years but only in the last decade has this technique come into widespread use; commercial test kits are now widely available. Some of the advantages and disadvantages of immunodiagnosis are summarized in Table 43–3. Because of the limitations of immunodiagnosis, it should be used in conjunction with conventional bacteriologic techniques whenever possible. Latex tests (Fig. 43–3), which require a minimum of equipment, are well suited for use in tropical developing countries and offer a means of establishing a bacterial cause of acute meningitis in small hospitals that lack a routine diagnostic bacteriology service. Their sensitivity is comparable to that of culture (Table 43–4).

Bacterial polysaccharide antigens can be demonstrated in the serum and urine, as well as in the CSF, of some patients with acute bacterial meningitis. Although detection of antigenemia is of little diagnostic value, it is of some prognostic significance, for prognosis is worse in a patient with one of the 3 main forms of bacterial meningitis who is serum antigen-positive than in a patient who is not.

TREATMENT

General Measures. Whenever possible, a patient with

TABLE 43–3. Advantages and Disadvantages of Immunodiagnosis of Acute Bacterial Meningitis

Advantages	Disadvantages
Easy to perform	May give false-negative results unless high-quality antisera are used
Little equipment required	Cannot differentiate between organisms with cross-reacting antigens (e.g., *E. coli* type K and *N. meningitidis* group B)
Gives a rapid diagnosis	Cannot detect infections by unusual organisms
	Gives no information on antibiotic sensitivity

acute bacterial meningitis should be managed in a hospital. An unconscious patient should be nursed in a position that maintains his or her airway and should be turned regularly to prevent bedsores. In hot countries, patients with acute meningitis often are severely dehydrated by the time they reach the hospital because they are febrile and have stopped drinking. Thus, the administration of intravenous or nasogastric fluids may be required. Headache may be severe, making a patient restless and difficult to nurse. Headache may be relieved by aspirin; some patients require stronger analgesics. Paraldehyde or diazepam may be needed to control convulsions. Early studies on the use of corticosteroids in the treatment of acute bacterial meningitis provided no evidence for a beneficial effect. However, recent studies in the United States and Egypt suggest that large doses may reduce the incidence of late complications.

Antibiotics. The choice of antibiotic and the dosage used to treat a patient with acute bacterial meningitis are governed mainly by the cause of the infection (Table 43–5). Thus, every attempt must be made to establish a bacteriologic diagnosis and antibiotic sensitivity as soon as possible. There is a considerable variation in the facility with which antibiotics cross the blood-brain barrier to enter the CSF. Chloramphenicol is a good antibiotic in this respect, because, when given by mouth or by intramuscular injection, CSF levels of up to 50% of blood levels are found. Penicillin and ampicillin enter the CSF much less readily than chloramphenicol unless the meninges are inflamed. Thus, the dose of penicillin should not be lowered as a patient improves on treatment, because this improvement is associated with a reduction in the permeability of the blood-brain barrier to this antibiotic. In general, bactericidal concentrations of most antibiotics can be achieved in CSF with intramuscular or intravenous therapy, and intrathecal treatment is seldom required.

Meningococcal Meningitis. Penicillin is the antibiotic of choice for the treatment of meningococcal meningitis. Chloramphenicol is a highly effective alternative for a patient who cannot be given penicillin, but this drug may cause aplastic anemia. The risk of this complication is reported to be of the order of 1:20,000 or less. Sulfonamides should not be used to treat meningococcal meningitis since many meningococci are resistant to sulfonamide. It usually is recommended that penicillin be given for 5 to 10 days for the treatment of meningococcal meningitis, but experience acquired during the

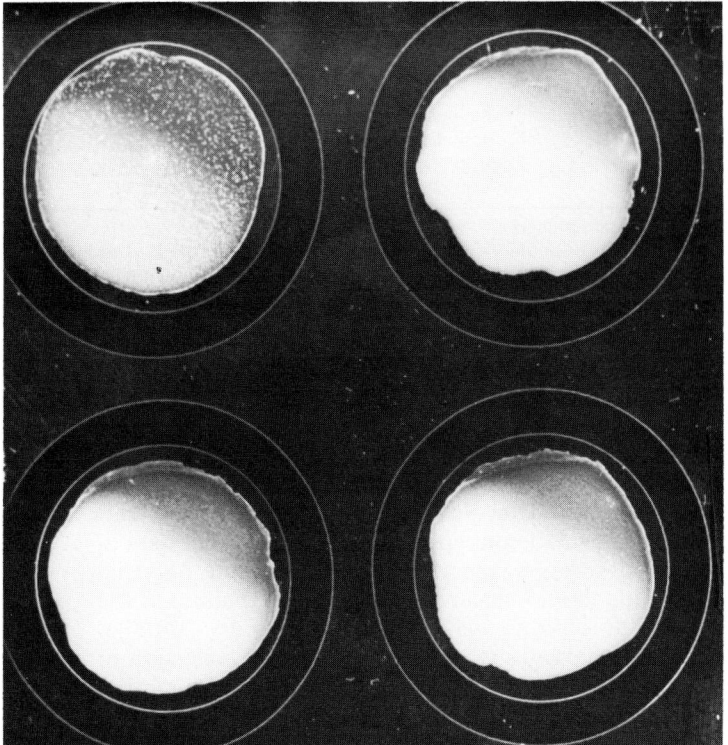

FIGURE 43–3. A latex test for the detection of bacterial antigens in CSF. A drop of CSF is mixed with latex particles coated with antibody to the meningococcus, pneumococcus, or *H. influenzae*. In this instance, agglutination (top left corner) has been produced by an antiserum to group A meningococcal capsular polysaccharide antigen.

management of major outbreaks of meningococcal meningitis (Chapter 42) suggests that such a course of treatment may be unnecessarily long.

Pneumococcal Meningitis. A patient with pneumococcal meningitis should be started on treatment with penicillin while the results of sensitivity tests are awaited. This must be given in high doses for at least 2 weeks to be effective. A number of penicillin-resistant strains of pneumococci have been isolated recently. Clinicians must be prepared to change from penicillin to another antibiotic if clinical or laboratory evidence of penicillin resistance is obtained. Most penicillin-resistant strains of pneumococci are sensitive to ampicillin. Strains of pneumococci have been identified, initially in South Africa, however, that are resistant to penicillin, ampicillin, tetracycline, chloramphenicol, and erythromycin and that are sensitive only to rifampicin, vancomycin, bacitracin, and fusidic acid. Fortunately, such multiple antibiotic-resistant strains are not widespread.

H. influenzae Meningitis. Chloramphenicol, rather than ampicillin, is the treatment of choice for *H. influenzae* meningitis because many strains of *H. influenzae* are now ampicillin-resistant, although the incidence of ampicillin resistance varies from area to area. If antibiotic sensitivity tests show that an isolate is ampicillin-

sensitive, a change to this antibiotic can then be made. Some pediatricians recommend that both ampicillin and chloramphenicol be given until the results of sensitivity tests are known. A few chloramphenicol-resistant strains of *H. influenzae* have been identified. Antibiotic treatment should be continued for 10 days.

E. coli Meningitis. A combination of intravenous chloramphenicol and intravenous gentamicin is recommended as the initial treatment for meningitis caused by gram-negative bacilli until the results of antibiotic sensitivity tests have been obtained. Controversy exists about the benefits obtained from gentamicin given by intrathecal injection.

Meningitis Without Bacteriologic Diagnosis. Chloramphenicol is the antibiotic of choice for the treatment of patients with acute bacterial meningitis in whom no bacteriologic diagnosis can be made, because this antibiotic penetrates well into the CSF and is effective against most isolates of meningococci, pneumococci, *H. influenzae*, and *E. coli*. No evidence suggests that a combination of penicillin and chloramphenicol is more effective than chloramphenicol alone.

New Antibiotics. Studies have shown that a number of third-generation cephalosporins are effective forms of treatment for acute bacterial meningitis because they

TABLE 43–4. Comparison of the Latex Test and Gram Stain and Culture in the Diagnosis of Acute Pyogenic Meningitis*

		Percentage Positive	
Diagnosis	Number of Samples Tested	*Latex Test*	*Routine Bacterial Culture and Gram Stain*
Meningococcal meningitis	126	88	79
Pneumococcal meningitis	87	82	67
H. influenzae meningitis	16	94	69
Not meningitis	162	0	0

*From Whittle HC, et al.: Lancet 2:619, 1974.

TABLE 43–5. Antibiotic Therapy Recommended for Initial Treatment of Patients with Acute Bacterial Meningitis*

Type of Meningitis	Antibiotic	Route	Dose		Duration (Days)
			Adults	*Children†*	
Meningococcal	Crystalline penicillin	IV or IM	2 megaunits every 6 hr	1 megaunit every 6 hr	5–7
Pneumococcal	Crystalline penicillin	IV then IM	4 megaunits every 6 hr	1–2 megaunits every 6 hr	14
H. influenzae	Chloramphenicol	IV or IM then PO	500 mg every 6 hr	25 mg/kg every 6 hr	10
Undiagnosed	Chloramphenicol	IV or IM then PO	500 mg every 6 hr	25 mg/kg every 6 hr	14

IM = intramuscular; IV = intravenous; PO = orally.
*The results of antibiotic sensitivity tests or a failure to respond to treatment may necessitate a change of therapy.
†Caution is required in the administration of chloramphenicol to infants. Neonates should not receive more than 50 mg/kg/day.

have a high level of activity against each of the three main causes of acute bacterial meningitis. Ceftriaxone is especially effective because it has a long half-life and it needs to be given only once per day. Unfortunately, ceftriaxone is too expensive for widespread use in most developing countries.

Assessment of the Response to Treatment. The temperature, level of consciousness, and neurologic state of a patient who is receiving treatment for acute bacterial meningitis should be carefully monitored. Failure of the patient to improve within 48 hours of the start of antibiotic therapy suggests that a localized collection of pus has formed or that an inappropriate antibiotic has been given. A patient who shows a deterioration in neurologic state during the course of treatment should be investigated for the presence of a space-occupying lesion by any of the available appropriate diagnostic means. If it is impossible to perform such investigations, and, if there are strong clinical grounds for suspecting an extradural collection of fluid or pus, exploratory bur holes should be made. Unfortunately, fluid collections are not always found in such patients; a late deterioration in neurologic state may be caused by a vascular occlusion.

A secondary rise in temperature during the course of treatment should suggest the possibility of an extradural abscess, the collection of pus at another site to which the causative organism has seeded, a drug reaction, or, in the case of a patient with meningococcal meningitis, the development of allergic complications.

Some physicians recommend that CSF changes should be monitored regularly throughout the course of treatment. It is uncertain, however, whether repeated examinations of CSF add much to the information that can be obtained by regular and careful clinical examination. Nevertheless, a second lumbar puncture should be performed in any patient who fails to improve after 48 hours of antibiotic treatment in case the initial bacteriologic diagnosis was incorrect or a resistant organism is present.

PROGNOSIS. The most important factor that determines the course and prognosis of acute bacterial meningitis is the cause. Most patients with meningococcal meningitis who are treated promptly with an appropriate antibiotic make a rapid and uneventful recovery. Hospital-based surveys in developing countries have shown that the overall mortality rate of treated cases is usually in the range of 5 to 10%. The mortality rate among untreated patients is approximately 50%. About 10% of patients with meningococcal meningitis develop allergic complications (Chapter 42). Some patients who

recover from meningococcal meningitis are left with a degree of deafness, but other residual neurologic defects are unusual.

In contrast to the good prognosis of patients with meningococcal meningitis, the outlook for patients with pneumococcal meningitis is poor. Surveys performed in various parts of the tropics have shown that the overall mortality rate for this infection is about 50%, even when treated appropriately, and that about half of the survivors are left with a serious neurologic defect. Severe impairment of consciousness, a short history, and associated pneumonia are all poor prognostic signs. A few patients with pneumococcal meningitis have turbid CSF containing bacteria but few white blood cells; such patients rarely recover. Why the prognosis of patients with pneumococcal meningitis is so much worse than that of patients with meningococcal meningitis is not understood.

The outlook for a patient with *H. influenzae* meningitis is closer to that of patients with meningococcal meningitis than to that of patients with pneumococcal meningitis.

PREVENTION AND CONTROL. The use of chemoprophylaxis and vaccine to control meningococcal disease is covered in Chapter 42.

Chemoprophylaxis. Chemoprophylaxis has been used less widely in the prevention of pneumococcal and *H. influenzae* infections than in the prevention of meningococcal disease. There is strong evidence, however, that penicillin gives some protection against pneumococcal infection in patients with sickle cell disease, and these patients should be given regular prophylaxis with penicillin until at least the age of 5 years. Because of the high risk of secondary infection in young children who have been in close contact with a patient with an *H. influenzae* infection, it has been suggested that they be given prophylaxis with rifampicin.

Vaccines. Pneumococcal polysaccharide vaccines that contain up to 23 different capsular polysaccharide antigens are commercially available. These vaccines protect against pneumococcal pneumonia and, almost certainly, against pneumococcal meningitis. Protection is achieved only against infection with organisms that belong to the vaccine serotypes. In most parts of the industrialized world, pneumococci that belong to the vaccine serogroups account for about 80% of all pneumococcal infections. This situation, however, may not necessarily apply in all parts of the tropics. Pneumococcal polysaccharide vaccines share many of the properties of meningococcal polysaccharide vaccines. They are poorly immunogenic in the young; they do not induce immunologic memory; and they are expensive. Consequently, pneumococcal capsular polysaccharide vaccines have not been used widely in developing countries where the main indication for their use would be the prevention of deaths from pneumococcal pneumonia in young children. A trial undertaken in Papua New Guinea, however, has shown that a pneumococcal capsular polysaccharide vaccine was effective in reducing overall mortality and mortality from acute respiratory infections even when given to infants. Further studies to confirm this important finding are needed. In the meanwhile, the use of pneumococcal capsular polysaccharide vaccines should be restricted to groups at risk such as patients with sickle cell disease, who should receive both pneumococcal vaccine, given at the age of 1 or 2 years, and penicillin prophylaxis.

A vaccine against *H. influenzae* prepared from the capsular polysaccharide of the bacterium is widely available. Unfortunately, this vaccine provides satisfactory protection only in older children and, in the United States, it is licensed for use only in children aged 24 months or older. This vaccine would be of little use in tropical developing countries where most cases of meningitis caused by *H. influenzae* occur before the age of 1 year. During the past few years, however, a number of new *H. influenzae* conjugated vaccines have been developed that comprise the capsular polysaccharide linked to a carrier protein. These vaccines are immunogenic in infants and induce immunologic memory. Encouraging results have been obtained in Finland with a diphtheria toxoid/polysaccharide conjugate given at the ages of 3, 4, and 6 months, and trials of other conjugate vaccines are in progress.

The pneumococcus, the meningococcus, and *H. influenzae* are major causes of mortality and morbidity among children in tropical developing countries. An urgent need exists, therefore, for effective vaccines against these bacteria that could be incorporated into existing infant immunization programs. Progress in the development of conjugate vaccines suggests that this is an achievable goal.

BIBLIOGRAPHY

Coonrod JD: Agglutination techniques for the detection of microbial antigens: methodology and overview. *In* Coonrod JD, Kunz LJ, Ferraro MJ (eds.): The Direct Detection of Microorganisms in Clinical Samples. Orlando, Academic Press, 1983, p 135.

Del Rio M de los A, Chrane D, Shelton S, et al.: Ceftriaxone versus ampicillin and chloramphenicol for treatment of bacterial meningitis in children. Lancet 1:1241, 1983.

Eskola J, Peltola H, Takala AK, et al.: Efficacy of *Haemophilus influenzae* type b polysaccharide-diphtheria toxoid conjugate vaccine in infancy. N Engl J Med 317:717, 1987.

Greenwood BM: The epidemiology of acute bacterial meningitis in tropical Africa. *In* Williams JD, Burnie J (eds.): Bacterial Meningitis. London, Academic Press, 1987, p 61.

Ingram DL: Bacterial meningitis symposium. Pediatrics 52:586, 1973.

Scheld WM, Quagliarello VJ, Lesse AJ: Selected aspects of the pathogenesis and pathophysiology of bacterial meningitis. *In* Williams JD, Burnie J (eds.): Bacterial Meningitis. London, Academic Press, 1987, p 1.

Shann F, Barker J, Poore P: Chloramphenicol alone versus chloramphenicol plus penicillin for bacterial meningitis in children. Lancet 2:681, 1985.

SECTION F

SEXUALLY TRANSMITTED BACTERIAL DISEASES

44. GONOCOCCAL INFECTIONS

Thomas A. Bell
and Peter L. Perine

DEFINITION. Gonorrhea is caused by *Neisseria gonorrhoeae* and is almost always transmitted sexually. In adults, infection is localized usually in the urogenital tract. The most common manifestation in men is purulent urethritis; in women, endocervicitis or vaginitis. Asymptomatic infections occur in both sexes. Complications include epididymo-orchitis, urethral stricture, batholinitis, salpingitis, perihepatitis, bacteremia, arthritis-dermatitis syndrome, chorioamnionitis, endocarditis, and meningitis. Proctitis and pharyngitis are common manifestations in male homosexuals. *N. gonorrhoeae* is transmitted readily to newborns at birth; manifestations include severe conjunctivitis, arthritis, and septicemia.

ETIOLOGY. *N. gonorrhoeae* is a gram-negative diplococcus. On "chocolate" agar, it forms small mucoid colonies. Presumptive identification may be made by gram-staining these colonies and testing them for oxidase. *N. gonorrhoeae* differs from other species of *Neisseria* by fermenting glucose but not lactose, maltose, or sucrose. Confirmatory tests include DNA-hybridization, coagglutination tests with monoclonal antibodies, determination of nutritional requirements, and analysis of enzymes. In most parts of the world, samples of isolates from patients should be tested for production of beta-lactamase and for susceptibility to tetracycline and penicillin.

The cell wall of *N. gonorrhoeae* contains lipopolysaccharide, protein, and phospholipid. Fimbriae or pili project from the cell wall and help the organisms attach to the host cell and resist phagocytosis by leukocytes.

Antigens and Immunity. Gonococcal fimbriae, lipopolysaccharide, and the outer membrane proteins are antigenic. Repeated infections by *N. gonorrhoeae* do not produce immunity to reinfection but may protect against recurrence of pelvic inflammatory disease (PID) caused by the same strain. Persons who lack terminal components of complement are particularly susceptible to repeated episodes of gonococcal bacteremia.

Strains of *N. gonorrhoeae* that cause bacteremia or disseminated infection are resistant to killing by pooled human serum complement. These strains usually require arginine, hypoxanthine, and uracil (A⁻H⁻U⁻) for growth and are especially susceptible to antibiotics. They are common in asymptomatic infections in North America and Europe but rare in the tropics.

Penicillin-Resistant Strains. Gonococcal plasmids that encode for production of beta-lactamases, which degrade penicillin, were detected in 1976. Penicillinase-producing *N. gonorrhoeae* is now common in Africa and Asia. The "African" and "Asian" plasmids have masses of 3.2 and 4.4 megadaltons, respectively. Other plasmids have appeared recently in other areas, and the original plasmids are now endemic in parts of North America and Europe.

EPIDEMIOLOGY

Distribution and Prevalence. Gonorrhea is common in the tropics and deserves more attention from public health agencies there. The social and economic costs of gonorrhea result from the blindness, infertility, ectopic pregnancy, and maternal deaths that it causes. The prevalence of asymptomatic gonorrhea in women in contraception clinics in Africa may be as high as 18%. The prevalence among female prostitutes in Asia is even higher. These women are an important source of gonorrhea for migrant male workers.

In parts of Africa, one third to one half of women are infertile from pelvic inflammatory disease, which is the most common reason for admissions to hospital gynecology services. In Sweden, the prevalence rates of involuntary infertility caused by pelvic inflammatory disease are 13%, 35%, and 75% after 1, 2, and 3 episodes of disease, respectively. Comparable data for tropical countries are not available. In comparison to tubal infections caused by other organisms, gonococcal disease is more acutely symptomatic and less likely to lead to infertility, perhaps because women seek treatment sooner.

Transmission. The current pandemic of gonorrhea is related to increased migration, more permissive sexual mores, and perhaps the use of oral contraceptives; increasing antibiotic resistance of *N. gonorrhoeae* to antimicrobials, changes in the social roles of women, who often resort to prostitution in economic desperation, and migration of male laborers to rapidly growing cities are perhaps the most significant causes of the increase of gonorrhea in subSaharan Africa. Even in developed countries, government agencies have failed to reduce the incidence of gonorrhea despite the availability of diagnostic and therapeutic resources.

The probability of a man's acquiring gonorrhea from a single sexual exposure to an infected women is 5 to 35%; the converse probability for a woman is 50 to 70%. Most women with gonorrhea develop symptoms within 2 menstrual cycles of infection. In both sexes, asymptomatic infections may last for months. Most gonorrhea is transmitted by persons who have mild or no symptoms, such as sexual consorts of women with gonococcal PID. Although they comprise a small pro-

portion of all persons with gonorrhea, asymptomatic carriers have great epidemiologic importance, because they are treated rarely unless they are named as a sexual contact by someone diagnosed with gonorrhea.

CLINICAL MANIFESTATIONS

Urethritis. In men, the usual manifestations of gonorrhea are a purulent urethral discharge and dysuria. The incubation period is usually 3 to 7 days. This anterior urethritis may spread to the paraurethral glands of Skene and Littré. Formation of a urethral stricture may cause fistulas between the urethra and perineum—the "watering can" perineum. Untreated gonococcal urethritis usually resolves within 6 months.

N. gonorrhoeae may spread to the prostate, epididymis, and testes. Before the advent of antibiotics, about 25% of men with gonorrhea developed epididymitis, a complication that is now rare if urethritis is treated promptly. Infertility may occur in 25% of unilateral and in 40% of bilateral cases of gonococcal epididymitis.

In women, gonococcal urethritis is manifested by dysuria rather than noticeable urethral discharge, and is one cause of "sterile" pyuria, or "urethral syndrome," when urine is only cultured on standard culture medium.

Endocervicitis. Gonococcal infection of the endocervix usually causes mild symptoms, such as vaginal discharge or bleeding. Pus is present often in the endocervical canal. It appears yellow or green on a white swab used to collect secretions from the endocervix. However, most women with cervicitis do not have grossly visible mucopus.

Pelvic Inflammatory Disease. Within 2 menstrual cycles after acquisition of *N. gonorrhoeae,* 10 to 20% of women develop infection of the endometrium, fallopian tubes, or other uterine adnexa. Signs and symptoms include fever, lower abdominal pain, dyspareunia, abnormal vaginal bleeding, pain with cervical motion, uterine and adnexal tenderness, and endocervical mucopus.

About one quarter of women have a second episode of PID. As with initial episodes of *N. gonorrhoeae* infection, facultative and anaerobic bacteria and *Chlamydia trachomatis* are associated with recurrences. Later, ectopic pregnancy and chronic pelvic pain are late sequelae in 2 to 5% of cases of PID.

Gonococcal Perihepatitis (Fitz-Hugh–Curtis Syndrome). In about 15% of cases of PID, the liver capsule becomes inflamed and adheres to the peritoneum. Signs and symptoms of perihepatitis include fever, right upper quadrant percussion-tenderness, and a friction rub. Blood levels of liver enzymes may be mildly elevated, but jaundice is rare. Gonococcal perihepatitis occurs almost exclusively in women.

Anorectal Infection. Most gonococcal infections of the anus and rectum are asymptomatic. Symptoms result from infection of the anal crypts and include mucopurulent anal discharge, rectal pruritus, and tenesmus. Gonococcal proctitis is common in homosexual men who practice passive anal intercourse, in whom anorectal gonorrhea is often associated with infection by other venereal and enteric pathogens. Women may become infected by spread of infected vaginal contents.

Gonococcal Bacteremia. Symptomatic gonococcal

bacteremia is rare. Women are more susceptible than men, especially during menses. Manifestations of disseminated gonococcal infection include fever and chills, tenosynovitis, and polyarthritis. The last usually affects no more than 3 joints asymmetrically. Painful pustular, hemorrhagic, or necrotic skin lesions develop on the distal extremities (Fig. 44–1). In about one half of cases, gonococci can be detected in these lesions by isolation or staining with fluorescent antibodies or Gram stain. Blood cultures yield *N. gonorrhoeae* in 50% of patients during the early stages of bacteremia if special culture medium without sodium polyanethol sulfonate is used. This syndrome usually resolves spontaneously without serious sequelae.

Gonococcal Arthritis. *N. gonorrhoeae* is the most common cause of septic arthritis in young adults. It may develop suddenly in 1 or 2 joints—usually the knee, elbow, ankle, or wrist—and without skin lesions. Fever is common. The joint contains a moderate amount of fluid and is painful when moved. Without treatment, the joint may be rapidly destroyed.

Other Septic Complications. Other complications of gonococcal bacteremia are now rare. They include peri-, myo-, and endocarditis, hepatitis, and meningitis.

Gonococcal Pharyngitis. Pharyngeal gonorrhea is asymptomatic usually and is found in persons who practice fellatio and cunnilingus. Transmission by kissing alone is extremely rare, and isolates from suspected cases should be rigorously differentiated from commensal flora such as *Neisseria cinerea.*

Neonatal Infections. Newborns may become infected via amnionic fluid or passage through an infected birth canal. The conjunctiva, pharynx, joints, leptomeninges, vagina, anus, joints, and blood may be infected also. Most cases of gonococcal conjunctivitis can be prevented by instillation of 1% silver nitrate eye drops, or 0.5% erythromycin ointment, or 1% tetracycline ointment given shortly after birth. Such prophylaxis does not prevent extraocular infection.

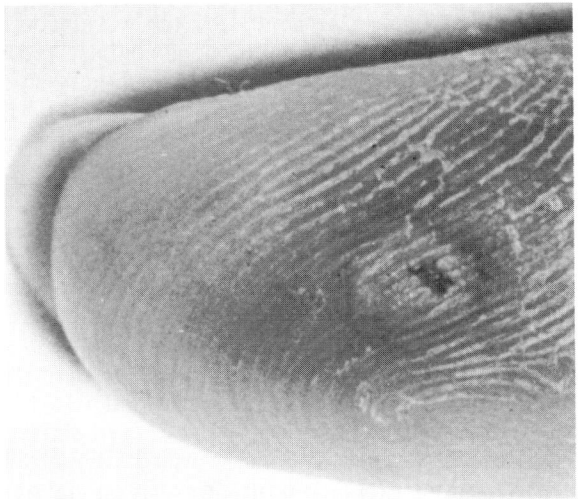

FIGURE 44–1. Gonorrhea. Painful, pustular skin lesion caused by *N. gonorrhoeae* bacteremia. The organisms can be identified in the biopsy tissue from such a lesion by Gram stain or by fluorescein-conjugated antibodies to *N. gonorrhoeae* but rarely by culture.

Neonatal gonococcal conjunctivitis is still a major cause of blindness in much of Africa and Asia. Symptoms in neonates usually begin 2 to 8 days after birth. The eyelids become red and swollen and exude copious pus (Fig. 44–2). Without treatment, the cornea may be destroyed in a few days. Adults may acquire gonococcal conjunctivitis by inoculation of their own or a consort's genital secretions.

Prepubertal Infections. Gonorrhea in prepubertal children is acquired almost always by sexual contact with infected adults—often members of, or visitors in, their household. Manifestations include urethritis in boys, vulvovaginitis in girls, and pharyngitis and proctitis in both sexes. Transmission by fomites in the tropics, where the ambient temperature and humidity may prolong survival of the *N. gonorrhoeae,* has been postulated, but such transmission should not be accepted until sexual abuse has been *rigorously* excluded.

DIAGNOSIS
The Gram Stain. The Gram stain is most useful for diagnosis of symptomatic urethritis and conjunctivitis and is almost perfectly specific for diagnosis of gonococcal urethritis in symptomatic men; the sensitivity is at least 95%. Only gram-negative intracellular diplococci with typical morphology are diagnostic (Fig. 44–3). If only extracellular organisms are seen, *N. gonorrhoeae* is probably not present. In women, the Gram stain is perhaps 60% sensitive compared to culture and is quite specific if evaluated properly. The Gram stain is not reliable for detecting pharyngeal infections.

Isolation. *N. gonorrhoeae* is usually cultured from the urethra or cervix with a medium that contains antibiotics (e.g., colistin, vancomycin, and nystatin) to inhibit growth of other bacteria and yeasts. Culture of endocervical specimens alone will detect about 85% of gonococcal infections in women. Another 5 to 10% more will be detected by culturing specimens from the anus also, and another 5% by urethral and pharyngeal cultures. The culture is negative in some infected patients of both sexes because the inoculum size is inadequate or, more commonly, because some strains are susceptible to the inhibitory antibiotics in the culture medium. Thus, a nonselective medium should be used for anatomic sites without competing flora, e.g., the conjunctiva. More than 2 hours' delay in placing an inoculated culture plate in an atmosphere of 5% carbon dioxide, e.g., a candle jar, or failure to incubate the culture at the proper temperature (35 to 37C) may invalidate the culture also.

In men, culture of first-voided urine is more sensitive than culture of urethral swabs. Urine cultures detect about 80% of cases in women with positive cervical cultures and are obtained more easily. Self-obtained vaginal cultures may be useful in some settings.

Serology. Commercial tests for gonococcal antibodies are not useful clinically because they do not distinguish current from prior infection.

DIFFERENTIAL DIAGNOSIS (Chapter 10)
Urethritis. Other causes of urethritis include *Chlamydia trachomatis* (Chapter 30), *Ureaplasma urealyticum,* and *Trichomonas vaginalis.* All may coexist with *N. gonorrhoeae.* The presence of dysuria and a urethral

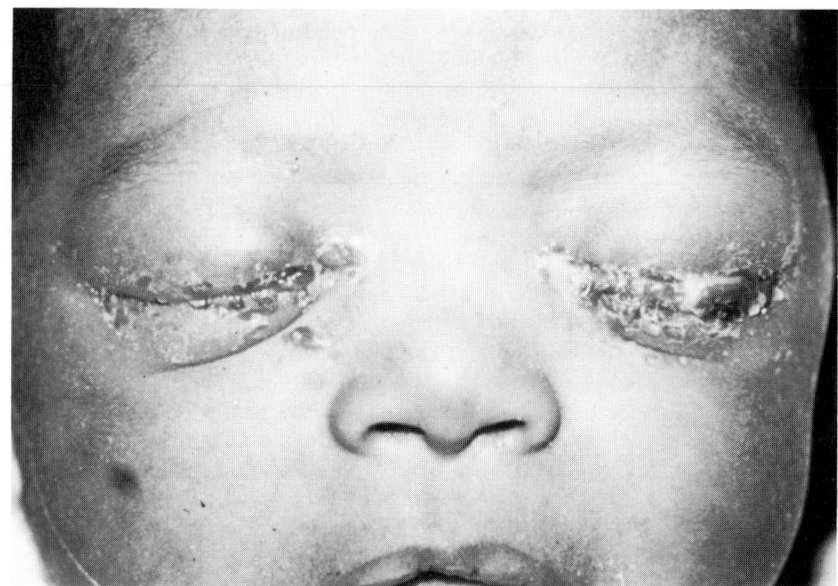

FIGURE 44–2. Gonorrhea. Gonococcal ophthalmia neonatorum, which almost always involves both eyes.

discharge that is spontaneous or can be expressed easily from the penis is characteristic of *N. gonorrhoeae.* Cultures for *N. gonorrhoeae* are warranted when the Gram stain of exudate from the urethra or cervix is negative or equivocal.

Cervicitis and Vaginitis. *N. gonorrhoeae* may coexist in the cervix with *C. trachomatis.* Cervical gonorrhea usually causes a mild vaginal discharge; more profuse discharges are likely to be caused by *T. vaginalis* (Chapter 72), bacterial vaginosis ("nonspecific vaginitis"), or *Candida albicans* (Chapter 64.3).

Pelvic Inflammatory Disease. A clinical diagnosis of PID based on only a few signs and symptoms is often

incorrect; in such cases laparoscopy often reveals only normal fallopian tubes or other diseases of the pelvis, such as acute appendicitis, ectopic pregnancy, ovarian cysts, or torsion. The accuracy of the clinical diagnosis increases with the number of abnormal findings present. Suspected cases with mild abnormalities should be treated vigorously to prevent sequelae.

Neonatal Conjunctivitis. In many tropical areas, *N. gonorrhoeae* is the most common cause of purulent conjunctivitis in newborns. Infants who receive silver nitrate prophylaxis often have chemical conjunctivitis in the first day of life. After that, time of onset within the first few weeks does not help distinguish among microbial etiologies. As with genital infections, *C. trachomatis* is often acquired concurrently but is manifested later (Chapter 28). Other important causes of neonatal conjunctivitis include unencapsulated *Haemophilus influenzae, Streptococcus pneumoniae, Staphylococcus aureus,* and enterococci.

TREATMENT. In recent years, the treatment of gonorrhea has been complicated by the worldwide dissemination of strains resistant to penicillins, tetracyclines, and spectinomycin. Such resistance may be mediated either by plasmids or the chromosome, and may become established in diverse strains after it is imported into a geographic area. Drugs such as ceftriaxone, which is now the treatment of choice in many industrialized countries, may not be affordable in developing countries. The recommendations mentioned here are attempts to achieve a balance between efficacy and economy. Their appropriateness should be considered only temporary, because the development of new drugs or new kinds of resistance in *N. gonorrhoeae* may make them obsolete. Where it can be afforded in tropical countries, ceftriaxone is probably the drug of choice for all gonococcal infections, unless susceptibility to less expensive antimicrobials can be shown. Regional health agencies should monitor the patterns of susceptibility of *N. gonorrhoeae* to antimicrobials and periodically revise recommendations for treatment.

Uncomplicated Infections. In much of Asia and Af-

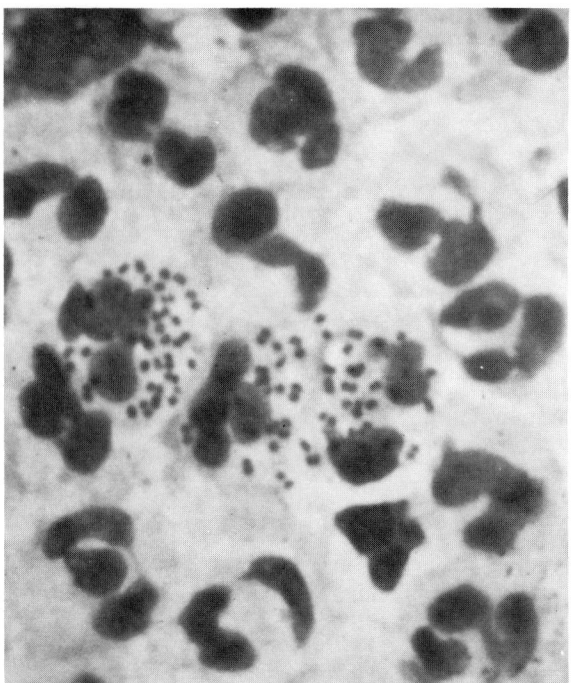

FIGURE 44–3. Gonorrhea. Gram stain of urethral exudate showing the gram-negative diplococci within the cytoplasm of polymorphonuclear leukocytes.

rica, *N. gonorrhoeae* is resistant usually to penicillins and tetracyclines. Other therapeutic considerations include the likelihood of the patient taking the drug as prescribed, the cost and availability of the drug, and the likelihood of concurrent infection. The following drug regimens are usually effective for treatment of uncomplicated gonorrhea caused by strains susceptible to penicillins:

- Aqueous procaine penicillin G, 4,800,000 units intramuscularly (half in each buttock), with 1 gm of oral probenecid.
- Ampicillin 3.5 gm or amoxicillin 3 gm, as a single oral dose with 1 gm of oral probenecid.
- Tetracycline hydrochloride 500 mg orally 4 times daily.
- Trimethoprim 720 mg/sulfamethoxazole 3600 mg once daily for 3 days.

Each of these regimens has disadvantages. Aqueous procaine penicillin has the best cure rate and aborts incubating syphilis, but carries the highest risk of anaphylaxis and may cause acute procaine toxicity. It is preferred for men with anorectal infection and for pregnant women. Pharyngeal infection is difficult to eradicate with any of these regimens, but may be treated with several days' treatment with amoxicillin or trimethoprim/sulfamethoxazole. Ampicillin and tetracycline may cause abdominal pain, anorexia, nausea, and emesis.

Therapy with tetracycline or sulfonamide is indicated if tetracycline is not used for treating the *N. gonorrhoeae* (Chapter 30). Tetracycline and trimethoprim/sulfamethoxazole are useful also for patients allergic to penicillins. Persons who cannot tolerate either drug may be treated with an intramuscular injection of 2 gm of spectinomycin hydrochloride. Treatment for concurrent *C. trachomatis* then would be with erythromycin 500 mg 4 times daily for 7 days. Sexual partners of patients with gonorrhea should be treated simultaneously, regardless of culture results.

Patients treated for uncomplicated gonorrhea should be re-evaluated 3 to 7 days after completing therapy. Initially, infected anatomic sites should be tested again for eradication of infection. Cultures or Gram stains positive for *N. gonorrhoeae* indicate treatment failure, reinfection, or possible infection by resistant strains. Patients in whom treatment with procaine penicillin, ampicillin, tetracycline, or trimethoprim/sulfamethoxazole is unsuccessful should be given intramuscular kanamycin or spectinomycin 2 gm or ceftriaxone 250 mg in 1% lidocaine. *N. gonorrhoeae* isolated after treatment should be tested for resistance to antimicrobials also.

Drug-resistant *N. gonorrhoeae*. Therapy of uncomplicated gonorrhea in areas where drug-resistant strains are prevalent—most of Southeast Asia and subSaharan Africa—poses a difficult choice among drugs that are not simultaneously efficacious, affordable, and safe. Spectinomycin and kanamycin are effective in such situations but lack activity against *Treponema pallidum* (Chapter 32.1) and *C. trachomatis* (Chapter 30). Chloramphenicol and its cogeners, tetracyclines, and trimethoprim/sulfamethoxazole are not optimally effective

against resistant strains of *N. gonorrhoeae,* and the last is ineffective against syphilis. Cephalosporins that resist beta-lactamase are expensive and ineffective against *C. trachomatis.*

Pelvic Inflammatory Disease and Other Complications. Complicated gonococcal infections require longer treatment. Women with pelvic infection with susceptible *N. gonorrhoeae* and without abscesses, ectopic pregnancy, or severe illness can be treated as outpatients with tetracycline 500 mg orally 4 times daily for 10 days, or with aqueous procaine penicillin, followed by oral ampicillin or amoxicillin 500 mg 4 times daily for a total of 10 days. Infections caused by drug-resistant *N. gonorrhoeae* should be treated with a single intramuscular dose of ceftriaxone, 250 mg diluted in 1% lidocaine and then with oral drugs for associated flora, especially *C. trachomatis.*

Empiric therapy of PID is complicated by the diversity of organisms that may be present simultaneously. The presence of *N. gonorrhoeae* in the cervix does not indicate that other organisms are not present in the fallopian tubes. The following 10-day oral regimens may be useful in developing countries:

- Chloramphenicol 500 mg and sulfisoxazole 500 mg, 4 times daily.
- Tetracycline 500 mg and metronidazole 500 mg, 4 times daily.
- Ampicillin (or amoxicillin) 500 mg, 4 (or 3) times daily, and sulfisoxazole 500 mg, 4 times daily.
- Chloramphenicol 500 mg and tetracycline 500 mg, 4 times daily.

Women with severe PID should be hospitalized. The following intravenous regimens may be used until the patient is ready for discharge or for an oral regimen to complete 10 days of therapy:

- Tetracycline 250 mg and clindamycin 600 mg every 6 hours.
- Ampicillin 500 mg and sulfisoxazole 25 mg/kg every 6 hours.
- Clindamycin 600 mg every 6 hours and gentamicin or tobramycin 1 mg/kg every 8 hours.
- Chloramphenicol 500 mg and tetracycline 250 mg every 6 hours.

Intrauterine devices should be removed for several months. Oral contraceptives may be desirable for several months after an episode of PID, because they reduce its likelihood and severity.

Epididymitis. The treatment of choice for epididymitis in young men is tetracycline, 500 mg, 4 times daily for 10 days. In older men, co-trimoxazole is probably the drug of choice and is a good alternative for younger men.

Disseminated Gonococcal Infections. These can be treated initially with oral ampicillin 3.5 gm or amoxicillin 3 gm, each with probenecid 1 gm, and then with either ampicillin or amoxicillin 500 mg orally 4 times a day for 7 days; or with spectinomycin 2 gm intramuscularly twice daily for 3 days; or with erythromycin 500 mg, 4 times daily for 5 days. Patients with gonococcal arthritis, meningitis, or endocarditis require high-dose intravenous penicillin or ceftriaxone. Chloramphenicol 2 to 4 gm daily initially given intravenously, or tetracycline 500 mg intravenously every 6 hours for 10 days, is useful for gonococcal meningitis in patients allergic to penicillin, but ceftriaxone should be used where available unless the patient is allergic to cephalosporins also. Intravenous penicillin is recommended also for gonococcal joint infections. Repeated aspiration of the fluid from the septic joint through a large-bore needle may relieve pain, but open surgical drainage and intra-articular antibiotics are unnecessary.

Infections in Infants and Children

Gonococcal Conjunctivitis. This potentially devastating infection should be treated with ceftriaxone 25 mg/kg, suspended in 1% lidocaine not to exceed 1 mg/kg. These may be given intramuscularly. A single dose is usually curative and thus avoids the need for hospitalization. A less effective alternative is kanamycin, in a single dose of 50 mg/kg. Topical antibiotics are not required when systematic treatment is given and are inadequate if given alone.

Children weighing less than 45 kg with uncomplicated gonorrhea can be treated by the following single-dose regimens: amoxicillin 50 mg/kg orally with probenecid 25 mg/kg (maximum 1 gm); or aqueous procaine penicillin G, 100,000 units/kg intramuscularly, plus probenecid orally. Children less than 8 years old who are allergic to penicillin should be treated with spectinomycin 40 mg/kg intramuscularly (maximum 2 gm). Older children may be treated with oral tetracycline, 40 mg/kg daily in 4 divided doses for 5 days. Children with complicated gonococcal infections should be treated with one of the drug regimens used to treat the same complications in adults with doses adjusted for their weight.

PREVENTION AND CONTROL. Control of gonorrhea is enhanced by identification and treatment of sexual contacts of persons with proven cases. Often, this is not possible with the limited resources of tropical countries. Patients with gonorrhea should be encouraged to refer their sexual partners for treatment. Index patients should not be given oral antibiotics for their sexual partners, because such medication often is taken inappropriately, saved for future use, sold, or discarded.

In developing countries, periodic screening of prostitutes, migrant workers, and military personnel will probably be the most productive gonorrhea control measures. This may be done by culturing first-catch urine or by first screening such urine for leukocytes or leukocyte esterase. Treatment of sexual partners of women with acute PID should decrease the reservoir of asymptomatic gonorrhea. Public education programs about gonorrhea and other venereal diseases, government control of the sale of antibiotics, education of health-care providers, and provision of facilities for free diagnosis and treatment are essential for control of the current pandemic of gonorrhea.

BIBLIOGRAPHY

Centers for Disease Control: Sexually transmitted disease treatment guidelines. 1989. MMWR 38(Suppl 8), 1989.

Fransen L, D'Costa L, Ronald AR, et al.: Single-dose kanamycin therapy of gonococcal ophthalmia neonatorum. Lancet 2:1234, 1984.

Laga M, Plummer FA, Piot P, et al.: Prophylaxis of gonococcal and chlamydial ophthalmia neonatorum: A comparison of silver nitrate and tetracycline. N Engl J Med 318:653, 1988.

Meheus A: Gonorrhea. Baillière's Clin Trop Med Comm Dis 2:17, 1987.

Plorde DS: Sexually transmitted diseases in Ethiopia: Social factors contributing to their spread and implication for developing countries. Br J Vener Dis 57:357, 1981.

45. CHANCROID

Thomas A. Bell
and Peter L. Perine

DEFINITION. Chancroid, or soft chancre, is an acute, autoinoculable, painful, ulcerative disease caused by *Haemophilus ducreyi*. Infection is usually sexually transmitted and localized to the anogenital area. It may be accompanied by suppurating inguinal buboes. Complications are local necrosis and destruction of anogenital tissue.

ETIOLOGY. *H. ducreyi* is a short, nonmotile, gram-negative rod with a characteristic streptobacillary "chaining" appearance on Gram stain. The organism is a facultative anaerobe and requires hemin for growth.

No virulence factors have been identified in *H. ducreyi*. Humans are the only natural host. Experimental infection can be produced in rabbits and monkeys by intradermal inoculation. Many strains do not produce lesions when inoculated into rabbits and are apparently nonpathogenic for humans as well.

PATHOGENESIS. Chancroid is autoinoculable, which suggests that *H. ducreyi* can penetrate the dermis, but the infection process is poorly understood. Minor skin trauma may facilitate infection. Other bacteria may be present in chancroid ulcers as contaminants or opportunistic pathogens. The degree to which these organisms contribute to formation of ulcers and destruction of tissue is unknown. No cellular toxins or endotoxins have been identified in *H. ducreyi* that would account for local tissue destruction. Consequently, *H. ducreyi* rarely causes bacteremia or other systemic complications, and it is rarely isolated in pure culture from buboes.

EPIDEMIOLOGY. Chancroid occurs worldwide. It is highly prevalent in much of tropical Africa and Asia and has recently increased in North America. Most clinical cases are diagnosed in men. Infected women may develop symptomatic genital ulcers, but most have no symptoms and may serve as the reservoir for infection. Mixed infections of chancroid and gonorrhea or other sexually transmitted diseases are common.

CLINICAL MANIFESTATIONS. The local genital lesion begins as an inflammatory papule at the site of the infection after an incubation period of 2 to 14 days, with an average of 5 days. The papule rapidly erodes to form a painful, nonindurated, irregular ulcer with slightly undermined edges (Fig. 45–1). The base of the ulcer is granular and is covered by a yellow-gray purulent exudate. The lesion bleeds easily when manipulated. Multiple ulcers are common. Through autoinoculation,

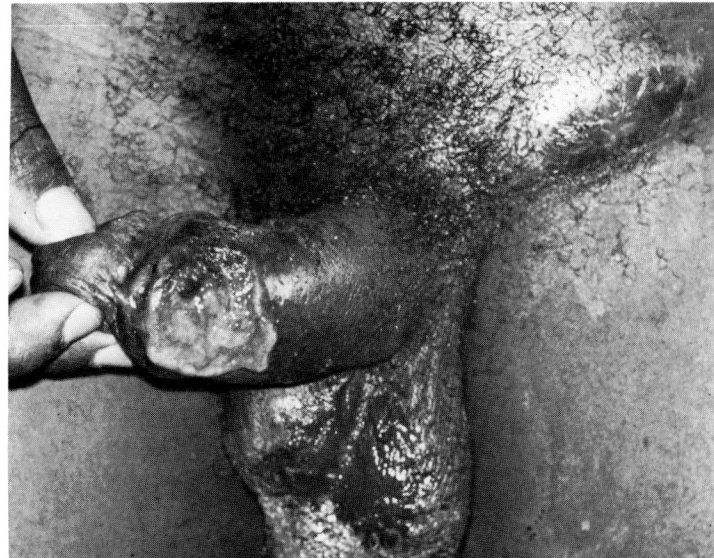

FIGURE 45–1. Chancroid. Large penile ulceration with a suppurative left inguinal bubo.

they proliferate if the disease remains untreated. The most common locations of the lesions in men are the shaft, prepuce, and frenulum and in the coronal sulcus of the penis. Autoinoculated lesions are common on the inner aspect of the thighs and on the scrotum. In women, the most frequent locations are the labia (Fig. 45–2), the vaginal fourchette, and the perianal region. Lesions may be autoinoculated anywhere on the body and are almost always accompanied by painful enlargement of the regional lymph nodes.

Inguinal lymphadenitis develops in 40 to 50% of men within 7 to 10 days after the appearance of the chancroidal ulcer; it is occasionally the initial manifestation of infection. The inguinal lymph nodes are acutely inflamed and tender and mat together to form a bubo. In 75% of cases, the bubo is unilateral and subsides without suppuration. Suppuration of the bubo often is associated with systemic manifestations such as fever, malaise, and

leukocytosis. Material aspirated from fluctuant buboes is thick and red in color and is usually sterile by Gram stain and culture. The suppurative bubo may spontaneously rupture and form a large inguinal ulcer, which heals slowly by fibrosis. There is no immunity to reinfection.

An alarmingly destructive "phagedenic" type of chancroid can destroy the skin and subcutaneous tissues of the genitalia. A single lesion of this type near the base of the penis can amputate the penis and scrotum within weeks or months. Whether such cases result from deficient host immunity or from infection with a particularly virulent strain of *H. ducreyi* is unknown. Fortunately, genital mutilation of this degree is rare today.

DIAGNOSIS

Isolation of Organisms. Definitive diagnosis of chancroid depends on the isolation of *H. ducreyi* from infected tissue; genital ulceration or other causes of inguinal lymphadenitis should be sought. Culture using a selective medium for presumptive identification of *H. ducreyi* is positive in 50 to 60% of clinically suspect ulcers. Optimal rates of isolation are obtained by using two media concurrently: gonococcal agar base containing bovine hemoglobulin 2% and Mueller-Hinton agar base with horse blood "chocolate" agar 5%; both media should contain 1% Isovitalex and vancomycin, 3 mg/L. Small, nonmucoid, yellow-gray translucent colonies appear on the surface of the agar after 2 to 9 days of incubation at 34°C in a candle-extinction jar: Gram staining of the colonies reveals gram-negative coccobacilli in short chains or in aggregates. Some organisms have bipolar staining. Staining of material from lesions is of little value because the polymicrobial flora of most ulcers interferes with the identification of *H. ducreyi*. The Gram stain diagnosis is more definitive when organisms with typical structures and parallel chains resembling schools of fish along strands of mucus are seen.

Differential Diagnosis. Most patients diagnosed as having chancroid in nonendemic areas are more likely to have genital herpes or secondarily infected traumatic lesions. Other diseases that should also be considered in the differential diagnosis of chancroid are primary

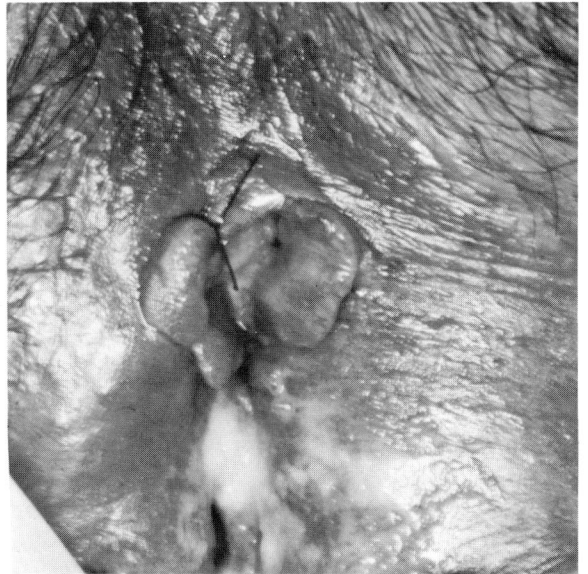

FIGURE 45–2. Chancroid. Labial lesion. (Courtesy of the Armed Forces Institute of Pathology, Photograph Neg. No. 82–9102.)

and secondary syphilis, lymphogranuloma venereum, and granuloma inguinale. Genital herpes usually presents with multiple vesicular lesions accompanied by nontender, bilateral, discrete, nonsuppurative inguinal lymphadenopathy. Genital chancroidal ulcers without inguinal lymphadenopathy, however, may be impossible to differentiate clinically from genital herpes. Syphilitic chancres have well-defined edges and are painless and indurated and contain spirochetes in darkfield microscopic specimens. The tender inguinal bubo of lymphogranuloma venereum is multilocular and is accompanied by constitutional symptoms such as fever, anorexia, and malaise. It usually occurs as the first manifestation of infection or after the evanescent primary genital lesion has healed. The genital ulcers of granuloma inguinale are painless, indurated, and chronic. The pseudobuboes of granuloma inguinale are subcutaneous masses of granulomatous tissue that overlie the inguinal nodes rather than a true lymphadenitis.

TREATMENT. Plasmids that confer resistance to antibiotics have spread widely in *H. ducreyi*. These plasmids are identical to those found in *Neisseria gonorrhoeae* and encode for production of β-lactamases. Penicillin-resistant *H. ducreyi* varies with locale, and treatment should be based on local patterns of susceptibility. The drug of choice is ceftriaxone in a dose of 250 mg diluted 1:1 with 1% lidocaine. Where its cost is prohibitive, treatment with 2 co-trimoxazole tablets, each containing 400 mg of sulfamethoxazole and 80 mg of trimethoprim, given twice a day for 7 to 10 days, or erythromycin, 500 mg given orally 4 times daily for 10 days is usually effective. Sulfamethoxazole alone or tetracycline is no longer recommended because of drug resistance. Fluctuant buboes should be aspirated with a large-bore needle and syringe to prevent rupture, since suppuration may progress despite effective antimicrobial therapy. Genital ulcers and ulcerating buboes can be treated with soaks containing a mild antiseptic such as a 1:4000 potassium permanganate solution.

PREVENTION. After cure, patients are susceptible to reinfection. Sexual partners should be treated concurrently. Condoms usually prevent transmission.

BIBLIOGRAPHY

Lubwama SW, Plummer FA, Ndinya-Achola J, et al.: Isolation and identification of *Haemophilus ducreyi* in a clinical laboratory. J Med Microbiol 22:175, 1986.
Nsanze H, Fast M, D'Costa LJ, et al.: Genital ulcer in Kenya: A clinical and laboratory study of 100 patients. Br J Vener Dis 57:378, 1981.
Nsanze H, Plummer FA, Maggwa ABN, et al.: Comparison of media for the primary isolation of *Haemophilus ducreyi*. Sex Transm Dis 11:6, 1984.
Schmid GP: The treatment of chancroid. JAMA 255:1757, 1986.

46. GRANULOMA INGUINALE

Peter L. Perine

DEFINITION. Granuloma inguinale (donovanosis, lymphogranuloma inguinale) is a chronic, superficial, granulomatous disease that affects primarily the anogenital area. It usually occurs in sexually active adults between the ages of 18 and 40 and is assumed to be a sexually transmitted disease. It is caused by *Calymmatobacterium granulomatis*, a gram-negative, pleomorphic bacillus found in the cytoplasm of large histiocytes in lesion biopsy specimens. The agent was thought to be a protozoan by Donovan, who discovered the organism in genital lesions in 1905. It has been known since as the Donovan body.

ETIOLOGY. The difficulty of growing *C. granulomatis* in vitro and the lack of an animal model have limited research on granuloma inguinale. Predominantly an intracellular parasite, it has a capsule, is nonmotile, and is antigenically related to certain species of *Klebsiella*. It has been recovered from the stool of asymptomatic persons.

Biopsy specimens or Giemsa-stained smears made from infected tissue reveal *C. granulomatis* within the cytoplasm of macrophages or histiocytes. The disease is limited to the skin and subcutaneous tissues and is autoinoculable. This indicates that the pathogenicity of the organism is limited and that it probably invades through small breaks in the skin or mucous membranes.

EPIDEMIOLOGY

Distribution and Incidence. Granuloma inguinale occurs worldwide, but its incidence is highest in the tropical areas of Africa, Asia, and Central and South America. It occurs predominantly among dark complexioned or black people. This is true even when the disease occurs in temperate climates, where it is rare. The highest reported occurrence of the disease, 10 to 35%, is in New Guinea.

Transmission. Poor personal hygiene and poverty favor infection. Genetic susceptibility may also be a contributing factor.

The anogenital area is the most common site of lesions. This location and sexual transmission may be related to the presence of *C. granulomatis* in normal stool. The skin of the genitals and perianal tissues might first be contaminated by *C. granulomatis* from stool, which is followed by invasion through skin or mucous membrane abrasions or lacerations as might be produced by trauma during sexual intercourse, anal intercourse, or close, nonsexual contact. Populations with a high incidence of granuloma inguinale may have high carrier rates for *C. granulomatis* in their stool or be genetically more susceptible to disease. Congenital transmission does not occur.

CLINICAL MANIFESTATIONS. The incubation period ranges from a few days to 3 months. The first lesion is a small, painless papule that erodes to form an indurated, slightly elevated ulcer. At first, the edges of the ulcer are elevated, and the surface glistens. As it enlarges, the base of the lesion becomes more granular and beefy-red and bleeds easily when scraped or manip-

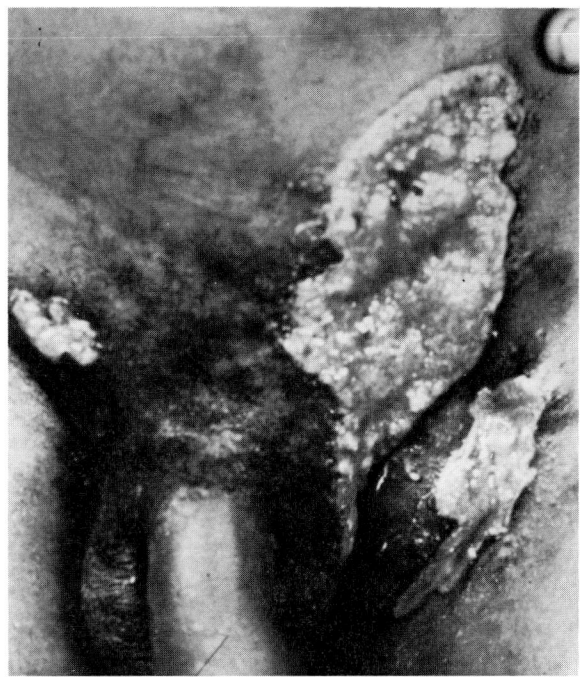

FIGURE 46–1. Granuloma inguinale. The subcutaneous granulomatous tissue has eroded through the skin in both inguinal areas. The surface of the granulation tissue glistens and is remarkably free of pus and necrotic debris.

ulated. Over several weeks or months, the ulcer grows several centimeters in diameter, extends to the fascia, and spreads subcutaneously into the groin or the perineum. Granulation tissue may project from the lesion, creating a grotesque but usually painless lesion that is well tolerated by the patient (Fig. 46–1). Many patients wait months before seeking treatment and do so only when the lesion becomes secondarily infected and pain-

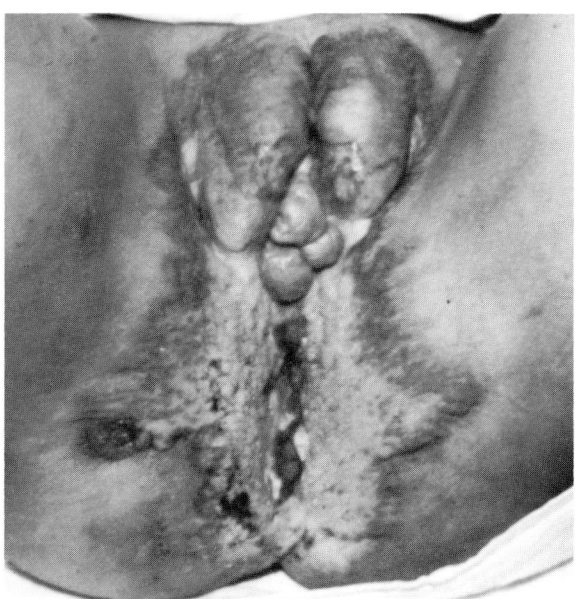

FIGURE 46–2. Granuloma inguinale. Involvement of the subcutaneous tissues of the groin, perineum, and perianal area. (Courtesy of the Armed Forces Institute of Pathology, Photograph Neg. No. 82–9105.)

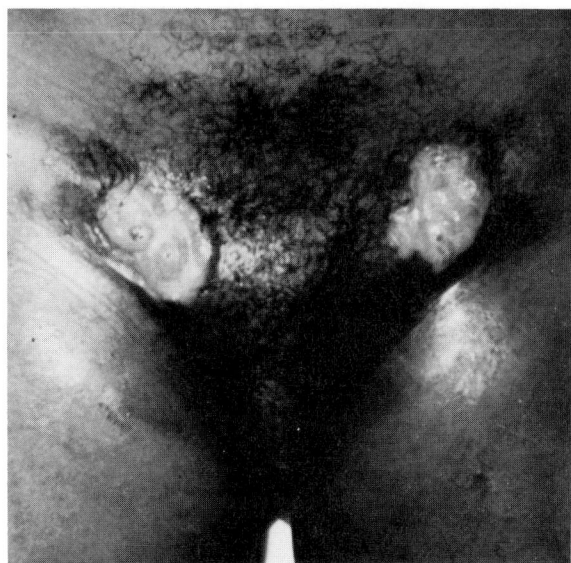

FIGURE 46–3. Granuloma inguinale. Broken-down inguinal pseudobuboes showing granulomatous subcutaneous tissue.

ful or when they become concerned about the destruction of genital tissue.

About half of the lesions of granuloma inguinale occur on the genitals; the remainder are found in the perineum and perianal area (Fig. 46–2) or in the inguinal region (Fig. 46–1). In men, the most common site of infection is the foreskin, where lesions may cause phimosis. Most genital lesions in women are on the labia or the vaginal fourchette and, less commonly, on the vaginal mucosa or the cervix. Subcutaneous lesions may form in the inguinal area over the inguinal lymph nodes to resemble inguinal buboes until the overlying skin ulcerates—the pseudobubo of granuloma inguinale (Fig. 46–3). These lesions usually do not involve the inguinal lymph nodes directly unless they become infected with other bacteria.

Extragenital lesions of granuloma inguinale may occur anywhere on the body by primary inoculation of these sites, by autoinoculation, or by direct spread from anogenital lesions. Like genital lesions, these also are mutilating if untreated. Not all lesions are progressive, but spontaneous healing is unusual and is accompanied by scarring.

Complications of granuloma inguinale include destruction of the external genitalia; local lymphatic obstruction, producing genital elephantiasis; fistula formation; and possible bacteremia. An association between granuloma inguinale and squamous cell carcinoma has been noted.

DIAGNOSIS. The diagnosis of granuloma inguinale is made by finding organisms with characteristic structure in a biopsy specimen or scraping taken from the active, granulating surface or the margin of a lesion. A small piece of tissue can be pressed ("spread") by the fingers between 2 glass slides, or a larger biopsy specimen can be fixed in 1 to 10% formalin. Wright-Giemsa or Leishman stains are commonly used. *C. granulomatis* stains bipolarly, often resembling a closed safety pin (Fig. 46–4). Tissue sections should be stained by silver impregnation because the organisms do not stain well with hematoxylin and eosin.

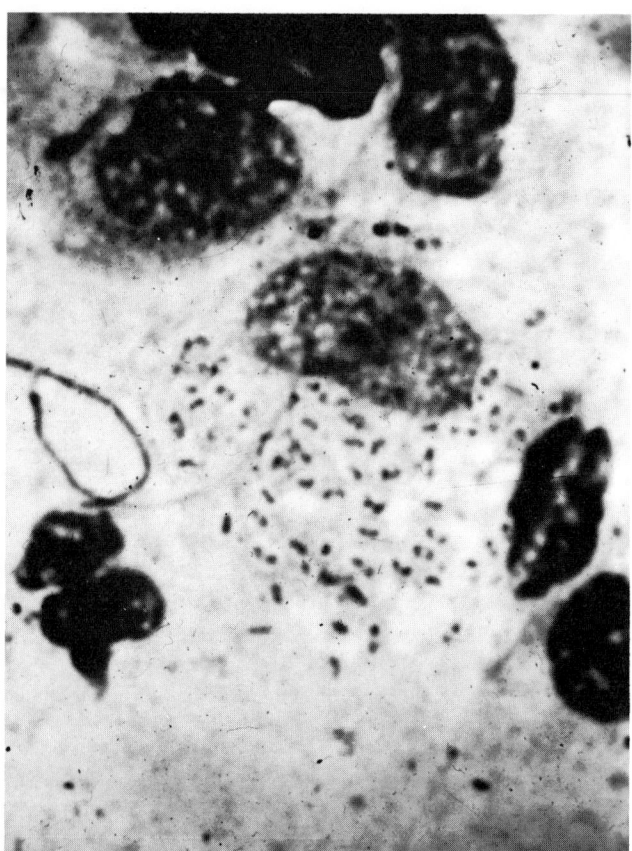

FIGURE 46–4. Granuloma inguinale. Donovan bodies in monocyte (Giemsa stain, × 2200). (Courtesy of the Armed Forces Institute of Pathology, Photograph Neg. No. TDS 106.)

Repeated examination of infected tissue is often necessary to find the organism in chronic lesions or in patients partially treated with antibiotics. Histologically, the lesion resembles squamous cell carcinoma. Granuloma inguinale usually can be differentiated from syphilis by darkfield microscopic examination and serologic tests for syphilis; from cutaneous amebiasis by biopsy and serologic tests; from lymphogranuloma venereum by tissue culture and serologic tests for *C. trachomatis*;

and from chancroid by culture of lesion material for *Haemophilus ducreyi*.

TREATMENT AND PREVENTION. Streptomycin, tetracycline, rifampin, chloramphenicol, and co-trimoxazole are effective treatments for granuloma inguinale. Reports suggest that some strains of *C. granulomatis* are resistant to streptomycin and tetracycline. Thus, co-trimoxazole or chloramphenicol may be the treatment of choice. Two tablets, containing 80 mg of trimethoprim and 400 mg of sulfamethoxazole, should be given orally twice a day for 14 days. The dose of chloramphenicol is 500 mg orally 4 times a day for 10 to 14 days.

Lesions may rapidly increase in size and number during pregnancy and can obstruct the birth canal. Pregnant women can be safely treated with the co-trimoxazole regimen.

Purulent lesions that show evidence of secondary infection usually heal faster if they are cleaned regularly with mild antiseptic solutions such as 1:4000 potassium permanganate in addition to antibiotics. Scarring from the lesion may be extensive. Surgical repair may be required to close fistulas and should not be attempted until healing is complete.

Regular sexual partners of patients with granuloma inguinale should be examined for the disease and treated if it is present. In the absence of lesions, prophylactic treatment is not indicated. Disease control in endemic areas with high incidence is based on active case finding to detect and treat all cases of clinically apparent infection.

BIBLIOGRAPHY

Davis CM: Granuloma inguinale: A clinical, histological, and ultra-structural study. JAMA 211:632, 1970.
Kuberski T: Granuloma inguinale (donovanosis). Sex Transm Dis 7:26, 1980.
Latif AS, Mason PR, Paraiwa E: The treatment of donovanosis (granuloma inguinale). Sex Transm Dis 15:27, 1988.
Maddocks I, Anders EM, Dennis E: Donovanosis in Papua New Guinea. Br J Vener Dis 52:190, 1976.
Rosen T, Tschen JA, Ramsdell W, et al.: Granuloma inguinale. J Am Acad Dermatol 1984:433, 1984.

SECTION G

INFECTIONS WITH SMALL PLEOMORPHIC GRAM-NEGATIVE BACTERIA

47. PLAGUE

Thomas Butler

DEFINITION. Plague is a bacterial infection of animals and humans caused by *Yersinia pestis*. The most common clinical form is acute regional lymphadenitis, called bubonic plague. Less common clinical forms include septicemic, pneumonic, and meningeal plague. Mortality is high in untreated cases, but antibiotic treatment administered early in the course of the disease markedly reduces fatalities. Plague has a widespread distribution in the world, with significant foci in the Americas, Africa, and Asia. The natural reservoirs of *Y. pestis* are predominantly urban and sylvatic rodents, and it is transmitted among animals and occasionally to humans by bites of infected fleas.

ETIOLOGY. The causative agent of plague, *Y. pestis*, belongs to the family of bacteria Enterobacteriaceae. It is an aerobic gram-negative bacillus that is readily cultured in broth or agar media, with an optimal growth rate at 28°C. *Y. pestis* is well adapted to a variety of mammalian hosts, especially rats, in which it maintains itself by flea transmission. The plague bacillus possesses a large number of antigens and toxins that have important roles in the virulence and pathogenicity of this bacterium. Virulence depends on plasmid-mediated V and W antigens, which confer a dependency of the bacterium on calcium for growth at 37°C. In the capsular envelope that surrounds the organism, there is a protein called fraction I antigen, which confers antiphagocytic activity and can activate complement proteins of the host. Fraction I is readily produced at 37°C but not at 28°C and below, indicating that this virulence factor develops while the bacteria are in their mammalian hosts but is absent while the bacteria are in fleas. In the cell walls of *Y. pestis* is a potent lipopolysaccharide endotoxin, which, like endotoxins of other gram-negative bacteria, produces fever, leukopenia followed by leukocytosis, disseminated intravascular coagulation, complement activation, and many kinds of tissue damage. In experimental systems, plague endotoxin causes local and generalized Shwartzman reactions, is mitogenic for B lymphocytes, and stimulates gelation of limulus lysate. In addition, *Y. pestis* elaborates exotoxins, which may play pathogenic roles. One of these is a protein called the murine toxin, which is cardiotoxic in animals and which causes β-adrenergic blockade, but the role of this exotoxin in human disease is unclear.

Another important protein secreted by *Y. pestis* is a coagulase enzyme that causes blood that is ingested by the flea to clot in the proventriculus, thus blocking the transit of the next blood meal into the stomach of the flea. These "blocked" fleas are efficient vectors for plague infection because they regurgitate *Y. pestis* into the bite wound while attempting to feed. The coagulase of *Y. pestis* is active at 28°C and below but is inactive at higher temperatures such as 35°C, thus explaining the cessation of plague transmission during the hot seasons in tropical countries.

HISTORY. *Y. pestis* has caused devastating pandemics throughout history with high mortality rates, in which pneumonic person-to-person transmission has occurred in addition to the usual flea-to-human spread. The fourth great pandemic in the world is currently underway. The first 3 are believed to have occurred in the following times: The first orginated in Egypt in 542 AD and spread to Turkey and Europe; the second pandemic started in the fourteenth century in Asia Minor and Africa and, on spreading to Europe, killed about one fourth of the continent's people; and the third also occurred in Europe during the fifteenth to eighteenth centuries. The present fourth pandemic began around 1860 in the Chinese province of Yunnan. It spread to the southern coast of China, reaching Hong Kong in 1894, when Yersin and Kitasato went there to discover the causative bacterium. Subsequently, plague was carried by ship to India and other Asian countries, Brazil, and California.

In the first half of the twentieth century, India was burdened with the largest share of reported plague in the world, with an estimated total of 10 million deaths. In the 1950s, plague ceased to occur in India, but a resurgence of plague was experienced in Vietnam in the 1960s, with as many as 10,000 deaths a year due to this disease. In the 1970s, Vietnam persisted in reporting the largest numbers of cases but was joined by Burma, Brazil, Kenya, and Sudan, all of which also experienced more than 100 cases per year at some time during this decade.

The plague bacillus is named after Alexandre Yersin (Swiss bacteriologist, 1863–1943), who spent most of his life in Indochina working on bacterial diseases and the production of antisera and vaccines. During an epidemic of plague in Hong Kong in June 1894, he identified bacteria in the tissues of autopsied plague victims and successfully obtained pure cultures of the organisms, which he showed to be lethal in experimental animals.

DISTRIBUTION AND INCIDENCE. Plague is endemic in several countries of Africa, the Americas, and Asia, as shown in Figure 47–1. The countries that reported more than 100 cases during 1980–1986 were Tanzania, 927 cases; Vietnam, 895 cases; Brazil, 649 cases; Peru, 512 cases; Uganda, 493 cases; Burma, 335 cases; Madagascar, 270 cases; Bolivia, 175 cases; and the United States, 148 cases.

In the United States, plague is geographically limited almost entirely to the southwestern states of New Mexico, Arizona, Colorado, Nevada, and California.

TRANSMISSION AND EPIDEMIOLOGY. Plague is primarily a zoonotic infection. It is transmitted among the natural animal reservoirs, which are predominantly urban and sylvatic rodents, by flea bites (Fig. 114–11), or by ingestion of contaminated animal tissues. A schematic depiction of the cycle of infection is shown in Figure 47–2 (also Fig. 110–1). Throughout the world, the urban and domestic rats *Rattus rattus* and *R. norvegicus* are the most important reservoirs of the plague bacillus. In sylvatic foci of plague, however, such as occur in the United States, the important reservoirs are the ground squirrel, rock squirrel, and prairie dog. Humans are accidental hosts in the natural cycle of plague when they are bitten by infected rodent fleas, and they appear to play no role in the maintenance of plague in nature. Only rarely, during epidemics of pneumonic plague, is the infection passed directly from person to person. Also, rarely, humans can develop infection by the direct handling of contaminated animal tissues.

In the classic theory of plague transmission, there are one or more relatively resistant small animal species that serve as the enzootic reservoir. There are also one or more relatively susceptible species that serve as epizootic hosts and may be involved in the so-called "rat die-offs" or "rat-falls." In urban plague, the same species of rats can be both the enzootic and epizootic species, whereas in rural or sylvatic plague, there are usually two or more species. For example, in India, Baltazard and Bahmanyar found that the field gerbil was resistant to plague and was the enzootic reservoir and that the domestic rat *R. rattus* was the liaison rodent

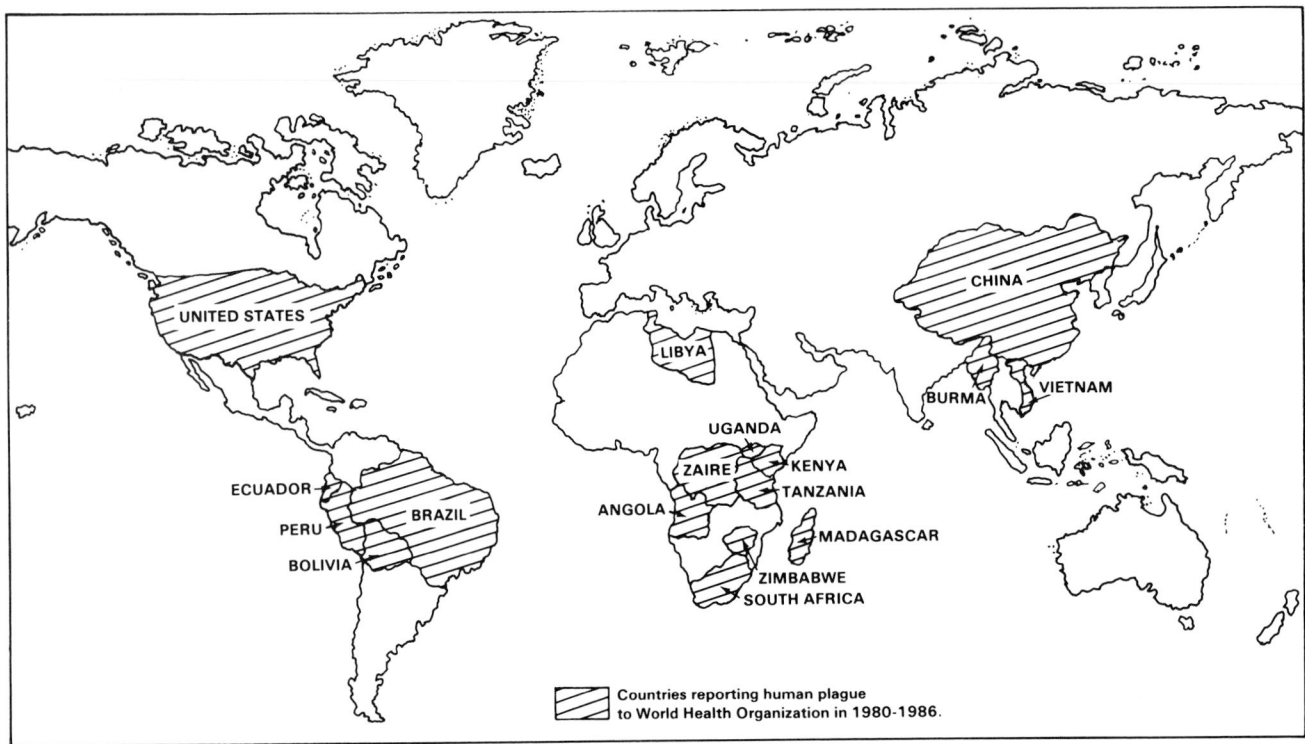

FIGURE 47–1. Geographic distribution of human plague by countries reporting cases to the World Health Organization 1980–1986.

carrying plague from gerbils to humans. Some of the fluctuations in plague occurrence have been related to changing populations of the rodent reservoirs. In Indian cities, Seal described replacement of *R. rattus* by the bandicoot rat at the same time plague infection was diminishing. Although both rodents were good hosts for *Y. pestis, R. rattus* were more heavily parasitized with the efficient flea vector *Xenopsylla cheopis* than were the bandicoot rats.

The occurrence of human plague is always linked to

the transmission of plague among the natural animal reservoirs. The incidence of plague in humans for any particular locality is, therefore, a function of both the frequency of infection in local rodent populations and the intimacy with which the people live with the infected rodents and their fleas. Although humans develop acquired immunity after plague infection, the role of immunity in determining host susceptibility of individuals in a population to infection appears to be small.

Two other epidemiologic features of plague infection

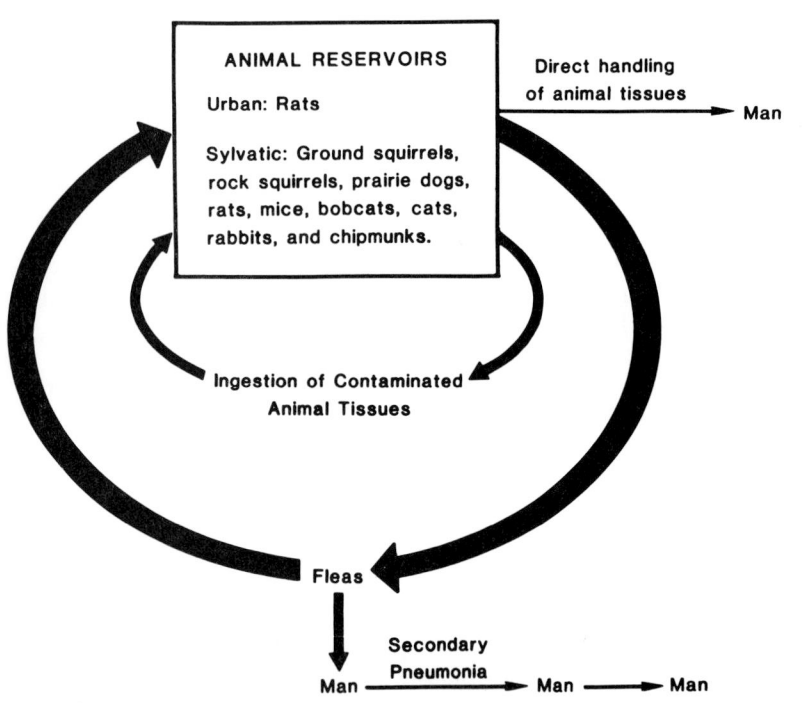

FIGURE 47–2. Transmission of plague. The wide arrows indicate the common or usual modes of transmission, the medium arrows indicate occasional transmission, and the thin arrows indicate rare kinds of transmission.

are its focalization and seasonality. Foci of active plague infection are typically limited to single villages and even to single city blocks, with the adjacent villages and blocks being entirely plague-free. This striking focalization of plague has been related to the parochial behavior of rats to stay near one food supply for extended periods. Only during transport of rodents by humans, such as on ships or trains, are infected rodents, and, thus, epidemics of plague, likely to spread to distant geographic areas.

Plague occurs predominantly in warm, tropical climates. Epizootics tend to occur during humid, warm seasons and are sharply curtailed during very hot seasons, when average daily temperatures exceed 30°C, and during very dry seasons. These seasonal fluctuations have been related to flea behavior and physiology. Humid conditions permit fleas longer periods between blood meals when they can survive off the bodies of their rodent hosts during their search for new hosts. At temperatures of 28°C and below, the coagulase enzyme of *Y. pestis* is active and causes blocking of the fleas, enabling them to be more efficient vectors for plague. Furthermore, during the best seasons for plague transmission, fleas proliferate on their hosts, and when the flea index (ratio of fleas to rodents) exceeds 1, the conditions are usually optimal for a plague epidemic.

PATHOGENESIS AND CLINICAL MANIFESTATIONS

Bubonic Plague. Although plague infection of humans can assume many and protean clinical forms, the most common presentation is bubonic plague, which presents a distinctive clinical picture. During an incubation period of 2 to 8 days after the bite of an infected flea, bacteria proliferate in the regional lymph nodes. Patients are typically affected by the sudden onset of fever, chills, weakness, and headache. Usually, at the same time, after a few hours, or on the next day, patients notice the bubo, which is signaled by intense pain in one anatomic region of lymph nodes, usually the groin, axilla, or neck. A swelling evolves in this area, which is so tender that the patients typically avoid any motion that would provoke discomfort. For example, if the bubo is in a femoral area, the patient characteristically flexes, abducts, and externally rotates the hip and walks with a limp to relieve pressure on the area. When the bubo is in an axilla, the patient abducts the shoulder or holds the arm in a splint. When a bubo is cervical in location, the patient tilts the heads to the opposite side.

The buboes of patients with plague are oval swellings that vary from about 1 to 10 cm in length and elevate the overlying skin, which may appear stretched or erythematous. They may appear either as a smooth, uniform, egg-shaped mass or as an irregular cluster of several nodes with intervening and surrounding edema. Palpation typically elicits extreme tenderness. There is warmth of the overlying skin and an underlying, firm, non-fluctuant mass. Around the lymph nodes, there is usually considerable edema, which can be either gelatinous or pitting in nature. Occasionally, a large area of edema extends from the bubo into the region drained by the affected lymph nodes. Although infections other than plague can produce acute lymphadenitis, plague is virtually unique for the suddenness of onset of the fever and bubo, the rapid development of intense inflammation in the bubo, and the fulminant clinical course that can produce death as quickly as 2 to 4 days after the onset of symptoms. The bubo of plague is also distinctive for the usual absence of a detectable skin lesion in the anatomic region in which it is located as well as for the absence of nearby ascending lymphangitis (Fig. 47–3).

The groin is the most common site of the buboes in plague. In clinical reports that have distinguished femoral from inguinal locations, the femoral site was found to be most common. Other common sites are the axillae and cervical region. The reason for a given distribution of buboes is presumed to be the distribution of flea bites, which inoculate the bacteria into the skin to migrate to the regional lymph nodes.

In uncomplicated bubonic plague, the patients are typically prostrate and lethargic and often exhibit restlessness or agitation. They occasionally are delirious with high fever, and seizures are common in children. Temperatures are usually elevated in the range 38.5° to 40.0°C, and the pulse rates are increased to 110 to 140 per minute. Because of extreme vasodilation, blood pressures are characteristically low, in the range of 100/60 mm Hg. Lower pressures that are unobtainable may occur if shock ensues. The liver and spleen are often palpable and tender.

The pathology of bubonic plague is unmistakable and is characterized by hemorrhage and necrosis. The border of the lymph nodes usually defined by the capsule is obliterated by the destructive inflammatory process, which involves the periglandular tissues as much as the lymph nodes themselves. The normal architecture that separates the cortex from the medulla is destroyed. The lymphoid cells of the medulla are all necrotic. There are large phagocytic cells, polymorphonuclear leukocytes, red cells, and a granular material that is a pure culture of plague bacilli. Blood vessels are thrombosed.

Most patients with bubonic plague do not have skin lesions; however, about one fourth of patients in Vietnam did show varied skin findings. The most common were pustules, vesicles, eschars, or papules near the bubo or in the anatomic region of skin that is lymphatically drained by the affected lymph nodes, and they presumably represent sites of the flea bites. When these lesions are opened, they usually contain white cells and plague bacilli. Rarely, these skin lesions progress to extensive cellulitis or abscesses. Ulceration, however, may lead to a larger plague carbuncle (Fig. 47–4).

Another kind of skin lesion in plague is purpura, which is a result of the systemic disease. The purpuric lesions may become necrotic, resulting in gangrene of distal extremities, the probable basis of the epithet Black Death attributed to plague through the ages. These purpuric lesions contain blood vessels affected by vasculitis and occlusion by fibrin thrombi, resulting in hemorrhage and necrosis (Fig. 47–5). These lesions resemble the local Shwartzman reaction in rabbits that is produced by an intradermal injection of endotoxin followed the next day by an intravenous injection of endotoxin. Accordingly, this necrotic purpura of plague has been attributed to an action of endotoxin from *Y. pestis*.

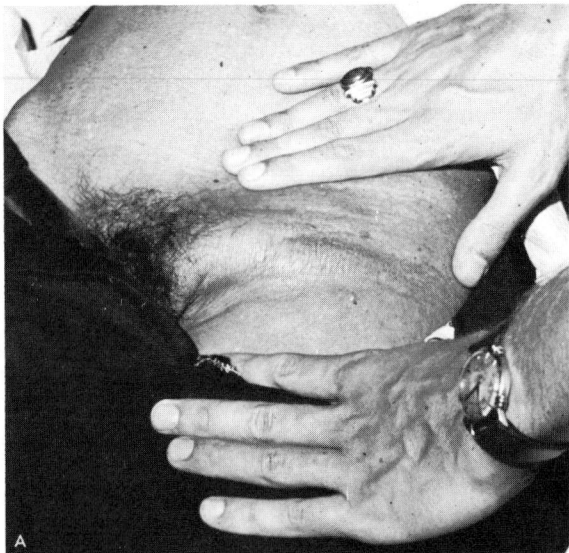

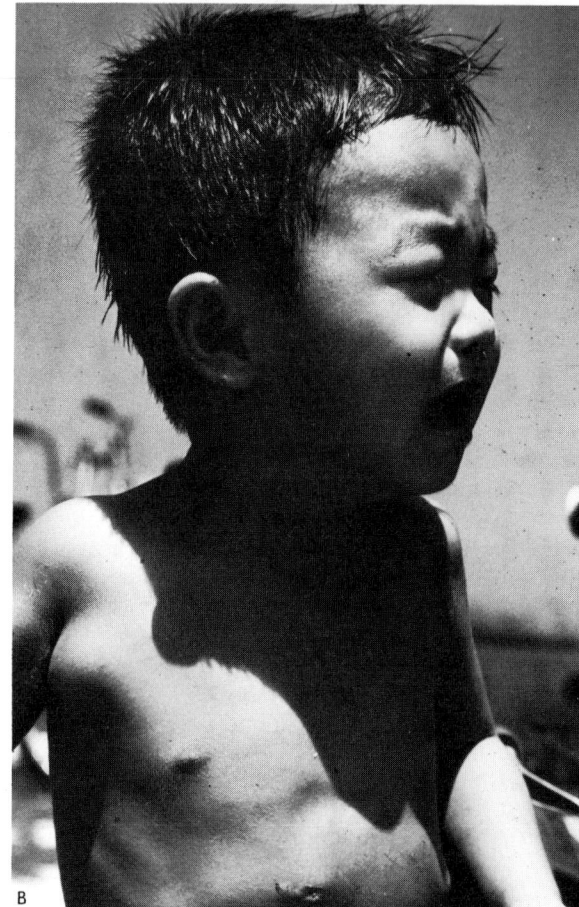

FIGURE 47–3. Buboes of bubonic plague. *A*, Cluster of inguinal lymph nodes with overlying erythema. *B*, Axillary bubo with purulent skin ulcer at presumed site of flea bite.

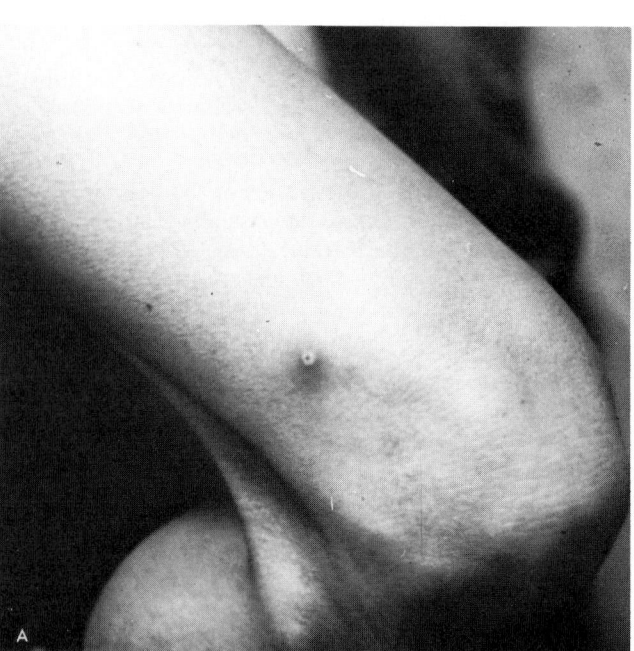

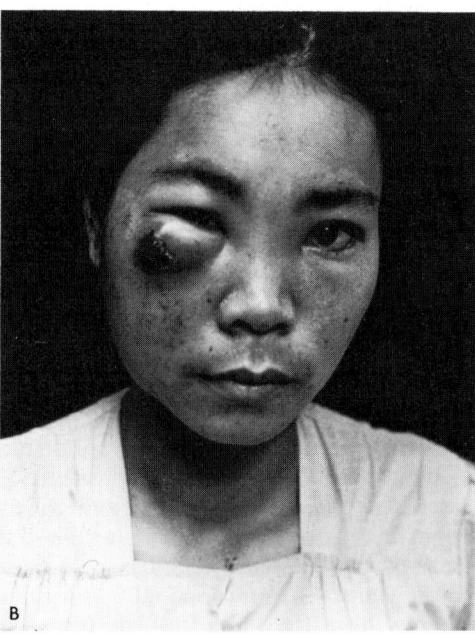

FIGURE 47–4. Skin lesions of bubonic plague. *A*, A pustule with a central eschar on the thigh of a patient who had a femoral bubo. The pus contained many *Y. pestis*. *B*, Suborbital abscess and carbuncle in a patient with a submandibular bubo.

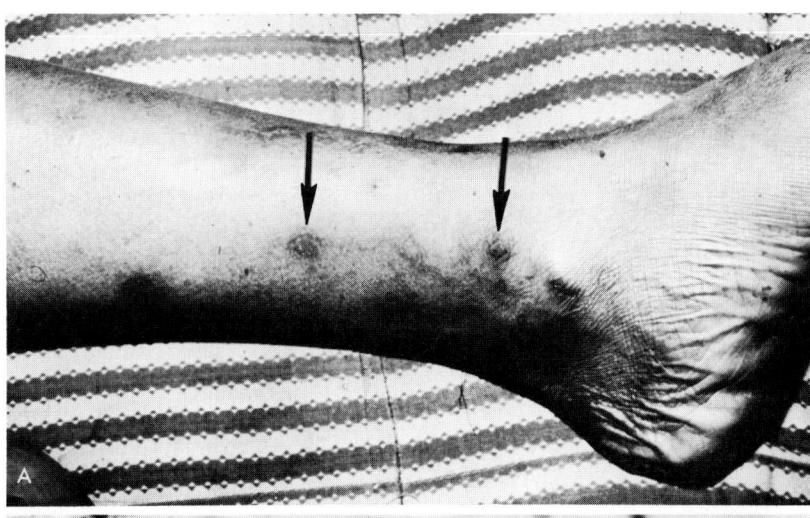

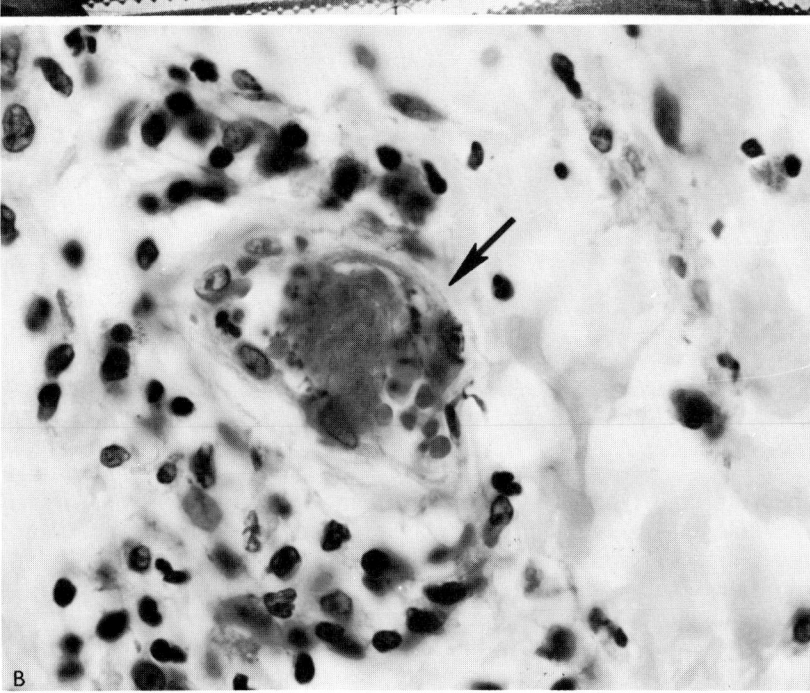

FIGURE 47–5. *A*, Purpuric skin lesions in bubonic plague *(arrows)*. *B*, Histologic examination revealed dermal hemorrhagic necrosis and fibrin thrombi occluding blood vessels in dermis. (From Butler T: Am J Med 53:268, 1972.)

Septicemic Plague. A distinctive feature of plague, in addition to the bubo, is the propensity of the disease to overwhelm patients with a massive growth of bacteria in the blood. In the early acute stages of bubonic plague, all patients probably have intermittent bacteremia. Single blood cultures obtained at the time of hospital admission in Vietnamese patients were positive in 27% of cases. A hallmark of moribund patients with plague is high-density bacteremia, so that a blood smear revealing characteristic bacilli has been used as a prognostic indicator in this disease (Fig. 47–6). In the pathogenesis of plague infection, bacteria sometimes are inoculated and proliferate in the body without producing a bubo. Patients may become ill with fever and actually die with bacteremia but without detectable lymphadenitis. This syndrome has been termed *septicemic plague* to denote plague without a bubo. This term, however, has given rise to confusion, because most patients with bubonic plague have bacteremia at some time in their clinical evolution, and some authors have called bubonic

plague with high-density bacteremia "bubonic-septicemic plague."

Pneumonic Plague. One of the feared complications of bubonic plague is secondary pneumonia. The infection reaches the lungs by hematogenous spread of bacteria from the bubo. In addition to the high mortality, plague pneumonia is highly contagious by airborne transmission. It presents in the setting of fever and lymphadenopathy as cough, chest pain, and often hemoptysis. Radiographically, there is patchy bronchopneumonia or confluent consolidation. The sputum is usually purulent and contains plague bacilli.

Primary inhalation pneumonia is rare but is a potential threat after exposure to a patient with plague who has a cough. It can be so rapidly fatal that persons reportedly have been exposed, become ill, and died on the same day. Plague pneumonia is invariably fatal when antibiotic therapy is delayed more than a day after the onset of illness.

Other Syndromes. Plague meningitis is a rarer com-

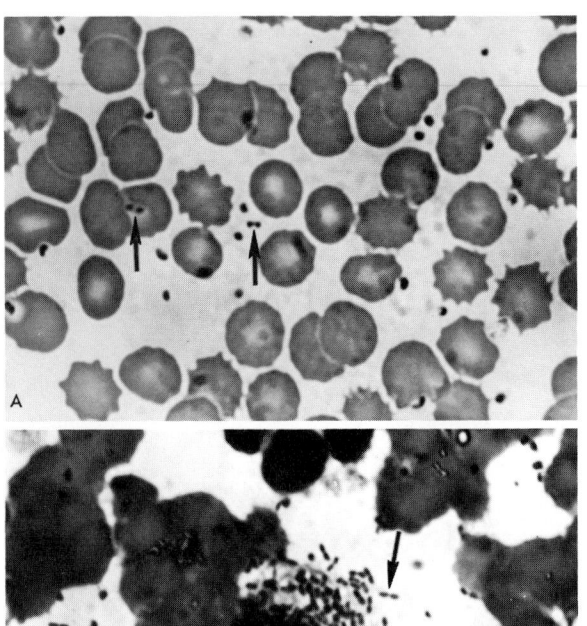

FIGURE 47–6. Blood smears in fatal bubonic plague showing bipolar bacilli. *A, Y. pestis (arrows)* are smaller than platelets and often have bipolar morphology. *B*, Bacilli emanating from circulating phagocyte *(arrow)*.

plication and typically occurs more than a week after inadequately treated bubonic plague. It results from hematogenous spread from a bubo and carries a high mortality rate compared with that of uncomplicated bubonic plague. There appears to be an association between buboes located in the axilla and the development of meningitis. Less commonly, plague meningitis presents as a primary infection of the meninges without antecedent lymphadenitis. Plague meningitis is characterized by fever, headache, meningismus, and pleocytosis with a predominance of polymorphonuclear leukocytes. Bacteria are frequently demonstrable with a Gram stain of spinal fluid sediment, and endotoxin has been demonstrated in spinal fluid with the limulus test.

Plague can produce pharyngitis that may resemble acute tonsillitis. The anterior cervical lymph nodes usually are inflamed, and *Y. pestis* may be recovered from a throat culture or by aspiration of a cervical bubo. This is a rare clinical form of plague that is presumed to follow the inhalation or ingestion of plague bacilli. In some cultures, plague pharyngitis has been noted predominantly in women and has been related to the practice of grooming each other's hair for lice or fleas that they kill by biting them between their teeth.

Plague presents sometimes with prominent gastrointestinal symptoms of nausea, vomiting, diarrhea, and abdominal pain. These symptoms may precede the bubo or, in septicemic plague, occur without a bubo and commonly result in diagnostic delay.

Laboratory Findings. The white blood cell count is typically elevated in the range of 10,000 to 20,000 cells/mm³, with a predominance of immature and mature neutrophils. Severely ill patients tend to have the higher white blood cell counts. Some patients, especially children, may develop myelocytic leukemoid reactions with white cell counts as high as 100,000/mm³. Examination of the white blood cells in the peripheral blood smear typically reveals cytoplasmic vacuolations, toxic granulations, and Döhle bodies that are characteristic of acute bacterial infections. Blood eosinophils are characteristically diminished or absent in the acute stage of infection but return to normal or elevated levels during convalescence. Blood platelets may be normal or low in the early stages of bubonic plague. Although patients with plague rarely develop a generalized bleeding tendency from profound thrombocytopenia, disseminated intravascular coagulation (DIC) is common in this infection. Fibrinogen-fibrin degradation products in the sera indicative of DIC were detected in elevated titers in most patients tested in Vietnam. Liver function tests, including serum aminotransferases and bilirubin, are frequently abnormally high. Renal function tests also may be abnormal in hypotensive patients.

DIAGNOSIS. Plague should be suspected in febrile patients who have been exposed to rodents or other mammals in the known endemic areas of the world. A bacteriologic diagnosis is readily made in most patients by smear and culture of a bubo aspirate. The aspirate is obtained by inserting a 20-gauge needle on a 10-mL syringe that contains 1 mL of sterile saline into the bubo and withdrawing it several times until the saline becomes blood-tinged. Because the bubo does not contain liquid pus, it may be necessary to inject some of the saline and immediately reaspirate it. Drops of the aspirate should be placed onto microscope slides and air-dried for both Gram and Wayson's stains. The Gram stain will reveal polymorphonuclear leukocytes and gram-negative coccobacilli and bacilli from 1 to 2 μm in length. Wayson's stain is prepared by mixing 0.2 gm of basic fuchsin (90% dye content) with 0.75 gm of methylene blue (90% dye content) in 20 mL of 95% ethyl alcohol. This mixture is then poured slowly into 200 mL of 5% phenol. A smear, after being fixed for 2 minutes in absolute methanol, is stained for 10 to 20 seconds in Wayson's stain, washed with water, and dried. *Y. pestis* appears as light blue bacilli with dark blue polar bodies (Fig. 47–7), and the remainder of the slide has a contrasting pink counterstain. Smears of blood, sputum, or spinal fluid can be handled similarly.

The aspirate, blood, and other appropriate fluids should be inoculated onto blood and MacConkey agar plates and into infusion broth. The organism is identified in triple sugar-iron agar by an alkaline slant and acid butt without gas or H₂S, by negative urease and indole reactions, by failure to use citrate, and by nonmotility. For definitive identification, cultures can be mailed in double containers to the Centers for Disease Control, Plague Branch, P.O. Box 2087, Fort Collins, Colorado, 80522 (telephone: [303] 482-0213). At this same laboratory, a serologic test, the passive hemagglutination test that uses fraction I of *Y. pestis*, can be performed

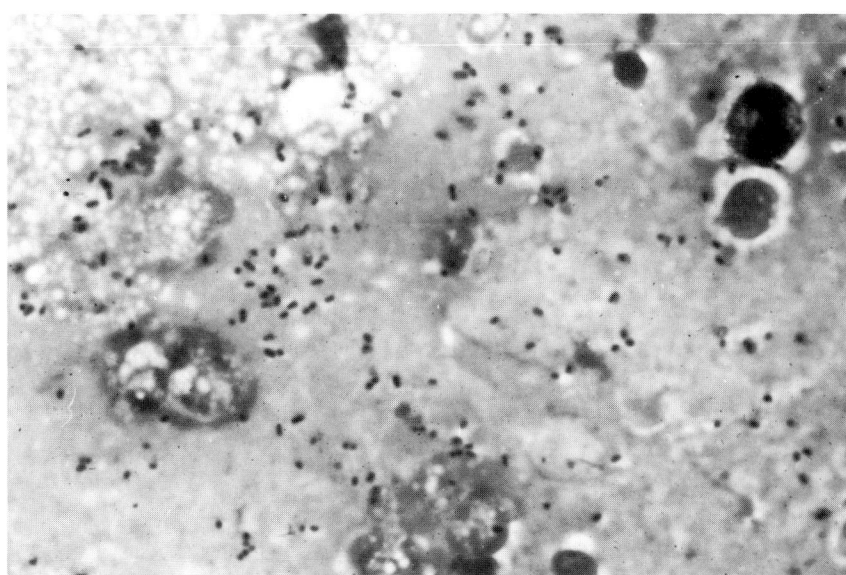

FIGURE 47–7. Wayson's stain of a bubo aspirate reveals bipolar bacilli among inflammatory cells.

on acute- and convalescent-phase serum. In patients with negative cultures, a fourfold or greater increase in titer or a single titer of at least 1:16 is presumptive evidence for plague infection.

TREATMENT AND PROGNOSIS

Antibiotics. Untreated plague has an estimated mortality rate of greater than 50% and can evolve into a fulminant illness complicated by septic shock. Therefore, the early institution of effective antibiotic therapy is mandatory following appropriate cultures. In 1948, streptomycin was identified as the drug of choice for the treatment of plague by reducing the mortality rate to less than 5%. No other drug has been demonstrated to be more efficacious or less toxic. Streptomycin should be administered intramuscularly in 2 divided doses daily totaling 30 mg/kg of body weight per day for 10 days. Most patients improve rapidly and become afebrile in about 3 days. The 10-day course of streptomycin is recommended to prevent relapses because viable bacteria have been isolated from buboes of patients with plague during convalescence. The risk of vestibular damage and hearing loss due to streptomycin is minimal. This antibiotic should be used cautiously, however, in pregnant women, in older patients who would have trouble adapting to vestibular damage, and in patients with previous hearing difficulty. In such patients, the course of streptomycin can be shortened to 3 days after the disappearance of fever. Renal injury as a result of streptomycin therapy is rare with this regimen; however, renal function should be monitored. If the serum creatinine rises significantly, the dose of streptomycin should be reduced. In mild renal failure, the recommended dose is about 20 mg/kg/day, and in advanced renal failure, it is 8 mg/kg every 3 days.

For patients allergic to streptomycin or in whom an oral drug is strongly preferred, tetracycline is a satisfactory alternative. It is administered orally in a dose of 2 to 4 gm/day in 4 divided doses for 10 days. Tetracycline is contraindicated in children younger than 7 years and in pregnant women because it stains developing teeth. It is also contraindicated in renal failure.

For patients with meningitis who require a drug with good penetration into the cerebrospinal fluid and for patients with profound hypotension in whom an intramuscular injection may be poorly absorbed, chloramphenicol should be administered intravenously. This is given as a loading dose of 25 mg/kg of body weight, followed by 60 mg/kg/day in 4 divided doses. After clinical improvement, chloramphenicol should be continued orally to complete a total course of 10 days. The dosage may be reduced to 30 mg/kg/day to lessen the magnitude of bone marrow suppression, which is reversible after completion of therapy. The irreversible bone marrow aplasia associated with chloramphenicol is so rare (estimated to occur in 1 in 40,000 patients) that its consideration should not deter the use of chloramphenicol in patients seriously ill with plague infection.

Other antimicrobial drugs have been used in plague with varying success. These include sulfonamides, trimethoprim–sulfamethoxazole, kanamycin, and ampicillin. These drugs all appear to be either less effective or more toxic than streptomycin and, therefore, should not be chosen.

Antibiotic resistance in human isolates of *Y. pestis* has never been reported, nor has resistance emerged during antibiotic therapy. The antibiotics streptomycin, tetracycline, and chloramphenicol given alone are clinically effective, and relapses are exceedingly rare. Therefore, there is no rationale for using multiple antibiotics to treat plague.

Supportive Therapy. Most patients are febrile with constitutional symptoms, including nausea and vomiting. Hypotension and dehydration are common. Therefore, intravenous 0.9% saline solution should be given to most patients for the first few days of the illness or until improvement occurs. Patients in shock require additional quantities of fluid with hemodynamic monitoring and the judicious use of epinephrine or dopamine. No evidence suggests that corticosteroids are beneficial in plague. Although DIC is commonly present and purpura occasionally develops in severely ill patients, therapy with heparin has no proven benefit in plague infections.

The buboes usually recede without need of local therapy. Occasionally, however, they may enlarge or become fluctuant during the first week of treatment, requiring incision and drainage. The aspirated fluid should be cultured for evidence of superinfection with other bacteria, but this material is usually sterile.

PREVENTION AND CONTROL. Plague is one of the 3 internationally quarantinable diseases, along with cholera and yellow fever. Accordingly, all patients who have suspected plague should be reported to the Health Department and to the World Health Organization. Patients with uncomplicated infections who are promptly treated present no health hazards to other persons. Those with cough or other signs of pneumonia must be placed in strict respiratory isolation for at least 48 hours after the institution of antibiotic therapy or until the sputum culture is negative. The bubo aspirate and blood must be handled with gloves and with care to avoid aerosolization of these infected fluids. Laboratory workers who process the cultures should be alerted to exercise precautions; however, standard bacteriologic techniques that safeguard against skin contact with and aerosolization of cultures should be adequate.

Vaccine. A formalin-killed vaccine, Plague Vaccine U.S.P. (Cutter Laboratories, Berkeley, California 94710) is available for travelers to epidemic or hyperendemic areas, for individuals who must live and work in close contact with rodents, and for laboratory workers who must handle live *Y. pestis* cultures. A primary series of two injections is recommended with a 1- to 3-month interval between them. Booster injections are given every 6 months for as long as exposure continues. In addition to vaccination, persons living in endemic areas should provide themselves with as much personal protection against rodents and fleas as possible, including living in ratproof houses, wearing shoes and garments to cover the legs, and applying insecticide dusts to houses.

Reservoir and Vector Control. The control of plague by health departments requires knowledge of the epidemiology of infected animals, vectors, and the contact of humans with these animals in any particular area. In the United States, the Plague Branch of the Centers for Disease Control in Fort Collins, Colorado, has a field team of entomologists, mammalogists, and epidemiologists to investigate cases of plague. A specific approach to each case should be chosen and usually consists of using insecticides around homes, trapping animals, and educating people to avoid contact with certain animals. Urban plague has been successfully controlled in many cities around the world by quarantine, rat control, and the use of insecticides. Sylvatic plague, however, defies most control measures because the wild rodent reservoirs are so widespread and diverse.

BIBLIOGRAPHY

Almeida CR, Almeida AR, Vieira JB, et al: Plague in Northeast Brazil: Two years of bacteriological and serological surveillance. Bull WHO 59:591, 1981.
Butler T: A clinical study of bubonic plague: Observations of the 1970 Vietnam epidemic with emphasis on coagulation studies, skin histology, and electrocardiograms. Am J Med 53:268, 1972.
Butler T: Plague and other *Yersinia* infections. New York, Plenum Medical Book Company, 1983.
Butler T, Bell WR, Linh NN, et al.: *Yersinia pestis* infection in Vietnam. I: Clinical and hematologic aspects. J Infect Dis 129:S78, 1974.
Butler T, Levin J, Linh NN, et al.: *Yersinia pestis* infection in Vietnam. II: Quantitative blood cultures and detection of endotoxin in the cerebrospinal fluid of patients with meningitis. J Infect Dis 133:493, 1976.
Hull HF, Montes JM, Mann JM: Septicemic plague in New Mexico. J Infect Dis 155:113, 1987.
Hull HF, Montes JM, Mann JM: Plague masquerading as gastrointestinal illness. West J Med 145:485, 1986.
Human Plague in 1986. Weekly Epidem Rec 40:299, 1987.
Mann JM, Martone WJ, Boyce JM, et al: Endemic human plague in New Mexico: Risk factors associated with infection. J Infect Dis 140:397, 1979.
Welty TK, Grabman J, Kampare E, et al: Nineteen cases of plague in Arizona: A spectrum including ecthyma gangrenosum due to plague and plague in pregnancy. West J Med 142:641, 1985.
Williams JE, Hudson BW, Turner RW, et al: Plague in Central Java, Indonesia. Bull WHO 58:459, 1980.

48. TULAREMIA

Jay P. Sanford

DEFINITION. Tularemia is an acute febrile illness caused by the gram-negative coccobacillus *Francisella tularensis*. It is a zoonotic disease to which humans are highly susceptible hosts.

ETIOLOGY. *F. tularensis* is a small, pleomorphic, obligate aerobic, nonmotile, nonsporulating, gram-negative coccobacillus. It grows well at 37°C on glucose-cystine blood agar, but selective media (incorporating cycloheximide and penicillin) facilitate isolation from respiratory secretions or skin ulcers. Exposure to a temperature of 56°C for 10 minutes kills the organisms. Organisms are not destroyed by freezing, however, and may remain viable in frozen animal carcasses for up to 3 weeks. All strains are serologically identical. Despite serologic homogeneity, there are 2 distinct varieties—strains that are highly virulent for humans (Jellison type A) and ferment glycerol, and strains that produce mild human disease, are avirulent for the rabbit (Jellison type B), and do not ferment glycerol.

EPIDEMIOLOGY. Tularemia is ubiquitous in the northern hemisphere between 30 and 71 degrees north latitude, disease having been documented in Japan, Russia, Canada, Mexico, and in all states of the United States except Hawaii. It has not been reported in South America or Africa. In the United States in 1988, Arkansas, Oklahoma, and Missouri were the states from which half of the cases are reported. Tularemia occurs throughout the year, with peaks in the summer (transmitted by ticks) and winter (associated with hunting and trapping).

Some 100 species of wild mammals, 25 species of birds, several species of fish and amphibians, and more than 50 arthropods have been found to be naturally infected. Humans are extremely susceptible; as few as 10 organisms of a virulent strain produced systemic disease in volunteers. Before 1945, most reported human infections followed direct contact with cottontail rabbits. Today, ticks (*Amblyomma americanum, Dermacentor variabilis, Dermacentor andersoni*) and tabanid flies (deer flies) are of greater importance as vectors. Water contaminated by voles, beavers, and muskrats has been responsible for outbreaks, with the portals of entry being the conjunctiva, oropharynx, or skin. Infections also may occur by aerosolization in laboratory workers or, occasionally, farm workers or others exposed to dust or threshings contaminated by voles or other rodents. A number of cases have been reported after cat bites, a circumstance that probably represents mechanical transmission from infected teeth or claws of a cat that have come into contact with an infected rabbit. Person-to-person transmission has not been documented.

CLINICAL MANIFESTATIONS. Tularemia is an extremely variable clinical entity; one patient may present with a low-grade fever and regional adenopathy, whereas another may present with a fulminant fatal infection. The incubation period may range from a few hours to 21 days, with a mean of 4.5 days. In most cases, disease is of abrupt onset with systemic symptoms—fever, chills, headache, bachache, malaise, and weakness. *F. tularensis* usually produces a marked reaction at the portal of entry. This has led to a classification that includes 6 clinical types: ulceroglandular, glandular, typhoidal, oculoglandular, oropharyngeal, and pulmonary.

Ulceroglandular Tularemia. Ulceroglandular tularemia cases constitute 70 to 80% of all cases. Within 2 days of onset of symptoms, patients complain of tender, firm, swollen, discrete lymph nodes, most commonly in the inguinal or axillary areas. Skin over the nodes may be inflamed. In half of untreated patients, the nodes suppurate and drain. Systemic manifestations may overshadow the portal of entry, which is a painful swollen papule that becomes pustular and then ruptures to form a shallow ulcer with raised edges (2 mm to 2 cm in diameter). In half of patients, a correlation exists between the vector and the ulcer site, (e.g., ticks—axillary, inguinal, perineal, and genital sites; rabbits or squirrels—sites distal to the wrist). Other signs may include mild, generalized lymphadenopathy and enlargement of the liver and spleen.

Glandular Tularemia. Glandular tularemia accounts for 10 to 15% of cases and is identical to the ulceroglandular type except that a primary lesion cannot be identified.

Typhoidal Tularemia. Typhoidal tularemia accounts for 10 to 15% of cases. These patients are extremely ill with fever, chills, headaches, severe sore throat, stupor, delirium, malaise, weakness, anorexia, abdominal pain, nausea, vomiting, diarrhea, and nuchal rigidity. Often, more than 1 family member may be affected. Typhoidal tularemia probably is acquired by inhalation of organisms during chewing of contaminated food. About a third of these patients have oropharyngeal involvement, and half have pneumonia or pleural effusion.

Oculoglandular Tularemia. Oculoglandular tularemia accounts for 1 to 5% of cases. Patients present with acute conjunctivitis, itching, lacrimation, and pain. If untreated, corneal ulceration may occur.

Oropharyngeal Tularemia. This category is less used, so that relative frequency is less defined. In 102 cases of typhoidal tularemia reviewed by Dienst, one third of the patients had oropharyngeal involvement. Findings are those of typhoidal tularemia, associated with an ulcerative pharyngitis with or without a gray, necrotic membrane that may involve the tonsils and oropharynx. Cervical nodes are involved, resembling the "bull neck" of diphtheria.

Pulmonary Tularemia. Primary pulmonary involvement is rare in naturally acquired infection. Lymphohematogenous spread to the lungs is the usual pathogenesis of pulmonary involvement. Symptoms include cough, which is usually dry, dyspnea, and pleuritic pain. On examination, cyanosis is uncommon. Signs include generalized moist rales (60%), dullness, bronchophony, and pleural friction rubs (40%). Radiographic findings (in order of decreasing frequency) are broncho-pneumonia, hilar adenopathy, pleural effusion, consolidation, apical infiltrates, and ovoid densities. Involvement is bilateral in two thirds of patients.

DIAGNOSIS. The demonstration of serum agglutinins for *F. tularensis* is a reliable method for confirming a clinical diagnosis. Agglutinins are usually detectable on the tenth to fourteenth day and increase to a maximum titer of about 1:2560 by the end of the third or fourth week. A serum titer of at least 1:160 is considered diagnostic. About half of patients present with such titers.

Culture of organisms should be attempted only by laboratory workers who have been immunized with the live attenuated vaccine. An intradermal test, using killed *F. tularensis*, gives tuberculin-type reactions in 92% of patients with tularemia as early as the first week, at a time when the agglutination test is still negative. This test is not generally available.

TREATMENT AND PROGNOSIS. Before streptomycin was introduced, the overall case-fatality rate was 7%. Today, it is rare for a treated patient to die of tularemia. Streptomycin, 7.5 mg/kg intramuscularly every 12 hours for 10 days, is still considered the regimen of choice by most clinicians. With streptomycin treatment, marked clinical improvement usually is seen within 72 hours. Gentamicin, 5 mg/kg/day intramuscularly for 10 days, is effective but no more so than streptomycin. Tetracycline and chloramphenicol (2 gm/day orally) are as effective as streptomycin; however, relapses occur if therapy is not continued for 15 days.

BIBLIOGRAPHY

Dienst FT: Tularemia: A perusal of 339 cases. J La State Med Soc 115:114, 1963.

Evans ME, Gregory DW, Schaffner W, et al.: Tularemia: A 30-year experience with 88 cases. Medicine 64:251, 1985.

Hopla CE: The ecology of tularemia. Adv Vet Sci Comp Med 18:25, 1974.

Overholt EL, Tigertt WD, Kadull PJ, et al.: An analysis of 42 cases of laboratory acquired tularemia. Am J Med 30:785, 1961.

Teutsch SM, Martone WJ, Brink EW, et al.: Pneumonic tularemia on Martha's Vineyard. N Engl J Med 301:826, 1979.

49. PERTUSSIS

Andrew M. Margileth

DEFINITION. Pertussis (whooping cough) is a highly communicable infection of the respiratory tract characterized by severe paroxysms of cough that end in a gasping, stridulous inspiratory "whooping" sound. It is caused by air drawn forcibly through a narrow glottis. The word "pertussis" means intensive cough. This designation is more appropriate than whooping cough, since not all patients with pertussis whoop.

ETIOLOGY AND HISTORY. Pertussis was first described by Baillou in 1578. Sydenham described several epidemics in England between 1670 and 1680. The genus, *Bordetella* first isolated by Bordet and Gengou in 1900, contains four species: *pertussis*, which causes human pertussis; *parapertussis*, which causes mild whooping cough disease in humans; *bronchiseptica*, which is primarily an animal pathogen but may infect humans; and *avium*, which causes respiratory disease in birds. DNA homology studies revealed that *B. pertussis*, *B. parapertussis*, and *B. bronchoseptica* are genetically similar. *B. pertussis* is a gram-negative coccobacillus, 0.2 to 0.8 μm in size, producing punctiform, convex, translucent, hemolytic colonies on Bordet-Gengou media at 35.5°C. Adenoviruses 1, 2, 3, and 5 have produced disease that mimics pertussis.

DISTRIBUTION AND INCIDENCE. Pertussis occurs worldwide and is a leading cause of sickness and death in children in developing countries in which immunization with pertussis vaccine is not practiced. The World Health Organization estimates that 600,000 deaths occur due to pertussis yearly. It is also prevalent in highly industrialized nations where no vaccine or ineffective vaccines are used. Pertussis is seen so infrequently in the United States that the diagnosis is often not considered unless the patient presents with the classic signs and symptoms of the disease. Yet, patients with pertussis were reported from almost every state in the United States in 1986.

Pertussis has a seasonal variation in incidence in some countries. A review of the reports in the United States over the past decade had shown it to be a year-round disease that continues to attack infants and young children primarily. The young infant under 6 months of age does not receive passive antibody protection against the disease from a mother who has had pertussis and is immune. In contrast to other childhood infectious diseases, pertussis is reported more commonly in girls than in boys.

TRANSMISSION AND EPIDEMIOLOGY. Pertussis is one of the most highly communicable diseases of humans. Transmission occurs by airborne droplets from infected persons, attack rates in unimmunized populations ranging from 25 to 50% in schools to 70 to 100% in susceptible household contacts.

Humans are the only natural reservoir of *B. pertussis* and *B. parapertussis* organisms. A healthy carrier state in humans is infrequent and transient in duration. Patients are most contagious during the preparoxysmal stage of the disease, at which time nasopharyngeal cultures may be positive for pertussis organisms in 80% of suspected cases. Cultures, remain positive for 3 or 4 weeks throughout the early paroxysmal stage.

Pertussis infection produces lasting immunity. Second attacks are more likely due to *B. parapertussis* infection or other agents that cause the whooping cough syndrome.

In developing countries, *B. pertussis* infection is responsible for more than 90% of cases of whooping cough, *B. parapertussis* accounting for only 5%. Pertussis vaccine affords protection only against *B. pertussis*. In some areas of the United States, use of this vaccine has resulted in *B. parapertussis* as the causative agent in as high as 20% of the cases of whooping cough.

PATHOGENESIS AND PATHOLOGY. Pertussis organisms are not invasive. Four steps are important in the pathogenesis of pertussis:

1. Attachment—*B. pertussis* organisms attach to the cilia of the ciliated epithelial cells. Both filamentous hemagglutinin (FHA) and lymphocytosis-promoting factor (LPF) play a role in attachment of the bacilli.

2. Evasion of host defenses—Adenylate cyclase and LPF adversely effect host immune effector cell function, contributing to propagation of the infection. Also, tracheal cytotoxin disrupts normal clearance mechanisms that allow infection to persist.

3. Local damage—Animal studies suggest that tracheal cytotoxin, dermonecrotic toxin, adenylate cyclase, and hemolysin contribute to local tissue damage in the respiratory tract. Profuse, tenacious mucous accumulates with stagnation of mucous flow, inspissation of air passages, and secondary infection.

Bronchitis is often severe, and areas of bronchopneumonia are common, patchy perihilar atelectasis producing a blurred cardiac border on a chest roentgenogram. Airway healing occurs slowly as secretory and humoral antibodies gradually eliminate the organism from respiratory passages.

4. Systemic disease—Weight loss and mild hypoglycemia are probably secondary to poor nutrition due to chronic anorexia. LPF produces leukocytosis and lymphocytosis but has not been shown to produce other systemic effects in humans.

The cause of encephalopathy is unknown but is probably related to transient anoxia associated with severe coughing paroxysms. Brain edema, with occasional perivascular and subarachnoid hemorrhages may be found, but massive hemorrhage is rare. Cerebrospinal fluid (CSF) pleocytosis is mild and is an inconsistent finding.

CLINICAL MANIFESTATIONS. After an incubation period of 7 to 10 days (range 5 to 20 days), clinical illness evolves in three stages: (1) the catarrhal stage (1 to 2 weeks); (2) the acute paroxysmal or spasmodic cough stage (1 to 4 weeks or longer); and (3) the convalescent stage (1 to 3 weeks).

Catarrhal Stage. The catarrhal stage is characterized by a period of 1 to several days of clear, serous, or mucoid rhinorrhea; nasal congestion; and sneezing followed by a mild cough. During this time, the disease resembles the common cold, and pertussis is seldom suspected unless clinical whooping cough has been observed in other family members or the local community. Fever is usually absent. Later, the cough grows more severe and persistent, particularly at night, and profuse nasopharyngeal secretions are thick and tenacious. There is heavy shedding of the *B. pertussis* organisms in these secretions. At this stage, the patient is most infectious and the organism is most easily cultured.

Paroxysmal Stage. The paroxysmal stage may begin abruptly without a preceding catarrhal stage. Violent, protracted bouts of coughing (30 to 40 forceful coughs per spasm) occur in distinct paroxysms lasting up to several minutes. There may be only 2 to 5 or up to 40 to 50 episodes a day. In children more than 6 months of age, the characteristic inspiratory whooping is often heard as the patient gasps for breath between cough paroxysms. Toward the end of these paroxysms, patients often vomit previously swallowed thick, ropy secretions. Afterward, patients appear to be refractory for a brief period to stimuli that provoke paroxysms such as feeding, suctioning, or examination of the pharynx. Severe cough may produce a marked florid venous engorgement of the head and neck with secondary facial petechiae, periorbital edema, and subconjunctival and scleral hemorrhages. Ulceration of the frenulum of the tongue may develop from frequent protrusion of the tongue over the lower incisors. In younger, weaker infants, severe cough paroxysms may not be associated with the characteristic inspiratory whoop but are more often terminated in exhaustion, vomiting, aspiration, apnea, cyanosis, and loss of consciousness. Without resuscitation, these episodes may result in significant hypoxia or death. In older children and adults with relatively larger upper airways, the characteristic whoop is often absent. The paroxysmal stage of pertussis usually lasts for a few days to 4 weeks. Coughing gradually decreases in frequency and severity until paroxysms are no longer present.

Convalescent Stage. The convalescent stage begins when a chronic cough replaces paroxysms. It usually lasts for 3 to 4 weeks with decrease in frequency and severity of the cough. Rarely, the convalescent stage may persist for months. In the young infant, failure to gain weight or weight loss may occur.

COMPLICATIONS

Suppurative Complications. Secondary infections of the respiratory tract should be suspected if the patient develops fever and toxicity, since uncomplicated pertussis is not associated with fever. Acute otitis media is common. Clinical and roentgenographic evidence of bronchopneumonia develops in about 10% of patients; roentgenogram-confirmed pneumonia has been reported in 20% of infants. This can be difficult to differentiate from atelectasis, which usually is present in varying degrees. Segmental or lobar atelectasis primarily affects the lower lobes, the right middle lobe, and the lingular segment of the left upper lobe. Serial roentgenograms often show frequent changes, as some segments re-aerate, whereas others collapse. Treatment of pneumonia and otitis media should be initiated against the more common bacterial pathogens *(Haemophilus influenzae, Streptococcus pneumoniae, Staphylococcus aureus, Streptococcus pyogenes)*.

Nonsuppurative Complications. Severe central nervous system (CNS) complications occur in 1.7 to 7% of patients with pertussis. Increased intrathoracic pressure that results from severe cough paroxysms, hypoxia, and persistent vomiting causes severe venous engorgement and hypoxemia with petechial hemorrhages, epistaxis, subconjunctival and scleral hemorrhages, and cerebral hemorrhages. Rarely, convulsions, transient hemiplegia, ataxia, aphasia, blindness, deafness, decerebrate rigidity, and coma occur. The CSF usually is normal or may show mild pleocytosis (<100 cells) or slight to moderate elevation of protein (<100 mg/dL).

Marked increase in intrathoracic and intra-abdominal pressure with cough paroxysms has been associated with interstitial, subcutaneous, or mediastinal emphysema, pneumothorax, umbilical and inguinal hernia, and rectal prolapse. Subdural hematoma and spinal epidural hematoma occur rarely. Intractable vomiting may produce severe metabolic alkalosis with tetany, aspiration pneumonia, and inanition.

DIAGNOSIS. The diagnosis of pertussis should be suspected in any child with severe cough and should be considered foremost if the cough occurs in severe paroxysms. It is helpful if there is a history of contact with a person known to have pertussis or if the disease is known to be prevalent in the community. Lack of prior immunization or only partial immunization against pertussis should further increase the likelihood of the diagnosis.

Differential Diagnosis. The differential diagnosis includes respiratory infections due to *B. parapertussis, B. bronchosepticum*, influenza, parainfluenza, and adenoviruses. Chlamydial pneumonia in young infants under 4 months of age may be confused with pertussis. Laryngeal foreign body and cystic fibrosis often are accompanied by persistent, severe bouts of cough. Spasmodic attacks of coughing may occur in infants with bronchiolitis and, more rarely, in patients with tuberculosis.

An elevated total white blood cell count with a lymphocytosis involving small, mature lymphocytes with counts ranging from 20,000 to greater than 50,000/mm³ usually is seen in the late catarrhal stage and throughout most of the paroxysmal stage. This characteristic lymphocytosis may not be present in infants less than 6 months of age or in partially immunized individuals. The erythrocyte sedimentation rate during this time is abnormally low.

Culture. The diagnosis is confirmed by identification of *B. pertussis* organisms in respiratory tract secretions. This is best accomplished by culture of the posterior nasopharynx with Dacron or calcium alginate swabs onto fresh Bordet-Gengou medium. An additional plate that contains penicillin (0.5 unit/mL) to reduce growth of other organisms should be inoculated. These plates should be streaked, sealed with masking tape to prevent drying, and incubated at 37°C for 3 to 7 days. Growth of *B. pertussis* organisms may appear at 72 hours as fine pinpoint-like colonies with a metallic luster. When growth is heavy and confluent, it may produce a silvery sheen that resembles aluminum foil. Maximal growth occurs after 5 days, but plates should not be discarded until after 7 days. Colonies may be further identified as *B. pertussis* by Gram stain, agglutination with specific antiserum, and staining with specific fluorescein-conjugated antiserum. Presumptive diagnosis may be made by direct examination of the nasopharyngeal smear on glass slides stained with fluorescein-conjugated *B. pertussis* and *B. parapertussis* antiserum.

Serology. Because all standard serologic tests depend on the demonstration of an antibody titer increase, no tests are available for early diagnosis.

TREATMENT AND PROGNOSIS

Clinical Management. Young infants should be hospitalized because the most important factor responsible for survival is efficient nursing care by experienced nurses in an intensive care setting. Infants under age 6 months may die of asphyxia if immediate resuscitation is not provided. During cough paroxysms, the infant should be positioned to facilitate drainage of secretions and to avoid aspiration of mucous that accumulates at the end of the paroxysm. Also, aspiration of vomitus by the already weakened and exhausted infant must be avoided. Judicious suctioning and oxygen administration are indicated. Stimulation of these patients should be avoided and a quiet environment maintained.

Active nursing care should be carried out immediately after a paroxysm when the patient is usually refractory to these stimuli. If possible, the parents should be instructed in the care of their child and allowed to stay at the bedside as much as possible. This may allow the infant or child to go home sooner when it is clear that the paroxysms, cyanotic episodes, and feeding problems can be safely managed at home.

Frequent small feedings should be provided daily with adequate fluids to maintain hydration and nutrition. To prevent choking and possible aspiration, solid foods should be avoided. Parenteral fluid therapy may be necessary. Mist therapy, cough suppressants, expectorants, and sedatives are not helpful. Also, hyperimmune pertussis globulin is without value in prevention or treatment.

Corticosteroids may reduce paroxysms. Hydrocortisone sodium succinate (Solu-Cortef) is given intramuscularly in a dose of 30 mg/kg/day for 2 days. The dose is then reduced gradually and discontinued by the eighth day.

Isolation. Strict isolation is recommended for 5 days after initiation of erythromycin therapy. If antimicrobial therapy is contraindicated, isolation of the patient is advised until 3 weeks after the onset of paroxysms. Therefore, early recognition of patients, especially infants with atypical signs and symptoms, is important.

Blood gas studies may be helpful in patients with dyspnea, tachypnea, unstable vital signs, or alterations in mental status. These patients may have atelectasis or bronchopneumonia. Well-humidified oxygen is necessary for some patients with sustained hypoxemia.

Antimicrobial Agents. Erythromycin is the most effective and least toxic antibiotic. Treatment is advised for 14 days to avoid relapses in shedding of the pertussis organism. The dose is 40 to 50 mg/kg/day in four doses (adults, 1 gm/day). Early administration of erythromycin to a susceptible child during the incubation period or catarrhal stage may prevent or modify the disease. If started after the paroxysmal cough has begun, patients in the treatment groups had significantly fewer whoops than did the control group. Erythromycin also may be considered for prophylaxis to exposed susceptible persons, especially infants or those children not completely immunized or with chronic respiratory disorders. Trimethoprim–sulfamethoxazole may be an alternative to erythromycin, but documentation of efficacy is inadequate.

Prognosis. The prognosis in uncomplicated pertussis is good. In the United States, of 5865 reported cases during 1984 and 1985, the mortality was 1%. In 1984 and 1985, 5 in 1000 patients with pertussis had encephalopathy. One third of these children died, one third survived with residua, and one third survived and appeared normal. Sequelae may include mental retardation, focal or generalized seizures, behavior and personality changes, and, rarely, focal paralysis.

Mortality is said to be greater in the tropics than in developed countries. Death frequently is due to secondary bacterial infections. Medical care, including the proper use of antibiotics, is limited, and children who die frequently have concomitant medical problems, (e.g., malnutrition, other infections).

PREVENTION AND CONTROL. Widespread active immunization using whole-cell vaccines standardized for potency has been dramatically effective in controlling pertussis in the United States. Protection is not complete or lasting, but field trials have shown that the attack rate in immunized exposed susceptible persons is reduced to about 20%, compared with 80 to 100% in unimmunized controls. The disease is also generally milder in both immunized and partially immunized individuals. This 80% effectiveness of pertussis vaccine is stable for 3 years and gradually decreases until 12 years, after which no protection can be demonstrated. After giving the basic series of three injections of pertussis vaccine, preferably with DPT (diphtheria-pertussis-tetanus) at 2, 4, and 6 months of age, protection is maintained if booster injections are given at 18 months and again at 4 to 6 years of age. Booster injections beyond 6 years of age appear to be associated with significant adverse reactions and are not recommended. Therefore, control of pertussis depends on maintaining a highly immunized population below age 6 years. If this is achieved, the major reservoir of the disease is so reduced that older, previously immunized individuals with waning immunity may be protected by lack of exposure.

A report by Baraff and colleagues revealed no serious neurologic damage as a result of a convulsion or a hypotonic hyporesponsive episode temporally associated with a prior DPT immunization. Whole-cell pertussis vaccine appears to be safe, immunogenic, and efficacious, and it rarely if ever produces permanent neurologic damage. It appears that the benefits of pertussis vaccination far outweigh its risks. Active immunization after exposure affords no protection. Control studies evaluating the effectiveness of prophylactic pertussis hyperimmune globulin for exposed susceptible household contacts have failed to show any benefit. Antimicrobial prophylaxis with erythromycin has been used successfully in some instances. Pending well-controlled prospective studies, erythromycin appears to afford some protection of susceptible individuals who have been exposed to pertussis. Therefore, a 2-week course of treatment is recommended.

BIBLIOGRAPHY

Aoyama T, Murase Y, Gonda T, et al.: Type-specific efficacy of acellular pertussis vaccine. Am J Dis Child 142:40, 1988.

Baraff LJ, Shields WD, Beckwith L, et al.: Infants and children with convulsions and hypotonic-hyporesponsive episodes following diphtheria-tetanus-pertussis immunization: Follow-up evaluation. Pediatrics 81:789, 1988.

Brooksaler F, Nelson JD: Pertussis: A reappraisal and report of 190 confirmed cases. Am J Dis Child 67:56, 1971.

Cherry JD: Vaccine encephalopathy: It is time to recognize it as the myth that it is. JAMA 263:1679, 1990.

Feigen RD, Cherry JD: Pertussis. In Feigen RD, Cherry JD (eds.): Textbook of Pediatric Infectious Disease, 2nd ed. Philadelphia: WB Saunders, 1987, p 1227.

Gordon JE, Hood RI: Whooping cough and its epidemiological anomalies. Am J Med Sci 222:333, 1951.

Griffen MR, Ray WA, Mortmer EA, et al.: Risks of seizures and encephalopathy after immunization with the diphtheria-tetanus-pertussis vaccine. JAMA 263:1641, 1990.

Linnemann CC Jr, Bass JW, Smith MHD: The carrier state in pertussis. Am J Epidemiol 88:422, 1968.

Morley D, Woodland M, Martin WJ: Whooping cough in Nigerian children. Trop Geogr Med 18:169, 1966.

Olson LC: Pertussis. Medicine 54:427, 1975.

50. BRUCELLOSIS

Stephen G. Wright
and Abdul Karem Al-Aska

DEFINITION. Brucellosis is a systemic infection with one of the species of *Brucella*, gram-negative coccobacilli: *B. abortus*, *B. melitensis*, and *B. suis*. This group of infections are zoonoses.

HISTORY. Brucellosis has been recognized in the Mediterranean litorral and the Red Sea basin for a long time. Hippocrates (460 to 357 BC) described a prolonged febrile illness that had a tendency to spontaneous, periodic defervescence in his treatise "On Epidemics." The disease was known by many local geographic names. Because brucellosis could not be distinguished clinically from other causes of prolonged fever (e.g., typhoid), the diagnostic accuracy was poor. Marston in 1861 was able to distinguish between brucellosis and typhoid in autopsy studies by the consistent involvement of Peyer's patches in typhoid and their normal appearance in brucellosis.

The island of Malta had considerable strategic importance in the nineteenth and early twentieth centuries. Brucellosis was common among both the military and civilian populations, including those among the large British garrison. In 1886, Bruce identified a "micrococcus" in fresh material from the spleen of a patient dying of the disease and in 1887 grew the organism from the spleen of another fatal case. In Copenhagen in 1895, Bang showed that contagious abortion in cattle was caused by a bacillus that he referred to as the "bacillus of abortion" and subsequently *Bacillus abortus*. This

organism was not then associated with human disease. The clinical features of brucellosis were clearly described by Hughes in his study "Mediterranean Fever" in 1897. The Mediterranean Fever Commission began its work as a result of the high incidence of brucellosis in the military and civilian populations of Malta, and its findings were published by the Royal Society of London between 1904 and 1907. This study is comprehensive, defining the clinical picture, the epidemiology, the etiologic agent, the reservoir of infection, the mode of transmission, and the means of control. Themistocles Zammit found both antibodies to the organism in high titer and later the organism in the blood and milk of a goat. When troops were prohibited from drinking local milk, the incidence of the disease declined dramatically.

Alice Evans in 1918 created a major stir in the bacteriologic world when she reported the similarities between *Bacillus abortus* and *Micrococcus melitensis*. She suggested that the former might be a human pathogen, and, in 1924, Keefer proved her correct. Subsequently, the genus was named *Brucella*.

ETIOLOGY. The members of the genus are small, gram-negative, aerobic, nonmotile coccobacilli. It is this variation in shape and size that led to the naming of the organism isolated by Bruce "*Micrococcus melitensis.*"

Species. *B. melitensis*, *B. abortus*, and *B. suis* are the species that cause disease in humans, and their virulence for humans decreases somewhat in the order given. Primarily a pathogen of dogs, *Brucella canis* occasionally causes human infections. *Brucella ovis*, a pathogen of sheep, and *B. neotomae*, which infects desert wood rats, are other members of the genus. These organisms are intracellular pathogens. The three principle species each have a number of biotypes; *B. melitensis* 3, *B. abortus* 9, and *B. suis* 5. This is the accepted classification, but DNA hybridization studies showed that the degree of homology among species and biotypes when compared with *B. melitensis* biotype 1 was so great as to raise questions about the validity of our views of *Brucella* taxonomy.

Culture, Biochemical Characteristics, and Antigens. Samples for culture are first inoculated into liquid medium such as trypticase soy broth. The organisms grow slowly in culture, and subcultures should be made every 5 days onto solid medium such as trypticase soy agar. Colonies are small, smooth, and circular. Growth is best at 37°C. An atmosphere containing 5 to 10% CO_2 is needed and is a distinguishing feature for most *B. abortus* isolates.

B. suis oxidizes l-arginine, dl-citrulline, l-lysine, and dl-ornithine, whereas *B. abortus* and *B. melitensis* do not. The latter two species can be distinguished by their oxidation reactions with ribose and galactose. These methods are used in reference laboratories. Phage typing is valuable in distinguishing species; the Tblisi phage lyses *B. abortus* but not *B. melitensis* or *B. suis*, whereas the Weybridge phage lyses *B. suis* and *B. abortus* but not *B. melitensis*.

Two antigens, *A* and *M*, have been defined in quantitative agglutination studies using smooth strains that are the forms isolated in initial culture. Rough strains cannot be used for these studies because they autoagglutinate. *A* antigen predominates in *B. abortus* and *B. suis*, whereas *M* predominates in *B. melitensis*. Serologic cross-reactivity exists between brucellae and *Escherichia coli* 0:116, *Francisella tularensis*, *Pseudomonas maltophila*, *Vibrio cholerae*, *Yersinia enterocolitica* serogroup 0:9, and *Salmonella urbana*.

EPIDEMIOLOGY

Reservoirs. Infected animals are the reservoirs from which humans are infected. The first pregnancy after infection of a cow ends in abortion, and the cow is likely to remain chronically infected thereafter. The animal's vaginal discharges, membranes, placenta, and fetus are all heavily contaminated with brucellae. Organisms survived for 20 weeks in fetal organs and placenta lying on the earth covered with leaves through winter and spring in the northeastern United States. In subsequent pregnancies, the cow can go to term but brucellosis recrudesces to infect the placenta, developing fetus, placental membranes, amniotic fluid, udders and, hence, the milk. Contamination of pastures and fodder from any of these sources infects other animals. Abortion rates up to 50% occur in newly infected herds. The cycle of transmission is similar in goats and sheep infected with *B. melitensis*. Among these animals, many recover spontaneously but those chronically infected may transmit the disease either congenitally or in the milk. Among pigs, infection localizes to the genitalia, and sows usually are infected from a common boar since brucellae are present in the semen. The economic effects of brucellosis in livestock are considerable, with reduced fecundity, fetal losses, and reduced milk production.

Transmission. Humans become infected by a variety of routes. Ingestion of organisms in contaminated foods is common. Milk and milk products are common sources of infection. Prolonged survival of the bacteria occurs if milk and milk products are stored under optimal conditions to prevent souring. Investigations in Malta clearly showed the relation between the amount of milk drunk and the risk of infection and the dramatic decline in incidence of the disease after prohibiting milk consumption.

Contact with infected animals or animal products also is important. Workers in the dairy industry, shepherds, farm workers, family members who have contact with animals around the home, abattoir workers, kitchen workers, and veterinarians are all at risk of infection. Cuts and abrasions on the hands and forearms are sites of entry of infected material. Aerosols of infected fluid also are sources of infection, and entry of organisms may take place across mucosal surfaces (e.g., the conjunctivae, oropharynx, or respiratory tract). Workers in microbiology laboratories who handle infected specimens are at particular risk. Accidental inoculation with the S19 *B. abortus* or Rev-1 *B. melitensis* vaccines causes brucellosis in humans.

The causes listed here account for most infections in humans. Brucellae are capable, however, of prolonged survival in the environment, so that viable organisms inhaled in dust may be infective. Blood transfusion, bone marrow transplantation, possibly kidney transplantation, and the placenta are sources of infection. Sexual transmission in semen may occur. Antacids and H2-receptor antagonists may increase the risk of infection by decreasing gastric acidity.

DISTRIBUTION AND INCIDENCE. Brucellosis has a worldwide distribution. The frequency of infection in animals is a guide to the likely occurrence in humans. Infection with the three species in animals is common in many parts of Africa, Asia (including the Middle East), and Central and South America. France and Spain have a moderate incidence of animal infections; in 1983, France had an incidence of 0.74 cases per 100,000 human population and Spain reported 1.04 cases per 100,000. Within France, the incidence is variable, ranging from 1.07 to 18.24 cases per 100,000 population in affected areas while many areas remain free of infection. The incidence in the United States has declined from 0.15 to 0.06 cases per 100,000 population over the decade to 1984. Brucellosis is common in the Middle East. The incidence reported from Kuwait has risen from 1.15 to 42.78 cases per 100,000 population over a similar period. This probably represents an increased awareness of the disease by physicians, improved reporting of cases, and a true increase as well. These figures take no account of frequent subclinical infections occuring in perhaps as many as half of the populations in endemic areas. Brucellosis is a major cause of morbidity in the endemic areas, but it has a low mortality. This infection is not commonly reported from Africa although it certainly exists there.

The disease is more common in males (male/female ratio, 1.6:1). Most cases occur in the second, third, and fourth decades, but no age is exempt. Cases in children under 10 years are not uncommon. About 6% of patients in a Kuwaiti series were aged 50 years or older.

PATHOGENESIS AND PATHOLOGY

Invasion. How brucellae penetrate the mucosal surface is not understood. Having crossed the epithelial surface, brucellae are phagocytosed by neutrophils and macrophages, which then pass to local lymph nodes. Organisms are retained in this site but replicate intracellularly, and bacteria from lysed cells can infect other cells or disseminate throughout the body.

Immune Response. Naturally occurring opsonins in normal human serum are important in promoting phagocytosis. Complement possesses considerable opsonic activity. Heating normal human serum to 56°C abolishes opsonization and destroys complement, but the addition of guinea pig serum, a rich source of complement, increases opsonizing activity to only 50% of the normal value. About half of *B. abortus* and avirulent *B. melitensis* are killed 4 hours after ingestion, but virulent *B. melitensis* are not killed. Macrophages become infected early in the course of infection. The macrophages of nude mice are capable of killing *B. abortus,* showing that these cells can become activated in the absence of T-cell stimulation. Studies of murine infections with *B. abortus* have shown that, at about 14 days after infection, the numbers of bacteria in the most heavily infected organs, the liver and spleen, decline markedly. This is thought to be due to T lymphocytes' activating macrophages. The specific subset of lymphocytes involved have a cytotoxic/suppressor phenotype. Thereafter, bacterial numbers decline further to minimal levels. When these bacteria are cultured in vitro and then injected again into mice, they show the same pattern of proliferation and decline as did the original population, suggesting that there is nothing peculiar about these "persisters." Rather, it is likely to be a defect in a population of macrophages, either failing to kill or to respond to stimuli from sensitized T cells. These persisters may be responsible for the protracted course of the illness in untreated patients.

The role of antibodies in containing infection is difficult to assess. This is in part due to the intracellular localization of organisms sequestered from the actions of antibody. When organisms are released by rupture of infected cells, they are exposed to antibrucella antibody. Murine antibodies to lipopolysaccharide and to peptidoglycan antigens were protective when injected into mice before intravenous bacterial challenge. Opsonization with antibrucella antibody reduced bacterial loads in the spleen and increased the hepatic load. Vaccine immunity may in part be mediated by these antibodies.

Pathology. The pathologic changes in brucellosis are characterized by granuloma formation in tissues (Fig. 50–1). All tissues and organs of the body can be involved, but liver and spleen are constantly affected. This applies to all three species that infect humans. The granulomas comprise epithelioid cells surrounded by lymphocytes and monocytes with fibroblasts. Giant cells are sometimes seen but caseation does not occur. Necrosis with pus formation may be present, most often with *B. suis,* less commonly with *B. melitensis,* and rarely with *B. abortus.* Abscesses can occur in any tissue, but lymph glands and the spine are the more usual sites.

CLINICAL MANIFESTATIONS. The incubation period, most accurately gauged in laboratory infections, is usually 3 to 4 weeks.

Acute Illness. The acute form is well recognized; fever, generalized aches and pains in the limbs, chills, night sweats, anorexia, and lethargy are typical features.

A number of authors have commented on the strong, moldy odor of the sweat, often noted by spouses and attendants rather than the patients themselves. The patient is unwell with these symptoms but may wait 3 weeks or more before seeking medical attention. Examination may show a febrile patient who is not very ill. Hepatosplenomegaly is common, being present in 27% of a large series with acute brucellosis.

Joint and Bone Involvement. Arthritis is common, often severe, and often disabling. The patient may be unable to walk because of back or hip pain. Large joints are commonly affected (i.e., lumbar spine, sacroiliac joints, hips, and knees). The cervical and thoracic vertebrae may be involved. Vertebral infection can produce an abscess that protrudes anteriorly, laterally, or posteriorly. Posteriorly sited abscesses can compress the spinal cord or cauda equina. A psoas abscess is seen occasionally. Involvement of other joints (e.g., wrist, elbow, sterno-clavicular joint) is well recognized. Inflammation at costochondral junctions also can occur. The nature of joint involvement is not always clear. Septic arthritis with organisms isolated from joint fluid occurs, and pre-existing degenerative joint disease is a predisposing factor in older patients. A reactive arthritis also is associated with this infection.

Other Localized Infections. Epididymo-orchitis is present in 5 to 9% of cases in different series. Pyelonephritis and glomerulonephritis have been documented, and brucellae can be excreted in the urine. Pulmonary involvement does not appear to be common. When it is present, it occurs early in the course of the illness, often in patients who have no history of milk drinking; this lends support to the notion of inhalation of contaminated dusts as the route of infection. Endocarditis that affects either a previously normal valve, usually the aortic, or a previously diseased valve, often the mitral, happens rarely. Pericarditis also is reported. Neurologic involvement has been reported in 2 to 7%

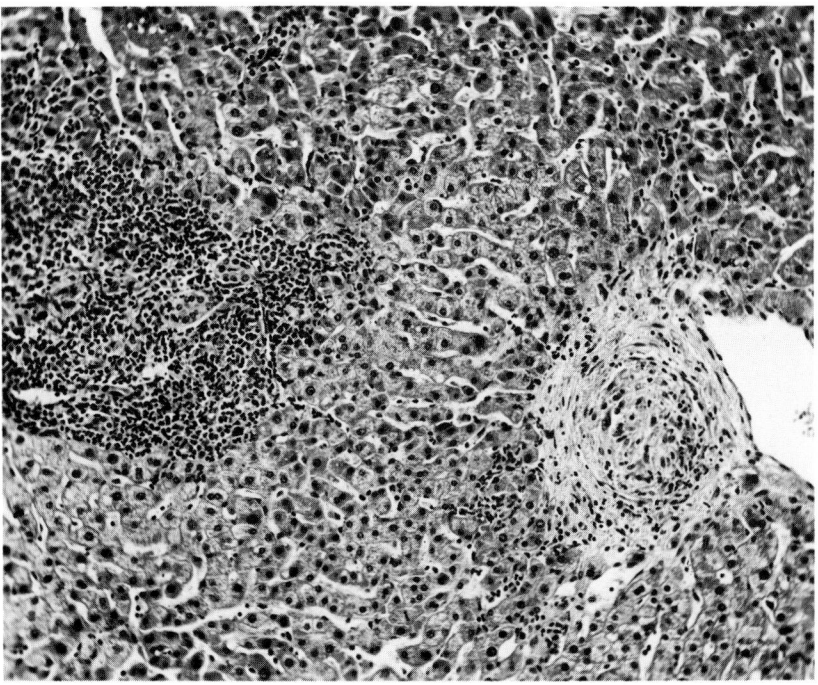

FIGURE 50–1. Brucellosis. Liver biopsy showing small epithelioid cell granuloma and a large periportal lymphocyte infiltrate (H & E, × 130). (Courtesy of the Armed Forces Institute of Pathology, Photograph Neg. No. 73–918).

of patients with a wide variety of manifestations (Table 50–1) and, like many of the clinical manifestations of brucellosis, can occur in the course of acute disease within days or weeks of the onset of symptoms or much later after months of disease in chronically infected cases. Lymphadenopathy is found in about 4% of cases, and abdominal lymphoid hyperplasia occasionally has led to surgery for appendicitis. Skin rashes are described, often papular lesions on the limbs and trunk. Ocular involvement, while uncommon, is recognized. Brucellosis in pregnancy can result in abortion, particularly in the first trimester of pregnancy. Whether this frequency (36%) is greater than that caused by any septicemic illness in early pregnancy is not clear.

Chronic Infection. In addition to the wide range of clinical manifestations, chronicity of infection adds to the complexity of the disease. Alice Evans, the American microbiologist, suffered relapses of the infection over many years. In a large series reported from Kuwait, 77% had symptoms for 2 months or less, 13% had symptoms lasting 2 to 12 months, and 10% had symptoms for over a year. The diagnosis in cases of protracted infection can be difficult. Fever may be present intermittently. Splenomegaly may be found. The history is particularly important with animal contact, occupational exposure, or raw milk drinking being valuable features that prompt further investigation.

Laboratory. Routine blood counts usually show a normal or slightly reduced hemoglobin level. White cell counts are below 4.0×10^9/L in a fifth of patients, and a lymphocytosis is present in almost half. Reduced platelet counts are seen in 10%, and disseminated intravascular coagulation has been seen. Liver function tests show moderate abnormalities with elevations of aminotransferases and alkaline phosphatase levels.

DIAGNOSIS

Culture. Blood culture is most commonly used to isolate the organism, yielding positive results in 14 to 30% of cases. If brucellosis is considered in the differential diagnosis, the laboratory must be informed so that the cultures are retained for up to 6 weeks to give

TABLE 50–1. Neurologic Syndromes in Brucellosis

Cerebral
Papilledema
Cranial neuritis
Focal or diffuse cerebritis
Meningoencephalitis
Parkinsonian syndrome
Cerebellar disorders
Encephalopathy
Transient ischemic episodes/cerebral
  vasculitis
Ruptured mycotic aneurysm

Spinal
Acute poliomyelitis-like syndrome
Spinal cord compression due to abscess
Cauda equina syndrome
Myelitis
Myelopathy

Peripheral
Monoradiculopathy ⎫
Polyradiculopathy ⎬ Motor/sensory or mixed
Sciatica   ⎭

TABLE 50–2. Serologic Responses in Brucellosis

Test	Clinical Status		
	Acute	*Chronic*	*Past Infection*
Agglutination	≥1/160	≤1/80	1/10–1/640
2-Mercaptoethanol	≥1/160	≤1/80	1/10–1/40
Anti–human globulin	Negative	≥1/160	1/10–1/80

the maximum chance of finding this slow-growing organism. Clot culture also is frequently positive, but manipulating infected material presents risks of laboratory infection. Bone marrow culture has given yields of up to 90%. Any pus or tissue taken during biopsy should be cultured as well.

Serology. Serologic testing contributes greatly to the diagnosis. The serum agglutination test (SAT) was developed in association with Almroth Wright who had used it in typhoid. A titer of over 1/160 is suggestive of disease, but results can never be interpreted without relevant clinical data. Titers usually rise fairly early in the course of infection and are positive by 21 days of illness. They remain elevated for long periods, even after treatment has started, although there is a downward trend in test results. In the main, agglutinating antibody is IgM. The prozone phenomenon can cause a false-negative result because of the presence of blocking, nonagglutinating antibody. This effect occurs at low titer and is readily overcome by diluting out test samples. Laboratories doing these tests routinely set them up at low and high dilutions to prevent this source of false-negative results.

The agglutination test also can be performed after treating the sample with 2-mercaptoethanol (2-ME), which inactivates IgM so that early in the course of disease the SAT is high but the 2-ME titer is much lower; the 2-ME titer is higher in patients with chronic infections. The antiglobulin Coombs test is positive in patients with chronic infections. The results of testing by several methods together with clinical assessment may be needed (Table 50–2). Complement fixation tests also have been used. Among more recent developments in serologic testing have been radioimmunoassay, which is not readily applicable in most endemic areas because of the need for isotopes and enzyme-linked immunosorbent assays using either whole organisms or subcellular fractions as antigen.

Radiology. Plain radiographs of affected bones and joints may show changes. The intervertebral disc space is narrowed, and there is bone destruction at the epiphysis. This is accompanied by sclerosis and formation of osteophytes and syndesmophytes (Fig. 50–2), which may firmly ankylose adjacent vertebrae. Soft tissue swelling, which may include an abscess, can be seen anterior or lateral to the bony lesion on plain radiographs. Computed tomographic scans show bone destruction and associated inflammation. They also show psoas abscesses. Technetium isotope scans show increased activity at the sites of bone or joint lesions (Fig. 50–3). This may be present before x-ray changes are evident, although abnormalities persist for a considerable time after treatment. Therefore, changes in scan appearances

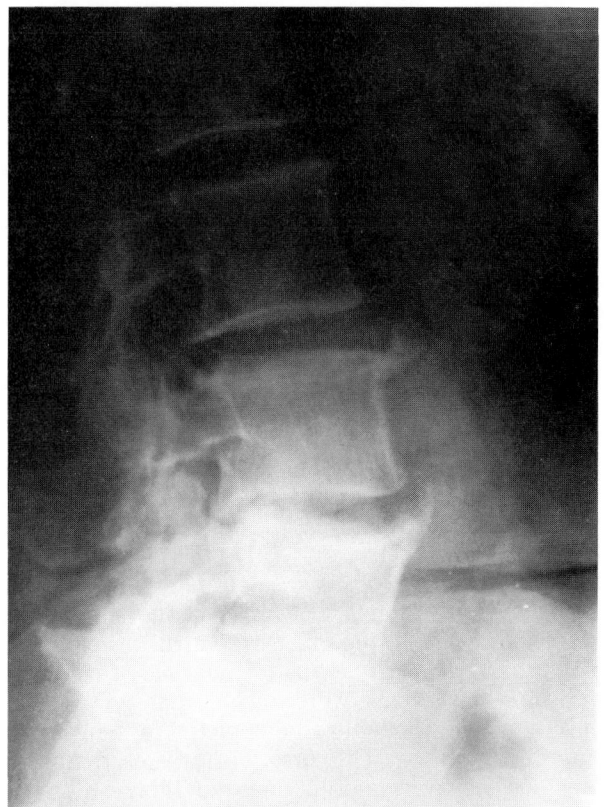

FIGURE 50–2. The fourth and fifth lumbar vertebrae are involved in this case of brucellar spondylitis. There is irregularity of affected vertebral bodies, loss of disc space, and osteophyte formation. There is also a soft tissue shadow in front of the spine.

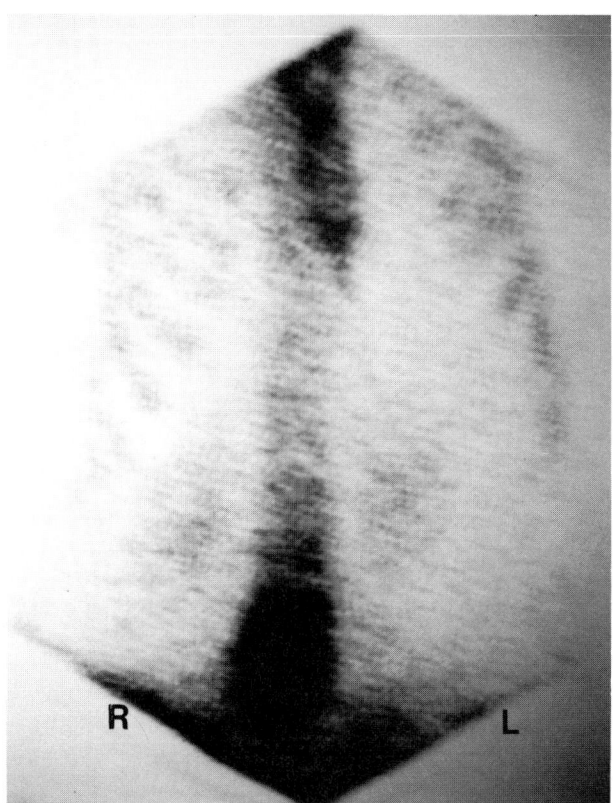

FIGURE 50–3. This is the technetium bone scan of the case illustrated in Figure 50–2. There is a marked increase in uptake of isotope in the lower lumbar spine. This nonspecific appearance is seen in any inflammatory spondylitis.

cannot be used to monitor the response. Gallium scanning also is abnormal, and some evidence suggests that resolution of gallium scan abnormalities may correlate with a good response to treatment.

Differential Diagnosis. The differential diagnosis is wide and includes tuberculosis (Chapter 61) and typhoid (Chapter 38). Gastrointestinal symptoms usually are more prominent in typhoid, and the duration of fever is less except when it occurs in patients with schistosomiasis. Bone and joint involvement are not common in typhoid fever. The wide range of manifestations of tuberculosis makes it difficult to distinguish from brucellosis. Bone and joint involvement are features common to both infections. The dorsal spine is more commonly the site of spinal disease in tuberculosis. Lumbar spine involvement is more common in brucellosis, but any part of the spine can be affected in both diseases. Sacroiliitis is common in brucellosis. Both diseases affect the nervous system. Meningitis in the two infections can be similar with similar changes in the cerebrospinal fluid (CSF). Protracted examination of CSF for tubercle bacilli may allow definitive diagnosis of tuberculous infection at the outset. Q fever is another condition capable of causing prolonged fever, hepatosplenomegaly with granulomatous liver disease, and epididymo-orchitis.

TREATMENT. Tetracyline and streptomycin (Table 50–3) are used most commonly in treatment. These drugs are effective and cheap. The main concern in

ensuring a successful outcome is patient compliance, which is difficult with multiple daily doses of drug. Doxycycline is a convenient alternative. Although once- or twice-daily dosing may increase compliance, its use increases the cost of treatment. This combination cannot be given to children under 8 years or to pregnant women. Alternatives are available but they are more expensive (Table 50–3). Trimethoprim–sulphamethoxazole (co-trimoxazole) alone gives good results, but there is a high relapse rate. Therefore, it must be used in combination with another drug such as rifampicin. Chloramphenicol is effective against brucellae, is cheap, and diffuses readily into the CSF but cannot be recommended for routine use in uncomplicated brucellosis. New cephalosporins, cefuroxime and ceftriaxone, are active against brucellae in vitro and are thought to be safe in pregnancy and so may find a place in special circumstances but again are expensive. The fluorinated quinolones also may prove to be useful in treatment.

Six weeks of chemotherapy is adequate for most infections when soft tissues are involved. Three months of treatment is needed when there is bone and joint involvement and when there is endocarditis, although surgical intervention to replace the infected valve may be necessary. Some authors suggest that patients with neurologic involvement require treatment for 3 months and that streptomycin, rifampicin, and a tetracycline should be given in combination. Surgical drainage of pus is needed when abscesses have formed. This may

TABLE 50–3. Antibiotic Treatment of Brucellosis*

Clinical Manifestations	Antibiotic Regimen
Systemic upset plus lymphadenopathy, enlargement of liver or spleen	Tetracycline, 500 mg q.i.d. for 6 wk *plus* Streptomycin, 1 gm IM daily for 2 wk **or** Doxycycline, 200 mg daily for 6 wk *plus* Streptomycin, 1 gm IM daily for 2 wk **or** Doxycycline, 200 mg daily for 6 wk *plus* Rifampicin, 600 mg daily for 6 wk
Localized disease such as neurologic involvement, osteoarticular disease, and endocarditis	Regimens as above but the 6-wk dosage period is extended up to 12 wk

*This is not an exhaustive list of regimens but indicates generally accepted approaches to treatment. Some authors have used 6-wk regimens successfully for treatment of localized disease. These regimens are not used in children under age 8 or in pregnant women.

be done at an open procedure, but percutaneous aspiration under imaging control may be possible, thus reducing the trauma to the patient.

The diversity of recommendations regarding drugs to be used and duration of regimens is such that there is a pressing need for well-controlled studies of treatment in brucellosis. In choosing antibiotics for study, it should be remembered that most brucellosis occurs in the poor areas of the world where expensive drugs are not available. Therefore, tetracycline and streptomycin should be one combination tried.

PREVENTION. Prevention of brucellosis can be achieved by boiling milk before it is drunk or used to prepare milk products. This seems easy, but, in many countries, it would require people to make a major change in their behavior. Pasteurization in commercial dairy practice achieves the same effect. Control of infection among the animal populations is of major importance and is achieved by testing animals to find which are infected, destroying infected animals with financial compensation to the farmer for loss of stock, vaccination of uninfected animals, and continued surveillance thereafter to ensure the herd remains free of infection. The vaccines used are attenuated strains of *B. abortus* (S19), *B. melitensis* (Rev-1), and *B. suis*.

BIBLIOGRAPHY

Acocella G, Bertrand A, Beytout J, et al.: Comparison of three different regimens in the treatment of acute brucellosis. J Antimicrob Chemother 23:433, 1989.
Araj GF, Lulu AR, Mustafa MY, et al.: Evaluation of ELISA in the diagnosis of acute and chronic brucellosis in human beings. J Hyg (Cambridge) 97:457, 1986.
Ariza J, Gudiol F, Valverde J, et al.: Brucellar spondylitis: A detailed analysis based on current findings. Rev Infect Dis 7:656, 1985.
Bashir R, Al-Khawi MX, Harder EJ, et al.: Nervous system brucellosis diagnosis and treatment. Neurology 35:1576, 1985.
Farrell ID, Robertson LR: The treatment of brucellosis. J Antimicrob Chemother 6:695, 1980.
How does *Brucella abortus* infect human beings? Lancet 2:1180, 1983.
Jayakumar RV, Al-Aska AK, Subesinghe NA, et al.: Unusual presentations of brucellosis. Postgrad Med J 64:118, 1988.
Lulu AR, Araj GF, Khateeb MI, et al.: Human brucellosis in Kuwait: A prospective study of 400 cases. Q J Med 66:39, 1988.
Mousa ARM, Koshy TS, Araj GF, et al.: Brucella meningitis: Presentation, diagnosis and treatment. Q J Med 60:873, 1986.

51. BARTONELLOSIS

F. Stephen Wignall

DEFINITION AND HISTORY. Bartonellosis is an often biphasic illness caused by *Bartonella bacilliformis*, a gram-negative bacteria transmitted by sandflies in inter-Andean valleys. The acute blood stage disease was first widely recognized at the end of the nineteenth century as the cause of a severe epidemic of fever, anemia, and thousands of deaths among workmen building the railway between Lima and Oroya, Peru, and was later dubbed "Oroya fever," though the disease does not actually occur there.

The same organism is responsible for the more chronic, benign, though disfiguring tissue stage of the disease that causes often-extensive verrucous cutaneous lesions or *verruga peruana* (Peruvian wart). The characteristic skin lesions were recognized by pre-Incan civilizations and thought to be depicted in their anthropomorphic pottery. The first written descriptions of analogous lesions are found in the literature of the Spanish conquest of Peru in the early sixteenth century.

The common origin of the two forms of the disease was established inadvertently at the end of the nineteenth century by a Peruvian medical student, Daniel Alcides Carrion. Carrion, trying to gather information on the prodromal phase of verruga peruana, was injected by a colleague with blood drawn from a patient's verrucous skin lesion; he had acute Oroya fever 3 weeks later. Three days before his death and nearly in a coma, he recognized that his disease was proof of the unitary origin of the previously distinct diseases. The disease complex caused by *B. bacilliformis* has been termed *Carrion's disease* in his honor.

In 1905, a Peruvian physician, Alberto Barton, described the presence of mobile intraerythrocytic organisms in patients with Oroya fever. Strong later confirmed Barton's observations and named the agent *Bartonella bacilliformis*. The organism was first cultured in vitro by Noguchi in 1926. Noguchi was able to produce septicemia experimentally in monkeys after intravenous inoculation and to produce skin lesions after intradermal inoculation of his cultured organisms.

The phlebotomine sandfly was first suspected as the vector by Townsend in 1912, who named the species *Lutzomyia verrucarum*. Hertig, traveling with Strong in 1913, confirmed this suspicion through exhaustive studies that have been continued by Herrer and other entomologists.

ETIOLOGY. *B. bacilliformis* is a small (0.2 to 0.5 μm × 1 to 2 μm), motile, pleomorphic, gram-negative coccobacillus with multiple unipolar flagella. Bacillary forms predominate in the early stages of the acute illness, with coccoid forms more prevalent during the verrucous phase and convalescence. The organisms occur within the cytoplasm of erythrocytes and endothelial cells, sometimes appearing to lie inside vacuoles or attached to the inner surface of the cell membrane. They bind to human erythrocytes in vitro and produce substantial, long-lasting deformations in erythrocyte membranes. *B. bacilliformis* appear as reddish violet rods and rounded forms with Giemsa or Romanovsky stain (Fig. 73–5*j*).

Bartonella-like hemotropic bacteria, often associated with febrile anemia or dermal nodules, have been reported from Thailand, Sudan, Niger, Pakistan, and the United States (Connecticut, Illinois, and Virginia). The relation of these organisms to *B. bacilliformis* is not clear. Other genera of close affinity include *Haemobartonella*, *Grahamella*, and *Eperythrozoon*, all pathogens of nonhuman hosts.

TRANSMISSION AND EPIDEMIOLOGY. Bartonellosis is confined in South America to the habitat of the phlebotomine sandfly vectors, *L. verrucarum* and a few other species. The disease is endemic in valleys of Peru, Ecuador, and Colombia on both slopes of the Andes from 800 to 2500 meters above sea level. The vector is intolerant of the low humidity at lower elevations. In Peru and Ecuador, *L. verrucarum* is the principal vector, and other species transmit the infection in Colombia.

Phlebotomine sandflies belong to the family Psychodidae of the order Diptera and transmit a variety of agents other than bartonella to humans. They are delicate, hairy insects that measure 2 to 5 mm in length, with distinctive upraised wings (Figs. 76–4 and 114–7). Although both sexes are crepuscular at temperatures above 11° to 13°C, only the females seek blood meals. Being weak flyers, their range is limited to a few hundred meters from the breeding site. Their activity is further deterred by wind and rain, hence the valleys in which they are found tend to be transverse to the prevailing Andean winds. They characteristically seek dark, humid crevices in dwellings and caves for shelter and breeding.

B. bacilliformis can be identified in the sandfly midgut adherent to the epithelium if they are fed on patients with lesions. Although this phenomenon is rarely seen in wild caught specimens, evidence suggests that at least mechanical if not biologic transmission occurs in the wild. Hertig estimated 20 to 50 bites per night for exposed persons in heavily infested areas and calculated from experimental evidence an infection rate of wild sandflies of 0.5 to 3.0%. There is no known reservoir other than the local human population in endemic areas where even 10 to 15% of asymptomatic persons have been reported as carriers with positive blood cultures.

CLINICAL MANIFESTATIONS AND COMPLICATIONS. The incubation period varies with the clinical presentation but is considered to be 7 to 100 days; typically it is 3 weeks in patients with Oroya fever; it often is longer in those who manifest only skin lesions or positive blood cultures. Asymptomatic infection is common in endemic areas.

Pathophysiology. After the inoculation of *B. bacilliformis* into the skin by the infected sandfly, initial proliferation occurs in the vascular epithelium with subsequent invasion of erythrocytes. In the acute febrile phase, virtually all of the peripheral erythrocytes of the severely ill patient may be infected, with individual cells showing as many as 20 bacilliform organisms. Hemolysis may be abrupt and profound. A significant erythroid hyperplasia results in an outpouring of nucleated cells, a macrocytosis, and very high reticulocyte counts that may approach 50%. Leukocyte counts are variable, but marked leukocytosis is rare. Thrombocytopenia may occur. Multiplication of bacilli in circulating erythrocyte cytoplasm leads to hemolysis and hepatosplenic erythrophagocytosis. Reticuloendothelial cells of the liver, spleen, and lymph nodes are engorged with organisms, erythrocytes, and hemosiderin. Hepatosplenomegaly, splenic infection, and centilobular hepatic necrosis may occur. Examination of the cerebrospinal fluid may show pleocytosis and organisms.

Oroya Fever. The acute blood stage disease may begin insidiously with anorexia, malaise, headache, and intermittent or remittent low fever (37.5° to 38°C) or abruptly with chills, high fever, profuse sweating, prostration, and altered consciousness. Musculoskeletal discomfort is common and often severe. As the anemia and febrile state progress, weakness, vertigo, and syncope are followed by complete prostration, often with delirium or psychosis. Pulmonary complaints and hemorrhage are infrequent. Physical findings include apathy, pallor, generalized nontender lymphadenopathy, jaundice, tachycardia, and hemic murmurs if anemia is prominent. Severely ill patients display dehydration, peripheral circulatory collapse, delirium, psychotic behavior, and bleeding diathesis if thrombocytopenia develops. In the presence of concomitant infection with malaria or *Salmonella*, hepatosplenomegaly may occur.

Death may occur in 10 days or less but often is delayed for 3 or 4 weeks. If the patient survives without complication, the fever abates and the anemia stabilizes and improves. Convalescence is slow, and the disease enters a latent stage that generally is followed by the development of cutaneous lesions or other late complications. Case-fatality rates vary but are reported to be 40 to 90% for untreated cases, two thirds being attributable to infectious complications.

Complications. Salmonellosis is the most important and predictable complication of bartonellosis, commonly appearing during convalescence from Oroya fever. Worsening of the patient's condition may be marked by renewed chills and prostration, high fever, gastrointestinal symptoms, and hepatosplenomegaly. The specific susceptibility of patients with acute hemolytic bartonellosis to intercurrent *Salmonella* infection may be related to reticuloendothelial blockade by erythrophagocytosis and interference with intracellular killing. Salmonellosis is reported in 40 to 50% of patients with acute bartonellosis, with an aggregate case-fatality rate of over 90% in the preantibiotic era.

Other infections that complicate bartonellosis are those common to endemic areas, including malaria, tuberculosis, brucellosis, bacterial pneumonia, and amebiasis.

Transition Phase. The interval between subsidence of the acute hemolytic disease and the eruption may be marked by various signs of continuing infection in a partially immune host: phlebitis, pleuritis, parotitis, meningoencephalitis, and erythemas. Transitory but often severe myalgias and arthralgias may occur, frequently with paresthesias and pruritus in this pre-eruptive stage.

Verrucous Phase. Skin lesions appear after 1 to several months have elapsed, arising as soft, round nodules beginning subcutaneously and evolving to erythematous papules that rapidly enlarge to their final size. The rapid growth phase is analogous to the rapid vascular proliferation within a pyogenic granuloma, which they resemble. The lesions are most frequently present on extensor surfaces of the extremities or on the face (Fig. 51–1), sometimes on the scalp or genitalia, and occasionally in a generalized distribution. Clinical designations are based on size and number: (1) miliary lesions are numerous, small (2- to 3-mm) papules resembling small pyogenic granulomas scattered over the body; (2) nodular lesions are fewer and larger and tend to occur over joints (Fig. 51–2); and (3) large tumors, often measuring several centimeters in diameter, that tend to ulcerate (often called "mular" after large, similar-appearing growths in mules) (Fig. 51–3). The three forms may be seen together because the lesions appear in successive crops. Mucosal lesions occur, and analogous lesions within the mesenchymal tissue of many organs have been reported at autopsy.

Verrucous lesions may bleed profusely after mild trauma and may become secondarily infected. All lesions regress over some months, and new lesions cease to arise. As healing occurs, they become less erythematous, flatten, and eventually leave a hypopigmented macule surrounded by a zone of hyperpigmentation.

DIAGNOSIS. A presumptive diagnosis of acute bartonellosis may be made in a patient with fever, progressive hemolytic anemia, and generalized lymphadenopathy on the basis of known nocturnal exposure to sandfly bites in the endemic area. Rapid confirmation can be obtained by demonstration of intraerythrocytic bacteria in a Giemsa-stained thin blood film (Fig. 73–5j). Definite diagnosis rests on isolation of *B. bacilliormis* from blood culture on appropriate media.

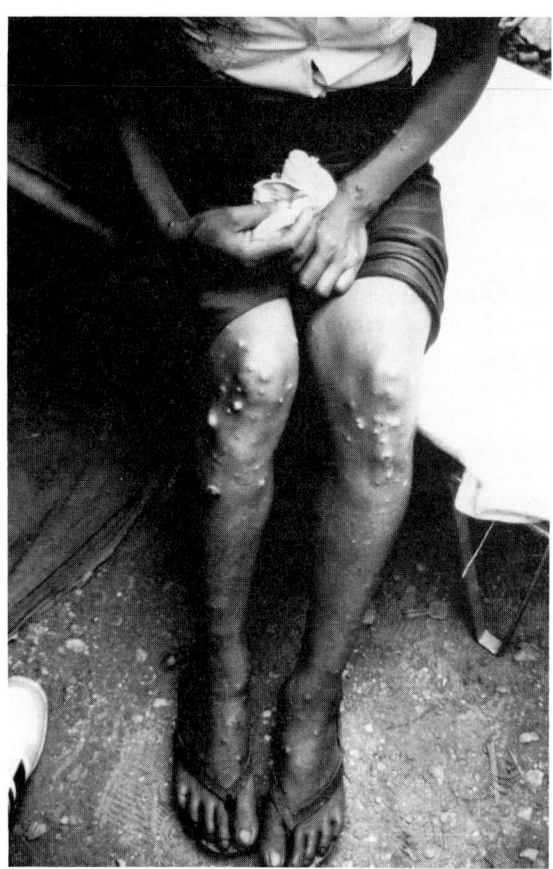

FIGURE 51–2. Bartonellosis. Numerous characteristic nodular lesions on the knees of a Peruvian woman.

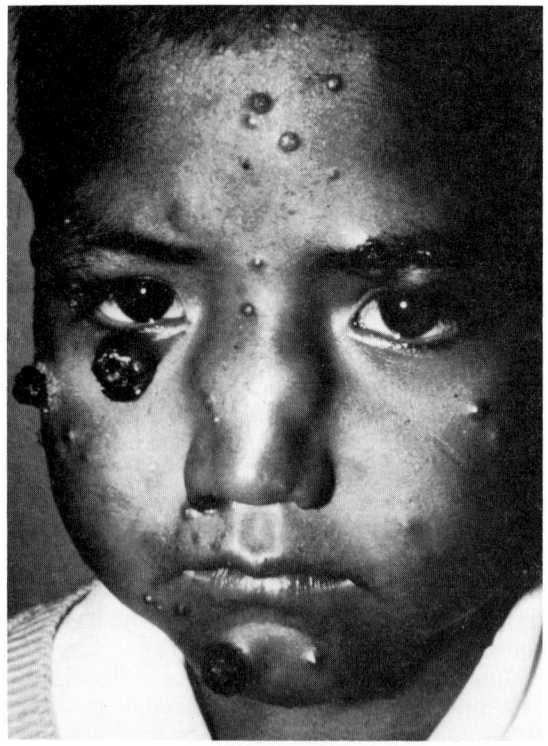

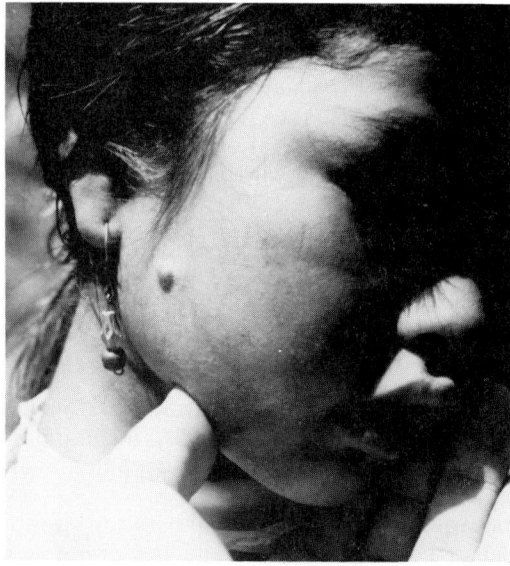

FIGURE 51–1. Bartonellosis. Characteristic papule on the face of young Peruvian girl.

FIGURE 51–3. Bartonellosis. Large "mular" lesions with ulcerations on the face of Peruvian boy.

During the chronic phase, a clinical diagnosis can be made when multiple hemangioma–like cutaneous papules, nodules, or tumors (Figs. 51–1 through 51–3) appear on a person who has been in the endemic area, with or without a history of febrile anemia. The differential diagnosis of a solitary lesion includes hemangioma, pyogenic granuloma, molluscum contagiosum, and spindle cell and epithelioid nevus of Spitz. Skin biopsy of a representative lesion with identification of characteristic Giemsa-stained organisms provides confirmation.

Asymptomatic carriers of *B. bacilliformis* may be identified by blood culture. Columbia agar with 5% defibrinated human blood or semisolid nutrient agar with 10% fresh rabbit serum and 0.5% rabbit hemoglobin is an appropriate aerobic growth medium; growth occurs best at 28°C, small colonies becoming apparent in 7 to 10 days. Identification of *Bartonella*-like bacteria that are sporadically encountered in blood films of patients outside the endemic foci in South America should be made at a referral center.

Some research laboratories offer serologic studies that use antigens prepared from cultured organisms for determination of antibodies by (beginning with the least sensitive) fluorescence antibody test, indirect hemagglutination, and enzyme immunoassay. Serologic investigations are useful in epidemiologic and confirmatory studies.

TREATMENT AND PROGNOSIS. A variety of antibiotics are effective against *B. bacilliformis*, including penicillin, tetracycline, streptomycin, and chloramphenicol. Chloramphenicol continues as the drug of choice for acute bartonellosis because of its efficacy against most strains of *Salmonella*. Blood transfusions and supportive measures are essential in severely anemic cases. With appropriate therapy, rapid defervescence occurs within 8 to 12 hours; organisms seen on blood films tend to become coccoid, and their numbers diminish rapidly. Blood cultures may continue to be positive in some patients after apparently adequate therapy, and a few may even develop verrucous skin lesions, but the course tends to be benign and recovery complete.

The chronic verrucous phase responds variably to antibiotic therapy. No antibiotics usually are needed. Excessively large or ulcerating tumors may require excision.

PREVENTION AND CONTROL. No vaccine is available. Individual protection depends on avoidance of nocturnal exposure to sandfly vectors in endemic areas, use of proper clothing and repellents, and screening. *L. verrucarum* penetrate ordinary screens and netting of 14 × 18 holes per inch but not those with 25 × 30 holes per inch. Residual spraying of homes with DDT or other insecticides is effective.

BIBLIOGRAPHY

Arias-Stella J, Lieberman PH, Garcia-Caceres U, et al.: Verruga peruana mimicking malignant neoplasms. Am J Dermatopathol 9:179, 1987.
Benson LA, Kar S, McLaughlin G, et al.: Entry of *Bartonella bacilliformis* into erythrocytes. Infect Immun 54:347, 1986.
Cuadra M: Salmonellosis complication in human bartonellosis. Tex Rep Biol Med 14:97, 1956.
Hertig M: Phlebotomus and Carrion's disease. Am J Trop Med Hyg 22(Suppl I):1, 1942.
Knobloch J, Solano LI, Alvarez O, et al.: Antibodies to *Bartonella bacilliformis* as determined by flourescence antibody test, indirect hemagglutination and ELISA. Trop Med Parasitol 36:183, 1985.
Knobloch J: Analysis and preparation of *Bartonella bacilliformis* antigens. Am J Trop Med Hyg 39:173, 1988.
Ricketts WE: Clinical manifestations of Carrion's disease. Arch Intern Med 84:751, 1949.
Schultz MG: A history of bartonellosis (Carrion's disease). Am J Trop Med Hyg 17:503, 1968.

52.   CAT SCRATCH DISEASE

Andrew M. Margileth

DEFINITION. Cat scratch disease (CSD), a regional lymphadenitis, occurs primarily in children and adolescents and is caused by a gram-negative bacterial infection. It is transmitted usually by cats; frequently, a skin, ocular, or mucous membrane inoculation lesion is found in the region of the lymphadenitis. Spontaneous resolution over a period of several weeks to months without sequela is the usual course. Recently this bacillus has been found to be the etiologic agent of liver, spleen, and bone infections, as well as causing systemic disease in older children and adults.

HISTORY AND ETIOLOGY. CSD was first recognized by Debré in France in 1931 in a 10-year-old boy with suppurative epitrochlear lymphadenitis. This child was thought to have tuberculous lymphadenitis, but after the disease healed spontaneously in several months, it was found that he slept with many cats and had multiple cat scratches. During the next 20 years, Dr. Debré saw other patients who had similar histories with regional lymphadenitis that resolved spontaneously. These observations were not reported until 1950.

In the United States in 1946, Rose performed a skin test on a fellow physician, Dr. Hanger, using material aspirated from his suppurative epitrochlear node. The cat scratch skin test was positive. Retrospectively, Dr. Hanger remembered a slowly healing lesion on his hand distal to the adenitis that may have been caused by the family Siamese cat. Almost simultaneously, Foshay developed a similar antigen for skin testing. Subsequently, it was found that both his and Rose's antigens gave positive reactions in patients with CSD in France.

By the mid-1950s there were many reports of cat scratch regional lymphadenitis. In 1954 MacMurray and Daniels reported 160 patients with CSD observed in private practice over a 4-year period who had positive cat scratch skin tests. In 1967 Warwick reviewed 567 references on CSD in the medical literature.

In 1983 Wear and colleagues reported detecting delicate pleomorphic bacilli in nodes removed from patients with CSD using the Warthin-Starry silver impregnation stain. The bacilli, 0.2 μm by 0.5 to 2.5 μm, were most readily found in the walls of vessels in the nonnecrotic areas of inflammation and in areas of suppurative necrosis (Fig. 52–1). The silver stain, deposited in several layers on the organisms, made them easier to visualize, whereas they were seen with difficulty using the gram-

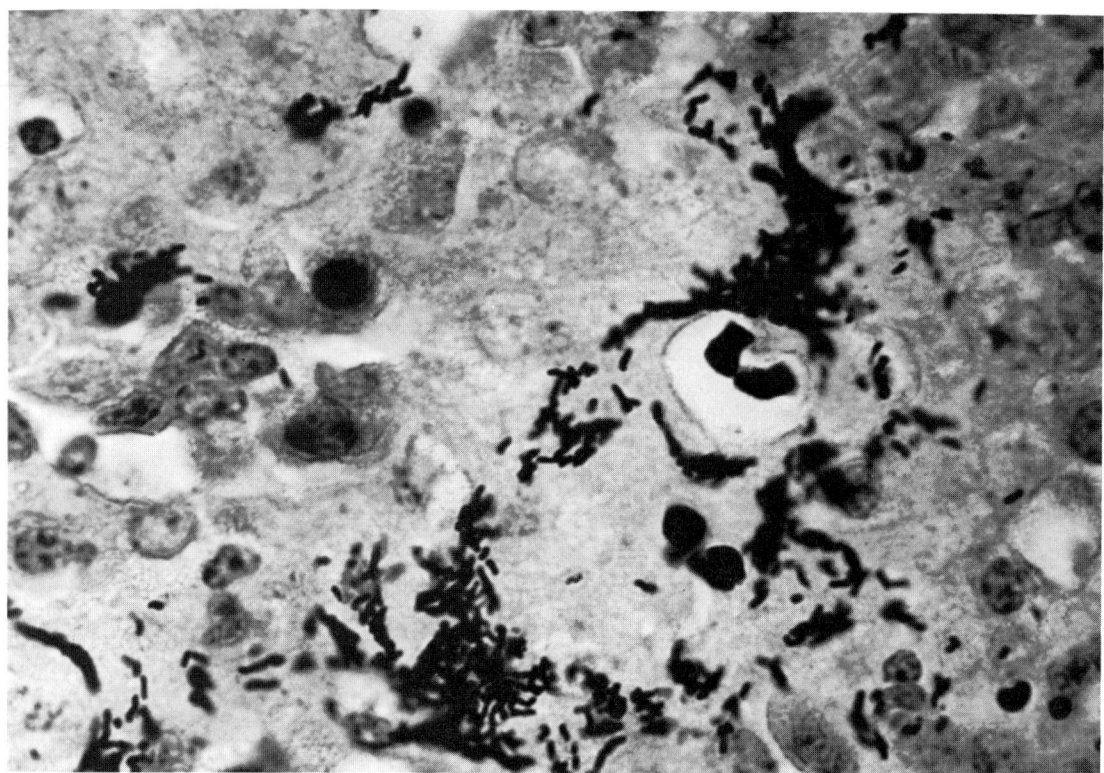

FIGURE 52–1. Warthin-Starry stained section of lymph node reveals many cat scratch bacilli clumped within vessel wall endothelial cells and free in necrotic debris. Two red blood cell fragments are present in the lumen of one vessel (× 290). (AFIP 83–C72. From Wear DJ, et al. Science 221:1403, 1983.)

negative Brown-Hopps stain and the hematoxylin-eosin stain. Serum from patients who had recovered from CSD showed reactions also with these organisms using an immunoperoxidase stain. On electron microscopy the organisms have distinct, thin cell walls characteristic of gram-negative organisms. Similar organisms have been found in biopsies from conjunctival granuloma, cutaneous inoculation lesions, and in liver and spleen biopsies from patients with CSD. The bacilli have been cultured from lymph nodes, blood, and other tissues from infected patients.

DISTRIBUTION AND INCIDENCE. More than 750 publications have reported over 3000 patients with CSD. Carithers calculated an incidence of 6.6 patients per 100,000 people in the United States. This was based on a survey of 1425 patients with a diagnosis of CSD who were discharged from 211 hospitals in the United States during a 10-year period. This figure is probably low, because CSD is a condition that rarely requires admission to a hospital. The disease occurs worldwide in all races, more often in males than in females. The author has studied between 100 to 150 patients each year during the past 5 years, whereas Dr. Carithers in Jacksonville, Florida has seen between 150 to 200 patients each year for the past decade.

TRANSMISSION AND EPIDEMIOLOGY. The mode of transmission is probably by direct cat or dog contact, because the adenopathy follows a scratch or lick, or in rare incidences, a bite, from a young cat. In our patients during the past 5 years, cat contact occurred in 95%, contact with a dog in 4%, while no history of animal contact occurred in 1% of patients. Animal scratches occur less often. About 76% of patients have had a cat scratch, 2% had a dog scratch or bite, and 22% of patients had no history of an animal scratch. Rarely, CSD followed a scratch from a thorn or wood splinter or was associated with insect bites. In almost every case the patient remembered that the cat licked the skin abrasion. Recently we have noted some association between mucous membrane lesions, such as canker sores, and regional lymphadenopathy in the head and neck. Human-to-human transmission has not been reported.

Of the 908 patients we observed between 1975 to 1986, 749 (83%) were less than 21 years of age. Out of 698 families with a member having CSD, 33 (4.7%) had a sibling (usually) or a parent who was infected also. Disease occurred in each family within a 2- to 3-week period, suggesting that the cat was infectious during a brief period.

PATHOGENESIS AND PATHOLOGY. Lymph node biopsies are performed most frequently in older patients with regional lymphadenopathy because of the concern of malignancy, and in patients under 18 years who have a prolonged or an atypical course of CSD. Pathologic sections of nodes removed from CSD patients show microabscesses and/or granulomas. Although these changes can occur with other infections and are not diagnostic of CSD, the combination of abscess and granuloma in the same specimen is consistent with CSD. The Warthin-Starry silver impregnation stain will reveal organisms singly, in chains, in clumps, or in filaments centered in areas of necrosis, in perivascular areas, or in collagen (Fig. 52–1). Bacilli can be found also in histiocytes or neutrophils, suggesting intracellular multiplication. The bacilli may be seen within areas of necrosis (80%) but are seen less often (40%) in association with giant cell granulomas. The bacilli are less likely to be detected in biopsies from skin inoculation sites, ocular granulomas, or lymph nodes taken more than a month after the onset of the disease. Cats implicated as causing CSD have been healthy and have shown no reaction to CSD skin tests. Recently, Kirkpatrick and Whiteley reported small, argyrophilic, pleomorphic bacilli in large macrophages and some vascular endothelial cells in a submandibular lymph node of a Siamese cat.

CLINICAL MANIFESTATIONS

Regional Lymphadenitis. For many years the disease was called cat scratch fever; however, only about one third of patients with CSD have fever greater than 101F. Less than 50% of patients have malaise; fatigue; headache; anorexia, with or without vomiting; sore throat; conjunctivitis; rashes; and rarely arthralgias and/or parotid swelling (Table 52–1). About 50% of children and adolescents have mild CSD presenting with adenopathy only for a few weeks, whereas nearly 75% of adults experience some of the above signs and/or symptoms.

Inoculation Lesion. Sixty to 93% of patients with CSD develop a 3 to 5 mm lesion 3 to 10 days after introduction of the organism into the skin. This may persist several days to several months. The lesion develops over a few days from a vesicle to a pustule, and finally to a papule, or more commonly, from a macule to a papule (Fig. 52–2). Careful examination of the skin, particularly the upper extremities, head, and scalp areas, may reveal a lesion that has been overlooked or mistaken for an insect bite. In 5 to 10% of patients, the inoculation lesion is in the conjunctiva, manifesting as a nonsuppurative conjunctivitis and/or an ocular granuloma. Inoculation lesions are nonpruritic and heal without scar formation.

Lymphadenopathy. Regional lymphadenopathy with either single or multiple nodes is a hallmark of the disease. Usually 2 weeks (range 7 to 50 days) after the scratch, enlarged tender lymph nodes appear proximal

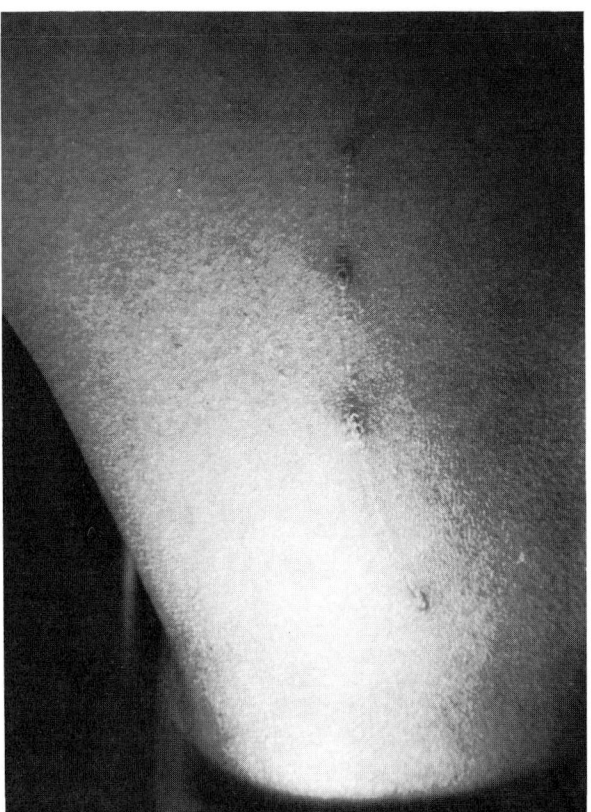

FIGURE 52–2. CSD in a 10-year-old boy with 4 crusted primary cat scratch inoculation papules on left knee for 2 weeks. Inguinal lymphadenitis present for 10 days resolved spontaneously in 2.5 months. Cat scratch skin test was positive.

to the inoculation site. Because the upper extremities, head, and neck are the most likely locations for scratches, over 80% of the involved nodes are in the axilla, epitrochlear, cervical, and supraclavicular areas (Fig. 52–3). Submandibular and preauricular lymphadenopathy is seen also and demands careful examination of the mucous membrane and ocular areas for a primary inoculation lesion. In about 66% of patients, the adenopathy consists of a single or several nodes in one region, whereas 30% will have enlarged nodes in multiple anatomical sites. If adenopathy is detected in more than one area, a search should be made for an additional inoculation lesion. Generalized lymphadenopathy is rare (< 5%) but has occurred in 22% of those with severe systemic CSD.

The majority of lymph nodes are 1 to 5 cm in diameter, but initially they may be as large as 10 cm. During the first 2 weeks of illness the nodes are almost always tender. Erythema of overlying skin may occur early in the disease and resolves as the node decreases in size. Cellulitis has been observed rarely.

The lymphadenopathy regresses generally over a period of 2 to 4 months, but in 1 to 2% of patients they have persisted for 1 to 2 years. Larger lymph nodes with erythema and tenderness regress slower usually and are more suppurative. Approximately 15% of nodes suppurate. Often the patient is not ill in spite of impressive lymphadenopathy.

Other Clinical Syndromes. In two large series of

TABLE 52–1. Cat Scratch Disease: Clinical Presentation of 1402 Patients During 30 Years (1 January 1957 to 1 July 1988)

Clinical Features	No.	%
Typical presentation	1230	87.7
Inoculation lesion (skin, eye, mucus membrane)	808	65
Unusual manifestation	172	12.3
Parinaud's oculoglandular syndrome	87	6.2
Encephalopathy	31	2.2
Systemic disease, severe, chronic	25	1.8
Erythema nodosum	11	0.8
Neuralgia, severe	4	0.3
Neuroretinitis	4	0.3
Atypical pneumonia	3	0.2
Thrombocytopenic purpura	3	0.2
Breast tumor	2	0.1
AIDS	2	0.2
Osteolysis	1	0.1

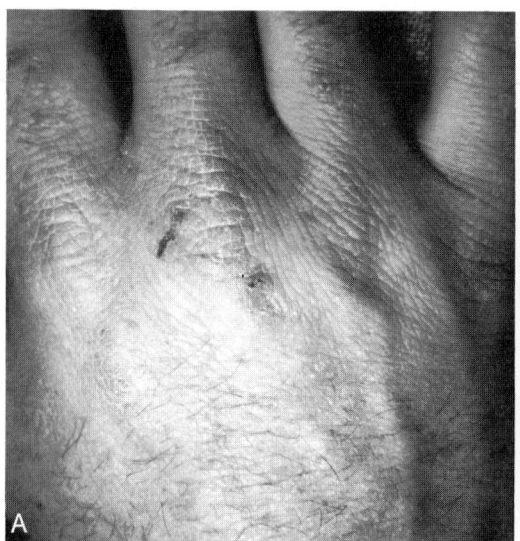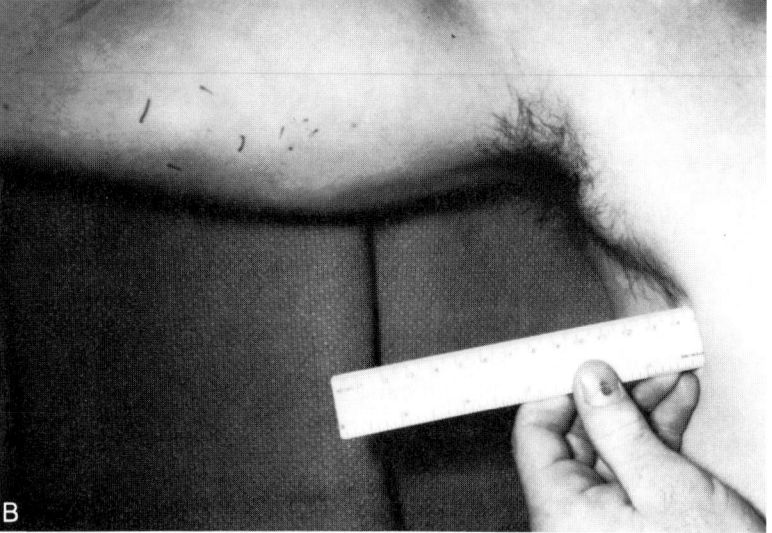

FIGURE 52–3. *A*, CSD in a 22-year-old male: 3 primary cat scratch inoculation papules on hand for 4.5 weeks. *B*, Epitrochlear, brachial, and axillary lymphadenitis was present for 3 weeks along with fever (100F), malaise, anorexia, and an 8-pound weight loss. Adenopathy resolved spontaneously in 6 to 7 months.

patients, 5 to 10% have had presentations other than regional lymphadenopathy (Table 52–2).

Oculoglandular Syndrome. The most frequent of the atypical forms of CSD is the oculoglandular syndrome, first described by Parinaud. This is manifested as a conjunctival granuloma at the inoculation site and pre-auricular lymphadenopathy (Fig. 52–4). The involved eye usually shows no discharge or pain. The swelling and associated discoloration may be impressive enough to cause concern about malignancy. Cat scratch bacilli have been found in the conjunctival granulomas. Usually patients with the oculoglandular syndrome have a spontaneous resolution of the lymphadenopathy within 2 to 4 months.

Neurologic Syndromes. In approximately 2% of patients, nervous system manifestations occur: encephalopathy, seizures, myelitis, radiculitis, polyneuritis, paraplegia, neuroretinitis, and cerebral arteritis. Neurologic symptoms begin usually within 1 to 6 weeks after the onset of lymphadenopathy, presenting with a sudden change in mental status and seizures. The cause of these abnormalities is unknown. Severe manifestations last 1 to 2 weeks, followed by a complete recovery in all cases. Rarely, patients with focal abnormalities noted by EEG or on CT scan may have recurrent seizures or neurologic

TABLE 52–2. Clinical Features in 1058 Patients with Cat Scratch Disease and a Positive Skin Test (April 1975 to July 1988)

Symptoms and Signs	No.	%	Duration in Days
Adenopathy	1058	100	14–365
Adenopathy only	517	49	14–365
Fever (38.3 to 41.1C)	333	31.5	1–60
Malaise/fatigue	324	30.6	1–21
Anorexia, emesis	157	15	3–30
Headache	140	13	1–7
Splenomegaly	119	11	7–30
Sore throat	87	8.2	1–5
Exanthem	48	4.5	5–17
Conjunctivitis	47	4.4	1–11
Parotid swelling	16	1.5	7–28

deficits. Cerebrospinal fluid may show pleocytosis, elevated protein, or both. Electroencephalograms are abnormal in most patients. Recovery may be gradual, taking 1 to 6 months, but sequelae are rare.

Systemic CSD. In recent years systemic illness due to CSD has been reported in both children and adults. These patients had a longer duration of fever, malaise and fatigue, more skin rashes, myalgias, and arthralgias than those with regional adenopathy. Also, these patients had more generalized lymphadenopathy, larger lymph nodes, and weight loss. All patients recovered eventually, although the severity of the disease was variable. We observed 6 patients with systemic CSD who had either neuroretinitis, pleurisy, arthralgia or arthritis, splenic abscesses, and mediastinal masses or enlarged nodes at the head of the pancreas. Others have reported children with CSD and associated granulomatous hepatitis. Three of these patients had high fever (39C) for more than 3 weeks, and 2 had no peripheral lymphadenopathy. The Warthin-Starry silver stain showed organisms consistent with the CSD bacillus in the liver, and a periaortic lymph node of 1 patient, the liver of the second patient, and the axillary lymph node of the third. All 3 children recovered without specific therapy.

Hematologic manifestations of CSD include hemolytic anemia with hepatosplenomegaly, thrombocytopenic purpura, nonthrombocytopenic purpura, and eosinophilia.

CSD in Immunocompromised Host. More recently, CSD has occurred as a severe illness in patients who are immunocompromised. An anergic renal transplant recipient developed refractory hypotension, severe metabolic acidosis, pulmonary infiltrates, and encephalopathy during an illness that began after kitten scratches. CSD bacilli were seen in histopathologic sections of the inoculum site and a lymph node. We have observed at least 1 AIDS patient with a severe form of systemic CSD. Recently, Knobler, et al. observed 4 patients with unique vascular skin lesions associated with human

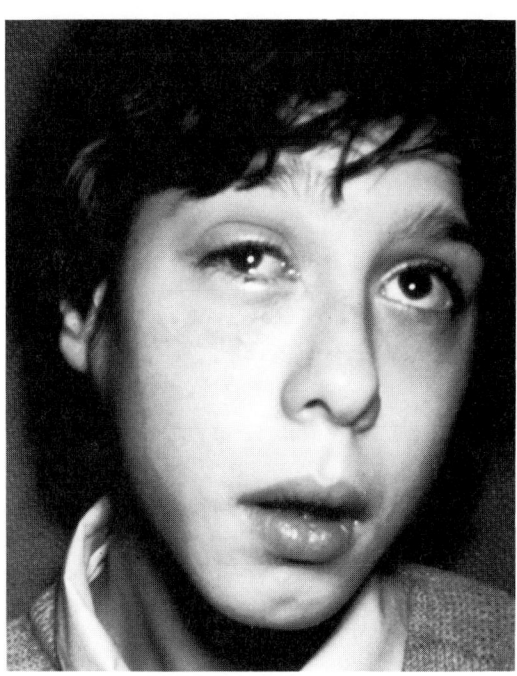

FIGURE 52–4. Oculoglandular syndrome of Parinaud in a 13-year-old; she had 2 weeks of fever, conjunctivitis, and a 5 mm ocular granuloma associated with preauricular adenitis. Adenopathy resolved after several months.

immunodeficiency virus. Biopsy material in 3 of these 4 patients demonstrated a positive Warthin-Starry stain, suggesting that the causative agent of the skin lesions was the cat scratch bacillus.

DIAGNOSIS. Often the diagnosis can be made on the basis of history of cat or kitten exposure, the clinical findings, exclusion of other causes of lymphadenopathy, and observation to resolution. Asking appropriate questions about contact with animals, particularly kittens, and looking carefully for an inoculation site are probably the most important means of diagnosing CSD. Criteria for a definitive diagnosis include the following: (1) contact with a cat, with the presence of a scratch or primary lesion of the dermis, eye, or mucous membrane; (2) a positive skin test for CSD; (3) negative laboratory results of serology, purified protein derivative (PPD-T and PPD-Battey) skin tests, and cultures of aspirated pus or lymph nodes performed for other causes of lymphadenopathy; and (4) characteristic histopathologic features in a biopsy specimen of skin, lymph node, or ocular granuloma. In clinical practice the diagnosis can be made when 3 of these 4 criteria are met.

Warthin-Starry Stain of Biopsy Specimen. In the atypical case of CSD the diagnosis can be confirmed by demonstrating small, pleomorphic bacilli in Warthin-Starry or Brown-Hopps stain section of lymph nodes, skin, or conjunctiva. Because a biopsy is expensive, often nondiagnostic, usually involves hospitalization, and may have complications, it is recommended only when the course of the disease is unusual enough to doubt the cause of the adenopathy.

Cat Scratch Skin Test. The skin test antigen, 0.1 mL, is injected intradermally on the flexor surface of the arm, and the site is circled. After 72 hours the exact amount of induration is delineated by carefully drawing a ballpoint pen held perpendicularly toward the area of induration. After several strokes of the pen in each of 4 quadrants, the maximum amount of induration is measured accurately. A positive reaction is induration of more than 5 mm, which usually fades over 3 or 4 days. Rarely, patients whose skin test is negative at 48 to 72 hours may have a positive test 7 to 10 days later.

The cat scratch skin test antigen reaction usually remains positive for many years, and the size of the reaction does not relate with severity of illness. Positive tests in patients without active disease are reported in family members of patients with CSD, animal workers (particularly veterinarians), cat lovers, healthy adults, and persons who have previously had the disease. False negative reactions occur if the test is done during the first 1 to 2 weeks of the illness or in patients who are anergic.

The preparation and safety of cat scratch antigen as a diagnostic test during 40 years was reviewed by Moriarty recently. Over 6000 doses of skin test material have been administered, and there have been no reports of associated disease transmission or serious reaction. Stored at −80C, the antigen is stable for years. Diagnostic sensitivity is 79 to 100%, specificity is 90 to 98%. Positive predictive values of 64 to 98% and negative predictive values of 78 to 100% have been calculated for the CSD skin tests.

Laboratory Tests. Laboratory tests are not diagnostic. Eosinophilia has been reported; a mild leukocytosis may occur at the onset of illness. The erythrocyte sedimentation rate is elevated usually during the first few weeks of adenopathy.

Culture of the CSD bacillus is still a research procedure. A 4-fold or greater rise in antibody titer against the vegetative cat scratch bacteria using serum from patients with recent CSD has also been demonstrated. Rabbit antiserum to cultured bacilli reacted in immunoperoxidase stains with vegetative, wall-defective cat scratch bacilli in lymph node, skin, or conjunctiva and with vegetative, wall-defective bacteria isolated from 10 patients. Vegetative bacteria produced lesions in the skin of an armadillo identical to early lesions in human skin and were recultured.

Differential Diagnosis. In 90% of patients with chronic regional lymphadenopathy, a healthy appearance and a history of exposure to and/or scratches by a cat and the presence of an inoculation lesion strongly suggest the diagnosis of CSD. If one of these features is missing, other infectious agents must be considered. Bacterial adenitis is commonly due to group A β-hemolytic strepococci, *Staphylococcus aureus*, anaerobes, atypical and human mycobacteria, and rarely *Franciscella tularensis* or *Brucella* species. Cytomegalovirus, EBV, HIV, and toxoplasma or fungi usually cause lymphadenopathy in 2 or more anatomic sites. A cystic hygroma or bronchogenic cyst should be considered in the differential diagnosis in children and adolescents. Neoplastic disease occurs more often in adolescents and adults.

The oculoglandular syndrome may be caused by chlamydial infection, or tularemia, tuberculosis, or syphilis.

Differential diagnosis of persistent skin papules or nodules with regional adenopathy include sarcoidosis, infection with typical or atypical mycobacteria or fungi, syphilis, and leishmaniasis.

TREATMENT. In the majority of patients, CSD resolves spontaneously over a 2- to 4-month period. Presently available oral antibiotics are not effective. However, English has shown that cat scratch bacilli are sensitive to cefoxitin, cefotaxime, gentamicin, amikacin, tobramycin, netilmicin, and mezlocillin in vitro.

Symptomatic treatment consists of local heat, analgesics, limitation of activity to avoid trauma to the node, and aspiration if it suppurates. If an abscess develops, it should be aspirated after preparing the skin with an antiseptic soap. An 18-gauge needle on a 20 to 30 cc syringe is advanced through 1 to 2 cm of normal skin before entering the enlarged node. This provides symptomatic relief and material for diagnosis. Aspiration is preferred to incision and drainage, because the latter may leave a scar and, sometimes, a draining fistula. Surgical excision of the node is indicated when the diagnosis is in doubt and when repeated aspirations fail to relieve pain or resolve the inflammatory process.

PROGNOSIS AND PREVENTION. The prognosis of most patients with CSD is excellent. Recurrence has been documented in 3 adults only; however, this is extremely rare.

Owing to the large number of household pets, at least 50 million cats in the United States, CSD will be difficult to prevent. Disposal of the suspect animal is not recommended, because the cat is invariably well and contagion is low. The patient with disease does not require isolation or quarantine. Active or passive protection is not available.

BIBLIOGRAPHY

Black JR, Harrington DA, Hadfield TL, et al.: Life threatening cat scratch disease in an immunocompromised host. Arch Int Med 146:394–396, 1986.

Bogue CW, Wise JD, Gray GF, Edwards KM: Antibiotic therapy for cat-scratch disease. JAMA 262:813–816, 1989.

Carithers HA: Cat Scratch Disease: An overview based on a study of 1200 patients. Am J Dis Child 139:1124–1133, 1985.

English CK, Wear DJ, Margileth AM, et al.: Cat scratch disease: Isolation and culture of the bacterial agent. JAMA 259:1347–1352, 1988.

Kirkpatrick CE, Whiteley HE: Argyrophilic, intracellular bacteria in the lymph node of a cat: Cat Scratch Disease bacilli? J Infect Dis 156:690–691, 1987.

Knobler EH, Silvers DN, Fine KC, et al.: Unique vascular skin lesions associated with human immunodeficiency virus. JAMA 260:524–527, 1988.

Koehler JE, LeBoit PE, Egberg BM, et al.: Cutaneous vascular lesions and disseminated Cat-Scratch Disease in patients with the Acquired Immunodeficiency Syndrome (AIDS) and AIDS-related complex. Ann Intern Med 109:449–455, 1988.

Lenoir AA, Storch GA, DeSchryver-Kecskemetik K: Granulomatous hepatitis associated with Cat Scratch Disease. Lancet 1:1132–1136, 1988.

Luddy RE, Sutherland JC, Levy BE, et al.: Cat scratch disease simulating malignant lymphoma. Cancer 50:584–586, 1982.

Margileth AM, Wear DJ, English CK: Systemic Cat Scratch Disease: Report of 23 patients with prolonged or recurrent severe bacterial infection. J Infect Dis 155:390–402, 1987.

Moriarty RA, Margileth AM: Cat scratch disease. Infect Dis Clin North Am 1:575–590, 1987.

Rizkallah M, Meyer L, Ayoub EM: Hepatic and splenic abscess in Cat Scratch Disease. Pediatr Infect Dis 7:191–195, 1988.

Schlossberg D, Morad Y, Krouse TB, et al: Culture-proved disseminated cat-scratch disease in acquired immunodeficiency syndrome. Arch Intern Med 149:1437–1439, 1989.

Warwick WJ: Cat Scratch Syndrome, many diseases or one disease? Prog Med Virol 9:256–301, 1967.

SECTION H

MISCELLANEOUS BACTERIAL INFECTIONS

53. ANTHRAX

Robert Longfield

DEFINITION. Anthrax is an acute bacterial zoonosis predominantly of herbivorous animals caused by *Bacillus anthracis* that may be transmitted to humans by inoculation, inhalation, or ingestion. In humans it primarily involves the skin or, rarely, the lungs or gastrointestinal tract. Cutaneous anthrax is characterized by the development of a black eschar surrounded by intense, local edema and may be complicated by septic shock and death in 5 to 20% of untreated cases. Pulmonary anthrax and gastrointestinal anthrax are fatal usually. Previously disease due to *B. anthracis* has been termed malignant pustule, malignant edema, malignant carbuncle, milzbrand, charbon, woolsorter's disease, rag-picker's disease, and splenic fever.

ETIOLOGY

Smear and Culture Characteristics. Anthrax bacilli are large (1.0 to 1.2 μm by 3 to 20 μm), nonmotile, gram-positive rods that possess a prominent capsule. Abundantly found in smears of blood and other tissues, bacilli occur singly, in pairs, and, occasionally, in long chains. Easily cultivated on sheep blood agar, 3- to 5-mm, gray-white, opaque, nonhemolytic colonies are evident within 24 hours and demonstrate the physical tenacity of beaten egg whites. On McFadyean's medium, typical curled or "Medusa's head" colonies are seen. *B. anthracis* is a facultative aerobe that prefers an atmosphere rich in CO_2, does not ferment lactose, and produces acid without gas from glucose. Anthrax is characteristically pathogenic for guinea pigs. Susceptibility to gamma bacteriophage or direct fluorescent antibody testing of isolated colonies may aid in identification also.

Spore Formation. *B. anthracis* develops central oval

spores in culture and in the soil but not in vivo. Spores are resistant to heat, and many disinfectants are destroyed by boiling for 10 minutes or by 140C dry heat for 3 hours. Anthrax spores remain viable for years in dry soil. Cattle have become infected by grazing in fields where animals died of anthrax decades before. Sporulating cultures represent a significant hazard to laboratory personnel.

EPIDEMIOLOGY

Incidence of Human Anthrax. Human infection with *B. anthracis* is infrequent and sporadic in the United States and most developed countries. Twenty thousand to 100,000 cases of human anthrax are estimated to occur annually throughout the world. Careful descriptive studies of its occurrence in many developing countries are lacking; however, anthrax appears ubiquitous in rural agricultural nations that are economically dependent on animal husbandry. Epidemics of human anthrax are rare; however, in April, 1979, inhalation anthrax was responsible for close to 1000 deaths in Sverdlovsk, USSR.

Zoonotic Anthrax. Anthrax is predominantly a disease of herbivores—cattle, sheep, horses, and goats. Animals are infected generally via the alimentary tract by grazing on contaminated pasture, rarely by direct contact with other infected animals. Prior to death, animals often contaminate the soil with infected saliva, urine, or feces. Soil, forage, and, to a lesser extent, ground water are the major reservoirs of anthrax.

Geographic Occurrence. Neutral or alkaline soils in areas characterized by early spring rains and warm summers are particularly conducive to perpetuating anthrax spores. Historically, Louisiana, Arkansas, Texas, Oklahoma, Oregon, and California were regions of endemic anthrax; however, owing to intensive surveillance and control procedures, animal anthrax has been virtually eliminated in the United States. In some areas of India, France, and Russia, zoonotic disease never appears to die out. In Great Britain, however, spore survival in soil is generally less than 1 year. *B. anthracis* spores germinate in soil at 20 to 44C in areas with humidity above 85%. Germinated bacilli are thought to be destroyed then by other soil microbes. Therefore, in many tropical regions, animal anthrax occurs predominantly in the dry season, with some persistence into the early wet season. Humans may be responsible for introducing anthrax into new areas by the importation of infected hides, hair, bristles, and bone, including bonemeal fertilizer. In certain areas, vultures may be responsible for the geographic dissemination of anthrax.

Transmission. Generally, human anthrax is traced to industrial, agricultural, or, rarely, laboratory acquisition. There is no evidence of direct human-to-human transmission. Owing to occupational exposure, males are more often infected than females (3:1), but anthrax has no predilection for age.

Industrially Acquired Anthrax. Industrial acquisition accounts for 78% of cutaneous anthrax and almost all respiratory anthrax, and occurs predominantly among tanners or leather workers and hair, wool, or bone-meal fertilizer workers. Subclinical infection and seroconversion among workers in these industries may be much more common than overt illness. Autochthonous infections in developed countries are acquired often industrially from contaminated animal hides, hair, or bones imported from developing countries. Goat hair and wool from China, India, Pakistan, and Iran are more commonly contaminated with spores than similar materials from Europe or Australia, reflecting the relative prevalence of zoonotic anthrax in these regions. Rough leather goods and bongo drums from Haiti and Morocco have been vehicles of anthrax transmission in the United States. In the past, facial lesions have been linked to natural-bristle shaving brushes and oral lesions to unsterilized toothbrushes.

Agriculturally Acquired Anthrax. Direct contact with infected animals by farmers, butchers, and veterinarians is implicated in 22% of cutaneous anthrax cases. Transmission by biting insects has been suspected but not conclusively demonstrated. Bone-meal fertilizer has been implicated in sporadic cases of inhalation anthrax among home gardeners.

Anthrax Acquired in Developing Countries. In developing countries, human anthrax is acquired usually from sick animals or from fomites contaminated with their blood or body fluids. In Gambia between 1970 and 1974, it was estimated that approximately 1.4% of the population of 1 area incurred cutaneous anthrax, most of the cases presenting in the dry season. Indirect human-to-human spread by the use of contaminated toilet articles or fomites was postulated also but not confirmed. Gastrointestinal anthrax was seen rarely, perhaps because the people refrain from eating the meat of sick or dying animals. Serum antibodies were present in some people who denied prior cutaneous lesions, suggesting that asymptomatic infections may occur. Anthrax caused more than 6000 human cutaneous infections and over 100 deaths in Zimbabwe and Ghana, and explosive outbreaks of gastrointestinal anthrax occur. Furthermore, in many developing countries, anthrax-contaminated meat may be sold to unsuspecting buyers by fraudulent vendors.

PATHOLOGY

Cutaneous Anthrax. Lesions demonstrate acute inflammation with irregular epidermal ulceration and underlying coagulation necrosis. A fibrinopurulent covering or membrane may be present, which, along with satellite bullous lesions, swarms with distinctive gram-positive bacilli; however, pus is not present unless superinfection occurs. Beneath the epidermis, edema and exudate are prominent, especially for lesions of the head and neck. Massive hemorrhage into the dermis and subcutaneous fat may be evident, but voluntary muscle is involved rarely. Neural infiltration and degeneration account for the characteristic hypalgesia of dermal anthrax. The blue-black eschar appears late and, rarely, may be inconspicuous.

Inhalation Anthrax. Woolsorter's disease is characterized by hemorrhagic edema of mediastinal lymph nodes and connective tissue. No endobronchial ulcers or eschars are evident. Bronchi reveal hemorrhage, desquamation of cellular debris, and abundant bacilli. Involved alveoli contain hemorrhage, proteinaceous debris, and bacilli, but polymorphonuclear leukocytes are absent usually. Alveolar capillaries have widespread fibrin thrombi. Hemorrhagic pleural effusions occur commonly. Hematogenous dissemination frequently ensues to other areas of the lung, the meninges, the spleen, and the intestine. Anthrax bacilli may disseminate also to the lung from cutaneous lesions, producing hemorrhagic pneumonitis.

Gastrointestinal Anthrax. In primary gastrointestinal anthrax, hemorrhage, edema, and ulceration of the stomach are noted. The intramural and regional lymphatics are involved extensively with hemorrhage and edema. Intestinal obstruction, perforation, and massive ascites follow.

Central Nervous System Anthrax. Hemorrhagic meningitis is characteristic of central nervous system infection by *B. anthracis*. The leptomeninges reveal scant inflammatory cell reactions but widespread hemorrhages. The brain has hemorrhages, and generalized cerebral edema is dramatic.

PATHOGENESIS

Cutaneous Anthrax. Cutaneous anthrax follows the inoculation of spores, usually into a minor abrasion or scratch. Then spores germinate, multiply, and elaborate a complex toxin. Hematogenous dissemination follows in 5 to 20% of untreated cases.

Inhalation Anthrax. Pulmonary anthrax follows the inhalation of spores 1 to 5 μm in diameter. Larger spores are cleared by the lung's mucociliary mechanism and generally fail to cause infection. Spore aerosols are encountered generally by workers handling contaminated batches of hair or wool and bone-meal fertilizer. The aerosol infective dose required for human infection appears to be high. In certain animal hair mills, air sampling studies have estimated that the average nonimmune worker inhaled between 150 and 700 infectious spores per 8-hour shift, yet clinical infection remained rare. Studies in primates indicate that inhaled anthrax spores are ingested initially by alveolar macrophages and are carried then to mediastinal lymph nodes, where they germinate. The initial necrosis of the germinal centers is followed quickly by generalized hemorrhagic lymphadenitis and early invasion of the blood stream. The complex toxin elaborated by the organism causes marked local vascular injury, with edema, hemorrhage, and thrombosis. No primary mucosal lesions, analogous to cutaneous eschars, are found within the respiratory passages.

Gastrointestinal Anthrax. Gastrointestinal anthrax follows the ingestion of spores, usually from poorly cooked, contaminated meat. There is no evidence that milk from infected animals transmits anthrax. Hemorrhagic abdominal lymphadenitis ensues in a fashion analogous to that encountered with inhalation anthrax.

Septicemic Anthrax. Generalized sepsis may follow cutaneous anthrax and almost invariably accompanies inhalation and gastrointestinal anthrax. Vascular injury results from both the exuberant proliferation of the organism in blood and the elaboration of complex toxin. Widespread capillary thrombosis, circulatory failure, shock, and death ensue. Several human cases have demonstrated adrenocortical hemorrhage.

Anthrax Toxin. Description of the complex toxin of *B. anthracis* has been an involved and, as yet, incomplete process. Owing to the abundance of bacilli in clinical specimens, microbial proliferation, aided by an antiphagocytic polypeptide capsule, is certainly important to pathogenesis. Experiments in laboratory animals have suggested that a toxic factor was involved in death and have established that bacteremia was not essential for death to ensue. During the 12 hours before demise, the number of bacilli in the blood of guinea pigs rises from 3×10^5 to 1×10^9 colony-forming units/mL. Antibiotic therapy when blood bacteria counts are less than 1/300 of the terminal level results in survival. Delayed therapy results in a massive reduction of bacteremia but 100% mortality. Injected extracts of killed anthrax bacilli are not toxic; however, sterile blood from doomed animals reproduces the syndrome and kills normal guinea pigs.

The protein exotoxin has been purified substantially by chromatographic techniques and is currently thought to be a synergistic complex of 3 heat-labile toxins: protective antigen (PA), edema factor (EF), and lethal factor (LF), which are produced by *Bacillus anthracis* in an inactive form. Anthrax toxin becomes activated following contact with heat-stable eukaryotic material. Studies suggest that 2 of the protein components of anthrax toxin, EF and PA, increase host susceptibility to infection by suppressing polymorphonuclear neutrophil function and impairing host resistance. The complex of EF and PA is thought to act as an adenylcyclase in dramatically elevating intracellular levels of cyclic AMP. LF in combination with PA induces lethality in laboratory animals and is toxic apparently to endothelial cell membranes, causing intense local vascular injury, platelet and leukocytic adherence, and thrombosis. Antitoxin is protective against these effects in primates only if injected before or less than 8 hours after injection of the toxin. Neurotoxic to rodents and primates, anthrax toxin may have direct central nervous system toxicity also and cause death from central respiratory failure. Hypoglycemia, hypoxia, and various electrolyte disturbances may follow its action. Other examples of synergistic toxin complexes include cholera enterotoxin, staphylococcal leukocidin, and the guinea pig toxin of *Yersinia pestis*. Antiphagocytic capsule and toxin production appear to be mediated by separate plasmids.

CLINICAL MANIFESTATIONS

Cutaneous Anthrax. Cutaneous anthrax accounts for 90% of human anthrax infections and commonly involves exposed areas of the face, neck, hands, and arms. The incubation period is from 12 hours to 7 days but averages 3 days. The initial lesion is a small erythematous macule or papule that resembles an insect bite or pimple. It turns brown subsequently and develops a surrounding ring of erythema and may form a pruritic vesicle or bulla. Vesicular satellite lesions may appear ("pearl wreath") (Fig. 53–1*A*). Vesicular fluid is initially clear but becomes blue-black by the third or fourth day (Fig. 53–1*B*), and organisms are abundantly evident on Gram stain and culture. The painless black eschar appears by the fifth to seventh day. Nonpitting, gelatinous edema may be prominent, extending occasionally to the iliac crest from lesions of the head and neck. "Malignant

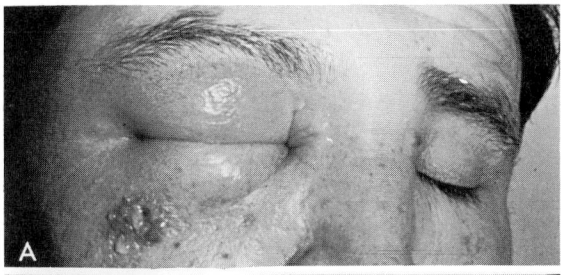

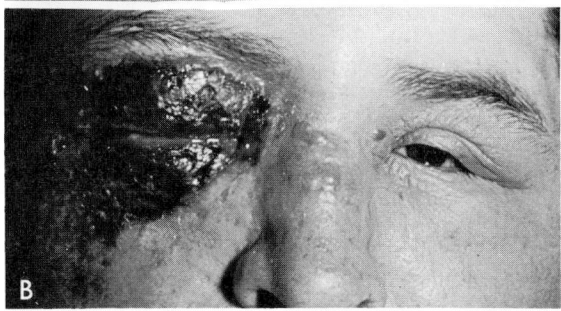

FIGURE 53–1. Cutaneous anthrax in a 45-year-old cattleman. *A,* Early facial lesion with prominent gelatinous edema and vesicular satellite lesions ("pearl wreath"), which revealed abundant anthrax bacilli on Gram stain and culture. *B,* Evolution of the cutaneous eschar despite antimicrobial therapy. (Courtesy of Dr. Alejandro Morales.)

edema," a rare and severe local reaction, usually involves the face and neck. An ulcer may form after several days and is typically painless. Tender regional lymphadenopathy, lymphangitis, and cellulitis are inconspicuous usually and should suggest secondary bacterial infection. Generally, patients have few symptoms, e.g., malaise and low-grade fever. A few will have a neutrophilic leukocytosis of 10,000 to 13,000/mm³. Blood cultures are often sterile.

Inhalation Anthrax. Inhalation anthrax (woolsorter's disease) accounts for 5% of reported cases and is characteristically a biphasic illness. In stage I, nonspecific symptoms of mild fever, malaise, fatigue, and myalgia ensue 1 to 5 days following exposure. Nonproductive cough and precordial oppression are often reported, and rhonchi may be heard. The patient may show actual improvement after several days. In stage II, sudden severe respiratory distress develops with dyspnea, cyanosis, diaphoresis, and tachycardia; a fever of 38 to 40C is present unless shock intervenes. Stridor may be dramatic if enlarged mediastinal nodes impinge upon the trachea. Diffuse rales and basilar dullness are present. Chest radiographs reveal symmetric mediastinal widening; patchy, nonsegmental infiltrates, and pleural effusions (Fig. 53–2). Massive superficial edema of the head and neck may occur. Unless meningitis is present, consciousness is maintained usually until death. Cultures of blood, sputum, pleural fluid, and cerebrospinal fluid are commonly positive.

Gastrointestinal Anthrax. Gastrointestinal anthrax accounts for 5% of cases. After an incubation period of 2 to 5 days, patients manifest generalized abdominal pain, anorexia, nausea, and vomiting. Severe prostration accompanies the development of bloody diarrhea, toxemia, and shock. Subcutaneous edema may extensively involve the lower trunk. Survival is rare.

Central Nervous System Anthrax. Anthrax meningitis, which constitutes less than 1% of anthrax cases, follows bacteremia from a cutaneous, pulmonary, or intestinal source. These critically ill patients present usually with fever, meningismus, and rapidly deteriorating mental status. Peripheral neutrophilic leukocytosis (10,000 to 80,000/mm³) is seen, and lumbar puncture reveals hemorrhagic spinal fluid. Bacteremia is documented in 70% of patients, and the usual survival is 2 to 4 days.

DIAGNOSIS

Differential Diagnosis. The epidemiologic background of an industrial or agricultural exposure, the evolution of a pruritic, then painless, lesion unassociated with cellulitis or lymphangitis, and the dramatic appearance of the eschar and extensive nonpitting edema help to distinguish anthrax from other bacterial skin infections. However, small, early skin lesions may be difficult to recognize. The initial stage of inhalation anthrax resembles influenza, bronchitis, or the common cold. The latter stage may mimic congestive cardiac failure or a cardiovascular catastrophe but is recognized by radiologic mediastinal widening in the setting of occupational exposure. Anthrax meningitis may be confused readily with subarachnoid hemorrhage or meningoencephalitis due to herpes simplex, Naegleria *species, Listeria monocytogenes,* syphilitic or rickettsial meningoencephalitis, or *Pseudomonas aeruginosa* meningitis. Intestinal anthrax with fever and severe abdominal pain may simulate typhoid fever with intestinal perforation or other intra-abdominal catastrophes.

Diagnosis by Direct Smear and Culture. In cutaneous anthrax, the encapsulated bacilli can be identified usually on Wright- or Giemsa-stained smears and cultured on sheep's blood or peptone agar. Nonpathogenic anthrax-like bacilli may be recovered also from suspicious skin lesions; therefore, animal inoculation or identification of isolates by specific bacteriophage lysis is advised.

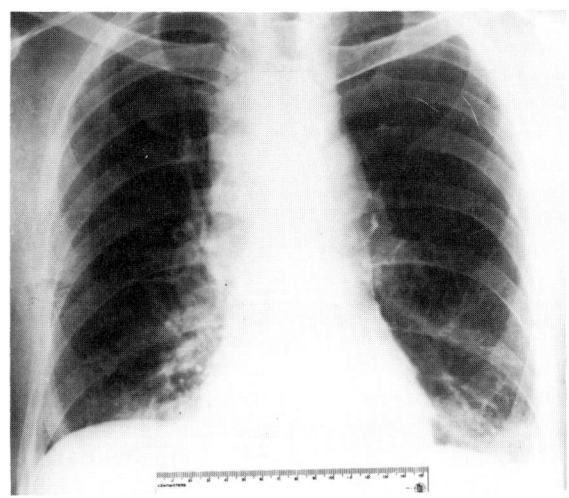

FIGURE 53–2. Chest radiograph on the second day of illness of a 51-year-old American laborer with occupational exposure to airborne anthrax. The combination of parenchymal infiltrate with striking mediastinal lymphadenopathy distinguishes pulmonary anthrax. (Courtesy of the Armed Forces Institute of Pathology, Photograph Neg. No. 71–12790–2.)

Bacilli may be abundant in Gram-stained smears of sputum and cerebrospinal fluid. As with other bacteremias, identification of anthrax bacilli on routine or centrifuged blood smears indicates high-grade sepsis (greater than 10^6 colony-forming units per mL) and a grave prognosis. Direct fluorescent antibody staining may enhance definitive, early identification of *B. anthracis* from vesicular fluid smears, tissue, or culture colonies.

Serologic Diagnosis. The anthrax indirect microhemagglutination (IMH) test has proved to be a less time-consuming and more sensitive test than the previously more widely used agar-gel precipitation test. In one study, IMH detected antibody in 93% of 91 patients receiving anthrax vaccine but in none of 100 controls. Anthrax serologic testing must be highly sensitive, because characteristically patients develop low levels of antibody.

THERAPY

Antimicrobial Therapy. The key to successful therapy is prompt administration of an antimicrobial at the first suspicion of anthrax.

Cutaneous Anthrax. Untreated cutaneous anthrax can be associated with local malignant edema and can progress with septicemia, shock, renal failure, and death in 5 to 20% of cases. Virtually all cutaneous anthrax lesions are cured by antimicrobial therapy. Penicillin, in daily doses of at least 1.2 million units, is the treatment of choice. Oral tetracycline, 2 gm/day, is an alternative for the penicillin-allergic patient and, although probably less effective than penicillin, regularly results in cure. Erythromycin, chloramphenicol, and streptomycin have been employed with success also.

Other Anthrax Syndromes. In adults, high-dose penicillin, 18 to 24 million units/day, plus streptomycin, 2 gm/day, may result in cure of inhalation anthrax if therapy is instituted during the first stage of the disease. One patient was reported to survive intestinal anthrax after treatment with high doses of intravenous ampicillin. Rare, sporadic patients surviving meningitis or bacteremia have also received early, intensive antimicrobial therapy.

Supportive Therapy. Although lesions are rapidly sterilized by treatment, the evolution of the anthrax pustule is not modified by antimicrobials; indeed, toxin mediated edema may increase during the first 24 hours of therapy. Malignant edema of the thorax or neck that interferes with breathing may require treatment with intravenous hydrocortisone, 100 to 200 mg/day. Twenty-four to 48 hours after the onset of therapy, swelling subsides usually, and constitutional symptoms lessen. Scarring of the local lesion is common and may require skin grafting.

Antianthrax Serum Therapy. Prior to the development of antimicrobials, antianthrax serum therapy was responsible for the dramatic reduction in mortality due to anthrax from 48 (24%) to 6 (4%). Anthrax antitoxin, although available for veterinary use in the United Kingdom, is no longer commercially available in the United States. Recent developments in our understanding of the pathogenic role of tripartite anthrax toxin and technological advances in passive immunotherapy may provoke renewed interest in adjunctive antitoxin therapy.

PROGNOSIS. Cutaneous anthrax is usually a self-limited disease. The 5 to 20% mortality rate of untreated patients is essentially eliminated by specific antimicrobial therapy. The progressive course of pulmonary or gastrointestinal anthrax with complicating bacteremia, meningitis, and circulatory collapse is so rapid that death occurs often within 24 to 48 hours, despite antimicrobial therapy.

PREVENTION

Zoonotic Anthrax. Disease should be diagnosed rapidly in animals; herds should be quarantined until 2 weeks after the last case; and all animals in the herd should be vaccinated. Recently, a cell-free vaccine of alum-absorbed protective antigen, available in the United States from Centers for Disease Control, Atlanta, Georgia, has replaced an attenuated vaccine.

Industrially Acquired Anthrax. Control of anthrax spores contaminating certain animal products would reduce human cases of anthrax. Sterilization of wool is not often economical or practical; however, bristles destined for shaving brushes may be sterilized readily prior to manufacture. Employee education, cleaning and disinfection of raw products, and routine vaccination of workers in the wool, hair, and bristle industries in Britain are thought to be responsible for the 4-fold decline in anthrax between the periods 1961 to 1965 and 1976 to 1980. Sporadic cases are reported still among transient factory workers, e.g., ventilation repair, and among hobbyists importing wool directly for their own use. Sterilization of bone-meal fertilizer is difficult and uneconomical; however, many nations require that bags carry warning labels recommending that gloves be worn when using the product. Veterinarians are another group who may benefit from routine vaccination.

Isolation of Patients. Although direct human-to-human transmission has not been demonstrated, wound and skin precautions should be observed for patients with skin lesions, and those with inhalation anthrax should be maintained in strict isolation until they are free of anthrax bacilli, as demonstrated by culture.

BIBLIOGRAPHY

Buchanan TM, Feeley JC, Hayes PS, et al.: Anthrax indirect microhemagglutination test. J Immunol 107:1631, 1971.

Dallforf FG, Kaufman AF, Brachmann PS: Woolsorter's disease: An experimental model. Arch Pathol 92:418, 1971.

Knudson GB: Treatment of anthrax in man: History and current concepts. Milit Med 151:71, 1986.

Leppa SH: Anthrax toxin edema factor: A bacterial adenylate cyclase that increases cyclic AMP concentrations in eukaryotic cells. Proc Natl Acad Sci USA 79:3162, 1982.

O'Brien JO, Friedlander A, Drier T, et al.: Effects of anthrax toxin components on human neutrophils. Infect Immun 47:306, 1985.

54. TETANUS

Sheldon M. Markowitz

DEFINITION. Tetanus is a potentially fatal neuro-paralytic disease caused by the action of a potent protein neurotoxin, tetanospasmin, which is produced by the vegetative form of *Clostridium tetani*.

ETIOLOGY AND PATHOGENESIS. *C. tetani* is a gram-positive, spore-forming obligately anaerobic bacillus that is widespread in nature. Disease is produced most commonly when spores of *C. tetani* are introduced into an unimmunized host under local tissue conditions that promote toxin production, e.g., traumatic, crush, and burn injuries. Tetanospasmin is a 150,000 dalton heat-labile protoplasmic protein that is released following autolysis of vegetative cells. The presence of necrotic tissue, foreign bodies, and other microorganisms lowers the oxidation-reduction potential (Eh), facilitating reversion of spore to vegetative forms. Tetanospasmin binds irreversibly to several ganglioside receptors located on the cell membranes of motor, sensory, and autonomic nerve cells. Tetanospasmin acts at the myoneural junction to inhibit the release of acetylcholine, but classic manifestations of tetanus result from the action of tetanospasmin within the spinal cord and brain stem. The neurotoxin is carried intra-axonally within membrane-bound vesicles at the rate of approximately 250 mm/day and, upon reaching the perikaryon of motor neurons, passes trans-synaptically to block release of neurotransmitters, such as gamma-aminobutyric acid (GABA) and glycine, from presynaptic terminals surrounding motor neurons. Blockage of the glycinergic inhibitory system results in unrestrained stimulation and sustained muscular contraction. Generalized tetanus may result from the uptake and retrograde transport of circulating neurotoxin from motor nerve terminals to the spinal cord and brain stem. The early involvement of the bulbar and paraspinous muscles is explained by their relatively short axons. Tetanospasmin is antigenically homogeneous and does not vary with the strain of *C. tetani* or geographic location.

Spores can be introduced into tissue by major trauma or by minor, often inapparent, skin injury. Tetanus-prone wounds include deep, neglected, and stellate or avulsed wounds related to missile, crush, burn, or frostbite injuries and often contain devitalized tissue and contaminants, such as dirt, feces, and soil. In contrast, nontetanus prone wounds are generally superficial, linear, and caused by sharp surfaces. Contaminants are absent. Any wound in a nonimmune person should be considered tetanus-prone. Ten to 30% of individuals have no trauma or acute injury by history or physical examination.

INCIDENCE AND DISTRIBUTION. Tetanus is a major worldwide health problem, especially in developing countries experiencing overcrowding, poor sanitation, economic deprivation, and a lack of compulsory immunization of children. The incidence of tetanus is determined by the immunization status of the population; where effective immunization is not likely to be achieved, tetanus is most likely to occur. Tetanus is estimated to cause over 600,000 deaths per year, occurring disproportionately in neonates. Lack of immunization in women of childbearing age, poor maternal care, and unhygienic practices, such as dressing the umbilical stump with dung, are factors leading to the high incidence of neonatal tetanus. Routine immunization of Allied troops during World War II prevented tetanus almost universally, despite the widespread exposure to spores of *C. tetani*.

Spores of *C. tetani* are widely distributed in soil, dust, the intestinal tracts of animals and humans, and their surrounding habitats and are highly resistant to many physical and chemical disinfectants, surviving in the soil for months to years if not exposed to sunlight. The recovery rate of *C. tetani* from soil samples varies from 20 to 65%, with recovery most common in cultivated soil, less frequent in grazing land and dairy yards, and least common in virgin soil. Recovery rates from the intestinal tracts of humans and the environment is increased in the presence of large animals and their feces. Vegetative forms of *C. tetani* are inactivated by heat, disinfectants, and many antibiotics.

CLINICAL MANIFESTATIONS. The incubation period, or time between inoculation of spores and the first clinical manifestations, varies from 3 days to 3 weeks and occasionally longer. Mortality rates for illness associated with short incubation periods (less than 7 days) or short periods of onset (less than 7 days for the time of onset of clinical illness to the first generalized spasm) are greater than for illness associated with longer periods of incubation or onset. Incubation periods are longer for illness associated with sites of injury distant to the spinal cord and brain stem, while central nervous system and head wounds produce symptoms after a shorter interval. Four forms of tetanus are recognized: local, cephalic, generalized, and tetanus neonatorum.

Local Tetanus. This form of tetanus usually affects an extremity bearing a tetanus-prone wound and is uncommon. Clinical expression is variable; in its severest form it includes intense, painful spasms in muscle groups near the wound. Local contractions may persist for weeks to months before diminishing and in some patients may progress to generalized tetanus. In the absence of generalized disease, the outlook for recovery is excellent, with a mortality rate of less than 1%.

Cephalic Tetanus. Cephalic tetanus is an extremely uncommon form of local tetanus characterized by a short incubation period (less than 3 days), dysfunction of multiple cranial nerves, and progression to generalized tetanus in two thirds of all patients. The most common presentation is a seventh cranial nerve palsy that often follows severe head injury; in developing countries it is associated often with chronic otitis media from which *C. tetani* can be isolated. The prognosis for this form of tetanus is poor, with mortality rates ranging from 15 to 30%.

Generalized Tetanus. Eighty percent of all cases of tetanus take this form. Usually, clinical manifestations follow an injury by 3 days to 3 weeks, but the incubation period may be as long as 60 to 90 days. Restlessness, irritability, difficulty in swallowing, and stiffness of jaw, facial, and neck muscles progressing to tonic contractions are present almost universally and often are presenting manifestations. Rigidity of abdominal and back muscles is common. Opisthotonos results from sustained contraction of back muscles, while the characteristic facial expression, risus sardonicus, follows persistent trismus (Fig. 54–1). Tetanic seizures are characterized by the sudden onset of opisthotonos, flexion and adduction of the arms, clenched fists, and extension of the legs, and are precipitated often by aural or tactile stimuli, although most are spontaneous. Temperature elevation greater than 38C occurs in 60% of patients. Autonomic instability occurs with severe tetanus and is an ominous and often life-threatening manifestation. Cardiac arrythmias, labile blood pressure, diaphoresis, and hypothermia may complicate management. Tetanic seizures and autonomic manifestations are associated with increased mortality from tetanus.

Tetanus Neonatorum. Neonatal tetanus has virtually disappeared in developed countries, but is a common cause of neonatal morbidity and death in developing countries, where a variety of contaminated materials are used to either sever or dress the umbilical cord of babies born to unimmunized mothers. Irritability and poor feeding are early signs, followed by trismus, facial rigidity, persistent flexion of the toes, and spasms that increase with stimulation. The usual incubation period is 7 days or less, with a mortality rate of 70% or greater. Neonatal tetanus claims an estimated 500,000 lives or more per year.

Complications and Residue. Complications of tetanus include fractures of the spine and clavicles, pulmonary emboli, autonomic dysfunction, laryngeal spasm and

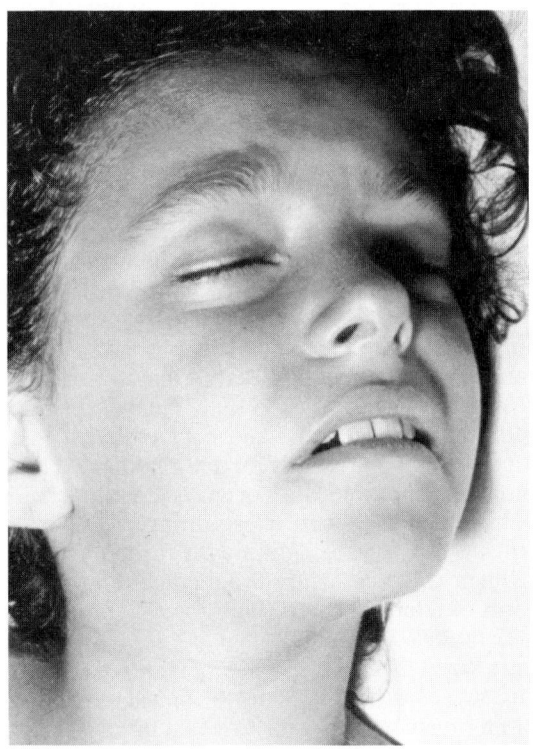

FIGURE 54–1. Risus sardonicus, or the sardonic smile, a grinning or sneering expression produced by spasm of the facial muscles and muscles of mastication.

edema, rhabdomyolysis and renal failure, coma, dehydration, and bacterial infections. Survivors may experience irritability, sleep disturbances, seizures, myoclonus, decreased libido, orthostasis, and electroencephalographic abnormalities as long-term complications.

DIAGNOSIS AND DIFFERENTIAL DIAGNOSES. No readily available diagnostic marker exists for tetanus despite the isolation of *C. tetani* from wounds in 30% of patients. The diagnosis is made usually on the basis of a history of injury followed by the development of the typical neurologic disease. A number of conditions can simulate one or more of the clinical findings of tetanus. Trismus may be caused by oral abscesses, mumps, trichinosis, temporomandibular joint disease, brain stem stroke, camphor poisoning, and phenothiazines. Dystonic muscle contractions, even opisthotonos, may be seen with strychnine poisoning, while confusion with tetanus may arise also with rabies, phenothiazine administration, hypocalcemic tetany, epilepsy, narcotic withdrawal, and hysterical reactions.

TREATMENT AND PROGNOSIS. The therapy of tetanus has 3 major goals: the neutralization of circulating neurotoxin and the prevention of further toxin elaboration; symptomatic and supportive therapy of neurologic and autonomic disease and prevention of complications; and finally, active immunization to provide subsequent protection.

Specific Therapy. Patients should be transferred to hospitals equipped with the intensive cardiopulmonary and support facilities required for the care of patients with tetanus. Human tetanus immune globulin (TIG) is administered intramuscularly at a dose of 3000 to 6000 units; equine tetanus immune globulin in a dose of 10,000 units is equally effective, but has a higher incidence of adverse reactions. Infiltration of the wound with a portion of the dose of antitoxin has been recommended but is of questionable efficacy. Intrathecal TIG has been used with benefit in patients with mild tetanus. Thorough surgical debridement of devitalized tissue, debris, and foreign bodies is essential to prevent further absorption of toxin. Penicillin G, given parenterally at a dose of 6 to 12 million units per day for 10 days, will kill the neurotoxin-elaborating vegetative forms of *C. tetani*, although the efficacy of antibiotics has never been proven in the treatment of tetanus. Cefazolin or tetracycline may be used in penicillin-allergic patients. Active immunization with alum-absorbed toxoid is desirable, because the lethal dose of tetanospasmin is lower than the dose required for immunization.

Supportive Therapy. Sedation and relief of painful muscle spasms can be achieved with the judicious use of diazepam, given intravenously at a dose of 5 to 20 mg intravenously every 4 to 6 hours as needed. Short-acting barbiturates may be useful also. Painful spasms may require the use of narcotic analgesics. External stimuli should be minimized.

A patent airway and effective ventilation should be maintained. Respiratory compromise and failure are the leading causes of death in tetanus. If respiratory dysfunction ensues because of chest wall muscle spasm or

TABLE 54–1. Recommendations for Wound Management for Prevention of Tetanus (Based on Immunization History)

Immunization Record	Wound*	Recommendation
Unimmunized, incomplete, or unknown	Low risk	Toxoid† followed by complete immunization
	Tetanus prone	Toxoid plus TIG, 250 to 500 units using separate syringe and injection sites; complete active immunization
Primary immunization but no booster in 10 years	Low risk	Toxoid
	Tetanus prone	Toxoid; use of TIG is arbitrary
Primary immunization with booster within 10 years	Low risk	—
	Tetanus prone	Toxoid if 5 years since booster

*Tetanus-prone wound indicates severe, neglected, or more than 24 hours old.
†Toxoid as DPT for children under 6 years old; DT for persons over 6 years old. TIG = tetanus immune globulin.

generalized tetanic seizures, endotracheal intubation or tracheostomy and control of ventilation are essential. Total skeletal muscle paralysis may be required with nondepolarizing neuromuscular blocking agents, such as D-tubocurarine, pancuronium bromide, or vecuronium. Dantrolene, which reduces muscle spasm by inhibiting the release of calcium from the sarcoplasmic reticulum, has been used successfully in a few patients. Adequate nutrition and hydration, as well as meticulous nursing care, are important for recovery. Additional measures include heparin for the prevention of thromboembolic disease, antacids or H_2–blockers to prevent stress ulceration, prevention of urinary retention, and the prudent use of beta-blockers to prevent autonomic complications.

Prognosis. Many of these measures are not available in less affluent, developing countries. Hence, mortality rates remain high in these areas. The overall death rate is 30 to 60% and tends to be highest when tetanus develops in neonates, narcotic addicts, the aged, and in those with short incubation periods, generalized seizures, and cephalic tetanus.

PREVENTION. Tetanus is universally preventable with primary immunization. However, even in developed countries where tetanus immunization is widely available, substantial segments of the population lack protective levels of neutralizing antibodies. Recommendations for primary immunization of children less than 7 years of age include 3 doses of tetanus toxoid (as part of the diphtheria, tetanus, and pertussis, or DPT, vaccine) given 4 to 8 weeks apart beginning at age 2 months, with a fourth dose given at 15 months. Booster doses at age 4 to 6 years and every 10 years thereafter maintain adequate immunity. For those 7 years of age and older, a series of 3 injections are given as tetanus-diphtheria (Td) toxoid, with the second injection given 4 to 8 weeks after the first, and the third 6 to 12 months after the second. Booster doses should be given every 10 years thereafter. Recommendations for wound management on the basis of immunization history are given in Table 54–1.

Prevention of wound contamination reduces the incidence of tetanus. Surgical removal of all dead tissue and foreign bodies is of paramount importance, as is the use of clean instruments and materials for circumcision and cutting of the umbilical cord. Tetanus toxoid is not teratogenic, and its use in unimmunized pregnant women will stimulate the formation of neutralizing antibodies that will provide passive protection for neonates. Pregnant women who are unimmunized and likely to deliver under unhygienic conditions should receive at least 2 doses of Td prior to delivery as part of the 3-dose primary immunization schedule. The immunization of women of childbearing age with tetanus toxoid can virtually eliminate neonatal tetanus.

BIBLIOGRAPHY

Bizzini B: Tetanus toxin. Microbial Rev 43:224–240, 1979.
Dowell VR: Botulism and tetanus: Selected epidemiologic and microbiologic aspects. Rev Infect Dis 6:S202–S207, 1984.
Faust RA, Vickers OR, Cohn I, Jr: Tetanus: 2,449 cases in 68 years at Charity Hospital. J Trauma 16:704–712, 1976.
Griffin JW: Local tetanus. Johns Hopkins Med J 149:84–88, 1981.
Gupta PS, Goyal S, Kapoor R, et al.: Intrathecal human tetanus immunoglobulin in early tetanus. Lancet 2:439–440, 1980.
Newell KW, Duenas Lehmann A, LeBlanc DR, et al.: Use of toxoid for prevention of tetanus neonatorum: Preliminary report of double-blind controlled field trial. Bull WHO 30:439–444, 1964.
Salimpour R: Cause of death in tetanus neonatorium: Study of 233 cases with 54 necropsies. Arch Dis Child 52:587–591, 1977.
Schofield FA, Tucker VM, Westbrook GR: Neonatal tetanus in New Guinea: Effect of active immunization in pregnancy. Br Med J 2:785–789, 1961.
Stanfield JP, Galazka A: Neonatal tetanus in the world today. Bull WHO 62:647–669, 1984.
Weinstein L: Tetanus. N Engl J Med 289:1293–1296, 1973.

55. OTHER CLOSTRIDIAL INFECTIONS

Sheldon M. Markowitz

GENERAL PRINCIPLES

The clostridia include a large number of obligately anaerobic gram-positive spore-forming bacilli that are found widely dispersed in soil and the gastrointestinal tract of mammals. At least 83 species of clostridia have been described, and whereas most are still considered harmless saprophytes, the list of human infections caused by the clostridia is impressive. Many clostridial diseases, including botulism, tetanus, food poisoning (due to *Clostridium perfringens*), and traumatic gas gangrene, are predominantly exogenous infections, whereas others, such as *C. difficile*-induced colitis and suppurative intra-abdominal and pelvic infections, are endogenous infections caused by the indigenous host flora. Disease is associated generally with the elaboration of a diverse group of exotoxins, including neurotoxins (botulism, tetanus), enterotoxins and cytotoxins

(C. perfringens, C. difficile), and histotoxins *(C. perfringens, C. novyi, C. bifermentans)*. Prior concepts of pathogenesis have required modification following the descriptions of wound and infant botulism, a botulism-like illness caused by neurotoxigenic species other than *C. botulinum*, nontraumatic gas gangrene, the association of *C. septicum* bacteremia with colonic carcinoma, and the nosocomial nature of *C. difficile*-induced colitis. The continuing evolution and expanding clinical spectrum of clostridial infections have been made possible by refinements in methods used to isolate anaerobic bacteria. Effective management and prevention of clostridial infections require an understanding of predisposing factors, disease mechanisms, and clinical presentations.

55.1. BOTULISM

DEFINITION. Botulism is a neuroparalytic illness of varying severity caused by neurotoxins produced by *Clostridium botulinum* and, rarely, other clostridia.

ETIOLOGY AND PATHOGENESIS

History. Outbreaks of botulism have been known in Europe since antiquity. In fact, the term botulism is derived from the early association with ingestion of spoiled sausages. In 1895, Van Ermengem isolated an anaerobic, spore-forming bacillus from raw ham and the post mortem tissues of persons who died during an outbreak of botulism. He postulated the presence of an extracellular toxin after he was able to reproduce the disease in animals following ingestion of the food vehicle or administration of culture filtrates. In parallel with the increase in commercial and home canning following World War I, numerous outbreaks of botulism were reported. Later, the ecology of *C. botulinum* was described, as well as the conditions favoring toxin production and those allowing destruction of toxin and spores during food processing. Application of these guidelines caused a dramatic decline, but did not eliminate, cases of botulism related to commercially prepared products. Today, food-borne botulism is associated most commonly with home-canned or home-processed food.

Organism and Toxins. *C. botulinum* is a diverse group of gram-positive, spore-forming obligate anaerobes that are widely distributed in nature. Although four biotypes have been described, *C. botulinum* is classified solely on the basis of the production of 8 antigenically distinct toxins (A, B, C1, C2, D, E, F, and G), each with a molecular size of 150,000 daltons. Production of toxins by types C1 and D depends on infection of *C. botulinum* by specific bacteriophages. Most human disease is caused by Types A, B, and E and rarely F and G. Types C1, C2, and D produce disease in mammals and birds. Each strain of *C. botulinum* produces but one toxin usually.

Spores of *C. botulinum* are ingested regularly by humans. During vegetative growth and lysis, the organism elaborates a neurotoxin that is among the most potent substances known. Some toxins, such as type E, may be elaborated in a precursor form that requires enzymatic activation. Spores, particularly types A and B, are heat-stable and resist boiling for hours, especially at high altitudes. However, the neurotoxins are heat-labile, providing the basis for the terminal heating of home-canned preparations. The neurotoxins are acid-stable and resistant to digestive enzymes and thus are able to survive the mammalian gastric acid barrier, but germination and elaboration of toxin are inhibited at a ph less than 4.5. Alkali readily destroys the toxins. Food containing toxins of types A and B may appear and taste normal or spoiled.

Once absorbed, the neurotoxin disseminates hematogenously to peripheral presynaptic terminals, binding irreversibly to block the release of the neurotransmitter acetylcholine. Intoxication may result from the ingestion of preformed toxin present in contaminated food or from absorption of toxin following vegetation growth of *C. botulinum* in the gastrointestinal tract or in an infected wound. Thus, at least 4 categories of botulism are now recognized: food-borne botulism, wound botulism, infant botulism, and botulism of undetermined classification.

DISTRIBUTION AND EPIDEMIOLOGY. Spores of *C. botulinum* are widely distributed in soil and aquatic environments throughout the world. Food-borne botulism occurs worldwide but is restricted generally to northern or temperate climates. The true incidence in developing countries is unknown because botulism may be misdiagnosed or under-reported. In the United States food-borne botulism has a distinctive distribution: over 80% of type A outbreaks have occurred west of the Mississippi River, 63% of type B outbreaks have occurred east of the Mississippi River, and over half of type E outbreaks have occurred in more northern areas, including the Great Lakes and Alaska. The distribution of clinical disease roughly parallels the distribution of *C. botulinum* spores in the soil.

Most cases in the United States are caused by *C. botulinum* types A, B, and E. From 1976 through 1984 124 outbreaks of botulism were identified involving 308 persons (or 2.7 persons per outbreak). Sixty-eight percent involved only 1 person; 20% involved 2 persons; and 12% involved more than 2 persons. Outbreaks were reported in 30 states, but most occurred in Alaska, Oregon, Washington, and California. *C. botulinum* types A, B, and E were identified in 60, 30, and 10% of outbreaks, respectively. Vegetables, usually home-canned, were implicated in 70% of cases and meat or fish in 30% of cases. Home-processed fish or meat from marine mammals were responsible for all type E outbreaks, over 90% of which occurred in Alaska, where dried or uncooked food is favored by the native populations. Meat and meat products are implicated most frequently in Europe, whereas dried fish is responsible most frequently in Japan, Scandinavia, and Russia.

Commercially canned foods accounted for 3% of outbreaks from 1970 to 1984, whereas only 4% were related to food served in restaurants. However, restaurant outbreaks accounted for 42% of all cases of botulism during this period. Newly identified vehicles of food-borne transmission were observed, including sauteed onions, potato salad, chopped garlic, beef stew, and meat loaf, among others.

Wound botulism, infant botulism, and botulism of undetermined source are usually caused by *C. botulinum* types A or B.

CLINICAL MANIFESTATIONS. Botulism is a neurologic disorder that classically manifests as a bilaterally symmetric descending paralysis or weakness with prominent bulbar and respiratory involvement.

Food-Borne Botulism. Symptoms of botulism begin usually 12 to 48 hours (range 6 hours to 8 days) following the ingestion of food containing preformed neurotoxins of *C. botulinum*. Symptoms of weakness, fatigue, and dizziness occur early. Sixty to 75% of those with disease due to type A or type B toxin have gastrointestinal symptoms, including nausea, vomiting, constipation, and abdominal cramps. Cholinergic blockade leads initially to bulbar dysfunction, with diplopia, dry mouth, dysphagia, dysphonia, and dysarthria. Although neurologic symptoms may be delayed for up to 3 days following the onset of illness, descending motor weakness and paralysis of the extremities develop with variable speed and severity. Respiratory muscles are involved, and breathing becomes difficult.

On physical examination, the patient is mentally alert and afebrile but may exhibit orthostasis. Ocular findings are prominent, with bilateral ptosis, fixed, dilated pupils, and cranial nerve palsies, especially weakness of the sixth cranial nerves leading to paralysis of lateral gaze (Fig. 55–1). The gag reflex is diminished. Mucous membranes and the tongue are dry and fissured. Motor dysfunction may be mild or severe. Deep tendon reflexes are variably affected, but sensation usually remains intact. Pathologic reflexes are absent. Ileus and urinary retention may be present. Progression of respiratory muscle weakness may be mild and abortive or rapid and life-threatening, requiring intubation and respiratory support. Recovery may be prolonged, with the patient plagued with persistent fatigue, constipation, or a sicca syndrome.

Wound Botulism. This form of botulism is rare but

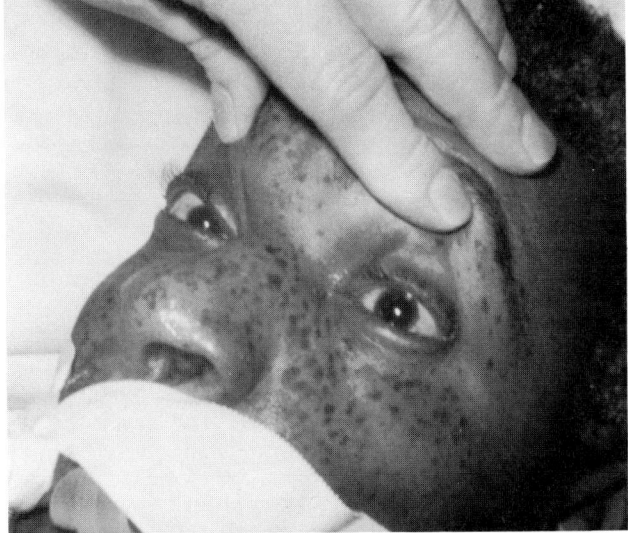

FIGURE 55–1. Bilateral palsies of the sixth cranial nerves and fixed, dilated pupils in an elderly woman on mechanical ventilation; the patient had lateral gaze paralysis bilaterally, although only left lateral gaze paralysis is shown.

probably underdiagnosed. Only 30 cases have been recorded since 1943, most occurring in the last 2 decades. Most patients have been young males who suffer a compound fracture or crush injury to an extremity with inoculation of *C. botulinum* spores. The incubation period ranges from 4 to 14 days (average, 10 days), gastrointestinal symptoms are infrequent, and single case outbreaks are characteristic. Otherwise, the clinical syndrome is similar to that of food-borne botulism. A variant of wound botulism has been described in chronic intravenous drug abusers. Although the portal of entry is presumed to be sites of drug injection, 50% of these patients have no obvious wound infection.

Infant Botulism. This form of botulism was first recognized in 1976 as a cause of the "floppy" infant syndrome. Infants age 3 weeks to 11 months have been affected primarily. The disease has a unique pathogenesis: germination, in vivo multiplication, and elaboration of botulinal toxin in the gastrointestinal tracts of infants who have ingested spores of *C. botulinum* and rarely *C. butyricum* and *C. barati*. Approximately 50 to 200 cases are estimated to occur annually in the United States, making it now the most common form of botulism. Clinical disease varies considerably, from "failure to thrive" to the sudden infant death syndrome (SIDS). Constipation, a feeble cry, poor sucking, lethargy, and pooled oral secretions presage the onset of cranial nerve palsies, generalized flaccid paralysis, and apnea. The source of *C. botulinum* is unknown in most instances, but honey contaminated with *C. botulinum* spores has been incriminated as a vector in some cases.

Botulism, Classification Undetermined. These are individuals greater than 12 months of age who develop botulism without an obvious source. It is likely that in some instances in vivo elaboration of toxin by *C. botulinum* colonizing the gut occurs in a manner similar to that seen with infant botulism. A few of these individuals have received antibiotics prior to the onset of illness, suggesting that alterations in the normal gut flora may have allowed proliferation of *C. botulinum*.

DIAGNOSIS. The diagnosis of botulism should be suspected in any person who develops a neurologic illness characterized by a descending flaccid paralysis associated with gastrointestinal symptoms following the ingestion of potentially contaminated food. Confirmation of the diagnosis depends on the isolation of *C. botulinum* from stool, gastric contents, antecedent wound, incriminated food, or the demonstration of botulinal toxin in the patient's serum, stool, gastric contents, or the incriminated food.

A sensitive enzyme-linked immunosorbent assay (ELISA) for type A toxin has been developed, but the most widely used method for assaying botulinal toxin is the mouse bioassay method. Identification of the toxin type and its quantitation may take up to 4 days and is performed usually in central or specialized laboratories. Therefore, presumptive clinical diagnosis is important for effective management but may be difficult. Lack of an obvious food vector, especially if not home-prepared, the absence of other cases, and atypical features may make clinical diagnosis difficult. Paresthesias, asymmetric paralysis and ptosis, nystagmus, normal pupils, elevated cerebrospinal fluid protein levels, and a positive response to edrophonium chloride (Tensilon) have been reported in 8 to 25% of patients with botulism. However, the diagnosis should be suspected strongly in an alert, afebrile patient who develops bilateral sixth cranial nerve palsies, dilated and fixed pupils, a descending paralysis with respiratory weakness, orthostasis, and dry mucous membranes, supported by the findings of a normal cerebrospinal fluid, typical changes on electromyography (an increase in the number of overall small amplitude action potentials, facilitation of muscle-action potential after tetanic stimulation or following rapid-repetitive stimulation, and muscle fibrillation), and a negative response to edrophonium chloride. Differential diagnostic considerations include the Guillain-Barré syndrome; myasthenia gravis; ingestion of anticholinergics, such as atropine or jimson weed; tick paralysis; paralytic poliomyelitis; the Eaton-Lambert syndrome; hypocalcemia; and paralytic shellfish poisoning.

TREATMENT AND PROGNOSIS

Supportive Therapy. Respiratory failure and superinfections are the principal causes of death in patients with botulism. Close monitoring of patients and early elective tracheal intubation or tracheostomy lowers the mortality rate for patients with diminishing vital capacities. The judicious use of antibiotics for nosocomial bacterial infections, nasogastric intubation and parenteral nutrition to relieve paralytic ileus, and bladder catheterization to relieve urinary retention are important to a successful outcome.

Toxin Neutralization. Efforts to remove neurotoxin from the gut and neutralize circulating toxin are indicated at any time during the course of illness, because toxin may persist in the gastrointestinal tract and serum for several weeks following onset. Cleansing enemas and cathartics given early may be beneficial in eliminating toxin from the body. The efficacy of equine trivalent botulinum antitoxin (containing antitoxins A, B, and E) has been questioned in the past; however, retrospective studies show a lowered mortality rate and a shorter duration of illness for botulism due to types A and B when antitoxin is administered early in the disease. Two vials of antitoxin are administered immediately, 1 intravenously and 1 intramuscularly; if the disease is severe or if it progresses, 2 additional vials are given in 4 hours. Hypersensitivity to horse serum should be determined prior to the administration of antitoxin, because 10 to 20% of patients will have an adverse reaction. Although *C. botulinum* is susceptible to penicillin, the use of antibiotics to treat food-borne botulism is not recommended now. The efficacy of antibiotic therapy for patients with wound botulism is unclear. In an experimental animal model of wound botulism due to *C. botulinum* type A, antitoxin was superior to antibiotics in decreasing mortality rates; both improved survival over control animals. Aqueous penicillin G, 10 to 20 million units/day, is given intravenously.

Prognosis. In the United States, recent mortality rates for food-borne botulism, wound botulism, and infant botulism have been 7.5, 12.5, and 2.7%, respectively. In those with the diagnosis of botulism of undetermined classification, the mortality rate is 29%, perhaps reflect-

ing a delay in diagnosis and the institution of appropriate therapy in the absence of an obvious source. Death is also more likely to occur in each of the following circumstances: age greater than 60 years, incubation period less than 36 hours, disease due to *C. botulinum* type A, delayed diagnosis, and 1-person outbreaks. Although mild cranial nerve dysfunction persists for a variable period during convalescence, the outlook for survivors is one of complete recovery.

PREVENTION. Although botulism is uncommon in the United States and mortality rates have declined over the past 30 years, the disease causes substantial mortality. Strict adherence to techniques of home canning will prevent food-borne botulism. Spores can be destroyed by heating food at 120C for 30 minutes under pressure. Terminal heating at 80C for 20 minutes or boiling for 1 minute will inactivate the neurotoxin. Germination of *C. botulinum* can be prevented by refrigeration, freezing, drying, or the addition of salt or sodium nitrite. Wound botulism is best prevented by the thorough surgical debridement of contaminated wounds and by avoiding chronic parenteral drug abuse. Some cases of infant botulism may be prevented by omitting honey from the diets of infants less than 12 months old.

BIBLIOGRAPHY

Arnon SS: Infant botulism: Anticipating the second decade: J Infect Dis 154:201–206, 1986.

Dowell VR, Jr: Botulism and tetanus: Selected epidemiologic and microbiologic aspects. Rev Infect Dis 6:5202–5207, 1984.

Hughes JM, Blumenthal JR, Merson MH, et al.: Clinical feature of types A and B food-borne botulism. Ann Intern Med 95:442–445, 1981.

MacDonald KL, Cohen ML, Blake PA: The changing epidemiology of adult botulism in the United States. Am J Epidemiol 124:794–799, 1986.

MacDonald KL, Rutherford GW, Friedman SM, et al.: Botulism and botulism-like illness in chronic drug abusers. Ann Intern Med 102:616–618, 1985.

Sakaguchi G: *Clostridium botulinum* toxins. Pharmacol Ther 19:165–194, 1983.

Schaffner W: Clostridium botulinum (botulism). *In* Mandell GL, Douglas RG, Jr, Bennett JE (eds.): Principles and Practice of Infectious Diseases, ed 2. New York, John Wiley and Sons, 1985, pp. 1359–1362.

Tacket CO, Shandera WX, Mann JM, et al.: Equine antitoxin use and other factors that predict outcome in type A foodborne botulism. Am J Med 76:794–798, 1984.

55.2. GAS GANGRENE

DEFINITION. Gas gangrene is a rapidly progressive, often life-threatening infection associated with myonecrosis due to a toxin or toxins elaborated by species of clostridia, usually *C. perfringens*. The term for gas gangrene is applied most accurately to a single entity, clostridial myonecrosis.

ETIOLOGY AND PATHOGENESIS. Over 150 species of clostridia have been recognized since the description of *C. butyricum* by Louis Pasteur in 1861. *C. welchii* was first recognized as a cause of gas gangrene in 1892 and later renamed *C. perfringens*. *C. perfringens* has been isolated subsequently from 80 to 90% of cases of gas gangrene, while 2 other histotoxic clostridia, *C. novyi* and *C. septicum,* have been implicated in 10 to 40% and 5 to 20% of cases, respectively. Patients may be infected with *C. histolyticum, C. bifermentans, C. fallax,* and *C. sporogenes,* but only rarely. These 7 species of clostridia produce over 22 exotoxins, of which the most important is alpha-toxin (alpha-lecithinase; phospholipase).

Toxins. *C. perfringens* is the most important histotoxic species of clostridia and, in addition to alpha-toxin, is known to produce at least 12 other tissue-active exotoxins. The species is divided into 5 types, designated A through E, on the basis of the production of 4 major toxins (alpha, beta, epsilon, and theta). All 5 serotypes produce alpha-toxin, but type A produces the greatest quantity. Alpha-toxin is oxygen stable and has a marked affinity for lipid membranes. As a result severe hemolysis, platelet destruction, and widespread alterations in capillary permeability occur. Other toxins, in particular the theta-toxin, contribute also to local tissue necrosis and systemic toxicity, including shock.

Local Tissue Factors. Clostridia thrive in tissues with low oxygen tension. When tissue is damaged, its vascular supply is compromised and tissue tension is lowered. Settings favoring toxin elaboration are seen with clostridial myonecrosis, which usually results from the contamination of traumatic or surgical wounds by histotoxic clostridia under conditions of a decreased oxidation-reduction potential (Eh). Blood vessel trauma, intense edema, the use of tourniquets, pressure dressings, and vasoconstrictors, and the presence of foreign bodies, devitalized tissue, and other microorganisms contribute to vascular insufficiency and tissue hypoxia and the resultant toxin-mediated liquefactive necrosis of muscle and surrounding tissue.

INCIDENCE. Estimates of the frequency of occurrence of gas gangrene vary widely. In a large review of major open wounds, the incidence of gas gangrene ranged from 0.03 to 5.2%, depending on the type of wound and treatment. The incidence following criminal abortion has been reported to be 0.5 to 1%. In the United States, 900 to 3000 cases per year are thought to occur. The incidence of gas gangrene in developing countries is likely higher.

DISTRIBUTION. The histotoxic clostridia are ubiquitous, exposure is universal, and infections occur worldwide. Soil samples universally harbor clostridia, including *C. perfringens,* at concentrations of 1000 organisms per gm or greater. *C. perfringens* is commonly present also in water, meat, clothing, dust, air samples, and agricultural products. Most animals and humans harbor *C. perfringens* in the gastrointestinal tract at a mean concentration of 10^8 to 10^9 organisms/gm of feces. Up to 80% of severe traumatic open wounds are contaminated with spores of *C. perfringens,* although gas gangrene occurs in less than 3%.

CLINICAL MANIFESTATIONS. Clinical settings associated with gas gangrene include the following: traumatic injuries and penetrating wounds; surgery, especially colonic resection or surgical wounds following a ruptured appendix, bowel perforation, or biliary tract surgery; uterine gas gangrene most commonly following septic abortion, less commonly normal delivery, and least commonly necrosis of uterine fibroid tumors; soft tissue infections associated with vascular insufficiency and occasionally diabetes mellitus; and spontaneous (or nontraumatic) gas gangrene, a variant that arises without an apparent source.

Symptoms and Signs. Clinical manifestations of gas gangrene begin 3 to 5 days following a traumatic wound or a surgical procedure, with a range of 8 hours to 3 weeks. The sudden appearance of severe pain and tense edema and tenderness at the wound site is observed early. Initial skin pallor gives way to a blue, purple, or bronze discoloration, often accompanied by large, tense, hemorrhagic bullae filled with dark red or purplish fluid and cutaneous necrosis. As the lesion evolves, the scant, thin, watery discharge is replaced by a thick, profuse, sweet-smelling, serosanguineous discharge that contains abundant gram-positive bacilli and a paucity of inflammatory cells on microscopic examination. Tissue gas may be present, but its occurrence is irregular and noted often in the late stages of disease. Fever is usually low-grade, but the pulse rate is increased usually far out of proportion to the temperature elevation. As the disease progresses, incisional or wound pain increases and circulatory collapse ensues with the development of hemolytic anemia, hemoglobinuria with renal failure, and profound systemic toxicity. Remarkably, patients remain unusually alert and aware of their surroundings despite their severe toxic state. Indifference and apathy or extreme apprehension and a sense of doom may be noted. Coma and shock are terminal events.

Uterine Gas Gangrene. Postabortal and postpartum clostridial uterine infections and postoperative gas gangrene are more prevalent in developing countries than in the United States and Europe. Uterine gas gangrene begins 1 to 3 days following septic abortion, with the early onset of jaundice and renal failure caused by the massive intravascular hemolysis mediated by alpha-toxin. Pigmenturia leads to acute renal cortical necrosis and anuria. Bacteremia is common, and hypotension and shock occur regularly. Pelvic findings may be minimal, although x-ray films may show uterine wall gas.

Spontaneous Gas Gangrene. Nontraumatic gas gangrene occurs without apparent source and is distinctive for the absence of trauma, its clostridial etiology, and its rapidly progressive course. Extensive soft tissue gas that spreads far beyond the borders of necrotic muscle is characteristic. Hemolysis, renal failure, and shock develop early, and patients may die within 2 or 3 days of onset. Spontaneous gas gangrene is usually caused by *C. perfringens;* however, *C. septicum* has been implicated in several patients, often in association with cryptic colonic carcinoma.

DIAGNOSIS AND DIFFERENTIAL DIAGNOSES. The diagnosis of gas gangrene is based usually on a combination of characteristic clinical manifestations and supporting microbiological studies. A history of trauma or surgery, the typical appearance of the wound in a severely toxic patient, the presence of acute hemolytic anemia, jaundice, and renal failure, and the observation of large gram-positive bacilli without spores on Gram's stain and *C. perfringens* on culture support the diagnosis of clostridial myonecrosis. Confirmation requires direct inspection of the involved muscle, which appears pale and edematous early in the disease. With progression the muscle becomes beefy red, black, or friable, and will eventually become gelatinous or even liquefy. Muscle contraction is absent on stimulation, and the cut surface fails to bleed. Radiographs of involved areas may show nonspecific gas collections. Blood cultures are positive in 15% of patients with gas gangrene, but the diagnosis can be established by the finding of myonecrosis at surgery or autopsy and typical organisms on Gram's stain.

Soft tissue gas may be seen with infections due to aerobic organisms, nonclostridial anaerobes such as *Bacteroides* species and peptostreptococci, and in mixed anaerobic infections. Noninfectious causes of soft tissue gas include the effects of trauma, hydrogen peroxide irrigation, barotrauma, and following extensive surgical procedures. Myonecrosis may be seen in streptococcal myositis and in a variety of synergistic and necrotizing infections involving both aerobes and nonclostridial anaerobes.

TREATMENT AND PROGNOSIS. Surgical exploration of the involved area with radical debridement of all necrotic tissue and delayed closure of open wounds are the most important therapeutic maneuvers. This usually involves excision of involved muscle, amputation of an extremity, or uterine curettage or hysterectomy. Although the efficacy of antibiotics in the treatment of established gas gangrene in humans is less well established, they are recommended as an adjunct to surgical debridement. Aqueous penicillin G should be given intravenously at a daily dose of 12 or 20 million units for 10 to 14 days; chloramphenicol, tetracycline, metronidazole, and clindamycin are effective alternatives and in murine models of gas gangrene have proved superior to penicillin G for prevention of disease. Cephalosporins have been shown to be inadequate in preventing gas gangrene following severe open trauma.

Hyperbaric Oxygen. The value of hyperbaric oxygen in the treatment of gas gangrene remains unsettled after many years of scrutiny and discussion. Support for its efficacy is derived mainly from anecdotal experiences and uncontrolled or noncomparative studies. Proponents cite the dramatic improvement in some patients and the arrest and demarcation of the disease process, which help to facilitate surgical debridement. Most authorities would advocate the use of hyperbaric oxygen if facilities were available, despite the problems of transferring critically ill patients to such centers. In experienced hands, oxygen toxicity has been minimal. Polyvalent gas gangrene antitoxin has proven worthless in the management of infected patients and is no longer available.

Prognosis. Supportive measures include fluid and electrolyte replacement, management of acidosis and hemolytic anemia, and measures to preserve renal function. Complications include superinfections, the adult respiratory distress syndrome, disseminated intravascular coagulopathy, acute tubular necrosis, myocardial irritability, thromboembolic disease, fat embolism, and

tetanus. Overall mortality rates range from 20 to 60%, with an average of 25%. It is highest in those patients with involvement of the abdominal wall, buttocks, myometrium, and in those with spontaneous (nontraumatic) gas gangrene and lowest in those with involvement of the distal extremity and the endometrium.

PREVENTION. If gas gangrene is suspected, early diagnosis and the avoidance of time-wasting and costly investigations is essential. Prompt and thorough debridement of traumatized tissue is a critical factor in the prevention of gas gangrene. Less delay in the institution of appropriate prophylactic antibiotics and prudent decisions regarding wound closure are important also. No effective means of active immunization exists.

BIBLIOGRAPHY

Gorbach SL: Other *Clostridium* species (including gas gangrene). *In* Mandell GL, Douglas RG, Jr, Bennett JE (eds.): Principles and Practice of Infectious Diseases, ed 2. New York, John Wiley and Sons, 1985, pp. 1362–1368.

Gorbach SL, Thadepalli H: Isolation of clostridium in human infections: Evaluation of 114 cases. J Infect Dis 131:S81–S85, 1975.

Hart GB, Lamb RC, Strauss MB: Gas gangrene: I. A collective review. J Trauma 23:991–995, 1983.

Heimbach RD: Gas grangene: Review and update. HBO Rev 1:41–51, 1980.

MacLennan JD: The histotoxic clostridial infections of man. Bacteriol Rev 26:177–276, 1962.

Smith LDS: The Pathogenic Anaerobic Bacteria, ed 2. Springfield, Illinois, Charles C Thomas, 1975, pp. 109–176, 322–24.

Stevens DL, Maier KA, Laine BM, et al.: Comparison of clindamycin, rifampin, tetracycline, metronidazole, and penicillin for efficacy in prevention of experimental gas gangrene due to *Clostridium perfringens*. J Infect Dis 155:220–228, 1987.

Stevens DL, Troyer BE, Merrick DT, et al.: Lethal effects and cardiovascular effects of purified alpha- and theta-toxins from *Clostridium perfringens*. J Infect Dis 157:272–279, 1988.

55.3. ENTERITIS NECROTICANS

DEFINITION. Enteritis necroticans, also known as "pig-bel" and "Darmbrand," is a necrotizing enteritis caused by beta-toxin produced by *Clostridium perfringens* type C.

HISTORY. The first systematic study of enteritis necroticans was conducted during and shortly after World War II. At that time, there were hundreds of cases of "Darmbrand" (meaning "firebowels") in Germany and Norway; most of these were in malnourished individuals who often had a history of sudden dietary overindulgence. The disease was limited to the early years following World War II, peaking in incidence in 1948, and disappearing thereafter. The etiology was debated, but the likely mechanism centered on a toxin produced by *C. perfringens*. These organisms were classified originally as type F and then reclassified as type C by Oakley, who also detected antitoxin to the beta-toxin produced by this organism in convalescing patients. Antitoxin therapy was proposed but not used, because the epidemic resolved with improved nutritional status around 1949. Interest in this disease revived in the early 1960s when the same disease process, known locally as "pig-bel," was found to be endemic in the highlands of New Guinea. Extensive studies of enteritis necroticans at this location have provided most of the current information concerning the pathology, pathophysiology, detection, treatment, and prevention of this disease.

DISTRIBUTION. The organism appears to be widely distributed in soil, has been found in asymptomatic carriers, and may be found in the stools of animals, including pigs. Acquisition of the disease depends on a complex combination of circumstances, including contact with the organism, dietary habits, and undernutrition. Since World War II, enteritis necroticans has been found occasionally in Western countries, but most cases occur in developing countries along the equator, e.g., Uganda, Indonesia, Thailand, Malaysia, and New Guinea. Serologic studies in the highlands of New Guinea in 1963 and 1964 showed a prevalence of 50 cases per 10,000 population with a mortality rate of 14 per 10,000 population. Enteritis necroticans is the most common cause of death in children over 12 months of age in this location, whereas over 86% of adults in the high-incidence region have circulating antibody to the beta-toxin.

PATHOGENESIS. In the highlands of New Guinea the disease is found commonly in children who have participated in pig and sweet potato feasts. The responsible toxin is a protein of approximately 48,000 daltons that is produced by *C. perfringens* type C. This exotoxin, which is produced in early logarithmic growth, is susceptible to destruction by proteases, including trypsin. The diet among inhabitants of the islands of Papua New Guinea is low in protein, with sweet potatoes accounting for up to 90% of calories. Contributory factors in the diet include a depression of proteolytic activity resulting from reduced protein consumption combined with trypsin inhibitors in the sweet potato staple. It is presumed that the organism is acquired by ingestion of contaminated pig or is present owing to prior colonization and that the toxin is not inactivated because of inadequate proteolysis. This theory is supported by the production of a similar disease in protein-deficient guinea pigs given sweet potato and a broth culture containing *C. perfringens* type C. Co-infection with intestinal parasites may be important also. *Ascaris lumbricoides,* present in 65% of cases of pig-bel, is a source of trypsin inhibitors, whereas another common intestinal helminth, *Strongyloides stercoralis,* may reduce intestinal motility, contribute to intestinal obstruction, or, by penetrating the intestinal mucosca, allow greater absorption of beta-toxin. Pig-bel is primarily a disease of children in New Guinea, with a peak incidence in children 4 years of age, apparently reflecting the fact that most adults have circulating antibody. The pathogenesis of enteritis necroticans may be different for disease occurring outside of New Guinea, especially when there is no history of pork or sweet potato ingestion or overeating.

PATHOLOGY. Enteritis necroticans is a segmental disease of the small bowel that may be restricted to a few centimeters or may involve the entire length of the small intestine. The external surface shows dilatation, with areas of erythema and fibropurulent exudate. The mucosa underlying segmental areas of peritonitis show green, necrotic pseudomembranes that may be restricted to the mucosa but are more frequently of full thickness. With more advanced lesions, the bowel wall becomes thinned, friable, and subject to perforation. Microscopic sections taken from involved segments show mucosal infarction with edema, hemorrhage, and infiltration by polymorphonuclear leukocytes. The membrane consists of necrotic mucosal epithelium containing numerous gram-positive bacilli. This inflamed segment is sharply demarcated, with small-vessel thrombi at the junctional zone, suggesting thrombotic necrosis.

CLINICAL MANIFESTATIONS. The usual presenting symptoms are abdominal pain and distention, vomiting, and passage of a bloody or black, tarry stool. The usual incubation period is 48 hours following ingestion of the dietary source of the toxin, but this may vary from 24 hours to 1 week. There is considerable variation in the severity of the disease. Some patients have a fulminant course and die within 24 hours following the onset of symptoms, whereas mild cases may be difficult to distinguish from common forms of gastroenteritis. Occasionally, patients present with malabsorption or intestinal obstruction months or years after the acute episode.

DIAGNOSIS. The diagnosis of enteritis necroticans in the endemic area is based usually on clinical observations, sometimes accompanied by the demonstration of typical pathologic changes at surgery or autopsy. The responsible organism, *Clostridium perfringens* type C, may be demonstrated in small bowel contents or stool using a fluorescein-stained antibody. Stool cultures are difficult to interpret, because the carrier rate of the putative agent in New Guinea is 50 to 100% for inhabitants of both the highland area, where the disease is endemic, and the coastal region, where the incidence is extremely low.

TREATMENT AND PROGNOSIS. Medical therapy includes intestinal decompression with nasogastric intubation, penicillin, or chloramphenicol given intravenously, and intravenous fluid support with appropriate monitoring of serum electrolytes and special attention to potassium depletion. The major indications for operative intervention are persistent toxicity, intestinal obstruction, suspected bowel perforation, and severe recurrent bleeding. Prolonged delays in therapy may result in a technically difficult operation, because the intestine becomes extremely friable with extensive adhesions. In New Guinea approximately 50% of patients require surgery. The usual procedure is small bowel resection, usually 50 to 200 cm of jejunum. The mortality rate, excluding mild cases, is reported to be 15 to 40%.

PREVENTION. There is little prospect for reversing the dietary and social habits in the highlands of New Guinea to alter the unique combination of circumstances that promotes enteritis necroticans. However, toxoid prepared from culture filtrates of the putative agent confers protection. This is based on analogous experience with this disease in veterinary medicine, the low incidence of the disease in the endemic area among adults with circulating antibody, and, most importantly, a vaccine trial that demonstrated efficacy.

Immunization. The current recommendation is to administer beta-toxoid to children in the highlands of New Guinea at 2, 4, and 6 months of age, and to children in other populations outside of New Guinea in whom the disease is active. A tattoo is the suggested recording method, because conventional methods of record-keeping have proved futile. The duration of protection is not known, and it is possible that booster injections may be needed.

BIBLIOGRAPHY

Johnson S, Taylor DN, Coninx R, et al.: Enteritis necroticans among Khmer children at an evacuation site in Thailand. Lancet 2:496–500, 1987.

Lawrence G, Cooke R: Experimental pigbel: The production and pathology of necrotizing enteritis due to *Clostridium welchii* type C in the guinea pig. Br J Exp Pathol 61:261–267, 1980.

Lawrence G, Shann F, Freestone DS, et al.: Prevention of necrotizing enteritis in Papua New Guinea by active immunization. Lancet 1:227–230, 1979.

Lawrence G, Walker PD: Pathogenesis of enteritis necroticans in Papua New Guinea. Lancet 1:125–126, 1976.

Lawrence G, Walker PD, Garap J, et al.: The occurrence of *Clostridium welchii* type C in Papua New Guinea. Papua New Guinea Med J 22:69–73, 1979.

Severin WPJ, de la Fuente AA, Stringer MF: *Clostridium perfringens* type C causing necrotising enteritis. J Clin Pathol 37:942–944, 1984.

55.4. *CLOSTRIDIUM DIFFICILE*-INDUCED COLITIS

DEFINITION. *Clostridium difficile* is a recently described enteric pathogen that is responsible for nearly all cases of antibiotic-associated colitis and approximately 20 to 25% of antibiotic-associated diarrhea.

HISTORY. Studies of antibiotic-associated colitis in the 1950s and early 1960s suggested that *Staphylococcus aureus* was the etiologic agent in most cases. Lack of histologic study, the presence of *S. aureus* in the fecal flora of healthy individuals, and the results of more recent studies cast doubt about the precise role of this microbe. In the early 1970s, the widespread use of endoscopy in patients with antibiotic-associated diarrhea permitted extensive studies of its incidence, pathology, and natural history. It was noted that *S. aureus* was rarely recovered from the stools of afflicted patients and that even when it was present, there was no clear cause-and-effect relationship. Studies in the later 1970s implicated *C. difficile* as the etiologic agent; a tissue culture assay was developed for detecting *C. difficile* toxin in stool, and vancomycin and cholestyramine became therapeutic modalities with established efficacy.

DISTRIBUTION. *Clostridium difficile* is found in soil samples and in the stools of a number of animals. The carrier rate in stools is 30 to 60% for newborn infants, which decreases to approximately 3% in adults and in children over the age of 8 months. The high carrier rate in infants, originally thought to be due to maternal-child transmission, is now considered linked to nosocomial spread.

TRANSMISSION AND EPIDEMIOLOGY. Anti-biotic-associated colitis due to *C. difficile* may occur sporadically or in epidemics. The latter occurs primarily in institutions, where there may be widespread contamination of the environment from stools of affected patients combined with extensive use of antibiotics. Environmental cultures near patients with *C. difficile*-induced diarrhea show that the organism is recovered in up to 30% of case-associated sites compared with only 1 to 3% of control sites. Recurrences of antibiotic-associated colitis due to *C. difficile* may in some instances be due to reinfection from environmental sources following successful elimination from the bowel. Outbreaks of disease have occurred in both acute and chronic care facilities.

Colitis most commonly follows parenteral or oral therapy with ampicillin, cephalosporins, and clindamycin, although most antibiotics, including antineoplastic antibiotics, have been implicated. Besides exposure to antibiotics, other risk factors include advanced age, female sex, antecedent bowel manipulations, and perhaps inflammatory bowel disease. Disease is rare in infants and in those with cystic fibrosis, even when they have large numbers of *C. difficile* and high titers of toxin in their stool. Lack of toxin receptors on the bowel mucosa or the presence of inhibitory substances, such as secretory antibody, may explain the low incidence in these groups.

C. difficile-induced colitis is recognized primarily in industrialized countries where toxin assays are available. It is assumed that this organism is also an important cause of enteric disease in developing countries where there is crowding of hospitalized patients and less stringent control of antibiotic utilization.

PATHOGENESIS AND PATHOLOGY. *C. difficile* is an enteric pathogen almost exclusively in the presence of antibiotic exposure. Endoscopy in patients with antibiotic-associated diarrhea shows a spectrum of pathologic changes ranging from an entirely normal colon to severe colitis, with the most characteristic lesion being pseudomembranous colitis (PMC). Typical findings in patients with PMC are multiple, elevated, yellowish-white plaques that vary in size from a few mm to 20 mm in diameter. Coalescence of these plaques, which consist of polymorphonuclear leukocytes, fibrin, epithelial cell debris, and mucin, produce the classic pseudomembrane. The intervening mucosa is normal or shows hyperemia and edema. In most instances, the entire colon is involved. Histologic studies show that the pseudomembrane arises from a superficial ulceration on an intact mucosa and an acute or chronic inflammatory infiltrate in the lamina propria.

C. difficile toxin assays implicate this organism in nearly all cases of antibiotic-associated PMC and in 20 to 25% of "simple diarrhea" related to antibiotic usage. The carriage rate among healthy adults increases with antibiotic exposure, presumably reflecting ingestion from environmental sources. Both colonization and toxin production are enhanced by suppression of the competing colonic flora. Support for the importance of the normal flora comes from clinical studies indicating a close association with antibiotic usage as well as from experimental studies in rodents indicating that typical disease is readily induced only in neonates, gnotobiotes, and animals given a variety of antibiotics. The common denominator in these seemingly diverse settings is reduced or altered colonic flora.

C. difficile Toxins. *C. difficile*-induced enteric disease is toxin-mediated. The putative agent produces 2 toxins, designated toxin A and toxin B, which are large-molecular-weight proteins produced during logarithmic growth of the vegetative forms. Toxin A causes fluid accumulation and a profound hemorrhagic inflammation in the rabbit ileal loop assay. Toxin B is a potent cytopathic toxin that is detected in tissue cultures in concentrations as low as 100 pg/mL. Toxins A and B are both present in the stools of patients with colitis and may act synergistically to produce disease. Toxin A may play a permissive role, interacting with gut mucosa to facilitate the exit of toxin B from the intestinal lumen. Toxin A damages villous tips and the brush border membrane, but has no demonstrable enzymatic activity. Toxin B activates guanylate cyclase and disrupts the cell's microfilament system. A motility-altering factor and adherence pili may be additional virulence factors.

CLINICAL MANIFESTATIONS. Nearly all antimicrobial agents that have an antibacterial spectrum of activity have been implicated in *C. difficile*-induced enteric disease. The diarrhea, which is generally large in volume and watery or mucoid, begins typically 5 to 7 days after the initiation of antibiotic therapy. It is first noted during antibiotic administration in two thirds of patients and up to 4 weeks following discontinuation of the implicated agent in the remaining third. Illness may be mild, but most patients with PMC experience abdominal cramps and tenderness, fever, and leukocytosis. Late and serious complications include severe dehydration, electrolyte imbalance, hypotension, hypoalbuminemia and anasarca, toxic megacolon, and colonic perforation. Without therapy, the illness abates generally 1 to 3 weeks after removal of the offending antibiotic.

DIAGNOSIS

Endoscopy. The typical mucosal plaque-like lesions are visualized by endoscopy. Less specific changes include hemorrhage, ulcerations, easy friability, erythema, and edema. These findings must be differentiated from those in other forms of colitis, e.g., idiopathic ulcerative colitis, shigellosis, and amebiasis.

Toxin Assays. The preferred method for confirming the diagnosis is to demonstrate *C. difficile* toxin or toxins in stool by observing in a tissue culture assay typical cytopathic changes that are neutralized by *C. sordellii* or *C. difficile* antitoxins. Toxin neutralization with antisera to *C. sordellii* represents an antigenic cross-reaction. Over 90% of patients with *C. difficile*-associated colitis have cytotoxic activity in their stools. Toxin is found much less frequently in the stool of those with colitis without pseudomembranes and in those with diarrhea only. Alternative methods for antigen detection include counterimmunoelectrophoresis or an ELISA procedure. Stool cultures may be done using a selective medium containing cycloserine and cefoxitin, but these are more laborious, may prove difficult in many clinical laboratories, and are less specific than the toxin assay.

TREATMENT AND PROGNOSIS. The natural course of the disease in patients with antibiotic-associated PMC is highly variable. Some patients have minimal symptoms that resolve rapidly when the implicated antibiotic is discontinued. Other patients have protracted or debilitating diarrhea with up to 30 stools/day. The overall mortality rate without specific therapy is approximately 20%. Therapeutic recommendations include antibiotics directed against the putative agent or anion exchange resins to bind *C. difficile* toxin. The most frequently used antibiotic is orally administered vancomycin, 125 to 500 mg, 4 times daily for 7 to 14 days. Nearly all patients respond, but approximately 20% relapse following discontinuation of this agent. Relapses may be due to the presence of *C. difficile* spores or due to reinfection with *C. difficile*. Relapses may be treated with an additional course of vancomycin, or with alternative antibiotics, such as metronidazole (1500 mg/day orally or intravenously) or bacitracin (500 mg orally 4 times/day). The latter antibiotics are considerably less expensive than vancomycin and deserve consideration as primary therapies, at least for those with mild to moderate disease. Cholestyramine and colestipol, 2 anion exchange resins that bind or inactivate *C. difficile* cytotoxin, may be given in doses of 4 gm, 3 times daily for 5 days. Compared with vancomycin, these resins have a less predictable response, but are also considerably less expensive, and patients who respond are less likely to have relapses.

PREVENTION AND CONTROL. The best control method is judicious use of antibiotics, especially those that are commonly associated with this complication. In view of evidence for spread within hospitals, it is recommended that hospitalized patients with *C. difficile*-induced disease be isolated and monitored with enteric precautions until diarrhea resolves or the toxin is eradicated in stools.

BIBLIOGRAPHY

Bartlett JG: Antibiotic-associated pseudomembranous colitis. Rev Infect Dis 1:530–539, 1979.

Chang TW, Laverman M, Bartlett JG: Cytotoxicity assay in antibiotic associated colitis. J Infect Dis 140:765–770, 1979.

Fekety R, Kim K-H, Brown D, et al.: Epidemiology of antibiotic-associated colitis: Isolation of *C. difficile* from the hospital environment. Am J Med 70:906–912, 1981.

Keighley MRB, Burdon DW, Cerabi Y, et al.: Randomized controlled trial of vancomycin for pseudomembranous colitis and postoperative diarrhea. Br Med J 2:1667–1669, 1978.

Lyerly DM, Krivan HC, Wilkins TD: *Clostridium difficile:* Its disease and toxins. Clin Microbiol Rev 1:1–18, 1988.

McFarland LV, Stamm WE: Review of *Clostridium difficile*-associated diseases. Am J Infect Control 14:99–109, 1986.

Young GP, Bayley N, Ward P, et al.: Antibiotic-associated colitis caused by *Clostridium difficile:* Relapse and risk factors. Med J Aust 144:303–306, 1986.

56. PSEUDOMONAS INFECTIONS: GLANDERS AND MELIOIDOSIS

Jay P. Sanford

56.1. GLANDERS

DEFINITION. Glanders is a serious infection of equine animals caused by a nonmotile gram-negative bacillus, *Pseudomonas mallei*. Occasional transmission to humans occurs.

EPIDEMIOLOGY. Glanders is a disease of horses, mules, and donkeys, but goats, sheep, cats, and dogs sometimes naturally contract the disease. Pigs and cattle are resistant. In horses, the disease may be systemic with prominent pulmonary involvement (glanders) or may be characterized by subcutaneous ulcerative lesions and lymphatic nodules (farcy). Glanders occurs in Asia, Africa, and South America. There has been no reported naturally acquired human case in the United States since 1938. In humans, the disease occurs primarily in individuals in close contact with infected horses, mules, or donkeys.

CLINICAL MANIFESTATIONS AND DIAGNOSIS. The incubation period is 1 to 5 days. The manifestations, which frequently overlap, have been categorized as acute localized suppurative, acute pulmonic, acute septicemic, and chronic suppurative. With systemic invasion, a generalized papular eruption that may become pustular is frequent. *P. mallei* can be cultured on most meat infusion nutrient media.

TREATMENT. The limited number of recent human infections has precluded evaluation of most antibiotic agents. Sulfadiazine, 100 mg/kg/day in divided doses, is effective in experimental animals and humans. In the absence of clinical experience and pending in vitro susceptibility studies, it seems prudent to use the regimens employed in treating melioidosis (see below).

BIBLIOGRAPHY

Howe C, Miller WR: Human glanders: report of six cases. Ann Intern Med 26:93, 1947.

56.2. MELIOIDOSIS

DEFINITION. Melioidosis is an infection of humans and animals caused by a motile aerobic gram-negative bacillus, *Pseudomonas pseudomallei*. Epidemiologically, melioidosis bears no relation to glanders, although the name melioidosis means "a resemblance to distemper of asses."

EPIDEMIOLOGY. Disease occurs worldwide, being recognized in countries between 20 degrees north and south latitude. Most human and animal cases have been recognized in Southeast Asia. Cases in humans or ani-

mals have been reported from Iran, Turkey, Madagascar, Kenya, and Central West Africa (Chad, Niger, Upper Volta, Ivory Coast, Gambia). In 1976, *P. pseudomallei* was isolated from animals in the Paris zoo and from horses in Madrid. Naturally acquired human melioidosis has been described only rarely in the Western Hemisphere (i.e., Panama, Ecuador, Mexico, Haiti, Brazil, Peru, Guyana) and the United States (a neonatal case in Hawaii, a case in Georgia, and a possible case in Oklahoma).

P. pseudomallei is a saprophyte that can be isolated from soil, stagnant streams, ponds, rice paddies, and market produce in endemic areas. It is capable of causing epizootics in sheep, goats, swine, horses, and dolphins. Although animals are susceptible, they apparently do not represent a reservoir for human disease. Humans may acquire melioidosis by soil contamination of skin abrasions. Ingestion and inhalation are other probable methods of acquisition. Person-to-person transmission is extremely rare; an instance of probable sexual transmission from an individual with *P. pseudonallei* prostatitis to his wife has been reported.

CLINICAL MANIFESTATIONS. The incubation period has not been defined; after a laboratory accident, it has been as short as 3 days. Infection may remain inapparent or latent for a number of years after an individual leaves an endemic area; an interval of 26 years has been reported in one patient.

Inapparent Infection. In Thailand, Vietnam, and Malaysia, 6 to 8% of healthy adult men have significant antibody titers against *P. pseudomallei*, with the prevalence reaching 20% in a group of Army recruits from the rice-growing states of western Malaysia. Ten per cent of serum specimens from inhabitants of a village in Upper Volta were positive, but clinical melioidosis was not recognized in this group.

Acute Localized Suppurative Disease. Infection by inoculation through a break in the skin usually results in a nodule with associated lymphangitis and regional lymphadenopathy.

Acute Pulmonic Disease. Acute pulmonic disease is the most commonly recognized form. Acute infection can vary in severity from mild bronchitis to overwhelming necrotizing pneumonia. Onset may be abrupt or gradual. Fever occurs in almost all patients, is often in excess of 39°C (102°F), and is associated with recurring rigors. Dull or pleuritic chest pain is common. Auscultatory findings may be absent or minimal but usually consist of rales in the area of involvement. The pneumonia usually involves upper lobes, with the appearance of consolidation. Although uncommon, pleural effusions and a pleural mass have been reported. In a serologic survey of 275 Chinese patients in a Hong Kong tuberculosis sanatorium, 14% had hemagglutinin titers of 1:80 or above.

Acute Septicemic Disease. Acute septicemic disease is the originally recognized form that occurred primarily in debilitated opium addicts. Subsequent reports have not shown a predilection for debilitated patients. In individuals with bacteremia, symptoms include disorientation, dyspnea, severe headache, pharyngitis, and watery diarrhea. High fever, extreme tachypnea, flushed skin, and cyanosis are other symptoms. Muscle tenderness may be striking. On auscultation the chest may be clear. The liver and spleen may be palpable. Signs of arthritis and meningitis may develop. Chest radiographs most commonly show irregular nodular densities.

Chronic Suppurative Disease. In many patients, secondary abscesses develop. Organs involved include skin, brain, lung, myocardium, liver, spleen, prostate, bones, joints, lymph nodes, and even the eye. Lung lesions may be indistinguishable radiographically from tuberculosis. Osteomyelitis is one of the more common manifestations.

Latent Recrudescent Disease. Late activation of infection that has been totally inapparent or quiescent or recrudescence of previous symptomatic disease may occur (in one case, 26 years later) and present with any of the aforementioned clinical features. In reported cases, surgery, trauma, intercurrent illness (e.g., severe influenzal pneumonia, diabetic ketoacidosis), alcohol excess, or radiation therapy appeared to act as triggering events.

DIAGNOSIS. *P. pseudomallei* grow on most bacteriologic media but may require 48 to 72 hours of incubation. Colonies develop a characteristic wrinkling within 72 to 96 hours. Identification is based on biochemical tests. Serodiagnosis includes use of hemagglutination and complement fixation tests. Single low titers with either test are difficult to interpret because of nonspecific responses. Hemagglutination tests are most widely used and titers of 1:80 or more suggest infection. A negative serologic test does not exclude infection.

TREATMENT. The treatment regimen should vary with the form of disease. Individuals with low titer–positive serologic tests but with no clinical evidence of disease do not require therapy. With active disease, the choice of antibiotics should be based on susceptibility studies, and treatment should be given for a minimum of 30 days. Unfortunately, the antimicrobial agents shown to be most effective are too costly to be used in many developing countries in which melioidosis is common. In patients with pneumonitis who are not seriously ill, effective oral regimens have included amoxicillin clavulanate, 750 mg 3 times daily, trimethoprim–sulfamethoxazole, TMP 10 mg and SMX 50 mg/kg/day (e.g., 2 tablets each containing 80 mg TMP and 400 mg SMX orally 4 times daily in a 70-kg adult), doxycycline, 4 mg/kg/day, or chloramphenicol, 50 mg/kg/day, for 60 to 150 days. In contrast to isolates of *P. pseudomallei* from most areas, fewer than 20% from Thailand are sensitive to trimethoprim–sulfomethoxazole. If the patient is moderately ill, the treatment of choice is ceftazidime, 120 mg/kg/day intravenously divided as 3 doses. Intravenous therapy should be given for at least 7 days, then followed by oral therapy as described for 30 to 120 days. If ceftazidime is not available, a regimen of 2 of these agents such as trimethoprim–sulfamethoxazole and doxycycline has been recommended. Regimens consisting of 2 to 4 agents have been used empirically because of poor initial responses and relapses with monodrug regimens. Dance and associates have shown in vitro antagonism between both trimethoprim and sulfamethoxazole and nonsulfonamide drugs, ceftazidime, doxy-

cycline, and chloramphenicol. Based on these observations, further clinical studies are clearly indicated. In the interim, empirical monodrug regimens seem more appropriate than equally empirical combined regimens. The mean interval for sputum cultures to become negative is 6 weeks. If sputum cultures remain positive at 6 months, surgery with lobectomy should be considered. In the septicemic form, antibiotics should be administered intravenously and ceftazidime is the agent of choice. When abscesses are present, the usual surgical principles of drainage should be followed.

PROGNOSIS. The mortality rate in all except the septicemic form is low. In septicemic melioidosis, however, even with appropriate antibiotics and vigorous supportive therapy including surgical drainage of lesions, the mortality remains high (37% being the lowest in a moderately sized series of patients). Among survivors, few patients have had long-term follow-up, but the incidence of late relapse is high.

BIBLIOGRAPHY

Ashdown LR, Guard RW: The prevalence of human melioidosis in northern Queensland. Am J Trop Med Hyg 33:474, 1984.
Dance DAB, Wuthiekanun V, Chaowagul W, et al.: Interactions in vitro between agents used to treat melioidosis. J Antimicrob Chemother 24:311, 1989.
Dance DAB, Wuthiekanun V, White NJ, et al.: Antibiotic resistance in *Pseudomonas pseudomallei*. Lancet 1:994, 1988.
Dodin A, Terry R: Recherche epidemiologigne du bacille de Whitmore en Afrique. Bull Soc Path Exot 67:121, 1974.
Everett ED, Nelson R: Pulmonary melioidosis, observations in 39 cases. Am Rev Resp Dis 112:331, 1975.
Schlech WF, Turchik JB, Westlake RE Jr, et al.: Laboratory-acquired infection with *Pseudomonas pseudomallei* (melioidosis). N Engl J Med 305:1133, 1981.
So SY, Chau PY, Aquinas M, et al: Melioidosis: A serological survey in a tuberculosis sanatorium in Hong Kong. Trans Roy Soc Trop Med Hyg 81:1017, 1987.
White NJ, Dance DAB, Chaowagul W, et al.: Halving of mortality of severe melioidosis by ceftazidime. Lancet 2:697, 1989.

57. DIPHTHERIA

Zoheir Farid

DEFINITION. Diphtheria is an acute infectious disease caused by virulent strains of *Corynebacterium diphtheriae*. It is characterized by the development of a membrane in the throat and production of an exotoxin that damages the heart muscle and nervous tissue. Infection is localized occasionally in the skin.

ETIOLOGY. The etiologic agent is a pleomorphic, gram-positive, nonmotile, nonsporulating, clavate bacillus. The 3 types of diphtheria bacillus—mitis, gravis, and intermedius—can be identified by colony morphology and biochemical properties. They are best grown aerobically on Loeffler's medium and are further differentiated on selective tellurite media. Most bacilli produce a protein exotoxin that is responsible for the clinical illness; however, diphtheria may follow infection with *C. diphtheriae* that do not produce exotoxin.

EPIDEMIOLOGY. Diphtheria has a worldwide distribution, being more common in temperate climates and endemic in developing countries where crowding, improper hygiene, and inadequate immunization prevail. Mass immunization against diphtheria has provided adequate population immunity in the more developed countries. Humans are the main reservoir, with infection transmitted directly or indirectly from a case or carrier by droplets and, in rare instances, by fomites or dust particles. Contaminated milk sometimes transmits the infection. *C. diphtheriae* infection of the skin, particularly in tropical areas, can be a source of a new infection. Skin infections, which are more infectious than throat infections, can be a major reservoir for transmission.

Immunity depends on the antitoxin level in the blood, acquired either naturally or by immunization. Infants under 6 months old are protected by antitoxins acquired from immunized mothers. Adults are usually protected by inapparent infection or by immunization. The disease in developing countries is therefore most common in children aged 1 to 6 years. However, there have been outbreaks of diphtheria in adults in Seattle, Denmark, and Sweden. Using a genetic probe, it was possible to show that the clinical and fatal cases of diphtheria in Scandinavia were caused by a single strain of *C. diphtheriae* that possibly had a virulence factor separate from toxigenicity. Antitoxin immunity has been shown to be inadequate in many adults who were immunized during childhood. Resistant factors may be important also, because many of those in the recent outbreaks were alcoholics and inhabitants of skid row. More diphtheria outbreaks in the future may be expected in populations who were highly immunized in childhood with no subsequent exposure.

In older children and adults, 0.1 mL of diphtheria toxin, injected intradermally and examined 48 hours later, is useful in indicating immunity (Schick test); a positive reaction indicates no immunity to diphtheria (no antitoxin in the blood to neutralize the injected toxin).

PATHOGENESIS. *C. diphtheriae* infection commonly occurs through the upper respiratory tract. Invasion of the epithelial cells of the pharynx by the organism results in formation of a thick, adherent membrane composed of bacteria, necrotic cells, phagocytes, and fibrin. The infection spreads occasionally to the larynx or nasal mucosa. The skin, genitalia, umbilical cord of newborns, eyes, and middle ears may be sites of infection, particularly in tropical countries. Exotoxin produced in the primary site of infection is absorbed into the circulation, causing toxic manifestations primarily involving the heart (myocarditis) or peripheral nerves (paralysis). The toxin is an acidic globular protein with a molecular weight of 62,000. It has a cellular site of action and a latent period before inhibiting cellular protein synthesis and is extremely potent.

CLINICAL MANIFESTATIONS

Pharyngeal Diphtheria. The incubation period is short (1 to 7 days). Onset may be gradual or sudden, the patient presenting with a low-grade fever, sore throat, and malaise. Twenty to 25% also have nausea and vomiting, headache, and/or pain on swallowing. The diphtheritic membrane appears then in the pharynx as small exudates, which unite and spread to invade the pharynx and tonsils. Later, the membrane, which is characteristically grayish green in color, thickens and adheres to underlying tissues; attempts to remove the membrane cause bleeding. The membrane may spread to involve the entire throat and mouth; the resultant cervical lymphadenitis and tissue edema lead to the "bull-neck" appearance. If membrane extension involves the larynx and trachea (laryngeal diphtheria), it may cause airway obstruction with cough and laryngeal stridor. In severe cases, pallor, tachycardia, and weakness may be prominent. Laryngeal diphtheria occurring without throat involvement must be differentiated from all other causes of "croup." Diphtheria is infrequently restricted to the nasal mucosa (nasal diphtheria), which usually leads to unilateral serosanguineous or thick mucopurulent nasal discharge.

Cutaneous Diphtheria. *C. diphtheriae* involving the skin is more common in tropical countries and areas of poor socioeconomic development. Cutaneous diphtheria may be secondary to organisms associated with wounds, burns, or infected insect bites, or it may be primary when the characteristic diphtheritic ulcer is confined to the extremities. The diphtheritic ulcer is shallow with rolled edges and is covered by a hard, adherent membrane. In rare instances, the genitalia, conjunctiva, and ears are invaded by *C. diphtheriae*.

COMPLICATIONS. The outcome of infection is dependent on the location and extent of the membrane, the amount of toxin absorbed, and the patient's immunity. Complications resulting from spread of the membrane to involve the pharynx, trachea, and, less frequently, the bronchioles lead to severe respiratory obstruction. The exotoxin can cause myocarditis with cardiac arrhythmias and, rarely, heart failure. Most ECG changes occur during the first week of illness, with the severity of illness and toxemia greater in patients with ECG abnormalities and acute circulatory failure. The toxin also often affects nervous tissue, causing peripheral neuritis and paralysis, usually of the lower limbs. The cranial nerves are occasionally involved, resulting in paralysis of the soft palate, blurred vision, or loss of accommodation. This may occur 1 to 4 weeks after onset of the disease.

PROGNOSIS. ECG abnormalities, particularly AV block and left bundle branch block, are associated with increased mortality. The single most important factor in preventing morbidity and complications is immunization. Immunized patients develop fewer complications and have a much lower fatality rate than nonimmunized patients. Delay in starting antitoxin therapy in infected patients increases the incidence of complications and death, and when antitoxin therapy is given later than 48 hours after clinical diphtheria begins, there is little effect.

DIAGNOSIS. The economic background and epidemiologic history of the patient and the characteristic clinical picture of a hard, adherent, bleeding membrane affecting mainly the pharynx are typical of diphtheria; differentiation must be made from acute viral and streptococcal tonsillitis and acute infectious mononucleosis. Laryngeal diphtheria with respiratory stridor in infants

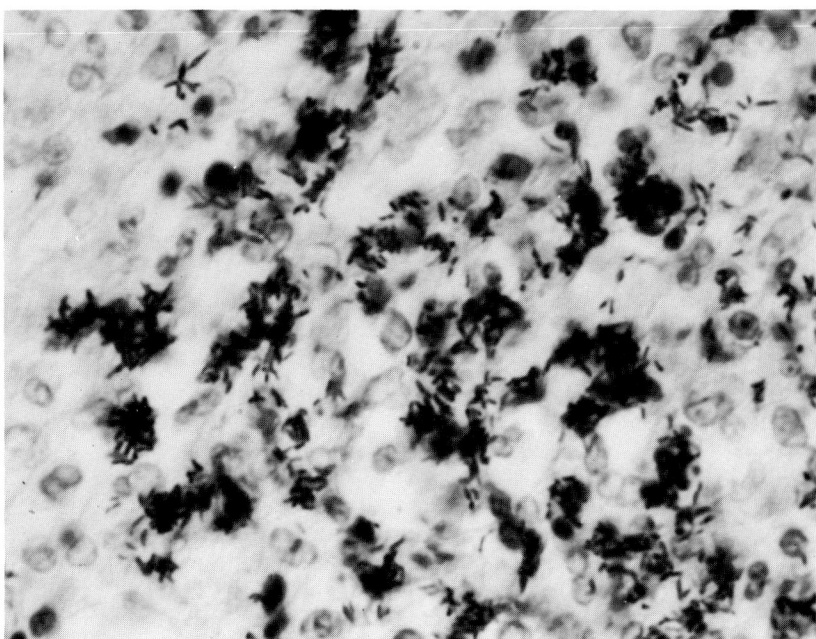

FIGURE 57–1. Cutaneous diphtheria of the scalp. Club-shaped *C. diphtheriae* gram-positive bacilli in the acute inflammatory reaction at the base of an ulcer (Brown and Brenn Gram stain. × 1200). (Courtesy of the Armed Forces Institute of Pathology. Photograph Neg. No. 76–7065.)

has to be differentiated from other causes of "croup." Specific diagnosis of diphtheria is made by detecting the bacilli in stained smears (Fig. 57–1) or by culture.

TREATMENT

Antitoxin. Clinically suspected diphtheria requires immediate specific treatment with antitoxin without waiting for laboratory confirmation. All patients must be tested for sensitivity to serum antitoxin by conjunctival and intradermal tests before the injection is given; desensitization may be necessary if either is positive. The antitoxin dose depends on the site, extent, and severity of infection. Mild early cases in which the membrane does not extend beyond the tonsil require 10,000 to 20,000 units of antitoxin administered intramuscularly or intravenously. More severe cases, particularly nasopharyngeal ones, require as much as 50,000 to 100,000 units, half of which is given intramuscularly and the rest intravenously in 200 mL of normal saline.

Antibiotics. Either procaine penicillin, 600,000 units intramuscularly every 12 hours, or erythromycin, 250 mg orally every 6 hours, is given for 10 days. In addition specific supportive therapy is indicated in patients who are severely toxic and in shock or to those with severe laryngeal obstruction. Patients with laryngeal obstruction may need intubation or tracheostomy. Careful nursing care is important to prevent secondary bacterial pneumonia.

Isolation. Patients with diphtheria should preferably be isolated and hospitalized. They should not be discharged before 2 successive cultures from the nose and throat are negative for *C. diphtheriae*.

Infected susceptible contacts are treated with 1000 to 2000 units of antitoxin and are given penicillin or erythromycin for 10 days. Later, active immunization is started. Throat carriers of *C. diphtheriae* are treated with antimicrobials (erythromycin or penicillin).

PREVENTION. Immunization with diphtheria toxoid prevents the disease. Immunization with diphtheria toxoid, pertussis vaccine, and tetanus toxoid (DPT) and oral poliomyelitis vaccine is usually given to infants under 1 year of age. The first dose of DPT is given at the age of 2 to 3 months and the second and third doses at 4- to 6-week intervals. Booster doses are given at 1 year of age and at school entry or at 5 years of age.

Primary immunizations in children over 6 years of age and adults should be with 3 doses of purified tetanus and diphtheria toxoid (Td). The second dose is given 6 weeks after the first, and the third dose is given 6 months after the second. Thereafter, booster doses of Td are given every 10 years.

Because of the waning levels of immunity in adults, it is recommended that those age 25 or older receive a single booster immunization with Td every 10 years. Because Central and South America, Africa, and Asia have high rates of endemic diphtheria, those traveling to these areas who have not been immunized within the past 10 years should be given a booster dose of Td.

BIBLIOGRAPHY

Bjorkholm B, Böttiger M, Christenson B, et al.: Antitoxin antibody levels and the outcome of illness during an outbreak of diphtheria among alcoholics. Scand J Infect Dis 18:235, 1986.

Chen RT, Broome CV, Weinstein RA, et al.: Diphtheria in the United States, 1971–81. Am J Public Health 75:1393–1397, 1985.

Christenson B, Böttiger M: Serological immunity to diphtheria in Sweden in 1974 and 1984. Scand J Infect Dis 18:227, 1986.

Karzon DT, Edwards KM: Diphtheria outbreaks in immunized populations. N Engl J Med 318:41–43, 1988.

Kjeldsen K, Simonsen O, Heron I: Immunity against diphtheria 25–30 years after primary vaccination in childhood. Lancet 1:900, 1985.

Pedersen AHB, Spearman J, Tronca E, et al.: Diphtheria on skid row, Seattle, Wash., 1972–1975. Public Health Rep 92:336, 1977.

Rappuoli R, Perugini M, Falsen E: Molecular epidemiology of the 1984–1986 outbreak of diphtheria in Sweden. N Engl J Med 318:12–14, 1988.

Simmons LE, Abbott JD, Macaulay ME, et al.: Diphtheria carriers in Manchester: Simultaneous infection with toxigenic and nontoxigenic mitis strains. Lancet 1:304, 1980.

58. PYOMYOSITIS

Joel D. Brown

DEFINITION. Pyomyositis is a purulent infection of skeletal muscle that occurs without penetrating trauma or spread from a contiguous septic focus. This disease is common in the tropics and rare in the temperate zones, hence the synonym "tropical pyomyositis." The infection often seems to appear spontaneously and can present a confusing diagnostic problem, particularly for physicians without experience in the tropics.

HISTORY. Pyomyositis was described in Japan by Scriba and Miyake at the turn of the century. *Staphylococcus aureus* was the usual pathogen, but streptococci and pneumococci were occasionally responsible. In the United States, William Osler wrote in 1892 of ". . . septic cases in which diffuse purulent infiltration of the muscles of different regions occurs," and indicated that the muscle may be the primary source of infection. In 1947 Traquir reviewed the history of pyomyositis and emphasized that it was endemic throughout the tropics. Most patients were indigenous to the tropics, but colonial Europeans were not spared. In 1971 the disease was reported in patients immigrating from the tropics to North America. Occasional cases have been recognized in temperate regions among persons who have not been in the tropics; some of these patients had other associated, immunocompromising diseases.

ETIOLOGY. *S. aureus* causes 95% of the cases. *Streptococcus pyogenes* and various streptococcus species account for most of the remaining. Other pyogenic bacteria, such as *Streptococcus pneumoniae* and gram-negative organisms, are rarely responsible for pyomyositis.

A variety of bacteria can infect open, traumatized wounds. Clostridia species cause myonecrosis in wounds and occasionally infect a muscle during bacteremia from intestinal sources. A focus of infection, e.g., osteomyelitis, intra-abdominal abscess, or necrotizing fasciitis, can invade contiguous skeletal muscle. However, these well-known muscle infections are not considered in the usual definition of pyomyositis.

DISTRIBUTION AND INCIDENCE. Pyomyositis is common throughout the tropics where it is familiar to local medical workers. Nearly 4% of all patients admitted to the surgical service of a major teaching hospital in Uganda, Africa had pyomyositis. This infection is reported primarily from tropical Africa and Asia, but it is common also in Oceania and the Caribbean. It occurs in Central and probably South America. Although initially described in Japan, pyomyositis has not been reported there recently. Most endemic regions are warm and humid, but pyomyositis occurs in warm, dry savannah regions as well. Most are young males, possibly because they encounter more trauma, but no age or gender is spared.

PATHOGENESIS. The mechanism by which bacteria establish infection in muscle, and the reasons for its predominance in the tropics, is unknown. Staphylococci, streptococci, and other pyogenic bacteria infect people throughout the world; however, these bacteria rarely infect normal skeletal muscle in patients outside the tropics, even during bacteremia.

Miyake designed an experimental rabbit model for staphylococcal pyomyositis. He injured a muscle by pinching, ligature venous stasis, or electrically induced tetanic spasm, then injected staphylococci intravenously. Animals that survived the initial septicemia developed abscesses only in the injured muscle. Clinical studies reveal a history of trauma to the involved muscle in up to two thirds of cases. Pyoderma is common in the tropics and could be a source of bacteremia, which may seed skeletal muscle, particularly previously abnormal muscle. Patients often have pyoderma distal to the infected muscle, suggesting that bacteria from the skin may reach the muscle via the lymphatics. The muscle abscess may be a manifestation of bacteremia with multiple metastatic infections, or it may be the source of bacteremia.

Pyomyositis has been associated with other tropical diseases that may invade or damage the muscle, such as dracunculiasis, filariasis, aberrant nematode larvae, leptospirosis, sickle cell disease, scurvy, thiamine deficiency, and viral myositis. It is likely that pyoderma, plus some form of muscle damage, is important in the pathogenesis of pyomyositis. In developed countries pyomyositis may occur in patients with diabetes, leukemia, aplastic anemia, asplenia, lupus erythematosis, Felty's syndrome, intravenous drug abuse, and the acquired immunodeficiency syndrome (AIDS). These case reports suggest that defects in host immunity may have a role in the pathogenesis.

PATHOLOGY. Pyomyositis usually involves 1 to several large skeletal muscles. The infection is subfascial usually but may be predominantly in the fascial space between the muscle groups. The muscle usually contains a solitary or multiloculated abscess with thick pus and necrotic muscle (Fig. 58–1). Occasionally the muscle is diffusely infiltrated and hard, grossly mimicking a soft tissue tumor such as rhabdomyosarcoma. The abscess may spread to contiguous structures and spaces leading to epidural abscess, meningitis, and peritonitis.

The histopathology consists of both acute and chronic inflammation, depending on the duration of the infection. Polymorphonuclear cells, lymphocytes, plasma cells, and eosinophils are present. The muscle may be diffusely infiltrated with inflammatory cells. It can have fibrosis or contain micro- and macroabscesses.

CLINICAL MANIFESTATIONS. The disease can be mild and confined to 1 muscle or associated with sepsis. Pain, swelling, and tenderness develop rapidly over a few days, or follow an indolent course over weeks. Fever is common but may be delayed for several days. A single large muscle of the lower extremity is usually involved, but there may be abscesses in multiple muscles of the arms or trunk. Skin redness and fluctuance of the muscle mass may not occur, or may appear later, as the infection spreads from the muscle towards the surface. Diffuse inflammation and infiltration of the muscle without abscess formation is seen occasionally. A hard, woody, tumor-like quality of the affected muscle is typical of pyomyositis. Laboratory findings include leukocytosis and perhaps positive blood cultures. Muscle enzymes are usually normal. Eosinophilia may be present but is probably due to endemic parasites. The diagnosis can be easy in the tropics but confusing outside the endemic areas.

DIAGNOSIS. A history of recent muscle trauma and pyoderma, particularly when the latter is distal to the affected muscle, suggests pyomyositis. Aspiration of the area with a large needle and bacterial culture and Gram stain of the pus can be diagnostic. If needle aspiration is unrewarding, ultrasonographic-guided aspiration or surgical exploration confirms the diagnosis often. Imaging with gallium and CT scans (Fig. 58–1) may be useful in confirming the diagnosis or in detecting other sites of infection that need drainage. Pyomyositis without macroabscess may require muscle biopsy with cultures and tissue stains for microorganisms.

Pyomyositis may mimic muscle hematoma, septic arthritis, osteomyelitis, deep venous thrombosis, appendicitis, cellulitis, or muscle tumor (Fig. 58–2). When the skin becomes inflamed, a misdiagnosis of superficial cellulitis may be made, but the history of muscle pain preceding the skin changes suggests pyomyositis.

PROGNOSIS. Pyomyositis is confined to the muscle usually, but some cases may be septic. In a recent series of children reported from Nigeria, 25% had osteomyelitis and 14% had metastatic infections to other organs. The fatality rate in Africa is less than 1.5% but can be higher in the more serious cases who have staphylococcal sepsis, endocarditis, pericarditis, pneumonia, or meningitis and are referred to larger hospitals. Rhabdomyolysis with acute renal failure may occur in severe infections.

TREATMENT. Drainage of pus and debridement of necrotic muscle is required. Percutaneous catheter drainage may suffice, particularly if ultrasound or CT imaging is available for guidance and re-evaluation. Diffuse myositis without abscess may respond to antimicrobial agents alone, but abscesses may develop eventually and require drainage. Antimicrobial agents effective against penicillin-resistant staphylococci should be administered parenterally before drainage. The total dose of the antimicrobial agent and duration of therapy depend on the severity of disease and presence of complications.

Metastatic infections to bone or heart require 4 to 6

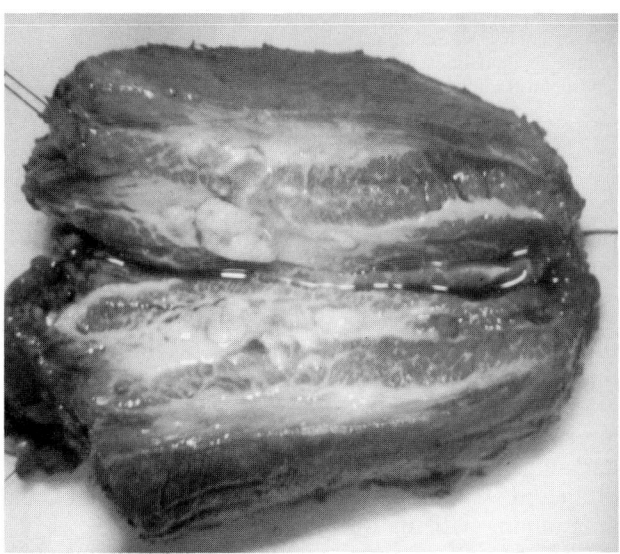

FIGURE 58–2. Infiltrating staphylococcal pyomyositis excised en bloc from a Samoan boy with a preoperative diagnosis of suspected rhabdomyosarcoma.

weeks of high dose parenteral therapy. An uncomplicated case can be treated initially with parenteral antimicrobials and drainage of pus; oral antimicrobials may be substituted as the patient improves. Therapy should be continued until the wound is clean, the leukocyte count is normal, and the patient has been afebrile for several days. Penicillin should be used for proven streptococcal infections; therapy for the less common agents should be directed by laboratory studies. If laboratory support is unavailable, and the patient fails to respond to initial antistaphylococcal management, broad spectrum agents, e.g., cephalosporins, are justified. When resources are limited, oral chloramphenicol may be appropriate broad spectrum therapy. Prognosis depends on severity of the illness. Most patients have minimal sequelae.

PREVENTION. There are no proven preventive measures. Primary prevention or early treatment of pyoderma would probably reduce the incidence of pyomyositis. Early recognition and treatment of the disease may prevent complications.

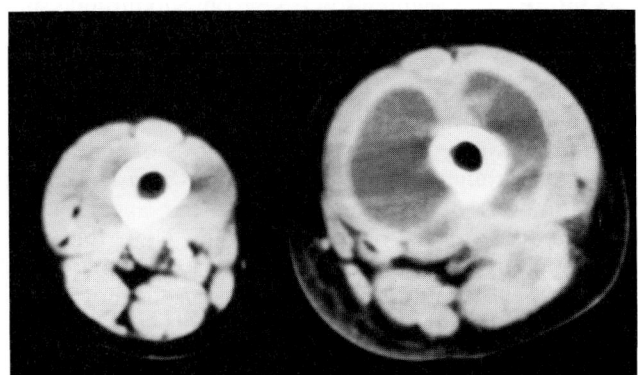

FIGURE 58–1. CT cross-sectional view of the thighs of a Micronesian boy who had fallen 1 month previously and developed staphylococcal abscesses in muscles of the arm and thigh.

BIBLIOGRAPHY

Brown JD, Wheeler B: Pyomyositis: Report of 18 cases in Hawaii. Arch Intern Med 144:1749–1751, 1984.

Chiedozi LC: Pyomyositis: Review of 205 cases in 112 patients. Am J Surg 137:255–259, 1979.

Echeverria P, Vaughn C: 'Tropical Pyomyositis': A diagnostic problem in temperate climates. Am J Dis Child 129:856–857, 1975.

Gaut P, Wong PK, Meyer RD: Pyomyositis in a patient with the Acquired Immunodeficiency Syndrome. Arch Intern Med 148:1608–1610, 1988.

Levin MJ, Gardner P, Waldvogel FA: 'Tropical Pyomyositis': An unusual infection due to *Staphylococcus aureus*. N Engl J Med 284:196–198, 1971.

Schlech WF III, Moulton P, Kaiser AB: Pyomyositis: Tropical disease in a temperate climate. Am J Med 71:900–902, 1981.

Traquir RN: Pyomyositis. J Trop Med Hyg 50:81–89, 1947.
Yousefzadeh DK, Schumann EM, Mulligan GM, et al.: The role of imaging modalities in diagnosis and management of pyomyositis. Skeletal Radiol 8:285–289, 1982.

59. NOCARDIOSIS

Donald W. R. Mackenzie
and Roderick J. Hay

DEFINITION. Nocardiosis is an acute or chronic suppurative infection caused mainly by the aerobic actinomycete *Nocardia asteroides*, although *N. brasiliensis* or *N. otitidis-caviarum* causes occasional cases. Primary infections are pulmonary, but the agent may spread hematogenously to affect other body sites, including brain and skin. Opportunistic infections are not uncommon among patients with impaired resistance.

ETIOLOGY. *N. asteroides* is widespread throughout the world. Its branching hyphae are delicate (1-μm diameter), gram-positive, and partially acid fast, eventually breaking up into bacillary or coccobacillary forms of varying lengths. It is distinguished from other species of *Nocardia* by a combination of morphologic and physiologic characteristics. *N. asteroides* is a soil inhabitant and can readily be isolated by using its ability to metabolize paraffin.

The first recorded case of nocardiosis in humans was described in 1890, but over the next 60 years only a small number of cases were reported in the literature. In the past 3 decades, it has been recognized more frequently, particularly in patients with chronic disorders such as Hodgkin's disease, malignant tumors, and leukemia.

EPIDEMIOLOGY. Nocardiosis occurs in all age groups, but is more common in older subjects. More males are infected than females. There are no occupational or racial susceptibilities. *N. asteroides* is thermophilic and can readily be isolated from compost heaps, where microbial fermentations create high temperatures. Although nocardiosis affects farmers and gardeners, there is no consistent association between systemic nocardiosis and outdoor occupations. The condition occurs sporadically throughout the world in both temperate and tropical climates.

PATHOGENESIS AND PATHOLOGY. The primary route of infection is respiratory, but access to tissues may be effected by ingestion or traumatic implantation. Once established, the agent appears in smears and sections as spreading delicate hyphae with no definite tendency to aggregate into the grains, which is such a characteristic feature of actinomycetoma. Lesions are suppurative, characterized by abscesses of varying size. Generally, these are multiple and confluent, and their walls may be partially lined by fibrosing granulation tissue. The reaction is almost exclusively pyogenic, with little evidence of granuloma formation or giant cells. Nocardiosis may be localized in the lungs, or lesions may occur in brain, meninges, peritoneum, subcutaneous tissues, or muscle. Sections of lung show abundant abscesses with areas of chronic pneumonia lying adjacent to areas of suppuration. Caseation and tubercle formation are not present. The gram-positive filaments are found within macrophages or lying free in the pus.

CLINICAL MANIFESTATIONS
Pulmonary Nocardiosis. Pulmonary nocardiosis is characterized by malaise, fever, weakness, night sweats, weight loss, dyspnea, and chest discomfort. Cough is unproductive initially, but mucopurulent sputum is eventually produced. Consolidation of one or more lobes is characteristic, and extension to the pleural space is common. The pleura may become markedly thickened, and the pleural space may be obliterated by suppuration. Cavitation may be prominent and associated with hemoptysis. Sinus tracts may be a prominent feature, occasionally penetrating the chest wall. The radiologic appearance may resemble upper lobe tuberculosis, unresolved pneumonia, bronchopneumonia, or metastatic tumors. Alternatively, small scattered opacities with cavitation may occur throughout both lung fields.

Disseminated Lesions. Metastatic spread to the brain is common, the presenting symptoms being those of a brain tumor or abscess (i.e., headache, nausea, and vomiting, leading to lethargy, mental confusion, convulsions, and paralysis). Other sites include the heart and kidney. Bone infections are uncommon. Subcutaneous abscesses may result from early metastasis. If untreated, these eventually rupture, leaving chronically draining fistulas.

N. asteroides has been implicated as a cause of actinomycetoma. In such cases, the infection, which originates by implantation, remains localized, causing tissue destruction and deformity at the affected site.

DIAGNOSIS. A positive diagnosis of nocardiosis depends on recognition of the discrete, slender, branching actinomycete hyphae in exudates or tissue sections and on the isolation and identification of *N. asteroides* in culture. Acid-fast stains should be made, using sulfuric acid for decolorization rather than acid alcohol.

Patients with systemic nocardiosis often have antibodies to *Nocardia,* which can be demonstrated by complement fixation or precipitin tests. Their presence and titer may help in making the diagnosis and in monitoring response to therapy. Cross-reactions with mycobacteria are common. Reagents, however, are not commercially available, and serologic tests therefore require the services of a special laboratory.

Culture. The agent grows well on Sabouraud's medium and on most media used by the bacteriology laboratory for isolation of tubercle bacilli. Identification of *N. asteroides* in the laboratory depends on the combination of morphologic and physiologic characteristics. Symptomatology and radiologic features of the disease are not pathognomonic. Presence of *N. asteroides* in sputum does not always implicate the agent as the primary cause of the patient's disorder. Nevertheless, it is strongly recommended that the repeated isolation of *N. asteroides* should be given the same diagnostic (but not prognostic) significance as the isolation of *Mycobacterium tuberculosis.*

Differential Diagnosis. Nocardiosis has many clinical forms and must be distinguished from a wide range of pulmonary, meningeal, cutaneous, and systemic diseases. Among these are tuberculosis, neoplasms, sarcoidosis, sarcoma, brain abscess, and actinomycosis.

TREATMENT. Sulfonamides have long been used as the treatment of choice, either alone or in combination with trimethoprim, ampicillin, or erythromycin. Drugs such as sulfadiazine or sulfisoxazole should be administered for at least 6 weeks after resolution or stabilization of the disease. Many authorities recommend 6- to 12-month courses of therapy to prevent relapse. Dosage should be sufficient to achieve blood levels of 10 mg/dL. Abscesses should be surgically drained. Sinus tracts should be explored and drained and excisions made of severely damaged tissues, when practicable. Minocycline has been used successfully in a few patients allergic to sulfonamides.

PROGNOSIS. The prognosis is most favorable when the diagnosis is made early, before metastasis to the brain. In view of the ubiquity of the organism, it is likely that humans have an innately high level of resistance.

Nocardiosis that is recognized early and treated promptly may be completely eradicated. However, the disease, particularly when disseminated, is often refractory to treatment and has a poor prognosis, with a survival rate of about 50%.

PREVENTION. Prevention is not practicable.

BIBLIOGRAPHY

Beaman RL, Burnside J, Edwards B, et al.: Nocardial infections in the United States, 1972–1974. J Infect Dis 134:286, 1976.

Conant NF, Smith DT, Baker RD, et al.: Manual of Clinical Mycology, 3rd ed. Philadelphia, WB Saunders, 1971, pp 37–61.

Frazier AR, Rosenow EC, Roberts GD: Nocardiosis: A review of 25 cases occurring during 24 months. Mayo Clin Proc 50:657, 1975.

Kurup PV, Randhawa HS, Gupta NP: Nocardiosis: A review. Mycopathol Mycol Appl 60:193, 1970.

60. ACTINOMYCOSIS

Donald W. R. Mackenzie and Roderick J. Hay

DEFINITION. Actinomycosis is a chronic, localized, suppurative, granulomatous bacterial disease caused by species of *Actinomyces*. It is characterized by the formation of abscesses and multiple draining sinus tracts, through which colonies (sulfur granules) are discharged onto the surface.

ETIOLOGY. The most common cause of actinomycosis in humans is *A. israelii*, although other species are recognized pathogens (i.e., *A. naeslundi*, *Arachnia propionica*, and *Bifidobacterium eriksonii*). They are anaerobic members of the normal human flora, growing on the surfaces of teeth and in the tonsillar crypts. They have not been recovered from other natural habitats, and infections are consequently endogenous rather than exogenous in origin. In the oral cavity and throat, the agents may consist of small bacilliform cells 0.5 to 1 μm in diameter or may be aggregated into small white or yellow clumps. In infected tissues, the agent appears as compact grains (sulfur granules) that are white or, more characteristically, yellow; rounded or lobulated; of a soft consistency; and up to 2 mm in diameter. Early stages of growth are by fine, branching hyphae, 0.5 to 1 μm in diameter, but the organisms may undergo extensive fragmentation in both tissues and cultures, so that their hyphal nature may not be readily recognized. Typically, they are closely associated with other anaerobic bacterial inhabitants of the colonized sites, including fusiform bacteria, anaerobic streptococci, and *Actinobacillus actinomycetemcomitans*. It is likely that these associated microorganisms act synergistically in establishing an infection.

Sulfur granules consist of interwoven and often fragmented hyphae together with cellular debris and associated microorganisms. Toward the periphery, hyphae are oriented radially and commonly have sheaths of eosinophilic material ("clubs").

Actinomycosis was first recognized in cattle in 1877 and in humans in 1880. The agents in both types of disease were originally thought to be identical, but they are now classified as different species.

EPIDEMIOLOGY. Actinomycosis occurs worldwide. Cases are sporadic and somewhat uncommon. Males are infected more frequently than females, but this sexual predilection has now become less evident with the recognition of a link between pelvic actinomycosis and intrauterine contraceptive devices. Any age group may be affected, but the disease is rare in children under 10 years of age and generally occurs between the ages of 15 and 40. No racial or occupational susceptibilities are evident, although individuals with poor standards of oral hygiene may be more likely to acquire the disease.

PATHOGENESIS AND PATHOLOGY. Because the causal agents are normal members of the microflora of mouth and throat, the most common form of actinomycosis is cervicofacial. Infection becomes established when the agents invade mucous membranes of the mouth and pharynx, presumably through the gums, teeth, or tonsils. Initial signs of actinomycosis may originate in the pharynx, but the disease more commonly is first seen in the lower jaw. A history of dental disease or extraction is common.

If the agents are aspirated, infection becomes established in the lung, with extension to the pleura and chest wall. Abdominal actinomycosis probably originates from the intestinal flora. Once established, infection may extend by the diaphragm to the chest cavity. Metastatic spread may set up focal infections in a wide range of body sites. The causes of susceptibility are not understood, but local or systemic predisposition can be inferred from the infrequency of actual disease, as opposed to colonization.

The gross pathology may vary according to the rate of infection, but the condition usually is characterized by chronicity, fibrosis, suppuration, and scar formation. Histopathologically, infected areas are characterized by abscesses of varying size and sinus tracts that often interconnect. Sulfur granules are surrounded by abundant neutrophils, and suppurative areas are limited by fibrosis and by granulation tissue with both acute and chronic inflammatory cells. Giant cells are uncommon.

Macrophages containing fat may be present in sufficient numbers to impart a yellow color to the lesion, which is visible on gross examination. Sulfur granules are distinctive and usually diagnostic, but they may not be abundant, and their detection may require a careful search of serial sections. They are clearly revealed in Gram-stained sections or in material stained by silver impregnation, but other fungal stains such as periodic acid–Schiff or Gridley stains are unsatisfactory.

CLINICAL MANIFESTATIONS

Cervicofacial Lesions. Tissue swelling is not prominent in the early stages of cervicofacial actinomycosis. Skin overlying the lesion soon becomes inflamed and develops an uneven surface, and the tumor becomes indurated and woody. Localized granulomas suppurate and drain through single and multiple sinus tracts, which may heal and reopen or be replaced by new ones. Extension to cranial bones, brain, and meninges may occur.

Thoracic Actinomycosis. Thoracic actinomycosis is characterized by areas of consolidation, usually in hilar or basal regions. Radiographs show large areas of consolidation, often containing small abscess cavities. In contrast to tuberculosis, infection often is confined to the bases of the lungs. Patients are anemic and complain of pleural pain. Common findings are cough, low-grade fever, weight loss, and night sweats; in addition, dysphagia may result from mediastinal invasion.

Abdominal Actinomycosis. Abdominal actinomycosis may initially mimic acute or subacute appendicitis, but primary lesions are usually palpable in the ileocecal region. As the infection progresses, there may be extension to the liver, ovaries, and urinary tract, with development of pyelonephritis or cystitis, or to the spine, resulting in compression of the cord and sometimes a psoas abscess. Sinus tracts may develop in the abdominal wall. The most common single finding is a tender, palpable mass in the region of the appendix or in other parts of the abdomen. Pelvic actinomycosis has been reported more frequently in recent years, particularly in women using intrauterine contraceptive devices for many years.

DIAGNOSIS. The diagnosis of actinomycosis is supported by detection of sulfur granules in pus or tissue sections and by the isolation and identification of the agent. Serologic tests are under development but are not yet consistently reliable. Cervicofacial actinomycosis or visceral forms of the disease that have progressed to the stage at which sinus tracts have appeared on the chest or abdominal wall usually present no difficulties with diagnosis. Abdominal or pelvic actinomycosis without abdominal wall involvement may be diagnosed only at laparotomy.

Differential Diagnosis. The condition may simulate several chronic diseases, including tuberculosis, osteomyelitis, carcinoma, and liver abscess.

TREATMENT. Penicillin is the drug of choice, the regimen depending on the extent and severity of the disease. High doses (5 to 10 million units daily) may be administered intramuscularly or intravenously for 6 weeks or until lesions have healed, followed by oral therapy with 2 to 5 million units of penicillin or 2 gm of tetracycline daily for 6 to 12 months. Patients allergic to penicillin may be given tetracycline, erythromycin, or possibly lincomycin. Surgical resection and incision and drainage of badly diseased tissues are valuable ancillary therapeutic procedures.

PROGNOSIS. Before the antibiotic era, the prognosis was very poor. Based on experience with penicillin, anticipated recovery rates are now about 90% for cervicofacial, 80% for abdominal, and 40% for thoracic forms for the disease. Prognosis is greatly improved when the condition is diagnosed early. Recovery with adequate penicillin therapy is common, but chronic abdominal infections and thoracic empyema may be difficult to eradicate.

PREVENTION. Prevention is not practicable.

BIBLIOGRAPHY

Brown JR: Human actinomycosis: A study of 181 subjects. Hum Pathol 4:319, 1973.
Gupta PK, Hollander DH, Frost JK: Actinomycetes in cervicovaginal smears: An association with I.U.C.D. usage. Acta Cytol 20:295, 1976.
Pollock, PG, Meyer DS, Fable WJ, et al.: Rapid diagnosis of actinomycosis by thin needle aspiration biopsy. Am J Clin Pathol 70:27, 1978.

■

SECTION I

MYCOBACTERIAL INFECTIONS

61. TUBERCULOSIS

Émile Fox

DEFINITION AND INTRODUCTION. Tuberculosis is a transmissible disease caused in humans by two bacilli of the genus *Mycobacterium*, *M. tuberculosis* and *M. bovis*. The disease is worldwide in distribution, but presents a much greater public health problem in poor countries and hot climates, as compared to the more developed countries, where the risk of infection has decreased markedly over the last 50 years. Infection is acquired usually through the lungs, but in some areas, the enteric route remains an important means of infection with the bovine bacillus, contained in unpasteurized milk from infected cattle. The clinical manifestations of the disease are protean and are caused by the host's immune response to the invading bacteria. Granulomas develop slowly and may undergo ulceration and cavitation through release of tumor necrosis factor by activated macrophages. Tuberculosis affects the lungs mainly in the form of a progressive destructive disease, but it may affect other parts of the body also (in particular, the bones, joints, kidneys, lymph nodes, and meninges) or become disseminated throughout the body.

Today, tuberculosis constitutes one of the most important aspects of medical practice in the developing world. New and exciting strategies are being devised for treating and controlling the disease worldwide, but unfortunately, the reasons for the ultimate failure of these methods are increasing. Causes for control failure include overcrowding, poor nutrition and sanitation, and shortage of funds and manpower needed to cope with the expense of diagnostic facilities, vaccinations, and mass chemotherapy. Recently, concern is mounting with the discovery of the pandemic caused by human immunodeficiency virus (HIV) and its startling relationship to infection by mycobacteria in the tropical environment.

ETIOLOGY AND BACTERIOLOGY

The Organism. *Mycobacterium tuberculosis* is a nonmotile slender rod, 2 to 4 μm in length and 0.2 to 0.4 μm in width. It is an obligate aerobe and does not produce spores. The high lipid content of the cell wall is responsible for the unique property, common to all mycobacteria, of "acid fastness" and "alcohol fastness," i.e., the retention of specific dyes despite subsequent exposure to acid and alcohol. In the diagnostic laboratory, the organisms are best stained by the Ziehl-Neelsen or Kinyoun stains. Under the light microscope, they appear as red bacteria on a blue or green background. They may appear as "solid" (evenly stained) or beaded (unevenly stained) in appearance. Under the fluorescence microscope, auramine-rhodamine staining as an alternative stain is more sensitive but less specific. It is useful when large numbers of specimens are to be tested.

Cultural Characteristics. The organisms grow slowly and require 3 weeks or more to develop colonies on solid media. In liquid media, the organism has a tendency to aggregate and form filaments or cords, which are associated with virulence. The most commonly used culture media are Löwenstein-Jensen (solid egg) or Middlebrook 7H-11. The temperature range for growth is from 33°C to 39°C. Maximum growth occurs at pH 6.6 to 6.8, a PO_2 of 120 mm Hg, and 5% of CO_2 in the atmosphere.

Mycobacteria species can be identified by biochemical tests. In contrast to the bovine bacillus, *M. tuberculosis* produces nicotinic acid (niacin), reduces nitrate to nitrite, and has weak catalase activity that is destroyed by heating. Phage typing of the organism is feasible and of potential usefulness in epidemiological studies and control attempts. Bacilli with properties intermediate between the typical human and bovine strains exist, like bacille *Calmette-Guérin (BCG)* and the so-called *M. africanum* strain, but these are not considered to be particular mycobacterial species.

In Vivo Growth Characteristics. *M. tuberculosis* can replicate extracellularly or inside phagocytic cells and has long generation times of 16 to 24 hours. It can infect man and other primates. Among laboratory animals, guinea pigs are particularly susceptible, and rabbits are particularly resistant to infection. Because tubercle bacilli are highly aerobic, they thrive best in tissues with a high oxygen tension. This aerophilia explains why certain body areas are so commonly involved in the chronic forms of the disease. Indeed, the highest PO_2 in the body is in the apices of the lungs, where tuberculosis is most frequent. Other organs commonly involved are the renal cortex and the growing ends of bones (where the PO_2 may reach 100 mm Hg). Organs with low oxygen tension, such as the spleen and the liver, are much less commonly affected, except in disseminated disease.

The tubercle organisms are resistant to heat and many disinfectants, but are killed easily by ultraviolet light.

Nontuberculous Mycobacteria. There are more than 40 known nontuberculous mycobacterial species, divided into 4 groups by Runyon in 1959 (Table 67–1). The most important are *M. kansasii* (group I), *M. scrofulaceum* (group II), *M. avium-intracellulare* (group III), and *M. fortuitum* (group IV). Laboratory diagnosis of nontuberculous mycobacteria requires multiple chemical tests and morphologic studies, which should be performed by persons experienced in mycobacteriology. The epidemiologic importance of nontuberculous mycobacteria is being re-evaluated; the designation "atypical mycobacteria" should be abandoned. Some 30 species occur as free-living organisms and are termed "environmental mycobacteria." The other 10 species are obligate or facultative pathogens of particular hosts. More than a dozen among the 40 nontuberculous mycobacterial species have been recognized as etiologic agents in human disease (Chapter 61.2). In addition to this role as potential agents of human disease, there is mounting evidence that immunologic recognition of environmentally acquired mycobacterial infection, whether it leads to disease or not, may determine the host's type of immune response to subsequent mycobacterial exposure (immune priming). Thus, environmental mycobacteria induce immune responses in humans that may cause reactivity on tuberculin skin tests, interfere with the efficacy of later vaccination with BCG, and perhaps be important natural vaccinators against tuberculosis and leprosy.

EPIDEMIOLOGY. Tuberculosis occurs all over the world, but its epidemiology varies in different regions. Spectacular results in the control of the disease have been achieved in the technically advanced countries, but there has been little or no improvement in most tropical countries, where over 85% of the world's tuberculosis now occurs (Table 61–1). Each year about 10 million people are thought to develop tuberculous disease in poor countries (5 million being highly infectious); at least 3 million die of the disease.

Source of Infection. *M. tuberculosis hominis* is transmitted primarily from persons with slowly smouldering cavitary lung disease who have close contact with nonimmune individuals. The typical situation in the tropical environment involves the grandmother who has a chronic tuberculous cough (while never seeking medical

TABLE 61–1. Tuberculosis Case Rates Per 100,000 Population from 1970 to 1974 for 15 Countries with the Highest, Middle, and Lowest Rates*

Highest			Middle			Lowest		
Country	*Year*	*Rate*	*Country*	*Year*	*Rate*	*Country*	*Year*	*Rate*
Macao	1973	469	St. Lucia	1972	64	Cuba	1972	14
Swaziland	1970	468	Austria	1973	62	United States	1974	14
Bolivia	1972	414	Kenya	1970	61	Martinique	1972	14
Gilbert and Ellice	1973	334	Italy	1970	61	Norway	1973	14
Islands			German Federal	1972	59	Denmark	1973	13
Mauritania	1970	332	Republic			Australia	1973	12
Philippines	1972	328	Angola	1970	58	Antigua	1973	11
Wallis and Futuna	1973	260	Madagascar	1970	57	Trinidad and	1972	11
Islands			Iran	1970	56	Tobago		
Republic of Korea	1973	249	Western Samoa	1973	55	Israel	1973	10
South Africa	1973	247	Ghana	1970	55	Virgin Islands (UK)	1971	9
New Hebrides	1973	223	Zaire	1970	54	Cameroon	1970	8
British Solomon	1973	215	France	1972	54	Virgin Islands (US)	1973	6
Islands			Venezuela	1973	54	Grenada	1972	5
Iraq	1970	214	Sri Lanka	1972	50	Faeroe Islands	1970	5
Brunei	1970	200	Equador	1973	50	St. Vincent	1972	2
Hong Kong	1973	196						
Pacific Islands, Trust	1973	175						
Territories								

*Adapted from Comstock GW: Am Rev Respir Dis 125 (Suppl):8, 1982.

treatment herself) and who gradually infects all her grandchildren. Caseum of tuberculous pulmonary cavities can contain large numbers of tubercle bacilli, from 10^7 to 10^9 organisms. Smear-positive persons constitute the most important source of infection. They are more contagious than culture-positive, smear-negative individuals, who are a threat mostly to persons living in prolonged close contact. Patients with tuberculous lung disease, but negative sputum examinations, are generally not infectious; neither are people with nonpulmonary tuberculosis.

The reservoir of *M. tuberculosis bovis* comprises infected cattle, cows, and buffalos.

Receptive Population. All humans are susceptible to infection by the tubercle bacilli, but some ethnic groups seem to be more vulnerable than others, perhaps due to natural selection from centuries of infection. Natural resistance is greater among Caucasians, Mongolians, and Jews, than among Africans, Eskimos, American Indians, Polynesians, and Melanesians. In the latter, the infection tends to be more acute and more often fatal, whereas in the former, it is more chronic and late recrudescence is more common. Within defined populations, it appears that innate host resistance and hereditary components may play an important role in the susceptibility to the disease. Associations have been described between tuberculosis and particular HLA antigens in various populations. Recently, a link has been described also between vitamin D deficiency and impaired host defense against *M. tuberculosis*. This hypothesis is attractive to help explain the high incidence of tuberculous disease among immigrants in industrialized countries, because these people often move from sunny regions to regions where the sunlight is much more limited.

Immune Population. Persons with tuberculous infection develop specific immunity that partially protects against further infection. Partial and transitory protection against tuberculous infection also can be achieved

through vaccination with BCG, and people exposed as children to high loads of certain environmental mycobacteria might also become immune to subsequent tuberculous infection. Immunity to tuberculosis is mediated through sensitized T lymphocytes that release lymphokines on stimulation by tubercle antigens. These lymphokines help activated macrophages to lyse the ingested mycobacteria. The role of immunoglobulins remains poorly understood, but specific IgA may be increased in patients with active tuberculosis. When people with previous tuberculous infection subsequently develop tuberculous disease, it is more often the result of a late recrudescence of infection than of a new infection.

Transmission

Airborne. Transmission of *M. tuberculosis* is mostly through aerosols. Bacilli in lung lesions become airborne in aerosols through coughing, sneezing, singing, and speaking (especially while pronouncing consonants). These airborne infectious particles are called "droplet nuclei" (Flügge's particles) and are of various sizes. Large droplet nuclei (more than 10 μm in size) are retained by the protective mucous epithelium of the bronchi and upper airways and are cleared without producing infection. Still larger droplets settle to the ground and are readily made harmless by adherence to dust, drying, and ultraviolet light and are not involved in the airborne transmission of the infection. However, the smaller droplet nuclei remain suspended in the air, remaining viable, and so are potentially infectious. Small particles measuring 5 to 10 μm in size and containing 2 to 3 bacilli may reach beyond the protective mucous blanket to the terminal bronchioles and alveoli, where, in a susceptible host, they may establish an infection. Because of the small probability of an infectious droplet of the right size to reach the periphery of a pulmonary lobule, exposure to airborne droplet nuclei in a closed environment must be relatively long for infection to occur. The number of organisms introduced into the air will depend on the frequency of cough and the concentration of bacilli in pulmonary secretions. These in turn depend on the extent of pulmonary involvement and the presence of lung cavities. Household contacts of a person with a smear-positive index case are at greatest risk of becoming infected, but only 25 to 50% of such individuals do acquire the infection, even in crowded environments.

Airborne transmission from humans to animal also occurs and is an important means of infecting animals kept in captivity. Tuberculosis does not befall free-living primates, but when a primate in a zoo or laboratory develops tuberculosis, it usually was infected at the tropical export station from a sputum-positive caretaker.

Milk. Infection with *M. bovis* is most commonly associated with consuming milk from infected cows. While this happens rarely in developed countries, owing to eradication of tuberculosis in cattle and pasteurization of milk, in tropical regions this remains a significant cause of human infection. Generally, milk and cattle control measures are not available in rural tropical areas. Animals such as cats and dogs also can acquire *M. bovis* infection from contaminated milk or meat.

Direct Transmission. Transmission of *M. tuberculosis* from open skin lesions or fistulas is extremely rare. Fomites, such as books, utensils, bed clothes, and dishes, play no role in the transmission of the disease and require no special attention. The risk of direct inoculation is confined primarily to pathologists and workers in the mycobacteriology laboratory.

Tuberculous Infection. Infection is not synonymous with disease. Infection defines the presence of multiplying microorganisms within a host, whereas disease describes the results from the progressive pathological changes that follow the multiplication of the invading organism and the host's response to it. Tuberculous infection is much more common than tuberculous disease, because a large proportion of infections are controlled by natural host defense mechanisms. Tuberculous infection can be identified through the visible changes related to the cellular immune response elicited from an infected host in whom mycobacterial antigens are injected into the epidermal layer of the skin (skin test).

Tuberculin Skin Test. The tuberculin skin test is an important tool for screening populations for tuberculous infection and also a valuable diagnostic test for evaluating patients with illnesses that are compatible with tuberculosis. In the past, the test was performed by injecting filtered broth from *M. tuberculosis* cultures (old tuberculin) into the skin. The test has now been better standardized to give a more precise and stable result by using purified protein derivative (PPD). The Mantoux test consists of the intradermal injection of 2 tuberculin units (TU) of PPD. An area of induration measuring 10 mm or more after 72 hours is called a positive reaction and is considered to indicate previous exposure. Because PPD contains many antigens common to many mycobacteria, including BCG and the nontuberculous environmental species, many cross-reactions occur, and classic Mantoux testing is said not to readily distinguish between infection by tubercle bacilli,

previous BCG vaccination, or sensitization by environmental mycobacteria. In fact, individuals with a small degree of tuberculin sensitivity seem to be protected from tuberculosis, whereas those with large reactions are less protected than those with no sensitivity at all. The difference between these two types of reactions is a protective, "prophylactic" cell-mediated immunity in the first case and a harmful, tissue-damaging "anaphylactic" hypersensitivity in the second case. To differentiate between these two types of reactions, it has been proposed recently that interpretation of skin tests should include the dynamic appearance of dermal induration as well as the appearance of macroscopic epidermal changes. Two types of Mantoux reactions can thus be differentiated: the Koch-type reaction (large-diameter, rapid, and long-lasting induration with reddish skin) is related to secretion of tumor necrosis factor by activated macrophages and may be detected in tuberculous disease or after infection with certain environmental mycobacteria, e.g., *M. kansasii* or *M. scrofulaceum*. The Listeria-type reaction (small-diameter, slow, short-living, colorless induration) is related to protective immunity and is found, for instance, after protective BCG vaccination. Some researchers now use more specific antigens for tuberculin testing (new tuberculins), with the hope of differentiating different hypersensitivity reactions elicited from different mycobacterial species.

Prevalence and Incidence of Tuberculous Infection

Developed Countries. BCG vaccination has not been employed in the United States, and PPD testing generally is considered a valuable tool for identifying the prevalence of tuberculous infection in the population. There are about 15 million tuberculin reactors, giving a prevalence of infection of 7000 per 100,000 population in the United States. This has decreased considerably since 1900, when 80% of the population was infected before the age of 20 years. Today, only a small percent of young adults are positive reactors, while in those aged 50 or older, the prevalence remains around 25%, with a rate of conversion back to "negative" of 5% per year.

In the Netherlands, by using the response to the first-strength PPD, 2 TU (adopted by the World Health Organization [WHO] as the standard dose), it was found that the annual incidence of infection had dropped from 11.3% in 1910 to 0.012% in 1989.

However, tuberculous infection cannot be eradicated easily in developed countries because of the unremitting arrival from underdeveloped countries of immigrants and refugees with tuberculous infection. Tuberculosis can be said to be eradicated from a country when the incidence of new cases drops below one per million inhabitants per year.

Developing Countries. Tuberculous infection is highly prevalent in most developing countries (see Table 61–1). Certain areas in Southern Asia, Africa, and Latin America have the highest prevalence of tuberculous infection in the world. However, determining the exact prevalence of infection by *M. tuberculosis* may be difficult in many tropical countries, because tuberculosis, sensitization to nontuberculous mycobacteria, and vaccination by BCG are common and can elicit a tuberculin reactivity. Methods for estimating the proportion of actual tuberculous infections among tuberculin reactors have been proposed and include determination of the cutting point for a positive reaction and performance of dual tests. Descriptions of the midpoint location (median, mean, mode) of the dermal induration are meaningful measures in the population of nonzero reactors to tuberculin; they usually display a normal Gaussian distribution. Despite these more complicated approaches, the various methods for estimation often yield wide-ranging results. For instance, among adult Nigerians, prevalence of tuberculous infection was found to range from 32% to 62%, depending on the different tests and criteria used. In some countries, 30% of children under 5 years of age and 90% of individuals above age 40 have a reactive tuberculin skin test. In certain populations, reactive tuberculin tests evolve in 2 stages. Initial reactivity is related to immunization to nontuberculous mycobacteria and is acquired early in life and at an annual rapid incidence (4%) until, by age 20, sensitivity is nearly universal. The indurations usually are in the 2 to 9 mm diameter range. The ensuing acquisition of large indurations (12+ mm) proceeds at a lower annual rate (1%), affects around 50% among middle-aged adults in many tropical countries, and is apparently more specific for tuberculosis.

The prevalence of tuberculous infection is not homogenous throughout a community. Much higher reactor rates are found among the contacts of tuberculous patients than in the general population. About 50% of children in contact with patients with positive smears have positive tuberculin reactions, compared with only 5% in nonhousehold contacts.

Prevalence and Incidence of Tuberculous Disease. The exact prevalence of tuberculous morbidity in tropical countries is difficult to assess, owing to under-use of health care facilities by tuberculous patients and insufficient epidemiologic data for smear-positive tuberculosis. Table 61–1 indicates the prevalence of disease in some countries where data are available. Average point prevalence of the disease is 250 to 350 cases per 100,000 population, with much higher prevalence rates in several countries in Asia and Latin America. This compares with less than 20 cases per 100,000 population in Western countries.

In the United States, the incidence of tuberculous disease was 9.4 per 100,000 population (22,768 cases) in 1986, a decrease from 24 per 100,000 in 1966 and 53 per 100,000 in 1953. From 1963 to 1985, the incidence rate of tuberculosis declined an average of 5.9% annually. Increases in the number of annual cases were reported in 1980 (influx of refugees from Vietnam and other Southeast Asian countries) and since 1986 (related to the spread of the HIV epidemic).

In developing countries, there has been an overall increase in the number of tuberculosis cases during the last 3 decades, which correlates with the increase of their populations. Unfortunately, reliable data are not available for most developing countries, since notification of cases is poorly done. Estimates of new tuberculous cases by the World Bank for 1990 range from about 1.6 million to 5.0 million.

Factors Influencing Disease Prevalence. There is a marked variation in the morbidity of tuberculosis related to age, sex, race, geography, and socioeconomic conditions. In the United States, more than 85% of new cases develop in persons over the age of 30; they occur twice as commonly in men than in women; and case rates in nonwhites are 4.5 times greater than those in whites. Likewise, the prevalence of the disease varies geographically within the United States, being lowest in Nebraska and highest in Hawaii. The prevalence of disease remains high among Eskimos, American Indians, and immigrant migrant workers. The case rate among immigrants from developing countries is considerably higher than that in the indigenous population, and the incidence of tuberculosis in a group of immigrants will be proportional to the incidence in the country of origin and not to that of the adopted country. In Europe, tuberculosis is more prevalent in the eastern countries than in western ones. Worldwide, socioeconomic factors play a major role in the prevalence of tuberculosis, which remains high in cities with populations of more than 250,000. Poverty, poor nutrition, minimal access to medical care, and overcrowded housing are all contributing factors. Socioeconomic improvements have reduced morbidity and mortality of tuberculosis in the West. The close relationship between the socioeconomic state of a country and the prevalence of tuberculosis indicates that a decline in incidence in the developing world will come only with the improvement in standards of living.

Factors Influencing Progression from Infection to Disease. Among persons infected with *M. tuberculosis*, the cumulative morbidity rate may be as high as 15%. The infection may progress to serious disease within 5 years in 5 to 10%, and a further 3 to 5% may develop late recrudescence at some time thereafter. In the United States it is proposed that early detection of the "conversion" from negative to positive tuberculin reaction should be followed by institution of isoniazid (INH) preventive therapy in an attempt to prevent both early and late development of disease in 90 to 95% of these tuberculin "converters." On the other hand, such a strategy appears unrealistic in the tropical environment, where a majority of the adult population reacts to tuberculin, owing to previous exposure to environmental bacteria, tubercle bacilli, or BCG. After infection, the risk of developing clinical tuberculosis is highest in infancy and next highest in young adults and adolescents. In the large majority of persons with a positive tuberculin reaction, the tuberculous lesion is latent or dormant ("healed"). However, the bacilli may remain dormant for years in the apical pulmonary scars and the hilar lymph nodes and may reactivate years or decades later to produce clinical tuberculosis. This may happen in other organs also, especially in areas of copious blood flow and high PO_2. Because this recrudescence occurs more often in the elderly, in the malnourished, and in persons with debilitating illnesses, it appears likely that the reactivation may be due to a waning of cellular immune surveillance. Accordingly, HIV infection, when acquired by a patient with latent tuberculous infection, may facilitate the progression to overt clinical tuberculosis (Chapter 61.1).

The risk of developing tuberculous disease in various individuals with a positive PPD reaction is presented in Table 61–2.

Mortality. In developed countries, the decline in tuberculosis had begun well before the advances in diagnosis and management of the disease that have taken place during the past 50 years. However, with the introduction of chemotherapy, the decline in mortality was greatly accelerated. In 1900, the mortality from tuberculosis in the United States was 202 per 100,000 population; in 1953, soon after the introduction of effective chemotherapy, the rate had decreased to 12.4 per 100,000. Since then, the decline has continued steadily to approach 1 per 100,000 population today.

In most developing countries, during this same period, there has been very little or no decline in tuberculosis mortality. In 1971, tuberculosis is said to have accounted for 3% of all deaths in Thailand, 10% in the Philippines, and up to 25% in several South American countries. In sub-Saharan Africa in 1990, overall mortality caused by tuberculosis was 6.7%. In Hong Kong, global death rates from tuberculosis were 9.7 per 100,000 in 1976 and 7.9 in 1980, whereas death rates from active tuberculous disease declined from 6.9 in 1975 to 4.3 in 1980.

PATHOGENESIS. Pathogenesis describes the sequence of events leading to the disease state characterizing clinical tuberculosis.

Primary Infection. Tubercle bacilli can enter the body by several routes (pulmonary, gastrointestinal, cutaneous), but the most frequent route of entry is through the lungs. When droplet nuclei are inhaled, the bacillus is deposited at the periphery of a pulmonary lobule beneath the pleura, most commonly in the lower two thirds of the lungs, where ventilation is greatest. In the nonimmune host, the bacilli are phagocytized by alveolar macrophages, but they are not killed intracellularly because of absent T-cell mediated immunity. Bacilli multiply intracellularly and are carried by infected macrophages throughout the host's body. Specific immunity to tubercle antigens develops slowly and in 3 to 6 weeks becomes sufficient to produce an exudative response and a nonspecific pneumonitis at the site of initial infection. This parenchymal and hilar lymph node involvement constitutes a primary (Ghon) complex (Fig. 61–1). With the development of acquired immunity, macrophages become activated by T lymphocytes to kill tubercle bacilli intracellularly, and the multiplication of the bacilli is usually brought under control. The characteristic tubercle granuloma with epithelioid cells, multinucleated giant cells, and caseation necrosis develops in the pulmonary lesion, regional lymph nodes, and any site to which bacilli have spread (Fig. 61–2). The tuberculous lesion usually heals with resolution, fibrosis, and calcification. A state of balance then becomes established between multiplying bacilli and intracellular macrophage killing. If the immune response fails, however, the infection may progress, overwhelm the patient, and produce disseminated tuberculosis.

Silent Dissemination. The bacillary dissemination occurring during the early course of the infection may be asymptomatic or associated with mild fever and "flu-like" symptoms, which may be overlooked unless the patient is observed closely after exposure. The bacilli are disseminated to other organs of the body and establish metastatic foci of infection where clinical tuberculosis may develop at a later date. The organs with high oxygen tension (90 mm Hg or more) are most suitable for growth of tubercle bacilli. Owing to uneven ventilation/perfusion in the apex of the lung when in the upright position, the P_{O_2} of this region is approximately 130 mm Hg, providing a particularly favorable environment for the bacilli. If these lesions heal by scarring, they are called Simon's foci, which are the most common source of later recrudescence of infection. Similarly, the growing ends of long bones and the renal cortex are more apt to support the growth of bacilli than are the liver and spleen, where the oxygen tension is much lower.

Latent (Dormant) Infection. If the tuberculous lesion

TABLE 61–2. Risk of Developing Tuberculosis in Infected Persons in the United States (Positive PPD Reactors)

Group	Risk
Children under 3 years of age	1 in 5
Reactors among close contacts of persons with active disease	First year: 1 in 20
Recent converters, unknown contact	First year: 1 in 20
Reactors between 5 and 25 years of age	Annual risk: 1 in 75
Reactors with scars of pulmonary tuberculosis and inadequate or no previous treatment	Annual risk: 1 in 75
Reactors with culture-negative pulmonary tuberculosis and inadequate or no previous treatment	Annual risk: 1 in 75
Reactors with special risk conditions (e.g., diabetes, blood and reticuloendothelial malignances, corticosteroid therapy, immunosuppressive therapy, HIV infection, silicosis, or post gastrectomy)	Increased 2- to 3-fold over other reactors
Other reactors over 35 years of age	1 in 1400

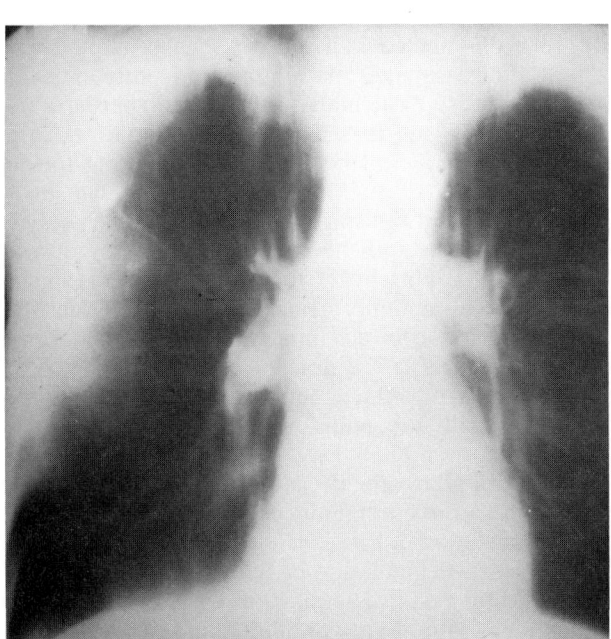

FIGURE 61–1. Primary infection. The chest tomogram shows a recent right primary (Ghon) complex.

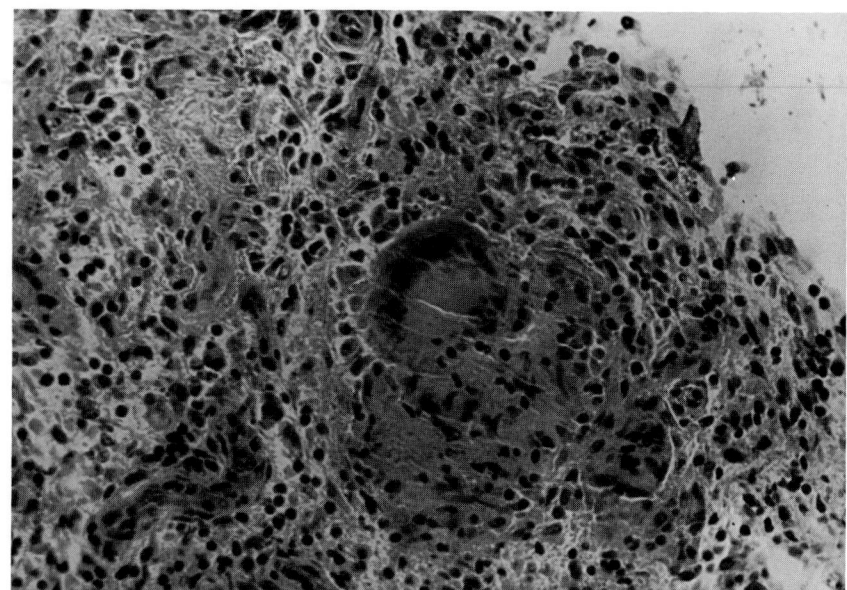

FIGURE 61–2. Caseating granuloma with multinucleated giant cells at the periphery.

regresses, the infection may remain dormant for years. At a later date, any dormant lesion may produce clinical tuberculosis when the balance between multiplying bacilli and killing macrophages becomes disturbed.

Clinical Tuberculosis. Most symptoms and lesions of tuberculosis are not caused by the invading and dividing bacilli, but by the host's immune response, which involves lymphocytic activation of macrophages and release of the monokine tumor necrosis factor/cachectin. This monokine is responsible for the chronic fever in tuberculosis and for the profound catabolic state accounting for the severe weight loss and cachexia of chronic tuberculosis. This monokine also leads to the caseation of the tubercle granulomas and the resulting severe destructive tissue disease. Tuberculous disease can begin after a few months, years, or decades following the initial infection. Development of disease soon after an infection (within 1 to 2 years) occurs in about 5 to 10% of infected individuals. Such prompt development of disease takes place more frequently in developing countries, particularly in children, perhaps because of poor nutritional state and large inocula. Another 5 to 10% will become diseased owing to late recrudescence of dormant lesions. Blood stream invasion may occur at any stage, resulting in miliary tuberculosis. In this instance, the host's immune response is incapable of coping with the multiplying organism, either because immunity against the bacillus is insufficient (e.g., in acquired immunodeficiency syndrome [AIDS]), or because the immune state is waning (e.g., in the elderly or after immunosuppressive therapy). Characteristically tuberculin testing is anergic in miliary tuberculosis.

In persons who are already infected with tubercle bacilli, considerable immunity is generally present. Subsequent inhalation of bacilli results in rapid mobilization of defenses and elimination of the bacilli before significant replication and dissemination can occur. Thus, in an individual with a reactive tuberculin test, the risk for tuberculosis comes from within the individual rather than from exposure to sputum-positive patients.

PATHOLOGY. Epithelioid granulomas are the hallmark of tuberculous lesions. They may be defined as chronic, focal, and compact collections of inflammatory cells in which mononuclear cells predominate and in which Langhans' giant cells and caseation necrosis may occur (Fig. 61–2). A granuloma is the result of the development of delayed hypersensitivity to the invading bacilli and is a dynamic lesion with recruitment of macrophages from the peripheral blood. Cell division, activation, and cell death occur simultaneously in a continuing process. Caseation is due to dissolution of bacteria and tissues by host secretions. The degree of caseous necrosis varies from one granuloma to another. Once the granuloma has developed, its regression leads to permanent structural change due to the fibrous reaction it causes. The pathology of the lesion of tuberculosis is the same regardless of the organ involved.

CLINICAL MANIFESTATIONS. The problems raised by tuberculosis in the tropical environment are exceedingly dissimilar from the developed countries. In the latter, tuberculosis is a relatively rare disease and often is a diagnosis of exclusion, while in the former, tuberculosis is so common that its differential diagnosis needs to be kept constantly in mind. Tuberculosis can present as a myriad of different clinical pictures and can also emerge behind clear-cut nontuberculous disorders. It may affect any organ of the body at any age.

Pulmonary tuberculosis is the most common disease presentation worldwide; in a recent survey in Nigeria, it accounted for 91.5% of all tuberculous patients. Only 0.6% of patients in that series had both pulmonary and extrapulmonary disease, and 7.9% had extrapulmonary tuberculosis alone, with lymph nodes most commonly affected (39%), followed by bone or joint disease (26%) and pleural effusions (19%). Other commonly affected sites are the central nervous system, intestinal and genitourinary systems. Statistics on organ involvement present many regional differences and are often related to the particular diagnostic skills of the physicians working in a particular area. It is commonly accepted that extrapulmonary tuberculosis and sputum-negative lung tuberculosis together are at least twice as numerous as the sputum-positive lung cases.

Primary Infection. Initial infection with tubercle bacilli does not produce symptoms often, or it causes only mild fever with malaise, which usually subsides without specific therapy. This phase of the infection commonly produces but slight roentgenographic abnormalities and often remains undetected. Occasionally, however, hilar and paratracheal lymph node enlargement may be visible on the chest radiograph (Fig. 61–3 A). In children, the lymphadenopathy may produce collapse of a lung segment or lobe due to compression of the bronchus (Fig. 61–3B). Although hematogenous and lymphogenous spread is the rule during this primary infection, disease generally remains self-limited following the development of specific immunity. On occasion, primary infection progresses directly to severe disease, either in the lungs or by dissemination through the blood stream. Hematogenous dissemination of bacilli may cause miliary and meningeal tuberculosis closely following primary infection. This usually occurs in children under 5 years of age and is more prevalent in malnourished children from developing countries. Progression of the initial infection to tuberculous pneumonia is associated with an abrupt high fever but is generally without great prostration. Initial tuberculous infection may also give rise to pleurisy with effusion or lymphadenitis. Erythema nodosum and phlyctenular conjunctivitis are possible manifestations of hypersensitivity heralding underlying primary tuberculous infection.

Pleuropulmonary Tuberculosis. Occasionally, primary tuberculous infection may, without interruption, lead to pulmonary disease, but lung tuberculosis more often results from a recrudescence of dormant infection, usually in the apices of the lungs (Simon's foci). The characteristics of this form of tuberculosis are chronicity, progressive worsening, cavitation, and fibrosis.

Usually the disease begins insidiously with few symptoms beyond a cough, which is often ascribed to smoking or a residual of a "cold." With progression of the disease, symptoms become constitutional, with malaise, low-grade fever, and loss of weight. Anorexia and abdominal pain may dominate the clinical picture. General malaise, depression, and fatigue occur usually at the end of the day. Night sweats due to defervescence at night or insensible fever may be quite troublesome. Cough can be productive or dry. When sputum is produced, it is classically green and sticky. Blood streaking from bronchial ulceration occurs, but production of a large quantity of blood is uncommon. Massive hemoptysis due to rupture of a branch of a pulmonary artery in a cavity wall may prove fatal, owing to either asphyxiation or exsanguination. Chest pain may occur if there is pleural involvement. Shortness of breath is generally due to extensive destruction of the lungs, rapidly developing tuberculous pneumonia, or a massive pleural effusion. Amenorrhea is common in young women with advanced disease. Inflammatory anemia often develops in long-standing disease.

Tuberculosis of the larynx, trachea, and bronchi is associated generally with advanced cavitary pulmonary disease. Blood-streaked sputum and expiratory wheeze suggest bronchial involvement. Rarely, the bronchial lumen may be blocked by granulomatous inflammation, but external compression by enlarged lymph nodes is more common, especially in children (see Fig. 61–3B). Involvement of the larynx produces hoarseness and painful swallowing. Occasionally, rupture of a mediastinal node into a lobar bronchus produces acute segmental tuberculous pneumonitis with high fever, shortness of breath, and marked weakness.

Pleurisy with effusion may occur within a few months of the initial infection or in association with late recrudescence of infection. Infection is either hematogenous or through involvement of the pleura by an underlying small subpleural tuberculous focus, which erodes the pleura and contaminates the pleural membrane. The development of pleurisy may give rise to a sharp pleuritic pain, and a large effusion may cause shortness of breath. Rupture of a large caseous lesion with massive contamination of the pleural space can lead to a bronchopleural fistula and a tuberculous empyema. This gives rise commonly to a subacute illness with fever, cough, expectoration, and general malaise, and requires prompt medical and surgical attention.

Extrapulmonary Tuberculosis. During the lymphogenous and hematogenous spread occurring during the initial infection, tuberculous bacilli are disseminated

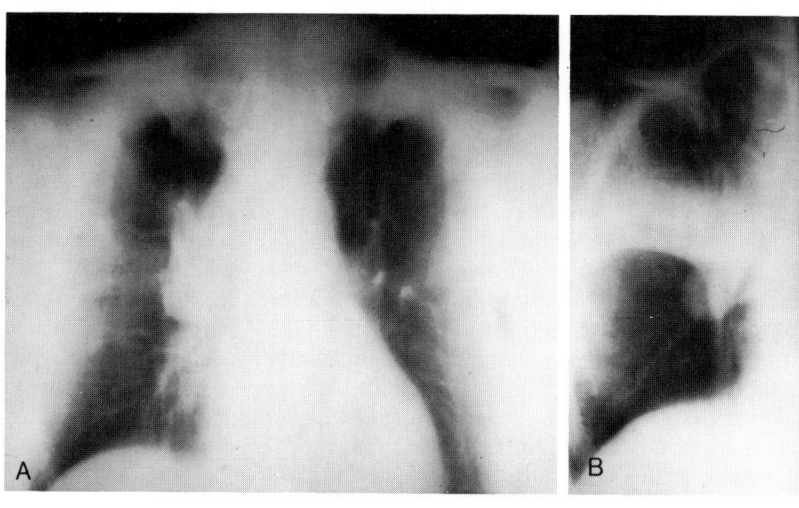

FIGURE 61–3. Adenopathy and bronchial obstruction. Chest tomograms show right hilar and paratracheal adenopathy *(A)* with right middle lobe collapse due to extreme pressure on the bronchi *(B).*

throughout the body inside infected macrophages, establishing infectious foci in many organs. Subsequently, if conditions will support the multiplying bacilli over the body's immune cells, disease can develop in a particular organ. This will occur mostly in those regions where tuberculous growth is sustained by a high oxygen content. Late generalized dissemination of bacilli may occur also through rupture of a caseous focus into the blood stream and concomitant anergy of the host.

Extrapulmonary forms of tuberculosis present numerous particularities in the various tropical regions. Causes are many but are badly understood, and comprise genetic, nutritive, environmental, and epidemiologic factors, in addition to concomitant nonmycobacterial infections, in particular, HIV (Chapter 61.1).

Tuberculous Adenitis. During the primary infection, the enlarged hilar lymph nodes may give rise to external compression of bronchi; in infants and children, it is more common for the right middle lobe bronchus to become compressed and to lead to collapse of the corresponding lobe ("middle lobe syndrome") (Fig. 61–3B), with later production of bronchiectasis. Enlarged hilar nodes may also erode a bronchial wall and discharge caseous material into the bronchus, producing a segmental tuberculous pneumonia.

Cervical adenitis is normally considered to be an uncommon presentation of tuberculosis in adults and typically occurs in the early course of infection in children (Fig. 12–4). However, in some countries, e.g., Djibouti and Papua New Guinea, lymph node involvement is a quite frequent presentation of adult tuberculosis, though no underlying reason has been detected. In some Central African countries, such as Rwanda, the recent emergence in adults of hitherto rare lymph node tuberculosis has been related to the spread of the AIDS epidemic. In a few developing countries, lymphadenitis can be due to *M. bovis,* but the vast majority of cases are due to *M. tuberculosis.* Nontuberculous mycobacteria, like *M. scrofulaceum* in Burma, may be the offending organisms also but can be identified only through isolation from a culture of pus or tissue. When involved by tuberculosis, lymph nodes become enlarged, firm, and matted with soft areas of fluctuation, which may burst open and discharge caseous material, leading to the formation of sinus tracts. Systemic symptoms may or may not be present. The tuberculin skin test is generally reactive. Abdominal lymph node involvement presents often as an inflammatory abdominal mass.

Osteomyelitis and Arthritis (Chapter 13). Ends of growing long bones, vertebral bodies, and joints are seeded often during the hematogenous dissemination that occurs during the initial infection in a subject who has not reached maturity. Bone or joint tuberculosis may result within 2 years of infection or as a late reactivation from a dormant lesion. Bone and joint tuberculosis usually starts during childhood and adolescence. Most commonly involved are the large joints, spine, hip, knee, wrist, elbow, and shoulder (Figs. 13–4 to 13–6). In the tropical environment, any monoarticular arthritis should raise the suspicion of tuberculosis. Pain in bones and joints is common, and in some patients, periosseous accumulation of the caseous ma-

terial occurs and leads to a "cold abscess." Radiographically, the bones show areas of rarefaction surrounded by sclerosis (Fig. 61–4A). In the spine, narrowing of the disk space is usually the earliest sign, but no abnormality can be detected when the radiograph is taken during the first few weeks after the onset of pain. Involvement of the articular surface and vertebral body occurs later. Finally, ventral collapse of the vertebral body and disk can occur, producing a gibbus or an angular kyphosis (Fig. 13–4). Compression of the spinal cord and nerve roots may lead to neurologic deficits. A soft tissue shadow of a paravertebral abscess may be visualized alongside the diseased vertebral bodies, and an abscess may even extend into the inguinal region. CT scanning can be used to better visualize the lesions (Fig. 61–4B), and confirmation of the diagnosis is obtained through biopsy and culture. In the absence of suggestive bacteriology, histopathological evidence with an evocative PPD reaction justifies treatment with antituberculous drugs.

Abdominal Tuberculosis. These are frequent problems in the tropical environment. Intestines and peritoneum can be infected from mesenteric glands, from infected fallopian tubes, and through hematogenous spread. Direct infection of the intestinal wall is possible after ingestion of unpasteurized milk or swallowing large quantities of bacilli from cavitary lung lesions. Endogenous reactivation occurring years after hematogenous spread is common, but the factors predisposing to the peritoneal disease remain obscure.

Tuberculous Peritonitis. Symptoms of tuberculous peritonitis are often nonspecific and insidious, and include abdominal pain, fever, malaise, night sweats, diarrhea, and increasing abdominal girth due to ascites. Clinical differentiation from other causes of ascites is usually difficult and, as a result, diagnosis is often delayed and mortality can be as high as 50%. Tuberculosis is claimed to have been responsible for 24% of all causes of ascites in Nigeria and 42% in Lesotho. Abdominal paracentesis is mandatory. Examination of the ascitic fluid usually reveals an exudative pattern with a protein level above 30 g/L, increased LDH, and a white cell count above 500/mm$_3$, predominantly lymphocytes. However, similar ascitic fluid abnormalities can be found in other peritoneal diseases, especially peritoneal carcinomatosis and uncomplicated cirrhosis. Measuring ascitic fluid glucose can be useful, especially if the ascitic/blood glucose ratio is determined; patients with tuberculous peritonitis have a ratio below 0.96, whereas patients with ascites of other etiology have a ratio higher than 0.96. Serosanguinous ascites is rare in tuberculosis and would suggest abdominal carcinomatosis. Percutaneous peritoneal biopsy during laparoscopy or even laparotomy greatly facilitates confirmation of the diagnosis, but often is not available in rural areas. A considerable proportion of patients have other organs affected by tuberculosis, especially pleura and pericardium. Tuberculin skin testing is considered unreliable by many clinicians, because severe disease is often accompanied by malnutrition and anergy.

Intestinal Tuberculosis. Intestinal wall involvement may produce chronic intestinal obstruction or melena.

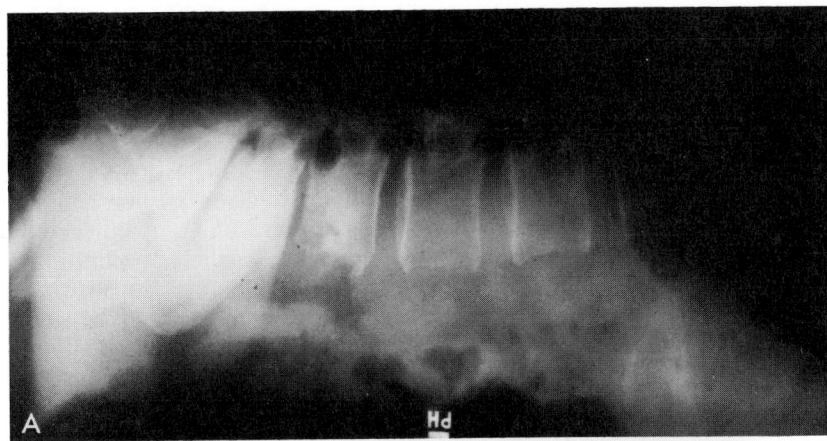

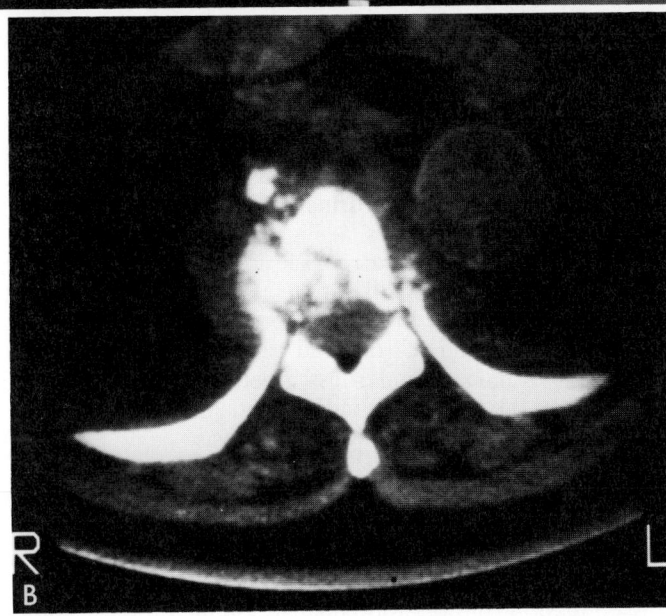

FIGURE 61–4. Pott's disease. *A*, Lateral roentgenogram of the spine shows destruction of the body of the fourth lumbar vertebra; *B*, CT scan of the fourth lumbar vertebra reveals considerable destruction.

Rectal bleeding is uncommon. The terminal ileum and the cecum are often involved and can be palpated sometimes as a mass. Malabsorption is a common complication and results in bulky stools and weight loss. Barium studies are helpful in the diagnosis of bowel involvement, but final incrimination of mycobacteria as the cause of an inflammatory bowel disease can be difficult. Optimally, clinical observations need to be supported by pathology results of biopsy material obtained through colonoscopy, which should be preceded by plain radiographic films of the abdomen; exploratory surgery sometimes is performed for a perplexing clinical picture and leads to an unexpected diagnosis of abdominal tuberculosis. Specific mycobacterial serologies proved to be of help in the diagnosis of intestinal tuberculosis in India.

Hepatic Tuberculosis. Tuberculosis of the liver may present as a diffuse involvement during miliary tuberculosis, with or without pulmonary disease, or more rarely as a tuberculoma (i.e., a focal or nodular lesion consisting of single or multiple tuberculomas or abscesses of the liver). Diagnosis is confirmed by liver biopsy, to be best performed under guidance by ultrasound or computed tomography (CT), if available. Drainage of an abscess may become necessary. Granu-

lomas on the surface of the liver can sometimes be visualized and biopsied during laparoscopy.

Pericarditis. The pericardium may become involved through contiguous spread from infected lymph nodes or pleuropulmonary tissue, or through hematogenous spread. As in pleural effusion, there is formation of a granuloma with exudation of effusion, followed by fibrosis. The patient usually complains of substernal pain and shortness of breath. Clinical signs of pericardial tamponade include distention of neck veins, hepatomegaly, edema, and paradoxical pulse, which consists of an inspiratory decrease in systolic arterial pressure greater than 10 mm Hg. The most important physical sign of pericarditis is the pericardial friction rub.

The condition is suspected usually when cardiac symptoms are associated with night sweats, malaise, and a positive PPD reaction. On chest radiographs, the cardiac shadow can be enlarged in the acute stage but may be normal or small in the chronic phase. The electrocardiogram can display the characteristic elevations of the ST segment. Ultrasound may be useful in the diagnosis, which is best confirmed by pericardial biopsy. The major complication of acute tuberculous pericarditis is cardiac tamponade, while constrictive pericarditis often complicates the chronic disease. Pericardiocentesis can be needed for diagnosis or as acute treatment to urgently relieve tamponade. Pericardial fluid shows an exudative response with lymphocytosis and often contains a significant number of red blood cells.

Genitourinary Tuberculosis. Another common site of involvement is the kidney, where the cortex can become infected during hematogenous dissemination. Concomitantly, the collecting system comprising ureters and bladder is often involved. Multiplying tuberculous bacilli may lead to severe tissue necrosis with excretion of large numbers of microorganisms in the urine. In the male, disease may also involve seminal vesicle, epididymis, and prostate. The symptoms tend to be insidious and include urinary frequency, dysuria, painful ejaculation, and pain and swelling of the epididymis. Fever, malaise, and flank pain may be present also.

When symptoms are accompanied by gross or microscopic hematuria or pyuria with a "sterile" urine, the possibility of urinary tract tuberculosis should be considered. Several separate early-morning specimens of urine should be cultured for tuberculosis, because culture is positive in 80% of patients with urinary tract tuberculosis. Radiological abnormalities are present usually, sometimes with calcification of a renal lesion. The retrograde pyelogram may show dilatation of the calyces or cavities and is more likely to show abnormalities than the intravenous pyelogram. Ultrasound can be of genuine diagnostic assistance. Tenderness, swelling, and a "craggy" feeling of the epididymis indicate inflammatory involvement, which requires biopsy for diagnosis.

Tuberculosis of the female genital tract is a rather uncommon presentation of extrapulmonary tuberculosis in many tropical countries, perhaps because of the difficulties of diagnosis. In the great majority of cases, genital tuberculosis in women is secondary to blood stream dissemination, but occasionally can follow intercourse with a man suffering from active genitourinary tuberculosis. The fallopian tubes are affected in nearly all cases, the endometrium in about 90%, the ovaries in 20%, the cervix in less than 1%, and the vagina and vulva practically never. The main presenting symptoms are infertility, pelvic pain, excessive menstrual loss, and amenorrhea. Vaginal discharge can contain young endometrial granulomas. Common complications include scarring of the fallopian tubes that may result in a later tendency toward ectopic pregnancy. Extension of the infection to the peritoneum may lead to generalized peritonitis or localized pelvic abscesses; adnexal masses are often palpable. The diagnosis is made by endometrial curettage, ultrasound, laparoscopy, or laparotomy.

Tuberculous Meningitis. The meninges may be involved during miliary dissemination of tubercle bacilli or by a caseous brain lesion discharging bacilli into the subarachnoid space. This may occur in infants during an overwhelming initial infection or in older persons during recrudescence of dormant lesions. Meningitis is seen more frequently in countries with a high prevalence of tuberculous disease and represents the most common cause of death from tuberculosis in children in many tropical countries. The diagnosis is based on clinical signs of meningeal irritation, including headache, vomiting, and irritability with restlessness or apathy and

refusal to play. With the progression of disease, neck stiffness, neurological signs, and coma will develop. These signs are associated with fever, malaise, night sweats, anorexia, and weight loss. In children with advanced disease, hydrocephalus due to obstruction of circulating cerebrospinal fluid is one of the most important causes of preventable neurological disability in the tropical environment. Because permanent brain damage occurs rapidly if therapy is delayed, early antituberculous treatment is important.

The slightest clinical suspicion of meningitis demands immediate funduscopy and investigation by lumbar puncture. However, examination of the cerebrospinal fluid (CSF) is often inconclusive. Spinal fluid pressure and total protein are generally elevated, but the hallmark of the infection is a lymphocytosis with a glucose level decreased to less than half the blood level. Direct smear examination of the CSF is often negative for acid-fast bacilli, while the culture results are received too late to assist in the decision regarding the start of chemotherapy. The PPD skin test may be negative, particularly in anergic patients. Early differentiation from other causes of chronic meningitis (particularly cryptococcosis and histoplasmosis) must be made as quickly as possible and empiric therapy with rifampin and isoniazid initiated, because any delay in therapy can cause permanent brain damage. Early diagnosis and initiation of therapy are more important than the choice of the drug regimen. Prognosis and survival are related directly to the clinical stage on admission, i.e., the time elapsed since the appearance of the first symptoms. Mortality remains high and affects about one third of patients; another third has neurological sequelae, and the remaining recover completely.

Tuberculosis of the Central Nervous System. Tuberculomas are a major cause of progressive space-occupying lesions of the brain in many tropical areas. Diagnosis is based on symptoms related to increased intracerebral pressure, chronic fever, and focal neurological signs. Invariably tuberculin testing is highly reactive. Brain tuberculomas can become calcified and need to be differentiated from the other causes of brain masses, in particular brain tumors and parasitic diseases affecting the brain, e.g., cysticercosis and toxoplasmosis. CT scanning has become a great help in the diagnostic work-up and in the follow-up during treatment.

Tuberculosis with Endocrine Dysfunction

Tuberculosis of Adrenal Glands. Hematogenous dissemination of tubercle bacilli localizes occasionally in the adrenal glands. The expanding granulomas can produce acute adrenocortical insufficiency (Addison's disease), which needs to be recognized early. Clinical diagnosis is based on progressive weakness, pigmentation of skin and mucosa, weight loss, anorexia, and hypotension. Serum sodium is reduced, and serum potassium is increased. Confirmation is based on decreased cortisol production and increased plasma ACTH levels. Differential diagnoses include other infectious diseases causing adrenocortical atrophy, e.g., histoplasmosis. Effective therapy of adrenal tuberculosis requires appropriate antituberculous chemotherapy, hormone replacement, and correction of electrolyte imbalance.

Inappropriate Secretion of Antidiuretic Hormone. This can occur during overwhelming pulmonary tuberculosis or meningitis, particularly in elderly patients. Signs include somnolence or coma associated with a low serum sodium level (below 120 mmol/L), a low plasma osmolality (below 270 mosmol/L), and the excretion of urine hypertonic relative to plasma. Therapy is based on water restriction. Demethylchlortetracycline interferes with the renal action of ADH and may be useful therapy in patients in whom fluid restriction is difficult.

Disseminated Tuberculosis. During the initial infection with tubercle bacilli, there is a consistent hematogenous dissemination of a small number of intracellular bacilli, which leads to seeding of most organs. These foci may later recrudesce to produce disease. Occasionally, a caseous tuberculous lesion containing large numbers of tubercle bacilli may erode a vein, and its contents may be emptied into the blood stream. This massive dissemination may occur soon after initial infection, or during the course of late recrudescence of the disease, and is called "miliary" tuberculosis (Fig. 61–5). With massive dissemination, the body's defense mechanisms are overwhelmed, and many organs are involved simultaneously. Alternatively, the miliary state can be precipitated by a primary anergy state caused by immune deficiency, as may occur in AIDS.

Acute Dissemination. Miliary tuberculosis is a grave clinical situation that is fatal if chemotherapy is not instituted immediately, pending bacteriological confirmation. The lesions are numerous but small (the size of millet seeds) and discrete, and are uniformly distributed throughout the organs. Tubercles are found in the liver, spleen, and bone marrow. Symptoms of miliary tuberculosis are nonspecific and consist of fever, weakness, sweats, and rapid loss of weight. Dyspnea is common

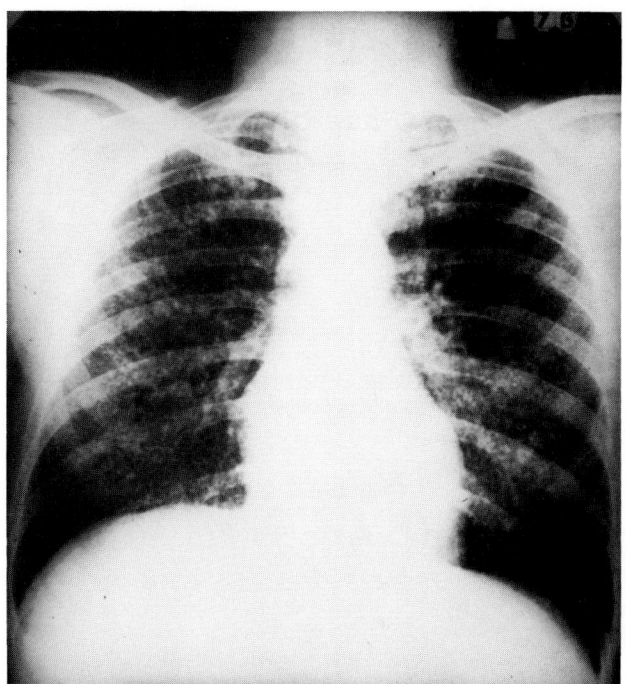

FIGURE 61–5. Miliary tuberculosis. Posteroanterior chest roentgenogram shows extensive bilateral miliary nodulations.

owing to stiffening of the lungs by the widespread tubercles. Meningitis and enlargement of the liver, spleen, and lymph nodes may be present. The diagnosis sometimes is suspected from the radiological picture of miliary nodules in the lungs. Acid fast bacilli are seldom detected in the sputum. The tuberculin skin test is often negative, owing to the host's inability to cope with the overwhelming infectious load or because of underlying immunodeficiency. The diagnosis can be made by biopsy and culture of the liver, bone marrow, or lung, and by histological demonstration of granulomas and tubercle bacilli. Diagnosis is complicated further by the fact that caseation is often scarce, and that many fungal infections can lead to similar clinical pictures that can be differentiated only by culture, histological examination, or serological tests. Other noninfectious diseases, e.g., hypersensitivity pneumonitis, collagen vascular diseases, and sarcoidosis, are often difficult to differentiate without open or transbronchial biopsy. In rare cases they can coexist with miliary tuberculosis. On ophthalmologic examination, tubercles are often seen in the choroid and suggest the diagnosis. The white cell count is usually normal, but a leukemoid reaction may occur.

Chronic Dissemination. The release of small numbers of bacilli intermittently may produce a subacute or chronic type of disseminated tuberculosis. The patient may present with a variety of clinical manifestations, including anemia, myelofibrosis, lymphadenopathy, leukemoid reaction, fever, effusion in pleural and peritoneal cavities, and headache with a chronic meningitis. The clinical manifestations of chronic dissemination are protean and can be bizarre. The tuberculin test may be negative. A high index of suspicion is necessary for an early solution of the clinical problem, because the prognosis is uniformly poor if the appropriate chemotherapy is not instituted early. Bone marrow biopsy and tissue examination from various sites are helpful in establishing the diagnosis.

Cryptogenic tuberculosis describes a chronic disease characterized by lassitude and weight loss. Isolation of the organism usually fails, and the diagnosis is made after a successful trial of antituberculous chemotherapy.

Congenital Tuberculosis. A fetus can become infected in utero through hematogenous infection via the umbilical vein or through fetal aspiration or ingestion of infected amniotic fluid. The affected child frequently is born prematurely and presents features of a severe generalized infection. Tuberculin skin tests are generally negative. Treatment should be started as soon as the diagnosis is suspected. Mortality is high for mothers and children. Despite its rarity, congenital tuberculosis must be considered, because prognosis depends on early diagnosis. In countries with a high prevalence of both tuberculosis and AIDS, congenital forms of these two diseases may become more frequent in the future.

DIAGNOSIS. In the tropical environment characterized by a high prevalence of tuberculous infection, physicians need to consider a diagnosis of tuberculosis when caring for any patient with an acute or chronic disease, regardless of the details of the clinical presentation of the patient. Fever, weight loss, and anemia are often present in acutely ill patients and in those with chronically advanced disease. Clubbing of fingers is rare in tuberculosis, and its presence should direct the search to other diseases.

Roentgenography. The most valuable diagnostic investigation in assessing the presence and extent of lung tuberculosis is plain roentgenography of the chest (PA and lateral films). Where old disease has been present, the early subtle changes indicative of activity can best be discerned by comparison of the radiograph with films taken months or years earlier. Evidence of pre-existing scars can be found on previous films in about 70% of persons with active tuberculosis. Hence, efforts to obtain old radiographs may allow recognition of an active process and initiation of therapy before further progression has occurred, including spread of infection to other parts of the lungs and to other persons.

A reticulonodular infiltrate in one or both upper lobes is the abnormality most commonly seen in lung tuberculosis (Fig. 61–6). The abnormality usually appears in the posterior segment of the upper lobe or in the apical segment of the lower lobe, although sometimes the upper lobe may be involved completely by the disease. Bilateral distribution of multiple infiltrates in the upper zones of the lungs is highly suggestive of tuberculosis. Liquefaction necrosis of the lesion is manifested as cavities that can be seen on the roentgenogram (Fig. 61–7). Extensive consolidation of the lung due to tuberculous pneumonia can be seen in acute development of the disease. Because the disease spreads to other parts of the lungs through the bronchi, "soft" alveolar filling infiltrates in the lower lung fields are common. Hilar lymphadenopathy and mid to lower lung infiltrates are seen commonly in children (Fig. 61–8) in developing countries. Tomograms of lung lesions can detect cavitation that is not apparent on the routine radiograph

(Fig. 61–7). A lordotic view helps in detecting infiltrates underlying apical ribs and the clavicle, and films taken in lateral and oblique positions are of value in visualizing the location and character of the lesion. A posteroanterior film taken with the patient in the lateral decubitus position, permitting the fluid to layer out along the lateral chest wall, can demonstrate a small or infrapulmonary pleural effusion.

Tuberculin Reaction. The tuberculin skin test (Mantoux) is performed by injecting 0.1 ml of diluent containing PPD intradermally. The amount injected varies from 1 to 250 TU, but 2 TU (known as intermediate-strength) is the accepted standard dose. The best method of reading the reaction is to approach the area from above and below with a felt-tip or ball-point pen and to measure between the points where the pen encounters the induration of the reaction. In healthy persons, Listeria-type reactions of less than 10 mm of induration after injection of 2 TU of PPD-T are often due to infection with nontuberculous mycobacteria or to vaccination with BCG. In 90% of persons with active tuberculous disease, a Koch-type induration of 10 mm or more in diameter is present 72 hours after injection. Unreactive tests may occur in up to 20% of patients with active tuberculosis if sensitized T cells are depleted or nonfunctional due to old age, debilitation, or an immunodeficiency state (e.g., AIDS). The tuberculin test is best performed simultaneously with tests for other common antigens, e.g., mumps, trichophytin, and streptokinase, to recognize these general anergic states.

Bacteriologic Examination. The only confirmatory proof of tuberculosis is the isolation of *M. tuberculosis* from body secretions or tissues. A stained smear of sputum, body fluid, or tissue can be used to identify acid-fast bacilli. In developing countries, where person-

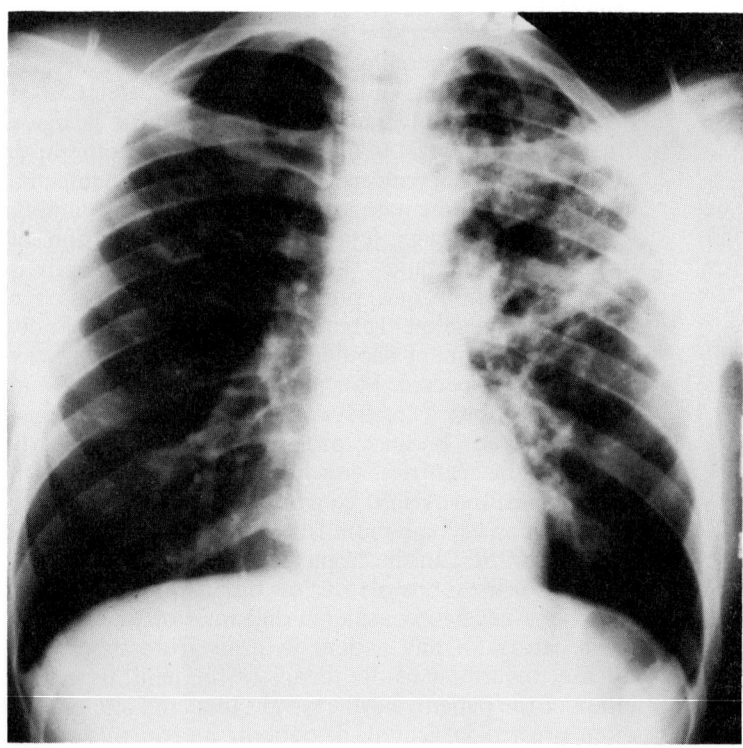

FIGURE 61–6. Adult recrudescent tuberculosis. Posteroanterior chest roentgenogram reveals nodular and linear infiltrates in the left and middle zones of the left lung.

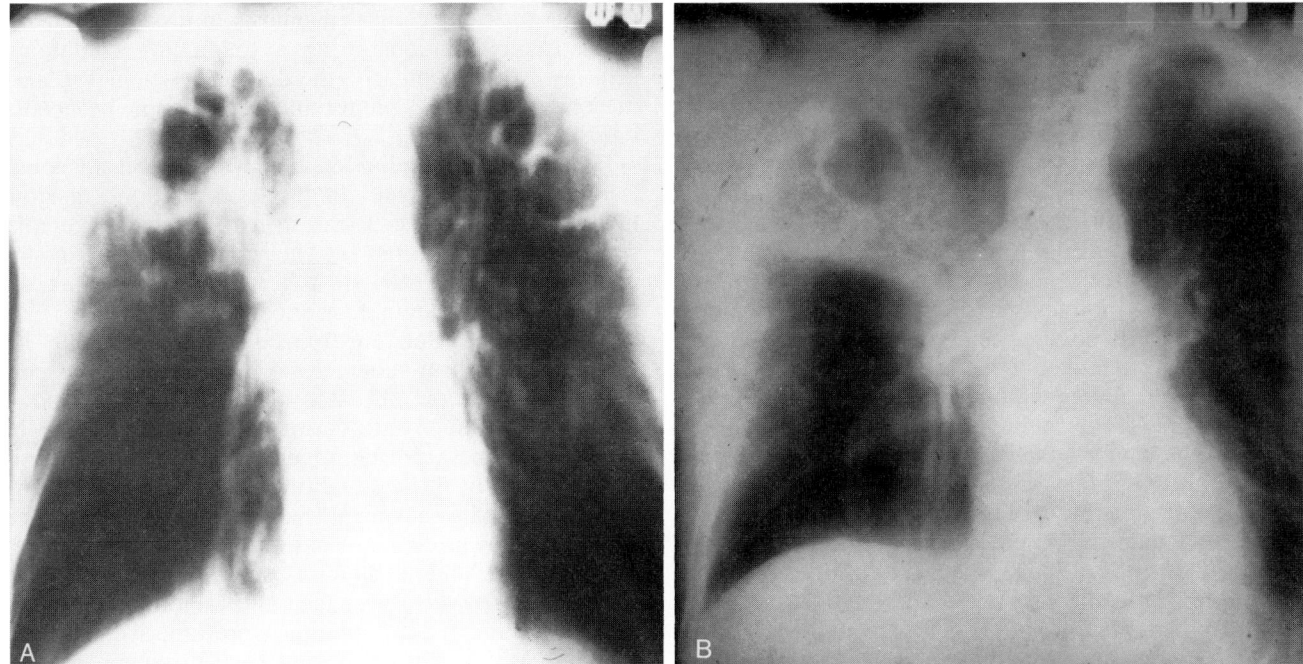

FIGURE 61–7. Chronic cavitary tuberculosis. The chest tomograms show tuberculous disease in both lungs *(A and B)*. It is more marked in both right lungs with cavitation at the apex.

nel and funds are in short supply, direct smear examination forms the basis of diagnosis and therapeutic response. A positive smear signifies the presence of large numbers of organisms. Results of the direct microscopy examination may be quantitated by observing the number of bacilli in, for instance, 300 separate

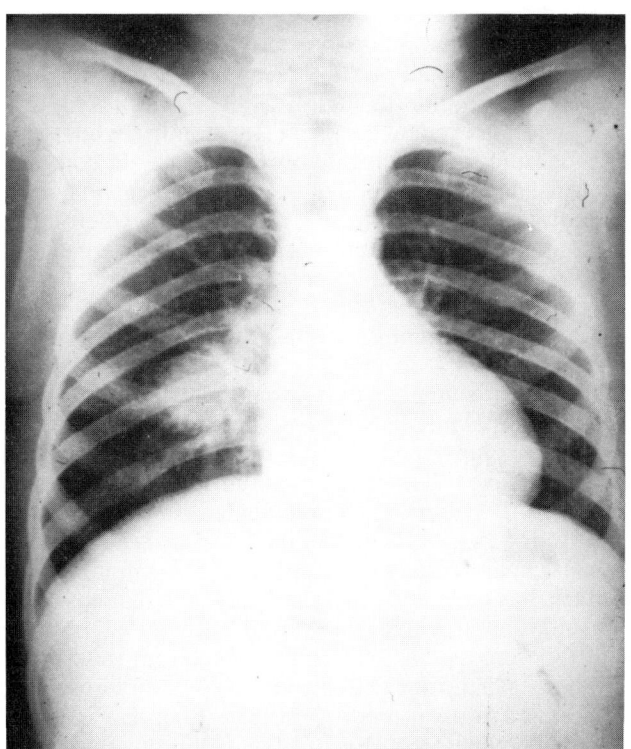

FIGURE 61–8. Primary infection. Posteroanterior chest roentgenogram shows an infiltrate in the periphery of the right middle zone of the lungs, with enlargement of lymph nodes in the right hilum.

microscope fields. However, not all workers agree that grading of the smears has any practical value. For identification of the bacillus to species level, investigation by culture is necessary. Many media have been described for the cultivation of *M. tuberculosis,* but there is no general agreement as to which of them is most appropriate for the isolation of this organism under routine diagnostic conditions. Except for specimens from sterile sites, most specimens need to be decontaminated before media can be inoculated. The most widely used techniques for decontamination are sodium hydroxide (4%,w/v) or sodium hydroxide/sodium dodecyl sulphate with Löwenstein-Jensen medium, sodium hydroxide/acetylcysteine with either egg or agar media and the trisodium phosphate/Zephiran technique. Because *M. tuberculosis* is a slow-growing organism, cultures will need to be incubated for 6 to 8 weeks before being considered negative and discarded. However, tuberculous bacilli from clinical specimens generally produce visible colonies after 2 to 4 weeks. *M. tuberculosis* presents a characteristic rough, buff to slightly yellow appearance of the colonies. This, together with a positive niacin test, is the minimum requirement as a speciation method. In depth bacteriologic work-up of mycobacteria and drug sensitivity testing are fields for specialized laboratories.

Polymerase chain reaction (PCR), a method that rapidly amplifies specific DNA sequences, has recently been successfully applied to the detection of mycobacterial DNA in clinical specimens, including peripheral blood samples from patients with disseminated tuberculosis. Synthetic oligonucleotides complementary to the DNA sequences that flank a portion of the gene encoding the mycobacterial 65 kD antigen are utilized with the PCR method to amplify this fragment of DNA from the bacterial genome.

Sputum. Spontaneously produced sputum is the specimen that is most often examined by smear and culture. Three early-morning specimens should be submitted fresh to the laboratory. A 24-hour collection is not recommended because of the problem of excessive contamination. When sputum is too scant to be produced spontaneously, nebulized water or hypertonic aerosol may be inhaled to increase bronchial secretion. Bronchial washing, bronchial brushing, and tracheal or pulmonary aspiration can be used to establish the diagnosis of tuberculosis. In young children and mentally handicapped persons who are unable to produce sputum, fasting gastric contents may be aspirated and cultured.

Body Fluids. Other materials that may be submitted for bacteriological examination are urine, CSF, serous effusion, pus, and synovial fluid. In urogenital tuberculosis, the urine reveals hematuria and pyuria without any bacterial growth on routine culture. Early-morning specimens should be submitted for tuberculosis culture.

Pleural Effusion. When a pleural effusion is present, thoracentesis must be performed and the fluid carefully examined. The pleural fluid is generally a clear, yellow exudate with a protein content above 3 gm/dL and has elevated LDH and ADA (adenosine deaminase activity) levels, cells that are predominantly mononuclear, and a pH between 7.0 and 7.25. Bacilli are not usually seen in the stained smear of the fluid because of their small number. Culture of the fluid for *M. tuberculosis* is positive in 30% of patients with tuberculous effusion. Pleural tissue obtained by percutaneous needle biopsy should be examined histologically and cultured for *M. tuberculosis* in a liquid medium. A presumptive diagnosis of tuberculosis is made if the biopsy reveals a granuloma and the PPD reaction is positive, even though the fluid fails to grow bacilli in culture. Similarly, when a peritoneal or pericardial effusion is present, a biopsy of the peritoneum or pericardial tissue should be cultured for tubercle bacilli. Therapy is initiated generally on the basis of a presumptive diagnosis made on histological examination showing caseating granulomas.

Cerebrospinal Fluid. Examination of the CSF in tuberculous meningitis usually reveals increased pressure, clear fluid with increased protein content, a reduced glucose level, and an increased white blood cell count with 90 to 95% monocytes. Because tubercle bacilli are found on direct smear in the CSF in less than 10% of initial samples, other diagnostic tests have been investigated with the aim of increasing early diagnosis of tuberculous meningitis. These tests comprise two nonspecific tests, the bromide partition test and the measurement of ADA in the CSF. More valuable are assays, which test for the presence of mycobacterial antigen or DNA in the CSF, such as the ELISA assay and the PCR technique. The latex particle agglutination assay has produced promising results, is inexpensive, does not require specialized equipment, and should be suitable for use in developing countries. When tuberculous meningitis is suspected but not confirmed on the patient's admission, therapy must be started without awaiting the culture results.

Histopathologic Examination. Biopsy of bone marrow, liver, and lymph nodes may be of great value in reaching an early clinical diagnosis in disseminated tuberculosis by demonstrating a granuloma containing acid-fast bacilli. Similarly, the diagnosis is achieved also in bones and joints, pleura and peritoneum, by needle biopsy.

Hematologic Examination. The white blood cell count is often normal, except in instances of bone marrow involvement, which can lead to leukopenia, leukemoid reaction, or pancytopenia. The white blood cell count may be increased in acute tuberculous pneumonia. In chronic cases, inflammatory anemia is usual.

Therapeutic Trial. In tropical countries it can be difficult to confirm tuberculosis in a patient with pulmonary infiltration or extrapulmonary disease and a positive reaction to intradermal PPD of more than 10 mm induration. A presumptive diagnosis of tuberculosis is acceptable in those situations, and empirical therapy may be started as a clinical trial. However, this practice often involves errors, and patients receiving such therapy must be evaluated clinically and radiographically for response to therapy. If clinical and radiologic improvement is definite at 2 to 3 months, a presumptive diagnosis of tuberculosis is justified, and the full course of chemotherapy should be completed.

A frequent but often unrecognized error is the failure to diagnose pulmonary aspergillomas in patients treated for cavitary lung tuberculosis, and who present with recurrent hemoptysis despite negative sputum examinations (Chapter 66.6). These patients are often treated repeatedly with antituberculous chemotherapy by a physician who considers that his patient does not comply or respond correctly to the given treatment regimens.

TREATMENT. The discovery of effective antituberculous drugs has revolutionized the practice of medicine in the tropics. In a follow-up study in India, of a cohort of tuberculosis patients not receiving treatment, 30% had died at 18 months and 49% by 5 years, and 42% continued to excrete bacilli at 18 months, while only 28% became sputum negative by that time. In contrast, the efficiency of well-applied chemotherapy can be illustrated by the results of a study in Holland, where after 24 months, 98% of sputum-positive patients were cured, only 1% remained sputum-positive, and 1% had died of their disease.

General Treatment Principles. Modern chemotherapy for tuberculosis is so effective that treatment in a hospital or sanatorium is now seldom indicated. Prolonged isolation of patients has become unnecessary. Initiation of chemotherapy renders the patient noninfectious in a few days, even though the sputum may still contain bacilli. The patient may be treated safely at home because the risk to family contacts diminishes readily as soon as chemotherapy is started. Infection among family contacts has occurred generally before the diagnosis and the initiation of chemotherapy. Treatment of patients with tuberculosis has been transferred from specialized hospitals (sanatoriums) to general community hospitals, clinics, and private medical offices. Bed rest is of no additional benefit to chemotherapy for the uncomplicated tuberculosis patient. Hospitalization is limited largely to patients with other medical conditions or for invasive diagnostic studies, and the stay is usually less than 2 weeks. Patients with tuberculosis can be safely admitted to a general hospital if the room has good ventilation and ultraviolet light for upper air sterilization to prevent the spread of infection to personnel and other patients. Adoption of this system is particularly important in developing countries, because sanatoriums are quite expensive to operate.

In the early days of the antituberculous era, therapy required 18 to 24 months for achieving cure of tuberculosis, and usually consisted of treatment with 2 drugs, which often had weak antituberculous action. Today, with the availability of more powerful drugs, the standard duration of therapy has been reduced to 9 months, with infrequent failures or relapses. Even shorter treatment regimens have been investigated and have given excellent results, especially when multiple drugs are combined. These short-term chemotherapy regimens have the additional advantage of improving the patient's compliance, a factor of primary importance in the tropical environment.

Antituberculous Drugs. Antituberculous drugs can be classified according to three characteristics: (1) the activity to rapidly kill large numbers of actively metabolizing bacilli defines their bactericidal action; (2) the activity to kill slowly metabolizing, semidormant bacilli—the so-called persisters—defines their sterilizing activity; and (3) their capability to prevent drug resistance. A list of drugs and their dosage, major side effects, and activity is presented in Table 61–3.

Isonicotinic Acid Hydrazid (INH). Isoniazid is a synthetic compound inhibiting the biosynthesis of mycolic acid in mycobacteria. INH is the most powerful, best tolerated, and least expensive antituberculous drug. It is absorbed rapidly and completely after oral dosage and readily penetrates through the tissues of the lung, into the CSF, and into pus. It is active against both extracellular and intracellular bacilli that have a high metabolic activity and are dividing rapidly. It has the best early bactericidal activity when given alone, and the bactericidal effects of other drugs is increased considerably if INH is combined with them during treatment. The drug is inactivated in the liver by acetylation. The rate of acetylation is under genetic control and quite stable in a given subject. Patients can be broadly divided into either rapid or slow acetylators. The proportion of the two phenotypes differs in populations from different parts of the world. Whereas some 50 to 60% of subjects of South Indian, European, or African origin are slow acetylators, the proportion of slow acetylators is from 5% to 22% in Chinese, Japanese, and Eskimos. The rate of INH inactivation in tuberculosis patients is of no prognostic significance when treatment is given daily, and only of doubtful importance when twice-weekly regimens are used. It is of considerable importance, however, in once-weekly treatment, since rapid acetylators respond less satisfactorily. For this reason, once-weekly regimens must be considered as unsuitable for general use in the tropics, unless the acetylator status of patients can be determined.

Dosage and Toxicity. The adult dose of INH is 5 to 10 mg/kg in a single daily dose, usually 300 mg; it is 10 to 20 mg/kg for children. For twice-weekly administration, the dose is 15 mg/kg (usually 900 mg for adults). Significant side effects occur in about 2% of patients. Direct toxic effects are due to competition with pyridoxine and occur after 1 to 4 months of INH therapy. They may result in sideroblastic anemia responsive to pyridoxine. Peripheral neuropathy is dose-related and occurs frequently in debilitated patients, such as alcoholics. Pyridoxine, added to INH in low doses (e.g., 30 to 50 mg), usually prevents these complications in such patients. The most important and serious side effect is hepatitis, which appears to be due to idiosyncrasy, but the role of toxic metabolic byproducts of isoniazid is not clear. The most common symptoms of toxic hepatitis are anorexia, nausea, vomiting, fever, and finally the appearance of jaundice. The best way to monitor for hepatitis is to acquaint each patient with the possible side effects (while emphasizing their rarity) and to determine the level of liver enzymes promptly if such symptoms develop. If the liver enzymes have increased persistently to 3 times their pretreatment values, hepatic toxicity due to isoniazid is likely, and administration of the drug is discontinued. A transient and harmless elevation of enzyme levels may occur without symptoms, particularly during the earlier part of therapy. Therefore, routine determination of these enzyme levels may create confusion and unnecessary withdrawal of the drug. The incidence of hepatitis is age-related, being higher in persons more than 45 years old than in younger persons.

Less common side effects are allergy to the drug (skin rashes, fever), abnormalities in behavior, and a clinical illness similar to systemic lupus erythematosus. About 20% of INH-treated patients develop antinuclear antibodies, usually without concurrent clinical signs. Hemolytic anemias have been described, some with a positive Coombs's test. Neutropenia, eosinophilia, thrombocytopenia, red cell aplasia, and agranulocytosis are possible but rare. Suicidal attempts by overdose produce convulsions, for which large doses of pyridoxine are helpful. Serious INH side effects are not more common in rapid acetylators, and assessment of the acetylator phenotype is unlikely to be of any value in trying to establish if any side effect occurring during treatment might be due to INH. It is equally unnecessary to determine the acetylator phenotype of tuberculous patients with impaired renal function.

Rifampin. This is a semisynthetic derivative of a naturally occurring antibiotic, produced by *Streptomyces mediaterranei.* It is a powerful bactericidal drug that inhibits DNA transcription and synthesis of all classes of RNA through acting on the bacterial DNA-dependent RNA polymerase. Rifampin is active against both extracellular and intracellular bacilli that are actively dividing or intermittently dividing. The latter action is remarkable in that the drug even kills organisms that show activity only episodically. Hence, its importance lies in the continuation phase of treatment to kill the last few viable bacilli (i.e., the sterilizing activity). Rifampin is absorbed rapidly when taken orally and is excreted in bile, with about 30% eliminated in the urine. It diffuses well into all fluid compartments of the body, the CSF, and the brain.

TABLE 61–3. Antituberculosis Drugs: Mode of Action, Dosage, and Side Effects

Drug	Activity	Dosage		Side Effects
		Daily	*Twice Weekly*	
Streptomycin	Active against rapidly multiplying bacilli in neutral or slightly alkaline extracellular medium	10–15 mg/kg (usually 0.5–1.0 gm) 5 days/week IM	20–25 mg/kg (usually 1.0–1.5 gm) IM	Vestibular or auditory nerve (VIII) damage, dizziness, vertigo, ataxia, nephrotoxicity, allergic fever, rash
Isoniazid (INH)	Acts strongly on rapidly dividing extracellular bacilli and acts weakly on slowly multiplying intracellular bacilli	5 mg/kg (usually 300 mg) PO or IM	15 mg/kg (usually 900 mg) PO	Peripheral neuritis, hepatotoxicity, allergic fever and rash, lupus erythematosus phenomenon
Rifampin	Acts on both rapidly and slowly multiplying bacilli, either extracellular or intracellular, particularly on slowly multiplying "persisters"	10 mg/kg (usually 450–600 mg) PO	10 mg/kg (usually 450–600 mg) PO	Hepatotoxicity, nausea and vomiting, allergic fever and rash, "flu-like" syndrome, petechiae with thrombocytopenia or acute renal failure during intermittent therapy
Pyrazinamide	Active in acid pH medium on intracellular bacilli	30–35 mg/kg (usually 1.5–2.5 gm) PO	45–50 mg/kg (usually 3.0–3.5 gm) PO	Hyperuricemia, hepatotoxicity, allergic fever and rash
Ethambutol	Weakly active against both extracellular and intracellular bacilli to inhibit the development of resistant bacilli	15–25 mg/kg (usually 800 to 1600 mg) PO	50 mg/kg PO	Optic neuritis, skin rash
Ethionamide	As above	10–15 mg/kg (usually 500–750 mg) in divided doses PO	—	Nausea, vomiting, anorexia, hepatotoxicity, allergic fever and rash
Cycloserine	As above	15–20 mg/kg (usually 0.75–1.0 gm) in divided doses with 100 mg of pyridoxine PO	—	Personality changes, psychosis, convulsions, rash
Para-aminosalicylic acid (PAS)	Weak action on extracellular bacilli; inhibits development of drug-resistant organisms	150 mg/kg (usually 12 gm) in divided doses PO	—	Nausea, vomiting, diarrhea, hepatotoxicity, allergic rash and fever
Thiacetazone (not available in the United States)	As above	150 mg daily PO	—	Allergic rash and fever, Stevens-Johnson syndrome, blood disorders, nausea and vomiting

Abbreviations: IM = intramuscular; PO = oral

Dosage and Toxicity. The dose is 10 mg/kg per day, usually 600 mg in adults. The same dose (600 mg) is used when given twice or thrice weekly, because raising it to 900 or 1200 mg increases hypersensitivity reactions. The drug may be hepatotoxic, with the hepatitis occurring more often during daily administration than during twice- or thrice-weekly therapy. Rifampin is an enzyme activator, and INH induced hepatotoxicity may worsen if the two drugs are given together. Intermittent administration of the drug may produce hypersensitivity reactions, including petechiae with thrombocytopenia, acute renal failure, often with demonstrable serum antibodies to the drug, and a "flu-like" syndrome, which could possibly be the first warning sign of intravascular hemolysis. Twice-weekly administration of 600 mg carries only a slight risk of toxicity, which is no more than that when it is administered on a daily basis. The excretion of rifampin colors the urine red, and the color may be noticed in other secretions, e.g., saliva, tears, and stool, a property useful for assessing patient compliance. Rifampin is still expensive, which limits its extensive use in developing countries. It is hoped that with international cooperation, the cost of the drug may be reduced, thus making it available for easier use in developing countries, because it is of vital importance in the short-course chemotherapy regimens.

Streptomycin (SM). This aminoglycoside antibiotic is isolated from *Streptomyces griseus*. It inhibits bacterial translation and interferes with protein biosynthesis through interacting with the 30S subunit of the bacterial ribosomes. SM is bactericidal for the large extracellular population of rapidly dividing bacilli in cavitary lesions. It is inactive in the acid environment within macrophages. Capreomycin and kanamycin have similar actions, but little cross-resistance and cross-hypersensitivity.

Dosage and Toxicity. The usual adult dose is 1 gm daily (5 days/week) intramuscularly, but it should be reduced to 0.5 gm in patients over age 60 or in persons with impaired renal function. In children, the dose is 20 mg/kg per day. The drug diffuses well into the body fluids, except the CSF. Important side effects are vertigo, ataxia, and diminution of hearing due to involvement of the eighth cranial nerve. Toxicity to the renal tubules can occur. All of these effects are dose-related but are uncommon in the recommended doses. Minor side effects include skin rash and fever. Slight dizziness and circumoral paresthesias are common immediately after injections but are usually of no clinical significance. SM is an inexpensive drug, but its use is limited presently, because more powerful and less toxic drugs have become available.

Pyrazinamide. This drug is related to nicotinamide; its mode of action remains unknown. It has a high killing activity against tuberculous bacilli dividing in the acid environment within macrophages but is not effective against extracellular organisms. For the past 30 years, the use of pyrazinamide was limited largely to drug-resistant cases, but recently, a central role has been found for it in intensive short-course regimens. It is absorbed rapidly after oral ingestion and is excreted in the urine.

Dosage and Toxicity. The drug is given once daily in a dose of 35 mg/kg of body weight and may also be administered twice or thrice weekly in doses of 45 to 50 mg/kg of body weight. In the past, liver toxicity has been overemphasized, probably because higher doses of the drug were used. In recent studies, liver toxicity was rare. A harmless hyperuricemia occurs regularly, but clinical gout is uncommon. Mild arthralgia may occur when the drug is given daily but is uncommon when it is given twice weekly. Pyrazinamide is still expensive, which limits its use in developing countries.

Ethambutol. This second-line drug is thought to act on the cell wall of mycobacteria. It has a relatively good early bactericidal activity. Its major indication is prevention of appearance of drug resistance, and it is used mostly as a companion drug with INH, because it inhibits the multiplication of mutants resistant to INH. The drug is well absorbed orally and is excreted in the urine. It is well tolerated and thus has replaced para-aminosalicylic acid (PAS) as the companion drug to INH.

Dosage and Toxicity. The starting dose of 25 mg/kg daily is reduced to 15 mg/kg daily after 2 months. Toxic reactions to the drug are few, but optic neuritis can occur with higher doses. Patients should be cautioned to watch for any reduction in visual acuity, and ophthalmic examinations are mandatory on follow-ups, because prompt withdrawal of the drug prevents permanent loss of vision. Because the cost of the drug is comparatively high, it cannot supplant the less expensive drugs, in particular thiacetazone, in developing countries.

Para-aminosalicylic Acid (PAS). The antituberculous action of this drug is thought to be due to interference with a function of salicylic acid. PAS is an antituberculous agent of low efficacy. In the past, it was used in combination with INH to avoid secondary INH resistance. It is still used in some developing countries, however, because of its low cost. It is absorbed orally and is excreted primarily in the urine.

Dosage and Toxicity. The adult dose is 12 gm daily, which must be given in divided doses. The most common side effects are nausea, vomiting, and diarrhea, which often require interruption of the therapy. Other side effects include fever, rash, hepatitis, and leukopenia. Goiter may occur with prolonged ingestion of PAS. However, the drug is better tolerated by children. There is little reason for use of PAS in tuberculosis today.

Cycloserine. This product of a streptomycete inhibits peptidoglycan synthesis in mycobacteria. It is a drug of modest efficacy, and its use is mostly confined to patients with complicated retreatment problems. The dosage is 15 mg/kg/day, usually 750 mg to 1 gm/day for adults. Side effects occur frequently, with central nervous system reactions of depression, psychosis, and convulsions. Pyridoxine, 100 mg with each dose, reduces the incidence of side effects.

Ethionamide. This inhibitor of mycolic acid synthesis is moderately effective. It is a useful second-line antituberculous drug and its principal use is in drug-resistant patients. However, a considerable incidence of gastric irritation limits its use. Nausea, vomiting, and a garlic-like taste are frequent complaints. The usual adult dose is 750 to 1000 mg in divided doses.

Thiacetazone. This drug is weakly bacteriostatic but is used extensively in many developing countries, because it is quite inexpensive. The adult dose is 150 mg/day. Side effects, especially gastrointestinal and skin reactions, are common. A severe hypersensitivity reaction may produce the Stevens-Johnson syndrome. Owing to its relative inefficacy and the toxic side effects, thiacetazone is not approved for use in the United States.

Principles of Chemotherapy. Bacilli in a tuberculous lesion are located either extracellularly in cavitary lesions or in closed caseous lesions, or intracellularly within macrophages (Fig. 61–9). The metabolic activity of the organisms depends largely on the oxygen supply and pH. Some drugs are most active against organisms that are replicating frequently, such as extracellular organisms in cavitary lesions where oxygen is plentiful (Table 61–4). Bacilli in closed lesions replicate slowly or infrequently, and different drugs are needed to eliminate them. As the cavities and caseous lesions communicate with the bronchi, a large actively multiplying extracellular bacillary population can be identified by a positive sputum smear. The slowly or intermittently replicating bacilli in closed lesions and within macrophages are captive and are not reflected in the sputum examination.

In a virginal population of bacilli, mutants resistant to rifampin occur at a frequency of 10^{-8}; mutants resistant to INH, streptomycin, ethambutol, kanamycin, or PAS at a frequency of 10^{-6}; and mutants resistant to ethionamide, cycloserine, and thiacetazone at a frequency of 10^{-3}. In tuberculosis with cavitary lesions and a positive sputum smear, the bacterial population is in the order of 10^9 organisms. Thus, there may be 1,000 to 100,000 organisms resistant to one drug, even when the organisms have never been exposed to that drug. However, if two drugs are combined, the probability of drug resistance becomes very low (e.g., 10^{-12}), and when 3 drugs are combined, the probability is practically nonexistent (10^{-18}). For this reason, 2 or 3 effective drugs

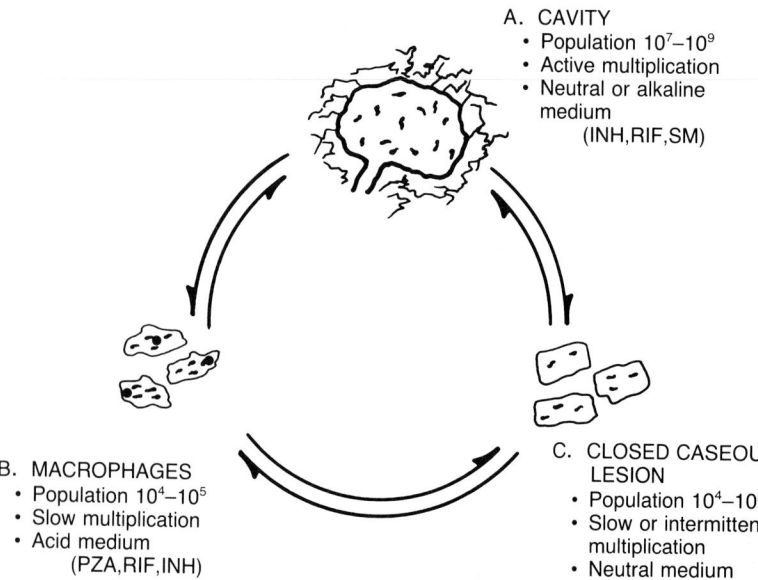

A. CAVITY
• Population 10^7–10^9
• Active multiplication
• Neutral or alkaline
  medium
  (INH,RIF,SM)

B. MACROPHAGES
• Population 10^4–10^5
• Slow multiplication
• Acid medium
  (PZA,RIF,INH)

C. CLOSED CASEOUS
   LESION
• Population 10^4–10^5
• Slow or intermittent
  multiplication
• Neutral medium
  (RIF,INH)

FIGURE 61–9. Bacterial populations in tuberculous lesions. *A*, Large and extracellular, actively multiplying in cavities. *B*, Small and intracellular, slowly multiplying inside macrophages. *C*, Small and extracellular, slowly or intermittently multiplying "persisters" in closed caseous lesions. (From Dutt AK, Stead WW: J Infect Dis 146:698, 1982.)

should be given simultaneously to avoid multiplication and emergence of drug-resistant mutants.

For chemotherapy to be effective, drugs must be capable of eliminating all 3 populations of bacilli without harming the host. Failure to eliminate the rapidly multiplying organisms in cavitary lesions results in continued positive culture, usually with drug-resistant organisms. However, if the large population is eliminated successfully but the slowly multiplying organisms located in closed lesions and within macrophages are not eradicated, late relapse may occur months after stopping chemotherapy, owing to late multiplication of these "persisters."

Drugs are selected to which the bacilli are expected to be susceptible. In developed countries, most of the newly diagnosed patients have tuberculosis caused by sensitive strains and pose little problem for therapy with INH and rifampin. In developing countries, initial resistance to drugs, particularly to INH, is common owing to improper use of the antituberculous drugs. A world atlas of initial INH-resistance has been compiled. Resistance rates are generally low in developed countries and high in developing countries, but greater than 20% in only a few countries.

Antituberculous medications should be given in a single dose before breakfast in order to achieve a single peak concentration of the drugs, which has a maximum

effect on the bacilli. Ethionamide, cycloserine, and PAS are exceptions because of their side effects and must be administered in divided doses.

A single drug should never be added to a failing regimen (no bacteriologic conversion to negative in 4 to 6 months), because it amounts to treatment with a single drug in a case in which resistance has developed to one of the drugs in use. This may result in accelerated development of drug resistance to the added drug. In such a situation, therapy with 2 or 3 new drugs should be instituted in full doses after stopping the drugs that have failed.

The use of 2 or more drugs with good early bactericidal activity reduces the extracellular bacterial population rapidly and avoids selection of drug-resistant mutants. SM acts best in a neutral or slightly alkaline medium and, therefore, kills most effectively the rapidly dividing extracellular bacilli in cavitary lesions (see Table 61–4). INH and rifampin act on both the rapidly multiplying extracellular bacilli and the slowly dividing bacilli in closed lesions and within macrophages. Pyrazinamide is effective in the acid environment within macrophages. INH and rifampin kill not only the extracellular bacilli but also the slowly dividing bacilli in closed lesions and within macrophages.

Treatment Regimens. Chemotherapy for tuberculosis has undergone revolutionary changes in recent years owing to the availability of a powerful new drug, rifampin, to use with INH, and to the reuse of an old drug, pyrazinamide. Many different types of regimens have been used for treating pulmonary tuberculosis, but two types of regimens have emerged as particularly successful and need to be considered in detail.

Isoniazid and Rifampin. The duration of treatment has now been reduced safely to 9 months for completing therapy for lung tuberculosis in developed countries, provided these two bactericidal drugs are used together for the total duration of therapy. When there is no suspicion of drug resistance to INH, therapy in adults should consist of INH and rifampin for 9 months. The addition of SM or ethambutol contributes little or noth-

TABLE 61–4. Action of Drugs Depending on the Metabolic Activity of the Bacilli*

	Rapidly Multiplying (Usually Extracellular)	Slowly Multiplying	
		At Acid pH (Intracellular)	At Neutral pH (Extracellular)
Streptomycin	+++	0	0
Isoniazid	++	+	±
Rifampin	++	+	+
Pyrazinamide	0	++	0
Ethambutol	±	±	0

*Modified from Grosset J: Clin Chest Med 1:231, 1980.

0 = none; + = minimal; ++ = modest; +++ = considerable.

ing to the efficacy of this regimen. Isoniazid, 300 mg, and rifampin, 600 mg, may be given daily for the full 9 months or may be given daily for 1 month, followed by rifampin, 600 mg, and INH, 900 mg, twice a week for the remaining 8 months.

Bacteriologic conversion to negative is quite rapid with bactericidal therapy, thus rendering the patient noninfectious to others. This rapid elimination of bacilli also greatly reduces the risk of selection of drug-resistant mutants. Relapses are rare, usually occurring within the first 6 months after completion of therapy and then only with bacilli still susceptible to drugs, indicating that these relapses are due to a replication of a few residual bacilli ("persisters") and not to the development of drug resistance.

Toxic side effects from the two bactericidal drugs are relatively uncommon. Hepatic toxicity occurs in about 2 to 4% of patients, primarily during daily administration of the drugs. Transient symptomatic elevations of enzyme levels are common with INH and rifampin therapy. Thus, routine monitoring of the enzymes during chemotherapy may cause confusion and unnecessary withdrawal of the drugs. If symptoms occur, the drugs should be stopped and a blood sample taken for the estimation of the enzyme levels. Elevation of liver enzymes to more than 3 times the baseline studies is presumed to be due to isoniazid. If a challenge dose is given later, it should be with only one drug at a time, in half dose, and the patient should be observed carefully. Hypersensitivity reactions such as petechiae with thrombocytopenia, the "flu-like" syndrome, and acute renal failure can occur with intermittent administration of the drug, often with demonstrable antibodies. These were overemphasized in the past when doses of 900 to 1200 mg of rifampin were used and when the drug was administered at 7-day intervals. When 600 mg of rifampin are administered twice weekly, these reactions occur in less than 1% of patients. When they do occur, rifampin should be withdrawn or the patient should be returned to the daily regimen.

Short-Course Chemotherapy with Four Drugs. One of the greatest advances in tuberculous control has been the introduction of the so-called short-course chemotherapy regimens. The aim of this modern treatment strategy is not only to kill rapidly the large numbers of actively metabolizing bacilli, but also to sterilize the lesions as quickly as possible by killing the slowly or intermittently metabolizing, semidormant bacilli. The duration of therapy can safely be reduced to 6 or even fewer months, even for patients with extensive, smear positive, cavitary disease. Regimens include initial daily therapy with several drugs, followed by twice- or thrice-weekly therapy for the rest of the treatment period. One successful short-course regimen consists of initial 4 daily drugs (streptomycin, isoniazid, rifampin, and pyrazinamide) during 2 months, followed by rifampin and INH daily for another 4 months. Reduction of the bacillary population is achieved rapidly through the early bactericidal action of INH. Slow-dividing, intracellular bacilli—the persisters—are killed mostly by pyrazinamide and rifampin, the 2 drugs with the highest sterilizing activity. Relapse rates are low, even in countries

where initial drug resistance is high. Ethambutol can be substituted for SM, thus giving a totally oral regimen for short-course chemotherapy. The 6-month daily rifampin regimen may be modified in 3 ways, all of which make it cheaper and more convenient to administer. First, isoniazid and rifampin may be given 3 times a week instead of daily during the continuation phase; second, the initial daily phase may be reduced from 2 months to 1 month; third, SM may be omitted from the 2 months' initial phase. Other regimens propose a continuation phase consisting of daily INH alone, for 4 to 6 months, or of a once weekly 4-drug combination. The role of pyrazinamide in the initial phase of treatment is beyond doubt, but its importance in the continuation phase is still under debate.

Numerous clinical studies of short-course chemotherapy regimens have been, and still are being, conducted in many developing countries. Concurrently, short-course regimens are applied widely in more and more parts of the world. In order to improve patient's compliance even further, fixed combinations of INH, rifampin, and pyrazinamide in 1 tablet have been proposed.

Other Regimens. Unfortunately, the cost of short-course regimens remains high, and in many of the developing countries, the least expensive yet effective regimen remains isoniazid, 300 mg, and thiacetazone, 150 mg, daily for 12 to 18 months, with SM, 0.75 to 1 gm daily, for the first 2 to 3 months in patients with positive smears.

National Antituberculous Programs and Their Costs. The aim of antituberculous therapy in developing countries is not only to cure the diseased patient, but also to interrupt the transmission of the disease. Therefore, physicians should not be allowed to prescribe a chemotherapy regimen of their own choice. They should prescribe only those regimens sanctioned by the national antituberculosis program. Otherwise, a country risks facing anarchy in its health services, confusion of its health-care personnel, and unacceptable expenses.

Most developing countries can devote only a small portion of their resources to health and to tuberculosis in particular. For instance, some years ago the Philippines spent only 5 cents per capita and 19 dollars per case of tuberculosis, versus 8 dollars and 31,000 dollars spent by Japan at the same time. Whereas in developed countries most of the tuberculosis budget is spent on hospitalization, in developing countries, most of this budget is allocated to BCG vaccination, case finding, and chemotherapy.

Whereas reduction of mortality and individual morbidity is often possible even with poor chemotherapy, the number of sources of infection are much more difficult to be reduced, and paradoxically this number can increase when national treatment regimens are inadequate. Singapore offers an example for a successful national program. Over a 24-year period, the rate of notification of new cases fell from over 300 per 100,000 to 85 per 100,000 in 1984.

Management of Extrapulmonary Tuberculosis. Now that there is an effective means of killing tubercle bacilli throughout the body, the treatment of extrapulmonary tuberculosis has become much improved. INH and rifampin are the cornerstones of treatment. They are often given with SM, pyrazinamide, and/or ethambutol. Treatment is extended usually to 12 months. There is no evidence that the short-term chemotherapy regimens used for pulmonary tuberculosis are efficacious treatment for extrapulmonary tuberculosis. Surgery is needed for draining pus, as in empyema or paraspinous abscess, and to correct residual damage from the disease in a few patients, e.g., constrictive pericarditis or hydrocephalus. Occasionally, a badly destroyed vertebra requires stabilization (Chapter 13). The indications for corticosteroids are heavily disputed, and there is no conclusive evidence that they relieve even the long-term effects of meningitis or pericarditis. Steroids may decrease the passage of antituberculous drugs through the blood-brain barrier.

Monitoring Treatment. Patient compliance and bacteriological response must be monitored closely during chemotherapy to assure its safety and effectiveness. In pulmonary tuberculosis, frequent bacteriological sputum examinations are the best and simplest way to monitor the therapeutic response, together with easy methods for following the patient's general improvement, like weight gain and normalization of the erythrocyte sedimentation rate. In developed countries, initially, cultures should be obtained at least once every month until 3 consecutive negative cultures have been reported, and thereafter every other month throughout therapy and for an additional 6 months. Sputum should be collected then every 3 months for another 6 months to detect any relapse. However, in developing countries, the diagnosis and follow-up studies are based often on smear examinations only. Cultural examinations are either too expensive, or the facilities are not available. A progressive reduction of the number of organisms on the smear examination is good evidence of response to therapy and compliance in taking the medication. Persistence of positive sputum by smear and culture after 3 months of treatment does not necessarily indicate failure of treatment, but does call for a check on patient compliance. The reappearance of bacilli in the sputum soon after conversion is a sign of failure of the treatment, often because of poor compliance. In such patients, drug susceptibility tests are indicated to detect development of resistance to the drugs. Frequent radiographic examinations of the chest contribute little if the bacteriological response is satisfactory. In economically poor countries, facilities for repeated roentgenographic studies are often unavailable. A better guide to therapy is repeated smear examination of the sputum. The patient must be seen frequently during the first 2 months of treatment to ensure compliance and to alert the physician to any problems. To be successful, many short-term chemotherapy regimens are intensive and fully supervised, i.e., patients take their medications under the continuous supervision of medical personnel. However, this is often difficult in countries with a high incidence of tuberculosis owing to the overwhelming number of patients, the shortage of transportation for the long distances to the clinics, and the shortage of

medical personnel. Attempts have to be made to follow patients with the help of nonmedical ancillary staff. Laboratory studies for routine monitoring for side effects are not necessary. The monitoring of side effects should be based on the development of symptoms of toxicity. After completion of therapy and a year of follow-up, the patient should be discharged from the clinic with the advice to return to the clinic if symptoms return. The policy of following patients for a longer period is unwarranted and only adds to the workload of clinics.

PREVENTION AND CONTROL

Case Finding and Chemotherapy. The most powerful strategy for controlling tuberculosis in developing countries consists of the combination of actively finding tuberculous cases and treatment of cases. These two activities must be developed simultaneously in order to break the chain of transmission. The essential of case finding is to discover all highly infectious individuals, i.e., those with positive sputum, by direct microscopy. Active case-finding campaigns may be useful, using health clinics or publicity media such as television, radio, posters, and leaflets. The aim of these campaigns is to encourage people with a cough of at least 1 month's duration to attend a health clinic for sputum examination. Sputum examination should become a routine examination in any community health institution.

In some developing countries, it is estimated that 0.5 to 1.0% of patients attending outpatient clinics have sputum positive for acid-fast bacilli. If these patients are treated with adequate drug regimens and compliance is assured, transmission of the infection can be halted. There is little value in spending scarce resources on hospital beds for tuberculosis, because ambulatory treatment is effective. It is not necessary to isolate tuberculous patients to check the dissemination of infection to noninfected persons. Transmission is best prevented by early treatment of all infectious individuals. This has been shown clearly in the Madras (India) study in 1956, in which the incidence of disease and infection in contacts during follow-up showed no statistical difference between the patients who were treated in the sanatorium and those who were treated at home, despite substandard living conditions. The infection of contacts had occurred before the initiation of chemotherapy in both groups of infectious patients. Chemotherapy rapidly reduces the cough and the number of bacilli in the sputum. Infectiousness drops rapidly within 2 weeks, even though the sputum may still contain bacilli on smear or culture.

A national case-finding and treatment program must ensure that supervision is assured even to persons in remote areas. The control program should be integrated into the primary health care system of the community.

Compliance with Antituberculous Chemotherapy in Tropical Countries. In order to interrupt the chain of transmission of tuberculosis in a country, effective chemotherapy needs to be given to the greatest possible number of sputum-positive patients. Noncompliance to treatment is less often due to the patient's failure to take the drugs correctly than to other factors, which include negligence or incompetence of people in charge of the antituberculous program at the national level, lack of standardization of chemotherapy, selection of regimens of doubtful efficacy, inefficient supply system, absence of supervision, absence of evaluation of drugs actually received, negligence of health service personnel, and poor reception at health clinics. It is only for a minority of patients that noncompliance is solely due to themselves or to their difficult social circumstances. Moreover, patient's apathy over the length of treatment is expected to decrease with the new short-term chemotherapy regimens.

Decontamination of the Environment. Hospital rooms can be decontaminated by intense ventilation with fresh air. This can be achieved by a one-way air control system, or alternatively, by open windows and exhaust fans. Because ultraviolet rays are lethal to the tubercle bacilli, ultraviolet irradiation of the upper air of the room, where the light droplet nuclei usually float, helps in the decontamination of the room. The intense sunlight in most tropical countries is rich in ultraviolet rays. Both of these methods are advised for decontamination of places where patients with known or suspected disease are housed. Patients can be safely hospitalized in general hospitals when necessary, if the precautions of ventilation of the rooms and hallways, use of ultraviolet light, training of patients, and prompt initiation of chemotherapy to proven infectious patients are taken.

BCG Vaccination. In 1921, after subculturing a virulent strain of *M. bovis* every 3 weeks for 235 times, two French scientists, Calmette and Guérin, managed to produce a strain of *M. bovis* that was avirulent for experimental animals. The organism came to be known as "bacille Calmette-Guérin," or BCG, and experiments showed that animals infected with a culture of this organism developed increased resistance to a later inoculation with virulent tuberculous bacilli.

BCG Trials. Despite the widespread use of BCG since 1921, controlled studies were not performed until the 1930s. Results of several recent trials have shown enormous differences in the degree of protection afforded by BCG, which has varied over a range from 0 to 80% (Table 61–5). For instance, BCG vaccination in children in England offered 78% protection for at least 10 years, whereas in South India, BCG failed to protect against culture-proven primary tuberculosis in the first 5 years of observation. The reason for this marked variation in effectiveness of BCG vaccination in different geographic areas is not entirely clear. It has been explained on theoretical grounds by errors in methods and differences in potency among the BCG strains used in various trials. Recent work suggests that "natural vaccination" due to contact with environmental mycobacteria might account for the striking differences in the protective efficacy of BCG from trial to trial. Two schools of thought have emerged, leading to contradictory attitudes toward the practice of BCG. The first school concludes that BCG achieves its full potential only in regions where the population is not exposed to environmental mycobacteria, and that elsewhere the observed effect of the vaccine is the difference between the potential effect and that of the "natural vaccination." According to this theory, individuals in those areas where BCG shows no protective effect are already protected maximally, and health authorities might abandon the costly procedure of BCG vaccination in the belief that the environment provides the same service. By contrast, the second school states that BCG affords protection when it elicits a Listeria-type reactivity in a person not exposed previously to mycobacteria, or when it boosts such a reaction in a person exposed to mycobacteria that have mounted this type of sensitivity response. In opposition, BCG proves ineffective or even harmful if it boosts a Koch-type response, which can follow certain environmental mycobacterial infections. In this case, vaccination cannot overcome the antagonistic immune reaction, and the vaccine will fail to protect the population. If this second theory is confirmed, BCG would need to be given in these regions early in life so as to induce protective immunity before the environment can have its adverse effects. Moreover, some form of immunotherapy aimed at reprogramming the immune response of Koch-type responders would be of real value. The resolution of the controversy between these two schools is one of the priorities in tuberculous research today, because the future of control of the disease depends on it.

BCG, Practical Aspects. In both developed and developing countries where BCG vaccination is practiced routinely, BCG is usually given at birth, in infancy, or in early childhood. Adult visitors to areas with a high endemicity of tuberculosis might benefit from receiving BCG vaccination prior to departure, if they are tuberculin unreactive and if they risk exposure to high loads of mycobacterial aerosols, e.g., physicians and nurses. A dose of 0.01 to 0.1 mg is injected intradermally and gives rise to a classical primary complex consisting of a cutaneous nodule at the site of injection and swelling of the regional lymph nodes. Adverse effects due to vac-

TABLE 61–5. Efficacy of BCG: Controlled Trials of BCG Vaccination Against Tuberculosis

Population Group	Age Range	No. of Subjects		TB Case Rates*		Protective Efficacy (%)
		Control	*Vaccinated*	*Control*	*Vaccinated*	
North American Indians	0–20 years	1457	1551	1563	320	80
Chicago infants	3 months	1665	1716	223	57	75
Georgia school children	6–17 years	2341	2498	11	17	0
Puerto Rico—general population	1–18 years	27338	50634	43	30	31
Illinois—school for mentally retarded	young adults	494	531	—	—	0
Georgia and Alabama—general population	5 years and older	17854	16913	13	11	14
Great Britain—urban population	14—15.5 years	12699	13598	128	28	78
South India—rural population	all ages	5808	5069	89	61	31

*Case rates/100,000 population.

cination are rare. Skin ulcerations and lymphadenitis in the vicinity of the injection site may occur in vaccinated children and may result in chronic suppuration. These complications seem to be more frequent in subjects exposed before vaccination to certain environmental mycobacteria (e.g., *M. scrofulaceum* in Burmese children). BCG-induced lesions may respond to oral treatment with isoniazid or erythromycin. Surgical drainage is seldom necessary. Meningitis after BCG and disseminated BCG infections resulting in death are reported rarely, but they are feared to increase with the spread of the AIDS epidemic, especially in African children.

Preventive Therapy. The rationale for preventive INH chemoprophylaxis differs markedly in countries with low and high prevalence of tuberculous disease. In the United States and in other countries with low incidence of tuberculosis, it is argued that identification of persons who are infected with tubercle bacilli through the use of the tuberculin test is important, because the development of clinical tuberculosis can be prevented effectively by a year of therapy with INH. Preventive therapy of contacts of infectious individuals may be important also in order to eliminate the risk of developing tuberculosis during old age. INH chemoprophylaxis (300 mg daily) of infected persons has shown protection of at least 80%. Persons less than 35 years of age have little risk (under 1%) of developing hepatitis from INH, whereas in those older than 50 years, the risk increases to 3%. For this reason, the chemoprophylaxis with INH is recommended only for persons in special risk groups. No prophylaxis is indicated for tuberculin reactors who have BCG scars.

In developing countries, the INH chemoprophylaxis approach for contacts and tuberculin-positive individuals is unrealistic. BCG use is widespread in tropical countries, and many individuals may react positive on tuberculin testing yet forget that they have been immunized previously. Household contacts of patients with active tuberculosis should be investigated for sputum positivity and treated accordingly. Persons with an abnormal nonprogressive chest radiograph and a positive PPD reaction, and whose sputum is bacteriologically negative, should be followed closely, and full treatment should be started in case they develop clinical disease and become sputum-positive. Persons who have documented conversion of the PPD reaction from negative to positive within the past 2 years (the so-called recent converters) should be evaluated for clinical disease and receive full treatment accordingly but not blindly, because many tuberculin conversions in tropical environments are due to infections by environmental mycobacteria and not tuberculous bacilli. Even tuberculin-positive persons with a "special risk" condition, e.g., long-term corticosteroid or immunosuppressive therapy, HIV infection, leukemia, Hodgkin's disease, diabetes mellitus, silicosis, or previous gastrectomy, might better be followed closely for signs of active disease, and then receive full treatment, rather than receiving blind INH prophylaxis.

Tuberculosis Control in Refugee Camps. Refugees living in camp settlements have become numerous over the last 10 years. Tuberculosis is one of the most serious health threats in many camps, owing to overcrowding,

poor nutrition, and increased transmission and susceptibility. For example, random sputum examinations indicated 3% prevalence of sputum positivity in Somali refugee camps. The control of tuberculosis in camps presents unique aspects, e.g., the uncertain time a refugee will remain in the camp and be accessible to health care. Patient defaulting is exceedingly high. During their stay, however, refugees usually have limited mobility and are easily accessible for case finding, contact tracing, and treatment. Refugee tuberculosis programs are best based on the national programs of the host government.

61.1. TUBERCULOSIS AND AIDS

Human immunodeficiency virus (HIV) is the etiologic agent of a severe immunodeficiency state with fatal outcome, the acquired immunodeficiency syndrome (AIDS) (Chapter 15.1). Over the last decade, HIV and AIDS have developed into a formidable pandemic, striking with particular ferocity the sub-Saharan countries on the African continent. Transmission of the virus is predominantly through heterosexual intercourse in tropical communities. HIV infects T-helper lymphocytes and leads to serious functional defects in the immune system, notably a failure to produce gamma interferon and other macrophage-activating lymphokines. This explains the high susceptibility of HIV-infected individuals to acquire disease by intracellular pathogens, like mycobacteria, which are normally controlled by T lymphocyte-macrophage cooperation. The risk of a person with HIV infection to acquire tuberculosis depends on the prevalence of tuberculosis in his community. In parts of Africa where HIV has become epidemic, there is also a high incidence of associated tuberculosis. In the tropical environment where people are exposed regularly to tuberculous bacilli, the highly pathogenic *M. tuberculosis* can lead to disease early in the course of HIV infection. Long before full-blown AIDS becomes manifest, only a small immune imbalance is needed to favor the mycobacterium against the macrophage. This explains why HIV infection is often common in populations of patients with tuberculosis. When tuberculous disease develops early in the course of immunodeficiency, granulomas may still be discernible, although relatively lymphocyte-depleted. Caseation is rare because of impaired production of the macrophage hormone tumor necrosis factor. Tuberculin reactions may still be seen in early disease, but usually are weak and will be lost with advancement of the degree of immunodeficiency. The clinical manifestations are often atypical and depend on the degree of immunodeficiency. In pulmonary tuberculosis, the upper lobes are often spared, whereas middle and lower lobes are mostly affected. Sputum examination may be positive in early HIV infection but become negative later. Diagnosis of the disease becomes increasingly difficult, and modern techniques (e.g., PCR) can be of great help. Pulmonary cavitation is rare. With progression of the immunodeficiency state, the tuberculous disease becomes gradually unreactive, and progressive dissemination occurs. Granulomas become poorly formed and often are completely absent; the tissues resemble those of lepromatous leprosy. Lungs are less often affected, and tuberculous lymphadenopathy becomes common, although it cannot be distinguished on clinical grounds from the lymphadenopathy of AIDS or the AIDS-related complex. Hilar and mediastinal lymph node enlargement is common. Other modes of presentation of tuberculosis in the advanced immunodeficiency state comprise miliary dissemination of tuberculosis with liver and bone marrow involvement, and central nervous system disease with tuberculomas, cerebral abscesses, and tuberculous meningitis. In this late state of severe immunodeficiency, nontuberculous mycobacteria of low virulence may also become pathogenic, such as *M. avium-intracellulare*. In countries where tuberculosis is rare, and in particular in the more developed countries of Europe and America, these opportunistic agents may be the most commonly encountered mycobacteria causing disease in the AIDS patient.

There seems to be no increased risk of disseminated BCG infection in the pediatric population with HIV infection, if immunization is carried out in early life without prior testing for HIV infection.

All persons with HIV infection should be given a tuberculin skin test, and if reactive, should be monitored closely for development of clinical tuberculous disease. As for chemotherapy in HIV-infected patients with clinical tuberculosis, the modern short-course regimens seem not to be appropriate treatment. Extended courses of triple or quadruple therapy followed by maintenance INH are generally indicated. Drug intolerance is common, and combined with drug resistance, often reduces the choice of agents, and these patients are overtaken finally by other opportunistic infections.

The HIV pandemic has jeopardized many of the achievements reached in tuberculosis control worldwide.

61.2. DISEASES CAUSED BY NONTUBERCULOUS MYCOBACTERIA

Among the more than 40 validly described species of mycobacteria, 17 can occasionally produce disease in humans, but they are less pathogenic than *M. tuberculosis*. Nontuberculous clinical disease is not a significant public health problem in the developing world, where it is eclipsed by the overwhelming problems produced by classic tuberculosis. Even where good laboratory support is available in tropical countries, nontuberculous bacilli are rarely isolated from clinical specimens. This low impact on the practice of clinical medicine contrasts with the importance that nontuberculous mycobacteria seem to have in the tropical world as agents of subclinical infections in humans, inducers of immunoresponses and "natural vaccinators."

The classification of nontuberculous mycobacteria as proposed by Wolinsky is most helpful for clinical purposes (Table 61–6). The usual route of entry of the organism appears to be through the respiratory tract,

TABLE 61–6. Classification of Mycobacteria Other Than *M. tuberculosis* and *M. lepra**

I. Slowly Growing Potential Pathogens
1. *M. kansasii*
2. *M. avium intracellulare* ⎤ (also known as the
3. *M. scrofulaceum* ⎦ *MAIS* complex)
4. *M. ulcerans*
5. *M. marinum*
6. *M. xenopi*
7. *M. szulgai*
8. *M. simiae*

II. Slowly Growing Nonpathogens
1. *M. gordonae*
2. *M. gastri*
3. *M. terrae* complex
4. *M. flavescens*

III. Rapidly Growing Potential Pathogens
1. *M. fortuitum*
2. *M. chelonei*

IV. Rapidly Growing Nonpathogens
1. *M. smegmatis*
2. *M. vaccae*
3. *M. parafortuitum* complex
4. *M. phlei*

*Adapted from Wolinsky E: Am Rev Respir Dis 119:107, 1979.

e.g., pulmonary involvement by *M. kansasii* and *M. avium-intracellulare*. The oropharyngeal mucous membranes may be the route to produce lymphadenitis, e.g., scrofula. *M. marinum* may cause granuloma of the skin and subcutaneous tissue by entering directly through skin abrasions. *M. kansasii*, the MAIS complex (which comprises *M. avium-intracellulare* and *M. scrofulaceum*), and the rapidly growing *M. chelonei* may rarely cause disseminated disease affecting several organs. Microscopic examination does not help in the differentiation between mycobacteria from different species. Cultural and biochemical tests are necessary. The service of a competent mycobacteriologist is essential for identification of these organisms. Skin testing with antigens prepared for various species has not yet proved helpful for clinical purposes but is helpful in epidemiological surveys. These antigens are not commercially available.

PULMONARY DISEASE. *M. kansasii* and the MAIS complex can cause pulmonary disease, although some other species may affect the lungs occasionally. The disease caused by these mycobacteria is often found in an abnormal lung where reduced pulmonary defenses allow establishment of infection. Obstructive lung disease is the most common underlying lung problem. Alternatively, these nontuberculous mycobacteria can cause lung disease in patients with generalized immunodeficiency, as happens for instance in HIV-infected patients with full-blown AIDS. The clinical presentation of lung disease due to nontuberculous mycobacteria resembles tuberculosis, i.e., slowly progressive cavitary lesions in the lungs with chronic productive cough. Tuberculin tests generally are only weakly reactive. Because nontuberculous mycobacteria are commonly present in the environment and have low virulence, differentiation between colonization and disease must be made more strictly than for *M. tuberculosis*. Indeed, these mycobacteria may be found as (1) saprophytic colonization in the respiratory tract; (2) infection without pathological manifestations; or (3) low-grade pathogens. Therefore, a definite diagnosis requires the presence of signs and symptoms of clinical disease compatible with tuberculosis, definite radiological features, and repeated isolation of the same species of mycobacteria from sputum in the absence of other pathogens.

LYMPHADENITIS. Adenitis due to nontuberculous mycobacteria is most frequent in children. The most common etiological organism is the MAIS complex, although *M. kansasii* and *M. fortuitum* may cause occasional cases. Submandibular and cervical nodes are usually involved. Lymphadenitis presents as swelling of discrete nodes without clinical symptoms. The nodes enlarge progressively, soften, and rupture with drainage. Healing eventually occurs slowly by fibrosis and calcification. Diagnosis is made by culture of the aspirated pus from the nodes. Histologic characteristics are identical to those caused by *M. tuberculosis.*

DISSEMINATED DISEASE. Rapidly progressive and disseminated disease is rare and usually occurs in immunocompromised hosts. Any organ can become involved. Dissemination may be encountered in one quarter of AIDS patients in the United States. The organism can be visualized often by Ziehl-Neelsen's stain of various body fluids, tissues, and stool. Rapid diagnosis can be made by blood-culture systems that use cell lysis and centrifugation. Blood cultures are positive in about 50% of AIDS patients with disseminated disease. Tissue biopsies characteristically show large numbers of mycobacteria with little granuloma formation and large, foamy macrophages loaded with acid-fast bacilli. Often, infection is progressive and fatal.

OTHER CLINICAL PICTURES. *M. marinum* and *M. ulcerans* cause disease in the skin and subcutaneous tissues (Chapter 63). *M. kansasii* and *M. avium-intracellulare* may involve bones, joints, tendon sheaths, the kidneys, and the meninges. Occasionally, disease may be caused by rapidly growing mycobacteria, like *M. chelonei* and *M. fortuitum.* The organisms involve preexisting chronic lung disease, e.g., bronchiectasis and silicosis, and produce progressive disease. Diagnosis is by cultural examination of tissue and clinical materials. Differentiation of *M. chelonei* from *M. fortuitum* may be helpful, as the latter is more susceptible to newer chemotherapeutic agents.

TREATMENT. Disease caused by nontuberculous mycobacteria is unfortunate for the patient, because there is inadequate knowledge regarding its pathogenesis and treatment. The disease should be clinically significant and progressive to justify therapy. Most nontuberculous mycobacteria manifest considerable in vitro resistance to antituberculous drugs. *M. avium-intracellulare* is generally completely resistant to antituberculous drugs. Absence of symptoms, especially in the AIDS patient, may signify that withholding treatment is the best option for the patient. In case of progressive disease, most authorities recommend a combination of 3 to 6 drugs, but there is no evidence that treatment prolongs life. Even with regimens containing 4, 5, and even 6 drugs, barely 50% of patients show benefit on long-term follow-up. The regimens usually contain 2 of the drugs to which some susceptibility is seen occasion-

ally, i.e., ethambutol (25 mg/kg of body weight), cycloserine, and ethionamide. Regimens containing rifampin have shown slightly better results. Most authorities include an injectable drug, such as SM, in the regimen. Investigational regimens include experimental drugs, e.g., rifabutine, clofazimine, ciprofloxacin, imipenem. If the disease is localized and pulmonary function permits, surgical resection of the diseased lobe may be considered as an adjunct to chemotherapy. The chemotherapy has to be given for 18 to 24 months. The disease is slowly progressive and may eventually lead to cor pulmonale and pulmonary insufficiency if it does not respond to chemotherapy.

M. kansasii may show some in vitro susceptibility to antituberculous drugs, and treatment is generally as effective as treatment of *M. tuberculosis.* A drug regimen containing isoniazid and rifampin generally produces conversion of sputum to negative, with clinical recovery.

M. chelonei and *M. fortuitum* are resistant usually to antituberculous drugs, and therapeutic results are disappointing. However, recent chemotherapeutic agents, such as amikacin, doxycycline, and sulfamethoxazole, have shown promising results in small numbers of patients. Some of these drugs are effective also in disease caused by *M. marinum* and *M. ulcerans.* Surgical excision of scrufula nodes may sometimes be necessary and is preferred over simple drainage, which tends to cause a chronic, open, draining sinus.

BIBLIOGRAPHY

Bishburg E, Sunderam G, Reichman LB, et al.: Central nervous system tuberculosis with the acquired immunodeficiency syndrome and its related complex. Ann Int Med 105:210, 1986.

Centers for Disease Control, U.S. Department of Health and Human Services: Diagnosis and management of mycobacterial infection and disease in persons with human immunodeficiency virus infection: Ann Intern Med 106:254, 1987.

Chaisson RE, Schecter GF, Theuer CP, et al.: Tuberculosis in patients with the acquired immunodeficiency syndrome. Clinical features, response to therapy, and survival. Am Rev Respir Dis 136:570, 1987.

Chaulet P: Compliance with anti-tuberculosis chemotherapy in developing countries. Tubercle 68(Suppl):19, 1987.

Comstock GW: Epidemiology of tuberculosis. Am Rev Respir Dis 125(Suppl):8, 1982.

Dutt AK, Stead WW: Present chemotherapy for tuberculosis. J Infect Dis 146:698, 1982.

East and Central African/British Medical Research Council Fifth Collaborative Study: Controlled clinical trial of 4 short-course regimens of chemotherapy (three 6-month and one 8-month) for pulmonary tuberculosis: Final report. Tubercle 67:5, 1986.

Editorial: BCG vaccination after the Madras Study. Lancet 1:309, 1981.

Ellard GA: The potential clinical significance of the isoniazid acetylator phenotype in the treatment of pulmonary tuberculosis. Tubercle 65:211, 1984.

Fox W: The current status of short course chemotherapy. Tubercle 60:177, 1979.

Fox W: Whither short course chemotherapy? Br J Dis Chest 75:331, 1981.

Girling DJ: The role of pyrazinamide in primary chemotherapy for pulmonary tuberculosis. Tubercle 65:1, 1984.

Glatt AE, Chirgwin K, Landesman SH: Treatment of infections associated with human immunodeficiency virus. N Engl J Med 318:1439, 1988.

Goldman KP: AIDS and tuberculosis. Br Med J 295:511, 1987.

Grange JM: Environmental mycobacteria and BCG vaccination. Tubercle 67:1, 1986.

Grzybowski S: Cost in tuberculosis control. Tubercle 68(Suppl):33, 1987.

Kiehn TE, Cammarata R: Laboratory diagnosis of mycobacterial infections in patients with acquired immunodeficiency syndrome. J Clin Microbiol 24:708, 1986.

Krambovitis E, McIllmurray MB, Lock PE, et al.: Rapid diagnosis of tuberculous meningitis by latex particle agglutination. Lancet 2:1229, 1984.

Menzies RI, Alsen H, Fitzgerald JM, et al.: Tuberculous peritonitis in Lesotho. Tubercle 67:47, 1986.

Mitchison DA: The action of antituberculosis drugs in short-course chemotherapy. Tubercle 66:219, 1985.

Pinching AJ: The Acquired Immunodeficiency Syndrome: With special reference to tuberculosis. Tubercle 68:65, 1987.

Pitchenik AE, Rubinson HA: The radiographic appearance of tuberculosis in patients with the acquired immune deficiency syndrome (AIDS) and pre-AIDS. Am Rev Respir Dis 131:393, 1985.

Pust RE, Erickson P: Determining *Mycobacterium tuberculosis* infection in high prevalence groups: A comparative study among Nigerian adults. Tubercle 65:263, 1984.

Ratledge C, Stanford JL: The Biology of the Mycobacteria, Vol. 1 & 2. New York, Academic Press, 1983.

Ramachandran P, Duraipandian M, Nagarajan M, et al.: Three chemotherapy studies of tuberculous meningitis in children. Tubercle 67:17, 1986.

Sutherland AM: Tuberculosis of the female genital tract. Tubercle 66:79, 1985.

Tanzanian/British Medical Research Council Collaborative Study: Tuberculosis in Tanzania—A national survey of newly notified cases. Tubercle 66:161, 1985.

For references published prior to 1981, see 6th edition, pp. 408–409.

62. LEPROSY

Wayne M. Meyers

DEFINITION. Leprosy is a chronic disease caused by *Mycobacterium leprae*. It affects the cooler parts of the body principally, especially the skin, upper respiratory tract, anterior segments of the eyes, superficial segments of peripheral nerves, and testes. The World Health Organization (WHO) estimates that there are 10 to 15 million patients with leprosy in the world.

LEPROSY AND SOCIETY. Comprehending the sources of the stigma of leprosy is essential to understanding the attitudes of society toward this disease and the effect that this stigma has on the leprosy patient. In Western cultures these attitudes are at least partially attributable to a misunderstanding of what is called "leprosy" in the Old Testament. Other cultures not influenced by Judaic laws and traditions, however, also have a similar tradition. For example, in China, possibly as early as the eighth century BC, people with a condition later recognized as leprosy were stigmatized.

The Hebrew word *tsara-ath* was rendered *lepra* when the Old Testament was translated into Greek about 200 BC. In preparing the Latin Vulgate version around 400 AD, St. Jerome perpetuated the use of the word *lepra*, and Wycliffe, translating from the Vulgate in 1384, changed the word *lepra* to *leprosy*. In the original text, *tsara-ath* was not a specific disease but a group of diseases with obscure identities, and the word referred more generally to ceremonial uncleanliness. Leprosy was common in Europe and Great Britain in the fourteenth century. To Wycliffe, leprosy in its most severe forms may thus have portrayed the physical image of an unholy and loathsome human condition. Old Testament *tsara-ath* as described in Leviticus 13 and 14, for example, had none of the distinctive features of leprosy. There is thus no rationale for including *tsara-ath*, as described in the Old Testament, in our understanding and care of leprosy patients today.

A continuing effort is being made to minimize the stigma peculiarly associated with leprosy. For example, the Fifth International Leprosy Congress in 1948 adopted a resolution to abandon the word *leper* for *leprosy patient*. Hansen's disease is preferred by some for leprosy. The U.S. Public Health Service Hospital for the treatment of leprosy patients at Carville, Louisiana, in 1981 was named the National Hansen's Disease Center, and is now called the Gillis W. Long Hansen's Disease Center. Because of the stigma of leprosy, physicians must carefully consider the social implications and assiduously avoid a casual diagnosis of this disease.

ETIOLOGY AND HISTORY. *M. leprae* is a species in the order *Actinomycetales* and the family *Mycobacteriaceae*. This bacillus was first seen by Hansen in Bergen, Norway, in 1873 in fresh mounts of scrapings from a leproma from a Norwegian leprosy patient, and it was the first reported bacterial pathogen of a chronic disease in humans. *M. leprae* is an acid-fast bacillus 0.3 to 0.5 μm wide by 4 to 7 μm long. The acid-fastness is weaker than that of other mycobacteria but, like other mycobacteria, is related to the mycolic acid in the cell wall. Viable undamaged *M. leprae* stain solidly; degenerating organisms first stain irregularly, then become granular, and eventually are fragmented. Serial evaluations of the staining quality thus provide a method for assessing therapeutic efficacy. All claims of in vitro cultivation of *M. leprae* are as yet unsubstantiated. In the absence of successful cultivation of *M. leprae*, identification depends on the results of a series of tests. The criteria for the identification of organisms as *M. leprae* are as follows: (1) organisms do not grow on routine mycobacteriologic media, (2) organisms infect the footpads of normal laboratory mice in a characteristic manner, (3) acid-fastness is extractable with pyridine, (4) suspensions of the bacilli oxidize DOPA, (5) organisms invade the nerves of hosts, and (6) killed suspensions of the bacilli produce a characteristic pattern of response when injected into the skin of patients with the various clinical forms of leprosy, i.e., tuberculoid patients react strongly and lepromatous patients are nonreactive.

M. leprae multiply slowly in experimental animals, with a generation time of 13 days in the logarithmic growth phase in the mouse footpad. This characteristic may account, at least in part, for the long incubation time of leprosy in humans. Localization of the heaviest infiltrations of leprosy to the cooler parts of the body, selective growth in the footpads of normal mice, and the high susceptibility of the armadillo (central body temperature 32 to 35°C) to disseminated infections all suggest that the optimal temperature for the growth of *M. leprae* is below 37C.

EPIDEMIOLOGY

Distribution and Incidence. Approximately half of all

patients with leprosy live in Africa and India (Fig. 62–1). By contrast, there are only approximately 6000 cases in the United States where 206 cases were reported in 1987. Most of these patients are immigrants, but there is indigenous leprosy in the United States, primarily in Louisiana, Texas, and Hawaii.

Transmission. The route or routes of the natural transmission of *M. leprae* are not known. The high frequency of single early lesions in skin that is usually covered by clothing argues against the local inoculation of *M. leprae* at the site of the lesion. Skin-to-skin contact was for many years considered the most important mode of transmission. This concept, although not abandoned, is now being challenged. Intact skin of patients with multibacillary leprosy regularly discharges small numbers of *M. leprae,* but open ulcers can be a source of large numbers of organisms. Thus, infection could take place by skin-to-skin contact or through fomites. The nasal mucosa of untreated lepromatous patients contains large numbers of *M. leprae* that are discharged regularly in the nasal secretions. *M. leprae* released in "nose-blows" and dried under ambient conditions remain viable for up to 1 week; the upper respiratory tract passages are thus a likely source of contagion. The experimental disseminated infections in immunosuppressed mice that follow the inhalation of aerosols containing *M. leprae* support this concept. Breast tissue and milk of mothers with lepromatous leprosy contain *M. leprae,* suggesting that infants could be infected during nursing. There is increasing evidence for placental transmission of leprosy. There are sporadic reports of leprosy in infants as young as 2 1/2 months old, and

fetal synthesis of antibodies to *M. leprae* has been documented. Natural transmission of leprosy by insects has not been proved.

Animal Reservoirs. With the discovery of naturally acquired leprosy in (1) armadillos in Louisiana and Texas, (2) a chimpanzee trapped in Sierra Leone, and (3) a mangabey monkey captured in West Africa, there is reason to believe that leprosy may be a zoonosis. In all three of these species the organisms causing the disease could not be distinguished from *M. leprae* of human origin.

Although the data are as yet fragmentary, there is anecdotal evidence that infected armadillos may transmit leprosy. By 1987 several hundred wild armadillos infected with *M. leprae* had been identified, and estimates are that 4 to 10% of wild armadillos in Louisiana and East Texas have acquired leprosy naturally.

Natural History of Infection. The spread of leprosy depends on the dissemination of the bacillus in a susceptible population. The prevalence of clinical disease in most populations rarely exceeds 5%. However, lymphocyte transformation studies in endemic areas demonstrate that approximately half of all close contacts (occupational and household) of leprosy patients are specifically sensitized, suggesting that exposure to *M. leprae* is frequent in these areas. The prevailing concept that repeated exposure is required to contract leprosy does not seem reasonable, because this concept is not valid for other infectious diseases. It may be true, however, that both the numbers of viable *M. leprae* being shed by the patient and the degree of susceptibility of the contact may vary, so that long periods of associ-

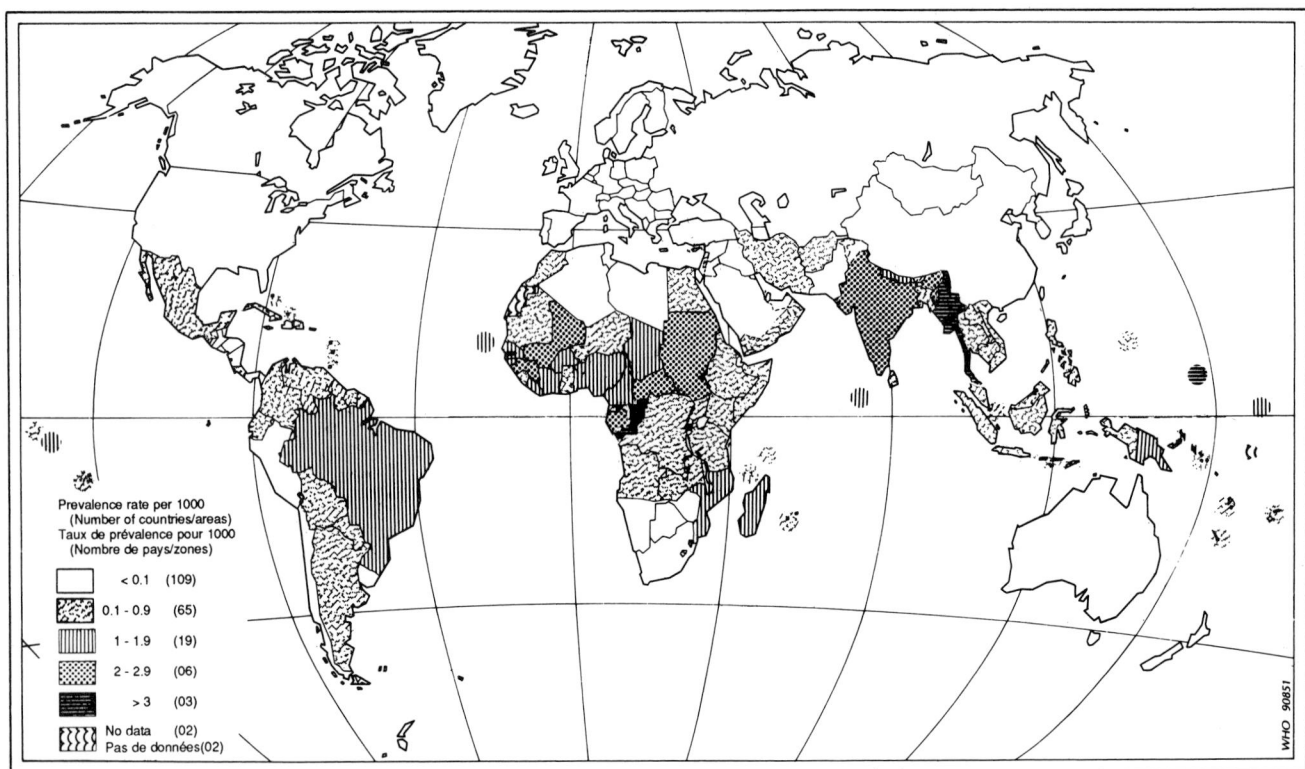

FIGURE 62–1. Prevalence of registered leprosy cases in the world as of 30 September 1990. (From Noordeen SK, Lopez Bravo L, Daumerie D: Global review of multidrug therapy (MDT) in leprosy. World Health Statistics Quarterly 44(1):2, 1991, Map 1. Reprinted by permission.)

ation would make optimal conditions for transmission in both patient and contact more likely.

Experimental infections can be established in the mouse footpad by the inoculation of a single viable *M. leprae*. Immunologically intact mice are partially resistant to leprosy; therefore, it would be expected that a susceptible person could be infected by a single or only a few viable *M. leprae*.

Geographic, ethnic, and socioeconomic factors may contribute to the spread of leprosy by affecting both the number of untreated or ineffectively treated bacillary-positive patients and the opportunity for exposure. In some Asian populations 50% or more of all leprosy patients have the lepromatous form, whereas in Africans this form occurs in only 5 to 10%. Socioeconomic factors are difficult to evaluate, and their relationship to prevalence or clinical severity is unknown. There is no convincing evidence that the prevalence of leprosy is unusually high in chronically malnourished populations, but in special situations nutrition and psychological trauma may influence the progress of the disease. Studies of patients in leprosaria in Malaysia and China showed that both the severity of leprosy and the mortality were increased in World War II during the occupation.

Improved living conditions have probably played an important role in diminishing the prevalence of leprosy. There is, for instance, no other satisfactory explanation for the virtual disappearance of leprosy from northern Europe after the Middle Ages and from Scandinavia in the twentieth century, well before the advent of effective chemotherapeutic agents. If transmission is airborne, the construction of dwellings that provide more spacious sleeping quarters could have contributed in a major way to the disappearance of leprosy in these geographic areas. Consistent with this concept is the existence of grossly inadequate housing in all geographic areas where leprosy is highly endemic now.

The widely presumed hypersusceptibility of children is difficult to establish and may represent only an early selection of susceptible individuals and/or increased exposure to contagious patients. The proportion of children in most samples of all detected patients is approximately 20 to 30%. For example, of the 615 leprosy patients diagnosed in Louisiana between 1855 and 1970, 5% had onset at 0 to 9 years and 19% at 10 to 19 years; also, of 2000 children who lived in one leprosarium in the Philippines prior to the chemotherapeutic era, 23% developed clinical leprosy. Of particular interest in this latter sample was the high proportion (75%) of those with early lesions that healed spontaneously; thus, approximately 6% of all children who were exposed developed active persistent leprosy.

In adults, leprosy is more common in males than in females (2:1 to 3:1), but in children the sex ratio is approximately 1:1. Genetic factors may influence susceptibility and control the form of disease that develops following infection.

PATHOGENESIS AND PATHOLOGY. No toxins have been identified in *M. leprae,* and the pathologic changes are most directly associated with the ability of this bacillus to survive in macrophages or to elicit delayed-type hypersensitivity reactions. If the macrophages of the host digest the bacilli early, either the disease is not detectable or only minor lesions develop. If macrophages are totally incapable of destroying the bacilli, widely disseminated lepromatous leprosy will follow. Survival of *M. leprae* in macrophages and the nature of the tissue response to antigens of the organisms depend on the immune response of the individual. Thus, knowledge of immunity to *M. leprae* is essential for understanding the pathologic changes of leprosy.

Immunity

Lepromin Reaction. The potential of an individual to resist leprosy is assessed by the reaction to an intradermal injection of suspensions of killed *M. leprae*. Classically, such suspensions were derived from lepromatous tissue from patients, but infected tissues from armadillos are now a ready and satisfactory source. The reagent is called "lepromin" and the response, the "lepromin reaction." This reaction, first studied in Japan by Hayashi and extensively evaluated by Mitsuda in 1919, has two components: an early response called the "Fernandez reaction," read 48 hours after inoculation, and a late response, the "Mitsuda reaction," read at 3 or 4 weeks. The Mitsuda reaction correlates most consistently with the immunologic status of the patient and, therefore, is used by clinicians as an aid in the classification of the form of leprosy and in the prognosis of the disease. Mitsuda reactions are strongly positive (more than 5 mm in diameter) in tuberculoid patients, weak or negative (0 to 2 mm) in lepromatous patients, and intermediate (3 to 5 mm) in borderline patients. The reactions are composed of epithelioid cell granulomas and, thus, are a direct assessment of the level of delayed-type hypersensitivity, or cell-mediated immunity (CMI), to antigens of *M. leprae*. It is important for the clinician, and sometimes helpful to the patient, to understand that the lepromin reaction is never diagnostic. The primary reason for this is that Mitsuda reactions are positive in more than 90% of most adult normal populations, even in areas nonendemic for leprosy.

Cell-mediated Immune Responses. Precise mechanisms are still being formulated, but there is abundant evidence that CMI to *M. leprae* is markedly suppressed in lepromatous patients. For example, modifications of the lepromin reaction, using concentrated lepromin, show that macrophages cannot clear *M. leprae* from the skin at the test site in lepromatous patients, whereas in tuberculoid patients the intracellular destruction of leprosy bacilli is highly efficient. Lepromatous patients have varying degrees of suppression of reactions to most skin test antigens, but the reactions are most consistently and most severely depressed to *M. leprae*. This suppression is less pronounced in clinical forms of the disease that are progressively more like tuberculoid leprosy.

There is a gradual decrease in the sensitivity of lymphocytes to *M. leprae,* proceeding from the tuberculoid to the lepromatous forms of the disease. Lymphocyte subsets in lesions of tuberculoid leprosy reveal T-helper lymphocytes distributed within the granulomas, with T-suppressor lymphocytes predominating in the mantle of the granuloma. In lepromatous lesions, T-helper cells are diminished markedly throughout the cellular infiltrates. Delayed-type hypersensitivity in the high resistance forms of leprosy is thought to be conferred by T-helper cells, and cloned T-helper cells recognize several protein antigens of *M. leprae.* Lepromin and the unique antigen of *M. leprae,* phenolic glycolipid-I, have been reported to induce suppressor T-cell activity in lymphocytes from lepromatous patients, but not those from tuberculoid patients; however, this finding is controversial. Thus, *M. leprae* contains both immunostimulating and immunosuppressive antigens and possibly previous sensitization to homologous antigens, or cross-reactive mycobacterial antigens determine the reactivity of T cells to *M. leprae* antigens. Interferon-gamma stimulates similar responses in macrophages from lepromatous patients and normal subjects, suggesting that the immunologic defect in lepromatous leprosy is not in the response of macrophages but in T lymphocytes. Interferon-gamma provokes features of delayed-type hypersensitivity in vivo in lesions of lepromatous leprosy, with apparent decreases in numbers of *M. leprae.* Lepromatous patients show defects in interleukin-2 (IL-2), and IL-2 restores T-lymphocyte proliferation in response to specific antigens.

There is genetic control of the type of leprosy that develops following infection, and this control resides in the HLA class II-linked genes. Ir genes regulating the immune response to *M. leprae* may code for restriction determinants that restrict and regulate the presentation of antigens of *M. leprae* to T-helper and T-suppressor cells. The majority of restriction determinants are thought to be in the polymorphic areas of HLA-DR molecules.

In advanced lepromatous patients, the thymus-dependent areas of lymph nodes and the spleen are heavily replaced by infiltrations of bacilli-laden macrophages, impeding the interactions of antigens and subpopulations of lymphocytes and macrophages and the circulation of T lymphocytes through these areas. This would be expected to contribute secondarily to suppression of CMI in such patients.

Antibody Responses. Immunoglobulin production (IgG, IgA, and IgM) and antibody to mycobacterial antigens are markedly elevated in lepromatous patients, but only slightly, if at all, in tuberculoid leprosy. These antibodies are not protective but do provide a basis for serologic detection of two *M. leprae* specific antigens: phenolic glycolipid-I, and an epitope of the 36kD protein. Nearly all untreated multibacillary leprosy patients have detectable antibody levels. Serologic testing, especially of contacts, may detect leprosy in a preclinical stage, and early treatment of these patients would prevent sequelae and help control the spread of leprosy.

Serologic abnormalities in lepromatous patients include (1) false-positive reactions for syphilis; (2) autoantibodies, e.g., rheumatoid factor, thyroglobulin antibodies, antinuclear antibodies, and cryoglobulinemia; (3) elevated C-reactive protein; and (4) elevated amyloid-related serum protein.

Histopathology. Biopsy specimens should be taken from the active border of well-defined lesions and fixed in neutral buffered 10% formalin or other suitable fixative. The Fite-Faraco staining method best demon-

strates *M. leprae* in tissue sections; however, the Ziehl-Neelsen method is not dependable for staining of *M. leprae* in such sections. The histopathologist must never make a diagnosis of leprosy unless the evidence is convincing. The essential features of the histopathologic changes in the skin are summarized in Table 62–1 and pictorially demonstrated in Figures 62–2 and 62–3.

Tissues other than the skin are affected to varying degrees in leprosy. The most frequently invaded structures are peripheral nerves, especially at sites where the nerves are near the body surface (Fig. 62–4). Lymph nodes in tuberculoid leprosy sometimes contain epithelioid cell granulomas and in lepromatous leprosy may be heavily replaced by bacilli-laden macrophages (Fig. 62–5). The liver and spleen may show similar cellular reactions. In addition to these changes, lepromatous infiltrations may invade the following structures: (1) upper respiratory tract from the nasal mucosa to the larynx; (2) the eye, which may show episcleritis, scleritis, keratitis, iritis, and iridocyclitis; and (3) the testis, in which the interstitial tissue and seminiferous tubules may be replaced completely.

CLINICAL MANIFESTATIONS. The incubation period is usually 2 to 5 years but may be as long as 20 years. There are no well-established prodromal symptoms, but some experienced clinicians may recognize focal paresthesias or itching prior to the appearance of lesions. The nature of the lesions and progress of disease depend on the immune response to *M. leprae.* Only minor strain variations in the etiologic agent have been observed, e.g., growth pattern in the mouse footpad. These strain differences probably do not influence disease patterns, except for those strains that are drug-resistant.

Most clinicians follow the classification schema outlined by Ridley and Jopling. Table 62–1 summarizes the criteria for classifying patients. Accurate classification is more than academic—it is fundamental for establishing treatment programs and for prognosis.

Indeterminate Leprosy. The indeterminate (I) lesion is frequently the earliest manifestation of leprosy and may heal spontaneously, remain unchanged for months or years, or progress toward the tuberculoid or lepromatous forms. Either a single macule or a few poorly defined ones occur in the skin. In more deeply pigmented skin the macule is mildly hypopigmented (Fig. 62–6) and is slightly erythematous in lighter skin. Skin texture, sensation, and sweating may be slightly altered, but these mild changes may be difficult to detect. Peripheral nerves are normal, and skin smears taken from lesions are either negative or contain only a few bacilli. Diagnosis based only on clinical findings is risky; histopathologic evaluations are advised.

Tuberculoid Leprosy. In tuberculoid leprosy (TT) there is a single lesion or a few randomly placed hypopigmented or erythematous lesions in the skin (Fig. 62–7). These lesions may arise de novo or develop from indeterminate macules. Lesions may be macular or infiltrated, but the edges are always sharply demarcated from the surrounding normal skin, and frequently the edges are finely papulated. The size of lesions ranges from less than 1 cm to those that cover entire body

TABLE 62–1. Criteria for Classification of Leprosy

Group	Clinical Features	Histologic Features	Lepromin Reaction (Mitsuda)	Bacillary Density in Skin
Tuberculoid (TT)	Single or a few anesthetic macules or plaques. Borders well defined. Peripheral nerve involvement common.	Epithelioid-lymphocyte granulomas, with or without giant cells, in skin and nerves. No subepidermal clear zone. Bacilli rarely found in nerves.	Strongly positive	Rare
Borderline tuberculoid (BT)	Lesions similar to TT but more numerous. Borders of lesions less distinct. Satellite lesions sometimes present around larger lesions. Peripheral nerve involvement common.	Granulomas similar to TT. Nerves are infiltrated. Bacilli frequently found in nerves.	Positive	Scanty
Borderline (BB)	More lesions than BT. Borders more vague. Satellite lesions often seen. Peripheral nerve involvement common.	Epithelioid cells and histiocytic infiltrations focalized by lymphocytes. Nerves show increased cellularity. Bacilli readily found in nerves.	Negative or weakly positive	Moderate
Borderline lepromatous (BL)	Lesions are numerous and similar to BB. Some nerve damage.	Histiocytic infiltrations show a tendency to evolve toward both epithelioid cells and foamy cells. Lymphocytes present. Nerves have less cellular infiltration. Bacilli plentiful in nerves.	Negative	Heavy
Lepromatous (LL)	Multiple, nonanesthetic, macular or papular, symmetrically distributed lesions. No neural lesions until late. Late complications of madarosis, leonine facies, testicular damage, etc.	Foamy histiocytes containing large numbers of bacilli. Bacilli in walls of blood vessels and arrector muscles. Few or no lymphocytes. Subepidermal clear zone. Numerous bacilli in nerves and perineurium without significant intraneural cellular infiltration.	Negative	Heavy
Indeterminate (I)	Vaguely defined hypopigmented or erythematous macule.	Often indistinguishable from "chronic dermatitis." Lymphocytes and histiocytes around skin appendages and nerves.	Weakly positive or negative	Rare or scanty

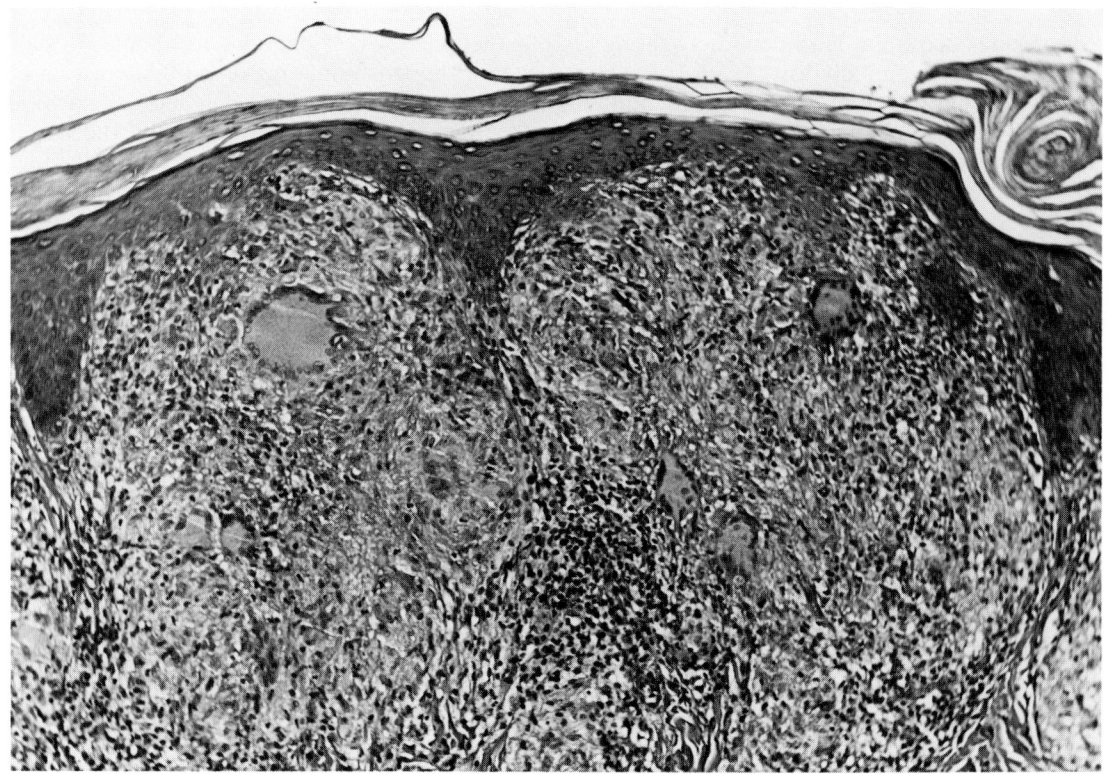

FIGURE 62–2. Tuberculoid leprosy showing a cellular infiltration of epithelioid cells, giant cells, and lymphocytes in the dermis. The infiltration invades the epidermis. (Hematoxylin-eosin stain. × 115.) (Courtesy of the Armed Forces Institute of Pathology. Photograph Neg. No. 72–12465.)

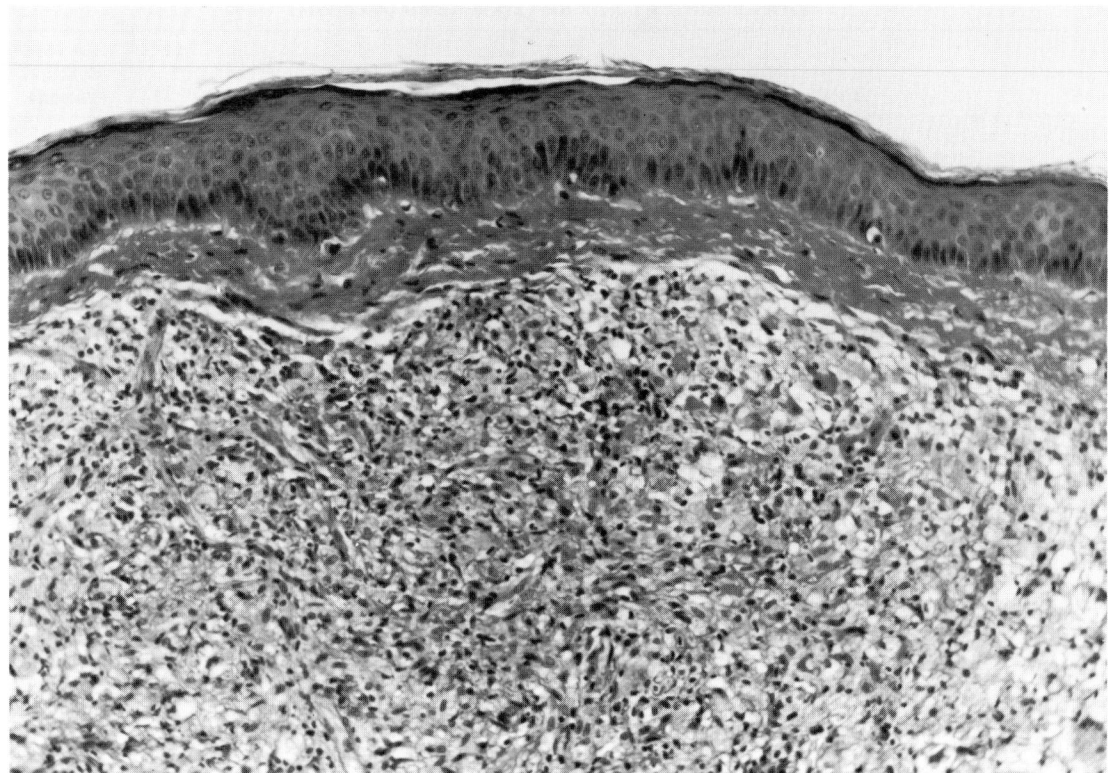

FIGURE 62–3. Lepromatous leprosy showing nearly complete replacement of the dermis by foamy histiocytes (macrophages), leaving a well-defined subepidermal clear zone. (Hematoxylin eosin stain, × 208.) (Courtesy of the Armed Forces Institute of Pathology, Photograph Neg. No. 65–1653.)

regions, such as the cheek, thigh, or buttock. Tuberculoid lesions may heal spontaneously or enlarge gradually, leaving a healed repigmented center.

Within the lesions sensation is impaired, sweating is diminished, and hair is eventually lost.

Damage to peripheral nerve trunks is common in tuberculoid leprosy, and enlarged cutaneous nerves can sometimes be palpated adjacent to or within lesions (Fig. 62–8). Enlarged or tender nerves should alert the clinician to the possibility of leprosy, particularly in endemic areas. Any readily palpable cutaneous nerve is most likely enlarged, but evaluation of nerve trunk size requires experience because of the wide range of normal sizes.

Borderline Leprosy. Borderline leprosy (BB), sometimes called dimorphous or intermediate leprosy, has features of both tuberculoid and lepromatous forms (Fig. 62–9). This is an unstable form of the disease that may evolve toward tuberculoid leprosy by reversal reactions or downgrade toward lepromatous leprosy. The salient features of the subgroups of the borderline form are described in Table 62–1.

Borderline patients are particularly prone to major damage to nerves, often early in the disease. Frequently, the patient consults a physician because of pain in nerves or neurotrophic sensory and/or motor changes, e.g., damaged hands or feet, clawing of the hands (Fig. 62–10), or footdrop. Important nerves most frequently enlarged or tender are the ulnar from the midarm to just distal to the olecranon groove, the median and radial nerves at or above the wrist, and the lateral popliteal just distal to the head of the fibula. Facial palsies lead frequently to exposure keratitis because the eyelids cannot be closed (lagophthalmos), and this is sometimes further aggravated by anesthesia of the cornea if the trigeminal nerve is affected.

Lepromatous Leprosy. The leprosy bacillus multiplies freely in lepromatous patients, and the disease disseminates widely, often before there are striking cutaneous manifestations. Lepromatous leprosy (LL) may evolve from indeterminate or borderline leprosy or may be the first recognized form.

Juvenile Leprosy. In its earliest form, lepromatous leprosy presents as "juvenile leprosy," a clinical entity delineated approximately 50 years ago from observations on large numbers of children in homes for children of leprosy patients in India. This form, also known as prelepromatous leprosy, is difficult to detect and is often unrecognized until a more advanced stage develops. Skin texture is usually not appreciably changed, and the vague macules with indistinct borders are seen only under appropriate lighting, preferably daylight. There are no alterations in sensation or sweating, and acid-fast bacilli are only infrequently seen in smears from the skin. Histopathologic analysis may confirm the diagnosis; if not, the patient should be followed closely until an explanation is found for the mild clinical changes. Failure to diagnose and treat leprosy at this stage often condemns the patient to the development of gross forms of lepromatous leprosy.

Macular Lesions. Early lepromatous leprosy, like the juvenile form, presents as vaguely hypopigmented or

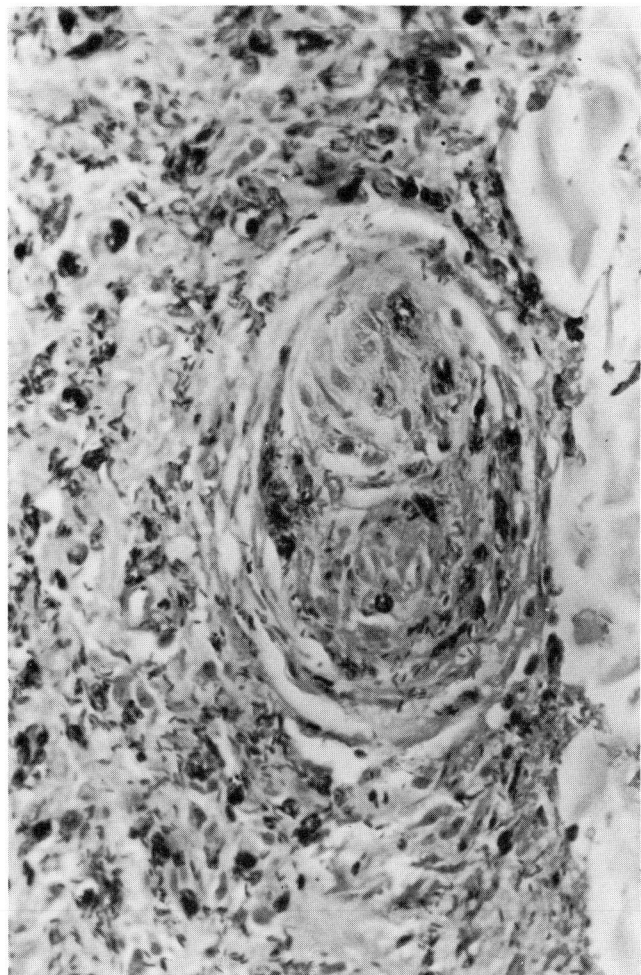

FIGURE 62–4. In lepromatous leprosy, there are large numbers of acid-fast bacilli (black clusters) in histiocytes and within nerves. Note that the dermal nerve is not severely damaged. (Fite-Faraco stain, × 524.) (Courtesy of the Armed Forces Institute of Pathology, Photograph Neg. No. 73–7532.)

slightly erythematous macules with slight or no sensory changes. These macules are small but may coalesce to cover large areas of skin, even most of the body. Clinical diagnosis is again difficult, but skin smears usually demonstrate acid-fast bacilli, and biopsy specimens are diagnostic.

Nodular Changes. If not treated in the macular stage, infiltrations of the skin gradually increase, and nodules may develop. The heaviest infiltrations are in the cooler areas, such as the ears (pinnae), face, exterior surfaces of the extremities, and buttocks (Fig. 62–11). At this stage, nerves are frequently enlarged, with sensory loss in the hands and feet. Eyebrows begin to thin at the lateral margins and may disappear completely. Pubic, axillary, and other body hair (except that on the scalp) is usually diminished.

The testes become atrophic at a late stage, leading to gynecomastia and sterility. The nasal mucosa is thickened frequently, causing a "stuffy" nose, and, if the larynx is infiltrated, the voice may change. There may be lepromas in the conjunctiva and sclera. Punctate or interstitial keratitis of the cornea and other ocular changes may be seen by the loupe and slit lamp.

Lucio Leprosy. Patients of Latin-American ancestry, especially those from Mexico, may develop a diffuse lepromatous form called Lucio leprosy. This is frequently so diffuse that the disease goes unrecognized until there are sensory changes and the eyebrows and other body hair begin to disappear. Advanced forms of Lucio leprosy are complicated by an obstructive vasculitis in the skin, producing dermal infarcts and irregular ulcers (Lucio phenomenon) (Fig. 62–12). These patients are prone to fatal septicemias.

Neuritic Leprosy. In rare cases, leprosy afflicts one or more major nerve trunks, unaccompanied by lesions in the skin. These patients have pain, anesthesia, paresis, or muscular atrophy in the affected area. Nerve trunks may be enlarged and tender. Histopathologically, this form of leprosy is usually either of the borderline or the tuberculoid form and may be confirmed by carefully taken biopsy specimens of a branch of the affected nerve.

Reactions. The course of leprosy, whether treated or not, is often interrupted by acute reactional episodes. These fall into two general categories: reversal reactions and erythema nodosum leprosum.

Reversal Reactions. Reversal reactions are seen in borderline leprosy and represent delayed-type hypersensitivity reactions with an upgrading of CMI to antigens of *M. leprae*. Lesions become erythematous and edematous, and frequently there is an acute neuritis (see Fig. 62–9). The disease tends to move toward the tuberculoid form. By this mechanism, patients, even with the near-lepromatous form, may be self-healing and produce the classic "burned-out" leprosy. The neuritis can cause severe sensory loss, and paralytic deformities such as clawhand, footdrop, and lagophthalmos are classic examples (Fig. 62–13). Completely anergic or polar lepromatous leprosy patients probably never experience reversal reactions spontaneously.

Erythema Nodosum Leprosum (ENL). ENL is an immune-complex reaction seen only in lepromatous and borderline lepromatous patients. Approximately half of all lepromatous patients have ENL after a few months of chemotherapy. There is a rapid onset of tender subcutaneous and intracutaneous nodules that become erythematous (Fig. 62–14). These reactions are accompanied by fever, frequently by iridocyclitis, and sometimes by synovitis. Biopsy specimens of ENL lesions show heavy infiltrations of polymorphonuclear leukocytes and sometimes an intense vasculitis. This reaction leads frequently to extensive ulceration of the skin. Glomerulonephritis sometimes complicates ENL, and secondary amyloidosis is a late sequela in some patients with repeated prolonged episodes.

DIAGNOSIS. The experienced clinician will diagnose most patients with advanced lesions accurately, purely on the physical findings. However, overconfidence may lead to mistaken diagnoses, especially in patients with early lesions. Histopathologic evaluation is strongly recommended for classification and for documentation (see Figs. 62–2 to 62–5).

Leprosy occurs in almost all geographic areas; an awareness of this will lessen the number of mistaken and delayed diagnoses. In the United States the average

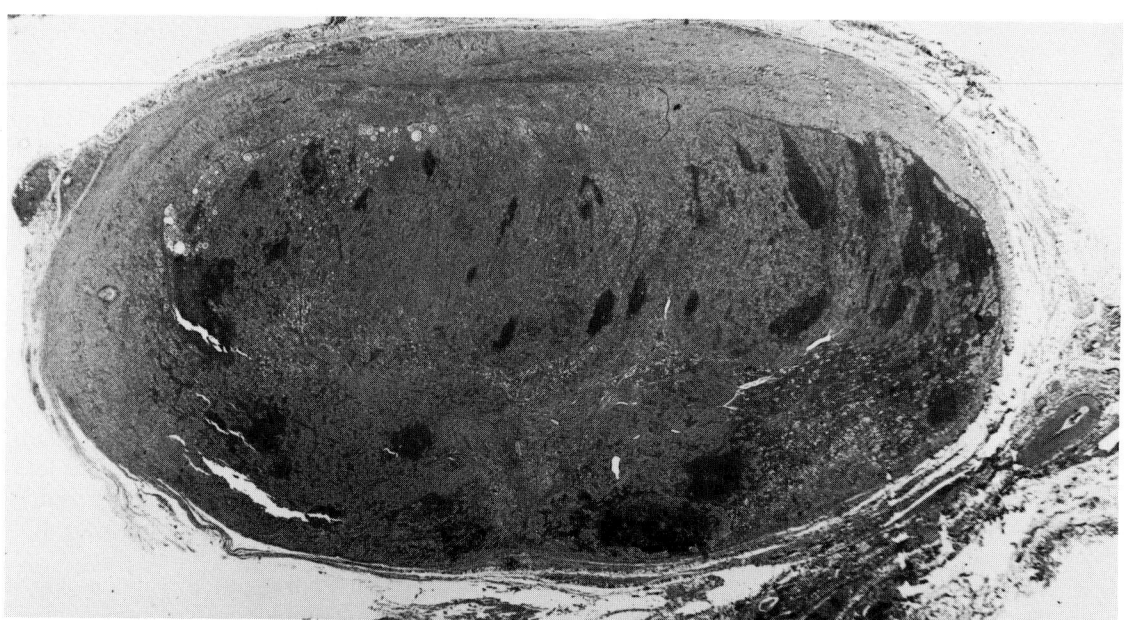

FIGURE 62–5. Section of peripheral lymph node from patient with advanced lepromatous leprosy showing early complete replacement of lymphoid elements. Replacement was by macrophages laden with acid-fast bacilli. (Hematoxylin eosin stain, × 11.) (Courtesy of the Armed Forces Institute of Pathology, Photograph Neg. No. 72–12502.)

delay between the first visit of the patient to a physician and diagnosis is 2 years.

The history may reveal contact with leprosy patients or residence in an endemic area, but many patients are unaware of any specific exposure. Sometimes a footdrop is the presenting symptom. Lepromatous patients may

first consult an otolaryngologist because of a chronic "stuffy" nose.

Physical Findings. Sensory evaluations of skin lesions must be executed carefully. Regional variations in the richness of the nerve supply to different body areas should be noted. For example, there must be extensive damage to dermal nerves of the face before sensory changes can be detected by routine testing; on the other

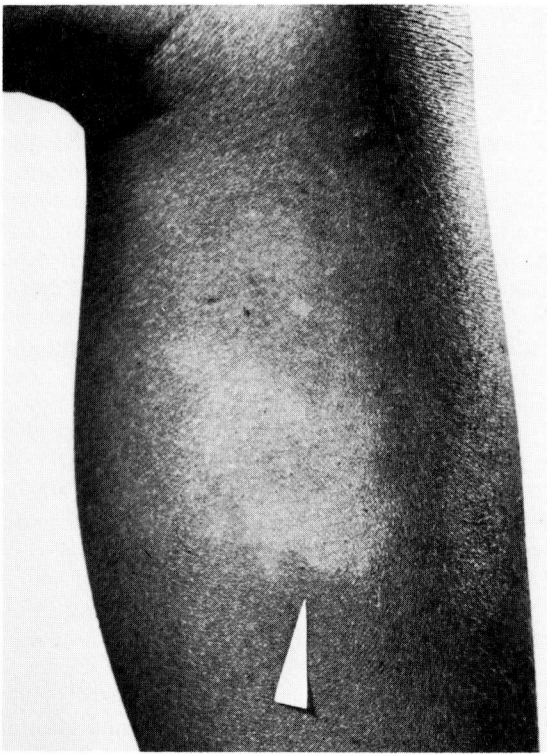

FIGURE 62–6. Lesion of indeterminate leprosy on calf of a Filipino patient. Note that the lesion is macular and mildly hypopigmented, with vaguely defined borders. (Courtesy of the Armed Forces Institute of Pathology, Photograph Neg. No. 74–9029–1.)

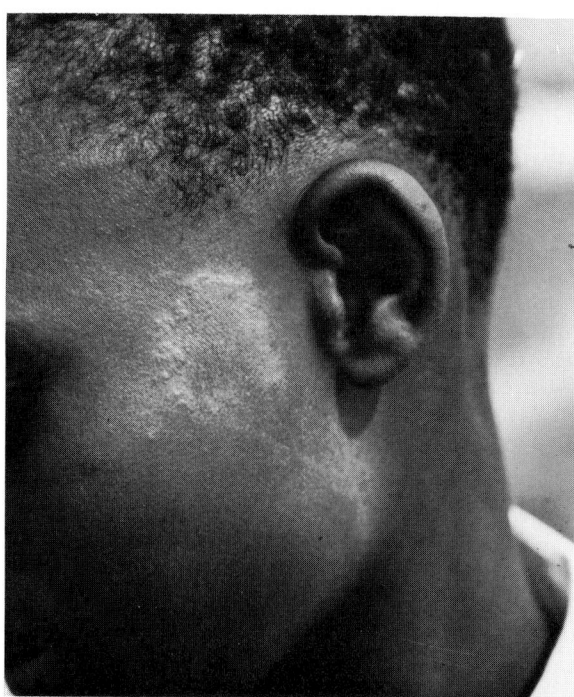

FIGURE 62–7. Early tuberculoid leprosy in an Angolan boy. The lesion is hypopigmented, and the borders are finely papulated. This was the only lesion. (Courtesy of the Armed Forces Institute of Pathology, Photograph Neg. No. 75–15598.)

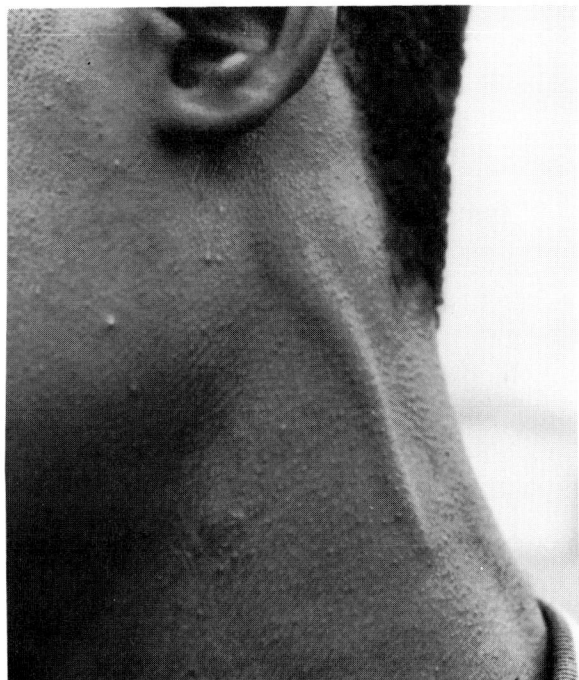

FIGURE 62–8. Enlarged great auricular nerve in a Zairian, with healed lesion of tuberculoid leprosy vaguely visible on adjacent cheek. (Courtesy of the Armed Forces Institute of Pathology, Photograph Neg. No. 77–9359–5.)

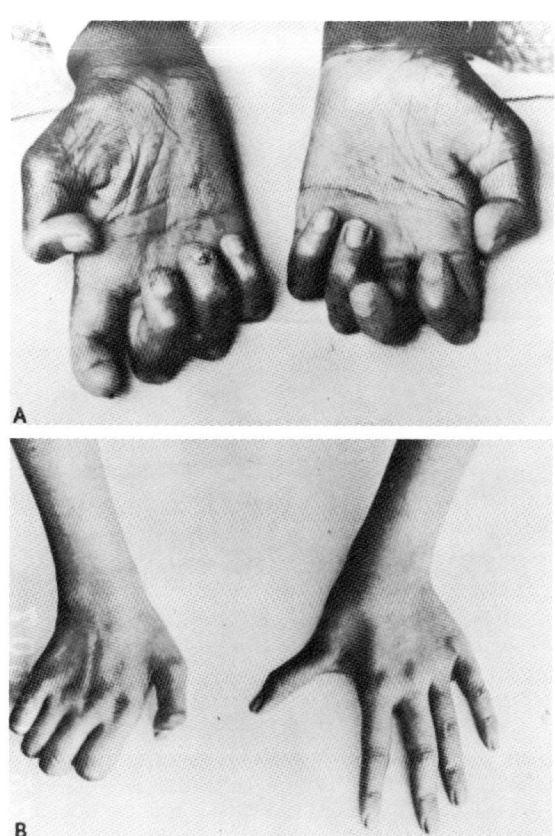

FIGURE 62–10. Clawing of hands in patients with long-standing borderline leprosy. Note wasting of thenar, hypothenar, and interosseous muscles. (Courtesy of the Armed Forces Institute of Pathology, Photograph Neg. No. 75–15807.)

hand, the skin over the knees, elbows, and greater trochanters is normally mildly hypoesthetic. A few fibers of cotton or fine nylon thread are used to test light touch, and heat-cold discrimination is tested by using warm and cold water in test tubes. Changes in spontaneous sweating can be observed directly or following induction with pilocarpine. Hair is preserved in early lesions but is lost in advanced lesions.

Main nerve trunks must be palpated for tenderness and enlargement, and the skin in areas of lesions is palpated for enlarged cutaneous nerves (see Fig. 62–8). Leprosy may be the most common cause of peripheral neuropathy in the world.

Skin Smears. Examination of smears for acid-fast bacilli is an important diagnostic procedure. Smears are taken from the edge of macules or plaques, nodules, ear lobes, and nasal mucosa. Smears from skin are made by lightly squeezing and holding a fold of skin between the thumb and forefinger to avoid blood in the smear and making a short, shallow slit in the skin with a razor or scalpel blade. The instrument is next turned at a right angle to the slit, and the edge of the incision is scraped lightly. The cells and fluid thus obtained are spread on a slide, heat fixed, and stained by the routine Ziehl-Neelsen method used to demonstrate mycobacteria. Evaluation of smears is best performed by those experienced in this procedure. An occasional acid-fast bacillus may, for example, be a harmless contaminant or a saprophytic organism.

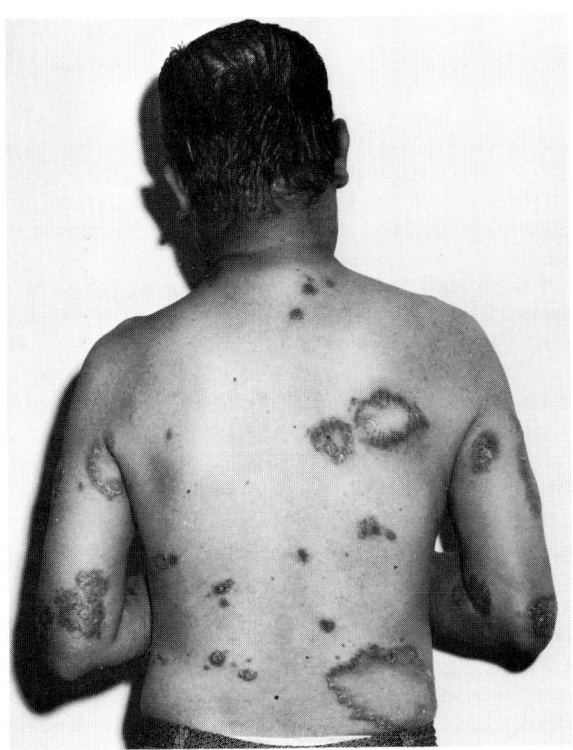

FIGURE 62–9. Borderline leprosy in a Filipino, with multiple erythematous annular lesions, plaques, and nodules. The lesions are in mild reversal reaction, and peripheral nerves were painful and tender. (Courtesy of the Armed Forces Institute of Pathology, Photograph Neg. No. 74–8485–2.)

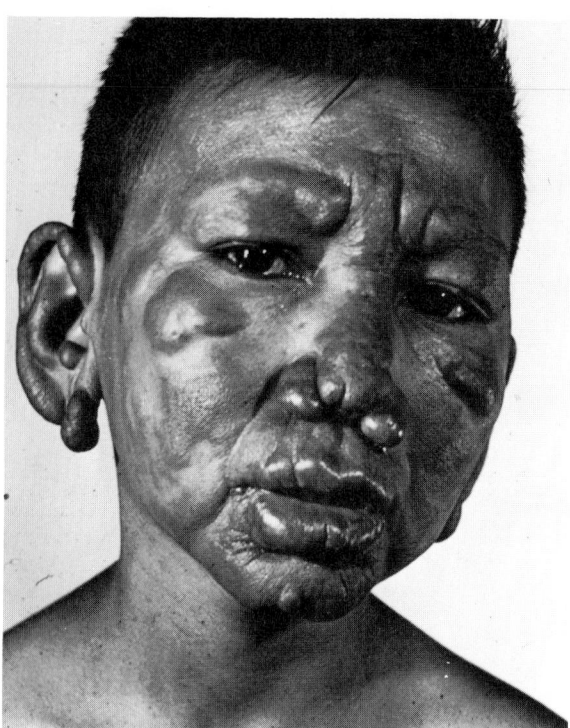

FIGURE 62–11. Advanced lepromatous leprosy in a Filipino adolescent, with nodular thickening of skin and loss of eyebrows. The heaviest infiltrations are over the central part of the face and ears—the coolest areas. (Courtesy of the Armed Forces Institute of Pathology, Photograph Neg. No. 77–9359–2.)

Differential Diagnosis. The differential diagnosis of leprosy is extensive, and the following partial lists serve only to stimulate the clinician to exercise every diagnostic precaution. Macular changes in pigmentation may be seen in scars, birthmarks, actinic dermatitis, dermatophytosis, and filariasis (especially streptocerciasis). Some infiltrated lesions of the skin that can resemble leprosy are leishmaniasis, granuloma annulare, granuloma multiforme, lupus erythematosus, psoriasis, pityriasis rosea, sarcoidosis, and neurofibromatosis. Periph-

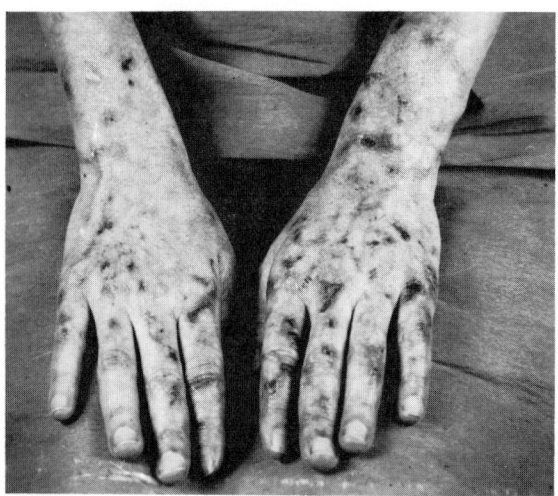

FIGURE 62–12. Lucio leprosy in patient of Mexican origin at USPHS Hospital, Carville, Louisiana, showing angular ulcers (Lucio phenomenon). (Courtesy of the Armed Forces Institute of Pathology, Photograph Neg. No. 74–9029–6.)

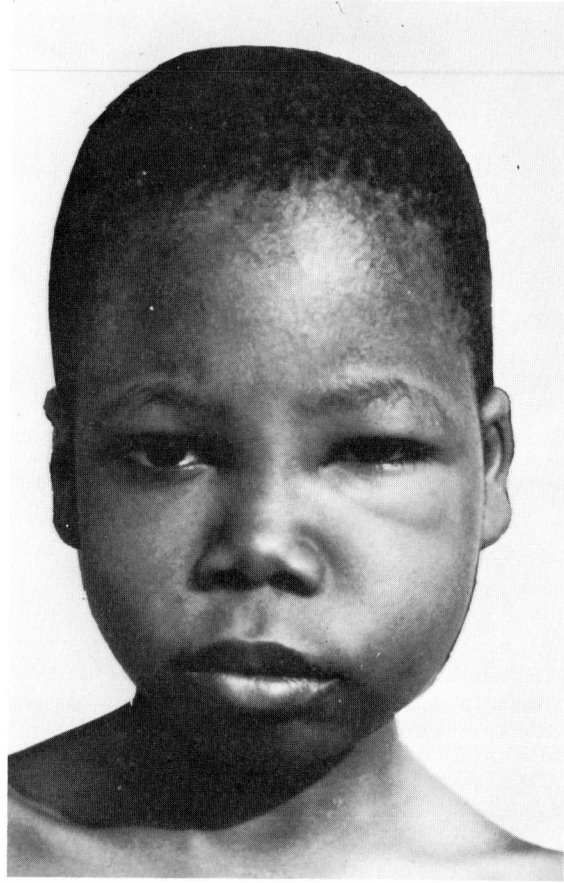

FIGURE 62–13. Zairian boy with borderline tuberculoid leprosy in reversal reaction. Left side of face is swollen, and there is a mild palsy resulting from damage to facial nerve. Patient responded rapidly to corticosteroid therapy. (Courtesy of the Armed Forces Institute of Pathology, Photograph Neg. No. 77–9359[A]–1.)

eral neuropathies that can be confused with leprosy are carpal tunnel syndrome, syringomyelia, lead toxicity, diabetes mellitus, primary amyloidosis of nerves, familial hypertrophic neuropathy, and congenital insensitivity to pain.

Serologic and Skin Tests. There are as yet no widely accepted skin or serologic tests for leprosy; however, this is an area of active study. The apparently unique phenolic glycolipid recently isolated from *M. leprae* is a promising reagent for the development of a specific serologic test. However, results to date, suggest that only patients with LL and BL disease are regularly positive. At least 50% of TT and BT patients are negative. Thus, antiphenolic glycolipid assays are not efficient in the diagnosis of nonlepromatous disease. The lepromin test is useless in the diagnosis of leprosy. Sera from lepromatous patients are often falsely positive for syphilis.

TREATMENT. The management of the patient with leprosy involves two primary principles: (1) specific chemotherapy for active disease, and (2) the prevention and correction of deformities or disability. Treatment should be on an outpatient basis. Patients should not be isolated and should be hospitalized only for complications, e.g., severe reactions or correction of deformities.

Chemotherapy. The three most commonly used drugs

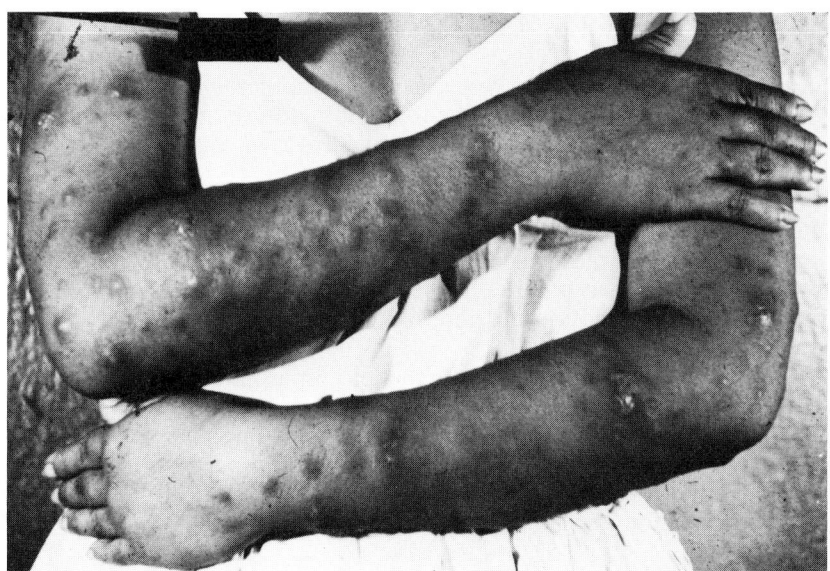

FIGURE 62–14. Erythema nodosum leprosum in a Filipino girl with lepromatous leprosy. (Courtesy of the Armed Forces Institute of Pathology, Photograph Neg. No. 74–9029–7.)

are dapsone (diaminodiphenylsulfone or DDS), clofazimine (Lamprene), and rifampin. Until recently, monotherapy with dapsone was used routinely; however, dapsone-resistant strains of *M. leprae* are being detected with alarming frequency. Secondary dapsone resistance has been reported in up to 9.3% of patients at risk and primary resistance in as many of 62.5% of patients presenting for the first time with leprosy.

Multiple Drug Regimens. Multibacillary patients, for the purpose of establishing therapeutic regimens, are defined as those with skin smears that are positive for acid-fast bacilli at one or more sites.

Field trials indicate that multiple drug therapy is effective, and relapse rates are at an acceptably low level. Treatment regimens are being changed, and multiple drug therapy is required. The current regimen recommended for adults by a WHO Study Group is as follows: (1) for multibacillary leprosy (BB, BL, and LL), dapsone 100 mg daily (self-administered), clofazimine 50 mg daily (self-administered), clofazimine 300 mg monthly (supervised), and rifampin 600 mg monthly (supervised); and (2) for paucibacillary leprosy (BT and TT), dapsone 100 mg daily (self-administered) for 6 months and rifampin 600 mg monthly (supervised) for 6 months. The regimen for multibacillary leprosy should be continued for at least 2 years or until skin smears are negative. Many clinicians will wish to continue the regimen for much longer periods, especially for the LL patient. Paucibacillary patients should be seen every 6 to 12 months to assure that there is no relapse.

Combined drug therapy should minimize the possibility of drug-resistant strains and perhaps eliminate "persisting" *M. leprae*. Persisting organisms are viable bacilli that can be isolated in small numbers from patients who are responding to treatment. These persisting organisms are drug sensitive when tested in the mouse footpad and may account for relapses when treatment is continued. Persisting *M. leprae* have been detected after as long as 5 years of rifampin, 6 years of clofazimine, and 12 years of dapsone therapy.

Dapsone Regimen. Dapsone monotherapy is never

recommended; however, because dapsone is relatively safe, stable, and inexpensive, it will probably continue to be used in monotherapy in many parts of the world. This drug is bacteriostatic and is given to adults at a dosage of 100 mg daily. The custom of following a schedule of graded drug increases is no longer in vogue. The effect of dapsone on *M. leprae* is slow, requiring 3 to 6 months treatment to render bacilli noninfectious for the mouse footpad. The duration of treatment is variable and there are no guidelines. The suggested duration for paucibacillary leprosy is 18 months after disease activity is no longer detectable. For multibacillary disease many clinicians treat the patient for life. An occasional patient is allergic to dapsone, resulting in a severe desquamating dermatitis. Other uncommon side reactions are anemia, hepatitis, peripheral neuropathy, and psychosis.

Clofazimine (Lamprene). This is a riminophenazine dye that has both antileprosy and anti-inflammatory activity, especially against ENL. When used as monotherapy, the adult dose is 100 to 300 mg daily; however, monotherapy is not recommended. The lesser amounts may be used for maintenance antileprosy therapy, whereas the larger doses may be required in patients with ENL. The major side reactions are hyperpigmentation of the skin and gastrointestinal manifestations. Occasionally, patients develop an adynamic ileus. These side reactions are reversible on discontinuing or lowering the daily dosage. Strains of *M. leprae* resistant to clofazimine are rare.

Rifampin. This drug is relatively rapidly bactericidal to *M. leprae*, rendering a highly positive lepromatous patient noninfectious within 1 week. Monotherapy with rifampin is not recommended.

Assessment of Chemotherapy. The efficacy of chemotherapy is readily assessed by serial evaluations of skin smears to determine the morphologic index (MI). The MI is the percentage of acid-fast bacilli uniformly stained by standardized procedures. With effective therapy, the bacilli first are stained irregularly, then become granular, and finally fragmented. Histopathologic evaluations also demonstrate this phenomenon, but in a less quantitative manner.

The physician unfamiliar with current chemotherapy of leprosy is advised to consult the relevant literature or a specialist in the field because of rapidly changing guidelines based on updated results of trials.

Treatment of Reactions. Reactions in leprosy are medical emergencies; however, early treatment will lessen the chances of developing deformities or disability. The patient is hospitalized if the reaction is severe. Specific chemotherapy is not interrupted during reactions.

Reversal Reactions. Reversal reactions in isolated skin lesions, without nerve involvement, are usually of little consequence, but the patient should be followed closely for signs of damage to nerves. Patients with painful, tender nerves should be assessed for impaired function of muscles. Analgesics are given, and the affected part is put at rest. If pain is severe and there is paresis or paralysis of muscles, corticosteroids in high dosage must be started, e.g., prednisone 40 to 60 mg daily. After clinical improvement the drug is tapered to a minimal effective dose until the reaction subsides. Appropriate physiotherapy must be instituted early.

Patients who are first seen with paralytic deformities, e.g., lagophthalmos or footdrop, of relatively recent onset but who are not currently in acute reaction, should be given a trial of corticosteroid therapy and physiotherapy. Some of these patients will recover function of the affected part.

Erythema Nodosum Leprosum. Mild ENL is treated with analgesics; more severe reactions require either thalidomide or corticosteroid therapy. Thalidomide is the drug of choice but is teratogenic and must not be administered to female patients who could potentially be pregnant. The initial adult dose of thalidomide is 100 to 400 mg daily, which is then tapered to the minimal effective dose. Corticosteroids, if employed, are given as for reversal reactions. If long-term corticosteroid therapy is necessary, some clinicians prescribe an alternate-day regimen to minimize side effects.

Clofazimine is effective against ENL and does not have the disadvantages of either thalidomide or corticosteroids. However, the anti-inflammatory action of clofazimine is not manifest until after 4 to 6 weeks of continuous use. Dosage is adjusted to the minimal effective level.

Iridocyclitis often accompanies ENL and requires emergency measures. Topical corticosteroids should be added to the systemic anti-inflammatory regimens and, if possible, ophthalmologic consultation obtained.

Management of Neurotrophic Complications. This is an extensive and complex problem, but there are several basic principles that can be followed: (1) the disease process should be explained to the patient so that insensitive hands, feet, and eyes are not unduly exposed to trauma; (2) the patient should be taught self-examination of the hands and feet and instructed to report the earliest signs of inflammation or trauma to the physician for treatment; (3) adequate footwear and gloves or other protective devices should be made available to those with insensitive or deformed feet and hands; (4) appropriate and early physiotherapy must be instituted; and (5) the patient should be referred to the appropriate specialist for evaluation and correction of deformity (Chapter 13).

Prognosis. Without chemotherapy the prognosis is potentially poor, except for those with limited and self-healing disease. Borderline and tuberculoid patients suffer mutilations frequently, and patients with the borderline form can downgrade to the lepromatous form. In lepromatous leprosy the disease is progressive; the patient frequently becomes debilitated and may die of laryngeal obstruction or renal failure. Blindness may result from exposure keratitis or repeated episodes of iridocyclitis. The patient with deformity is frequently stigmatized and cannot be gainfully employed. With effective chemotherapy and control of reactions, prognosis is good in nearly all patients. If treatment is started early, prognosis is excellent and mutilations can be prevented.

PREVENTION AND CONTROL. The control of leprosy is based on the early detection and treatment of patients. Candidate antileprosy vaccines are now under development, and some are being tested under field conditions. These vaccines are composed of either heat-killed *M. leprae* alone or in combination with live BCG. Heat-killed *M. leprae* plus BCG is known to increase CMI to *M. leprae* in lepromatous patients and has an immunotherapeutic effect. A highly immunogenic cell wall protein-peptidoglycan complex of *M. leprae* offers promise for a purified vaccinogenic product for leprosy. Because of the potentially long incubation periods of leprosy, the efficacy of candidate leprosy vaccines will probably not be known before the year 2000. Chemoprophylaxis with sulfone may be used for individuals who are at risk; however, wide application is not feasible.

BIBLIOGRAPHY

Binford CH, Meyers WM, Walsh GP: Leprosy—state of the art. JAMA 247:2283–2292, 1982.

Edwards D, Kirkpatrick CH: The immunology of mycobacterial diseases. Am Rev Respir Dis 134:1062–1071, 1986.

Fritschi EP: Reconstructive Surgery in Leprosy. Bristol, John Wright and Sons, 1971.

Gaylord H, Brennan PJ: Leprosy and the leprosy bacillus: Recent developments in characterization of antigens and immunology of the disease. Ann Rev Microbiol 41:645–675, 1987.

Hastings RC (ed.): Leprosy. New York, Churchill Livingstone, 1985.

Meyers WM, Binford CH, McDougall AC, et al.: Histopathologic responses in 60 multibacillary leprosy patients inoculated with autoclaved *Mycobacterium leprae* and live BCG. Int J Lepr 56:302–309, 1988.

Meyers WM, Binford CH, Walsh GP, et al.: Animal models in leprosy. *In* Microbiology 1984. Washington, American Society for Microbiology, 1984, pp 307–311.

Ridley DS: Skin Biopsy in Leprosy. Histological Interpretation and Clinical Application. 2nd ed. Documenta Geigy, Basel, CIBA-GEIGY, 1985.

Ridley DS, Jopling WH: Classification of leprosy according to immunity. A five group system. Int J Lepr 34:255–273, 1966.

63. ATYPICAL MYCOBACTERIA SKIN INFECTIONS

Wayne M. Meyers

Robert Koch identified *Mycobacterium tuberculosis* in 1882 and thus established the tubercle bacillus as the "typical" mycobacterium. There are two major types of infection of the skin by *M. tuberculosis*: primary tuberculosis, such as is seen occasionally in those who perform autopsies on patients with tuberculosis (prosector's paronychia), and reinfection tuberculosis, as characterized by the common lesion of lupus vulgaris. Approximately 75% of patients with lupus vulgaris have tuberculosis of other organs (Chapter 61); therefore, this is a common problem in some developing countries.

In the decades following the identification of *M. tuberculosis*, mycobacteria were isolated that differed from *M. tuberculosis*, and these became known as "atypical" mycobacteria.

In 1954, Timpe and Runyon first classified the variety of atypical mycobacteria into four groups on the basis of their growth characteristics (Table 63–1). Each of the Runyon groups is composed of multiple species. The following species or species complexes of atypical mycobacteria causing lesions in the skin have been reported: *M. leprae, M. ulcerans, M. marinum, M. kansasii, M. avium-intracellulare, M. scrofulaceum, M. fortuitum* complex, *M. haemophilum, M. gordonae,* and *M. szulgai.*

Leprosy, caused by *M. leprae,* is a common infection of the skin afflicting perhaps 15 million people (Chapter 62).

63.1. *MYCOBACTERIUM ULCERANS* INFECTION (Buruli Ulcer)

DEFINITION AND ETIOLOGY. *Mycobacterium ulcerans* is a slow-growing mycobacterium that infects the skin and subcutaneous tissues, giving rise to indolent ulcers. *M. ulcerans* grows optimally on routine mycobacteriologic media at 32C and elaborates a necrotizing immunosuppressive cytotoxin. Large ulcers almost cer-

tainly caused by *M. ulcerans* were first described by Cook in Uganda in 1897; however, the etiologic agent was not isolated and characterized until 1948 in Australia by MacCallum and associates.

Mycobacteria biochemically similar to *M. ulcerans* have been isolated from the environment in Zaire, but they are not pathogenic for mice, the usual animal model.

EPIDEMIOLOGY. The source of *M. ulcerans* in nature is not known; however, typical infections were reported recently in koalas in southeastern Australia by Mitchell, et al. Because all major endemic foci are in swampy terrain or subtropical countries, environmental factors are thought to play an essential role in the survival of the organism. The disease is rarely transmitted from patient to patient. Infection is probably most frequently the result of the introduction by trauma of *M. ulcerans* from surface-contaminated skin. The inciting trauma has been as slight as a hypodermic needle puncture or as severe as gunshot or exploding land mine wounds. Individuals of all ages are affected, but the highest frequencies of infection are in those in the second and third decades. The largest concentrations of patients are in Uganda and Zaire, but there are significant foci in nearly all countries in Central Africa, in Southeast Asia, and in Australia, and there are a few patients in Central and South America.

PATHOGENESIS AND PATHOLOGY. Following inoculation into the skin, *M. ulcerans* proliferates and elaborates a toxin that causes necrosis of the dermis, panniculus, and deep fascia. Early lesions are closed, but as the necrosis spreads, the overlying dermis and epidermis become infarcted and eventually ulcerate, leaving undermined edges and a necrotic slough in the base of the ulcer. Histopathologic sections reveal a contiguous coagulation necrosis of the deep dermis and panniculus, with destruction of nerves, appendages, and blood vessels. There is interstitial edema. Clumps of extracellular acid-fast bacilli are plentiful and are limited frequently to the base of the ulcer and adjacent necrotic subcutaneous tissue. Bone is occasionally involved. In active lesions, inflammatory cells are conspicuously few, presumably as a result of the immunosuppressive activity of the toxin. With healing, there is a granulomatous response, and eventually the ulcerated area is replaced by a depressed scar.

CLINICAL MANIFESTATIONS. Lesions are usually single and begin as firm, painless, nontender, movable, subcutaneous nodules 1 to 2 cm in diameter. Many patients complain of itching in the lesion. In 1 or 2 months, the nodule becomes fluctuant and ulcerates, leaving an undermined edge that often extends 15 cm or more (Fig. 63–1). The skin adjacent to the lesion, and often that of the entire corresponding limb, may be indurated by edema. Ordinarily, there is no regional lymphadenopathy or systemic manifestations. Ulcers may remain small and heal without treatment or may spread rapidly, undermining the skin over large areas, even an entire leg, thigh, or arm. Rarely, important structures, such as an eye, may be lost. Most lesions heal spontaneously but frequently leave extensive scarring, with deformity and lymphedema (Fig. 63–2).

TABLE 63–1. Classification of Atypical Mycobacteria Causing Disease in Skin of Man

Runyon Group	Pigmentation	Growth Rate	Species
I	Photochromogens[a]	Slow	*M. kanasasii* *M. marinum*
II	Scotochromogens[b]	Slow	*M. scrofulaceum* *M. szulgai*
III	Nonphotochromogens[c]	Slow	*M. avium* *M. intracellulare*
IV	Variable	Rapid	*M. fortuitum* *M. chelonae*
Other[d]		Slow	*M. ulcerans*

[a]Pigment produced only on exposure to light.
[b]Pigment produced in dark or light.
[c]Nonpigmented.
[d]*M. ulcerans* has not been classified in the Runyon system.

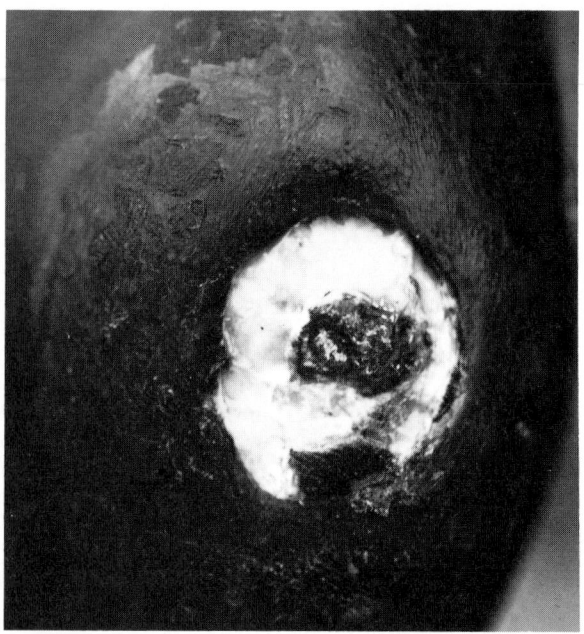

FIGURE 63–1. *Mycobacterium ulcerans* infection in the deltoid area of a Zairian boy. The patient presented with this lesion 3 months after a hypodermic injection at this site. Note induration of adjacent skin and undermined border of the ulcer with a necrotic base. (Courtesy of the Armed Forces Institute of Pathology, Photograph Neg. No. 76–11034–5.)

DIAGNOSIS. Smears from the necrotic base of ulcers stained by the Ziehl-Neelsen method usually reveal clumps of acid-fast bacilli. Biopsy specimens that include the necrotic base and the undermined edge of lesions with subcutaneous tissue are nearly always diagnostic. *M. ulcerans* can be cultured from a high percentage of lesions, either from exudates or biopsy specimens, but visible growth often requires 6 to 8 weeks of incubation at 32C. There are no specific serologic or skin tests.

TREATMENT. Preulcerative lesions are excised en bloc, and the skin is closed primarily. Ulcers are widely excised and skin grafts applied. Continuous local heating to 40C, e.g., by circulating water jackets, will promote healing without excision. Amputation of limbs is rarely

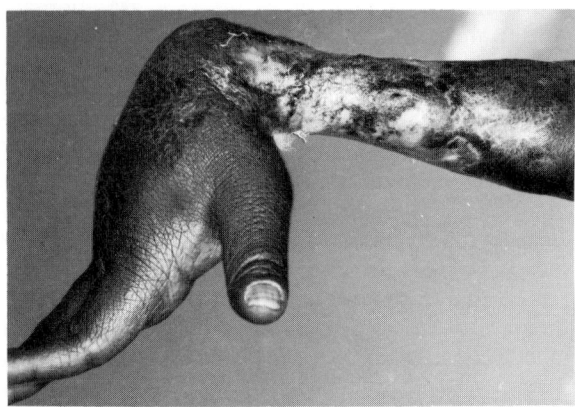

FIGURE 63–2. Healed *Mycobacterium ulcerans* infection of the forearm and wrist. Scar has caused contraction deformity with subluxation of the wrist and lymphedema of the hand. (Courtesy of the Armed Forces Institute of Pathology, Photograph Neg. No. 65–2982–1.)

necessary. Rifampin promotes healing of preulcerative lesions or early ulcers but is not effective for extensive lesions. Appropriate physiotherapy is important when contracture deformities are likely to develop.

PREVENTION. No effective prophylactic measures have been demonstrated, but bacille Calmette-Guérin (BCG) vaccination may produce protection or delay of onset for approximately 6 months.

63.2. *MYCOBACTERIUM MARINUM* INFECTION

DEFINITION AND ETIOLOGY. *M. marinum* was first identified in 1926 in marine fish in an aquarium in Philadelphia but was first isolated from a group of patients who had used a common swimming pool in Sweden in 1954. These lesions are thus often known as swimming pool granulomas. *M. marinum*, also known as *M. balnei,* grows on routine mycobacteriologic media incubated at 30 to 32C, but not at 37C.

EPIDEMIOLOGY. *M. marinum* is presumed to be ubiquitous, and lesions have been reported in many countries. Many patients have been in contaminated swimming pools. The infection is acquired occasionally from tropical fish aquaria or by fishermen or those who work or swim in bayous, rivers, or coastal or brackish water. The organisms are introduced into the skin at sites of trauma. Person-to-person transmission is not known. In nature, water-dwelling animals become infected and shed *M. marinum* into water. The "water flea" *Daphnia* can serve as a host. Because of the cross-reactivity of *M. marinum* with antigens from many other mycobacteria, epidemiologic studies based on skin testing are not valid.

PATHOGENESIS AND PATHOLOGY. Incubation periods vary slightly but are usually from 1 to 6 weeks. The low temperature growth requirement limits infection to the skin, usually to the area of inoculation, but occasionally there is regional proximal lymphatic spread resembling that seen in sporotrichosis. There are rare instances of disseminated infections in immunosuppressed patients. Histopathologically, in early lesions there are pyogranulomatous infiltrations, but in older lesions there are tuberculoid granulomas with caseation necrosis. Acid-fast bacilli are few and are usually located in the granulomas.

CLINICAL MANIFESTATIONS. The earliest sign is erythema with tenderness at the inoculation site, followed by a papule or violaceous nodule that ulcerates and drains pus (Fig. 63–3). Older lesions may be verrucous. The cutaneous surfaces of the hands, elbows, and knees are preferred sites, and bursae of the elbows and knees are sometimes invaded. A sporotrichoid spread of lesions is uncommon. Spontaneous cure in 3 months to several years is the rule, but lesions have persisted for up to 17 years.

DIAGNOSIS. Histopathologic findings are not specific, even when acid-fast bacilli are seen in tissue sections, making cultivation of the organism necessary for diagnosis. There are no serologic tests, and skin tests are nonspecific.

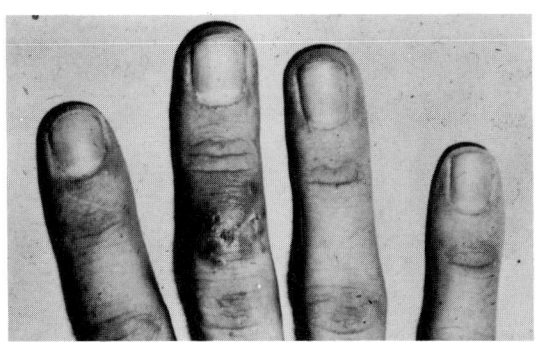

FIGURE 63–3. *Mycobacterium marinum* infection, "swimming pool granuloma," on the dorsum of the middle finger. There is an ulcer in the center of the nodule. (Courtesy of the Armed Forces Institute of Pathology, Photograph Neg. No. 75–12395.)

TREATMENT. Most lesions will heal spontaneously, but because of the protracted course of the disease, many patients seek therapy. When possible, surgical excision or curettage and electrodesiccation have been recommended. Antituberculous drugs, even with multidrug regimens, are not regularly successful. Treatment with tetracycline, 1 to 2 g daily, or minocycline, 100 mg twice daily, plus sulfamethoxazole, 800 mg twice daily, and trimethoprim, 60 mg twice daily, sometimes leads to healing of the cutaneous lesions. Others recommend combined therapy with rifampin and ethambutol until the lesion is healed.

PREVENTION. Adequate maintenance of swimming pools interrupts epidemics, but sporadic cases can be prevented only by avoiding potentially contaminated sources.

63.3. MYCOBACTERIUM KANSASII INFECTION

DEFINITION AND ETIOLOGY. *Mycobacterium kansasii* commonly infects the lungs (Chapter 61.2), and only occasionally causes lesions of the skin. *M. kansasii* grows at 37C.

EPIDEMIOLOGY. In nature, *M. kansasii* is found most frequently in tap water but occasionally in cows and swine. The organism apparently has a worldwide distribution, but in the United States, it is most common in the Midwest and Southwest. Pulmonary infections are acquired by inhalation and are probably transmissible. The mode of primary infection of the skin is unknown but is most likely by direct inoculation.

PATHOGENESIS AND PATHOLOGY. The incubation period is unknown, but 1 reported lesion developed 1 year after specific trauma. Histopathologic sections show granulomas with caseation, and acid-fast bacilli are usually scarce. Immunosuppressed patients with primary infections elsewhere sometimes have secondary spread to the skin. These lesions show a variable acute and chronic inflammatory response, and acid-fast bacilli may be numerous.

CLINICAL MANIFESTATIONS. The primary lesion in the skin may be a single nodule or there may be sporotrichoid spread. Some nodular lesions are preceded by tender erythematous swellings. Lesions have been reported to last as long as 22 years. Patients with disseminated disease with spread to the skin have erythema, induration, abscesses, cellulitis, and ulcers.

DIAGNOSIS. Diagnosis requires cultivation of *M. kansasii* from exudates or biopsy specimens. There are no serologic reactions or specific skin tests.

TREATMENT. Chemotherapy should be based on results of in vitro sensitivity tests on the isolated *M. kansasii*. Primary lesions have healed after 4 months of combined therapy with isoniazid, para-aminosalicylate, and streptomycin. Rifampin is frequently used in combined regimens.

PREVENTION. No prophylactic measures are known.

63.4. INFECTION BY "RAPID-GROWING" MYCOBACTERIA

DEFINITION AND ETIOLOGY. This group of mycobacteria grows within 5 days, frequently in 48 hours, even on many of the routine bacteriologic media, at 32 to 37C. The nomenclature of the "rapid growers" is imprecise, and some employ the term *M. fortuitum* complex for all members of this group, whereas others separate them into 2 species—*M. fortuitum* and *M. chelonae*. The two species are now divided into 5 subgroups: *M. fortuitum* into 3 biovariants, and *M. chelonae* into the subspecies *abscessus* and *chelonae*. (Note: *M. chelonae* was formerly spelled *M. chelonei*.)

EPIDEMIOLOGY. These ubiquitous mycobacteria are common saprophytes in soil and water. *M. fortuitum* was first identified as the cause of an injection abscess in 1938 in Brazil. Penetrating wounds of the skin, including surgical incisions and hypodermic injections, are frequent methods of introducing these infectious agents. These organisms may cause disease in amphibians, rodents, and other animals, but there are no epidemiologic data to suggest that these animals are sources of human infection. Infections have been traced to hot tubs and hydrotherapy pools.

PATHOGENESIS AND PATHOLOGY. Incubation periods range from 2 to 7 months. The earliest clinical lesion is a fluctuant abscess that usually forms 1 or more sinuses that drain pus. A study of specimens in The Registry of Geographic Pathology has shown a striking and unique histopathologic reaction to this group of organisms. The reaction is characterized by a pyogranulomatous response containing clear spaces. These clear spaces are spherical, vary from 20 to 300 μm in diameter, and contain acid-fast bacilli (Fig. 63–4). The bacilli are sometimes clumped and aligned and at other times randomly scattered. The surrounding inflammatory cells are a mixture of neutrophils, epithelioid cells, histiocytes, and Langhan's giant cells. At the perimeter of these inflammatory foci are varying amounts of scar tissue with lymphocytes, plasma cells, and Russell bodies. The number of neutrophils varies. In some lesions, they predominate and form abscesses; in other foci, the

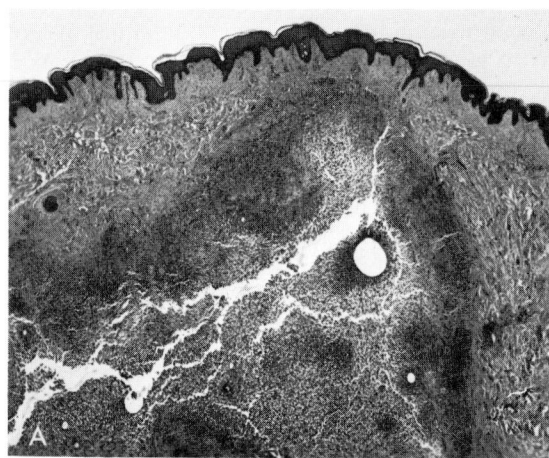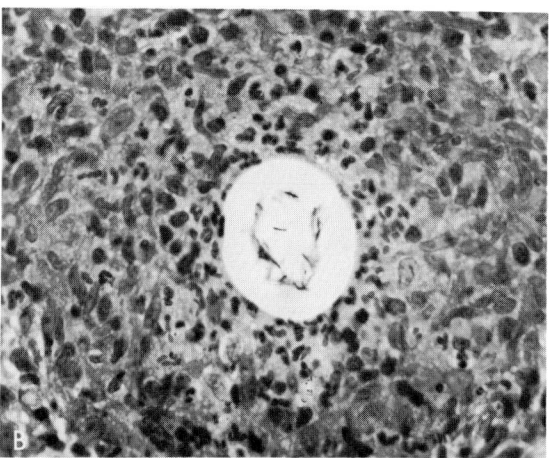

FIGURE 63–4. Skin from patient with *M. chelonae* infection. *A*, There is a large area of necrosis, suppuration, and granulomatous reaction within the dermis. At this level, the process has not penetrated to the surface of the skin, but in other areas, sinuses have already formed. Within the necrotic area are numerous scattered, circumscribed, spherical vacuoles in which special stains reveal acid-fast bacilli. (H & E stain, × 25.) (Courtesy of the Armed Forces Institute of Pathology, Photograph Neg. No. 81–13874.) *B*, Higher magnification of a vacuole. It is circumscribed, spherical, surrounded by a mixed suppurative and granulomatous reaction, and contains discrete and clumped acid-fast bacilli in a delicate matrix. (Ziehl-Neelsen stain, × 630.) (Courtesy of the Armed Forces Institute of Pathology, Photograph Neg. No. 81–13871.)

granulomatous component—epithelioid cells, histiocytes, and Langhan's giant cells—predominates. In larger lesions, multiple small pyogranulomatous foci appear to coalesce. Although the acid-fast bacilli are concentrated in the clear central vacuoles, occasional bacilli are seen in the adjacent and surrounding histiocytes. The origin and nature of these clear central vacuoles are obscure but may be derived from enlarging phagolysosomes. Most lesions remain localized to the site of inoculation. Spread is rare but has been reported in immunosuppressed patients.

CLINICAL MANIFESTATIONS. Mild local erythema and tenderness develop within a few days at the site of an injection or injury. These changes are usually so minor that the patient does not consult the physician until there is a subcutaneous nodule, fluctuation, or ulceration, sometimes with associated regional lymphadenopathy. Sites of predilection are the deltoid areas and buttocks (usual sites of injections) (Fig. 63–5). Larger lesions may have multiple sinuses.

DIAGNOSIS. Frequently, there is a history of trauma at the site of the lesion. Diagnosis depends on the cultivation and identification of the etiologic agent. In closed lesions, exudates may be obtained by aspiration. Smears stained by the Ziehl-Neelsen method will usually demonstrate acid-fast organisms. Positive cultures are obtained from a high percentage of active lesions.

TREATMENT. Most lesions heal following incision if drainage is maintained. Preulcerative nodules caused by *M. chelonae* have been excised and closed primarily without recurrence. *M. fortuitum* and *M. chelonae* are frequently resistant to antibiotics and chemotherapy, but in vitro drug sensitivity tests should be performed and appropriate therapy initiated. Successful treatment with amikacin, doxycycline, minocycline, erythromycin, sulfonamides, and the quinolones has been reported, but the results are variable.

PREVENTION. Infection acquired by hypodermic injection or wound contamination is completely preventable by using sterile equipment and aseptic proce-

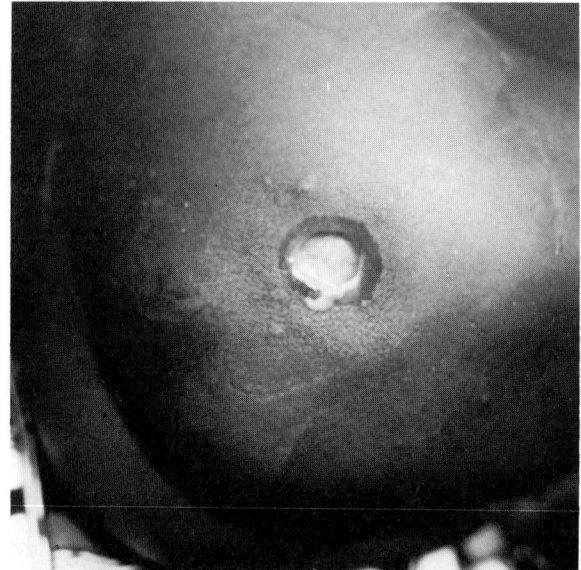

FIGURE 63–5. Injection ulcer caused by *Mycobacterium fortuitum* in buttock of Zairian child who had a hypodermic injection at this site 2 months previously. (Courtesy of the Armed Forces Institute of Pathology, Photograph Neg. No. 78–3306.)

dures. Periodic examination of hydrotherapy pools and other water baths for rapid-growing mycobacteria may help control hospital-acquired infections.

63.5. MISCELLANEOUS MYCOBACTERIAL INFECTIONS

Of the more than 50 commonly recognized mycobacterial species, perhaps half of them have caused disease in humans. There is increasing evidence that, given a large enough inoculum and a sufficiently immunosuppressed host, most mycobacteria would be pathogenic.

MYCOBACTERIUM AVIUM-INTRACELLULARE-SCROFULACEUM COMPLEX. *M. scrofulaceum* is a common saprophyte and a frequent contaminant in cultures obtained from human tissues; hence, the causal relationship of this organism to lesions must be accepted cautiously. *M. scrofulaceum* is a common cause of cervical lymphadenitis and scrofuloderma in children (Fig. 63–6) but is rarely the etiologic agent of primary lesions in the skin. Combined isoniazid and rifampin therapy has been reported to be successful.

M. avium-intracellulare has been reported as the cause of only a few primary skin lesions. One reported patient had extensive ulcerated lesions that developed over 11 years over 20 to 30% of the body surface. Combined therapy with isoniazid, cycloserine, or ethionamide, and streptomycin has been effective.

Patients with acquired immune deficiency syndrome (AIDS) have been reported to be unusually susceptible to *M. avium-intracellulare* infections, but cutaneous lesions are rare in these patients.

MYCOBACTERIUM GORDONAE COMPLEX. *M. szulgai* and *M. gordonae* are in this complex of slow-growing scotochromogenic mycobacteria and have been reported as rare causes of cutaneous lesions. The lesions were single or multiple and were nodules, abscesses, or cellulitis. Some were in immunosuppressed patients. Lesions have responded to rifampin therapy.

MYCOBACTERIUM HAEMOPHILUM. This slow-growing organism is so named because iron-supple-

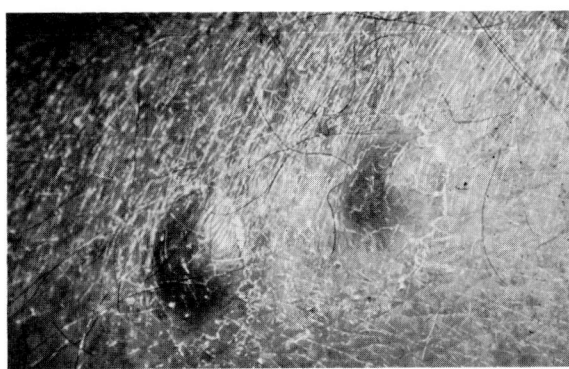

FIGURE 63–7. Two of many similar papules in skin of 51-year-old American who was under immunosuppressive therapy following an organ transplant. The nodule was caused by an unidentified acid-fast bacillus. (Courtesy of the Armed Forces Institute of Pathology, Photograph Neg. No. 75–12220–1.)

mented media are required for cultivation. Approximately 12 patients with cutaneous lesions caused by *M. haemophilum* are known. The patients usually have multiple nodules, abscesses, or ulcers. While most patients have been immunosuppressed, immunocompetent individuals are susceptible.

LESIONS CAUSED BY UNIDENTIFIED ACID-FAST BACILLI. From 1957 to 1971, a benign disease was observed in 29 patients in the northern central United States and Canada who had indurated erythematous papules (Fig. 63–7), primarily of the limbs, and regional lymphadenopathy. These lesions ulcerated and contained large numbers of acid-fast bacilli that could not be cultured but were not *M. leprae*. The files of the Armed Forces Institute of Pathology contain several similar additional cases, some in immunosuppressed patients. The etiologic agent of these lesions has not been identified.

BACILLE CALMETTE-GUÉRIN (BCG). Occasionally, vaccination with BCG (an attenuated *M. bovis*) causes progressive disease. Large lupus vulgaris-like lesions develop at the inoculation site, accompanied by regional lymphadenopathy. Immunosuppressed patients may rarely develop systemic infections. Most progressive infections caused by BCG respond to isoniazid therapy.

BIBLIOGRAPHY

Chapman JS: The Atypical Mycobacteria and Human Mycobacteriosis. New York, Plenum Medical Book Company, 1977.

Connor DH, Meyers WM, Krieg RE: Infection by *Mycobacterium ulcerans. In* Binford CH, Connor DH (eds.): Pathology of Tropical and Extraordinary Diseases. An Atlas. Vol. 1. Washington, D.C., Armed Forces Institute of Pathology, 1976, pp 226–235.

Cox SK, Strausbaugh LJ: Chronic cutaneous infection caused by *Mycobacterium intracellulare.* Arch Dermatol 117:794–796, 1981.

Cross GM, Guill MA, Aton JK: Cutaneous *Mycobacterium szulgai* infection. Arch Dermatol 121:247–249, 1985.

Dalovisio JR, Pankey GA, Wallace RJ, et al.: Clinical usefulness of amikacin and doxycycline in the treatment of infection due to *Mycobacterium fortuitum* and *Mycobacterium chelonei.* Rev Infect Dis 3:1068–1074, 1981.

Davidson PD: Treatment of infections due to atypical mycobacteria. *In* Remington JS, Swartz MN (eds.): Current Clinical Topics in Infectious Diseases. Vol 3. New York, McGraw-Hill Book Co., 1982.

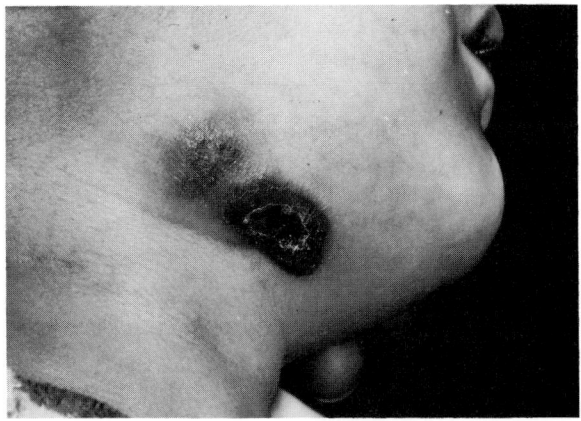

FIGURE 63–6. Scrofuloderma in a child. The ulcer and sinus tract in the skin communicated with an underlying cervical lymphadenitis. (Courtesy of the Armed Forces Institute of Pathology, Photograph Neg. No. 53–11701.)

Feldman RA, Hershfield E: Mycobacterial skin infections by an unidentified species. A report of 29 patients. Ann Intern Med 80:445–452, 1974.

Gengoux P, Portaels F, Lachapelle JM, et al.: Skin granulomas due to *Mycobacterium gordonae*. Int J Dermatol 26:181–184, 1987.

Lester TW: Drug-resistant and atypical mycobacterial disease. Bacteriology and treatment. Arch Intern Med 139:1399–1401, 1979.

MacCallum P, Tolhurst JC, Buckle G, et al.: A new mycobacterial infection in man. J Pathol Bacteriol 60:93–122, 1948.

Meyers WM, Shelly WM, Connor DH: Heat treatment of *Mycobacterium ulcerans* infection without surgical excision. Am J Trop Med Hyg 23:924–929, 1974.

Mitchell PJ, McOrist S, Bilney R: Epidemiology of *Mycobacterium ulcerans* infection in koalas *(Phascolarctas cinereus)* on Raymond Island, southeastern Australia. J Wildlife Dis 23:386–390, 1987.

Pimsler M, Sponsler TA, Meyers WM: Immunosuppressive properties of the soluble toxin from *Mycobacterium ulcerans*. J Infect Dis 157:577–580, 1988.

Ratledge C, Stanford J (eds.): The Biology of the Mycobacteria. Vol. 1 & 2. London, Academic Press, 1982. (1098 pages)

Timpe A, Runyon EH: The relationship of "atypical" and acid-fast bacteria to human disease: A preliminary report. J Lab Clin Med 44:202–209, 1954.

Wallace RS: Recent clinical advances in knowledge of the nonleprous environmental mycobacteria responsible for cutaneous disease. Arch Dermatol 123:337–339, 1987.

Wayne LG: The "atypical" mycobacteria: Recognition and disease association. CRC Critical Rev in Microbiol 12:185–222, 1985.

Wolinsky E: Nontuberculous mycobacteria and associated diseases. Am Rev Respir Dis 119:107–158, 1979.

PART IV

THE MYCOSES

GENERAL PRINCIPLES

Donald W. R. Mackenzie

Mycoses are diseases caused by fungi, which are among the most common microorganisms in man's environment. Fungi represent a highly successful life form and affect man both indirectly and directly. As agents of spoilage and destruction, they cause serious losses to crops and stored foodstuffs and to a wide range of manufactured materials. Some of the toxins produced by fungi are highly potent carcinogens and teratogens, and outbreaks of mycotoxicoses are not unknown among individuals in the tropics who are forced by necessity to eat grain or other produce that has become moldy. Many fungi produce spores, sometimes in astronomic quantities, and these may sensitize atopic subjects, causing symptoms of respiratory allergy after inhalation. Apart from their toxigenic and allergenic potentials, several fungi are capable of causing disease directly, by invasion of man's external or internal body surfaces. The type of infection caused varies from localized and entirely superficial colonization of hair shafts to serious, invasive disease with a high mortality.

DISTRIBUTION AND MEDICAL IMPORTANCE. Some mycoses are restricted to certain geographic areas; others are distributed worldwide. Their recognition may be comparatively simple in some instances, but the full spectrum of investigative diagnostic aids, principally microscopy, culture, and serology, may have to be used before a fungal etiology can be recognized. Mycoses are common particularly in the tropics, where they constitute an important public health problem. Fungi do not rank with parasites or bacteria as causes of mortality, but they are widespread and common causes of morbidity, and individual patients may suffer greatly as a result of progressive or disseminated disease. Although most fungal infections are acquired exogenously from a source in nature, some mycoses, e.g., candidosis, are initiated by fungi that are normal members of man's microflora.

With few exceptions, mycotic disease is seen more frequently in males than in females. In some conditions, the male-to-female ratio may be high, exceeding 30:1. Although occupational exposure may account in part for this sexual predilection, it can often be demonstrated that, although both sexes may have equal rates of infection, the disease is manifested more commonly in males. In tropical countries, mycologic expertise is often lacking, and accurate knowledge of the prevalence of individual mycoses fragmentary.

MORPHOLOGY. The basic vegetative organization of most pathogenic fungi is filamentous. In substrates supporting their growth, they take the shape of cylindric, branching hyphae, usually about 3 to 5 μm in diameter. They are bound by a rigid cell wall and may or may not have cross walls along their length. Hyphae increase in length only at their tips. Because they frequently send out side branches, new growing tips are constantly formed, and the rate of colonization of substrates therefore increases rapidly. Once established in their normal habitat, the vegetative phase in most fungi is followed by a reproductive phase. Fungi produce an enormous range of spore types. These are of value to the mycologist in distinguishing between different species or groups of fungi but are also the means whereby the pathogen may gain access to its host. Many spores (conidia) are dispersed aerially, and infection is therefore commonly established by the respiratory route. Some fungi have adopted a unicellular habit and reproduce by budding (yeasts). The range of morphologic expression among many fungi is wide. In several of the more important pathogenic species, they may assume one form when growing in their natural habitat (e.g., soil, decaying vegetation) or in laboratory culture media, and a different form in parasitized tissues. The saprophytic and pathogenic phases in several species, e.g., *Histoplasma capsulatum* and *Blastomyces dermatitidis*, correspond to filamentous (hyphal) and yeast-like (budding) growth, respectively. This phenomenon (dimorphism) is characteristic of some, but not all, pathogenic fungi.

DIAGNOSIS. Isolation and identification of the causal agent are valuable laboratory procedures. Serologic tests may also be helpful, although they sometimes yield equivocal results. Direct microscopy of skin fragments or examination of tissue sections stained with special fungal stains (e.g., methenamine silver Grocott modification of periodic acid—Schiff (PAS) stain) can provide direct and unequivocal evidence of fungal etiology and identity.

A feature of most types of mycoses is the acquisition of hypersensitivity, and in some instances, the development of antibodies. Immunologic tests may therefore be of value in epidemiologic studies (using skin tests to assess previous infection) and in diagnosis (using serologic procedures to detect and quantitate specific antibodies).

The acquisition of elementary mycologic skills in the form of direct microscopy is comparatively simple and pays dividends in the form of improved diagnostic capability. Most fungi are readily seen in superficial infections, and positive microscopy is one of the most reliable of all laboratory diagnostic procedures. Other laboratory procedures, such as isolation and identification, and serologic testing, require the expertise of trained personnel.

DISEASE CLASSIFICATION. Traditionally, mycoses have been classified according to their mode of establishment and the body region involved.

Superficial Mycoses (Chapter 64). These mycoses, e.g., pityriasis versicolor, affect only the dead, fully keratinized portions of the epidermis and its appendages. Living tissues are not invaded, and the infections are of cosmetic rather than pathologic significance.

Cutaneous Mycoses (Chapter 64). These mycoses, e.g., tinea, although also confined to keratinized parts of the body, may elicit acute or chronic inflammatory changes in the skin, which can be painful, unsightly, or disfiguring. Invasion of nails may result in dystrophy. Cutaneous mycoses may be acute or chronic, inflammatory or noninflammatory, and—unusual among fungal infections—acquired by contagion.

Subcutaneous Mycoses (Chapter 65). These diseases, e.g., mycetoma, are introduced through the skin surface by a penetrating wound, such as a thorn prick or splinter wound. The agents are usually environmental saprophytes. Once established they provoke an intense and destructive host response. The lesions tend to be localized and progressive, usually without any tendency to heal spontaneously.

Systemic Mycoses (Chapter 66). These mycoses, e.g., histoplasmosis, are acquired by inhalation of airborne spores, and the initial site of multiplication is the lung. Most infections are self-limiting, but serious progressive or disseminated disease occurs in a small proportion of patients.

Opportunistic Mycoses (Chapter 67). These infections, e.g., mucormycosis, owe their origins more to the susceptibility of the host than to the inherent pathogenicity of the infecting fungus. They are commonly associated with patients whose normal defenses have been compromised by primary debilitating diseases, e.g., AIDS, leukemia, diabetes, and malnutrition; by defects in the immune system; or by treatment with steroids or broad-spectrum antibiotics.

BIBLIOGRAPHY

Baker RD: The Pathologic Anatomy of Mycoses: Human Infections with Fungi, Actinomycetes and Algae. New York, Springer-Verlag, 1971.

Chandler FW, Kaplan W, Ajello L: A Color Atlas and Textbook of the Histopathology of Mycotic Diseases. London, Wolfe Medical Publications Ltd., 1980.

Emmons CW, Binford CH, Utz JP, et al.: Medical Mycology. 3rd ed. Philadelphia, Lea & Febiger, 1977.

Rippon JW: Medical Mycology: The Pathogenic Fungi and the Pathogenic Actinomycetes. 3rd ed. Philadelphia, W. B. Saunders Company, 1988.

64. CUTANEOUS MYCOSES

Roderick J. Hay

64.1.   DERMATOPHYTE INFECTIONS
(Ringworm, Tinea)

DEFINITION. The dermatophyte fungi cause infections that are confined to the superficial stratum corneum as well as keratinized structures, such as hair or nail arising from skin. Deep invasion occurs only rarely. The infections caused by these organisms are known collectively as ringworm. Alternatively, the word tinea followed by the Latin term for the appropriate part of the body involved is used, such as tinea capitis for ringworm of the scalp.

ETIOLOGY. In humans, dermatophyte infections are seen in both tropical and temperate climates, although the predominant pattern of invasion may differ in these areas. For instance, in Europe and the United States, tinea pedis affecting the interdigital spaces on the feet is the most common symptomatic form of ringworm, whereas in the tropics, groin, body, and scalp infections are more prevalent. Infections are derived from 3 main sources—man (anthropophilic), animals (zoophilic), and soil (geophilic). Those originating from the soil are not common. Zoophilic infections tend to produce lesions of the scalp or body and are often highly inflammatory. In contrast, the anthropophilic organisms may be found in lesions in any site and often, depending on the species involved and the site of invasion, the inflammatory response is minimal.

The natural course of a human infection is frequently self-limiting, although infections of certain sites, including the toenails, soles, and, in some instances, scalp, or by certain organisms, such as *Trichophyton rubrum* or *T. concentricum*, may be chronic. The condition of the host is also important in determining the course of infection. Atopic subjects are more likely to develop persistent infections.

The organisms that cause dermatophyte infections in humans are confined to 3 genera, *Trichophyton, Microsporum,* and *Epidermophyton* (Table 64–1). Each is characterized by the pattern of growth and production

TABLE 64–1. Most Common Dermatophyte Fungi of the Tropics

Genus	Species	Source
Trichophyton	*T. rubrum*	Humans
	T. mentagrophytes	Rodents, cats, dogs
	T. interdigitale	Humans
	T. tonsurans	Humans
	T. concentricum	Humans
	T. schoenleinii	Humans
	T. violaceum	Humans
	T. soudanense	Humans
Microsporum	*M. audouinii*	Humans
	M. canis	Cats, dogs
	M. ferrugineum	Humans
	M. gypseum	Soil
Epidermophyton	*E. floccosum*	Humans

of spores (macro- or microconidia). Different species can be distinguished on the basis of colonial morphology, spore production, and nutritional requirements in vitro.

EPIDEMIOLOGY. The epidemiology of dermatophyte infections is incompletely understood. However, various trends have emerged over the years. The most common cause of ringworm throughout the world is *T. rubrum*. In the early part of the century, infections with this organism were most prevalent in the Far East. However, since then considerable spread has taken place, and in many areas of the tropics *T. rubrum* is the major cause of groin or body infections. Asymptomatic involvement of the sole may occur also in any climate. Scalp infection caused by this organism is rare, however. In temperate areas, toenail and toe web invasion are seen often. *T. violaceum* is an organism that has been isolated predominantly from patients in India and the Far and Middle East. *T. violaceum* also causes ringworm in other sites, including the body.

Ringworm of the Scalp. The distribution of the agents of ringworm of the scalp throughout the tropical world is complex. In Europe, parts of the United States, and South America, *Microsporum canis*, whose natural host is the cat or dog, is the most important cause of ringworm of the scalp. This contrasts with some areas of the southern United States and Mexico, where *T. tonsurans* is the main agent in this infection. In Africa, there is considerable variation in the main types of scalp ringworm seen.

Frequently, small pockets of infection with distinct organisms can be noticed, e.g., *M. audouini* in Nigeria and *T. violaceum* in North Africa. In India and the Middle East, *T. violaceum* is the major cause of ringworm of the scalp. The factors underlying the occurrence of small endemic foci of ringworm of the scalp include the stability of the population, absence of control measures, and, on occasion, spread via external agents such as hairdressers' equipment.

Favus. *T. schoenleini* is the major cause of the scalp infection known as favus, which is characterized by the formation of perifollicular crusts (scutula) that may amalgamate to form a dense mat on the scalp. Favus, once common in Europe, is now found normally in small endemic foci, often involving a single family or a group of families. Such clusters of cases have been described, for instance, in Guatemala and southern Brazil. However, larger numbers of cases have also been seen in North Africa, South Africa, and parts of the Middle East. The organism is noted for its persistence and may involve all of the female members of one family. Infection acquired in childhood may persist in females into adult life.

Tinea Imbricata. *T. concentricum* is the cause of the infection known as tinea imbricata or tokelau. It is characterized by the appearance of homogenous sheets or concentric rings of scaling that may cover large areas of the body (Fig. 64–1). Tinea imbricata is best known in the Pacific Islands and Melanesia, but scattered reports of the disease in isolated populations, often living in primitive conditions, have been reported from Malaysia, India, Brazil, and Mexico.

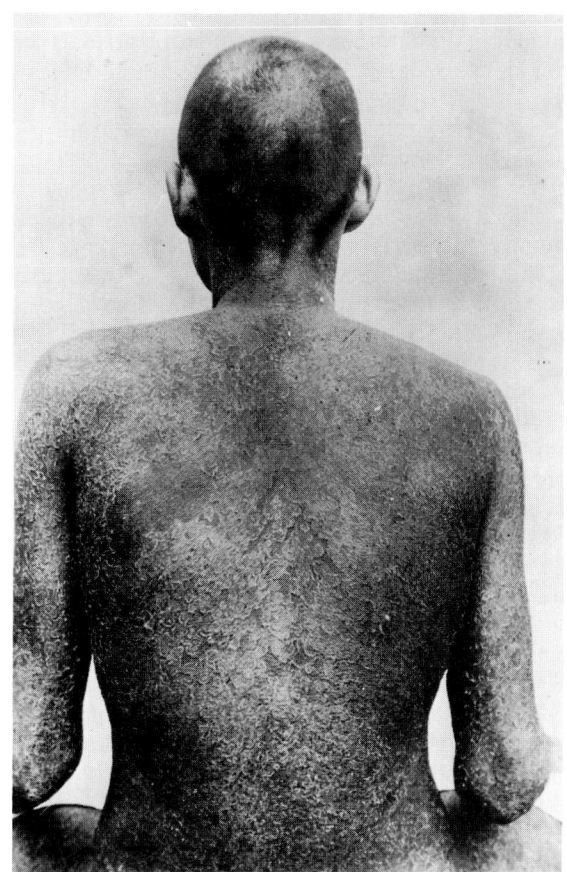

FIGURE 64–1. Tinea imbricata, caused by *T. concentricum*, is characterized by concentric rings of scales. (Courtesy of the Armed Forces Institute of Pathology, Photograph Neg. No. 39237.)

PATHOLOGY AND PATHOGENESIS. In many forms of dermatophytosis, the organisms are confined to the stratum corneum. There is minimal hyperkeratosis and acanthosis and a sparse infiltrate of lymphocytes around upper dermal blood vessels. In severe forms of animal ringworm, a dense infiltrate of polymorphonuclear leukocytes and lymphocytes can be found in the upper dermis. In a late stage of this process, lymphocytes and histiocytes predominate in the infiltrate.

Resistance to dermatophytosis depends on a number of nonspecific and immunologic factors. Serum from uninfected individuals contains a factor(s) that is inhibitory to the growth of dermatophyte fungi. Unsaturated transferrin, for instance, can inhibit the organisms. Sebaceous material may be inhibitory also. Changes in the fatty acid composition of sebum may explain the common observation that ringworm of the scalp is rare after puberty. When it does occur in an older age group, it almost always affects women.

The rate of epidermal turnover in an infected area increases, and this may explain the appearance of scaling. It is not clear, however, if this is directly triggered by the organism or involves some immunologic mechanism. The roles of complement and phagocytosis are not well established in dermatophyte infections. Polymorphs, for instance, are not common in the inflammatory response to ringworm except in kerion in the dermis or favus in the epidermis, but they have been shown to destroy dermatophyte hyphae in vitro. The production of antibodies in dermatophytosis is highly variable. Persistent *T. rubrum* infections or favus is more likely to be associated with positive serologic reactions. However, transfer of immune serum in animals is not associated with clearance of lesions. In contrast, the appearance of delayed-type hypersensitivity (DTH) as a measure of T lymphocyte-mediated immunity correlates well with the clearance of lesions in some infections, and immunity can be transferred in mice with sensitized lymphocytes. In addition to these responses, the clearance of infection is affected also by the site of invasion and the organisms. Certain organisms, such as *T. rubrum*, are usually associated with poor lymphocyte transformation responses, although, again, this varies with the site of infection. Some organisms appear to be more prominent than others in chronic infections by virtue of their weak immunogenicity.

CLINICAL MANIFESTATIONS. The main clinical features of dermatophytosis depend on the site of infection. In temperate areas occluded surfaces such as groins, toe webs, and axillae are most often infected, but in the tropics any site may be involved.

Tinea Pedis. Athlete's foot is a term used to describe scaling and maceration accompanied by itching between the toes, particularly the fourth interdigital space. It is a syndrome that may be caused by *Candida* species, erythrasma, or other bacteria as well as by dermatophytes. In dermatophyte infections, the cracked area between the toes may be wet or dry and, in some infections, particularly those caused by *T. interdigitale*, vesicular. The infection is sometimes self-limiting, or it may persist for considerable periods. Involvement of the dorsum of the foot or the sole may occur. *T. rubrum* infection is often responsible for a dry type of invasion over the sole and sides of the foot in a "moccasin type" of distribution. Symptoms may be minimal. Nail invasion, although not common in the tropics, may accompany this type of infection.

Tinea pedis is not the predominant form of dermatophytosis in the tropics; however, it is seen in certain situations. It is more common in people who wear shoes and socks and is therefore associated with urban development in tropical areas. Individuals from temperate climates with intermittently active or persistent tinea pedis nearly always have an exacerbation of their infection in the tropics. The asymptomatic dry form of sole infection caused by *T. rubrum* is also being recognized more frequently in the tropics.

Tinea pedis in tropical areas must be distinguished from other conditions, particularly pompholyx and, less commonly, plantar psoriasis. The possibility of the toe web infections being caused by *Candida* or bacteria should be considered. The interplay between bacteria and fungi is poorly understood, but in the tropics secondary gram negative bacterial infection on top of interdigital dermatophytosis may occur.

Tinea Cruris (Ringworm of the Groin). Dermatophyte infections of the groin are seen frequently in the tropics. A ring of erythema with a scaling margin radiates from the groin down the inner border of the thigh (Fig. 64–2). It is intensely itchy. The eruption may be accom-

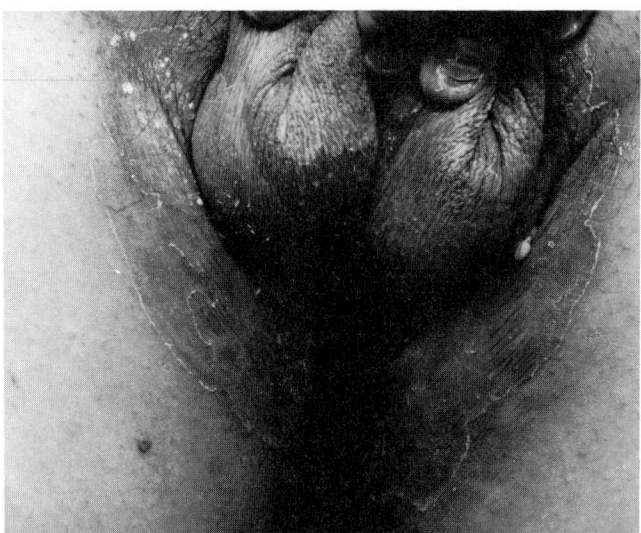

FIGURE 64–2. Tinea cruris caused by *T. rubrum*. (Courtesy of St. John's Hospital for Diseases of the Skin, London.)

panied by marked folliculitis. Tinea cruris is more common in males and may extend posteriorly to include the natal cleft. In women in tropical areas, an extensive form of ringworm may be found in the waist area that involves a large part of the skin surface around the hip girdle. Coexistent patches of tinea corporis are frequently seen with this type of infection.

Common causes of dermatophytosis in this site are *T. rubrum* and *Epidermophyton floccosum*, but *Candida intertrigo* may closely resemble tinea cruris.

Tinea Corporis (Ringworm of the Body). The characteristic lesion of dermatophyte infection on trunk or limbs is an annular plaque with a varying degree of erythema and a prominent edge (Fig. 64–3). Scaling is most prominent at this margin. However, the appearance of this lesion varies with the organism and host. Zoophilic dermatophytes such as *M. canis* may produce highly inflammatory lesions. In their most florid form, inflammatory ringworm plaques on the body or scalp become indurated and pustular (kerion). At the other end of the spectrum, inflammation may be minimal, and single or multiple plaques on the body or face may be accompanied by few symptoms. Particularly in the Far East, *T. rubrum* is often associated with persistent and minimally inflammatory tinea corporis.

Discoid eczema, impetigo, psoriasis, and discoid lupus erythematosus may all be mistaken for ringworm.

Tinea Capitis (Ringworm of the Scalp). Invasion of scalp hairs is seen in certain dermatophyte infections. They can be divided into 3 main groups—endothrix infections, in which spores (arthrospores) are formed within the hair matrix; ectothrix infections, in which sporulation occurs around the hair; and favus. All 3 types of infection are more common in childhood (Fig. 64–4). Those that spread from person to person are likely to occur in overcrowded conditions, including refugee camps, and can spread rapidly to achieve epidemic proportions. Chronically infected patients may develop some permanent alopecia; persistent infections are much more common with certain organisms, including *T. tonsurans* and *T. schoenleini*.

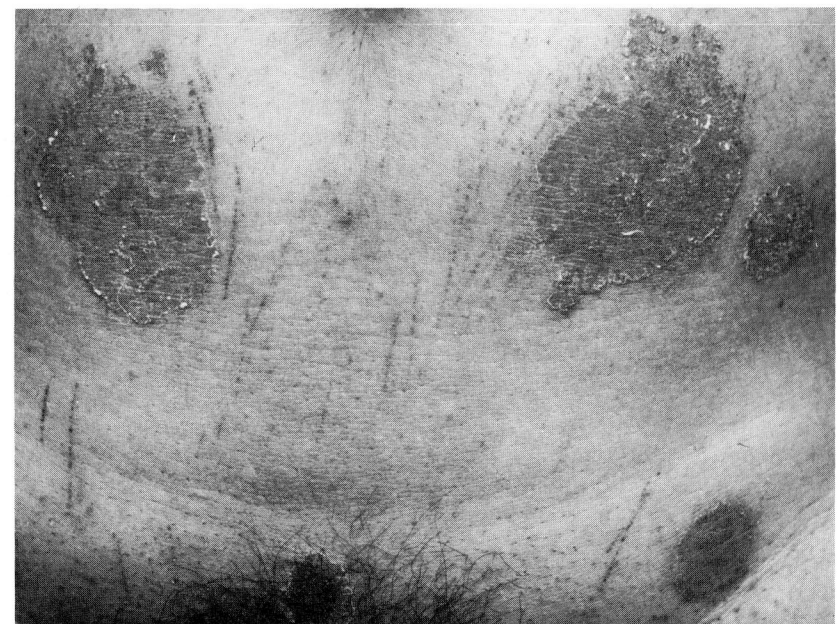

FIGURE 64–3. Tinea corporis caused by *T. rubrum*. (Courtesy of St. John's Hospital for Diseases of the Skin, London.)

Endothrix and Ectothrix Infections. In ectothrix infections, scalp hairs may break at any level, but often this occurs several millimeters above the skin surface. There is often considerable exudation and erythema. In endothrix infections, the onset is often more insidious. Hairs break at scalp level usually, and inflammation may be minimal. However, kerion may develop with either type, although it is more common with the former. The organisms that cause scalp infections have been discussed in the section on epidemiology.

Favus. Favus presents with hair loss accompanied by the formation of crusts or scutula. These tend to coalesce to form a dense mat on parts or all of the scalp. The infected scalp has a peculiar odor. Atypical forms that are more prevalent in adults may be accompanied by minimal crust formation. In an area where favus is endemic, female patients presenting with cicatricial alopecia, for instance, should be examined for scalp infection. Family infections with favus are often seen. Hairs invaded by *T. schoenleini* have a characteristic appearance, with air spaces within the infected shaft.

The diagnosis of tinea capitis is facilitated by filtered ultraviolet light examination (Wood's light), although not all organisms fluoresce under these conditions (Table 64–2).

Ringworm of the scalp must be distinguished from seborrheic dermatitis, psoriasis, or cicatricial alopecia. The last may be produced in end-stage favus.

Onychomycosis. Dermatophyte invasion of the nails is more common in temperate areas and the subtropics but is seen with a number of organisms, particularly *T. rubrum*. The nail plate is invaded from the distal border and lateral surfaces, usually from the underside. The affected nail becomes thickened and opaque, with a varying degree of onycholysis. Patients with onychomycosis often have infection of other sites such as the soles or toe webs.

In addition to psoriasis, other fungal infections e.g., candidosis or *Hendersonula* infections, must be differentiated from onychomycosis.

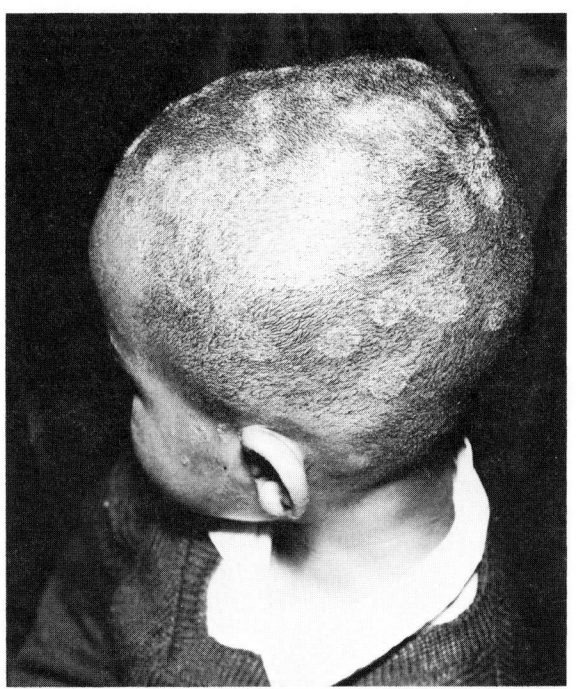

FIGURE 64–4. Tinea capitis, caused by *Microsporum audouini*, presents as multiple patches of alopecia with scaling in this little boy. (Courtesy of the Armed Forces Institute of Pathology, Photograph Neg. No. 57–6860.)

TABLE 64–2. Ringworm of the Scalp: Effect of Wood's Light

Hair usually fluorescent:
M. canis, M. audouinii, M. ferrugineum, M. distortum
Hair not fluorescent:
M. gypseum, T. verrucosum, T. tonsurans, T. violaceum,
T. soudanense, T. yaoundei, T. gourvilii
Dull fluorescence:
T. schoenleinii

Dermatophytosis of Other Sites. Dermatophyte infection of the beard area (tinea barbae) may be highly inflammatory and persistent. Involvement of the palms is most commonly seen with *T. rubrum* infection. Often only one hand is involved, and the fingernails on that side may be invaded also. The palm shows mild scaling similar to the dry type of sole infection.

LABORATORY DIAGNOSIS. The laboratory diagnosis of dermatophytosis is entirely dependent on local facilities. However, the identification of the organism, although not absolutely essential, is helpful for several reasons. First, the likely source of the infection can be recognized. Second, certain organisms show different patterns of infection and responses to treatment, and recognition of the organism will assist the physician in determining the likely course of the infection. Finally, appropriate control mechanisms depend on the identification of the organism, particularly in zoophilic infections.

There are several methods of laboratory recognition of dermatophyte infections:

Direct Examination. Scrapings can be taken from the lesion using a blunt scalpel and examined with a microscope after being mounted in 10% potassium hydroxide on a glass slide. The presence of dermatophyte hyphae can be demonstrated in infected material or hairs.

Wood's Light Examination. Examination of infected scalps using a source of filtered ultraviolet radiation is extremely helpful in screening large numbers of potentially infected children, e.g., in schools. Certain, but not all, dermatophytes fluoresce green under Wood's light (see Table 64–2).

Culture. Scrapings or hairs may be placed directly onto Sabouraud agar. Colonies develop in 7 to 28 days. Their gross and microscopic appearance, as well as nutritional requirements, can be used in identification.

TREATMENT. Most dermatophyte infections require treatment. However, the advisability of prolonged therapy in nail or sole infection must be weighed against the symptoms experienced by the patient (often minimal) and the low rate of success.

Topical Therapy. Dermatophytoses can be treated topically by a number of different methods. Certain simple compounds, including dyes, are known to have weak antifungal properties that may be sufficient to treat certain types of dermatophytosis, e.g., tinea cruris. Gentian violet and magenta paint are examples. A second therapeutic approach is promotion of the exfoliation of stratum corneum by compounds known as keratolytic agents. Salicylic acid in concentrations of 5 to 20% in ointment base is an effective keratolytic agent. Whitfield's ointment (BPC), which contains 3% salicylic acid and 3% benzoic acid, a weak antifungal agent, is an inexpensive and effective method of treating all dermatophyte infections apart from scalp or nail disease or kerion. It may be prescribed in half strength for sensitive areas. Although the newer specific antifungal compounds may result in a more rapid response and be less irritative, there is little evidence that they are more effective. They are also more expensive.

Specific Antifungals. The specific antifungal compounds that can be used against dermatophytes include the imidazole compounds (miconazole, clotrimazole, econazole, and tioconazole) as well as a miscellaneous group of antifungal drugs such as tolnaftate and haloprogin. All are available for topical therapy in 1 to 2% concentration. Many are effective against candidosis and pityriasis versicolor.

Systemic Therapy. For nail and scalp disease or severe infections, including kerion, the topical agents have less value, and systemic treatment with griseofulvin or ketoconazole is required. Griseofulvin is given in a daily dose of 500 to 1000 mg in adults or 10 mg/kg in children. The drug is best prescribed in microcrystalline form and is usually well absorbed when given with a meal. Side effects, such as headache, nausea, or urticaria, occur in less than 5% of those treated. Of patients with toenail infections, 20 to 40% fail to respond to courses of griseofulvin given over 1 to 2 years. There is good evidence that for scalp infections effective treatment in large numbers of children can be attained by giving intermittent supervised therapy, e.g., 30 mg/kg at 3-week intervals. Ketoconazole is also beneficial in treating some scalp and nail infections. It is given in a dose of 200 to 400 mg daily. The new oral antifungals itracarazole (a triazole) and terbinafine (an allylamine) show considerable promise in the treatment of dermatophytosis.

Removal of Infected Tissues. Surgery is occasionally recommended for resistant nail infections. However, an alternative to this is application of a 40% urea ointment to the nail under occlusion for 1 week. The nail can be removed painlessly by excision after this treatment.

Systemic corticosteroids are rarely required in dermatophyte infections. In patients with animal ringworm or kerion, however, examination is advisable within 3 to 5 days of starting griseofulvin therapy, as a severe generalized allergic reaction may take place. This may require concurrent therapy with topical or systemic corticosteroids.

64.2. DERMATOPHYTE-LIKE INFECTIONS CAUSED BY *SCYTALIDIUM* AND *HENDERSONULA*

Two nondermatophyte organisms have been found to cause infections that closely resemble the dry type of palmar or plantar and nail infections caused by *T. rubrum* (Fig. 64–5). Their prevalence in the tropics is unknown, although they have been shown to cause sole infections in the Caribbean and are not uncommon in immigrants from the tropics living in Europe.

ETIOLOGY. *Hendersonula toruloidea* is a plant pathogen found in many parts of the tropics. It is a black mold without obvious distinguishing features that may easily be mistaken for a laboratory contaminant, and its growth is inhibited by cycloheximide, which is often used in mycologic media. *Scytalidium hyalinum* is similar but is white to gray in color.

TREATMENT. The treatment of these infections is extremely difficult, because the organisms are not gen-

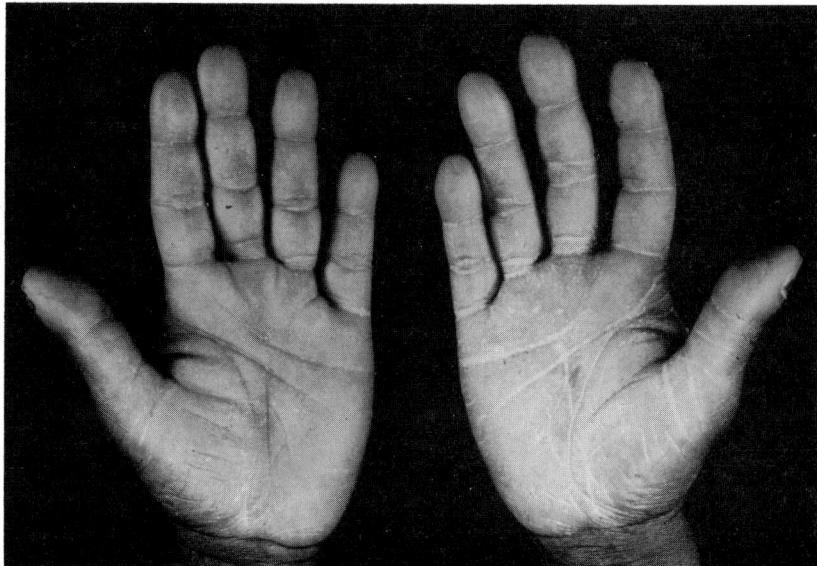

FIGURE 64–5. *Hendersonula toruloidea* infection of the palms mimicking a "dry" type of dermatophyte infection. (Courtesy of St. John's Hospital for Diseases of the Skin, London.)

erally sensitive to the commonly used specific antifungal agents. Whitfield's ointment is probably the treatment of choice. Many affected patients also have eczema or plantar keratoderma in addition to the fungal infection. The laboratory diagnosis depends on culture on cycloheximidefree media.

64.3.   SUPERFICIAL CANDIDOSIS (Candidiasis)

DEFINITION. Superficial infections caused by species of the genus *Candida* are common in all parts of the world. They include conditions such as thrush and vaginal candidosis as well as interdigital candidosis. The pattern of *Candida* infections in the tropics differs from that seen in temperate areas. This is in part due to different trends in medical therapy and also to differences in the prevalence of underlying disease states, such as diabetes mellitus.

ETIOLOGY AND EPIDEMIOLOGY. *Candida albicans* is the most common organism to be associated with superficial candidosis. However, other species such as *C. tropicalis* or *C. guilliermondi* may be involved. *C. albicans* is a common saprophyte on mucosal surfaces, particularly the mouth, gastrointestinal tract, and vagina. Oral colonization may originate early in infancy, although its incidence is increased by a number of factors, including hospitalization and bottle feeding. However, predisposing conditions in the tropics are largely unexplored. For instance, the effect of malnutrition on oral carriage of *Candida* is unknown. *C. albicans* may be isolated also from the environment, particularly where contact with humans is frequent, e.g., washbasins, drinking bowls.

PATHOGENESIS. *C. albicans* usually, but not always, causes infection as opposed to colonization in individuals with predisposing factors (Table 64–3). Some of these factors are systemic, and others relate to local conditions on the skin or mucosa. The effect of climate on infection is unknown, although a number of studies have confirmed the high incidence of saprophytic carriage of *Candida* species in the tropics.

CLINICAL MANIFESTATIONS. The clinical manifestations of superficial candidosis vary with the site of infection.

Oral Candidosis (Thrush). This is a common condition, particularly in the elderly, infants, and denture wearers. It may also follow immunosuppression or antibiotic therapy. The infection presents with solitary or confluent white plaques on the oral mucosa. Alternatively, the mucosa may appear glazed and erythematous. Persistent oral candidosis may be a problem in the elderly in particular. One of the earliest features of oral candidosis is the appearance of cracking at the angles of the mouth, angular cheilitis. Other causes, such as vitamin or iron deficiency, should be considered. Oral candidosis is a common feature of AIDS in the tropics and is often accompanied by esophageal infection.

Vaginal Candidosis. Vaginal infection with *Candida* species is common, and although it is particularly associated with diabetes and the third trimester of pregnancy, the majority of those affected have no obvious underlying abnormality. It has been suggested, without objective evidence, that the widespread use of oral contraceptives may also be a predisposing factor.

The symptoms of vaginal candidosis are irritation and discomfort associated, in many cases, with a creamy discharge. The rash in the groin is erythematous with a

TABLE 64–3. Predisposing Factors in Superficial Candidosis

Infancy, pregnancy, old age
Occlusion of epithelial surfaces, e.g., by dentures, occlusive dressings
Disorders of immune function
   a. Primary, e.g., chronic granulomatous disease
   b. Secondary, e.g., leukemia, corticosteroid therapy
Chemotherapy
   a. Immunosuppressive
   b. Antibiotic
Endocrine disease, e.g., diabetes mellitus
Carcinoma
Miscellaneous, e.g., damaged nail folds

prominent border. Small "satellite" pustules or crusts are often seen outside this border. As with oral infections, the vaginal mucosa may be covered with small white plaques or may become red and friable. This infection must be distinguished from *Trichomonas* infections and gonorrhea.

Paronychia and *Candida* Onychomycosis. Infection of the nail folds by *Candida* species is one cause of paronychia. The periungual skin is raised and painful, and a prominent gap develops between the fold and the nail plate. Pus may be discharged. More rarely, invasion of the nail plate with onycholysis occurs.

Certain bacteria, such as *Staphylococcus aureus*, also play a role in the formation of paronychia, and the condition is best regarded as being caused by a number of factors, although women with heavy domestic responsibilities (washing, cooking) seem to be predisposed. Patients with abnormal nail folds associated with skin disease, such as hand eczema or contact dermatitis, may also be infected.

Interdigital Candidosis. *Candida* may cause scaling and maceration between the toes (athlete's foot). In addition, a superficial erosion on the hand between the fingers on the dorsal web space may also be caused by *Candida* infection. This type of interdigital erosion is seen much more frequently in warm climates.

Intertrigo. Intertrigo is the name given to a painful or irritative inflammatory dermatosis confined to body folds to which secondary bacterial or *Candida* infections may contribute. Treatment of *Candida* infection alone rarely produces a cure. The infection is most common in overweight or diabetic individuals.

Diaper rash is mainly a problem of the colder latitudes but may occur elsewhere if diapers are used on infants. Secondary infection with *Candida* may occur in this area on top of an irritative dermatosis caused by urine.

Chronic Candidosis. Chronic *Candida* infections of the mouth (Fig. 64–6), vagina, nails, or other skin surfaces are rare but may persist despite treatment. The most extreme example, chronic mucocutaneous candidosis, is a rare condition that occurs worldwide. It is usually recognized in infancy or childhood, and there are frequently underlying genetic, endocrine, or immunologic features. Severe oral and nail infection as well as widespread infection and granuloma formation on other surfaces may develop. There is some tendency for the condition to improve in adult life if the affected individual does not succumb to intercurrent illness.

LABORATORY DIAGNOSIS. The laboratory diagnosis can be confirmed by demonstration of the organism in potassium hydroxide wet mounts. Yeast and hyphal forms are seen in the same area. The organism can be cultured on Sabouraud's agar.

TREATMENT. Topical treatment with gentian violet is effective in some patients. However, locally applied amphotericin B, nystatin, or an imidazole preparation is preferable. Creams, lozenges, suspensions, or pessaries (vaginal tablets) are available. The only practicable systemic treatment for superficial candidosis is ketoconazole. Its use is best reserved for severe oral or chronic forms of candidosis. AIDS patients with oral candidosis may respond to topical therapy, but in many cases it is necessary to use ketoconazole or fluconazole.

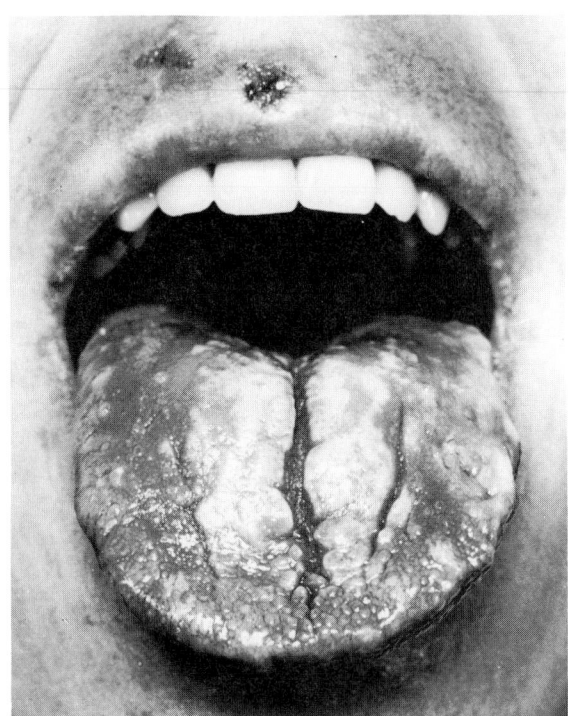

FIGURE 64–6. Chronic oral candidosis of the tongue. (Courtesy of St. John's Hospital for Diseases of the Skin, London.)

Vaginal infections respond to intensive topical therapy given for 3 to 5 days using a combination of cream and pessaries. Amphotericin B, nystatin, or an imidazole such as miconazole is usually successful. If the initial treatment is unsucessful, the male partner should be treated as well.

Control measures are rarely practicable. However, patients at risk for oral or systemic candidosis may be given topical nystatin suspension or amphotericin B lozenges. These include patients with neutropenia or leukemia and those receiving high doses of corticosteroids.

64.4. PITYRIASIS (TINEA) VERSICOLOR

DEFINITION. This common infection is widespread in the tropics and may affect over 60% of the population in certain areas. It is caused by the lipophilic yeast *Malassezia furfur.*

ETIOLOGY. *Malassezia furfur* may be present on normal skin, where it exists as a saprophyte in its yeast form, known previously as *Pityrosporum orbiculare.* The development of detectable lesions is usually, but not invariably, accompanied by the formation of short, stubby pseudohyphae (Fig. 64–7). In temperate areas, pityriasis versicolor is seen most often in patients returning from an overseas vacation. Rarely, it may occur in immunocompromised individuals, in particular those with Cushing's syndrome.

EPIDEMIOLOGY. Pityriasis versicolor is seen throughout the world and is extremely common in the tropics.

PATHOLOGY AND PATHOGENESIS. *M. furfur*

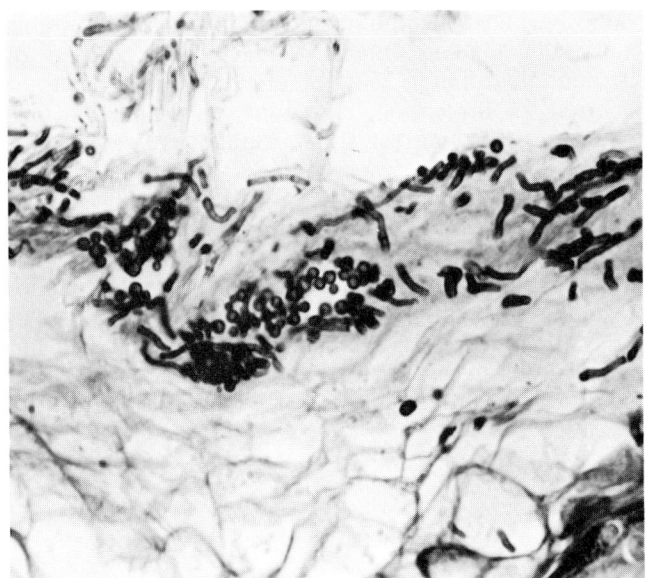

FIGURE 64–7. The causative organism of tinea versicolor *(Malassezia furfur)* is seen in the stratum corneum as multiple spores and relatively short, wavy hyphae. (PAS stain, × 633.) (Courtesy of the Armed Forces Institute of Pathology, Photograph Neg. No. 75–5301.)

normally inhabits the superficial layers of keratin, particularly around the orifices of hair follicles. The sequential development of hyphal forms can be observed during the course of immunosuppressive therapy, which suggests that immune factors play a role in preventing the infection. However, the high prevalence of the disease in normal people in the tropics indicates that other factors are involved. Exposure to sunlight, heat, and humidity as well as locally applied oils have all been cited, but without objective proof.

CLINICAL MANIFESTATIONS. The lesions of pityriasis versicolor are small, scaling macules that are hypopigmented or hyperpigmented (Fig. 64–8). Scaling is rarely prominent but can be elicited by scratching affected areas. This feature is important in distinguishing this infection from other types of macular pigmentary disorders, e.g., vitiligo. Under Wood's light, the patches

fluoresce pale yellow, but this sign is often unreliable. The areas most commonly infected are the upper trunk, neck, and upper arms. In the tropics, the infection may extend beyond these areas to involve the face, abdomen, lower arms, and penis. The rash is rarely symptomatic but may cause concern because of its superficial resemblance to certain types of leprosy.

LABORATORY DIAGNOSIS. The appearance of well-defined macules with fine scaling is distinctive usually. However, the diagnosis can be confirmed by demonstration of the clusters of yeasts and hyphae in potassium hydroxide mounts. Recognition of the fungi is facilitated by the addition of equal quantities of blue ink (Parker Quink) to the potassium hydroxide.

TREATMENT. Applications of 20% sodium thiosulfate or 2.5% selenium sulfide twice daily for 7 to 10 days are usually effective. The response to a topical imidazole may be more rapid, and some studies show that a single 400 mg dose of ketoconazole will clear infection. No control measures are practicable.

64.5. MISCELLANEOUS FUNGAL INFECTIONS

BLACK PIEDRA. Black piedra is an uncommon persistent infection confined to hair shafts and is seen in small endemic foci in the tropics, e.g., Latin America or Central Africa. Individual or clusters of cases may occur. The infection is seen most often on the hairs of the scalp. The hallmark of this condition is the presence of small, gritty nodules on the hair shafts. These represent areas of hyphal invasion in which the characteristic spores (ascospores) of the organism *Piedraia hortae* may be found.

WHITE PIEDRA. White piedra is caused by the yeast *Trichosporon beigelii*, which, on rare occasions, may also cause systemic infections. The clinical appearances are similar to those of black piedra, although the swellings are "softer" and pale. The infected areas may involve hair on the scalp, groins, or, rarely, the axillae.

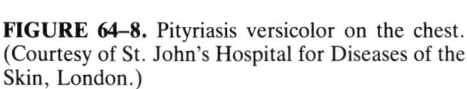

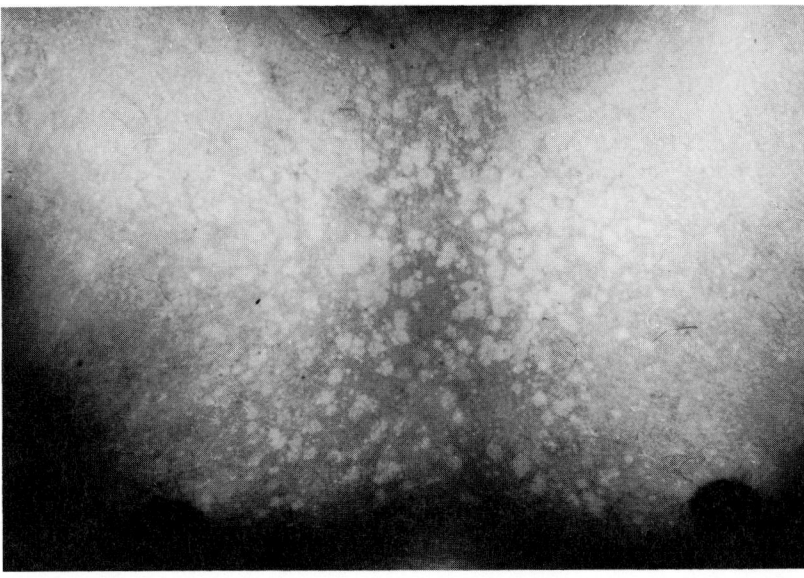

FIGURE 64–8. Pityriasis versicolor on the chest. (Courtesy of St. John's Hospital for Diseases of the Skin, London.)

Infections are not common but have been recognized in different climates from temperate to tropical areas.

TINEA NIGRA. Tinea nigra is the superficial infection caused by a black yeast, *Exophiala werneckii*, which is associated with the appearance of focal areas of hyperpigmentation, usually on the palms or soles. It is seen exclusively in the tropics and subtropics and is never common. The infection has been recognized primarily in Central and South America as well as in the Far East.

Patients rarely complain of symptoms directly attributable to the infection. Characteristically, the lesion is a dark brown or black stain that appears on the palms or the soles and, on rare occasions, elsewhere. There is little scaling, and multiple lesions are rare. The diagnosis can be confirmed by demonstration of the characteristic darkly pigmented arthrospores in scrapings. The infection responds well to Whitfield's ointment.

BIBLIOGRAPHY

Faergemann J, Bernander S: Tinea versicolor and *Pityrosporum orbiculare*: A mycological investigation. Sabouraudia 17:171, 1979.

Hildick-Smith G, Blank H, Sarkany I: Fungus Diseases and Their Treatment. Boston, Little, Brown and Co., 1964.

Jones HE, Rinehardt JH, Rinaldi MG: Acquired immunity to dermatophytes. Arch Dermatol 109:840, 1974.

Kamalam A, Thambiah AS: Tinea capitis in Madras. Sabouraudia 11:106, 1973.

Kouek P, Ouankou MD: Les épidermomycoses à Yaounde: Aspects cliniques et thérapeutiques. Med Afr Noire 25:449, 1978.

Moore MK: Skin and nail infections by non-dermatophytic filamentous fungi. Mykosen (Suppl 1):128, 1978.

Rebell G, Taplin D: Dermatophytes: Their Recognition and Identification. Miami, Florida, University of Miami Press, 1970.

Roberts SOB: Treatment of the superficial and subcutaneous mycoses. *In* Speller DC (ed.): Antifungal Chemotherapy. New York, John Wiley and Sons Ltd., 1980.

Soyinka F: Epidemiologic study of dermatophyte infections in Nigeria (clinical survey and laboratory investigations). Mycopathologia 63:99, 1978.

65. SUBCUTANEOUS MYCOSES

Donald W. R. Mackenzie

DEFINITION. Subcutaneous mycoses are chronic fungal infections resulting from the percutaneous inoculation of the causal agents from an exogenous source. Therefore, they are acquired by *implantation* rather than by inhalation or contagion. The primary site of multiplication is the skin, and although lesions generally remain localized to the site of inoculation, there is usually a slow and inexorable spread to surrounding tissue. Several different mycoses with this pathogenesis are grouped together, each with its distinctive clinical features. As a rule, lesions do not undergo spontaneous remission. If unchecked, tissue destruction may be severe. Dissemination is rare and has been recorded only for chromomycosis.

ETIOLOGY. The principal forms of subcutaneous mycoses are mycetoma, sporotrichosis, and chromomycosis. Less common are the subcutaneous zygomycoses,

rhinosporidiosis, and phaeohyphomycosis. Exceptionally, subcutaneous infections have been caused by dermatophyte fungi. Multiple etiologies have been recognized for mycetoma, chromomycosis, and phaeohyphomycosis. In contrast, the subcutaneous zygomycoses, sporotrichosis, and rhinosporidiosis are caused by single species of pathogenic fungi.

EPIDEMIOLOGY. The normal habitat of the fungi causing subcutaneous mycoses is soil or vegetation. Man is an accidental and nonessential host, with infection resulting from the fortuitous introduction into the skin of a fungus that is equipped with the qualities and mechanisms necessary to defy nonspecific and specific defenses of the body.

65.1. MYCETOMA
(Maduromycosis)

DEFINITION. Mycetoma is a chronic, localized, slowly progressive, subcutaneous infection caused by species of actinomycetes or fungi. It is characterized by destructive granulomatous and suppurative responses, by the production of tumefaction, by deformity, and by draining sinus tracts that may communicate with each other and with the skin surface. In affected tissues, the causal agents form compact *grains* or *granules,* which are often characteristic of the infecting species. The infection becomes established by traumatic implantation of the agent from an exogenous source. Lesions are localized initially to the inoculation site but spread slowly to involve contiguous tissues, including muscle and bone.

ETIOLOGY. Mycetoma has multiple etiologies, with more than 20 species of fungi or bacteria being commonly implicated. About 60% of infections are caused by actinomycetes (actinomycetoma) and 40% by filamentous fungi (eumycetoma). Predominant causes vary markedly in different parts of the world. Species most prevalent in the tropics include the actinomycetes *Streptomyces somaliensis, Actinomadura madurae, A. pelletieri,* and *Nocardia brasiliensis* and the fungi *Madurella mycetomatis, M. grisea, Leptosphaeria senegalensis, Pseudallescheria boydii,* and species of *Fusarium, Acremonium,* and *Aspergillus.*

HISTORY. The disease was reported initially from India almost 140 years ago and was named "madura foot," after the district in which it appeared to be prevalent. The preferred disease name "mycetoma" was introduced in 1861 to distinguish the disease from other tumors. Later reports established the widespread occurrence of mycetoma throughout the world and the wide range of causal organisms.

EPIDEMIOLOGY. Mycetoma is endemic in many tropical countries and is most commonly reported from Africa, Central and South America, India, and the Far East. Although sporadic cases occur in temperate countries, the condition is seen most frequently between latitudes 15 degrees S and 30 degrees N, typically in regions with a short rainy season of 4 to 6 months, a daily temperature range of 30 to 37C, and a relative humidity of 60 to 80%, alternating with a dry season with relative humidities of 12 to 30% and daily temperatures ranging from 45 to 50C during the day and 15 to 18C at night. Geographic distribution of the individual agents causing mycetoma is determined principally by rainfall rather than by other climatic factors. Areas of endemicity are characterized by savannah or forest and by the presence of thorny trees or bushes. Many of the agents causing mycetoma have been isolated from soil, which is considered to be the natural habitat for all species, and in several instances organisms have been recovered from acacia thorns, which are responsible for intracutaneous inoculation of the pathogen. In some areas, males are more frequently affected than females, but there is no consistent differential sex distribution. The disease can affect all age groups but is most commonly reported in young adults. Many patients are field laborers or herdsmen whose occupation exposes them frequently to soil and minor penetrating wounds.

PATHOGENESIS AND PATHOLOGY. Infection is initiated by traumatic implantation, often by the piercing of skin or mucosal surfaces with thorns or wood splinters. On several occasions, agents of mycetoma have been isolated in culture from thorns and other vegetable matter. Mycetoma may involve any part of the body but is most common on the feet, particularly among those who are habitually barefoot, followed by the hands and other parts of the body that come into contact with the soil or vegetation during working, sitting, or lying. Other sites commonly affected include the back, neck, and back of the head, often in individuals who routinely carry wood or loads contaminated with soil.

Once introduced subcutaneously, the agent begins to grow in the tissues, eliciting a suppurative inflammatory response that is predominantly neutrophilic and may be accompanied by a granulomatous reaction with varying proportions of epithelioid cells, plasma cells, lymphocytes, and giant cells. Other pathologic features include fibrosis, local endarteritic changes, and the formation of dense scar tissue. The agent appears in infected tissues as compact grains or granules up to 5 mm in diameter whose appearance may be diagnostic of the species involved. These are often invested with refractile eosinophilic material (Splendore-Hoeppli phenomenon).

At the margin of each grain, the intensity of the host-parasite reaction results in local necrosis, multiple abscesses, osteitis, and osteomyelitis, and the formation of sinuses and fistulas that interconnect and erupt onto the skin surface. Different agents induce different pathologic changes of bone. In some, the dominant feature may be bone resorption; in others, osteoblastic activity toward the periphery of the lesion may result in the encasement of grains by bone. In a third type, bone regeneration is incomplete, resulting in spicule formation. The most common and most distinctive radiologic appearance is focal bone destruction with cavity formation. Cavities are generally small and abundant in cases of actinomycetoma and larger and less numerous in eumycetoma.

Regional extension with destruction of deep tissues is slow, inexorable, and, at times, extensive. Spread may occur proximally as well as distally, but the process involves only the lymphatics or the blood stream.

CLINICAL MANIFESTATIONS. In tropical countries, patients most commonly present with long-standing infections. The initial lesion, which appears several months after the traumatic incident, is a small, firm, painless subcutaneous nodule or plaque that increases progressively in size.

Subsequent evolutions of eumycetoma and actinomycetoma may differ. In the former, lesions remain localized and the condition progresses slowly. Neither swelling nor destruction of adjacent anatomic structures is marked until late in the course of the disease. The tumor is usually firm and round but may be soft and lobulated. Skin nodules break down to form ulcerated areas discharging sanguineous, seropurulent, or purulent exudates (Fig. 13–10). As it progresses, the condition is characterized by marked swelling and deformity, and the production of draining sinus tracts through which fungal grains are expelled onto the surface of the skin (Fig. 65–1). As old sinus tracts heal, fresh ones appear.

In actinomycetoma infections, lesions may have less well-defined margins and tend to merge with surrounding tissue. Progression is often more rapid and involvement of bone earlier and more extensive (Fig. 65–2).

Most mycetomas are painless, even when well established. Although the patient may appear wasted and anemic, this is usually caused by other processes, such as malnutrition, unrelated to mycetoma. The latter may result in loss of function of an affected limb and consequent inability to work. Systemic disturbances, when present, are related not to mycetoma, but to other concurrent disease.

Evidence is accumulating to suggest that infected subjects have defects of cellular immunity. For instance, in Sudan, it has been shown that only 25% of patients with mycetoma react to intracutaneous tuberculin, in contrast to 70% of subjects in a control group. The condition does not remit spontaneously, although temporary improvement is not unknown. Spread tends to follow fascial planes, but nerves and tendons are resistant; hence, neurologic symptoms are lacking. The foot is the most common site involved, with about 70% of infections affecting the lower limbs. Other sites include the buttocks and perineum, hands, back, and scalp, although many other localizations are encountered.

DIAGNOSIS

Histopathology. Grains produced by different agents are so distinctive that a definite diagnosis can be made usually by examination of tissue sections stained with hematoxylin and eosin (Fig. 65–3). Fungal grains have a coarser texture, consisting of a dense mass of interwoven filaments (hyphae) 2 to 5 μm in diameter. Many are pigmented, being permeated by a dark-brown cement-like material, which confers a gritty texture to the grains. In tissue sections, individual hyphae or vesicular swellings can always be distinguished. Actinomycete grains, in contrast, are more finely textured, the hyphae being 1 μm or less in diameter and not individually distinguishable. They are never black. Distinctive histopathologic features of the most common causes of mycetoma are indicated in Table 65–1, which indicates both macroscopic and microscopic features.

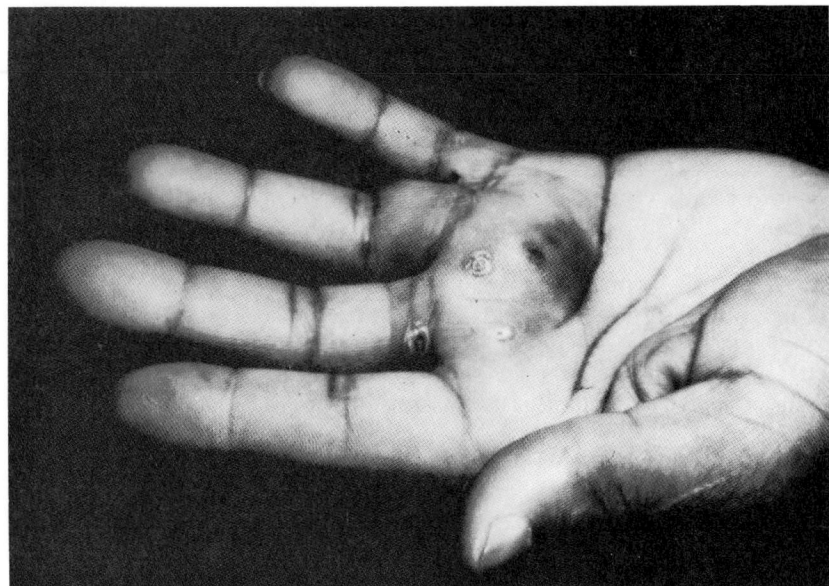

FIGURE 65–1. Mycetoma (eumycetoma) affecting the palm. (Courtesy of St. John's Hospital for Diseases of the Skin, London.)

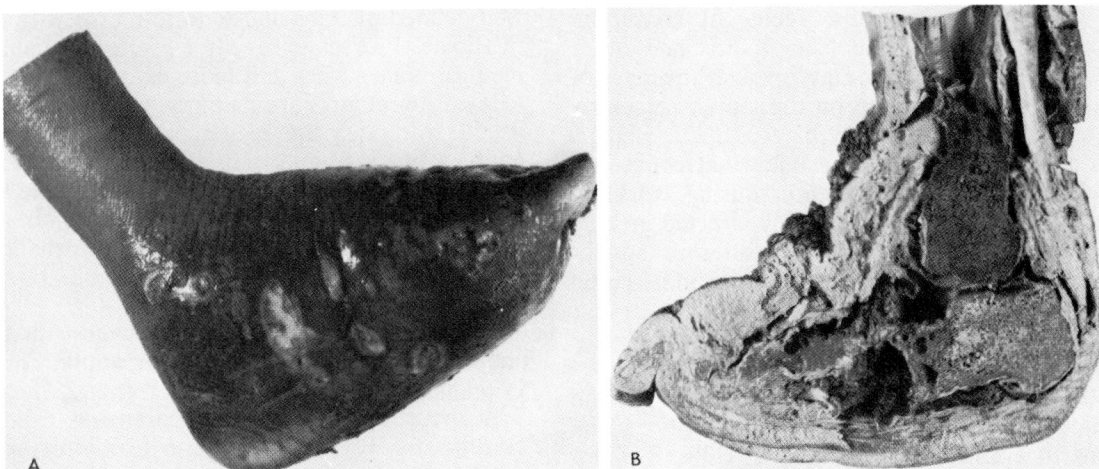

FIGURE 65–2. *A*. Mycetoma of the foot. Nocardia species were cultured, and branching gram-positive filaments were present in the granule. *B*. Hemisection through the foot. There is advanced destruction of the bones, and empty spaces contained purulent material. (Courtesy of the Armed Forces Institute of Pathology, Photograph Neg. No. N–77646.)

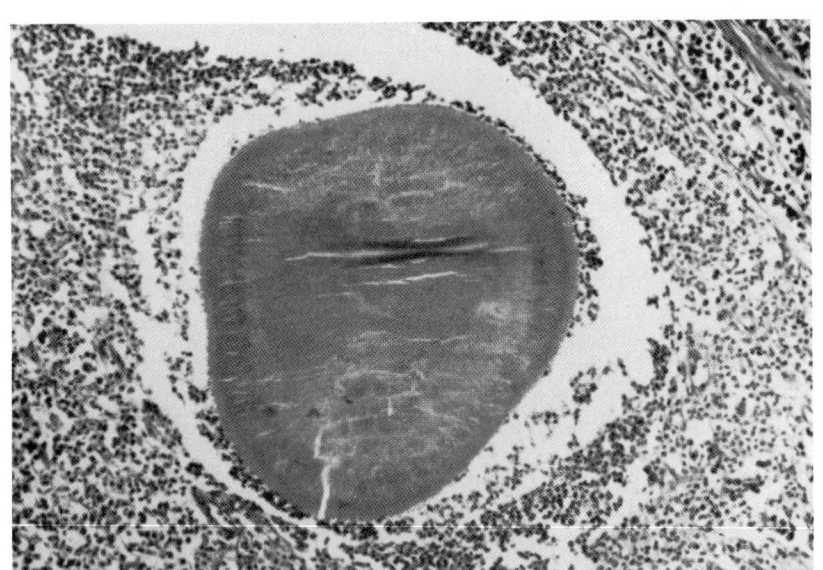

FIGURE 65–3. Grain of *Streptomyces somaliensis* surrounded by acute inflammatory cells (H & E stain, × 360). (Courtesy of St. John's Hospital for Diseases of the Skin, London.)

TABLE 65–1. Macroscopic and Histopathologic Features of Mycetoma Grains

	Size (mm)	Texture	H & E Section
Eumycetoma			
1. Dark grains			
Madurella mycetomatis	0.2–5.0	Hard, brittle	Cement, compact, vesicles sometimes prominent
M. grisea	0.3–0.5	Soft	Cement lacking, compact outer layer
Leptosphaeria senegalensis	0.4–0.6	Soft	Cement, dark periphery with vesicular center
Exophiala jeanselmei	0.2–0.3	Soft	Cement absent, often hollow
Pyrenochaeta romeroi	0.3–0.6	Soft	Cement lacking, compact outer layer
2. Pale grains			
Fusarium species			Compact, pigment lacking, interwoven fungal filaments
Acremonium species			
Pseudallescheria boydii	0.1–2.0	Soft	
Aspergillus nidulans			
Neotestudina rosatii			
Actinomycetoma			
1. Pale (white to yellow) grains			
Actinomadura madurae	0.1–0.5	Soft	Variegated
Nocardia brasiliensis	0.04–0.1	Soft	Small, pale blue, eosinophilic
2. Yellow to brown grains			
Streptomyces somaliensis	0.2–0.6	Soft	Grains fractured, basophilic
3. Red to pink grains			
Actinomadura pelletieri	0.06–0.2	Soft	Small, basophilic

Direct Examination. Exudates should be examined for the presence of grains. Their size, texture, and color provide clues to the etiology of the infection. Removal of crusted material plugging a sinus tract may reveal the grains on the undersurface. Differentiation of fungal and actinomycete grains is readily achieved by crushing the grain between 2 glass slides and examining it microscopically for broad (fungal) or narrow (actinomycete) filaments.

Culture. A tentative diagnosis can be made by consideration of the characteristics of the grain in relation to the predominant species for any one geographic area. A definitive diagnosis, however, requires isolation of the agent in culture and its identification. In view of the multiple etiology, a range of culture media and conditions of incubation should be employed. Different genera and species are distinguished by their morphologic and physiologic characteristics.

Serology. Precipitins are usually present in the sera of patients with long-standing mycetoma. Their detection requires the services of a specialized laboratory because of the wide range of potential antigens and their lack of availability from commercial sources. Precipitin tests can be helpful in the early stages of infection, when sinus tracts are lacking. Cross-reactions are common between different fungal species and between different actinomycete agents, but not between fungal and actinomycete agents.

Differential Diagnosis. Chronic osteomyelitis of bacterial etiology, e.g., syphilitic, actinomycotic, or tuberculous, may resemble mycetoma, particularly in the early stages. Cases of mycetoma lacking sinus tracts may resemble soft tissue tumors such as lipomata, or cystic lesions, e.g., cold abscess or implantation dermoid. Botryomycosis, in which persistent bacterial infection is associated with granule and sinus formation, must be distinguished also. This pattern of infection is seen most often in immunologically deficient individuals.

TREATMENT. The distinction between a fungal and actinomycete etiology is of critical importance because of the different responses of the 2 conditions to chemotherapy.

Eumycetoma. As a rule, eumycetoma is unresponsive, and management should be directed toward early diagnosis and radical surgical removal. Because eumycetoma infections are generally well circumscribed and progress rather slowly, excision is often successful, particularly if there has been no invasion of bone. Arteriography may demonstrate the extent of infection. In advanced cases of eumycetoma, amputation was initially thought to offer the only real hope of eradication. All traces of infection have to be removed, otherwise relapse is inevitable; recurrence rates of 80% have been recorded. If the disease is only slowly progressive and if the patient can be reviewed regularly, the decision about surgical intervention can be deferred for several years. More recently, encouraging results have been obtained in eradicating infections caused by *Madurella mycetomatis* with oral ketoconazoles.

Actinomycetoma. Medical treatment is often effective in cases of actinomycetoma. Good results have been obtained with a combination of dapsone (100 mg twice daily) and streptomycin (1 gm daily for 1 month). Perhaps the most effective combination is trimethoprim-sulfamethoxazole (co-trimoxazole) and streptomycin or rifampicin. One of the last 2 drugs is usually given for the first 3 to 4 months of therapy. The dapsone regimen is usually preferred because the drug is inexpensive. The average duration of treatment is about 9 months, and responses to chemotherapy are generally good, even when there has been involvement of bone.

PROGNOSIS. Provided the diagnosis is established early, the prognosis for both types of mycetoma is good. In advanced cases with sinus formation and bone involvement, the outlook is bleak, particularly when the etiology is fungal.

Apart from the mutilation resulting from amputation, loss of function can render the afflicted subject unemployable. Moreover, the recurrence rate can be high. When lesions affect the back, abdomen, neck, scalp, or other site where excision or amputation is impracticable, little practical aid can be offered.

With actinomycetoma, the prognosis is reasonable, with improvement or cure likely in about 70% of patients. Clinical response involves reduction of swelling, closing of sinuses, formation of new bone, and healing of skin abnormalities. If practicable, serial monitoring of serum precipitin levels provides objective measure of response to management.

PREVENTION. Unfortunately, preventive measures are impracticable in view of the widespread occurrence of the agents in nature and the frequency with which minor skin wounds occur in endemic areas.

BIBLIOGRAPHY

Mahgoub ES: Medical management of mycetoma. Bull WHO 54:303, 1976.
Mahgoub ES, Murray IG: Mycetoma. London, William Heinemann, 1973.
Mahgoub ES, Gumaa SA, El Hassan AM: Immunological status of mycetoma patients. Bull Soc Pathol Exot 70:48, 1977.
Mahgoub, ES, Gumaa SA: Ketoconazole in the treatment of eumycetoma due to *Madurella mycetomii*. Trans R Soc Trop Med Hyg 78:376, 1984.
Mariat F: Sur la distribution géographique et la répartition des agents des mycetomes. Bull Soc Pathol Exot 56:35, 1963.
Peyron JP, Herouin P, Lesquere C, et al.: Intérêt de la radiologie dans le diagnostic des mycetomes. Med Trop 39:27, 1979.

65.2. SPOROTRICHOSIS

DEFINITION. Sporotrichosis is a chronic fungal infection principally affecting the skin, lymphatics, and subcutaneous tissues. Pulmonary and disseminated forms occur less frequently, with involvement of the lungs, osteoarticular and musculoskeletal tissues, viscera, mucous membranes, and central nervous system. Lesions may be nodular, pustular, or ulcerative but exhibit a wide morphologic range.

ETIOLOGY. Sporotrichosis is caused by a single species of fungus, *Sporothrix schenckii,* which is widely distributed throughout the world. It is a common saprophyte and can be readily isolated from soils particularly of those rich in organic matter or vegetable debris, or from a wide range of plants and plant materials.

The fungus has a filamentous vegetative organization consisting of fine, branching hyphae on which minute unicellular spores are formed. In common with many other pathogenic fungi, it is dimorphic, being mold-like or yeast-like, depending on the growth environment. In infected tissues, the agent is yeast-like.

HISTORY. The first description of sporotrichosis and its causal agent was reported in 1898. Many of the earlier reports originated in France, but it is now uncommon there. One of the most remarkable outbreaks occurred in the gold mines of Witwatersrand in the 1940s, when almost 3000 cases were recorded, the source of infection being heavy growth of *S. schenckii* on the surface of timber used as pit props.

EPIDEMIOLOGY. Sporotrichosis occurs worldwide but is most common in warm, temperate, or tropical countries. In temperate countries, infections are sometimes associated with minor gardening traumas from rose thorns or splinters. Most cases are sporadic, but epidemics may occur in endemic areas. In Guatemala, 53 cases were diagnosed during a 3-year period. Many of the patients became infected after handling a fish that burrows near the edge of a lake and presumably comes into contact with soil. There is no sex, age, or race predilection. The disease affects individuals whose occupation brings them into contact with soil, plants, or plant materials such as straw, wood, or reeds. It is most commonly reported from Central and South America, Africa, and Australasia.

PATHOGENESIS AND PATHOLOGY. Once introduced into the dermis, the fungus provokes a granulomatous response with foci of suppuration and necrosis. Associated with localized lesions are foci of neutrophils, histiocytes, and epithelioid cells. Langerhans' giant cells may be present. In some lesions, there are circumscribed microabscesses surrounded by tissue infiltrated with lymphocytes, neutrophils, and plasma cells. In skin lesions, pseudoepitheliomatous hyperplasia associated with a mixed pyogenic-granulomatous reaction may be seen. Rete pegs are elongated and broadened.

Unusual amongst the mycoses, the causal agent is rarely seen in histopathologic material from primary infections. When present, it appears as small, round, oval, or cigar-shaped budding yeast cells 2 to 3 μm wide by 3 to 8 μm long. In some instances, a central fungal cell is surrounded by radiating eosinophilic material (asteroid body), or rarely there may be slender strands of hyphae.

CLINICAL MANIFESTATIONS. Sporotrichosis has a wide range of clinical expression. It is not contagious and is acquired from the environment, usually by implantation through the skin. Although inhalation with the resultant establishment of a primary pulmonary infection is a recognized mechanism of pathogenesis, the most common route of entry is by minor traumatic subcutaneous inoculation, or via an abrasion. The incubation period usually varies from 1 to 4 weeks, exceptionally up to 6 months. About 75% of infections affect an upper extremity.

Primary Lymphatic Sporotrichosis. The most common and familiar form of sporotrichosis is primary cutaneous lymphatic sporotrichosis, in which a small, firm, movable subcutaneous nodule develops at the site of inoculation. The nodule later becomes soft and breaks down to form a persistent friable ulcer or chancre. Subsequently, additional nodules develop along the lymphatics draining the area, which, in turn, progress to ulceration (Fig. 7–5). The lymphatic vessels connecting the nodules may become acutely inflamed or indurated and cord-like. The presence of a persistent ulcer on a finger or hand and a chain of swollen lymph nodes extending up the arm is suspicious, but this may be caused by other organisms. If untreated, the lesions may persist for years. In about 23% of cutaneous infections, the initial lesion remains "fixed," without lymphatic spread. Such infections are common in children and in Latin Americans. Facial lesions also often behave in this way.

Pulmonary Sporotrichosis. Primary pulmonary infection was originally thought to be rare, but it may not be uncommon in endemic areas. In most cases, it is asymptomatic, but a residual infection may occur in individuals with a low level of immunity and lead to disseminated disease.

Disseminated (Secondary) Sporotrichosis. This is uncommon and is generally seen in subjects with underlying diseases or predisposition. It is always endogenous, originating by hematogenous spread from primary skin or lung foci. Multiple cutaneous nodules that eventually ulcerate may develop over the body surfaces. Other sites affected include joints, the lungs, bone, mucous membranes, and the central nervous system.

DIAGNOSIS. Classic cutaneous lymphatic sporotrichosis is clinically distinct, but the complexity and variability of other forms of the disease may make the clinical diagnosis difficult. Direct examination of pus or skin scales is seldom helpful, and *S. schenckii* is usually absent or rare in tissue sections. Immunofluorescence may assist in visualizing single fungal cells, but culture and serologic testing are of the greatest value as ancillary diagnostic procedures. *S. schenckii* is readily isolated from clinical material on a variety of culture media. It normally appears 3 to 10 days after inoculation and is identified by the colonial and microscopic morphology and by the demonstration of dimorphism in vitro.

Serology. Serologic procedures may be of value, although they are not always reliable. Antibodies may not be demonstrable in patients with proven infection, and existing serodiagnostic reagents lack specificity. Nevertheless, the demonstration of antibodies to *S. schenckii* by double diffusion, agglutination, or immunofluorescence may provide a valuable clue in disseminated sporotrichosis, and where practicable, the services of a specialized mycologic laboratory should be recruited.

Differential Diagnosis. Apart from cutaneous lymphatic sporotrichosis, the condition must be distinguished from other mycoses and from a range of infective skin lesions such as tularemia, leishmaniasis, anthrax, tuberculosis, and pyogenic bacterioses. Lymphatic spread similar to that of sporotrichosis may also occur in atypical mycobacterial infections and some South American forms of leishmaniasis.

TREATMENT. The most reliable treatment is orally administered potassium iodide (KI) in saturated solution, which usually produces a cure within 3 months. An adult can be given 1 ml of KI 3 times daily, with drops in incremental increases to a maximum of 4 to 6 ml 3 times daily after 1 month. To increase palatability, the drug may be administered in milk. Treatment should be continued for 3 to 4 weeks after clinical cure. This form of treatment is most effective for cutaneous sporotrichosis. In cases of disseminated disease or patient intolerance to iodide, amphotericin B is the drug of choice (Chapter 67). An intriguing and apparently effective treatment is the use of externally applied heat. In one series of 9 patients with cutaneous sporotrichosis reported from Uruguay, cure was effected by repeated application of hot compresses several times daily, with or without rubefacients.

PROGNOSIS. The prognosis is excellent for cutaneous forms of the disease but is less satisfactory for patients with disseminated sporotrichosis, particularly if associated with another severe underlying disease.

PREVENTION. As with other subcutaneous mycoses in which the agent is widely distributed in nature, epidemiologic control is not practicable.

BIBLIOGRAPHY

Galiana J, Conti-Diaz IA: Healing effects of heat and a rubefacient on nine cases of sporotrichosis. Sabouraudia 3:64, 1963.

Kaplan W, Gonzalez-Ochoa A: Application of the fluorescent antibody technique to the rapid diagnosis of sporotrichosis. J Lab Clin Med 62:835, 1963.

Lurie HI: Sporotrichosis. *In* Baker RD (ed.).: Human Infections with Fungi, Actinomycetes and Algae. New York, Springer-Verlag, 1971, pp 614–675.

Mariat F: The epidemiology of sporotrichosis. *In* Wolstenholme GEW, Porter R (eds.): Systemic Mycoses. London, J. & A. Churchill, 1968, pp 144–159.

Mayorga R, Caceres A, Toriello C, et al.: Étude d'une zone d'endemic sporotrichosique au Guatemala. Sabouraudia 16:185, 1978.

65.3. CHROMOMYCOSIS

DEFINITION. Chromomycosis (chromoblastomycosis) is a chronic mycosis affecting skin and subcutaneous tissues characterized by the development of slow-growing verrucous nodules that eventually coalesce and form hyperkeratotic masses.

ETIOLOGY. The condition is caused by several species of related fungi, the most common and widespread of which are *Fonsecaea pedrosoi*, *F. compacta*, *Phialophora verrucosa*, and *Cladosporium carrionii*. *Wangiella dermatitidis* has more restricted distribution, occurring in the Far East. Irrespective of the causal species, all have an identical appearance in infected tissues, i.e., single or clustered, rounded or angular, thick-walled, dark-brown bodies ("sclerotic cells"). In culture, considerable variation exists in the types and

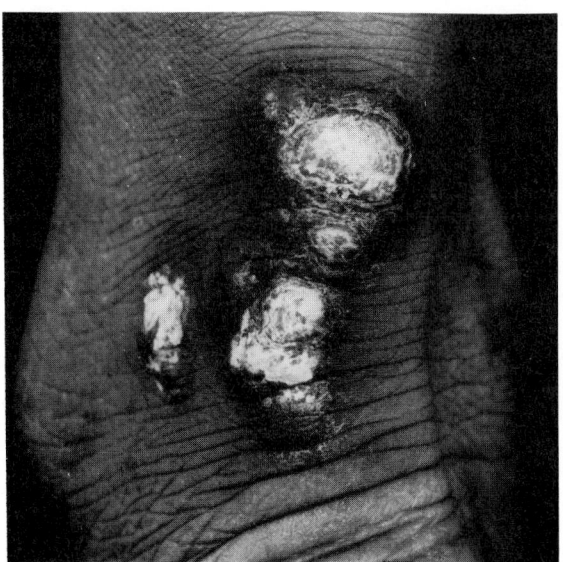

FIGURE 65–4. Chromomycosis. An early lesion on the ankle. (Courtesy of St. John's Hospital for Diseases of the Skin, London.)

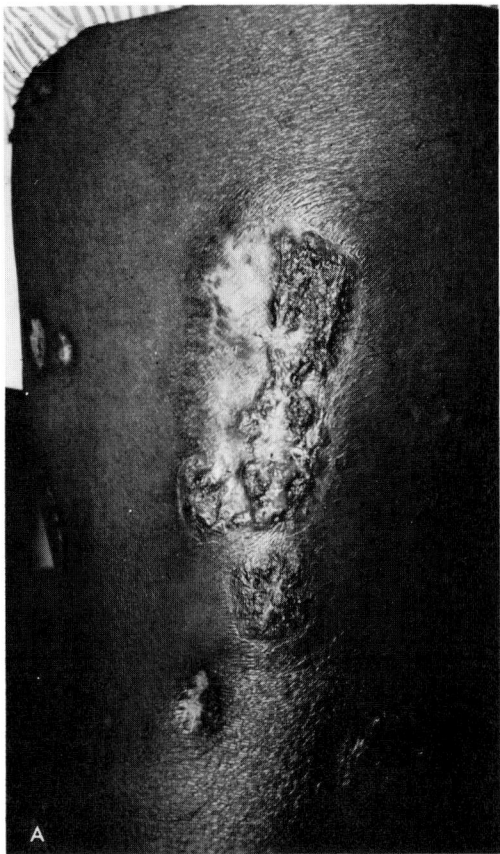

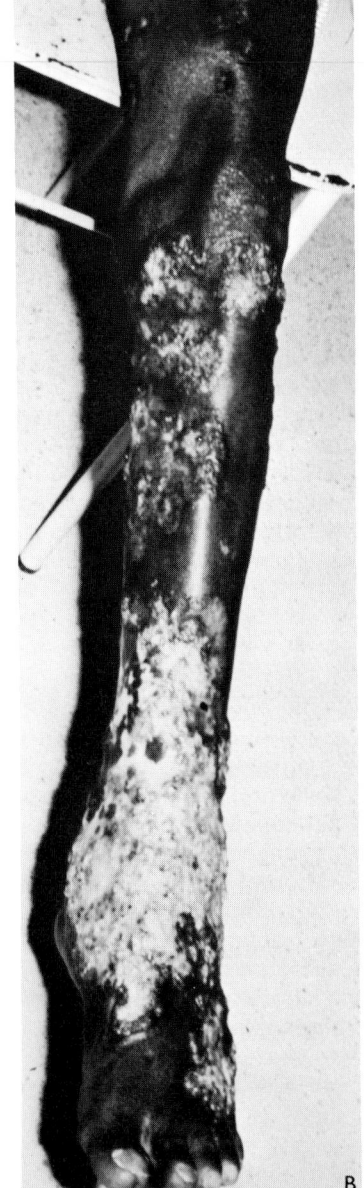

FIGURE 65–5. Chromomycosis. These scarred verrucous lesions of the thigh (*A*) and leg and foot (*B*) had persisted for 6 years in a 53-year-old Brazilian man. (Courtesy of the Armed Forces Institute of Pathology, Photograph Neg. No. 74–12824.)

predominance of spore forms, and considerable controversy exists among mycologists as to their nomenclature. The organisms are commonly found in soil and wood as saprophytes. The first case was reported from the United States in 1915, but it was subsequently shown to be a disease of tropical and subtropical countries.

EPIDEMIOLOGY. Chromomycosis is diagnosed more commonly in males than in females. Because, in common with other types of subcutaneous mycoses, infection is from an exogenous source, lesions occur most frequently among those whose occupation exposes them to thorn pricks, splinters, and other penetrating wounds. Therefore, the disease is more prevalent in rural than in urban dwellers and among those who work barefoot rather than those who wear shoes. All races are affected. Curiously, the condition is uncommon among children. Although experimental infections can

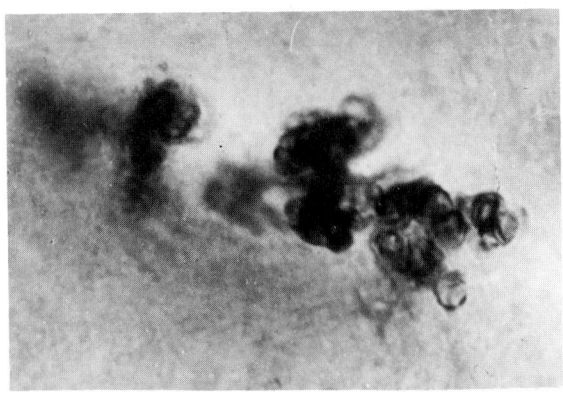

FIGURE 65–6. Scraping of chromomycosis mounted in 20% potassium hydroxide. Note the thick-walled pigmented fungal cells. (Courtesy of St. John's Hospital for Diseases of the Skin, London.)

be established in animals, they are not normally naturally infected.

There are some indications that climate affects the prevalence of different species. Thus, in Madagascar, Brygoo and Segretain (1960) showed that infections with *C. carrionii* occurred in areas of low rainfall (50 to 60 cm annually), in contrast to infections caused by *F. pedrosoi*, which are characteristic of areas with a high rainfall (220 to 300 cm annually). The disease has a worldwide distribution and has a particularly high prevalence in Costa Rica (1:21,000 population) and Madagascar (1:30,000 population).

PATHOGENESIS AND PATHOLOGY. In some instances, there is a history of trauma, but usually the patient can remember no specific incident that preceded development of the primary lesion. The sites affected most frequently are the feet and legs, but other exposed parts of the body, such as the hands, arms, buttocks, back, neck, and face, may be involved. Early primary lesions are rarely seen or recognized as such, and the patient does not usually seek medical attention until the lesion has been present for 15 years or more.

Lesions are usually hyperkeratotic and characterized by pseudoepitheliomatous hyperplasia with microabscess formation. Granulomatous nodules are present in the dermis and are composed of epithelioid cells, with occasional giant cells, surrounded by plasma cells, macrophages, eosinophils, and lymphocytes. Fibrosis of the dermis and subcutaneous tissue is a prominent feature. The fungal cells are 5 to 12 μm in diameter, common in some sections and rare in others. They may be associated with giant cells. Their distinctive dark-brown color, thick walls, and multiplication by splitting rather than by budding are diagnostic. Secondary bacterial infection is often present.

CLINICAL MANIFESTATIONS. The initial lesion is a warty papule that enlarges slowly to form a verrucoid plaque (Fig. 65–4). In some instances, the primary lesion is a pustule, a flat plaque, or an ulcer. As the infection progresses, ulceration and serous exudation can become features (Fig. 65–5B). Eventually, the lesion becomes dry and crusted, with a roughened surface and raised margin (Fig. 65–5A). Some lesions may be pedunculated. Large hyperkeratotic plaques up to 3 cm thick with central scar formation may be formed. Characteristically, the lesion does not spread peripherally, although there may be spread by autoinoculation and via the lymphatics to adjacent areas. The condition is not painful but may itch. Superinfection may be responsible for lymph stasis and resultant elephantiasis, and secondary infected lesions have an unpleasant smell.

Lesions of chromomycosis are almost always confined to the skin and subcutaneous tissues. Rarely, *F. pedrosoi* and *Wangiella dermatitidis* have been isolated from the brain, suggesting that hematogenous spread and systemic infection are possible.

DIAGNOSIS. Clinical history and manifestations are often diagnostic. Early or atypical lesions can be recognized by direct microscopy, the distinctive brown fungal cells being readily distinguished in 20% potassium hydroxide mounts of skin scrapings (Fig. 65–6). Cells seen in tissue sections are also diagnostic. Culture and identification of the specific etiologic agent can be time-consuming and should always be entrusted to a specialist laboratory, because the polymorphic appearance of many isolates makes their positive identification difficult. Serologic tests have not been reliable indicators of infection. Antibodies are produced during the course of infection, but neither presence nor titer is diagnostic.

Differential Diagnosis. Chromomycosis may resemble blastomycosis, and in parts of the world where the latter is endemic, a differentiation between the two diseases must be made (Chapter 66.3). Other conditions that may simulate chromomycosis include cutaneous tuberculosis and leishmaniasis, syphilis, and yaws.

TREATMENT. In advanced cases with multiple extensive lesions, amputations are sometimes considered to be necessary. No simple antifungal regimen is universally satisfactory, although 5-fluorocytosine has been effective in many cases. Resistance to this drug may occur, and in extensive lesions amphotericin B should be given intravenously (Chapter 67) at the outset of treatment in addition to 5-fluorocytosine. Encouraging results have been obtained with the newer imidazoles, e.g. itraconazole. Local excision of early lesions or destruction by cautery or diathermy may be effective, emphasizing the importance of an early diagnosis. Surgery may be effective also in treating local spread of the infection.

PROGNOSIS. Chromomycosis progresses slowly and usually remains localized. Since hematogenous spread is such a rare event, the condition is not life-threatening. Moreover, in contrast to mycetoma, chromomycosis does not invade the deeper tissues with attendant destruction and loss of function. The principal clinical problems relate to the pain, tissue damage, and elephantiasis associated with bacterial superinfection. Cures are rare in patients with advanced disease.

PREVENTION. This is not practicable.

BIBLIOGRAPHY

Brygoo ER, Segretain G: Étude clinique épidemiologique et mycologique de la chromoblastomycose á Madagascar. Bull Soc Pathol Exot 53:443, 1960.
Cameron HM, Gatei D, Bremner AD: The deep mycoses in Kenya: A histopathological study. 3. Chromomycosis. East Afr Med J 50:406, 1973.
Zaias N: Chromomycosis. J Cutan Pathol 5:155, 1978.

65.4. RHINOSPORIDIOSIS

DEFINITION. Rhinosporidiosis is a chronic, localized granulomatous infection of nasal and other mucosal surfaces, conjunctiva, and skin that is characterized by hyperplasia and development of polyps.

ETIOLOGY. The causal agent is *Rhinosporidium seeberi*. In infected tissues, it forms abundant sporangia up to 350 μm in diameter and containing large numbers of spores. Details of its ecology and life cycle are unknown. It has not been cultivated in vitro, nor have experimental infections of animals been established.

DISTRIBUTION. The disease has been reported from many tropical and temperate countries throughout the world, but 90% of reported cases are from India and Sri Lanka.

PATHOGENESIS AND EPIDEMIOLOGY. The mechanism by which infection is acquired is not known. Rhinosporidiosis is most common in children and young adults, but any age group may be affected. Males are more commonly affected than females (3:1). The disease is not contagious, and infection is thought to be exogenous. The high proportion of patients with a history of long exposure to fresh water does suggest that *R. seeberi* may occur naturally in rivers or lakes, possibly as a pathogen of fish or insects, and that humans become infected by continued contact with such contaminated environments. Because of the localized nature of the condition and its presumed exogenous origin, rhinosporidiosis can provisionally be regarded as a mycosis of implantation.

The most common site of rhinosporidiosis is the nose (70% of infections), with sessile or pedunculated polyps affecting one or both nostrils. Lesions may affect the conjunctiva also and, more rarely, the larynx, genitals, and skin. Dissemination has been reported but is exceptional.

PATHOLOGY. Examination of H & E—stained tissue sections reveals hyperplasia and a chronic inflammatory reaction with neutrophils, lymphocytes, plasma cells, and occasional foreign-body giant cells and abundant globular sporangia of varying sizes and stages of development.

DIAGNOSIS. Polyps of rhinosporidiosis can be recognized by their pink or purple color and friable consistency and by the presence of small, white sporangia on the polyp surface. Diagnosis is confirmed by examination of biopsy sections and the detection of the distinctive sporangia. Culture, serologic tests, and animal inoculation procedures are not helpful in establishing or confirming a diagnosis.

Differential Diagnosis. Rhinosporidiosis must be differentiated from nasal polyps. Lesions in other sites, particularly on the genitalia or anal region, must be distinguished from warts, condylomata, and hemorrhoids.

TREATMENT. Chemotherapy is of little proven value. The treatment of choice is surgical excision, with or without cauterization.

BIBLIOGRAPHY

Mohapatra LN: Rhinosporidiosis. *In* Baker RD (ed.): Human Infection with Fungi, Actinomycetes and Algae. New York, Springer-Verlag, 1971, pp 676–683.

65.5. SUBCUTANEOUS ZYGOMYCOSIS

DEFINITION. Subcutaneous zygomycosis (subcutaneous phycomycosis, entomophthoromycosis due to *Basidiobolus*) is a localized mycotic infection causing a firm, progressive swelling of the subcutaneous tissues and characterized by eosinophil infiltration and granuloma formation.

ETIOLOGY. The causal fungus is *Basidiobolus haptosporus,* which is a common saprophyte in decaying vegetation overlying soil. It has also been reported to be found in the intestines of frogs, toads, lizards, and other small reptiles, in the absence of pathologic conditions.

EPIDEMIOLOGY. The disease was first described in Indonesia in 1956, but it is most commonly reported from Africa. Sporadic cases have also been reported from India, the Middle East, Asia, and Europe. Unusual among subcutaneous mycoses, the condition affects children and adolescents rather than adults, and boys rather than girls.

PATHOGENESIS AND PATHOLOGY. The mode of entry of the fungus has not been clearly established but is most likely implantation from an exogenous source via percutaneous inoculation. Once established, the lesion affects mainly subcutaneous tissues, largely replacing fat. It is characterized, particularly towards the margins of the tumor, by microabscesses in which eosinophils predominate. Strands of broad (5 to 15 μm), thin-walled, branching, and generally nonseptate hyphae are found toward the edge of the lesions, each surrounded by a distinctive eosinophilic sheath several micrometers wide (Splendore-Hoeppli phenomenon). In subacute stages, hyphae may be surrounded by epithelioid and plasma cells. Giant cells may also be present, together with varying quantities of "fibrinoid" material. In later stages fibrosis and necrosis are prominent, along with a variable cellular infiltration.

CLINICAL MANIFESTATIONS. The subcutaneous swelling is firm, movable, and well defined; satellite lesions may be palpable at the advancing margins. The masses are disk-shaped, with the consistency of rubber. The overlying skin is usually intact and may be tense, edematous, hyperpigmented, or normal (Fig. 65–7). Ulceration is uncommon, and regional lymph nodes are rarely affected. Pain and tenderness are usually absent. Any part of the body may be affected, but the most common sites are the limbs, buttocks, trunk, and neck. Penetration of deeper tissues and viscera has been reported but is uncommon.

DIAGNOSIS. The clinical picture is usually characteristic, but a firm diagnosis requires histopathologic confirmation. The agent can be cultivated readily and has distinctive colonial and microscopic features. Serologic tests have not been developed to the point where they constitute a diagnostic aid.

Differential Diagnosis. At presentation, subcutaneous malignant lymphoma may have clinical similarities to subcutaneous zygomycosis, but it is characterized by more rapid growth. Clinical characteristics should serve to distinguish it from sarcoma, mycetoma, or bacterial cellulitis. Lymphatic edema and elephantiasis are differentiated by the absence of a clear margin and by the tendency to affect the extremities.

TREATMENT. The most effective treatment is orally administered potassium iodide, in saturated solutions, in doses up to 10 ml 3 times daily for 3 months. Not all patients respond well, and combined therapy with iodide

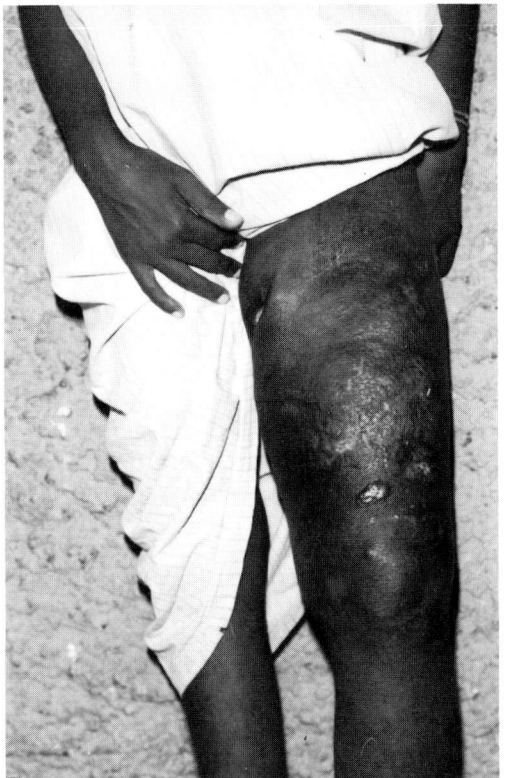

FIGURE 65–7. Subcutaneous phycomycosis in the thigh of an Ugandan woman. (Courtesy of the Armed Forces Institute of Pathology, Photograph Neg. No. 70–11661.)

and trimethoprimsulfamethoxazole (co-trimoxazole) (14 mg/kg of sulfamethoxazole twice daily) has been used with some success. Amphotericin B has been used in patients refractory to treatment. The rare patient is unresponsive to chemotherapy, inevitably leading to a consideration of amputation.

PROGNOSIS. The infection generally pursues a slow and benign course, with increasing lateral extension of the initial tumor. Spontaneous recovery occasionally occurs, but in untreated cases the condition may persist for years.

PREVENTION. This is not practicable.

BIBLIOGRAPHY

Cameron HM, Gatei D, Bremner AD: The deep mycoses in Kenya: A histopathological study. 2. Phycomycosis. East Afr Med J 50:396, 1973.

Clark BM: The epidemiology of phycomycosis. *In* Wolstenholme GEW, Porter R (eds.): Systemic Mycoses. London, J. & A. Churchill, 1968.

Clark BM, Edington GM: Subcutaneous phycomycosis and rhinoentomophthoromycosis. *In* Baker RD (ed.): Human Infection with Fungi, Actinomycetes and Algae. New York, Springer-Verlag, 1971, pp 684–690.

65.6. RHINOENTOMOPHTHOROMYCOSIS

DEFINITION. Rhinoentomophthoromycosis (entomophthoromycosis due to *Conidiobolus*) is a chronic, localized, subcutaneous fungal infection affecting tissues of the nose, cheek, and upper lip. It is also called nasofacial phycomycosis.

ETIOLOGY. The condition is caused by *Conidiobolus coronatus,* a ubiquitous saprophyte in tropical rain forest areas. Clark (1968) isolated it most commonly from soil and decaying vegetation in Nigeria during September and October, when rainfall was regular but not excessive. Unlike *Basidiobolus,* no association with reptilian or amphibian intestines has been recognized.

The disease was reported initially in 1961, affecting horses. The first reported human cases were by Martinson in 1963 in Nigeria, but the agent was isolated in culture from a patient in the Congo in 1965. Earlier isolated reports in the literature suggest that the condition existed a decade or more earlier but had not been recognized as a new disease entity.

EPIDEMIOLOGY. In striking contrast to subcutaneous zygomycosis, rhinoentomophthoromycosis is a disease of young adults rather than children. Males are more commonly affected than females. Most cases affect men 20 to 40 years old who work outdoors in tropical forest areas. Most infections are reported from West Africa, particularly Nigeria, but cases have been recognized in India and South America. The geographic range is probably explained in part by climatic factors, the agent failing to grow well at temperatures below 15C.

PATHOGENESIS AND PATHOLOGY. The mode of infection is unknown but is probably inoculation of contaminated soil or vegetable matter through minor trauma or insect bites. The initial site of infection is the region of the inferior turbinates.

Respiratory epithelium may show transitional or squamous metaplasia, but ulceration is uncommon. The condition affects subepithelial tissue and muscle. Bone is not affected, but radiographs may show evidence of soft tissue swelling. Tomography has been useful in establishing the extent of infection, particularly in demonstrating the involvement of ethmoidal air cells. Histopathologic features are identical to those already described for subcutaneous zygomycosis, both in the types of tissue responses and the appearance of the pathogen.

CLINICAL MANIFESTATIONS. Infection apparently originates in the nasal mucosa, leading to nasal obstruction, which may be unilateral. Tissue swelling becomes pronounced, affecting the nose and nasolabial folds, cheeks, and upper lip and eventually producing gross facial distortion (Fig. 65–8). The infected areas have distinct margins, but the mass is not movable over the underlying tissues. As the condition progresses, infection may spread rarely to the paranasal sinuses, palate, and pharynx. Satellite lesions may be detectable at the margins. The overlying skin becomes stretched but does not ulcerate. The reason for the curiously restricted anatomic distribution is unknown.

There are few symptoms. Nasal discharge is an early finding, but pain, tenderness, and constitutional upset are rare. Pharyngeal involvement may result in dysphagia. The most serious effect on the patient may result from the severe and, at times, grotesque distortion of perinasal areas.

DIAGNOSIS. The clinical features are highly distinc-

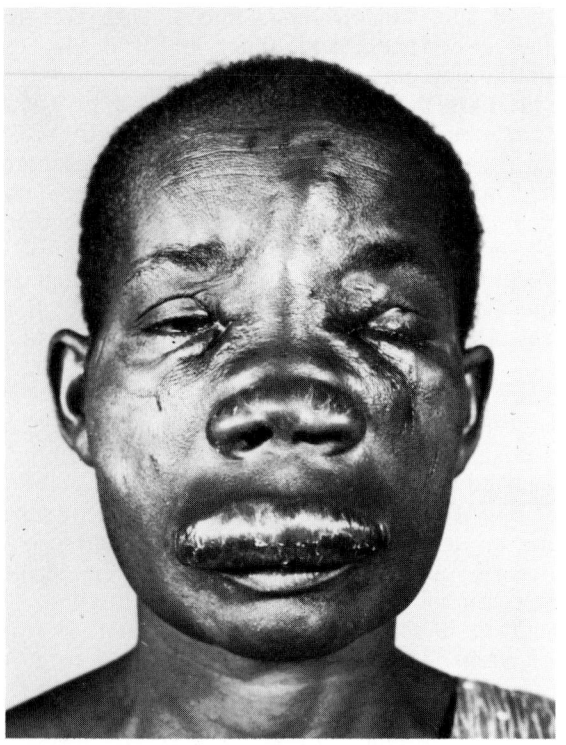

FIGURE 65–8. Nigerian woman with nasofacial phycomycosis (rhinoentomophthoromycosis) involving the entire nose, cheeks, eyelids, forehead, and upper lip. (Courtesy of the Armed Forces Institute of Pathology, Photograph Neg. No. 76–6165.)

tive, i.e., localized swelling of the nose and face in tropical countries. Biopsy may be definitive when the characteristic hyphae are present and associated with an eosinophilic sheath and eosinophilic granuloma. Positive diagnosis may depend on culture and identification of the etiologic agent. Serologic tests have not been developed.

Differential Diagnosis. Rhinoentomophthoromycosis can be differentiated from subcutaneous zygomycosis by the anatomic localization and the lack of mobility of the infected mass over underlying tissues. Other conditions that may resemble rhinoentomophthoromycosis include rhinosporidiosis, nasal polyps, and regional carcinoma or sarcoma.

TREATMENT. Treatment is the same as for subcutaneous zygomycosis (Chapter 65.5).

PROGNOSIS. Spontaneous remission is unknown. Surgical intervention may be required to alleviate nasal obstruction or to reduce gross deformities. The response to therapy is less satisfactory than that in subcutaneous zygomycosis.

PREVENTION. None is practicable.

BIBLIOGRAPHY

Clark BM: The epidemiology of phycomycosis. *In* Wolstenholme GEW, Porter R (eds.): Systemic Mycoses. London, J. & A. Churchill, 1968, pp. 179–192.
Clark BM, Edington GM: Subcutaneous phycomycosis and rhinoentomophthoromycosis. *In* Baker RD (ed.): Human Infection with Fungi, Actinomycetes and Algae. New York, Springer-Verlag, 1971, pp 684–690.

Cockshott WP, Clark BM, Martinson FD: Upper respiratory tract infection due to *Entomophthora coronata*. Radiology 90:1016, 1968.
Martinson RD: Rhinophycomycosis. J Laryngol Otol 77:691, 1963.

65.7. OTHER SUBCUTANEOUS MYCOSES

PHAEOHYPHOMYCOSIS

DEFINITION AND ETIOLOGY. This is a catchall term to describe infections with dark-pigmented fungi that are distinct clinically and pathologically from chromomycosis or mycetoma. Within this heterogeneous group is a wide range of uncommon subcutaneous mycoses that have been described in the literature under many disease names. These include cladosporiosis, subcutaneous mycotic cyst, phaeosporotrichosis, and cystic chromomycosis. The range of causal organisms is also a wide one, embracing some 16 genera and almost 30 species. Phaeohyphomycosis is an uncommon disease, and its prevalence in the tropics is unknown.

CLINICAL MANIFESTATIONS AND TREATMENT. Lesions are usually solitary and circumscribed, occurring on the feet, legs, hands, and other body sites. As with all subcutaneous mycoses, entry of the pathogen is assumed to occur by a penetrating wound, the site of the injury being contaminated with the pathogen. Over a period of months or years, the lesions may increase in size, producing a crusted or cystic mass that remains localized. Rarely, phaeohyphomycosis may affect the brain, producing symptoms and pathology of cerebral abscesses. Diagnosis depends on the recognition of brown fungal elements by direct microscopy or in tissue sections, which may be filamentous, irregularly swollen, or yeast-like, and by isolation and identification of the agents in a specialist laboratory. The treatment for localized forms of the disease is surgical excision. Recurrence may result from inadequate or careless excision. The prognosis in cerebral forms of the disease is poor.

LOBO'S DISEASE

DEFINITION. Lobo's disease is a chronic, localized mycosis of skin and subcutaneous tissues characterized by keloidal or verrucoid lesions that contain abundant round or lemon-shaped cells.

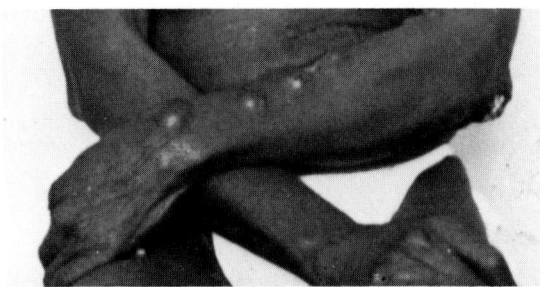

FIGURE 65–9. Lobo's disease. Nodules on the left forearm of a man. Initial lesion occurred 30 years previously following minor injury to the foot. (Courtesy of the Armed Forces Institute of Pathology, Photograph Neg. No. 75–771.)

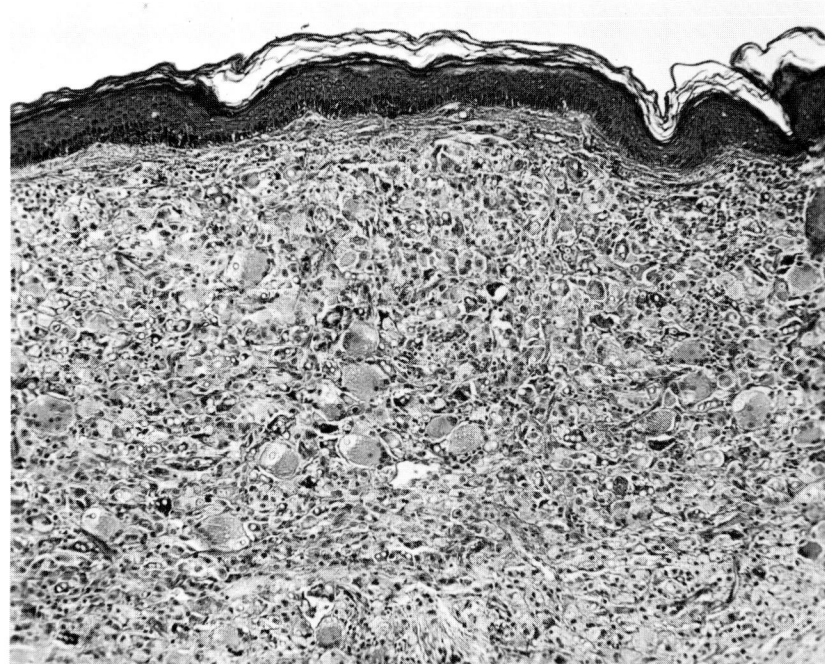

FIGURE 65–10. Biopsy from the lesion on forearm (Fig. 65–9) showing giant cell granulomas of dermis containing many yeast-like cells. The stroma is not collagenous (× 70). (Courtesy of the Armed Forces Institute of Pathology, Photograph Neg. 61–6506.)

ETIOLOGY. The agent has been named *Loboa loboi*. In infected tissues, its cells are yeast-like, 9 to 10 μm in diameter, round, thick-walled, elliptical or lemon-shaped, and numerous, with largely unbranched budding chains, giving the appearance of a string of beads in tissue reactions. In preparations stained with methenamine silver, adjacent cells are sometimes seen to be joined by a narrow connecting tube. The agent has never been isolated in culture, but experimental infections have been achieved in the armadillo. It is considered by some authorities to be related to *Paracoccidioides brasiliensis*.

DISTRIBUTION. Lobo's disease was first described in 1931 from the Amazon Valley and has been reported sporadically since then from the State of Amazonas in Brazil, Surinam, Panama, Venezuela, Colombia, French Guiana, and Costa Rica. Several hundred cases have been described in Brazil. Curiously, the condition has also been reported in Atlantic bottle-nosed dolphins off the coast of Florida.

PATHOGENESIS AND EPIDEMIOLOGY. Little information is available on the ecology of the pathogen and the likely mechanism of its entry into human tissues. In view of the chronic and localized nature of the lesions and the evidence available from studies of native communities in endemic areas, it would seem likely that infection is acquired from an exogenous source and that the mycosis is acquired by implantation. Lesions have been induced experimentally in a human volunteer following percutaneous inoculation of material obtained from a natural infection.

PATHOLOGY AND CLINICAL MANIFESTATIONS. Cutaneous lesions have been called keloidal blastomycosis because they are characteristically erythematous, hard, and shiny (Fig. 65–9). It is slowly progressive over decades and never involves the mucosa or internal organs. Lesions are nodular, fungating, or tu-mor-like, sometimes with involvement of mucosa or lymphatics. Autoinoculation may lead to the development of secondary elevated, crusted plaques that resemble primary lesions. Normal dermis becomes replaced by granulomatous tissue characterized by giant cells, histiocytes, and abundant fungal cells (Fig. 65–10). Silver stains show that giant cells are supported by a network of reticular and collagen fibers. Plasma cells and lymphocytes are scarce, and ulceration per se is uncommon. At the advancing margins of tumor-like lesions, the epidermis often shows hyperplasia, sometimes with pseudoepitheliomatous hyperplasia.

DIAGNOSIS. The diagnosis is made by recognition of a combination of clinical and histopathologic features. The presence of a persistent skin granuloma consisting of giant cells, macrophages, and numerous fungal cells provides a distinctive histopathologic syndrome, strongly suggestive of Lobo's disease. The presence of large numbers of fungal cells in the affected areas immediately distinguishes Lobo's disease from hypertrophic scars and keloids.

TREATMENT. Antimycotic agents, including ketoconazole, are ineffectual. The condition progresses slowly and is not life-threatening. In some circumstances, particularly early lesions, surgical excision is feasible.

BIBLIOGRAPHY

Ajello L: Phaeohyphomycosis: Definition and Etiology. Washington, D.C., Pan American Health Organization, Publication 304, 1975, pp 126–133.
Baruzzi RG, Marcopito LF, Vincente LS, et al.: Jorge Lobo's disease (keloidal blastomycosis) and tinea imbricata in Indians from the Xingu National Park in Central Brazil. Trop Doct 12:13, 1982.

65.8. PROTOTHECOSIS

Ann M. Nelson
and Ronald C. Neafie

DEFINITION AND DISTRIBUTION. Protothecosis is a rare infection caused by achlorophyllic algae belonging to the genus *Prototheca*. Infections have involved skin, subcutaneous tissue, olecranon bursa, and rarely, lymph nodes or deep organs. Less than 50 cases have been reported in the world literature, but they have come from both temperate and tropical areas of all continents.

ETIOLOGY. The index case of protothecosis in humans (Fig. 65–11) was caused by *Prototheca zopfii*. All other infections in humans, with one exception, where speciation was done, have been caused by *Prototheca wickerhamii*. *P. wickerhamii* and *P. zopfii* are ubiquitous achloric algae usually found in soil and contaminated water. Both organisms are spherical unicellular organisms, 3 to 30 μm in diameter with hyaline sporangia and asexual reproduction by internal septation and cytoplasmic cleavage, *Prototheca* are thought to be mutant strains of chlorophyllic (green) algae. *P. wickerhamii* divides to form characteristic morulas (Fig. 65–12), a form not produced by *P. zopfii*. Infections by both organisms have been reported in a variety of animals.

Chlorella is similar to *Prototheca* and must be differentiated in tissue sections. Both *Prototheca* and *Chlorella* are distinct from fungi and bacteria by size, morphology, and type of reproduction. In addition,

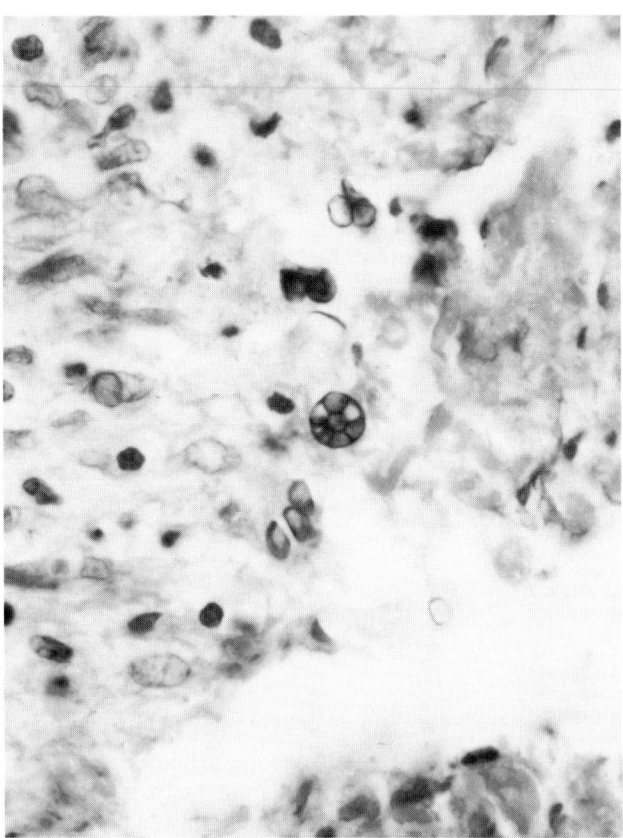

FIGURE 65–12. Characteristic morula of *P. wickerhamii* in subcutaneous tissue of wrist. (Courtesy of the Armed Forces Institute of Pathology, Photograph Neg. No. 86–7088.)

Prototheca and *Chlorella* lack the glucosamine of the fungal cell wall and the muramic acid of bacteria. *Prototheca* do not have chloroplasts, whereas *Chorella* do. Although infections by *Chorella* have been described in several animals, there is only one published report involving humans.

CLINICOPATHOLOGIC FEATURES. There are two clinical syndromes associated with prototheca infection: a localized infection of the olecranon bursa in patients with normal immunity and an eczematoid dermatitis in immunosuppressed individuals. Some infections have been associated with trauma and/or contact with contaminated water.

Protothecosis of the olecranon bursa develops usually several weeks after injury to the elbow. The lesion is localized to the bursa, but there may be epithelial hyperplasia and overlying sinus tracts. The bursa is thickened, and histopathologic changes include areas of caseation necrosis surrounded by granulation tissue, Langhan's giant cells, and fibrosis. Prototheca organisms are scattered throughout the areas of caseation.

In the cutaneous and subcutaneous forms, there are single or multiple lesions on the skin or within the subcutaneous tissue, usually over an exposed portion of the body, such as a limb or the face. The lesions are papulomacular to plaque-like and may have an overlying crust or focal ulceration; they spread slowly often in a centrifugal pattern and do not resolve. The inflammatory response varies from minimal to necrotizing granulo-

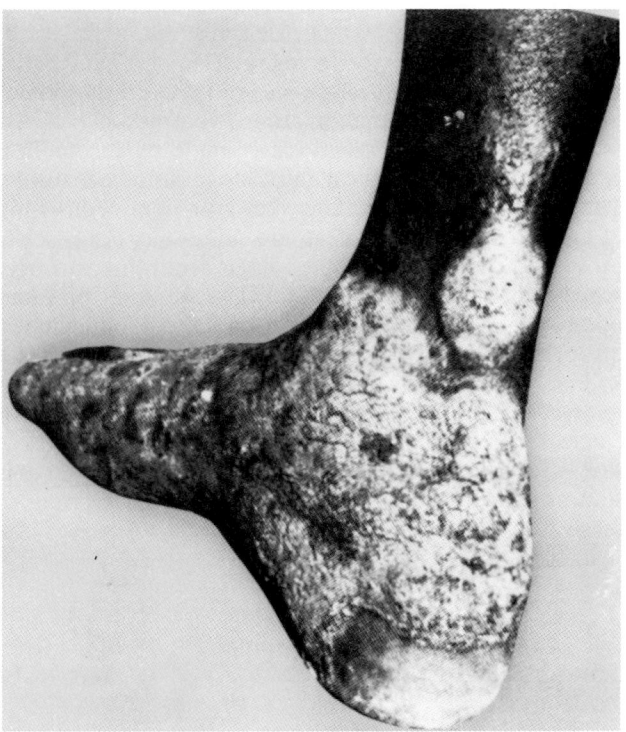

FIGURE 65–11. Protothecosis of the foot of a rice farmer from Sierra Leone. The lesion began as a papule on the instep 9 years earlier. It now encircles the foot, and there is a satellite lesion. (Armed Forces Institute of Pathology, Neg. No. 75–12872–2. Photograph courtesy of Dr. P. O. Wakelin.)

matous reaction and appears related to the depth of invasion. The organisms may be in any or all layers of the skin and may be single or in clusters, extracellular or within giant cells. These lesions must be differentiated from other chronic granulomatous diseases of the skin.

DIAGNOSIS. Scraping of the skin, biopsy specimen, and aspirates can all be cultured on Sabouraud's medium and require 1 to 2 days for growth. Typical sporulating forms can be identified on stained wet-mounts. Although the organisms are usually apparent with routine staining by hematoxylin-eosin (H&E), they are much better seen with fungal stains, such as Gomori methenamine-silver (GMS), periodic acid-Schiff (PAS), and Gridley fungus (GF). *Prototheca* species are distinguished from *Cryptococcus, Coccidioides, Blastomyces,* and other fungi by the type of division. Fluorescent immunoassay aids in speciation. Specific antisera for each of the *Prototheca* species are available and can be used on either fresh or formalin-fixed tissue.

TREATMENT. Simple bursectomy cures protothecosis of the olecranon bursa. The cutaneous lesions in immunosuppressed patients resist treatment and may persist for several years, eventually spreading to other sites. Topical medicaments, including Castellani's paint, saturated copper sulfate, potassium permanganate, and amphotericin B, as well as systemic griseofulvin, penicillin, emetine hydrochloride, and pentamidine isothionate, have not been effective. In vitro studies have demonstrated sensitivity to amphotericin B and tetracycline, and combined therapy with these two drugs has been reported to be effective.

BIBLIOGRAPHY

Connor DH, Gibson DW, Ziefer AM: Diagnostic features of three unusual infections: Micronemiasis, pheomycotic cyst, and protothecosis. *In* Majno G, Cotran RS (eds.): Current Topics in Inflammation and Infection. Baltimore, William and Wilkins, 1982, pp 205–239.

Naryshkin S, et al.: *Prototheca zopfii* isolated from a patient with olecranon bursitis. Diagn Microbiol Infect Dis 6:171–174, 1987.

Nelson AM, Neafie RC, Connor DH: Cutaneous protothecosis and chlorellosis, extraordinary "aquatic-borne" algal infections. *In* Mandojan RM (ed.): Clinic in Dermatology (Aquatic Dermatology). Philadelphia, J.B. Lippincott, 1987, vol 5, pp 76–87.

66. SYSTEMIC MYCOSES

The systemic mycoses are a group of fungal infections that involve the internal organs such as the lungs or brain. Some of the systemic fungal infections are primarily respiratory illnesses caused by organisms that are confined to recognized endemic areas. In some infections, subclinical disease is the most common form, recognized only by the development of a delayed-type skin reaction to an intradermal injection of specific antigen. In contrast, other systemic infections, the opportunistic mycoses, occur predominantly in immunocompromised individuals. The portal of entry is variable and may involve lung as well as the gastrointestinal tract, skin, or other sites. These infections are worldwide in distribution.

66.1. HISTOPLASMOSIS

Roderick J. Hay

DEFINITION. The term histoplasmosis is used to describe 2 related but different disease states—classic or small-form histoplasmosis and African histoplasmosis. The former is more common and more widespread and is a disease in which pulmonary and/or reticuloendothelial involvement is the major feature. The causative organism, *Histoplasma capsulatum,* is characteristically present in tissue in the form of small ovoid yeasts that are 2 to 4 µm in diameter. African histoplasmosis has a more restricted range, being confined to the African continent. Cutaneous and bone infections are the predominant clinical forms, and the causative agent, *H. capsulatum* var. *duboisii,* although identical in culture to *H. capsulatum,* produces much larger yeast forms (8 to 15 µm in diameter) in tissue. However, the word histoplasmosis is commonly used to describe the more common small form of the disease.

CLASSIC OR SMALL-FORM HISTOPLASMOSIS

ETIOLOGY AND EPIDEMIOLOGY. *H. capsulatum* is dimorphic, being present in the environment or on primary isolation as a mold but in tissue in yeast phase. The organism is found in soil, particularly in sites contaminated by bird or bat excreta. The relationship between birds and *H. capsulatum* has been most closely investigated in the United States, where starlings, grackles, and chickens are particularly associated with the presence of the organisms. Buildings or roosting sites sheltering these birds are consistent sources of the fungus. However, in the tropics, the majority of positive isolations have originated from sites where bats have nested, including caves and under trees. Bats are widely distributed throughout the tropical world, making exposure to *H. capsulatum* a relatively frequent occurrence.

PATHOLOGY AND PATHOGENESIS. Histoplasmosis is primarily a disease of inhalation with secondary spread from the primary site in the lung. This secondary dissemination occurs early, but in the majority of those affected it is easily controlled by the patient's inflammatory response. An alternative site of entry is via direct implantation, although in this case the infection is usually localized to the skin and subcutis, with local lymphadenopathy (primary cutaneous histoplasmosis).

Yeast forms of *H. capsulatum* are difficult to distinguish in hematoxylin-eosin-stained tissue sections. They are small, oval, and intracellular (Fig. 66–1A). Periodic acid-Schiff or methenamine silver stains will outline the organisms. Small forms of *Cryptococcus* or *Blastomyces* may resemble *H. capsulatum.* However, normally some more representative cells of the former organisms can be found.

CLINICAL MANIFESTATIONS. The main forms of the infection recognized in the tropics are the acute epidemic and chronic disseminated varieties.

Acute Epidemic Histoplasmosis. This normally fol-

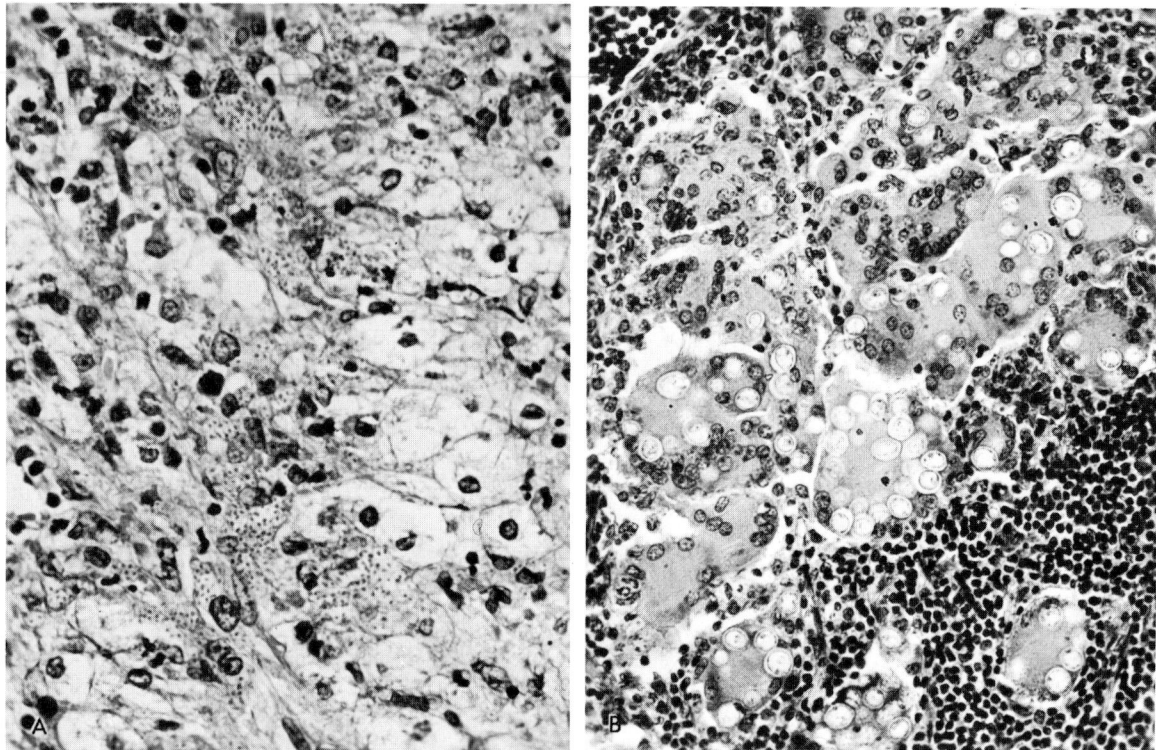

FIGURE 66–1. *A*, Histoplasmosis. *H. capsulatum* in many macrophages (H & E stain, × 400). (Courtesy of the Armed Forces Institute of Pathology, Photograph Neg. No. 54–17185.) *B*, African histoplasmosis. *H. capsulatum* var. *duboisii* in giant cells within a lymph node (H & E stain, × 310). (Courtesy of the Armed Forces Institute of Pathology, Photograph Neg. No. 54–19426.) Compare the difference in size of the two fungi.

lows exposure to a source of the organism such as a bat-infested cave; group exposure is common. The symptoms develop within 8 to 15 days of exposure. Cough, breathlessness, headache, and lassitude are common. Less frequently, allergic phenomena such as arthralgia or erythema multiforme or erythema nodosum develop. The process is self-limiting in the majority of those exposed. However, in some patients, progressive pulmonary incapacity or mediastinitis may occur. Dissemination may follow this form of infection, particularly in the elderly or immunosuppressed.

Chest radiographs show a variety of features, including hilar lymphadenopathy, consolidation, and, in some individuals, bilateral mottling.

Normally, acute epidemic histoplasmosis is managed conservatively with rest. However, in patients who develop severe or prolonged symptoms or progressive hypoxia or in those with severe underlying diseases such as lymphoma or with serologic titers suggestive of dissemination, specific chemotherapy with amphotericin B or ketoconazole is advised (Chapter 67).

Residua of pulmonary histoplasmosis, e.g., focal granulomas, solitary or multiple, may remain after primary infection or be discovered coincidentally. They are usually discovered at operation for suspected carcinoma.

Chronic Pulmonary Histoplasmosis. This is rare in the tropics, possibly because it is associated with the presence of chronic bronchitis and emphysema. It may be undiagnosed because it can be easily confused with tuberculosis. The symptoms of chronic pulmonary histoplasmosis, e.g., cough, malaise, and weight loss with

pyrexia, are similar to those of tuberculosis. Chest pain is a frequent complaint. The main site of infection in the lung is usually apical, with the development of segmental wedge-shaped shadows. These may heal, leaving fibrotic scars, or alternatively, they may cavitate (Fig. 66–2). Progressive extension of the fibrocavitary infiltrate is a serious and frequent complication. Secondary dissemination is rare in this type of infection.

Early cases may respond to bed rest. However, a trial of chemotherapy with ketoconazole or amphotericin B is normally given in established disease. Surgical removal of infected lobes is ineffective usually in eradicating the infection.

Disseminated Histoplasmosis. In infants, the elderly, or immunosuppressed patients, particularly those with lymphoma or AIDS, a rapidly progressive disseminating form of histoplasmosis may develop, with predominant invasion of reticuloendothelial cells of the bone marrow, liver, and spleen. Patients present with fever and hepatosplenomegaly. Purpura may be present. Other sites of invasion are the lungs, gastrointestinal tract, and heart valves. Evidence of bone marrow involvement, such as neutropenia and thrombocytopenia, may be found. Such cases are normally fatal unless treated.

Disseminated forms of histoplasmosis in normal adults may progress at a much slower rate. The first recognized lesions may present up to 30 years after the patient leaves an endemic area. This chronic disseminated form of infection may be seen in the tropics or in patients returning from those areas, particularly Southeast Asia. Oral involvement and adrenal involvement are the most

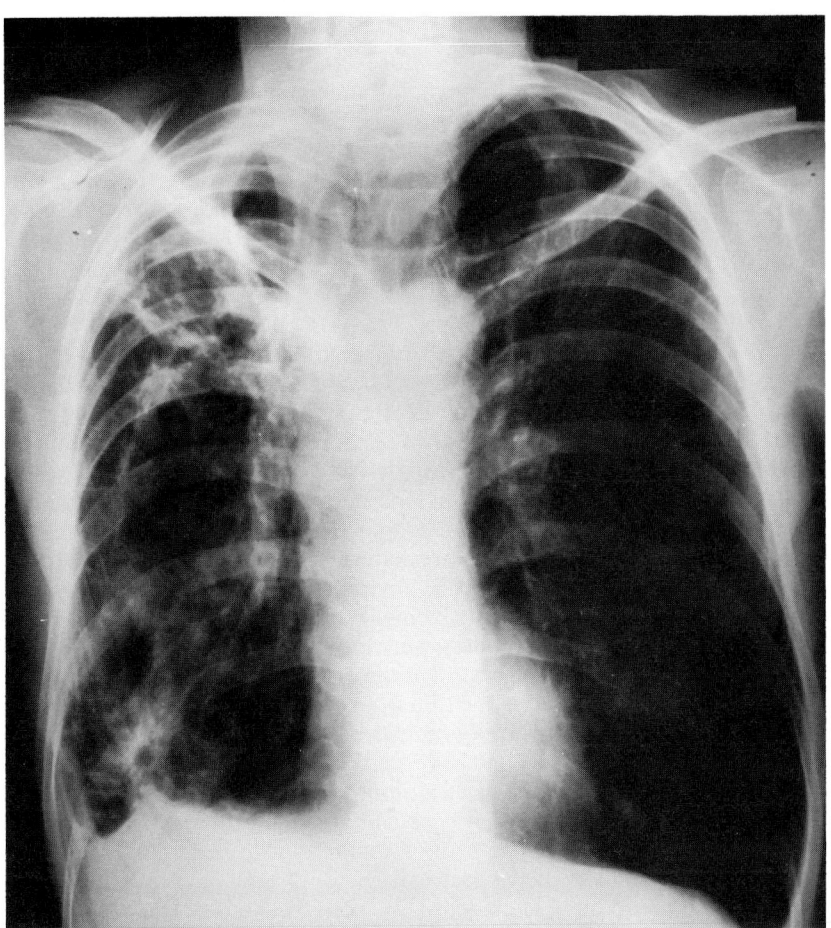

FIGURE 66–2. Chronic pulmonary histoplasmosis with extensive involvement of the left lung. (Courtesy of Dr. John Bennett.)

common clinical forms of this variant of histoplasmosis. Laryngeal ulceration with secondary stricture formation may occur also. The ulcers in the mouth are usually shallow individual lesions that may heal spontaneously, although progressive enlargement is more likely to occur. Adrenal infiltration is often occult, but patients may present with established Addison's disease.

DIAGNOSIS

Laboratory Techniques. The diagnosis can be confirmed by isolation of the organism on Sabouraud's or enriched agar at room temperature. Serologic changes suggest the diagnosis in many instances; the double diffusion and complement fixation tests are the most widely used techniques. However, in acute pulmonary forms of the infection, serologic conversion usually develops slowly over 3 to 6 weeks, and tests may remain negative. In about half the cases of chronic disseminated histoplasmosis, serologic tests are only positive in low titer or remain negative. The histoplasmin skin test has little value in diagnosis, because the reaction may be due to prior exposure (infection) and not to the present illness. It may remain negative in patients with disseminated histoplasmosis and may also cause false-positive serologic reactions.

Differential Diagnosis. Acute epidemic histoplasmosis may be confused with other acute pulmonary processes, e.g., influenza or mycoplasmal pneumonia. Chronic pulmonary histoplasmosis is similar in presentation to tuberculosis (Fig. 66–2). In the rapidly progressive disseminated forms of disease, the presence of large histiocytes may be confused with lymphoma cells unless special fungal stains are used (Fig. 66–1A). The latter are helpful also in distinguishing between *Histoplasma* and *Leishmania,* which are similar in size. However, *Histoplasma* do not have kinetoplasts and stain with PAS (periodic acid-Schiff) or methenamine silver reagents.

TREATMENT. The treatment of choice in histoplasmosis is amphotericin B (Chapter 67). In the majority of those requiring treatment, a total dose consisting of at least 2 gm of the drug is usually necessary, although in those patients with acute epidemic histoplasmosis who require treatment, lower doses (800 to 1200 mg) may be adequate. Oral ketoconazole or, more recently, itraconazole have proved useful in chronic disseminated and pulmonary forms of histoplasmosis. The latter drug also appears to be effective in patients with AIDS. For other patients, intravenous amphotericin B should be used.

PREVENTION. There is no effective practicable environmental control, although it is useful to post warning notices in caves known to contain the organism. Spraying contaminated soil with 3% cresol or formalin may eliminate viable organisms.

AFRICAN HISTOPLASMOSIS

ETIOLOGY AND EPIDEMIOLOGY. As its name suggests, African histoplasmosis is restricted to the African continent and has not been recognized north of the Sahara desert or in countries south of the Zambesi river. It is most prevalent, although still uncommon, in countries of West Africa. The portal of entry is presumed to be respiratory, although cases with pulmonary involvement are rare in African histoplasmosis. It is also not possible to use histoplasmin surveys to estimate the risk of subclinical exposure, as the small form of histoplasmosis can be endemic in the same areas and both organisms are closely related antigenically.

CLINICAL MANIFESTATIONS. The most common clinical sites of involvement in African histoplasmosis are skin and bone. Skin lesions present as small papules that often develop an umbilicated center, nodules, abscesses, or ulcers. With larger lesions, underlying bone deposits are common. Solitary skin lesions may also occur. Bone deposits of African histoplasmosis are well circumscribed and lytic. Long bones and the skull are typical sites of invasion. Patients presenting with lesions of African histoplasmosis should be investigated radiologically for occult bone foci. Involvement of other sites, including the lung lymph nodes, and gastrointestinal tract, are less common. However, multiorgan invasion occurs rarely and is associated with a poor prognosis.

DIAGNOSIS. The diagnosis is made by biopsy and smears taken from skin or bone lesions. These may also be cultured on Sabouraud's agar, although *H. duboisii* cannot be distinguished from *H. capsulatum* by culture. Microscopically, *H. duboisii* appears as numerous large, round or oval, thick-walled yeast cells 8 to 15 μm in diameter that are in large giant cells (Fig. 66–1B). These cells are much larger than the *H. capsulatum* cells, which are 2 to 4 μm in diameter. The place of serology in African histoplasmosis has not been clearly established.

TREATMENT. Solitary cutaneous lesions may be removed surgically and in many cases do not recur. Oral ketoconazole (400 to 800 mg daily) is useful in most cases, either on its own or in addition to surgery. However, in widespread infections amphotericin B may be necessary (Chapter 67). In some cases reasonable responses have been seen with sulphonamides. Relapse after therapy is common.

BIBLIOGRAPHY

Ajello L, Manson-Bahr PEC, Moore JC: Amboni caves, Tanganyika, a new epidemic area for *Histoplasma capsulatum.* Am J Trop Med Hyg 9:33, 1960.
Alford RH, Goodwin RA: Variation in lymphocyte reactivity to histoplasmin during the course of chronic pulmonary histoplasmosis. Am Rev Respir Dis 108:85, 1973.
Cockshott WP, Lucas AO: *Histoplasma duboisii.* Q J Med 33:223, 1964.
Cole ACE, Ridley DS, Wolfe HRI: Bowel infection with *Histoplasma duboisii.* J Trop Med Hyg 68:92, 1965.
Goodwin RA, des Prez RM: Pathogenesis and clinical spectrum of histoplasmosis. South Med J 66:13, 1973.
Larabee WF, Ajello L, Kaufman L: An epidemic of histoplasmosis on the isthmus of Panama. J Trop Med 27:281, 1977.
Symmers WS: Histoplasmosis in southern and south-eastern Asia. A syndrome associated with a peculiar tissue form of histoplasma: A study of 48 cases. Ann Soc Belg Med Trop 52:435, 1972.
Vanbreuseghem R: Les manifestations cutanées de l'histoplasmose africaine. Ann Soc Belg Med Trop 44:1037, 1964.

66.2.   COCCIDIOIDOMYCOSIS

Edward C. Oldfield, III

DEFINITION. Coccidioidomycosis is a fungal infection with a broad clinical spectrum ranging from asymptomatic skin test conversion, through benign, self-limited pulmonary infection, to chronic fatal disseminated disease. There are an estimated 100,000 new cases each year in the United States alone, with 70 deaths annually.

HISTORY. In 1892, Alejandro Posadas, while still an intern, first described the disease in an Argentinian soldier with the disseminated form. Rixford and Gilchrist named the organism *Coccidioides immitis* in 1896, Coccidioides because of its resemblance to the protozoan Coccidia and "immitis" meaning "not mild." It was Ophuls, in 1900, who determined that the etiologic agent was a fungus and delineated its life cycle.

ETIOLOGY. The disease is caused by the dimorphic fungus *Coccidioides immitis.* This fungus grows in soil and in the laboratory as a mold with white aerial mycelium, whereas in human tissues it takes the form of endosporulating spherules.

The septate mycelium is composed of arthroconidia, which are barrel-shaped and 2 to 5 μm in length. These arthroconidia are the infectious agents. They are readily detached and become airborne. Experimental studies in primates have shown that as few as 10 arthroconidia may lead to infection.

Once inhaled, the arthroconidium swells into a spherule. Internal cleavage of the cytoplasm leads to the formation of endospores. The mature spherule ruptures, releasing its endospores, each with the capacity to grow into another spherule (Fig. 66–3). Neither spherules nor endospores are infectious by aerosol. Coccidioidomycosis has been transmitted from person to person only by direct inoculation, such as cutaneous infections acquired by pathologists during autopsy on infected cases. Humans are not required in the life cycle and are only infected incidentally.

EPIDEMIOLOGY AND TRANSMISSION. Coccidioidomycosis is acquired by inhalation of airborne arthroconidia produced by this normally saprophytic soil fungus. The distribution of *C. immitis* is limited to the Western Hemisphere. Endemic areas in the United States are in the Southwest and include Arizona, California, New Mexico, Southwestern Texas, Southwestern Utah, and Nevada. The areas of highest endemicity are found in Arizona and the San Joaquin Valley of California (Fig. 66–4). Most of these areas have in common a semi-arid climate with a short but intense rainy season.

Mexico has 3 areas of high endemicity, including the northern area bordering the United States, the Pacific littoral zone, and the northern central area. In Central America, there are small areas of endemicity in Guatemala and Honduras, with only rare cases in El Salvador. In South America, Venezuela appears to have the areas of greatest endemicity. There are also areas in the Chaco regions of Paraguay and in Argentina. A few cases have been reported from Colombia and Bolivia.

Any activity that is associated with disturbance of soil can lead to arthroconidia becoming airborne and an

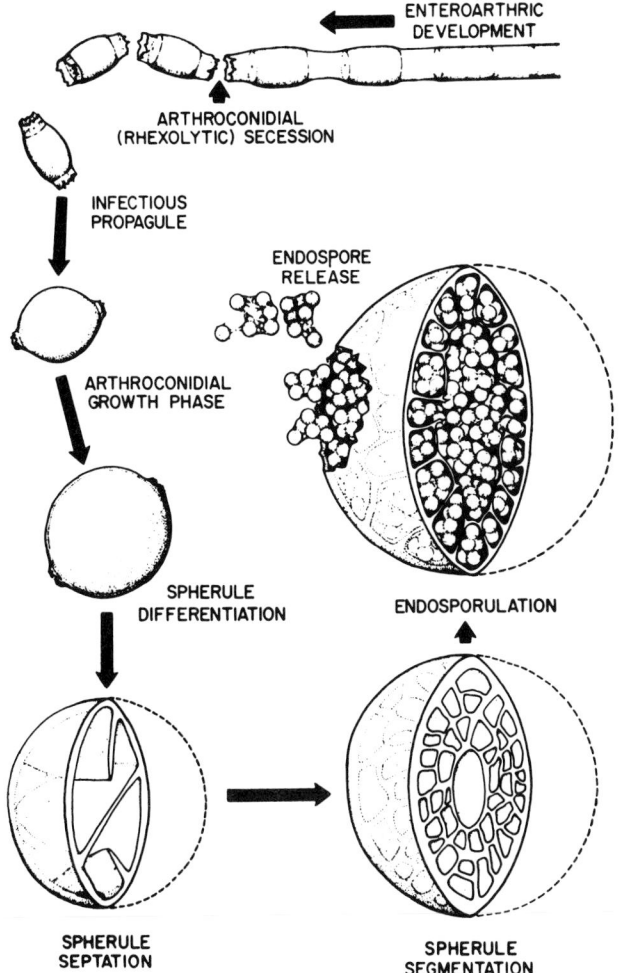

FIGURE 66–3. Life cycle of *Coccidioides immitis*. (From Cole GT, Sun SH: Arthrocomidium-spherule-endospore transformation in *Coccidioides immitis*. *In* Szaniszlo PJ (ed.): Fungal Dimorphism. New York, Plenum Press, 1985.)

increased incidence of infection. These include the dusty conditions associated with construction work, archeologic digs, and wind storms. However, extensive exposure is not required; in fact, cases have been reported to occur after merely driving through endemic areas. Fomites have been noted to transmit disease also, as with cotton shipped from an endemic area to other parts of the world.

Many species of animals are infected with *C. immitis*, including fatal infections in primates in zoos in the endemic area. Animals are not involved in transmission to humans.

PATHOGENESIS AND PATHOLOGY. The tissue reaction to *C. immitis* is most often granulomatous but may be suppurative also. Most commonly, there is a mixed reaction: to intact spherules it is believed to be granulomatous, whereas to the endospores it is believed to be suppurative with polymorphonuclear leukocytes. *C. immitis* appears in tissue as large spherules (10 to 80 μm) with doubly refractile walls, containing endospores from 2 to 5 μm in diameter (Fig. 66–5). Immature spherules may be seen without endospores but are diagnostically much less specific and may be confused

easily with artifacts. The spherules usually stain well with hematoxylin and eosin or periodic acid-Schiff stain. However, the most suitable stain for diagnosis is Grocott-Gomori methenamine silver.

CLINICAL MANIFESTATIONS AND COMPLICATIONS. The most common result of infection is asymptomatic skin test conversion in 60% of infected individuals.

Pulmonary Coccidioidomycosis. Primary pulmonary infection is manifested after a 7- to 28-day incubation period, with cough (usually nonproductive) in 89% of patients, fever in 82%, and chest pain in 70%, which is often pleuritic and of acute onset. Headache, myalgias, night sweats, and chills are common also. Toxic erythema, a fine, diffuse, erythematous rash with a macular component covering the trunk and extremities, occurs in 10% of patients.

Erythema nodosum and erythema multiforme are seen commonly with primary coccidioidomycosis and usually occur at the same time that delayed hypersensitivity develops. Erythema nodosum occurs in conjunction with a violent skin test reaction to coccidioidin and sometimes with arthralgias and conjunctivitis. It is associated with a good prognosis, although dissemination has rarely been noted in patients with previous erythema nodosum.

The chest radiograph is abnormal in 80% of infections requiring hospitalization. The infiltrates, single or multiple, are associated with ipsilateral hilar adenopathy in 20%. Small pleural effusions may be noted in 20% of patients, but significant pleural effusions are rarely seen. The usual clinical course in untreated patients with primary pulmonary disease is complete resolution in 2 to 3 weeks.

Those patients who have not clinically improved in 6 to 8 weeks are often said to have persistent pulmonary coccidioidomycosis. This may take the form of a progressive pneumonia, the formation of cavities, or miliary disease. These patients' condition may progress further to a chronic form of disease resembling tuberculosis, with apical fibronodular lesions and cavities.

The primary pneumonia may resolve with formation of a solitary pulmonary nodule, or it may progress to cavity formation. Coccidioidal cavities are most often single (90%), in the upper lung fields (70%), and thin-walled, with a tendency toward rapid fluctuations in size. In 5% of cases, the cavities have been noted to cross fissures. Long-term follow-up has revealed that although hemoptysis is reported in 20 to 50% of patients, the prognosis is benign, with spontaneous closure of cavities in 50% within 2 years.

Disseminated Coccidioidomycosis. The most serious form of coccidioidomycosis is extrapulmonary dissemination. Race has been consistently noted to bear a strong influence on the likelihood of dissemination. Mexicans are 3.4 times as likely to develop dissemination as whites, whereas blacks and Filipinos are 10 times more likely to develop disseminated disease. It has been estimated that 1 in 100 white males with clinical disease will progress to dissemination, whereas only 1 in 500 white females will develop dissemination. Coccidioidomycosis is also adversely affected by pregnancy; the

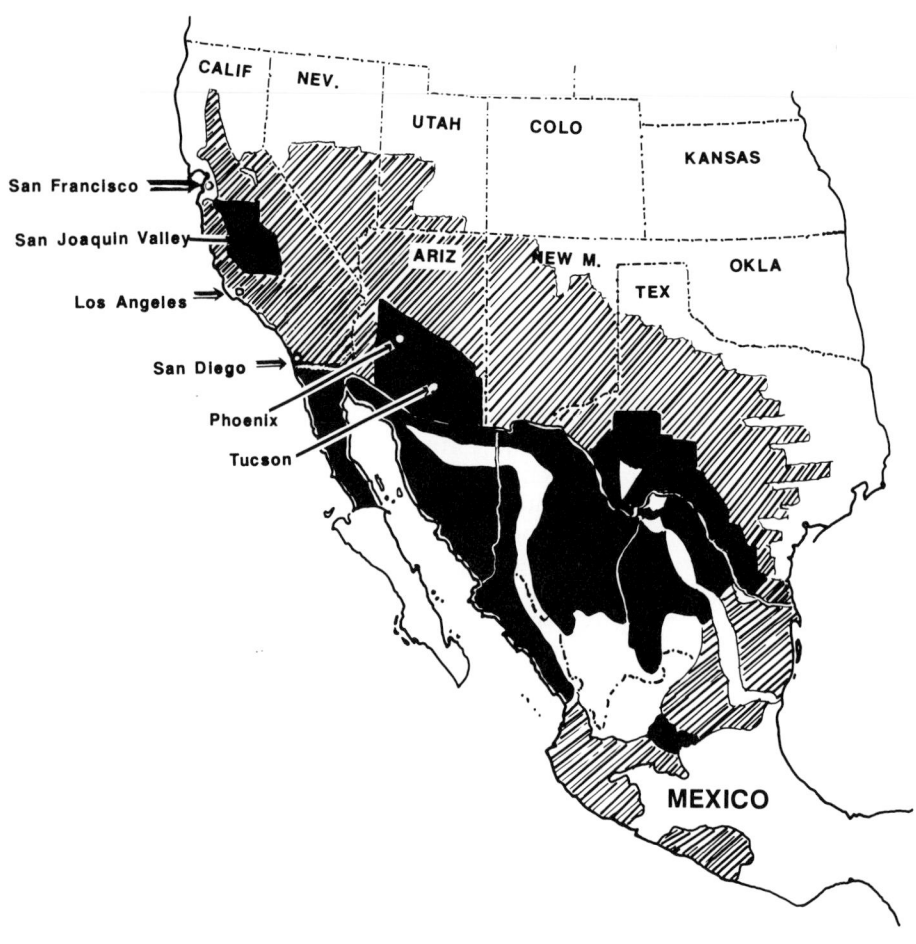

FIGURE 66–4. Endemic areas of coccidioidomycosis in North America: ■ 30–70% and ▨ 6–30% of the population with positive skin test to coccidioidin.

later infection occurs during pregnancy, the more likely it is that dissemination will occur, usually with a fatal outcome for the mother. The role of diabetes mellitus in the outcome of coccidioidomycosis is less clear, but it may have an adverse effect.

Patients with a diagnosis of disseminated coccidioidomycosis should have a baseline bone scan, gallium scan, and lumbar puncture to better define the extent of dissemination.

Dissemination usually occurs in the first few months after infection and is most likely to involve the skin, bones and joints, meninges, and genitourinary tract. It may involve almost any organ system in the body, except the gastrointestinal tract, which is rarely involved. The skin lesions may take many forms, including verrucous granulomas, "cold" subcutaneous abscesses, indolent ulcers, and small papules.

Bone Lesions. Osseous involvement occurs particularly in the vertebrae, tibia, skull, metacarpals and metatarsals, femur, and ribs. The lesions may be single (59%) or multiple. The vertebral lesions are noted for a propensity to spare the disk, to involve all portions of the vertebra, and to be associated with paraspinous abscesses. Radiographically, lesions are usually lytic. The most commonly involved joints are the knees and ankles, often with negative synovial fluid culture but positive cultures from biopsy specimens of synovial membrane.

Meningitis. Meningitis occurs in about 30% of cases of disseminated coccidioidomycosis. The onset is subtle usually, with malaise, personality change, and headache. The nonspecific nature of the early symptoms are the reason for a lumbar puncture in the work-up of all patients with disseminated disease. Involvement is limited usually to the meninges, rarely the brain. Examination of the cerebrospinal fluid (CSF) reveals elevated protein, decreased glucose, and increased cells with a mononuclear predominance. CSF eosinophilia may provide a clue to the coccidioidal nature of the process. Without treatment, the meningitis is almost invariably fatal.

Immunosuppression. Disseminated coccidioidomycosis has been reported in a variety of immunosuppressed patients from endemic areas, including patients on steroids and those with hematologic malignancies and AIDS. In Arizona, coccidioidomycosis is the most common single etiologic agent of infection in renal transplants, with 6.9% of all patients becoming infected and 75% of these patients disseminating.

DIAGNOSIS. The *sine qua non* of diagnosis is the demonstration of spherules with endospores in tissue or recovery of the fungus in culture.

Culture. *Coccidioides immitis* grows rapidly on almost all routine laboratory media. Growth usually occurs by the third or fourth day, and sporulation occurs by the tenth to the fourteenth day. Because of the abundant

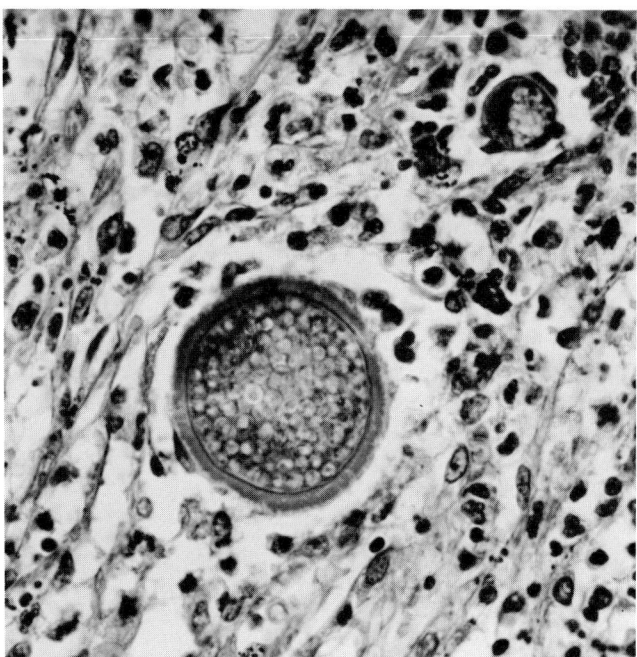

FIGURE 66–5. Mature *C. immitis* sporangium in the lung. The material on the outer surface of the thick wall is a precipitate containing immune complexes (Splendore-Hoeppli phenomenon). (× 530.) (Courtesy of the Armed Forces Institute of Pathology, Photograph Neg. No. 59–5706.)

mycelial growth and the ease with which arthroconidia become airborne, laboratory identification of *C. immitis* can be hazardous. The clinician should warn laboratory personnel when he or she suspects a clinical case of coccidioidomycosis. Extreme care should be taken to avoid aerosolization of the mycelial phase, and work with suspected *C. immitis* should be performed under a ventilated safety hood. There have been over 200 cases of laboratory-acquired disease reported in the literature. Accurate identification of *C. immitis* is difficult because of the marked cultural variability among strains and the resemblance to other nonpathogenic strains. Therefore, the production of endosporulating spherules must be confirmed to assure the diagnosis. This can be accomplished by animal inoculation, special in vitro techniques to induce endospore formation, or immunologic tests for antigens specific to *C. immitis*. Cultures of expectorated sputum are positive in 12 to 32% of patients with active pulmonary disease. This yield can be increased to 69% with fiberoptic bronchoscopy.

Skin and Serologic Tests. The proper interpretation of skin and serologic tests is of critical importance from both a diagnostic and a prognostic perspective. The standard skin test is a 1:100 dilution of coccidioidin, which is prepared from culture filtrates of the mycelial phase of *Coccidioides immitis*. A skin test is considered positive when there is 5 mm of induration at 24 or 48 hours. Reactivity should be measured at both times. A positive skin test indicates only that a patient has been infected at some time in the past and does not necessarily indicate that the patient's present symptoms are due to infection with *C. immitis*. However, documentation of skin test conversion from negative to positive does indicate that infection occurred during that time interval.

Fortunately, even repeated skin testing has no effect on the results of serologic testing.

In cases of primary pulmonary disease, the skin test usually becomes reactive soon after the onset of symptoms, with 99% positive by the third week. With disseminated disease, the skin test is negative in 70% of cases and serves more as a prognostic indicator than as a diagnostic test. Of those with disseminated disease and a positive skin test, 75% survived; of those with a negative skin test, only 16% survived prior to the introduction of amphotericin B.

Spherulin, derived from the spherule phase, appears to be a more sensitive skin test antigen than coccidioidin at comparable dilutions in epidemiologic studies. The two skin tests appear comparable in detecting clinical disease.

Serologic tests are also of diagnostic and prognostic significance. The tube precipitin (TP) and latex particle agglutination (LPA) tests both measure primarily IgM; thus, a positive test indicates a recent infection. The LPA test is more sensitive and more easily performed, becoming positive in the first 1 to 3 weeks after onset of symptoms and then rapidly returning to negative. These 2 tests are of no value in the diagnosis of central nervous system (CNS) infections. There is also a 6 to 10% false-positive rate with the LPA test. Therefore, all positive tests must be confirmed by a more specific test.

The complement fixation (CF) test measures IgG antibodies and is reported as a specific titer. The CF test has been shown consistently to be an important prognostic indicator. Those patients who develop asymptomatic skin test conversion usually do not develop elevated CF titers, whereas titers greater than 1:16 or 1:32 are associated with but not diagnostic of dissemination. The complement fixation test has been noted to be positive in 99% of patients with disseminated disease. False negatives have been noted in AIDS and renal transplant patients. A fall in the CF titer during therapy indicates a good response to therapy. Chronic persistence of low titers is common. A positive CF antibody in the cerebrospinal fluid is diagnostic of meningitis, with the rare exception of parameningeal infections. However, the CF test may be negative in the CSF of a minority of documented cases of coccidioidal meningitis.

Eosinophilia, usually in the range of 3 to 10%, is common in coccidioidomycosis, peaking during the second and third weeks of illness.

TREATMENT AND PROGNOSIS. The treatment of coccidioidomycosis remains a formidable clinical challenge. The drug of choice for life-threatening infections is amphotericin B (Chapter 67). Amphotericin B is fungistatic for *Coccidioides immitis* with most isolates appearing to be sensitive in vitro. Isolates recovered during relapses almost always remain sensitive.

Patients with uncomplicated primary pulmonary disease do not usually require therapy. Likewise, cavitary disease is usually not an indication for therapy, because treatment has not been shown to enhance cavity closure. Therapy is not indicated usually for pulmonary nodules, either before or after surgical resection.

Patients with persistent pulmonary infection longer than 6 weeks with continued systemic toxicity and those with chronic progressive pulmonary disease may benefit from therapy to limit symptoms or extension of disease. Therapy should be considered also for those with rising complement fixation titers (especially if 1:16 or greater), which may indicate incipient dissemination. Patients with negative skin tests are also of serious concern because of their poor host defenses and increased risk of dissemination. Infancy, pregnancy, immunosuppression, and race (Filipino, black) all increase the risk of dissemination and add to the consideration of treatment.

All cases of dissemination outside the lung require treatment. Skin and bone lesions respond the best, while lesions of the joints and meninges respond less well. Treatment with amphotericin B is increased usually to a maintenance dose of 1 mg/kg, not usually exceeding 50 mg, and given daily until the patient becomes clinically stable. At this point, the patient is changed often to a thrice weekly maintenance schedule that can be administered as an outpatient. Specific total doses of amphotericin B are difficult to recommend because of the unpredictable nature of the disease and the interaction with the patient's immune system. A course of 2 to 3 gm of amphotericin B is required often and rarely as high as 10 to 15 gm. The actual dose is determined by the clinical response, which can be monitored by diminished clinical symptoms, improvement in lesions, a fall in complement fixation titer, weight gain, and decrease of erythrocyte sedimentation rate. Conversion of skin test from negative to positive suggests an enhanced immune response, whereas a persistently negative skin test is more likely to require prolonged therapy and indicate an increased chance of relapse. In addition, bone lesions may require debridement, joint lesions may require synovectomy, and abscesses may require drainage.

Coccidioidal meningitis requires intrathecal (IT) amphotericin B. This is administered initially via the lumbar route, but toxicity and arachnoiditis usually require alternative methods, such as administration via lateral cervical puncture, cisternal puncture, or an Ommaya reservoir. A total dose of 40 mg or more of IT amphotericin B and rapid escalation to IT doses of 0.75 to 1.5 mg has been associated with improved outcomes. The limiting factor in therapy is most commonly management of the complications of IT amphotericin B and hydrocephalus from the basilar meningitis. An Indium III radionuclide CSF flow study or computerized axial tomography should be performed to assess CSF dynamics and to detect hydrocephalus. Rarely, oral ketoconazole and intraventricular miconazole have been used to treat coccidioidal meningitis.

Ketoconazole is being used increasingly in nonmeningeal, nonlife-threatening coccidioidal infections in the immunocompetent individual. Ketoconazole has been used to maintain remissions in patients who were treated initially with amphotericin B but appeared to be at high risk of relapse (negative skin test, elevated complement fixation test, persistent skin or bone lesions) or who developed significant nephrotoxicity to amphotericin B before completion of therapy. Ketoconazole is only

fungistatic for *Coccidioides immitis,* with MICs in the range of 1.6 to 3.2 µg/ml. However, serum levels and MICs have not correlated with success. There has been no evidence of resistance developing during prolonged therapy.

The starting dose of ketoconazole commonly has been 400 mg once per day. Patients who fail at 400 mg may respond to higher doses, but the incidence of toxicity increases with increasing dose. Infections in soft tissue respond most rapidly, whereas pulmonary and skeletal infections respond more slowly. Relapses have been a problem, and can occur even after years of apparently successful disease suppression.

The triazoles, itraconazole and fluconazole, are being investigated currently for use in the treatment of coccidioidomycosis. Fluconazole may play a role in the treatment of coccidioidal meningitis.

BIBLIOGRAPHY

Bouza E, Dreyer JS, Hewitt WL, et al.: Coccidioidal meningitis. An analysis of 31 cases and review of the literature. Medicine 60:139–155, 1981.
Bronnimann DA, Adam RD, Galgiani JN, et al.: Coccidioidomycosis in the acquired immunodeficiency syndrome. Ann Intern Med 106:372–379, 1987.
Drutz DJ: Amphotericin B in the treatment of coccidioidomycosis. Drugs 26:337–346, 1983.
Drutz DJ, Catanzaro A: Coccidioidomycosis. Am Rev Respir Dis 117:559–585, 727–771, 1978.
Fiese MJ: Coccidioidomycosis. Springfield, Illinois, Charles C. Thomas, 1958.
Galgiani JN, Stevens DA, Graybill JR, et al.: Ketoconazole therapy of progressive coccidioidomycosis. Am J Med 84:603–610, 1988.
Graybill JR: Azole antifungal drugs in treatment of coccidioidomycosis. Semin Resp Inf 1:53–60, 1986.
Labadie EL, Hamilton RH: Survival improvement in coccidioidal meningitis by high-dose intrathecal amphotericin B. Arch Intern Med 146:2013–2018, 1986.
Shehab ZN, Britton H, Dunn JH: Imidazole therapy of coccidioidal meningitis in children. Pediatr Infect Dis 7:40–44, 1988.
Stevens DA: Coccidioidomycosis, A Text. New York, Plenum Press, 1980.

66.3. BLASTOMYCOSIS

Robert W. Bradsher

DEFINITION. Blastomycosis is the infection caused by the fungus *Blastomyces dermatitidis.* Infection typically presents as either an acute or indolent pneumonia or as a chronic skin lesion. The terminology of "North American" blastomycosis has been abandoned because of increasing reports of this infection from other continents and the acceptance of paracoccidioidomycosis rather than the outdated terminology of "South American" blastomycosis for disease due to *Paracoccidioides brasiliensis.*

ETIOLOGY. *B. dermatitidis* is a dimorphic fungus that grows at room temperature as a mold and at 37C as a budding, yeast-like cell. The mold grows well, if slowly, on a wide range of culture media, including Sabouraud's agar. The white to tan colony is composed of hyphae measuring approximately 2 µm in diameter and smooth, round or oval microconidia measuring from 2 to 10 μm in diameter. The mold closely resembles *Histoplasma capsulatum,* except for presence of tuberculate macroconidia and the finely roughened microconidia of *H. capsulatum.* Blastomyces yeast-like cells are multinucleate, round, and 8 to 15 μm in diameter and have broad-based buds between mother and daughter cells. *B. dermatitidis* may exist in one of two mating types. Co-culture of isolates having opposite mating types results in formation of distinctive structures called ascocarps, which contain ascospores. These sexual structures classify the perfect state of this fungus as an ascomycete, called *Ajellomyces dermatitidis.*

EPIDEMIOLOGY. Most reported cases of blastomycosis have been from the United States and central or eastern Canada. Occasional cases have been reported from Africa, Mexico, and Central America. In the United States, endemic areas include states surrounding the Mississippi and Ohio Rivers with greatest numbers in Kentucky, Arkansas, Mississippi, North Carolina, Tennessee, Louisiana, Illinois, and Wisconsin. A few common-source outbreaks have been described. Although most investigators have not been successful in recovering the organism from soil, Klein and co-workers provided strong evidence of the location of *B. dermatitidis* in microfoci in soil by isolating the organism in association with an epidemic of infection. Because a majority of patients in that outbreak were not ill, the investigations also supported the concept of subclinical infection as is found frequently in histoplasmosis and coccidioidomycosis. Infection has occurred in animals such as dogs, cats, and cows, but spread to humans has not occurred. The only documented case of person-to-person transmission was that of a male with genitourinary disease causing pelvic blastomycosis in the wife.

Although there is no occupational or medical predisposition to developing blastomycosis, many persons have exposure to soil associated with animals or bodies of water. Whether water or animals are the primary factors for the microfoci in soil or simply represent an area with greater potential for exposure because of

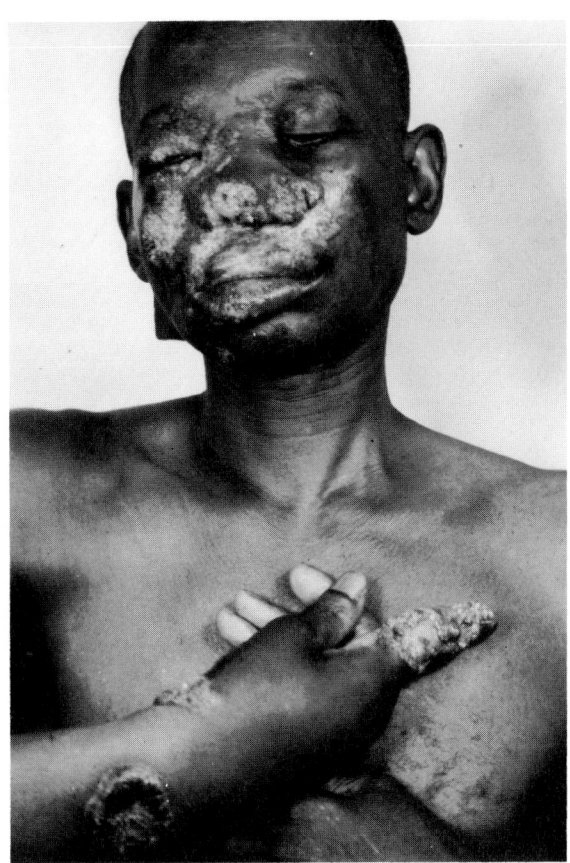

FIGURE 66–7. Cutaneous blastomycosis in a 50-year-old patient in the USPHS Hospital, New Orleans. Louisiana. No pulmonary lesions were visible radiographically. (Courtesy of the Armed Forces Institute of Pathology, Photograph Neg. No. 75–9748.)

occupational or recreational activities is not yet clear. A review of 1114 cases from the literature revealed that 87% of patients were between 20 and 69 years old. Infection of prepubertal children is rare but well documented. The ratio of males to females is approximately 6:1.

PATHOGENESIS AND PATHOLOGY. The portal of infection is the lung, although pulmonary infection may cause few symptoms and may heal spontaneously with cure or subsequent signs of infection at distant

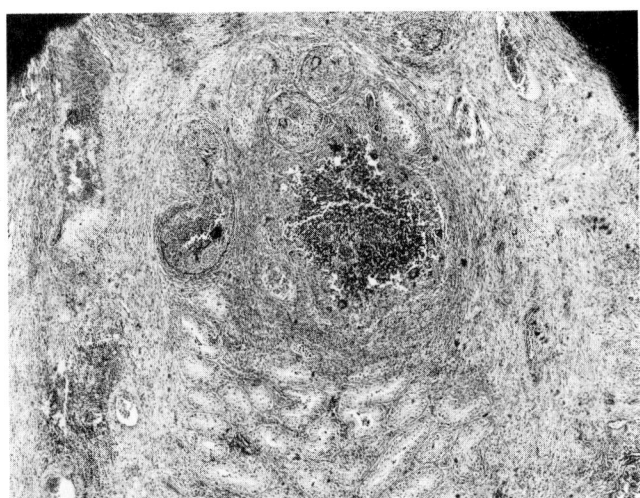

FIGURE 66–6. Testicular blastomycosis (H and E, × 23). Note microscopic abscess surrounded by granulomatous inflammation.

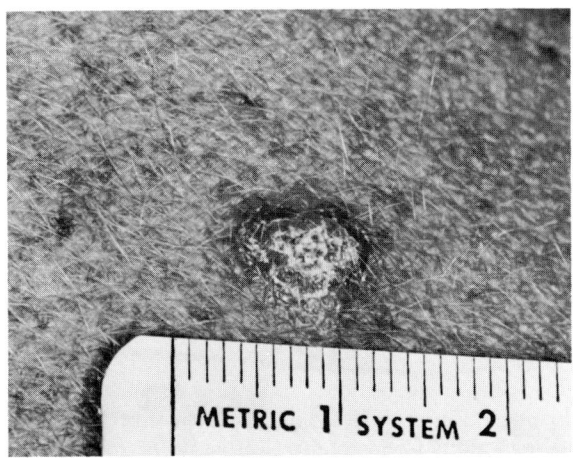

FIGURE 66–8. Small hyperkeratotic skin lesion of blastomycosis.

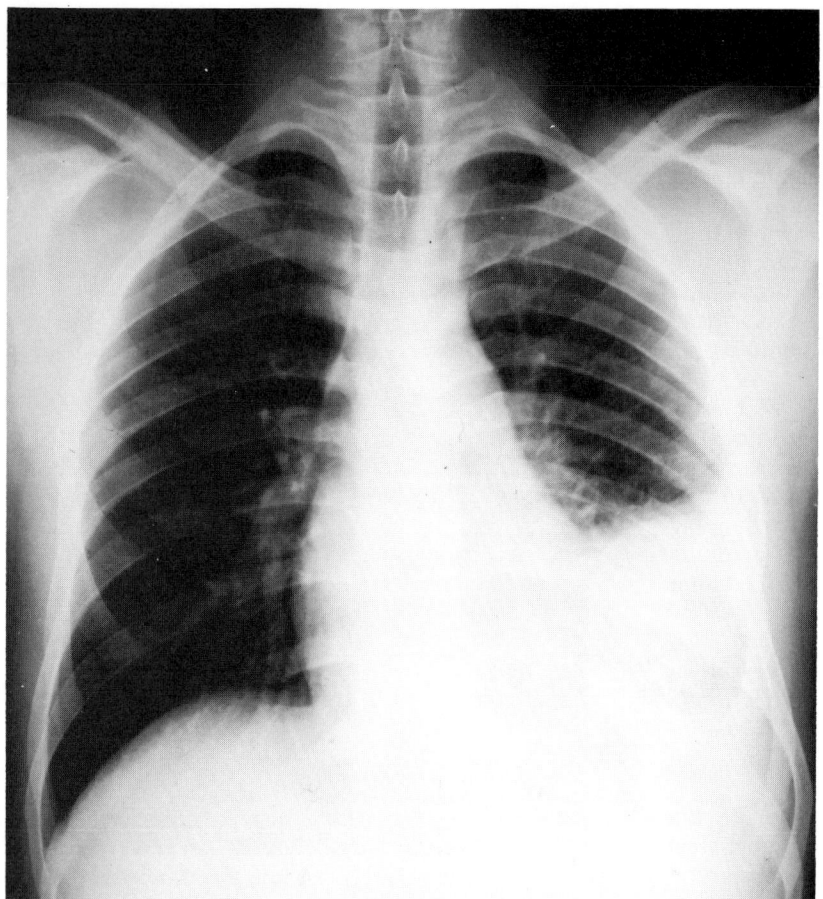

FIGURE 66–9. Blastomycosis of left lower lobe.

sites. Presenting signs and symptoms are generally nonspecific but referable to sites of hematogenous seeding in the skin, bone, prostate, epididymis, or other organs. The inflammatory response is a mixture of granulomatous and pyogenic elements. Collections of neutrophils range in size from microscopic to large abscesses (Fig. 66–6). Pseudoepitheliomatous hyperplasia and acanthosis is found in skin and mucous membrane lesions, which has prompted misdiagnosis of squamous cell carcinoma or kertoacanthoma in some patients.

CLINICAL MANIFESTATIONS

Skin Lesions. Approximately one third to one half of the patients have skin lesions at the time of diagnosis, making this accessible site the best diagnostic clue. Lesions are often multiple and tend to be located on the face and extremities (Fig. 66–7), and they are typically painless, erythematous, well-circumscribed hyperkeratotic, crusted nodules or plaques that enlarge over weeks; these may ulcerate to leave an undermined edge (Fig. 66–8). Some central healing can occur in chronic cases, forming a hypopigmented, atrophic, fibrotic area. Lesions may occur in the mucous membranes of the nose, lips, larynx, and vagina.

Lung Lesions. Pulmonary findings are present radiologically in half of the patients. The infection may either resemble bacterial pneumonia in radiologic appearance in patients who present more acutely (Fig. 66–9), or as a mass lesion in patients with a more indolent course. Chronic pulmonary lesions may show fibrosis and cavitation. Calcification, pleural effusion, or hilar adenopathy is rarely encountered.

Bone Lesions. Osteomyelitis occurs in one fourth of the patients, affecting almost any bone. Osteolytic lesions and an adjacent cold abscess are typical features. Almost every organ has been reported to be infected. In the majority, either concomitant skin or lung infection allows the diagnosis to be easily made.

Systemic Infections. Once infection has progressed beyond the lung, spontaneous remission is rarely observed. After a period ranging from weeks to years, chronic infection may disseminate to multiple organs and cause death. Systemic symptoms of fever and weight loss are mild early in the course but become progressively more severe with extension of the disease.

DIAGNOSIS. Culture for fungus should be performed on sputum, pus, and prostatic secretions or urine. Direct microscopic examination of clinical material following digestion of human tissue with 10% potassium hydroxide added to exudate on the microscope slide is the most rapid and effective means for diagnosis. Cytologic specimens stained by the Papanicolaou method have allowed the diagnosis. Skin lesions can be biopsied for culture and histopathologic section. The best tissue stains are Gomori methenamine silver and periodic acid-Schiff stains. Serologic tests and skin tests are not helpful.

Differential Diagnosis. Skin lesions may be mistaken for basal or squamous cell carcinoma. Nasal lesions resemble leishmaniasis and paracoccidioidomycosis. Laryngeal lesions mimic epidermoid carcinoma both clinically and pathologically. Pulmonary blastomycosis may suggest bronchogenic carcinoma symptomatically and radiographically.

TREATMENT. The vast majority of patients coming to medical attention will require chemotherapy (Chapter 67). The drug of choice for all patients was amphotericin B in the past as it continues to be for those with life-threatening blastomycosis or those with CNS infections. It is given intravenously as 0.5 mg/kg daily or double that dose on alternate days. Eight weeks of therapy is curative in most cases, but cavitary lung lesions and severe multiorgan disease may require 10 to 12 weeks of therapy to prevent relapse. Toxicity often limits the amount of drug which can be given.

Ketoconazole has replaced amphotericin B in the majority with blastomycosis based on the reported efficacy in 2 large trials and the low incidence of serious toxicity compared to amphotericin B. Cure rates of approximately 90% were achieved in those who took ketoconazole for the entire treatment period. At a dose of 400 mg/day for 6 months this agent should replace amphotericin B as therapy in compliant patients with less than overwhelming or life-threatening blastomycosis. Itraconazole appears promising in the treatment of the rare relapse of infection after ketoconazole.

PREVENTION. No means of prevention are known.

BIBLIOGRAPHY

Berkowitz I, Diamond TH: Disseminated *Blastomyces dermatitidis* infection in a non-endemic area. S Afr Med J 71:717–719, 1987.
Bradsher RW: Water and blastomycosis: Don't blame beaver. Am Rev Respir Dis 136:1324–1326, 1987.
Bradsher RW, Rice DC, Abernathy RS: Ketoconazole therapy of endemic blastomycosis. Ann Intern Med 103:872–879, 1985.
Craig MW, Davey WN, Green RA: Conjungal blastomycosis. Am Rev Respir Dis 102:86, 1970.
Furcolow ML, Chick EW, Busey JD, et al.: Prevalence and incidence studies of human and canine blastomycosis cases in the United States 1885–1968. Am Rev Respir Dis 102:60, 1970.
Halvorsen RA, Duncan JD, Merten DF, et al.: Pulmonary blastomycosis: Radiologic manifestations. Radiology 150:1–5, 1984.
Klein BS, Vergeront JM, Weeks RJ, et al.: Isolation of *B. dermatitidis* in soil associated with a large outbreak of blastomycosis in Wisconsin. N Engl J Med 314:529–534, 1986.
NIAID Mycoses Study Group: Treatment of blastomycosis and histoplasmosis with ketoconazole. Ann Intern Med 103:861–872, 1985.
Witorsch P, Utz JP: North American blastomycosis: A study of 40 patients. Medicine 47:169, 1968.

66.4. PARACOCCIDIOIDOMYCOSIS

Roderick J. Hay

DEFINITION. Paracoccidioidomycosis (also called South American blastomycosis) is an uncommon infection found in parts of South and Central America caused by the organism *Paracoccidioides brasiliensis*. Pulmonary and mucocutaneous lesions are prominent in this infection, which usually follows an indolent course. Patients may also present with paracoccidioidomycosis many years after they have left an endemic area.

ETIOLOGY. *P. brasiliensis* has only rarely been found in the natural environment. It has been reported on isolated occasions to be present in soil as well as in bat excreta, but its distribution in the latter is much less widespread as *Histoplasma capsulatum* (Chapter 66.1). *P. brasiliensis* is a dimorphic organism that exists as a yeast form in the infected animal but grows as a mold on primary isolation on Sabouraud's agar at room temperature. The yeast phase of the organism characteristically forms multipolar buds that may be arranged concentrically around the parent cell. Hyphae are only rarely found in tissue.

EPIDEMIOLOGY. Paracoccidioidomycosis is strictly a New World infection. Cases have been found in southern Mexico, Central America, and South America, and infected patients have been reported from all countries of South America except Chile and Guyana. The area of highest prevalence is around São Paulo, Brazil. Rural workers are most commonly affected, and the disease is strikingly more prevalent in males. Skin test surveys have shown that in endemic areas a substantial proportion of the normal population, up to 30%, may have sensitization to the organism, suggesting that subclinical infection is common.

PATHOLOGY AND PATHOGENESIS. The primary route of infection is almost certainly respiratory, although the frequent occurrence of mucocutaneous forms of the infection has led some workers to suggest that direct implantation may occur. However, as infection may be present in other sites, particularly the lung, in individuals with isolated mucous membrane lesions, it is likely that the latter represent focal sites of dissemination from a primary pulmonary focus.

The inflammatory reaction to *P. brasiliensis* is primarily granulomatous, although focal areas of necrosis and polymorphonuclear leukocyte infiltration may develop. The organism is present in tissue in yeast phase (Fig. 66–10). Rudimentary hyphae are rarely, if ever, seen.

CLINICAL MANIFESTATIONS. As with other systemic pathogenic mycoses, there are a number of forms of paracoccidioidomycosis. These include subclinical, acute, and chronic pulmonary, as well as acute or chronic disseminated forms of disease. Alternatively, the infection may be classified on the basis of the site affected into pulmonary, mucocutaneous, lymphatic, or mixed forms. If the former classification is used, most cases of paracoccidioidomycosis fall into the chronic pulmonary or chronic disseminated forms of disease.

Pulmonary Paracoccidioidomycosis. The presentation of pulmonary paracoccidioidomycosis is usually insidious, with slow evolution of symptoms such as cough, weight loss, and malaise. Only on rare occasions does the onset occur rapidly over a few days. Scattered areas of consolidation can be demonstrated radiologically in either or both lung fields, particularly the middle and lower zones. Although apical infiltrates may occur, this is not the most common site of pulmonary infection. Miliary infiltration may be seen in widely disseminated forms of the disease.

Disseminated Paracoccidioidomycosis. Ulcerative mucocutaneous lesions are the most frequently recognized forms of disseminated disease. These occur predominantly within the mouth or nose or on adjacent

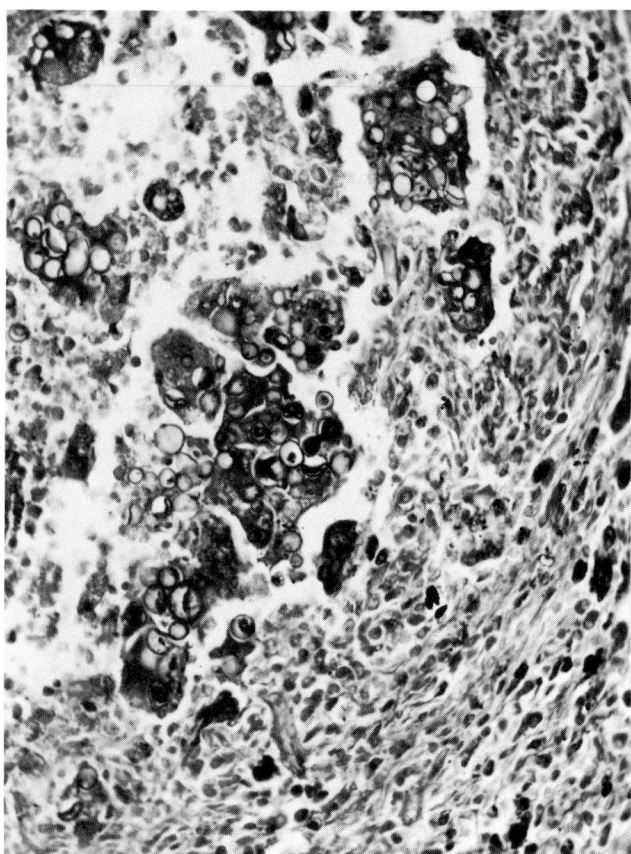

FIGURE 66–10. Paracoccidioidomycosis of the lung. Clusters of *P. brasiliensis* in giant cells. No peripheral buds are seen. (PAS stain, × 275.) (Courtesy of the Armed Forces Institute of Pathology, Photograph Neg. No. 73–3048.)

skin surfaces. Conjunctival or perianal lesions may also develop, and in chronic cases palatal perforation or laryngeal strictures may occur. The ulcers are large, irregular, and often painful. Fleshy granulomas may also be seen. The disease may present with lymph node enlargement. Overlying skin, particularly in the cervical region, may be involved also, giving an appearance of scrofuloderma. Enlarged lymph nodes may be painful.

Less common sites of involvement include skin, bone, or the gastrointestinal tract. In rapidly progressive cases, enlargement of the liver and spleen occurs in association with multiple skin lesions, e.g., ulcers or acneiform granulomas. Lung involvement may occur in any of the forms of disseminated paracoccidioidomycosis.

DIAGNOSIS. The characteristic yeast forms of *P. brasiliensis* may be visualized microscopically or cultured from smears, sputum, or biopsy (Fig. 66–10). In rapidly spreading forms, the small yeast forms of *P. brasiliensis* may closely resemble *Histoplasma*. However, with careful searching, the larger and characteristic budding cells are usually seen. Complement fixation or immunodiffusion tests are helpful in following the course of infection during treatment and in predicting relapse.

TREATMENT. Treatment of paracoccidioidomycosis is a lengthy process, and relapse is common. Treated patients should be examined at regular intervals. The treatment of choice in most cases is ketoconazole in doses of 200 to 400 mg daily (Chapter 67). Recent work

with itraconazole suggests that it is equally, if not more, effective. The initial course of treatment with ketoconazole is normally about six months in duration. In some cases it may be necessary to use intravenous amphotericin B. Cures are difficult to assess, particularly where there is considerable fibrosis, e.g., in pulmonary infections, and patients should be followed up carefully after initial induction of remission.

BIBLIOGRAPHY

Borelli D: Some ecological aspects of paracoccidioidomycosis. *In* Paracoccidioidomycosis. Proceedings of the 1st Pan-Am. Symposium. Washington, D.C., PAHO Scientific Publications, 1972, p 59.
Cuce L, Wroclawski EL, Sampaio SAP: Treatment of paracoccidioidomycosis with ketoconazole. Rev Inst Med Trop São Paulo 23:82, 1981.
Negroni R: Anfotericina B, farmacologia, terapeutica y su aplicacian en la blastomycosis sudamericana. Rev Assoc Med Argent 77:505, 1963.

66.5. CRYPTOCOCCOSIS

Roderick J. Hay

DEFINITION. Crytococcosis is an infection caused by the encapsulated yeast *Cryptococcus neoformans*. The most common clinical form of the disease is meningitis. Other clinical varieties, including lung and skin infections, are seen also.

ETIOLOGY. *Cryptococcus neoformans* is a yeast found widely in nature in association with accumulations of pigeon droppings. There are 4 serotypes of the organism (A, B, C, and D), although there are no established clinical correlates of infection with these varieties.

Cryptococcus neoformans is represented by two different varieties, *C. neoformans neoformans* and *C. neoformans gattii,* which can be distinguished in the laboratory by growth on canavarine bromthymol blue agar. The *neoformans,* but not the *gattii,* variety is found widely in nature in association with accumulation of pigeon droppings. The birds themselves are not affected by the organism. *C. neoformans,* which is resistant to many environmental changes, particularly desiccation, may reach high concentrations in urban areas. Small-size yeasts (2 to 4 μm) may be aerosolized and will penetrate to the terminal alveoli to establish infection.

The budding yeast cells of *C. neoformans* are characterized by the production of typical polysaccharide capsules in vivo or in vitro. The presence of the capsule is believed to affect the capacity of certain cells of the phagocyte series to ingest the organism.

EPIDEMIOLOGY. *C. neoformans* is found in both temperate and tropical areas. In the tropical areas throughout South America, Africa, India, and the Far East, it has been isolated from the environment or infected patients. Most human cases of cryptococcosis have been recorded in the United States, where, in certain areas, *C. neoformans* may be present in large concentrations in the environment, e.g., pigeon droppings. However, large numbers of cases have been recorded in Australia and South Africa, and cryptococcosis is regularly recognized elsewhere in the tropics, particularly in Malaysia. The *gattii* variety is most commonly associated with tropical infections, the *neoformans* variety with infections in temperate climates and infections in AIDS patients.

PATHOLOGY AND PATHOGENESIS. The primary site of infection is the lung, and although cases of isolated cutaneous infection may occur, the organism can only rarely cause disease by implantation in man. In both the United States and India, the organism has been isolated from the sputum of noninfected patients, showing that carriage without invasion may occur. In addition, skin test surveys have suggested subclinical infection in significant numbers of apparently normal individuals. Cryptococcal infections in the tropics may occur in both healthy patients and those with diseases with defective T-lymphocyte function, e.g., AIDS.

Although the main histologic response to cryptococcal infection is granulomatous, large numbers of organisms may be found also in clusters resembling tiny cystic spaces (Fig. 66–11). The yeasts show varying degrees of encapsulation and considerable variation in size. In addition to conventional fungal stains, cryptococci stain red with mucicarmine, which highlights the capsular material.

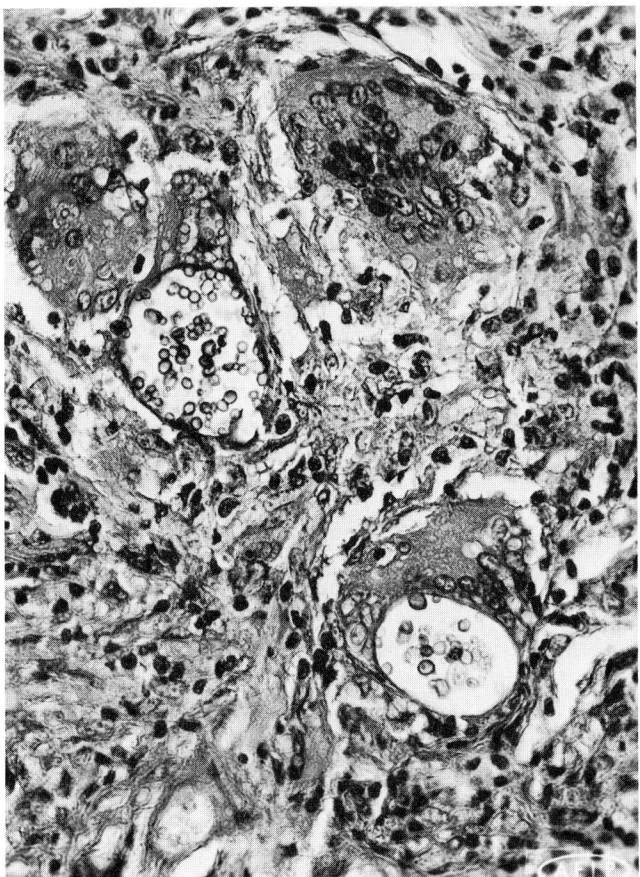

FIGURE 66–11. Small forms of *C. neoformans* in giant cells in a primary pulmonary nodule. These organisms were mucicarmine stain–positive. (× 350.) (Courtesy of the Armed Forces Institute of Pathology, Photograph Neg. No. 61–6700.)

CLINICAL MANIFESTATIONS. The main clinical forms of cryptococcosis are pulmonary and disseminated infections, of which meningitis is the major clinical problem.

Pulmonary Infections. Pulmonary infections without dissemination caused by *C. neoformans* are not common and have been reported most frequently from the United States. However, in many instances, they are self-limiting. The patient may be asymptomatic or may present with fever, dull chest ache, or cough. The radiologic features are highly variable, although bilateral middle or lower lobe foci of consolidation are seen most frequently (Fig. 66–12). More occasionally, cavitation, lobar pneumonitis, hilar lymphadenopathy, or pleural effusion may develop. Extensive miliary shadowing is highly suggestive of a rapidly advancing disseminated infection. In the majority of cases, there is slow resolution of pulmonary infiltrates, although a "walled off" granuloma or cryptococcoma may remain. This may be difficult to differentiate from a pulmonary neoplasm without surgical removal.

Patients presenting with pulmonary lesions who have serious underlying diseases such as lymphoma are more likely to develop a disseminated infection. However, all patients with established pulmonary cryptococcosis should be followed closely with a culture of CSF and urine, and serum antigen, radiologic, and serologic tests and repeat radiologic examinations; if there is evidence of progression of the disease, treatment should be instituted immediately.

Cryptococcal Meningitis. This is the most frequently diagnosed form of cryptococcosis. The onset is usually slow and closely resembles other forms of chronic meningitis such as tuberculosis. A dull occipital headache, pyrexia, drowsiness, and disturbance of the conscious state or behavior may be presenting features. Visual impairment may develop also. On examination, stiffness of the neck is often found, and focal neurologic defects may be elicited. Progression is slow in most cases, but the process is ultimately fatal if the patient is not treated. In patients with AIDS, signs and symptoms of meningitis are often minimal.

Cerebrospinal fluid is often under pressure, and a variable pleocytosis is found; lymphocytes are usually in excess, but sometimes polymorphonuclear leukocytes are the predominant cells. A high protein content and, in half the cases, a low sugar content complete the picture. If available, a CAT scan will demonstrate the presence or absence of significant hydrocephalus.

A solid cryptococcoma sometimes develops in the central nervous system. It presents as a cerebral tumor with focal neurologic signs or a raised intracranial pressure.

Other Sites of Infection. Other sites of dissemination include skin, bone, the prostate, and the retinas. Cutaneous cryptococcosis occurs in 10 to 15% of patients. Even in the absence of clinical signs, approximately half of these patients have or will develop meningitis. Cutaneous lesions include ulcers, granulomas, nodules, and cellulitis. Osseous cryptococcosis is often slightly painful, and lytic lesions are seen on the radiograph. Invasion of the liver, spleen, and kidneys occur mainly in widely

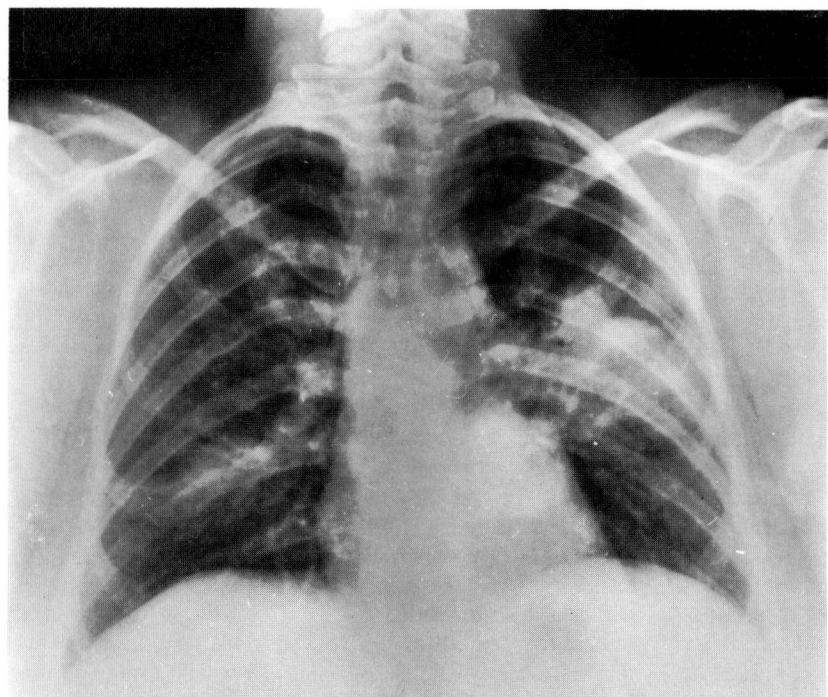

FIGURE 66–12. Pulmonary cryptococcosis with multiple bilateral pulmonary infiltrates. (Courtesy of Dr. John Bennett.)

disseminated infections, although isolated lesions in the last are seen occasionally.

DIAGNOSIS. The diagnosis of cryptococcosis can be confirmed by demonstration or isolation of the organisms. These can be shown in centrifuged sediment of CSF using India ink or nigrosin preparation, both of which highlight the capsule. These techniques are not easy to use and can be misinterpreted. The organisms normally grow readily on Sabouraud's agar, but repeated attempts at isolation should be made if initial efforts are unsuccessful.

If available, the latex test for demonstration of CSF or serum cryptococcal antigen is helpful. The presence of high titers is a poor prognostic sign, and the reduction in titer can be monitored as evidence of progress in treatment. Patients with AIDS frequently show persistently elevated serum antigen titers indicating an incomplete response to therapy. A number of methods are available for antibody detection, but these lack specificity and are usually positive in less than 30 to 40% of those tested.

TREATMENT. The treatment of choice in most cases of crytococcosis is the combination of amphotericin B (0.3 mg/kg daily) and 5-fluorocytosine (150 mg/kg daily in 4 divided doses) (Chapter 67). For localized pulmonary, bone, or skin disease requiring treatment, a short course of amphotericin B alone (about 2 gm) is usually sufficient. The combination of amphotericin B and 5-fluorocytosine must be monitored carefully, and adjustments must be made to the dosage of the latter if there is renal impairment. Local instillations of amphotericin B into the CSF via intrathecal injection or intraventricular reservoir are occasionally required, but side effects such as arachnoiditis are frequently seen. Permanent remission is achieved rarely in patients with AIDS, and long-term suppressive therapy with intermittent ampho-

tericin B or oral fluconazole or itraconazole may be necessary.

Early results with fluconazole and itraconazole as primary treatment of cryptococcosis in AIDS patients have been encouraging.

BIBLIOGRAPHY

Bennett JE, et al.: A comparison of amphotericin B alone and combined with flucytosine in the treatment of cryptococcal meningitis. N Engl J Med 301:126, 1979.
Campbell GD: Pulmonary cryptococcosis. Am Rev Respir Dis 94:236, 1966.
Chu AC, Hay RJ, MacDonald DM: Cutaneous cryptococcosis. Br J Dermatol 103:95, 1980.
Diamond RD, Bennett JE: Prognostic factors in cryptococcal meningitis. Ann Intern Med 80:176, 1974.
Pillay N, Simjee AE: Cryptococcal meningitis. S Afr Med J 50:1604, 1976.

66.6.   SYSTEMIC OPPORTUNISTIC MYCOSES

Roderick J. Hay

Opportunistic organisms are those that cause invasive disease in the presence of some deficiency in host defense. These infections are extremely rare in normal individuals. However, distinction between these mycoses and those caused by the primary pathogens is one of convenience, and opportunism in the latter group occurs quite frequently. For instance, patients with AIDS are prone to develop the disseminated form of histoplasmosis in an endemic area.

In the United States, Europe, and other temperate areas, opportunistic infections are well recognized in patients under treatment for carcinoma or leukemia as well as in those who have received transplanted organs. The immunosuppressive effects of the underlying disease or its treatment are important in determining the likelihood and occurrence of these infections. In the tropics, the pattern is largely unexplored. However, in these areas certain conditions such as diabetes mellitus may be more prevalent, whereas organ transplantation is less frequent. Underlying disease such as malnutrition and tuberculosis may also be associated with systemic fungal infections in the tropics.

ASPERGILLOSIS

DEFINITION. The term aspergillosis covers a group of infectious and allergic conditions caused by fungi of the genus *Aspergillus*. It includes invasive infections seen in immunocompromised patients, as well as allergic bronchopulmonary aspergillosis, a form of intrinsic allergic asthma, and aspergilloma. These conditions are well recognized in temperate areas but are worldwide in distribution.

ETIOLOGY. Aspergilli are common saprophytic molds readily isolated in the laboratory as contaminants. The species most commonly involved with human infections is *Aspergillus fumigatus*, which has been implicated in invasive and allergic bronchopulmonary aspergillosis as well as aspergilloma. *A. flavus* is less commonly isolated from cases of invasive disease and aspergilloma, although it is the main cause of the tropical infection paranasal aspergilloma. *A. niger* is another cause of aspergilloma, as well as otomycosis, in the tropics. Other species of *Aspergillus* are implicated occasionally in these infections.

EPIDEMIOLOGY. The distribution of these organisms is worldwide. However, there are subtle variations. For instance, in Europe *A. fumigatus* is the species most often isolated from sinus washings. In Sudan, the predominant organism is *A. flavus*. Such changes in the predominance of different organisms may possibly influence the distribution of the syndromes that comprise aspergillosis.

PATHOGENESIS, CLINICAL MANIFESTATIONS, AND TREATMENT. The clinical symptoms and subsequent progress of aspergillosis infections depend on the site, method of entry, and underlying condition of the host. In severely ill or compromised patients, invasion and dissemination may occur. However, aspergillosis may also proliferate in large quantities in dilated bronchial airways, lung cavities (aspergilloma), or the external ear. In atopic subjects and some nonatopic subjects, chronic carriage of *Aspergillus* in the bronchial tree leads to an allergic condition associated with considerable edema and peribronchial inflammatory infiltrates. Allergic bronchopulmonary aspergillosis has features of both type I and a type IV hypersensitivity response.

Allergic and Bronchopulmonary Aspergillosis. This is a persistent form of intrinsic asthma associated with chronic carriage of aspergilli within the airways. In early cases, airway obstruction is reversible, although the patient may expectorate mucoid plugs. In chronically affected patients, secondary destructive changes such as bronchiectasis may be found. The condition is diagnosed by demonstration of the characteristic clinical pattern of disease associated with a positive intradermal skin test to *Aspergillus,* eosinophilia, and on occasion, antibodies to the organism.

Treatment is directed toward relief of airway obstruction, using bronchodilators or systemic corticosteroids. The use of antifungal agents has been disappointing because of the frequency of relapse and recolonization.

Aspergilloma. An aspergilloma is a solid mycelial mass caused by the growth of *Aspergillus* species within a cavity, usually within the lung. The latter is most commonly the result of a previous tuberculous infection. Although the patient may be asymptomatic, cough is frequent and severe hemoptysis may occur.

The diagnosis is confirmed by the demonstration of a mobile intracavitary mass on the radiograph. Although cultures are often negative, patients frequently have high titers of antibody to *Aspergillus*.

Treatment is usually conservative, although surgical removal is the only reliable method of curing the aspergilloma. Spontaneous expectoration of the fungal mass may occur.

Invasive Aspergillosis. Although it occurs most commonly in immunocompromised neutropenic patients, e.g., those with leukemia, *Aspergillus* can also cause invasive disease following severe concurrent infection or, in children, in association with congenital neutrophil defects. The most common site of infection is the lung (Fig. 66–13), although metastatic brain or kidney abscesses, among others, may develop.

The development of a focal pulmonary lesion with cavitation in an immunosuppressed patient is a typical, but not universal, radiologic feature of invasive aspergillosis. Culture and serologic tests are often negative in this form of disease.

Amphotericin B is given in full dosage (Chapter 67). In addition, predisposing factors should be relieved when possible, e.g., by leukocyte transfusions or by modification of steroid dosage.

Chronic Necrotizing Pulmonary Aspergillosis. *Aspergillus* may cause an indolent lung infection, usually in patients with pre-existing cavitary or fibrotic lung disease associated with limited invasion of lung parenchyma. The main symptoms are chronic cough, weight loss, and fever, but complications such as aspergillus empyema or aspergilloma may develop. The diagnosis is difficult to establish, but the presence of persistent positive sputum cultures, positive serology, and persistent localized pulmonary shadowing in an ill patient should arouse suspicion. A lung biopsy, if feasible, will confirm the diagnosis. Treatment is difficult, but successes have been seen with amphotericin B or oral itraconazole.

Paranasal Aspergilloma. This is a sclerosing granuloma that originates in the paranasal sinuses. The causative organism is usually *Aspergillus flavus*. The infection is seen in Sudan, India, and the Middle East but may be more widespread in the tropics. Early symptoms

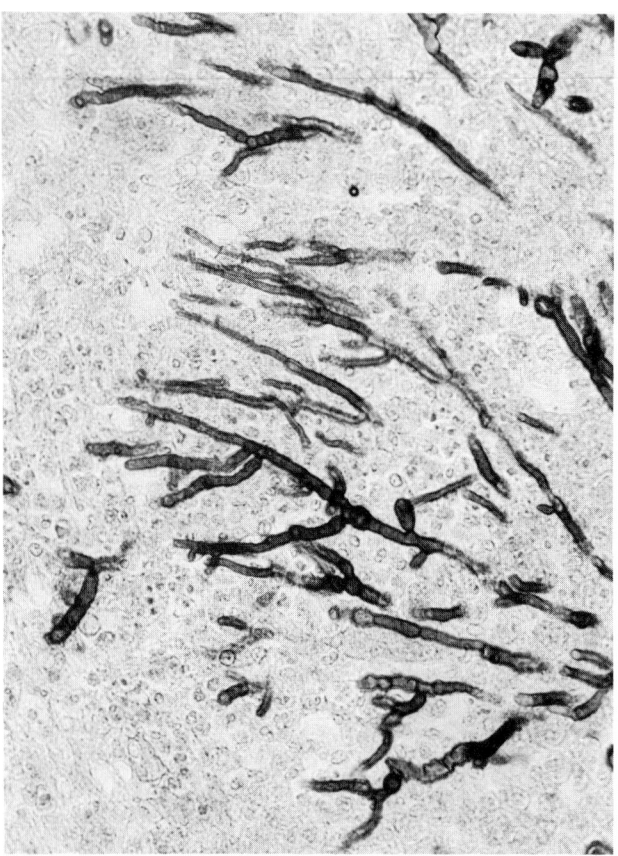

FIGURE 66–13. *Aspergillus* in lung. Acute infection with dichotomous branching of hyphae. (Gridley fungus stain, × 400.) (Courtesy of the Armed Forces Institute of Pathology, Photograph Neg. No. 61–6516.)

include unilateral nasal obstruction and facial pain or headache. Later, proptosis associated with orbital invasion may develop, or more persistent headache with evidence of meningismus may herald central nervous system involvement. Subsequently, tumor seedlings may occur within the central nervous system, giving rise to focal neurologic signs.

Patients presenting in the early phases of this condition are commonly investigated and treated for chronic sinusitis, and the diagnosis is made after biopsy of the sinus lesion. On radiographic examination, opacification of the sinuses may be found. The most frequent site of infection is the maxillary sinus, followed by the ethmoids. There may be considerable periosteal thickening in these areas, and in late lesions lytic zones may be distinguished.

When this diagnosis is suspected the organism is readily cultured. Alternatively, the histologic examination of the lesion shows a sclerosing granuloma in which hyphal fragments are sparsely scattered. It is important to combine histologic and cultural investigations, as *A. flavus* can be isolated from sinuses without granuloma formation. Serologic tests for *A. flavus* in infected patients are often positive.

The first line of treatment is surgical removal. The tumor should be removed as completely as possible, with the patient receiving intravenous amphotericin B in full dosage (Chapter 67). Relapse occurs frequently, and the condition may progress relentlessly to death.

BIBLIOGRAPHY

Black JM: Pulmonary aspergillosis. Proc R Soc Med 53:974, 1960.
Kilman JW, Ahn C, Andrews NC, et al.: Surgery for pulmonary aspergillosis. J Thorac Cardiovasc Surg 57:642, 1969.
Milošev B, el-Mahgoub S, Aal OA: Primary aspergilloma of paranasal sinuses in the Sudan. Br J Surg 56:132, 1969.
Turner-Warwick M: *Aspergillus fumigatus* and lung disease. Postgrad Med J 55:642, 1979.

SYSTEMIC CANDIDA INFECTIONS

DEFINITION. *Candida* species are capable of causing both superficial and deep infections, although the onset of the former only rarely presages the development of the latter. A number of different clinical patterns of systemic infection are seen. Infections may be focal and confined to a body cavity such as the peritoneum or to the CSF. Infection of the lower urinary tract may occur also. Alternatively, where blood stream spread develops, the disease may follow a benign self-limiting or progressive invasive course. Endocarditis caused by *Candida* usually follows homograft valve surgery but may occur in drug addicts.

ETIOLOGY. *Candida albicans* is the most common cause of systemic candidosis, but other species may be involved also. *C. tropicalis,* for instance, is not uncommonly isolated from patients with deep candidosis. *Candida* species other than *C. albicans,* particularly *C. parapsilosis,* are isolated in almost half of the patients with *Candida* endocarditis.

EPIDEMIOLOGY. Little is known about the distribution and importance of systemic *Candida* infections in the tropics. However, the rate of saprophytic carriage is high, and it is likely that invasive candidosis may contribute to the morbidity and mortality of a number of conditions, from malnutrition to carcinoma and AIDS.

PATHOLOGY AND PATHOGENESIS. The organisms causing systemic *Candida* infections gain entry via a number of routes. In many instances, blood stream spread follows penetration of the gut wall by organisms within the gastrointestinal tract. Alternative routes of invasion include the bladder, the lung, or intravenous lines. The organisms may be implanted also directly following surgery or the insertion of peritoneal dialysis catheters. The factors affecting invasion are not clear. However, as with superficial infections, deep candidosis is nearly always seen in compromised patients, particularly those with leukemia and those receiving immunosuppressive therapy. Patients with prolonged periods of neutropenia and particularly those who have been receiving systemic antibiotic therapy are prone to infection with *Candida.*

CLINICAL MANIFESTATIONS. There are a number of different clinical varieties of deep candidosis.

Candidemia. Although *Candida* species may be isolated from blood, this finding is not necessarily accompanied by invasion of internal organs or progressive disease. Candidemia may occur in the presence of indwelling intravenous catheters, in postoperative states, or in immunosuppressed patients. Such patients may be managed conservatively by the removal of intravenous catheters and the monitoring of successive blood cultures. They should be investigated also for evidence of invasive candidosis. In a substantial proportion of patients, candidemia is transient. However, in severely ill or immunosuppressed individuals, treatment may still be advisable.

Systemic Candidosis. Deep invasive *Candida* infections, with or without positive blood cultures, are less common than candidemia. Sites of invasion include the kidneys, liver, muscle, skin, brain, and retina. Contrary to a widely held belief, the lung is not a common site for invasive *Candida* infections, and if involved, the radiologic appearance may be unexceptional because of the diffuse nature of the invasive process. Endocarditis is seen more commonly as a distinctive form of the disease and is discussed later.

In many patients with systemic candidosis, there is considerable difficulty in confirming the laboratory or clinical diagnosis unless retinopathy is present or there are lesions accessible for biopsy. Both fungal cultures and serologic tests are negative in a substantial proportion of patients.

Candida Endocarditis. This is seen most frequently following homograft valve surgery or in drug addicts. The mitral or aortic valves are involved most commonly, often producing large vegetations. Emboli from these can obstruct major blood vessels. The diagnosis is confirmed by culture and serologic testing. High titers of antibody may occur in this form of candidosis.

Deep Focal Invasion. This may follow surgery or local injury. The main areas involved are the peritoneum (after peritoneal dialysis or gastrointestinal perforation) and the meninges (following surgery). The infection usually remains localized. *Candida* urinary tract infections are not uncommon and are seen most frequently in patients with urinary tract obstruction, indwelling bladder catheters, and diabetes mellitus. The appearance of *Candida* in the urine is not necessarily an indication for treatment unless the patient experiences symptoms (e.g., pain on urination or frequency), or unless, in severely ill patients, there is risk of dissemination.

TREATMENT. The main treatment for systemic candidosis is amphotericin B (Chapter 67). In severe or retinal infections, 5-fluorocytosine is added usually to the regimen. There is a little evidence that ketoconazole, itraconazole, or fluconazole may be helpful in some forms of systemic candidosis. In urinary infections caused by *Candida,* fluconazole may be used alone for 7 to 10 days.

BIBLIOGRAPHY

Ellis CA, Spivack ML: The significance of candidemia. Ann Intern Med 67:511, 1967.

Hyun BH, Collier FC: Mycotic endocarditis following intracardiac operations. N Engl J Med 263:1339, 1961.

Kozinn PJ, Hasenclever, HF, Taschdjian CL, et al.: Problems in the diagnosis and treatment of systemic candidosis. J Infect Dis 126:548, 1972.

Myerowitz RL, Pazin GJ, Allen CM: Disseminated candidosis. Changes in incidence, underlying diseases and pathology. Am J Clin Pathol 68:29, 1977.

Stone HH, Geheber CE, Kolg LD, et al.: Alimentary tract colonization by Candida albicans. J Surg Res 14:273, 1973.

MUCORMYCOSIS

DEFINITION. Mucormycosis (zygomycosis, systemic hycomycosis) is a systemic fungal infection caused by certain Zygomycetes fungi of the genera *Rhizopus, Absidia,* or, on rare occasions, *Cunninghamella* and *Saksenaea.*

ETIOLOGY AND PATHOGENESIS. There are a number of sites of primary invasion in mucormycosis, including the paranasal sinuses, skin, lungs, and gastrointestinal tract. The organisms are common environmental saprophytes in most parts of the world. However, they only produce invasive disease in compromised patients, such as those with leukemia, diabetic ketoacidosis, burn injuries, or malnutrition. This infection has not been widely described from the tropics. There are scattered reports of cases in South Africa and the Far East, however, and its distribution is likely to be worldwide.

CLINICAL MANIFESTATIONS. There are a number of different clinical varieties of mucormycosis.

Rhinocerebral Mucormycosis. This form is most often seen in patients with poorly controlled, insulin-dependent diabetes mellitus. The presenting features are most commonly those of an orbital cellulitis, with unilateral facial swelling, proptosis, and orbital pain. Alternatively, palatal perforation may be found. The process is rapidly progressive, and invasion of adjacent structures, including the optic nerve, cranium, and other sinuses, may occur. The infection is accompanied often by extensive infarction, as blood vessel invasion is a prominent feature. Secondary spread to other areas such as the lung may occur.

Pulmonary Mucormycosis. Lung invasion may occur in any affected group but is found most often in immunosuppressed or leukemic patients. Extensive pulmonary infection is associated often with disseminated infection elsewhere.

Other Sites of Invasion. Invasion of burns or postoperative wounds with secondary spread and extensive thrombosis has been described. It has also been recognized that contaminated dressing packs may be associated with this pattern of infection. Severe gastrointestinal hemorrhage or perforation may be the presenting feature of gastrointestinal invasion. The stomach and jejunum are the sites invaded most frequently. This form of mucormycosis has been described in malnourished patients.

DIAGNOSIS. Mucormycosis may be manifested by distinctive clinical features that aid in establishing the diagnosis. However, cultures are frequently negative, and serologic testing is unhelpful. The distinctive broad aseptate hyphae may be seen in biopsy specimens or smears taken from infected areas. Biopsy is normally the best method of establishing the diagnosis and should be performed early in the course of the infection.

TREATMENT. When possible, extensive surgical

débridement of infected areas should be performed, combined with administration of amphotericin B, given in high dosage (0.8 to 1.0 mg/kg daily) (Chapter 67). Treatment is continued until clinical remission is achieved.

BIBLIOGRAPHY

Kahn LR: Gastric mucormycosis: Report of a case with a review of the literature. S Afr Med J 37:1265, 1963.
Lehrer RI, Howard DH, Sypherd PS, et al.: Mucormycosis. Ann Intern Med 93:93, 1980.
Meyer RD, Armstrong D: Mucormycosis—changing status. CRC Crit Rev Clin Lab Sci 4:421, 1973.
Tanphaichitra D: Rhinocerebral mucormycosis with emphasis on clinical diagnosis, altered host defence mechanisms and management. Postgrad Med J 55:622, 1979.

67.   TREATMENT OF THE DEEP MYCOSES

Edward C. Oldfield, III

The treatment of the systemic mycoses remains a clinical challenge. The infections are chronic, with a tendency to relapse, and the standard therapy, amphotericin B, has multiple toxicities. From the 1950s until recently, there were few significant new antifungal agents. With the introduction of the imidazole class, especially the oral agents ketoconazole, fluconazole, and itraconazole, there is the promise of relatively nontoxic long-term therapy. The purpose of this chapter is to discuss the properties and use of the major antifungals: amphotericin B, flucytosine, ketoconazole, fluconazole, itraconazole, miconazole, and hydroxystilbamidine. For specific indications to institute therapy for a particular systemic fungal infection, duration of therapy, and parameters indicating response, refer to the chapter on the particular systemic mycosis.

AMPHOTERICIN B. Amphotericin B is a member of the class of antibiotics called macrolide polyenes and is a product of *Streptomyces nodosus*. Despite its formidable and essentially unavoidable toxicities, amphotericin B remains the standard therapeutic agent for most of the deep mycoses.

Mechanism of Action. The polyene structure of amphotericin B is responsible for both its therapeutic and its toxic properties. All cells susceptible to polyenes contain sterols in their cell membranes. Amphotericin B interacts with membrane sterols, leading to an alteration in the integrity of the cell membrane, with subsequent leakage of intracellular contents. In the fungi, the interaction is with ergosterol and results in inhibition of fungal growth, whereas in human cells, the interaction is with cholesterol, resulting in toxic side effects.

Sensitive Organisms. Most of the fungi responsible for systemic mycotic infections are sensitive to amphotericin B. These include *Coccidioides immitis*, *Cryptococcus neoformans*, *Histoplasma capsulatum*, *Blasto-*

myces dermatitidis, *Candida* species, *Torulopsis glabrata*, *Aspergillus* species, *Paracoccidioides braziliensis*, and the causative agents of mucormycosis. Activity has been noted also against a number of protozoan pathogens: trichomonads, *Entamoeba*, *Naegleria*, *Leishmania*, and trypanosomes. Intrinsic resistance has been reported among many species; however, these data are difficult to interpret because of a lack of standardization among laboratories and the variance between in vitro and clinical results. At present, there seems little to be gained from in vitro susceptibility testing or measurement of serum levels of amphotericin B.

The development of acquired resistance during therapy has not been a problem. As a rule, the fungi isolated from patients who have been treated and subsequently relapsed have been as sensitive as the initial isolates.

Synergism of amphotericin B with a number of agents has been noted. This effect has had the most clinical promise with flucytosine and is discussed in the section on that drug. Amphotericin B has been noted to be synergistic with agents not normally believed to have intrinsic antifungal activity, i.e., rifampin, tetracycline, and minocycline. The clinical importance of this interaction remains untested.

Pharmacologic Properties. Peak serum concentrations of amphotericin B with standard therapeutic doses are 0.5 to 2.0 µg/ml. The fate of the drug is unknown, and no metabolites have been identified. There is a biphasic excretion of drug from the body, with a rapid elimination half-life of 24 hours, followed by a prolonged terminal half life of 15 days. Renal excretion accounts for only 3 to 5% of total drug elimination. For this reason, there is no accumulation of amphotericin B in serum during renal failure, and no dosage adjustment is required, even in the anephric patient. A dosage reduction may be needed to avoid further nephrotoxicity, but it should be noted that this will result in decreased serum levels. Amphotericin B is not removed by peritoneal dialysis or hemodialysis. Biliary excretion has been noted to be 19%, but it has not been believed that hepatic disease necessitates a dosage change.

Cerebrospinal fluid penetration has been poor even with inflamed meninges. The levels of amphotericin B in the CSF are 30 to 50 times lower than concomitant serum levels. Urine concentrations are similar to those in serum. Levels in the aqueous humor are about two thirds of those in serum, and poor vitreous humor penetration has been noted. Levels of amphotericin B in pleural, peritoneal, and synovial fluid are also about two thirds of serum levels.

Preparations. Amphotericin B (Fungizone, Squibb) is available as a sterile powder for intravenous use in vials containing 50 mg of amphotericin B and 41 mg of desoxycholate, which creates a colloidal dispersion of the insoluble antibiotic. It is reconstituted with 10 ml of sterile water without additives and then added to 5% dextrose in water. The addition of even minimal amounts of sodium or chloride will reduce bioactivity and induce the prompt appearance of turbidity in the infusion bottle. Therefore, amphotericin B should not be mixed with electrolytes or acidic solutions.

Amphotericin B is light-sensitive, but during a 24-

hour period there is no appreciable loss of activity. Therefore, no special precautions, such as wrapping the bottle with aluminum foil, are necessary.

The drug is poorly absorbed from the gastrointestinal tract; oral doses as high as 5 gm result in inadequate serum levels.

Therapeutic Usage

Intravenous Therapy. Therapy with amphotericin B is initiated with a 1-mg test dose in 5% dextrose in water infused over 20 minutes to evaluate the extent of the commonly encountered febrile response. Vital signs should be monitored closely. Subsequent dosage increments to the full therapeutic dose of 0.3 to 0.7 mg/kg are determined by the severity of the toxic reactions encountered and the severity of the fungal infection. If the toxic reactions are minimal or the fungal infection is fulminating, rapid attainment of a full therapeutic dose can be achieved. If the toxic reactions are severe or the fungal infection is chronic, a more gradual institution of therapy may be desirable. For chronic infections, the dose may be increased daily until the desired level is reached. For instance, the daily dose of amphotericin B may be increased from the 1-mg test dose on the first day to 5-, 10-, 20-, and 40-mg doses in 500 ml of 5% dextrose in water on days 2, 3, 4, and 5, respectively. The duration of infusion is commonly 2 to 3 hours, although some have noted decreased toxicity with infusions of 1 hour. Infusions of less than 1 hour's duration should be avoided, as cardiac arrhythmias have been noted in dogs when rapid infusions are used. In cases in which the fungal disease is more severe, rapid attainment of therapeutic levels is desirable. In this situation, the full therapeutic dose (usually 20 to 50 mg) may be put in 500 ml of 5% dextrose in water. The equivalent of 1 mg is then infused over 20 to 30 minutes. If no severe reactions are encountered, the remainder is infused over 2 to 3 hours, with monitoring of vital signs.

If toxic reactions are noted, hydrocortisone, 25 mg, may be added to the infusion bottle. Hydrocortisone decreases the frequency but not the severity of fever and chills. Increasing the dose of hydrocortisone does not provide additional benefit. Premedication with acetylsalicylic acid and diphenhydramine may further ameliorate the toxicity. As the infusions are continued, many patients will develop tolerance to the amphotericin B, and the addition of hydrocortisone may be discontinued. Intravenous meperidine hydrochloride, in an average dose of 45 mg, has been shown to be effective in terminating rigors and chills during an infusion. For patients with severe rigors, the meperidine may be given prophylactically just prior to the amphotericin B infusion. Ibuprofen administered prior to the infusion has been noted also to decrease severe chills. However, there is a potential to enhance the nephrotoxicity of amphotericin B with ibuprofen, which also decreases renal blood flow and has tubular toxicity. Heparin, 500 to 1000 U, is commonly added to the infusion solution to decrease the incidence of phlebitis.

The usual recommended maintenance dose is 0.3 to 0.7 mg/kg/day, not exceeding 50 mg/day. During maintenance therapy, it is best to remove the intravenous needle after each infusion to decrease the incidence of phlebitis. The use of a double dose on alternate days (usually not exceeding 70 mg) has been shown to be as efficacious as daily therapy. The trough concentrations are similar on the off day to those obtained with daily therapy, and the peak concentrations with either regimen tend to reach a plateau at doses exceeding 50 mg. With the alternate-day regimen, prolonged out-patient therapy is greatly facilitated, and the patients feel better on the off day. The renal toxicity is equivalent with either regimen.

During prolonged therapy, toxicity is to be expected but can be monitored with twice weekly serum creatinine, blood urea nitrogen, potassium, magnesium, and hematocrit determinations. The total duration of therapy is variable and depends on the particular fungus being treated, the anatomic site of involvement, and the clinical response.

Other Routes of Administration. Intrathecal therapy may be required for fungal meningitis because of the poor penetration into cerebrospinal fluid. Only selected cases of cryptococcal meningitis will require intrathecal therapy, whereas all cases of coccidioidal meningitis will require this form of therapy. An initial dose of 0.1 mg is followed by increments of 0.1 mg until a total daily dose of 0.5 to 1.0 mg is attained. The dose is usually administered by the lumbar route on a thrice weekly schedule. Toxic reactions are common and include radicular pain, paresthesias, urinary retention, monoparesis, and acute toxic delirium. Hydrocortisone hemisuccinate (10 to 25 mg) is usually added to the injection to decrease radicular pain.

As therapy is continued, an arachnoiditis commonly develops at the lumbar site of injection. This may necessitate cisterna magna injections, with their potential for serious complications in inexperienced hands. Another approach is the implantation of subcutaneous siliconized-rubber reservoirs connected by tubing to the lateral ventricles. Although ease of administration is greatly enhanced, there has been a high incidence of side effects, including bacterial meningitis, hemiparesis, intracranial hemorrhage, and nonfunctioning tubing.

Intraperitoneal administration has been recommended at a dose of 1 mg of amphotericin B added to 1000 ml of dialysis fluid. Intra-articular use has been reported at doses ranging from 5 to 25 mg per injection. Bladder irrigation may be accomplished with 50 mg in 1000 cc of sterile water. Ocular penetration is poor with intravenous administration, but direct intravitreous administration in rabbits has led to retinal necrosis and detachment. For a more detailed discussion of the use of amphotericin B in ophthalmology, see Havener WH, 1983.

Toxicity. Amphotericin B is noted for its formidable and essentially unavoidable toxicity. However, with appropriate management, most patients can complete a course of therapy and the side effects can be minimized. On occasion, with chronic indolent infections, toxicity may preclude the successful completion of therapy, and alternate therapeutic regimens may be required.

General Toxicity. Toxicity associated with the infusion of amphotericin B has been noted in up to 93% of patients. This includes fever, occasionally in excess of 40C, rigors, headaches, anorexia, nausea, vomiting, dyspnea, and hypotension.

Nephrotoxicity. The most severe form of toxicity is renal. During the therapeutic use of amphotericin B, it is common for the creatinine level to rise to the range of 2.0 to 3.0 mg/dL. In many patients, the creatinine will reach a plateau at this level and therapy may be continued. However, in others, the creatinine level will continue to rise. Once the creatinine rises above 3.0 mg/dL, it is advisable to reduce the dose or temporarily withhold the infusion to prevent a further decrease in glomerular filtration. In some series, more than 80% of patients developed a significant alteration of renal function. In those patients who receive a total dose of less than 4 gm, the renal insufficiency is usually reversible. However, once the total dose exceeds 5 gm, most patients will exhibit some degree of persistent renal insufficiency.

The mechanism of renal toxicity appears to be due to a combination of direct tubular damage, primarily distal, and renal artery constriction. Pathologically, there are degenerative changes of the tubules, with intratubular and interstitial calcifications. Glomerular involvement is minimal. Functionally, there are consistent decreases in glomerular filtration rate and renal blood flow. There is also a consistent impairment of distal tubular function, with an increased renal clearance of potassium, and an impairment of renal hydrogen excretion, with the development of renal tubular acidosis. There is usually an absence of red blood cells, red blood cell casts, and significant proteinuria in the urine sediment, but cylindruria is common.

Renal toxicity is enhanced by intravascular volume depletion secondary to low sodium intake, diuretics, vomiting, diarrhea, or cirrhosis with ascites. Correcting volume depletion is essential for successful therapy by rehydration, high salt diet, discontinuation of diuretics, or volume expansion.

Hematologic Toxicity. Anemia is a common side effect. A decrease in hematocrit of 10 units can be expected in three fourths of patients, and one third will have a reduction of 15 units or greater. There is no correlation between the total dosage of amphotericin B or degree of azotemia and the magnitude of the anemia. The anemia is normochromic and normocytic, without a reticulocytosis. The hematocrit decreases early in therapy and then stabilizes. Transfusions have not been beneficial, as the hematocrit will return gradually to the pretransfusion level. Thrombocytopenia and neutropenia have been noted rarely.

Hypokalemia. Renal potassium wasting commonly results in decreased levels of serum potassium. Oral supplementation will be necessary in 25% of patients. Hypomagnesemia has also been noted.

Allergic Reactions. Allergic reactions are remarkably absent with amphotericin B. Because well-documented reports of drug eruptions are so rare, when a rash appears during therapy, it can be attributed usually to some other cause.

Hepatotoxicity. Alterations in hepatic function have been extremely rare.

Pregnancy. Amphotericin B has been used in pregnancy without evidence of teratogenesis or persistent toxicity in infants. Treatment of a pregnant woman should not be considered an indication for termination of pregnancy.

Therapeutic Indications. For specific indications, dosage, duration, and synergism, refer to the chapter on the particular systemic fungal infection.

FLUCYTOSINE (5-FLUOROCYTOSINE). Flucytosine is a fluorinated pyrimidine that was first synthesized as an antitumor agent in 1957. The drug has a narrow spectrum of activity and is used primarily because of its synergism with amphotericin B against certain fungi.

Mechanism of Action. Flucytosine is deaminated within the fungal cell to 5-fluorouracil, which is a commonly used antitumor agent. The 5-fluorouracil is then incorporated into fungal RNA as 5-fluorouridine triphosphate and leads to faulty protein synthesis and subsequent growth inhibition. Flucytosine also blocks thymidylate synthetase, leading to a decrease in DNA synthesis. The toxicity of flucytosine may be low because human cells lack the enzyme cytosine deaminase required to convert flucytosine to 5-fluorouracil.

Sensitive Organisms. Flucytosine is active against *Cryptococcus neoformans, Candida albicans,* some other *Candida* species, *Torulopsis glabrata,* and the causative agents of chromomycosis. Primary resistance is rare with *Cryptococcus neoformans* and *Torulopsis glabrata.* The sensitivity of *Candida albicans* varies from 50 to 90%, depending on the method used. When flucytosine is used alone, the development of secondary resistance during therapy has been a more serious problem. This is the primary reason why flucytosine is rarely used alone. As many as two thirds of isolates obtained during therapy have been resistant; however, they remain sensitive to amphotericin B.

Synergism with amphotericin B has been noted for *Cryptococcus neoformans* and for *Candida* species. An additive effect is commonly seen with *Candida* even if the isolate exhibits partial in vitro resistance to flucytosine.

Pharmacokinetics. Oral absorption of flucytosine is excellent, even in renal failure. Administration with meals does not decrease total absorption. Penetration of tissue is excellent, resulting in levels in the liver, kidneys, spleen, heart, and lungs that are equal to or greater than those in serum. The concentration of flucytosine in CSF averages 75% of simultaneous serum levels. The drug is concentrated in the urine with levels of 1000 to 2000 µg/ml, and lesser but adequate levels are maintained with renal insufficiency.

Excretion is primarily by the kidneys, with only minimal metabolism. The half-life of flucytosine with normal renal function is 3 to 4 hours, but even minor decreases in renal function will lead to prolongation. Both peritoneal dialysis and hemodialysis remove significant amounts of the drug.

Dosage and Administration. Flucytosine (Ancobon, Roche) is manufactured in tablets or capsules of 250- or 500-mg strength. The standard daily dose is 150 mg/kg divided into 4 equal doses of 37.5 mg/kg. It is critical that the dosage be adjusted in the presence of renal insufficiency, as even mild azotemia may lead to significant increases in serum levels. In order to avoid accumulation of toxic levels in serum, i.e., greater than 100 μg/ml, a number of dosage adjustments have been recommended. One commonly used regimen maintains a normal dose of 37.5 mg/kg but prolongs the interval between doses, with a 12-hour interval for creatinine clearance between 20 and 40 ml/min and a 24-hour interval for creatinine clearance between 10 and 20 ml/min. For patients on hemodialysis, a dose of 37.5 mg/kg after each dialysis may be used.

During treatment, it is essential to monitor serum creatinine, blood urea nitrogen, liver function, and platelet and white blood cell counts. Particular caution must be used when there is pre-existing renal insufficiency, decreased platelet count, neutropenia, or liver disease.

Toxicity. As a rule, flucytosine is well tolerated. In one large series, 18% of patients experienced gastrointestinal, 7% hepatic, and 18% hematologic complications. The gastrointestinal toxicity usually takes the form of nausea, vomiting, and diarrhea. This is usually not severe; however, severe colitis with multiple colonic perforations may develop. Hepatitis may occur and is usually nonprogressive. The abnormalities resolve usually with discontinuation of the drug.

Neutropenia has been the most common hematologic toxicity. There may also be thrombocytopenia or a combination of the two. The bone marrow toxicity resolves usually with decreased dosage or discontinuation of flucytosine. However, fatal bone marrow suppression has been reported. This hematologic toxicity correlates with serum levels of 100 to 125 μg/ml or greater, usually with associated renal insufficiency. When available, serum levels should be monitored to avoid toxic levels.

Less commonly reported toxicity has included maculopapular rashes and eosinophilia. Flucytosine should be used with caution in women of childbearing age because of teratogenicity noted in experimental animals.

Therapeutic Indications. The combination of amphotericin B and flucytosine is the treatment of choice for cryptococcal meningitis; it improves cure rates and decreases relapses when compared with therapy with amphotericin B alone. This combination is indicated also in disseminated cryptococcal disease and severe infections with *Candida* species and *Torulopsis*. The combination will allow a decreased dose of amphotericin B (0.3 mg/kg) and, hence, a decrease in renal toxicity. The presence of amphotericin B decreases the emergence of flucytosine resistance but may lead to an increase in flucytosine toxicity. Chromomycosis may be an indication for flucytosine alone, and some have used the drug alone to treat urinary candidiasis.

KETOCONAZOLE. The synthetic imidazole ketoconazole is an oral broad-spectrum antifungal agent introduced in 1977. It, along with the triazoles, is the most promising addition to the antifungal armamentarium since the introduction of amphotericin B.

Mechanism of Action. Ketoconazole is a potent inhibitor of the major membrane sterol of fungi, ergosterol. A concentration of drug 600 times higher is required to inhibit mammalian sterols and may account for the limited toxicity.

Sensitive Organisms. Ketoconazole has a broad range of antifungal activity that includes the dimorphic fungi, yeasts, and dermatophytes. The most promising activity in invasive fungal disease has been noted with *Paracoccidioides braziliensis*, *Histoplasma capsulatum*, *Coccidioides immitis*, and *Candida* species. Activity has also been noted against *Leishmania*, *Plasmodium falciparum*, and *Trypanosoma cruzi*. Synergism with other antifungal agents does not seem to be clinically important. The development of resistance during therapy has not been a problem to date.

Pharmacokinetics. Peak serum concentrations after a 200-mg dose of ketoconazole are in the range of 2 μg/ml and occur 2 to 4 hours after administration. Gastric acidity is critical for adequate absorption of the drug. Any agent that lowers gastric acidity, e.g., cimetidine, antacids, and anticholinergics, will lower serum levels. Conversely, administration of ketoconazole with a meal has been noted to provide higher and more consistent serum levels as well as to decrease associated nausea and vomiting.

Ketoconazole is metabolized extensively. The half-life is biphasic, with a first phase of 1.4 to 2.2 hours and a second phase of 7 to 10 hours. The half-life has not been prolonged with renal insufficiency, and no dosage adjustments have been recommended. The urinary concentrations are low, about 0.4 μg/ml. The need for adjustment with hepatic disease has not been determined. Cerebrospinal fluid concentrations have been low, 2 to 4% of serum levels.

Rifampin and isoniazid have been noted to decrease serum levels of ketoconazole. The clearance of cyclosporin, methylprednisolone, quinidine, warfarin, and chlordiazepoxide have all been decreased by ketoconazole.

Toxicity. Ketoconazole has been a remarkably safe and well-tolerated drug. Nausea, vomiting, pruritus, and abdominal pain are the most frequent side effects, occurring in 2 to 3% of patients. The incidence increases as the dose is increased but usually subsides with continued use and when the drug is administered with meals. Less common side effects include fatigue, diarrhea, dizziness, somnolence, rash, hypertension, anaphylaxis, hemolytic anemia, and headache. Toxicity is dose related and required discontinuation of therapy in 6, 17, 23, and 56% of patients at doses of 400, 800, 1200, and 1600 mg/day.

Hepatitis is the most serious toxicity associated with ketoconazole use. About 1 in 15,000 patients will develop a symptomatic hepatitis, which has rarely resulted in fatalities. In addition, mild asymptomatic reversible elevations of liver function tests have been noted in 12% of patients. Monitoring of liver function tests is recommended every 2 weeks for the first 2 months and then monthly or bimonthly. If there is a rise in transaminases of 3 to 5 times normal or the development of clinical symptoms or jaundice, ketoconazole should be discontinued immediately.

Multiple interactions with the endocrine system have

been noted, which are dose dependent and usually reversible. The inhibition of testosterone synthesis may lead to gynecomastia, decreased libido, impotence, and azoospermia, and has led to the use of ketoconazole in the treatment of prostatic cancer and precocious puberty. Inhibition of steroid synthesis has rarely led to adrenal insufficiency, but usually occurs at doses higher than those used to treat fungal infections.

Teratogenic and embryotoxic effects have been noted in rats. The drug is contraindicated in pregnancy.

Therapeutic Uses. Ketoconazole (Nizoral, Janssen Pharmaceutical) is supplied as a 200-mg tablet. The response of paracoccidioidomycosis has been most impressive. The remission rate with a dose of 200 mg has been 79%, and another 16% of patients have markedly improved. Skin and mucosal lesions have responded more rapidly than pulmonary lesions. The results with histoplasmosis and blastomycosis in the immunocompetent patient without meningitis have been excellent, but amphotericin B remains the drug of choice in the immunocompromised patient and in meningeal and life-threatening infections. In the treatment of coccidioidomycosis with ketoconazole, some encouraging results have been noted. The response has been best with skin lesions, including abscesses, with an 80% response rate. However, there is often only a suppression of clinical symptoms, with relapses occurring even after years of apparently successful therapy. Some patients must be placed on lifelong therapy.

Ketoconazole has become the drug of choice for chronic mucocutaneous candidiasis, and some success has been noted in the treatment of *Pseudallescheria boydii*, which is resistant to amphotericin B. There have also been reports of successful therapy in chromomycosis, entomophthoromycosis, and mycetoma due to a variety of fungi.

TRIAZOLES. There are two new triazoles, fluconazole and itraconazole. Fluconazole, approved by the FDA in 1990, is water-soluble, weakly protein-bound, attains high CSF levels (60 to 80% of serum levels), and is excreted unchanged in the urine. Fluconazole may prove useful especially in the treatment of fungal meningitis and urinary tract infections. The dose should be decreased by 50% with a creatinine clearance of 21 to 50 cc/min and by 75% with one of 11 to 20 cc/min. Fluconazole may increase serum levels of warfarin, phenytoin, sulfonylurea hypoglycemics, and cyclosporine.

Itraconazole is highly protein-bound with high tissue levels. Antimycotic activity is similar to ketoconazole, but additional activity has been noted against the causative agents of chromomycosis, cryptococcosis, sporotrichosis, and aspergillosis.

MICONAZOLE. Miconazole is a member of the imidazole class of broad-spectrum antifungal agents that is available only as an intravenous preparation with a carrier of polyethoxylated castor oil. The usual dose is 600 to 3000 mg/day in 3 divided doses in 5% dextrose, which is infused over 1 hour. Toxicity has included anemia, hyponatremia, thrombocytopenia, hyperlipemia, and rouleaux formation of erythrocytes. Thrombophlebitis has been noted in up to 70% of patients and

may cause problems with venous access. This may be reduced by administration through a central venous catheter.

Because miconazole requires hospitalization and intravenous administration and has more toxicity than ketoconazole or the triazoles, there are no primary indications for the drug. Its use should be reserved for treatment failures that occur with ketoconazole and amphotericin B.

2–HYDROCYSTILBAMIDINE. 2–hydroxystilbamidine is a narrow-spectrum synthetic antifungal agent used only in the treatment of blastomycosis. However, amphotericin B is more effective and appears to be the drug of choice except in mild or limited disease.

The usual dose of 2-hydroxystilbamidine is 225 mg given intravenously once daily, to a total of 8 gm. The usual infusion time is 5 to 6 hours to avoid the hypotension associated with rapid infusions. The solution must be protected from light. Toxicity has commonly included anorexia, malaise, and vomiting. Rashes and hepatotoxicity have been reported also.

BIBLIOGRAPHY

Bennett JE: Treatment of cryptococcal, candidal and coccidioidal meningitis. *In* Remington JS, Swartz MN (eds.): Current Clinical Topics in Infectious Disease. New York, McGraw-Hill Book Co, 1980, pp 54–67.

Bennett JE, Dismukes WE, Duma RJ, et al.: A comparison of amphotericin B alone and combined with flucytosine in the treatment of cryptococcal meningitis. N Engl J Med 301:126, 1979.

Bindschadler DD, Bennett JE: A pharmacologic guide to the clinical use of amphotericin B. J Infect Dis 120:427, 1969.

Burks LC, Aisner J, Fortner CL, et al.: Meperidine for the treatment of shaking chills and fever. Arch Intern Med 140:438, 1980.

Butler WT, Bennett JE, Alling DW, et al.: Nephrotoxicity of amphotericin B: Early and late effects in 81 patients. Ann Intern Med 61:175, 1964.

Cutler RE, Blair AD, Kelly MR: Flucytosine kinetics in subjects with normal and impaired renal function. Clin Pharmacol Ther 24:333, 1978.

Daneshmend TK, Warnock DW: Clinical pharmacokinetics of ketoconazole. Clin Pharmacokinet 14:13–34, 1988.

Drouhet E, Dupont B: Laboratory and clinical assessment of ketoconazole in deep-seated mycoses. Am J Med 74 (1B):30–47, 1983.

Drutz DJ: In vitro antifungal susceptibility testing and measurement of levels of antifungal agents in body fluids. Rev Infect Dis 9:392–397, 1987.

Engelhard D, Stutman HR, Marks MI: Interaction of ketoconazole with rifampin and isoniazid. N Engl J Med 311:1681–1683, 1984.

Gigliotti F, Shenep JL, Lott LL, et al.: Induction of prostaglandin synthesis as the mechanism responsible for the chills and fever produced by infusing amphotericin B. J Infect Dis 156:784–789, 1987.

Havener WH: Ocular pharmacology. St. Louis, CV Mosby, 1983, pp 133–137.

Heidemann HT, Gerkens JF, Spickard WA, et al.: Amphotericin B nephrotoxicity in humans decreased by salt repletion. Am J Med 75:476–481, 1983.

Ismail MA, Lerner SA: Disseminated blastomycosis in a pregnant woman. Am Rev Respir Dis 126:350–353, 1982.

Lewis JH, Zimmerman HJ, Benson GD, et al.: Hepatic injury associated with ketoconazole therapy. Gastroenterology 83:503–513, 1984.

NIAID Mycoses Study Group: Treatment of blastomycosis and histoplasmosis with ketoconazole. Ann Intern Med 103:861–872, 1985.

Restrepo A, Stevens DA, Gomez I, et al.: Ketoconazole: A new drug for the treatment of paracoccidioidomycosis. Rev Infect Dis 2:633, 1980.

Saag MS, Dismukes WE: Azole antifungal agents: Emphasis on new triazoles. Antimicrob Agents Chemother 32:1–8, 1988.

Shadomy S, White SC, Yu HP, et al.: NIAID Mycoses Study Group: Treatment of systemic mycoses with ketoconazole: In vitro susceptibilities of clinical isolates of systemic and pathogenic fungi to ketoconazole. J Infect Dis 152:1249–1256, 1985.

Sohn CA: Evaluation of ketoconazole. Clin Pharmacol 1:217, 1982.

Sonino N: The use of ketoconazole as an inhibitor of steroid production. N Engl J Med 317:817–818, 1987.

Stamm AM, Diasio RB, Dismukes WE, et al.: Toxicity of amphotericin B plus flucytosine in 194 patients with cryptococcal meningitis. Am J Med 83:236–242, 1987.

Sugar AM, Alsip SG, Galgiani JN, et al.: Pharmacology and toxicity of high-dose ketoconazole. Antimicrob Agents Chemother 31: 1874–1878, 1987.

Utz JP, Bennett JE, Brandriss MW, et al.: Amphotericin B toxicity. Ann Intern Med 61:334, 1964.

Wise GJ, Kozinn PJ, Goldberg P: Flucytosine in the management of genitourinary candidiasis. 5 years of experience. J Urol 124:70–72, 1980.

PART V

PROTOZOAL INFECTIONS

GENERAL PRINCIPLES

G. Thomas Strickland

PARASITISM

DEFINITIONS. Parasite comes from the Greek word *parasitos* and is defined as "a plant or an animal which lives upon or within another living organism at whose expense it obtains some advantage." Parasitism is a type of *symbiosis,* in which an intimate and obligatory relationship exists between two heterospecific organisms. The *parasite,* generally the smaller of the two, is usually metabolically dependent on its host. This association may be beneficial to both *(mutualism),* beneficial to one with little effect on the other *(commensalism),* or beneficial to one and detrimental to the other *(parasitism).* The term parasite is generally reserved for animal species of protozoa, helminths, and arthropods.

NATURAL HISTORY

Host. The organism on or within which the parasite lives is called the *host.* The life cycle of the parasite may take place in a single host species (e.g., *Entamoeba histolytica*—man), in two host species (e.g., *Plasmodium vivax*—man and mosquito), or in more than two host species (e.g., *Clonorchis sinensis*—man, snail, and cyprinoid fish).

A *definitive host* (e.g., man for *Taenia saginata*) is one in which a parasite undergoes sexual reproduction. Man may be the only definitive host for some parasites (e.g., *Trichomonas vaginalis*), whereas others may have several definitive hosts (e.g., bushbuck, other game animals, and man for *Trypanosoma brucei rhodesiense*). Animals that harbor a parasite that is pathogenic for other animals are called *reservoir hosts* (e.g., dogs for *Leishmania tropica*). Parasites that have reservoir hosts (e.g., *Brugia malayi*) are more difficult to eradicate than those that do not (e.g., *Wuchereria bancrofti*); the reservoir host serves as an alternate in the life cycle, thus increasing the chance of transmission and survival.

The animal in which the larval or asexual stage habitates (e.g., freshwater snail for *Schistosoma* species) is known as the *intermediate host.* A *transfer or paratenic host* (e.g., large predator fish for *Diphyllobothrium latum*) is not necessary for the completion of the life cycle of the parasite but is utilized as a temporary refuge and vehicle for reaching the obligatory or definitive host. An *incidental host* is one that is accidentally infected and is not required for the parasite's survival or development (e.g., man for *Toxoplasma gondii*).

Vector. A *vector* (from the Latin *vehere,* to carry), usually an arthropod, transfers an infectious agent from one host to another. The parasite may develop or multiply within the body of the vector before becoming infective, in which case the vector is called a *biologic vector.* Biologic vectors are actually hosts—definitive hosts in the case of anopheline mosquitoes for human *Plasmodium* species or intermediate hosts in the case of *Cyclops* species for *Dracunculus medinensis.* A *mechanical vector* carries a parasite from one host to another but is not essential for the parasite's life cycle (e.g., houseflies for *Entamoeba histolytica*).

PROTOZOA

DEFINITIONS. *Protozoa,* derived from the Greek words *protos,* meaning first or primary, and *zoon,* meaning animal, is a phylum comprising some of the morphologically simplest organisms of the animal kingdom. Most species are unicellular and range in size from submicroscopic to macroscopic; most are free-living, but some have commensalistic, mutualistic, or parasitic relationships. Approximately 10,000 of the described living species are parasitic. Protozoa infect most vertebrate and invertebrate species and have developed the capacity to adapt to living in most host organs.

The parasitic protozoa, unlike almost all helminths, can replicate (sexually, asexually, or both ways) within the host's body—a phenomenon that largely explains their survival as well as the overwhelming infections that develop from single exposures.

CLASSIFICATION. It remains convenient to divide protozoa pathogenic to man into four phyla or subphyla (or superclasses in the case of the sporozoa) according to their type of locomotion: (1) Sarcodina (amebae); (2) Mastigophora (flagellates); (3) Ciliophora (ciliates); and (4) Sporozoa.

Sarcodina. *Ameboid* movements produce pseudopods in the Sarcodina. Reproduction is almost exclusively asexual, usually by binary fission. Amebae that infect man include *Entamoeba histolytica* (Chapter 68). Other species of Sarcodina that can be either parasitic (e.g., *Naegleria fowleri,* normally a free-living organism) or mutualistic or commensalistic (e.g., *Entamoeba hartmanni* and *Entamoeba coli*) are covered in Chapters 71 and 80. Most are parasites or commensals of the gastrointestinal tract.

Mastigophora. *Flagella* produce a whiplike motion. Most species, like those of the Sarcodina, have both *cysts* (transmission stage) and *trophozoites* (proliferative stage). Flagellates that infect man include *Giardia lamblia* (Chapter 69), *Trichomonas vaginalis* (Chapter 72), *Trypanosoma brucei gambiense, T. b. rhodesiense,* and

T. cruzi (Chapters 74 and 75), and *Leishmania* species (Chapter 76). Species in this group are capable of infecting many different tissues and cells.

Ciliophora. *Cilia* supply the motion in this subphylum. They have two kinds of nuclei, a macronucleus and a micronucleus. Reproduction is by asexual transverse binary fission and sexual conjugation. *Balantidium coli,* the largest intestinal parasite of man, is a ciliate (Chapter 71.1).

Sporozoa. Protozoa in this subphylum typically have no locomotor organs in the adult stage(s) and reproduce alternately by asexual multiplication (schizogony) and sexual multiplication (sporogony). They are exclusively parasitic. Pathogens of man in this group include *Plasmodium* species (Chapter 73), *Toxoplasma gondii* (Chapter 78), and *Isospora* and *Sarcocystis* species (Chapters 71.2 and 81). Based upon ribosmal gene analysis, *Pneumocystis carinii* (Chapter 79) is now considered by most to be a fungus. However, it obviously still remains somewhere between protozoa and fungi and can best be covered among the former.

PHYSIOLOGY. With the exception of the Sarcodina trophozoites, which have an ectoplastic covering, protozoa have cell membranes.

Ectoplasm. Across this membrane, nutrients can be actively transported, phagocytized, or moved by pinocytosis. Some species have a peristome through which food passes directly into the cytosome and cytopharynx to the endoplasm.

Endoplasm. Protozoa are eukaryotic; some have multiple nuclei. Cytoplasmic inclusions and a variety of organelles are responsible for metabolic, reproductive, and protective functions.

Reproduction. Asexual or binary fission–type reproduction is characteristic of the Sarcodina, Mastigophora, and Ciliophora. In some species, asexual reproduction is more complex. Sexual reproduction in the Sporozoa always takes place in the definitive host (e.g., mosquito for malarial parasites, cat for *T. gondii*); it results in the formation of a zygote. Asexual reproduction occurs in the intermediate host (e.g., man for malarial parasites and for *T. gondii*).

TRANSMISSION

Intestinal Protozoa. These are usually transmitted from host to host by the fecal-oral route via food and water. Many species have a cystic stage that is capable of resisting adverse environmental conditions (e.g., drying, heat, and cold). *Toxoplasma gondii* is also transmitted by ingestion of undercooked meat (contaminated with cysts) or materials containing cat feces (contaminated with oocysts).

Blood and Tissue Protozoa. Most of these have two hosts—vertebrate (man) and an invertebrate vector (arthropod). The parasite is usually transmitted by the vector's bite (e.g., in infections with *Plasmodium* species, *T. b. gambiense* and *T. b. rhodesiense, Leishmania* species, or *Babesia* species) or by exposure to contaminated vector feces (e.g., in infections with *T. cruzi*).

MAGNITUDE OF THE HEALTH PROBLEM. Protozoal infections cause man more disease and misery than any other group of infectious agents.

In the Tropics

Malaria. Infections with *Plasmodium* species may be the greatest cause of mortality and morbidity in the world today, particularly in children under 5 years of age and in pregnant women. The World Health Organization (WHO) has given up the goal of global eradication of malaria and has set a realistic long-term aim of control: control of transmission with drugs and insecticides in areas where this is feasible, and control of disease with selective chemoprophylaxis and/or chemotherapy where transmission control is not possible (e.g., most of sub-Saharan Africa). Malaria was a greater global medical problem in the 1980s than it was in the 1970s and will be even more of a scourge in the 1990s. The continuing development of resistance to insecticides by the anopheline vectors has meant that new chemicals are required, and these are too expensive to be used by those who need them.

Multiple drug–resistant *P. falciparum* has spread from Southeast Asia into the Indian subcontinent and the Western Pacific. It is widespread in most malaria-endemic areas of South America and during the past 10 years has covered much of sub-Saharan Africa. Estimates of the numbers infected and dying from malaria are totally inaccurate. In endemic areas, most individuals exposed to infectious bites have low levels of parasitemia. Many, frequently children, have relatively high intensity of parasitemias that are often associated with illness (Chapter 73).

African Trypanosomiasis. Infection with either *Trypanosoma brucei gambiense* or *T. b. rhodesiense* almost always causes severe human illness. If untreated, it is fatal; fortunately, however, relatively few people are infected. (Although information is limited, there has been an epidemic of sleeping sickness in Uganda during the past few years.) *Trypanosoma brucei brucei,* which is morphologically identical to the subspecies causing human sleeping sickness (Chapter 74), causes infection in cattle (nagana) across much of Central and East Africa. Thus, cattle raising is limited, greatly interfering with economic development and with the nutritional status of the entire area. The prospects for reducing the impact of African trypanosomiasis are slim: (1) There are no efficacious and safe chemotherapeutic agents available; (2) control of transmission is difficult because of the habits of the tsetse fly; and (3) vaccine development is hampered by the ability of the parasite to evade the immune response by varying its antigens.

American Trypanosomiasis. *Trypanosoma cruzi* affects as many as 15 million people living in South and Central America. Although acute infections may be fatal, most infections are not even detected (Chapter 75). Unfortunately, chronic complications years later often lead to severe disability and death from Chagas' cardiopathy and the "mega" syndromes. The poor who live in crudely built huts infested with the vector, "the kissing bug," contract Chagas' disease. If adequate housing were available, this major parasitic disease would become a minor problem. However, prospects for the poor of Latin America to obtain improved housing in the near future are not good. Furthermore, infection can be transmitted transplacentally from mother to fetus and by blood transfusion. There are still no efficacious and safe drugs for treating the infection, particularly the chronic form. The large and varied animal reservoirs make transmission control more difficult, and vaccine development remains in the future.

Amebiasis and Giardiasis. *Entamoeba histolytica* (Chapter 68) and *Giardia lamblia* (Chapter 69) normally infect the gastrointestinal tract. Each parasite has a trophozoite proliferative stage and a cystic transmissible stage, but the majority of the millions infected do not have clinical illness. What causes illness in some and not in others is unknown. Studies of *E. histolytica* isoenzymes are showing that identical-appearing organisms have differences that correlate with their pathogenicity. Neither parasite appears to cause increased illness in those infected with HIV virus. In many areas of the world, disease caused by *E. histolytica* appears to be decreasing.

Leishmaniasis. *Leishmania* species also infect millions worldwide and cause clinical syndromes varying from a minimal, single, self-healing chronic ulceration (urban oriental sore [Chapter 76.2]) to a severe and often fatal generalized febrile illness (kala-azar [Chapter 76.1]). *Leishmania* species causing these different syndromes appear morphologically identical. Strain differences can be detected, however, by using biochemical, immunologic, and other techniques that correlate with epidemiologic and clinical differences. Better diagnosis has demonstrated more cases of subclinical and mild infections than of the characteristic diseases.

In Temperate Climates. All of the above noted protozoal infections are potential dangers to travelers to endemic areas from more developed countries (Chapter 121), and all should be suspected in emigrants from developing countries (Chapter 120). Amebiasis, giardiasis, and toxoplasmosis are also transmitted within temperate climates, where they are becoming more common medical problems. The first two occur with increasing frequency in promiscuous male homosexuals but usually do not cause illness. Pneumocystosis, cryptosporidiosis, primary amebic meningoencephalitis, and babesiosis also are more common in patients who are immunosuppressed.

Trichomoniasis. *Trichomonas vaginalis* is one of the most common causes of vaginal irritation and discharge among women in temperate climates (Chapter 72). Infection with this organism is very contagious and sexually transmitted and can cause nongonococcal urethritis in both males and females. Nitroimidazole drugs provide the best means of cure. There is still no evidence that these compounds cause congenital malformations in pregnant women treated for trichomoniasis; the recommendation that treatment be withheld during pregnancy should be reconsidered.

NEW DEVELOPMENTS. There have been several exciting developments in protozoology since the last edition of this book was published.

Malaria Vaccine. Considerable progress continues to be made in basic malaria research: The gene coding for the *P. falciparum* circumsporozoite (CS) protein has been cloned and sequenced; the antigen was produced synthetically and by genetic engineering and shown to be safe and immunogenic in animals and human volunteers. When immunized individuals were challenged by bite from *P. falciparum*–infected anopheline mosquitoes, only two volunteers were fully protected. Most peptide-immunized volunteers produced antibodies, but there was no booster effect from multiple doses. For optimal protection, future malaria sporozoite vaccines must not only contain the B cell epitope but must also induce T-helper cells and cytotoxic T cells, which have been shown to inhibit the development of liver stage parasites.

The parasite can evade the immune response by several mechanisms, of which antigenic variation is believed to be one of the most important. The existence of these evasive mechanisms makes malaria vaccine development very difficult. Vaccine candidates are being developed from three stages of the malaria parasites, for both *P. falciparum* and *P. vivax:* (1) the sporozoite stage (to prevent infection); (2) the asexual blood stages (to prevent clinical disease); and (3) the gamete stage (to prevent transmission to the feeding vectors). The workable vaccine will probably be a "cocktail" of several antigens from two or three of the parasite stages.

Chemotherapy. There have been some accomplishments in the chemotherapy of protozoa in the past 5 or 6 years.

Leishmaniasis. United States Army investigators, their Kenyan colleagues, and others, during the 1980s, worked out a new and safe dose schedule for using pentavalent compounds, the therapeutic mainstays for treating leishmaniasis for the past 70 years. By doubling the daily dose and making the course twice as long, they have increased the primary response rate and reduced relapses without encountering increased toxicity in the treatment of visceral leishmaniasis. Other studies evaluating the efficacy of allopurinol have been mostly discouraging. Newer research on the application of local heat to treat leishmanial skin lesions and the formulation of drugs so that they would be taken up by macrophages (e.g., liposomal encapsulation of Pentostam) appear promising.

Malaria. The spread of multidrug-resistant falciparum malaria in Sourtheast Asia and the presence of strains resistant to chloroquine in Africa (Chapter 73) have increased the difficulty and the cost of treating and controlling that disease.

Mefloquine is now available for treatment and prophylaxis in many areas having multiple drug–resistant *P. falciparum.* However, its use should be limited because of cost (which is considerably more than for chloroquine) and potential for toxicity and for the parasite to develop resistance to its action. Other drugs that appear to be useful for treating chloroquine-resistant *P. falciparum,* i.e., halofantrine and ginghaosu and its derivative artemesenine, are undergoing extensive clinical trials. The latter compounds have a rapid onset of action and high relapse rate; they are being tested in China with the assistance of the WHO.

Some excellent clinical pharmacologic studies have recently been performed with the standard antimalarial drugs as well as with the newer compounds. For instance, safer and more effective ways have been demonstrated to use parenteral chloroquine, and this drug has been shown to be still useful for treating the local population in many areas where chloroquine-resistant *P. falciparum* is endemic.

Pneumocystis Pneumonia. Either trimethoprim-sulfamethoxazole or pentamidine isethionate is usually effective for treating and preventing *Pneumocystis carinii* pneumonia. (The latter is best given by inhalation when used in prophylaxis.) However, fatality rates are high in those who fail initial treatment with these agents, and the incidence of adverse effects is 50 to 80% in patients with AIDS. Trimetrexate, used for treating certain malignancies, binds 1500 times greater than trimethoprim to *Pneumocystis* dihydrofolate reductase. In a recent clinical trial, trimetrexate with concomitant leucovorin to reduce bone marrow toxicity gave good results in about 90% of AIDS patients with pneumocystis pneumonia. This provides an additional regimen for treating AIDS patients with *Pneumocystis carinii* pneumonia.

Other Protozoal Infections. There is still no effective treatment for cryptosporidiosis (Chapter 70) or for babesiosis (Chapter 77). The treatment currently available for African (Chapter 74) and American (Chapter 75) trypanosomiasis has limited effect and is frequently toxic. However, evaluation of potential new therapeutic agents for treating these infections is continuing.

Acquired Immunodeficiency Syndrome (AIDS). Infection with the immunodeficiency viruses (HIV) impairs cellular immunity and leads to opportunistic infections (Chapter 15.1). Some of these are included among the criteria for diagnosing AIDS.

Endogenous Infections. *Pneumocystis carinii* pneumonitis is the most common opportunistic infection in AIDS patients; it is the index diagnosis in 60% of AIDS patients in the United States and occurs at least once in an additional 20% (Chapter 79).

Cerebral toxoplasmosis is the most common infection involving the central nervous system in AIDS patients and occurs in about 30% of those with *Toxoplasma* antibodies (Chapter 78). Since about 50% of Americans have *Toxoplasma* antibodies by adulthood, cerebral toxoplasmosis occurs in about 1 in 6 or 7 American AIDS patients; it would occur more frequently in places with greater prevalence of positive serology to *T. gondii,* e.g., in France or most developing countries.

Visceral leishmaniasis has been reported with increasing frequency in HIV-positive patients living in South America and countries bordering the Mediterranean. HIV infection depresses T-cell and macrophage function, which is required for protective immunity to *Leishmania* (Chapter 76.1).

Exogenous Infections. Cryptosporidiosis (Chapter 70) and isosporiasis (Chapter 71.2) have been reported with increasing frequency in patients with AIDS. Ingested *Cryptosporidium* oocysts attach to microvilli in the small intestine (Fig. 70–4) and cause a secretory diarrhea. Patients with impaired immunity are unable to eradicate the infection and are almost impossible to cure. *Isospora belli,* another coccidian parasite, has been reported to cause a similar watery diarrhea, most frequently in Haitian patients with AIDS. Fortunately, it can be cured with trimethoprim-sulfamethoxazole.

Infection Without Illness. Both *Giardia lamblia* (Chapter 69) and *Entamoeba histolytica* (Chapter 68) are commonly found in male homosexuals. However, neither appears to cause increased illness in AIDS patients or in those who are HIV positive. The reason for this is unclear; it cannot be fully explained by the fact that nonpathogenic zymodemes of *E. histolytica* are usually isolated from male homosexuals. The immune defects produced by HIV infection do not appear to favor ameba invasion or *Giardia* pathogenicity. Malaria also does not cause illness more frequently in AIDS or in HIV-positive individuals.

Mechanisms. *Pneumocystis carinii, Toxoplasma gondii,* and *Leishmania donovani* cause endogenous disease in those who have HIV infections, whereas *Cryptosporidium* and *Isospora* cause exogenous infections. An HIV-induced defect in the immune response can interfere with containment of chronic asymptomatic infections. The pathology occurs where the latent stages of the parasite primarily persist: *P. carinii* in the lung, *T. gondii* in the brain, and *L. donovani* in the liver, spleen, and bone marrow.

Opportunistic parasitic infections are not as frequent as expected in developing countries. This may be because many HIV-positive individuals die of more virulent agents causing bacterial septicemias, pneumonias, and meningitis before their immune response is suppressed sufficiently for endogenous opportunistic agents to become pathogenic. For example, *Salmonella typhosa* is frequently transmitted and is often nonpathogenic in developing countries (Chapter 38). It would be of interest to compare mortality rates in HIV-negative and HIV-positive individuals exposed to S. *typhosa.*

BIBLIOGRAPHY

Allason-Jones E, Mindel A, Sargeaunt P, Williams P: *Entamoeba histolytica* as a commensal intestinal parasite in homosexual men. N Engl J Med 315: 353–356, 1986.

Berenguer J, Moreno S, Cercenado E, et al: Visceral leishmaniasis in patients infected with human immunodeficiency virus (HIV). Ann Intern Med 111: 129–132, 1989.

De Hovitz JA, Pape JW, Boncy M, Johnson WD Jr: Clinical manifestations and therapy of *Isospora belli* infection in patients with the acquired immunodeficiency syndrome. N Engl J Med 315: 87–90, 1986.

Hopewell RC: *Pneumocystis carinii* pneumonia: Diagnosis. J Infect Dis 157: 1115–1119, 1988.

Kovacs JA, Masur H: *Pneumocystis carinii* pneumonia: Therapy and prophylaxis. J Infect Dis 158: 254–259, 1988.

Lockwood DNJ, Weber JN: Parasite infections in AIDS. Parasitol Today 5: 310–317, 1989.

Luft BJ, Remington JS: Toxoplasmic encephalitis. J Infect Dis 157: 1–6, 1988.

McCabe R, Remington JS: Toxoplasmosis: The time has come. N Engl J Med 318: 313–315, 1988.

Nussenzweig RS, Nussenzweig V: Antisporozoite vaccine for malaria: Experimental basis and current status. Rev Infect Dis 11:S579–S585, 1989.

Sattler FR, Allegra CJ, Verdegem TD, et al: Trimetrexate-leucovorin dosage evaluation study for treatment of *Pneumocystis carinii* pneumonia. J Infect Dis 161: 91–96, 1990.

Soave R, Johnson WD Jr: *Cryptosporidium* and *Isospora belli* infections. J Infect Dis 157: 225–229, 1988.

White NJ, Krishna S: Treatment of malaria: some considerations and limitations of the current methods of assessment. Trans R Soc Trop Med Hyg 83: 767–777, 1989.

SECTION A

INTESTINAL AND GENITAL INFECTIONS

68. AMEBIASIS

Martin S. Wolfe

DEFINITION. Amebiasis is an infection caused by the ameba *Entamoeba histolytica*, the *Entamoeba* of humans, growing in vitro only at 37C and producing 4-nucleate cysts measuring approximately 10 to 15 μm in diameter. Intestinal amebiasis has a variable clinical picture and may cause acute or chronic symptoms. At one extreme of the clinical spectrum is acute amebic dysentery, which can be life-threatening. At the opposite extreme is the asymptomatic cyst passer, whose infection may possibly be caused by nonpathogenic strains of the parasite. The majority of those infected with amebiasis have a nondysenteric intestinal infection, which may cause frequent unformed stools, lower abdominal cramps, fatigue, and intermittent constipation and diarrhea with excessive abdominal distention and gas. Serious complications may follow symptomatic or asymptomatic intestinal infection, including amebic liver abscess, pleuropulmonary amebiasis, amebic pericarditis, ameboma or amebic stricture, and rarely, cerebral, genital, or skin amebiasis.

HISTORY. *E. histolytica* was first described by Lösch in St. Petersburg, Russia, in 1875 after studying a case of acute dysentery. Later investigations by Kartulis in Cairo in 1886, Hlava in Prague in 1887, and Councilman and Lafleur in Baltimore in 1891 related this ameba to a particular type of dysentery and liver abscess. The cyst stage was discovered by Quincke and Roos in 1893. Schaudinn in 1903 first named the species *E. histolytica* and differentiated it from the related nonpathogenic ameba *Entamoeba coli*. Rogers in 1912 in Calcutta reported successful treatment of both intestinal and hepatic amebiasis by injections of emetine salts. Nitroimidazoles, the present drugs of choice for invasive amebiasis, were first used in 1966.

ETIOLOGY. *E. histolytica* is the most important of the intestinal amebae of humans. The 3 distinct stages in the life cycle are the trophozoite, precyst, and cyst (Fig. 68–16). The cyst, the infective stage, is ingested in fecally contaminated food, water, or fingers. Both young uninucleate and more mature quadrinucleate cysts are infective. Ingested cysts pass through the stomach, and excystation occurs in the lower small bowel. A metacystic ameba containing the 4 cystic nuclei emerges from each cyst. Cytoplasmic division occurs and 8 small metacystic trophozoites are formed, which grow to full size. Cysts thus provide for both transmission and reproduction. The uninucleate trophozoite is the actively growing and multiplying stage, having a single nucleus and pseudopods. These pass along the intestinal canal until conditions favorable for colonization are found. This can occur anywhere in the large bowel, but happens most frequently in the cecal area. Multiplication is by rapid and repeated binary fission. Depending on various parasite and host factors, trophozoites may invade the tissue of the large intestine, probably by both lytic and physical means, and may also metastasize to the liver and other extraintestinal sites. In the presence of dysentery or diarrheic unformed stools, trophozoites do not become encysted during their evacuation. However, if bowel passage is not rapid, with semiformed or formed stools, as trophozoites are carried toward the rectum, they eliminate food vacuoles and other cytoplasmic inclusions and become precysts. The precyst then forms a cyst wall and develops from a uninucleate into a mature quadrinucleate cyst. These cysts constitute the transmission state to the next host. Cysts form only in the intestinal lumen, although immature cysts may mature outside the body under favorable conditions.

DISTRIBUTION AND PREVALENCE. *E. histolytica* has a worldwide distribution, being found in arctic, temperate, and tropical climates. It is more prevalent in tropical areas, where invasive disease is frequent and symptoms tend to be severe. This is no doubt related to poorer sanitation and nutrition and decreased resistance in those living in tropical climates, as well as other poorly understood factors.

It is difficult to determine the true prevalence of amebiasis accurately. Populations surveyed may differ, and the prevalence in certain groups is higher than in the general population, e.g., in families of infected patients, in male homosexuals, and in persons in mental hospitals, prisons, and institutions for children. Differences in laboratory techniques, competence of laboratory personnel, stool collection methods, and number of specimens examined from each person may lead to either under- or overdiagnosis. In some earlier surveys, the now recognized nonpathogen *E. hartmanni* was included with *E. histolytica* in prevalence figures. A difference of opinion as to what constitutes amebic disease also clouds attempts at establishing valid geographic prevalence data. Some tend to include all unidentified dysenteries in the amebic category. Walsh has estimated that approximately 10% of the world population carries the parasite, although a much smaller percentage have disease. An excellent discussion of the variables and problems in determining valid worldwide prevalence figures for amebiasis has been given by Elsdon-Dew.

Recognized high-risk areas for acquiring amebiasis, include Mexico, the western portion of South America, West Africa, South Africa (particularly in the black population), parts of the Middle East, and South and Southeast Asia. Invasive disease is more common in these areas. Many of the cases identified in North America and in Europe are imported, but a level of endemicity is present and occasional water-borne epi-

550

demics have occurred. Approximately 40 years ago, it was estimated that 5 to 10% of the population of the United States were passing amebic organisms in their stools. The generally accepted figure presently is less than 3% but is higher among institutionalized individuals, male homosexuals, and Indians on reservations, and in some lower socioeconomic areas of the country.

EPIDEMIOLOGY

Infectious Stage. Motile trophozoites passed with diarrheal or dysenteric stools can survive only briefly outside the body, are destroyed by gastric secretions, and therefore play no role in transmission.

Cysts are relatively hardy and can survive outside the body long enough to be ingested. They are sensitive to desiccation and to temperatures above 40C or below −5C and are killed almost immediately by boiling. They are relatively resistant to chlorine, not being destroyed by concentrations usually used for water purification. Cysts may remain viable for 1 month at 4C in both sewage and natural surface water. Viable cysts may be recovered from the intestines and feces of flies and cockroaches. Cysts have been found to survive for up to 48 hours at 20 to 25C on foods such as cheese, bread, green salads, and fruits.

Transmission. Animal reservoirs of *E. histolytica* include monkeys, dogs, and pigs, but these have a very minor role in transmission in comparison to humans, the principal reservoir of infection. Infection by cysts usually occurs by either direct person to person transmission or contamination of water or food. In institutionalized groups, e.g., in homes for the mentally retarded, old age homes, and prisons, transmission is often by direct fecal contamination of the environment. Daycare centers for young children have been implicated in the transmission of giardiasis and, to a lesser extent, amebiasis. Male homosexuals have high rates of infection with *E. histolytica* and other fecally transmitted organisms. Transmission occurs during oral-anal sexual practices and is related to sexual promiscuity.

In underdeveloped areas where supplies of pure water are inadequate and often fecally contaminated, amebiasis and other enteric infections have high prevalences. Remarkable water-borne epidemics of amebiasis have also occurred in the United States. In some areas, contaminated water or sewage is used to grow or freshen vegetables before selling them. Human excreta, or night soil, is used as a fertilizer in growing vegetables, making ingestion of leafy and root vegetables especially hazardous. Contaminated water can be used in making salads and cold drinks, and contamination of cold foods can occur from the fecally soiled fingers of food handlers. The extent of the latter problem is difficult to quantitate, but is thought to be considerable in developing countries and may occur to a lesser extent in the developed world. Where flies and cockroaches are numerous and have access to feces and then to unprotected foodstuffs, these insects may cause individual or group infections.

Persons of all ages are susceptible to infection, but the rate is lower in infants and young children. Females are as likely to be infected as males, but invasive amebiasis is much more common in males. Racial differences in prevalence and pathogenicity appear to be determined less by genetic factors than by socioeconomic status.

PATHOGENESIS AND PATHOLOGY. Following ingestion of cysts, excystment occurs in the small intestine; it is influenced by the host digestive enzymes, the quantity of food ingested, and the velocity of intestinal transit. The resulting small metacystic trophozoites are carried in the fecal stream into the cecum, where various factors allow colonization and tissue invasion by *E. histolytica* strains with virulent capabilities. If trophozoites are abundant, there is an increased chance that some will make contact with the mucosa long enough to grow, multiply, and eventually invade the tissues. Colonization is decreased with bowel hypermotility. Amebae develop only under conditions of very low oxygen tension, as is present in the colon. A suitable enteric bacterial flora must also be present to lower the oxidation reduction potential and to provide necessary metabolic requirements for amebae remaining outside the tissues on the bowel mucosa or in the glandular crypts.

Strains of *E. histolytica*. *E. histolytica* is unique among the amebae of humans in its ability to invade tissue. Strains of *E. histolytica* vary in their ability to invade the colonic mucosa. *E. hartmanni*, formerly known as "small race" *E. histolytica*, is now considered a separate nonpathogenic species. Although morphologically identical, *E. histolytica* and *E. hartmanni* are differentiated on the basis of cyst size, distinct antigens, and noninvasiveness of the latter species.

Laredo-like strains are also considered nonpathogenic. The differences between these amebae and the "classic" *E. histolytica* have been summarized by Goldman. In cultures, the optimum growth temperature for the "classic" *E. histolytica* is 37C, whereas Laredo-like amebae grow at 25 to 30C. "Classic" *E. histolytica* can be maintained only in isotonic medium, whereas Laredo-like strains can grow in a diluted medium. Most significantly, no isolate of Laredo-like ameba has clearly come from an individual with symptomatic amebiasis; all come from asymptomatic cyst passers.

Sargeaunt has shown that *E. histolytica* occurs worldwide as a spectrum of zymodemes (strains separated by characteristic isoenzyme patterns). Isoenzymes, particularly phosphoglucomutase and hexokinase, allow for consistent differentiation among pathogenic *E. histolytica* zymodemes obtained from persons with symptomatic amebiasis, and nonpathogenic zymodemes obtained from persons with asymptomatic infection. It is suggested that genetic differences are reflected in isoenzyme patterns. Similar findings have been obtained from *E. histolytica* isolates from homosexual men; zymodemes in isolates from asymptomatic homosexual men were similar to other nonpathogenic zymodemes and differed from those from pathogenic isolates. A third group of asymptomatic subjects in South Africa harbored pathogenic zymodemes, but had serologic (amebic gel diffusion test) responses analogous to those in patients with invasive disease; this implies subclinical tissue invasion in this group. Studies with cloned isolates indicate that nonpathogenic zymodemes can be converted to pathogenic zymodemes in vitro by exposure to lethally irradiated bacteria. The clinical controversy raised by these currently confusing findings is whether nonpathogenic zymodemes, such as those found in homosexual men, require treatment. Because amebic culture and isoenzyme electrophoresis required for zymodeme identification are currently research techniques, zymodeme classification is not readily available for clinical use.

Characteristics of Virulence. In addition to the pathogenic potential of the strain of ameba, a number of other parasite and host factors influence tissue invasion. The number of amebae ingested is directly related to the frequency and magnitude of intestinal lesions. Pathogenic *E. histolytica* contain surface adhesins that allow attachment to the colonic epithelium and appear to be important in pathogenesis. Pathogenic strains of *E. histolytica* have multiple mechanisms available by which they damage tissue and become invasive. These include secreted proteolytic enzymes, release of cell-free cytotoxins, contact-dependent cytolysis, and phagocytosis. Of the host factors, the nutritional status of the host is often mentioned as a contributing element, but it is not certain how nutrition influences either the capacity of the parasite to cause tissue damage or the susceptibility of the host to the parasite. Some observations supporting a nutritional role are that invasion is more common in the Bantu of South Africa, whose diet is mainly corn, and that the addition of cholesterol, an important nutritional factor for amebae, to the diet of guinea pigs increases the frequency and size of ulcerous bowel lesions. It is speculated that nutritional deficiencies facilitate disease by means of atrophy of the mucosa, leading to increased susceptibility to lysis and penetration by amebae. Stress may also play a role in the pathogenesis of amebiasis. Thus, asymptomatic female carriers may develop severe amebiasis during pregnancy and the puerperium. Some synergism between amebae and the intestinal bacteria might be necessary to produce pathologic effects.

Pathology

Colonic Lesions. The initial lesions of amebic invasion begin as small foci of necrosis in the large bowel mucosa. These foci progress to form ulcers; some remain small and discrete, whereas others expand to form broad geographic patterns. Undermining of the ulcer margin and confluence of one or more ulcers lead to sloughing of mucosa and development of broad ulcers with irregular outlines. Amebic ulcers may be disseminated throughout the colon, but more frequently are limited to one region, particularly the cecum. Lesions are sometimes limited to the ascending, transverse, descending, or sigmoid colon or to the rectum. Amebic ulcers of the terminal ileum rarely occur. The typical amebic ulcer is undermined and is sharply defined, without ragged edges (Fig. 68–1). The crater contains gray necrotic tissue composed of fibrin, cellular debris, and amebic trophozoites. The exudate often raises the undermined mucosa, producing the characteristic flask, bottle neck, or larger "sea anemone" ulcer (Fig. 68–2). The mucosa between ulcers may be coated with mucus. Initially there is little edema and inflammatory response, but as the ulcers widen, secondary bacterial infection occurs, leading to accumulation of neutrophils, lymphocytes, histiocytes,

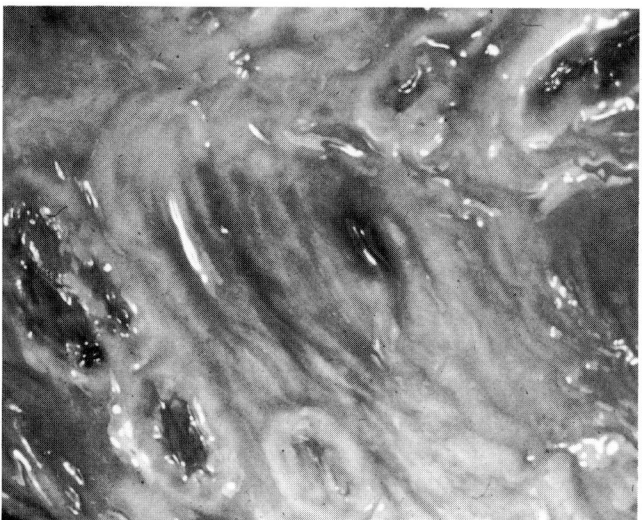

FIGURE 68–1. Amebic ulcers of the large intestine. Note raised margins of ulcers. (Courtesy of the Louisiana State University School of Medicine, New Orleans.)

plasma cells, and sometimes eosinophils in the ulcer crater and surrounding tissue. If eosinophils are present, Charcot-Leyden crystals may appear in the stool or dysenteric exudate. Trophozoites may be present on the mucosal surface, in the exudate, in the crater, and frequently in the submucosa, muscularis, serosa, and blood vessels (Fig. 68–3).

Complications of Intestinal Amebiasis. In addition to extraintestinal amebiasis, which originates from initial intestinal involvement, complications of intestinal amebiasis may include perforation with or without peritonitis, intra-abdominal abscess, amebic appendicitis, hemorrhage, and ameboma and amebic stricture.

Perforation of the Intestine. This occurs most often in the cecum and next most commonly in the rectosigmoid; it is the most frequent complication of intestinal ame-

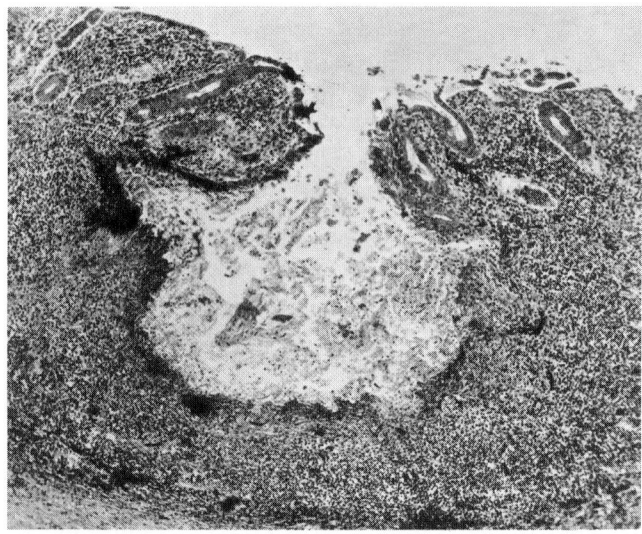

FIGURE 68–2. Section of colon showing flask-shaped chronic amebic ulcer involving the mucosa and submucosa. The neutrophilic infiltration of the border of the lesion suggests secondary bacterial invasion. (From Medical Museum Collection, Armed Forces Institute of Pathology.)

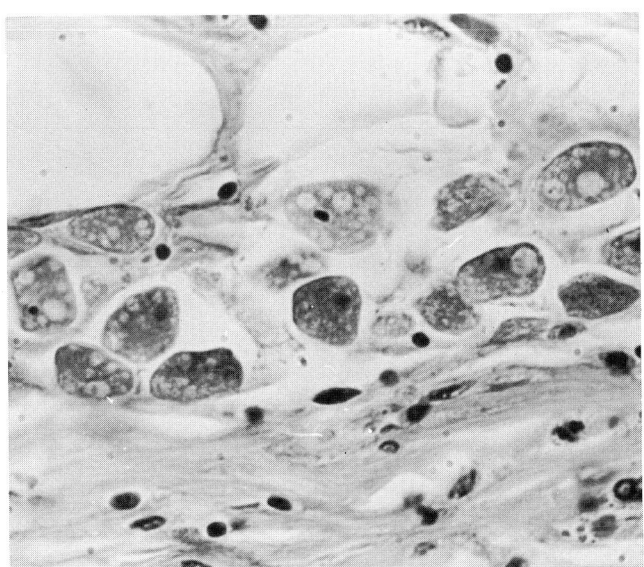

FIGURE 68–3. Trophozoites of *E. histolytica* in submucosa of the colon. (Courtesy of the Louisiana State University School of Medicine, New Orleans.)

biasis. Slow leakage into the peritoneal cavity is more common than the more dramatic acute perforation. Peritonitis or intra-abdominal abscess follows either of these situations. Perforation may also occur from the primarily involved colon into other hollow organs in the abdominal cavity.

Amebic Appendicitis. This almost always occurs as a complication of severe colonic amebiasis. The amebic appendix is slightly thickened, tends to be gangrenous, and has an apparently intact mucosa except for a gray sanguineous slough covering irregular superficial ulcers. Microscopic changes resemble those in the colon.

Massive Hemorrhage. Fortunately, this is rare. It results from the erosion of a large artery by an ulcer. Superficial ulceration may lead to the oozing of numerous small blood vessels in the mucosa.

Amebomas. These are inflammatory thickenings of the bowel wall that are firm, hard, well-defined lesions resembling a carcinoma (Fig. 68–4). They occur in about 1% of patients with colonic amebiasis. Amebomas occur in any area of the colon but are most common in the cecum. They are typical granulomas, consisting of a mass of fibroblasts, collagen, and chronic inflammatory cells, with an obliterating vasculitis, numerous eosinophils and Charcot-Leyden crystals, and relatively few amebae.

Amebic Strictures. These are also caused by granulation tissue, usually without fibrosis. They are generally single, but occasionally there may be 2 or more. Strictures are most commonly observed in the anus, rectum, or sigmoid colon. *E. histolytica* trophozoites are present in the lesion.

Hepatic Lesions. Amebic trophozoites may enter the radicles of the portal vein and metastasize to the liver, where colonies of trophozoites become established (Fig. 68–5B). As the colonies increase in size, lysis of liver tissue occurs and leukocytes then infiltrate.

Abscess. One or more of these initial lesions may enlarge into a single or multiple amebic abscesses (Fig. 68–5A). Three zones may be recognized by gross and microscopic examination: (1) a center containing yellow or gray opaque liquid material—this is amorphous and necrotic, but does not contain leukocytes as the term "abscess" would suggest; (2) a median zone consisting only of stroma; and (3) a shaggy, fibrinous outer wall invaded by trophozoites clustered in the fibrin next to viable hepatic tissue. The surrounding liver is edematous and may be infiltrated with mixed chronic inflammatory cells. Most abscesses develop in the right lobe of the liver.

"Amebic Hepatitis." This describes a hypothetical diffuse spread of trophozoites throughout the liver that causes microscopic inflammatory lesions, a presuppurative phase of amebic liver abscess. This condition has not been proved histologically, and its existence is denied by most investigators.

Other Extraintestinal Lesions

Pleuropulmonary Amebiasis. Next to the liver in frequency of extraintestinal sites of amebiasis is pleuropulmonary involvement. This is usually a direct extension of a liver abscess through the diaphragm, but may also develop via vascular spread, leading to both pleural and pulmonary involvement. Rupture into the pleural space leads to an amebic empyema or effusion. Rupture into the lung may result in consolidation, abscess formation, or a hepatobronchial fistula. Microscopically, pulmonary amebiasis shows no significant differences from the amebic process in the liver or other organs.

Amebic Pericarditis. This usually results from extension of a left lobe liver abscess through the diaphragm into the pericardium. Much more rarely, it may originate from a right lobe abscess or a lung abscess or empyema. Direct trauma and strenuous activity are two possible precipitating factors. Prior to actual rupture of the abscess, irritation of the pericardium may lead to a serous effusion, described as the "presuppurative" phase; with rupture into the pericardial sac, "suppurative" pericarditis develops. This may be followed by constrictive pericarditis, cardiac tamponade, and cardiac failure.

Cerebral Amebiasis. This form is hematogenous in origin, is usually associated with a liver or lung abscess, and is fortunately a rare occurrence. Cerebral lesions may be single or multiple and may localize in any area of the brain, although the left hemisphere is predominantly involved. Small lesions appear grossly as minute areas of softening with petechial hemorrhages. Larger lesions are necrotic and contain yellowish-green material with hemorrhage (Fig. 68–6). Meningeal involvement resembles other types of acute purulent meningitis. Microscopically, the lesions show all the features of amebic destruction seen in other organs.

Cutaneous Amebiasis. This form is also rare, may develop from a hepatic abscess fistula, by extension of rectal amebiasis to the perianal or genital area, by infection of the penis from anal intercourse, or via external inoculation. Grossly, the lesions are deep ulcerations with a raised border and are covered with necrotic material (Fig. 68–7).

Other Lesions. Cases of secondary amebic infections

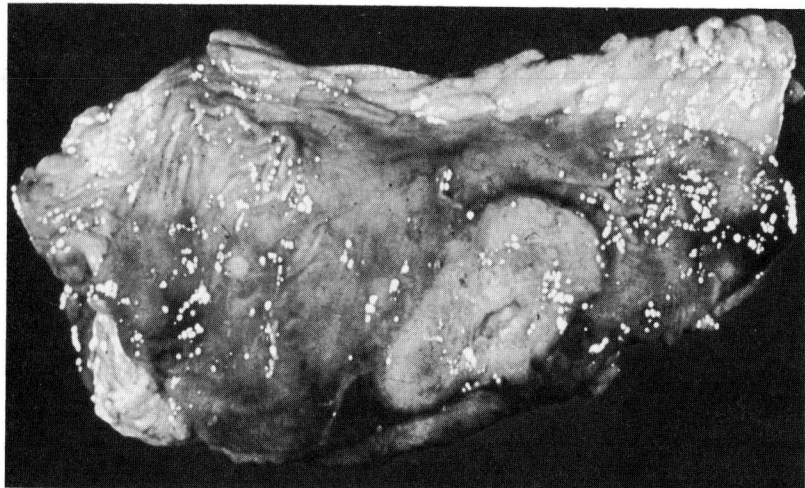

FIGURE 68–4. Amebic granuloma or ameboma in the cecum. (Courtesy of the Louisiana State University School of Medicine, New Orleans.)

of the urinary tract, genital tract, and other organs have very rarely been described.

CLINICAL MANIFESTATIONS. There is a variable clinical response to amebiasis, depending on the pathogenicity of the strain of *E. histolytica*, the intensity of infection, the bacterial flora, a number of host factors, and the site and extent of tissue damage. Invasive amebiasis leading to dysentery, liver abscess, pleuropulmonary involvement, or, less commonly, involvement of other organs occurs in only a small percentage of

amebic infections. The majority of patients have either nondysenteric intestinal amebiasis with mild to moderate symptoms or are asymptomatic cyst passers. Infection with this parasite may persist for many years.

Amebic Dysentery (Acute Amebic Colitis). The incubation period is usually about 7 to 21 days, and onset is often sudden. Acute dysenteric symptoms may also develop in individuals who have had long-standing mild symptoms or who have been asymptomatic cyst passers. Typical acute symptoms and signs include severe abdom-

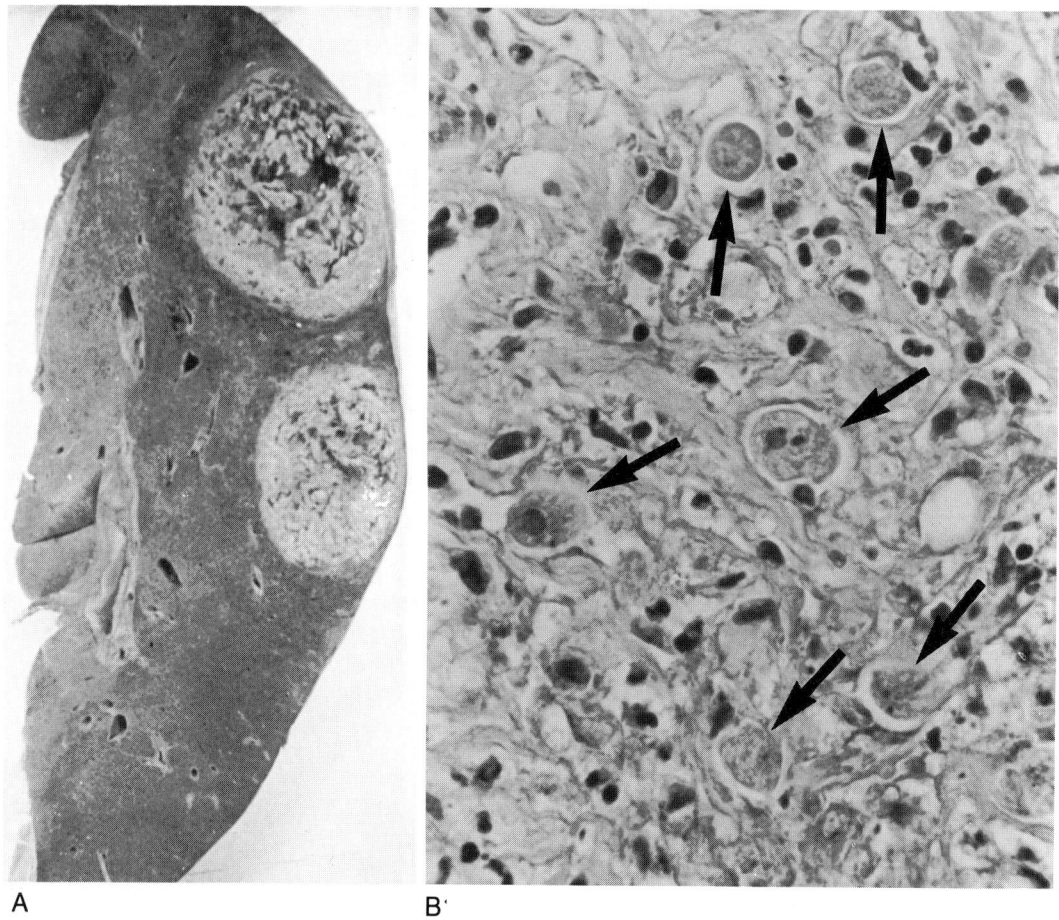

A   B

FIGURE 68–5. *A*, Multiple amebic abscesses of the liver. *B*, Trophozoites *(arrows)* of *E. histolytica* in the liver.

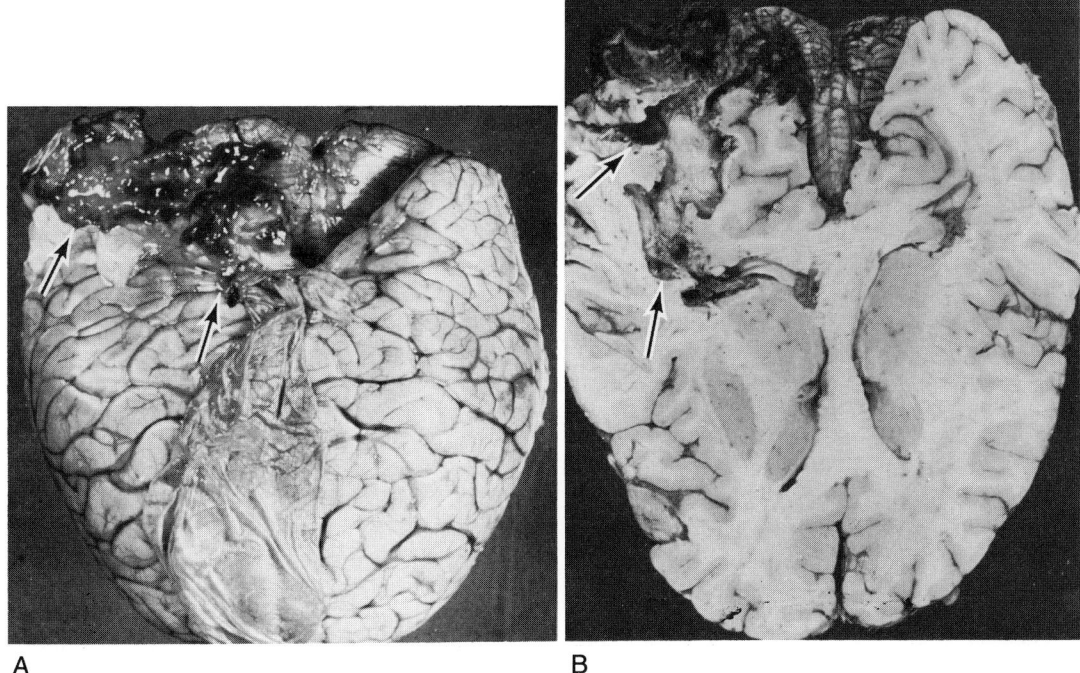

A   B

FIGURE 68–6. Amebic brain abscess. *A*, External view. *B*, Coronal section. (Courtesy of the Louisiana State University School of Medicine, New Orleans.)

inal cramps, chills, fever, prostration, nausea, headache, and tenesmus. Dehydration may occur with prolonged diarrhea. The stools are liquid and contain bloody mucus, but leukocytes are not as prevalent as in bacterial dysenteries. The peripheral white blood cell count is often elevated, with a polymorphonuclear leukocytosis. Anemia is not a feature unless disease is long-standing. In severe fulminant cases, extensive colonic involvement may lead to massive destruction of the mucosa, hemorrhage, and perforation and peritonitis. These complications may be fatal. Some patients with severe intestinal amebiasis may have enlarged, tender livers without abscess formation that respond to appropriate treatment of the intestinal infection.

Ulcerative Postdysenteric Colitis. As a sequel to acute amebic dysentery, some patients may develop a post-

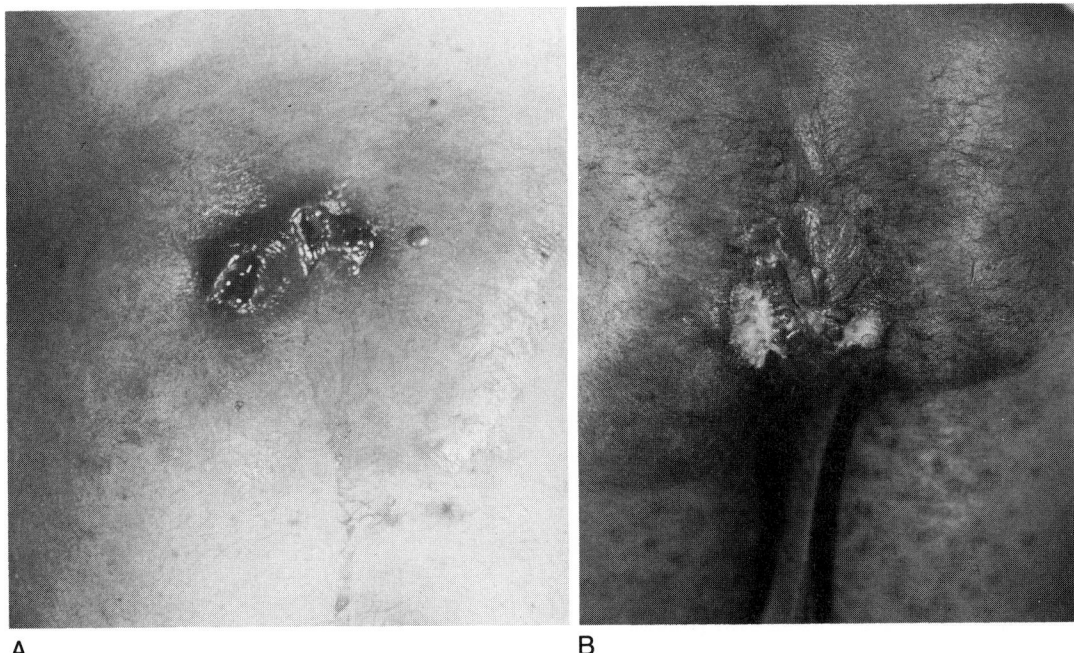

A   B

FIGURE 68–7. Amebiasis cutis. *A*, Lesions of anterior abdominal wall resulting from extension of an amebic liver abscess. *B*, Two lesions lateral to the anus that communicated by sinus tracts with the rectum. (Courtesy of the Louisiana State University School of Medicine, New Orleans.)

dysenteric colitis. Two forms have been described: (1) patients with mild symptoms and no colonic ulceration, i.e., "functional postdysenteric colonic irritability," and (2) those with colonic ulceration and more severe symptoms, i.e., "ulcerative postdysenteric colitis." Amebic trophozoites are not present, and further antiamebic treatment is of no value. Clinically, it is difficult to differentiate this entity from ulcerative colitis, and the proctoscopic appearance is similar. Treatment with steroids or sulfasalazine (Azulfidine) is useful in both conditions, but it is essential to rule out active amebic infection, which can be exacerbated by these drugs.

Nondysenteric Intestinal Amebiasis. A spectrum of symptoms is seen with nondysenteric amebiasis, ranging from totally asymptomatic individuals; to those with increased numbers of soft stools, intermittent constipation, distention and flatulence, and increased fatigue; to more severely infected individuals who do not have frank amebic dysentery but show clinical evidence of some localized invasion of the bowel wall, as manifested by frequent watery to mushy stools, lower abdominal cramps (often localized over the cecum or sigmoid), weight loss, anorexia and nausea, marked asthenia, and, occasionally, urticaria. The white blood cell count and differential count are usually normal.

Asymptomatic Cyst Passers. These make up the majority of amebic infections seen in temperate climates. Some infections are due to nonpathogenic Laredo-like strains, which appear to be more resistant to treatment. Others are caused by nonpathogenic zymodemes of "classic" *E. histolytica*, which usually remain asymptomatic but might change into symptomatic or invasive infections and be the source of infection for others.

Complications of Intestinal Amebiasis

Perforation and Peritonitis. With acute perforation there is sudden pain at the perforation site, and signs of an acute abdomen are present. Slow leakage does not present as dramatically, but should be suspected in a seriously ill patient whose condition gradually deteriorates along with the development of increased distention and signs of ileus.

Appendicitis. It is difficult clinically to differentiate amebic from other causes of inflammatory involvement of the appendix. Amebic appendicitis should be considered in the presence of other signs of amebic colitis, and antiamebic drug treatment should then be administered prior to any surgery.

Ameboma. Amebomas may cause pain, a tender mass, and rarely, intussusception. They often occur during the course of proven amebic dysentery, justifying a presumptive diagnosis. When not associated with amebic dysentery or the presence of ulcers, amebomas may easily be confused with adenocarcinoma or annular carcinoma when recognized after barium enema examination or at sigmoidoscopy or colonoscopy.

Amebic Stricture. A stricture develops either during an attack of amebic dysentery or later. Amebic strictures are often symptomless, although they may rarely produce abdominal or rectal pain, partial obstruction, and difficulty in defecation.

Cutaneous Amebiasis. There is rapid growth of amebic skin lesions, which are characteristically painful.

With prompt diagnosis and appropriate treatment, the lesions heal rapidly.

Amebic Liver Abscess. Liver abscess may occur in the presence or absence of intestinal symptoms. Often it develops after a latent period following earlier diarrhea or other intestinal disorders, particularly in patients with a history of prior travel to or residence in endemic areas. Only about 20% of patients with amebic liver abscess will have *E. histolytica* present on stool examinations. The right lobe is more often involved than the left, in a ratio of about 5:1 or 6:1. Although pus aspirated from an amebic abscess is classically described as having the appearance of "anchovy paste," owing to a mixture of blood and necrotic material, it can also be creamy white or yellow in color. Material from the abscess is usually bacteriologically sterile, although secondary infection may develop in 2 to 3%. Amebic aspirates are not foul smelling, unlike most material from bacterial abscesses.

Onset of symptoms can be either insidious or acute. Clinical findings may vary, but typically there is fever, pain in the right lower anterior chest or right hypochondrium, tenderness over an enlarged liver, and a moderate leukocytosis. These symptoms and signs should alert the physician to the possibility of amebic liver abscess, and liver scanning and amebic serologic tests should be promptly performed. Other signs may include referred pain to the right shoulder, a visible mass with a large abscess, and a nonproductive cough. In many cases, abscesses extend upward to involve the diaphragm, leading to diaphragmatic elevation and immobility and compression of the right lower lobe of the lung. This, in turn, may cause decreased diaphragmatic excursion, dullness to percussion over the lower lobe of the lung, atelectasis, right-sided pleural effusion, cough, and dyspnea. Chills and profuse sweats may be present. Jaundice occurs only with large abscesses and is a poor prognostic sign. The alkaline phosphatase level may be elevated, but liver enzymes are usually normal. There is often a leukocytosis with left shift, an elevated sedimentation rate, and a normochromic, normocytic anemia. Occasionally, the abscess may rupture into the peritoneum, lung, pericardium, or abdominal wall.

Pleuropulmonary Amebiasis. Most patients complain of pain, cough, hemoptysis, and dyspnea. Pain typically occurs in the lower right area of the chest and may be pleuritic. Cough may be nonproductive, but more often produces a small amount of whitish or reddish material. If the abscess drains into a bronchus, large amounts of abscess material may be coughed up, which may be reddish-brown, dirty-brown, purulent, or frank amebic pus. Chills, fever, and leukocytosis are frequently present.

Amebic Pericarditis. As with other forms of pericarditis, amebic pericarditis may present with generalized deterioration in the patient's condition, left or retrosternal chest pain, dyspnea, a fast pulse, pulsus paradoxus, a pericardial friction rub, or shock. If associated point tenderness of the liver and other signs and symptoms of liver abscess are present, amebic involvement of the pericardium and/or pleuropulmonary space should be seriously suspected.

Amebic Brain Abscess. The onset of symptoms is abrupt and the course is fulminant, resembling that of a pyogenic brain abscess. Headache, fever, seizures, and coma may be present. Cerebral amebiasis is almost always fatal.

DIAGNOSIS

Intestinal Amebiasis. Definitive diagnosis of intestinal amebiasis is by demonstration of *E. histolytica* parasites in the stool. There is a tendency to overdiagnose intestinal parasites, particularly *E. histolytica*, by mistakenly identifying nonpathogenic amebae, macrophages, or white blood cells as *E. histolytica*. The physician must be certain that the laboratory is using correct procedures in collecting and examining specimens and that the examinations are performed by experienced parasitology technicians.

Stool Specimen Collection. E. histolytica cysts may remain viable for some time in unpreserved stools; trophozoites, occurring with dysenteric and diarrheal stool specimens, are labile and may disappear from a fresh stool within 30 minutes of passage. Refrigeration, freezing, or incubation at 37C of liquid or formed stools often has a deleterious effect on both trophozoites and cysts. It is preferable to collect specimens in preservatives, which will retain the structure and characteristics of cysts and trophozoites until the specimen can be examined. A number of commercial collection kits are available (Chapter 124).

There is some rationale for collecting a series of 3 stool specimens on alternate days. Amebic cysts and trophozoites are passed intermittently in the stool, and the diagnostic yield will be higher in specimens collected over a 6-day rather than a 3-day period. Approximately 70 to 90% of infections should be diagnosed by this series of examinations. At least 3 negative, adequately performed examinations carried out on alternate days should be accomplished before attempting to rule out amebiasis or going on to more specialized techniques, if warranted by the clinical condition (Chapter 122).

Many preparations, including antibiotics and antiparasitic drugs, sulfa drugs, antacids, kaolin products, paregoric, bismuth subsalicylate, most enema products, oily laxatives, and barium, can cause a transient inhibition of multiplication of amebic organisms or can interfere with their recognition. When searching for amebae, it is recommended to wait at least 7 days after a course of anti-infective drugs or barium examination and at least 3 to 4 days after use of other preparations.

When spontaneously passed specimens are not sufficient to confirm the presence of *E. histolytica*, purged specimens may be obtained following a saline cathartic. This requires that the liquid specimen be examined immediately for the labile trophozoites. Although purging may allow for some additional diagnoses to be made, it is not an easy procedure for the patient.

Examination of Stool Specimens. With fresh stools, flecks of mucus, with or without blood staining, should be searched for, and if found, a particle is placed on a slide, diluted with normal saline, covered with a coverglass, and immediately examined. Alternatively, particles of stool are similarly examined. *E. histolytica* trophozoites have glasslike pseudopodia, progressive motility, and may contain ingested red blood cells if blood is present in the stool (Fig. 68–8) (Tables 68–1 and 71–3). An iodine-stained smear is also made to assist in differentiating *E. histolytica* from nonpathogenic amebic cysts (Table 71–2). A concentration test should also be performed; the formalin-ethylacetate method is particularly useful. Smears of mucus or fecal material can also be made immediately from fresh stool for later permanent staining. Permanent stained smears may be necessary for definite confirmation of *E. histolytica* parasites (Figs. 68–9, 68–10, and 71–7). (See Chapter 124 for details of the above procedures.)

Charcot-Leyden crystals may be present in the stools of patients with amebiasis. Although associated with amebiasis, these crystals are not pathognomonic, as they may also be present in other colonic diseases and in infections with *Trichuris trichiura* and *Schistosoma* species. Stools from patients with amebic dysentery uncomplicated by secondary bacterial infection seldom contain more than a few leukocytes, in contrast to the sheets of leukocytes usually seen with acute shigellosis and *Campylobacter* infections.

Culture. Laboratories experienced in culture techniques for *E. histolytica* may increase the diagnostic yield by utilizing this supplemental procedure (Chapter 122). Culturing at both 37 and 25C can also be used to differentiate "classic" *E. histolytica* from nonpathogenic Laredo strains.

Proctoscopic Examination. In dysenteric amebiasis, typical ulcerative lesions are often visualized, and scrapings may be obtained through the proctoscope for immediate examination or fixation for later examination. Cotton swabs are not recommended for this purpose, as they will absorb liquid material. A glass tube and rubber bulb may be used to aspirate liquid material. Scrapings can be taken with a biopsy forceps or long-handled Volkmann spoon; Turner has described a special rectal spoon developed for diagnosis of schistosomiasis that is particularly useful for this purpose.* Proctoscopic examination, and specimens thereby obtained, will rarely be of value in nondysenteric amebic cases. Biopsies from ulcers or suspected amebomas or amebic strictures may be obtained. Hematoxylin-eosin slides are prepared, and these should be examined by a pathologist experienced in the identification of *E. histolytica* trophozoites in tissue (Figs. 68–3 and 68–9*B*). *E. histolytica* in rectal biopsies may be detected more easily in ethanol-fixed tissues stained with either a fluorescent antibody or with periodic acid-Schiff (PAS).

Barium X-ray Examination. This is seldom useful in nondysenteric cases and must not be performed before a sufficient number of stools have been examined or proctoscopy has been performed, as barium will interfere with identification of parasites. In acute dysenteric cases, evidence of ulceration, spasm, loss of haustral pattern, narrowing, or a cone- or V-shaped deformity of the cecum may be seen. When amebic colitis is diffuse, it roentgenographically resembles diffuse inflammatory bowel disease. The risk of perforation from a barium enema must be considered in patients with

---

*Turner JS: Am J Trop Med Hyg 11:620, 1962.

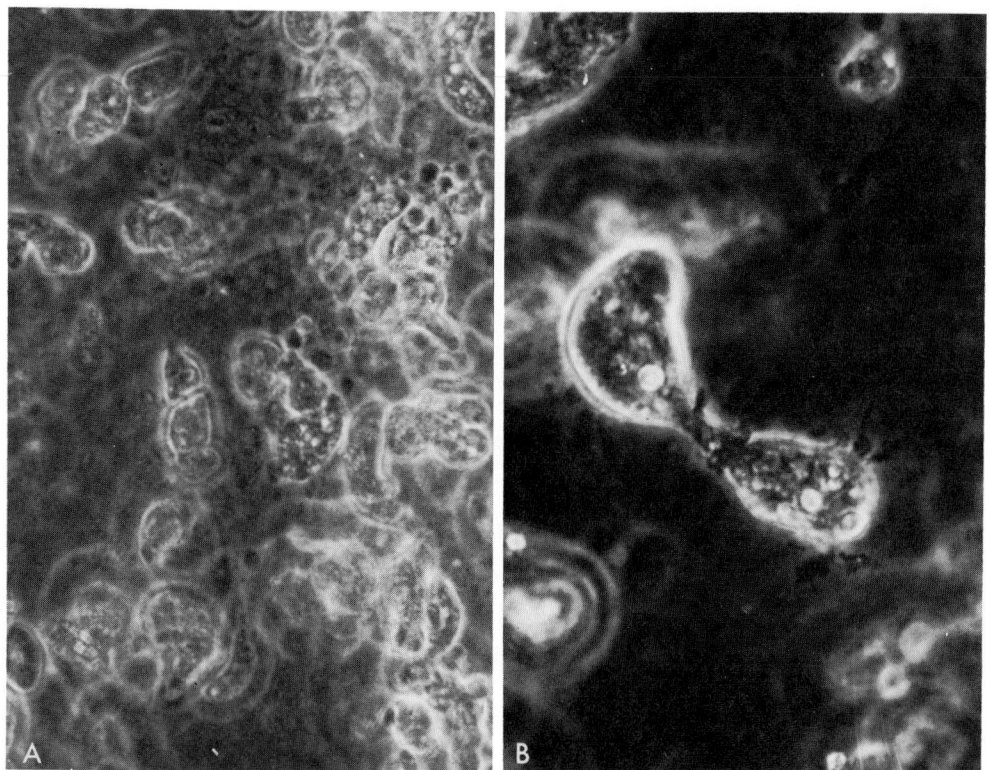

FIGURE 68–8. *E. histolytica* trophozoites in the stool from an Indonesian woman with severe amebic dysentery. *A,* Lower magnification showing numerous trophozoites with engulfed erythrocytes. *B,* Higher magnification showing trophozoite with pseudopods and many engulfed erythrocytes. Unstained fresh preparation with phase contrast. (Courtesy of Dr. James Palmieri.)

possible toxic megacolon. Amebomas or amebic strictures, initially recognized by barium enema, must be differentiated from carcinoma by biopsy and serologic tests.

Serologic Tests. Serum antibodies reflect amebic invasion and do not correlate with protective immunity. In patients clinically suspected of having amebic dysentery, liver abscess, pericarditis, ameboma, or other less common forms of invasive amebiasis, a positive serologic response with a reliable, well-evaluated test (such as the indirect hemagglutination test, or IHA) is good evidence of an amebic etiology (Chapter 125). Conversely, a negative serologic test makes the diagnosis of amebic liver abscess or ameboma almost untenable and makes the diagnosis of amebic colitis unlikely. The IHA is positive in approximately 96% of patients with amebic liver abscess and in about 85% of those with dysentery. The IHA is particularly useful in the important differential diagnoses between amebic dysentery and inflammatory bowel disease, amebic and pyogenic liver abscess, and ameboma and colonic carcinoma. Because of

the sensitivity of this test, false-positive reactions may persist in some patients for years after clinical and parasitologic cure of invasive amebiasis in the absence of reinfection. Rarely, in early invasive amebiasis, the IHA test may be negative. Immunofluorescence (IF) testing may become positive earlier than IHA, but this is technically more difficult to perform. A major drawback is the general unavailability of reliable IHA testing, since it is performed only at specialized laboratories. Other relatively simple but often somewhat less reliable techniques include latex agglutination, the gel diffusion precipitation test, and counterimmunoelectrophoresis. An enzyme-linked immunosorbent assay (ELISA) is also available. A variation of the ELISA technique has been evaluated for detecting antigen to *E. histolytica* in fecal, serum, and abscess samples.

Amebic Liver Abscess. Clinical suspicion of amebic liver abscess can best be confirmed by a reliably performed positive amebic serologic test in conjunction with a positive radioisotopic, sonographic, or radiologic procedure, followed by a response to specific therapy.

TABLE 68–1. Diagnostic Characteristics of *Entamoeba histolytica*

	Form	Where Found	Morphology
Liquid stools	Trophozoites	Blood-stained mucus or feces	Progressive motion; glasslike pseudopodia; sluglike shape; may contain red blood cells
Formed stools	Cysts	In the fecal mass	Saline preparation: Blunt-ended chromatoidals may be visible; nuclei not visible except after formalin fixation Iodine preparation: 1–4 nuclei at different levels; chromatoidals usually not visible except after formalin fixation
Semiformed stools	Cysts and/or trophozoites	In the fecal mass	Same as above

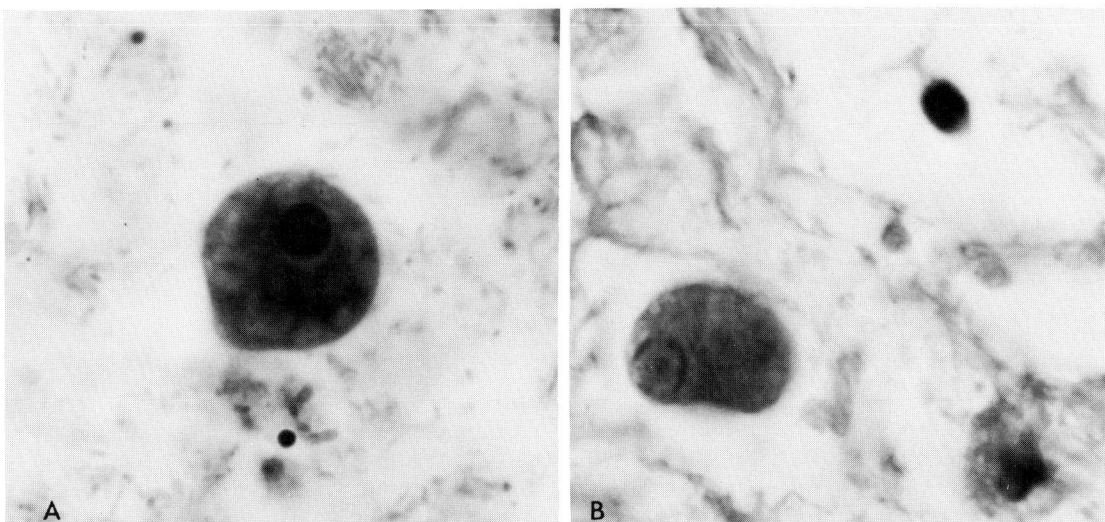

FIGURE 68–9. Trophozoites of *E. histolytica. A*, Fecal smear. Note the irregular ameboid outline, the coarse cytoplasm, the spherical nucleus, and the tiny central karyosome. (Iron-hematoxylin stain, × 1980.) (Courtesy of the Armed Forces Institute of Pathology, Photograph Neg. No. 72–17635.) *B*, Section of colon shows the nuclear and central karyosome of an invading trophozoite (× 1440). (Courtesy of the Armed Forces Institute of Pathology, Photograph Neg. No. 75–11539.)

Scans. Noninvasive procedures to demonstrate a hepatic abscess include ultrasonography (Fig. 68–11), technetium scan (Fig. 68–12), gallium scan, computed tomography (Fig. 68–13), and magnetic resonance imaging. When a technetium scan is positive, ultrasound scanning can distinguish between cystic and solid lesions. The finding of increased gallium activity (with a ^{67}Ga scan) at the periphery of a large "gallium-negative" lesion has been described as useful in the diagnosis of an amebic liver abscess, but large neoplasms with central necrosis may also show this feature.

Chest X-ray Film. This will frequently show elevation of the right diaphragm, right pleural effusion, and right parenchymatous densities (Fig. 68–14). These are frequent findings when the abscess is in the superior portion of the right lobe of the liver, as is common. Similar left-sided changes may be seen with left lobe abscesses.

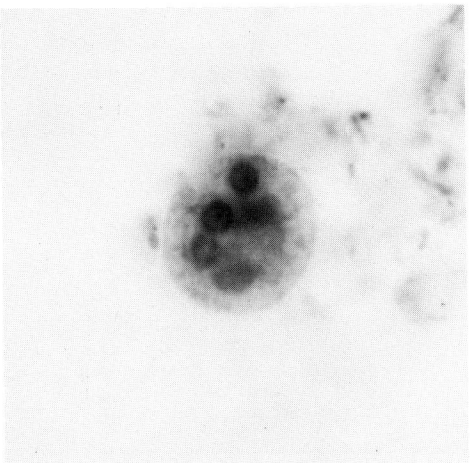

FIGURE 68–10. Cyst of *E. histolytica* in fecal smear. The cyst is spherical and contains clearly visualized nuclei, each having a central karyosome. (Iron-hematoxylin stain, × 1980.) (Courtesy of the Armed Forces Institute of Pathology, Photograph Neg. No. 72–17636.)

Signs of pericardial effusion may also be seen radiologically or sonographically.

Aspiration. Diagnostic aspiration may occasionally be needed to differentiate between amebic and pyogenic abscesses. If possible, aspiration should be carried out using ultrasound guidance. Percutaneous needle aspiration should be performed at the site of maximal tenderness or over the area of maximum dullness to percussion. If these localizing signs are not present, the site of choice is along the anterior axillary line in the ninth interspace. A number 20 needle equipped with a stop is initially used and is introduced medially and cephalad. When the abscess is located, this is changed to a wider bore needle for aspiration.

Amebic aspirates are often chocolate, reddish, or grayish brown, but may also be yellowish or white. Amebic abscesses do not have the foul odor of pyogenic abscesses. Amebic trophozoites are rarely present in the central necrotic contents of the abscess cavity itself, but can sometimes be seen in the terminal few milliliters of aspirated fluid, which is believed to be from the advancing abscess wall (Fig. 68–15). Ten units of streptodornase should be added to each milliliter of fluid, which is then incubated for 30 minutes at 35C, centrifuged for 5 minutes at 1000 rpm, and then examined in saline wet mounts and in stained preparations. Gram stain and both aerobic and anaerobic cultures should also be performed on all aspirates to detect a possible bacterial etiology for the abscess.

Metronidazole is highly effective against invasive amebiasis, as well as anaerobic bacteria, a leading cause of bacterial liver abscess. When a suspected liver abscess is confirmed by scan or sonography and while awaiting serologic confirmation of an amebic etiology, treatment with metronidazole can lead to rapid improvement of most amebic or anaerobic bacterial abscesses and may obviate the need for a diagnostic needle aspiration. However, if satisfactory clinical improvement is not obtained in about 3 days, aspiration should be per-

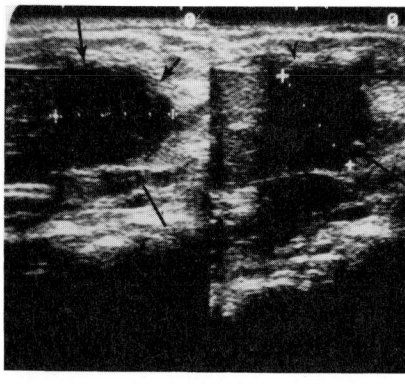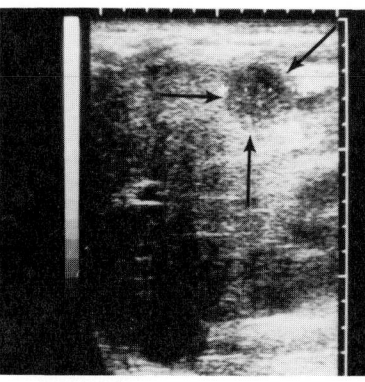

FIGURE 68–11. Rapid resolution demonstrated by ultrasonography of a 5 × 5 cm abscess in the left lobe of the liver (left frame). Two weeks later the abscess is much smaller and has increasing echogenicity (right frame). Four months later a sector scan of the same area of the liver showed complete resolution of the abscess. (Courtesy of Dr. Laila Ahmed.)

formed. Some workers always recommend pretreatment diagnostic aspiration when the etiology is not clear.

Stool Examinations. These reveal amebic parasites in only about 20% of cases of amebic liver abscess.

Blood Tests. A leukocytosis of 12,000 to 20,000/mm³ and normochromic, normocytic anemia are usually present. Eosinophilia is not a feature of either hepatic or intestinal amebiasis. The erythrocyte sedimentation rate is frequently elevated. Alkaline phosphatase is the most useful liver function test, as levels are elevated in up to 75% of patients. Aminotransaminase elevations, when they occur, are minimal; they are present in less than 50% of patients. Bilirubin levels are seldom elevated, except with large abscess cavities that may cause biliary obstruction.

TREATMENT

Drugs. Drugs available in the United States and other parts of the world include chloroquine phosphate, eme-

tine hydrochloride, iodoquinol, metronidazole (Flagyl), and paromomycin (Humatin). Dehydroemetine and diloxanide furoate (Furamide), readily available in many countries, are investigational drugs in the United States and are available from the Parasitic Disease Drug Service of the Centers for Disease Control (CDC). Tinidazole (Fasigyn), a widely used and effective antiamebic drug, is not available in the United States, but has certain advantages over metronidazole (e.g., longer half-life and relatively fewer side effects).

Metronidazole, tinidazole, emetine, and dehydroemetine are tissue amebicides that act on bowel, liver, and other sites of invasive amebiasis. Chloroquine is amebicidal in the liver. Iodoquinol, paromomycin, and diloxanide furoate are all poorly absorbed, primarily luminal-acting drugs (Fig. 68–16).

A number of other amebicides previously used have no particular place in modern day treatment. These include oral emetine and bismuth iodide; arsenicals, e.g., carbarsone, diphetarsone, and glycobiarsol (Milibis); and niridazole (Ambilhar). Tetracycline is indirectly amebicidal in the bowel and has no advantage over other available drugs. Erythromycin has some direct amebicidal action but is also not a drug of choice today.

Following are commonly used antiamebic drugs, listed

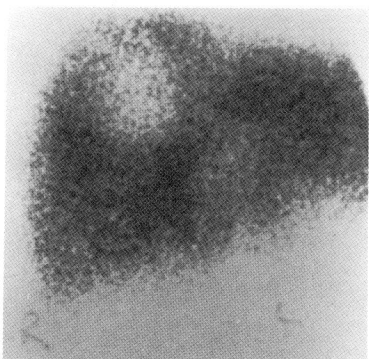
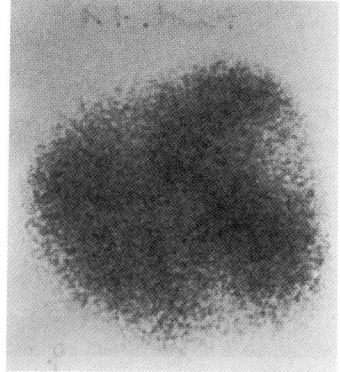

FIGURE 68–12. Amebic abscess of the liver. Hepatic nucleotide scan demonstrating a large filling defect in the anterosuperior portion of the right lobe.

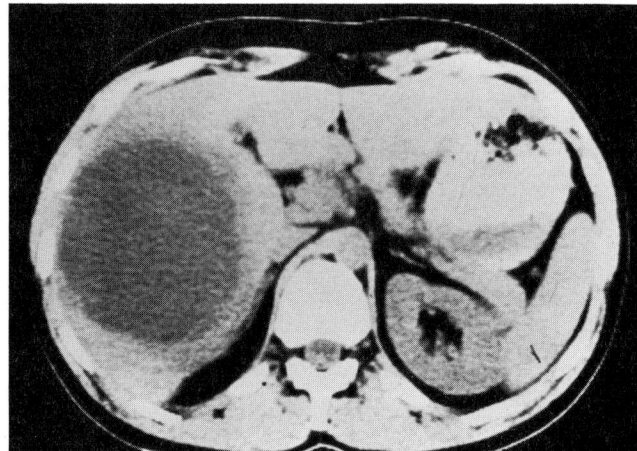

FIGURE 68–13. CT scan of the abdomen showing almost complete replacement of the right lobe of the liver by an amebic abscess that is 10 cm in diameter. The patient was a 42-year-old male who had been stationed in the Philippines from 2 to 4 years prior to his present illness. (Courtesy of the National Naval Medical Center, Bethesda.)

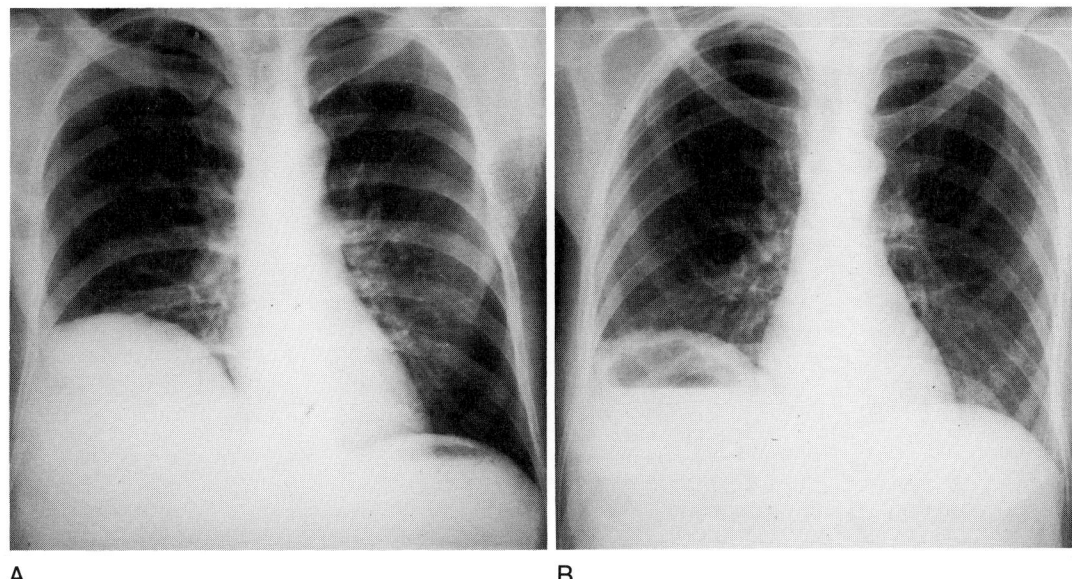

A   B

FIGURE 68–14. Chest radiographs in amebic liver abscess. *A,* Marked elevation of the right hemidiaphragm. (Courtesy of the Veterans Administration Hospital, New Orleans.) *B,* Outline of abscess cavity (air injected) with fluid level after closed aspiration. (Courtesy of the Louisiana State University School of Medicine, New Orleans.)

alphabetically by generic name, with specific information on their use in amebiasis, side effects, contraindications, and significant drug interactions. Adult and pediatric dosages for treatment of various types of amebic disorders are summarized in Table 68–2.

Chloroquine phosphate (Aralen, Nivaquine). Chloroquine can be used in treatment of amebic liver abscess. In the United States, chloroquine is marketed as 500-mg salt (300-mg base) Aralen tablets. It is also available in the United States as the generic product in 250-mg salt (equal to 150-mg base) tablets. A chloroquine hydrochloride salt, Aralen hydrochloride, is a parenteral solution for intramuscular use. Chloroquine is almost completely absorbed from the gastrointestinal tract, is deposited in the tissues (including the liver) in considerable amounts, and is slowly excreted. It is therefore

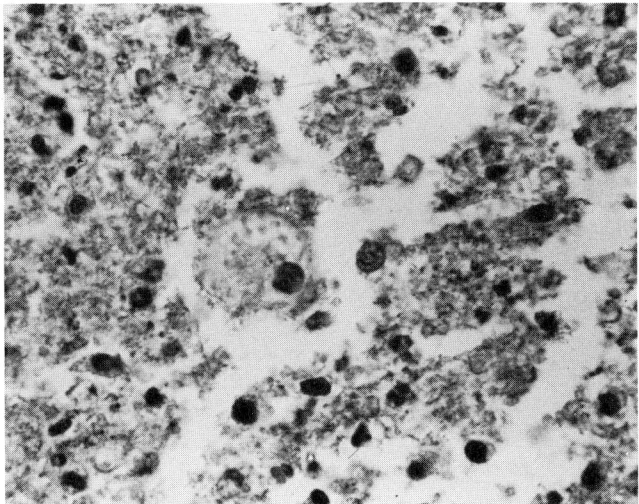

FIGURE 68–15. Smear made from material removed by needle aspiration from a patient with an amebic liver abscess. The large cell in the center is an *E. histolytica* trophozoite with nucleus and central karyosome and partially digested erythrocytes. (Courtesy of the Armed Forces Institute of Pathology, Photograph Neg. No. 82–7637.)

particularly effective in hepatic amebiasis, but has no activity against amebae in the large bowel or elsewhere. Although chloroquine has been shown to be effective when used alone for amebic abscesses, most workers prefer to use it in combination with emetine, dehydroemetine, or metronidazole. It is also advocated by some as adjunctive therapy for intestinal amebiasis when only amebicides without liver activity are used. The standard adult course of treatment for hepatic amebiasis is 600-mg base daily for 2 days, followed by 300-mg base daily for an additional 14 to 28 days. Pediatric dosage is 10-mg base/kg daily. Side effects may include gastrointestinal upset, headache, dizziness, and blurred vision. Chloroquine should not be used in patients with psoriasis or porphyria, nor in the presence of retinal abnormalities. The drug appears to be safe when it is required during pregnancy.

Diloxanide furoate (Furamide). This substituted acetanilid is produced in England in 500-mg tablets and is available in the United States only from the CDC. It is poorly absorbed and is effective alone in the asymptomatic cyst passer and in mildly symptomatic noninvasive amebiasis and as follow-up treatment to tissue-active amebicides. The only frequently observed side effect is excessive flatulence, although other mild gastrointestinal symptoms occasionally occur. Dosage for adults is 500 mg given 3 times daily for 10 days. Pediatric dosage is 30 mg/kg/day divided into 3 doses for 10 days. Diloxanide furoate is not recommended in pregnancy because little is known concerning possible teratogenic effects.

Emetine and Dehydroemetine. Emetine is a salt of an ipecac alkaloid used in treatment of invasive amebiasis. It is a white crystalline powder and is administered by deep subcutaneous or intramuscular injection. Emetine has a direct lethal action on *E. histolytica* and is more effective against trophozoites than against cysts. Local reactions to emetine are common. Systemic toxic effects are frequent and include cardiac arrhythmias, precordial pain, muscle weakness, diarrhea, and vomiting. Patients should be hospitalized and remain in bed during treat-

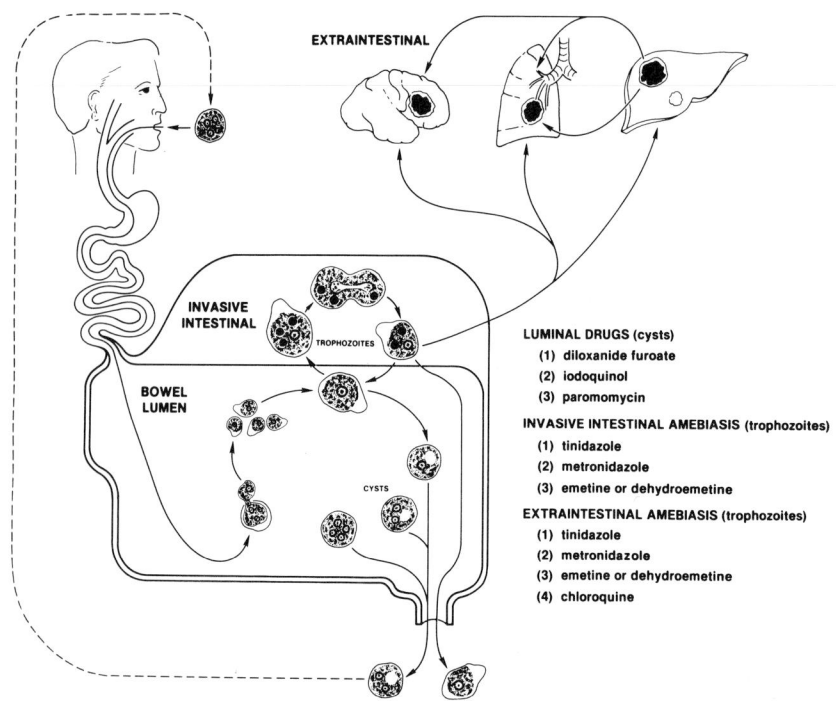

EXTRAINTESTINAL

INVASIVE
INTESTINAL

TROPHOZOITES

BOWEL
LUMEN

CYSTS

LUMINAL DRUGS (cysts)
(1) diloxanide furoate
(2) iodoquinol
(3) paromomycin

INVASIVE INTESTINAL AMEBIASIS (trophozoites)
(1) tinidazole
(2) metronidazole
(3) emetine or dehydroemetine

EXTRAINTESTINAL AMEBIASIS (trophozoites)
(1) tinidazole
(2) metronidazole
(3) emetine or dehydroemetine
(4) chloroquine

FIGURE 68–16. Modified life cycle of *E. histolytica* showing transmission and sites of infection and actions of chemotherapeutic agents.

TABLE 68–2. Summary of Drug Treatment of Amebiasis

Drugs	Adult Dose	Pediatric Dose
Amebic Dysentery or Ameboma		
Metronidazole	750 mg tid × 10 days	50 mg/kg/day in 3 doses × 10 days
or: Tinidazole	600 mg bid × 5 days	50 mg/kg/day (max, 2 gm) in single dose × 3 days
followed by either: Iodoquinol	650 mg tid × 20 days	40 mg/kg/day in 3 doses × 20 days
or: Paromomyoin	500 mg tid × 7 days	30 mg/kg/day in 3 doses × 7 days
or: Diloxanide furoate	500 mg tid × 10 days	30 mg/kg/day in 3 doses × 10 days
Alternatives: Emetine	1 mg/kg/day IM (max, 65 mg) × 10 days	1 mg/kg/day IM (max, 65 mg) in 2 doses × 10 days
or: Dehydroemetine	1 to 1.5 mg/kg/day IM (max, 90 mg) × 10 days	1 to 1.5 mg/kg/day IM (max, 90 mg) in 2 doses × 10 days

To be followed by either paromomycin, iodoquinol, or diloxanide furoate, as above

Moderately Severe Nondysenteric Amebiasis		
Metronidazole	500 mg tid × 10 days	35 mg/kg/day in 3 doses × 10 days
or: Tinidazole	600 mg bid × 5 days	50 mg/kg/day (max, 2 gm) in single dose × 3 days

To be followed by either paromomycin, iodoquinol, or diloxanide furoate, as in treating amebic cyst passers

Mildly Symptomatic Nondysenteric Amebiasis		
Paromomycin	500 mg tid × 7 days	30 mg/kg/day in 3 doses × 7 days
or: Diloxanide furoate	500 mg tid × 10 days	30 mg/kg/day in 3 doses × 10 days
Asymptomatic Cyst Passer		
Paromomycin	650 mg tid × 20 days	40 mg/kg/day in 3 doses × 20 days
or: Iodoquinol	500 mg tid × 7 days	30 mg/kg/day in 3 doses × 7 days
or: Diloxanide furoate	500 mg tid × 10 days	30 mg/kg/day in 3 doses × 10 days
Amebic Liver Abcess		
Metronidazole	750 mg tid × 10 days	50 mg/kg/day in 3 doses × 10 days
or: Tinidazole	800 mg tid × 5 days	60 mg/kg/day (max, 2 gm) in single doses × 3 days
Alternatives: Emetine	1 mg/kg/day IM (max, 65 mg) × 10 days	1 mg/kg/day IM (max, 65 mg) in 2 doses × 10 days
or: Dehydroemetine	1 to 1.5 mg/kg/day IM (max, 90 mg) × 10 days	1 to 1.5 mg/kg/day IM (max, 90 mg) in 2 doses × 10 days
plus: Chloroquine	600 mg base daily × 2 days, then 300 mg base daily × 14–28 days	10 mg base/kg/day (max, 300 mg) × 2 to 4 weeks

All to be followed by either paromomycin, iodoquinol, or diloxanide furoate as in treating amebic cyst passers ment and should have daily electrocardiographic monitoring. Emetine is contraindicated in those with heart and kidney disease and should be used cautiously in the debilitated and aged. A course of emetine therapy should not be continued for more than 10 days, the total dose should not exceed 650 mg, and a course should not be repeated until a rest period of at least 6 weeks has intervened. In treatment of acute amebic dysentery and amebic liver abscess, adults should receive 1 mg/kg/day for 10 days (up to a maximum of 65 mg/day). Pediatric dosage is 1 mg/kg/day in 2 divided doses for up to 10 days. When used in treating amebic liver abscess, emetine should be given along with chloroquine. In severe invasive amebiasis, it may be given with a nitroimidazole drug. In invasive amebiasis, it should always be followed by a luminal amebicide.

Dehydroemetine hydrochloride is identical to emetine except for the absence of hydrogen atoms at positions 2 and 3 and is also used in treating invasive amebiasis. It is manufactured in Switzerland and is supplied in 2-ml ampules containing 30 mg/ml in solution for intramuscular injection. In the United States, it must be obtained from the CDC. Dehydroemetine has amebicidal properties similar to those of emetine but has less cardiotoxicity. Nevertheless, it must be used with the same cautions as those for emetine described above. Its indications and the need for combined and sequential use of other antiamebic drugs are similar to emetine. The dose for adults is 1 to 1.5 mg/kg/day for up to 10 days (maximum 90 mg/day) and for children 1 to 1.5 mg/kg/day in 2 divided doses for up to 10 days.

Iodoquinol. This halogenated oxyquinoline was formerly known as diiodohydroxyquin and as Diodoquin, but is presently available in the United States only as the generic preparation in tablets of 650 mg and as Yodoxin in 210-mg and 650-mg tablets. Iodoquinol acts against amebae in the intestinal lumen only and is ineffective in invasive amebiasis. Because so little of the drug is absorbed, it has only minimal toxicity, e.g., abdominal pain, diarrhea, and rash. It may interfere with results of thyroid function tests for several months and is contraindicated in patients with iodine intolerance or hepatic damage.

A related compound, iodochlorhydroxyquin (Cloquinol, Mexaform, Entero-vioform) has caused the syndrome of subacute myelo-optic neuropathy (SMON) and should not be used. In doses recommended for treating intestinal protozoa, iodoquinol does not cause optic atrophy.

Used alone in treatment of asymptomatic amebiasis or used following a tissue-active amebicide in symptomatic amebiasis, the dosage of iodoquinol in adults is 650 mg 3 times daily for 20 days. Children should receive 40 mg/kg/day in 3 divided doses for 20 days.

Metronidazole. This nitroimidazole compound is marketed as tablets and as an intravenous preparation. Metronidazole is amebicidal and is highly effective in invasive amebiasis; it is the usual drug of choice for more severe infections. Because it is so well absorbed, it does not work well as a luminal-acting drug, and relapse rates are relatively high when it is used alone. Common side effects include nausea, headache, and a metallic taste. Dizziness, vomiting, abdominal cramps, and diarrhea are less common. The urine may become dark from a metabolite of the drug. Overgrowth of *Candida* in the mouth, vagina, or intestine may occur. Metronidazole may potentiate the anticoagulant effect of coumarin. It has a disulfiram (Antabuse) effect and should not be used with alcohol. Extensive clinical experience and epidemiologic data show that the risk of carcinogenicity and mutagenicity in humans is negligible to nil. Some workers prefer not to use the drug during pregnancy because of earlier studies showing it to be carcinogenic in some rodents and mutagenic to bacteria.

For acute amebic dysentery and amebic liver abscess, adults should receive 750 mg 3 times a day and children 50 mg/kg/day in 3 divided doses for 10 days. For symptomatic nondysenteric intestinal amebiasis, adults should receive 500 mg 3 times a day and children 35 mg/kg/day in 3 divided doses, for 10 days. Outside the United States, single daily doses of 2 to 2.4 gm for 1 or 2 days have been used. Intravenous metronidazole may be given as a loading dose of 1 gm, followed by 500 mg every 6 hours, until oral metronidazole can be taken. To prevent relapses from persistent cysts, metronidazole should always be followed by a luminal-acting drug.

Paromomycin (Humatin). This broad-spectrum antibiotic is marketed as a 250-mg capsule and in some countries (but no longer in the United States) as a pediatric syrup. Paromomycin is poorly absorbed after oral administration; nearly all of the drug is recoverable in the stool. It is most effective in treating asymptomatic cyst passers and patients with mildly symptomatic intestinal amebiasis. It is equally effective as other luminal-acting drugs in clearing cysts from the lumen in the follow-up to treatment of invasive amebiasis with tissue-active drugs. Nausea, abdominal cramps, and diarrhea may occur. The drug should be used with caution in persons with ulcerative lesions of the bowel. The adult dose is 500 mg 3 times daily for 7 days. Children should receive 30 mg/kg/day in 3 divided doses for 7 days.

Tinidazole (Fasigyn). This synthetic nitroimidazole derivative is marketed outside the United States in tablets of various formulations. Its action is similar to that of metronidazole, but in comparative studies it appears to be more effective and better tolerated when given as a short course in divided or single daily doses for invasive intestinal and hepatic amebiasis. Intestinal amebiasis has been treated with 600 mg twice daily for 5 to 10 days; single daily doses of 2 gm have also been used for 2 to 6 days. For amebic liver abscess, the more successful regimens have been 800 mg 3 times daily for 5 days or a single daily dose of 2 gm repeated for 3 days. As with metronidazole, it is prudent to follow these regimens with a luminal amebicide to decrease the possibility of relapse, because tinidazole is also not very active against the cyst stage. Single daily doses for children are approximately 50 to 60 mg/kg, with a maximum dose of 2 gm. Precautions are similar to those for metronidazole.

Treatment of Amebic Dysentery and Ameboma. Amebic dysentery implies tissue invasion. Initial treatment therefore requires a potent, well-absorbed tissue-active drug, e.g., metronidazole and tinidazole, followed by a luminal-acting drug to prevent relapse (Table 68–2). In severe dysentery with imminent or proven bowel perforation, combined parenteral metronidazole and emetine or dehydroemetine is often recommended. Supportive management is also essential. Severe diarrhea requires correction of water and electrolyte loss. Hemorrhage, a rare occurrence, may require blood transfusion. Gastric suction may be needed. On rare occasions, surgery may be necessary for patients with acute bowel perforation with peritonitis and for those with fulminating amebic colitis not responding to chemotherapy and medical supportive measures.

It is essential to attempt to differentiate acute amebic colitis from ulcerative colitis before administering corticosteroids. In amebiasis, corticosteroids may cause fulminant infection and perforation. Amebomas and amebic strictures are treated similarly to amebic dysentery.

Treatment of Nondysenteric Intestinal Amebiasis. Moderately severe symptoms may be present without blood or mucus in the stool. In this situation, metronidazole or tinidazole should be given initially, followed by a luminal-acting drug (Table 68–2). Those with mildly symptomatic amebiasis may be given paromomycin or diloxanide furoate alone; if this fails, a more vigorous retreatment regimen may be tried, such as for moderately severe cases.

Treatment of Asymptomatic Cyst Passers. Differences of opinion exist over the need to treat the asymptomatic cyst passer. Some workers believe that the presence of cysts in an asymptomatic individual indicates a commensal nature of the parasite or that the parasite is one of the Laredo-like or nonpathogenic zymodeme strains that are considered nonpathogenic and are perhaps more resistant to treatment. However, the asymptomatic cyst passer is a potential public health hazard, and long-term carriage might possibly lead to later acute invasive disease. Other workers therefore recommend that all infected persons be treated with a luminal-active drug (Table 68–2). Further investigations on and ready availability of zymodeme identification will be helpful in resolving this current controversy.

Treatment of Amebic Liver Abscess. Oral or intravenous metronidazole or tinidazole should lead to rapid clinical improvement of an amebic liver abscess. Multiple abscesses or complicated cases may benefit from the addition of chloroquine. Emetine or dehydroemetine plus chloroquine is an alternative regimen, but is now seldom used. Whatever initial regimen is used, it should be followed by a luminal-active drug (Table 68–2).

Aspiration. There is controversy over the specific indications for therapeutic aspiration of an amebic liver abscess, either percutaneously or surgically. In the developing world, where patients often present with long-standing large abscesses associated with risk of imminent rupture, most workers employ therapeutic aspiration. In Durban, South Africa, where there has been considerable experience with amebic liver abscess, all abscesses that can be reached percutaneously are aspirated. The majority of amebic liver abscesses seen in the United States are diagnosed earlier and are relatively small, usually responding to drug therapy alone. Percutaneous

aspiration is then reserved for abscesses that may potentially rupture, for abscesses not responding promptly to drugs alone, and for abscesses of uncertain etiology. Open surgical drainage may be indicated when needle aspiration is unsuccessful, when an abscess cannot be safely aspirated with a needle (as in some left lobe abscesses), or when the patient's condition is deteriorating with drug treatment.

Serial liver scans and sonograms (Fig. 68–11) have shown that most liver abscesses completely heal gradually over 4 to 8 months following chemotherapy. Occasionally, the resolution time may be 1 year or longer for large abscesses. Relapses that do occur usually happen within 2 months.

Complications of Amebic Liver Abscess. When extension into the thorax causes hepatobronchial fistula, pleural effusion and empyema, lung abscess, or pulmonary consolidation, treatment includes a tissue amebicide, aspiration of the liver abscess when possible, and aspiration of the pleural effusion or abscess. Repeat aspirations, closed thoracotomy, or surgery may be required in some advanced cases. Amebic peritonitis is treated by surgical drainage and a tissue amebicide. Amebic pericarditis is treated by adequate drainage of the pericardial sac using needle aspiration and occasionally by surgery, along with a tissue amebicide. In Durban, it has been suggested that 2 tissue amebicides used in combination (emetine and chloroquine or metronidazole and dehydroemetine) may be better than 1 agent.

PREVENTION AND CONTROL. Prevention should be directed toward education concerning transmission of amebiasis and methods of avoiding infection. Infected food handlers should be identified and treated. Food handlers must also wash their hands, and appropriate sanitary facilities must be made available. Infected individuals in institutions and daycare centers should be identified and treated. Homosexual males should be made aware of transmission by oral-anal sexual practices and of the relation of infection to sexual promiscuity, and those found to be infected should be treated. Follow-up stool examinations should be performed in all those treated. Contamination of food by flies may be prevented by screening and use of insecticides. In endemic areas it is necessary to avoid cold foods and salads. Vegetables can be infected from night soil, sewage, or contaminated water; therefore, before eating they should be washed with a weak detergent, rinsed in potable water, soaked with strong concentrations of chlorine or iodine, and then rinsed again with water. Fruits in endemic areas should be peeled before eating.

Water sources should be protected from fecal contamination and made safe by both proper filtration and chlorination. Boiling of water destroys amebic cysts almost immediately. Water can be effectively treated with iodine water purification tablets such as Globaline or Potable-Aqua, with tincture of iodine or Lugol's solution, or with liquid chlorine laundry bleach. The Walbro Water Purifier cup is also effective. Only ice prepared from treated water should be used.

Certain antiamebic drugs are recommended by some for prophylactic use. These include iodochlorhydroxyquin (Entero-vioform, Clioquinol, Mexaform) and iodoquinol. The prophylactic effectiveness of these drugs has never been scientifically proved, and the use of the former has been associated with the syndrome of subacute myelo-optic neuropathy, a blinding and paralytic disorder.

BIBLIOGRAPHY

Adams EB, MacLeod IN: Invasive amebiasis. I. Amebic dysentery and its complications. Medicine 56:315, 1977.

Adams EB, MacLeod IN: Invasive amebiasis. II. Amebic liver abscess and its complications. Medicine 56:325, 1977.

Ahmed L, Selama ZA, El Rooby A, Strickland GT: Ultrasonographic resolution time for amebic liver abscess. Am J Trop Med Hyg 41:406, 1989.

Ahmed L, El Raoby A, Kassem MI, et al. Ultrasonography in the diagnosis and management of 52 patients with amebic liver abscess in Cairo. Rev Infect Dis 12:330, 1990.

Alkan WJ, Kalmi B, Kalderon M: The clinical syndrome of amebic abscess of the left lobe of the liver. Ann Intern Med 55:800, 1961.

Elsdon-Dew R: The epidemiology of amebiasis. Adv Parasitol 6:1, 1968.

Feingold SM: Metronidazole. Ann Intern Med 93:585, 1980.

Goldman M: *Entamoeba histolytica*-like amoebae occurring in man. Bull WHO 40:355, 1969.

Grundy MS, Voller A, Warhurst D: An enzyme-linked immunosorbent assay for detection of *Entamoeba histolytica* antigens in faecal material. Trans R Soc Trop Med Hyg 81:627, 1987.

Guerrant RL: Amebiasis: Introduction, current status, and research questions. Rev Infect Dis 8:218, 1986. (Also see other papers of series in this issue.)

Ibarra-Perez C: Thoracic complications of amebic abscess of the liver. Report of 501 cases. Chest 79:672, 1981.

Imperato PJ: A historical overview of amebiasis. Bull NY Acad Med 57:175, 1981.

Jackson TFHG: *Entamoeba histolytica* cyst passers—to treat or not to treat? S Afr Med J 72:657, 1987.

Katzenstein D, Rickerson V, Braude A: New concepts of amebic liver abscess derived from hepatic imaging, serodiagnosis, and hepatic enzymes in 67 consecutive cases in San Diego. Medicine 61:237, 1982.

Knight R: The chemotherapy of amebiasis. J Antimicrob Chemother 6:577, 1980.

Kovaleski T, Malangoni MA, Wheat LJ: Treatment of an amebic liver abscess with intravenous metronidazole. Arch Intern Med 141:132, 1981.

Lamont NMcE, Pooler NR: Hepatic amebiasis. A study of 250 cases. Quart J Med 107:389, 1958.

Mathews HM, Moss DM, Healy GR, Mildvan D: Isoenzyme analysis of *Entamoeba histolytica* isolated from homosexual men. J Infect Dis 153:793, 1986.

Patterson M, Healy GR, Shabot JM: Serologic testing for amoebiasis. Gastroenterology 78:136, 1980.

Powell SJ, Wilmot AJ: Ulcerative post-dysenteric colitis. Gut 7:438, 1966.

Ralls PW, Henley DS, Colletti PM, et al: Amebic liver abscess: MR imaging. Radiology 165:801, 1987.

Ralls PW, Quinn MF, Boswell WD, et al: Patterns of resolution in successfully treated hepatic amebic abscess: Sonographic evaluation. Radiology 149:541, 1979.

Ravdin JI (ed): Amebiasis. Human Infection by *Entamoeba histolytica*. New York, Wiley & Sons, 1988.

Sargeaunt PG: Zymodemes of *Entamoeba histolytica*. *In* Ravdin JI (ed): Amebiasis. Human Infection by *Entamoeba histolytica*. New York, Wiley & Sons, 1988, pp 370–387.

Sargeaunt PG, Williams JE, Grene JD: The differentiation of invasive and noninvasive *Entamoeba histolytica* by isoenzyme electrophoresis. Trans R Soc Trop Med Hyg 72:519, 1978.

Sukov RJ, Cohen LJ, Sample FW: Sonography of hepatic amebic abscesses. Am J Roentgenol 134:911, 1980.

Thompson JE, Forlenza S, Verma R: Amebic liver abscess: A therapeutic approach. Rev Infect Dis 7:171, 1985.

Tucker PC, Webster PD, Kilpatrick ZM: Amebic colitis mistaken for inflammatory bowel disease. Arch Intern Med 135:681, 1975.

Walsh JA: Problems in recognition and diagnosis of amebiasis: Estimation of the global magnitude of morbidity and mortality. Rev Inf Dis 8:228, 1986.

Wilmot AJ: Clinical Amoebiasis. Oxford, Blackwell Scientific Publications, 1962.

Wolfe MS: The treatment of intestinal protozoan infections. Med Clin North Am 66:707, 1982.

69. GIARDIASIS

Stephen G. Wright

DEFINITION. Giardiasis is infection of the lumen of the small intestine with the flagellate protozoan *Giardia lamblia*, also called *Lamblia intestinalis*. Many infected persons have no symptoms, whereas a smaller proportion have diarrheal disease that varies in severity.

HISTORY. In the late seventeenth century, Van Leeuwenhoek, using his microscope, saw trophozoites of *G. lamblia* in his own stool. In the nineteenth century, Vilem Lambl found parasites in the stools of children. Giardiasis was recognized as a common cause of diarrhea among troops repatriated from various areas of Europe during World War I. Interest in giardiasis declined after World War II but has increased markedly during the past 2 decades. A major factor in the increased interest in this parasite has been the advent of axenic culture of *G. lamblia* described by Meyer in 1976.

INCIDENCE AND DISTRIBUTION. Giardiasis occurs in all parts of the world, not only in warm climates. The highest levels of endemicity occur in areas where sanitation and sanitary practices are poor and fecal contamination of the environment is common. These conditions prevail in many countries in the tropics and subtropics. Prevalence is low in developed countries, although Leningrad, Russia, and several countries in Eastern Europe are endemic areas. Water-borne outbreaks of giardiasis have occurred in towns in the United States, e.g., Aspen, Colorado, and Rome, New York, and in England. Infections have occurred in holiday visitors to Madeira, Italy, Sardinia, and other areas of the Mediterranean littoral.

TRANSMISSION. Infection follows ingestion of viable cysts of the parasite in contaminated food or water. Cysts may also be transported to the mouth on fingers, particularly of children, as a result of contact with feces on the ground around the home. Person to person spread also occurs in children. As few as 100 cysts produced infection in prison volunteers. More recent volunteer studies have been carried out using 2 different strains, both derived from human sources with diarrhea. Trophozoites were lavaged directly into the small intestine. One strain infected all 10 volunteers, whereas none of the 5 receiving the other strain became infected. The prepatent period averaged 7.5 days. Cyst excretion showed considerable variation from large numbers to occasional, and on some days, no cysts passed. Half of those infected developed symptoms, with 40% showing the typical clinical features of giardiasis.

Studies of water-borne outbreaks of giardiasis in the United States have usually shown defective water treatment plants with malfunctioning filters that do not retain giardia cysts. The cysts in surface water sources sometimes come from beavers. A variety of mammals, including dogs, can become infected and excrete cysts. Reservoirs such as these may be important in the outbreaks occurring in backpackers and others visiting rural areas of the United States. The role of animal reservoirs may be greater in temperate regions where pets live in close proximity to their owners. This issue is not resolved. In the tropics high levels of environmental contamination may be the dominant factor in transmission.

Both sexes seem equally susceptible to infection. In the tropics, children are more often infected than adults, and symptomatic disease is probably more common among children, although indigenous adults may have diarrhea due to giardiasis. Although there has been an emphasis on *Giardia* as a cause of diarrhea in children and adults, *Giardia* as a cause of diarrhea in the elderly must not be overlooked. In this group there may be relative immune deficiency owing to involution of the immune system.

Parasite Resistance. Heating to 50C kills the encysted trophozoite; the survival ratio of cysts stored at 37C in water is low. At 21C, some cysts remain viable for up to 20 days. A high proportion of cysts stored at 8C in tap water are viable for up to 5 weeks. *Giardia* cysts are not killed by chlorine concentrations used for disinfection of domestic water supplies. Tincture of iodine (2% solution) can be used to purify drinking water in endemic areas; add 5 drops (0.05 ml/drop) to 1 L of clear water and 10 drops to 1 L of cloudy water and allow the water to stand for 30 minutes.

Predisposing Factors. Children who are malnourished may be prone to giardiasis. Children attending daycare centers, residents of homes for the mentally retarded, and homosexuals all have an increased risk of giardiasis from person to person spread. Reduced gastric acid secretion due to malnutrition, atrophic gastritis, antacid treatment, or surgery predisposes to giardiasis. Adults and children with hypogammaglobulinemia often have giardiasis as a cause of diarrhea. Giardiasis does not appear to be important as a cause of diarrhea in human immunodeficiency virus (HIV) infection and acquired immunodeficiency syndrome (AIDS). There is no association with any particular group of the ABO blood grouping system, but an association between HLA-B12 and giardiasis has been reported.

Parasitology. Exposure to gastric acid followed by the alkaline duodenal contents containing bile and proteolytic enzymes allows excystation of the quadrinucleate trophozoite, which then divides asexually, producing binucleate trophozoites. Parasite populations then rise rapidly in a phase of logarithmic growth.

Restriction endonuclease analysis has shown that there are numerous strains of the parasite. These variations are stable both in vitro and in vivo, for example in the volunteer studies referred to above. In gerbils, cross-protection between strains is evident.

Morphology. The cyst is oval and measures 8 × 12 × 8 μm. The median body is easily seen, and 4 nuclei may be identified. Electron microscopy reveals fine

detail of the cyst. The pear-shaped trophozoite measures about 15 μm long, 10 μm wide, and 2 to 4 μm thick (Figs. 69–1 and 71–10). It has a curved dorsal surface and a concave ventral surface, much of which is taken up by a disk with regular striations termed the sucker disk (Figs. 69–2 and 71–10). Two of the 8 flagella emerge near the midline on the ventral surface of the organism, and the others emerge symmetrically around the periphery, 3 on each side. The beating of the flagella produces the trophozoite's spiraling motion and may cause a suction force that can maintain the trophozoite in a position closely applied to the microvilli of the gut epithelium. The extent of small bowel colonization in humans is not certain. *Giardia muris* colonizes the proximal quarter of the mouse small intestine.

Scanning and transmission electron microscopy confirm the appearances seen on light microscopy but give much clearer definition of parasite fine structure (Fig. 69–2). Studies of the cytoskeleton of *Giardia* have shown that it diverged as a species at an early stage in evolutionary history. Ribosomal RNA, which is highly conserved among related species, provides evidence for this. The cytoskeletal proteins and β giardin constitute the microribbons of the ventral sucker disk; they are linked to cross-bridges and microtubules. There are contractile proteins around the edge of the sucker disk. *G. lamblia* in the gerbil and *G. muris* in the mouse leave a cookie cutter–shaped "footprint" of the sucker disk in the microvillous carpet of the enterocytes at sites of attachment, although this is not seen in humans.

Parasite Kinetics. Comparatively little is known about the kinetics of infection in humans, at least as far as trophozoite populations are concerned. Cyst excretion can vary markedly among infected populations, with extreme variations even in the same person. The median duration of infection in children was 2 months with a range of up to 11 months. Using cultured trophozoites, encystation was induced by increasing concentrations of bile.

Mouse giardiasis (caused by *G. muris*) has been studied extensively. Following infection with 1000 cysts, trophozoite populations rise to peak at about 10^6 organisms 2 weeks after infection. There is a progressive decline in parasite numbers over the next 4 weeks and most strains of mice eradicate the infection in 4 to 8 weeks. The mechanisms of this process are poorly understood, but some strains of mice reduce parasite numbers much more efficiently than others, indicating that genetically determined factors may be important. Nude mice deficient in T cells, mice deficient in mast cells, and C3H/He mice have prolonged infections.

G. lamblia is an aerotolerant anaerobe. Glucose can stimulate respiration. This is not sensitive to cyanide, malonate, and 2,4-dinitrophenol. Glucose is converted to carbon dioxide, ethanol, and acetate under aerobic or anaerobic conditions, irrespective of the source of glucose, which may be exogenous or endogenous. There is no oxidative phosphorylation mediated by cytochromes nor a tricarboxylic acid (Krebs) cycle. Both free-living and encysted trophozoites carry out these metabolic activities. The parasite is not capable of synthesizing phospholipid and derives its supplies from

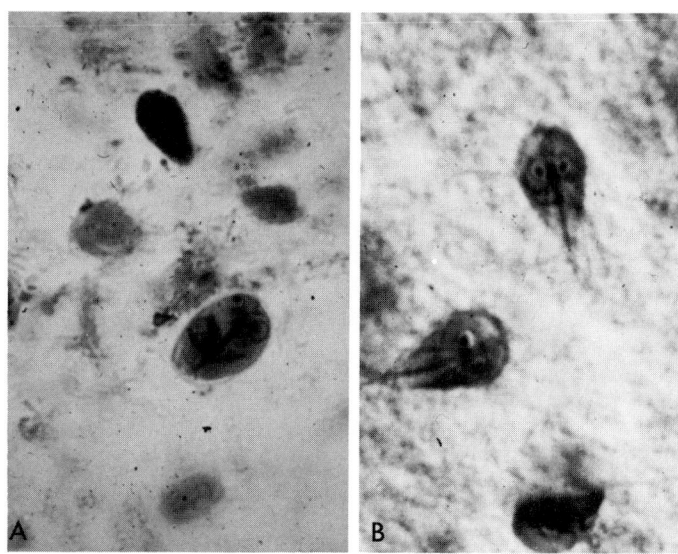

FIGURE 69–1. *Giardia lamblia. A*, Cyst. *B*, Trophozoite. (From Smith JW, McQuay RM, Ash LR, et al: Diagnostic Medical Parasitology: Intestinal Protozoa. Chicago, The American Society of Clinical Pathologists, 1976.)

host biliary phospholipid; in association with this, it also actively takes up bile salts. This requirement for phospholipid may determine its predilection for the proximal jejunum.

PATHOGENESIS. The sequence of events leading to infection with *G. lamblia* is similar to that described for other intestinal pathogens that cause diarrhea: ingestion, colonization, and adhesion. Strain variation among parasites may contribute to variations in clinical manifestations. However, within 1 family, presumed to be exposed to a common strain, the whole range of pathogenicity may occur, from asymptomatic to severe diarrhea.

Colonization and Adhesion. Events in the stomach are not clearly understood. On the one hand, acid provides a chemical barrier to the entry of pathogens, unless they are acid resistant, and reduced gastric acid predisposes to this and other infections. On the other hand, at least in vitro, exposure to acid is essential for excystation (hydrochloric acid at pH 2.0). Probably not all those who develop giardiasis have permanently reduced acid secretion, although one could speculate about the role of other infections, e.g., *Helicobacter pylori*, which are capable of inducing temporary hypochlorhydria in increasing risk of giardia infection.

A large infecting dose increases the risk of infection, as shown by Rendtorff's volunteer studies. This may also increase the probability of symptomatic infection through more rapid build-up of trophozoite populations. Parasite adhesion has been investigated using cultured trophozoites. There are at least 2 mechanisms involved. One is mechanical and relates to the beating of the two ventral flagella, perhaps aided by contractile elements in the ventral sucker disk. The other mechanism is mediated by a lectin on the surface of the parasite. The lectin allows mannose-dependent adhesion of parasites

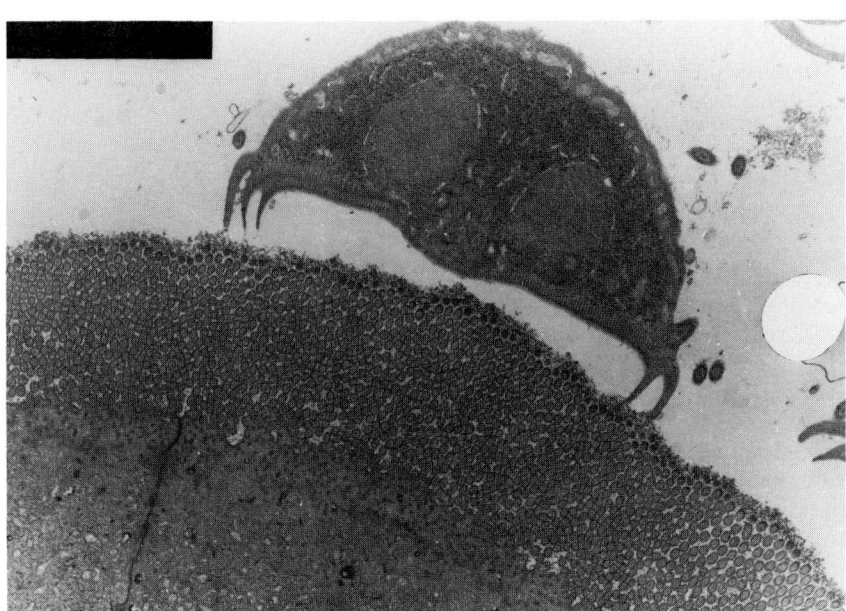

FIGURE 69–2. A *Giardia* trophozoite close to the microvillous border of a jejunal epithelial cell. The tips of microvilli beneath the trophozoite are more densely stained, probably representing damage to these structures caused by the parasite. (Electron micrograph reproduced by permission of Prof. G. N. Tytgat and Dr. K. Huibregtse, University of Amsterdam.)

to mammalian red blood cells experimentally. The lectin is located intracellularly, where it is in the form of a prolectin, which is modified by host protease when it is expressed on the surface membrane. The nature of the enterocyte receptor is not clear but it is located in the parasite's basolateral regions.

Mechanism for Diarrhea. The cause of diarrhea in giardiasis is not understood; it seems likely that there is no single cause for the absorptive defects observed. Electron microscopic studies show damage at the microvillous border, the site of much terminal digestive and absorptive activity (Fig. 69–2). Absorption of actively transported substrates such as glucose and amino acids is markedly reduced in animals infected with *G. lamblia*. Brush border disaccharidase levels decline with infection and lowest levels of enzyme activity relate to peak trophozoite populations, suggesting that microvillous damage is proportional to parasite numbers. When parasites move about on the surface of the small intestine, lectin adhesion to enterocytes is continually being made and broken. Breaking adhesion sites may disrupt enzymes and surface membranes of microvilli. Failure to absorb nutrients may lead to the accumulation of osmotically active molecules in the gut lumen, which would then cause diarrhea.

Luminal events may also affect digestive processes. It is possible that the active uptake of bile salts by trophozoites alters micelle formation sufficiently to cause malabsorption of fat. Alterations in bile salt concentrations may influence the activity of pancreatic lipase to impair fat digestion. Bile salt deconjugation is a recognized cause of fat malabsorption. However, in vitro this does not occur and results of clinical studies have not been consistent. There is small bowel overgrowth of bacteria in patients with giardiasis, but the microflora comprises facultative anaerobes and not the obligate anaerobes associated with the bile salt deconjugation of jejunal diverticulosis and intestinal strictures. These organisms secrete enterotoxin and alcohol, which may contribute to intestinal damage. Patients with severe malabsorption caused by giardiasis and tropical sprue have prolonged intestinal transit time. This may be a factor by allowing microbial colonization.

Immunopathology. More severe degrees of functional upset are associated with increasingly severe degrees of morphologic change in the jejunum. Villi are shortened, crypts are deeper, and there is an increase both in interepithelial lymphocyte counts and in the lamina propria infiltrate with lymphocytes and plasma cells (Fig. 69–3). These findings are common to many mucosal diseases of the gut. The significance of the changes in relation to functional impairment is uncertain, but there is increasing evidence that the changes in mucosal architecture relate to the stimulatory effects of T-cell products on the crypt cell population. One or more *Giardia* antigens or food antigens entering through a leaky mucosa may have this stimulatory effect. This would explain the crypt hypertrophy but not the reduction in villous height because stimulatory effects from T cells in the crypts should not change to cytotoxic effects on the villi. Enterocyte damage caused by *Giardia* trophozoites may impair intercellular adhesion and allow

increased cell desquamation into the gut lumen. The distribution of *Giardia* trophozoites is predominantly intervillous (Fig. 69–3), and crypts are rarely colonized. Therefore, for *Giardia* antigen to drive this, a secreted or excreted antigen would have to diffuse down into the crypt region. The absence of a major role for *G. lamblia* in the enteropathy of AIDS suggests that immune responses mediated by CD4+ cells are not a major influence in protection.

Protective Immunity. Nonspecific and specific host responses are important in controlling the parasite population. A bile salt–dependent breast milk lipase is toxic to *Giardia* in vitro and may be important in protection before weaning.

Humoral responses are best characterized. Antibody responses to *Giardia* were followed in volunteers infected with trophozoites of 1 of 2 strains. Serum antibody was detected in *all* 10 who received the strain producing patent infections but in *none* of the 5 who received the other strain, suggesting that strain variation in infectivity, and not humoral immunity, is important in some cases. All infected subjects showed IgM antibody when either of the challenge strains was used as antigen. Most had detectable antibody by day 14. Serum IgG and IgM antibodies were present in 70% and 60%

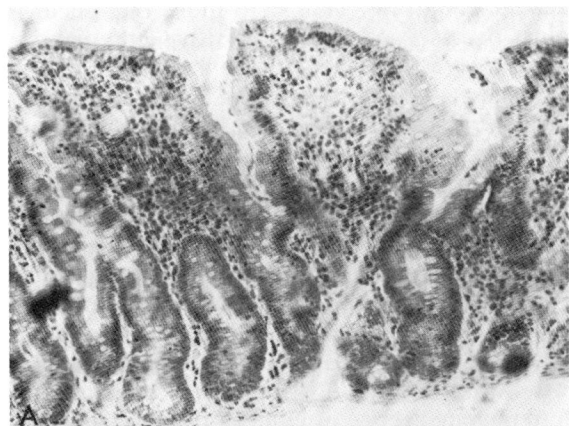

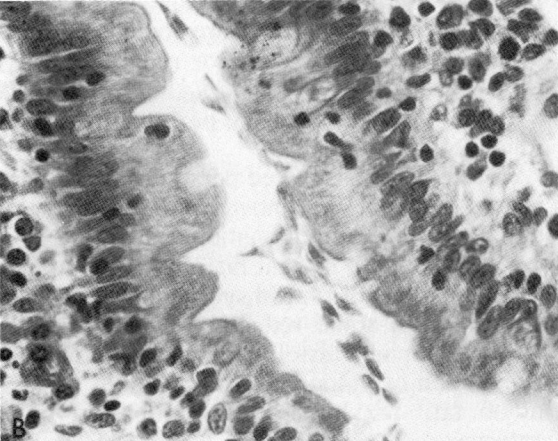

FIGURE 69–3. Jejunal biopsy section from a patient with symptomatic giardiasis. *A*, There are definite abnormalities, with shortened villi, deepened crypts, and an increased inflammatory infiltrate in the lamina propria. *Giardia* trophozoites are seen in the intervillous spaces. *B*, With greater magnification, the characteristic morphologic features of the parasites can be seen.

of infected volunteers with a similar time course. Five of 10 had detectable antigiardia IgA in jejunal fluid. IgM antibody titers in serum declined within weeks of effective treatment, unlike IgG antibody, which persisted up to 6 months after treatment.

A range of antigens evoking antibody responses have been identified. A surface antigen with a molecular weight of 82 to 88 kDA has been defined. The giardins, a family of proteins of which 2 are presently described, are antigenic and are localized to the sucker disk. An interesting surface antigen with a molecular weight of 170 kDA seems to be capable of variable expression.

In vitro antibody agglutinates trophozoites, immobilizing and killing them by binding to flagella. IgM antibody with complement activation by the classic pathway will kill parasites. Both secretory IgA and IgM could cause these effects in the gut lumen. Antibody-dependent cytotoxicity has also been observed.

PATHOLOGY. Infected persons have a range of severity of functional and morphologic changes. Persons who are asymptomatic usually have normal absorption and normal histologic appearance of the jejunal mucosa. Mild symptoms are usually associated with some reduction in D-xylose absorption and minor histologic abnormalities without reduction of villous height. Impaired absorption of fat, D-xylose, and vitamin B_{12} and hypolactasia are common in those severely affected. There is obvious reduction in villous height, increase in crypt depth with increased numbers of mitotic figures, and an increased infiltrate of plasma cells and lymphocytes in the lamina propria (Fig. 69–3A). Interepithelial lymphocyte counts are increased. *Giardia* trophozoites may be seen in the intervillous spaces and on the microvillous border of epithelial cells (Figs. 69–2 and 69–3).

Severe villous atrophy due to *G. lamblia* alone has been reported, but it is exceptional. When such severe histologic changes are found, celiac disease should be suspected; serial biopsies after eradication of *Giardia*, gluten withdrawal, and gluten challenge are needed to confirm this diagnosis. Giardiasis causes severe diarrhea in those patients whose celiac disease had been covert. Folate deficiency causing macrocytosis and megaloblastic anemia occasionally occurs. Protein-losing enteropathy has been found in giardiasis.

CLINICAL MANIFESTATIONS. Symptoms in acute infections begin after an incubation period of about 2 weeks. Usual symptoms are anorexia, nausea, lassitude, and diarrhea, with frequent passing of offensive yellow stools. Systemic upset does not occur. Abdominal distention and discomfort, a bad taste in the mouth, and flatulence are usual at this stage; weight loss occurs because of the anorexia and diarrhea. These symptoms may persist for several weeks and then start to resolve spontaneously with return of appetite, regaining of weight and resolution of diarrhea.

After infection, a variety of outcomes are possible: (1) an acute diarrheal illness that resolves spontaneously, with eradication of the infection by natural means; (2) continuing diarrhea with weight loss and continuing infection; (3) resolution of diarrhea with continuing cyst excretion.

Complications. A proportion of those infected remain markedly symptomatic with no tendency toward spontaneous resolution. Weight loss in this group suggests malabsorption, confirmed by abnormal tests of absorption. When symptoms have been present for several months, the patient may have glossitis, indicating folate deficiency although this is not common. Instances of food allergy apparently brought on by symptomatic giardiasis have been reported. When the infection is treated, the food allergy disappears. It is possible that the offending allergen enters through a mucosa that is more permeable to macromolecules. Colonization of the biliary tract has been reported in symptomatic patients. The frequency of this event is uncertain. As endoscopic examination of the biliary tract becomes more widely practiced in endemic areas, more information on this may become available.

The main complications of giardiasis relate to the effect of the infection on nutritional status of the host. Recurrent symptomatic giardiasis in children can cause failure to thrive and may play a part, with other gastrointestinal infections, in causing overt malnutrition in the tropics. Specific nutritional deficiencies are not as common as they are in tropical sprue.

DIAGNOSIS

Demonstration of the Parasite. This depends on finding the parasite (Fig. 69–1). Cysts are usually found by microscopy of concentrated stool samples (Chapter 122). It may be necessary to examine several samples because of the considerable variations in cyst excretion from day to day. A fecal smear of fluid stools should be examined directly for cysts and trophozoites.

If *Giardia* have not been found in several stools in a symptomatic patient, particularly if there is a clinical suspicion of malabsorption, sampling the upper gastrointestinal tract by intubation, jejunal biopsy, or string test is indicated (Chapter 123). Flecks of mucus adhering to the biopsy fragment or capsule should be mounted in saline for microscopic examination, and mucosal impression smears should be made from the epithelial surface of the biopsy specimen. Trophozoites can be seen on or near the epithelial surface in histologic sections stained with hematoxylin and eosin (Fig. 69–3). When the parasite cannot be found by any of these methods but giardiasis is still suspected on clinical grounds, drug treatment may be indicated.

Antigen Detection. This is an area of great promise in parasitologic diagnosis and there have been studies showing the technique to be applicable in giardiasis. Indirect fluorescent antibody (IFA) techniques, enzyme-linked immunosorbent assay (ELISA), and coagglutination using *Staphylococcus aureus* coated with antigiardia antibody are some of the methods used. Using an ELISA technique, 76 of 77 positive specimens were correctly identified with no false-positive results. Antigen was detected for 2 days after the parasite could no longer be detected by conventional methods following treatment. These methods may become widely available in the future.

Serology. Serum antibodies to *G. lamblia* have been found using IFA and ELISA techniques, and cyst or, more recently, trophozoite antigens. About 80% of symptomatic patients have detectable antibodies. Anti-

TABLE 69–1. Drugs and Dosages Used in Treating Giardiasis

	Metronidazole	Tinidazole	Quinacrine
Adult Dose			
Long course	200–250 mg 3 times daily for 14 days		100 mg 3 times daily for 5–10 days
Short course	2.0 gm daily for 3 days	2.0 gm once	—
Pediatric Dose			
Long course	10–15 mg/kg/day in 3 divided doses for 14 days		5 mg/kg/day in 3 divided doses for 5–10 days
Short course	35–40 mg/kg daily for 3 days	50 mg/kg once	—

bodies persist in circulation for about 6 months after eradication of the infection. In an area where there is little giardiasis, antibodies in a symptomatic patient may indicate infection and should prompt further diagnostic tests. In an endemic region antibodies may only indicate past infection, although the occurrence of serum IgM responses in symptomatic patients in endemic areas and the relatively rapid decline in titer after eradication may have practical value.

Radiographic Changes. Radiologic changes in an upper gastrointestinal series comprise dilatation of small bowel loops and thickening of mucosal folds. These changes occur in patients with malabsorption from many causes and are not specific for giardiasis.

TREATMENT

Drugs. Metronidazole, tinidazole, and quinacrine are the agents most often used for treatment of giardiasis. Long courses at low dose or short courses at high dose can be used (Table 69–1).

Both metronidazole and tinidazole interact with alcohol like disulfiram; therefore patients should not drink alcohol while taking either drug. Their other side effects include nausea, a metallic taste in the mouth, headache, and drowsiness. These are not usually noticeable at lower dosages and resolve quickly after treatment is completed. Because of occasional drowsiness with high-dose regimens, patients should be advised not to ride a bicycle, drive a car, or operate any dangerous machinery during treatment. Side effects seem to be less marked with tinidazole, which also has the advantage of twice-daily dosage in the long-course regimen and single dosage in the short-course regimen, allowing for a greater likelihood of patient compliance.

The common side effects of quinacrine include nausea, vomiting, abdominal pain, and temporary yellow staining of the skin. Psychosis also occurs occasionally. Quinacrine is contraindicated in patients with psoriasis.

Drug Resistance. This has been suspected clinically in those relatively few patients who remain persistently infected despite the use of currently available drugs in optimal dosage. In vitro sensitivity testing has shown variations in drug sensitivity among strains as well as drug-resistant strains. As yet there is not an agreed on method for general application.

Response to Therapy. Diarrhea usually stops within 1 to 2 weeks of completing treatment, occasionally within a day or so. Cyst excretion ceases 2 days after initiation of treatment. Abnormalities of intestinal function and morphology resolve within 1 to 2 months of treatment. Persistent symptoms respond, in most cases, to a low-lactose diet and avoidance of alcohol, herbs, and spices. If giardiasis persists, further courses of treatment should be given.

PREVENTION AND CONTROL. Clean drinking water, proper disposal of excreta, and clean hands would prevent most transmission of giardiasis. Heating drinking water to over 50C kills cysts. A 2% solution of iodine kills cysts and can be used by travelers to endemic areas to sterilize drinking water. Filters are also available to purify drinking water. Avoiding salads, uncooked foods, and unpeeled fruits is also helpful. Thoroughly cooked foods and boiled water in drinks are safe.

BIBLIOGRAPHY

Ament ME, Rubin CE: Relationship of giardiasis to abnormal intestinal structure and function in gastrointestinal immunodeficiency syndromes. Gastroenterology 62:216, 1972.

Belosevic M, Faubert GM, Maclean JD: Disaccharidase activity in the small intestine of gerbils (*Meriones unguiculatus*) during primary and challenge infections with *Giardia lamblia*. Gut 30:1213, 1989.

Danciger M, Lopez M: Numbers of *Giardia* in feces of infected children. Am J Trop Med Hyg 24:237, 1975.

Dykes AC, Juranek DD, Lorenz RA, et al: Municipal waterborne giardiasis: An epidemiologic investigation. Ann Intern Med 92:165, 1980.

Earlandsen SL, Meyer EA (eds): Giardia and Giardiasis. New York, Plenum Press, 1984.

Farthing MJG: Host-parasite interactions in human giardiasis. Q J Med 70:191, 1989.

Ferguson A, Gillon J, Thamery D: Intestinal abnormalities in murine giardiasis. Trans R Soc Trop Med Hyg 74:445, 1980.

Gilman RE, Marquis GS, Miranda E, et al: Rapid reinfection by *Giardia lamblia* after treatment in a hyperendemic third world community. Lancet 1:343, 1988.

Green EL, Miles MA, Warhurst DC: Immunodiagnostic detection of *Giardia* antigen by a rapid visual enzyme-linked immunosorbent assay. Lancet 1:691, 1985.

Keystone JS, Kradjens S, Warren MR: Person to person transmission of *Giardia lamblia* in day care nurseries. J Can Med Assoc 119:241, 1978.

Meyer EA, Jarroll EL: Giardiasis. Am J Epidemiol 111:1, 1980.

Nash TE, Herrington DA, Losonsky GA, Levine MM: Experimental human infections with *Giardia lamblia*. J Infect Dis 156:974, 1987.

Peattie DA: The giardins of *Giardia lamblia*: Genes and proteins with promise. Parasitol Today 6:52, 1990.

Rendtorff RC: The experimental transmission of human intestinal protozoan parasites. II. *Giardia lamblia* cysts given in capsules. Am J Hyg 59:209, 1954.

Roberts-Thomson IC: Giardiasis: The role of immunological mechanisms to host-parasite relationships. *In* Marsh MN (ed): Immunopathology of the Small Intestine. Chichester, Wiley, 1987, pp 209–222.

Wright SG, Tomkins AM, Ridley DS: Giardiasis: Clinical and therapeutic aspects. Gut 18:343, 1977.

70. CRYPTOSPORIDIOSIS

Gordon C. Cook

DEFINITION. Cryptosporidiosis consists of an intestinal infection, involving most importantly the jejunum, with *Cryptosporidium* sp.—an intracellular protozoan parasite, which has a broad distribution in the animal kingdom; it is not host specific. Clinical manifestations vary from a self-limited, relatively trivial traveler's diarrhea–like illness to a life-threatening disease with torrential diarrhea often associated with malabsorption and severe weight loss in immunosuppressed individuals, especially those with the acquired immunodeficiency syndrome (AIDS).

HISTORY. *Cryptosporidium* sp. was first recognized in the stomach and small intestine of asymptomatic mice by Tyzzer in 1907. Extensive data have since accumulated on infection in both small and large mammals (the calf and lamb in particular), as well as many other animal species, including fish, reptiles, and birds. In 1955 *Cryptosporidium* was implicated as a cause of diarrhea in turkeys. The first report of a human infection, which followed exposure to farm animals, was made in 1976. An explosive increase in the literature relating to this parasite has arisen since 1982, when *Cryptosporidium* sp. was firmly shown to be an important opportunistic organism in patients with AIDS.

INCIDENCE AND DISTRIBUTION. Most of the early human cases had been infected by calves and other farm animals. Domestic water supplies contaminated with sewerage of animal or human origin are, however, a more important source of infection and community epidemics of diarrhea have occurred. Many outbreaks have now been described in daycare centers and less frequently in family groups; person to person transmission (via fecal contamination) is more common than zoonotic sources. *Cryptosporidium* is an important cause of acute diarrhea in infants and children in developing countries; in some areas up to 15% of acute gastroenteritis is caused by this organism. Infection is less common in breastfed infants. It is also an important cause of traveler's diarrhea. Simultaneous infection with *Giardia lamblia* has been reported from several countries, especially the Soviet Union.

PARASITOLOGY

Taxonomy. The coccidia constitute an extremely ancient subclass of organisms that belong to the class Sporozoea of the phylum Apicomplexa; Cryptosporidiidae (to which *Cryptosporidium* sp. belongs), Eimeriidae, and Sarcocystidae are families belonging to the suborder Eimeriina of the order Eucoccidiida. Following the first description, some 18 species of *Cryptosporidium* were named; this, however, presupposed that each was host specific, as is the case with the closely related coccidia assigned to the genus *Eimeria* of the suborder Eimeriidae. Several alternative classifications have since been made. The organisms have recently been subdivided into 4 species: *C. nasorum* (fish), *C. crotali* (reptiles), *C. meleagridis* (birds), and *C. muris* or *C. parvum* (mammals). However, cross-transmission studies have demonstrated little host specificity for isolates from calves, lambs, and humans, and a number of investigators consider this to be a single-species genus.

Life Cycle. *Cryptosporidium* has an apical complex but possesses neither cilia nor flagella. Although intracellular—the oocyst is 2 to 8 μm—(existing within the enterocyte), it lies immediately beneath the surface membrane and is thus extracytoplasmic. Investigation of the development of human and calf isolates of *C. parvum* in mice, chicken embryos, and cell culture have shown that, as with other true coccidia, the life cycle of *Cryptosporidium* involves 6 major stages (Figs. 70–1 to 70–4): excystation (infective sporozoites are released from the oocysts), merogony (asexual replication), gametogony (gamete formation), fertilization, oocyst wall formation, and sporogony (sporozoite formation). Unlike other coccidian species, the cycle can be completed in cell culture. The life cycle has been reproduced at 35, 37, and 41C and this reflects the varying temperatures of fish and snake, mammals, and avian hosts. Internal autoinfection seems likely in vivo.

PATHOGENESIS. The size of the infecting dose required to produce human disease is unknown; infant macaques develop a self-limited illness after an inoculation with 10 oocysts. Most knowledge concerning the pathogenesis of human cryptosporidiosis has resulted from histologic studies of intestinal biopsy material obtained from infected immunodeficient individuals (usually AIDS patients). Developmental stages have been detected in the pharynx, esophagus, stomach, duodenum, jejunum, ileum, appendix, colon, and rectum of humans, mice, and calves; at postmortem examination, the jejunum is usually most severely affected. Histologic lesions include villous atrophy, an increase in crypt length, and mild to moderate infiltration (consisting of mononuclear cells) in the lamina propria. These abnormalities are similar to those in experimentally infected mice, pigs, and lambs and in germ-free calves that have been infected with *C. parvum*.

The pathophysiology of the diarrhea and malabsorption (which is usually confined to the immunosuppressed individual) is not clear. In the calf, the structural (histologic) abnormalities in both small intestine and colon seem important; in AIDS patients, however, the diarrhea is characteristically watery and presumably results from hypersecretion. More clinical investigations directed to the mechanism(s) of pathogenicity are clearly required. Does malabsorption result from physical brush border damage, toxins, or metabolites released by *Cryptosporidium* or from an immunologic reaction? The reason for the cell loss is also unclear.

Immunology. Immune competence is important in human infections. Whereas the disease usually runs a short course (less than 2 weeks) in the otherwise normal individual, in AIDS patients (and those receiving corticosteroids and with hypogammaglobulinemia) a prolonged life-threatening infection involving not only the intestinal but also the respiratory and biliary tracts is well documented. It is probable that both humoral and cell-mediated immunity (CMI) are involved, although the latter seems to be more important. Normal T-cell function has been reported in some hypogammaglobulinemic patients with a severe infection; also a high *Cryptosporidium* antibody titer has been demonstrated in some AIDS patients with severe infection. Measles (which suppresses CMI) has been implicated as a predisposing factor in developing countries. Most immunocompetent individuals possess *C. parvum*–specific serum antibodies for several months (and as long as 2

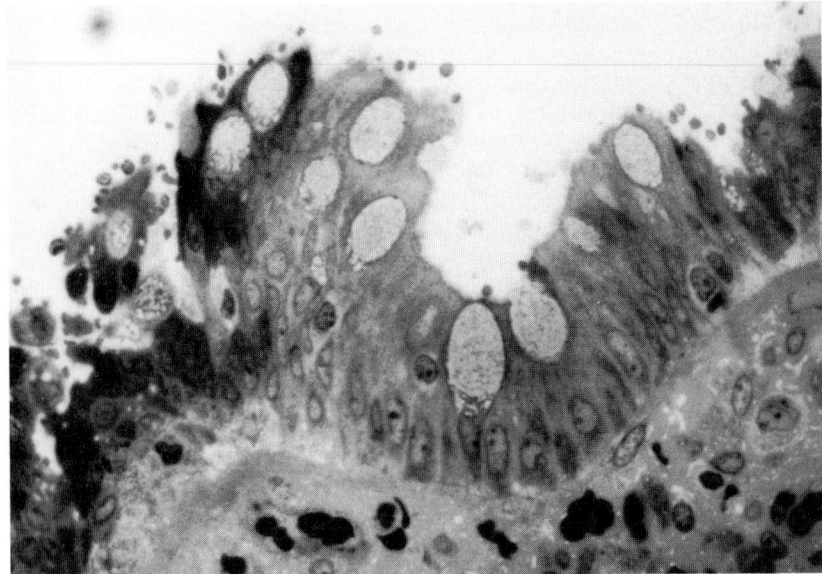

FIGURE 70–1. Light micrograph of a rectal biopsy specimen from an AIDS patient showing endogenous stages of *Cryptosporidium* sp. Toluidine blue–stained section. (Courtesy of D. P. Casemore.)

years) after recovery from gastrointestinal cryptosporidiosis. In the immunointact individual, *Cryptosporidium* is localized to the microvillous region of the enterocyte (Figs. 70–1 to 70–4). This makes it difficult to understand how serum antibodies can play a major role in the production of acquired immunity. A more plausible explanation is that local antibodies (intestinal IgA and IgG) coupled with CMI mechanisms are required for parasite clearance from the enterocyte. The importance of T cells in recovery of an experimental *Cryptosporidium* infection is also unclear; however, in T-cell deficient nude white mice, diarrhea (with continuing oocyst excretion) persists much longer than in immunocompetent littermates.

In experimental studies, an age-dependent factor is important in resistance to infection. Thus, suckling rodents develop heavy intestinal infections following an oral inoculation with calf or human isolates of *Cryptosporidium;* however, in adults if an infection occurs it is mild. In addition, infection in cattle usually occurs when they are calves.

EPIDEMIOLOGY. Presence of *Cryptosporidium* in the enterocyte is usually, but not always, associated with overt symptoms; however, a study in India demonstrated a 10% rate of infection in an asymptomatic control group. Although common in AIDS, it is unusual in male homosexuals. During the past decade, evidence for reservoirs of zoonotic foci of *Cryptosporidium,* person to person transmission, and water-borne spread via domestic supplies has accumulated. There are close parallels with *G. lamblia* transmission, and these 2 protozoan parasites can be transferred simultaneously.

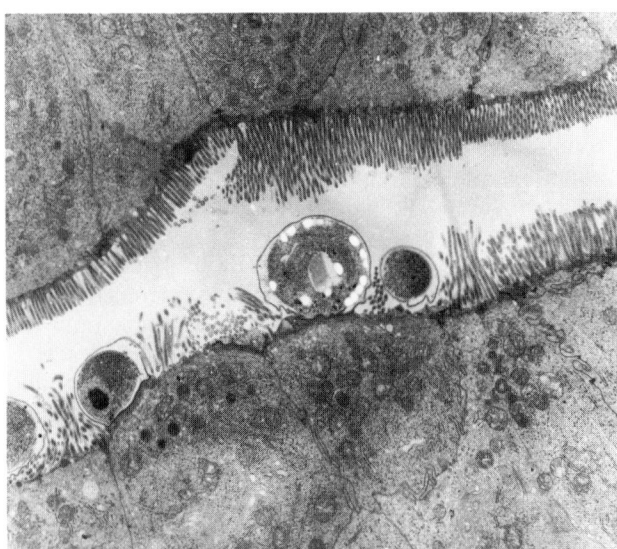

FIGURE 70–2. Electron micrograph of mouse intestine showing *C. parvum*. A uninucleate meront (trophozoite) with prominent nucleolus within a parasitophorous vacuole is shown with a macrogamete; parts of two other meronts are also present (× 6000). (Courtesy of D. P. Casemore.)

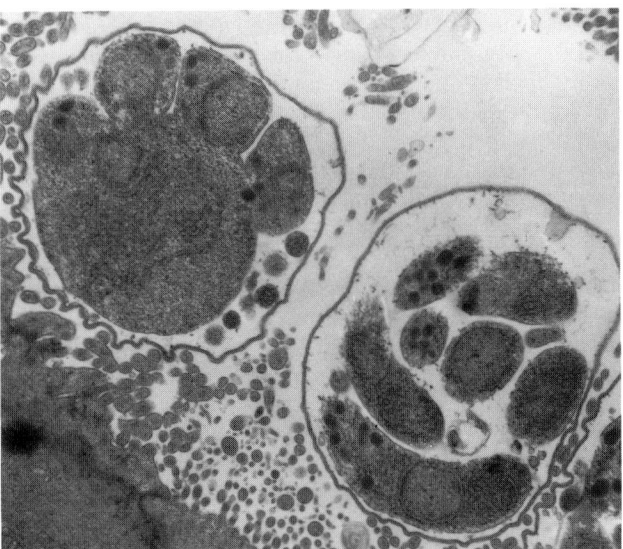

FIGURE 70–3. Electron micrograph showing schizonts (types I and II meronts [trophozoites]) of *Cryptosporidium* sp.; one contains 4 partly developed, and the other parts of 8 fully developed, merozoites that have budded into the parasitophorous vacuole (× 16,000). (Courtesy of D. P. Casemore.)

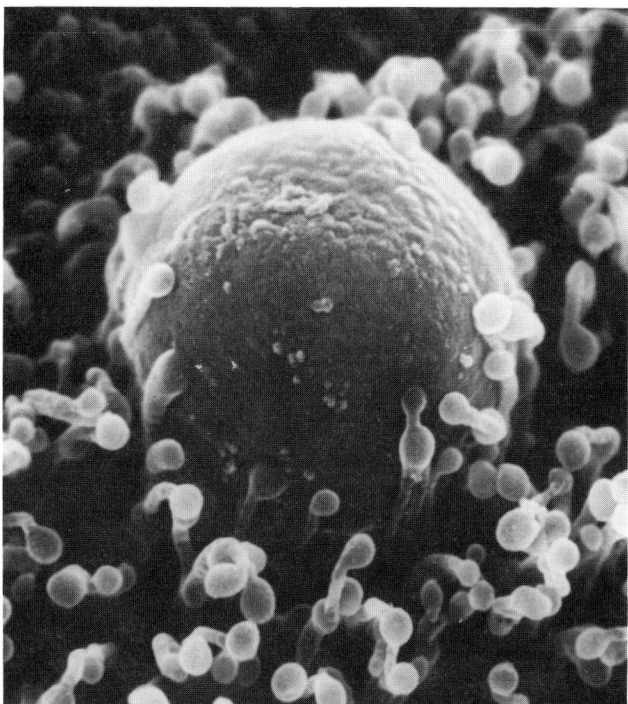

FIGURE 70–4. Scanning electron micrograph showing oocyst of *Cryptosporidium* sp. surrounded by intestinal microvilli in an AIDS patient infected with HIV-2 (× 40,000). (Courtesy of the Electron Microscopy Laboratory, London School of Hygiene and Tropical Medicine.)

Calves are a source of human infection. Whereas farm animals are undoubtedly important in transmission in rural areas, person to person (e.g., in daycare centers) and water-borne transmission are more important in an urban setting. Using immunofluorescence detection, *Cryptosporidium* oocysts can frequently be identified in filtered samples of river water in both developing and developed countries. There are also reports suggesting airborne (which might account for respiratory infection in AIDS) and perinatal transmission. Food-borne disease has not been well documented. Studies in many countries (both developed and developing) have given estimates for the importance of *Cryptosporidium* as a cause of acute diarrhea in both infants and adults. A higher prevalence has been demonstrated in the tropics in the wetter, humid, warmer months of the year. Oocysts can be excreted in feces for up to 2 weeks (and rarely up to 3 months) after cessation of diarrhea, a factor of considerable importance in infection control.

Physicians and other medical personnel require a higher index of suspicion for *Cryptosporidium* infection, and veterinarians should more readily recognize disease in farm animals so that individuals at high risk of serious infection can be warned of this hazard. Rodents, puppies, and kittens are other reservoir hosts that are probably important.

Experimental investigations in both farm and laboratory animals have demonstrated transmission of *C. parvum* oocysts, which are fully sporulated and infective; these cysts (which can remain viable for 9 to 12 months in vitro) are resistant to most commonly used disinfectants, but are readily destroyed by 5% ammonia, commercial bleach (sodium hypochlorite), 10% formol saline, freeze drying, and exposure at −20C or greater than 65C for 30 minutes. Pasteurization of raw milk also renders the oocysts noninfective. Routine chlorination of drinking water has no effect on the infectivity of *Cryptosporidium* oocysts.

CLINICAL MANIFESTATIONS. In most human infections, presentation between the immunointact and immunodeficient individual varies markedly; however, this is not always so and documentation of mild or asymptomatic infection in immunodeficient, and conversely severe diarrhea (of several months' duration) in the immunointact, has been made.

Acute Diarrheal Illness. A self-limited attack of cholera-like diarrheal disease (incubation period 1 to 2 weeks) with a duration of 3 to 12 days constitutes the usual course in the immunointact; bloody diarrhea has not been described and a fecal sample does not contain leukocytes or red blood cells. Most cases occur in children, young adults, and travelers to developing countries. A transient "influenza-like" illness may also be present. Abdominal cramps (colic), nausea, vomiting, low-grade fever, anorexia, weight loss, and headache are occasional associated features. Bloating and flatus are less common than in a *G. lamblia* infection. Shedding of oocysts continues for 8 to 50 days (mean 12 to 14 days); a carrier state and relapse seem unusual in the immunointact.

Chronic Diarrheal Illness. In individuals with AIDS or hypogammaglobulinemia and those receiving immunosuppressive chemotherapy, diarrhea (often accompanied by malabsorption) is frequently torrential and a major factor leading to death; passage of up to 17 liters of fluid feces daily has been recorded. Anorexia, abdominal pain, vomiting, weakness, malaise, low-grade fever, and marked weight loss may also be present. In the immunodepressed, infection is not always confined to the gastrointestinal tract. *Cryptosporidium* has been associated with the "slim disease" of Africans with AIDS.

Extraintestinal Illness. Biliary tract disease, including acute and gangrenous cholecystitis, has been reported; the gallbladder epithelium may be severely involved. Sclerosing cholangitis in AIDS patients has been recorded in mixed *Cryptosporidium* and cytomegalovirus (CMV) infections. Respiratory tract involvement presenting with a chronic cough, dyspnea, bronchiolitis, and pneumonitis has also been reported in immunodeficient individuals.

DIAGNOSIS

Ova in Stool. Failure to recognize *Cryptosporidium* as a cause of human disease until 1976 was in large part associated with the use of inappropriate staining techniques to identify fecal oocysts (in both human and animal hosts). Infected patients with diarrhea excrete much higher numbers of oocysts than those with formed stools. Assuming the infection is large enough to produce moderate oocyst excretion, an acid-fast staining technique is adequate for a reliable diagnosis. The Ziehl-Neelsen or modified Kinyoun carbolfuchsin technique is appropriate (Chapter 122). Negative staining techniques are less reliable. Increased sensitivity can be achieved by the use of a concentration technique, e.g., the formalin-ethylacetate sedimentation or Sheather's sucrose flotation method (Chapter 122). Atypical oocysts occasionally fail to stain by these standard methods. Indirect fluorescent and monoclonal antibody techniques, which have a high degree of sensitivity and specificity, have also been used to detect fecal oocysts; they can also be used for detection of oocysts in contaminated water. *Cryptosporidium* oocysts should be distinguished from yeasts (by an iodine wet mount or acid-fast stain), which are commonly present in fecal samples, often concurrently. All diagnostic laboratories should possess at least 1 technician who has had considerable practice at identifying *Cryptosporidium* and other coccidial oocysts in a fecal specimen; a test sample can be maintained for 12 months if stored cold (4C) in either 2.5% potassium dichromate or 10% formalin.

Biopsies. Light or electron microscopy can detect the developmental stages of *Cryptosporidium* in jejunal, ileal, or colonic biopsy specimens; they can be visualized in the microvillous region of the enterocyte (Fig. 70–1). Serial biopsy techniques can delineate the region of the intestinal tract that is most affected. Other fecal pathogens may also be present concurrently, especially in the presence of AIDS and in developing countries. Oocysts can also be detected in lung biopsy material or sputum (in AIDS).

Serologic Diagnosis. Serum antibody to *Cryptosporidium* can be detected by using an indirect immunofluorescence technique (IFA). An enzyme-linked immunosorbent assay (ELISA) using calf-derived oocysts as antigen has been developed for detecting IgG and IgM; this is of value in both immunointact and immunodeficient individuals, but is not yet available on a commercial basis.

MANAGEMENT

Chemotherapy. Chemotherapeutic agents are not indicated in individuals with an intact immune response; infection is self-limited, but oral rehydration may be required in the acute phase of the illness. When the immune response is depressed (as in AIDS), chemotherapy is indicated but is usually ineffective. The macrolide antibiotic, spiramycin (1 to 3/gm daily for 2 weeks or longer) is the only agent established to be of any value; however, even when temporarily successful, recurrence is usual in the presence of AIDS. At least 70 other agents (given either alone or in combination) have been tested or administered, including co-trimoxazole, erythromycin, furazolidone plus tetracycline, diloxanide furoate, amprolium, polyamines, quinine plus clindamycin, amphotericin B plus flucytosine, α-difluoromethylornithine, interferon-α, and interleukin-2. Unlike other coccidia, *Cryptosporidium* is not sensitive to folate antagonists. The value of azidothymidine (AZT) is presently unclear but promising results have been reported. Development of in vitro culture systems will facilitate testing potentially useful therapeutic agents. Delay in initiating immunosuppressive chemotherapy until after a mild or subclinical *Cryptosporidium* infection has been eliminated may prevent a life-threatening diarrheal illness.

General Measures. Rehydration and measures for symptomatic relief may both be necessary even in the immunointact individual. Codeine phosphate, diphenoxylate, or loperamide may be required to control severe diarrhea in AIDS. Somatostatin has also been used. Hyperimmune bovine colostrum (containing IgG antibodies) has recently been administered orally but with contradictory results. Bovine transfer factor has been of value in the management of cryptosporidiosis associated with AIDS. Immunomodulation, or passive transfer of antibodies or lymphocytes, might also have a place in the treatment of *Cryptosporidium* infection in immunodeficient patients. There is no effective vaccine.

PREVENTION AND CONTROL. A low incidence of infection has been reported in breastfed infants compared with those fed an artificial diet; this suggests that there might be effective lactogenic immunity (although this has not been convincingly demonstrated in either mice or calves). Improved methods for inactivation of infective oocysts would be of value. Elimination of disease from farm animals, especially calves, should be attempted. Standard enteric precautions should be used for those in close contact with infected animals or humans. Filtration of domestic water supplies will help to eliminate infection by this route; however, the small size of the oocysts may limit the usefulness of commonly used filters. Special precautions are required to prevent infection in immunosuppressed patients and those with AIDS. Similarly the potential risk of contracting an infection from an AIDS patient (which seems to be high) should be appreciated; standard enteric precautions are indicated. When traveling, avoidance of exposure to untreated water and uncooked vegetables is important.

BIBLIOGRAPHY

Casemore DP: Human cryptosporidiosis. *In* Reeves DS, Geddes AM (eds): Recent Advances in Infection. Edinburgh, Churchill Livingstone, 1989, pp 209–236.

Casemore DP, Sands RL, Curry A: *Cryptosporidium* species: a "new" human pathogen. J Clin Pathol 38:1321, 1985.

Cook DJ, Kelton JG, Stanisz AM, Collins SM: Somatostatin treatment for cryptosporidial diarrhea in a patient with the acquired immunodeficiency syndrome (AIDS). Ann Intern Med 108:708, 1988.

Cook GC: *Cryptosporidium* sp and Other Intestinal Coccidia: A Bibliography. London, Bureau of Hygiene and Tropical Diseases, 1987, pp v–xiv.

Cook GC: Opportunistic parasitic infections associated with the acquired immune deficiency syndrome (AIDS): Parasitology, clinical presentation, diagnosis and management. Q J Med 65:967, 1987.

Cook GC: Small-intestinal coccidiosis: An emergent clinical problem. J Infect 16:213, 1988.

Cook GC: Parasitic Disease in Clinical Practice. London, Springer Verlag, 1990, pp 77–90.

Current WL: The biology of *Cryptosporidium*. *In* Leech JH, Sande MA, Root RK (eds): Parasitic Infections. Edinburgh, Churchill Livingstone, 1982, pp 109–132.

Fayer R, Ungar BLP: *Cryptosporidium* spp. and cryptosporidiosis. Microbiol Rev 50:458, 1986.

Hart A, Baxby D. Management of cryptosporidiosis. J Antimicrob Chemother 15:3, 1985.

Janoff EN, Reller LB: *Cryptosporidium* species, a protean protozoan. J Clin Microbiol 25:967, 1987.

O'Donoghue PJ: *Cryptosporidium* infections in man, animals, birds and fish. Aust Vet J 62:253, 1985.

Soave R, Ma P: Cryptosporidiosis: Traveler's diarrhea in two families. Arch Intern Med 145:70, 1985.

Tzipori S: Cryptosporidiosis in perspective. Adv Parasit 27:63, 1988.

Ungar BLP, Soave R, Fayer R, Nash TE: Enzyme immunoassay detection of immunoglobulin M and G antibodies to *Cryptosporidium* in immunocompetent and immunocompromised persons. J Infect Dis 153:570, 1986.

Wolfson JS, Richter JM, Waldron MA, et al: Cryptosporidiosis in immunocompetent patients. N Engl J Med 312:1278, 1985.

71. MISCELLANEOUS INTESTINAL PROTOZOA

Martin S. Wolfe

This chapter covers less common intestinal protozoa that are proven or probable pathogens for humans, as well as other nonpathogenic intestinal protozoa that must be differentiated morphologically from those of medical significance (Table 71–1).

Most of the intestinal protozoa pass through trophozoite and cyst stages. The trophozoites are motile, multiply by binary fission, and actively feed. Cysts are less susceptible to changes of environment, can survive better outside the intestinal tract, and are primarily responsible for transmission of the infection.

Identification of specific protozoa is based on certain characteristics of the cyst (Table 71–2) and trophozoite (Table 71–3). Distinguishing features of the trophozoite include the type of motility, food inclusions, and the number and structure of the nuclei. Cysts are distinguished by size and shape, nuclear number and structure, type of chromatoidal bodies when present, and amount and distribution of glycogen. All these features are best demonstrated by permanently stained fecal smears, which should be performed along with unstained

and iodine-stained smears of direct and concentrated stool specimens (Tables 71–2 and 71–3; Chapter 122). Certain intestinal protozoa may be isolated and maintained in artificial culture media (Chapter 122).

71.1. BALANTIDIASIS

DEFINITION. Balantidiasis is caused by *Balantidium coli*, a large pathogenic ciliated protozoan that in rare instances infects humans and produces intestinal symptoms.

DISTRIBUTION AND PREVALENCE. *B. coli* has a worldwide distribution. It has most commonly been reported from various parts of Latin America, the Far East, and New Guinea, but such reports are rare. Prevalence is highest in areas of poor hygiene and nutrition and where pigs and humans have close contact.

TRANSMISSION AND EPIDEMIOLOGY. *B. coli* is widespread in the animal world. Infection is particularly common in pigs, which tolerate the parasite well and are the main source of transmission to humans. In one review, more than 50% of human cases had contact with pigs. The handling and slaughtering of pigs and the use of pig excrement for fertilizing vegetables favor increased transmission. Person to person contact occurs through fecal contamination. Water-borne epidemics have also occurred. Cysts are the infective stage and may remain viable for weeks in moist feces. Excystation occurs in the bowel, and the trophozoites live in the large intestine, where they either remain in the lumen or invade the intestinal mucosa. Encystation occurs either as fecal material is being moved down the bowel or after passage of a semiformed stool.

PATHOGENESIS AND PATHOLOGY. *B. coli* trophozoites can penetrate the mucosa, producing necrosis and ulceration. Masses of *B. coli* trophozoites can then be found in the submucosa, with or without an associated inflammatory reaction (Fig. 71–1). Following mucosal invasion, secondary bacterial invasion may occur, leading to cellular infiltration. Multiplication of balantidia in the tissues leads to ulcers or subsurface abscesses. The ulcers are similar to those caused by *Entamoeba histolytica*, i.e., discrete and round or irregular with undermined edges. The intervening mucosa may be normal or swollen and hemorrhagic. The gross appearance resembles amebic ulceration of the bowel.

B. coli, like *E. histolytica*, may exist for a limited period in the lumen of the large bowel without producing symptoms. Without evidence of invasion, the mucous membrane may be hyperemic and show superficial necrosis. Metastatic spread is extremely rare. The appendix may be invaded by balantidia.

CLINICAL MANIFESTATIONS. As in amebiasis, symptomatology ranges from the asymptomatic carrier state; to chronic symptoms with intermittent diarrhea and constipation, abdominal pain, and weight loss; to a dysenteric form with blood and mucus in the stool, anorexia, nausea, tenderness over the colon, weight loss, and weakness. Fulminating dysentery, although rare, may lead to intestinal perforation, hemorrhage,

TABLE 71–1. Some Important Intestinal Protozoa of Humans

Organism	Potentially Pathogenic	Stages of Organism	
		Trophozoite	*Cyst*
Amebae:			
Entamoeba histolytica	+	+	+
E. hartmanni	−	+	+
E. coli	−	+	+
E. polecki	+	+	+
Iodamoeba bütschlii	−	+	+
Endolimax nana	−	+	+
Flagellates:			
*Dientamoeba fragilis**	+	+	−
Chilomastix mesnili	−	+	+
Pentatrichomonas hominis	−	+	−
Giardia lamblia	+	+	+
Retortamonas intestinalis	−	+	+
Enteromonas hominis	−	+	+
Ciliates:			
Balantidium coli	+	+	+
Sporozoa:			
Isospora belli	+	−	+
Sarcocystis species	+	−	+
Cryptosporidium species	+	−	+
Other:			
Blastocystis hominis†	?	−	?

*Considered an ameba-like flagellate.
†Some workers continue to recognize this as a yeast.

TABLE 71–2. Salient Features of Cysts of Some Intestinal Protozoa of Humans

Parasite	Usual Shape	Usual Size (μm)	Number Nuclei	Nuclear Karyosome	Glycogen Mass (in Iodine)	Chromatoidal Bodies	Other Characteristics
Entamoeba histolytica	Round	10–15	1–4	Small granule	Diffuse, brown. In young cysts	Rod-shaped or thick bars	In fresh unstained cyst: nuclei not visible; chromatoids conspicuous when present
E. hartmanni	Round	<10	1–4	Small granule	Similar to *E. histolytica*	Similar to *E. histolytica*	Similar to *E. histolytica*
E. coli	Round	15–20	1–8	Coarser than in *E. histolytica*	Large, deep brown. In young cysts	Splinterlike or filamentous	Nuclei usually visible in unstained cyst; cyst wall heavy
E. polecki	Round	12–14	1; rarely 2	Large, massed	—	Rod-shaped or spherical; ends angular, pointed, or round	Spherical, ovoid, or irregular inclusion body may be present
Iodamoeba bütschlii	Ovoid; round	6–15	1–2	Bulky, round	Large or small, sharply delimited, deep brown	None	Usually granular mass next to karyosome
Endolimax nana	Ovoid; round	7–10 × 6–7	1–4	Eccentric mass	Occasionally present in young cysts	None	Often cytoplasmic volutin granules confused with karyosomes
Chilomastix mesnili	Lemon-shaped	7–9 × 4.5–6	1	Mass at 1 pole	Sometimes present	None	Oral apparatus beside nucleus
Giardia lamblia	Ovoid	8–12 × 6–10	4	Punctiform, central	None	None	Nuclei at anterior pole; fibrils in cytoplasm
Retortamonas intestinalis	Pear-shaped	4–7 × 3–5	1	Slightly eccentric	None	None	Cyst wall appears double in fresh preparations; margin of cytostome may show when stained
Enteromonas hominis	Elongate; ovoid	6–8 × 4–6	1–4	Small; central	None	None	1 or 2 nuclei at each end; well defined cyst wall
Balantidium coli	Round	50–65	1 macronucleus 1 micronucleus	—	None	None	Macronucleus kidney-shaped, large, conspicuous; contractile vacuole present
Sarcocystis spp.	Ovoid	Sporocyst 10 × 15	—	—	None	None	Oocyst wall usually absent; sporocysts single or paired
Isospora belli	Ovoid	Oocyst 12 × 30	—	—	None	None	Oocyst wall present; 2 sporocysts 9 × 11 μm each within oocyst wall
Cryptosporidium spp.	Spherical	Oocyst 5 × 6	—	—	None	None	Phase-contrast microscopy shows 1 to 6 prominent dark granules and numerous fine dark granules; after sporulating, oocysts contain 4 sporozoites and a spherical residium
Blastocystis hominis	Round	10–15	1–8	—	None	None	Nuclei marginal between inner and outer wall

and shock. Chronic symptoms may persist for many years. A characteristic fetid breath odor has been noted in some patients, resembling that of a pigpen.

DIAGNOSIS. Diagnosis depends on demonstrating *B. coli* in the stool by direct or concentration examinations. Large trophozoites (Fig. 71–2) have been found in about 90% of cases, with cysts being seen only infrequently (Fig. 71–8). *B. coli* trophozoites can be cultured with bacteria in media used for *E. histolytica*.

TREATMENT. The treatments of choice are tetracycline, 500 mg 4 times a day for 10 days, or iodoquinol, 650 mg 3 times a day for 20 days. Other drugs found useful are nitrimidazine (Naxogin) and paromomycin. Mixed results have been reported with metronidazole.

71.2. ISOSPORIASIS

DEFINITION. Isosporiasis is caused by *Isospora belli*, a protozoan of the subphylum Sporozoa, that has alternating generations, one sexual (sporogony) and one asexual (schizogony), in the small bowel mucosa. *Isospora hominis*, formerly grouped together with *I. belli*, is now recognized as a *Sarcocystis* species.

DISTRIBUTION AND PREVALENCE. *I. belli* has a worldwide distribution, but is rarely reported in humans. It is most prevalent in South America and Africa and is usually reported in residents of or returnees from these and other tropical areas. In recent years, *I. belli*

TABLE 71–3. Salient Features of Viable Trophozoites of Some Intestinal Protozoa of Humans

Parasite	Size (μm) Living	Normal Motility	Pseudopodia	Stained Nucleus	Other Characteristics
Entamoeba histolytica	10–25 (rounded forms)	Active, progressive, streaming; cytoplasm flows into pseudopod	Tonguelike, explosively formed	Round; minute karyosome; fine chromatic lining of membrane; ringlike	Living nucleus not visible
E. hartmanni	<12			Similar to *E. histolytica*	
E. coli	20–30 (rounded forms)	Sluggish, not progressive	Blunt, hemispheric, semilunar	Round; coarse karyosome; coarse chromatic lining of membrane; ringlike	Living nucleus visible
E. polecki	16–18 (rounded forms)	Usually sluggish	Rounded, extruded slowly, occasionally 2 or more	Round; karyosome usually small; nuclear membrane thin; ringlike	Living nucleus occasionally seen
Iodamoeba bütschlii	9–13 (rounded forms)	Like *E. coli*	Like *E. coli*	Round; large round karyosome	
Endolimax nana	8–12 (rounded forms)	Usually nonmotile; occasionally slightly progressive	Round, budlike	Round; large irregular karyosome	
Dientamoeba fragilis	5–20 (rounded forms)	Usually sluggish or nonmotile	Triangular (tentlike), rectangular, veil-like, cloverleaf	2 (or 1) nuclei, with mass of chromatin granules embedded in clear matrix	
Chilomastix mesnili	13–24 × 6–11	Flagellate; spiral; body rigid	—	Round; small eccentric or central karyosome	Body pear-shaped; buccal structures prominent; spiral twist in body
Pentatrichomonas hominis	10–15 × 5–8	Flagellate; continuous, jerky, wobbly; body plastic	—	Round or oval; karyosome more or less central	3–5 anterior flagella; undulating membrane and axostyle present
Giardia lamblia	9–21 × 5–15	Active; tumbling and turning like falling leaves; spinning	—	Right and left nuclei; ovoid with prominent irregular karyosomes	Has sucking disk, 8 flagella
Retortamonas intestinalis	4–9 × 3–4	Flagellate; jerky and progressive	—	Round; membrane delicate; karyosome eccentric	2 anterior flagella and 2 blepharoplasts near nucleus
Enteromonas hominis	4–10 × 3–6	Similar to *R. intestinalis*	—	Ovoid; membrane delicate; karyosome large	Body pear-shaped; 3 anterior flagella and 1 along flattened surface and extending free posteriorly
Balantidium coli	50–70 × 30–60	Ciliate; strong progressive swimmer; rapid, gliding	—	Macronucleus sausage-shaped; micronucleus ovoid or round	V-shaped peristome; anus at posterior end

has been increasingly recognized as an opportunistic infection in immunosuppressed male homosexuals in the United States. It is also being found more frequently in those from Haiti and Africa with chronic diarrhea associated with acquired immunodeficiency syndrome (AIDS) (Chapter 15.1).

TRANSMISSION AND EPIDEMIOLOGY. Infection occurs from oral ingestion of ripe oocysts. The oocyst is ovoid, has a thin, translucent cyst wall, and contains 2 spherical sporocysts, which in turn each contain 4 crescent-shaped uninucleate sporozoites (Fig. 71–3). Following ingestion, excystation of these sporulated oocysts occurs in the proximal small intestine. The released sporozoites invade epithelial cells and become round trophozoites. These forms enter the asexual stage, schizogony, and enlarge into mature schizonts contain-

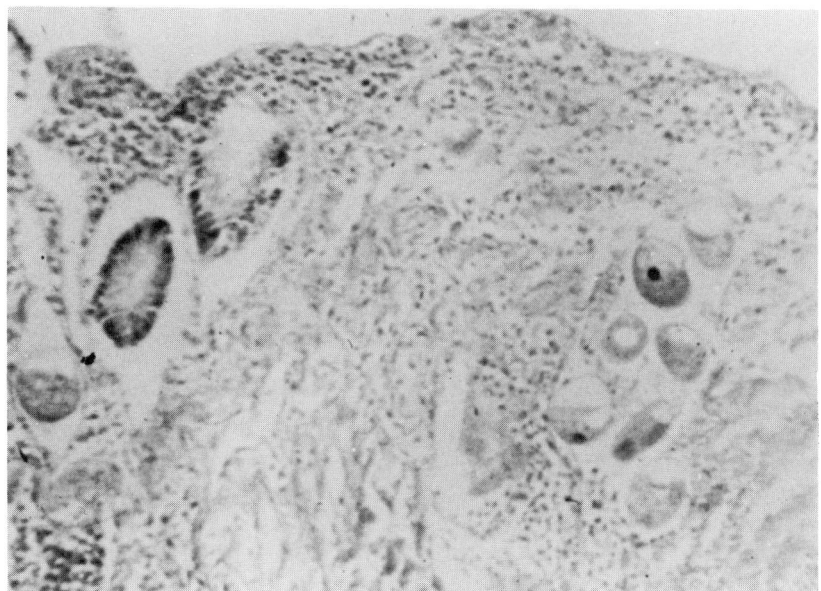

FIGURE 71–1. *Balantidium coli.* Tissue section of colon biopsy specimen showing ulcer with inflammatory response, necrosis, and *B. coli* trophozoites. (H & E stain.)

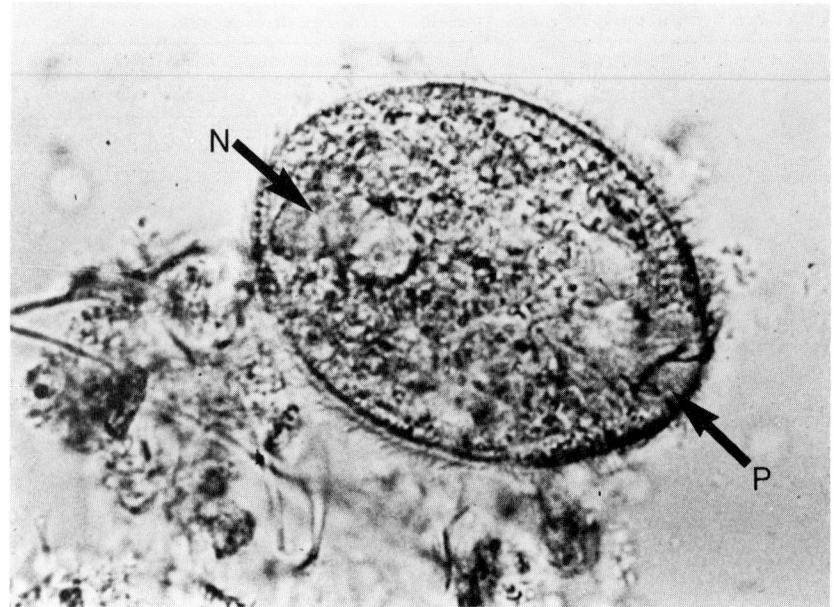

FIGURE 71-2. *Balantidium coli* trophozoite in stool. Note peristome *(P)*, kidney-shaped macronucleus *(N)*, and cilia. (× 400.) (From Smith W, McQuay RM, Ash LR, et al: Diagnostic Medical Parasitology: Intestinal Protozoa. Chicago, The American Society of Clinical Pathologists, 1976.)

ing merozoites. The host cell then ruptures, releasing the merozoites, which invade other epithelial cells. This process may continue for weeks or months and, rarely, for many years. Some merozoites may become sexual gametocytes, either multicellular male microgametocytes or unicellular female macrogametocytes. Male microgametocytes rupture and release flagellated microgametes that fertilize the female macrogametocytes. The fertilized macrogametocytes become unsporulated oocysts that are liberated into the bowel lumen and eliminated in the feces. Stool oocysts usually mature within 48 hours following evacuation from the body, and are then infective.

Infection occurs from ingestion of food or water contaminated with feces containing ripe oocysts. In experimental infections in humans, symptoms developed in 1 week and oocysts were recovered 9 to 15 days after ingestion. There is no evidence of an animal reservoir of *I. belli*.

PATHOGENESIS AND PATHOLOGY. The mechanism by which the invading parasites produce mucosal lesions is unclear. Pathologic changes have been best described in the biopsy specimens of 6 patients studied by Brandborg and associates. The pathology of the small bowel mucosa varied, but none of the patients had a normal mucosa. The 2 most severely ill patients, both of whom died, had a flat mucosa. Another had elongated crypts with stubby residual villi, and yet another had tall villi with focal fusion and flattening. The least severely ill patient had a patchy abnormality, with some biopsies showing only a mild nonspecific abnormality. The epithelium in all 6 patients was often normal, except that all the specimens had foci of vacuolization not necessarily related to the parasites. The parasitized cells were destroyed, but the adjacent cells often appeared normal. The lamina propria contained increased numbers of lymphocytes, plasma cells, and eosinophils. The mucosa was said to be sufficiently damaged to account for the diarrhea and steatorrhea, which are often found in patients infected with *I. belli*.

Little is known of host susceptibility in *I. belli* infections, but immunologic deficiency predisposes to enteritis. Isosporiasis with diarrhea persisting for longer than 1 month is an indicator of the diagnosis of AIDS in a human immunodeficiency virus (HIV)–positive individual.

CLINICAL MANIFESTATIONS. Some *I. belli* infections are asymptomatic, but others may lead to significant disease. Symptoms include diarrhea, abdominal colic, flatulence, malaise, anorexia, weight loss, and low-grade fever. The clinical picture resembles giardiasis or cryptosporidiosis. The stools are often pale and may contain undigested food, mucus, and Charcot-Leyden crystals. Some patients, particularly those with AIDS, may be ill for months or years, but most are symptomatic for only 2 or 3 weeks. Peripheral eosinophilia may be present.

DIAGNOSIS. Oocysts are usually scanty in the stool. Zinc sulfate or sugar flotation is the most sensitive stool concentration technique (Chapter 122). Duodenal drain-

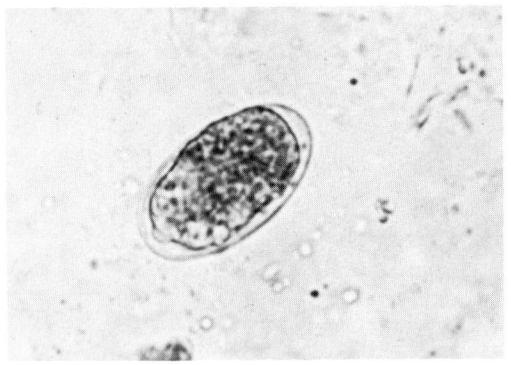

FIGURE 71-3. *Isospora belli* immature oocyst in stool (30 × 12 μm). (Courtesy of the Armed Forces Institute of Pathology.)

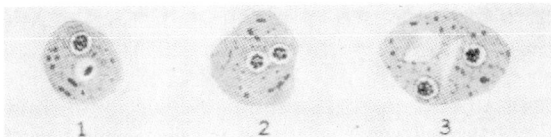

FIGURE 71–4. *Dientamoeba fragilis*. *1*, Uninucleate. *2* and *3*, Binucleate. (After Dobell and O'Connor. From Craig CF: Amebiasis and Amebic Dysentery. Springfield, IL, Charles C Thomas, 1934.)

age and intestinal mucosal biopsy may detect infections not found by stool examinations. It is often necessary to examine multiple serial biopsy sections to find organisms, which may be in both sexual and asexual stages.

TREATMENT. No effective drug treatment was available until recent years, when combined therapy with pyrimethamine and sulfadiazine for 7 weeks was found curative. Subsequently, trimethoprim (160 mg)-sulfamethoxazole (800 mg), every 6 hours for 10 days, then twice a day for 3 weeks, was found curative. Nitrofurantoin and furazolidone may also be useful.

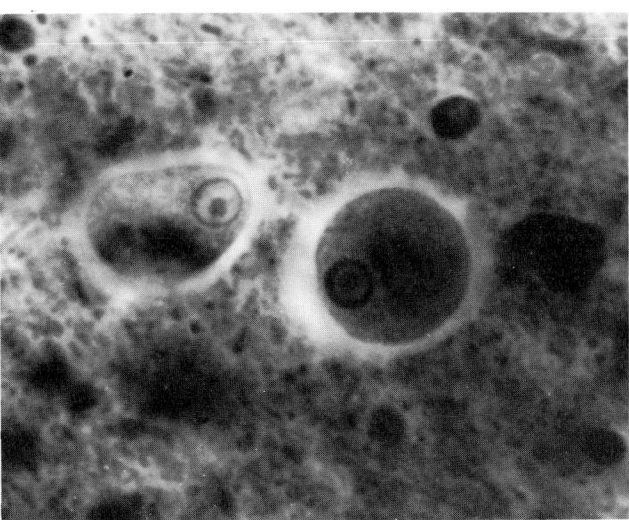

FIGURE 71–5. *Entamoeba polecki*. Uninucleate cysts in stool. Note prominent karyosome and nuclear membrane. (12 × 14 μm.)

71.3. *Dientamoeba fragilis* INFECTION

DEFINITION. *Dientamoeba fragilis*, formerly thought to be an ameba occurring only in a labile trophozoite form, has more recently been considered an ameba-like flagellate more closely related to the genera *Histomonas* and *Trichomonas*.

DISTRIBUTION AND PREVALENCE. *D. fragilis* has a worldwide distribution. When only fresh stool examinations are performed, it is generally considered a rare parasite. Its prevalence is higher in surveys employing preserved stool specimens, permanently stained fecal smears, and multiple stool examinations. The highest prevalence figures have been reported from residents of mental institutions and some missionary groups in the tropics. In recent years *D. fragilis* has become a more commonly recognized parasite in the general American population.

TRANSMISSION AND EPIDEMIOLOGY. The mode of transmission remains uncertain. There is some epidemiologic evidence of water-borne and person to person transmission. A close correlation has been found between the incidence of *Enterobius vermicularis* and *D. fragilis* infections. The combination of these 2 parasites observed in a study in Canada was about 9 times higher than expected on the basis of random distribution. It has therefore been postulated that pinworm eggs or larvae may be a transmitting agent of *D. fragilis*.

PATHOGENESIS AND PATHOLOGY. The ability of *D. fragilis* to invade the host has not been demonstrated; it appears that irritation of the intestinal mucosa is the most likely cause of the symptoms found in infected individuals. Fibrosis was present in appendices infected with *D. fragilis*, and it was postulated that the parasite released an irritant responsible for this. In some cases the parasite has been found in human bile ducts.

CLINICAL MANIFESTATIONS. *D. fragilis* has been considered a nonpathogen by some, and many of those infected are asymptomatic. Symptoms present in others include intermittent diarrhea, abdominal pain,

anorexia, and fatigue. Symptoms reported less commonly include fever, irritability, weight loss, and vomiting. A number of workers have reported a low-grade eosinophilia in infected individuals in the absence of associated pinworm or other helminthic infections; particularly striking was a 50% incidence of eosinophilia in 28 infected children in California. Generalized tenderness to abdominal palpation is present in some infected individuals, but physical examination is otherwise usually unremarkable.

DIAGNOSIS. *D. fragilis* is diagnosed by finding trophozoites in the stool (Fig. 71–4). The presence of the

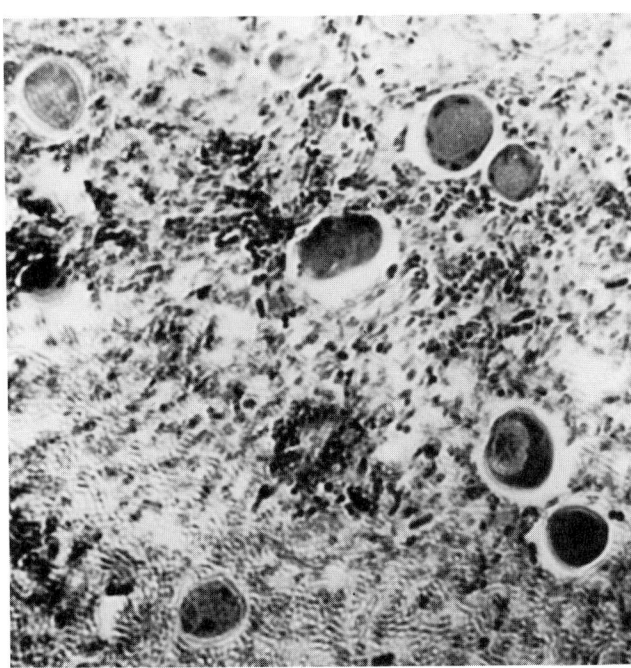

FIGURE 71–6. *Blastocystis hominis*. Stool smear from patient with diarrhea. (H & E stain, × 800.) (Courtesy of Dr. C. H. Zierdt.)

labile trophozoite will often be missed if only fresh stool specimens are examined. Collection into various preservatives immediately on passage of a stool and the preparation and careful examination of stained fecal smears will lead to higher recovery rates (Chapter 122). Some workers report that examination of a purged stool is more productive. *D. fragilis* may also be isolated by culture techniques. Examination of multiple specimens passed on alternate days has also been found useful in diagnosis, as the excretion of parasites may fluctuate markedly from day to day.

TREATMENT. Tetracycline and iodoquinol, alone or in combination in doses used for amebiasis, are often mentioned as the drugs of choice, but careful scrutiny of the literature indicates that cure rates are not high with these drugs. Paromomycin, in a dosage of 500 mg 3 times a day for 5 to 7 days, appears to be more effective. Metronidazole, furazolidone, and diloxanide furoate deserve further evaluation against *D. fragilis*. In earlier studies, good cure rates and clearance of symptoms were obtained with arsenicals, which are no longer in vogue.

71.4. *ENTAMOEBA POLECKI* INFECTION

DEFINITION. *Entamoeba polecki* is an ameba common in the intestine of pigs and monkeys but is rarely reported in humans. It is usually, but not always, nonpathogenic.

DISTRIBUTION AND PREVALENCE. The majority of cases reported in humans have been found in Papua New Guinea, but the distribution appears to be worldwide. It is likely that *E. polecki* is not infrequently mistaken for the much more common and similar-appearing *Entamoeba histolytica*, unless careful examination of permanently stained fecal smears is performed.

TRANSMISSION AND EPIDEMIOLOGY. *E. polecki* occurs in both trophozoite and cyst forms. The most likely source of infection is transmission via cysts from pigs and monkeys to humans, although human to human transmission may also occur.

CLINICAL MANIFESTATIONS. The great majority of recognized cases have been asymptomatic. However, at least 3 patients with heavy infections had intestinal symptoms, including anorexia, diarrhea, mucoid stools, abdominal cramps, malaise, and eosinophilia.

DIAGNOSIS. *E. polecki* cysts are the usual form found in stool examinations (Fig. 71–5). The cysts are consistently uninucleate, and the persistence of uninucleate cysts in multiple stool examinations should raise a strong suspicion of *E. polecki*. Differentiating characteristics in permanently stained fecal smears are described in Tables 71–2 and 71–3.

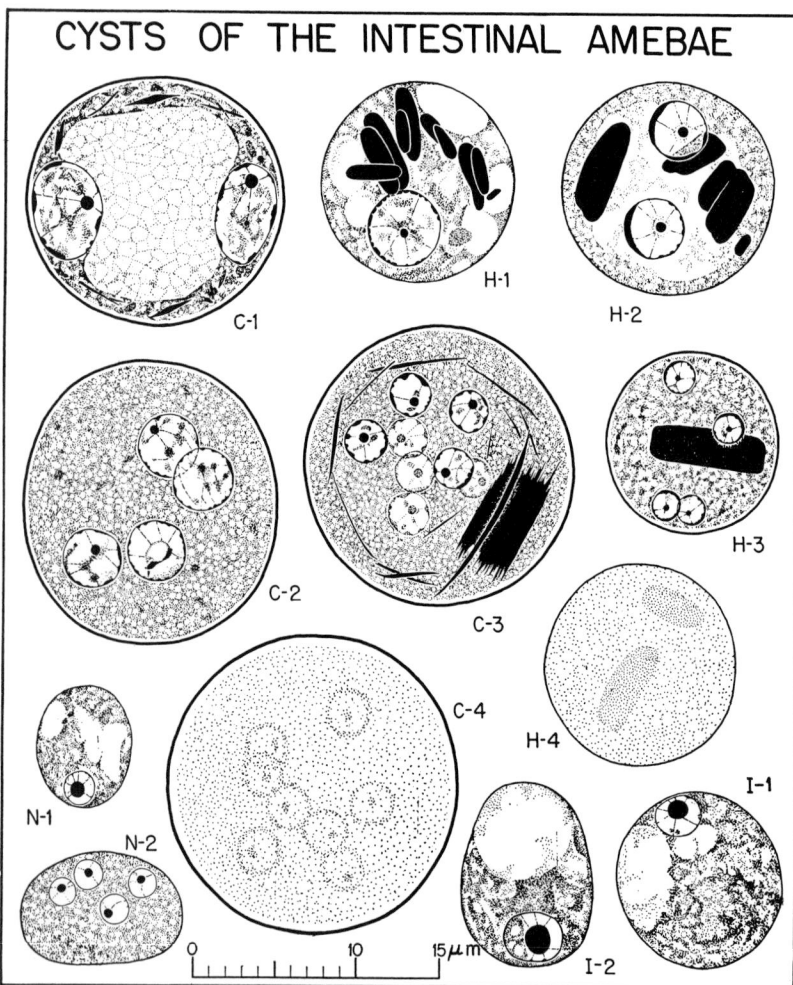

CYSTS OF THE INTESTINAL AMEBAE

FIGURE 71–7. *C-1*, Iron-hematoxylin–stained binucleate cyst of *Entamoeba coli*. *C-2*, Iron-hematoxylin–stained quadrinucleate cyst of *E. coli*. *C-3*, Iron-hematoxylin–stained mature cyst of *E. coli*. *C-4*, Unstained mature cyst of *E. coli*. *H-1*, Iron-hematoxylin–stained uninucleate cyst of *Entamoeba histolytica*. *H-2*, Iron-hematoxylin–stained binucleate cysts of *E. histolytica*. *H-3*, Iron-hematoxylin–stained mature cyst of *E. histolytica*. *H-4*, Unstained cyst of *E. histolytica* showing chromatoidal bars. *N-1*, Iron-hematoxylin–stained uninucleate cyst of *Endolimax nana*. *N-2*, Iron-hematoxylin–stained mature cysts of *E. nana*. *I-1* and *I-2*, Iron-hematoxylin–stained mature cysts of *Iodamoeba bütschlii*.

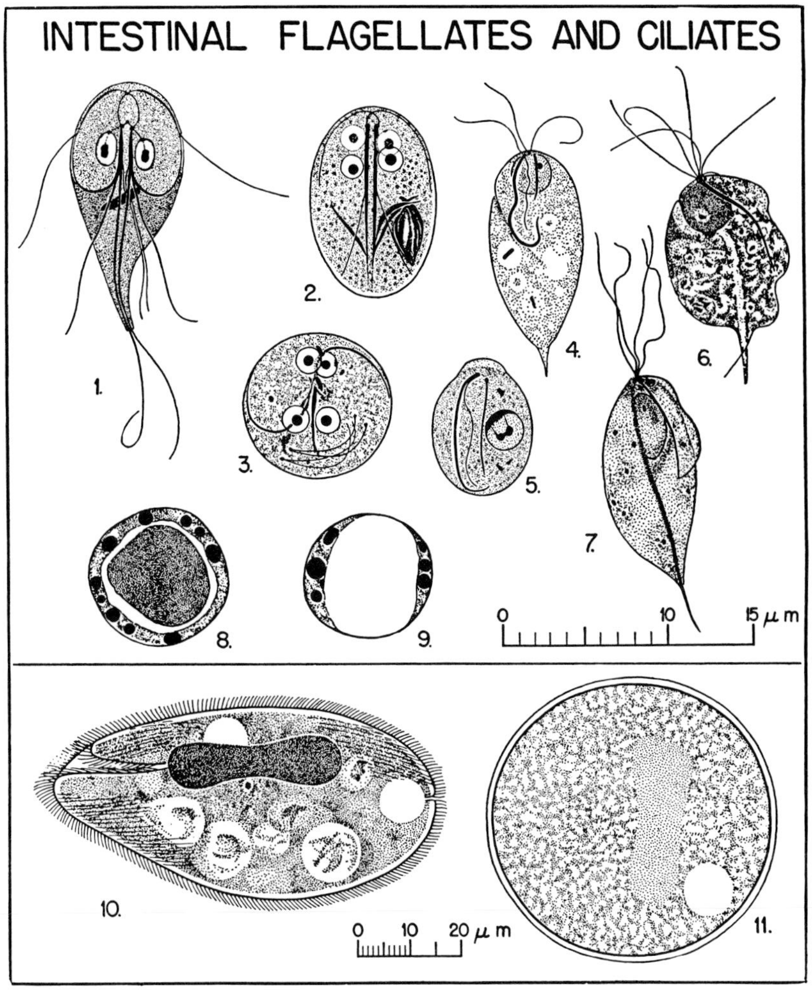

FIGURE 71–8. *1*, Iron-hematoxylin–stained trophozoite of *Giardia lamblia*. *2*, Iron-hematoxylin-stained cyst of *G. lamblia*. *3*, End view of iron-hematoxylin-stained cyst of *G. lamblia*. *4*, Iron-hematoxylin-stained trophozoite of *Chilomastix mesnili*. *5*, Iron-hematoxylin-stained cyst of *C. mesnili*. *6*, Iron-hematoxylin-stained trophozoite of *Pentatrichomonas hominis*. *7*, Iron-hematoxylin-stained trophozoite of *Trichomonas vaginalis*. (*T. vaginalis* dwells in the genitourinary tract and cannot survive in the alimentary canal.) *8*, Iron-hematoxylin-stained *Blastocystis hominis*. *9*, Unstained *B. hominis*. *10*, Trophozoite of *Balantidium coli*. *11*, Unstained cyst of *B. coli*.

TREATMENT. Numerous antiamebic drugs are ineffective against *E. polecki*, but a symptomatic case was cured with only metronidazole, 750 mg 3 times a day for 10 days, followed by diloxanide furoate, 500 mg 3 times a day for 10 days. Another study reported 6 of 8 patients successfully treated with a single course of metronidazole in a regimen similar to that used for *E. histolytica*.

71.5. *Blastocystis hominis* INFECTION

Blastocystis hominis is a common inhabitant of the human intestinal tract. In some stool surveys it has been reported in 10 to 15% of subjects. For many years, most workers regarded *B. hominis* as a harmless yeast. Studies by Zierdt offer convincing evidence that it is a protozoan, but not all protozoan classifications accept it as such. A number of reports in recent years have attributed pathogenicity to *B. hominis*, particularly when the number of organisms present is consistently more than 5 per oil immersion field (Figs. 71–6 and 71–8). When the organism is present in numbers less than this, Zierdt disregards it as a possible agent of disease; in these instances the organism appears uniformly small.

Reported symptoms associated with heavy *B. hominis*

infection in the absence of other recognized pathogenic organisms include mild diarrhea, nausea, anorexia, and fatigue. It remains unclear whether *B. hominis* itself is the cause of these symptoms or if it is only a marker of some other unidentified pathogen. Markell and Udkow have given an interesting perspective to the controversy over the pathogenicity of *B. hominis*. In 32 subjects initially found with *B. hominis* alone, or in combination with nonpathogenic protozoa, an additional series of stool specimens up to a total of 6 were examined. In 27 of these 32 patients, at least 1 known pathogen, in addition to *B. hominis*, was found. *B. hominis* persisted, but symptoms improved in all 27 patients treated specifically for these other pathogens. They concluded that *B. hominis* was not a pathogen and that treatment with common antiprotozoal drugs does not eliminate it from the stool; that "symptomatic blastocystosis" was attributable to either an undetected parasite or parasites in some patients or functional bowel problems in others.

On the basis of these findings, it is recommended that symptomatic patients with heavy infection with *B. hominis* have repeated stool specimens tested by concentration and thorough stained slide examination. With this extra effort, one of the recognized pathogenic protozoa may be found. However, because it remains possible that heavy *B. hominis* infections could cause symptoms, an alternative is to treat with an antiprotozoal drug that has been used with mixed results in *B. hominis* (i.e., iodoquinol, metronidazole, tinidazole, or furazolidone). However, it must be recognized that a symptomatic response could represent the elimination of some other undetected pathogen.

71.6. NONPATHOGENIC INTESTINAL PROTOZOA

A number of nonpathogenic amebae (Fig. 71–7) and flagellates (Fig. 71–8) are frequently found on stool examination, indicating fecal contamination by the host. If intestinal symptoms are present, further search should be made for recognized pathogens.

AMEBAE

Entamoeba hartmanni. Formerly known as "small race" *Entamoeba histolytica*, this organism is morphologically identical to *E. histolytica* and is differentiated primarily on the basis of size (Tables 71–2 and 71–3). Trophozoites in wet preparations measure less than 12 μm and cysts less than 10 μm; on permanent stained smears, trophozoites measure less than 11 μm and cysts measure less than 9 μm.

Entamoeba coli. This is a rather common intestinal protozoan; young cysts can sometimes be difficult to distinguish from *E. histolytica*. Most mature cysts will have at least 5 nuclei visible and be about 15 μm in diameter (Table 71–2 and Fig. 71–7). *E. coli* and *E. histolytica* trophozoites may also pose some difficulty in differentiation (Table 71–3). *E. coli* usually do not have progressive motility nor contain ingested red blood cells.

Endolimax nana. This is perhaps the most common intestinal protozoan. *E. nana* trophozoite and cyst stages are smaller than *E. histolytica*, and the nuclear structure is characteristic (Tables 71–2 and 71–3 and Fig. 71–7).

Iodamoeba bütschlii. This organism is primarily distinguished by the highly vacuolated cytoplasm of the trophozoite and the large glycogen vacuole of the cyst (Tables 71–2 and 71–3 and Fig. 71–7).

FLAGELLATES. The commonly seen flagellate *Chilomastix mesnili* can be differentiated from *Giardia lamblia* by its pear or lemon shape and single nucleus (Tables 71–2 and 71–3 and Fig. 71–8). *Pentatrichomonas hominis*, another flagellate, occurs only in the trophozoite stage and has a single nucleus (Table 71–3 and Fig. 71–8). *Enteromonas hominis* and *Retortamonas intestinalis* are uncommon flagellates and are often overlooked when present. They are usually identified by "ruling out" everything else (Tables 71–2 and 71–3).

BIBLIOGRAPHY

Babcock D, Houston R, Kumaki D, et al: *Blastocystis hominis* in Kathmandu, Nepal. N Engl J Med 313:1419, 1986.
Brandborg LL, Goldberg SB, Breidenbach WC: Human coccidiosis—a possible cause of malabsorption. The life cycle in small-bowel mucosal biopsies as a diagnostic feature. N Engl J Med 283:1306, 1970.
De Hovitz JA, Pape JW, Boncy M, et al: Clinical manifestations and

therapy of *Isospora belli* infection in patients with the acquired immunodeficiency syndrome. N Engl J Med 315:87, 1986.
Garcia LS, Voge M: Diagnostic clinical parasitology. II. Identification of the intestinal protozoa. Am J Med Technol 46:821, 1980.
Gay JD, Abell TL, Thompson JH, et al: *Entamoeba polecki* infection in Southeast Asian refugees. Multiple cases of a rarely reported parasite. Mayo Clin Proc 60:523, 1985.
Kean BH, Malloch CL: The neglected ameba: *Dientamoeba fragilis.* A report of 100 "pure" infections. Am J Dig Dis 11:735, 1966.
Markell EK, Udkow MP: *Blastocystis hominis*: Pathogen or fellow traveler? Am J Trop Med Hyg 35:1023, 1986.
Salaki JS, Shirey JL, Strickland GT: Successful treatment of symptomatic *Entamoeba polecki* infection. Am J Trop Med Hyg 28:190, 1979.
Soave R, Johnson WD: *Cryptosporidium* and *Isospora belli* infections. J Infect Dis 157:225, 1988.
Spencer MJ, Garcia LS, Chapin MR: *Dientamoeba fragilis*. An intestinal pathogen in children? Am J Dis Child 133:390, 1979.
Swartzwelder JC: Balantidiasis Am J Dig Dis 17:173, 1950.
Trier JS, Moxey PC, Schimmel EM, et al: Chronic intestinal coccidiosis in man: Intestinal morphology and response to treatment. Gastroenterology 66:923, 1974.
Yang J, Scholten TH: *Dientamoeba fragilis*: A review with notes on its epidemiology, pathogenicity, mode of transmission, and diagnosis. Am J Trop Med Hyg 26:16, 1977.
Zierdt CH: *Blastocystis hominis*, an intestinal protozoan parasite of man. Public Health Lab 36:147, 1978.
Zierdt CH: *Blastocystis hominis*, a protozoan parasite and intestinal pathogen of human beings. Clin Microbiol Newslett 5:57, 1983.

72. TRICHOMONIASIS

Michael F. Rein

DEFINITION. Trichomoniasis is a specific genitourinary tract infection with *Trichomonas vaginalis*. The organism is highly site specific. *T. tenax* is sometimes found in the mouth, often in association with gingivitis, and *Pentatrichomonas hominis* is sometimes isolated from the colon of patients with diarrhea, but the pathogenicity of neither organism is established. Trichomoniasis is defined by the presence of the organism whether or not the patient is symptomatic.

HISTORY. Donné described the organism in 1836, making it the first sexually transmitted pathogen to be specifically recognized. However, the organism was for a long time regarded as a harmless commensal. Its pathogenicity was established early in the twentieth century through inoculation studies. Therapy was inadequate until the development of metronidazole in the 1960s.

ETIOLOGY. The organism is generally oval and 10 to 20 μm wide. Its characteristic twitching motility is provided by 4 anterior flagella and a recurrent flagellum embedded in an undulating membrane, which runs along two thirds of the cell (Figs. 71–8(7) and 72–1). There is a large, single nucleus and a highly developed Golgi complex. An axostyle, composed of microtubules, projects from the anterior end. Hydrogenosomes replace the mitochondria found in most other organisms. The organism is actively phagocytic, and optimal growth occurs under moderately anaerobic conditions. *T. vaginalis* reproduces by binary fission; cysts are not formed. Individual strains vary in surface antigens and vary in virulence both in vitro and in vivo.

DISTRIBUTION AND INCIDENCE. Trichomoniasis occurs worldwide, in both urban and rural settings. Because it is not reportable, data on incidence and prevalence are unreliable. Figures given for various groups are highly dependent on selection biases. It is crudely estimated that some 3 million infections are acquired annually in the United States. In the 1970s, the World Health Organization estimated a worldwide annual incidence of 180 million cases. The prevalence in tropical populations has ranged from 3.1% among university students in Manila to 15 to 20% among various clinic populations in Asia and Africa, and up to 80% among some prostitutes. The prevalence of trichomoniasis among women in sexually transmitted disease clinics ranges from 7 to 32%.

The prevalence of infection is significantly associated with the nonuse of barrier contraceptives.

Information on the incidence and prevalence of infection in men is essentially nonexistent. The disease is frequently self-limited in men.

TRANSMISSION AND EPIDEMIOLOGY. The venereal nature of trichomoniasis is now unquestioned and is supported by (1) high prevalence among the sexual partners of infected individuals (90 to 100% of women; 30 to 70% of men); (2) highest prevalence among groups with high level of sexual activity; (3) established coprevalence with other sexually transmitted diseases (e.g., the prevalence of gonorrhea among women with trichomoniasis is twice as high as the prevalence of gonorrhea among women without trichomoniasis in the same groups); (4) an increased cure rate if sexual partners are treated simultaneously; and (5) failure, with few exceptions, of the disease to appear in household contacts who are not sexual partners. Recognizing the sexually transmitted nature of the infection is extremely important because patients with trichomoniasis should be screened for other sexually transmitted diseases that may be clinically silent but of greater eventual medical significance.

The organism can survive for several hours in a suitably moist environment, and the possibility of nonvenereal transmission is often raised. Nonvenereal acquisition of T. vaginalis by adults is extremely rare. Perinatal acquisition of disease, however, is reported in about 5% of female babies vaginally delivered by infected mothers.

Fewer than 10^4 trichomonads can produce infection in women, and 4×10^6 protozoa can cause infection in men.

PATHOGENESIS AND PATHOLOGY. The mechanisms by which T. vaginalis causes disease are not well understood. The organism is isolated from the vagina in more than 95% of infected women and from the urinary tract alone in less than 5%. Squamous, but not columnar, epithelium is infected, and organisms are rarely isolated from the endocervix. The urethra is, however, involved in 90% of cases, and organism have been isolated from bladder urine. Rarely, trichomonads have been recovered from the epididymis and identified in the prostate.

Trichomoniasis in women ranges from asymptomatic carriage to severe inflammation. Initially asymptomatic disease frequently becomes symptomatic, supporting the need to treat asymptomatic carriers. Trichomoniasis in men is almost always asymptomatic, but T. vaginalis causes some cases of tetracycline-resistant nongonococcal urethritis.

Trichomonal vaginitis elicits vaginal discharge containing large numbers of polymorphonuclear neutrophils (PMNs). Organisms are found free in the vaginal cavity or adhering to the epithelium. Tissue invasion does not occur. Colposcopy reveals microscopic hemorrhages in about 50% of cases, but these are visible to the naked eye only in 1 to 2% of cases.

In vitro, trichomonads destroy epithelial cells with which they make direct contact. In biopsies of human infection, microulcerations are observed under clumps of trichomonads.

Low titers of serum antibody are detected in human infections, but the humoral response cannot be used for diagnosis. Local IgA is detected in most infections. Delayed hypersensitivity can be demonstrated by skin testing in many infected women. PMNs and macrophages are capable of killing Trichomonas.

CLINICAL FEATURES

Disease in Women. In various series, 50 to 90% of women with trichomoniasis have symptoms, but this observation depends on the way in which the series are collected. Many women with trichomoniasis have other sexually transmitted infections, and it is sometimes difficult to attribute specific clinical features to trichomoniasis alone. Vaginal discharge is described by 50 to 75% of infected women, but the discharge is considered malodorous by only 10%. One quarter to one half of infected women note vulvar irritation or pruritus, and up to 50% suffer dyspareunia. Dysuria, usually "internal," is sometimes present but usually mild.

Lower abdominal discomfort is described by only 10% of women, and its presence, particularly if accompanied by adnexal tenderness on bimanual examination, should suggest the possibility of coincident salpingitis of a different cause.

Some women report that symptoms began or were exacerbated immediately following a menstrual period. In experimentally induced infection, the incubation period reportedly ranges from 3 to 28 days.

The vulva is erythematous in less than one third of patients. On speculum examination, excessive discharge is noted in 50 to 75% of infected women. A yellow vaginal discharge suggests trichomoniasis, but the classically yellow or green, frothy discharge is seen in only a minority of patients. Indeed, bubbles are present in only 8 to 50% of infected women in various series, and bubbles are also seen in bacterial vaginosis, so their presence is nonspecific.

Vaginal wall erythema is observed in 20 to 75% of cases, and punctate hemorrhages are rarely observed on the vaginal walls or the exocervix.

Disease in Men. Most infected men are asymptomatic and come to treatment as sexual contacts of infected women. T. vaginalis causes some cases of nongonococcal urethritis (NGU), which are usually recognized because they fail to respond to standard therapies. When symptomatic, such infections resemble NGU of other etiologies. The organism can be recovered from 70% of men who have had sex with an infected woman within the past 48 hours. Rarely, involvement of the epididymis and prostate are encountered.

Disease in Children. Perhaps 5% of babies born to infected women contract trichomoniasis. Infected children may be febrile and fussy. Trichomoniasis in older children may indicate sexual abuse.

COMPLICATIONS. Trichomoniasis is a relatively benign disease. Older studies suggested a relationship to premature rupture of the fetal membranes and a postpartum endometritis syndrome, but these associations are poorly documented. Likewise, early attempts to relate trichomoniasis to cancer of the cervix were uncontrolled for other sexually transmitted agents of much higher malignant potential (e.g., human papillomavirus).

DIAGNOSIS. The definitive diagnosis of trichomoniasis rests on demonstration of the parasite (Fig. 72–1). The clinician is often confronted with a symptomatic woman who presents for evaluation of some combination of vaginal discharge, vulvar irritation, or odor. A history of contact with a new partner supports the diagnosis of sexually transmitted vaginitis. Recent use of antibiotics, on the other hand, increases the likelihood of a candidal etiology. The presence of odor without much irritation is somewhat more consistent with bacterial vaginosis than with trichomoniasis, in which irritation is more prominent.

Physical Examination. The female patient is examined in the lithotomy position. The vulva should be carefully evaluated for lesions of other sexually transmitted diseases. The presence of *satellite lesions*, small papulopustules beyond an area of erythema, suggests vulvovaginal candidiasis.

Some women with trichomoniasis are sufficiently tender so that the speculum cannot be inserted without

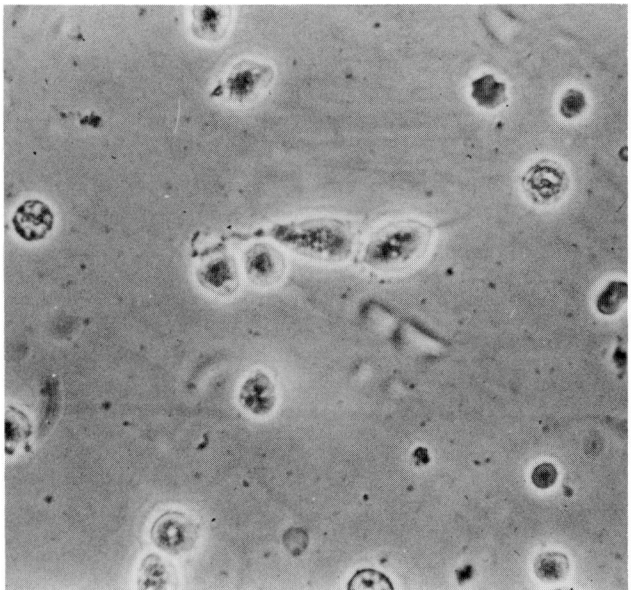

FIGURE 72–1. Trichomoniasis. Wet mount of vaginal discharge showing several round polymorphonuclear neutrophils and two ovoid trichomonads. Anterior flagella are visible. (Phase contrast, × 1000.)

undue discomfort. In such women, a swab gently inserted into the vagina can be used to recover material for evaluation. If the diagnosis of trichomoniasis is thereby made, such women should be asked to return for re-evaluation after the infection has resolved, so that coincident sexually transmitted diseases can be sought.

On insertion of the speculum, the vaginal walls may be erythematous and edematous. Vaginal wall inflammation is seen with trichomoniasis and candidiasis but not with bacterial vaginosis. The amount and nature of vaginal discharge is noted. A frankly yellow discharge supports a diagnosis of trichomoniasis, but bubbles are also seen with bacterial vaginosis. It is important to examine the cervix for evidence of cervicitis and purulent or mucopurulent discharge. Cervical discharge is dumped into the vaginal pool. After wiping off the exocervix, cervical material is recovered for appropriate laboratory examination. Vaginal discharge is then obtained by swabbing the vaginal fornices. The specimen can be transferred directly to a microscope slide, or (preferably) the swab may be agitated in a tube containing about 1 ml of saline.

T. vaginalis can be cultured in a variety of media. A swab of vaginal discharge can be agitated in a tube of liquid medium.

Laboratory Evaluation. After completing the physical examination, it is useful to determine the pH of vaginal secretions. This is conveniently accomplished by inserting a strip of indicator paper into the vaginal discharge pooled in the lower lip of the speculum. The normal vaginal pH of 4.5 or less is maintained in most patients with vulvovaginal candidiasis. The vaginal pH is elevated above 4.5 in three fourths or more of women with trichomoniasis. An elevated pH is also seen in most women with bacterial vaginosis and is not specific. The pH of vaginal material may be artifactually elevated if contaminated with cervical discharge, which has an elevated pH. Recent coitus can elevate the apparent pH because semen is considerably more alkaline than normal vaginal secretions.

After the pH has been determined, several drops of 10 to 20% potassium hydroxide should be added to the discharge in the speculum. The clinician then seeks the elaboration of a pungent, fishy, amine-like odor. This positive "whiff test" is manifested by 75% of women with trichomoniasis but is also seen in most women with bacterial vaginosis. The whiff test is not positive in vulvovaginal candidiasis.

Microscopic Evaluation. Bedside techniques tend to separate infectious vaginitides into candidiasis on the one hand, and trichomoniasis or bacterial vaginosis on the other. Final differentiation is based on microscopic examination of the vaginal discharge. A drop of the wet mount preparation is examined microscopically under a coverslip, with the substage condenser racked down and the substage diaphragm closed to increase contrast.

In bacterial vaginosis, the normal flora of rods is replaced by clumps of coccobacilli. Few PMNs are observed, with 1 PMN per epithelial cell being considered normal. The epithelial cells are encrusted with coccobacilli, so-called clue cells.

In trichomoniasis, on the other hand, the flora consists of rods or coccobacilli. The epithelial cells are clean (unless bacterial vaginosis is coincidentally present), and there are usually larger numbers of PMNs. Motile trichomonads are seen in 40 to 80% of infected women, with most studies yielding a sensitivity of approximately 67%. The organisms are best recognized by their characteristic twitching motility, but this motility decreases in older, cooled preparations.

Presumptive Diagnosis. Trichomonads are not recognized in the vaginal discharge of about one third of infected women. The presence in a sexually active woman of an abnormal discharge, particularly if it is yellow; an elevated vaginal pH; a positive whiff test; and excess PMNs in the wet mount (assuming the patient does not have a purulent cervical discharge) can be presumptive evidence of trichomonal infection. On the other hand, clue cells and the absence of PMNs argue for a diagnosis of bacterial vaginosis.

Diagnosis in Men. Trichomonal infection is difficult to diagnose in men. Occasionally, the wet mount of urethral discharge reveals motile organisms. The most effective way to make the diagnosis is by culture, optimally of the urine sediment obtained following prostatic massage. Most men are "epidemiologically" treated for trichomoniasis because they have had sexual contact with infected women.

Stains. Trichomonads may be detected in genital discharge with a variety of stains. The Giemsa stain is approximately 50% sensitive, and an acridine orange stain will detect organisms in about 60% of cases. New fluorescent antibody techniques have a sensitivity of 80 to 90% compared to culture. The routine Papanicolaou stain of a cervical specimen is said to detect organisms in 60 to 70% of cases. The Gram stain is useless.

Culture. Culture techniques are not widely used but appreciably increase the detection of trichomoniasis. Trichomonads grow best in anaerobic environment at about 37C; the addition of antibiotics allows for selective growth. Several media are used, and cultures are usually read daily for 7 days before being discarded as negative. The sensitivity of the culture exceeds 95%.

Serodiagnosis. Although serum antibodies can be detected in many infected patients, serologic diagnosis is experimental and adds nothing to the management of the individual case.

TREATMENT. The treatment of trichomoniasis was revolutionized by the development of the 5-nitroimidazoles. *T. vaginalis* is not susceptible to many other antimicrobial agents.

Susceptibility testing of trichomonads is not standardized. Still, most strains of *T. vaginalis* are highly susceptible to metronidazole and related drugs, with minimal inhibitory concentrations of 1 μg/ml or less. Minimum trichomonacidal concentrations range from 0.25 to 16 μg/ml. Recently, isolates of *T. vaginalis* with relatively high levels of resistance to metronidazole have been obtained from patients who were not cured by repeated courses of the drug. Testing under aerobic conditions enhances the difference between susceptible and resistant organisms. Resistance should be considered a possible explanation for repeated treatment failures.

The recommended treatment of trichomoniasis in women consists of 2.0 gm of metronidazole administered as a single oral dose (or another 5-nitroimidazole in equivalent dosage). This regimen cures about 85% of infected women; if sexual partners are treated simultaneously, the cure rate exceeds 95%. An older regimen consisting of 250 mg orally 3 times daily for 7 days is at least as effective but requires a larger total administration and is highly dependent on patient compliance.

The 7-day regimen is highly effective in curing men, but the single-dose regimen, although probably effective, has not been extensively evaluated. Asymptomatic male sexual partners of infected women should be treated.

Treatment of trichomoniasis in pregnancy is unsatisfactory. The 5-nitroimidazoles should be avoided during the first trimester, and symptomatic women might be treated with clotrimazole, 100 mg intravaginally at night, which relieves symptoms in many cases but, in a 7-day course, cures only about 20%. After the first trimester, women can probably be given metronidazole safely.

Side effects of metronidazole include nausea and vomiting. When taken with alcohol, metronidazole may produce a disulfiram-like effect manifested as flushing, headache, nausea, vomiting, vertigo, dyspnea, and tachycardia. Some treated women subsequently develop candidiasis. Metronidazole and similar drugs potentiate the effects of anticonvulsants and warfarin. Reversible neutropenia is sometimes observed.

Because they have been associated with unacceptably high failure rates, the wide variety of topical therapies proposed over the years are not considered effective primary therapy for this infection.

PROGNOSIS. Severe complications of trichomoniasis are essentially unreported. Putative associations with salpingitis and cervical carcinoma probably result from the coprevalence of other sexually transmitted diseases.

PREVENTION AND CONTROL. Nonoxynol 9, a spermaticide found in many vaginal preparations, is trichomonacidal. The degree of actual protection provided by such preparations is undefined. Appropriately used condoms will prevent the transmission of trichomoniasis. No effective vaccine strategy has been developed.

BIBLIOGRAPHY

Honigberg BM (ed): Trichomonads Parasitic in Humans. New York, Springer-Verlag, 1989.

Krieger JN: Urologic aspects of trichomoniasis. Invest Urol 18:411, 1981.

Krieger JN, Tam MR, Stevens CE, et al: Diagnosis of trichomoniasis. Comparison of conventional wet-mount preparation with cytologic studies, cultures, and monoclonal antibody staining of direct specimens. JAMA 259:1223, 1988.

Latif AS, Mason PR, Marowa E: Urethral trichomoniasis in men. Sex Transm Dis 14:9, 1987.

Lossick JG, Muller M, Gorrell TE: In vitro drug susceptibility and doses of metronidazole required for cure in cases of refractory vaginal trichomoniasis. J Infect Dis 15:17, 1988.

Muller M, Lossick JG, Gorrell TE: In vitro susceptibility of *Tricho-*

moniasis vaginalis to metronidazole and treatment outcome in vaginal trichomoniasis. Sex Transm Dis 15:17, 1988.
Rein MD, Muller M: *Trichomonas vaginalis. In* Holmes KK, Mardh PA, Sparling PF, et al (eds): Sexually Transmitted Diseases, 2nd ed. New York, McGraw-Hill, 1990, pp 481–492.

Robbie MD, Sweet RL: Metronidazole use in obstetrics and gynecology: A review. Am J Obstet Gynecol 145:865, 1983.
Wolner-Hanssen P, Krieger JN, Stevens CE, et al: Clinical manifestations of vaginal trichomoniasis: Implications for strategies for diagnosis and of the infection. JAMA 264:571, 1989.

SECTION B

INFECTIONS OF THE BLOOD AND RETICULOENDOTHELIAL SYSTEM

73. MALARIA

G. Thomas Strickland

DEFINITION. Malaria is an acute and chronic disease caused by obligate intracellular protozoa of the genus *Plasmodium*. The 4 species that cause human malaria are *P. malariae* (Laveran, 1881), *P. vivax* (Grassi and Feletti, 1890), *P. falciparum* (Welch, 1897), and *P. ovale* (Stephens, 1922). The parasites are cyclically transmitted to humans by female mosquitoes of the genus *Anopheles*. The clinical course is characterized by paroxysms of high fever, chills, anemia, and splenomegaly. *P. falciparum* often causes serious or fatal complications.

ETIOLOGY. The zoologic family Plasmodidae contains protozoal parasites found in the blood of birds, reptiles, and mammals. These organisms undergo 2 types of asexual division called schizogony in the vertebrate host and undergo a single sexual multiplication termed sporogony in the mosquito host. As noted previously, human malaria parasites belong to the genus *Plasmodium*. In this genus, one cycle of asexual division called exoerythrocytic schizogony occurs in the parenchymal cells of the liver of the vertebrate host; the mosquito vector is a species of *Anopheles*.

There are more than 100 species of plasmodia, including 82 of birds and reptiles and 22 of nonhuman primates. Some of the latter parasites are closely related to human plasmodia and can produce disease in man under both natural and experimental conditions. However, such infections are rare and of no epidemiologic significance.

HISTORY. Few diseases have had a greater impact on human social and economic development than malaria. Prehistoric man was subject to malaria; it is probable that the disease originated in Africa. Fossil mosquitoes have been found in geologic strata 30 million years old. The infection was probably spread throughout the warmer regions of the globe long before the dawn of history.

Although the disease was not named until the eighteenth century by the Italians (*mal aria*—foul air), the first references to periodic fevers can be found in early Hindu and Chinese writings. In the fifth century B.C., the Greek physician Hippocrates was the first to describe

clinical manifestations and some complications of malaria and to logically relate the appearance of the disease to the seasons of the year or the places where his patients lived. The association of periodic fevers and splenomegaly with exposure to stagnant waters and swamps led the Greeks, and later the Romans, to undertake various methods of drainage—still an effective method of malaria control.

In the early seventeenth century, the bark of the Peruvian guina-guina (cinchona) tree was successfully used for treatment of intermittent fever. However, the alkaloid quinine, the active ingredient, was not isolated until 1820 by Pelletier and Caventou in France.

The first major breakthrough in understanding the etiology of the disease came in 1880, when Laveran, a French army surgeon in Algeria, first described exflagellated gametocytes of *P. falciparum* in a fresh blood film from a patient with malaria. Five years later, Golgi reported in detail the asexual forms of *P. vivax* and *P. malariae*. The polychrome staining method developed by Romanowsky in 1891 permitted more detailed morphologic studies.

Transmission remained a mystery until the 1880s, when Patrick Manson discovered that filariasis was transmitted by mosquitoes and postulated that malaria was similarly transmitted. In 1897, Ronald Ross, a British army surgeon in India, found a developing form of the malaria parasite in the gut of a mosquito that had previously fed on a malarious patient. In 1898, Ross conclusively established the major features of the life cycle of plasmodia by a careful series of experiments in naturally infected sparrows. The complex cycle of development was confirmed as the result of further studies by Bignami, Bastianelli, and Grassi in Italy in 1898 and 1899, and by Patrick Manson and his colleagues in London and Rome in 1900. The exoerythrocytic (E-E) cycle of *P. cynomolgi* was described by Shortt and Garnham in 1948. In 1980, Krotoski and Garnham demonstrated a dormant liver stage in *P. cynomolgi*, termed a hypnozoite, postulated to be responsible for late relapses.

During the twentieth century, progress has been made in vector control technology and in the development of potent synthetic antimalarial compounds. Larvicides in the form of oil and Paris green were introduced; these and other methods of mosquito reduction proved useful in controlling malaria and yellow fever in Panama and

Cuba. In the late 1930s, Paul Muller in Switzerland discovered the potent insecticidal activity of dichlorodiphenyltrichloroethane (DDT). From 1942 to 1946, new synthetic residual insecticides, including hexachlorocyclohexane (BHC), dieldrin, and chlordane, were developed.

The difficulties of securing inexpensive supplies of quinine during war stimulated research aimed at discovering synthetic antimalarial compounds. These investigations resulted in the discovery of pamaquine (1924), quinacrine (1930), chloroquine (1934), chlorguanide (1945), amodiaquine (1946), primaquine (1950), and pyrimethamine (1951).

In 1955, encouraged by the high potency of DDT and other residual insecticides against mosquitoes as well as their low toxicity, ease of application in rural areas, and low cost, the World Health Assembly (WHA) adopted the idea of global eradication. Two years later, a program of worldwide malaria eradication was launched by the World Health Organization (WHO).

The development of resistance to DDT by some vectors, as well as resistance to chloroquine by strains of *P. falciparum*, severely impaired the success of this program. In 1969, WHO revised the eradication strategy to stress the need for further research and for greater involvement of general health services in the program. During the last 20 years, there has been an increase of malaria in many areas. In 1978, the WHA endorsed a strategy of malaria control based on assessment of localized control potential. This ranges from a reduction in morbidity and elimination of mortality in poorly developed areas of malarial hyperendemicity (mainly using chemotherapy) to a comprehensive campaign stressing personal protection and vector reduction through community-based bioenvironmental interventions (rather than dependence on insecticide spraying).

DISTRIBUTION AND INCIDENCE. Malaria transmission occurs in more than 100 countries throughout Africa, Asia, Oceania, and Latin America, on certain Caribbean islands, and in Turkey (Fig. 73–1). More than 1.6 billion inhabitants of these areas are exposed to risk of malarial infection. The estimated annual global incidence of malaria is 200 million clinical cases. In sub-Saharan Africa alone, there are more than 100 million cases each year, with an estimated 1 million deaths, mostly in infants and young children.

Malaria transmission has been interrupted in the United States and Canada, Europe including the USSR, parts of South America, the Caribbean excepting Haiti and the Dominican Republic, Israel, Lebanon, Réunion, Singapore, Hong Kong, Japan, Korea, Taiwan, Brunei, and Australia. However, many cases are imported into these countries, with the United States receiving around 1000 annually, and Europe 5000.

P. falciparum and *P. malariae* are found in most malarious areas. *P. falciparum* is the predominant species in Africa, Haiti, and New Guinea. *P. vivax* predominates in Latin America. *P. falciparum* and *P. vivax* are both common in South America, the Indian subcontinent, Southeast Asia, and Oceania. *P. ovale* occurs mainly in Africa, with rare cases reported from other continents. *P. vivax* is rare in Africa because most black persons are genetically resistant to this parasite.

TRANSMISSION. Malaria is transmitted by the bite of an infected female *Anopheles* mosquito or through direct inoculation of infected red blood cells, i.e., congenital malaria, transfusion malaria, and malaria from contaminated needles.

Life Cycle. The life cycle of malaria is complex (Fig. 73–2), and certain aspects differ according to the *Plasmodium* species involved (Table 73–1). The infective stages of plasmodia, called *sporozoites* (Fig. 73–3), are injected during feeding from the salivary glands of the infected mosquito into the blood stream through subcutaneous capillaries. After 30 minutes, the sporozoites disappear from the blood.

Exoerythrocytic Phase. Some sporozoites are destroyed by phagocytes, but many enter the parenchymal cells of the liver (hepatocytes), where they multiply asexually in a process known as *exoerythrocytic schizogony* (Fig. 73–4A and B, Plate I). There the nucleus undergoes repeated division, resulting in the formation of thousands of uninucleate *merozoites*, each measuring 0.7 to 1.8 μm in diameter. The nucleus of the liver cell is displaced, but there is no inflammatory reaction in the surrounding liver tissue.

After 6 to 16 days from the time of infection, the hepatic cell containing the tissue schizont ruptures and the merozoites enter the circulation. In infection due to *P. falciparum* and *P. malariae*, the tissue schizonts all rupture at about the same time, and none persists in the liver. In contrast, *P. vivax* and *P. ovale* have 2 types of exoerythrocytic forms. A primary type develops and ruptures within 6 to 9 days. In addition, there is a secondary type, the hypnozoite, that may remain dormant in the liver for weeks, months, or up to 5 years before developing and resulting in *relapses* of erythrocytic infection. The first hypnozoites identified were those of *P. cynomolgi*, a simian parasite resembling *P. vivax* (Fig. 73–4A and B, Plate I).

P. falciparum and *P. malariae* have no persistent exoerythrocytic phase, and therefore relapses do not occur in infections with these species; recurrent parasitemia is due to proliferation of persistent erythrocytic forms and is known as recrudescence. The prolonged, delayed recrudescences occasionally seen with *P. malariae* are due to erythrocytic parasites that have persisted in the tissue microcapillary circulation. The following facts support the contention that true relapses do not occur in *P. malariae* infection: (1) *P. malariae* infection can be cured by blood schizonticides alone; (2) no exoerythrocytic schizonts have been found in the liver of chimpanzees or humans after the primary cycle; and (3) parasites persist in the blood for prolonged periods, as evidenced in some cases of transfusion malaria.

Erythrocytic Phase. Merozoites released from tissue schizonts invade erythrocytes. Invasion depends on the interaction of a specific receptor on the red blood cells, glycophorin, and the merozoite. At least one glycophorin-binding protein has been isolated, characterized, and studied. The anterior end of the merozoite attaches to the erythrocyte membrane. The membrane of the merozoite thickens and joins with the plasma membrane of the erythrocyte, and then invaginates, forming a vacuole within which the parasite lies. As the merozoite

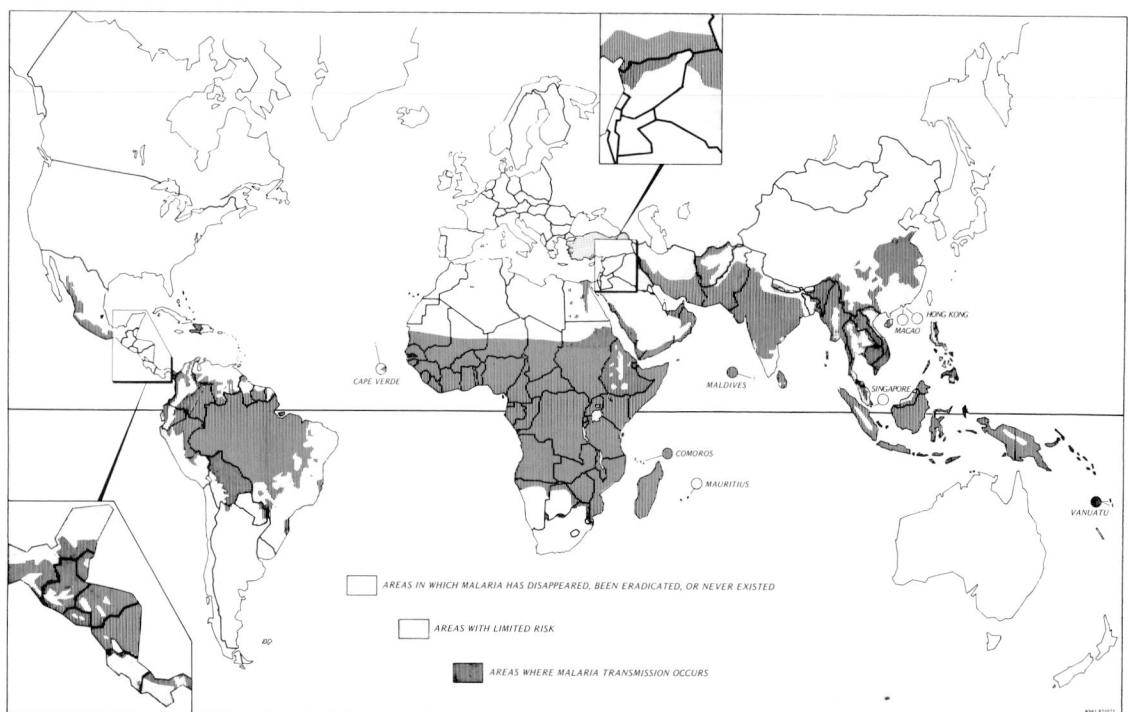

FIGURE 73–1. Epidemiologic assessment of status of malaria. Reproduced with permission of WHO. (Courtesy of the Director General and Joachim H.-G. Hempel. Epidemiological Methodology and Evaluation, Malaria Action Programme.)

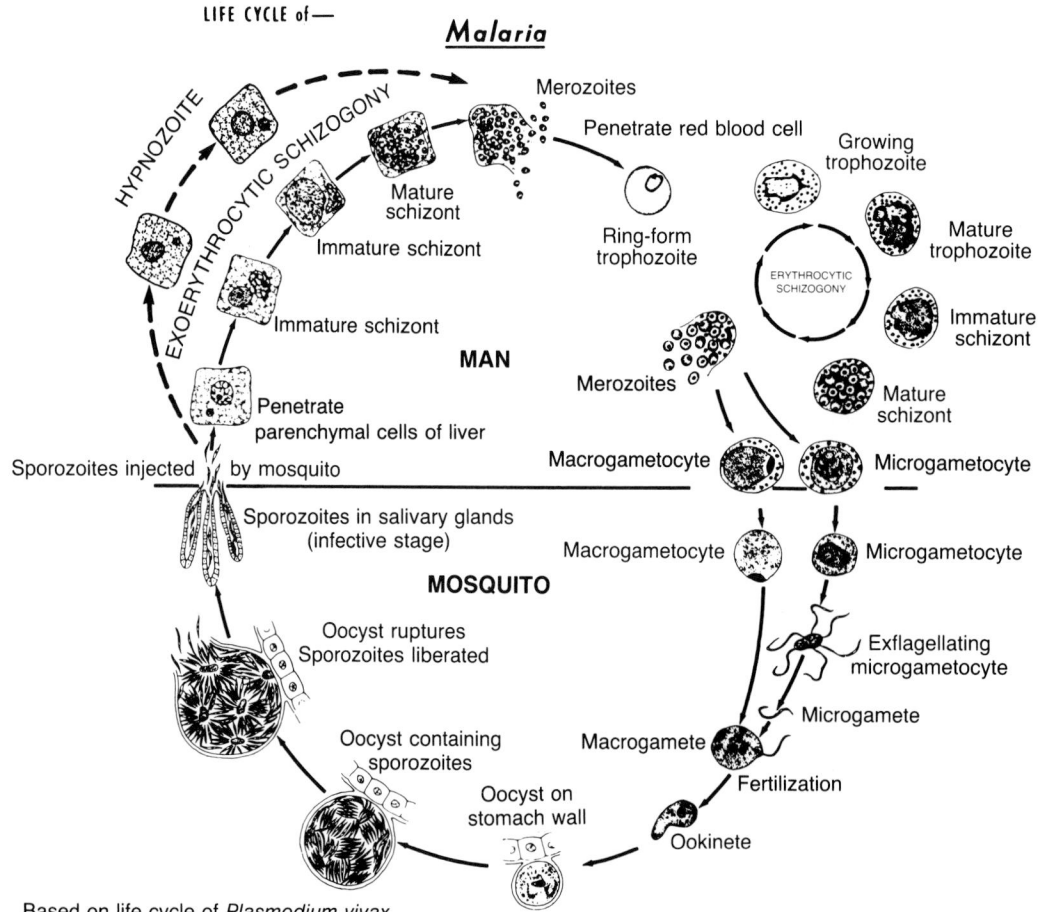

FIGURE 73–2. Life cycle of malaria (based on cycle for *Plasmodium vivax*). The dormant hypnozoite stage is believed to be present in *P. vivax* and *P. ovale* and to be responsible for relapsing infections. (Modified from Melvin DM, et al.: Common Blood and Tissue Parasites of Man. Life Cycle Charts. Atlanta, Georgia, Centers for Disease Control, 1979.)

TABLE 73–1. Selected Characteristics of Four Species of Human Malaria*

	P. falciparum	*P. vivax*	*P. ovale*	*P. malariae*
Exoerythrocytic cycle (days)	5½–7	6–8	9	12–16
Erythrocytic cycle (hours)	48	42–48	49–50	72
Prepatent period (days)	9–10	11–13	10–14	15
Usual incubation period in days (range)[1]	12 (9–14)	13 (12–17) or up to 6–12 months	17 (16–18) or longer	28 (18–40) or longer
Earliest appearance of peripheral gametocytes (days)	10	3	?	?
Secondary exoerythrocytic cycle	none	present	present	none
Average number of merozoites per tissue schizont	40,000	10,000	15,000	2000
Size of tissue schizont	60 μm	45 μm	70 μm	45 μm
Duration of untreated infection (years)	1–2	1½–4	1½–4	3–50
Average parasitemia (per mm)[2]	20,000 or greater	10,000	9000	6000
Minimum duration (and range) of sporogony cycle in mosquito in days[3]	9 (9–22)	8 (8–16)	12 (12–14)	16 (16–35)
Severity of primary attack[2]	severe in nonimmune	mild to severe	mild	mild
Usual periodicity of febrile attacks (hours)	none	48	48	72
Duration of febrile paroxysm (hours)	16–36 or longer	8–12	8–12	8–10

*Modified from Bruce-Chwatt LJ: Essential Malariology. London, William Heinemann Medical Books Ltd., 1980.
[1] Patterns in different strains vary.
[2] Influenced by level of immunity.
[3] Temperature-dependent.

enters, its surface coat appears to be pinched off. The entire process takes about 30 seconds (Fig. 73–5).

Asexual Stages. The youngest stages in the blood are small, rounded trophozoites, known as *ring forms* (Fig. 73–7 [Row 1]). As the parasites grow, they become irregular and ameboid *trophozoites* (Fig. 73–7, Rows 2 and 3). During development, the parasites utilize hemoglobin, leaving as the product of digestion an iron-containing pigment, hematin or hemozoin, which can be seen in the cytoplasm of the parasite as dark granules. After a period of growth in the red blood cell, the *schizont* stage (Figs. 73–6 [Row 4] [Plate III] and 73–7) begins when the parasite undergoes nuclear division and culminates in segmentation to form *merozoites*. This process of asexual multiplication is called erythrocytic schizogony. The infected erythrocytes rupture, liberating merozoites, which must invade new red cells. The erythrocytic cycle of schizogony is repeated over and over again. The periodicity of schizogony differs according to species (Table 73–1).

Sexual Stages. From 3 to 15 days after the onset of symptoms, subpopulations of merozoites differentiate into sexual forms, gametocytes, i.e., female *macrogametocytes* (Fig. 73–6 [Row 5] [Plate III]) and male *microgametocytes* (Fig. 73–6 [Row 6] [Plate III]). The duration of gametocytogony is assumed to be 4 days in *P. vivax* infections and 10 or more days in *P. falciparum* infections.

Vector Phase

Exflagellation. While feeding on an infected human, the female anopheline mosquito (Fig. 73–8) ingests gametocytes, which undergo further development in the stomach of the mosquito. The nucleus of the male gametocyte divides into 4 to 8 nuclei, each of which combines with cytoplasm to form a long, threadlike flagellum measuring 20 to 25 μm in length. These exflagellated *microgametes* shoot out from the original cell, lash about, and then break free (Fig. 73–9). This process of *exflagellation* takes only a few minutes at the appropriate temperature.

The microgametes move actively toward and through small projections that form on the female parasites, now known as macrogametes, and mitosis takes place. The product, zygotes, within 18 to 24 hours elongate to 18 to 24 μm and become motile ookinetes.

Sporogony. The ookinete forces its way between the epithelial cells to the outer surface of the stomach (midgut) and rounds up into a small sphere within an elastic membrane; at this point, it is called an *oocyst*. The number of oocysts on the stomach of an infected *Anopheles* may vary between a few and several hundred (Fig. 73–10).

The oocyst appears as a semitransparent globular body that grows to 40 to 80 μm in size and contains grains of pigment whose distribution, size, and color are characteristic for a given species of plasmodia. The oocyst enlarges progressively, up to 500 μm in diameter, as the nucleus divides repeatedly, obscuring the pig-

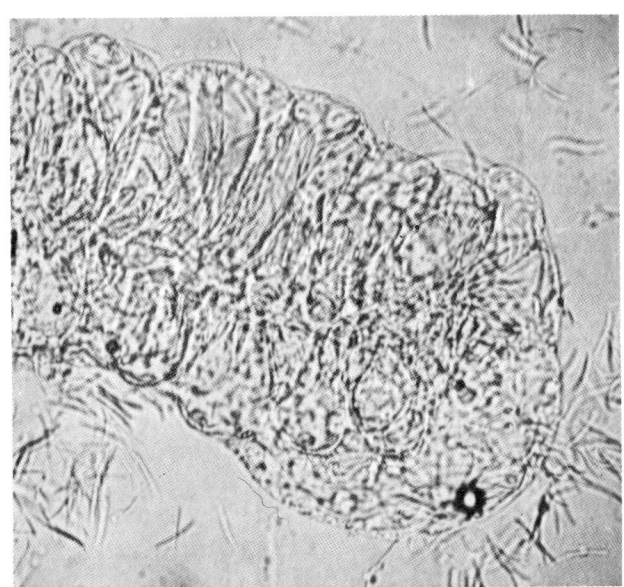

FIGURE 73–3. Sporozoites.

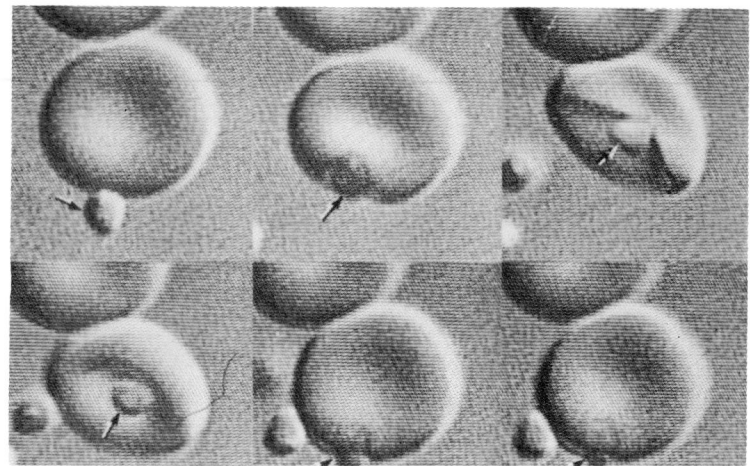

FIGURE 73–5. This inverted microscope sequence shows (from upper left to lower right) the invasion of a red blood cell by a malaria parasite *(arrow)*. Following attachment of the parasite to the red blood cell, there is a marked distortion of the red blood cell, followed by the relatively slow invasion of the red blood cell by the parasite. (From Plocinik B: The NIH Record, March 25, 1975.)

ment. The divided nuclei form finger-like processes, at the periphery of which develop large numbers of elongated, fusiform *sporozoites*. All plasmodial sporozoites seem to have the same structure. The oocyst ruptures, liberating thousands of motile sporozoites into the body cavity; from there they migrate to the salivary glands (Fig. 73–3). The female mosquito is now infective.

Sporogony, the progress of the malarial parasite in the mosquito from gametocyte maturation until the appearance of infective sporozoites, varies from 8 to 35 days, depending on external temperature and on the species (Table 73–1).

EPIDEMIOLOGY. Transmission requires the interaction of 4 epidemiologic factors: the human host, the malarial parasite, the anopheline vector, and the environment (physical, biologic, and socioeconomic). The level of transmission is determined by (1) the prevalence of infection in man (the reservoir) and the seasonal incidence; (2) characteristics of the indigenous vector mosquitoes, including their relative abundance, feeding and resting behavior, susceptibility to infection, and effectiveness as a vector; (3) the presence of a susceptible human population; and (4) local climatic and environmental features that affect vector breeding and the rate of sporogony. There are definite annual fluctuations, and a particular sequence exists in the times at which malaria appears in different areas; these patterns of transmission are dependent on seasonal variations of temperature, humidity, and rainfall. Other controlling influences probably exist, because in many areas the prevalence of malaria exhibits cyclic increases and recessions that are not well understood.

The Parasite. To survive, the parasite must be present in human blood long enough to produce viable gametocytes at a time when environmental conditions are suitable for transmission. In addition, the parasite must be naturally adapted to a vector capable of transmitting the infection. Specific adaptive characteristics to the human host and to the vector differ for each species and affect disease manifestations and transmission.

P. falciparum is the species that most often causes death. When *P. falciparum* is compared with the 3 other species (Table 73–1), the duration of infection is the shortest, exoerythrocytic schizonts release 2.5 to 20 times as many merozoites, and the rate of development of the exoerythrocytic stage is fastest. In contrast, *P. malariae* has the longest duration of infection and is almost a commensal infection in some adults.

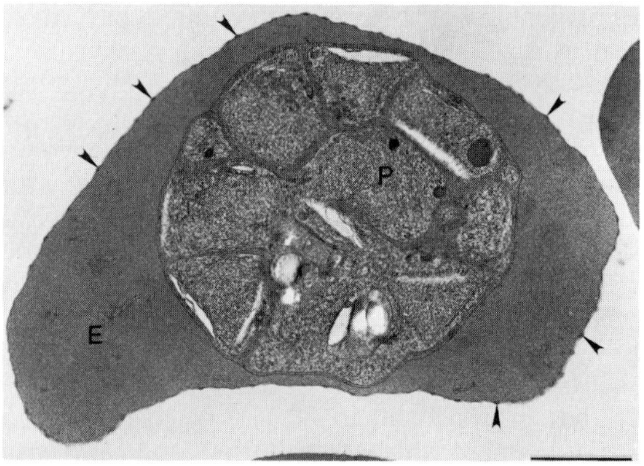

FIGURE 73–7. Segmenting schizont of *Plasmodium falciparum* (P) in an erythrocyte (E). The surface of the erythrocyte has been altered by the parasite, resulting in dense structures or "knobs" *(arrows).* The bar represents 1 μm. (Courtesy of Susan G. Langreth.)

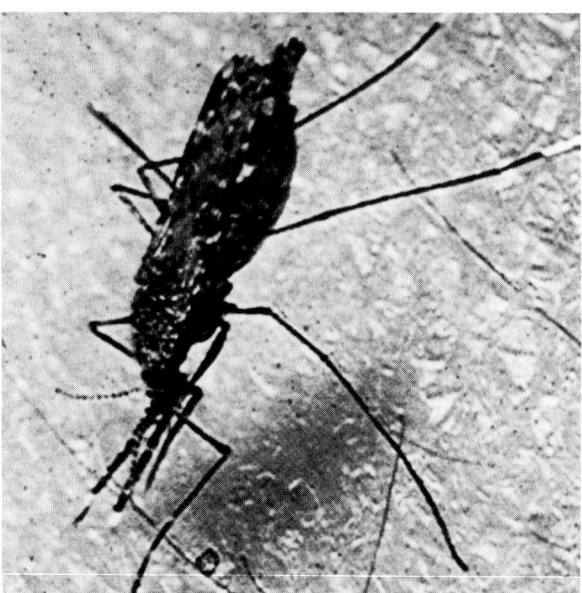

FIGURE 73–8. Feeding female anopheline mosquito.

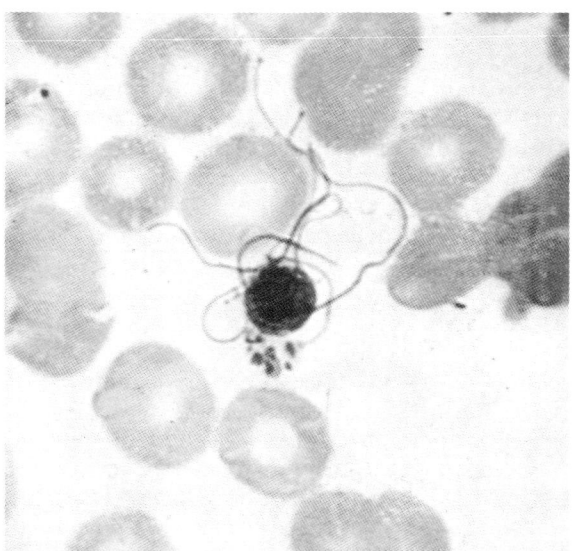

FIGURE 73–9. Exflagellation of male gametocyte.

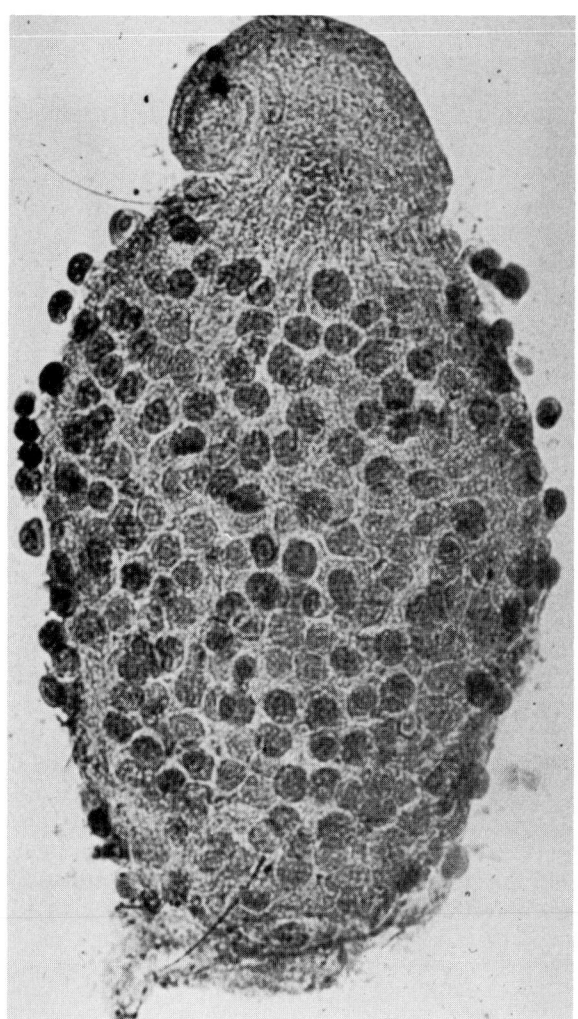

FIGURE 73–10. Many oocysts on the stomach of a heavily infected mosquito.

Studies of *P. falciparum* indicate a periodicity and strictly limited duration of infectivity of gametocytes that coincide exactly with the period of highest biting activity of the vector. Gametocytes appear late in falciparum malaria, never before 10 to 15 days after the onset of patency.

The age of erythrocytes is an important determinant of parasitemia. *P. vivax* and *P. ovale* tend to invade only young red cells, the reticulocytes. *P. malariae* invades only aging erythrocytes. Parasitemia by these species is therefore limited in density (maximum 1% to 7%), and morbidity is low. In contrast, *P. falciparum* can invade all erythrocytes, resulting in extremely high levels of parasitemia.

Each species of human plasmodia consists of a number of different strains that are indistinguishable morphologically but have different features, reflecting a process of natural selection. Strains of a species of malarial parasite will infect local vectors but may not be infective for vectors from other areas. Geographic strains of *P. falciparum* and *P. vivax* demonstrate different response curves to antimalarial drugs. Relapse patterns of *P. vivax* from various regions differ and frequently reflect local environmental conditions. Long incubation periods in vivax malaria are seen in temperate climates, where the transmission season is short. This is presumably due to a greater number of hypnozoite stages in the liver and assures parasite survival during the colder season.

Host Factors. Sex and age do not affect the incidence or severity of malarial infection except as they relate to the frequency of exposure and the development of immunity. Occupation, social behavior, and migration all affect vector-human interaction.

Immunity. In general, populations continuously exposed to malaria in endemic areas develop a degree of immunity to infection. Clinical manifestations, parasitemia, and probably the production of gametocytes also are reduced by immunity. In holoendemic and hyperendemic areas, malaria prevalence and gametocyte production are highest among infants and young children,

groups with the least developed immunity. Adults have high malarial antibody titers and very low levels of circulating parasites and have developed a degree of immunity. Individuals with fever and other clinical manifestations are not necessarily those most responsible for transmission. Asymptomatic persons with gametocytemia may be more responsible for infecting mosquitoes. During late pregnancy, resistance to malaria decreases, frequently resulting in severe infections. Latent malaria may become symptomatic.

Genetic Factors. These are important determinants of susceptibility to malaria. The development of *P. falciparum* is suppressed in the presence of fetal hemoglobin, hemoglobin S, and perhaps other abnormal hemoglobins as well. In vitro studies have demonstrated that *P. falciparum* parasites do not survive in cells with SA or SS hemoglobin when oxygen tension is decreased. Heterozygotic persons with sickle cell trait (SA) have less severe falciparum malaria infections and do not suffer from lethal sickle cell disease. The high frequency of hemoglobin S in certain parts of Africa is due to the selective advantage of this balanced polymorphism. Similar evidence has been presented in beta-thalassemia and for persistence of fetal hemoglobin (HbF). The protective action of a genetic deficiency of the erythrocytic enzyme glucose-6-phosphate dehydrogenase (G-6-PD) for falciparum malaria has been postulated but not proved. Hereditary ovalocytosis also provides some protection (Chapter 5).

Persons whose red cells lack the Duffy a and b (Fy^a and Fy^b) blood group determinants (Duffy-negative blood type) are resistant to infection with *P. vivax*. The specific receptors for invasion of vivax merozoites are absent. The low incidence of *P. vivax* in Africa is explained by the fact that most Africans are Duffy-negative.

Congenital Malaria. This is rare, and its occurrence is associated with low immunity in the mother. Therefore, most cases of congenital malaria either appear in areas where the prevalence of malaria is low or involve nonimmune mothers. Passive transfer of antibody across the placenta helps protect neonates for the first 6 months of life. Malaria is an important cause of spontaneous abortions, stillbirths, and low birth weight as well as neonatal and infant mortality.

Nutritional Factors. Minimal to modest malnutrition is commonly believed to potentiate malarial infections, probably because of the immunosuppressive effects of malnutrition. Investigations using experimental animals and studies of populations during famine suggest that hosts with diets deficient in certain factors required for the growth of the parasite, such as para-aminobenzoic acid (PABA) and iron, are protected from fatal or severe falciparum infections. Susceptibility returns after restitution of the nutritional deficit. Breast milk, deficient in PABA, provides a similar protection.

Vector. The effectiveness of a vector in transmitting malaria depends on (1) its presence in adequate numbers in or near human habitation, (2) marked preference for human blood (anthropophilic) rather than animal blood (zoophilic), (3) sufficient longevity to complete sporogony and then transmit the infection, and (4) a preference to bite and rest outdoors (exophilic) or indoors (endophilic). Temperature and humidity greatly affect the rate of parasite development in the vector.

There are about 400 species of anophelines, of which some 80 are proven vectors. However, only 27 are considered effective vectors. Anophelines that are excellent vectors of a malaria strain from one area may not transmit strains from another, and in each area often only 1, and usually not more than 2 or 3 species, can be considered important vectors.

Environment. Malaria transmission is profoundly influenced by climate. The optimal conditions for transmission occur when the temperature is 20° to 30°C and the mean relative humidity is at least 60%. Sporogony does not occur below 16°C or above 33°C. Water temperature regulates the duration of the aquatic breeding cycle. A high relative humidity increases mosquito longevity and therefore increases the probability of the mosquito becoming infective. The observed association of increased malaria incidence with rainfall is due both to an increase in breeding sites and to the increased survival rates of female anophelines because of the rise in relative humidity. Excessive rainfall may be deleterious to vector larvae and pupae. Conversely, droughts

in dry seasons may reduce the size and flow rates of rivers, resulting in more suitable breeding sites.

The proximity of human habitation to breeding sites is directly related to vector-human contact and therefore to transmission. The stability of breeding places is influenced by water supply, soil, vegetation, and so on. Irrigation schemes, dams, and other manmade changes can radically alter stable patterns of malaria transmission (see section entitled "Epidemics" further on in this chapter).

Epidemiologic Terminology. *Stable endemic malaria* is present when natural transmission occurs over many successive years and there is a predictably constant incidence of cases. Transmission is generally high and epidemics unlikely. In *unstable malaria,* the amount of transmission varies from year to year, collective immunity is low, and epidemics are therefore likely. *Autochthonous malaria* is contracted locally. Malaria is *indigenous* when naturally present in an area or country. *Imported malaria* is acquired outside a given area. Secondary cases are those derived from imported cases and are referred to as *introduced malaria.* Malaria acquired by blood transfusions, sharing of needles, intentional inoculation, or accidental laboratory infections is known as *induced malaria.*

A number of parameters are commonly used to classify malaria in an area. Descriptive terms include:

1. *Malaria incidence*—the number of new cases occurring over a given period of time.

2. *Malaria prevalence*—the number of cases, both new and existing, over a given time interval or the total number of cases at one point in time.

3. *Spleen rate*—the proportion of children 2 to 9 years of age with enlarged spleens. Other population groups may be used, e.g., the adult spleen rate, but these should be specified.

4. *Parasite rate*—the proportion of persons in a defined age group or on a given date with microscopically proven parasitemia.

5. *Transmission index*—the proportion of infants less than 1 year of age with parasitemia.

The degree of endemic malaria is determined by examination of a statistically significant population sample and is assessed and classified as follows:

1. *Hypoendemic*—spleen rate or parasite rate of 0% to 10% in children 2 through 9 years old.

2. *Mesoendemic*—spleen rate or parasite rate of 11% to 50% in children 2 through 9 years old.

3. *Hyperendemic*—spleen rate or parasite rate consistently over 50% in children 2 through 9 years old; the adult spleen rate is also high.

4. *Holoendemic*—spleen rate or parasite rate of more than 75% in children 2 to 9 years old. The adult spleen rate is low, and the parasite rate in infants (less than 1 year old) is high.

Mathematical models have been applied to malaria, but caution is indicated in their predictive value in making decisions for intervention measures. Social conditions, for example, are subject to wide variation and change. The cost of obtaining data for verification may often be prohibitive in developing countries.

The *natural index of infection* is the proportion of

mosquitoes with stomach wall oocysts or sporozoite infection in the salivary glands. A salivary gland index as low as 0.1% may indicate an important vector when the species is abundant. Higher rates may be encountered.

Epidemics. Epidemics of malaria with high mortality rates are less frequent now than in the past. However, the epidemic potential continues to exist. An epidemic occurs when malaria is introduced to a population in whom the disease was previously unknown or when a seasonal or unexpected increase in cases occurs in a known malarious area. The genesis of epidemics involves one or more of the following factors: (1) an increase in susceptibility of the human population; (2) the introduction of new vector or new strain of parasite; (3) changes in patterns of vector–human contact; and/or (4) increased effectiveness of the local vector in transmitting the disease.

Increased susceptibility of populations generally occurs when a large number of nonimmune individuals move into a malarious area. Inadvertent introduction of a more efficient vector, such as the importation of *A. gambiae* into Brazil in the 1930s by ship from Africa, can result in explosive outbreaks. Similarly, introduction of new strains of the parasite can result in epidemics. Changes in human behavior, housing conditions, or other factors that result in increased man-vector contact may cause epidemics. Manmade dams and irrigation schemes cause an increase in vector density. Changes in climate can affect both the numbers and the longevity of vectors. Finally, a decrease in the numbers of animals in an area will force a previously predominantly zoophilic mosquito to use man as the primary source of blood meals, resulting in increased transmission.

Imported Malaria. The increase in international air travel has resulted in importation of malaria and other diseases to nonendemic areas. Regions where malaria has been eradicated are at continuing risk of imported cases. Patients often arrive during the incubation period and may not become ill until reaching home. Delays in diagnosis, misdiagnosis, and inappropriate treatment may occur, resulting in excessive morbidity and mortality. Physicians and public health officials must remain aware of the possibility of imported malarial infections.

PATHOPHYSIOLOGY. Pathophysiologic changes in malaria are primarily associated with impairment of local blood flow resulting from sticking of parasitized erythrocytes to the venular endothelium. These changes are rapidly reversible in those who survive. In some circumstances, adherent leukocytes may be responsible for capillary damage. The role of various humoral mediators is still uncertain, but they appear to be involved in the pathogenesis of fever and inflammation. Exoerythrocytic schizogony may cause an inconsequential local leukocytic and phagocytic reaction, whereas sporozoites and gametocytes do not induce pathophysiologic changes.

Etiology. The pathophysiology of malaria is multifactoral and includes the following:

Erythrocyte Destruction. Erythrocytes are destroyed not only when parasitized cells are ruptured but also through phagocytosis of infected and noninfected erythrocytes. Anemia and tissue anoxia result. With severe intravascular hemolysis ("blackwater fever"), the resulting hemoglobinuria may contribute to renal failure.

Endotoxin-Macrophage Mediators. At the time of schizogony, parasitized erythrocytes induce endotoxin-sensitive macrophages to release a range of mediators. These mediators appear to account for some of the pathophysiologic changes associated with malaria.

Endotoxin is not present in malaria parasites; its source may be from the gut lumen, and malaria parasites themselves can lead to release of tumor necrosis factor (TNF). TNF, a monokine, has been detected in the circulation of humans and animals infected with malarial parasites. Recombinant TNF produces symptomatology and laboratory findings typical of malaria following inoculation into nonmalarious subjects. TNF and other related cytokines produce fever, hypoglycemia (secondary to hyperinsulinemia and interference with hepatic gluconeogenesis), and adult respiratory disease syndrome (ARDS) with neutrophil sequestration in pulmonary blood vessels. It can also destroy *P. falciparum* parasites in vitro and may increase adhesiveness of parasitized red cells to vascular endothelium.

Serum concentrations of TNF in children with acute falciparum malaria correlate directly with mortality, hypoglycemia, hyperparasitemia, and severity of illness. The theory that TNF acts with other polypeptide mediators to cause some of the pathophysiology of malaria is not accepted by all and requires further study. However, it is enticing for several reasons: (1) It explains some pathologic mechanisms that are difficult to associate with sludging of parasitized erythrocytes; (2) it provides a mechanism to explain the pathophysiology of infection with the malaria species in which sludging does not occur; (3) it relates to the pathophysiology caused by sludging in that TNF might increase endothelial adherence; (4) it is based upon an immunologic process that is both protective and causes illness; and (5) it provides a theory to explain premunition, tolerance to infection. Premunition could result from the development of tolerance to the effects of TNF. Therefore, the individual having malarial parasitemia might have minimal or no symptoms owing to the fact that he or she has developed a tolerance to the pathologic effects of TNF and other cytokines.

Sequestration of Infected Erythrocytes. Erythrocytes infected with the later stages of *P. falciparum* may develop "knobs" on their surface (Fig. 73–7). These "knobs" contain malarial antigens and react with malarial antibodies. They are associated with affinity of *P. falciparum*–infected erythrocytes for the vascular endothelium of capillaries in the internal organs, causing schizogony to occur in the deep rather than the peripheral circulation. The infected erythrocytes attach to vascular endothelium and form sludged masses blocking capillaries in the vital organs. Leakage of protein and fluid through the abnormally permeable capillary membranes then follows, resulting in further anoxia and edema of the tissues. If there is sufficient tissue anoxia, death ensues. Histidine-rich *P. falciparum* proteins have been localized in these knobs; at least 3 endothelial cell cytoadherence proteins for *P. falciparum*–infected erythrocytes, thrombospondin, ICAM-1, and CD 36, have been identified.

Biochemical and Electrolyte Changes

Hyponatremia. Both urine water and sodium excretion are reduced during the acute phase of falciparum malaria. Hyponatremia is due to decreased free water clearance and should not be treated by sodium loading. Orthostatic hypotension is a common occurrence during acute falciparum malaria. An increased plasma volume is associated with the decreased effective blood volume and generalized vasodilation. In response, aldosterone and antidiuretic hormone secretion is increased to conserve sodium and water. During recovery, the integrity of the capillary system is re-established, vasodilation is diminished, and effective circulating blood volume is restored. A reduction in aldosterone secretion and natriuresis follow.

Pituitary function and adrenal function are normal in acute falciparum malaria, although algid malaria may resemble an addisonian crisis. Serum albumin and total protein can be reduced by the fluid retention.

Hypoglycemia. Hypoglycemia occurs in some patients with severe falciparum malaria and markedly increases both morbidity and mortality. It has been shown to be a consequence of parenteral quinine therapy (i.e., as a result of quinine-induced hyperinsulinemia). In a recent study, most patients had hypoglycemia before treatment, which was associated with elevated plasma concentrations of lactate, alanine, and 5'-nucleotidase—all of which suggest that impaired hepatic gluconeogenesis contributes to the pathogenesis of hypoglycemia in malaria. Hypoglycemia is associated with cerebral malaria and is more common in young children and pregnant women. TNF may be one of the inducers of hypoglycemia.

Hematologic Changes.

Anemia, leukopenia, and thrombocytopenia are often prominent features of acute malarial infections. Red cell mass, as measured with ^{51}Cr-tagged erythrocytes, is either normal or reduced, depending on the extent of hemolysis. Anemia may persist after appropriate treatment.

Hemolysis. During the acute phase of the illness, the survival of ^{51}Cr-tagged erythrocytes is reduced in both infected and noninfected erythrocytes. Sequestration and destruction of erythrocytes occur in the spleen. The extent of sequestration correlates with splenic size and not with the presence of antimalarial antibodies. In some patients, the hemolysis is out of proportion to the parasitemia, suggesting an autoimmune component to the anemia. Studies to detect antibodies against normal erythrocytes in patients with falciparum malaria have yielded variable results. A minority have demonstrated positive Coombs' reactions between erythrocytes from infected patients and anticomplement sera and with antisera to C3d, C3b, and, rarely, IgG. Immune complexes have also been described in acute malaria. The role of nonspecific activation of the reticuloendothelial function by the parasite infection in hemolysis is apparent. It is still uncertain whether hemolysis is antibody- or complement-mediated, although blackwater fever almost certainly has an autoimmune etiology.

Bone Marrow Depression.

Erythrocyte production is impaired. Incorporation of ^{59}Fe into red blood cells is depressed during the period of parasitemia. The reticulocyte count is inappropriately normal or low. During the acute phase of illness, iron sequestration, erythrophagocytosis, and dyserythropoiesis occur. Maturation defects are usually present in the bone marrow, and the serum iron is reduced. Bone marrow cellularity and the myeloid:erythroid ratio are initially normal, but both usually fall during recovery in association with a reticulocytosis.

Gastrointestinal Changes.

Reduced blood flow to the liver caused by constriction of the hepatic venous system results in edema and vascular congestion. Hepatomegaly, hepatic tenderness, and abnormalities in liver function tests may be present. Small bowel malabsorption, documented to D-xylose, vitamin B_{12}, and fats, is secondary to vascular congestion and obstruction from sludging of parasitized erythrocytes in the mucosal venules and capillaries (Fig. 73–11).

Reticuloendothelial System (RES) Phagocytic Function Changes.

The reduced hepatic blood flow causes a slight delay in clearance of macroaggregated human serum albumin. However, the major effect of malaria is a marked enhancement of phagocytic activity.

Pulmonary Changes.

Acute pulmonary edema can be precipitated by excessive parenteral fluid therapy causing circulatory overload. In most cases, however, it develops in patients with normal or low pulmonary

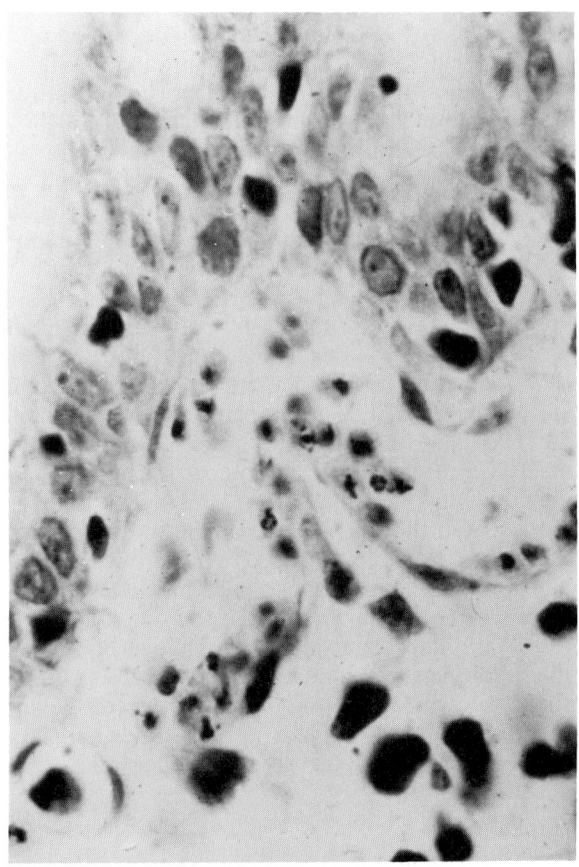

FIGURE 73–11. Acute falciparum malaria. Jejunal biopsy specimen demonstrating edema and capillaries packed with schizont-infected erythrocytes in the lamina propria. (Courtesy of Walter Karney.)

PLATE I

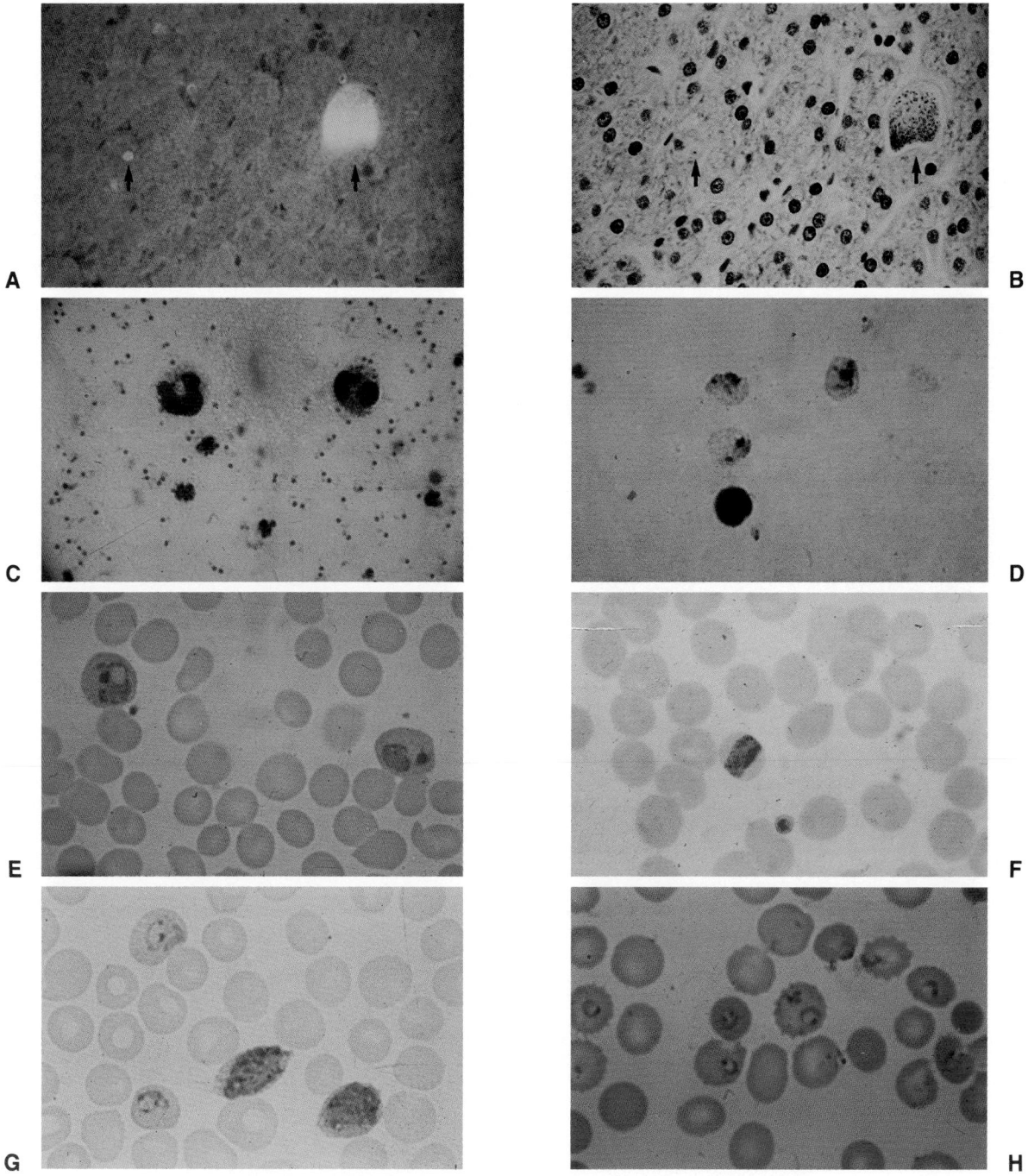

FIGURE 73–4. All blood smears are stained with Giemsa stain. *A* and *B*, Schizont *(right arrow)* and hypnozoite *(left arrow)* of *Plasmodium cynomolgi bastianellii* in a liver biopsy specimen taken from a rhesus monkey that was inoculated intravenously with 12 million sporozoites 7 days before. *A*, Indirect immunofluorescence staining, using rhesus antibody to disrupted blood stages and a fluorescein-conjugated rabbit anti-rhesus IgG. *B*, After restaining with Giemsa-colophonium. The schizont is approximately 30 μm in diameter; the hypnozoite has a diameter of 5 μm (× 500). (Courtesy of W. A. Krotoski.) *C*, Thick blood smear from a patient with heavy *Plasmodium falciparum* infection. Note the leukocytes, platelets, and numerous ring forms of the parasite. *D*, Thick blood smear from a patient with *Plasmodium vivax* infection. Note the three ameboid trophozoites and smaller ring form. Lymphocyte nucleus assists in estimating size of parasites. *E*, Thin blood smear from a patient with *P. vivax* infection. Note the ameboid trophozoites and Schüffner's dots in the enlarged erythrocytes. *F*, Thin blood smear from a patient with *Plasmodium malariae* infection. Note the band-shaped trophozoite in the normal-sized erythrocyte. *G*, Thin blood smear from a patient with *Plasmodium ovale* infection. Note the two ameboid trophozoites in the enlarged stippled erythrocytes and the two schizonts in oval (or elongated) erythrocytes. *H*, Thin blood smear from a patient with heavy *P. falciparum* infection. Note the normal-sized erythrocytes with multiple infections with small ring trophozoites and accolé forms (parasite present on the margin of the erythrocyte) (× 290).

PLATE II

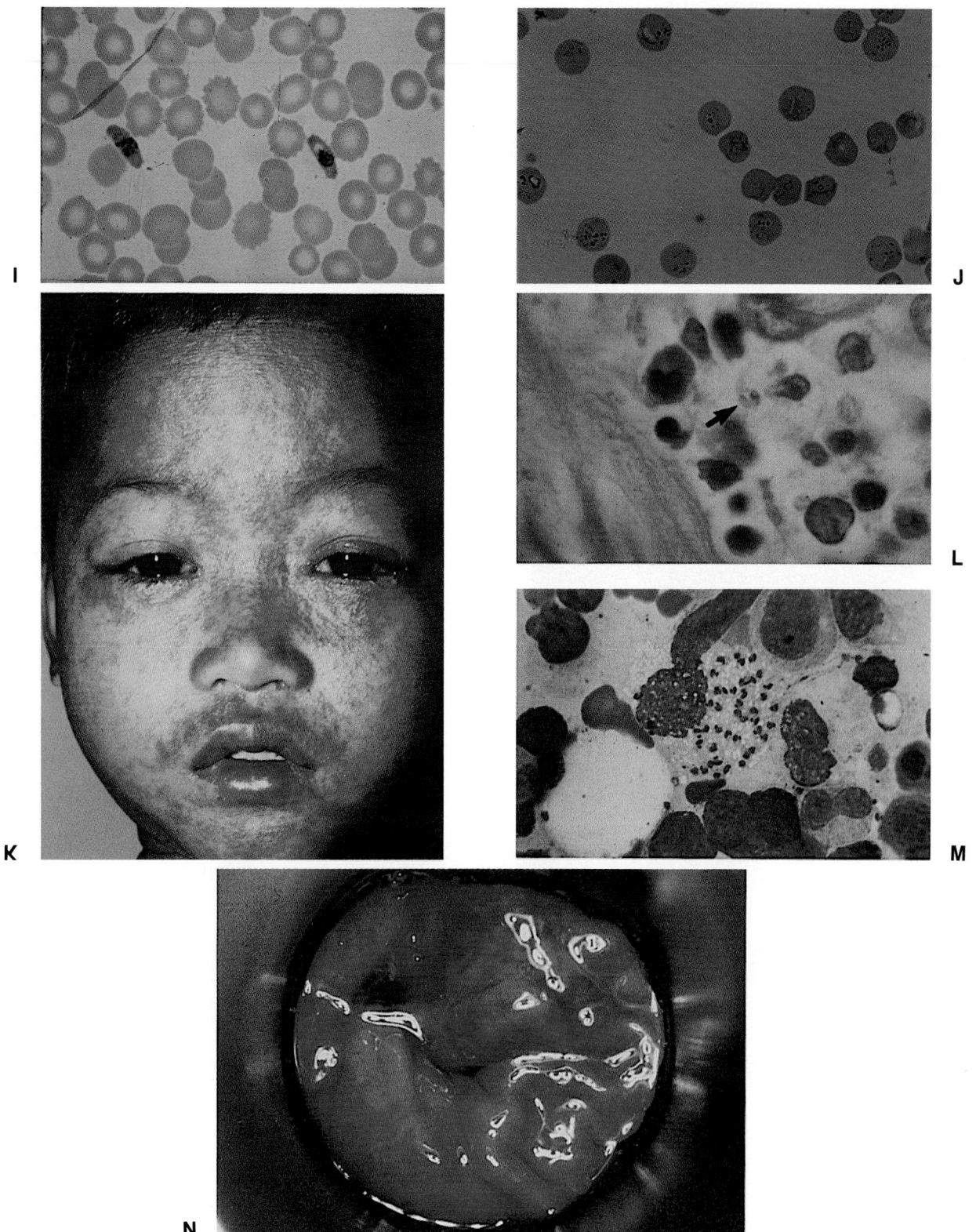

FIGURE 73–4 *(Continued)*. *I*, Thin blood film showing *P. falciparum* microgametocyte *(left)* and macrogametocyte *(right)*. *J*, *Bartonella* in a peripheral blood film. (Courtesy of Evan R. Farmer, M.D.) *K*, Asian child with erythematous rash, conjunctivitis, and coryza of measles. *L*, Skin biopsy specimen from a patient with cutaneous leishmaniasis. An amastigote is present in tissue macrophage *(arrow)*. Note the nucleus and kinetoplast (H & E stain, × 2600). (Courtesy of Ronald Neafie and the Armed Forces Institute of Pathology, Photograph Neg. No. 74-11632.) *M*, Bone marrow aspirate from a patient with visceral leishmaniasis. Note the numerous amastigotes in macrophage (Giemsa stain). (Courtesy of the Armed Forces Institute of Pathology.) *N*, Sigmoidoscopic view of the rectum of a patient with shigellosis. Note the ulcerations and erythema. (Courtesy of M. Levine.)

PLATE III

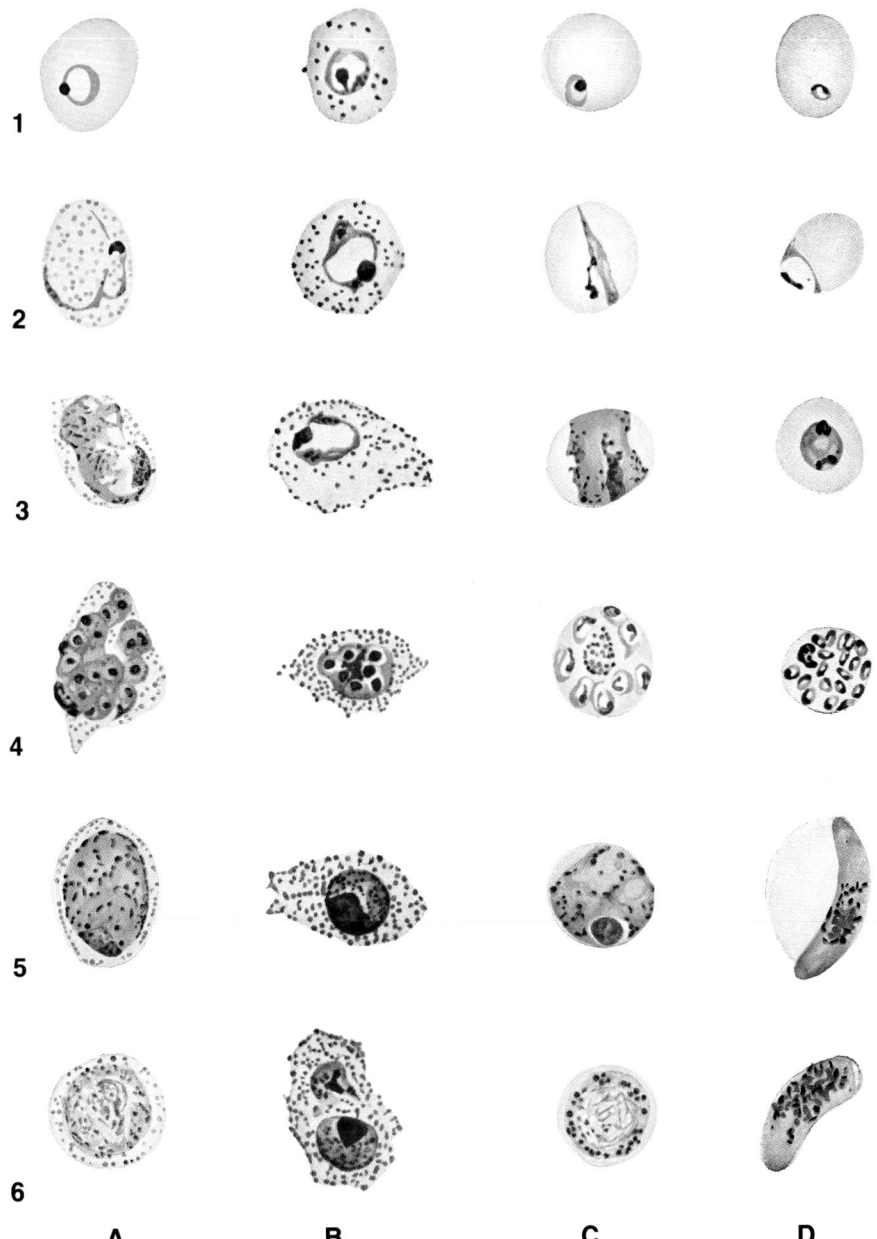

FIGURE 73–6. Rows *A, Plasmodium vivax; B, P. ovale; C, P. malariae; D, P. falciparum.* Rows *1,* Young trophozoites; *2,* growing trophozoites; *3,* mature trophozoites; *4,* mature schizonts; *5,* macrogametocytes; *6,* microgametocytes. (From Wilcox A: Manual for the Microscopical Diagnosis of Malaria in Man. Bulletin No. 180, National Institute of Health, 1942.)

arterial wedge pressures. Increased pulmonary capillary permeability, as occurs in ARDS, is the cause of pulmonary edema in these patients. In this circumstance, adherent leukocytes releasing cytokines and other potentially toxic substances could be responsible for the changes.

Neurologic Changes. *P. falciparum*–infected red cells (particularly schizont-infected erythrocytes) adhere to the cerebral venular endothelium. The binding takes place between knobs protruding from the surface of the parasitized erythrocyte and a ligand in the endothelium. This impedes cerebral blood flow. In some cases, other factors (e.g., agglutination of parasitized erythrocytes, fibrin microthrombi, altered rheologic properties of the parasitized red cells, and vascular endothelial changes) contribute to the microvascular obstruction. The mechanisms causing the symptomatology (e.g., coma, seizures, upper motor neuron dysfunction) are metabolic rather than mechanical and are rapidly reversible in those who survive.

Renal Changes. Mild renal abnormalities, including slightly elevated urea nitrogen and creatinine levels, proteinuria, and an abnormal urine sediment, are common in malaria. A reduced glomerular filtration rate and renal plasma flow, circulating immune complexes, and minimal changes on renal biopsy are associated.

Acute renal insufficiency is common in severe falciparum malaria with high parasitemia and marked intravascular hemolysis.

PATHOLOGY. Death from malaria is almost always due to infection by *P. falciparum*. Vivax, ovale, and quartan malaria are seldom fatal in an otherwise healthy person. Therefore, the pathologic changes described in this section are those caused by *P. falciparum*.

Central Nervous System. Brains of patients dying of cerebral falciparum malaria are edematous, with broadened and flattened gyri. The arachnoid blood vessels are congested, and the cut surface shows congestion and petechiae in the white matter. Ring hemorrhages surround capillaries and arterioles centrally blocked with parasitized erythrocytes (Fig. 73–12). In older hemorrhages, midzonal necrosis is surrounded by proliferating small glial cells, a Durck's granuloma.

Bone Marrow. During the acute infection, the bone marrow is often hyperemic, with parasitized erythrocytes and hemozoin in the reticuloendothelial cells. Many of the marrow sinusoids appear blocked by parasitized erythrocytes that are bound to the endothelium at their knobs. A normoblastic or megaloblastic hyperplasia occurs, even in the absence of peripheral reticulocytosis.

Spleen. The spleen is enlarged and tense, and the cut surface is slate gray with prominent malpighian corpuscles. The blood vessels, Billroth cords, and sinusoids are engorged with parasitized erythrocytes. There is reticuloendothelial hyperplasia, and the macrophages lining the sinusoids contain malarial pigment and parasitized and nonparasitized erythrocytes. Hemorrhages and infarcts may be present. The organ is often friable; it occasionally ruptures, causing death. The development of immunity in endemic areas is associated with a greatly enlarged spleen during childhood that gradually becomes smaller, darker, and fibrotic and contains foci of mineralization.

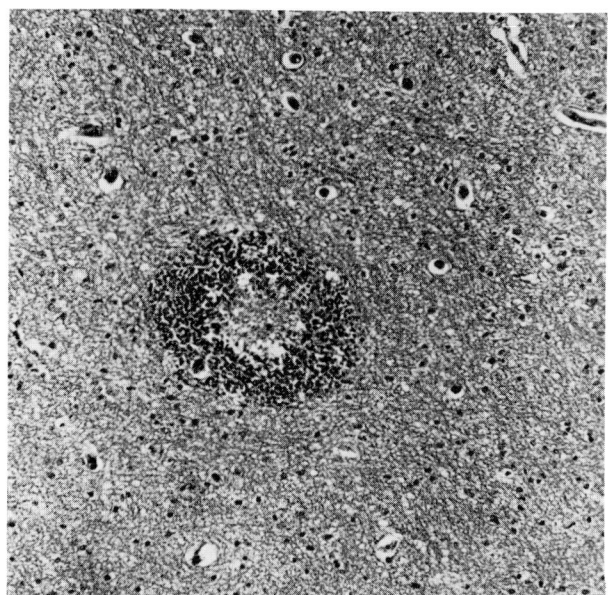

FIGURE 73–12. Acute falciparum malaria. Patient dying of cerebral malaria has ring hemorrhage surrounding obstructed arteriole (H & E stain, × 130.) (Courtesy of the Armed Forces Institute of Pathology, Photograph Neg. No. 66–2329.)

Liver. The liver is enlarged and is usually slate gray. During the acute infection, Kupffer cells are enlarged and increased in numbers. They contain malarial pigment, parasites, and parasitized and nonparasitized erythrocytes (Fig. 73–13). Lymphocytic infiltrations are common in the portal tracts.

Kidneys. The kidneys are usually slightly enlarged and congested. Punctate hemorrhages may be present in the pelvis, cortex, or medulla. Malarial pigment is prominent within the glomeruli, and the capillaries often contain parasitized erythrocytes. Monocytes and lym-

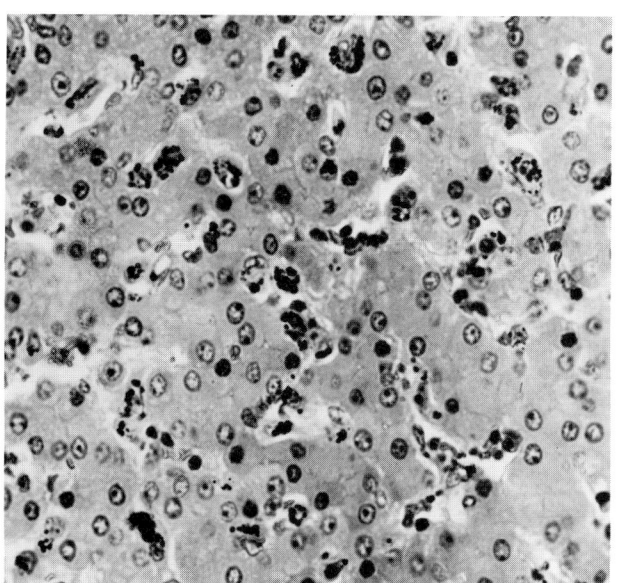

FIGURE 73–13. Acute falciparum malaria. Kupffer cells of liver contain grains of malaria pigment (darker spots). (H & E stain, × 395.) (Courtesy of the Armed Forces Institute of Pathology, Photograph Neg. No. 66–1426.)

phocytes collect in the small vessels of the medulla (Fig. 73–14).

The kidneys of patients dying of blackwater fever are dark, enlarged, and edematous. The cut surface is pale and shows cortical swelling and hemorrhages and medullary congestion. The striking microscopic change is tubular necrosis with hemoglobin casts and an interstitial lymphocytic infiltration.

Acute glomerulonephritis with proliferative changes and basement membrane thickening rarely occurs in patients with falciparum malaria. Focal small deposits in the glomerular mesangial areas have been shown to contain IgM, IgG, and components of complement. The glomerular immune complexes usually disappear with treatment. On rare occasions, however, lesions persist; these are believed to be of autoimmune etiology rather than of antigen-antibody disposition.

Lungs. The lungs are frequently congested and edematous, with parasitized erythrocytes within pulmonary capillaries. Chronic inflammatory cells may be present in the thickened alveolar walls. Interstitial edema of alveolar septa with damaged capillary endothelium is present. More severe changes include hyaline membrane formation and focal intra-alveolar hemorrhages (Fig. 73–15).

Heart. Cardiac changes are usually minimal. Capillaries may be congested and occluded with parasitized erythrocytes. Sometimes, edema and a lymphocytic and monocytic infiltrate of the interstitial tissues are present.

Gastrointestinal Tract. The intestinal mucosa is frequently edematous and congested. Small blood vessels of the mucosa contain parasitized erythrocytes (Fig. 73–11).

Placenta. Abortion and premature labor can be precipitated by the large numbers of parasitized erythrocytes, usually containing developing and mature schiz-

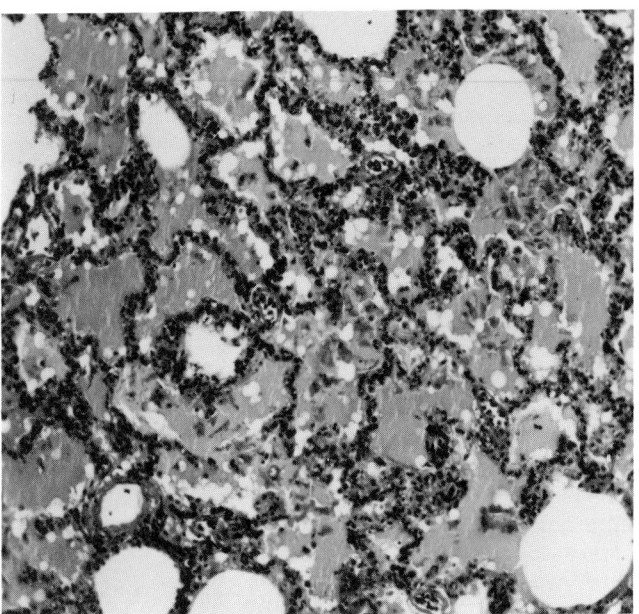

FIGURE 73–15. Acute falciparum malaria. Patient died with pulmonary edema with chronic inflammatory cells and parasitized erythrocytes in thickened aveolar walls. (H & E stain, × 95.) (Courtesy of the Armed Forces Institute of Pathology, Photograph Neg. No. 66–7186.)

onts, in the maternal placental sinusoids (Fig. 73–16). An infected placenta, being black, is easy to recognize at delivery.

IMMUNE RESPONSE. The immune response in malarial infection is complex. Both cellular and humoral components are involved.

Antibodies. In vivo and in vitro studies suggest that much of the protective immune response is mediated by antibody. Protective antibody is mainly IgG. It enhances parasite recognition and phagocytosis by macrophages by binding to sporozoites, free merozoites, parasitized erythrocytes, or the macrophages themselves. Complement does not appear to play a role in parasite destruction, although levels may be depressed in acute malarial infections. Antibodies to the circumsporozoite protein (CSP) of *P. falciparum* are present in those living in areas endemic for malaria. Mean titers increase with age and correlate with in vitro tests showing immunity to sporozoites. However, until now, immunization with a subfraction of CSP has protected only a very few human volunteers who were subsequently challenged with infectious sporozoites. Antibody-mediated phagocytosis of merozoites during their brief extracellular period is probably the major means of reducing parasitemia in individuals with some immunity. Antibody-coated merozoites are inhibited in their ability to penetrate red blood cells. Specific malarial antibodies have been shown to inhibit merozoite dispersals from schizonts and to agglutinate merozoites. Malarial antibodies and antigens have been demonstrated on the surfaces of infected and, less frequently, noninfected erythrocytes.

Acute malarial infections also cause production of nonspecific antibodies. Malarial antigens and sera from malaria-infected patients contain nonspecific mitogens that stimulate lymphocytes in vitro. The high levels of

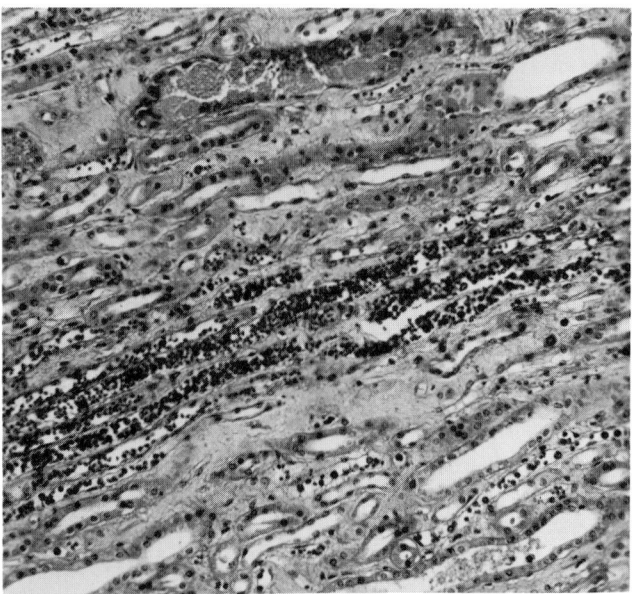

FIGURE 73–14. Acute falciparum malaria. Patient died with renal failure with acute tubular necrosis. Note the monocytic and lymphocytic collections in the medulla. (H & E stain, × 130.) (Courtesy of the Armed Forces Institute of Pathology, Photograph Neg. No. 67–2239.)

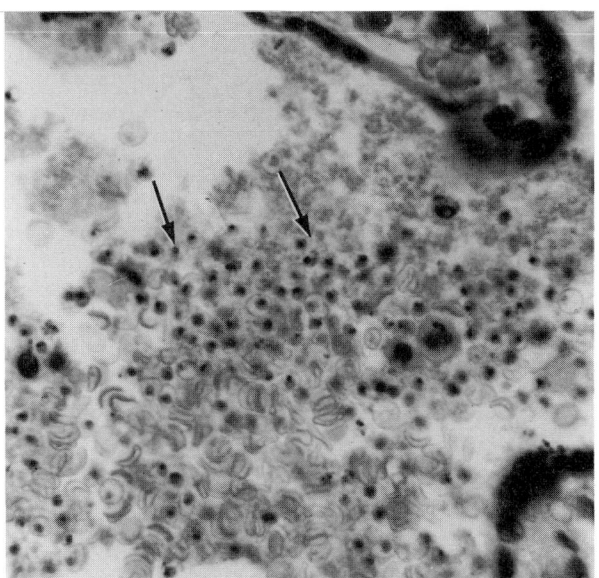

FIGURE 73–16. Section of placenta from a patient with *P. falciparum* infection. Numerous red blood corpuscles in the intervillous space (maternal side) are parasitized *(arrows)*; the corpuscles in the chorionic villus (fetal side) are not parasitized. (Courtesy of the Louisiana State University School of Medicine, New Orleans.)

polyclonal antibodies observed in malaria are probably due to this phenomenon.

Nonspecific Protection. Mechanisms of host defense against malaria other than antibody-mediated phagocytosis occur during the crisis stage of infection. These mechanisms are induced by antigenic materials but do not have immunologic specificity. They include reticuloendothelial cell activation, splenic hypertrophy, and the production of increased autoantibodies to modified or enzymatically exposed host erythrocyte membrane materials. This activated phagocytic-autoantibody system destroys erythrocytes with damaged membranes, including those induced by parasite penetration, by absorption of enzymes of host or parasite origin, and by antigen-antibody complexes. Erythrocyte destruction coincidentally destroys parasites.

Other Immunologic Mechanisms. Lymphokines and monokines, including interferon, may be involved in parasite destruction inside the erythrocytes. Cell-mediated destruction of parasites or parasitized erythrocytes by T cells, natural killer cells, and null cells (K cells), either alone or in association with antibody, has been proposed. Removal of parasitized red cells by the spleen is probably not an important immunologic mechanism.

Development of Immunity. Complete immunity to malaria seldom occurs, even after repeated infections. A partial homologous immunity develops that is species- and strain-specific. The individual becomes partially or totally resistant to reinfections by the same strain. There is no cross-immunity between species. The adult from an area endemic for malaria is asymptomatic but often has very low levels of circulating parasites, which are at times undetectable. Such immunity, dependent on a persisting latent infection, is known as *premunition,* and the person is considered to be "semi-immune." Premunition is slowly acquired; many children living in areas

endemic for malaria do not live to acquire it. *Tolerance* is the initial step in the development of this immunity and is expressed by cessation of clinical symptoms and signs despite little change in levels of parasitemia.

Children. Infants in endemic areas are protected from malaria during the first months of life by passive transfer of antibodies from semi-immune mothers, both across the placenta and in breast milk. Following this period, the child has repeated bouts of malaria. In highly endemic areas, splenomegaly is almost universal; anemia is common; febrile periods are frequent; and parasites can usually be found in peripheral blood smears. Malarial infection may prove fatal in young children if untreated, particularly when occurring together with measles, severe gastroenteritis, or malnutrition. If the child survives, clinical symptoms become less frequent, and the spleen eventually becomes smaller. Parasitemia may occur intermittently, often unassociated with fever.

Adults. Both specific malarial antibodies and IgM, IgG, and IgA immunoglobulin levels increase from early childhood during the period of repeated exposure to malaria. The primary cause of elevated immunoglobulin levels in endemic areas is malaria. Much of the antibody is IgM and is not protective. The semi-immune adult from malarious areas characteristically has high titers of circulating malarial antibodies, low to undetectable parasitemia without associated symptoms, and a spleen of normal size. If the individual leaves the area or receives malaria chemoprophylaxis, exposure to blood-stage parasites is reduced, and immunoglobulin levels and specific malaria immunity diminish over a period of months to years. On reinfection, the individual is susceptible to a severe bout of clinical malaria.

High-risk groups for severe, often fatal, malarial infections, particularly with *P. falciparum,* include young children, pregnant women, and nonimmune immigrants or visitors to malarious areas. Splenectomy in the tropics, including that performed for the tropical splenomegaly syndrome, can result in fatal malarial infections.

Vaccine Development. The in vitro cultivation of *P. falciparum* by Trager and Jensen in 1976 and advances in genetic engineering and monoclonal antibody technology have improved the potential for development of a malaria vaccine. Current vaccine research is directed at 3 developmental stages of the parasite—the sporozoite, the merozoite, and the gamete.

Human safety, immunogenicity, and protective efficacy trials of two candidate *P. falciparum* sporozoite vaccines have been reported. One vaccine is a synthetic peptide construct simulating repeat portions of the natural circumsporozoite antigen, and the other is a recombinant DNA–derived immunogen expressed in *Escherichia coli*. The results, however, have been disappointing. A recombinant *P. vivax* sporozoite immunogen expressed in yeast is inadequately immunogenic in human trials, but a synthetic merozoite vaccine simulating portions of an infected erythrocytic surface antigen (RESA) is undergoing human trials, with encouraging results. Extensive field trials of a merozoite vaccine are being conducted in Colombia and Venezuela at this time (1990). The principal constraints to the sporozoite vaccines tested so far appear to be inadequacy of the adjuvant in the vaccines and difficulty in identifying T-cell epitopes necessary for stimulation of the CMI component of the immune responses.

CLINICAL MANIFESTATIONS. Clinical symptoms and signs of malaria are associated with the release of merozoites, malarial pigment, and debris into the circulation following rupture of infected erythrocytes. Semi-immune patients are less likely to develop severe manifestations and complications when they become infected.

Prodromal Symptoms. Some patients have vague prodromal symptoms before parasites can be detected in the blood. These manifestations, i.e., malaise, myalgia, headache, anorexia, and slight fever, may persist for 2 or 3 days before an acute paroxysm begins. The incubation period, or time from exposure to onset of symptoms, can be prolonged by partial immunity or by incomplete chemosuppression.

Periodicity. In primary attacks, 2 or 3 days are usually required before the rhythm of parasitic schizogony is determined. During this time, the fever is irregular and intermittent. After 5 to 7 days, *P. vivax, P. malariae,* and *P. ovale* infections often become synchronous and cause periodic febrile paroxysms (Figs. 73–17 and 116–2*C*). Periodicity may be less apparent in falciparum malaria, although sometimes pronounced synchronicity is present and most patients infected with this parasite have a waxing and waning of symptoms. In vivax and ovale malaria, the schizonts of each brood of parasites mature every 48 hours (tertian periodicity), whereas in *P. malariae* infections, schizonts mature at 72-hour intervals, causing a quartan periodicity.

The typical paroxysm has an abrupt onset with a feeling of coldness and a chill. The teeth chatter, and the patient covers himself. Within 30 to 60 minutes, the patient feels hot and has profuse sweating, usually a headache, malaise, and myalgia, along with a varying degree of other symptoms, e.g., nausea, vomiting, flushed face, dry and burning skin, and convulsions. Temperatures of 40° to 41°C (104° to 106°F) are usual in primary falciparum infections, whereas peak fevers in infections with the other 3 species of plasmodia are usually lower, i.e., 39° to 40°C (102° to 104°F). The hot

stage lasts from 2 to 6 hours. The sweating stage, in which the patient's temperature falls rapidly, lasts 2 to 3 hours. The entire paroxysm, which often begins in the early afternoon, averages 9 to 10 hours. Between paroxysms, the patient may feel well.

Symptoms. Generalized constitutional symptoms include fever, chills, dizziness, backache, myalgia, malaise, and fatigue. Gastrointestinal symptoms, i.e., anorexia, nausea, vomiting, abdominal pain, and diarrhea, can be prominent, causing confusion with gastroenteritis. The patient sometimes complains of a dry cough and shortness of breath. Young children and semi-immune individuals may have fever and headache as only symptoms.

Signs. Physical examination usually demonstrates a fever, tachycardia, and warm, flushed skin. The spleen is often palpable in acute malaria and is commonly so in later attacks of the infection. It is usually soft and may be tender. The liver is frequently enlarged and tender. Orthostatic hypotension often occurs during initial infections. Mental confusion, jaundice, and cyanosis are not unusual. Some patients have recurrent herpes simplex infections ("fever blisters").

Laboratory Findings. Anemia, leukopenia, and thrombocytopenia are usual but may not be obvious on initial examination, because they often occur following the institution of chemotherapy and clearance of parasitemia. The reticulocyte count is usually normal despite hemolysis and becomes elevated only after the fever and parasitemia have cleared. Urinalysis reveals albuminuria, urobilinogen, and increased conjugated bilirubin in many patients.

Abnormalities in liver function tests may cause diagnostic confusion with viral hepatitis. Serum transaminases, e.g., ALT and AST, are usually elevated. Both the direct and the indirect bilirubin can be elevated. The prothrombin time can be prolonged. Serum albumin is frequently depressed, and globulins, particularly in repeat infections, are elevated.

Malaria causes a polyclonal increase in immunoglobulins, both IgM (in acute attacks) and IgG. This is associated with a rapid appearance of specific malarial

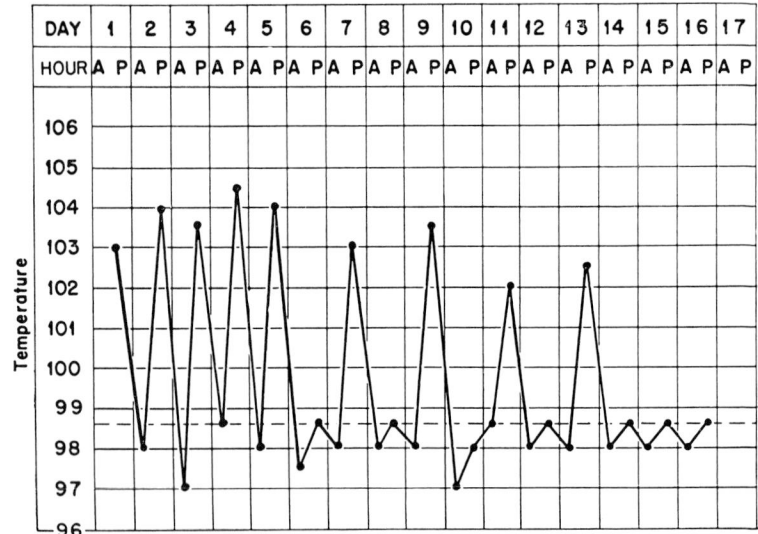

FIGURE 73–17. Fever chart in a *P. vivax* infection showing an initial quotidian tendency becoming tertian. No specific therapy. (A = A.M.; P = P.M.) (From Russell, West, Manwell, et al.: Practical Malariology, 2nd ed. London, Oxford University Press, 1963.)

antibodies and reduced complement levels. False-positive serologic tests for syphilis (VDRL), rheumatoid factors, heterophil agglutinins, and cold agglutinins may be present.

Hyponatremia and decreased serum osmolality occur in severe malarial infections associated with urinary sodium retention and a reversal of the urinary sodium/potassium ratio. Transient increases in the serum creatinine and blood urea nitrogen frequently occur. Hypoglycemia occurs in severe falciparum infections and in women who either are pregnant or have recently delivered; it is also caused by the use of quinine.

Vivax Malaria. In the nonimmune individual, the incubation period is usually 12 to 18 days, but occasionally, with certain strains, it can be much longer, i.e., 5 to 13 months. Relapses are common within 6 months of an acute attack. Vivax malaria is usually less severe than falciparum malaria. Parasitemia rates are lower. Deaths have been reported occasionally following rupture of an enlarged spleen, either spontaneously or after trauma. In some individuals, e.g., children in India, high parasitemias and death have been associated with the reticulocytosis following anemia.

In the initial phase of illness, the fever can be erratic or continuous. If the infection continues for 3 to 4 days, a synchronous cycle may develop with afternoon temperature elevations approximately every 48 hours, the classic benign tertian periodicity (Figs. 73–17 and 116–2C). The fever can be as high as 40°C (104°F), and the patient often feels worse than with falciparum malaria.

Physical findings usually include an enlarged, tender spleen by the second week of infection and a palpable liver. Anemia is common in chronic infections.

Ovale Malaria. Infection with *P. ovale* is clinically very similar to infection with *P. vivax. P. ovale* is frequently found in conjunction with *P. falciparum.*

Quartan Malaria. Quartan malaria is the mildest and most chronic of all the human malarial infections. Invasion of erythrocytes builds up slowly. Therefore, anemia is less pronounced, parasitemias are low, and the diagnosis may be difficult to confirm. However, *P. malariae* can cause relatively severe acute illness and may be associated with persistent ill health with recurrent attacks of fever, malaise, headaches, fatigue, and sweating. The incubation period can be as short as 18 days but is often many weeks. Recrudescences can occur even after 30 to 50 years, and the infection has been transmitted by blood transfusion from donors with subpatent infections.

The patient may have had several febrile paroxysms before parasites are seen in the peripheral blood. As in vivax and ovale malaria, the paroxysms commonly occur during the day, usually in the afternoon, and, classically, every 72 hours. Splenomegaly is common.

Falciparum Malaria. *P. falciparum* causes the most severe form of malarial infection. It may kill up to 25% of nonimmune adults within 2 weeks of a primary attack unless appropriate treatment is given. The initial attack often follows mild prodromal symptoms. The incubation period is usually 10 to 14 days but may be longer. The fever is irregular at first but occurs daily. Paroxysms are irregular, unlike those often seen in the other malarial

infections. The fever spikes are often higher, i.e., 40.5° to 41°C (105° to 106°F), than those in vivax malaria. Complications are more common, including confusion, drowsiness, urinary incontinence, cough, vomiting, diarrhea, and abdominal pain.

Physical examination often demonstrates hepatosplenomegaly and pallor. Some patients have pulmonary basilar rales. The pulse may be rapid, e.g., 100 to 120 pulsations per minute, and the blood pressure is often low, e.g., 90 to 100 mm Hg/50 to 60 mm Hg. On standing, there is frequently a further increase in the pulse and a drop in the blood pressure. The patient complains of lightheadedness and may faint. Abdominal tenderness, especially over the liver and spleen, is frequently present. Jaundice occurs in 10 to 15% of patients with high parasitemia.

Patients who have had many previous attacks of falciparum malaria have partial immunity and thus have milder or asymptomatic infections.

Mixed Infections. Mixed infections, usually with *P. falciparum* and another species, are common in certain malarious areas. Management should include maximum consideration given to the most serious parasite. However, treatment to prevent relapses from persistent E-E forms of *P. vivax* and *P. ovale* must also be given.

Malaria in Children. In nonimmune children, the primary attack can vary widely. Common symptoms are drowsiness, refusal of food, thirst, headache, nausea, vomiting, and frequent loose stools. There may be no rigor, but the temperature can be greater than 40°C (104°F). Physical findings often include pallor, cyanosis, and, later, hepatosplenomegaly. Convulsions are frequent, and cerebral malaria is the major complication. Anemia can be a major clinical problem in children with repeated malarial infections. The mortality rate is high in infants and children with complicated *P. falciparum* infections.

Infants in endemic areas have some immunity to malaria. Symptoms, when they occur, are often more insidious, e.g., anemia, restlessness, loss of appetite, easy fatigue, sweating, and intermittent fever.

When malaria occurs in association with other clinical insults, e.g., anemia, malnutrition, diarrhea, pneumonia, measles, intestinal parasites, or schistosomiasis, mortality and serious morbidity are increased. "Malarial cachexia" is characterized by stunting of growth, wasting, anemia, and hepatosplenomegaly.

Malaria in Pregnancy

Malaria in the Mother. Recrudescences and relapses of malaria are frequent during the second half of pregnancy, probably because of the immunosuppression associated with pregnancy. Malaria can potentiate anemia. Acute renal insufficiency and hypoglycemia sometimes occur as complications of falciparum malaria in pregnancy.

Low birth weight has been associated with placental infection with malarial parasites, particularly in primigravidas. In communities with incomplete immunity, epidemic malaria is an important cause of abortions, miscarriages, stillbirths, and neonatal deaths.

Congenital Malaria. Congenital infection can occur with all 4 species causing human malaria but is more commonly due to *P. vivax* and *P. malariae*. The incubation period is usually 9 to 30 days, consistent with infection occurring at parturition. Congenital malaria is rare when the mother has solid immunity because of transplacental passive transfer of protective IgG antimalarial antibodies.

The signs and symptoms are often subtle and insidious. The classic malarial paroxysm of chills and sweats is absent, although fever is usual. The infant feeds poorly and is restless and drowsy. Vomiting, diarrhea, pallor, and cyanosis may be present. Jaundice and hepatosplenomegaly should make one suspect the diagnosis of malaria, particularly when the mother has malaria or has been exposed to it. Because there are no exoerythrocytic hepatic stages in congenital *P. vivax* and *P. ovale* infections, radical cure with primaquine is unnecessary.

Transfusion Malaria. Any of the 4 types of human malaria can be transmitted directly, from a blood donor, from accidental infection by a contaminated needle, or from drug addicts sharing needles. The incubation period following the injection is as short as a few days for *P. falciparum* to 40 days or longer for *P. malariae*. As in congenital malaria, radical cure to prevent relapses is not necessary.

COMPLICATIONS

Splenic Rupture. Splenic rupture may occur in acute infections with all species. Often following a latent period, the patient develops circulatory collapse with rapid weak pulse and low blood pressure along with pain and fullness in the left upper quadrant of the abdomen. There may be referred pain in the left shoulder and abnormalities in the left lung base on the chest radiograph. Rupture can be spontaneous but usually follows trauma, including overly aggressive palpation of the spleen. A subcapsular hematoma is often the initial event, leading to a capsular tear. Rupture of an enlarged, friable spleen is a medical emergency requiring blood transfusion and surgical removal of the organ.

Cerebral Malaria. A frequent cause of mortality, especially in children and nonimmune adults, is cerebral malaria. It usually develops slowly over several days but may occur early in the illness. A severe headache appears. The patient becomes increasingly drowsy and confused and, if not treated rapidly, becomes delirious and then comatose. Hallucinations occur, and the patient may appear drunk.

The results of neurologic examination may be normal, or there may be extensive findings. Abnormalities encountered include contracted and unequal pupils, absent or exaggerated deep tendon reflexes, and a Babinski sign. Convulsions are frequent. The patient may also have muscular twitching and jerky or rhythmic movements of the head, neck, and extremities. Electroencephalographic abnormalities are nonspecific and are present in patients with minimal cerebral symptoms and signs. Examination of the cerebrospinal fluid shows increased pressure and protein with minimal or no pleocytosis.

In patients with cerebral malaria, very high fever, i.e., 41° to 42°C (106° to 108°F), can occur. The skin is often flushed and dry, as in heat stroke. Hyperpyrexia requires immediate treatment to reduce the fever.

Hypoglycemia. This complication more commonly occurs in patients receiving quinine therapy and in young children and pregnant women. It is associated with increased mortality and neurologic sequelae. Altered consciousness is the principal manifestation, and it will be mistakenly believed to be due to cerebral malaria if a blood sugar test is not performed.

Renal Failure. Mild proteinuria, azotemia, and oliguria occur frequently in heavy *P. falciparum* infections. Acute renal failure often complicates severe falciparum infections with high parasitemia and marked hemolysis; an acute tubular necrosis results from renal anoxia, a reduced renal blood flow, and deposition of hemoglobin in the renal tubules. Anuria is a poor prognostic sign, requiring peritoneal dialysis or hemodialysis.

Immunohemolytic Anemia. Severe hemolysis, hemoglobinuria, and renal failure make up the clinical triad of "blackwater fever." This syndrome is less common now than in the past, when it was associated with intermittent quinine therapy, with *P. falciparum* infection in nonimmune individuals, or with interrupted exposure in partially immune individuals. The clinical findings consist of severe hemolytic anemia, hemoglobinuria, oliguria, and jaundice. The urine is dark brown (caused by methemoglobin) if acid, or red (oxyhemoglobin-related) if alkaline or neutral. Other signs of serious difficulty with renal function, e.g., hemoglobin casts and proteinuria, develop rapidly as well. Patients with blackwater fever also have the usual symptoms and signs of severe falciparum malaria. The parasitemia rate is usually low, i.e., less than 1%. Another cause of intravascular hemolysis and hemoglobinuria in patients with malaria is the destruction of G-6-PD–deficient erythrocytes by oxidant antimalarial drugs, e.g., primaquine.

Pulmonary Failure. Acute pulmonary edema can develop rapidly, has been associated with excessive intravenous fluid administration, and is often fatal. Hyperpnea, dyspnea, a nonproductive cough, and scattered moist rales and rhonchi over the lungs are usually present. Chest radiographs may show increased bronchovascular markings. Arterial blood gases show hypocapnia and alkalosis due to hyperventilation and hypoxia. Signs of DIC have been reported in patients dying of severe pulmonary failure.

Algid Malaria. In some patients, the blood pressure is low, i.e., 80 to 90 mm Hg/40 to 50 mm Hg, and there is actual vascular collapse, resembling acute adrenal insufficiency. These patients have pale, cold, and clammy skin with shallow breathing. The blood volume must be expanded to prevent death.

Gastrointestinal Symptoms. Most patients with falciparum malaria have anorexia and nausea. However, additional gastrointestinal symptoms, e.g., vomiting, abdominal pain, watery diarrhea, and jaundice, may be present and may be so severe that the illness is diagnostically confused with gastroenteritis or hepatitis.

DIAGNOSIS

Blood Smears. Definitive diagnosis of malaria depends on microscopic demonstration of parasites in the peripheral blood film. For detection of organisms, the thick blood film is superior because it concentrates the red blood cells by a factor of 20 to 40 times (Fig. 73–

4C and D on Plate I). Identification of species in the thick film is difficult because the red cells are lysed in the staining procedure and there is alteration of the morphologic features of the parasites. For positive identification of species, a thin blood film is often necessary (Figs. 73–4E–I [Plate II] and 73–6). A thick film will yield 3 to 4 times as many positive findings as a thin smear and will reveal plasmodia in virtually all active clinical cases. Thick and thin films can be made on the same slide. In doubtful cases, it may be necessary to repeat the thick blood smears every 4 to 6 hours until the diagnosis is made. Symptoms may precede detectable parasitemia by 1 to 2 days. Timing of blood smears is less important than obtaining several smears daily in order to make the diagnosis. Quantitation of parasitemia is useful in following the response to therapy. Blood smears should be stained with Giemsa stain (Chapter 123). Leishman's stain and Wright's stain can also be used but are not as good. Rapid staining may be done with Field's stain, although this stain is less permanent.

The most important initial distinction to make is whether *P. falciparum* is present, because this parasite is frequently life-threatening. Species identification may require expert opinion; many physicians are not sufficiently experienced in morphologic differentiation. *P. falciparum* is suggested by criteria such as small ring size, accolé forms (Fig. 73–4H [Plate I]), banana-shaped gametocytes (Fig. 73–4I), multiple parasites in a single erythrocyte, parasitemia greater than 2% of the red blood cells (Fig. 73–4H), and predominance of rings with few trophozoites and no schizonts (Fig. 73–4C and H) (Table 73–2).

The presence of granular brownish pigment in monocytes or leukocytes should alert physicians to malaria even in the absence of demonstrated parasitemia.

Parasites may also be demonstrated in a bone marrow specimen, but this is rarely required.

Differential Diagnosis. The clinical diagnosis of malaria is frequently difficult. Early symptoms may mimic influenza. Malaria may be confused with febrile illnesses, including kala-azar, gastroenteritis, hepatitis, amebic liver abscess, relapsing fever, yellow fever, typhoid fever, tuberculosis, brucellosis, endocarditis, pyelonephritis, trypanosomiasis, blood disorders, poliomy-

elitis, and the pre-rash stages of many viral diseases. In endemic areas, the diagnosis requires clinical judgment to distinguish infection from disease. The presence of a few malarial parasites in the blood film of a semi-immune person from an endemic area proves that he or she is infected with malaria but does not necessarily determine the actual disease responsible for symptoms.

Serologic Tests. Serologic methods cannot replace parasitologic examination in clinical diagnosis because they do not distinguish present infection from past experience. However, serologic testing is extremely important in epidemiologic surveys and in screening potential blood donors. With appropriate sampling techniques, serologic data can help determine the occurrence and intensity of transmission as well as the change in transmission patterns over time for a given area.

The most standardized serologic test is the indirect fluorescent antibody (IFA) test using species-specific antigens. The enzyme-linked immunosorbent assay (ELISA) has been adapted to *P. falciparum* using parasites from in vitro cultivation. The indirect hemagglutination (IHA) test and immunoprecipitin tests are less satisfactory. For serologic testing, blood can be collected by finger prick into heparinized microcapillary tubes, placed on filter papers, and later eluted.

These methods do not distinguish between protective and nonprotective antibody. Tests to detect antisporozoite antibodies, including the circumsporozoite precipitin (CSP) reaction, the IFA test, the ELISA, and tests for inhibition of sporozoite and merozoite development (in hepatocyte and erythrocyte stage cultures, respectively), are being used in some field surveys.

The ELISA and radioimmune assays have been used successfully to detect parasite antigens in mosquitoes and in human blood. DNA probes for detecting infection with *P. falciparum* and *P. vivax* in the blood have been developed and are used in some research projects but are not yet clinically available.

PROGNOSIS. Prognosis is excellent for complete recovery from primary attacks of *P. vivax*, *P. ovale*, and *P. malariae*. Falciparum malaria carries a good prognosis if diagnosed rapidly and treated appropriately, although mortality may still occur. If *P. falciparum* infection goes untreated, mortality is high. The prognosis of *P. falcip-*

TABLE 73–2. Differential Characteristics of Human Malarial Parasites in Stained Thin Blood Films

Characteristics	P. falciparum	P. vivax	P. ovale	P. malariae
Infected erythrocyte enlarged	−	+	±	−
Infected erythrocyte fimbriated* and/or oval	rare	rare	frequent	rare
Infected erythrocyte decolorized	−	+	+	−
Infected erythrocyte with Schüffner's dots (stippling)*	−	+	+	−
Infected erythrocyte with Maurer's dots*	+	−	−	−
Multiple parasites in a single erythrocyte*	+	rare	−	−
Parasite, all forms in peripheral blood	−	+	+	+
Parasite, large coarse rings	−	+	+	+
Parasite, double chromatin dots*	+	rare	−	−
Parasite, accolé forms*	+	rare	−	−
Parasite, band forms*	−	−	−	+
Parasite, sausage-shaped gametocytes	+	−	−	−
Number of merozoites in an erythrocytic schizont	8–24	12–24	8–12	6–12

*Not invariable but suggestive when seen.

arum infection is directly related to the proportion of red blood cells parasitized when therapy is instituted. When parasitemia is greater than 100,000 per mm^3 and the hematocrit is less than 30%, the patient is at grave risk of complications and death. Advanced age and associated complications also increase the risk of fatal outcome with *P. falciparum* infection. However, with proper use of antimalarials, radical cure of malaria is possible in the great majority of cases.

BIBLIOGRAPHY

Aikawa M: Human cerebral malaria. Am J Trop Med Hyg 39:3, 1988.

Aikawa M, Miller LH, Johnson J, et al: Erythrocyte entry by malaria parasites. A moving junction between erythrocyte and parasite. J Cell Biol 77:72, 1978.

Brooks MH, Malloy JP, Bartelloni PJ, et al: Pathophysiology of acute malaria. 1. Correlation of clinical and biochemical abnormalities. Am J Med 43:735, 1967.

Bruce-Chwatt LJ: Essential Malariology. 2nd ed. London, William Heinemann Medical Books, 1985.

Campbell GH, Aley SB, Ballou WR, et al: Use of synthetic and recombinant peptides in the study of host-parasite interactions in the malarias. Am J Trop Med Hyg 37:428, 1987.

Clark IA: Monokines and lymphokines in malarial pathology. Ann Trop Med Parasitol 81:577, 1987.

Clark IA: Cell-mediated immunity in protection and pathology of malaria. Parasitol Today 3:300, 1987.

Clark IA, Chaudhri G, Cowden WB: Role of tumor necrosis factor in the illness and pathology of malaria. Trans R Soc Trop Med Hyg 83:436, 1989.

Drugs for parasitic infections. Med Lett Drugs Ther 30:15, 1988.

Friedman MJ, Trager W: The biochemistry of resistance to malaria. Sci Am 244:154, 1981.

Gilles HM, Lawson JB, Sibelas M, et al: Malaria, anaemia and pregnancy. Ann Trop Med Parasitol 63:245, 1969.

Grau GE, Taylor TE, Molyneux ME, et al: Tumor necrosis factor and disease severity in children with falciparum malaria. N Engl J Med 320:1586, 1989.

Hoffman SL, Wistar R, Ballou WR, et al: Immunity to malaria and naturally acquired antibodies to the circumsporozoite protein of *Plasmodium falciparum*. N Engl J Med 315:601, 1986.

Karney WW, Tong MJ: Malabsorption in *Plasmodium falciparum* malaria. Am J Trop Med Hyg 21:1, 1972.

Krotoski WA, Bray RS, Garnham PCC, et al: Observations on early and late post-sporozoite tissue stages in primate malaria. II. The hypnozoite of *Plasmodium cynomolgi bastianellii* from 3 to 105 days after infection, and detection of 36- to 40-hour pre-erythrocytic forms. Am J Trop Med Hyg 31:211, 1982.

Krotoski WA, Garnham PCC, Bray RS, et al: Observations on early and late post-sporozoite tissue stages in primate malaria. I. Discovery of a new latent form of *Plasmodium cynomolgi* (the hypnozoite), and failure to detect hepatic forms within the first 24 hours after infection. Am J Trop Med Hyg 31:24, 1982.

Looareesuwan S, Merry AH, Phillips RE, et al: Reduced erythrocyte survival following clearance of malarial parasitaemia in Thai patients. Br J Haematol 67:473, 1987.

Luzzatto L: Genetics of red cells and susceptibility to malaria. Blood 54:961, 1979.

MacPherson GG, Warrell MJ, White NJ: Human cerebral malaria. A quantitative ultrastructural analysis of parasitized erythrocyte sequestration. Am J Pathol 119:385, 1985.

Malloy JP, Brooks MH, Barry KG: Pathophysiology of acute falciparum malaria. II. Fluid compartmentalization. Am J Med 43:745, 1967.

Marsh K, Greenwood BM: The immunopathology of malaria. Clin Trop Med Comm Dis 1:91, 1986.

McGregor IA: Malaria: Nutritional implications. Rev Infect Dis 4:798, 1982.

McGregor IA: The development and maintenance of immunity to malaria in highly endemic areas. Clin Trop Med Comm Dis 1:29, 1986.

Miller LH, Haynes JD, McAuliffe FM, et al: Evidence for differences in erythrocyte surface receptors for the malaria parasites *Plasmodium falciparum* and *Plasmodium knowlesi*. J Exp Med 146:277, 1977.

Miller LH, Mason SJ, Clyde DF, et al: The resistance factor to *Plasmodium vivax* in blacks: The Duffy-blood-group genotype. FyFy. N Engl J Med 295:302, 1976.

Miller LH, Usami S, Chien S: Alterations in the rheologic properties of *Plasmodium knowlesi*–infected red cells. J Clin Invest 50:1451, 1971.

Molyneux MX, Taylor TE, Wirima JJ, Borgstein A: Clinical features and prognostic indicators in pediatric cerebral malaria: a study of 131 comatose Malawian children. Q J Med 71:441, 1989.

Nussenzweig V, Nussenzweig RS: Development of a sporozoite malaria vaccine. Am J Trop Med Hyg 35:678, 1986.

Phillips RE, Looareesuwan S, Warrell DA, et al: The importance of anaemia in cerebral and uncomplicated falciparum malaria: role of complications, dyserythropoiesis and iron sequestration. Q J Med 58:305, 1986.

Phillips RE, Warrell DA: The pathophysiology of severe falciparum malaria. Parasitol Today 2:271, 1986.

Punyagupta S, Srichaikul T, Nitiyanant P, et al: Acute pulmonary insufficiency in falciparum malaria. Am J Trop Med Hyg 23:551, 1974.

Quinn TC, Strickland GT: Clinical manifestations of malaria. Clin Trop Med Comm Dis 1:127, 1986.

Rosenberg EB, Strickland GT, Yang S-L, et al: IgM antibodies to red cells and autoimmune anemia in patients with malaria. Am J Trop Med Hyg 22:146, 1973.

Spencer HC: Epidemiology of malaria. Clin Trop Med Comm Dis 1:1 1986.

Spencer HC, Kaseje DCO, Mosley WH, et al: Impact on mortality and fertility of a community-based malaria control programme in Saradidi, Kenya. Ann Trop Med Parasitol 81 (Suppl 1):36, 1987.

Taylor TE, Molyneux ME, Wirima JJ, et al: Blood glucose levels in Malawian children before and during the administration of intravenous quinine for severe falciparum malaria. N Engl J Med 319:1040, 1988.

Warrell DA: Pathophysiology of severe falciparum malaria in man. Parasitology 94:553, 1987.

Warrell DA, Looareesuwan S, Warrell MJ, et al: Dexamethasone proves deleterious in cerebral malaria: A double-blind trial in 100 comatose patients. N Engl J Med 306:313, 1982.

Warrell DA, White NJ, Veall N, et al: Cerebral anaerobic glycolysis and reduced cerebral oxygen transport in human cerebral malaria. Lancet 2:534, 1988.

White NJ: Pathophysiology (of malaria). Clin Trop Med Comm Dis 1:55, 1986.

White NJ, Miller KD, Marsh K, et al: Hypoglycemia in African children with severe malaria. Lancet 1:708, 1987.

White NJ, Warrell DA, Chanthavanich P, et al: Severe hypoglycemia and hyperinsulinemia in falciparum malaria. N Engl J Med 309:61, 1983.

Williamson WA, Greenwood BM: Impairment of the immune response to vaccination after acute malaria. Lancet 1:1328, 1978.

World Health Organization: Severe and complicaed malaria. Trans R Soc Trop Med Hyg 80 (Suppl):1, 1986 and 84 (Suppl 2):1–65, 1990.

World Health Organization: WHO Expert Committee on Malaria, 18th Report. Geneva, WHO Tech Rep Ser 735, 1986.

World Health Organization: The biology of malaria parasites. Geneva, WHO Tech Rep Ser 743, 1987.

73.1.   TREATMENT AND CONTROL OF MALARIA

GENERAL PRINCIPLES

Definitions. Antimalarial drugs have a selective action on different phases of the life cycle of the parasite. *Blood schizonticides* destroy asexual parasites in the red blood cells and are effective in the treatment of a clinical attack. *Tissue schizonticides* act on the exoerythrocytic stages to prevent relapses of *P. vivax* and *P. ovale* infections. Some antimalarials prevent transmission by the vector. *Gametocidal drugs* destroy the sexual forms of the parasite, whereas *sporonticidal drugs* inhibit the development of oocysts on the stomach wall of the mosquito.

Certain drugs have a suppressive and prophylactic action to prevent the occurrence of infection or clinical manifestations. *Causal prophylactics* act on tissue forms of the malarial parasite. Other compounds are *suppressive* or *clinical prophylactics* because they prevent clinical symptoms by destroying malarial parasites as they enter the blood; all blood schizonticides are clinical prophylactics.

Some antimalarials exert more than one of these effects; thus, they may be put to several uses. However, no single antimalarial compound demonstrates all of these actions.

Modifying Factors. Blood schizonticides alone cure *P. falciparum* and *P. malariae* infections, but for complete (radical) cure of vivax and ovale malaria, a tissue schizonticide is necessary as well.

The state of immunity may influence drug use. Persons living in holoendemic or hyperendemic malarious areas acquire a degree of immunity to local strains and can often be cured or protected with less drug than can nonimmune individuals.

The sensitivity of the local malarial parasites is a prime consideration in drug selection. The resistance of *P. falciparum* strains from many geographic areas to 4-aminoquinolines is the most important example of this phenomenon.

Antimalarial Compounds. The chemical groupings of the most important antimalarial compounds are presented below and are divided into those in current use and those undergoing clinical trials. The following compounds are in current use:

1. 4-Aminoquinolines—chloroquine, amodiaquine
2. Cinchona alkaloids—quinine, quinidine
3. 4-Quinoline-carbinolamines (quinolinemethanols)—mefloquine
4. 8-Aminoquinolines—primaquine
5. Diaminopyrimidines—pyrimethamine
6. Sulfonamides and sulfones—sulfadoxine, sulfalene, dapsone
7. Tetracyclines—tetracycline, doxycycline
8. Biguanides—chlorguanide (proguanil)

The following compounds are undergoing clinical trials:

1. Sesquiterpene lactones—artemisinin (qinghaosu)
2. Phenanthrene-methanols—halofantrine

ANTIMALARIAL PHARMACOLOGY

Chloroquine. This drug is marketed for oral administration as a diphosphate or sulfate salt and for intramuscular or intravenous injection as the dihydrochloride.

Antimalarial Actions. Chloroquine is a 4-aminoquinoline with marked, rapid blood schizonticidal activity against susceptible strains of malarial parasites. The drug is not effective against exoerythrocytic forms in the liver. Chloroquine is gametocidal against *P. vivax*, *P. ovale*, and *P. malariae* and is effective against immature

but not mature gametocytes of *P. falciparum*. The action of chloroquine is rapid, with parasitemia disappearing in 48 to 72 hours after the standard regimen has been administered.

Pharmacology and Metabolism. The drug is rapidly and almost completely absorbed from the gastrointestinal tract, following which it is localized in the tissues, mainly concentrated in cell lysosomes. The drug is metabolized by alkylation in the liver and excreted slowly by the kidneys, with a half-life of from 3 to 6 or 7 days in a normal healthy adult, depending on the amount and frequency of drug intake. Following daily administration of chloroquine, about 10% appears in the feces and about 60% in the urine, of which approximately two thirds is the parent compound. With therapeutic doses given orally, an effective blood concentration is usually reached within minutes. Acidification of urine increases renal excretion.

Toxicity. At doses used for suppression and treatment of malaria, toxic manifestations are rare with chloroquine. Minor reported side effects include nausea, vomiting, dizziness, headache, blurred vision, fatigue, diarrhea, and confusion. Gastrointestinal symptoms may be reduced by taking the drug after meals. Pruritus is sometimes a problem in individuals, particularly blacks, taking therapeutic doses who have taken the drug before. These symptoms usually disappear after the drug has been discontinued.

In prolonged high daily doses such as those used in the treatment of rheumatoid arthritis, chloroquine may cause a severe, often irreversible, retinopathy characterized by loss of central visual acuity, pigmentation of the macula, and retinal artery constriction. However, retinopathy has never been reported following treatment for malarial infection at recommended doses.

There are no reports of teratogenic effects in humans when chloroquine has been used as an antimalarial drug; therefore, it may be administered during pregnancy. Hypotension, acute circulatory failure, and respiratory and cardiac arrest have been reported following parenteral administration of chloroquine, *particularly in infants and young children*. Transient high blood concentrations induce hypotension and sometimes sudden death. Therefore, intravenous chloroquine should always be given slowly and never as a bolus. Gastric lavage and intramuscular injections are safer than the intravenous route for treating severely ill patients.

Dosage reduction may be required in patients with severe renal and hepatic disease, although some authorities recommend a standard therapeutic regimen for these patients.

Uses. Chloroquine is the drug of choice for treatment and prevention of infections with *P. vivax*, *P. ovale*, *P. malariae*, and sensitive *P. falciparum* strains.

Amodiaquine. This drug is marketed as the dihydrochloride dihydrate. The efficacy, side effects, recommendations, and precautions for amodiaquine are essentially the same as those for chloroquine, with a few exceptions.

Pharmacology and Metabolism. Amodiaquine is also a 4-aminoquinoline. There is no parenteral preparation for amodiaquine. There are in vivo and in vitro data suggesting that amodiaquine is more active than chloroquine against some strains of *P. falciparum* resistant to chloroquine. However, this increase in activity is not of a magnitude to support recommending the use of amodiaquine in known chloroquine-resistant infections.

Toxicity. Amodiaquine has side effects similar to those of chloroquine. In addition, there have been recent reports of agranulocytosis and severe hepatitis associated with its use. Amodiaquine is not licensed or marketed in the United States. It is unlikely to become a replacement for chloroquine because of several reports showing that it has no greater therapeutic effect in some geographic areas than chloroquine, and, most important, because of rare, but severe, toxicity.

Uses. Amodiaquine has been used in place of chloroquine.

Quinine. Quinine is marketed for oral administration as the sulfate salt. Quinine dihydrochloride is available for intravenous use.

Quinine has been a traditional antimalarial compound for centuries. The drug is customarily isolated from the bark of the cinchona tree; it can also be synthesized, although with difficulty.

Antimalarial Actions. Quinine is active against asexual erythrocytic stages of all forms of human malarial parasites. The drug does *not* affect exoerythrocytic forms. The gametocytes of *P. vivax, P. ovale,* and *P. malariae* and immature gametocytes of *P. falciparum* are sensitive to quinine. Mature gametocytes of *P. falciparum* are not susceptible. Quinine is regarded by many experienced clinicians as the most rapidly acting drug for treatment of severe cases of falciparum malaria.

Pharmacology and Metabolism. Quinine is quickly and almost completely absorbed from the intestinal tract. Peak plasma concentrations occur within 2 to 3 hours after a single oral dose. Most of the drug is bound to plasma proteins, although it is also concentrated in the liver, spleen, and kidneys. Less than 5% of quinine is excreted unchanged in the urine. In patients with normal liver function, most of the drug appears in the urine as hydroxyl derivatives. The usual half-life of 5.7 to 10 hours is often prolonged in patients with liver disease or sustained fever. There is no accumulation in the tissues, even with continued administration. Monitoring of blood levels is recommended in patients with impaired renal or hepatic function and may be particularly useful in young children. Quinine readily crosses the placenta, but cerebrospinal fluid levels are 1/20 to 1/50 of those in plasma. Acidification of urine increases renal excretion.

Toxicity. Quinine has a bitter taste. A common syndrome known as cinchonism (tinnitus, headache, nausea, abdominal pain, minor visual disturbances, transient loss of hearing, and tremors) occurs in many patients taking the drug. These symptoms may appear during the first 2 to 3 days of therapy and subside quickly when the drug is stopped. Very rare but more serious toxic effects include urticaria; "asthma" attacks in susceptible individuals; angioedema of the face, mucous membranes, and lungs; deafness; blindness; hemolytic anemia; and agranulocytosis. Severe poisoning results in convulsions, delirium, depressed respiration, coma, circulatory failure, and death. Quinine is a local irritant, sometimes causing gastric pain, nausea, and vomiting when given orally. For the same reason, it is associated with thrombophlebitis with sclerosis of veins following intravenous administration and damage to the renal tubules. Quinine can cause hypoprothrombinemia, which is prevented by administration of vitamin K.

There are reports of a limited risk of induced abortion with the use of quinine in pregnancy. However, because falciparum malaria also can cause abortions, it is difficult to implicate quinine toxicity as a cause of abortions. Pregnant women may be susceptible to acute hemolytic anemia or thrombocytopenia due to the drug, and quinine may accentuate hypoglycemia already produced by falciparum malaria in these women.

Uses. Quinine is more toxic than most other antimalarials. Its major uses are for persons with *P. falciparum* malaria resistant to chloroquine and for critically ill patients requiring parenteral medication.

Quinidine. Quinidine, a dextrorotary optical isomer of quinine, was found to be effective against *P. falciparum* over 100 years ago in India. However, it has been almost completely ignored for this purpose until the past 10 years, when investigators in Thailand began to show that it was at least as effective and safe as quinine in treating severe chloroquine-resistant malaria. Its use is particularly important in the United States, where intravenous quinine is not readily available. Most hospitals have a supply of quinidine for intravenous treatment of cardiac arrhythmias.

Antimalarial Actions. These are apparently similar to those of quinine. Quinidine has a lower MIC for *P. falciparum* in Thailand than quinine and is effective against quinine-resistant strains.

Pharmacology and Metabolism. Absorption and disposition appear to be similar to those of quinine. Mean plasma levels are slightly lower than with equivalent doses of quinine. Peak plasma levels after a single oral dose occur in 1.5 to 4.0 hours. Food decreases the rate but not the extent of absorption and may reduce side effects. Quinidine is 80% to 90% bound to plasma proteins, but protein binding may be decreased in patients with impaired hepatic function. It is present in breast milk in quinidine-treated mothers. Metabolism and elimination are primarily (60 to 85%) hepatic, but 15% to 40% appears in the urine as unchanged drug. The elimination half-life is not prolonged in nonmalarious patients with renal failure. Severe malaria may delay metabolism and elimination.

Toxicity. This is similar to the toxicity of quinine and is dose-related. Severe cardiovascular reactions are more likely to occur after parenteral administration. Intramuscular injections are painful, increase serum creatine phosphokinase levels, and are erratically and incompletely absorbed. Diarrhea, nausea, and vomiting (due to a direct irritant effect) are the most common adverse effects. Fever, hepatitis, manifestations of cinchonism, and thrombocytopenic purpura may occur. Severe hypotension due to peripheral vasodilation may occur after rapid parenteral administration; the hypotension should be treated with volume replacement and administration of vasopressor amines. Large doses of quinidine depress myocardial contractility and aggravate or induce heart failure. Quinidine may produce A-V block. Syncopal episodes and sudden death during quinidine therapy may be due to ventricular fibrillation, probably as a result of a markedly prolonged QT interval.

Hypotension and disturbance in cardiac conduction are related to serum concentrations. Therefore, when it is used intravenously, quinidine should be given with careful monitoring, preferably in the hospital. It is best to determine the serum quinidine levels after the initial loading dose and at least daily.

Uses. Quinidine can be used either intravenously or orally to treat chloroquine-resistant *P. falciparum*. It is particularly useful when an intravenous preparation of quinine is not available and to treat infections acquired in Thailand, where *P. falciparum* is becoming increasingly resistant to quinine. *In vitro* studies of *P. falciparum* isolates in Thailand have shown the parasite to be 2 or 3 times more sensitive to quinidine than to quinine. Quinidine sulphate, gluconate, and polygalacturonate are available as tablets and capsules containing 100 to 324 mg of the drug. Quinidine gluconate is available in 10 ml vials containing 80 mg/ml for parenteral therapy. In the treatment of severe or complicated malaria, quinidine is best given as a continous intravenous infusion (Table 73–4).

Mefloquine. Mefloquine is a 4-quinoline-carbinolamine developed by the United States Army malarial chemotherapy program. Mefloquine represents a major advance in the treatment of multidrug-resistant *P. falciparum* infections.

Antimalarial Actions. The exact mechanism of action of mefloquine is not known. Some similarity to the activity of quinine or quinine-related drugs is supposed by the fact that mefloquine, like quinine, inhibits or reverses chloroquine-induced hemozoin clumping in *P. berghei* trophozoites. However, unlike chloroquine and quinine, mefloquine does not intercalate with DNA but binds strongly to membranes, which may be the cause of its lethal action. Chloroquine-resistant plasmodia take up mefloquine, a difference that provides an explanation for the effectiveness of mefloquine against chloroquine-resistant malaria.

Pharmacology and Metabolism. Mefloquine is structurally related to quinine. After a single dose, peak plasma levels are reached between 2 and 12 hours. The drug binds extensively to plasma proteins but gives high concentrations in the lungs, gallbladder, liver, spleen, and kidneys. It is metabolized primarily to one component devoid of antiplasmodial activity and accumulates in the plasma. It undergoes extensive biliary and gastric secretion, followed by reabsorption. Most of the drug and its metabolites eventually appear in the feces. It has a long but variable elimination half-life, ranging from 13 to 24 days.

Toxicity. Single oral doses are well tolerated. Large amounts produce transient dizziness and nausea. Other undesirable effects include vomiting, soft stools and diarrhea, abdominal discomfort, anorexia, headache, bradycardia, skin rash and pruritus, and asthenia. Repeated high doses have caused histologic abnormalities in the retinas of laboratory animals.

Recently, neurologic and psychiatric reactions have been reported following the therapeutic and prophylactic use of mefloquine both alone and in combination with other antimalarials. Milder reactions have included ataxia, fatigue and asthenia, headache, nausea and vomiting, dysequilibrium, poor concentration, memory disturbances, and sleep disturbances. Some individuals have had vertigo, anxiety, depression, poor coordination, and agitation and confusion. More serious reactions have included severe depression with suicidal tendencies, anxiety neurosis, hallucinations, acute psychosis, seizures, mutism, manic behavior, delirium, and disturbed consciousness (stupor, coma). The incidence of these adverse effects may be on the order of 1% of those receiving mefloquine therapy. Although the adverse effects have occurred following all dosages, they appear to be more common following treatment doses above 1000 mg. No serious events have been reported in prophylactic drug trials of mefloquine. Limited evidence suggests that neurologic toxicity may be related to the accumulative prophylactic dose. Additional associated risk factors, e.g., sex, age, other antimalarial drugs, and prior neuropsychiatric illness, are uncertain at this time.

Uses. Mefloquine has been effective in the treatment and prevention of multidrug-resistant *P. falciparum*. Mefloquine is also active against *P. vivax*. In vitro studies have demonstrated varying response patterns of *P. falciparum* strains to mefloquine, and resistance has been developed during in vitro culture in the presence of the drug. Recent reports of neuropsychiatric toxicities have tempered the recommendations for using mefloquine. Therefore, it is mandatory that mefloquine be used judiciously and according to WHO guidelines. The drug should not be given to persons involved with activities requiring fine coordination and special performance, e.g., airplane crews, and operators of heavy or dangerous equipment. It should not be administered concurrently with chloroquine, quinine, or guinidine. If these drugs are used in the initial treatment of malaria, mefloquine administration should be delayed for at least 12 hours after the last dose. Relative contraindications include pregnancy, the concomitant use of β-blocker drugs, and neurologic illness. Also, for the time being, therapeutic doses of 15 mg/kg or 1250 mg, whichever is less, should not be exceeded.

Primaquine. Primaquine tablets contain the diphosphate salt.

Antimalarial Actions. Primaquine is an 8-aminoquinoline derivative. The drug is gametocidal and sporonticidal for all species of human malaria. It is a poor blood schizonticide but is effective against exoerythrocytic hypnozoites and will usually prevent relapses due to *P. vivax* and *P. ovale*.

Pharmacology and Metabolism. Primaquine is rapidly absorbed and excreted after oral adminstration. Peak plasma levels occur within 30 to 60 minutes and fall rapidly. The half-life is about 4 hours. The drug is probably rapidly metabolized, but metabolites have not been identified. Very little drug is fixed in the tissues.

Toxicity. There are 2 major types of toxic manifestations. The first is related to the gastrointestinal tract and includes anorexia, nausea, epigastric pain, and, sometimes, severe abdominal cramps. Intravascular hemolysis, the most important toxic reaction, relates to the genetic background of the individual. Individuals with erythrocyte glucose-6-phosphate dehydrogenase (G-6-PD) deficiency may have an acute hemolytic episode following administration of the drug (Chapter 5); G-6-PD deficiency is an inherited X-linked trait occurring most frequently in blacks and person of Mediterranean and Asian extraction. Intravascular hemolysis occurs when erythrocytes are exposed to oxidant stress. The severity of hemolysis depends on which variant is present. In most blacks, hemolysis is self-limited, even when drug administration is continued. In the Mediterranean variant and the Canton variant present in some persons of Chinese ancestry, however, hemolysis is more severe and does not appear to be self-limited, even after the drug is withdrawn. Therefore, it is generally recommended that a test for G-6-PD deficiency be performed before administering the drug in full doses. Other very rare untoward effects from primaquine include methemoglobinuria, hemoglobinuria, and, rarely, agranulocytosis, granulocytopenia, and leukopenia. Primaquine can produce marked methemoglobinemia in persons with congenital deficiency of nicotinamide-adenine dinucleotide (NAD) methemoglobin reductase.

Primaquine should not be administered to pregnant women because its safety in pregnancy has not been established.

Uses. Primaquine is used to prevent relapses of *P. vivax* and *P. ovale* infections. Its excellent gametocidal and sporonticidal action makes it potentially useful in combination with a blood schizonticide to prevent transmission in endemic areas.

Pyrimethamine

Antimalarial Actions. Pyrimethamine is a 2,4-diaminopyrimidine. The drug is a slow but effective blood schizonticide. It is also active against the primary tissue forms of *P. falciparum* and, to a lesser extent, *P. vivax* and is an excellent sporonticidal agent. The drug is not effective for radical cure of vivax and ovale malaria because it is inactive against latent exoerythrocytic stages.

Pharmacology and Metabolism. Pyrimethamine has a prolonged half-life of about 92 hours. It is slowly but completely absorbed from the intestinal tract and then firmly bound to proteins in the tissues. Pyrimethamine localizes in the liver, spleen, kidneys, and lungs. It is excreted in the urine and gives stable and prolonged plasma levels following single doses. The drug is excreted in the milk of nursing mothers. Pyrimethamine is a selective inhibitor of the plasmodial enzyme dihydrofolate reductase and therefore interferes with nucleic acid metabolism.

Toxicity. When given for malaria chemoprophylaxis or as treatment at recommended doses, no significant toxic symptoms have been reported for pyrimethamine. Some experts recommend that pyrimethamine not be given during pregnancy because teratogenic effects were reported in animal experiments. However, congenital defects associated with the use of pyrimethamine for chemoprophylaxis of malaria in recommended doses have not been reported, despite extensive use of the drug in endemic areas.

Uses. Pyrimethamine is not indicated for treatment of acute malarial infections except in combination with sulfonamides or sulfones. These combinations are used for treatment and prophylaxis of chloroquine-resistant falciparum malaria.

Sulfonamides and Sulfones

Antimalarial Actions. Sulfonamides and sulfones are highly effective blood schizonticides for *P. falciparum* but are less active against the asexual blood forms of other malarial parasite species. Like pyrimethamine, their action is too slow for them to be used alone. These drugs are used in combination with pyrimethamine or proguanil for the treatment of malaria.

Pharmacology and Metabolism. There is considerable variation in the rates of absorption and excretion of different compounds. They are excreted in the urine mainly as metabolites. The estimated half-lives of those frequently used as antimalarials are as follows: sulfadoxine, 100 to 200 hours; sulfalene, 65 hours; and dapsone, 28 hours. Failures with sulfonamides may be due to host differences in ability to acetylate the drug rather than to drug-resistant parasites. Sulfonamides and sulfones inhibit plasmodial dihydropteroate synthetase, an earlier step in the folate pathway than that affected by pyrimethamine.

Toxicity. These drugs are generally well tolerated. The sulfonamides may occasionally cause urticaria, Stevens-Johnson syndrome, and other hypersensitivity reactions. Hepatitis occurs but is rare. Agranulocytosis has also been reported but is very rare. Both sulfonamides and sulfones may precipitate hemolysis in persons with G-6-PD deficiency and methemoglobinemia in patients with hereditary NAD methemoglobinemia reductase deficiency. Acute hemolytic anemia may be produced in otherwise healthy persons, particularly black individuals. These compounds are contraindicated in persons with a previous history of hypersensitivity and in premature or newborn infants during the first month of life. Sulfadoxine and sulfalene are generally avoided during the first trimester of pregnancy. However, like pyrimethamine, teratogenic effects have never been proved. Because of danger to the newborn, sulfones and sulfonamides are contraindicated for pregnant women near term.

Uses. The sulfonamides and sulfones are used in combination with pyrimethamine and proguanil for treatment and prophylaxis of *P. falciparum* resistant to chloroquine.

Tetracycline. Tetracycline is manufactured as the hydrochloride salt for oral use.

Antimalarial Actions. Tetracycline has a very slow blood schizonticidal activity in man. Activity against tissue schizonts of chloroquine-resistant *P. falciparum* has also been demonstrated. Doxycycline and minocycline are as effective as tetracycline but are more expensive and have as many or more side effects.

Toxicity. Major side effects of tetracycline include permanent discoloration of teeth, hypoplasia of tooth enamel, and impaired bone growth in children less than 8 years of age. For these reasons, tetracycline should not be used in young children or pregnant women.

Gastrointestinal complaints, including nausea, vomiting, abdominal pain, and diarrhea, are common with the use of this drug. Overgrowth of *Candida* in the mouth, gut, vagina, or skin is a frequent problem in those taking tetracyclines. Rarely, a *Campylobacter* enteritis complicates tetracycline or doxycycline therapy. Doxycycline commonly causes photosensitivity, a real problem with its use in tropical areas.

Uses. Tetracycline and doxycyline are used as antimalarials for treatment of chloroquine- and pyrethamine-sulfonamide-resistant *P. falciparum* infections. Resistance by the parasites to tetracycline has never been proved. Since the action of these drugs against *P. falciparum* is so slow, they should always be used in combination with a rapid-acting blood schizonticide such as quinine.

Proguanil. Proguanil is formulated in tablets of the hydrochloride salt.

Antimalarial Actions. Proguanil has a slow schizonticidal action on erythrocytic forms. However, the drug is effective against the primary tissue phase of *P. falciparum.* Thus, it provides excellent causal prophylaxis against *P. falciparum* and is sporonticidal against this species. Proguanil is less active against *P. vivax,* and many patients on proguanil prophylaxis develop vivax malaria after the drug is discontinued.

Pharmacology and Metabolism. Proguanil is rapidly absorbed through the upper gastrointestinal tract. Its antimalarial action is accounted for by its rapid conversion to a dihydrotriazone derivative known as cycloguanil. Proguanil is eliminated slowly, mainly in the urine and feces, in which about 40% appears as the parent compound. The half-life of the dihydrotriazine derivative is much shorter than that of proguanil itself. Cycloguanil is a powerful inhibitor of dihydrofolate reductase. Like pyrimethamine, the binding affinity of cycloguanil is much greater for this enzyme in the parasite than in mammalian cells.

Toxicity. The advantage of this drug is its safety. Even at high doses, the only reported adverse effects are abdominal discomfort, loss of appetite, vomiting, diarrhea, and, rarely, hematuria.

Uses. Proguanil is used for causal prophylaxis, particularly of falciparum malaria in areas where parasites are not resistant to the drug. Resistance to pyrimethamine and resistance to proguanil frequently coexist because of the similar modes of action of these drugs. It is being extensively used for prophylaxis in areas of Africa where chloroquine-resistant *P. falciparum* is present. It appears to be more useful in East Africa than in West Africa, but resistance in *P. falciparum* strains is extensive. The combination of proguanil with dapsone or short-acting sulfonamides is being evaluated for prophylaxis in Southeast Asia, where it appears to have efficacy. Clinical response of an established infection is slow, and the use of proguanil for treatment of malaria is not recommended.

Artemisinin. Artemisinin (qinghaosu) is a sesquiterpene lactone extracted in 1972 at the Chinese Institute of Materia Medica from a medicinal herb *(Artemisia annua),* sweet wormwood. It has a very rapid onset of action but has a rather high recrudescence rate. Several artemisinin derivatives are currently being evaluated by the Chinese: artemether administered by intramuscular injection; artesunate, which can be given intravenously or by suppository; and arteether. These compounds and others being chemically synthesized are potentially excellent candidates for treating severe chloroquine-resistant *P. falciparum* infection.

Antimalarial Actions. Qinghaosu is a blood schizonticide. In humans, the drug is active against *P. vivax* and chloroquine-sensitive and -resistant strains of *P. falciparum.* There is no evidence of activity against exoerythrocytic stages or gametes.

Pharmacology and Metabolism. The drug is rapidly absorbed in animals. The half-life is about 4 hours. The high rate of recrudescence reported after initial treatment is reduced when the drug is administered intramuscularly in an oil suspension.

Toxicity. No significant side effects have been reported to date.

Uses. Artemisinin is proving useful in China in the treatment of chloroquine-resistant *P. falciparum* disease. It is not available for general use, but because of its rapidity of action against most strains of *P. falciparum,* its absence of cross-resistance with other antimalarials, and its apparent safety it may become a very valuable drug to treat resistant parasites. Because of the high rate of recrudescence, it may best be given with another, slower-acting antimalarial, e.g., doxycycline.

Halofantrine. Halofantrine hydrochloride (Halfan) is a phenanthrene-methanol, which has not previously produced an antimalarial compound. Like mefloquine, it was initially developed by Walter Reed Army Institute of Research. Because of its relatively short half-life and unique chemical identity, it offers hope that the development of drug resistance by the parasite will be delayed.

Antimalarial Actions. Halofantrine is a blood schizonticide with an unknown mode of action. It has no effect against the hepatic stages of the parasite.

Pharmacology and Metabolism. Absorption after oral administration is incomplete and variable. Peak plasma levels of the parent drug occur in 6 hours; the principal, desbutyl, metabolite peaks at 12 hours. Excretion is primarily in the feces, and the half-life for the compound is about 24 hours. There is no parenteral formulation of the drug.

Toxicity. Halofantrine is generally well tolerated. It is embryotoxic and is excreted in the milk in animals; it therefore is not recommended for treatment during pregnancy or breast-feeding. Abdominal pain, diarrhea, pruritus, skin rash, and elevated transaminases have been reported in some individuals taking the drug.

Uses. Clinical studies have shown that 500 mg of halofantrine every 6 hours for 3 doses cured 85% to 95% of those infected with any of the four species of *Plasmodium. P. falciparum* was very responsive, even in areas where parasites resistant to other drugs were common. Fever and parasitemia cleared rapidly, both usually responding by 2 or 3 days from the initiation of treatment. The pediatric dose is 8 mg/kg three times at 6-hour intervals. The drug is available as a suspension (5 ml contains 100 mg) and as a 250 mg tablet. It is not available in the United States. It is useful for treating clinical malaria in areas where multiple drug–resistant strains of *P. falciparum* are present.

Combination Drugs. When a sulfonamide or sulfone is given together with a dihydrofolate reductase inhibitor, a potentiating effect against malarial parasites is observed. The synergy is often so marked that the combination is effective against strains of *Plasmodium* resistant to the individual component drugs. The use of combinations permits lower doses of each component to be given and may help reduce the development of resistance to the individual compounds. The potentiating effect of these two classes of drugs occurs because they block sequential steps in the folate pathway, leading to de novo synthesis of purines and pyrimidines by plasmodia. Mammalian cells are permeable to folate and can use preformed folate, whereas bacteria and protozoa cannot. In general, these combinations are more effective against *P. falciparum* than against the other 3 species.

Pyrimethamine-Sulfadoxine. This combination, Fansidar, is marketed in tablets containing 500 mg of sulfadoxine and 25 mg of pyrimethamine. Toxic manifestations are rare. Those reported include headache, nausea, vomiting, abdominal pain, and skin reactions. Other side effects to sulfonamides may occur. Severe cutaneous reactions (erythema multiforme, Stevens-Johnson syndrome, and toxic epidermal necrolysis) have been reported in travelers using this drug for malaria prophylaxis. It has been calculated that fatalities occurred in 1 in 11,000 to 1 in 25,000 users. This explains the recent modification in recommendations for malaria prophylaxis. The safety of the combination in pregnancy has not been established. However, this drug has been used to treat malarial infection in large numbers of pregnant women without apparent adverse effects to the fetus. Pyrimethamine-sulfadoxine is used in the treatment and prophylaxis of chloroquine-resistant falciparum malaria. Because the action of this combination may be slow, a rapid-acting blood schizonticide such as quinine may also be given to acutely ill patients during the first 3 days of treatment.

Pyrimethamine-Sulfalene. This drug is considered equivalent to pyrimethamine-sulfadoxine in efficacy and toxicity. Each tablet contains 25 mg of pyrimethamine and 500 mg of sulfalene.

Pyrimethamine-Dapsone. This combination, which contains 12.5 mg of pyrimethamine and 100 mg of dapsone, is used for causal prophylaxis. There are no data demonstrating this drug to be more effective than pyrimethamine-sulfadoxine.

Mefloquine-Pyrimethamine-Sulfadoxine. This combination, Fansimef, is available in some areas, including Thailand. One tablet contains 250 mg of mefloquine (as the hydrochloride), 500 mg of sulfadoxine, and 25 mg of pyrimethamine. All components are odorless, white, crystalline powders. The combination's purpose is to protect mefloquine from the development of resistant strains of *P. falciparum*. This combination was used because all components have relatively long half-lives and allow for single-dose treatment and because mefloquine has an entirely different mode of action from the other two compounds. Therefore, no cross-resistance between mefloquine and pyrimethamine-sulfadoxine should exist.

The difficulty with this combination is that it is unusable if toxicity to any of its components develops. The chances of this happening, particularly to the long-acting sulfonamide, are good. It is accordingly preferable to use mefloquine and pyrimethamine-sulfadoxine separately as needed.

Trimethoprim Plus Short-Acting Sulfonamides. These combinations are not recommended for use in malaria, although some activity against malarial parasites has been demonstrated. Trimethoprim is less active against plasmodia than is pyrimethamine or proguanil. These combinations are pharmacologically balanced for treatment of bacterial infections, not for malaria, and overuse may accelerate the development of bacterial resistance.

THERAPEUTIC REGIMENS. The recommended treatment for malaria is outlined in Table 73–3, and the dosages of antimalarial drugs are given in Table 73–4. The first steps are to establish the diagnosis, identify the species of malarial parasite, and establish the parasite density, the immune status of the patient, the places where infection could have occurred, and the severity of the clinical illness. Species identification determines which drug is selected and is best accomplished by examination of a Giemsa-stained thin blood smear. Determination of where infection took place helps predict drug response by identifying the possibility of drug resistance. The severity of the illness and parasite density are important parameters in determining choice of drug and route of administration (Table 73–3). Parasitemia involving more than 1% or 2% of the erythrocytes indicates severe disease, as do complications and potentially life-threatening clinical manifestations. If the patient cannot take oral medication or the disease is severe, an intravenous drug is indicated.

Treatment of Falciparum Malaria. The chemotherapy of falciparum malaria is complicated by the problem of drug resistance. Hospitalization is often required because the patient is very ill. Frequent blood smears are made to assess parasitologic response. Failure of a drug to reduce parasitemia within 48 hours indicates the possibility of drug failure. Recommendations for therapy are based on patterns of drug sensitivity (Chapter 121).

P. falciparum Infections with Exposure in Areas Where Resistance to 4-Aminoquinolines Is Established. These areas include South America, the Indian subcontinent, Southeast Asia, Indonesia, China, some islands of the Pacific, including New Guinea and the Philippines, and sub-Saharan Africa (Chapter 121). The recommended treatment for uncomplicated chloroquine-resistant malaria in those areas where resistance to the combination drug pyrimethamine-sulfadoxine has not yet developed is Fansidar (Table 73–3). This combination is often effective even when *P. falciparum* isolates are resistant to pyrimethamine, but resistance is already common in Southeast Asia, East Africa, and Brazil and is rapidly increasing.

If Fansidar resistance is locally present, if the clinical condition of the patient is severe, or if parasitemia is high, quinine sulfate or quinidine gluconate should be given concomitantly for 2 to 5 days. The shorter dose is generally given to individuals with partial immunity. Quinine usually acts more rapidly in clearing parasites than the pyrimethamine-sulfonamide combination. The intravenous route may be required. Quinine plus tetracycline or doxycycline is a suitable alternative, as is quinine alone. If given alone, quinine should be given for 7 days. Quinidine is an effective substitute for quinine. Mefloquine is also effective in such cases.

TABLE 73–3. Recommended Drugs for Treatment of Malaria

Type	Parasitemia Clinical Illness	Recommended Drugs (Route)	Alternative Drugs (Route)
A. *P. falciparum*			
1. Exposure in areas where chloroquine resistance is established *or*	severe[2]	quinine or quinidine (IV) *plus* pyrimethamine-sulfadoxine[4] (oral)	quinine or quinidine (IV) *plus* tetracycline[5] (oral) *or* mefloquine (oral)
Infection known to be chloroquine-resistant[1]	not severe[3]	quinine or quinidine (oral) *plus* pyrimethamine-sulfadoxine[4] (oral)	quinine or quinidine (oral) *plus* tetracycline[5] (oral) *or* mefloquine (oral)
2. Exposure only in areas without known chloroquine resistance	severe[2]	quinine or quinidine (IV) *followed by* chloroquine (oral)	chloroquine (IV or IM[7]) *followed by* chloroquine (oral)
	not severe[3]	chloroquine (oral)	amodiaquine (oral)
3. Exposure in areas with known chloroquine and pyrimethamine-sulfadoxine resistance *or*	severe[2]	quinine or quinidine (IV) *plus* tetracycline[5] (oral)	quinine or quinidine (IV) *followed by* mefloquine (oral)
Infection known to be resistant to both drugs[8]	not severe[3]	quinine or quinidine (oral) *plus* tetracycline[5] (oral)	
4. Exposure area unknown		as in A-3	as in A-3
B. *P. malariae*		chloroquine[6] (oral)	amodiaquine[6] (oral)
C. *P. vivax* and *P. ovale*		chloroquine[6] (oral) *followed by* primaquine (oral)	amodiaquine[6] (oral) *followed by* primaquine (oral)
D. Species unknown	severe[2] not severe[3] }	Treat as if *P. falciparum*, as outlined in Section A.	
E. Mixed infections with 2 or more species	severe[2] not severe[3] }	Initiate treatment for *P. falciparum*, as outlined in Section A. Then treat other species as necessary.	

[1]Chloroquine prophylaxis treatment failure.

[2]Parasitemia ≥1% and/or clinical manifestations severe and/or complications present, or if patient is unable to take oral medication.

[3]Parasitemia <1%, clinical manifestations not severe, and no complications present.

[4]Pyrimethamine-sulfalene considered equivalent to pyrimethamine-sulfadoxine.

[5]Doxycycline can be used instead.

[6]If illness is life-threatening, if there are complications, or if the patient is unable to take oral medication, IV quinine or quinidine is preferred. Otherwise, oral chloroquine or amodiaquine can be given.

[7]Intramuscular (IM) or slow IV drip route preferred. Parenteral chloroquine can cause severe toxicity in infants and young children.

[8]Prophylaxis or treatment failure with both drugs.

Chloroquine-Sensitive P. falciparum Infections. Falciparum malaria contracted in areas with no reports of chloroquine resistance should be treated initially with chloroquine or amodiaquine unless intravenous medication is required (Table 73–3). No asexual parasites should be detectable on smears 4 to 5 days after completion of a course of chloroquine; persistence implies treatment failure. However, gametocytes may persist in the blood for weeks after asexual forms have been successfully eliminated; their presence does not imply treatment failure.

Multidrug-Resistant P. falciparum Infections. There have been reports of *P. falciparum* infections that are resistant to both chloroquine and pyrimethamine-sulfadoxine (Chapter 121). These infections have responded to quinine or quinidine plus tetracycline or doxycycline for 7 days alone. Tetracycline has very slow activity against *P. falciparum* and should not be used alone or in pregnant women or young children. Patients less than 8 years old with these multidrug-resistant infections can be treated with a full course of quinine or quinidine alone. Alternatively, mefloquine may be used.

Treatment of Complicated P. falciparum Infections.

P. falciparum infection is potentially life-threatening. Clinical management includes early diagnosis, rapid institution of effective antimalarial chemotherapy by appropriate route of administration, recognition of and therapy for complications, and monitoring of the clinical and parasitologic responses to treatment. It is imperative to determine where the patient acquired his or her infection. High-risk groups for complications include pregnant women, infants, young children, and nonimmune individuals.

Antimalarial Therapy. If chloroquine-resistant falciparum malaria cannot be excluded, the patient should be treated accordingly (Table 73–3). Frequent examinations of blood smears should be performed during treatment. Lack of clinical and/or parasitologic response to therapy should alert the physician to the possibility of drug resistance.

Even patients with falciparum malaria who appear clinically stable may deteriorate rapidly if treatment is not instituted quickly. Complications often appear during treatment. Patients should receive parenteral therapy if they are suffering from major complications of falciparum malaria, including severe anemia, renal fail-

TABLE 73–4. Dosages for Antimalarial Drugs

Drug	Adult Dose				Pediatric Dose			
	Treatment	*Route*	*Prophylaxis*[1]	*Route*	*Treatment*	*Route*	*Prophylaxis*[1]	*Route*
Amodiaquine dihydrochloride[2]	600 mg of *base* initially, then either 400 mg of *base* at 24 and 48 hours, or 300 mg of *base* at 6, 24, and 48 hours	oral	see text		10 mg/kg of *base*[3] initially, then 5 mg/kg of *base* at 6, 24, and 48 hours	oral	see text	
Chloroquine phosphate *or* Chloroquine sulfate *or* Hydroxychloroquine sulfate	600 mg of *base*[3] initially, then 300 mg of *base* at 6, 24, and 48 hours	oral	300 mg of *base*[3] weekly (heavier individuals could be given drug every 5 or 6 days)	oral	10 mg/kg of *base*[3] initially, then 5 mg/kg of *base* at 6, 24, and 48 hours	oral	5 mg/kg of *base*[3] weekly	oral
Chloroquine dihydrochloride	300 mg of *base*[3] every 8 to 12 hours	IM	not indicated		3.5 mg/kg of *base*[3] every 6 hours,[4] to total of 25 mg/kg	IM or SC	not indicated	
Doxycycline	100 mg twice daily for 7 days	oral	100 mg once daily	oral	2 mg/kg twice daily for 7 days	oral	2 mg/kg once daily for those >8 years of age	oral
Halofantrine	500 mg every 6 hours for 3 doses; repeat in 7 days	oral	not indicated		8 mg/kg every 6 hours for 3 doses; repeat in 7 days	oral	not indicated	
Mefloquine	750 to 1250 mg in a single dose	oral	250 mg weekly	oral	15 mg/kg in a single dose	oral	<1 year = 31 mg 1–4 years = 62 mg 5–12 years = 125 mg (all given weekly)	oral
Pyrimethamine-sulfadoxine	3 tablets in a single dose (each tablet contains 25 mg of pyrimethamine plus 500 mg of sulfadoxine)	oral	see text		0.5–4 years = ½ tablet 5–8 years = 1 tablet 9–14 years = 2 tablets (in a single dose)	oral	see text	
Pyrimethamine-sulfalene	3 tablets in a single dose (each tablet contains 25 mg of pyrimethamine plus 500 mg of sulfalene)	oral	see text		as with pyrimethamine-sulfadoxine	oral	see text	
Primaquine	15 mg of *base* daily for 14 days *or* 45 mg of *base* weekly for 8 weeks	oral	as in treatment[6]	oral	0.25 mg/kg of *base* daily for 14 days *or* 0.75 mg/kg of *base* weekly for 8 weeks	oral	as in treatment[6]	oral
Proguanil (Paludrine)	not indicated		200 mg daily	oral	not indicated		<2 years = 50 mg daily 2–6 years = 100 mg daily 7–10 years = 150 mg daily >10 years = 200 mg daily	oral
Quinidine sulfate *or* Quinidine gluconate	600 to 650 mg of base 3 times daily for 3 to 7 days[7]	oral	not indicated		10 mg/kg 3 times daily for 3 to 7 days[7]	oral	not indicated	
Quinidine gluconate	10–15 mg/kg (salt) loading dose in 500 ml of isotonic saline with glucose over 1 to 2 hours; then 1.0 to 1.5 mg/kg per hour by constant infusion for a maximum of 72 hours[4, 8]	IV	not indicated		same as adult dose	IV	not indicated	

TABLE 73–4. Dosages for Antimalarial Drugs *Continued*

Drug	Adult Dose				Pediatric Dose			
	Treatment	*Route*	*Prophylaxis*[1]	*Route*	*Treatment*	*Route*	*Prophylaxis*[1]	*Route*
Quinine dihydrochloride	500 mg in 500 ml of isotonic saline with glucose over 2 to 4 hours every 8 to 12 hours[4, 8]	IV	not indicated		5–10 mg/kg in 10 ml/kg of isotonic saline with glucose over 3 to 4 hours every 8 to 12 hours[4, 8]	IV	not indicated	
Quinine sulfate	650 mg 3 times daily for 3 to 7 days[7]	oral	not indicated		10 mg/kg 3 times daily for 3 to 7 days[7]	oral	not indicated	
Tetracycline	250 or 500 mg 4 times daily for 7 days[5]	oral	not indicated		10 mg/kg 4 times daily for 7 days[5]	oral	not indicated	

[1] Except for primaquine, chemoprophylactic regimens are begun prior to entering, continued during, and for 4 weeks after leaving a malarious area. The drug should be taken on the same day each week.

[2] Amodiaquine dosage varies because some tablets contain 150 mg of *base* and others 200 mg of *base*.

[3] Dose for 4-aminoquinolines, amodiaquine, and chloroquine is expressed as *base*, not the salt. Ensure that correct amount of *base* is given.

[4] Switch to oral medication as soon as possible. Reduce dose by one third if used parenterally for more than 72 hours. Parenteral chloroquine may be given with care intramuscularly, subcutaneously, or intravenously by slow constant infusion (see text).

[5] Tetracyclines should be used only in combination with quinine or quinidine to treat severe *P. falciparum* infections in those 8 years of age or older who were infected in areas where resistance to both chloroquine and pyrimethamine-sulfadoxine is present. They are toxic to younger children.

[6] Terminal prophylaxis with primaquine is to be given with last 2 weeks of chemoprophylaxis after leaving the malarious area.

[7] Duration of quinine and quinidine treatment is shorter if they are given with another drug (e.g., doxycycline) or if the patient has partial immunity to malaria. They act rapidly and are administered for initial 2 to 4 days of combined therapy.

[8] The higher loading dose may be given to treat those who acquired their infections in Thailand.

ure, pulmonary edema, and cerebral dysfunction, or if they are unable to take oral medication.

Quinine. Intravenous quinine is the drug of choice. When given parenterally, 10 mg/kg of body weight (500 to 1000 mg for an adult) of quinine dihydrochloride is diluted in about 10 ml/kg of isotonic saline solution (500 ml for an adult). The intravenous infusion is given slowly over 2 to 4 hours, and it may be repeated within 12 to 24 hours. The volume of infusion fluid can be adjusted according to the state of hydration of the patient. Direct intravenous injection of quinine by syringe is to be avoided, even if given slowly in a dilute solution. Intramuscular injection of quinine is also not recommended because it is painful and frequently causes sterile abscesses and because absorption of the drug is erratic.

Quinine dihydrochloride in a loading intravenous dose of 20 mg/kg was used for the treatment of cerebral malaria in adult Thais. This regimen gave a therapeutic level of quinine (i.e., plasma concentration > 10 mg/L) in 13 of 15 patients within 4 hours. It was associated with a more rapid ability to be roused and to regain full consciousness and a more rapid clearance of fever and parasitemia than quinine in the standard intravenous dose of 10 mg/kg, which was administered to a control group. There was no increased toxicity in the group receiving the loading dose, and quinine levels in the blood were the same in the two groups after 2 days of therapy. The loading dose is not recommended except for patients with severe complications, and more extensive studies will be needed before it can be used in children and in areas where the parasite strains show less drug resistance.

Once complications have been controlled and the patient can take medication by mouth, oral preparations of quinine, chloroquine, or an alternative drug can be given (Table 73–3). Most patients respond to a single

quinine infusion and then can be switched to oral medication. However, some patients may require 2 or 3 infusions. The dosage should be reduced in severely ill patients with hepatic or renal insufficiency. Close monitoring is warranted, because occasionally, hypotension or cardiac arrhythmias have been reported.

Quinidine. In areas with known chloroquine-resistant *P. falciparum* infections, when quinine is not available and parenteral medication is required, severely ill patients should be treated with quinidine. Quinidine can be given in a continuous intravenous infusion. A loading dose of 10 mg of quinidine gluconate (salt) per kg of body weight is given over 1 or 2 hours. This is followed by 1.0 to 1.5 mg/kg per hour, up to a maximum of 72 hours. The drug is mixed in isotonic saline and dextrose at a concentration to ensure that the patient does not receive excessive intravenous fluids. Blood pressure should be monitored every 5 to 10 minutes during the loading dose and every 15 to 20 minutes while intravenous quinidine is continued. An electrocardiographic monitor tracing should be taken every hour, if the equipment is available. The quinidine infusion should be temporarily slowed or stopped in the case of a QT interval of more than 0.6 second, a QRS complex wider than 50% of baseline, hypotension unresponsive to a moderate fluid challenge, or a serum quinidine level above 7 µg/L (21 µmol/L). The infusion should be discontinued permanently in the event of persistent severe hypotension (systolic pressure < 80 mm Hg), evidence of immediate hypersensitivity, or clinically important cardiac arrhythmia. In many circumstances it would be impossible to monitor IV quinidine therapy so closely. However, it appears to be a safe drug if given slowly and not in excess. Common sense must rule the situation.

Chloroquine. Chloroquine dihydrochloride may be

used parenterally in areas where *P. falciparum* isolates are known to be sensitive to this drug. Parenteral chloroquine can cause hypotension, shock, and sudden death, particularly in infants and young children.

Severely ill patients can usually be satisfactorily treated with chloroquine given by nasogastric tube at a dosage of 10 mg/kg followed by 5 mg/kg at 6, 24, and 48 hours. Absorption is rapid and reaches therapeutic levels within 2 hours. Intramuscular chloroquine is best given at more frequent intervals than previously recommended (i.e., 5 mg/kg of base every 6 hours), since cardiovascular toxicity is related to high blood levels associated with less frequent administration of higher doses. For the same reason, intravenous therapy should be given as a continuous infusion. The most current regimen (1990) is 0.83 mg of base/kg per hour for 30 hours.

Supportive Therapy. Dexamethasone increases morbidity and has no effect on mortality in cerebral malaria. Therefore, steroids are to be avoided. Fluid replacement should be judiciously instituted to prevent precipitation of the adult respiratory distress syndrome (ARDS). Hyponatremia usually is the result of decreased free water clearance, not sodium loss, and therefore should not be treated with sodium loading. All severely ill patients should have a blood sugar test performed. If hypoglycemia is present, it should be treated with an infusion of 50% glucose. It is appropriate to give all those requiring intravenous therapy a 5% dextrose infusion. Pulmonary edema signifies poor prognosis, regardless of therapy. Cerebral malaria should be managed by fluid restriction and vigorous antimalarial chemotherapy. A single intramuscular dose of phenobarbital, 200 mg for adults or 3.5 mg/kg for those weighing less than 60 kg, has been shown to markedly reduce the incidence of convulsions in those with cerebral malaria.

Transfusion of packed red blood cells or whole blood for severe anemia may be required. Treatment of coagulopathies, when present, is controversial. Heparin, with or without fresh frozen plasma, and low molecular weight dextran have been used. However, there is no evidence that patient survival has improved; conservative management without heparin but with vigorous treatment of the underlying malarial infection is probably indicated when DIC is present.

Exchange Transfusion. In extreme cases, exchange transfusion has been successful. A proportion of the patient's red cells are removed and are replaced with fresh noninfected ones. Using sterile technique, whole blood is removed from the patient and replaced with blood products equivalent to whole blood. This may be repeated as necessary. If available, an automated cell separator may be used. This process prolongs survival and permits the chemotherapy to cure the patient. It has been used in severely ill patients.

Exchange transfusions should be considered in patients with complications (e.g., cerebral malaria, renal failure, ARDS, sepsis) and/or high parasitemias (e.g., parasitemia rate > 10% or 100,000/mm³ of blood). The exchange transfusion removes parasitized erythrocytes and red cell debris that contribute to sludging and the resultant pathology. The greatest reduction in circulating infected red cells usually occurs with exchange of the first 2 or 3 units, and parasitemia levels are reduced to 1% or less in most patients following exchange of 8 or 10 units. Careful monitoring of the patient's parasitemia will provide the information required to decide when the exchange transfusion can be discontinued.

Treatment of Malaria Due to *P. vivax*, *P. ovale*, and *P. malariae*. Chloroquine is the drug of choice because chloroquine resistance has never been described in these species (Tables 73–3 and 73–4). Patients can generally be treated with oral therapy as outpatients. Clinical response is generally rapid. Amodiaquine is the recommended alternative. Its dosage efficacy, mode of action, and toxicity are almost identical to those of chloroquine.

Patients with *P. vivax* and *P. ovale* infections should be given primaquine to prevent relapses from persistent exoerythrocytic stages in the liver (Table 73–3). Primaquine has no effect on the blood forms. Primaquine may cause hemolytic anemia in persons with G-6-PD deficiency (Chapter 5). At standard doses, hemolysis is usually subclinical in blacks with G-6-PD deficiency because it is limited to old erythrocytes. Patients with the more severe Mediterranean and Canton variants of G-6-PD deficiency should be treated with chloroquine for each relapse rather than be given primaquine. The incidence of side effects is reported to be lower with the weekly dosage. Primaquine is not required for *P. malariae* or *P. falciparum* infections because these species do not have hypnozoite stages. In addition, patients infected with *P. vivax* and *P. ovale* by direct blood inoculation do not require primaquine.

Up to 30% of patients with *P. vivax* infection who are treated with chloroquine and primaquine may still undergo relapse, depending on the locality where the infection is acquired. These patients should receive a second course of chloroquine and primaquine.

Treatment of Malaria When Species and/or Exposure Area Is Unknown. If the species of malarial parasite is unknown, the patient should be treated as though *P. falciparum* is the organism. If the exposure area is unknown and falciparum malaria is diagnosed or is a possibility, the infection must be considered to be chloroquine-resistant and the patient should be treated accordingly.

Treatment of Mixed Infections. In mixed infections, therapy for *P. falciparum* should be rapidly initiated. Other species can then be treated as necessary.

Treatment of Malaria in Children. In general, the treatment of malarial infections in children is essentially the same as that for adults. The diagnosis of acute malaria in young children is often difficult. The disease may present as a medical emergency. Certain drugs such as tetracyclines and intramuscular chloroquine should be avoided in infants and young children. Oral drugs are the safest in this age group. Parenteral therapy is often necessary but it should be administered with extreme caution. Intravenous quinine is the drug of choice and should be given very slowly in glucose saline. Parenteral chloroquine should not be given unless absolutely necessary. Injections of antimalarials should not be given to febrile children without slide demonstration of the parasites.

There is no simple way of precisely calculating pediatric dosages of antimalarials. The presence of fever, malnutrition, dehydration, or acidosis may affect drug metabolism in infants and young children. Calculation of the appropriate dose from determination of body surface area is too complicated for ordinary purposes in many malarious areas. Two methods used for dose determination in children, body weight and age, are presented in Table 73–5.

CHEMOPROPHYLAXIS. Chemoprophylaxis for malaria is given to nonimmune persons entering areas endemic for malaria. Anyone traveling to malarious areas, even for brief visits, is at risk of acquiring malaria; chemoprophylaxis reduces but does not totally prevent this risk.

Chemoprophylaxis may also be appropriate for certain high-risk groups living in malarious areas, e.g., infants, young children, pregnant women, and immigrants from places that are malaria-free. Most studies in Africa have failed to demonstrate that chemoprophylaxis of children living in endemic areas reduces malarial morbidity or mortality. However, Greenwood et al. recently reported that treatment of presumptive episodes of clinical malaria with chloroquine combined with fortnightly chemoprophylaxis with pyrimethamine-dapsone by village health workers reduced both morbidity and mortality in young Gambian children. This requires confirmation in other areas before chemoprophylaxis of young children can be routinely recommended.

Drug prophylaxis does not prevent infection but aborts or modifies the clinical attack. Thus, an individual may acquire malaria even if taking prescribed medication. If given for a sufficient time after the person leaves the malarious area, chemoprophylaxis may result in suppressive cure because medication is continued long enough to exceed the duration of the exoerythrocytic stage of the species of malarial parasite.

Selection of a particular drug for chemoprophylaxis depends on the distribution and intensity of transmission, the pattern of drug resistance, and the planned duration of residence in the area. Special problems include prophylaxis for infants, very young children, and pregnant women and the balance between short-term individual protection and long-term community welfare.

Areas Where Only Chloroquine-Sensitive Malaria Is Present

Suppressive Prophylaxis. Chloroquine phosphate is highly effective for suppression of infections caused by *P. vivax*, *P. ovale*, *P. malariae*, and chloroquine-sensitive strains of *P. falciparum*. Amodiaquine hydrochloride is essentially equivalent to chloroquine. Administration should be initiated before entering a malarious area and should be continued for 6 weeks after leaving the area. Doses are given in Table 73–4.

Chloroquine has potential ophthalmic toxicity. Severe, irreversible retinopathy has been described in individuals taking high *daily* doses for prolonged periods for treatment of nonparasitic diseases. However, large numbers of people have used chloroquine as malarial chemoprophylaxis for many years without complications, and there is no evidence that data from studies of individuals using high daily doses of chloroquine can be applied to those taking weekly doses. Some authorities recommend periodic ophthalmologic examinations after the total cumulative chloroquine dose exceeds 100 gm of *base*. This amount would be attained in about 6½ years at the recommended dose for chemoprophylaxis. Chloroquine is safe in pregnancy and for young children.

In some cases drug failures may be related to insufficient doses for large individuals. It might be reasonable to adjust the dosage for the patient's weight. For instance, individuals weighing more than 75 kg might be better protected by taking a 300 mg tablet of chloroquine every 5 or 6 days rather than once weekly.

Alternative drugs are the antifolates chlorguanide (proguanil) or pyrimethamine (Table 73–4). These drugs have no significant toxicity in prophylactic doses. However, their use in many areas is limited by the high incidence of parasite resistance to the drugs.

Terminal Prophylaxis. Relapses of *P. vivax* and *P. ovale* infections can be prevented by single daily doses of primaquine during the last 2 weeks of or just following a course of suppressive therapy with chloroquine or a comparable drug. Primaquine should not be given until after leaving the malarious area. Terminal prophylaxis with primaquine is not indicated for all travelers. The decision should be made on an individual basis, taking into account the intensity and duration of the exposure to *P. vivax* and *P. ovale* and the status of the patient's G-6-PD enzyme.

Areas Where Chloroquine-Resistant Strains of P. falciparum Are Present. For suppression of chloroquine-resistant *P. falciparum* malaria, the recommended drug has been the fixed combination of pyrimethamine (25 mg) with sulfadoxine (500 mg) or sulfalene (500 mg). This combination has been widely used for chemoprophylaxis, but adverse reactions are increasingly being reported. For this reason, it is now advocated that chloroquine be ingested routinely by travelers and other designated individuals, and a therapeutic dose of pyrimethamine-sulfadoxine be carried for use should fever develop and definitive diagnosis not be available immediately. In the increasing number of areas where *P. falciparum* malaria is resistant to 4-aminoquinolines and to pyrimethamine-sulfadoxine (notably in Thailand, Kampuchea, and Brazil (Chapter 121), short-term nonimmune travelers (excluding children younger than 8 years and pregnant women) might be advised to ingest doxycycline 100 mg (adult dose) daily and for 4 weeks after departure from those areas.

An alternative is pyrimethamine-dapsone. A combination of proguanil 200 mg daily and chloroquine 300

TABLE 73–5. Determination of Antimalarial Dosages in Children by Weight and Age

Weight of Child in kg	Percentage of Adult Dose	Age of Child	Proportion of Adult Dose
4.5	15.0	less than 2 years	⅛ to ¼
10.0	25.0	2 to 6 years	¼ to ½
15.0	33.3	6 to 12 years	½ to ¾
23.0	50.0	greater than 12 years	¾ to 1
30.0–40.0	75.0		
45.0–65.0	100.0		

mg weekly is being used with variable efficacy in some areas of Africa. Proguanil is also undergoing evaluation in combination with either dapsone or short-acting sulfonamines. Another alternative is to use mefloquine at a weekly dose of 250 mg. This is taken up to 4 weeks following the last exposure. This is currently a very effective way of preventing malaria in travelers to areas where multiple drug–resistant *P. falciparum* is present.

PREVENTION AND CONTROL

For Individuals. There is no single method to prevent malarial infection. However, a number of precautions can be taken to reduce the risk. Malaria transmission usually occurs between dusk and dawn. The chance of being infected is reduced by remaining in well-screened areas during these hours and by sleeping under mosquito netting. The most cost-effective means of preventing malaria infection is to sleep under a bed net that has been treated with pyrethroids, e.g., permethrin.* Most studies evaluating insecticide-impregnated bed nets have shown substantial reduction in sporozoite inoculation rates and reduced incidence of malaria attacks. Outdoor exposure to mosquito bites can be reduced by wearing clothing that covers the arms and legs and by applying mosquito repellent to thin clothing and exposed areas of the skin. The most effective repellents are *N,N*-diethyltoluamide (DEET) and dimethyl phthalate (DIMP), which are ingredients in many commercially available insect repellents. All visitors to malarious areas should receive malaria chemoprophylaxis.

For Populations. During the 1970s, following the failure of malaria eradication, the WHO adopted a revised strategy of malaria control based on a realistic assessment of an individual country's epidemiologic conditions and potential for effective control. Unlike eradication, a malaria control program is of indefinite duration and has recurring costs. It attempts to reduce, not eliminate, transmission. An integrated control program involves the simultaneous use of several control methods based on the epidemiologic characteristics of transmission in the area involved and the availability of resources. The tactical approaches to such a program were consolidated by WHO in 1986, two substantially different approaches being identified depending on local development, economic capability, and epidemic potential. These are: (1) Improve the general health services to ensure adequate diagnosis, accessibility to care, and treatment for individual patients; and provide protection for communities by promoting personal and environmental health measures—this would not interfere fundamentally with transmission. (2) Establish long-term control of transmission by implementing antiparasite and antivector measures that would change the epidemiologic equilibrium and lead to malaria eradication.

Insecticide-Impregnated Mosquito Nets. The community-wide use of insecticide-treated mosquito nets is currently being extensively evaluated. This can effectively reduce exposure to biting mosquitoes and other insects. Mosquitoes are killed; infective bites are reduced. In some circumstances, community malaria prev-

alence rates and malaria morbidity are reduced. This is not always the case, since in highly endemic areas hungry anophelines find other ways to feed on people or are channeled to those who are not using bed nets. In communities where vectors are more zoophilic or in places or seasons in which malaria transmission is less intense, impregnated bed nets appear to be effective in reducing parasite rates.

Measures for Prevention of Malaria in Individuals and for Large-Scale Control of the Disease. These measures can be divided according to a modified classification of that proposed by Russell in 1952:

1. Measures to prevent mosquitoes from feeding on humans, e.g., permethrin-treated nets, protective clothing, repellents, screening, and site selection for new housing.

2. Measures to prevent or reduce the breeding of mosquitoes by eliminating the collections of water or altering the environment at breeding sites, e.g., source reduction, drainage, and filling.

3. Measures to destroy mosquito larvae, e.g., larvicides, larvicidal oil, increasing or decreasing the degree of salinity, shading, and introduction of pathogens or predators (e.g., fish).

4. Measures to destroy adult mosquitoes, e.g., residual and space spray insecticides, use of permethrin-treated bed nets.

5. Measures to eliminate the malarial parasites in the human host or to prevent transmission to mosquitoes, e.g., mass drug therapy campaigns, diagnosis and early treatment of cases, presumptive therapy based on symptoms, and use of gametocidal and sporonticidal drugs.

6. Measures to protect the susceptible host, e.g., chemoprophylaxis, immunoprophylaxis.

Malaria control should involve integration of available technology with knowledge from epidemiologic evaluation of the situation in each area.

BIBLIOGRAPHY

Boudreau EF, Pang LW, Dixon KE, et al: Malaria: Treatment efficacy of halofantrine (WR 171 669) in initial field trials in Thailand. Bull WHO 66:227, 1988.

Bradley AK, Greenwood BM, Greenwood AM, et al: Bednets (mosquito nets) and morbidity from malaria. Lancet 2:204, 1986.

Bruce-Chwatt LJ, Black RH, Canfield CJ, et al: Chemotherapy of Malaria. 2nd ed. Geneva, World Health Organization, 1986.

Centers for Disease Control: Recommendations for the prevention of malaria in travelers. MMWR 37:277, 1988.

Clyde DF: Recent trends in the epidemiology and control of malaria. Epidemiol Rev 9:219, 1987.

De Souza JM, Sheth UK, Wernsdorfer WH, et al: A phase II/III double-blind dose-finding clinical trial of a combination of mefloquine, sulfadoxine, and pyremethamine (Fansimef) in falciparum malaria. Bull WHO 65:357, 1987.

Greenwood BM, Greenwood AM, Bradley AK, et al: Comparison of two strategies for control of malaria within a primary health care programme in the Gambia. Lancet 1:1121, 1988.

Hoffman S: Treatment of malaria. Clin Trop Med Comm Dis 1:171, 1986.

Larrey D, Castot A, Pessayre D, et al: Amodiaquine-induced hepatitis. A report of seven cases. Ann Intern Med 104:801, 1986.

---

*A portable bed net (La Mosquette) is available from IAMAT, 40 Regal Road, Guelph, Ontario NIK 1B5, Canada.

Lobel HO, Campbell CC: Malaria prophylaxis and distribution of drug resistance. Clin Trop Med Comm Dis 1:225, 1986.

Miller KD, Greenberg AE, Campbell CC: Treatment of severe malaria in the United States with a continuous infusion of quinidine gluconate and exchange transfusion. N Engl J Med 321:65, 1989.

Molineaux L, Gramiccia G: The Garki Project. Research on the Epidemiology and Control of Malaria in the Sudan Savanna of West Africa. Geneva, World Health Organization, 1980.

Nevill CG, Watkins WM, Carter JY, Munafu CG: Comparison of mosquito nets, proguanil hydrochloride, and placebo to prevent malaria. Br Med J 297:401, 1988.

Pearlman EJ, Doberstyn EB, Sudsok S, et al: Chemosuppressive field trials in Thailand. IV. The suppression of *Plasmodium falciparum* and *Plasmodium vivax* parasitemias by mefloquine (WR 142, 490, a 4-quinoline methanol). Am J Trop Med Hyg 29:1131, 1980.

Phillips RE, Warrell DA, White NJ, et al: Intravenous quinidine for the treatment of severe falciparum malaria: clinical and pharmacokinetic studies. N Engl J Med 312:1273, 1985.

Rouveix B, Bricaire F, Michon C, et al: Mefloquine and an acute brain syndrome. Ann Intern Med 110:577, 1989.

Rozendaal JA: Impregnated mosquito nets and curtains for self-protection and vector control. Trop Dis Bull 86:R1, 1989.

Rozendaal JA: Self-protection and vector control with insecticide-treated mosquito nets (a review of present status). WHO/VBC/89:965, 1989.

Snow RW, Rowan KM, Greenwood BM: A trial of permethrin treated bednets in the prevention of malaria in Gambian children. Trans R Soc Trop Med Hyg 81:563, 1987.

Strickland GT: The control of malaria. Clin Trop Med Comm Dis 1:243, 1986.

Watkins WM, Lury JD, Kariuki D, et al: Efficacy of multiple-dose halofantrine in treatment of chloroquine-resistant falciparum malaria in children in Kenya. Lancet 2:247, 1988.

White NJ, Looareesuwan S, Phillips RE, et al: Single dose phenobarbitone prevents convulsions in cerebral malaria. Lancet 2:64, 1988.

White NJ, Looareesuwan S, Warrell DA, et al: Quinidine in falciparum malaria. Lancet 2:1069, 1981.

White NJ, Looareesuwan S, Warrell DA, et al: Quinine pharmacokinetics and toxicity in cerebral and uncomplicated falciparum malaria. Am J Med 73:564, 1982.

White NJ, Looareesuwan S, Warrell DA, et al: Quinine loading dose in cerebral malaria. Am J Trop Med Hyg 32:1, 1983.

White NJ, Miller KD, Churchill FC, et al: Chloroquine treatment of severe malaria in children. Pharmacokinetics, toxicity, and new dosage recommendations. N Engl J Med 319:1493, 1988.

White NJ, Watt G, Bergqvist Y, et al: Parenteral chloroquine for treating falciparum malaria. J Infect Dis 155:192, 1987.

Wirima J, Khoromana C, Molyneaux ME, Gilles HM: Clinical trials with halofantrine hydrochloride in Malawi. Lancet 2:250, 1988.

73.2. SYNDROMES ASSOCIATED WITH CHRONIC MALARIA

HYPERREACTIVE MALARIAL SYNDROME

DEFINITION AND ETIOLOGY. Hyperreactive malarial syndrome (HMS), formerly called tropical splenomegaly syndrome (TSS), is an immunologic disorder related to chronic malaria. The diagnosis is based on the presence of massive splenomegaly, high circulating titers of malarial antibodies, elevated IgM levels, lymphocytic infiltration of the hepatic sinusoids, hematologic findings of hypersplenism, and exclusion of other diagnostic possibilities. Pathogenesis is unknown but appears to involve genetic susceptibility and chronic exposure to malaria.

DISTRIBUTION AND INCIDENCE. Although HMS may be widespread in the tropics, most investigations of idiopathic splenomegaly have been performed in Uganda, Zambia, Nigeria, and New Guinea. The reported incidence of HMS varies from 0.5% to 80% of the adult population. There is a close geographic association between HMS and malaria endemicity, although genetic and tribal factors within a given area affect the incidence.

IMMUNOLOGIC FINDINGS. Patients with HMS have a polyclonal macroglobulinemia, circulating immune complexes, and autoantibodies, including isohemagglutinins, rheumatoid factor, antinuclear factor, cold agglutinins, and cryoprotein. High titer IgM malarial antibodies are present, and a correlation between IgM levels and spleen size has been described. IgM levels fall promptly following splenectomy or more gradually following malarial prophylaxis.

Patients with HMS do not appear to have any defects in cell-mediated immunity. However, antibody response following certain immunizations, e.g., *Salmonella adelaide* flagellin or monovalent influenza vaccine, is depressed.

PATHOGENESIS AND PATHOLOGY. In areas where HMS occurs, a proportion of children fail to have a regression of splenomegaly with the development of immunity to malaria. Hypertrophy of the reticuloendothelial elements in the liver and spleen progresses with exposure to malaria. It has been hypothesized that HMS is the result of chronic stimulation of the splenic and hepatic reticuloendothelial system by circulating antigen-antibody complexes that are triggered by a nonspecific mitogen from the malarial parasite. Both a complement-fixing lymphocytotoxin in the sera and a reduction in the number of suppressor T-lymphocytes in the blood have been described in patients with HMS.

On microscopic section, the spleen has normal architecture, with dilated sinusoids containing erythrocytes and lymphocytes. Large macrophages ingesting erythrocytes and granulocytes are in abundance. Malarial parasites and pigment are absent. There is lymphocytic infiltration of the hepatic sinusoids (Fig. 73–18). Kupffer cells are hyperplastic and hypertrophied.

CLINICAL MANIFESTATIONS. Most patients have huge spleens (to the level of the umbilicus or below) and complain of a dragging left-sided abdominal pain (Fig. 73–19). Anemia with an increased reticulocyte count is universal. Thrombocytopenia is usual, but patients seldom have a tendency to bleed. The liver is also enlarged and smooth, with a prominent left lobe. There may be an increased susceptibility to bacterial infections, but other clinical complications are unusual. Neutropenia may be present. Occasionally, life-threatening episodes of hemolytic anemia occur in HMS, particularly in pregnant or lactating women. The bone marrow shows hypercellularity with hyperplasia of both the erythroid and the myeloid series. Splenic sequestration of erythrocytes as well as a greatly expanded plasma volume has been demonstrated.

TREATMENT AND PROGNOSIS. Chronic (life-long) antimalarial prophylaxis is the treatment of choice for HMS; splenectomy is no longer recommended. There is an increased risk of surgical morbidity and mortality. Long-term follow-up of patients treated with splenectomy demonstrates a compensatory hepatomeg-

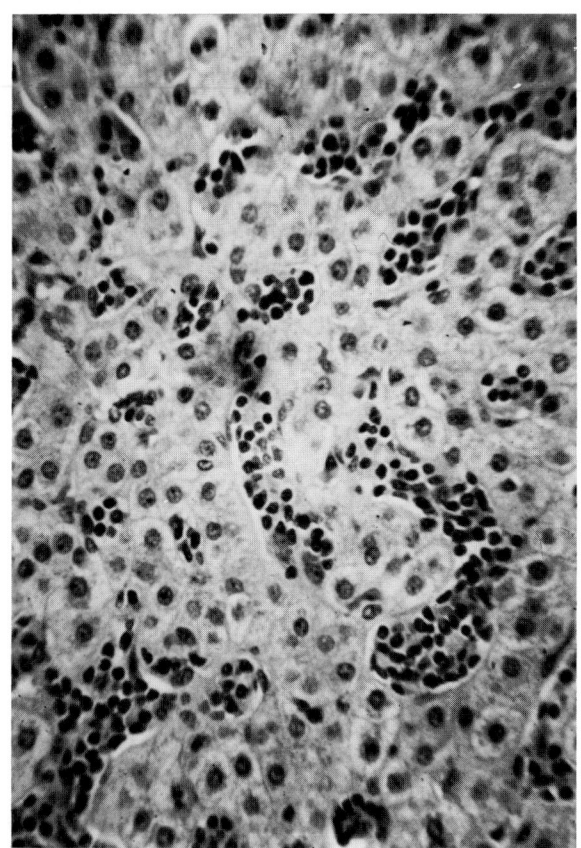

FIGURE 73–18. Hyperreactive malarial syndrome. Hypertrophy of Kupffer cells and increased chronic inflammatory cells in the hepatic sinusoids. (H & E stain.) (Courtesy of Dr. Michael Hutt.)

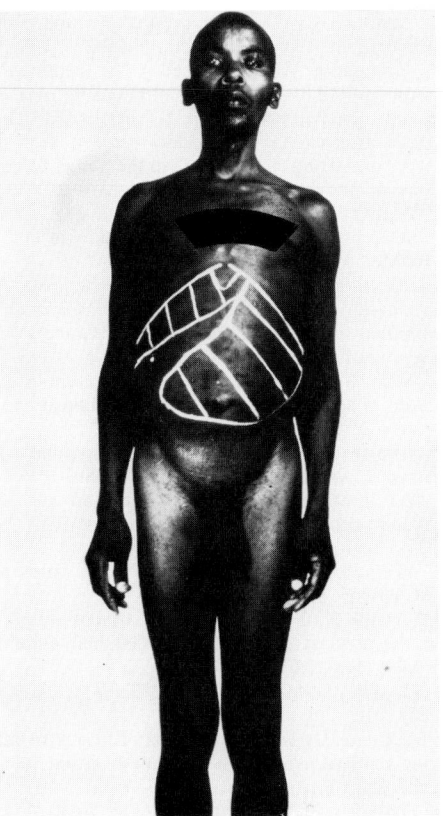

FIGURE 73–19. Ugandan patient with hyperreactive malarial syndrome with a very large spleen and liver. (Courtesy of Dr. Patrick Hamilton.)

aly and an increased susceptibility to severe infections, including malaria itself. Following appropriate treatment, hepatosplenomegaly and elevated IgM levels regress.

NEPHROTIC SYNDROME (Chapter 6)

DEFINITION AND ETIOLOGY. The high incidence of nephrotic syndrome (NS) occurring in some tropical areas has been attributed to quartan malaria. NS is more common in areas where malaria is endemic, and patients with NS have increased infection rates with *P. malariae*. Induced infections with *P. malariae* in man and monkeys have produced NS.

DISTRIBUTION AND INCIDENCE. Detailed studies have described NS associated with quartan malaria in Uganda in East Africa; Nigeria, the Ivory Coast, and Senegal in West Africa; and Papua New Guinea. In the past, the association has been reported in Southeast Asia, India, and Guyana. The entity disappeared in areas where *P. malariae* was eradicated, such as Guyana.

PATHOLOGY AND PATHOGENESIS. Pathologic lesions are variable. A common lesion in children consists of localized or diffuse thickening in the capillary wall of the glomeruli tuft with PAS-positive material, segmented sclerosis of peripheral capillary loops, and increased mesangial cells (Fig. 6–2). Progression to total glomerular sclerosis and secondary tubular atrophy may

occur. A proliferative glomerulonephritis has been described in adults.

Immunofluorescence studies of biopsy specimens taken early during the disease demonstrate granular deposits of IgG and IgM in virtually all glomeruli, C3 component of complement in two thirds of the glomeruli, and *P. malariae* antigens in one fourth of the glomeruli. Specific *P. malariae* antibodies were confirmed in most samples. Biopsy specimens taken more than 3 months after the onset of renal symptoms usually still had antibodies and complement but not *P. malariae* antigens. The depositions vary from a coarse to a fine granular pattern. The coarse granular pattern correlates with the presence of electron-dense material localized within the glomerular basement membrane (Fig. 6–3).

CLINICAL MANIFESTATIONS. Approximately half of those with quartan malaria NS have their first symptoms before the age of 15 years. The classic findings of NS, including persistent heavy proteinuria, hypoalbuminemia, edema, and ascites, are usually present (Fig. 6–1). Hypertension, azotemia, and hematuria are rare in children, although the first two are not uncommon in adults. Most patients have poorly selective proteinuria. Blood smears in children, but not adults, are likely to demonstrate *P. malariae*. The most common clinical course includes transient remissions, persistent symptomless proteinuria, slowly progressive deterioration of renal function, and hypertension.

TREATMENT AND PROGNOSIS. Patients with quartan malaria NS do not respond to antimalarial therapy. The response to corticosteroids, cyclophosphamide, and azathioprine is variable. Remission of abnormalities with treatment occurs almost exclusively in those with only mild proliferative changes on the initial renal biopsy.

BURKITT'S LYMPHOMA

Endemic cases of Burkitt's lymphoma have been causally related to Epstein-Barr virus infection (Chapter 11). Among other etiologic factors may be immunologic suppression by chronic malaria because of the geographic coincidence of hyperendemic or holoendemic malaria with Burkitt's lymphoma.

ENDOMYOCARDIAL FIBROSIS

Exposure to malaria has been associated with this cardiomyopathy (Chapter 2).

BIBLIOGRAPHY

Crane CG: Tropical splenomegaly. Part 2: Oceania. Clin Haematol 10:976, 1981.

Fakunle YM: Tropical splenomegaly. Part 1: Tropical Africa. Clin Haematol 10:963, 1981.

Hendrickse RG, Adeniyi A, Edington GM, et al: Quartan malarial nephrotic syndrome. Lancet 1:1143, 1972.

Piessens WF, Hoffman SL, Wadee AA et al: Antibody-mediated killing of suppressor T lymphocytes as a possible cause of macroglobulinemia in the tropical splenomegaly syndrome. J Clin Invest 75:1821, 1985.

Stuiver PC, Ziegler JL, Wood JB, et al: Clinical trial of malaria prophylaxis in tropical splenomegaly syndrome. Br Med J 1:426, 1971.

Wing AJ, Hutt MSR, Kibukamusoke JW: Progression and remission in the nephrotic syndrome associated with quartan malaria in Uganda. Q J Med 16:273, 1972.

74. AFRICAN TRYPANOSOMIASIS

James D. Bales, Jr.

INTRODUCTION. Members of the family Trypanisomatidae, genus *Trypanosoma*, include the etiologic agents responsible for 2 important diseases of humans: American trypanosomiasis (Chagas' disease) and African trypanosomiasis (sleeping sickness). These organisms are digenetic parasites whose life cycle involves 2 hosts: a definitive mammalian host and an intermediate host, an arthropod vector, which transmits the infection to a new vertebrate. Normally, the blood stream forms that are ingested by the insect while feeding undergo a cycle of development in the intermediate host that culminates in the production of special infective forms known as metacyclic trypanosomes, which are then transmitted to a new mammalian host. Trypanosomes have been classified according to the localization of their development in the vector and other characteristics.

STERCORARIA. This group comprises species with the developmental cycle in the insect vector occurring in the hindgut (posterior station). Organisms are present in the feces. Transmission is by fecal contamination during biting. This group includes the subgenus *Schizotrypanum* and contains 1 pathogen, *Trypanosoma (Schizotrypanum) cruzi*, the causative agent of Chagas' disease.

SALIVARIA. These are species in which the developmental cycle in the insect vector (tsetse fly of *Glossina* species) is completed in the salivary glands (the anterior station) and transmission is by inoculation through the hypopharynx. The subgenus *Trypanozoon* is found in this group and includes the species infecting humans, *Trypanosoma (Trypanozoon) brucei*. Because it is unclear if the 2 agents causing African trypanosomiasis in humans are in fact different species, they are often considered as nosodemes of the "*brucei* complex" and therefore are referred to as the subspecies *Trypanosoma (Trypanozoon) brucei gambiense* and *T. (T.) b. rhodesiense*. The etiologic agent of the animal disease nagana, which is morphologically identical, is accordingly classified as *T. (T.) b. brucei* and is the third subspecies of the species *T. (T.) brucei*.

PARASITE STAGES. Trypanosomes are characterized at some stage in their life cycle by the presence of a free flagellum arising from the kinetoplast, an organelle containing DNA and associated with the mitochondrion. During development, these organisms multiply and pass through a number of different stages (Fig. 74–1) in which they resemble other genera in the family, such as *Leishmania*.

The flagellum and undulating membrane give motility to trypanosomes. Locomotion is usually in the direction of the free flagellum.

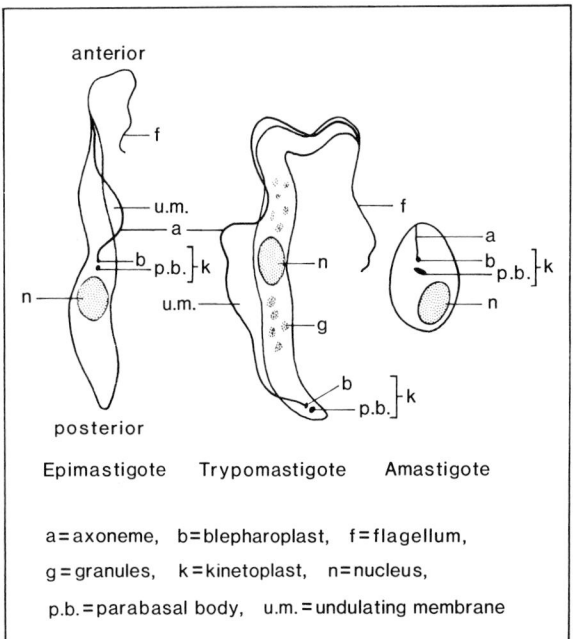

FIGURE 74–1. Morphologic stages of trypanosomes. (Modified from Ash LR, Orihel TC: Atlas of Human Parasitology, 2nd ed. Chicago, American Society of Clinical Pathologists, 1984.)

Multiplication occurs by longitudinal binary fission. The kinetoplast and the nucleus divide before the cytoplasm. The flagellum does not divide, but a new one develops rapidly from the new kinetoplast.

Epimastigote. The epimastigote stage occurs in the insect vector. This form is slender and elongated with a central vesicular nucleus. The kinetoplast is close but anterior to the nucleus. The flagellum passes along the border of a short undulating membrane to the anterior end of the parasite, where it becomes free. The epimastigote is not infective for humans but changes in the anterior or posterior station to the infective, metacyclic trypanosome, which is short and stumpy with a centrally placed nucleus and a posterior kinetoplast and is considered to be a form of young trypomastigote.

Trypomastigote. This is the long and slender mature form that is 17 to 30 µm in length and found in the blood of the mammalian hosts. The nucleus is centrally located, and the kinetoplast is subterminal. The flagellum initially is contiguous to the body of the parasite, is attached by desmosomes, and helps to form the undulating membrane. The free flagellum lies anteriorly. Polymorphic trypomastigotes may be present, particularly associated with high parasitemia. These forms exhibit morphologic differences and vary with respect to size, position of the nucleus, and length of the flagellum. If all individual trypomastigote forms possess a free flagellum, the species is monomorphic, e.g., *T. (S.) cruzi*. If some organisms do and some do not, the group is polymorphic, e.g., *T. (T.) b. gambiense* and *T. (T.) b. rhodesiense.*

Amastigote. The amastigote is the stage in which the organism exists as a round or ovoid intracellular body measuring 1.5 to 5 µm in diameter. There is no external flagellum, but a spherical nucleus and small kinetoplast are present. This form is found intracellularly in the tissues in persons infected with *T. (S.) cruzi.*

The geographic distribution of sleeping sickness and that of Chagas' disease do not overlap. *T. (S.) cruzi* is found only in North, Central, and South America, and *T. (T.) b. gambiense* and *T. (T.) b. rhodesiense* are found only in sub-Saharan Africa. Although they are included in the same family and genus and have similar morphologic features, these agents have little else in common. Differences in geographic distribution, transmission, development, pathogenesis, pathology, clinical characteristics, and therapy distinguish American and African trypanosomiasis.

DEFINITION. African trypanosomiasis (sleeping sickness) is an acute and chronic disease caused by the morphologically identical hemoflagellate protozoans *T. (T.) b. gambiense* and *T. (T.) b. rhodesiense*. The parasites are transmitted cyclically by various species of tsetse flies of the genus *Glossina*. The early acute disease is a systemic illness characterized by hemolymphatic involvement with intermittent fever, rash, and transitory edemas. Later, invasion of the central nervous system (CNS) occurs, with resultant meningoencephalitis leading to mental and physical lethargy, coma, and, ultimately, death if untreated. Infection with *T. (T.) b. rhodesiense* most often appears initially as a severe acute illness. *T. (T.) b. gambiense* infection usually presents as a chronic illness with meningoencephalitis.

ETIOLOGY. The agents responsible for human sleeping sickness, *T. (T.) b. gambiense* and *T. (T.) b. rhodesiense,* are polymorphic salivarian trypanosomes that are morphologically identical to *T. (T.) b. brucei,* an organism infecting animals but not humans. These 3 African trypanosomes are considered subspecies belonging to the family Trypanosomatidae, genus *Trypanosoma,* subgenus *Trypanozoon,* species *brucei,* according to the classification of Hoare. Taxonomy of the nominate subspecies is controversial and is based on differences in infectivity, pathogenicity, or virulence to humans, geographic distribution, drug sensitivity, and dyskinetoplasty. *T. (T.) b. brucei* is separated from the purely human parasite *T. (T.) b. gambiense* because of its epizootiologic features and its inability to infect humans. The position of *T. (T.) b. rhodesiense* is not as clear. This parasite is identical to *T. (T.) b. brucei* zoologically except that its hosts include people. However, *T. (T.) b. rhodesiense* is medically more closely related to *T. (T.) b. gambiense,* because both cause human sleeping sickness. They differ only in type and virulence of disease produced. The quadripartite names are used throughout this chapter for convenience, although *T. (T.) b. rhodesiense* may not be a separate subspecies.

HISTORY. In 1880, Griffith Evans discovered that trypanosomes might be pathogens by finding them in the blood of animals. This was the key to subsequent investigations incriminating these organisms in both animal and human disease. The most important contribution was made in 1895 by David Bruce, who discovered trypanosomes to be the cause of nagana, cattle trypanosomiasis. The new species was named *T. brucei* by Plimmer and Bradford in 1899. The first scientific evidence of human trypanosomiasis was provided in 1902 by Dutton, who recognized trypanosomes in the blood of a European patient from Gambia under the care of Forde. These organisms were designated *T. gambiense* by Dutton. The pathogenicity was first demonstrated in 1903 by Castellani, who associated trypanosomes with sleeping sickness by finding them in the cerebrospinal fluid (CSF) of a Ugandan patient. In 1909, the German scientist Kleine proved that the trypanosomes had to undergo a cycle of development in the tsetse fly vector to be infective, and in 1913, Robertson described in detail the morphologic transformations of the trypanosomes in the vector. In 1910, Stephens and Fantham identified *T. rhodesiense* as a separate species based on higher parasitemias, the occurrence of posteronuclear forms, and a more acute infection in humans.

Early in this century, the high mortality rates of human sleeping sickness were dramatically illustrated in a series of epidemics. The only available control measure was evacuation of large areas. An epidemic in Zaire between 1896 and 1906 was said to have killed 500,000 people. Another along the shores of Lake Victoria resulted in the deaths of two thirds of the population—approximately 250,000 persons. Trypanosomiasis in cattle has been a major obstacle to economic development in Africa. The importance of human sleeping sickness in regard to public health lies not in the annual incidence, but in its potential for the development of explosive epidemics.

DISTRIBUTION AND INCIDENCE. Human African trypanosomiasis occurs in West, Central, and East Africa (Fig. 74–2). In general, the location is determined by the distribution of the tsetse fly vectors. However, sleeping sickness is a focal disease, and there are areas where the vectors are present but there is no transmission. Thirty-six countries of subSaharan Africa with some 200 foci are considered to be endemic for sleeping sickness, with some 50 million people at risk. Approximately 7 to 10 million km² of Africa are infested with tsetse, limiting cattle production to 20 million head in areas with 140 million head capacity. Vast areas of Africa cannot be used for breeding of domestic animals owing to the high incidence of the animal disease. Although some 20,000 new human cases are reported annually, this is almost certainly an underestimate due to under-reporting, poor surveillance, and a shortage of trained health care personnel. Sleeping sickness is considered to be a major health problem in many African countries. Epidemics are not uncommon, usually resulting from an increase in human-fly contact from population movements, changes in vegetation or climate, interruption of systematic medical surveillance, the introduction of new virulent strains of the parasite, or, in some instances, a natural periodicity, perhaps related to the susceptibility of humans. The recent outbreak in Uganda produced more than 4000 new cases in 1986.

TRANSMISSION

Life Cycle. The trypanosomes are transmitted cyclically by blood-sucking flies of the genus *Glossina* (Fig. 74–3). Trypomastigotes are ingested during the blood meal. In the midgut of the fly, the ingested blood forms lose their surface antigenic coat and begin to multiply. Long, slender forms are produced, which then move to the salivary glands and form epimastigotes. In turn, these epimastigotes change into short, stumpy, infective, metacyclic trypanosomes, which enter the bite wound through the hypopharynx. Flies become infective 18 to 35 days (usually approximately 21 days) after feeding on an infected host, depending on the temperature and humidity. The intratsetse cycle is complex and is completed probably less than 10% of the time. Mechanical transmission can theoretically occur when any biting fly, including the tsetse fly, probes an infected host, is disturbed while feeding, and, before the blood on the mouth parts has dried, bites again, inoculating trypanosomes into the second host. The epidemiologic significance of this mode is unknown. Congenital transmission has been reported with *T. (T.) b. gambiense* but is rare. Transmission by blood transfusion is possible but is unusual.

Vector. The genus *Glossina* contains more than 22 species of tsetse fly, all restricted to Africa, of which only a few are of importance in the transmission of sleeping sickness (Fig. 74–4). Both sexes feed on mammalian blood and inflict painful bites. Tsetse flies are viviparous and produce mature larvae that pupate after burrowing into sandy soil. They live in hot, dark, moist places in proximity to blood meals. The flies that transmit *T. (T.) b. gambiense* and *T. (T.) b. rhodesiense* have different ecologic requirements that relate to the epidemiologic differences of the 2 types. Less than 1% of flies are naturally infected in an endemic area, with no more than 5% being infected in epidemic areas. A fly remains infective for life. Experimental evidence suggests that a minimum of approximately 350 trypanosomes must be injected for the infection to "take" in humans.

EPIDEMIOLOGY. West African *(gambiense)* trypanosomiasis and East African *(rhodesiense)* trypanosomiasis are epidemiologically distinct. Major differences are presented in Table 74–1. Overlap of distribution occurs in a few areas.

West African *(Gambiense)* Trypanosomiasis. West

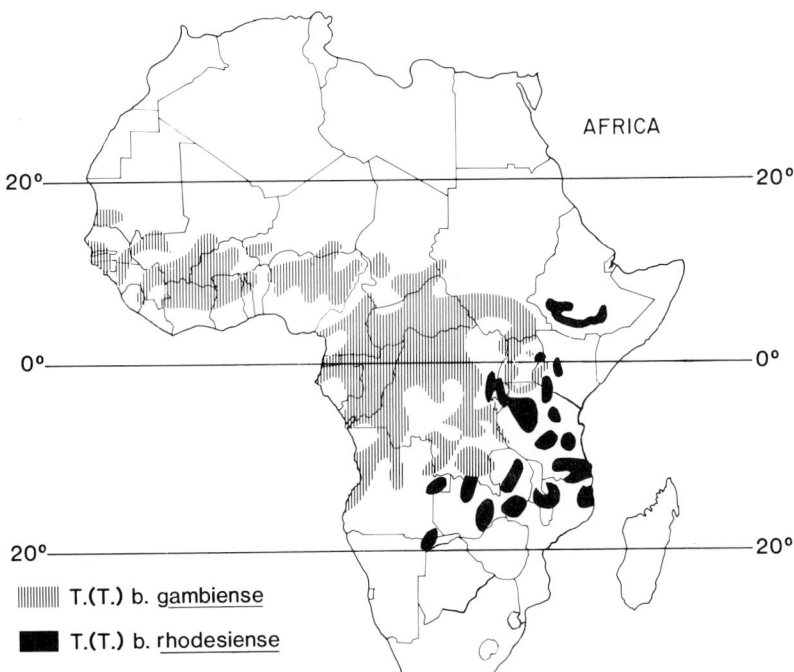

FIGURE 74–2. Distribution of *Trypanosoma (Trypanozoon) brucei gambiense* and *T. (T.) b. rhodesiense*.

▨▨▨ T.(T.) b. <u>gambiense</u>

■■ T.(T.) b. <u>rhodesiense</u>

LIFE CYCLE of –

Trypanosoma (Trypanozoon) brucei
T. (T.) b. gambiense and T. (T.) b. rhodesiense

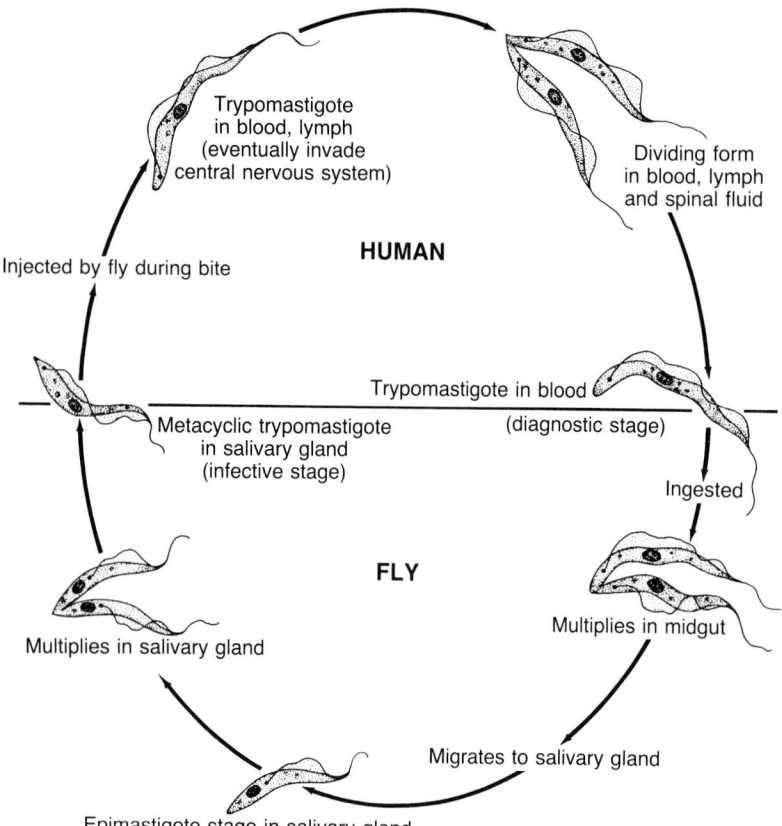

FIGURE 74–3. Life cycle of *Trypanosoma (Trypanozoon) brucei—T. (T.) b. gambiense* and *T. (T.) b. rhodesiense*. (Modified from Melvin DM, et al: Common Blood and Tissue Parasites of Man. Life Cycle Charts. Atlanta, GA, Centers for Disease Control, 1979.)

African trypanosomiasis is caused by *T. (T.) b. gambiense*. The common vectors are the "riverine" tsetse flies of the *palpalis* group (subgenus *Nemorhina*), *Glossina palpalis, G. tachinoides,* and *G. fuscipes*. The principal habitat of these tsetse flies is dense vegetation along rivers and forests, where proper conditions of temperature, moisture, and light are combined with the availability of blood meals. Distribution is focal. These flies readily adapt to whatever source of blood is available. Humans, the preferred hosts, are a variable source of food (8 to 40%) and are frequently bitten at water sites, particularly during the dry season, when many sources of water disappear, thereby increasing human-fly contact. Humans are the only important reservoir. An animal reservoir has not been proved, although several species of animals have been infected experimentally. The incidence of the disease is determined by exposure, not by sex, age, or race characteristics. The long incubation period and chronicity of the disease reflect the high degree of adaptation of the parasite to humans as hosts and are important in the transmission. Many infected persons are almost symptom free. They are ambulant, lead normal lives, can infect flies, and are primarily responsible for spread of the disease. Asymptomatic carriers may play a role in the interepidemic reservoir of infection but the existence of such an asymptomatic state is controversial. The disease is a rural one because of the characteristics of the vector and reservoir, and tourists are rarely infected.

East African (Rhodesiense) Trypanosomiasis. East African sleeping sickness is caused by *T. (T.) b. rhodesiense* and is transmitted by tsetse of the *morsitans* group (subgenus *Glossina* spp.), *G. morsitans, G. pallidipes,* and *G. swynnertoni*. These vectors are widely distributed through the woodland and thickets of East African lakes and savanna. These tsetse flies are zoophilic and are less

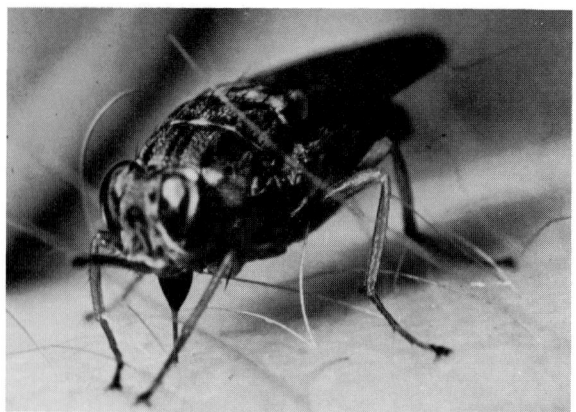

FIGURE 74–4. Tsetse fly biting. (Courtesy of Dr. J. Patana and the Wellcome Museum of Medical Science.)

TABLE 74–1. Differences Between Gambian and Rhodesian Sleeping Sickness

	Gambiense (West African)	*Rhodesiense* (East African)
Agent	T. (T.) b. gambiense	T. (T.) b. rhodesiense
Main vectors	G. palpalis group (riverine tsetse)	G. morsitans group (savanna tsetse)
Distribution	West and Central Africa	East and Central Africa
Location	Around water holes and rivers	Savanna and recently cleared bush
Main reservoir	Humans	Antelope and cattle
Type	Anthroponosis	Anthropozoonosis
Disease	Chronic—late CNS invasion	Acute—early CNS invasion
Duration	Several months to years	3–9 months
Development in laboratory rodents	Poor	Good
Parasitemia	Low	High
Diagnosis	Lymph node aspirate	Peripheral blood examination
	CSF examination	Animal inoculation
		CSF examination
Population at particular risk	Rural population in endemic areas	Tourists to game parks
		Special occupational groups
		Population in endemic areas

flexible in their choice of blood meals than the *G. palpalis* group. The disease is a zoonosis, and humans are only incidentally infected. Antelope, particularly bushbuck *(Tragelaphus scriptus)* and hartebeest *(Alcelaphus),* are important reservoirs. Cattle are the only proven domestic reservoirs. Many other animals can become infected but are not as effective reservoirs because either parasitemia is transient or the animal quickly succumbs to the disease. Carnivores such as the lion and hyena act as reservoirs.

Rhodesiense sleeping sickness is an occupational hazard, e.g., of fishermen and game wardens. The dependence of the *G. morsitans* group of tsetse flies on game means that they are generally confined to country away from human habitation. People become infected by traveling into fly-infested country or when vegetation and humidity favor the establishment of human-fly contact close to homesteads (adaptation to the peridomestic habitat). Full use of land, the presence of game, and the presence of tsetse flies are not compatible. Vast areas in Africa are unused because of the presence of tsetse flies. Age, sex, and race have no influence on the risk of infection except as they relate to exposure. Sporadic cases are often seen, and the disease is a special threat to visitors to the game reserves of East Africa. The acute nature of the disease and the risk of spread from an enzootic focus imply that epidemics are always possible.

PATHOGENESIS AND PATHOLOGY

Pathogenesis. Our understanding of the pathogenesis of sleeping sickness is still inadequate. Most theories implicate immunopathologic processes. Immune complexes formed between variant antigens and antibodies frequently associated with complement have been demonstrated both in the circulation and deposited in target organs. Hypocomplementemia occurs with increased immunoconglutinin and an activated kinin system. Anemia can be severe, and the resulting anoxia could contribute to tissue destruction. The production of autoantibodies is a prominent feature, and these, directed against antigenic components of red blood cells, brain, and heart, could cause damage. Although eosinophilia is not seen in untreated sleeping sickness, eosinophil counts may rise during therapy. The urticaria and pruritus that are sometimes present could be caused by a type I immediate hypersensitivity reaction directed toward the trypanosomes. However, the classic clinical and pathologic features of this disease cannot be readily explained by any of the 4 types of immunopathologic reactions. A direct role for a toxin produced by the organism has not been proved. Similarly unknown is the pathologic importance of metabolic changes induced by the pharmacologically active substances such as kinins that are known to be increased in the disease. A theory suggests that the observed polyclonal proliferation of B lymphocytes in lymph nodes, brain, and heart could lead to tissue damage from an as-yet-unknown mechanism. Advances in immunologic and culture techniques should be helpful in elucidating these mechanisms in the future.

Immune Response. The African trypanosome survives in the mammalian host by periodically altering its surface antigenic coat, thereby aborting the developing immune response of the host. These variant antigenic types mark the identity of different subpopulations of trypanosomes. Acquired immunity is type specific only. Therefore, sleeping sickness is characterized by recurring parasitemia, with each new wave of parasites representing the selection of an immunologically distinct antigenic variant. Experimental evidence suggests that the surface antigens are a matrix of identical glycoproteins, that a single organism contains all the necessary information to produce variants, and that antigenic variants do not arise by mutation but are genetically determined. Variants apparently have a definable order of priority but no strict sequence of appearance. Some estimates suggest that a single clone can produce more than 100 variable antigenic types.

Pronounced immunologic changes occur during the course of the disease. In the acute phase, there is marked reactivity of the lymphoid tissue with predominant plasma cells. Later, the immune system becomes depleted of lymphocytes and plasma cells, which are replaced by histiocytes. Polyclonal hypergammaglobulinemia, particularly increased immunoglobulin M (IgM), is striking and a constant feature. Little of the IgM produced is specific antitrypanosome antibody. Heterophile antibody, rheumatoid factor—like substance, and anti-DNA autoantibodies are also produced.

A stage of relative immunosuppression develops. Impairment of both cellular and humoral immunity occurs, as evidenced by a reduced reaction to a variety of skin test antigens and diminished response to bacterial and viral vaccines.

Pathology. The dominant pathologic changes of African trypanosomiasis are present in the lymphatic, cardiac, and central nervous systems. In the early stages, lymphocytic and histiocytic proliferation occur in the spleen and lymph nodes, which are enlarged and may contain trypanosomes. Later, fibrosis may occur. Leukocytes contain cellular debris, erythrocytes, and trypanosomes. Cellular degeneration is found in association with a marked infiltration of monocytes, macrophages, lymphocytes, large lymphoid cells, and plasma cells. In the chronic stages, an endarteritis appears, with endothelial proliferation involving small vessels accompanied by perivascular infiltration of plasma cells and lymphocytes. The liver shows Kupffer cell hyperplasia, portal tract infiltrates, and fatty degeneration. Glomerulonephritis has been noted.

Cardiac involvement and polyserositis are prominent features of *rhodesiense* disease. A pancarditis has been described involving all layers of the heart, including mural and valvular endocardium; the myocardium, including the conducting system; and the epicardium, including the autonomic nervous system. The pathologic changes observed have consisted of marked cellular infiltration, including plasma and morular cells, as well as myocytolysis and fibrosis. The pancarditis may cause death in patients with *rhodesiense* disease before major CNS damage has developed.

CNS involvement results in meningoencephalitis or meningomyelitis. Perivascular infiltration associated with prominent neuroglial proliferation is present and is most marked in the pia-arachnoid of the brain and spinal cord (Fig. 74–5). Edema, hemorrhages, and granulomatous lesions are present in the brain. Thrombosis as a result of endarteritis is a major cause of cerebral degeneration. Two cytotoxic abnormalities suggestive of sleeping sickness may be found—lymphophagocytosis and the so-called morular or Mott cells (Fig. 74–6). The latter are modified plasma cells (up to 20 μm in diameter) with large eosinophilic inclusions that have been shown to consist of IgG. These cells may play an important role in the local production of IgM in the cerebrospinal fluid. These cells have also been found in the heart. Demyelinization is minimal.

CLINICAL MANIFESTATIONS AND COMPLICATIONS. Sleeping sickness is characterized clinically by the development of a lesion at the site of the infected tsetse bite, followed by parasitemia, fever, and hemolymphatic involvement and then by CNS invasion, with meningoencephalitis and death. Clinical manifestations may vary greatly and are not pathognomonic. *Rhodesiense* disease is usually an acute disease with chancre, fever, early CNS involvement (within 3 to 4 weeks), no clear distinction between early and late stages, often prominent cardiac involvement, and death within weeks to months. In contrast, *gambiense* sleeping sickness is characterized by prominent involvement of lymph glands, late CNS invasion, and a chronic progressive course that may last months to years before death ensues.

Chancre. A primary lesion (the trypanosomal chancre) may develop within 5 to 15 days at the site of the tsetse bite. Shorter and longer incubation periods have been described. The chancre appears as a painful, circumscribed, rubbery, indurated, dusky-red papule 2 to 5 cm in diameter that subsides spontaneously in 2 to 3 weeks. The frequency of the primary lesion is inconstant, but it occurs more often in non-Africans and may be more common with *T. (T.) b. rhodesiense* infection. The lesion may be associated with local lymph gland enlargement. Prominent cellulitis may occur and mask the chancre.

Early Stages (Hemolymphatic Involvement). Within a few hours to days after the appearance of the chancre or, if there is no chancre, within about 1 to 3 weeks after the infected bite occurred, invasion of the blood

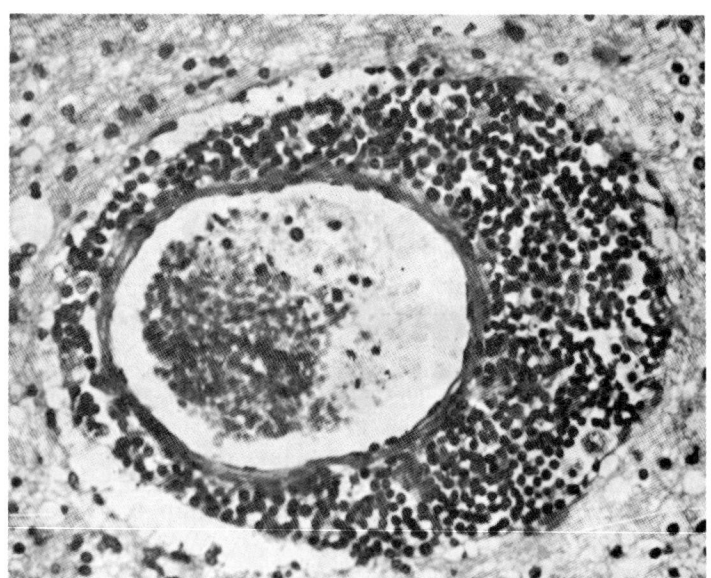

FIGURE 74–5. African sleeping sickness. Section of brain showing perivascular infiltration (cuffing) and edema.

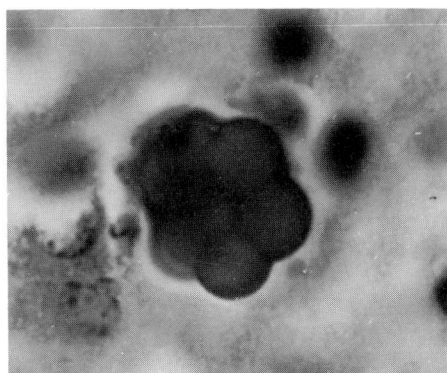

FIGURE 74–6. Morular cell of Mott (× 2000). (Courtesy of the Wellcome Museum of Medical Science.)

stream is heralded by an attack of high fever lasting 1 to 7 days. In West Africa, the onset may be more gradual, and several years may pass before the onset of clinical symptoms.

Non-Africans tend to have acute onsets. Following the initial febrile episode, the early stage of the disease is characterized by intermittent bouts of fever separated by remissions during which the patient feels well. Symptoms and signs are nonspecific, irregular, and inconsistent. Malaise, persistent headache, dizziness, joint pain, weight loss, weakness, general itching, and tachycardia all may be present.

Irritability, insomnia, loss of ability to concentrate, personality change, and even somnolence are characteristic early features, especially in non-Africans. These symptoms may be present long before there are detectable changes in the CSF and are not diagnostic of CNS involvement.

An irregular, circinate, evanescent rash that is more easily demonstrated in white persons may appear. This rash is most commonly observed on the trunk, shoulders, and thighs as scattered, oval, pinkish, erythematous areas often 3 to 4 inches in diameter with clear centers. Pruritus and painful local edemas of the hands, feet, and periorbital and joint regions are frequent and transient. Deep hyperesthesia (Kerandel's sign) is reported to occur in 20% of Europeans but is uncommon in Africans and results in delayed, intense pain when soft tissues are compressed, e.g., by a sharp blow or squeeze.

Generalized lymph node enlargement follows as the disease progresses. In *gambiense* disease, the supraclavicular and posterior cervical lymph nodes are often enlarged. Characteristic of *gambiense* disease is visible enlargement of the glands of the posterior cervical triangle (Winterbottom's sign) (Fig. 74–7). Classically, the lymph nodes are discrete, freely movable, nontender, and rubbery. Later, fibrosis occurs. The spleen and liver may be mildly enlarged.

Later Stages (Central Nervous System Invasion). Involvement of the CNS may occur within weeks to a few months in the clinical course (*rhodesiense* disease) or may not develop until months or even years later (*gambiense* disease). Onset of this stage is usually insidious, with gradual, progressive involvement. The clinical manifestations are protean, and early changes may be subtle, involving alterations in personality and behavior. In general, the symptoms are those associated with a diffuse meningoencephalomyelitis with predominant involvement of the base of the brain. The common presenting symptom is gradually increasing indifference and lassitude. Most impressive is daytime somnolence, often alternating with insomnia at night. Extrapyramidal signs occur frequently, with tremors of the tongue and fingers, fasciculations of the muscles of the limbs, face, lips, and tongue, choreiform or oscillatory movements of the arms, head, neck, and trunk (especially in children), and increasing tonicity or muscular rigidity. Speech becomes indistinct and difficult to follow. There is usually a considerable element of cerebellar ataxia, leading to problems in walking. Headache and papilledema reflect cerebral edema. Backache and neck stiffness may be present. Parkinson's disease may be mimicked by shuffling gait, muscular rigidity, tremors of the tongue and muscles, and slurred speech. Further neurologic abnormalities appearing in the later stages include epileptiform seizures, sometimes followed by local paralyses, euphoria, maniacal changes, and somnolence. The patient becomes indifferent to his or her environment. Cranial nerve palsies and long tract signs are uncommon.

The final stage is one of progressive mental deterioration and classic sleeping sickness. There is intolerable pruritus, generalized wasting, and dribbling of saliva. The patient is difficult to arouse and lies immobile in the hut or hospital bed. Initially, the person can be aroused to take food and water, but he or she never speaks or takes food spontaneously. Later, coma ensues. Death results from the sleeping sickness itself, intercurrent infection, or malnutrition. In acute *rhodesiense* disease, death may occur before CNS involvement develops, perhaps as the result of cardiac arrhythmia or cardiac failure from the pancarditis.

Pediatric Age Group. Children are not usually infected under normal circumstances, mainly because of decreased risk of exposure. However, African trypanosomiasis in children is often fulminant, with early CNS involvement. Diagnosis is often delayed, and the child

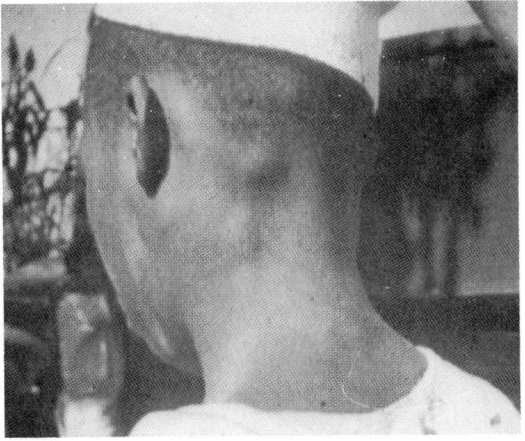

FIGURE 74–7. Enlargement of posterior cervical lymph nodes— Winterbottom's sign. (Courtesy of Dr. James R. Busvine, London School of Hygiene and Tropical Medicine.)

presents with choreiform movements, psychomotor retardation, seizures, and/or coma.

Laboratory Test Abnormalities. The main abnormalities associated with sleeping sickness that are revealed by laboratory tests include anemia, abnormal liver function, coagulation abnormalities, thrombocytopenia, hypocomplementemia, and increased plasma kinins. Laboratory features of disseminated intravascular coagulation (DIC) may be prominent. None of these changes is pathognomonic. The most characteristic laboratory feature is increased serum and CSF (after CNS invasion) IgM. White blood cells, mainly mononuclear, are also present in the CSF. Morular cells of Mott may be seen. The anemia is mainly hemolytic, but impaired erythropoiesis and increased reticuloendothelial destruction may play a role. Anemia, abnormal liver function tests, thrombocytopenia, and DIC are more marked in *rhodesiense* disease than in *gambiense* disease. IgM heterophile antibodies may also be present.

DIAGNOSIS. Diagnosis depends on demonstration of trypanosomes from the chancre, in blood, in aspirate from enlarged lymph nodes, or in the CSF (Fig. 74–8). Serologic tests are helpful in epidemiologic surveys but are not diagnostic. Clinical manifestations are nonspecific. Malaria, kala-azar, tuberculosis, brucellosis, viral encephalitis, tick typhus, syphilis, lymphoma, CNS tumors, psychoses, and causes of meningitis with a mononuclear response are all included in the differential diagnosis. Therefore, a high index of suspicion is necessary, particularly for persons presenting in nonendemic areas. Lumbar puncture should be done in all patients, both those with suspected and those with proven hemolymphatic disease.

Direct Demonstration of the Parasite. Trypanosomes may be found in the chancre before their appearance in the peripheral blood. The chancre is punctured. A drop of the serous exudate is then examined for motile trypanosomes as a wet preparation.

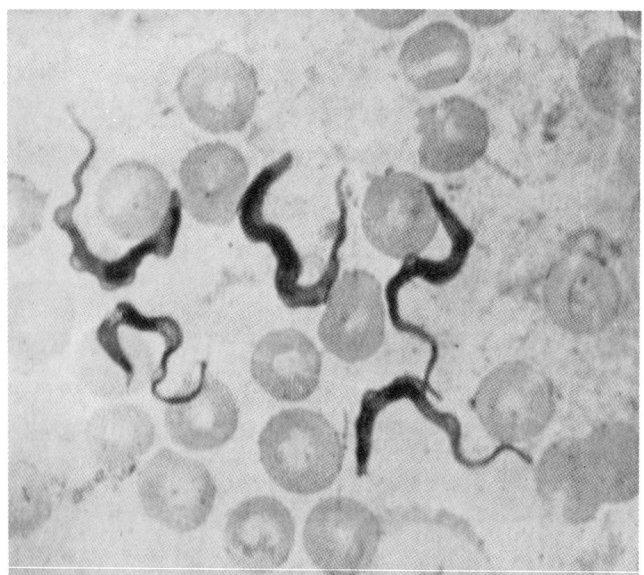

FIGURE 74–8. *Trypanosoma (T.) b. gambiense* in stained blood film.

Examination of stained thick and thin peripheral blood films is a sensitive method of detection of *T. (T.) b. rhodesiense*. Giemsa is the best stain, but Wright's and Leishman's stains may also be used. Microscopic examination of blood is less useful in identifying *T. (T.) b. gambiense* because these parasites are scanty in the peripheral circulation. Blood is more often positive in the early stages of infection. It is advisable to examine multiple daily specimens, because parasites occur in waves and parasitemia may be below detectable levels at one particular time.

Several methods increase the yield of blood examination. A sensitive technique is filtration of blood samples through anion-exchanger DEAE-cellulose, followed by centrifugation or membrane filtration. Concentration methods may be useful, utilizing 6% sodium citrate in 0.9% saline. The buffy coat layer of centrifuged venous or microcapillary blood can be stained or examined as a wet preparation directly, using a darkfield microscope, or with an ultraviolet microscope, after the addition of a fluorescent drug, e.g., homidium.

The most dependable diagnostic procedure in *gambiense* trypanosomiasis is examination of a stained smear of fluid aspirated from an enlarged, soft lymph node. A prolonged search is often necessary. This technique is not of value in later stages when the nodes have become hard and fibrotic. Motile trypanosomes may be seen on examination of a wet preparation. In *rhodesiense* disease, lymph node enlargement is less prominent, and aspiration is less rewarding.

Examination of CSF. Examination of the CSF is mandatory. Demonstration of increased white blood cells (>5 per mm³) and/or protein (>25 mg/dl) (by the turbidimetry method) indicates invasion of the CNS. Double centrifugation and examination of the sediment may increase detection of trypanosomes. The first detectable abnormality is usually an increased cell count. Later, CSF pressure increases, and IgM and total protein levels become elevated. Demonstration of increased IgM and/or increased cells in the CSF can be regarded as pathognomonic of CNS invasion if trypanosomes have been demonstrated peripherally. A high level of IgM in the CSF with only a modest increase in CSF total protein is also suggestive. The inflammatory cells are predominantly mononuclear, mostly small lymphocytes. IgM levels in the CSF may remain elevated for long periods of time after successful treatment.

Animal Inoculation. The most sensitive method for diagnosis of *T. (T.) b. rhodesiense* infection is still intraperitoneal inoculation of 0.5 ml of heparinized blood or CSF into 2 mice. Parasitemia usually develops in 4 to 7 days and almost always within 2 weeks. *T. (T.) b. rhodesiense* also readily infects other laboratory rodents such as rats and guinea pigs. *Gambiense* trypanosomes will infect rodents only with difficulty or not at all.

Culture. Blood, CSF, or lymph fluid can also be inoculated into GLSH (glucose, lactalbumin, serum, and hemoglobin) culture medium. Modified systems using different fibroblast feeder layers and various media have been successful in growing infective blood forms and may prove useful in primary isolation.

Bone marrow examination and culture may be of use in individual patients in whom trypanosomes cannot be demonstrated by other methods.

Serologic Tests. Although at present no serologic test provides sufficiently definitive information for treatment of a patient without demonstration of the organism, these techniques are useful in population studies and provide valuable ancillary information to parasitologic surveys. The capillary indirect hemagglutination test is suitable for the field. Others include the indirect fluorescent antibody test (IFA), the enzyme-linked immunosorbent assay (ELISA), and the defined antigen substrate spheres (DASS) system. These tests measuring antibodies to trypanosomes are more specific than are methods for detecting increased serum or IgM levels in CSF. Advances in hybridoma and DNA technology and the in vitro tissue culture technique could be useful to serologic methodology in the future through production of more specific antigens.

TREATMENT. There are 2 classes of drugs for treatment of African trypanosomiasis: (1) those useful in the early stages of the disease prior to invasion of the CNS and (2) those effective in advanced stages in which CNS invasion has already occurred. To insure detection of CNS invasion, a lumbar puncture must be performed prior to instituting therapy, periodically during treatment, 3 months after treatment, and then every 6 months for 2 years.

In the United States, these drugs can be obtained from the Parasitic Diseases Division, Center for Infectious Diseases, Centers for Disease Control, Atlanta, GA 30333 (telephone number: day—[404] 329-3311; night—[404] 329-3644).

Early Stages (Hemolymphatic Involvement). Suramin and the pentamidines are the standard drugs used for treatment of the disease prior to CNS invasion.

Suramin. Suramin (Bayer 205, Germanin, Naganol, Moranyl, Fourneau 309, Belganyl, Naphuride, Antrypol) is the drug of choice for the early stages of both *T. (T.) b. gambiense* and *T. (T.) b. rhodesiense* infections when the CSF is normal. This drug will clear the blood of trypanosomes, and a full course will cure nearly 100% of early cases. However, because suramin does not cross the blood-brain barrier in appreciable amounts, it will not cure the disease once CNS invasion has occurred, although it will clear trypanosomes in blood and lymph nodes.

Suramin is administered by slow intravenous injection as a freshly prepared 10% aqueous solution. Once reconstituted, the drug must be used within 30 minutes. Intramuscular injection causes local irritation, is painful, and is not advised. Suramin binds to plasma proteins and can persist at low concentration for as long as 3 months. Metabolic destruction is negligible, and the drug is excreted virtually unchanged through the kidneys.

The usual dose is 20 mg/kg body weight given intravenously to a maximum single dose of 1.0 gm. A test dose of 200 mg (or 5 mg/kg) is given to identify patients who show an idiosyncratic reaction to the drug, followed by full doses on days 1, 3, 7, 14, and 21, or weekly until a total of 5.0 gm is achieved. A single course for an adult should not exceed 7.0 gm.

Suramin is a toxic drug, requiring close supervision. Approximately 1 person in 20,000 appears to have an idiosyncratic reaction to suramin. Concomitant onchocerciasis increases the risk of this complication. In these persons, injection is followed immediately by nausea, vomiting, seizures, shock, and collapse. Although the patient usually recovers, fatalities have been reported. Less severe reactions are common, including joint pain, fever, pruritus, urticaria, photophobia, papular eruption, conjunctivitis, paresthesia, and cutaneous hyperesthesia of the palms and soles. These are usually transient and are not indications for discontinuation of the drug.

Kidney damage is the most important toxic effect. The drug is deposited in the renal tubules. Usually, renal damage is manifested only by albuminuria, which clears within a few weeks and is not an indication for suspension of treatment. However, if albuminuria increases or if casts or red blood cells are seen in the urine sediment, alternative therapy should be given. The urine should be examined prior to administration of each dose of suramin, and the drug should not be given to any patient with pre-existing renal disease. Severe exfoliative dermatitis, agranulocytosis, hemolytic anemia, relative adrenal insufficiency, jaundice, hepatitis, fulminating diarrhea, and death have all been reported, although rarely, following suramin therapy.

Pentamidine. Pentamidine (M & B 800, Lomidine) is an aromatic diamidine. Two preparations are in common use: the isethionate (1.74 mg of salt equivalent to 1 mg of base) and the dimethane sulfonate (1.56 mg of salt containing 1 mg of base). The actions, effects, and toxicity of these 2 compounds are similar. Pentamidine is effective in early cases of *gambiense* disease. However, cure rates are lower than those with suramin, and *T. (T.) b. rhodesiense* infections often do not respond to this drug.

Pentamidine isethionate is supplied in vials containing 200 mg of *salt* and should be freshly prepared by dissolution in sterile distilled water, not saline solution. Pentamidine dimethane sulfonate comes already prepared as a 4% solution of *base.*

The dosage, 3 to 4 mg/kg body weight, calculated on the pentamidine *base,* is given intramuscularly daily or cn alternative days for 10 doses. The calculated daily dose should be dissolved in no more than 3 ml of sterile distilled water.

Intravenous administration causes profound hypotension and occasional collapse. Therefore, the drug is given intramuscularly, as noted. Pentamidine achieves its highest concentration in the kidneys and is excreted unchanged mainly in the urine over an extended period of time. Both the liver and kidneys store the drug for months. The drug does not penetrate the CSF.

Even intramuscular injection can cause hypotension, nausea, vomiting, and tachycardia. Although bothersome, these toxic manifestations invariably disappear after 10 to 30 minutes. Elevating the legs often shortens the duration of symptoms. These side effects will frequently recur to the same degree after each injection, but if tolerated by the patient, they are not sufficient cause to discontinue therapy. These reactions may be minimized by keeping the patient supine. Local reactions, including necrosis and sterile abscess formation, can occur in debilitated or immunosuppressed patients.

Reversible renal lesions have been associated with the use of the drug in a proportion of patients. Hypoglycemia has been reported. The greatest depression of blood sugar usually occurs between the fifth and seventh days of therapy. Paradoxically, pentamidine may aggravate diabetes mellitus and may even produce hyperglycemia in nondiabetic patients.

Diminazene aceturate. Diminazene aceturate (Berenil) has been reported to be successful in treating early cases of trypanosomiasis in East Africa. However, this compound is manufactured for veterinary use only. In addition, severe polyneuropathy and ascending polyneuritis have been associated with its use.

Later Stages (CNS Invasion)

Melarsoprol. Melarsoprol (Mel B, Arsobal), a combination of melarsen oxide and BAL, will cure all stages of sleeping sickness. This is the drug of choice when CNS invasion has occurred and is also indicated in early disease after treatment with suramin and/or pentamidine has failed. Because of its toxicity, melarsoprol is never the first choice for treatment of early sleeping sickness.

Melarsoprol contains 18.8% arsenic and is supplied as a clear, sterile 3.6% solution in propylene glycol. The drug must be given only intravenously, and care must be taken to avoid leakage into the tissues. Melarsoprol is rapidly excreted in the urine. A small but therapeutically important amount enters the CSF.

The drug is given in 3 courses of 3 successive- or alternate-day intravenous injections with 1 week between each course. One accepted regimen for adults weighing 60 kg or more is 3 daily doses of 2.5 ml, 3.0 ml, and 3.5 ml, followed after a 5- to 7-day interval with doses of 3.5 ml, 4.0 ml, and 4.5 ml on successive or alternate days, then a third course of 3 daily injections of 5.0 ml after another 5- to 7-day interval. The maximum daily dose is 5 ml (180 mg). The total dose is 20 mg/kg. For patients weighing less than 60 kg, the maximum daily dose is 3.6 mg/kg (to 180 mg). The first course consists of daily intravenous injections of 1.8 mg/kg, 2.1 mg/kg, and 2.4 mg/kg, the second of 2.7 mg/kg, 3.0 mg/kg, and 3.3 mg/kg, and the third of 3 daily injections of 3.6 mg/kg. A 7-day interval separates each course. Other treatment schedules can be found in the World Health Organization's Technical Report Series, No. 739, 1986.

Patients with advanced meningoencephalitis or those who are acutely ill, febrile, or wasted should be treated first with 2 to 4 doses of suramin, 250 to 500 mg on alternate days, prior to receiving melarsoprol. However, if there is no immediate improvement, melarsoprol should be administered.

Melarsoprol is also the drug of choice after treatment with suramin or pentamidine has been unsuccessful. For relapse with hemolymphatic involvement only (normal CSF), 3 daily doses of 3.6 mg/kg are given and are repeated after an interval of 1 to 2 weeks. If CNS invasion has occurred, 3 courses of 3 daily injections of 3.6 mg/kg are given, with each course separated by 1 week.

Like all arsenicals, melarsoprol displays significant toxicity in many patients receiving the drug. Extravasation during intravenous injections may lead to intense local reactions. A Jarisch-Herxheimer–type reaction has been reported. However, the most important toxic reactions involve the CNS. Reactive encephalopathy occurs, in 18% of patients in some series; it may be fatal and usually develops during the first course. The onset may be sudden, or the condition may develop slowly. The reaction is characterized clinically by premonitory headache, tremor, difficulty in speech, hyperpyrexia, convulsions, and, finally, coma. Reactive encephalopathy is believed to be due to the interaction of the drug, diseased brain, and trypanosomes. It seemingly occurs at random, although it is rare in patients with minimal CNS involvement. Incidence and fatality rates have been ascribed to the initial condition of the patient, overdosage, or batch of the drug. As clinical experience with melarsoprol has increased, the mortality due to drug toxicity has decreased. At the first sign of encephalopathy, the drug should be stopped. Therapy can be cautiously reinstituted with small doses a few days after recovery. Dimercaprol (BAL) and corticosteroids have been recommended for treatment of reactive encephalopathy.

A rare, almost invariably fatal, hemorrhagic encephalopathy has been reported with melarsoprol. Other toxic effects suggestive of heavy metal toxicity occur. Abdominal pain and vomiting may appear and can be reduced by injecting the drug slowly with the patient in the supine position. Albuminuria with casts and hepatic dysfunction may occur, necessitating modification of treatment. Exfoliative dermatitis is a rare complication. Despite these difficulties, melarsoprol is a valuable drug and is the only agent available for routine treatment of patients with sleeping sickness with CNS involvement.

Melarsonyl potassium. Melarsonyl potassium (Mel W, Trimelarsen) is similar to melarsoprol. Its sole advantage is that it is water soluble and can be given intramuscularly or subcutaneously; this is useful when the intravenous route cannot be used. Toxicity may be greater than that of melarsoprol, and the drug is less effective against *T. (T.) b. rhodesiense*.

DFMO. α-Difluoromethylornithine (Elfornithine, DFMO) is an irreversible inhibitor of ornithine decarboxylase and inhibits the biosynthesis of polyamines and subsequently RNA and DNA in *T. (T.) b. brucei*. In a large series from West Africa *gambiense* disease refractory to arsenicals was successfully treated with DFMO intravenously, orally, or via both routes. Dosage is 400 mg/kg/day intravenously for 2 weeks followed by oral administration for an additional 2 to 4 weeks. DFMO therapy of arsenical refractory cases of *rhodesiense* disease has not been successful.

Nitrofurazone. This drug is useful in infections proven resistant to melarsoprol. In adults nitrofurazone is administered orally at a dose of 0.5 gm 3 or 4 times daily for 5 to 7 days. Three courses may be given, with 1 week between each course. Polyneuropathy and reversible degeneration of the seminiferous tubules are the most frequent side effects. A hemolytic anemia may occur in patients with glucose-6-phosphate dehydrogenase deficiency.

Nifurtimox. Nifurtimox (Bayer 2502, Lampit) has been used successfully in a small number of arsenical refractory cases of *gambiense* disease. The dosage used was 15 mg/kg/day orally for 21 to 30 days. Toxicity is similar to that of nitrofurazone.

PROGNOSIS. Untreated sleeping sickness is almost invariably fatal. There have been a few case reports of chronic asymptomatic *gambiense* infections, but these are rare. A matter for serious concern is the emergence of drug resistance. With increasing frequency, infections are not responding to conventional therapy. The prognosis is good if there is no CNS involvement or if only minimal changes are present in the CSF at the time treatment is instituted. A CSF protein concentration greater than 40 mg/dl at the time the patient begins treatment is a poor prognostic sign. Some of these patients may not respond to any drug.

Following appropriate treatment, there is usually a marked improvement in the patient's condition unless the therapy is obviously going to fail. To determine if therapy has been effective, periodic examinations of the CSF must be performed during and after treatment. A favorable sign is continued decrease in the CSF protein concentration and cell count. The first sign of a relapse will generally be a rise in the cell count followed by an increase in protein (particularly IgM). At this time, the patient may still be asymptomatic. Nonspecific complaints such as headache, malaise, fever, and weakness should increase suspicion of a relapse. Although trypanosomes may be seen in the CSF early in a relapse, either a rising CSF cell count *or* protein concentration is *sufficient alone* to indicate the need for further treatment. Two points of caution are necessary: Cell count and protein level may rise immediately after treatment with melarsoprol and not begin to fall for 2 or 3 months. High CSF IgM levels may persist for an extended period of time.

PREVENTION AND CONTROL. Extensive rapid international travel has facilitated the importation of exotic diseases to nonendemic countries. Although the risk to tourists of acquiring sleeping sickness is low, cases have been documented in persons visiting the game parks of East and Central Africa. Patients may have stopped only briefly in endemic areas. Symptoms are often nonspecific, and the travel history may be the only clue to the diagnosis. *Unde venis?* "Where have you been?" should be a standard question in the workup of every febrile illness. Rapid diagnosis and appropriate treatment are vital in preventing unnecessary mortality and morbidity.

Routine Preventive Measures. These should include avoidance of known foci of sleeping sickness and/or tsetse infestation, wearing of wrist- and ankle-length clothing in endemic areas, use of insect repellents, the routine use of mosquito nets, advance contact with medical personnel in areas on the itinerary where sleeping sickness is endemic, and close monitoring and prompt medical attention for any febrile illness occurring while in an endemic area or after return home. The flies are attracted to moving objects and will follow a car for long distances. They can bite through thin clothing easily. Motor vehicles should be inspected for flies. Care should be taken to avoid areas known to be heavily infested with tsetse flies.

Case Detection. Medical surveillance and case detection by means of mobile teams who diagnose and treat patients early in their illness constitute an efficient control method in areas of *gambiense* disease. Because *rhodesiense* sleeping sickness is an acute disease, the majority of patients attend hospitals and/or health centers. Therefore, strengthening the personnel and equipment of the primary health care delivery system is more efficient. However, case detection and surveillance also have a role in control in special circumstances. Where possible, persons living in endemic areas should avoid known sleeping sickness and tsetse-infested areas.

Chemoprophylaxis. Suramin and particularly pentamidine have been reported to be effective chemoprophylactic agents for *gambiense* disease. However, chemoprophylaxis is *not* recommended for individuals traveling to endemic areas except under unusual circumstances. Resistance develops to the drug used. Most tourists are exposed to *rhodesiense* disease. The efficacy of chemoprophylaxis for this form of sleeping sickness has not been proved. However, the most disquieting hazard associated with chemoprophylaxis is the tendency to mask symptoms until CNS invasion occurs. The result is induction of advanced cryptic cases in which organisms are not found in the blood or lymph nodes but are present in the CSF at diagnosis. Chemoprophylaxis may be considered only for individuals who will have constant, heavy exposure to the tsetse fly over an extended period in areas with known transmission of *gambiense* disease.

Vector Control. Permanent control requires that human-fly contact be reduced by application of insecticides, use of insecticide-impregnated targets or traps, destruction of tsetse habitats by selective clearing of vegetation, and/or restriction of population movement into known infected areas. In zones of the *G. morsitans* group, the food source—animals—can be depleted by fencing, selective game control, or opening land to agriculture. Another potentially profitable area of research involves biologic control methods. There are few data available on the practicability of tsetse control with known predators, parasites, and microbial pathogens, but some of these could be useful control measures. The release of male tsetse flies sterilized by irradiation or chemical means to decrease fertility of wild females is being evaluated. Finally, the potential for development of a vaccine has been vastly increased by new techniques, including tissue culture of infective blood forms and hybridoma technology.

BIBLIOGRAPHY

Baker JR: Epidemiology of African sleeping sickness. Ciba Found Symp 20:29, 1974.

Barrett-Connor E, Ugoretz RJ, Braude AI: Disseminated intravascular coagulation in trypanosomiasis. Arch Intern Med 131:574, 1973.

Buyst H: The diagnosis of sleeping sickness. Trop Doc 3:110, 1973.

Cross GAM, Holder AA, Allen G, et al: An introduction to antigenic variation in trypanosomes. Am J Trop Med Hyg 29(Suppl):1027, 1980.

Donelson JE: Antigenic variation in African trypanosomes. Contrib Microbiol Immunol 8:138, 1987.

Duggan AJ, Hutchinson MP: Sleeping sickness in Europeans: A review of 109 cases. J Trop Med Hyg 69:124, 1966.

Dukes P, Rickman LR, Killick-Kendrick R, et al: A field comparison of seven diagnostic techniques for human trypanosomiasis in the Luangwa Valley, Zambia. Tropenmed Parasitol 35:141, 1984.

Ford J: The Role of the Trypanosomiases in African Ecology. Oxford, Clarendon Press, 1971.

Gibson WC: Will the real *Trypanosoma b. gambiense* please stand up. Parasitol Today 2:255, 1986.

Greenwood BM, Whittle HC: Cerebrospinal fluid IgM in patients with sleeping sickness. Lancet 2:525, 1973.

Greenwood BM, Whittle HC: The pathogenesis of sleeping sickness. Trans Soc Trop Med Hyg 74:716, 1980.

Hirumi H, Doyle JJ, Hirumi K: African trypanosomes: Cultivation of animal-infective *Trypanosoma brucei in vitro*. Science 196:992, 1977.

Jordan AM: Recent developments in the ecology and methods of control of tsetse flies *(Glossina)* spp. (Dipt., *Glossinidae)*: a review. Bull Ent Res 63:361, 1974.

Mahmoud AAF, Warren KS: Algorithms in the diagnosis and management of exotic diseases. XI. African trypanosomiasis. J Infect Dis 113:487, 1976.

Molyneux DH, Ashford RW: The Biology of *Trypanosoma* and *Leishmania,* Parasites of Man and Domestic Animals. London, Taylor and Francis, 1983.

Molyneux DH, deRaadt P, Seed JR: African human trypanosomiasis. *In* Gilles HM (ed): Recent Advances in Tropical Medicine 1. London, Churchill Livingstone, 1984, pp 39–62.

Mulligan HW, Potts WH (eds): The African Trypanosomiases. London, George Allen and Unwin, 1970.

Newton BA (ed): Trypanosomiasis. Br Med Bull 41:103, 1985.

Poltera AA: Immunopathological and chemotherapeutic studies in experimental trypanosomiasis with special reference to the heart and brain. Trans R Soc Trop Med Hyg 74:706, 1980.

Robertson DHH: Chemotherapy of African trypanosomiasis. Practitioner 188:80, 1963.

Schechter PJ, Sjoerdsma A: Difluoromethylornithine in treatment of African trypanosomiasis. Parasitol Today 2:223, 1986.

Spencer HC, Gibson JJ, Brodsky RE, et al: Imported African trypanosomiasis in the United States. Ann Intern Med 82:633, 1975.

Taylor AER: Trypanosomiasis I. Salivaria. Trop Dis Bull 83:R1, 1986.

Tizzard I (ed): Immunology and Pathogenesis of Trypanosomiasis. Boca Raton, FL, CRC Press, 1985.

Vickerman K: Antigenic variation. Nature 273 (Parasitology Suppl):613, 1978.

Voller A: Serology of African trypanosomiasis. Ann Soc Belg Med Trop 57:273, 1977.

75. AMERICAN TRYPANOSOMIASIS

Marco Tulio A. Garcia-Zapata, Patrick B. McGreevy, and Philip D. Marsden

DEFINITION. American trypanosomiasis, or Chagas' disease, is an acute, subacute, or chronic disease produced by infection with *Trypanosoma cruzi.* Human infection with *T. cruzi* has a parasitemic acute phase lasting only weeks and a chronic phase that is lifelong. The parasite multiplies in humans in the amastigote stage in the tissues, particularly of the heart and other muscles, causing cardiac syndromes in a minority of patients. *T. cruzi* is a zoonotic parasite infecting many vertebrates and is transmitted by true bugs of the subfamily Triatominae.

In endemic areas the prevalence of human infection with *T. cruzi* is often high, whereas clinically detectable disease is infrequent. In Latin America, there are 24 million seropositive people, representing 8% of the population (Fig. 75–1). Between 10 and 30% will develop clinical syndromes of Chagas' disease, depending on the strains of *T. cruzi* present in the geographic area. Like mucocutaneous leishmaniasis, severe disease is more frequent as one moves south from Texas to central Brazil. The infected people are typically poor subsistence farmers residing in remote homesteads in rural areas who rarely travel outside their country.

HISTORY. In 1921, Carlos Chagas reiterated his important discoveries with a definition of the disease that differed little from that given here. Chagas was a gifted scientist who not only discovered the etiologic agent of American trypanosomiasis, but also documented the insect vectors and reservoir hosts. In the 1930s, Mazza of Argentina published a long series of observations that confirmed Chagas' earlier findings and aroused new interest in the disease. The first epidemiologic study was conducted in Bambui, Minas Gerais, where Emmanuel Dias demonstrated that spraying of houses with the residual insecticide benzene hexachloride was an effective way to control bug populations and suppress transmission. In the 1960s, Fritz Koberle and his group clarified the gut "megasyndromes" (megaesophagus and megacolon) due to aperistalsis as the result of parasympathetic denervation. The past two decades have seen a remarkable increase in research on Chagas' disease.

BIOLOGY OF THE ORGANISM. *T. cruzi* is a polymorphic trypanosome with an indirect life cycle (Fig. 75–2). There are 2 developmental stages of *T. cruzi* in the vertebrate host, infective trypomastigotes

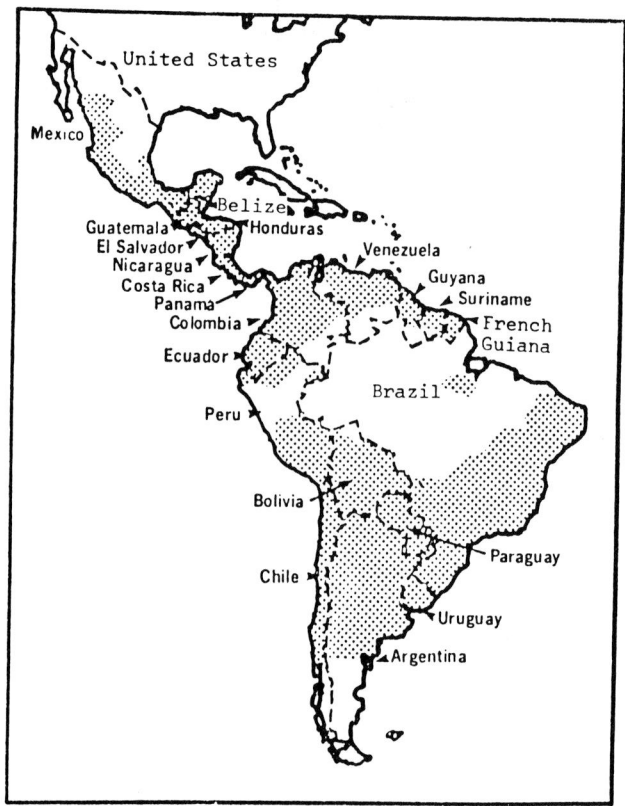

FIGURE 75–1. Distribution of American trypanosomiasis. (PAHO, 1984.)

LIFE CYCLE of –

Trypanosoma cruzi

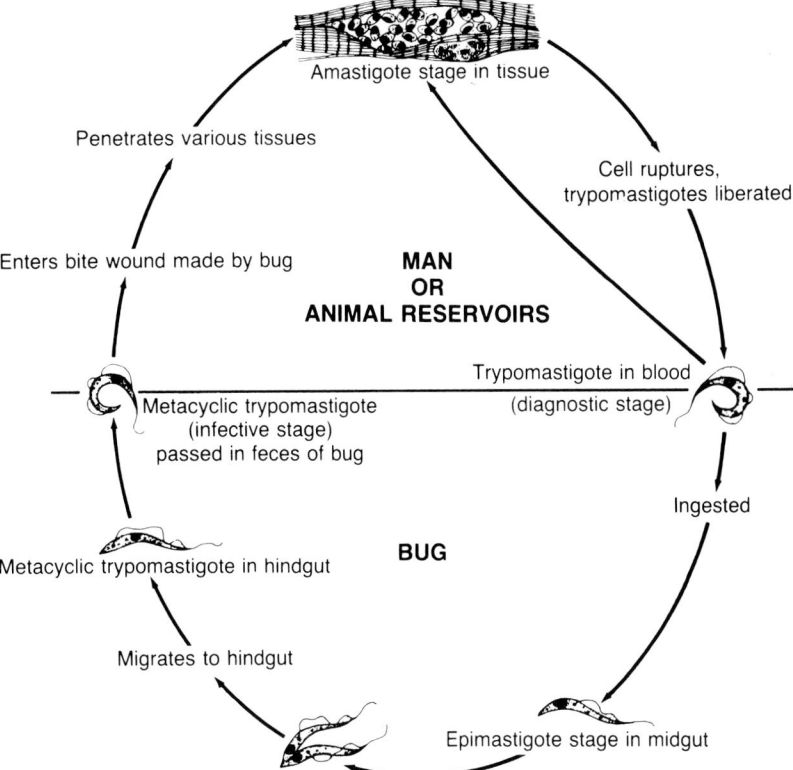

Amastigote stage in tissue

Penetrates various tissues

Cell ruptures, trypomastigotes liberated

Enters bite wound made by bug

MAN OR ANIMAL RESERVOIRS

Trypomastigote in blood (diagnostic stage)

Metacyclic trypomastigote (infective stage) passed in feces of bug

Ingested

Metacyclic trypomastigote in hindgut

BUG

Migrates to hindgut

Epimastigote stage in midgut

Multiplies in midgut

FIGURE 75–2. Life cycle of *Trypanosoma cruzi*. (Modified from Melvin DM, et al: Common Blood and Tissue Parasites of Man. Life Cycle Charts. Atlanta, GA, Centers for Disease Control, 1979.)

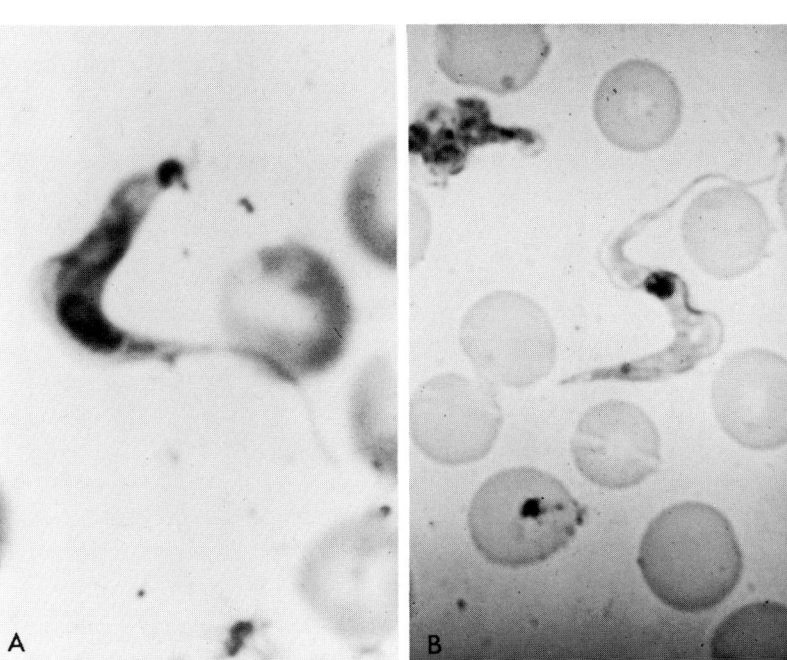

A

B

FIGURE 75–3. *A*, Giemsa-stained trypomastigote of *T. cruzi* showing large kinetoplast. *B*, Giemsa-stained trypomastigote of *T. rangeli* showing a small kinetoplast (× 1200).

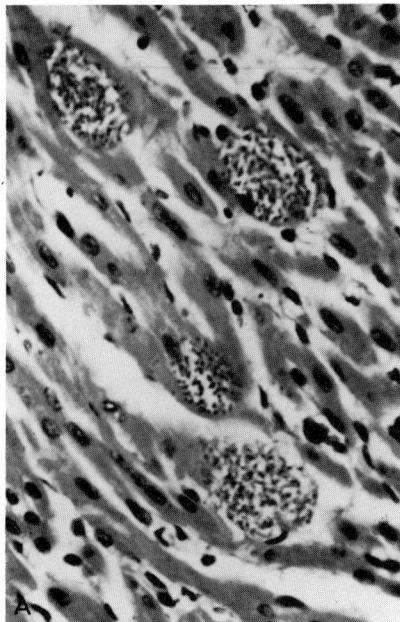
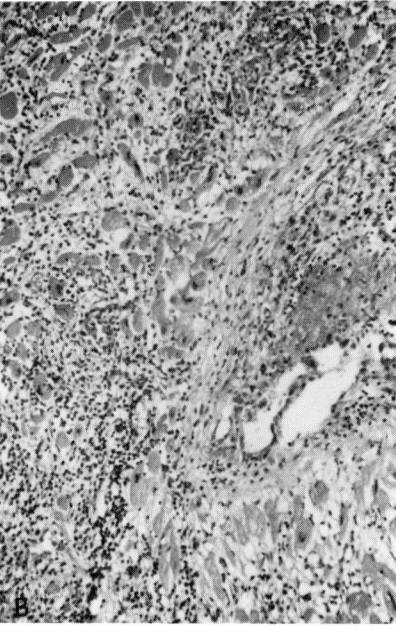

FIGURE 75–4. *A*, Myocardium in the acute phase of infection showing pseudocysts containing many amastigotes without inflammatory response (× 400). *B*, Chronic chagasic myocarditis with extensive inflammatory cell infiltrate, fragmentation of muscle fibers, and hemorrhage but no visible parasites (× 250).

and dividing amastigotes (Figs. 75–3 and 75–4). Trypomastigotes are flagellated forms measuring 15 to 20 μm in length with a posterior kinetoplast. They circulate in the blood and are infective to muscle, nerve, and other host cells. As intracellular parasites, they develop into oval amastigotes about 3 μm in diameter, which multiply by binary fission. Daughter amastigotes develop into trypomastigotes, which are released on rupture of the host cell and enter the circulation. The time from trypomastigote penetration of a cell to its rupture is thought to be about 5 days, but varies according to cell size and strain differences. This process of amastigote multiplication in the tissues and trypomastigote dissemination continues indefinitely. Circulating trypomastigotes are also infective to the insect vector. Triatomine bugs are obligate blood feeders measuring 5 to 45 mm in length, depending on the species (Fig. 75–5). They aspirate blood directly from capillaries and become infected by ingestion of circulating trypomastigotes (Fig. 75–3). These transform into epimastigotes, flagellated forms measuring 20 μm in length with an anterior kinetoplast near the nucleus. The epimastigotes divide in the midgut by binary fission. Daughter epimastigotes migrate to the hindgut where they develop into metacyclic trypomastigotes, which are infective to the vertebrate host (Fig. 75–2). Metacyclic trypomastigotes appear as early as 20 days after infection. Bugs usually remain infective for life and transmit *T. cruzi* for up to several years.

Humans are infected usually by fecal contamination of the skin from bugs that defecate during or shortly after engorgement. Infective metacyclic trypomastigotes in the feces penetrate the slightest break in the skin or intact mucosal tissue to infect local tissue histiocytes. Intracellular amastigotes develop and multiply, giving rise to blood trypomastigotes that rupture the histiocytes and disseminate in the circulation to invade other tissue cells. By the time, during the acute phase, blood trypomastigotes reach detectable levels, amastigotes are already present in the heart.

Blood trypomastigotes are intensely antigenic and antibodies are often present during the first month of infection. The immune response suppresses parasitemia to levels undetectable by direct microscopy; this low-level parasitemia persists for life. Although the concentration of trypomastigotes in blood during the chronic phase is low, there are often sufficient numbers to infect the vector bugs.

EPIDEMIOLOGY

Reservoir Hosts. *T. cruzi* has been found in over 100 species of mammals, representing 24 families of the following orders: Marsupialia, Edentata, Chiroptera, Carnivora, Lagomorpha, Rodentia, and Primates. One of the most primitive groups of mammals, marsupials of the genus *Didelphis,* have a high prevalence and an unusual tolerance to infection. The broad host specificity and ability to infect primitive mammals indicate that *T. cruzi* is an ancient infection that occurred long before humans arrived in the New World.

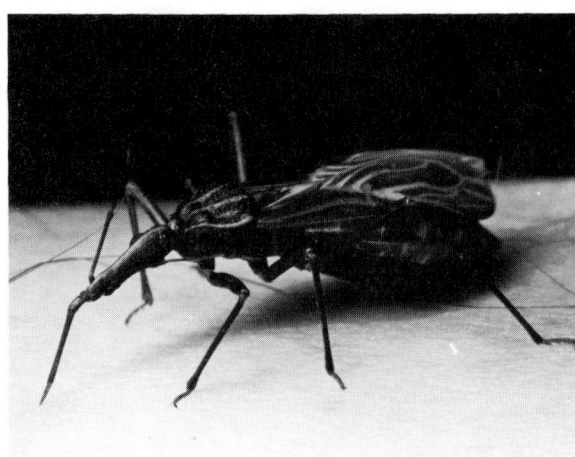

FIGURE 75–5. An adult reduviid bug—*Rhodnius prolixus* (× 2). (Courtesy of Dr. Robert Wirtz, Walter Reed Army Institute of Research.)

Domestic animals are frequently infected, and typical prevalence rates may reach 80% for dogs, 60% for cats, 90% for mice, 60% for rats, and 60% for guinea pigs. In view of the wide host specificity and broad geographic distribution of *T. cruzi* in the Americas, eradication of this parasite is impossible.

Human Chagas' disease is rare in the southern United States where *T. cruzi* usually circulates between opossums and armadillos. Human infections are infrequent because the local bugs rarely enter high-quality American homes and people do not infringe on the sylvan cycle. However, the absence of positive serology in animal trappers in Louisiana suggests that northern strains of *T. cruzi* have low infectivity for humans.

Vector. Chagas' disease is restricted to Central and South America where more than a hundred of the known triatomine species exist. A few bug species, because of their adaptation to houses, are important vectors and determine the distribution of human *T. cruzi* infections. *Triatoma infestans* is the most important species because it is the principal vector in Chile, Argentina, Brazil, Paraguay, Uruguay, Bolivia, and Peru. *Panstrongylus megistus* is also an efficient vector in Brazil. In Venezuela, Colombia, and parts of Central America, *Rhodnius prolixus* (Fig. 75–5) is the principal triatomine involved in transmission. In contrast to the 2 vectors mentioned above, *R. prolixus* frequently transmits *Trypanosoma rangeli*, which is infective but not pathogenic for humans. Wild caught bugs may contain both *T. cruzi* and *T. rangeli*, which can be distinguished by the site of multiplication in the bug and by flagellate morphology (Chapter 75.1). Other species have local importance, e.g., *Triatoma dimidiata* in Ecuador and *Rhodnius pallescens* in Panama.

Each of the 5 instars of the juvenile triatomines requires a blood meal to molt, and adults feed several times. All of these developmental stages can be infected with *T. cruzi*. However, to be important vectors of human disease the bugs must colonize houses and prefer human blood. To transmit, the bugs must defecate while feeding so that adequate numbers of metacyclic trypomastigotes are deposited on the skin. The period that the trypomastigotes survive on the skin depends on humidity and the rate of desiccation of the fecal drop. Humid conditions allow more time to scratch the bite site and spread contaminated feces to the mucosa and the puncture wound that remains in the skin after withdrawal of the bug's proboscis. Human vectors frequently feed on the face, facilitating transmission via the mucosa when the awaking child rubs bug feces into his or her eye.

Sylvan and Domestic Cycles. American trypanosomiasis is an anthropozoonosis. Sylvan transmission occurs independently of humans. However, people are at risk for infection when they enter the sylvan cycle, and the sylvan cycle of *T. cruzi* serves as a source of infection for domestic transmission. Perhaps the most important link between the sylvan and domestic cycles is the opossum because it is a peridomiciliary nester and enters houses in search of food. Similarly, synanthropic rodents invade the domestic environment.

Triatomine bugs have become domiciliated as a result of humans' impact on their environment with destruction of their natural habitats by deforestation and cultivation. As natural habitats disappear, a few species of bugs such as *T. infestans, R. prolixus,* and *P. megistus* "move in" with humans. Often, a transitory step for a bug to enter the domestic environment is the initial colonization of outhouses harboring chickens and other domestic animals. These colonization events explain why Chagas' disease is largely a disease of poor, rural, subsistence farmers.

The center of domestic transmission is the house because it provides the bugs a place to hide during the day and a source of frequent blood meals (Fig. 75–6). Bugs prefer houses constructed of mud and wattle with cracked walls and thatched roofs, which provide ideal cover during the day. At night, the bugs prey on their human hosts and their domestic animals. If a convenient blood source is available, the bugs will remain in the wall fabric near that source resulting in a patchy distribution throughout the house.

Dogs constitute an important reservoir of human infection because they live in close contact with humans and sleep around the house at night when the bugs are actively feeding. The role of cats in human transmission is not clear because they are rarely home at night and their availability to domestic bugs is limited. Perhaps, *T. cruzi* is passed from infected bugs via mice to cats by the food chain. Goats (Argentina) and guinea pigs (Peru and Bolivia) are important reservoirs in certain situations.

Direct Transmission. Although transmission by triatomine bugs accounts for most human infections, there are other modes of transmission.

Blood Transfusions. In Brazil, it is estimated that 20,000 infections occur each year by blood transfusion. Transfusion transmission is a significant problem in rural endemic areas where the poor sell their blood. It is a growing problem in metropolitan areas as the rural poor from endemic areas migrate to urban centers in search of economic opportunity. Transfusion transmission has also been reported in the United States, but the prevalence of infection in the donor population has not been studied. In view of increasing immigration from endemic areas of Central and South America, it is likely that the

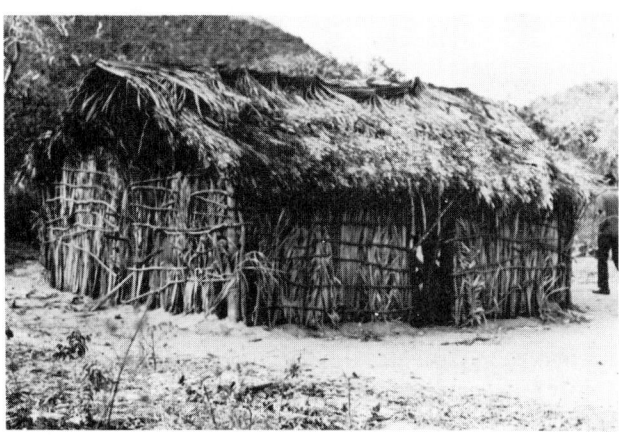

FIGURE 75–6. A palm thatch house in Mambai Goiás, Brazil, which at demolition contained over 1000 *Triatoma infestans*.

frequency of transfusion transmission in the United States will increase.

Person to Person. Congenital transmission is estimated to occur in about 1% of deliveries of serologically positive mothers. Transmission via maternal milk to infants has been documented. Transmission via contaminated food to adults has also been recorded. In Brazil, 58 people were infected in 4 outbreaks linked to cold soup and sugar cane contaminated with animal urine and feces from bugs. In the state of Nayarit, Mexico, *Triatoma phyllosoma* is eaten for its supposed aphrodisiac properties. More than 50 laboratory infections in research workers have occurred, usually from pipetting suspensions of *T. cruzi* by mouth or from an accident while inoculating animals. Finally, *T. cruzi* has been transmitted by organ transplant.

PATHOGENESIS. A number of mechanisms have been postulated on the pathogenesis of Chagas' disease. These are dependent on various factors that qualitatively and quantitatively interfere with the development of *T. cruzi* infection. In general, these are parasite dependent (i.e., polymorphism, cell tropism, virulence, antigenicity, size of inoculum) and host dependent (i.e., genetic constitution, sex, age, species, route of infection, immune response, reinfection, nutrition).

Parasite Factors. *T. cruzi* strain differences probably explain geographic morphologic polymorphism and geographic differences in frequency of "megasyndromes," tissue tropisms, virulence in animal hosts, and chemotherapeutic responses in humans. Isoenzyme studies have identified at least 5 zymodemes of *T. cruzi,* and kinetoplastic DNA analyses suggest many variants will be distinguished. *T. cruzi* infecting humans can be classified into 3 main strains or principal zymodemes: Z1, Z2, and Z3. Isoenzyme data on *T. cruzi* are available from Brazil, Bolivia, Chile, Venezuela, Colombia, Peru, Paraguay, French Guiana, and Central America. With 1 exception, zymodeme Z2 has only been reported south of the Amazon basin and multiple-banded Z2 patterns are especially common in southern regions of South America (Bolivia, Chile, Paraguay, Peru).

Immune Response. Research has focused on mechanisms by which trypomastigotes and amastigotes avoid the immune response to persist for years in their vertebrate hosts. Both metacyclic trypomastigotes from the bug and circulating trypomastigotes from the vertebrate host resist serum killing by the alternate complement pathway. These trypomastigotes shed a glycoprotein that inhibits the formation of complement C3 convertases and accelerates their decay. Presumably, this inhibitory protein blocks trypomastigote lysis by the alternate complement pathway in the immunologically naive host. However, in the immunologically responsive host, antibodies are generated that neutralize this regulatory glycoprotein, exposing the trypomastigotes to complement-mediated lysis. These antibodies probably play an important role in the suppression of circulating trypomastigotes in patients with chronic infections.

After they are in the circulation, trypomastigotes must identify and infect susceptible host cells. This probably occurs through receptor-ligand–mediated endocytosis. Macrophages and monocytes, as well as trypomasti-

gotes, have fibronectin receptors; this molecule enhances both parasite-cell binding and parasite uptake. The receptor-ligand system that facilitates infection of cardiac muscle, nerve cells, and other cells are not known.

As intracellular parasites, the trypomastigotes must evade intracellular killing mechanisms, particularly the lethal effects of the oxidative burst. A proportion of trypomastigotes pass through the phagosomal membrane to infect the cytoplasm, a privileged site free from lysosomal enzymes. In heart and nerve cells, trypomastigotes develop into amastigotes that multiply. Differentiation of amastigotes into trypomastigotes in the host cells occurs about 24 hours before cell rupture, but many parasites do not achieve full differentiation and are killed by the surrounding inflammatory cells, neutrophils, eosinophils, monocytes, and macrophages. Parasite transmission from 1 cell to the other depends on the transformation of the daughter amastigotes into infective trypomastigotes, which are able to successfully infect other cells.

Pathology

Acute Phase. Acute Chagas' disease usually occurs in children. During this phase circulating trypomastigotes and amastigote nests can usually be found with ease. Although *T. cruzi* can infect many cell types (histiocytes, fibroblasts, and nerve and muscle cells), the best place to look is in the heart, particularly the right auricle, and the smooth muscle of the gut. Early in the infection, these intracellular parasites promote little inflammatory reaction (Fig. 75–4*A*). After the first generation of amastigotes, immunologically competent lymphocytes and plasma cells rapidly make their appearance. As the infection progresses, parasites are more difficult to find and inflammatory cells become common (Fig. 75–4*B*). The acute phase terminates after several weeks to months.

The acute myocardial inflammatory changes in Chagas' disease are probably the most severe of all known forms of myocarditis. There is intense infection of cardiac cells, which rupture and release amastigotes into the interstitium. Focal inflammatory reactions against these parasites and disrupted tissues also destroy nearby normal tissue, including the cardiac conducting system. The lesions of the esophagus and gastrointestinal tract are predominantly located in the muscle layers and in the intramural nerve plexus. As in the heart, focal myositis is observed around degenerated amastigotes in the interstitium. The lesions of the sympathetic and parasympathetic nervous systems include periganglionitis, ganglionitis, neuritis, perineuritis, chromatolysis, and death and necrosis of nerve fibers.

The congenital form of the disease is similar to acute Chagas' disease. In addition, parasitism of the conceptus has been associated with abortion, premature birth, pneumonitis, meningoencephalitis, and diffuse dermal granulomas of the newborn. Recently, intracranial calcifications, megaesophagus, and metaphysitis have also been described in newborn children with Chagas' disease.

Chronic Phase. The acute phase is usually followed by the indeterminate phase, an asymptomatic period that may last for decades, before signs of heart or gut disease appear. Chronic Chagas' myopathy shows the following lesions: chronic inflammation, fibrosis, constant degenerative processes of muscle cells, damage of the heart impulse conductivity system, injury of the pericardium and the subpericardial fatty tissue, and destruction of the intracardial nervous system. The new anatomic character in this phase is fibrosis. This is focal or diffuse and is associated with the inflammatory foci. No other type of cardiopathy develops fibrosis so intensely as chronic Chagas' disease.

In spite of many studies, the most controversial problem in the pathogenesis of Chagas' disease is the identification of mechanisms by which chronic lesions occur in different organs after a long latent period when parasites are scarce. Some pathologists argue that tissue-dwelling amastigotes are difficult to detect in the heart and that the prevalence of infected cells and the number of intracellular parasites is higher than believed. It is also possible that amastigotes are sequestered in tissues other than the heart and gut; the muscle wall of the suprarenal vein was recently described as a site of amastigote proliferation.

Antoimmunity. Other pathologists argue that infection with *T. cruzi* stimulates autoimmunity, which results in chronic pathologic changes in the absence of parasites. Autoantibodies against endocardium, interstitium, and blood vessels (EVI antibodies) have been described from sera of chagasic patients. Autoimmune lymphocytes have also been reported from chagasic patients. *T. cruzi* shares common antigens with heart tissue, and it has been speculated that these parasite antigens stimulate autoimmunity. An alternative hypothesis is that damage to host tissue exposes previously "covered" antigens, which stimulate autoimmunity. All of these observations on autoimmunity are controversial. It is extremely important to establish without doubt if infection with *T. cruzi* causes autoimmunity and to clarify the pathogenic mechanisms. The development of vaccines rest on the resolution of this point!

CLINICAL MANIFESTATIONS

Acute Phase. Often the acute phase is asymptomatic, and only about 10% of infected people experience clinical disease. In our hospital service in the state of Goias, Central Brazil, acute Chagas' disease was frequently seen in the first decade of life, but now it is seldom seen because of control programs.

Romaña's Sign. At the site of inoculation a visible lesion is seen in about half of the patients. Contamination of the conjunctiva occurs when infected bug feces are rubbed into the eye. Local inflammation to the proliferating parasites produced the commonly called Romaña's sign (Fig. 75–7). This is characterized as bipalpebral, unilateral, chronic edema, which may be associated with local lymph gland enlargement. Trypomastigotes can sometimes be found in tears. The fact that the Romaña sign lasts for weeks differentiates it from most other causes of unilateral bipalpebral edema.

Chagoma. An inoculation granuloma or chagoma may follow infection through abraded skin. A chagoma presents as a dusky, erythematous, indurated lesion covered with scaling skin. Motile trypomastigotes can often be

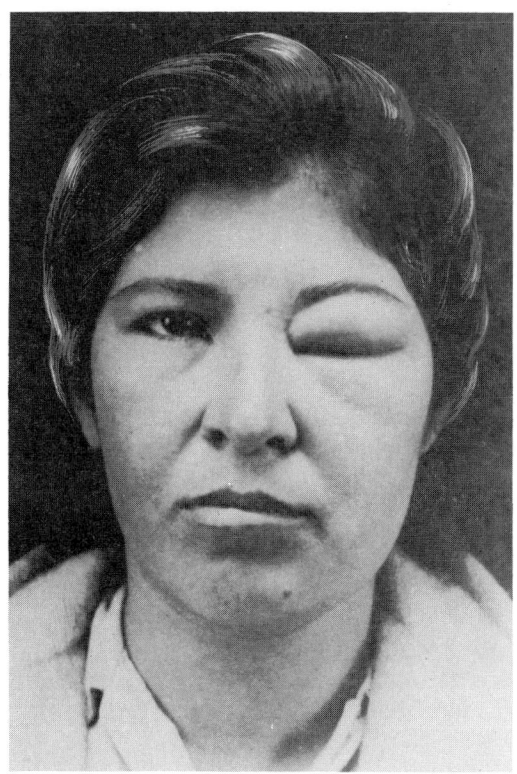

FIGURE 75–7. Unilateral orbital edema. (Romaña's sign in acute Chagas' disease). (Courtesy of Dr. Ramon S. Freire, Chaco, Argentina.)

demonstrated in wet mount preparations of needle aspirates taken from chagomas.

Other Findings. Constitutional signs are mild fever (95 to 100%), disproportional sinus tachycardia (40%), edema (60%), lymphadenopathy (50%), hepatomegaly (50%), and splenomegaly (30%). Electrocardiographic alterations are alterations in ventricular repolarization (40%), low QRS complex (35%), rise in electrical systole (14%), and first-degree atrioventricular block (14%). On x-ray film, varying degrees of cardiomegaly may be detected, and heart failure (a sign of poor prognosis) may be present. Meningoencephalitis is another cause of mortality in the acute phase, but it is uncommon.

Chronic Phase. The chronic form of the infection is most frequently encountered in endemic areas.

Asymptomatic Period. Most patients never develop clinical signs of Chagas' disease. They remain permanently in the indeterminate phase characterized by positive serology in all and positive xenodiagnosis in about 50%, but without signs and symptoms. However, 10 to 30% of these patients in the indeterminate phase will develop chronic Chagas' disease over the ensuing decades.

Cardiomyopathy. Many patients show only electrocardiographic changes, but chagasic cardiomyopathy presents as primary heart muscle failure, arrhythmias, and/or thromboemboli. Patients in this phase can die suddenly and without warning, probably owing to ventricular fibrillation or sudden cardiac arrest. Cardiomyopathy with enlarged heart (Fig. 75–8) usually appears

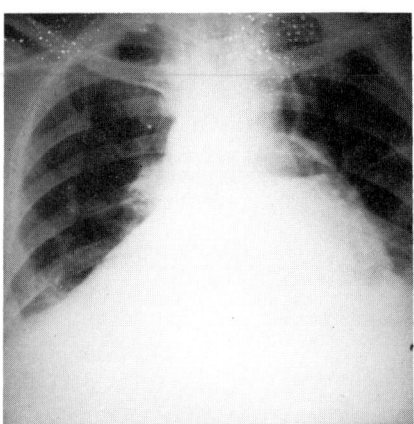

FIGURE 75–8. Anteroposterior radiograph of the chest showing a generally enlarged heart and a fluid level in a megaesophagus behind the heart in a patient with chronic Chagas' disease.

in adult life and is more often seen in males, probably because of increased cardiac work. An embolus, either pulmonary or systemic, due to intracardiac mural thrombosis may be responsible for the first hospital admission. The electrocardiogram shows abnormal cardiac conduction in more than 50% of patients. Extrasystoles and first-degree heart block are common, and the combination of complete right bundle branch block and left anterior hemiblock is suggestive of Chagas' disease. Atrial fibrillation and left bundle branch block are rarer lesions. Progression of the damage to the Purkinje fibers may lead eventually to complete heart block with Stokes-Adams attacks.

Megasyndromes (dilation of tubular organs, Fig. 75–9). The frequency of megasyndromes varies with the country under consideration (up to 10% of positive seroreactors). For example, in 1 study megaesophagus occurred in 17% of those who were seropositive on the high plateau of Central Brazil but was unknown in Venezuela. They are rarely lethal but cause considerable morbidity owing to difficulty in swallowing (megaesophagus) or constipation (megacolon). Because of the retention of solid residues, aperistalsis of the organ results in dilation. The symptoms are characteristic. Difficulty in swallowing is progressive and may reach a point at which solid food cannot be ingested. Barium contrast radiologic studies enable the degree of dilation to be classified. Four grades of esophageal dysfunction have been defined, from cardiospasm to dolichomegaesophagus, with an enormous viscus on top of the diaphragm. In advanced cases, esophagitis is common, and food overspill may lead to frequent aspiration and pulmonary infections. This can be aggravated by pressure on the lungs from the dilated viscus' interfering with lung drainage. Frequently, to provide saliva for lubrication, the parotid gland hypertrophies. This, coupled with wasting due to malnutrition, is responsible for the "cat facies" seen in advanced megaesophagus (Fig. 75–10). In megacolon, severe constipation and fecal impaction are common, and volvulus may present as an acute emergency. Megasyndromes of other organs occur but usually are not detected clinically. In 1 study, a concomitant chagasic chronic cardiopathy was observed in 50% of the cases displaying esophageal dysperistalsis.

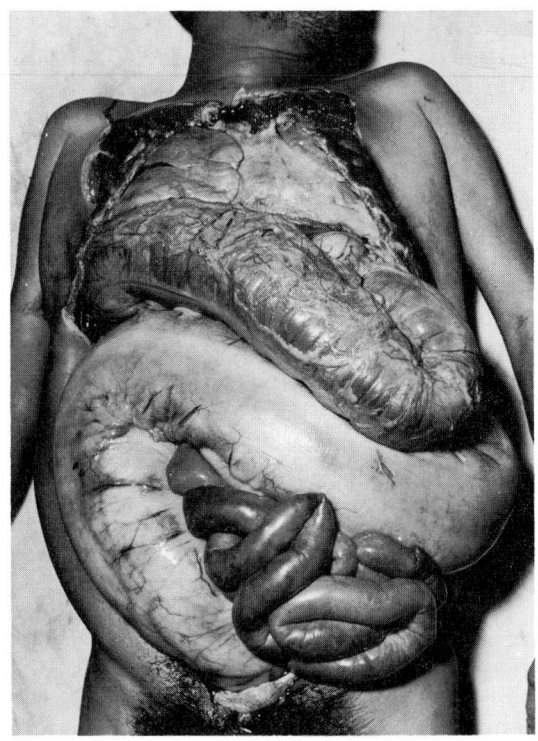

FIGURE 75–9. Megacolon in chronic Chagas' disease. (Courtesy of Dr. Fritz Köberle, São Paulo, Brazil. J Trop Med 61:21, 1958.)

Other Lesions. Myositis also occurs in skeletal muscles in this disease, and dysfunction of the motor end plate and the lower motor neuron pathway is demonstrated by absent knee and ankle deep tendon reflexes. Animal studies show a diminution in the number of anterior horn cells of the spinal cord. The possible occurrence of other central nervous system lesions (first suggested by Chagas) is under investigation at present. There is some evidence of exocrine and endocrine gland dys-

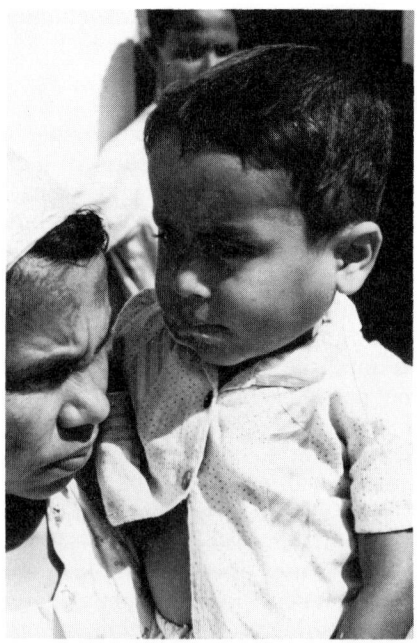

FIGURE 75–10. Child with advanced megaesophagus. Note the parotid enlargement producing the so-called cat facies.

function in chronic infections, as well as an abnormal, hormonal regulation of gut function. Such a widespread lesion of the vegetative peripheral nervous system is likely to have subtle clinical effects that may yet await detection.

Congenital Infections. Congenital Chagas' disease can be associated with the newborn's being small for gestational age, premature birth, and stillbirth.

In the majority, hepatosplenomegaly is present at birth. The most severe cases have hemorrhagic symptoms (i.e., petechiae, ecchymosis, bleeding). Some infants die during the first week of life and others show meningoencephalitic symptoms (from slight tremor to generalized convulsions). A few have jaundice, or disseminated chagomas (hemorrhagic and even necrotic lesions of the skin and mucous membranes). Occasionally, metaphysitis, intracranial calcifications, and ocular lesions have been described.

DIAGNOSIS. The diagnosis of Chagas' disease must include epidemiologic, serologic, and parasitologic factors.

Epidemiology. Epidemiologic data include travel to endemic areas, contact with bugs, blood transfusion, and laboratory accidents occurring at anytime throughout life. Clinics in endemic areas must have preserved triatomine bugs to show patients for establishing contact with the vector.

Laboratory Diagnosis. The selection of a particular laboratory test depends on the phase of the disease. During the acute phase when the level of parasitemia is high, trypomastigotes can be detected by direct blood examination or by blood concentration techniques, e.g., Strout's method (Chapter 123). During the chronic phase parasitemia is subpatent and the diagnosis is usually made from positive serology associated with a compatible clinical picture. Patients with indeterminate Chagas' disease are usually detected serologically during blood bank or epidemiologic screens. Both indeterminate and chronic infections may be confirmed by xenodiagnosis, hemoculture, or animal inoculation.

Microscopy. Motile trypomastigotes can be detected and the density of parasites determined in wet mount preparations of blood during the acute phase. However, it is better to concentrate the parasites after clot retraction and centrifugation at 640 G. The trypomastigotes of *T. cruzi* are distinguished morphologically from those of *T. rangeli* by microscopic examination of Giemsa-stained blood films. Infection with *T. cruzi* is indicated if the trypomastigotes appear C shaped, are less than 30 μm in length, and have a central nucleus and a large subterminal kinetoplast at the posterior end (Fig. 75–3A). Infection with *T. rangeli* is indicated if the blood trypomastigotes are greater than 30 μm in length, the posterior kinetoplast is small, and dividing forms are seen (Fig. 75–3B).

Chagas' disease can also be diagnosed from histologic sections of infected tissue, but this method is insensitive. Typically, clusters of amastigotes are seen in muscle cells surrounded with acute or chronic inflammation (Fig. 75–4A and B).

Xenodiagnosis. Triatomine bugs (Fig. 75–5) are extremely susceptible to infection and this characteristic makes them valuable in xenodiagnosis. This is a sensitive test in which 40 laboratory-reared juvenile bugs are fed on the patient. A month later their feces and hindgut contents are examined for infection with flagellates. The level of parasitemia, species of bug, method of examination, and frequency of bug examination determine the sensitivity of the test. Circulating trypomastigotes can be detected in up to 50% of chronic patients with a positive serology by xenodiagnosis. In areas with sympatric *T. rangeli*, the parasites can be distinguished by the site of multiplication in the bug and by the morphology of the epimastigote stage. *T. rangeli* is larger and its kinetoplast smaller relative to *T. cruzi* (Chapter 75.1).

Culture. Facilities for xenodiagnosis are frequently not available outside Latin America. Culture using media (e.g., NNN, Warren, or Lit) can detect circulating parasites, but not with the sensitivity of xenodiagnosis. Cultures should be inoculated at 26C and examined weekly for 4 weeks for epimastigotes.

Animal Inoculation. Blood from patients can be inoculated into laboratory animals, which become patent with circulating trypomastigotes between 5 and 15 days.

Serology. The clinician is dependant on reliable serology for a presumptive diagnosis of Chagas' disease. Antibodies appear during the acute phase of Chagas' disease and persist for life. Unfortunately, available serologic tests do not fulfill all criteria required for use in rural, poor, endemic areas where laboratory equipment and immunologic expertise are scarce or nonexistent. The optimal test must be fast, simple, sensitive, specific, and cheap. Three tests were developed in the 1960s and have been used extensively: indirect hemagglutination test (IHA), indirect fluorescence test (IFA), and complement fixation test (CF). Recently, the direct agglutination test has received attention because of its simplicity and the enzyme-linked immunosorbent assay (ELISA) because of its superior sensitivity, but these tests have not been evaluated adequately in the field. All of these serodiagnostic tests use intact flagellates or heterogeneous extracts as antigens and all cross-react with varying frequencies with sera from patients with leishmaniasis, *T. rangeli*, and sometimes, tuberculosis and leprosy. Species-specific antigens have been isolated from *T. cruzi*, but their large-scale production has not been realized.

Differential Diagnosis

Acute Infections. The Romaña sign (Fig. 75–7) must be differentiated from local allergic edema, such as that due to insect bite, which resolves much more rapidly. Other ocular alterations such as severe conjunctivitis or trauma must be considered. Chagas' disease must be considered together with typhoid fever, kala-azar, schistosomiasis, brucellosis, infectious mononucleosis, toxoplasmosis, malaria, and glomerulonephritis as a cause for unexplained fever with or without signs of a portal of entry in an endemic area.

Chronic Infection. Cardiac failure in Chagas' disease is biventricular without acute pulmonary edema. The dilated heart with weak muscle force may promote functional tricuspid incompetence. Myocarditis and pericarditis may be due to other causes, such as rheumatic fever or viral myocarditis. Endomyocardial fibrosis may closely mimic chagasic cardiomyopathy, but serology is negative. Other forms of cardiomyopathy, particularly alcoholic, must be considered.

TREATMENT

Specific Chemotherapy. Only 2 drugs are available for specific treatment, nifurtimox (Lampit, Bayer 2502) from 1967, and benznidazole (Rochagan, R07-1051, Radinil) from 1973. Both usually abolish parasitemia and one can be recommended for all patients in the acute phase. Their use in chronic phase infections, particularly in infected children or in adults up to 2 years after infection, may improve prognosis by minimizing parasite invasion of vital tissues and diminishing inflammatory responses that damage the heart muscle and the peripheral autonomic nervous system. Strains of *T. cruzi* from Argentina and Chile seem more sensitive to nifurtimox than Brazilian strains. Neither of these drugs are licensed in the United States.

Nifurtimox. This is a nitrofuran that is active against both trypomastigotes and amastigotes. It interferes with the parasite's carbohydrate metabolism by inhibiting pyruvic acid synthesis. The drug is given orally 3 times a day after meals. The dose for adults is 8 to 10 mg/kg body weight. Children tolerate the drug better than adults and they can take 15 mg/kg. Therapy must be given for 90 days and under strict medical supervision because serious side effects may occur. The peak plasma concentration occurs 1 to 3 hours after treatment. The concentration of the drug in tissues and urine is low. Peripheral neuritis (30%) and psychosis are dose dependent and appear near the end of treatment. Hemolysis may occur in patients with glucose-6-phosphate dehydrogenase deficiency. Tremors, excitation, insomnia, anorexia, and weight loss are frequent. Polyneuropathy is the most serious adverse effect, but it usually disappears when treatment is stopped. In the United States, nifurtimox is available from the Center for Disease Control (CDC), Parasitic Disease Division, Atlanta, GA.

Benznidazole. This nitroimidazole is more trypanocidal than nifurtimox and also acts against the amastigote stage. It is given orally 2 times a day. In adults, the daily dose is 5 mg/kg body weight while in children it is 5 to 10 mg/kg. Therapy must be given for 60 days under strict medical supervision. The drug is rapidly absorbed and distributed throughout the body. More than 40% of the drug binds to protein and more than 70% of the metabolites are excreted in the urine. About half of the patients develop light-sensitive rashes that rarely progress to exfoliative dermatitis. Peripheral neuritis, anorexia, weight loss, hematologic alterations (neutropenia, agranulocytosis, thrombocytopenia), and depressed thymus-dependent immunity (in rabbits) are also common complications. In South America, especially Brazil, this drug is the first choice for specific therapy.

Criteria of Cure. The effect of therapy on acute disease is measured by the remission of signs and symptoms and the elimination of parasitemia. The antibodies detected by conventional serology (IFA, IHA, CF) are not useful in the evaluation of treatment. Recently, it has been suggested that antibodies detected against living trypomastigotes by complement-mediated lysis may be a more reliable marker of ongoing infections, whereas their absence indicates cure.

Symptomatic Treatment. This is all that can be offered to patients with chronic chagasic syndromes. Heart failure initially responds to digitalis and diuretics. Arrhythmias may require emergency therapy, but β-blocking agents are contraindicated. The following drugs are recommended in these cases: amiodosome (300 to 600 mg/day), propaphenane (300 mg/day), and procainamide (500 mg/day). Complete heart block causing bradycardia and low cardiac output responds to a pacemaker, which may allow the patient to return to normal activity. Patients with large hearts, indicating dilation and thinning of ventricular muscle, do poorly with pacemakers. Megaesophagus can be treated initially with balloon dilation, although a return of symptoms necessitates surgery. A Tal operation, entailing simple excision of the spastic cardia, is currently favored. An enormously dilated esophagus can be excised and replaced with a segment of intestine. Megasigmoids can be excised.

PROGNOSIS. Sufficient data are still not available to formulate an accurate prognosis for patients with chronic infections. Generally, it is dependent on the clinical state, intensity of parasitism, and early institution of treatment. Usually, 70 to 90% of those infected with *T. cruzi* having lifelong positive serology never develop clinical Chagas' disease. Approximately 25% of the seroreactors develop electrocardiographic abnormalities and 1% may develop detectable megaesophagus in a 10-year period. Cardiac failure usually appears between 20 and 50 years of age, and life expectancy after its onset is less than 2 years. Overall, expectation of life of people living in endemic areas is estimated to be 9 years less than that of people in nonendemic areas.

CONTROL. In the absence of specific therapy and without a vaccine, the only way to control Chagas' disease is to prevent its transmission. Prevention is focused on the elimination of domiciliated bugs in houses, elimination of infected blood in blood banks, and reduction of congenital transmission.

Vector Control. The nidus of natural infection is the house, and the principles of vector control are based on the behavior of the domiciliated bugs. Under the cover of darkness, the bugs leave their refuge and travel across the surface of the walls to reach their human prey. It is during this walk that the bugs make contact with residual insecticides sprayed on the walls. Benzene hexachloride, dieldrin, and malathion have been used extensively in the past because they are cheap and kill bugs up to 3 to 4 months after application. The new generation of insecticides, the synthetic pyrethroids (deltamethrin and cypermethrin), are more expensive, but they are applied in low concentrations and last up to 9 months. Insecticide resistance in bugs has only been reported for dieldrin in Venezuela.

National Control Programs. There are 3 countries with national programs to control the transmission of Chagas' disease: Argentina, Brazil, and Venezuela. Typical control programs include 3 operational phases. During the preparatory phase, seroprevalence is determined and each house is examined for bug infestation. This information is used to estimate required resources: money, personnel, insecticide, equipment, and transport. During the attack phase, insecticide is sprayed on the inside and outside walls, roof, and furniture of all houses and outhouses. The effective dose of insecticide depends on factors such as climate, sunlight, porosity of the sprayed surface, and the method of application. Sprays are not completely effective because they do not kill eggs or well-fed bugs hiding deep in the walls and do not prevent reinvasion from the peridomicile. To maintain vector suppression, house to house searches for bugs are conducted to find houses with persistent infestations for repeat spraying. This "evaluation-spray cycle" is repeated until the frequency of infested houses is reduced to 5% or less. During the vigilance phase, the responsibility for detecting bug-infested houses is passed to the community. Public health teams teach the residents to identify and capture bugs and to take them to the local health post where their identification is confirmed by an expert. Houses with persistent infestation often require structural improvement, including the plastering of walls to eliminate bug hiding places. Without public health education and community participation, the prospects of permanent control would be bleak.

Results from the national control programs in Brazil show that the seroprevalence of school children has been reduced from 20 to 40% to 0 to 2% in many endemic areas. In view of this success, it is sad that other endemic countries have not implemented these model programs. There are 6 million infected people living in 17 countries with either precarious or no national control programs. Most of these countries lack the political stability and financial strength to assist their rural subsistence farmers with Chagas' disease.

Residual Insecticides. New insecticide delivery systems under development promise to decrease the cost and improve the efficacy of bug control. Most impressive are fumigant canisters, which debug houses immediately, and slow-release formulations of insecticide incorporated into paints, which can kill bugs for up to 2 years. Because these delivery systems can be used by the homeowner, they eliminate the need for backpack sprayers and technical personnel.

The use of insecticide is an inexpensive way to control Chagas' disease. In rural Brazil, it costs $0.20 to $1.50 to investigate a house for bug infestation and $5.00 to $14.00 to spray. However, insecticides must be considered for only the short term.

Improved Housing. The long-term solution is elimination of domiciliated bugs through improved housing. In endemic areas of Brazil, the average cost of a traditional earth house that will stand for 10 years is $1,100, whereas a "bug-proof" brick house with a tile roof that will stand for 20 to 30 years is only $2,000. Durable bricks can be produced with local materials at an acceptable price. However, political decisions must be made to place this cottage industry in endemic areas. Finally, there is a need for public health education to convince local residents of the value of bug-proof architecture. In one area of Venezuela, local residents preferred to live in their traditional mud huts rather than in modern brick houses provided free by the government.

Small changes in human behavior can also reduce transmission. Sleeping in a hammock under a mosquito net with a cloth roof will reduce the chances of contact with bugs and their feces. However, bugs congregate near the retaining hooks in the wall and run along the net. Bugs do not like light and night illumination is a deterrent. Better hygiene and, particularly, the banishing of all animals (e.g., chickens and dogs) from the house will diminish the risk of bug invasion.

Control in Blood Banks. The prevention of transmission of *T. cruzi* in blood banks requires a diagnostic test to screen donors and a method of killing the trypanosomes in infected blood. The serologic test in common use is the IFA. There is a need to develop, evaluate, and implement other tests in rural blood banks that are simple, inexpensive, and rapid, e.g., the DOT-ELISA and direct agglutination tests. However, false-negative results occur with all serologic tests, and a screening program will eliminate most, but not all, transmission. The usual practice in endemic areas is to treat all blood with gentian violet at a concentration of 0.25 gm/L for 24 hours in the refrigerator before use. Although this procedure is safe, the quality of the blood is often questioned by the patient because of its purple color. The development of colorless compounds as blood sterilants would be helpful.

Preventing Vertical Transmission. Women with acute infections must not nurse until they have been treated with benzidazole. For mothers with chronic infections, there is little recourse because of the risk of neonatal malnutrition and death. Children nursing from infected mothers should be monitored for infection.

BIBLIOGRAPHY

Brener Z: Pathogenesis and immunopathology of chronic Chagas' disease. Mem Inst Oswaldo Cruz 82(Suppl):205, 1987.

Brener Z: Recent advances in the chemotherapy of Chagas' disease. Mem Inst Oswaldo Cruz 79(Suppl):149, 1984.

Brener Z, Andrade, Z (eds): *Trypanosoma cruzi* e Doenca de Chagas. Rio de Janeiro, Guanabara Koogan, 1979, p 463.

Brenner RR, Stoka AM: Chagas' Disease Vectors. Vol 1, Taxonomic, Ecological and Epidemiological Aspects; Vol 2, Anatomic and Physiological Aspects; Vol 3, Biochemical Aspects and Control. Boca Raton, FL, CRC Press, 1987.

Chagas C: American trypanosomiasis. Study of the parasite and of the transmitting insect. Proc Inst Med Chicago, 3:220, 1921.

Dias E: Um ensaio de profilaxia de molestia de Chagas. Rio de Janeiro, Imprensa Nacional, 1945, p 116.

Dias JCP: Control of Chagas' disease in Brazil. Parasitol Today 3:336, 1987.

Garcia-Zapata MTA, Marsden PD: Chagas' disease. Clin Trop Med Comm Dis 1:557, 1986.

Koberle F: Chagas' disease and Chagas' syndromes: The pathology of American trypanosomiasis. Adv Parasitol 6:63, 1968.

World Health Organization: Meeting on research needs in the field of Chagas' disease vector control, Panama City, 28 September–2 October 1987. Rev Argent Microbiol 20(Suppl), 1988.

75.1. *TRYPANOSOMA RANGELI* INFECTIONS

Philip D. Marsden

ETIOLOGY, HISTORY, AND DISTRIBUTION. In 1920, while examining intestinal contents of *Rhodnius prolixus* in Venezuela, Tejera found flagellates with long epimastigote forms and a small kinetoplast different from *T. cruzi* epimastigotes. In 1942, a trypanosome with a small subterminal kinetoplast was found in the blood of Guatemalan children (Fig. 75–3). Both of these were forms of *Trypanosoma rangeli*. This organism has been reported in humans primarily from Venezuela, Brazil, Colombia, Costa Rica, Guatemala, Panama, and El Salvador, with occasional reports of *T. rangeli*–like organisms from many other South American countries. Proper identification is not always possible, as it requires studies in animals, bugs, and culture.

CLINICAL MANIFESTATIONS AND DIAGNOSIS. *T. rangeli* does not produce clinical symptoms in humans. In 2 experimentally infected volunteers, parasitemia continued erratically for years. Late in the infection, it is only detected by xenodiagnosis. The mode of multiplication in the vertebrate host is unknown. *T. rangeli* and *T. cruzi* share common antigens; thus, serology for Chagas' disease could be misleading in endemic areas. Specific monoclonal antibodies for the 2 species have been developed.

TRANSMISSION AND LIFE CYCLE. *T. rangeli* makes interpretation of flagellate infections in wild caught bugs more difficult. Sometimes, *T. cruzi* and *T. rangeli* coexist in the same bug. *T. rangeli* escapes into the hemolymph and invades the salivary glands, so that flagellates found in these locations in a live bug indicate the presence of *T. rangeli* infection. It is often pathogenic for bugs, causing a shortened life span. Members of the genus *Rhodnius* are the usual vectors—*R. prolixus* in most countries, *R. pallescens* in Panama, and *R. ecuadoriensis* in Peru.

The transmission of *T. rangeli* to humans and animals is by bite of the bug, i.e., by inoculation of infected saliva, rather than through excreta, because the infectious metacyclic trypanosome assumes an anterior station. A large number of isolations of *T. rangeli*—like trypanosomes have been made from sylvatic animals, but their taxonomic status is still under investigation.

BIBLIOGRAPHY

Anthony RL, Lody TS, Constantine NT: Antigenic differentiation of *Trypanosoma cruzi* and *Trypanosoma rangeli* by means of monoclonal-hybridoma antibodies. Am J Trop Med Hyg 30:1192, 1981.

D'Alessandro A: Biology of *Trypanosoma (Herpetosoma) rangeli*—Tejera. 1920. *In* Lumsden WHR, Evans DA (eds): Biology of the Kinetoplastida, Vol I. New York and London, Academic Press, 1976, pp 328–370.

76. LEISHMANIASIS

76.1. GENERAL PRINCIPLES

Jeffrey D. Chulay

DEFINITION. Leishmaniasis is a group of infections of the viscera, skin, and mucous membranes caused by protozoa of the genus *Leishmania* that are transmitted by sandflies of the genera *Phlebotomus* (Old World leishmaniasis) and *Lutzomyia* (New World leishmaniasis).

HISTORY. Increasingly precise descriptions of parasites from lesions of cutaneous leishmaniasis were made by Cunningham (1885), Borovsky (1898), and Wright (1903). The organism in visceral leishmaniasis was first described in 1903 by Leishman, who examined the spleen of a British soldier with kala-azar who had been stationed at Dum Dum near Calcutta (hence, the name "Dumdum fever"). Later the same year, Donovan also identified the parasite in splenic tissue, and the organism is often called a Leishman-Donovan or L-D body. In 1904, Rogers observed the conversion of amastigotes to promastigotes in culture, and promastigotes were found in sandflies by Adler and Theodor in 1925. Transmission of Oriental sore by infected sandfly bite was achieved by Wenyon in Baghdad (1911) and Sergent in Algeria (1921). The leishmanin skin test was described by Montenegro in 1926, and in 1942, the British Commission in India experimentally transmitted kala-azar to human volunteers by sandfly bite.

ETIOLOGY

Life Cycle. *Leishmania* have a relatively simple life cycle (Fig. 76–1). Promastigotes in the proboscis of a female sandfly are introduced into the skin of a vertebrate host during a blood meal. The promastigotes invade reticuloendothelial cells, transform into amastigotes, multiply within phagolysosomes, and invade other reticuloendothelial cells. Sandflies feeding on infected individuals ingest parasitized cells, and the amastigotes transform into promastigotes, which multiply in the gut and migrate to the proboscis, completing the cycle.

The Organism

Amastigote Stage. The amastigote, found within reticuloendothelial cells in the vertebrate host, is a round or oval organism measuring 2 to 5 μm in greatest diameter (Figs. 73–5*L* and *M*, 74–1, and 76–8). In Wright- or Giemsa-stained preparations, the pale blue cytoplasm is surrounded by a plasma membrane and contains a large dark-purple nucleus and a small purple kinetoplast. A delicate thread connects the kinetoplast to a dotlike basal body, from which an axoneme arises and extends to the anterior end of the organism. Multiplication is by binary fission, and mitotically dividing forms may be seen in spleen smears.

Promastigote Stage. The promastigote, found in culture and in the sandfly digestive tract, measures 1.5 to 3.5 by 15 to 20 μm and has a single free flagellum 15 to 28 μm long (Figs. 76–2 and 74–1). Old cultures may contain short, broad forms and rounded forms 4 to 5

LIFE CYCLE of—

Leishmania

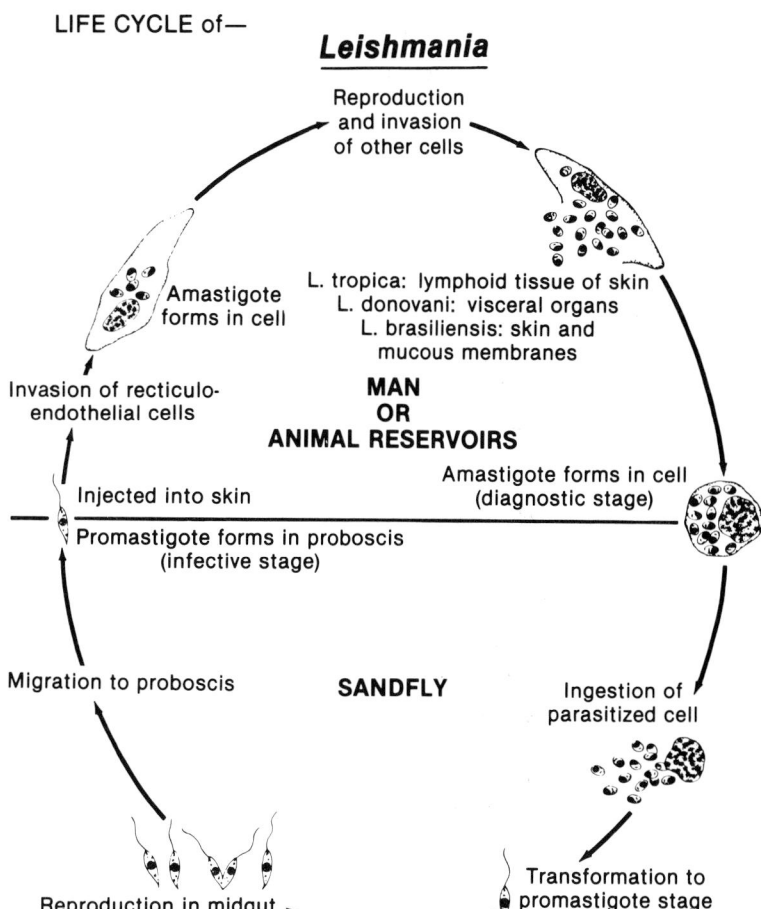

FIGURE 76–1. The life cycle of *Leishmania*. (Modified from Melvin DM, et al: Common Blood and Tissue Parasites of Man. Life Cycle Charts. Atlanta, GA, Centers for Disease Control, 1979.)

μm in diameter with long flagella centrally directed to form rosettes. Ultrastructurally, the organism is surrounded by a trilaminar plasma membrane, beneath which is a row of microtubules. The cytoplasm contains a large central nucleus, ribosomes, rough and smooth endoplasmic reticulum, a Golgi apparatus, various vesicles, and a single mitochondrion. The kinetoplast is a complex body and appears as an electron-dense granular band with a distinct fibrillar pattern, lying within an extension of the mitochondrion. The axoneme, which arises from the basal body, and a paraxial rod are contained within the flagellar sheath.

Culture and Animal Inoculation. Promastigotes can be grown in a variety of media at 22 to 25C. A biphasic medium such as NNN (Nicolle's modification of Novy and MacNeal's medium) is often used. Schneider's *Drosophila* medium supplemented with fetal bovine serum is often more effective in primary isolation from New World cutaneous lesions. When animal or human specimens are being cultured, penicillin and streptomycin should be added with the inoculum to prevent bacterial overgrowth. 5-Fluorocytosine can be used to inhibit fungal contamination, but amphotericin B should not be added because it may inhibit growth of *Leishmania*. Promastigotes are generally found 2 to 7 days after inoculation of amastigotes into Schneider's medium and after 7 to 21 days in NNN medium. The golden hamster *(Mesocricetus auratus)* is susceptible to infection with

Leishmania donovani amastigotes, and after intraperitoneal inoculation, the parasites multiply geometrically until the death of the animal in 6 months. Hamster inoculation is useful for detecting small numbers of parasites in aspirates and tissues.

Taxonomy. The taxonomy of *Leishmania* is confusing, and there is no single generally agreed on classification. One taxonomic classification is presented in Table 76–1. The species that infect humans are difficult to distinguish morphologically, although subtle differences in size and ultrastructure are sometimes detected. Isolates have usually been assigned to species and subspecies based on their geographic origin, the clinical syndrome they produce, and ecologic characteristics. Parasites of the *L. mexicana* complex have been differentiated from those of the *L. braziliensis* complex by the location at which they develop in the sandfly, their growth in culture, and the pattern of disease produced in hamsters.

Serologic and Biochemical Classification. A variety of serologic and biochemical tests have also been studied as potential aids in speciating *Leishmania* isolates, including agglutination tests, serotyping of factors excreted into culture media, fluorescent staining with monoclonal antibodies, measuring buoyant density of nuclear and kinetoplast DNA in cesium chloride gradients, identifying parasite isoenzymes, and characterizing parasite metabolism by radiorespirometry.

Clinical Classification. A simplified clinical classifi-

TABLE 76–1. *Leishmania* **Infecting Humans and Their Clinical Syndromes, Distribution, Reservoirs, and Vectors**

Species	Clinical Syndrome	Geographic Distribution	Major Reservoirs	Major Vectors
L. donovani complex				
L. donovani	Visceral	India, Pakistan, Nepal	Humans	*Phlebotomus argentipes*
		SubSaharan Africa, East Africa	Rodent, dog, ? humans	*P. orientalis, P. martini*
L. infantum	Visceral (infantile)	Mediterranean littoral	Dog, fox	*P. perniciosus, P. major*
		Central Asia, Middle East	Fox, jackal, dog	*P. caucasicus, P. major*
		China	Dog	*P. chinensis, P. sergenti*
L. chagasi	Visceral	South and Central America	Dog, fox	*Lutzomyia longipalpis*
L. tropica complex				
L. tropica	Cutaneous (dry, urban Oriental sore)	Middle East, Mediterranean littoral, Southwest Asia	Dog, humans	*P. sergenti, P. papatasi*
L. major	Cutaneous (moist, rural Oriental sore)	Middle East, Southwest Asia, subSaharan Africa	Gerbil	*P. papatasi, P. caucasicus*
L. aethiopica	Cutaneous; DCL*	Ethiopia, Kenya	Hyrax	*P. longipes, P. pedifer*
L. mexicana complex				
L. mexicana	Cutaneous; DCL rare	Mexico, Guatemala, Belize	Rodent	*Lutzomyia olmeca olmeca*
L. amazonensis	Cutaneous; DCL	Amazon basin of Brazil	Rodent, marsupial	*Lu. flaviscutellata*
L. venezuelensis	Cutaneous	Venezuela	Unknown	*Lu. olmeca bicolor*
L. braziliensis complex				
L. braziliensis	Cutaneous; MCL†	Brazil, Peru, Ecuador, Bolivia, Venezuela, Paraguay, Colombia	Rodent	*Lu. wellcomei*
L. panamensis	Cutaneous; MCL rare	Panama, Costa Rica, Colombia	Sloth	*Lu. trapidoi*
L. guyanensis	Cutaneous	Guyana, French Guyana, Surinam, Brazil	Sloth, anteater	*Lu. umbratilis*
L. peruviana	Cutaneous	Peru, Argentina	Dog	*Lu. peruensis, Lu. verrucarum*

*DCL = diffuse cutaneous leishmaniasis.
†MCL = mucocutaneous leishmaniasis.

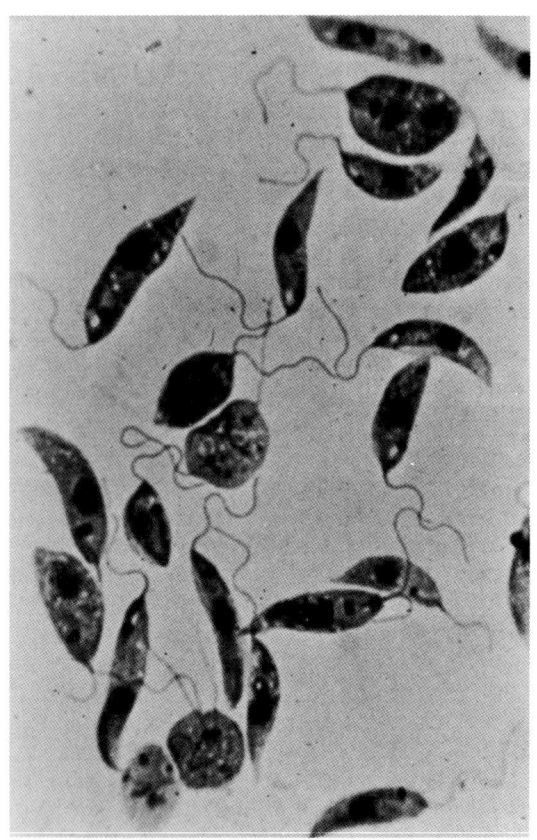

FIGURE 76–2. Promastigotes of *Leishmania donovani* from culture.

cation separates leishmaniasis into 3 syndromes: (1) visceral leishmaniasis, characterized by hepatosplenomegaly and anemia and caused by *L. donovani;* (2) cutaneous leishmaniasis, characterized by ulcerative skin lesions and caused by *L. tropica, L. mexicana,* or *L. braziliensis;* and (3) mucocutaneous leishmaniasis, caused by *L. braziliensis* and characterized by a primary cutaneous lesion that may be followed months to years later by destructive nasopharyngeal lesions (espundia). The geographic distribution of these 3 forms of leishmaniasis is indicated in Figure 76–3.

TRANSMISSION AND EPIDEMIOLOGY

The Vector. The phlebotomine sandflies that transmit leishmaniasis are small (1.5 to 2.5 mm), hairy flies that are recognized by their characteristic hopping movement and the position of the wings, which are held in a nearly erect V configuration over the body (Fig. 76–4). Less than 10% of the 600 known species of sandflies are thought to be involved in the transmission of human leishmaniasis. The female requires one or more blood meals for each batch of eggs to mature. Males feed on fruit juices and do not suck blood. Sandflies are generally inactive in daylight, seeking shelter in dark, moist places. They breed in dark, damp places rich in organic matter, e.g., leaf litter in tropical rain forests, rubble and loose earth, caves, and rock holes. Eggs are laid in batches of 15 to 80. The 4 wormlike larval instars feed on particulate organic matter and require high humidity. Pupation occurs in a drier environment. Soon after adult emergence, males become sexually active and are capable of inseminating females, who store sufficient

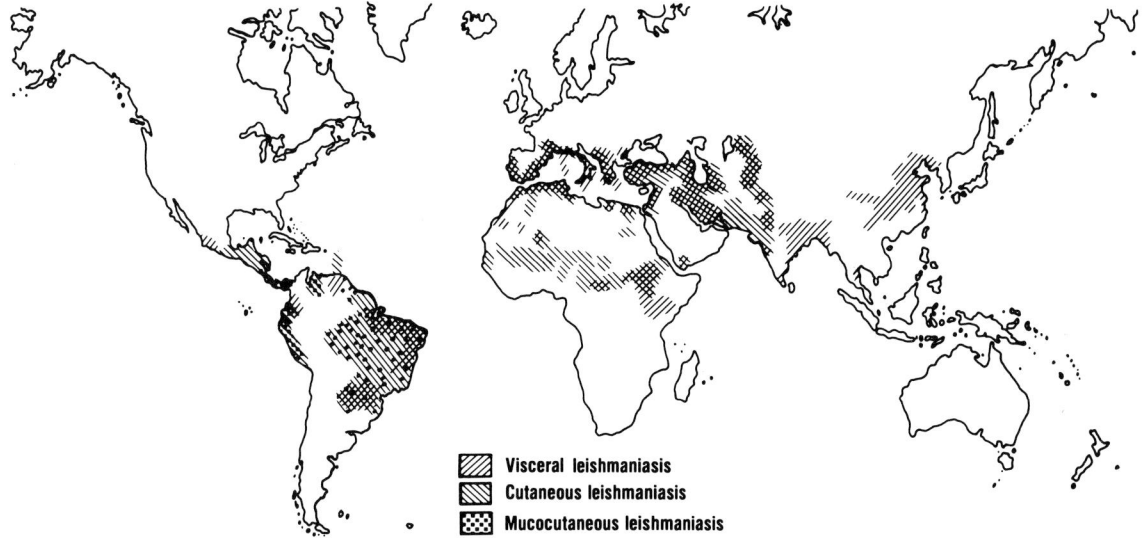

FIGURE 76–3. Geographic distribution of leishmaniasis.

sperm to fertilize eggs at intervals throughout their lives. Under favorable conditions, the life cycle is completed in 2 to 3 months.

Female sandflies feed on a variety of warm- and cold-blooded hosts, including humans, cats, dogs, rodents, cattle, bats, birds, and lizards. They can acquire *Leishmania* with their first blood meal and are capable of disease transmission 7 to 10 days later. They then remain infective throughout adult life, which is usually only a few weeks. *Leishmania*-infected sandflies have abnormal feeding behavior, probing more while attempting to take a blood meal. This behavior may facilitate transmission to the vertebrate host.

The Reservoir. The *Leishmania* that infect humans usually have canine or rodent reservoirs, in which they may cause inapparent or mild infections, cutaneous lesions only, or severe visceral disease. They are generally zoonotic, occurring in completely wild or peridomestic situations. The epidemiology of various forms of leishmaniasis is discussed in Chapters 76.2, 76.3, and 76.4.

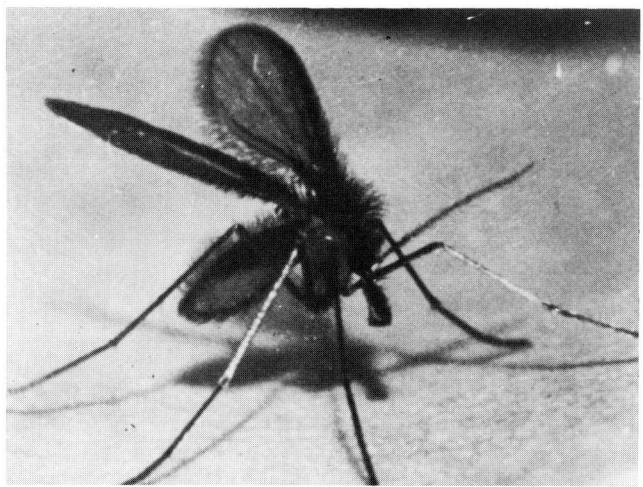

FIGURE 76–4. A sandfly, *Phlebotomus longipes*. (Courtesy of Dr. Gemetchu, Geneva.)

IMMUNOLOGY. The protective immune response to leishmaniasis is primarily cell mediated. High titers of antibodies detected in visceral leishmaniasis appear to play no part in defense against the parasite, and naturally occurring antibodies that cause complement-mediated lysis of promastigotes in vitro do not prevent acquisition of disease. In contrast, a positive leishmanin skin test correlates with resistance to leishmaniasis. It is negative during active visceral leishmaniasis, becoming positive after recovery. In addition, some patients with subclinical, self-curing visceral leishmaniasis have had positive leishmanin skin tests associated with well-developed tuberculoid granulomas demonstrated in liver biopsies. Cell-mediated immune responses are not entirely beneficial, as they also cause tissue destruction. The onset of ulceration correlates with the development of a positive leishmanin skin test in cutaneous leishmaniasis, and in mucocutaneous leishmaniasis, the reaction to the leishmanin skin test is much larger in individuals with more severe mucosal damage. Two subsets of T-helper lymphocytes have been identified in mouse models of leishmaniasis, one of which confers protective immunity while the other exacerbates the disease.

Spectrum of Clinical Disease. In all forms of leishmaniasis, there is a spectrum of clinical disease similar to that observed in leprosy. In cutaneous leishmaniasis, the spectrum varies from a nonhealing infection to a form with exaggerated hypersensitivity in which severe tissue damage is mediated by the immune response (espundia and leishmaniasis recidivans). In visceral leishmaniasis, many infections are subclinical and self-healing, although they can be activated by malnutrition or an immunosuppressive process. In those who develop the syndrome of kala-azar, delayed hypersensitivity is suppressed specifically to leishmanial antigens and nonspecifically to tuberculin and other unrelated antigens, and there is proliferation of reticuloendothelial cells and an exaggerated humoral immune response with the production of polyclonal, nonprotective immunoglobulins. Defective cell-mediated immunity in patients with leishmaniasis has been associated with increased suppressor cell activity and defective production of interferon-γ, interleukin-1, and interleukin-2 by peripheral blood mononuclear cells.

The Leishmanin Skin Test. The Montenegro test measures delayed sensitivity to antigens prepared from promastigotes. Cultured organisms are washed in 0.5% phenol saline, diluted to 1×10^6/ml, and 0.1 ml is injected intradermally. The injection site is examined 48 hours later, and induration of 5 mm or greater constitutes a positive test. The test is generally positive in cutaneous and mucocutaneous leishmaniasis but negative in visceral leishmaniasis. Although *Leishmania* share common antigens with mycobacteria and trypanosomes, the leishmanin skin test is not positive in pulmonary tuberculosis, leprosy, African trypanosomiasis, or Chagas' disease. Occasional false-positive reactions have been noted in patients with glandular tuberculosis and systemic fungal infections.

A positive leishmanin test denotes present or past infection with *Leishmania*, but protective immunity generally exists only against the homologous species that has caused the positive reaction. However, with certain species, there may be a degree of cross-reactive immunity between species that is not reciprocal. In a small number of experimentally infected individuals, infection with *L. mexicana* did not protect against *L. braziliensis*, although infection with *L. braziliensis* did protect against *L. mexicana*. Experimental studies and clinical experience suggest that infection with *L. major* protects against *L. tropica* but not vice versa. Reinfection with *L. tropica* has occasionally been observed many years after initial infection with the same species, often following an illness or therapy that causes immunosuppression.

BIBLIOGRAPHY

Lainson R, Shaw JJ: Evolution, classification and geographical distribution. *In* Peters W, Killick-Kendrick R (eds): The Leishmaniases in Biology and Medicine. London and New York, Academic Press, 1987.

Glew RH, Saha AK, Siddhartha DAS, et al: Biochemistry of the *Leishmania* species. Microbiol Rev 52:412, 1988.

Pearson RD, Wheeler DA, Harrison LH, Kay HD: The immunobiology of leishmaniasis. Rev Infect Dis 5:907, 1983.

Peters W, Killick-Kendrick R (eds): The Leishmaniases in Biology and Medicine. London and New York, Academic Press, 1987.

World Health Organization: The leishmaniases. Report of a WHO Expert Committee. WHO Tech Rep Ser 701, 1984.

76.2.　VISCERAL LEISHMANIASIS (Kala-azar)

Charles N. Oster
and Jeffrey D. Chulay

DEFINITION. Visceral leishmaniasis is a chronic infectious disease caused by *Leishmania donovani* and characterized by irregular fever, enlargement of the spleen and liver, weight loss, anemia, leukopenia, and hypergammaglobulinemia. The disease is also known as kala-azar (Hindi for black sickness), Dumdum fever, and ponos (Greek for hurt).

ETIOLOGY. Visceral leishmaniasis is caused by one

of three species of the *L. donovani* complex (Table 76–1) that occur in different parts of the world: (1) *L. donovani* (India); (2) *L. infantum* (Mediterranean littoral, Middle East, Africa, China); and (3) *L. chagasi* (South America). There are currently no morphologic or serologic methods for distinguishing the species, but differences in biochemical characteristics, epidemiology, clinical features, and response to treatment suggest that distinct species are involved. Organisms with biochemical characteristics of *L. tropica* have occasionally been isolated from bone marrow cultures of patients with visceral leishmaniasis (Chapter 76.1).

DISTRIBUTION AND INCIDENCE. Visceral leishmaniasis is widely distributed (Fig. 76–3). Mediterranean or infantile kala-azar is found in Portugal, France, Italy, Greece, Yugoslavia, North Africa, the Mediterranean islands, Lebanon, Iraq, Iran, Saudi Arabia, Yemen, southern Russia, central Asia, and northern China. Indian kala-azar occurs in the eastern part of India (Assam, Bengal, Bihar, Uttar Pradesh, Madras, Sikkim) and Bangladesh. African kala-azar is common in Kenya and Sudan, but sporadic cases occur in Chad, Upper Volta, Central African Republic, Uganda, Zaire, Zambia, and Ethiopia. American kala-azar occurs in northeastern Brazil, Paraguay, Argentina, Venezuela, Colombia, Guatemala, El Salvador, Honduras, and Mexico.

Precise incidence figures are not available, but it is likely that tens of thousands of cases of visceral leishmaniasis occur each year throughout the world.

TRANSMISSION AND EPIDEMIOLOGY. *L. donovani* is transmitted by phlebotomine sandflies (Fig. 76–4) of the genera *Phlebotomus* in the Old World and *Lutzomyia* in the New World (Table 76–1). The epidemiology depends on the interaction of sandflies, reservoir hosts, and susceptible humans.

Reservoir Hosts

Humans. In India, where the domestic sandfly vector *P. argentipes* feeds solely on humans, people appear to be the only reservoir, and large epidemics occur that can often be traced to migration of an infected individual into a new locality. The possibility of an animal reservoir that maintains the cycle in interepidemic periods has not been excluded.

Dogs. Around the Mediterranean, dogs are the main reservoir and the disease is urban, transmitted by *P. perniciosus*, *P. major*, *P. simici*, and *P. longicuspis*. Human disease in this area usually occurs in infants and young children. Young dogs and certain breeds (foxhounds and beagles) are especially susceptible to infection with *L. infantum* and develop overt disease that is often fatal. Dogs are also important reservoirs in China, where the main vector is *P. chinensis*, and in South America, where the main vector is *Lu. longipalpis*. Biochemical studies indicate that *L. chagasi* and *L. infantum* are very similar, and it is possible that the organism was brought to the New World by the dogs of the conquistadors.

Wild Canines. In southern France and central Italy, foxes with inapparent infection are the reservoir, *P. ariasi* and *P. perfiliewi* are the vectors, and visceral leishmaniasis is primarily a rural disease affecting older children and adults. Foxes are also reservoirs in Brazil, and jackals are probably an important source of the sporadic, mainly rural cases that occur in the Middle East and central Asia.

Multiple Hosts, Rodents. The epidemiology of visceral leishmaniasis in Africa is incompletely understood. In Kenya, where *P. martini* is the probable vector, epidemics of kala-azar occurred in the 1950s and 1970s, suggesting a human reservoir, but domestic dogs have occasionally been found infected with *L. donovani.* In Sudan, epidemics of visceral leishmaniasis also occurred in the 1950s and in 1988 and 1989, but the disease usually occurs sporadically in nomads who occupy temporary villages in the dry season near patches of scrub that harbor the vector *P. orientalis. L. donovani* has been isolated from *Arvicanthis niloticus* and other rodents in Sudan, and rodents are probably important in maintaining enzootic foci in interepidemic periods. Parasite isolates from Sudan, Ethiopia, and Kenya appear to be more closely related biochemically to *L. donovani* than to *L. infantum.*

Unusual Routes of Transmission. *L. donovani* can be transmitted by means other than sandfly bite, such as blood transfusion or sexual contact, but these events occur rarely. Organisms have been demonstrated in nasal mucus, but it is unlikely that direct transmission occurs. Animals can become infected after eating infected carcasses. Experimentally, humans can develop kala-azar following intradermal inoculation of *L. donovani* promastigotes.

PATHOGENESIS AND PATHOLOGY. Following inoculation by the sandfly, promastigotes enter reticuloendothelial cells and multiply. At the site of inoculation, a granuloma develops, consisting of histiocytes filled with amastigotes and surrounded initially by epithelioid cells and later by giant cells as well. Parasites spread to local lymph nodes and then hematogenously within macrophages to the liver, spleen, and bone marrow, where they stimulate a granulomatous cellular immune response that results in subclinical disease and spontaneous resolution, or where they multiply further and cause the clinical syndrome of kala-azar.

Spleen. Patients with progressive disease develop marked splenomegaly due to hyperplasia of reticuloendothelial cells that are filled with parasites, and splenic infarcts are common. In acute cases, the spleen is smooth and friable, but it is firm in the more usual chronic cases.

Liver. The liver is usually enlarged and contains numerous amastigote-laden Kupffer cells, with little or no cellular reaction (Fig. 76–5). In subclinical cases, noncaseating granulomas with few parasites are scattered throughout the liver.

Lymph Nodes. Lymph nodes may be enlarged and contain macrophages filled with amastigotes, usually with few surrounding lymphocytes. Tonsillar lymphoid tissue may also contain *Leishmania.* In subclinical cases or in lymphatic leishmaniasis, there is a granulomatous and giant cell reaction closely resembling tuberculosis but without caseation.

Mouth and Nasopharynx. In the Sudan, East Africa, and India, visceral leishmaniasis is sometimes associated with oral and nasopharyngeal lesions. The histologic appearance of these lesions varies from numerous parasitized histiocytes to granulomas with few parasites. Parasites are more abundant in oral lesions than in nasopharyngeal ones but may be demonstrated in nasal and pharyngeal secretions.

Gastrointestinal Tract. In the gastrointestinal tract, there is proliferation of reticuloendothelial cells in the duodenum and jejunum, infiltration of the submucosa with parasitized cells, and sometimes, villous atrophy with hyperplasia of crypt cells. Small ulcerations may occur in which parasites can be demonstrated.

Other Organs. The bone marrow usually contains numerous parasite-laden macrophages. The skin may contain *Leishmania,* and in fatal cases, all levels beneath the epidermis are often heavily infiltrated, with masses of parasitized cells concentrated around the sweat glands and arterioles. Parasites have also been identified in heart muscle, the adrenal glands, and the parotid glands. The kidneys may show an interstitial nephritis or a mild proliferative glomerulonephritis and may contain immune complexes. Renal amyloidosis is an uncommon late complication.

CLINICAL MANIFESTATIONS

Symptoms. The incubation period is generally 2 to 6 months, although disease occasionally occurs many years after the patient has left an endemic area. The patient usually does not recall the primary skin lesion. The onset of the disease is occasionally acute, especially in migrants and visitors to an endemic area, with high fever, chills, and malaise. More often, the onset is gradual, with intermittent fever, progressive enlargement of the spleen and liver, and vague abdominal discomfort. Other common symptoms include weight loss, epistaxis, diarrhea, and cough. Appetite is generally well maintained.

Signs. The patient is often weak and emaciated, with the abdomen distended by a markedly enlarged spleen and a moderately enlarged liver (Fig. 76–6). In rare cases of acute kala-azar, the spleen may not be palpably enlarged. In chronic cases, there is generally little malaise or apathy. Femoral and inguinal lymphadenopathy are often noted, especially in African kala-azar, and generalized lymphadenopathy is a feature of lymphatic leishmaniasis (see below). Trophic changes of the hair (thinning, dryness, hypopigmentation, and loss of curl) and of the skin on the lower legs are common. Hemic heart murmurs are often present, and edema of the legs, jaundice, petechiae, and purpura may sometimes be noted.

Skin. Cutaneous abnormalities are commonly associated with kala-azar. Many patients, especially in India, acquire an earth-gray color of the skin, which gave rise to the name kala-azar (black sickness). The primary lesion at the site of inoculation appears as a small papule or a cutaneous ulcer that may be mistaken for a basal cell epithelioma, although this has almost always resolved by the time the patient seeks medical care. Skin lesions may also occur simultaneously with visceral leishmaniasis, especially in Africa. Such lesions are polymorphic, although often they appear as diffuse, warty, nonulcerated lesions in which variable numbers of par-

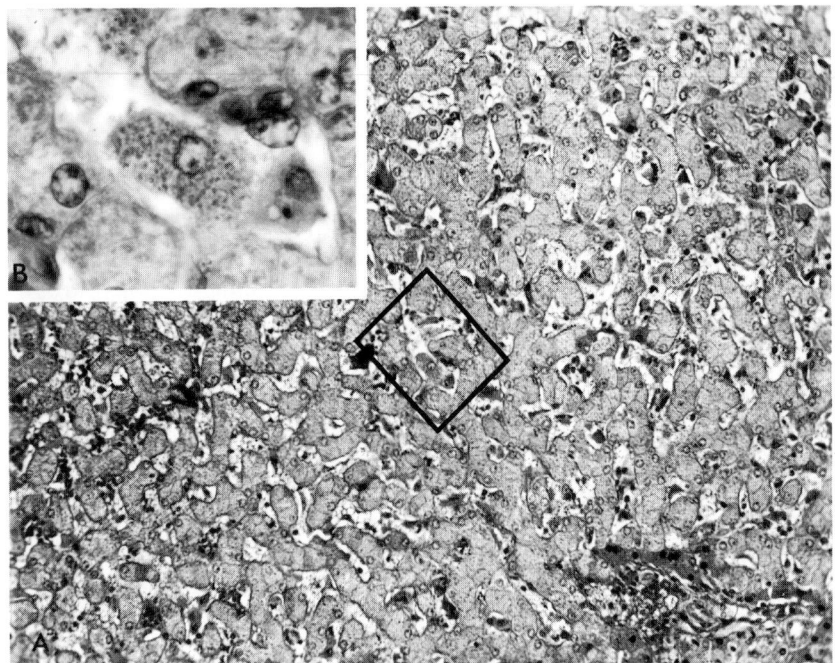

FIGURE 76–5. Visceral leishmaniasis. *A*, Section of liver showing dilated sinusoids and greatly enlarged Kupffer cells (× 165). (Courtesy of the Armed Forces Institute of Pathology, Photograph Neg. No. 70–7723.) *B*, Kupffer cell in *A* magnified to × 1800. The cytoplasm contains numerous *Leishmania* amastigotes. (Courtesy of The Armed Forces Institute of Pathology, Photograph Neg. No. 70–7722.)

asites are found. Lesions of post–kala-azar dermal leishmaniasis (PKDL) are usually not present during active visceral infection (see later discussion).

Oral and Nasopharyngeal Lesions. Mucosal lesions are occasionally seen in patients with visceral leishmaniasis in Sudan and rarely in patients in East Africa and India. Oral lesions appear as nodules or ulcers of the gum, palate, tongue, or lip. Lesions of the nasal mucosa may cause perforation of the septum. Nasopharyngeal and laryngeal lesions present with mucosal swelling and hoarseness. These lesions may be associated with active visceral infections or with PKDL. They respond well to antimony therapy and may be due to an exaggerated nonhealing immune response.

Other Findings. Other unusual manifestations of visceral leishmaniasis include retinal hemorrhages, massive hepatic necrosis, pancytopenia without splenomegaly, and lymphatic leishmaniasis, in which generalized lymphadenopathy occurs without hepatosplenomegaly, resembling tuberculosis or sarcoidosis. The diagnosis of lymphatic leishmaniasis is made by finding noncaseating granulomas and amastigotes in a lymph node biopsy specimen.

Laboratory Abnormalities

Hematologic. Anemia is invariably present and often severe, with hemoglobin levels of 6 to 8 gm/dl being common. The anemia is multifactorial. Erythrocyte survival time is shortened owing to hypersplenism and possibly autoimmune mechanisms. Bone marrow depression is indicated by a reticulocytosis lower than expected for the degree of anemia. Coexistent iron deficiency may be present. The Coombs test is usually positive, with both C3 and IgG present on red blood cells, but does not correlate with the severity of the anemia. Leukopenia is also characteristic, with white blood cell counts often below 3000/mm³. The neutrophil survival time is shortened, and the white blood cell

differential demonstrates neutropenia, relative lymphocytosis, and an almost complete absence of eosinophils. Agranulocytosis is rare. Moderate thrombocytopenia (50,000 to 100,000/mm³) is common.

Others. Liver enzymes (ALT more than AST) are mildly elevated in the majority of patients, but elevations of serum bilirubin are uncommon. The prothrombin time is usually 2 to 4 seconds longer than that in controls, and serum albumin is generally less than 3 gm/dl. A polyclonal hypergammaglobulinemia of 5 to 10 gm/dl, most of which is IgG, is usual. In some reports, albuminuria is common, but in others, the urinalysis is normal, as are tests of renal function.

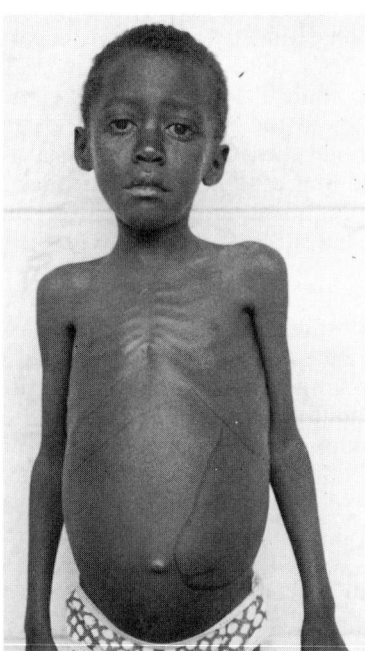

FIGURE 76–6. A young Kenyan girl with visceral leishmaniasis.

Complications. Bacterial pneumonia may be present on admission or may develop during treatment. Pulmonary tuberculosis is a common complication of visceral leishmaniasis, and it should be suspected in any patient responding poorly to antimony therapy. Cancrum oris, a necrotizing oral infection, occurs late in the course when neutropenia is severe. Hepatic cirrhosis is an uncommon sequela of visceral leishmaniasis, and portal hypertension may cause persistent splenomegaly, despite successful treatment of kala-azar. Uveitis can occur after apparent recovery from visceral disease. Rare complications include disseminated intravascular coagulation, immune complex–mediated glomerulonephritis, and renal amyloidosis presenting with a nephrotic syndrome.

Subclinical Infections. In areas endemic for visceral leishmaniasis, many inhabitants develop a positive leishmanin skin test without clinical disease, and such individuals appear to be resistant to naturally occurring and experimental infection with *L. donovani*. In a prospective study in Brazil, 28 of 86 children with antibodies to *L. donovani* developed classic visceral leishmaniasis within a few weeks to 15 months after the positive serology. Twenty others remained asymptomatic during observation for up to 5 years, and 38 had a prolonged subclinical illness, manifested by mild constitutional symptoms and intermittent hepatomegaly, that resolved without antileishmanial treatment after an average of 35 months. These observations help to explain the fact that apparently healthy individuals have occasionally transmitted infection via blood transfusion.

Infections in Immunocompromised Hosts. In the past several years, there have been reports of visceral leishmaniasis' occurring as an opportunistic infection in patients with human immunodeficiency virus (HIV) infection, with or without the acquired immunodeficiency syndrome (AIDS) (Chapter 15.1). These patients often differ from non–HIV-infected patients in that they may have a shorter duration of symptoms, no fever or splenomegaly, negative serologic tests for leishmaniasis, a poor response to treatment, a higher rate of relapse after treatment, and a higher mortality. Fever or hepatosplenomegaly in an HIV-infected patient who has resided in or visited an area endemic for visceral leishmaniasis should prompt an examination of the bone marrow, with both smears and cultures for *Leishmania*. Visceral leishmaniasis may also occur as an opportunistic infection in renal transplant recipients and other patients receiving immunosuppressive therapy.

Post–Kala-azar Dermal Leishmaniasis. PKDL was first described in India using the term dermal leishmanoid. It occurs in up to 20% of patients with visceral leishmaniasis in India, but it is uncommon (approximately 2%) in East Africa and rare in China. In India, skin lesions usually appear 2 to 10 years after successful treatment of visceral leishmaniasis, but in East Africa, they often appear within a few months of treatment. The lesions occur predominantly on the face and to a lesser extent on the extensor surfaces of the arms, the trunk, and, occasionally, the legs. Initially, they appear as small hypopigmented patches, which enlarge and may progress to nodules that sometimes resemble leprosy

(Fig. 76–7). Histologically, there is a spectrum of cellular response, varying from numerous parasites with few inflammatory cells to a granulomatous reaction containing few parasites. Occasionally, a xanthomatous form occurs, with raised, orange-colored, nonulcerated plaques. Parasites isolated from patients with PKDL are serologically and biochemically identical to *L. donovani* isolated from patients with visceral leishmaniasis. Since PKDL may persist for up to 20 years, such patients may act as a chronic reservoir of infection.

DIAGNOSIS. Splenomegaly and anemia in a patient who has lived in an area endemic for visceral leishmaniasis suggest the diagnosis. The diagnosis is unlikely if the absolute eosinophil count is above 100/mm^3, the serum albumin is above 3 gm/dl, or the serum globulin is less than 4 gm/dl.

Demonstration of Parasites. Splenic aspiration is the surest method of confirming the diagnosis. However, deaths have occurred after splenic aspiration, presumably owing to splenic laceration, and careful observation after the procedure is mandatory. In recent experience in Kenya with more than 3000 splenic aspirations in more than 400 patients, 3 patients developed shock and died within 24 hours after splenic aspiration, and intraabdominal bleeding was diagnosed in another 4 patients who recovered with conservative, nonsurgical therapy. Contraindications to splenic aspiration are a soft spleen in acute disease, a prothrombin time 5 seconds or more longer than the normal control, or a platelet count below 40,000/mm^3. In patients less than 5 years old, splenic aspiration should be performed only by a physician fully experienced with the procedure. The procedure uses a 21-gauge needle attached to a 5-ml syringe, which is inserted just under the skin over the middle of the spleen. As suction is applied, the needle is rapidly inserted into the spleen and withdrawn, with the needle remaining in the spleen only a fraction of a second. The small amount of splenic tissue and blood in the needle is expressed into culture medium and onto slides for

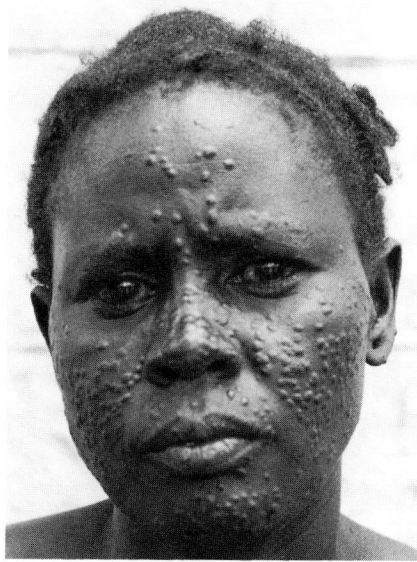

FIGURE 76–7. Nodular lesions of post–kala-azar dermal leishmaniasis in a Kenyan woman.

thin smears. Splenic smears stained with Giemsa or Leishman's stain demonstrate amastigotes in 98% of cases and can give the diagnosis within an hour (Fig. 76–8). Promastigotes are generally found after incubation at 25C for 2 to 7 days in Schneider's medium or 7 to 21 days in NNN medium.

Bone marrow aspiration is preferred in many areas because of concern about the hazards of splenic aspiration. Bone marrow smears usually contain fewer amastigotes, and parasites are found in only 80 to 85% of cases (Fig. 73–5M). Amastigotes are also found frequently in liver biopsy specimens (Fig. 76–5) or aspirates and in lymph node aspirates. Buffy coat smears often demonstrate amastigotes in Indian and Kenyan kala-azar, but it is unusual to make the diagnosis by this method.

Serologic Tests. A variety of serologic tests are helpful in suggesting the diagnosis of visceral leishmaniasis. The formol-gel test, which detects high levels of IgG or IgM from any cause, is of limited value because it becomes positive late in the course of visceral leishmaniasis and false-positive tests are common. It may be useful in field situations or rural health centers where other serologic tests are unavailable. The complement fixation test, using antigen prepared from *L. donovani* or from the cross-reactive *Mycobacterium phlei* (Kedrowsky's bacillus), has also been replaced by tests with greater sensitivity and specificity. The indirect fluorescent antibody test (IFA) using promastigotes as antigen is positive in more than 95% of patients with visceral leishmaniasis, generally with titers above 1:256. These are readily distinguishable from the low-titer positive tests that occur occasionally in malaria, typhoid fever, and other diseases. The enzyme-linked immunosorbent assay (ELISA) test using soluble promastigote antigens appears to be as sensitive and specific as the IFA, and because of economy and technical practicality, it is especially useful for large-scale epidemiologic studies of human and canine leishmaniasis. Both the IFA and the ELISA test can be performed on sera eluted from filter papers impregnated with 50 μl of capillary blood. The specificity of serologic tests for visceral leishmaniasis can be improved by using a competitive binding assay, in which the binding of *L. donovani*–specific monoclonal antibodies is inhibited by antibodies present in the sera of patients with visceral leishmaniasis, or by using specific leishmanial proteins purified from parasites or recombinant DNA expression systems.

Leishmanin Skin Test. The Montenegro test is uniformly negative in active visceral leishmaniasis but becomes positive in 90% of patients 6 weeks to 1 year after recovery. Tuberculin sensitivity usually is similarly depressed during active kala-azar, indicating a broad defect in cell-mediated immunity. In vitro lymphocyte blastogenesis responses to leishmanin and tuberculin are also depressed. A positive leishmanin skin test in a patient with fever, anemia, and splenomegaly excludes the diagnosis of visceral leishmaniasis as the cause of the illness.

Differential Diagnosis. The differential diagnosis of visceral leishmaniasis includes malaria, African trypanosomiasis, hepatosplenic schistosomiasis, brucellosis, typhoid fever, bacterial endocarditis, generalized histoplasmosis, chronic myelocytic leukemia, Hodgkin's disease and other lymphomas, sarcoidosis, hepatic cirrhosis, and tuberculosis. Tropical splenomegaly syndrome is especially difficult to differentiate, although high titers of antimalarial antibodies and a characteristic histologic appearance of the liver suggest this disease. Patients with multiple myeloma and Waldenström's macroglobulinemia have monoclonal hypergammaglobulinemia.

TREATMENT. Patients should receive a nutritious diet. Antimicrobial agents are given when concurrent pneumonia, tuberculosis, or other bacterial infections are present. Patients with chronic disease generally tolerate anemia well, but blood transfusion may be needed if the hemoglobin level falls below 6 gm/dl. Coexistent iron or vitamin deficiency requires specific treatment.

Pentavalent Antimonials. Antimonial drugs are the initial treatment of choice for all forms of visceral leishmaniasis. Sodium stibogluconate (Pentostam) is used in Asia, much of Europe, and English-speaking parts of Africa, whereas meglumine antimoniate (Glucantime) is used in Latin America and French-speaking parts of Africa and Europe. They can be administered intravenously or intramuscularly.

Sodium Stibogluconate. This drug is provided as a solution containing 100 mg of antimony (Sb) per ml. In the United States, sodium stibogluconate is available under an Investigational New Drug (IND) application from the Centers for Disease Control. The recommended treatment regimen is 20 mg of Sb/kg/day, to a maximum daily dose of 850 mg, for at least 20 days. Studies in India and Kenya have demonstrated that higher doses (20 mg/kg/day versus 10 mg/kg/day) and longer courses of therapy (30 or 40 days versus 20 days) increase the rate of initial response to chemotherapy and decrease the rate of relapse. These longer courses of treatment are well tolerated.

Sodium stibogluconate is a safe drug. Intramuscular injections are moderately painful. Intravenous injections

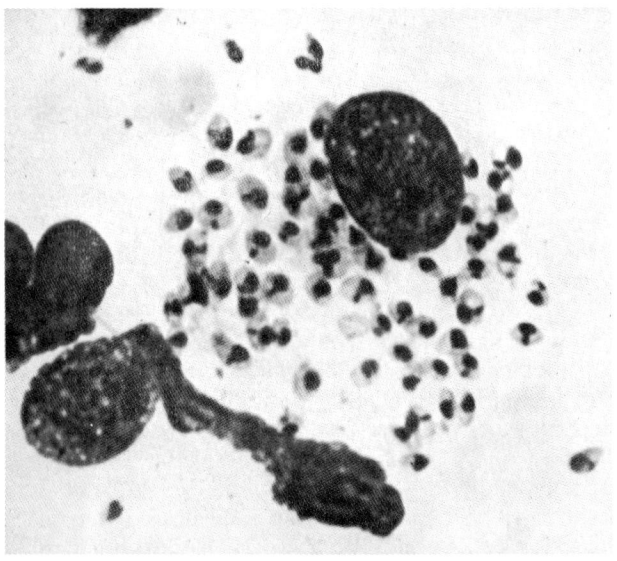

FIGURE 76–8. Amastigotes of *Leishmania donovani* in a splenic aspirate smear.

should be given slowly through a 23- to 26-gauge needle, or diluted at least 1:10 with 5% dextrose in water, to reduce the incidence of local thrombosis. Nausea, anorexia, malaise, and lethargy are uncommon, except when high dosages (more than 20 mg of Sb/kg/day) are administered. Electrocardiographic (ECG) abnormalities, including nonspecific ST- and T-wave changes and T-wave flattening or inversion, occur in more than one half of patients receiving sodium stibogluconate, and the frequency of these changes is proportional to the total daily dose and the duration of therapy. One patient treated in Kenya with sodium stibogluconate at a dosage of 20 mg of Sb/kg 3 times daily for disease unresponsive to lower doses developed a prolonged QT interval after 2 weeks of treatment and died suddenly on treatment day 23. If doses above 20 mg of Sb/kg/day are used, an electrocardiogram should be obtained once or twice weekly, and treatment should be suspended if the corrected QT interval (the measured QT interval divided by the square root of the RR interval) becomes prolonged beyond 0.50. T-wave inversion, the most common ECG abnormality during antimony administration, is not an indication to stop treatment.

Meglumine Antimoniate. This agent is provided as a solution containing 85 mg of Sb per ml. The recommended dosage is 20 mg of Sb/kg/day, to a maximum dosage of 850 mg of Sb/day, for at least 20 days. The side effects of meglumine antimoniate are similar to those of sodium stibogluconate.

Treatment of Relapses. Patients who relapse after initial therapy usually respond to additional treatment with pentavalent antimonials, but if they are treated with the same regimen used to treat initial infections, they have a high risk of subsequent relapse and eventual unresponsiveness to antimony. Patients who undergo relapse should therefore be treated with pentavalent antimonials in higher doses (20 to 30 mg of Sb/kg/day) for longer periods of time (60 to 90 days). Failure to respond to initial antimony therapy is uncommon in previously untreated patients.

Diamidines. In patients unresponsive to antimony, treatment with one of the diamidines is usually given. Pentamidine is the diamidine most generally available. Pentamidine (as the isethionate or methane sulfonate salt) is provided as a sterile powder that must be dissolved in sterile water and administered by intramuscular or slow intravenous injection. The recommended dose of 4 mg/kg body weight daily for 10 to 14 days is often toxic (frequency too great) and ineffective (duration too short). Experience in Kenya indicates that 3 doses per week for 4 to 6 months is often effective with little risk of serious toxicity. Common side effects include pain, induration, and sterile abscesses at the injection sites, as well as immediate hypotensive reactions if the drug is given too rapidly intravenously. Both hypoglycemia and diabetes may occur. Renal insufficiency, which is common when pentamidine is used to treat *Pneumocystis carinii* pneumonia, is uncommon in patients with visceral leishmaniasis.

Stilbamidine may be more effective than pentamidine, but delayed toxicity (neuropathy, especially of the trigeminal nerve) has limited its use. Hydroxystilbamidine is an excellent drug but is not generally available. It has been used in an adult dose of 250 mg by slow intravenous infusion daily for 10 days, repeated twice after a 7-day interval to a total of 7.5 gm.

Amphotericin B. This drug has also been used successfully in cases of visceral leishmaniasis resistant to other medications. It is administered by slow intravenous infusion over 4 to 6 hours, starting at 0.1 mg/kg body weight daily and gradually increasing to 1 mg/kg body weight every 2 days until a total dose of 1 to 2 gm has been given. Serum creatinine and blood urea nitrogen levels should be monitored and the dosage reduced or the drug stopped if they rise above 4 mg/dl or 50 mg/dl, respectively. Other side effects include fever, thrombophlebitis, anorexia, nausea, anemia, and hypokalemia. (See Chapter 67 for additional information about the use of amphotericin B.)

Allopurinol. Because allopurinol inhibits *L. donovani* in vitro, it has been used in patients with visceral leishmaniasis. Cures have not been achieved when allopurinol was used alone in previously untreated patients, and a controlled trial in Kenya of sodium stibogluconate alone (20 mg of Sb/kg/day) versus sodium stibogluconate plus allopurinol (21 mg/kg/day), each given for 30 days, demonstrated no advantage of the combination. Allopurinol has apparently been useful when used in combination with pentavalent antimonials in a few patients whose disease had relapsed.

Immunotherapy. Combined treatment using recombinant interferon-γ (100 μg/m^2 body surface area) plus meglumine antimoniate (20 mg of Sb/kg/day) for 10 to 60 days was effective in 6 of 8 patients with visceral leishmaniasis unresponsive to multiple courses of pentavalent antimonials alone. A similar regimen given for 10 to 20 days was effective in 8 of 9 previously untreated patients, but definition of the role of interferon in the initial management of visceral leishmaniasis must await the results of controlled clinical trials comparing combined treatment versus antimonials alone.

Splenectomy. Splenectomy is occasionally employed in patients with visceral leishmaniasis who are resistant to other forms of treatment. There is usually a prompt rise in hemoglobin levels and white blood cell and platelet counts after splenectomy, but additional chemotherapy is necessary, because cure is unlikely otherwise. Splenectomized patients are at increased risk of overwhelming sepsis due to pneumococci and other encapsulated bacteria and should receive antipneumococcal vaccination before splenectomy. Because malaria is often fatal in splenectomized individuals, lifelong antimalarial prophylaxis is essential in countries where malaria occurs.

Post–Kala-azar Dermal Leishmaniasis. Treatment of PKDL with adequate doses of pentavalent antimonials usually causes improvement in the skin lesions, although pigmentary changes may persist indefinitely. In Africa, PKDL usually clears without treatment.

PROGNOSIS. Infection with *L. donovani* comprises a spectrum of diseases, and spontaneous cure of inapparent infection is more common than was formerly realized. In contrast, the established syndrome of kala-azar is almost always fatal in the absence of specific chemotherapy. Response to treatment should be monitored by daily assessment of temperature, weekly assessment of hemoglobin levels and spleen size, and splenic or bone marrow aspirate smear and culture at the end of treatment. In most patients, fever disappears within 7 days, the hemoglobin level rises and the spleen becomes smaller within 2 weeks, and parasites disappear by the end of treatment. When fever persists and the general condition does not improve during treatment, concomitant tuberculosis should be suspected. Within 6 to 12 months, the spleen usually becomes nonpalpable and elevated immunoglobulin levels and serologic tests become normal. Persistent splenomegaly after otherwise successful treatment may be due to portal hypertension.

Follow-up examination is important for the early detection and treatment of relapses. Relapse is suggested by an increase in spleen size, a fall in hemoglobin levels, and a decrease in eosinophil counts to fewer than 50/mm^3 and should be confirmed by the demonstration of parasites. Relapse occurs in 3 to 7% of patients in China, 0.5 to 13% in India, and 5 to 30% in Kenya. Relapses are most common during the first 2 to 6 months after finishing treatment, but occasionally, they occur several years later, particularly in patients who become immunocompromised by disease or medication.

PREVENTION AND CONTROL

Treatment of Cases. In epidemics of visceral leishmaniasis in which humans are the reservoir (India and perhaps Kenya and Sudan), case finding and treatment may possibly help interrupt the epidemic.

Reservoir Control. Identification and destruction of infected dogs have been successful in reducing the incidence of visceral leishmaniasis in areas where the dog is the reservoir (the Mediterranean, China, and South America).

Vector Control. In India during the early part of this century, houses known to be microfoci were burned. During the malaria eradication campaigns, visceral leishmaniasis virtually disappeared from India, but since spraying of DDT has stopped, the incidence of visceral leishmaniasis has again increased to high levels.

Immunization. Intradermal inoculation of a rodent strain of *Leishmania* from East Africa gave protection against experimental inoculation of *L. donovani,* but a field trial with this parasite failed to demonstrate protection, perhaps because of loss of virulence of the rodent parasite with subculture. There is continued interest in developing a method for immunization against visceral leishmaniasis, but this goal is unlikely to be achieved in the near future.

BIBLIOGRAPHY

Badaro R, Falcoff E, Badaro FS, et al: Treatment of visceral leishmaniasis with pentavalent antimony and interferon gamma. N Engl J Med 322:16, 1990.
Badaro R, Jones TC, Carvalho EM, et al: New perspectives on a subclinical form of visceral leishmaniasis. J Infect Dis 154:1003, 1986.
Badaro R, Jones TC, Lorenco R, et al: A prospective study of visceral leishmaniasis in an endemic area of Brazil. J Infect Dis 154:639, 1986.

Berman JD: Chemotherapy of leishmaniasis: Biochemical mechanisms, clinical efficacy and future strategies. Rev Infect Dis 10:560, 1988.
Bryceson ADM, Chulay J, Mugambi M, et al: Visceral leishmaniasis unresponsive to antimonial drugs. II. Response to high dosage sodium stibogluconate or prolonged treatment with pentamidine. Trans R Soc Trop Med Hyg 79:705, 1985.
Bryceson ADM: Therapy in man. *In* Killick-Kendrick R, Peters W (eds): The Leishmaniases in Biology and Medicine. London and New York, Academic Press, 1987, p 847.
Chulay JD, Bryceson ADM: Quantitation of amastigotes of *Leishmania donovani* in smears of splenic aspirates from patients with visceral leishmaniasis. Am J Trop Med Hyg 32:475, 1983.
Chulay JD, Spencer HC, Mugambi M: Electrocardiographic changes during treatment of leishmaniasis with pentavalent antimony (sodium stibogluconate). Am J Trop Med Hyg 34:702, 1985.
Jaffe CL, McMahon-Pratt D: Serodiagnostic assay for visceral leishmaniasis employing monoclonal antibodies. Trans R Soc Trop Med Hyg 81:587, 1987.
Jaffe CL, Zalis M: Use of purified parasite proteins from *Leishmania donovani* for the rapid serodiagnosis of visceral leishmaniasis. J Infect Dis 157:1212, 1988.
LeBlancq SM, Peters W: *Leishmania* in the Old World: 4. The distribution of *L. donovani sensu latu* zymodemes. Trans R Soc Trop Med Hyg 80:367, 1986.
Montalban C, Martinez-Fernandez R, Calleja JL, et al: Visceral leishmaniasis (kala-azar) as an opportunistic infection in patients infected with the human immunodeficiency virus in Spain. Rev Infect Dis 11:655, 1989.
Meleney HE: The histopathology of kala-azar in the hamster, monkey and man. Am J Pathol 1:147, 1925.
Thakur CP, Kumar M, Kumar P, et al: Rationalization of regimens of treatment of kala-azar with sodium stibogluconate in India: A randomised study. Br Med J 296:1557, 1988.
World Health Organization: Report of the workshop on the chemotherapy of visceral leishmaniasis. WHO Document TDR/CHEM LEISH/VL/82.3, 1982.

76.3.   CUTANEOUS LEISHMANIASIS OF THE OLD WORLD

Jeffrey D. Chulay

DEFINITION. Cutaneous leishmaniasis of the Old World is an infection characterized by nodular and ulcerative skin lesions caused by *Leishmania tropica, L. major,* or *L. aethiopica.* Local names for this disease include Oriental sore, Baghdad boil, Delhi boil, Biskra button, and Aleppo evil.

ETIOLOGY. There are at least 3 species in the *L. tropica* complex that can be distinguished on ecologic, biochemical, and serologic grounds (Table 76–1). *L. major (L. tropica major)* is a parasite of desert rodents that occasionally infects humans as a rural zoonosis. *L. tropica (L. tropica minor* or *L. tropica tropica)* is a parasite of dog and humans that occurs in an urban environment. *L. aethiopica (L. tropica aethiopica)* is a parasite of the hyrax, found in the Rift Valley of Ethiopia and Kenya, which infects people when they encroach on the environment after deforestation of mountain slopes. *L. major* strains isolated from West Africa, Sudan, and Ethiopia have a common excreted factor serotype that differs from that of Middle Eastern strains. (See Chapter 76.1 for a detailed description of the parasite.)

DISTRIBUTION AND EPIDEMIOLOGY (Fig. 76–3)

***Leishmania major* Infections.** Rural cutaneous leishmaniasis caused by *L. major* is primarily an infection of desert rodents. The giant or great gerbil *(Rhombomys opimus)* lives in dry desert areas of central Asia, in southern Russia, throughout Iran, and in parts of Iraq and northwestern India. These gerbils may have an infection rate of 30%, with cutaneous lesions on relatively hairless parts of the body, chiefly the head, ears, and base of the tail (Fig. 76–9). Other rodents in these areas play a secondary role in maintaining the infection. In Libya and Israel, the fat rat *(Psammomys obesus)* is an important host. Infection in all these areas is maintained by *Phlebotomus caucasicus* and *P. papatasi,* although only the latter transmits the infection to humans. Other vectors of lesser importance are *P. mongolensis, P. alexanderi,* and *P. ansarii.* Inhabitants of villages near gerbil burrows may have infection prevalence rates of 100%, and other groups of people who enter the ecosystem, e.g., travelers, hunters, military patrols, may also have high attack rates. The peak incidence of disease occurs in late summer and autumn, and most children in endemic areas acquire a sore between 2 and 3 years of age, rarely reaching maturity without a scar.

Cutaneous leishmaniasis caused by *L. major* is also found in a wide area of subSaharan Africa between the tenth and thirteenth parallels north, from Senegal in the West to the Sudan and Kenya in the East. The Nile rat *(Arvicanthis niloticus)* is a major host, although infection has also been demonstrated in other rodents. Human disease is also a rural zoonosis, and the main vector is *P. papatasi* in Sudan and *P. duboscqi* elsewhere.

***Leishmania aethiopica* Infections.** Cutaneous leishmaniasis in Africa can also be caused by *L. aethiopica.* The parasite is found in mountain valleys of the Rift Valley in Ethiopia and Kenya. It infects the rock hyrax *(Procavia habessinica)* and the tree hyrax *(Heterohyrax brucei),* and humans are infected when their homesteads encroach on deforested mountain slopes. The vectors are the high-altitude sandflies *P. longipes* (Ethiopia) and *P. pedifer* (Kenya). Human disease caused by *L. aethiopica* is usually self-healing, but a small percentage of infected individuals develop nonhealing diffuse cutaneous leishmaniasis.

The situation in Namibia superficially resembles that in Ethiopia and Kenya because sporadic human cases of cutaneous leishmaniasis occur and *Leishmania* have been isolated from hyrax and from *P. rossi* near hyrax burrows. However, the parasites from humans and *P. rossi,* although identical, were biochemically different from parasites isolated from hyrax, and both parasites were different from *L. aethiopica.*

***Leishmania tropica* Infections.** Urban cutaneous leishmaniasis is a natural infection of dogs and humans caused by *L. tropica.* The parasite has been demonstrated in cutaneous lesions on the ears, lips, nose, and inner canthus of the eyes of dogs in Iran, Iraq, and India, where it is transmitted by *P. sergenti.* In southern France, Italy, and some Mediterranean islands, *P. papatasi* is the vector. The infection was formerly common in many large cities of the Middle East (Baghdad, Teheran, Aleppo, and Damascus) and in southern Italy, Greece, Pakistan, and northwestern India. In the first half of the twentieth century, 40 to 70% of Europeans living in Delhi became infected. With residual insecticide spraying for malaria control, there has been a marked decrease in the sandfly populations and a concomitant decline in the incidence of urban cutaneous leishmaniasis.

PATHOLOGY AND PATHOGENESIS. At the site of inoculation, parasites enter macrophages and induce a cell-mediated immune response. A varying histologic appearance results from the interplay of host and parasites. In a typical case, lymphocytes, plasma cells, and large mononuclear cells surround the infected macrophages in a poorly organized granulomatous reaction. As the parasites are eliminated, epithelioid and giant cells appear, usually associated with tissue necrosis. Healing occurs with fibrosis. Small granulomas with central fibrinoid necrosis containing numerous parasites may be found, principally when disease is acquired in countries bordering the Mediterranean or in West Africa. In rural cutaneous leishmaniasis caused by *L. major,* granulomas may be found in nodules along the lymphatics or in local lymph nodes.

Nonhealing Forms. In leishmaniasis recidivans, there is healing with fibrosis in the center of the lesion but failure to heal peripherally, where a granulomatous reaction without caseation is seen. Parasites are scanty, and the histologic changes are similar to those of lupus vulgaris. In diffuse cutaneous leishmaniasis (DCL), there is a defect in the cell-mediated immune response, and numerous macrophages filled with amastigotes are seen with no cellular reaction or only a few surrounding lymphocytes.

Although *Leishmania* have been found in the peripheral blood of a few patients infected with *L. major,* visceral lesions do not occur in this disease.

CLINICAL MANIFESTATIONS. After experimental inoculation of human volunteers, the incubation period of cutaneous leishmaniasis is generally 2 to 8 weeks, but in exceptional cases, the incubation period may be as long as 3 years. Different forms of cutaneous leishmaniasis vary in some of their clinical features. The lesions of rural disease caused by *L. major* tend to be multiple and are accompanied by marked inflammation and crusting. They mature rapidly and heal relatively quickly, lasting a few months. The lesions of urban disease caused by *L. tropica* tend to be single, develop more slowly, and persist for a year or more. The lesions of cutaneous leishmaniasis caused by *L. aethiopica* are the least inflamed and most chronic, generally lasting several years.

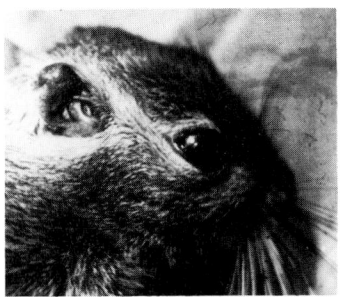

FIGURE 76–9. Lesion of *Leishmania major* on the ear of a gerbil *(Rhombomys opimus).*

The clinical appearance of the lesions reflects the degree of the host's immune response and may vary from small papules to nonulcerated plaques to large ulcers with well-defined, raised, indurated margins. When multiple lesions are present, they are usually similar in appearance and enlarge and heal together (isophasic reaction). The lesion begins as a small, often pruritic papule that enlarges with an infiltrated border. It may persist as a flattened plaque or may progress after a few days or weeks, with the surface becoming covered with fine, papery scales (Fig. 76–10), which are white and dry at first but later become moist and adherent, uncovering a shallow ulcer as they fall off. As the ulcer enlarges, it oozes serous fluid and may become covered with a thick crust. The edge of the ulcer is surrounded by a raised, indurated area with a characteristic dusky discoloration. Satellite lesions are common (Fig. 76–10) and may ultimately merge with the parent lesion. After a few months to more than a year, healing begins with central granulation tissue that spreads peripherally. The resultant depressed white or pink scar is often cosmetically disfiguring, especially when on the face. *L. major* infections may be associated with severe scarring, which can cause disability if located at critical sites such as the wrist or elbow.

Multiple lesions are common, especially in rural cutaneous leishmaniasis, and occasionally, more than 100 lesions may be counted on an individual patient. Lesions usually occur on exposed parts of the body such as face, hands, feet, arms, and legs, but rarely on the trunk and never on the palms or soles or hairy scalp. Uncommon sites of ulcers include the ears, tongue, and eyelids. Fever has occasionally preceded the appearance of multiple nodules. Lymphatic spread may occur in *L. major* infections, with subcutaneous nodules in a linear distribution and regional lymphadenopathy. When the primary lesion is on the hand, this may resemble sporotrichosis. Secondary bacterial infection of an ulcer is unusual. It may cause pain and, rarely, bacteremia.

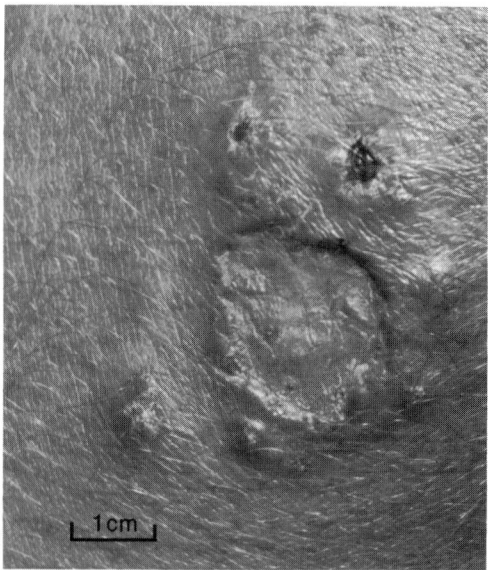

FIGURE 76–10. Oriental sore caused by *Leishmania major*. Note the satellite lesions.

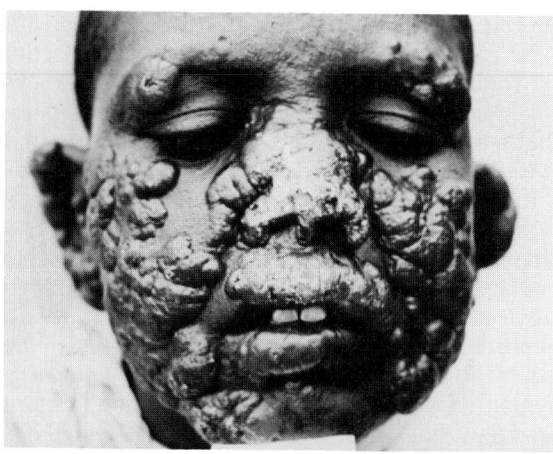

FIGURE 76–11. Nodular lesions of diffuse cutaneous leishmaniasis caused by *Leishmania aethiopica*. (Courtesy of Dr. A. D. M. Bryceson.)

Leishmaniasis Recidivans. Also known as lupoid leishmaniasis, leishmaniasis recidivans is an unusual chronic form of cutaneous leishmaniasis that is found primarily in Iran and Iraq and may persist for 20 to 40 years. The lesion often begins on the face and enlarges relentlessly, healing in the center and advancing at the periphery, analogous to some forms of cutaneous tuberculosis. Mucous membrane involvement may lead to nasal destruction. The dense scar tissue in the center of the lesion contains small granulomas, whereas the nodules and papules at the periphery resemble the "apple jelly" nodules of lupus vulgaris. Organisms are extremely difficult to demonstrate in biopsy specimens but can more often be isolated by culture or animal inoculation. The leishmanin skin test is strongly positive.

Diffuse Cutaneous Leishmaniasis. DCL is an uncommon result of infection with *L. aethiopica* in Ethiopia and Kenya. Patients with DCL lack specific cell-mediated immune responses to leishmanial antigens, although delayed hypersensitivity to tuberculin and other antigens appears normal. This is similar to the specific anergy that occurs in lepromatous leprosy. DCL usually begins as a single, nodular, nonulcerating lesion, often on the face, which enlarges and is followed by multiple similar lesions scattered over the entire body, especially on the face and nose, limbs, and buttocks (Fig. 76–11). The lesions do not ulcerate and may coalesce to form plaques. *Leishmania* have been recovered rarely from blood and bone marrow, but visceral lesions do not develop. The leishmanin skin test is persistently negative unless and until recovery occurs.

DIAGNOSIS

Differential Diagnosis. On clinical grounds, the lesions of cutaneous leishmaniasis must be distinguished from diphtheritic or veldt sores, tropical ulcer, tertiary syphilis, yaws, lupus vulgaris, blastomycosis, basal cell epithelioma, and other causes of chronic nodules and ulcers. Although the leishmanin skin test is sometimes helpful, definitive diagnosis depends on demonstration or isolation of the organism.

Demonstration of the Organism. Organisms can sometimes be identified in slit skin smears prepared as for diagnosing leprosy. The margin of the lesion is squeezed between the thumb and forefinger until bloodless; a scalpel blade is used to make a small incision; the cut edge of the incision is scraped with the blade; and the tissue juice on the blade is spread on a clean glass slide and stained with Giemsa or Leishman's stain. Alternatively, a small biopsy specimen may be removed from the edge of the lesion and an impression smear made by pressing the cut surface lightly against a slide. A portion of the biopsy specimen is macerated and cultured in NNN or Schneider's medium, and the remainder is fixed for pathologic examination. Varying numbers of organisms can be identified in histologic sections according to the immune status of the individual. Amastigotes in sections must be differentiated from yeast cells and the intracellular forms of *Histoplasma capsulatum* and *Toxoplasma gondii*. Organisms are especially difficult to find in biopsy specimens of leishmaniasis recidivans, and culture of biopsy specimens must be undertaken in suspected cases. Tissue juice aspirated from the margin of lesions can also be cultured. Cultures generally become positive within 2 to 7 days in Schneider's medium but may take longer (up to 21 days) to grow in NNN medium.

Skin Test. The leishmanin skin test becomes positive within 3 months of the onset of skin lesions and remains positive for life. Skin test–positive individuals may have skin lesions for which the etiology is not leishmaniasis. The skin test is strongly positive in leishmaniasis recidivans but remains negative in DCL.

Serologic Tests. Immunoglobulin levels are normal in cutaneous leishmaniasis. Low titers of antileishmanial antibodies are detected in more than half of patients with cutaneous leishmaniasis, but these tests are generally of little diagnostic help.

TREATMENT. The majority of lesions are self-healing, requiring a few months to a few years to heal completely.

Chemotherapy. Antileishmanial drugs should be given to patients with large or multiple lesions, especially if they are secondarily infected, and to patients with lesions in functionally or cosmetically important areas such as the wrist or face. Pentavalent antimonials (sodium stibogluconate and meglumine antimoniate) are usually effective if given in adequate dose for an adequate duration. Treatment with 10 to 20 mg of Sb/kg/day for 2 to 4 weeks or longer may be needed. Toxicity is unusual with this treatment regimen (Chapter 76.2). Various other drugs have been used to treat cutaneous leishmaniasis, but the lack of controlled trials makes evaluation of their efficacy impossible. Local infiltration of 0.3 to 0.8 ml of sodium stibogluconate or a 5% solution of mepacrine has been used with some success and merits further evaluation, especially for early non-ulcerated lesions. The use of toxic or unusual drugs in the treatment of cutaneous leishmaniasis of the Old World is seldom indicated.

Heat Therapy. Because members of the *L. tropica* species complex do not survive at temperatures above 37C, local heat therapy may be useful in treating unresponsive lesions. This can be accomplished with an ordinary infrared heating lamp or by using a specially fitted prosthesis that can be molded to fit closely against the lesion. The intralesional temperature should be raised to 40 to 42C for 12 hours at a time to achieve a rapid response.

Leishmaniasis Recidivans. The lesions of leishmaniasis recidivans are resistant to ordinary antileishmanial therapy, but some success has been achieved using intralesional emetine, locally applied heat, or injections of transfer factor. The use of higher doses of sodium stibogluconate, e.g., 20 mg of Sb/kg once or twice daily, for a prolonged period (30 to 60 days or longer) should also be considered.

Diffuse Cutaneous Leishmaniasis. DCL is also quite refractory to treatment. Pentavalent antimonials appear to be of no value in Ethiopia. Pentamidine has been helpful in many patients, although it must be administered for many months and lesions usually reappear when the drug is stopped. Pentamidine, given as a single weekly injection of 4 mg/kg body weight for at least 4 months longer than it takes to eliminate parasites from slit skin smears, appears to offer the best compromise between maximal efficacy and minimal toxicity. Diabetes has developed in 10% of Ethiopian patients with DCL treated with pentamidine. (See Chapter 76.2 for additional details about pentamidine toxicity.)

PREVENTION AND CONTROL

Vector Control. Reducing the vector population can decrease the incidence of cutaneous leishmaniasis. Improved general sanitation and removal of refuse and rubble in which sandflies breed reduce the incidence of urban cutaneous leishmaniasis. Residual spraying with DDT for malaria control had eliminated cutaneous leishmaniasis in many areas, although it has returned with the cessation of spraying.

Reservoir Control. In the central Asian republics of the Soviet Union, disease incidence has been reduced by poisoning gerbil burrows with picrotoxin or by deep plowing on irrigation projects to destroy burrows and eliminate gerbils from the area.

Immunization. Vaccination against cutaneous leishmaniasis has been used for many years in Russia, Israel, and Jordan. Live, virulent promastigotes from cultures of *L. major* are inoculated intracutaneously, and a lesion is allowed to develop and run its natural course. This results in a single scar in a cosmetically acceptable location, and the immunity that develops is comparable to that following a natural infection. There is a small risk of a leishmaniasis recidivans lesion's developing at the site of immunization.

BIBLIOGRAPHY

Bryceson ADM: Diffuse cutaneous leishmaniasis in Ethiopia. I. The clinical and histological features. Trans R Soc Trop Med Hyg 63:708, 1969.

Bryceson ADM: Diffuse cutaneous leishmaniasis in Ethiopia. II. Treatment. Trans R Soc Trop Med Hyg 64:369, 1970.

Bryceson ADM: Diffuse cutaneous leishmaniasis in Ethiopia. III. Immunological studies. IV. Pathogenesis. Trans R Soc Trop Med Hyg 64:380, 1970.

Chulay JD, Anzeze EM, Koech DK, Bryceson ADM: High-dose sodium stibogluconate treatment of cutaneous leishmaniasis in Kenya. Trans R Soc Trop Med Hyg 77:717, 1983.

Nadim A, Javadian E, Tahvildar-Bidruni G, Ghorbani M: Effectiveness of leishmanization in the control of cutaneous leishmaniasis. Bull Soc Pathol Exot Filialies 76:377, 1983.

Ridley DS, Ridley MJ: The evolution of the lesion in cutaneous leishmaniasis. J Pathol 141:83, 1983.

Sharquie KE, Al-Talib KK, Chu AC: Intralesional therapy of cutaneous leishmaniasis with sodium stibogluconate antimony. Br J Dermatol 119:53, 1988.

76.4. CUTANEOUS LEISHMANIASIS OF THE NEW WORLD

Jeffrey D. Chulay

DEFINITION. Cutaneous leishmaniasis of the New World is a zoonosis caused by parasites of the species complexes *Leishmania mexicana* and *L. braziliensis*, transmitted by sandflies and characterized by ulcerative skin lesions. Some persons with *L. braziliensis* infection develop destructive oral, nasal, or pharyngeal lesions, called mucocutaneous leishmaniasis or espundia. Local names for cutaneous leishmaniasis of the New World include uta (Peru), chiclero ulcer or bay sore (Mexico), úlcera de Baurú (Brazil), and pian bois, or forest yaws (Guyana). Collectively, these diseases are also referred to as American cutaneous leishmaniasis.

ETIOLOGY. There are presently 3 organisms in the *L. mexicana* complex and 4 in the *L. braziliensis* complex that are known to infect humans (Table 76–1). Members of the *L. mexicana* complex develop only in the midgut and foregut of their sandfly vectors, whereas members of the *L. braziliensis* complex develop in the hindgut as well as the midgut and foregut. *L. chagasi* has also been isolated from lesions of cutaneous leishmaniasis on rare occasions. (See Chapter 76.1 for a detailed description of the parasite.)

DISTRIBUTION AND EPIDEMIOLOGY
(Fig. 76–3)

Leishmania mexicana **Infections.** The parasite causing chiclero ulcer is common throughout southern Mexico, Belize, and Guatemala and has probably been responsible for the rare cases of cutaneous leishmaniasis acquired in the southern United States. It is transmitted among forest rodents by *Lutzomyia olmeca olmeca*, which is not highly attracted to humans. However, the prolonged exposure of "chicleros," who live for many months in the forest collecting chewing gum latex from chicle trees, explains the high incidence of infection in these workers, i.e., 30% during the first year of employment. Timber cutters, road builders, and agricultural workers are also commonly infected.

Leishmania amazonensis **Infections.** This parasite occurs in the Amazon region of Brazil and neighboring countries. It is primarily a disease of forest rodents, but marsupials and foxes can be secondary hosts. Infection rates of 20% occur in some rodent species in Brazil, but human disease is rare because the vector, *Lu. flaviscutellata*, is nocturnal and not very anthropophilic and lives in swampy areas of the forest seldom frequented by people.

Leishmania venezuelensis **Infections.** This parasite has been isolated only from humans with cutaneous leishmaniasis in Venezuela. Like other members of the

L. mexicana complex, it grows rapidly in hamsters and develops in the hindgut of sandflies. It is atypical, however, in its poor long-term growth in blood agar medium. *Lu. olmeca bicolor* is the probable vector. The mammalian host has not yet been discovered.

Leishmania braziliensis **Infections.** *L. braziliensis*, which primarily causes infection of forest rodents, causes cutaneous and mucocutaneous leishmaniasis in humans. Human infection occurs mainly in Brazil but has also been recorded in Peru, Ecuador, Bolivia, Venezuela, Paraguay, and Colombia. The major vector, *Lu. wellcomei*, avidly bites humans and rodents and, unlike most sandflies, feeds during daylight hours. The other vectors, *Lu. intermedius* and *Lu. pessoai*, are also anthropophilic. Disease is common among persons living in farming communities in newly cleared forest areas and in road construction and mining workers.

Leishmania panamensis **Infections.** This parasite is found in Panama and adjacent areas of Central America and Colombia. The principal reservoir is the sloth *Choloepus hoffmanni*. Other sloths, procyonids, and forest primates are secondary hosts. The major vector, *Lu. trapidoi*, usually lives in the forest canopy in close contact with the known reservoirs. However, at certain times of the year, when rainfall is moderate, it can be found close to the ground, where it can bite humans. Human disease is common in rural agricultural workers, especially in the first year after settlement before deforestation is complete, and in military personnel participating in jungle warfare maneuvers.

Leishmania guyanensis **Infections.** Pian bois or forest yaws, the human disease caused by *L. guyanensis*, occurs in the Guyanas and northern Brazil. Because the principal vector, *Lu. umbratilis*, has a high infection rate (up to 7%) and readily bites humans in the daytime when disturbed from its resting sites on tree trunks, disease is common among forest workers. The major reservoirs of *L. guyanensis* are the 2-toed sloth *Choloepus didactylus* and the lesser anteater *Tamandua tetradactyla*.

Leishmania peruviana **Infections.** *L. peruviana* is found only at 900 to 3000 m above sea level in the Peruvian Andes and the highlands of Argentina, where dogs with inapparent infection are the reservoir hosts. Human disease (uta) is contracted in and around the home, and in some villages 90% of people are infected or scarred. *Lu. verrucarum* and *Lu. peruensis* are the probable vectors.

Infections Caused by Other *Leishmania* Species. Parasites have been cultured from lesions of cutaneous leishmaniasis in various parts of South America that have isoenzyme patterns and growth characteristics in culture and laboratory animals that are different from those of known species of *Leishmania*. The parasites isolated from persons with diffuse cutaneous leishmaniasis in the Dominican Republic are also biochemically distinct. Species names have not yet been proposed for these parasites. *L. pifanoi*, suggested as a name for the parasite causing diffuse cutaneous leishmaniasis in Venezuela, seems to be identical to *L. amazonensis*.

PATHOLOGY. Lesions of American cutaneous leishmaniasis demonstrate a variety of pathologic changes. Early skin lesions generally show hyperplasia of the epidermis and necrosis of the dermis, with scattered neutrophils, eosinophils, and mononuclear cells. As the disease progresses, there is heavy infiltration with plasma cells and lymphocytes, followed later by epithelioid cells and Langhans giant cells. Long-standing lesions usually contain well-formed granulomas. Variable numbers of parasites are found within macrophages and free in the tissues (Fig. 73–5L).

Mucosal lesions show necrotizing granulomatous inflammation with a paucity of organisms. In contrast, the lesions of diffuse cutaneous leishmaniasis contain large numbers of amastigote-laden macrophages but very few lymphocytes.

CLINICAL MANIFESTATIONS

Cutaneous Disease. The lesions of cutaneous leishmaniasis of the New World are generally similar to those of Old World disease. A few weeks to several months after infection, an erythematous, often pruritic papule develops at the site of inoculation. This may become scaly or gradually enlarge, developing a raised indurated margin with central ulceration (Fig. 76–12). Verrucous and acneiform lesions are uncommon. The lesions are usually painless, unless secondarily infected. The natural history varies, depending on the infecting species, location of the lesion, and host immunity. *L. mexicana* infections generally have one or a few lesions, which heal spontaneously within 6 months, but lesions on the ear occur in 40% of patients and are chronic, lasting many years (Fig. 76–13). Simple cutaneous lesions caused by parasites of the *L. braziliensis* complex generally require 6 to 18 months for spontaneous healing but sometimes persist much longer. Multiple skin lesions due to metastatic spread along lymphatics are common with *L. guyanensis* infections, and subcutaneous lymphatic nodules resembling sporotrichosis are often seen in *L. panamensis* infections.

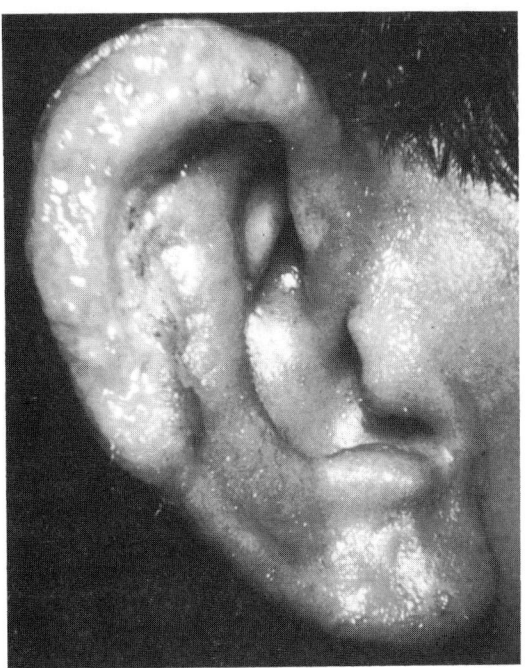

FIGURE 76–13. Chiclero ulcer. (Courtesy of the Louisiana State University School of Medicine, New Orleans.)

Mucosal Disease. Many persons infected with *L. braziliensis* develop metastatic spread of disease to the nasal, pharyngeal, and buccal mucosa, known as espundia. Mucosal lesions appear several months to many years after the initial cutaneous lesion, which has usually healed. Erythema and edema of the involved mucosa are followed by ulcerations that are covered with a mucopurulent exudate. There is often mutilating destruction of the nasal septum (Fig. 76–14), palate, lips, pharynx, and larynx. The lesions are chronic and progressive, and death can be caused by aspiration or inanition. Mucosal lesions occur rarely in *L. panamensis* infections.

Diffuse Cutaneous Leishmaniasis (DCL). In Venezuela, Brazil, Mexico, and the Dominican Republic, a diffuse form of cutaneous leishmaniasis occurs that is similar to DCL in Ethiopia (Fig. 76–11). The initial lesion is usually a macule, papule, or nodule (rarely an ulcer). Because of an immunologic defect in the host, the parasite spreads locally and hematogenously to cause generalized nodular lesions consisting of heavily parasitized macrophages. The nasal mucosa and laryngopharynx are sometimes involved, but visceral lesions do not occur. As in patients with DCL in Ethiopia, there is specific anergy to leishmanin but not to unrelated antigens such as tuberculin.

DIAGNOSIS

Demonstration of the Organism. As in other forms of leishmaniasis, definitive diagnosis requires demonstration of the parasite. The methods are the same as those for diagnosis of cutaneous leishmaniasis of the Old World (Chapter 76.3). Organisms are generally numerous in smears and biopsy specimens (Fig. 73–5L) of lesions of diffuse cutaneous leishmaniasis and cutaneous leishmaniasis caused by *L. mexicana* but are often scanty in *L. braziliensis* infection of both the skin and mucous

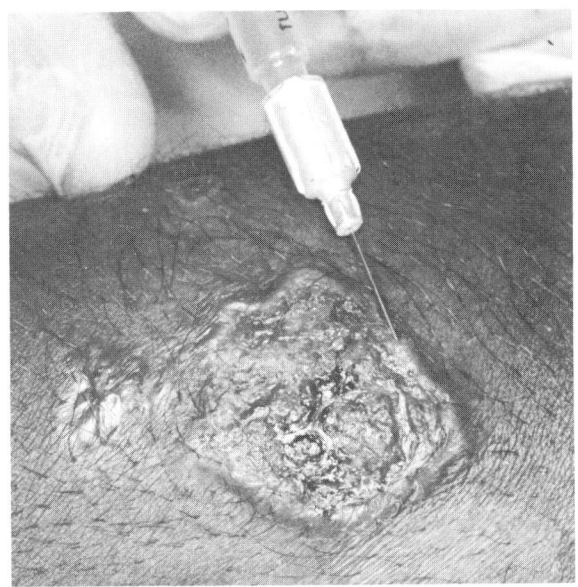

FIGURE 76–12. Cutaneous leishmaniasis due to *Leishmania panamensis.* Note the elevated margin and the satellite lesion. The picture also demonstrates the technique of aspirating tissue fluid for parasite culture. (Courtesy of Dr. L. D. Hendricks, Walter Reed Army Institute of Research, Washington, DC.)

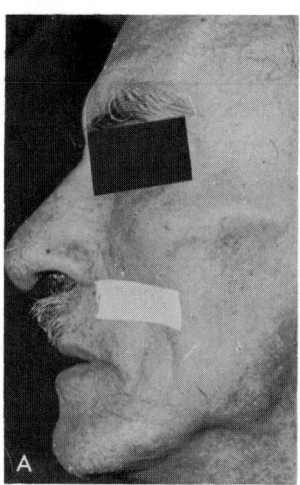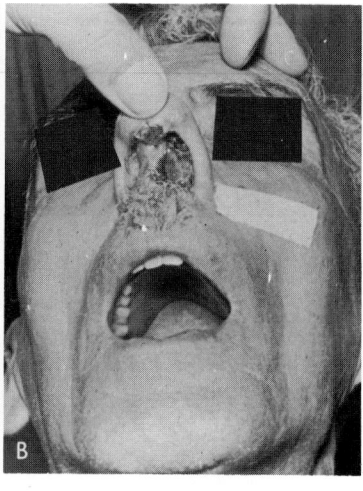

FIGURE 76–14. Mucocutaneous leishmaniasis in a Costa Rican patient who had the disease for more than 15 years. *A*, Lateral view showing the tapir nose. *B*, Destruction of the nasal septum. (Courtesy of the Louisiana State University School of Medicine, New Orleans.)

membranes, especially in long-standing disease. Cultures of tissue juice aspirated from the indurated margin of a skin lesion (Fig. 76–12) or cultures or hamster inoculation of biopsy specimens of skin or mucosal lesions are more likely to confirm *L. braziliensis* infection.

Skin Test. The leishmanin skin test is positive in almost all patients with active cutaneous and mucocutaneous leishmaniasis, although it may be negative during the first few months. Treatment is occasionally justified despite the failure to demonstrate parasites in persons with typical lesions and a positive skin test, especially in those with espundia. In DCL, the skin test is uniformly negative, and in vitro lymphocyte blastogenesis in response to leishmanial antigens does not occur. Adherent suppressor cells (monocytes) have been found in patients from the Dominican Republic with DCL.

Serologic Tests. A large number of tests for antibodies against *Leishmania* have been developed, but none is ideal for diagnosing cutaneous and mucocutaneous leishmaniasis. The most commonly used are an indirect fluorescent antibody test using amastigotes, a direct agglutination test using promastigotes, and an enzyme-linked immunosorbent assay (ELISA) using antigens obtained from promastigotes. All are positive in only 70 to 80% of cases and are especially likely to be negative early in the course of the disease. Serial measurement of antibody may be helpful in evaluating the response to treatment in patients who have a positive test initially.

Differential Diagnosis. Cutaneous leishmaniasis must be distinguished from sporotrichosis, blastomycosis, yaws, syphilis, cutaneous tuberculosis, and *Mycobacterium marinum* infection. Diseases that may resemble espundia include paracoccidioidomycosis, histoplasmosis, tuberculosis, syphilis, malignant tumors, and lethal midline granuloma. Diffuse cutaneous leishmaniasis must be differentiated from lepromatous leprosy.

TREATMENT. In patients with espundia, adequate nutrition must be ensured, and destructive or obstructive lesions may require ventilatory support or treatment, as in aspiration pneumonia. Plastic surgery may be required after parasitologic cure in patients with extensive tissue destruction from espundia.

In contrast to Old World cutaneous leishmaniasis, systemic chemotherapy is generally indicated in American cutaneous leishmaniasis because of the risk of subsequent mucosal disease (*L. braziliensis* infections), the multiplicity of lesions (*L. guyanensis* infection), the chronicity of untreated disease (*L. mexicana* ear lesions and *L. braziliensis* complex infections), or invariable progression of mucosal disease in the absence of chemotherapy.

Pentavalent Antimonials. Antimony is the treatment of choice for all forms of New World cutaneous leishmaniasis. In Latin America, meglumine antimoniate (Glucantime) is used because sodium stibogluconate (Pentostam) is not generally available. In the United States, sodium stibogluconate is available under an Investigational New Drug (IND) application from the Centers for Disease Control. A randomized controlled trial in patients with *L. panamensis* infections showed that treatment with sodium stibogluconate at a dosage of 20 mg of Sb/kg/day for 20 days gave a significantly higher cure rate than did a dosage of 10 mg of Sb/kg/day for 20 days. This dosage and duration are also recommended for other forms of simple American cutaneous leishmaniasis. Serious toxicity is unusual with such a treatment regimen (Chapter 76.2). If toxicity does occur at the higher doses, the drug should be withheld until it resolves and treatment resumed at a slightly lower dose once or twice daily.

Espundia usually responds to treatment with pentavalent antimonials, but relapse is common unless dosages of 20 mg of Sb/kg/day are administered for at least 30 days. Relapses have been successfully treated with 20 mg of Sb/kg/day for 60 to 90 days.

In contrast to Ethiopian DCL, Venezuelan DCL usually improves after initial treatment with pentavalent antimonials, although relapse is invariable and patients who relapse often do not respond to additional antimony treatment. Although untested, it would seem reasonable to treat newly diagnosed DCL patients with 10 to 20 mg of Sb/kg once or twice daily until apparent clinical and parasitologic cure is achieved and for several months thereafter.

Other Drugs. In patients unresponsive to pentavalent antimonials, amphotericin B is often effective. It is administered by slow intravenous infusion in gradually increasing doses to 1 mg/kg, at which level it should be given on alternate days. Prolonged treatment to a total of 2 to 3 gm is generally required. (See Chapters 67 and 76.2 for additional details about the toxicity and use of amphotericin B.)

Ketoconazole at a dosage of 600 mg once daily for 28 days appears to be as effective (70% cure rate) as a low dosage of sodium stibogluconate (10 mg of Sb/kg/day) in patients with cutaneous leishmaniasis caused by *L. panamensis*. Because it can be given orally, ketoconazole may thus have a role in some patients for whom parenteral therapy is not possible. Ketoconazole is not effective for *L. braziliensis* infections.

Pentamidine should also be considered in patients unresponsive to antimonials. Although experience is lacking, prolonged treatment with pentamidine at a dosage of 4 mg/kg 3 times weekly for many months, as described in Chapter 76.2 for visceral leishmaniasis, is recommended.

Immunotherapy. Studies in Venezuela have shown that treatment with 3 injections of heat-killed *L. amazonensis* promastigotes mixed with viable bacille Calmette-Guérin (BCG) given intradermally every 6 to 8 weeks is as effective as meglumine antimoniate in achieving clinical cures of localized cutaneous leishmaniasis caused by *L. braziliensis,* and either of these treatments is more effective than BCG alone. Treatment with chemotherapy plus combined immunotherapy was also variably effective in 8 of 9 patients with DCL. Because of its low cost and suitability for administration by unsophisticated primary health care workers, immunotherapy may be an especially useful treatment modality in less developed countries where leishmaniasis is endemic.

PROGNOSIS. Cutaneous lesions usually heal within 1 month after initiation of treatment with pentavalent antimonials, although large ulcers may require a longer healing time. Mucosal disease caused by *L. braziliensis,* which may appear many years after the primary cutaneous lesion has resolved, is progressive unless treated. The risk of espundia appears to be reduced in persons whose primary cutaneous lesions are treated with adequate dosages of pentavalent antimonials. Diffuse cutaneous leishmaniasis is characteristically a relapsing or chronically progressive disease.

PREVENTION AND CONTROL. Vaccines and chemoprophylactic drugs are not available. Because of the forest location of vectors and reservoirs, control of American cutaneous and mucocutaneous leishmaniasis is not possible. The only exception is uta, which, because of its domiciliary nature, can be controlled by spraying houses with insecticides. Insect repellents, long-sleeved shirts, and fine-mesh bed netting may reduce the risk of infection for individuals.

BIBLIOGRAPHY

Ballou WR, McClain JB, Gordon DM, et al: Safety and efficacy of high-dose sodium stibogluconate therapy of American cutaneous leishmaniasis. Lancet 2:13, 1987.

Berman JD: Chemotherapy of leishmaniasis: Biochemical mechanisms, clinical efficacy and future strategies. Rev Infect Dis 10:560, 1988.

Bryceson A: Therapy in man. *In* Peters W, Killick-Kendrick R (eds): The Leishmaniases in Biology and Medicine. London and New York, Academic Press, 1987, p 847.

Cerf B, Reed SG, Netto EM, et al: Epidemiology of American cutaneous leishmaniasis due to *Leishmania braziliensis braziliensis.* J Infect Dis 156:73, 1987.

Convit J, Castellanos PL, Ulrich M, et al: Immunotherapy of localized, intermediate, and diffuse forms of American cutaneous leishmaniasis. J Infect Dis 160:104, 1989.

Hendricks LD, Wright N: Diagnosis of cutaneous leishmaniasis by *in vitro* cultivation of saline aspirates in Schneider's *Drosophila* medium. Am J Trop Med Hyg 28:962, 1979.

Marsden PD: Mucosal leishmaniasis ("espundia" Escomel, 1911). Trans R Soc Trop Med Hyg 80:859, 1986.

Marsden PD, Sampaio RN, Carvalho EM, et al: High continuous antimony therapy in two patients with unresponsive mucosal leishmaniasis. Am J Trop Med Hyg 34:710, 1985.

Ridley DS, Marsden PD, Cuba CC, et al: A histological classification of mucocutaneous leishmaniasis in Brazil and its clinical evaluation. Trans R Soc Trop Med Hyg 74:508, 1980.

Shaw JJ, Lainson R: Ecology and epidemiology: New World. *In* Peters W, Killick-Kendrick R (eds): The Leishmaniases in Biology and Medicine. London and New York, Academic Press, 1987, p 291.

77. BABESIOSIS

Trenton K. Ruebush II

DEFINITION. Babesiosis, or piroplasmosis, is a hemoprotozoan infection of animals characterized by fever, hemolytic anemia, hemoglobinuria, and renal failure. It is transmitted by ixodid ticks. Occasional human infections with *Babesia* species occur when humans intrude into the zoonotic cycle between the tick vector and its vertebrate host.

ETIOLOGY AND HISTORY. Organisms of the genus Babesia are intraerythrocytic protozoan parasites of a wide variety of domestic and wild animals. Morphologically, *Babesia* closely resemble malaria parasites but can be distinguished from them by the absence of pigment in infected red blood cells. More than 70 different species of *Babesia* have been described, including *B. bigemina, B. argentina,* and *B. divergens* in cattle; *B. caballi* and *B. equi* in horses; *B. canis* in dogs; and *B. microti* and *B. rodhaini* in rodents. At present, identification of different species of *Babesia* is based largely on their morphology and the vertebrate host in which the parasite is found. This practice has led to considerable confusion in taxonomy because the morphologic characteristics of a single strain of *Babesia* may vary in different hosts and the host range of some species is quite broad. In some cases, the same organism may even carry 2 or more different names.

Babesiosis is important historically because *B. bigemina,* the cause of Texas cattle fever, was the first organism shown to be transmitted by an arthropod. This finding in 1893 by Smith and Kilborne predated by several years the discovery of the routes of transmission for malaria, filariasis, and yellow fever.

DISTRIBUTION AND INCIDENCE. *Babesia* infections in wild and domestic animals occur worldwide and are well known in veterinary medicine. In many countries, they are responsible for serious economic losses to the livestock industry.

Human babesiosis, in contrast, is somewhat of a medical curiosity. Fewer than 100 cases have been reported, all of them from Europe and North America. The European cases were acquired in Yugoslavia, France, Ireland, Great Britain, the Soviet Union, and Spain and are thought to have been caused by *B. divergens*, a parasite of cattle. *B. microti*, an organism that normally infects rodents, has been responsible for most of the North American cases. The majority of these infections were acquired on a chain of islands that lie off the coast of New England, including Nantucket and Martha's Vineyard, Massachusetts, and Long Island and Shelter Island, New York, although cases have also been reported from Wisconsin.

Cases of human babesiosis in which the species of the infecting organism could not be identified have been reported from California, Georgia, and Mexico.

TRANSMISSION. Babesiosis is transmitted in nature by ixodid, or hard-bodied, ticks (Fig. 77–1). Organisms are ingested by the tick when it feeds. The parasites then multiply within the epithelial cells of the tick's gut and spread throughout its body. In some species of ticks, *Babesia* organisms invade the ovaries and are passed through the egg to the developing larval stage (transovarial transmission). In such cases, the tick may serve as both vector and reservoir for the parasite. In other tick species, infections are acquired during the larval or nymphal stage and are transmitted by the subsequent stage after the tick has molted (trans-stadial passage).

EPIDEMIOLOGY. Human babesiosis is a zoonotic disease. Infection is acquired accidentally when humans intrude in the natural cycle of the parasite between the tick vector and its domestic or wild animal host. Epidemiologically, several differences are apparent between the cases of human babesiosis acquired in Europe and those reported from North America. The European cases have been sporadic in occurrence and widely distributed geographically. The causative organism is a parasite of cattle, *B. divergens*. All of the infections occurred in persons who had previously had splenectomies, a factor that is believed to have increased their susceptibility to this parasite. In contrast, the majority of cases reported from North America were acquired in a circumscribed area along the northeastern coast of the United States. The infections were caused by a parasite of rodents, *B. microti*, which has a much broader host

range than *B. divergens* and is capable of infecting human beings with functioning spleens.

The vector in the European cases is probably *Ixodes ricinus*, the tick responsible for transmission of the parasite among cattle. *I. dammini*, a tick that feeds on rodents during its larval and nymphal stages and on deer as an adult, is the vector of *B. microti*.

Cases of human babesiosis occur only in situations in which the following factors are present: a parasite infective for humans, a tick vector that feeds on humans, and opportunity for contact between humans and the infected vector. Because of the wide geographic distribution of *Babesia* infections in wild and domestic animal populations, contact between human beings and infected ticks is probably a frequent occurrence. Thus, the host ranges of the parasite and tick vector appear to be of greater importance in determining whether or not human babesiosis will occur in an area. In the case of *B. microti* infections in the northeastern United States, *I. dammini* readily feeds on humans, and the parasite has a wide host range, ensuring relatively frequent human infections. In contrast, in Europe, where *B. divergens* is apparently infective only for splenectomized persons, human infections are likely to be sporadic because of the low risk of contact between an infected tick and a splenectomized patient. The absence or rarity of recognized cases of human babesiosis from other parts of the world may be due to even more restricted vector and parasite host ranges. However, it is possible that such infections do occur but do not come to medical attention or are not recognized as babesiosis. Underdiagnosis may be the major reason for the limited geographic distribution of human *B. microti* infections, because the parasite has been identified in rodent populations in many parts of the United States and the range of the vector extends north into Canada and at least as far west as Wisconsin.

Babesia may also be transmitted by blood transfusion. This route of infection is particularly likely in the case of human *B. microti* infections because of the tendency of this parasite to cause prolonged asymptomatic parasitemias.

PATHOGENESIS AND PATHOLOGY. Babesia is an intraerythrocytic parasite. No evidence for an exo-erythrocytic stage, such as occurs in malaria, has been found. *Babesia* multiplies asexually by budding within red blood cells, usually forming 2 or 4 daughter parasites. When the infected red blood cell ruptures, other erythrocytes are invaded, and the cycle is repeated. The major clinicopathologic features of babesiosis, including hemoglobinemia, hemoglobinuria, jaundice, and renal insufficiency or failure, are the result of the multiplication of organisms within the red blood cells and the subsequent destruction of those cells.

Babesia infections in animals frequently persist for many years after the acute illness. These prolonged parasitemias are thought to be due to the ability of the parasites to change the specificity of their surface antigens in response to exposure to specific antibody, a phenomenon known as antigenic variation. After each passage through the tick vector, the parasites apparently revert to a common antigenic type.

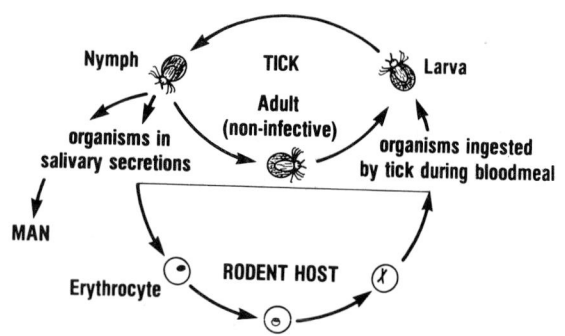

FIGURE 77–1. Life cycle of *Babesia microti*.

Several factors influence the response of a vertebrate host to *Babesia* infection. Different species of *Babesia* vary markedly in their virulence for different animals, and the susceptibility of a particular vertebrate host may be affected by its age and the presence or absence of a spleen. In cattle and horses and perhaps also in *B. microti* infections in humans, severity of infection appears to be related to host age. Infections in older animals are usually quite severe, whereas younger animals tend to have mild or even asymptomatic infections. The spleen also plays an important role in immunity to *Babesia*. Splenectomized patients are more susceptible to infection than persons with intact spleens, and in animals splenectomy frequently causes a recurrence of parasitemia and symptoms.

CLINICAL MANIFESTATIONS

***Babesia microti* Infections.** Human *B. microti* infections range in severity from asymptomatic to prolonged severe illness. Most patients have a gradual onset of irregular fever, chills, diaphoresis, generalized myalgia, and fatigue. There is no periodicity of symptoms. The incubation period varies from 1 to 4 weeks, although most patients do not remember a tick bite.

On physical examination, the only constant finding is fever. Mild hepatosplenomegaly occurs occasionally. Most patients have a mild to moderately severe hemolytic anemia and a normal or slightly depressed white blood cell count. In about half of the patients, there are slight elevations of liver enzymes and bilirubin.

The illness may last from a few weeks to several months. Although relapses, such as are seen in malaria, have not been observed in *B. microti* infections, complete recovery is often delayed by prolonged weakness and malaise. Parasitemia may persist at low levels with or without symptoms for up to 4 months after the onset of illness.

Splenectomized patients infected with *B. microti* generally have higher levels of parasitemia and more severe hemolytic anemia than persons with functioning spleens.

***Babesia divergens* Infections.** Human *B. divergens* infections are characterized by chills, high fever, nausea, vomiting, and severe hemolytic anemia, which progress rapidly to jaundice, hemoglobinemia, hemoglobinuria, and renal insufficiency or failure. All patients studied had undergone splenectomies before becoming infected for reasons that included trauma, surgical accidents, portal hypertension, and lymphoma. Fever, hypotension, and jaundice are the major findings on physical examination. Anemia is generally severe, with elevated reticulocyte counts and nucleated red blood cells on peripheral blood smears. Marked elevations of bilirubin, liver enzymes, blood urea nitrogen, and creatinine levels are common. Most human *B. divergens* infections are fatal.

DIAGNOSIS

Parasite Identification. The diagnosis of human babesiosis requires the identification of characteristic intraerythrocytic parasites on Giemsa-stained thin or thick blood smears (Fig. 77–2). Examination of repeated blood smears may be necessary because of the low-level parasitemia seen in some patients. The morphologic characteristics of *Babesia* parasites are variable, and the same species or strain of *Babesia* may produce morphologically distinct forms in different vertebrate hosts. In humans, *B. microti* usually appears as a small ring form indistinguishable from young trophozoites of *Plasmodium falciparum*. Older stages have more abundant cytoplasm and chromatin. Unlike *Plasmodium* species, no pigment is produced in erythrocytes infected with *Babesia* parasites. Dividing parasites, made up of 4 daughter cells held together by thin strands of cytoplasm, are rarely seen in human blood films.

B. divergens in human blood smears range from round, oval, or piriform in shape to small ring forms. Dividing parasites usually consist of 2 daughter cells.

Differential Diagnosis. Babesiosis should be considered in any patient with a fever and a history of a tick bite or exposure to ticks. Hemolytic anemia is usually present but may be quite mild. Even though all reported cases of human babesiosis have been acquired in Europe and North America, the diagnosis of human babesiosis should not be ruled out in patients from other parts of the world, because *Babesia* infections in lower animals are worldwide in distribution.

Serologic Tests. Several serologic tests for babesiosis have been developed and may aid in suspected cases but should not be considered a substitute for parasitologic diagnosis. Serologic cross-reactions occur with other species of *Babesia* and with malaria parasites, but antibody titers are generally highest to the infecting organism.

Isolation in Animals. In cases in which organisms are difficult to detect in blood smears, intraperitoneal or intravenous inoculation of small laboratory animals such as hamsters or gerbils has been helpful in diagnosis. *B. microti* parasitemia usually appears in inoculated animals within 2 to 4 weeks. Although *B. divergens* seems to have a narrower host range than *B. microti*, attempts to infect gerbils have been successful, indicating that inoculation of this animal might also be used as an aid to diagnosis.

TREATMENT AND PROGNOSIS. Evaluation of treatment regimens for human babesiosis has been complicated by the small number of cases and the fact that *Babesia* is resistant to most antiprotozoal drugs used in human medicine. In many of the reported cases, it is not clear whether the therapeutic regimen was effective or whether the patient would have recovered spontaneously.

Human *B. microti* infections are generally self-limited, although symptoms and parasitemia may persist for several months. Because no completely effective drugs have been identified for the treatment of these infections, symptomatic therapy is probably sufficient in the majority of patients. Chloroquine, which was initially reported to be effective in human *B. microti* infections, seems to act primarily as an anti-inflammatory agent, reducing fever and myalgia, rather than as an antibabesial drug. Pentamidine isethionate has been reported in several cases to reduce fever and parasitemia; however, organisms were not eradicated from the blood. In asplenic patients and in patients with functioning spleens who have severe infections, quinine (650 mg orally 3 times daily) and clindamycin (600 mg orally 3 times

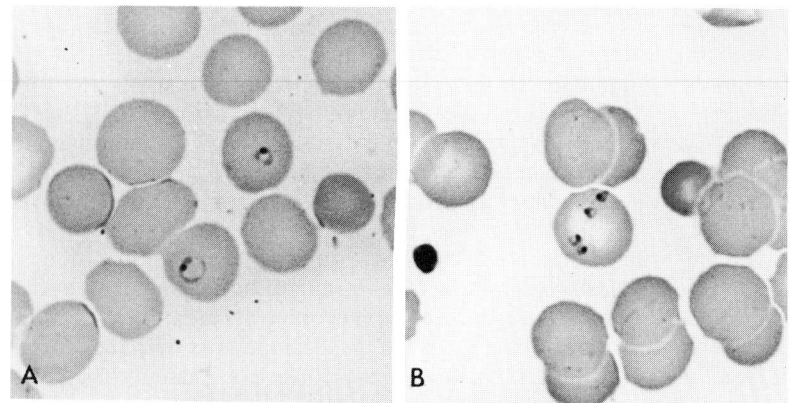

FIGURE 77–2. *Babesia microti* in human blood film (× 1250). *A*, Young trophozoites. *B*, Dividing form made up of 4 daughter parasites. (From Ruebush TK II: Babesia. *In* Mandel GL, Douglas RG, Bennett JE: Principles and Practice of Infectious Disease. New York, Wiley & Sons, 1979.)

daily or 600 mg parenterally twice daily) for 5 to 10 days is currently the treatment of choice. Exchange blood transfusion has been used successfully in several splenectomized patients with severe *B. microti* infection, but this technique should be considered only when all other therapy has failed.

The treatment of human *B. divergens* infections is extremely difficult owing to the fulminant course of the disease. The only patients who have recovered have been aggressively managed with blood transfusions and renal dialysis. No chemotherapeutic agents have been shown to be effective; however, pentamidine is a logical choice for treatment, because it is known to be effective against several species of *Babesia* in animals.

PREVENTION AND CONTROL. *Babesia* infections can be prevented by avoiding exposure to ticks. If this is not feasible, it is recommended that ticks be removed as soon as possible after they have attached, because there is evidence to suggest that the tick does not transmit infective organisms until it has been feeding

for at least 12 hours. Blood transfusion–induced babesiosis can be prevented only by careful screening of prospective donors, excluding all persons from endemic areas who have a history of fever in the preceding 1 to 2 months.

BIBLIOGRAPHY

Garnham PCC: Human babesiosis: European aspects. Trans R Soc Trop Med Hyg 74:153, 1980.
Healy GR, Ruebush TK II: Morphology of *Babesia microti* in human blood smears. Am J Clin Pathol 73:107, 1980.
Jacoby GA, Hunt JV, Kosinski KS, et al: Treatment of transfusion-transmitted babesiosis by exchange transfusion. N Engl J Med 303:1098, 1980.
Rowin KS, Tanowitz HB, Wittner M: Therapy of experimental babesiosis. Ann Intern Med 97:556, 1982.
Rowin KS, Tanowitz HB, Rubinstein A, et al: Babesiosis in asplenic hosts. Trans R Soc Trop Med Hyg 78:442, 1984.
Ruebush TK II: Human babesiosis in North America. Trans R Soc Trop Med Hyg 74:149, 1980.

SECTION C

TISSUE INFECTIONS

78. TOXOPLASMOSIS

Jacob K. Frenkel

DEFINITION. Toxoplasmosis is a generalized infection of animals and humans produced by the sporozoan *Toxoplasma gondii*. The infection may be asymptomatic or may be accompanied by fever or symptoms of lung, liver, heart, brain, lymph node, or eye involvement; during pregnancy, fetal infection may result. Immunity is associated with chronic infection, which may recrudesce when a patient is immunosuppressed, particularly causing encephalitis in patients with acquired immunodeficiency syndrome (AIDS). Death may result from acute or recrudescent infection. The infection is transmitted by oocysts shed in the feces of cats, the definitive host, usually via contaminated soil, by tissue cysts from infected meat, and rarely, by tachyzoites in blood.

ETIOLOGY AND HISTORY

Discovery of the Organism. *Toxoplasma* was discovered first in laboratory animals and simultaneously in 2 tropical countries in 1908 long before it was appreciated as a pathogen of humans and domestic animals. Charles Nicolle and Louis Manceaux described a *Leishmania*-like parasite in the gondi, a small North African rodent used in research on leishmaniasis and typhus fever at the Pasteur Institute in Tunisia. Alfonso Splendore described it from laboratory rabbits at the Portuguese hospital in São Paulo, Brazil. The name *Toxoplasma gondii* was given to the parasite by Nicolle and Manceaux in 1909 after they differentiated this new tissue parasite from *Leishmania* and *Piroplasma*.

Human Disease. The first well-documented human case of toxoplasmosis was described in 1923 by Josef Janku in Prague in a congenitally infected baby with retinochoroiditis due to what was believed to be *En-*

cephalitozoon (Chapter 81.2). Toxoplasmosis became recognized as a human disease through the clinical and pathologic descriptions of babies with the congenital infection by Abner Wolf, David Cowan, and Beryl Paige from New York, together with the isolation of *Toxoplasma*. The first adult case of toxoplasmosis was diagnosed in 1940 by Henry Pinkerton and David Weinman in a Peruvian patient with concomitant bartonellosis. The development of diagnostic tests, especially the dye test by Albert Sabin and Harry Feldman in 1948, was an important milestone. The recognition of ocular toxoplasmosis in humans was aided by the development of the skin test.

Life Cycle. Numerous animals were found infected, e.g., dogs, cats, sheep, pigs, rats, pigeons, and zoo animals. It became clear that ingestion of raw or undercooked meat could lead to infection, but it remained a mystery how herbivorous "meat animals" became infected. Attempts at transmission of *Toxoplasma* through arthropods were not successful. There was no evidence of sexually transmitted infection. In 1967, William Hutchison showed that cats that had eaten *Toxoplasma*-infected mice shed an infectious stage in their feces. Although first associated with eggs of the nematode *Toxocara cati*, this transmission hypothesis was soon "dewormed" and linked to a new stage, the *Toxoplasma* oocyst, in 1970.

Parasite Stages. Recognition of the coccidian oocyst in the life cycle of *Toxoplasma* explained its transmission to herbivores. It also led to the recognition of the 2-host coccidian life cycle (Fig. 78–1). An enteroepithelial cycle was identified in the intestine of cats with 5 types of multiplicative stages, followed by the development of macrogametocytes and microgametocytes, by gametogony, and by oocysts, which are shed in the feces.

The oocyst is ovoid and measures 9×13 μm (Fig. 78–2D). It sporulates in the feces or soil, differentiating into 2 sporocysts, each with 4 sporozoites.

Previously, 2 tissue forms had been known. The tachyzoites are 2 to 4 μm $\times$ 6 to 7 μm ovoid organisms that multiply rapidly during the acute infection (Fig. 78–2A). The bradyzoites in tissue cysts are found during chronic infection, principally in muscles and brain (Fig. 78–2B and C). Tachyzoites and tissue cysts occur in all animals now recognized as intermediate hosts and also in cats, the final host, which may be regarded as a complete host (Fig. 78–1).

The incubation, or prepatent, period in cats until oocyst shedding varies with the infecting stage. After infection with tissue cysts, almost 100% of cats will shed oocysts, and the prepatent period is 3 to 10 days. However, after the ingestion of oocysts or tachyzoites, only 16 to 20% of cats shed oocysts, and the prepatent period ranges from 19 to 48 days. The cyst stage, defined as giving rise to a short prepatent period, is reached 3 to 5 days following infection with tachyzoites, 7 days after infection with cysts, and 9 days after infection with sporozoites. It takes longer for bradyzoites and cysts to become resistant to pepsin or for cysts to become morphologically recognizable by their cyst wall or by the presence of large periodic acid-Schiff-positive cytoplasmic inclusions.

DISTRIBUTION AND PREVALENCE. *Toxoplasma* is spread worldwide principally by the millions of oocysts shed by cats. Theoretically, birds can carry *Toxoplasma* to an area lacking cats, such as islands; however, the purely carnivorous transmission to one or a few predators at a time is unlikely to maintain the infection.

The incidence of *Toxoplasma* infection in humans

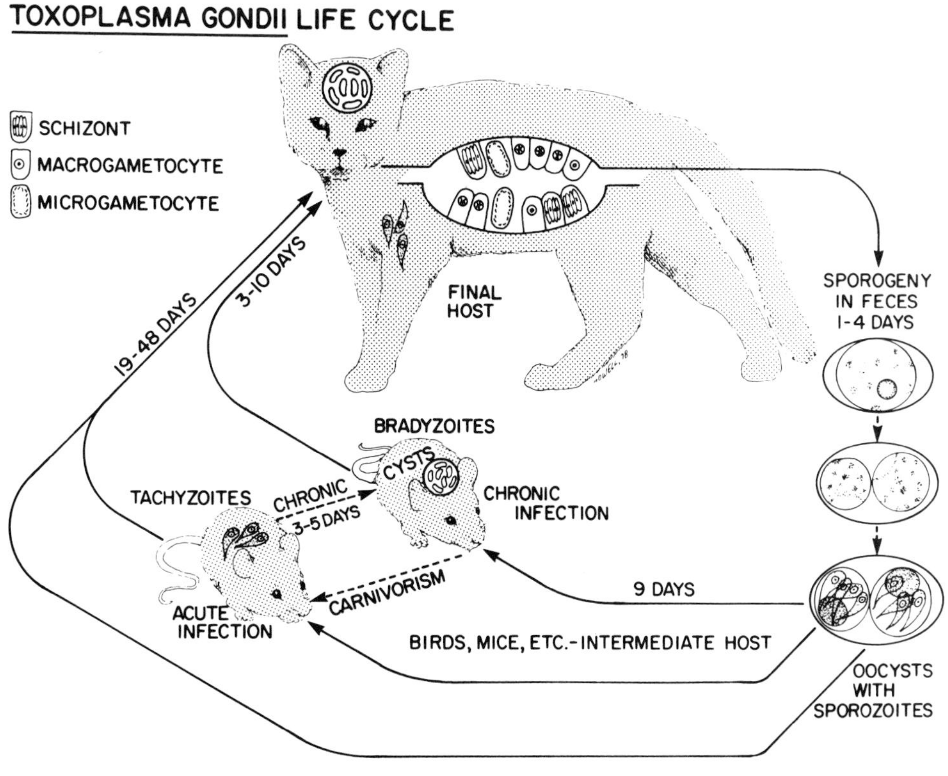

TOXOPLASMA GONDII LIFE CYCLE

FIGURE 78–1. Life cycle of *Toxoplasma gondii*; details in text. (From Frenkel JK: *In* Montali RJ, Migaki G (eds): The Comparative Pathology of Zoo Animals. Washington, DC, Smithsonian Institution Press, 1980, pp 329–342.)

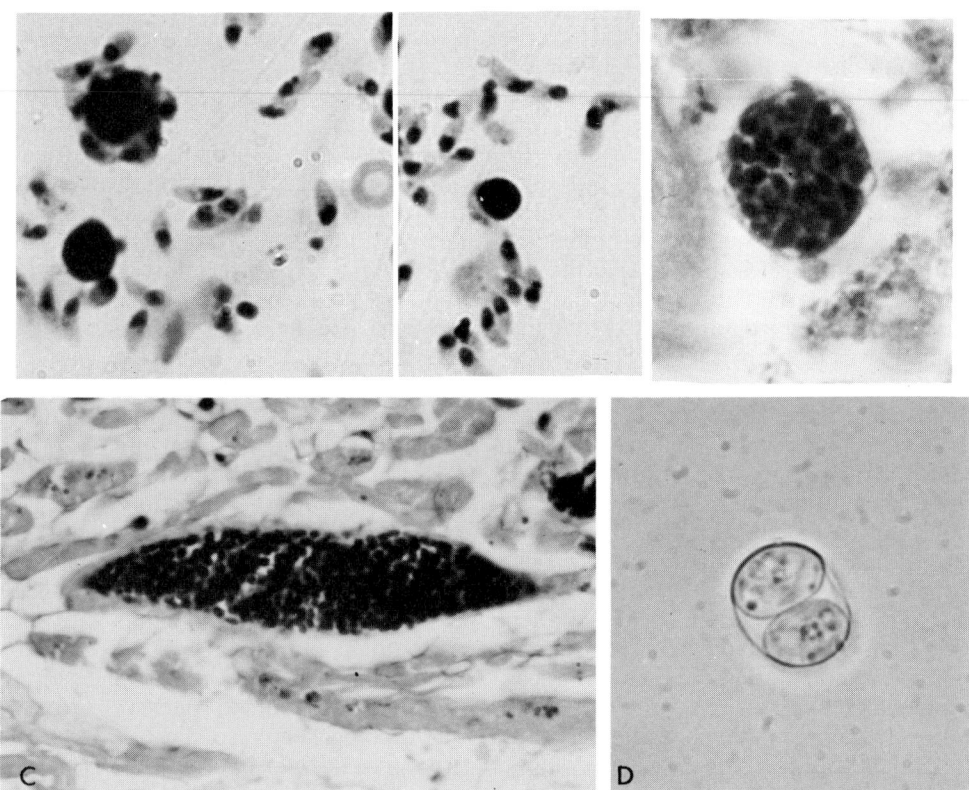

FIGURE 78–2. *A,* Tachyzoites of *Toxoplasma* in mouse peritoneal fluid (× 1000). (Courtesy of The Louisiana State University School of Medicine, New Orleans.) *B,* Tissue cyst of *T. gondii* containing bradyzoites in section of brain. (Courtesy of Dr. Paul A. McGarry, Louisiana State University School of Medicine, New Orleans.) *C,* Tissue cyst of *T. gondii* containing bradyzoites in heart muscle (periodic acid-Schiff, hematoxylin stain, × 700). (From Marcial-Rojas RA: Pathology of Protozoal and Helminthic Diseases, Baltimore, Williams & Wilkins, 1971.) *D,* Oocyst of *T. gondii* from feces of cat, containing 2 sporocysts with 4 sporozoites in each (unstained, × 1500).

varies widely, and as shown by Feldman, the prevalence increases with age. Prevalence rates in individuals 15 to 25 years old are 14% in the United States, 50% in Colombia, 56% in Brazil, 61% in Costa Rica, 27% in New York City and in London, 81% in French Parisians, but only 53% in Spanish, North African, and Portuguese persons living in Paris. Other ethnic differences have been found by Wallace in Hawaii. Within the United States, rates were highest in the eastern and central areas (18 to 20%) and lowest in the mountain and Pacific areas (3 to 8%). Dryness limits the survival of oocysts in soil. Low prevalence rates may also result from a low density of cats and intermediate hosts, giving rise to great variations from one locality to another. In a survey of settlements of Alaskan Eskimos and Indians by Donald R. Peterson and associates, prevalence rates were found to vary between 5 and 50%, and cats were found in up to 50% of habitations. The high antibody prevalence rates found in France and Germany probably stem from local customs of eating undercooked meat, especially mutton. Prevalence rates of infection in humans and other mammals can generally be estimated serologically, because antibody persists for years and possibly for life; however, for birds, tissues would have to be passaged, because many avian species do not develop an antibody that is detected in the common serologic tests.

TRANSMISSION. The modes of transmission rec-

ognized and the stages involved were, first, transplacental transmission by tachyzoites, followed by carnivorism via tissue cysts, and then, in 1970, fecal-oral spread by oocysts. However, the biologic frequency and importance of those modes follow the reverse order.

Oral Transmission

Oocysts. A cat that has eaten a single infected bird or mouse may shed millions of oocysts capable of infecting theoretically a similar number of intermediate hosts; transplacental or carnivorous transmission can infect only one or few animals at a time. Oocysts persist in moist soil for weeks and months. Deposits of infected cat feces remained infectious to mice for a year in Costa Rica and for 18 months in Kansas. Rain, earthworms, dung beetles, and cockroaches may be instrumental in slightly spreading the oocysts from where the feces have been deposited. After 2 weeks, oocyst-contaminated moist soil cannot be recognized, except by inoculation into susceptible animals. Therefore, humans, especially children, can become infected with oocysts from seemingly clean soil (Fig. 78–3). Outbreaks of toxoplasmosis in a riding stable in Atlanta, Georgia, and in a group of soldiers in jungle warfare training in Panama have been circumstantially traced to oocyst contamination of soil and water, respectively.

Tissue Cysts. Most intermediate hosts though infected by oocysts will transmit the infection with their tissue cysts when eaten by a carnivore. Ground-feeding birds

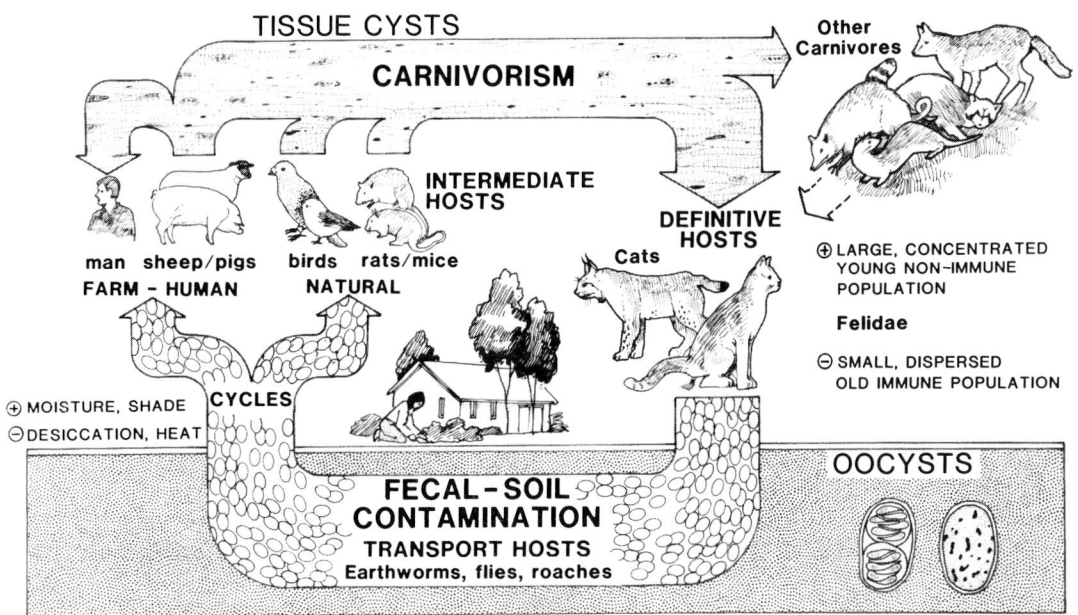

FIGURE 78–3. Transmission of toxoplasmosis. The 3 important reservoirs are cats, soil, and intermediate hosts. Oocysts from cats, the final host, feed the soil reservoir. Ground-feeding birds and rodents constitute the intermediate hosts of the natural cycle; sheep, pigs, and humans are the intermediate hosts of the farm-human cycle. Tissue cysts of bradyzoites are found in all intermediate hosts as well as in cats. Cats become infected from the tissue cysts of the intermediate hosts and close the cycle by shedding oocysts. Other carnivores become infected but are dead-end hosts as are humans. (Modified from Frenkel JK, Ruiz A: Am J Epidemiol 113:254, 1981.)

and rodents are probably the most important intermediate hosts, because they in turn transmit the infection to cats, thereby closing the natural transmission chain (Fig. 78–3). Sheep and pigs transmit the infection to humans, who are essentially a dead-end host (Fig. 78–3).

Carnivorism is the manner by which cats are infected naturally. Kittens may be infected by prey brought by their mothers. Other carnivores also become infected but are of little importance in the transmission chain because they are rarely preyed on and do not shed oocysts. Meat-related outbreaks have been attributed to mutton, hamburgers, and steak tartare. In northern Germany, raw pork (Hackepeter) is a favorite repast, made possible by the eradication of *Trichinella*. In parts of the Arab world, ground lamb mixed with spices (kibbe) is eaten as a delicacy.

Transplacental Transmission. Transplacental infection occurs in humans, sheep, and goats when first infection occurred during pregnancy. Only in mice and goats has transmission in successive pregnancies been recognized. However, transplacental transmission during chronic infection has been observed in immunosuppressed women. Infection-immunity or premunition prevents transmission to the fetus by immunocompetent mothers.

Congenital transmission to the fetus occurs in 30 to 40% of women first infected during pregnancy. This is statistically most likely when infection rates average 3% per year; with higher infection rates, more women are immune by the time they become pregnant; with lower infection rates, few contract infection during pregnancy. High infection rates have been found in infants of immigrants from North Africa, an area of low incidence, to France, who acquire local habits of eating undercooked meat, especially mutton and steak tartare.

Uncommon Types of Transmission. Transmission by kissing has been suggested, but there is little to support this idea. Sexual transmission is unlikely; data by Price indicate that antibody is found as commonly in one marital partner as in both. Experimental leukocyte transfusions with blood from immunosuppressed leukemic donors have served to transmit the infection, and *T. gondii* has been isolated from peripheral blood of symptomatic patients. However, blood from asymptomatic carriers is generally safe. Transplanted hearts of seropositive donors transmit toxoplasmosis because *Toxoplasma* cysts are common in the heart. These cysts are rare in the kidneys.

EPIDEMIOLOGY. Epidemiologic studies are generally based on serologic tests that show increasing prevalence rates with age. In humans and practically all animals studied, these antibody prevalence rates appear to be cumulative, although the titers generally decline. Only in cattle is antibody prevalence not cumulative, because infections are short lived. In birds, epidemiologic studies need to be based on passage, unless it is demonstrated that antibodies can be measured by the tests chosen and that they persist in the species to be studied.

Tropics and Subtropics. In much of the tropics, where the highest incidence of infection is during childhood, oocysts in contaminated soil around the house are believed to be the major sources of infection. For example, in Costa Rica, up to 30% of children have been infected prior to 5 years of age during their crawling and dirt-eating stages, and there is a 61% prevalence of infection at age 25. The ingestion of undercooked eggs and meat could be excluded as a major cause of acquiring infection. Toxoplasmosis is also commonly acquired in childhood in Hawaii and other Pacific Islands studied by

Wallace, in Japan, tropical Africa, Tahiti, Brazil, Colombia, and Panama, from where detailed studies are available.

Developed Countries. In North America, seroconversion rates are generally lower, with seroconversion either being evenly distributed by age or occurring predominantly during adulthood. Although the exact sources of infection cannot be stated definitively, the ingestion of infective meat as a source can be circumstantially inferred. Eating undercooked meat is a habit that is individually acquired. Contact with contaminated soil appears to be less important during childhood or adult life in the United States.

In part of Europe, undercooked meat (often mutton) is consumed, and the juice of raw meat is sometimes given to children for its supposed nutritional qualities. This combination of factors is believed to account for the high incidence rates of toxoplasmosis in French children. Although cats may also be prevalent in developed countries, young children spend more time indoors there than in tropical areas.

PATHOGENESIS AND PATHOLOGY. *Toxoplasma* is generally acquired by ingestion and causes enteritis in experimental animals infected with large doses of oocysts or tissue cysts. In humans, the usual dose of infection is low, and the enteric phase of infection is either asymptomatic or unrecognized. From the gut, tachyzoites disseminate via lymphatics to regional lymph nodes and by blood to the liver, lungs, and rest of the body. Antibody usually develops in a week or two, so that by the time lesions and clinical symptoms are produced, a proportion of extracellular *Toxoplasma* are destroyed in the blood stream. Much of the dissemination is from cell to cell or hematogenously inside monocytes and granulocytes. Four pathogenetic mechanisms can be recognized: necrosis of individual cells, delayed hypersensitivity, antigen-antibody reaction, and infarction.

Active Infection. Tachyzoites multiply probably in all nucleated cell types and destroy their host cells, entering adjacent cells, and eventually give rise to focal necrosis. The organisms divide every 5 to 12 hours, and 16 to 32 organisms are sufficient to destroy most cells; therefore, significant cell destruction may take place prior to the time effective immunity can be acquired.

Autopsies in adults show interstitial pneumonia, focal hepatitis, myocarditis, myositis, and encephalitis associated with tachyzoites and a few cysts. Biopsy of enlarged lymph nodes shows preservation of architecture, reticular cell hyperplasia, prominent histiocytes infiltrating the germinal center, absence of necrosis, slight periadenitis, and a paucity of *Toxoplasma* organisms; cysts have been found occasionally in serial tissue sections, and the organism has been isolated by inoculation into mice. Placental lesions are usually microscopic in humans, but macroscopic necrosis has been reported in animals.

Recrudescent lesions in the brain and lungs in immunosuppressed patients show huge numbers of tachyzoites in target-like focal lesions, usually only in 1 organ, e.g., the brain, retina, or lung, where cellular immunity is most compromised. Hematogenous dissemination is probably inhibited by circulating antibody.

Chronic Infection. Bradyzoites persist in tissue cysts during chronic infection, mainly in the brain, retina, and skeletal and cardiac muscle. Because delayed-type hypersensitivity is usually acquired with immunity, rupture of these cysts with liberation of bradyzoites results in a type IV allergic reaction, which is characterized by tissue necrosis and chronic inflammation. This is clinically important in the retina, where function is highly concentrated, and sometimes leads to focal encephalitis or myositis, which is self-limited. Antibody and cellular immunity are usually sufficient to destroy the released bradyzoites; however, in the immunosuppressed patient, there is renewed proliferation of tachyzoites, as mentioned previously.

Congenital Infection. At autopsy in congenitally infected infants, either generalized or central nervous system lesions predominate. Pneumonia, hepatitis, and myocarditis are usually most severe, with mononuclear inflammatory reaction and tachyzoites at the periphery of the lesions. Generalized lesions later subside, leaving areas of fibrosis. However, active encephalitis persists as a consequence of the reduced immunity in the brain, with necrosis of infected cells, microglial nodules, small scattered infarcts, and periventricular necrosis.

The third mechanism of pathogenesis results in the periventricular zone of necrosis seen in babies with congenital toxoplasmosis. A spread of *Toxoplasma* to the brain eventually leads to infection of ependymal cells and to dissemination within the ventricular system. Ependymitis in the aqueduct leads to aqueductal obstruction and the accumulation of *Toxoplasma* antigen in the lateral and third ventricles. Seepage of this *Toxoplasma* antigen through ependymal ulcerations is accompanied by vasculitis and thrombosis, resulting in infarction necrosis of periventricular tissues. This has been interpreted as an antigen-antibody, or type III allergic, reaction. The high titers of intravascular antibody are transferred from the mother and in part elaborated by the infants themselves.

A fourth pathogenic mechanism is infarction necrosis, resulting from vascular thrombosis adjacent to foci of *Toxoplasma* infection in the brain, spleen, and other areas where single arterial supply with few anastomoses and end arteries are found.

CLINICAL MANIFESTATIONS AND COMPLICATIONS. Although it is usually asymptomatic, toxoplasmosis can produce illness. This will be discussed under 4 headings: acute acquired infection, neonatal toxoplasmosis, ocular toxoplasmosis, and infection in the immunocompromised host.

Acute Acquired Toxoplasmosis

Signs and Symptoms. The range of signs and symptoms of acute acquired toxoplasmosis is best illustrated by people infected in outbreaks. The following symptoms were reported by Teutsch and associates in an outbreak involving 37 patrons of a riding stable in Atlanta, Georgia, which was attributed to the ingestion of oocysts: 89% of the individuals had fever, 84% had headache and lymphadenopathy (usually, the cervical lymph nodes were enlarged, firm, and discrete but not markedly tender), 60% had myalgia (occasionally diagnosed as polymyositis), 54% had stiff neck and/or anorexia, and 20% had a macular or urticarial rash (generally accompanied by fever and confusion). Arthralgia (24%) and hepatitis (11%) were less common findings. In all, 95% of those acquiring infection were considered to have been symptomatic. Although 25 of the 37 individuals visited a physician, only 3 were diagnosed as having toxoplasmosis. Miller and coworkers reported the development of *Toxoplasma* antibody in laboratory workers after they began to work with oocysts. In this group of scientists, only 3 of 7 reported symptoms: swelling of midcervical lymph nodes, which persisted for 4 months, a mild influenza-like episode, and fatigue and malaise without objective symptoms. Four infections were asymptomatic.

Following infection with tissue cysts, the incubation period could also be determined. Of 5 students reported by Kean and colleagues with common exposure to undercooked hamburger in New York, all had headache, fever, and myalgia, with enlarged lymph nodes persisting for 3 months. Three had a fleeting erythematous macular rash of limited distribution during the first week, and 3 had splenomegaly for up to 4 months. The incubation period was 10 to 12 days. In another meat-related outbreak, reported by Masur, the incubation period was 7 to 17 days, with 5 of 7 individuals being symptomatic and 1 developing retinochoroiditis.

There are sporadic reports of single patients with symptoms of myocarditis, encephalitis, hepatitis, and pneumonia, some of whom died; the manner of their infection is unknown.

Lymphadenopathy. This most commonly follows acute infection, whether accompanied by symptoms or not. It is 3 times as common in women as in men and is usually located in the neck. This lymphadenopathy, which coincides with the appearance of immunity, is accompanied by high titers of IgG and IgM antibody. On biopsy, reticular cell hyperplasia is seen, and occasionally a *Toxoplasma* cyst.

Laboratory Tests. These show normal or slightly reduced leukocyte counts, often with lymphocytosis or monocytosis with rare atypical cells. The early hematocrit is normal, but prolonged illness may be accompanied by anemia. Lymph node biopsy shows reticular hyperplasia. Chest films are normal or show interstitial pneumonia. Serum aminotransferase may be slightly elevated. Heterophil tests are negative. Antibody titers to *Toxoplasma*, both IgG and IgM, are high or rising.

Neonatal Toxoplasmosis. Up to 60% of babies infected in utero are asymptomatic at birth, as shown in a large prospective study of Desmonts and Couvreur in Paris. Other infected babies may be aborted or stillborn. Many are born prematurely. Eichenwald classified 152 babies with symptomatic toxoplasmosis into 44 with predominantly generalized illness and 108 with predominantly neurologic illness. In the former group, the most frequent findings were splenomegaly (90%), jaundice (80%), fever (77%), anemia (77%), hepatomegaly (77%), lymphadenopathy (68%), pneumonia (40%), and rash (25%). All reflect generalized infection, contracted via the umbilical vein. Associated findings were abnormal spinal fluid (84%), retinochoroiditis (66%), hypothermia (20%), and convulsions (18%), indicating

early central nervous system involvement. Babies with prominent neurologic involvement showed retinochoroiditis (95%), abnormal spinal fluid (55%), anemia (50%), convulsions (50%), intracranial calcifications (50%) (Fig. 78–4), internal hydrocephalus (28%), fever (25%), splenomegaly (21%), lymphadenopathy (16%), hepatomegaly (16%), and microcephaly (30%). In both groups, the mortality rate was about 12%, and the sequelae observed over a 4-year period (100 patients), included mental retardation (86%), convulsions (81%), spasticity and palsies (70%), severely impaired sight (63%), hydrocephalus or microcephaly (42%), and deafness (16%); only 11% of the children were considered normal. Most of Eichenwald's patients were referred to him for illness; therefore, the more severe aspects of the disease are represented.

Alford, Stagno, and Reynolds observed the mildest symptoms in a prospective study on intrauterine infection. They found 10 infected infants among 7500 live births screened at the University of Alabama Medical Centers. Findings of interest for the diagnosis of milder illness were gestational prematurity (5), intrauterine growth retardation (2), abnormal spinal fluid (8), IgM elevations (9), and IgM antibody (10). Follow-up studies of this group and some others for up to 11 years showed that retinochoroiditis developed in about 75% of the children.

In babies with clinically active congenital toxoplasmosis, the retinal lesions are usually bilateral and usually involve the macular area, although often obscured by the intense vitreous inflammatory exudate. The lesion appears as a fuzzy white area, the size of the disk or larger, surrounded by orange, normal-appearing fundus. Because the maculae are involved in about two-thirds of these infants, visual impairment is great. In neonates infected in the second trimester, trophic cataracts and microphthalmia, nystagmus, and cerebral calcification are commonly found (Fig. 78–4); IgG and IgM antibody titers are generally high.

Ocular Toxoplasmosis. Retinochoroiditis found in children or adults is usually a unilateral, painless, focally

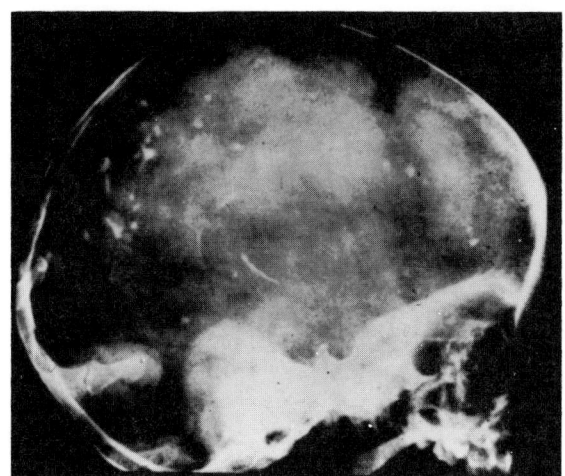

FIGURE 78–4. Cerebral calcifications in a radiograph of a 7-week-old baby who died with congenital toxoplasmosis. (Courtesy of Dr. Jack Beverley, University of Sheffield Medical School, Sheffield, England.)

necrotic retinal lesion with fuzzy outlines (Fig. 78–5). It is accompanied by a whitish vitreous exudate that sometimes obscures the lesion and causes marked blurring of vision. Circumscribed white or pigmented healed scars are often present in either eye. Sometimes, a new lesion arises from the edge of an old one. Because the organisms and the lesions are in the retina, retinochoroiditis is the proper designation. Most of these patients have stable low IgG titers, suggesting that these may be late sequelae of congenital or pediatric infection. In rare instances, however, these lesions are preceded by symptoms of generalized illness, in which case antibody titers are high compared with those in the general population. The lesions are often recurrent, but the majority are of limited duration. With clearing of the vitreous exudate, visual acuity may return to what it was before if the lesion is away from the macula. However, prolonged smoldering lesions have been described; occasionally, they follow treatment with corticosteroids that is not covered by antitoxoplasmal therapy, and others are in patients with lymphomas. Progressive lesions may result in blindness and glaucoma.

Associated with retinochoroiditis may be edema of the retina and optic nerve, optic neuritis, iridocyclitis, and, in rare instances, panuveitis.

Toxoplasmosis in the Immunocompromised Host. Two types of infection are seen—recrudescent chronic infections and severe primary infections. With relapse, encephalitis is most common (Figs. 78–6 and 78–7), and retinochoroiditis, myocarditis, and focal pneumonia are rare manifestations. Most cases are relapses of chronic infection caused by the acquired immune deficiency syndrome (AIDS) or immunosuppressive drugs that impair cellular immunity, especially corticosteroids and cyclophosphamide. The lesions are characteristically focal and often simulate an abscess or tumor, although they may be multicentric. IgM antibody is rarely present. IgG antibody titers are elevated and tend to be stable.

Primary infections occur in the immunosuppressed patient by natural routes, by heart transplant, or by leukocyte transfusion. They are generalized and involve multiple organs, as described for acute acquired toxo-

plasmosis, but tend to be more severe. The usual predisposing factors are that the patient has been receiving immunosuppressive drugs and, rarely, early undiagnosed leukemia, lymphoma, or AIDS are present. IgG antibody titers are elevated and rising, or stable, and IgM titers are usually high.

DIAGNOSIS. Diagnostic techniques consist of the identification of *Toxoplasma*, histopathologic examination, tests for antibody, and tests for antigen and for delayed-type hypersensitivity.

Identification of the Parasite. *Toxoplasma* tachyzoites (Fig. 78–2A) can be demonstrated on tissue imprints that are dried, fixed with methanol, and stained with Giemsa as 7- × 3-μm ovoid organisms possessing a red nucleus and a blue cytoplasm. In tissue sections, tachyzoites are best demonstrated by hematoxylin and eosin stain, are ovoid or rounded, and measure 3 to 4 μm. Bradyzoites are of similar size but are more closely packed, and hence, their size is not easily determined in tissue sections (Fig. 78–2B and C). They are distinguished by containing a form of glycogen. Therefore, they stain prominently with the periodic acid-Schiff (PAS) technique. On tissue imprints, they are well stained with Giemsa. Whereas the finding of cell or tissue necrosis with tachyzoites (and cysts) establishes the presence of active infection, the presence only of cysts would indicate only chronic infection, except in the placenta and the newborn. Staining with specific antibody marked with fluorescein or enzyme and the ultrastructural features demonstrated by electron microscopy facilitate identification of the organisms.

Parasite Isolation. Ventricular fluid, placenta, biopsy or autopsy tissues, or the buffy coat of a centrifuged blood specimen may be inoculated intraperitoneally into mice (especially athymic, nude mice), hamsters, or cell culture. Contaminated material may be mixed with penicillin (1000 units/ml) and streptomycin (100 μg/ml) for half an hour before injection subcutaneously. Identification of tachyzoites in the peritoneal fluid is sometimes possible after 4 to 8 days (Fig. 78–2A). If the animals survive, they are examined after 4 to 6 weeks for the presence of tissue cysts in the brain, using stained tissue imprints (Giemsa) or tissue sections (PAS) (Fig. 78–2B), and for the development of *Toxoplasma* antibody, which should be absent in uninoculated control mice. The cells of inoculated cultures can be stained, or the supernatants are spun down and the Giemsa-stained sediment examined for tachyzoites (Fig. 78–2A).

Serology

Interpretation of Results. When seeking a serologic diagnosis, it is important to distinguish pre-existing antibody and passively transferred antibody from antibody related to the illness. Although numerous techniques for measurement for *Toxoplasma* antibody have been described, it is best to become familiar with one or two available tests. Most diagnoses can be made with one test for IgG, and almost all diagnoses can be made with an additional test for IgM. IgM antibody is developed first during infection and persists for 6 months in the conventional test but up to 6 years in the capture test. IgM is not transferred by the intact placenta and, if leaking across a break, has a half-life of 3 to 5 days.

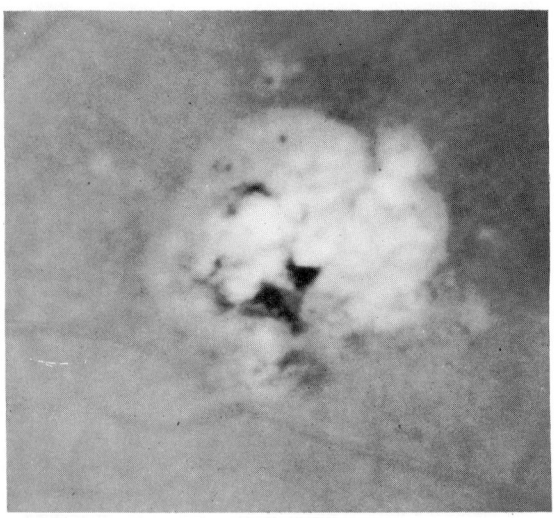

FIGURE 78–5. Presumed toxoplasmic retinochoroiditis. (Courtesy of the University of Florida College of Medicine, Gainesville.)

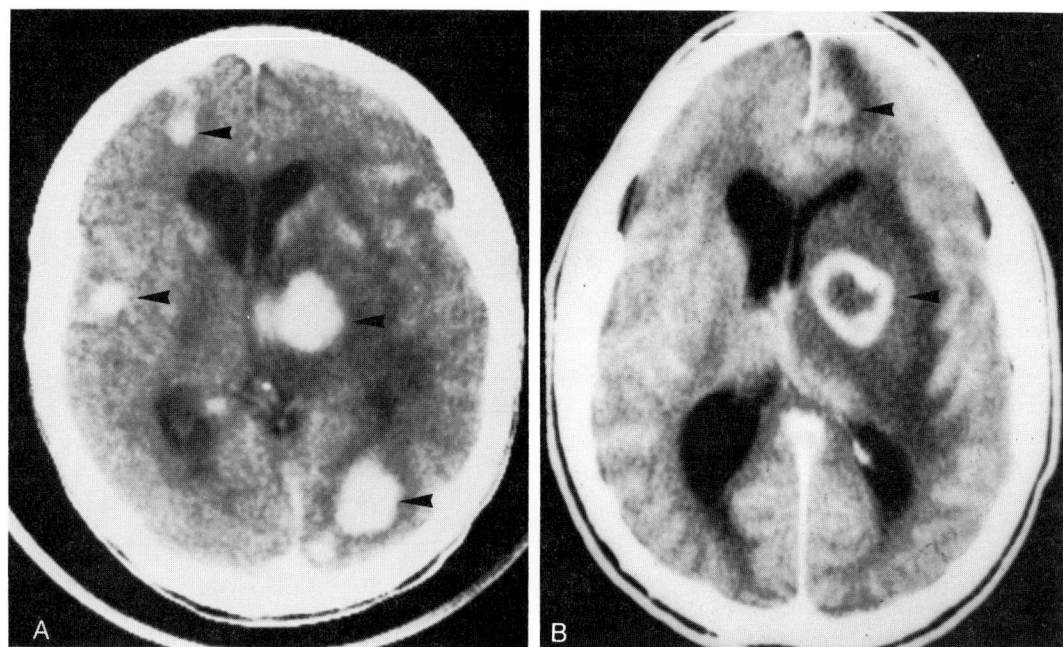

FIGURE 78–6. Recrudescent toxoplasmic encephalitis in two patients with AIDS. *A,* CT scan of brain with multiple enhancing lesions in right and left cerebral hemispheres and cerebellum. There is extensive edema with subfalcial herniation and left to right shift of the midline and left ventricle. (Courtesy of Dr. George Hensley, University of Miami School of Medicine.) *B,* CT scan of brain with a more advanced ring-enhancing lesion, indicating central necrosis in the right basal ganglia. There is compression of the right lateral ventricle and a shift to the left. A smaller lesion is present in the frontal lobe. Generalized edema is present. (Courtesy of Dr. Charles Poser, Harvard University Medical School.)

Determination of the IgM fraction is therefore useful to separate lower antibody titers of early infection (in which IgM would be present) from those of late chronic infection (in which IgM would be absent) and to distinguish actively acquired antibody (IgM present) from passively transferred antibody (IgM absent) in a baby.

Serologic diagnosis may be based on demonstration of a rise in antibody titers (IgG) between 2 or more specimens tested in the same test run (Table 78–1). The presence of elevated IgM titers can be considered presumptive evidence of recent infection. To support the diagnosis of acute febrile toxoplasmosis, a 4-tube antibody rise is required. If the specimens are taken during

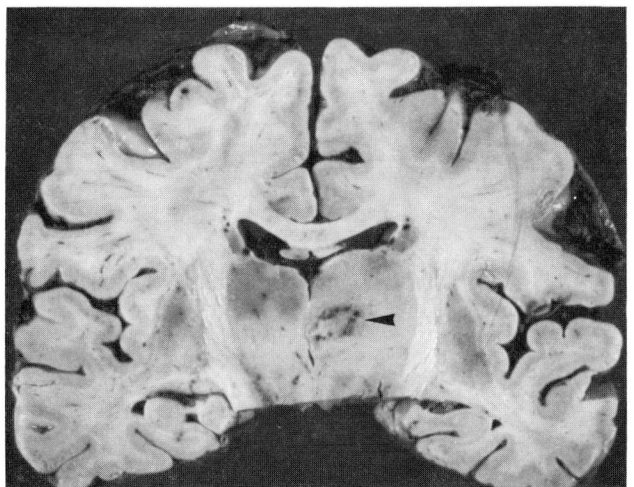

FIGURE 78–7. Recrudescent toxoplasmic encephalitis. In this cross-section of the brain, a spherical necrotic lesion surrounded by hemorrhage is seen in the right thalamus. (Courtesy of Dr. George Hensley, University of Miami School of Medicine.)

the late illness or for the presence of lymphadenopathy, titers in excess of 1:1000 should be present. In many tropical areas such titers are common in the normal population, presumably because of frequent reinfections. Stable antibody titers are usually associated with immunity and when found during the first trimester of pregnancy would predict protection of the fetus (Fig. 78–8*A*).

For the diagnosis of congenital toxoplasmosis, a titer of over 1:1000 can be considered tentatively diagnostic, subject to confirmation by findings of antibody in the IgM fraction, the exclusion of rheumatoid factor and antinuclear antibody, and the isolation of *Toxoplasma,* if possible. Passively transferred antibody shows a tenfold decay every 3 months, whereas in the presence of infection, high antibody titers are stable or increase. An international standard has been prepared and is used by some laboratories. International units are approximately one-fourth of the reciprocal of the titers expressed here as fractions (Fig. 78–8*C*).

Toxoplasmic retinochoroiditis, which is usually a manifestation of chronic toxoplasmosis, generally is accompanied by stable low antibody titers. Any titer, even in undiluted serum, is sufficient to support a presumptive diagnosis with a compatible lesion. However, in areas of high antibody prevalence, such serologic support becomes correspondingly less certain (see Fig. 78–8*D*).

Recrudescent toxoplasmosis may be accompanied by high, low, and, rarely absent antibody titers. The possibility of antibody's having been transfused must be kept in mind. Diagnostic help should be sought from biopsy and isolation. The cerebrospinal fluid of patients with toxoplasmic encephalitis often contains antibody, which is helpful diagnostically.

Serologic Tests. IgG and IgM antibodies can be de-

TABLE 78–1. Guide to Interpretation of Serologic Tests for Toxoplasmosis
(Dye Test or Indirect Fluorescent Antibody Test for IgG)†

Clinical Problem	Titer				
	0	*1:2–1:16*	*1:32–1:128*	*1:256–1:512*	*1:1024+*
None (asymptomatic)	Susceptible to infection	Remote infection, probably immune			Recent infection or reinfection
Pregnancy	Susceptible to infection	Remote infection, probably immune			Need to follow newborn baby for infection
Newborn, asymptomatic or with jaundice	Incompatible	Incompatible	Unlikely (can be found in babies treated for toxoplasmosis)	Unlikely	Possible*
Newborn with encephalitis	Incompatible	Incompatible	Incompatible	Unlikely	Likely if titer is stable or rises*
Lymphadenopathy	Incompatible	Incompatible	Incompatible	Unlikely	Possible
Fever with pneumonia, myocarditis, or hepatitis	Incompatible	Incompatible	Unlikely	Unlikely	Possible*
Retinochoroiditis	Incompatible	Possible	Possible	Possible	Possible
Encephalitis	Incompatible	Incompatible	Unlikely	Unlikely	Possible*
Encephalitis in patient who is immunosuppressed	Nondiagnostic	Unlikely (possibly transfused)	Possible	Possible	Likely*

*Tests for *Toxoplasma* antibody in the IgM fraction may be informative.
†Modified from Frenkel KJ: *In* Prier JE, Friedman H (eds): Opportunistic Pathogens. Baltimore, University Park Press, 1974.
Incompatible: With such a titer, toxoplasmosis should not be diagnosed.
Unlikely: The lowest titers found in typical forms of the syndrome.
Possible: A characteristic titer, but not necessarily diagnostic.

termined by means of antihuman IgG and antihuman IgM, labeled with either fluorescein (IFA) or an enzyme that later colors an added substrate (ELISA). In "conventional tests" *Toxoplasma* tachyzoites on a slide are overlaid with the patient's serum, followed by antihuman IgG or IgM, depending on what one wishes to measure. The result of an IgM titer may be falsely positive with presence of antinuclear antibody or rheumatoid factor. These test results may be negative when large quantities of IgG compete for binding with IgM, and rarely vice versa. These problems are avoided by the "IgM capture test." Antihuman IgM attached to wells of a test plate or to test tubes when overlaid with a patient's serum "captures" the patient's total IgM. The content of *Toxoplasma* antibody is then measured by the amount of *Toxoplasma* antigen the "captured" IgM binds. The *Toxoplasma* antigen can be supplied in several forms: whole tachyzoites or soluble antigen (either free or attached to latex beads or red blood cells). In the "double sandwich IgM-ELISA," the *Toxoplasma* antigen is identified by means of anti-*Toxoplasma* serum linked to alkaline phosphatase, which imparts color to an added substrate. In the "reverse IgM ELISA," the *Toxoplasma* antigen itself is labeled with enzyme, and only the appropriate substrate is added. In the immunosorbent agglutination assay (ISAgA or the IgM-ISA), *Toxoplasma* tachyzoites are agglutinated in a distinctive carpet-like pattern. In the "latex IgM-ISA," soluble *Toxoplasma* antigen-coated latex particles are also agglutinated in a carpet-like pattern. In the "HA IgM-ISA," red blood cells coated with soluble *Toxoplasma* antigen are agglutinated.

The dye test of Sabin and Feldman is the standard test; it depends on lysis of *Toxoplasma* by the patient's antibody in the presence of complement, simulating the presumed mechanisms of humoral immunity in the body. It is highly specific and is particularly useful when testing sera of many species of animals, because no species-specific antiglobulin is required. However, the dye test requires living *Toxoplasma*, and it does not separate IgG from IgM. The antigens for the indirect hemagglutination test (IHA) (using *Toxoplasma* antigen-coated red blood cells), the latex agglutination test (LAT), and the direct agglutination of *Toxoplasma* (HA) may be available in kits. The usefulness of complement-fixation and precipitin tests is limited.

Detection of Toxoplasma Antigens. A test for antigenemia is under investigation; it would be promising for a rapid, direct diagnosis of active infection, with the exception of isolated ocular lesions. This test circumvents dependence on antibody responses, which are unreliable in immunosuppressed patients, and may distinguish between low titers in acute and chronic infections. In tissue sections the peroxidase-antiperoxidase technique is invaluable for the demonstration of small numbers of tachyzoites. Known *Toxoplasma* antiserum from an animal and (preinoculation) control serum are necessary. Immune peroxidase kits can be adapted as long as the antiserum came from a species that reacts with the antispecies serum in the kit.

Skin Tests. Delayed-type hypersensitivity responses are positive in a majority of people with antibody. The skin test is useful for population surveys and can be used to support a clinical diagnosis of toxoplasmic retinochoroiditis where no serologic tests are available. Skin test positivity is used in some countries to identify pregnant women who are immune and need not be concerned about contracting infection during pregnancy.

Differential Diagnosis. The signs and symptoms of toxoplasmosis are usually so nonspecific that they are not diagnosed. Most illnesses are mild and often are not recorded. In the study by Teutsch and colleagues, if there were any days absent from work or school, they were not ascertained, and none of the 5 students in Kean and associates' study became ill enough to be "incapacitated." However, patients have been recorded

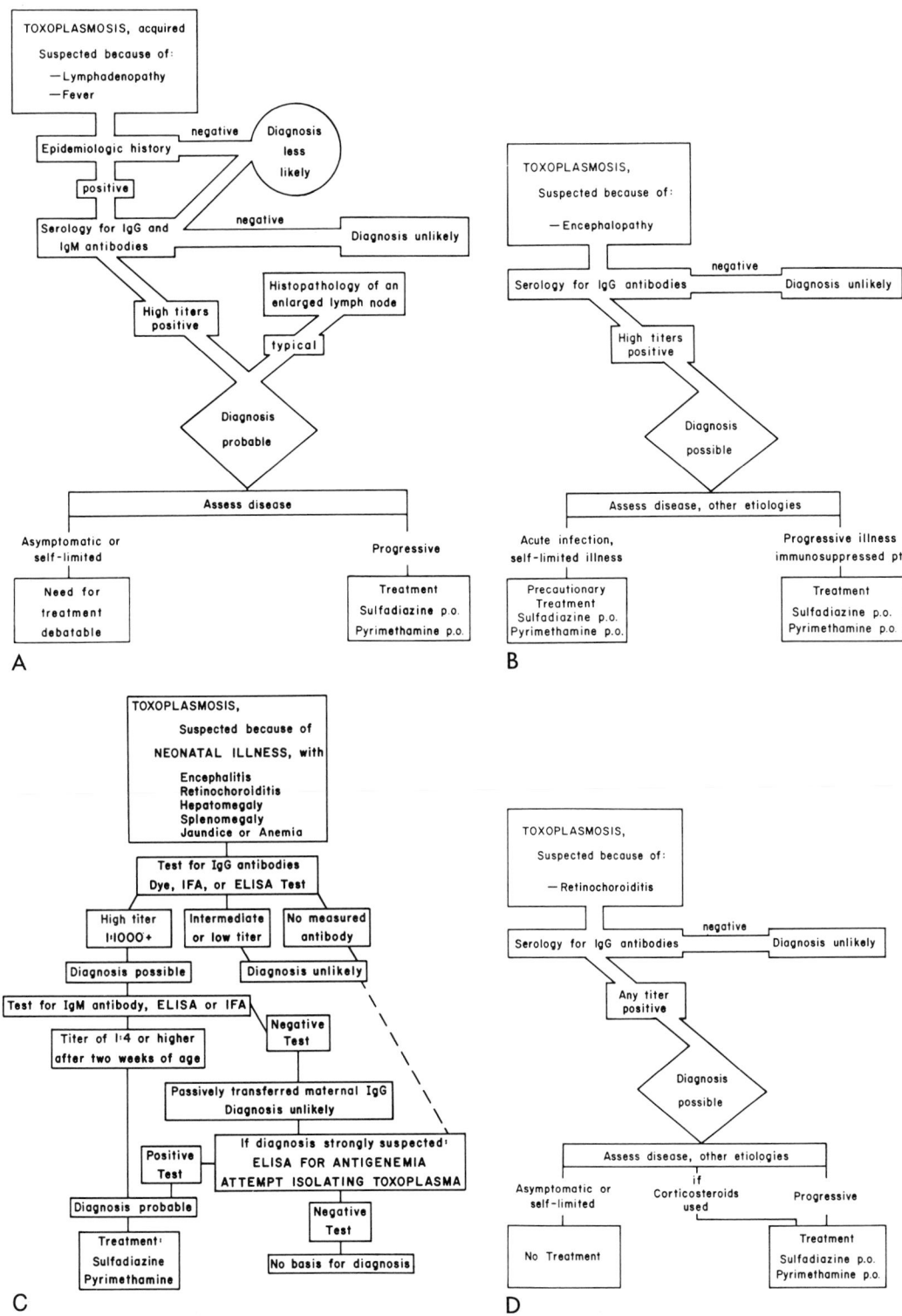

FIGURE 78–8. Algorithms for the diagnosis and treatment of toxoplasmosis: *A,* In the presence of fever or lymphadenopathy. *B,* In the presence of encephalopathy. *C,* In the presence of neonatal illness. *D,* In the presence of retinochoroiditis. (Modified from Mahmoud AAF, Warren KS: J Infect Dis 135:493, 1977.)

with a fever up to 39.5C and marked malaise lasting for 2 months, sometimes with myalgia and sore throat, suggesting infectious mononucleosis or cytomegalovirus infections, which must be excluded. The persistent lymphadenopathy, sometimes with splenomegaly and a Coombs' test–negative hemolytic anemia, may suggest

a lymphoma; lymph node biopsy is diagnostic. The algorithms presented in Figure 78–8 outline diagnostic steps to be followed with several presenting symptoms.

Although retinochoroiditis is often due to *Toxoplasma,* isolated anterior ocular segment inflammatory disease is unlikely to be due to toxoplasmosis. The differential diagnosis includes cytomegalovirus infection, syphilis, brucellosis, leptospirosis, tuberculosis, visceral larva migrans, and retinoblastoma.

TREATMENT. Indications for treatment are diagnosed clinical illness, active lesions (e.g., in the eye), congenital infection (whether the infant is symptomatic or not), and symptoms and signs compatible with toxoplasmosis in immunosuppressed patients. Treatment of a pregnant woman who acquired the infection during pregnancy is controversial, because only a third of the babies become infected and because of possible toxic drug effects on the fetus. The mere presence of a high antibody titer is *not* an indication for treatment.

Chemotherapy (Table 78–2)

Sulfonamides and Pyrimethamine. The most effective treatment for toxoplasmosis consists of sulfadiazine and pyrimethamine because the considerable individual inhibitory effect of each drug acts synergistically in combination. In the combined treatment regimen, sulfadiazine (or sulfamerazine, sulfamethazine, sulfapyrazine, sulfalene, or sulfadoxine) is given to adults in 500-mg doses, 4 times daily and to children in doses of 25 to 35 mg/kg 4 times daily. For pyrimethamine (Daraprim, Chloridin, Malocide), the adult dose is 75 mg daily for 3 days, followed by 25 mg/day. Children are given 1 mg/kg/day with meals, and if they are asymptomatic, the dose can be reduced to half that after 3 days. If pyrimethamine induces vomiting, one of the mentioned sulfonamides can be given alone for a few days.

The sulfadiazine-pyrimethamine combination is effective principally on the actively multiplying tachyzoites. Chronic infections with bradyzoites probably persist in most instances unless treatment was maintained for several months. It is important to continue treatment until there is circumstantial evidence that the patient may have developed immunity and can control chronic infection. No drug-resistant strains of *Toxoplasma* have been encountered while testing 44 isolates requiring sulfadiazine in mice.

Toxicity of the sulfadiazine-pyrimethamine combination consists of bone marrow depression, first manifested by thrombocytopenia and leukopenia. This is relieved by *folinic acid* or yeast without impairing the chemotherapeutic effect. Folic acid should not be used!

Patients with AIDS often develop manifestations of hypersensitivity to sulfonamides and need to be treated with high doses of pyrimethamine only, or with an alternate drugs.

TABLE 78–2. Chemotherapy for Toxoplasmosis—Daily Drug Doses

Drug	First 3 Days		Fourth Day Onward	
	Adult	Children	Adult	Children
Pyrimethamine (once daily)	75 mg	2 mg/kg	25 mg	1 mg/kg
Sulfadiazine* (4 times daily)	500 mg	25 mg/kg	500 mg	25 mg/kg
Antagonists†				
Folinic acid (leucovorin),			3–10 mg	1 mg
or baker's yeast			5–10 gm	100 mg

*Certain other sulfonamides, as mentioned in the text, may be substituted.

†To be given if platelet counts are below 100,000/mm³, or if twice weekly platelet counts are not feasible. Antagonists of toxicity may be given prophylactically with the treatment.

Folinic Acid. Platelet and white blood cell counts should be performed weekly, if possible. When this is not possible or with the decline of platelets to below 100,000/mm³, an antagonist is given together with sulfadiazine-pyrimethamine: Folinic acid (Calcium Leucovorin) is administered in a dose of 3 to 10 mg daily orally for adults and 1 mg daily for children. When folinic acid is not available, fresh baker's or brewer's yeast can be substituted; 5 to 10 gm daily for adults and 100 mg daily for children are mixed with food or formula.

Other Antitoxoplasmal Agents. Concerning the sulfamethoxazole-trimethoprim combination (Bactrim, Septra, Septrin), effectiveness has been shown only for sulfamethoxazole; hence, the presence of synergism is uncertain. This combination could be used when sulfadiazine and pyrimethamine are not available. Clindamycin is effective against *Toxoplasma* but does not penetrate well into the central nervous system, except in the presence of encephalitis. It has been considered useful in treatment of encephalitis in patients who did not tolerate sulfonamides. Possible side effects of clindamycin (antibiotic-associated colitis) militate against its use for long-term prophylaxis of toxoplasmosis.

Spiramycin, a relative of erythromycin, has been recommended to treat women infected during pregnancy because of less potential long-term toxicity. Spiramycin (Rovamycin) is given in a dose of 500 to 750 mg 4 times daily for adults or 50 to 100 mg/kg twice daily for children. Treatment for 4 to 6 weeks has been advised. This drug is said to be concentrated in the placenta but not to cross it freely, and drug levels in the newborn are low. Spiramycin has been used in congenitally infected infants alternating with sulfadiazine-pyrimethamine treatment.

5-Fluorouracil inhibited *Toxoplasma* in cell culture and potentiated the effect of pyrimethamine.

New drugs are being tested. Among these are arprinocid, a purine analogue, which had been used as an anticoccidial agent in chickens; trimetrexate, a pyrimethamine analogue used in tumor chemotherapy; and polyether ionophores, such as monensin and lasalocid, which are effective in the cat intestine, but not in the tissue infections because they are not appreciably absorbed.

Corticosteroids. Anti-inflammatory corticosteroids may be used to inhibit manifestations of hypersensitivity such as that in retinochoroiditis. Because anti-inflammatory doses are also immunosuppressive, corticosteroids should always be used with the sulfadiazine-pyrimethamine combination. Prednisone, 50 to 75 mg/day, is given until signs of acute vitreous inflammation have started to diminish, which usually occurs after 5 to 10 days. The dose is then tapered by 5 mg/day to 0, whereas sulfadiazine-pyrimethamine is continued for a total of 4 to 6 weeks.

PROGNOSIS. The outlook for immunocompetent patients with acute toxoplasmosis is good. However, acute infection, especially in the fetus and young child, may be followed by single or repeated attacks of retinochoroiditis. Prolonged treatment for several months appears to reduce the frequency of these attacks.

The risks for the fetus of both toxoplasmosis and treatment suggest that abortion should be considered when a woman acquires acute toxoplasmosis early during pregnancy. This would be suggested by rising IgM titers. However, the presence of high IgG titers by IFA test or dye test titers in the second month of pregnancy generally indicates that infection had occurred prior to pregnancy, in which case the risk of the fetus' acquiring toxoplasmosis is virtually nil. Subsequent babies born to mothers who previously delivered infected infants can be expected to be free from congenital toxoplasmosis.

Chronic asymptomatic *Toxoplasma* infection, as indicated by a persistent antibody titer, prevalent in many populations, is generally benign and accompanied by immunity. However, if such people are immunosuppressed, recrudescent toxoplasmosis must be anticipated, and should be mitigated by chemoprophylaxis, although relapsing toxoplasmosis is rare when compared with the frequency of recurrence of cytomegalovirus infection.

PREVENTION AND CONTROL

Soil Transmission. *Toxoplasma* oocysts remain viable in moist and shaded soil for a year or longer. Oocysts are ingested by geophagia, whether compulsive (pica) or inadvertent, similar to ingestion of *Ascaris* eggs. Hands should therefore be washed after contact with soil potentially contaminated by cat feces. Oocysts are destroyed by exposure to heat over 60C, but the usual chemical disinfectants are ineffective.

Meat Transmission. Tissue cysts that have persisted for months or years in the animal remain viable in pork, mutton, and other meat for days at room or refrigerator temperatures. Most of the organisms are destroyed when meat is frozen and thawed but are destroyed more effectively when it is heated to 60C, indicated by a change in the color of the meat. Hands should be washed after contact with raw meat. Soap and water, alcohol, and chemical disinfectants inactivate bradyzoites from tissue cysts on the skin.

Neonatal Transmission. Prevention of *Toxoplasma* infection is most important during pregnancy and early childhood, when the consequences of infection tend to be more severe. The admonition to wash hands after contact with cats, soil, and raw meat and before eating or touching the face and to cook meat thoroughly should be incorporated into the general instructions for pregnant women. Work gloves should be used when handling soil potentially contaminated by cat feces.

Because infection of older children, especially young girls, is of value for immunization and the risk of appreciable illness is small, prevention becomes less important in this group. A vaccine to protect seronegative women during pregnancy is under investigation. This vaccine would also be useful to protect seronegative heart transplant candidates, to prevent a primary infection, transferred with the heart, from occurring during a period of immunosuppression. Many specialists are offering chemoprophylaxis to those with HIV infection who have *Toxoplasma* antibodies.

The Cat. Only control of the spread of oocysts by cats would ultimately reduce transmission to fewer animals and humans (Fig. 78–3). To interrupt the natural cycle in wild and stray cats would be impractical at present. The opportunities for intervention in the farm-human cycle depend to a large degree on local conditions and beliefs. Where cats are pets, it may sometimes be possible to keep them indoors and to control their diet, feeding them only dry, canned, or cooked food. A vaccine that immunizes cats without oocyst shedding has been developed, and vaccination of cats is theoretically feasible. Whatever opportunities exist locally should be used to separate stray cats from human habitation and to control infection of meat animals, especially where their meat is eaten undercooked or raw (e.g., steak tartare, churrasco, kibbe, Schabefleisch, Hackepeter).

BIBLIOGRAPHY

Alford CA, Foft JW, Blankenship WJ, et al: Subclinical central nervous system disease of neonates: a prospective study of infants born with increased levels of IgM. J Pediatr 75:1167, 1969.

Benenson MW, Takafuji ET, Lemon SM, et al: Oocyst-transmitted toxoplasmosis associated with ingestion of contaminated water. N Engl J Med 307:666, 1982.

Desmonts G, Couvreur J: Congenital toxoplasmosis. A prospective study of 378 pregnancies. N Engl J Med 290:1110, 1974.

Eichenwald HF: A study of congenital toxoplasmosis with particular emphasis on clinical manifestations, sequelae and therapy. In Siim J (ed): Human Toxoplasmosis. Copenhagen, Munksgaard, 1960, pp 41–49.

Frenkel JK: Toxoplasmosis. Mechanisms of infection, laboratory diagnosis and management. Curr Top Pathol 54:28, 1971.

Frenkel JK, Ruiz A: Human toxoplasma and cat contact in Costa Rica. Am J Trop Med Hyg 29:1167, 1980.

Frenkel JK, Ruiz A: Endemicity of toxoplasmosis in Costa Rica. Transmission between cats, soil, intermediate hosts and humans. Am J Epidemiol 113:254, 1981.

Juliao-Ruiz O, Corredor-Arjona A, Moreno-Moreno GS: Toxoplasmosis en Colombia. Instit Nacional de Salud, A.A. 80080, Bogota, Colombia, 1983, 1–67.

Kean BH, Kimball AC, Christensen WN: An epidemic of acute toxoplasmosis. JAMA 208:1002, 1969.

Luft BJ, Remington JS: Toxoplasmic encephalitis. J Infect Dis 157:1, 1988.

Masur H, Jones TC, Lempert JA, et al: Outbreak of toxoplasmosis in a family and documentation of acquired retinochoroiditis. Am J Med 64:396, 1978.

Miller NL, Frenkel JK, Dubey JP: Oral infections with Toxoplasma cysts and oocysts in felines, other mammals, and in birds. J Parasitol 58:928, 1972.

Mitchell CD, Erlich SS, Mastrucci MT, et al: Congenital toxoplasmosis occurring in infants perinatally infected with human immunodeficiency virus 1. Pediatr Infect Dis J 9:512, 1990.

Peterson DR, Cooney MK, Beasley RP: Prevalence of antibody to *Toxoplasma* among Alaskan natives: Relation to exposure to the Felidae. J Infect Dis 130:557, 1974.

Ruiz A, Frenkel JK: *Toxoplasma gondii* in Costa Rican cats. Am J Trop Med Hyg 29:1150, 1980.

Ruiz A, Frenkel JK: Intermediate and transport hosts of *Toxoplasma gondii* in Costa Rica. Am J Trop Med Hyg 29:1161, 1980.

Ruskin J, Remington JS: Toxoplasmosis in the compromised host. Ann Intern Med 84:193, 1976.

Sousa OE, Saenz RE, Frenkel JK: Toxoplasmosis in Panama: A 10-year study. Am J Trop Med Hyg 38:315, 1988.

Teutsch SM, Juranek DD, Sulzer A, et al: Epidemic toxoplasmosis associated with infected cats. N Engl J Med 300:695, 1979.

Wallace GD: The role of the cat in the natural history of *Toxoplasma gondii*. Am J Trop Med Hyg 22:313, 1973.

Welch PC, Masur H, Jones TC, et al: Serologic diagnosis of acute lymphadenopathic toxoplasmosis. J Infect Dis 142:256, 1980.

Wilson CB, Remington JS, Stagno S, et al: Development of adverse sequelae in children born with subclinical congenital *Toxoplasma* infection. Pediatrics 66:767, 1980.

79. PNEUMOCYSTOSIS

Walter T. Hughes

DEFINITION. Pneumocystosis is an acute pneumonitis caused by the protozoan-like microbe *Pneumocystis carinii*. With rare exception, the organism and the disease it causes remain localized to the lung.

ETIOLOGY AND HISTORY. The taxonomy for *P. carinii* has not been clearly established. When first discovered, it was believed to be a form of *Trypanosoma cruzi*; however, recognition as a separate entity soon followed. The organism is found in infected tissue as cystic and extracystic forms. The cyst is 4 to 6 μm in diameter (Fig. 79–1) and may contain up to 8 intracystic cells (referred to as sporozoites). These intracystic structures are pleomorphic nucleated cells measuring 1 to 2 μm in diameter (Fig. 79–2). The extracystic cell is a thin-walled, round to crescent-shaped, nucleated structure measuring about 1.5 to 4 μm in diameter (referred to as a trophozoite). The trophozoite is believed to be an excysted sporozoite.

DISTRIBUTION AND INCIDENCE. *P. carinii* has been identified in the lungs of humans and animals from most countries of the world. The latent organisms may be sparsely dispersed as foci in the alveoli without causing clinical manifestations. This asymptomatic form is recognized only in biopsy or autopsy specimens of the lung. In unselected autopsy studies in the United States, *P. carinii* has been found in from 0.2 to 4.0% of cases. Serologic surveys in the United States and the Netherlands indicate that 75% of children have acquired antibody to *P. carinii* by approximately 4 years of age.

Overt pneumonitis occurs almost exclusively in debilitated and malnourished infants, children with congenital immune deficiency disorders, individuals with cancer, patients receiving immunosuppressive drugs, those with the acquired immunodeficiency syndrome (AIDS), and those with severe protein-calorie malnutrition. In addition, 7% of African children with kwashiorkor have been found to have foci of *P. carinii* in the lungs. The impact of *P. carinii* pneumonitis on undernourished

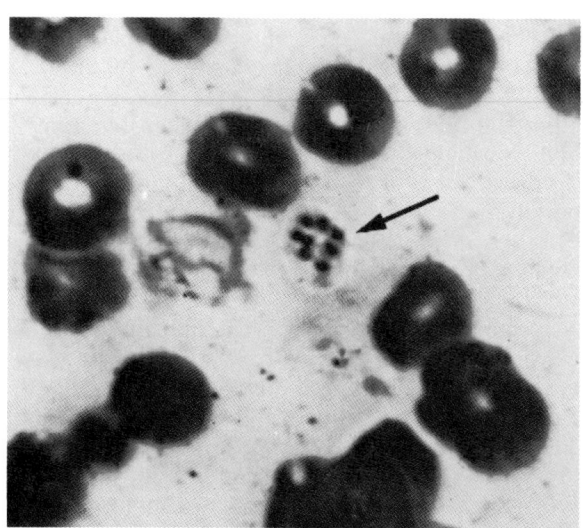

FIGURE 79–2. A Giemsa stain of a needle aspirate specimen from an infected lung showing the intracystic structures (sporozoites) of *P. carinii (arrow)*. The cyst wall is unstained. Comparison for size can be made with adjacent red blood cells.

populations has not been studied. However, from 60 to 80% of children with marasmus, marasmus-kwashiorkor, or kwashiorkor have evidence of impaired cell-mediated immunity, indicating susceptibility to infections such as *P. carinii*. There are no data to compare attack rates between tropical and nontropical populations.

Although *P. carinii* has been discovered in a variety of animals, the species have been limited to wild and domesticated mammals, especially rodents.

TRANSMISSION AND EPIDEMIOLOGY. The natural habitat and mode of transmission of *P. carinii* are unknown. Person to person and animal to person transmission have not been precisely documented. Animal to animal transmission by the airborne route has been demonstrated in laboratory experiments. Endemics and epidemics of *P. carinii* pneumonitis have been described in nurseries and nursing homes for debilitated infants in Europe. A few reports of clustering of cases in cancer hospitals further suggest a contagion pattern for humans.

PATHOGENESIS AND PATHOLOGY. In some asymptomatic individuals small numbers of *P. carinii* may persist as latent forms in the lung. Either single isolated cysts or small clusters of the organism are encountered with careful searching through lung sections. The organisms are located on the alveolar septal wall, which shows little or no evidence of inflammatory reaction. Some cysts are in the cytoplasm of alveolar macrophages undergoing various stages of digestion.

As clinical manifestations of *P. carinii* infection evolve, the number of organisms increases, causing massive infestation. In the immunosuppressed child and adult, the lung becomes noncompliant and liver-like. There is desquamation of alveolar cells into the lumina, where large numbers of organisms exist (Fig. 79–3). With extensive disease, mononuclear cells infiltrate the alveolar septa. In the infantile type, seen in certain European outbreaks, the histopathologic response is

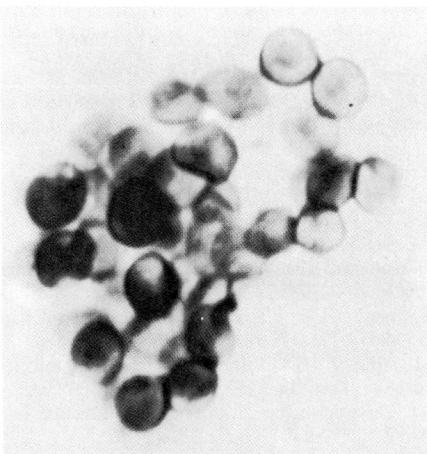

FIGURE 79–1. A toluidine blue O stain of specimens obtained from needle aspirate of infected lung. Only the cyst form of *P. carinii* is seen as a structure 4 to 6 μm in diameter.

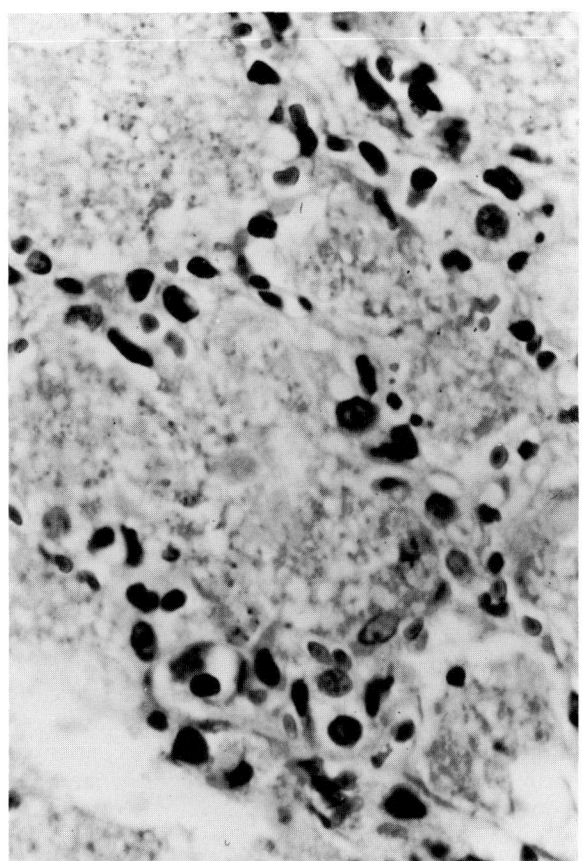

FIGURE 79–3. A lung section from a fatal case of *P. carinii* pneumonitis of the child and adult type. The hematoxylin and eosin-stained section shows the extensive desquamative alveolopathy, with alveoli filled with the characteristic foamy "proteinaceous"-like material. *P. carinii* is not visible with this stain but requires special stains, such as those shown in Figures 79–1 and 79–2, to be recognized.

that of a pronounced interstitial plasma cell infiltration. The thickness of the alveolar septa may be increased to 5 to 10 times the normal size. Hyaline membranes are sometimes seen.

Only with rare exception are *P. carinii* organisms found at extrapulmonary sites. Even in fatal cases, the organisms and the disease remain localized to the lung.

CLINICAL MANIFESTATIONS AND COMPLICATIONS. The clinical features of the pneumonitis in immunosuppressed children and adults are remarkably uniform. The onset is usually abrupt. Fever is usually present early in the course, and tachypnea is pronounced. Cough is dry and nonproductive. Intercostal retractions, flaring of the nasal alae, and cyanosis occur in severe cases. Rales are usually absent. In the infantile type, seen in children from 2 to 6 months of age, the onset is insidious. Tachypnea becomes increasingly pronounced, fever is usually absent, and crepitant rales can usually be heard. Diarrhea may precede the pneumonitis in some cases.

The chest radiograph reveals a bilateral diffuse pneumonitis usually more intense in the mid and lower lung fields than in the upper portions. Air bronchograms may reveal further evidence of disease (Fig. 79–4).

The arterial oxygen tension is reduced, the carbon dioxide level is usually normal and the arterial pH is normal or increased.

Either the child-adult or the infantile type may occur in malnourished individuals, and the clinical features are related more to age than to the cause of immunocompromise.

DIAGNOSIS. A definitive diagnosis requires the identification of *P. carinii* in specimens obtained directly from the lung. Samples of secretions obtained by tracheal aspiration, expectorated sputum, hypopharyngeal swabs, and gastric aspiration may sometimes yield the organism, but these are not dependable approaches to diagnosis. Invasive techniques such as lung biopsy, fiberoptic bronchoscopy with bronchoalveolar lavage, or needle aspiration of the lung are the most precise methods for diagnosis. If invasive diagnostic techniques are not feasible or not available, the diagnosis can be suspected on clinical features alone when other causes of pneumonitis are not apparent. Under these circumstances, the relatively nontoxic agent trimethoprim-sulfamethoxazole can be used, and the patient should be observed for a cause-effect response. However, certain bacterial and chlamydial infections may also respond to this therapy.

After specimens are obtained, several staining procedures are available. Preferably each specimen should be examined by at least 3 methods: the Gomori-Grocott methenamine-silver nitrate stain, toluidine blue O stain, and Giemsa stain. The Gomori stain provides the easiest preparation for locating *P. carinii* cysts. The cyst stains brownish-black, and background tissues are green. Only the cyst forms are stained, and the trophozoites and intracystic structures are not visible. The 4- to 6-μm cyst may appear cup shaped, round, oval, or crescent shaped. The toluidine blue O stain is quickly and simply done, and the organism appears similar to the Gomori-stained cyst, except that it is lavender or blue rather than

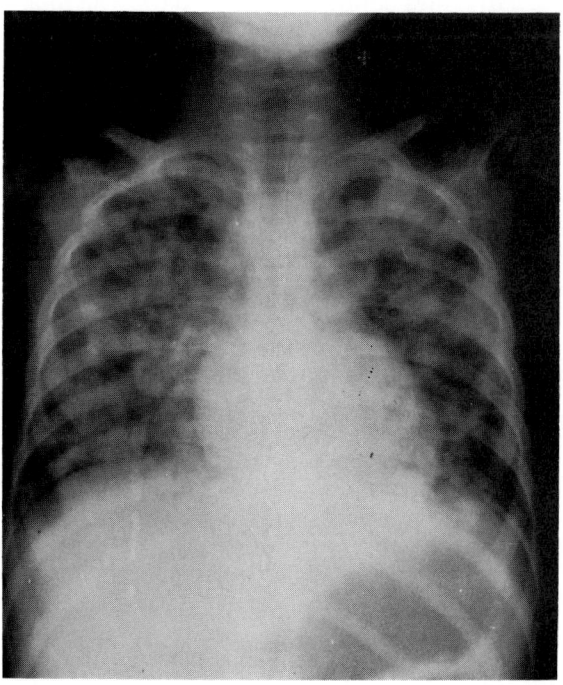

FIGURE 79–4. Chest radiograph of a patient with extensive *P. carinii* pneumonitis. Bilateral diffuse alveolopathy is evident with air bronchogram.

brownish-black (Fig. 79–1). The Giemsa stain reveals the organism more fully than the other 2 stains (Fig. 79–2). This polychrome stain does not identify the cyst wall, but does stain the intracystic structures (sporozoites) and trophozoites.

Serologic tests are of little diagnostic help in *P. carinii* pneumonitis. An indirect immunofluorescent antibody test and complement-fixation tests have been used, but are hampered by the high proportion of normal children and adults who have detectable antibody, presumably from subclinical infection early in life.

TREATMENT

Chemotherapy. Trimethoprim-sulfamethoxazole and pentamidine isethionate are equally effective in the treatment of *P. carinii* pneumonitis; however, trimethoprim-sulfamethoxazole is the drug of choice because of its lower toxicity and fewer adverse effects.

Trimethoprim-Sulfamethoxazole. This is given orally in the dosage of 20 mg of trimethoprim and 100 mg of sulfamethoxazole/kg/day. The total daily dose is divided by 4 and administered at 6-hour intervals. An intravenous preparation is available in most countries and can be given to those who cannot take the oral tablet or suspension. The parenteral dosage is 15 mg of trimethoprim and 75 mg of sulfamethoxazole/kg/day in 4 divided doses. A course of 14 days is usually adequate. The adverse effects are essentially those of sulfonamides.

A combination of pyrimethamine and a sulfonamide (Fansidar) has been used successfully in some cases, but extensive evaluation of this treatment has not been done.

Pentamidine. In contrast to previous practices, recent studies have shown that intravenous administration is preferred because severe adverse effects are less likely by this route than by the intramuscular route. A single daily dose of 4 mg/kg is given intravenously or intramuscularly for a period of 10 to 14 days. The total dose should not exceed 56 mg/kg. Adverse effects include nephrotoxicity, hypoglycemia, injection site reaction, hypotension, anemia, thrombocytopenia, leukopenia, tachycardia, hyperkalemia, hypocalcemia, and alteration in liver function.

Supportive Therapy. Oxygen should be administered as needed to maintain the PaO$_2$ above 70 mm Hg. However, care should be taken to avoid oxygen toxicity by keeping the fraction of inspired oxygen below 50 volumes % as long as possible.

Because bacterial, viral, or fungal infections sometimes accompany *P. carinii* pneumonitis, efforts should be made to identify and treat these infections.

Prognosis. Without treatment the pneumonitis is usually fatal in the compromised host. With either trimethoprim-sulfamethoxazole or pentamidine, the mortality rate has been reduced to about 25%. After treatment is begun fever, tachypnea, and pulmonary infiltrates usually persist unchanged for 4 to 6 days. If no improvement is apparent after 1 week of treatment, the alternative drug should be used and a search made for an associated infection.

After recovery, if an immunodeficiency exists, recurrence can be expected at a later date in at least 10 to 15% of cases. In AIDS patients, recurrence can be expected in more than 30% of cases.

PREVENTION AND CONTROL. *P. carinii* pneumonitis can be prevented by the administration of trimethoprim-sulfamethoxazole. The prophylactic dosage is 5 mg of trimethoprim and 25 mg of sulfamethoxazole/kg daily in 2 divided doses. Recent studies show that this drug combination given only 3 consecutive days per week is as effective as daily doses, provided compliance in administration is sound. Protection is afforded only as long as the patient receives the drug. Such a regimen is recommended for individuals who are at unusually high risk for the disease. Severely malnourished patients whose dietary deficits might not be restored could benefit from this prophylaxis. However, correction of the nutritional state should receive first priority. Aerosolized pentamidine has been approved by the FDA for adults with AIDS, but studies in children have not been reported. The adult dose is 300 mg of pentamidine administered by a Respirgard II nebulizer once monthly.

Several experimental drugs are in various stages of development for the treatment and prevention of *P. carinii* pneumonitis. Dapsone, trimetrexate plus leukovorin, a hydroxynaphthoquinone (566C80), and difluoromethylornithine have been reported to be efficacious, but none has been accepted for general use at this time. These may offer an alternative approach to patients who cannot take parenteral pentamidine or trimethoprim-sulfamethoxazole.

BIBLIOGRAPHY

Dutz W: *Pneumocystis carinii* pneumonia. Pathol Annu 5:309, 1970.

Gajdusek DC: *Pneumocystis carinii*—etiologic agent of interstitial plasma cell pneumonia of premature and young infants. Pediatrics 19:543, 1957.

Hughes WT, Feldman S, Chaudhary SC, et al: Comparison of pentamidine isethionate and trimethoprim-sulfamethoxazole in the treatment of *Pneumocystis carinii* pneumonia. J Pediatr 92:285, 1978.

Hughes WT, Price RH, Sisko F, et al: Protein-calorie malnutrition: A host determinant for *Pneumocystis carinii* infection. Am J Dis Child 128:44, 1974.

Hughes WT: *Pneumocystis carinii*. Boca Raton, FL, CRC Press, 1987, Vol 1, p 131, Vol 2, p 136.

Masur H, Kovacs JA: Treatment and prophylaxis of *Pneumocystis carinii* pneumonia. Infect Dis Clin North Am 2:419, 1988.

80. FREE-LIVING AMEBIC INFECTIONS

Richard J. Duma

DEFINITION. Free-living amebic (FLA) infections are caused by invasive amebae, principally of the genera *Naegleria* and *Acanthamoeba,* which are ubiquitous in nature and readily found free-living in soil and water. These infections are to be distinguished from those caused by the parasite *Entamoeba histolytica* (amebiasis), especially when secondary spread occurs from the liver or lung to the central nervous system (CNS). Primary amebic meningoencephalitis (PAM) is the most frequently reported FLA infection, followed by ocular and, rarely, pulmonary, sinus, and otitic involvement.

ETIOLOGY AND EPIDEMIOLOGY. PAM, first described by Fowler and Carter in Australia in 1967, is an infection of the CNS. It is almost always fatal and may be classified as *acute, subacute,* or *chronic,* depending on the responsible pathogen involved, the incubation period of the disease, and the length of illness. Although fewer than 150 cases have been reported worldwide thus far (Table 80–1), evidence suggests that this may be only a small proportion of those actually occurring. Most reports are from developed countries and probably reflect good identification and surveillance techniques rather than a peculiarly high incidence.

Acute PAM. This is most often caused by *Naegleria fowleri,* but on occasion may be caused by *Acanthamoeba.* When caused by *N. fowleri,* intimate patient contact with warm fresh water has almost always been noted (although on 1 occasion dust-borne spread was suspected), and common source epidemics may occur. The incubation period is 5 to 7 days. When acute PAM is caused by species of *Acanthamoeba,* no clues are generally available as to the source of the organism or the mode of transmission, epidemics are not known to occur, and infection is more commonly seen in immunosuppressed individuals than in otherwise healthy people.

Subacute or Chronic PAM. This is usually caused by *Acanthamoeba* (principally *A. castellanii* or *A. polyphaga*), although other as yet unidentified free-living amebae may be responsible. The incubation period is more than 7 days, and the clinical course varies from weeks to months. This form also occurs more commonly in immunosuppressed people. To date, all cases of *Acanthamoeba* PAM have been fatal.

Other FLA Infections. FLA infections of the eye are due to acanthamoebae. Generally, these infections follow minor trauma to the eye or are associated with the presence of a foreign body (especially soft contact lens).

TABLE 80–1. Approximate Number of Cases of PAM Reported Worldwide (1967–1987)

Country	No. Cases	Probable Organism*		
		Naegleria	*Acanthamoeba*	*Unknown*
Australia	13	13	0	0
Barbados	1	0	1	0
Belgium	6	6	0	0
Czechoslovakia	17	17	0	0
England	6	5	1	0
India	11	8	3	0
Ireland	1	1	0	0
Korea	1	1	0	0
Mexico	1	1	0	0
New Guinea	1	1	0	0
New Zealand	7	7	0	0
Nigeria	6	5	1	0
Peru	1	0	0	1
Puerto Rico	1	0	0	1
Venezuela	2	1	1	0
Uganda	1	1	0	0
United States	58	30	25	3
Total	134	97	32	5

*Based on clinical picture, epidemiologic history, and/or identification of organism by immunologic or cultural methods.

The precise source of organisms and mode of transmission are unknown, but contamination of the eye by water or soil containing the amebae is believed to occur. Usually, the infection remains confined, but spread to the CNS (as in PAM) can result. Pulmonary, otitic, and sinus FLA infections occur only rarely and are poorly documented. Most are believed due to acanthamoebae, and spread to the CNS may or may not result. The epidemiology of these infections is obscure.

PATHOLOGY AND PATHOGENESIS. The histopathology of FLA infections depends on the acuteness or chronicity of the infection. Only the trophozoite stage of the ameba is invasive.

Acute PAM. In acute infections, a polymorphonuclear cell response is seen, generally with an absence of eosinophils. Amebae invade via the olfactory mucosa and migrate along the fila olfactoria through the cribriform plate to the olfactory nerve and eventually to the brain. Early invasion of the subarachnoid space is noted, and additional cerebral invasion of gray matter occurs from without via the Virchow-Robin spaces. Acute, purulent, hemorrhagic necrosis is the rule, and amebae are readily seen within and in advance of involved areas. Amebae commonly collect in large numbers around small vessels (Fig. 80–1). Trophozoites are readily stained with hematoxylin and eosin; however, in fixed sections of tissue they are often mistaken for macrophages. Iron hematoxylin is a better stain for identification purposes, and characteristically a large single karyosome surrounded by a clear halo is noted. Nevertheless, such stains and fixation cannot be used to distinguish *Acanthamoeba* from *Naegleria,* and immune specific fluorescent staining techniques are employed for this purpose.

Subacute or Chronic PAM. In subacute or chronic PAM, lymphocytes, monocytes, epithelioid cells, plasma cells, scattered neutrophils, and giant cells may be seen in the inflammatory response, depending on the chronicity of the infection. Multiple areas of granulomatous cerebritis may occur, often involving midbrain structures such as the thalamus, pons, and corpus callosum. Amebic cysts can occasionally be found, as the responsible organisms are usually acanthamoebae.

Other FLA Infections. The histopathology depends on the organisms present and the length of time of involvement. Necrosis is commonly seen. In ocular infections the cornea is principally involved and destroyed early, a purulent exudate is commonly found in the anterior and posterior chambers, and uveitis may be present.

CLINICAL MANIFESTATIONS

Acute PAM. Acute PAM resembles acute purulent bacterial meningitis and in the early stages cannot be readily distinguished from this entity. Acute PAM usually begins abruptly with severe, unrelenting bifrontal headache associated with fever and often with nausea and vomiting. Either generalized or focal seizures are common, and in some instances abnormalities in taste or smell may be present (olfactory involvement) in the early stages. Marked nuchal rigidity occurs, with positive Kernig and Brudzinski signs. Focal or diffuse cerebral involvement is manifest by 48 hours, and the patient

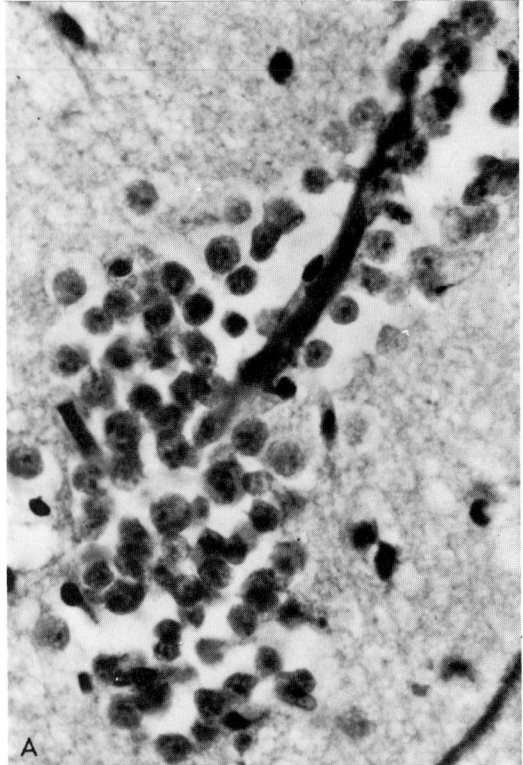

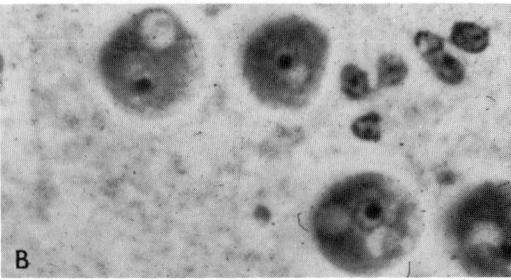

FIGURE 80–1. *A,* Cluster of amebae in perivascular space of formalin-fixed brain of patient with PAM; note rounding up of amebae (× 400). *B,* Higher magnification of same amebae. Note the single contractile vacuole and characteristic nucleus with a large, dark karyosome surrounded by a clear halo and a fine nuclear rim (× 1000). Cultures and fluorescent antibody tests were positive for *N. fowleri.*

may be confused, obtunded, or frankly comatose. If the olfactory tract is involved, PAM should be highly suspected. When infection is due to *Naegleria,* amebae are readily seen in and isolated from the cerebrospinal fluid (CSF), and bacteria are notably absent. The CSF glucose level may be extremely low (<10 mg/dl); white blood cells may number from 100 to 10,000/mm³ with neutrophils predominating. Red blood cells are occasionally present. Serologic tests are of no value in the diagnosis of acute infections.

Subacute or Chronic PAM. The clinical picture in subacute or chronic PAM is that of single or multiple brain abscesses. Headache occurs early and is insidious. Fever is present, but is sporadic and generally of low grade. Seizures, especially focal, occur later than in acute PAM, and a wide variety of localizing neurologic signs, depending on the area(s) of brain involved, sooner

or later appear. The CSF may contain as many mononuclear cells as neutrophils. The glucose level may be normal, and amebae are seldom seen in or isolated from the CSF. Midbrain lesions in the absence of olfactory involvement are common. Computed tomography (CT) may be valuable in identifying and locating such lesions.

Other FLA Infections. FLA infections of the eye or other structures generally cause chronic, progressively destructive lesions. Trauma preceding ocular infection is common. Amebae may be seen or isolated in clinical specimens. Rising serologic titers are occasionally useful in confirming the diagnosis.

DIAGNOSIS. For isolation of FLA, specimens should be kept at room temperature (23C). They should not be frozen or refrigerated, as amebae will be destroyed. Generally, amebae are easily isolated on plain agar plates seeded with gram-negative bacilli such as *Escherichia coli,* or they are grown axenically in a variety of liquid media or on tissue cultures. Identification is not difficult and is based principally on the morphology of the various stages. *Naegleria* possesses a flagellate stage; *Acanthamoeba* does not. In living preparations *Naegleria* appears limax in form with blunt pseudopodia, a single nucleus and contractile vacuole are present, and the organism is highly motile. On the other hand, *Acanthamoeba* possesses acanthapodia and is extremely sluggish. In tissues, both organisms become round, are about 12 to 20 μm in diameter, and have trophozoite stages that are virtually indistinguishable from one another. In such situations, immunofluorescent techniques are extremely useful in identification. Optimal growth is achieved aerobically and at temperatures between 33 and 37C, *Naegleria* being the more thermophilic of the 2 organisms.

TREATMENT. The treatment of acute PAM due to *Naegleria* is with intravenous amphotericin B. High CSF drug levels must be achieved rapidly; thus, the patient should be receiving 1 mg/kg/day by the second day of therapy. Intrathecal, intracisternal, and intraventricular modes of therapy are hazardous, and these routes should be approached with extreme caution because of the frequent occurrence of marked cerebral edema. Therapy should be continued for about 10 days. Amphotericin B should be solubilized in D₅W and *not* in salt solutions (which cause it to precipitate), and each intravenous dose should be administered slowly over a period of *not less than* 1 hour. A rise in the serum creatinine level will occur, reflecting some degree of renal failure, but this should not deter continuation of therapy in this otherwise fatal disease. Also, serum potassium levels usually fall and may require correction. Miconazole and rifampin have been recommended and used, but their value is unproved. In 1 case, the combination of miconazole and amphotericin B appeared to be synergistic; however, because imidazoles inhibit sterol synthesis, they may also antagonize amphotericin B.

No satisfactory therapeutic agents are available for treating acanthamoebic CNS infections. If a single lesion is present, surgical excision may be the only hope for cure. Unfortunately, lesions in cerebral infections are often multiple and located deep in the midbrain, thus being inaccessible to surgery. Flucytosine and sulfa have been used, but their value is unproved. For ocular infections, enucleation and/or corneal transplants are often necessary. Topically applied polymyxin, hamycin (Primamycin) paromomycin, hydroxystilbamidine isethionate, and/or clotrimazole may be tried, but there are few clinical data regarding effectiveness.

PREVENTION. No vaccines are available for any of these infections, and no other methods of prevention are known. When *Naegleria* infection is a possibility, every effort should be made either to avoid the suspected water source or to keep the water containing the amebae away from the nasal, and thus the olfactory, structures. The most likely source for this organism is warm, fresh water, whether artificially or naturally heated; thus, local health authorities should pay careful attention to a history of neurologic or infectious diseases associated with particular warm springs, hot baths, freshwater lakes, or heated pools.

BIBLIOGRAPHY

Carter RF: Primary amoebic meningo-encephalitis. Trans R Soc Trop Med Hyg 66:193, 1972.
Duma RJ, Ferrell HW, Nelson CE, et al: Primary amebic meningo-encephalitis. N Engl J Med 281:1315, 1969.
Duma RJ, Rosenblum WI, McGehee RF, et al: Primary amebic meningoencephalitis caused by *Naegleria*. Ann Intern Med 74:923, 1971.
Jones DB, Visvesvara GA, Robinson NM: *Acanthamoeba* polyphaga keratitis and *Acanthamoeba* uveitis associated with fatal meningo-encephalitis. Trans Ophthal Soc UK 95:221, 1975.
Ma P, Willaert E, Jeuchter KB, et al: A case of keratitis due to *Acanthamoeba* in New York, New York, and features of 10 cases. J Infect Dis 143:662, 1981.
Martinez AJ, Sotelo-Avila C, Garcia-Tamayo J, et al: Meningoencephalitis due to *Acanthamoeba* sp. Pathogenesis and clinico-pathological study. Acta Neuropath 37:183, 1977.
Seidel JS, Harmatz P, Visvesvara GS, et al: Successful treatment of primary amebic meningoencephalitis. N Engl J Med 306:346, 1982.

81. OTHER TISSUE PROTOZOAN INFECTIONS

Jacob K. Frenkel

81.1. SARCOSPORIDIOSIS

DEFINITION. *Sarcocystis* is a 2-host coccidian. It forms muscle cysts containing bradyzoites in the intermediate host, or host of prey, and undergoes sporogony in the intestine of a definitive or predatory host. Humans function as definitive host for some *Sarcocystis* species, which give rise to enteritis and to sporocysts in the feces, and an intermediate host for others, which form muscle cysts, causing myositis when they disintegrate.

ETIOLOGY AND HISTORY. *Sarcocystis* infections were first described in the nineteenth century with the finding of sporozoan cysts in heart or skeletal muscle of animals and humans. Transmission remained obscure because the infection could not be reproduced by passage. During the mid-1970s, the coccidian affinity of

Sarcocystis was recognized, and the transmission cycles in several animal species were shown to involve 2 hosts. More than 100 *Sarcocystis* species have been described from the skeletal muscle and heart of various animals, but the definitive hosts generally remain to be identified, except for some domestic species (Fig. 81–1).

TRANSMISSION AND EPIDEMIOLOGY. Humans can serve as an accidental intermediate host for several *Sarcocystis* species and as a regular final host for at least 2 species (Fig. 81–1). Humans with muscle cysts are an aberrant host for species of *Sarcocystis* that normally live in the muscle of prey animals, e.g., a monkey, transmitted by unidentified predatory carnivores, e.g., a python. Humans are presumably infected by ingesting sporocysts from the feces of the carnivore, usually with contaminated soil.

Humans are the regular definitive host of certain *Sarcocystis* species of cattle and pigs; after the ingestion of raw or undercooked meat, the liberated bradyzoites enter the intestinal mucosa and develop into gametes, which after fertilization develop into oocysts. Unlike those in the 1-host coccidia, the oocysts sporulate in the mucosa, so that *Sarcocystis bovihominis* and *S. suihominis* are shed as sporulated sporocysts. These sporocysts were formerly called *Isospora hominis* when they were believed to be 1-host coccidia (Chapter 71.2) of a single species.

DISTRIBUTION AND INCIDENCE. The ease with which the cycle is maintained determines distribution and incidence. For example, *S. bovicanis* (Fig. 81–1) is distributed worldwide because cattle and dogs live in close proximity, dogs are fed slaughter wastes, and cattle eat dog feces.

S. bovihominis and *S. suihominis* (Fig. 81–1) occur where people eat raw or undercooked beef, pork, or venison, and where human feces are accessible to cattle or pigs.

Sarcocystis in skeletal muscle of humans has been described so rarely and sporadically as to suggest accidental parasitism. Beaver and colleagues have analyzed the morphology of sarcocysts and their location in cardiac or skeletal muscle in about 40 human cases and found that 4 types of organisms identified in skeletal muscle resembled a species commonly found in local monkeys. The organisms of 13 infections probably acquired in Southeast Asia resembled a *Sarcocystis* species found in *Macaca fascicularis;* in 8 infections probably acquired in India, the organism resembled *Sarcocystis* species found in *Macaca mulatta;* and in 1 of 4 infections probably acquired in Africa or Europe, the organism resembled the *Sarcocystis* found in *Cercopithicus talapoin.* Among 3 types of cysts found in human hearts, the organism of 1 resembled *S. bovicanis.* The causative organism of 3 infections acquired in the United States could not be identified. One of these was in a Kansas farmer who had a hobby of keeping exotic animals. *Sarcocystis lindemanni* is of doubtful validity because it apparently describes a nonparasitic object.

PATHOGENESIS AND PATHOLOGY. Intact sarcocysts in skeletal or cardiac muscle of humans measure up to 100 μm in diameter and 325 μm in length and generally are not accompanied by inflammatory reaction

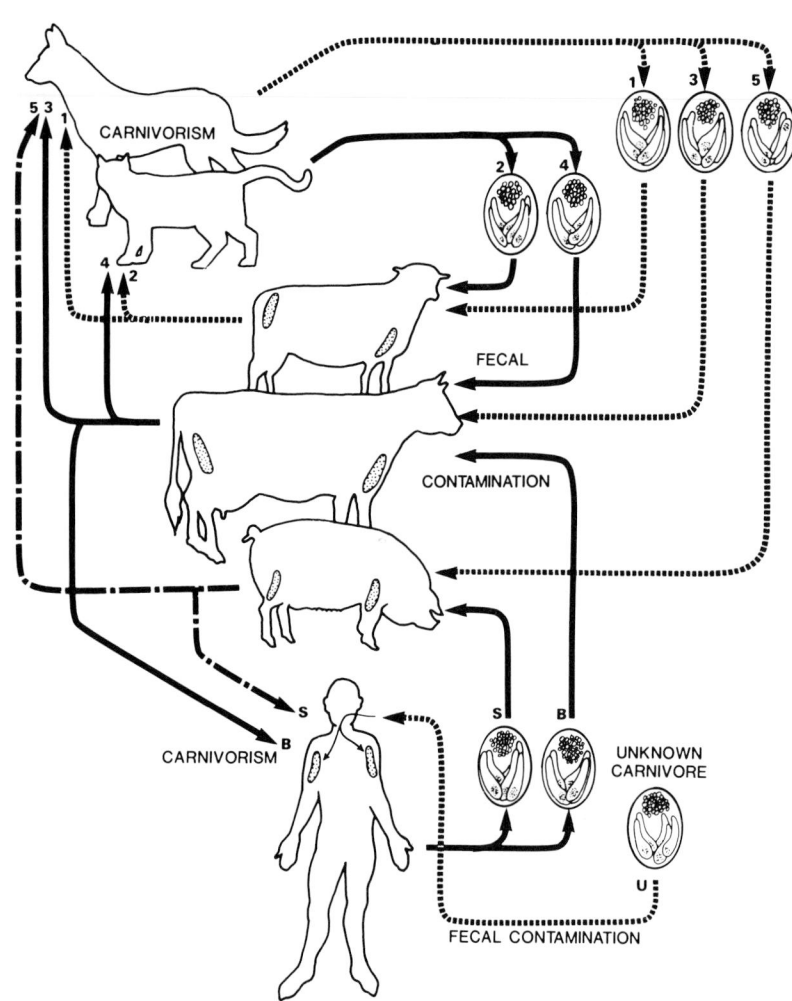

FIGURE 81–1. *Sarcocystis* transmission cycles involving humans and some domestic animals. Humans are the definitive host of *S. bovihominis (B)* and *S. suihominis (S)*, the two intestinal sarcosporidia. Humans are the accidental intermediate host with *Sarcocystis* of unknown species *(U)*, where skeletal and heart muscles are parasitized. Also indicated are the cycles of *S. ovicanis (1)*, *S. ovifelis (2)*, *S. bovicanis (3)*, *S. bovifelis (4)*, and *S. suicanis (5)*. (From Frenkel JK: *In* Mehlhorn H (ed): Parasitology in Focus. Berlin, Springer, 1988, p 549.)

(Fig. 81–2). Each sarcocyst contains numerous bradyzoites measuring 7 to 16 μm in length, depending on the species (Fig. 81–2B). Inflammation follows disintegration of these cysts; after the death of the intracystic bradyzoites, probably from antibody and complement, neutrophils, eosinophils, and lymphocytes accumulate, followed by plasma cells and, later, focal fibrosis. Vasculitis is commonly present in the muscle and subcutaneous tissues. This may stem from an earlier phase of intravascular schizogony, which has been observed in experimental animals but not in humans, or from nearby inflammation. Histopathologic diagnoses are myonecrosis and myositis with vasculitis.

The finding of sporulated oocysts or sporocysts, probably *S. bovihominis*, in the lamina propria of the small intestine was observed in 6 resected specimens of segmental eosinophilic necrotizing enteritis in Thailand. Although in 5 patients the focally obstructive inflammatory lesions were possibly related to the numerous gram-positive bacilli present, the intense tissue eosinophilia in 4 patients, one of whom demonstrated no evidence of bacteria, strongly suggests a relationship to the sporocysts of *Sarcocystis*.

CLINICAL MANIFESTATIONS

Muscle Infection. Painful muscle swellings, measuring 1 to 3 cm in diameter, initially associated with erythema of the overlying skin in various parts of the body, occurring episodically, and lasting for 2 days to 2 weeks,

were present in most of the patients. In some, these lesions were accompanied by fever, diffuse myalgia, muscle tenderness, weakness, eosinophilia, and bronchospasm. No clinical findings had been noted in patients in whom myocardial *Sarcocystis* infection was found accidentally by autopsy.

Enteric Infection. Following the ingestion of pork containing *S. suihominis,* volunteers developed diarrhea, vomiting, chills, and diaphoresis, starting 6 to 24 hours after ingestion and continuing for 12 to 24 hours. Sporocysts were shed between 11 and 71 days after the meal. Consumption of beef containing *S. bovihominis* was followed by abdominal discomfort and, in some volunteers, by nausea and diarrhea; sporocyst shedding started between 13 and 39 days after the meal and continued for 9 to 179 days. Eosinophilic enteritis and ulcerative obstructive enterocolitis may be occasional complications. Cases of enteritis after eating venison have been described in Europe.

DIAGNOSIS. Diagnosis of *Sarcocystis* myositis is by muscle biopsy (Fig. 81–2). Other cyst-forming organisms, e.g., *Toxoplasma gondii* and *Trypanosoma cruzi,* must be differentiated. Sarcocysts are often septate, and the cyst wall is distinct ultrastructurally. Bradyzoites of *Sarcocystis* and *Toxoplasma* are periodic acid–Schiff–positive, but *T. cruzi* is not. Serologic reactions have not been investigated in detail. They appear to be specific for the genus, but nonspecific as to species.

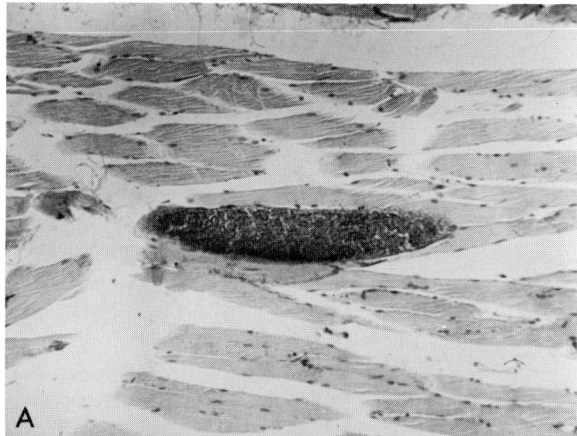

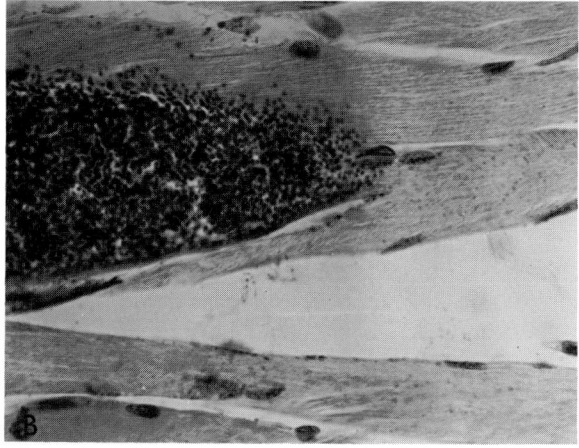

FIGURE 81–2. Sarcocyst in human skeletal muscle (PAS stain, × 150 *[A]* and × 600 *[B]*).

Intestinal sarcosporidiosis is diagnosed by finding already sporulated sporocysts, each containing 4 sporozoites, in freshly voided stool specimens with the aid of flotation procedures. Eosinophilia is often present.

TREATMENT AND PROGNOSIS. Because *Sarcocystis* in muscle and intestine are fully formed terminal stages when diagnosed and no new cells are parasitized, specific treatment of the muscle and enteric infection is unsatisfactory. However, corticosteroids should palliate the allergic inflammatory reactions episodically occurring after cyst rupture. Because the intracystic bradyzoites are not capable of infecting new cells in the host, there is no risk of recrudescence.

PREVENTION. Muscle involvement can be prevented by avoiding food and water that are potentially contaminated with feces of predatory carnivores. Enteric infection can be prevented by avoiding the ingestion of raw beef and pork; most frozen (− 20C) and well-cooked meats are safe, however.

BIBLIOGRAPHY

Beaver PC, Gadgil RK, Morera P: Sarcocystis in man: A review and report of five cases. Am J Trop Med Hyg 28:819, 1979.
Bunyaratvej S, Bunyawongwiroj P, Nitiyanant P: Human intestinal sarcosporidiosis—report of 6 cases. Am J Trop Med Hyg 31:36, 1982.
Dubey JP, Speer CS, Fayer R: Sarcocystosis of Animals and Man. Boca Raton, FL, CRC Press, 1988, pp 1–215.
Frenkel JK, Heydorn AO, Mehlhorn H, et al: Sarcocystinae: *Nomina dubia* and available names. Z Parasitenkd 58:115, 1979.
Levine ND, Tadros W: Named species and hosts of *Sarcocystis* (Protozoa: Apicomplexa: Sarcocystidae). Systematic Parasitology 2:41, 1980.
McLeod R, Hirabayashi RN, Rothman W, et al: Necrotizing vasculitis and *Sarcocystis:* A cause-and-effect relationship. South Med J 73:1380, 1980.
Mehlhorn H, Heydorn AO: The Sarcosporidia. Life cycle and fine structure. Adv Parasitol 16:43, 1978.
Piekarski G, Heydorn AO, Aryeetey ME, et al: Clinical, parasitologic, and serologic studies of sarcosporidiosis *(Sarcocystis suihominis)* of man. Immun Infekt 6:153, 1978.

81.2. MICROSPORIDIOSIS

DEFINITION. Microsporidia are parasitic protozoa characterized by spores containing a polar filament arranged in a spiral visible by electron microscopy (Fig. 81–3). Human infection has been described with 4 genera: *Encephalitozoon* with a uninucleate spore in a cytoplasmic vacuole; *Enterocytozoon*, uninucleate organisms in direct contact with host cell cytoplasm in the enterocyte; *Pleistophora,* a pansporoblastic organism forming multiple spores from individual sporants within cytoplasmic vacuoles; and *Nosema* with a binucleate spore free in the cytoplasms. All multiply in various tissues. The size of the spores varies from 2 to 3 μm.

ETIOLOGY AND HISTORY. The microsporidia are obligate intracellular protozoa, parasitizing a wide variety of lower animals. Economically important and well studied are *Nosema bombycis* of silkworms and *N. apis*

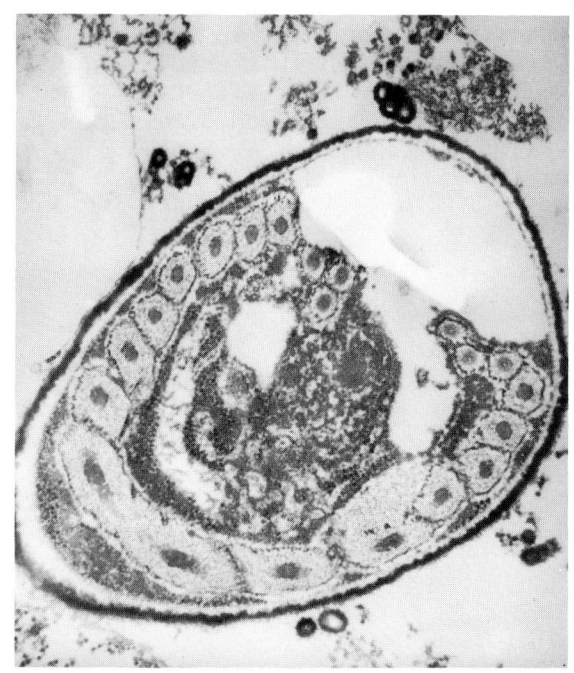

FIGURE 81–3. Ultrastructure of a microsporidian showing diagnostic polar filament arranged in a spiral (× 30,000). (Courtesy of Drs. Daniel Connor and Ann Cali and the Armed Forces Institute of Pathology, Photograph Neg. No. 71–11521–4.)

of bees. Laboratory mice, rats, hamsters, and rabbits are often asymptomatically infected with *Encephalitozoon cuniculi;* this has given rise to erroneous interpretations when these animals were used in attempts to isolate an infectious agent.

The history of human infection is marked by uncertainty, because microsporidia used to be confused with *Toxoplasma* and other small organisms and because some of the older reports were poorly documented. The taxonomy had been confusing but has been clarified by ultrastructural analysis, cultivation, and experimental cross-infections.

DISTRIBUTION AND INCIDENCE. Because only a few human cases have been well documented, it is likely that these obligatory parasites are contracted from more commonly infected natural hosts; whether these hosts are vertebrate or invertebrate is as yet unknown. Infection of laboratory rodents and rabbits and of domestic and wild animals appears to occur worldwide, but little is known about the prevalence of the infection in the latter. As noted, the disease is rare in humans; only 4 cases had been described up until recent years. Recently, the infection has been diagnosed in a few patients with acquired immunodeficiency syndrome (AIDS). Because more than one-half of the laboratory rabbits and mice from a given colony may be infected, asymptomatic infection of humans must be suspected.

TRANSMISSION. The spores of the microsporidia are shed in the urine of rabbits and mice and are excreted in the feces of the insect species. The spores are somewhat resistant to the environment, favoring contaminative transmission. Usually, after ingestion, the polar filament everts, injecting the sporoplasm with its nuclear material into an adjacent cell in the intestine; here it multiplies and is disseminated. Because the infection has been found in cesarean-derived, barrier-sustained mice, the occurrence of transplacental transmission has been suspected in laboratory animals.

PATHOGENESIS AND PATHOLOGY. The first 4 cases of microsporidiosis reported are as follows: A disseminated infection with *N. connori* (Fig. 81–4),

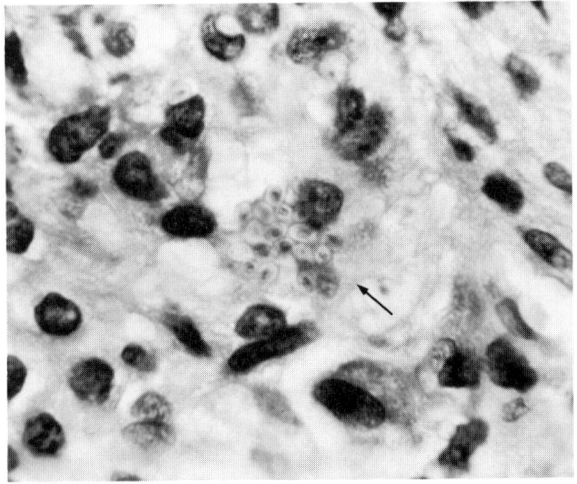

FIGURE 81–4. Microsporidia *(arrow)* *(Nosema connori)* in a human infant (× 1260). (Courtesy of Drs. Daniel Connor and Ann Cali and the Armed Forces Institute of Pathology, Photograph Neg. No. 71–5882.)

involving the muscles of stomach, bowel, arteries, diaphragm, and heart and the parenchymal cells of liver, lungs, and adrenals, was found in a 4-month-old infant. Mononuclear cell inflammation was present. This patient also had thymic alymphoplasia and advanced *Pneumocystis* infection of the lungs. In another instance, microsporidia were found in the cerebrospinal fluid and urine of a 9-year-old Japanese boy with encephalitis who recovered; no biopsy material was obtained. The organism was recovered from mice injected with patient specimens, whereas none were found in control mice.

The corneal biopsy specimen from an 11-year-old Ceylonese boy showed keratitis with central necrosis associated with acute inflammation. Abundant refractile oval bodies interpreted as *Nosema* were present. Another case of ocular nosematosis was found in a 26-year-old woman from Botswana, Africa; she had a necrotizing keratitis that caused perforation, and the blind, painful eye was enucleated 5 months after onset of the infection.

Intestinal microsporidiosis has been observed in several patients with AIDS. Inflammation was minimal, and the diagnosis was made ultrastructurally. Microsporidial myositis was reported in another patient with AIDS. Scarring and inflammation with plasma cells, lymphocytes, and histiocytes were accompanied by atrophic and degenerating microsporidia-infected muscle fibers in 1 AIDS patient. The patients with AIDS had general symptoms, including diarrhea, none of which could be specifically attributed to microsporidiosis in view of the additional infections present. Some investigators believe that African slim disease results from microsporidial infection.

CLINICAL MANIFESTATIONS AND COMPLICATIONS. Symptoms varied widely in the few reported patients with microsporidiosis. The 4-month-old boy was immunologically compromised; exhibited diarrhea, vomiting, malabsorption, and hypogammaglobulinemia; and died after an illness of 22 days. The 9-year-old Japanese boy presented with vomiting, convulsions, recurrent fever, headaches, and loss of consciousness. His spinal fluid showed 116 to 336 leukocytes/mm³; a direct smear of the sediment on the fifth and eighth days of illness showed oval bodies measuring about 3 × 1.5 µm. Similar bodies were seen in urine sediment on the eleventh to thirteenth days of illness. The patient was considered recovered after 24 days except for persisting headaches. The AIDS patients had diarrhea (attributed to a concurrent *Giardia* infection) and general muscle weakness. The 11-year-old Ceylonese boy developed keratitis 6 years after he had been gored by a goat and suffered a lacerated eyelid. The woman from Botswana had a 4-month history of a painful left eye with a corneal ulcer, keratouveitis, and hyphemia. Light perception had been lost.

DIAGNOSIS. In sections, both the proliferating organisms and the spores are ovoid, measuring 1 to 2 µm × 2 to 4 µm in size. Intracellular accumulation of these organisms reaches up to 30 µm (Fig. 81–4). On staining with hematoxylin and eosin, a defined nuclear mass is seen in a clear cytoplasm. The spores sometimes appear refractile. With periodic acid–Schiff staining, an intensely red–staining polar granule is seen in each organism (Fig. 81–3). The walls of the spores stain variably with Gomori and Wilder's silver stains and show variable Gram staining and acid fastness. The Goodpasture acid-fast method of staining (carbolfuchsin decolorized with 37% formaldehyde and counterstained with picric acid) and Weil's myelin stain demonstrate *Encephalitozoon* but not *Toxoplasma*. The encephalitozoa of laboratory animals can be cultured in fibroblasts, rabbit or dog kidney cells, canine embryo cells, and rabbit choroid plexus cells. Spontaneous infection of the Yoshida ascites tumor has been observed. Mice injected intraperitoneally with infectious material generally develop ascites after 2 to 5 weeks; organisms can be demonstrated in peritoneal macrophages in Giemsa-stained smears. Brain from control mice should be passaged to check for the presence of spontaneous infection. Serologic tests and skin tests have been developed using cell culture–grown antigen. Indirect fluorescent antibody, complement-fixation, and enzyme-linked immunosorbent assay (ELISA) techniques have been used for antibody detection; an India ink immunoreaction test is available in kit form from Testman, Box 9020, S75009, Uppsala, Sweden, for the diagnosis of the infection in rabbits. Antibody has been found in a variable percentage of rabbits and in a small percentage of humans—supposedly with a higher prevalence in those in contact with rabbits.

TREATMENT AND PROGNOSIS. Fumagillin (Fumadil-B) in concentrations of 5 μg/ml in cell culture inhibited 2 isolates of *Encephalitozoon cuniculi* obtained from a rabbit and from a spontaneously infected puppy. No trials in mice were reported. Because fumagillin inhibited toxoplasmosis in mice when given in doses of 10 mg/gm of body weight, there is evidence for the absorption of this drug in effective concentrations.

PREVENTION AND CONTROL. The usual sanitary measures that prevent contamination of food and water with urine and feces of animals should decrease the chance for systemic infection. Hand washing and general hygienic habits may possibly reduce the chance for contamination of the conjunctiva and cornea.

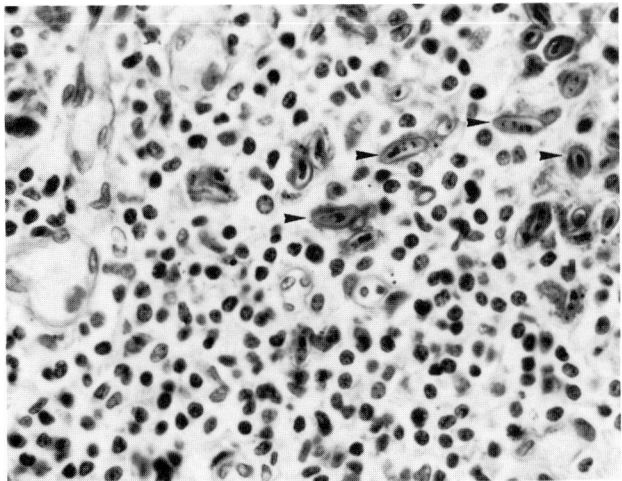

FIGURE 81–5. Unizoic cysts of *Cystoisospora belli* in mesenteric lymph node *(arrowheads)* of an AIDS patient (× 600, periodic acid–Schiff hematoxylin). (Courtesy of Dr. Carlos Restrepo.)

Shadduck JA, Greeley E: Microsporidia and human infections. Clin Microbiol Rev 2:158, 1989.
Vavra J, Blazek K, Lavicka N, et al: Nosematosis in carnivores. J Parasitol 57:923, 1971.
Waller T: The India-ink immunoreaction: A method for the rapid diagnosis of encephalitozoonosis. Lab Anim 11:93, 1977.
Wilson JM: Biology of *Encephalitozoon cuniculi*. Med Biol 57:84, 1979.

81.3. CYSTOISOSPORIDIOSIS

Isospora belli has been considered to undergo only a classic coccidian cycle with schizogony and gametogony in the small intestinal epithelium (Chapter 71.2). However, a new stage was found, individual encysted zoites, so-called hypnozoites (Fig. 81–5). These were present in the lamina propria and lymph nodes of a patient with the acquired immunodeficiency syndrome (AIDS). Similar cysts had previously been found in rodents capable of serving as intermediate hosts that were experimentally infected with feline isosporiasis. The genus *Cystoisospora* was created for such 2-host coccidia with hypnozoites, previously classified in the genus *Isospora*. The presence of unizoic cysts indicates that the human *I. belli* would be better classified as *Cystoisospora belli*. It is suggested that this organism has an intermediate host and that infection can be contracted by ingestion of meat. In this patient, an intense inflammatory reaction, including plasma cells, lymphocytes, neutrophils, and eosinophils, accompanied the tissue cysts in gut and lymph nodes (Fig. 81–5).

BIBLIOGRAPHY

Ashton N, Wirasinha PA: Encephalitozoonosis (nosematosis) of the cornea. Br J Ophthalmol 57:669, 1973.
Desportes I, Le Charpentier Y, Gallian A, et al: Occurrence of a new microsporidian: *Enterocytozoon bieneusi* n.g., n. sp., in the enterocytes of a patient with AIDS. J Protozool 32:250, 1985.
Ledford DK, Overman MD, Gonzalvo A, et al: Microsporidial myositis in a patient with the immunodeficiency syndrome. Ann Intern Med 102:628, 1985.
Margileth AM, Strano AJ, Chandra R, et al: Disseminated nosematosis in an immunologically compromised infant. Arch Pathol 95:145, 1973.
Matsubayashi H, Koike T, Mikata I, et al: A case of *Encephalitozoon*-like body infection in man. Arch Pathol 67:181, 1959.
Orenstein IH, Chiang J, Steinberg W, et al: Intestinal microsporidiosis as a cause of diarrhea in human immunodeficiency virus–infected patients. A report of 20 cases. Hum Pathol 21:475, 1990.
Pinnolis M, Egbert PR, Font RL, et al: Nosematosis of the cornea. Arch Ophthalmol 99:1044, 1981.

BIBLIOGRAPHY

Frenkel JK, Dubey JP: Rodents as vectors for feline coccidia, *Isospora felis* and *Isospora rivolta*. J Infect Dis 125:69, 1972.
Restrepo C, Macher AM, Radany EH: Disseminated intestinal isosporiasis in a patient with the acquired immune deficiency syndrome. Am J Clin Pathol 87:40, 1987.

PART VI

HELMINTHIC INFECTIONS

GENERAL PRINCIPLES

G. Thomas Strickland

DEFINITIONS. *Helminth* is derived from the Greek word *helmins* and means worm. As usually interpreted, the word connotes several groups of parasitic worms. In comparison with the small unicellular protozoa, the helminths are large multicellular organisms with complex tissues and organs.

CLASSIFICATION. There are 3 groups of helminths that parasitize humans: (1) annelids (segmented worms), (2) nematodes (roundworms), and (3) platyhelminths (flatworms).

Annelida. The Hirudinea (leeches [Chapter 103.2]) is the only class of annelids of medical importance.

Nematoda. Members of this phylum are nonsegmented roundworms. They are characterized by longitudinally oriented muscles and by a triradiate esophagus. They are bilaterally symmetrical and have a complete digestive tract, and the sexes are usually distinct. Most species are free-living and inhabit soil and water. Most of the 80,000 species parasitic to vertebrates have developed a biologic dependence on a single host (Chapters 82 to 95). The word nematode is derived from the Greek *nema* for thread and *eidos* for form.

It is useful to divide nematodes into groups according to the body organ of humans in which they reside.

Adults That Reside in the Gut. This group includes human parasites of the following species: *Ascaris lumbricoides* (Chapter 83), *Ancylostoma duodenale* and *Necator americanus* (Chapter 84.1), *Trichuris trichiura* (Chapter 82.2), *Enterobius vermicularis* (Chapter 82.1), *Strongyloides stercoralis* (Chapter 84.2), *Capillaria philippinensis* (this nematode has apparently recently adapted to parasitizing humans) (Chapter 82.3), and *Trichostrongylus orientalis* (Chapter 82.4).

Adults That Reside in the Blood or Lymphatic or Subcutaneous Tissues. This group includes human parasites of the following species: *Wuchereria bancrofti* (Chapter 85.1), *Brugia malayi* (Chapter 85.2), *Brugia timori* (Chapter 85.3), *Loa loa* (Chapter 86), *Onchocerca volvulus* (Chapter 87), *Mansonella ozzardi*, *M. perstans*, and *M. streptocerca* (Chapter 88), and *Dracunculus medinensis* (Chapter 89).

Larval Stages That Cause Human Pathologic Conditions in Various Tissues. These, with the exception of *Trichinella spiralis*, are nonhuman parasites that are unable to develop to adults in humans, an aberrant host. In general, these nematodes follow the same migration pattern here as in their definitive host, except that it is interrupted.

Infections That Are Usually Limited to the Skin and Subcutaneous Tissues. Creeping eruption is primarily caused by the dog and cat hookworms (i.e., *Ancylostoma braziliense*, *A. caninum*, and *Uncinaria stenocephala* [Chapter 94]) as well as other rare animal parasites that infect by skin penetration. Skin penetration by human hookworms (Chapter 84.1) and *Strongyloides* (Chapter 84.2) sometimes causes similar findings. Some *Dirofilaria* parasites of various animals (Chapter 88.4) cause subcutaneous nodules in man.

Infections Primarily Involving the Muscles. The larvae of *Trichinella spiralis* can migrate through many tissues, including the heart and brain, before encysting in muscle (Chapter 90).

Infections Causing a Visceral Larva Migrans Syndrome. The larval stages of the dog and cat ascarids, *Toxocara canis* and *T. cati*, and *Capillaria hepatica* (Chapter 91) commonly cause lesions in multiple organs, principally the liver, brain, lungs, and eyes.

Angiostrongylus costaricensis (Chapter 93.2) and marine ascarids (i.e., the anisakids and eustrongylids) (Chapter 95) primarily cause abdominal lesions.

Angiostrongylus cantonensis, the rat lungworm, causes eosinophilic meningitis (Chapter 93.1). *Gnathostoma spinigerum*, a stomach worm of domestic and wild cats and dogs, can cause a creeping eruption, an abdominopulmonary hypereosinophilic syndrome, and an eosinophilic myeloencephalitis (Chapter 92).

The dog heartworm, *Dirofilaria immitis*, sometimes causes pulmonary nodules in humans following bites from infectious mosquitoes (Chapter 88.4). A pulmonary hypereosinophilia syndrome can be caused by migrating human ascarid (Chapter 83), hookworm (Chapter 84.1), and *Strongyloides* (Chapter 84.2) larvae and microfilariae of *W. bancrofti*, *B. malayi*, and various animal filariae (Chapter 85.4).

Platyhelminthes. Flatworms are usually dorsoventrally flattened, are bilaterally symmetrical, and have 3 body layers lacking a body cavity. They include the trematodes and cestodes. The word is derived from the Greek *platys*, meaning broad, and *helmins*, meaning worm.

Trematoda. This class includes the flukes that are parasitic to humans and animals. They are usually hermaphroditic, and a digestive canal is present except in the sporocyst stage of digenetic species. Trematode eggs are excreted in the stool, urine, or sputum of the definitive host. All flukes require a mollusk as their first intermediate host. The larval stage that escapes from the mollusk may then enter a second intermediate host (fish, crustacean), encyst on vegetation, or penetrate directly into the skin of the definitive host. Infection generally results from the ingestion of insufficiently cooked fish, crustaceans, and vegetation (Fig. VI D-1).

The important trematodes of humans belong to the following genera: (1) adults that live in the venous system—*Schistosoma* (Chapter 96); (2) adults that live in the intestines—*Fasciolopsis, Echinostoma, Heterophyes, Gastrodiscoides,* and *Metagonimus* (Chapter 97); (3) adults that live in the biliary system—*Clonorchis, Opisthorchis, Fasciola,* and *Dicrocoelium* (Chapter 98); and (4) adults that live in the bronchi—*Paragonimus* (Chapter 99).

Cestoda. This is a subclass of Cestoidea comprising the true tapeworms, which have a head (scolex) and segments (proglottids). Adults are all parasitic and hermaphroditic and live in the intestinal lumen of vertebrate hosts. Those that can infect humans include *Diphyllobothrium latum* and *D. pacificum* (Chapter 100.1), *Taenia saginata* and *T. solium* (Chapter 100.2), *Hymenolepis nana* and *H. diminuta* (Chapter 100.3), and *Dipylidium caninum* (Chapter 100.4). Their larval stages (hydatid, cysticercus, sparganum, coenurus) may be found in various organs and tissues of humans (Chapter 101) and other intermediate hosts (Chapters 100 and 101).

ANATOMY AND PHYSIOLOGY. Helminths are complicated multicellular organisms. Those infecting humans range in length from 0.3 mm (e.g., *Toxocara canis* [Chapter 91] and *Ancylostoma braziliense* [Chapter 94] larvae) to 12 m (e.g., adult *Taenia saginata* [Chapter 100.2]). They are round (nematodes) or flat (flukes and tapeworms). They all have an outer coating, the cuticle, which provides protection and is involved in active transport of water, electrolytes, and other substances.

Almost all helminths are unable to multiply in their host. The reproductive organs make up a large portion of the body cavities. The nematodes are sexually distinct, with separate males and females. The trematodes and cestodes are both diecious (schistosomes) and monoecious (other flukes and the tapeworms). The monoecious trematodes reproduce by self-fertilization or by cross-fertilization. Among the tapeworms, each proglottid possesses both male and female sex organs. Usually, sperm is transferred between adjacent mature proglottids of the worm. (See the individual sections in Chapters 82 to 101 for the details of the muscular, nervous, digestive, excretory, and reproductive systems.)

TRANSMISSION. Parasitic worms infect humans in almost all regions of the world, but there is a particular abundance in the tropics of both parasite species and infected individuals. This is the result of climatic and sociologic factors. Many of these parasites require special conditions of temperature and humidity for survival and multiplication. Others require particular vertebrate or invertebrate hosts such as fish, snails, crustaceans, or insects for the completion of their life cycles. The intermediate hosts, particularly insect vectors, gain ready access to humans in tropical regions owing to the lack of preventive measures by the indigenous populations.

Oral Transmission. The distribution of intestinal nematodes whose eggs are passed in human feces (Chapters 82 to 84) is affected by climatic conditions (e.g., rainfall, temperature, and humidity) as well as sanitary practices. The customs in many regions of using human excreta (night soil) for fertilizer and of indiscriminate defecation result in widespread pollution of soil, water supplies, and foods (particularly vegetables). This results in a high prevalence of fecally transmitted nematodes in most of the tropics and subtropics.

Eating habits account for the transmission of other nematodes. Ingestion of undercooked or raw meat (*Trichinella spiralis* [Chapter 90], *Taenia* species [Chapter 100.2]) or fish (anisakid larvae [Chapter 95], *Diphyllobothrium latum* [Chapter 100.1], and *Clonorchis sinensis* and *Opisthorchis* species [Chapter 98]) infected with larval stages of the parasite transmits some helminths. Other helminthic infections follow the ingestion of larvae-contaminated water (*Dracunculus medinensis* [Chapter 89]), raw snails (*Angiostrongylus* species [Chapter 93]), raw or undercooked crabs (*Paragonimus westermani* [Chapter 99]), and aquatic plants (*Fasciola hepatica* [Chapter 98.3] and *Fasciolopsis buski* [Chapter 97.1]).

People are infected with *Toxocara canis* (Chapter 91) and *Echinococcus granulosus* (Chapter 101.2) following the ingestion of substances contaminated with dog feces containing the helminth eggs.

Transmission by Skin Penetration. Larval stages of hookworm parasites (Chapter 84.1) and *Strongyloides stercoralis* (Chapter 84.2) in the soil cause infection when they penetrate the intact skin. Third-stage larvae of dog and cat hookworms can penetrate unbroken skin but cannot develop fully in humans. They cause a creeping eruption (Chapter 94). Cercariae of *Schistosoma* species penetrate the skin of those exposed to contaminated water (Chapter 96). Those species not capable of developing in humans cause a rash, called swimmer's itch.

Transmission by Bite of a Vector. The filarial parasites (Chapters 85 to 88) develop within the biologic vector, which is also an intermediate host. These can be mosquitoes (*Wuchereria bancrofti* [Chapter 85.1] or *Brugia malaya* [Chapter 85.2]), black flies (*Onchocerca volvulus* [Chapter 87]), or Chrysops flies (*Loa loa* [Chapter 86]).

MAGNITUDE OF THE HEALTH PROBLEM
In The Tropics and Subtropics
Prevalence of Infection. Because many people are infected with more than 1 species of helminth, there are more different species of helminths infecting people than there are people in the world. The numbers infected with hookworms, *Ascaris, Trichuris,* pinworm, schistosomes, onchocerca, and filariae are each in the hundreds of millions. A common trinity of intestinal helminthiasis includes ascariasis, hookworm infection, and trichuriasis.

Intensity of Infection. Some helminth infections (i.e., schistosomiasis, hookworm disease, and onchocerciasis) are among those medical conditions that cause major human suffering in the world. It is difficult to document morbidity in the vast majority of those infected with these parasites and with other helminth infections (e.g., clonorchiasis, taeniasis, ascariasis, trichuriasis, enterobiasis, and filariasis).

The magnitude of disease caused by helminths is related to the intensity of infection. Individuals with light infections have a tendency to have few or no abnormal findings, whereas those with heavy and prolonged infections often have clinical symptoms and signs and develop complications. This is well documented in schistosomiasis, hookworm disease (versus infection), onchocerciasis, and filariasis.

Hookworm Disease. The major cause of death in Puerto Rico prior to Bailey K. Ashford's treatment campaign during the first decade of the twentieth century was anemia from hookworm disease (Chapter 5). Hookworm disease is still a major cause of iron deficiency anemia in children and pregnant and lactating women in the tropics and subtropics (Chapter 84.1). Iron deficiency is still one of the major nutritional problems in these areas (Chapter 108.1). Even *Trichuris trichiura* can cause anemia, malnutrition, and diarrhea in children with heavy infections (Chapter 82.2).

Schistosomiasis. It has been said that it is difficult to demonstrate increased morbidity or mortality due to schistosomiasis (Chapter 96). Although, admittedly, the data are still incomplete, some points about that disease in Egypt are well worth noting: (1) Hemorrhage from esophageal varices secondary to the portal hypertension of schistosomiasis mansoni is considered the most common cause of death in adult Egyptian males. (2) Bladder carcinoma in association with *S. haematobium* infection is the most commonly diagnosed malignancy in adult Egyptian males. (3) The association of anemia and hypoproteinemia with heavy *S. mansoni* infection of the colon is common in rural Egyptian children and adolescents. (4) Decreased work capacity and dyspnea on exertion have been shown to occur in farmers having schistosomal cor pulmonale, which is generally associated with heavy and prolonged infections with *S. mansoni* and/or *S. haematobium* along with portal hypertension. (5) The interaction between hepatosplenic schistosomiasis and the complications of viral hepatitis results in a huge, and as yet still unmeasured hepatic morbidity and mortality in the adult population. (6) Individuals with either *S. mansoni* or *S. haematobium* infection are prone to have the chronic salmonellosis syndrome consisting of prolonged and intermittent fever and chronic and recurring bacteremia with *Salmonella* species. (7) Hydronephrosis, chronic pyelonephritis, and renal failure are complications of chronic and heavy *S. haematobium* infections.

Abdominal ultrasonography is proving to be an excellent means of detecting morbidity in schistosomiasis, not only in individuals in hospitals and clinics, but also in groups directly in their communities. The technique is inexpensive and noninvasive. It can accurately detect hepatosplenomegaly, urinary tract obstruction, hepatic periportal fibrosis, and bladder polyps and masses. Sonography is being used to demonstrate morbidity in communities and is showing that many individuals, even those with a paucity of symptoms, have detectable schistosomal morbidity.

Onchocerciasis. It is estimated that 40 million people are infected with *Onchocerca volvulus,* 39 million of these in Africa alone (Chapter 87). The majority of those infected have dermatitis and lesions involving the subcutaneous tissues, which cause considerable discomfort, interfering with their ability to work. Moreover,

250,000 to 500,000 are blind from this parasite, and more have eye lesions that have not yet progressed to blindness. Often, those blinded are young adult males—fathers and former providers for the family. Those who are afflicted with onchocerciasis are often illiterate subsistence farmers who frequently live in isolated communities. The parasite does not normally infect city dwellers and is not transmitted in developed countries, nor is it much of a threat to travelers.

Although there are no good cost effective means to control transmission by the vector, there is now an excellent new drug, ivermectin, that can reduce both morbidity and transmission.

Dracontiasis. This helminthic infection (Chapter 89) is particularly important because it could be so easily eradicated by providing communities with clean water, and yet it causes significant morbidity in millions of people annually. Individuals with open, draining lesions on their lower extremities, often having superinfections with bacteria, have considerable misery and are limited in their ability to work in the fields and households.

Cysticercosis. During 1972 and 1973, medical officers working in West Irian (New Guinea) began seeing an epidemic of severe burns from rolling into open fires. This had not previously been a medical problem. In 1971, the natives had received a gift of pigs from the Indonesian government. Unlike the native pigs of New Guinea, these gift pigs from Bali were heavily infected with the larval stage of *Taenia solium (Cysticercus cellulosae)*. The New Guinea tribesmen became infected from eating the undercooked pork, following their habitual way of preparing the meat. The resultant adult tapeworms caused no symptoms (Chapter 100.2), but the eggs passed in the feces infected pigs and humans alike with the larval stage of the parasite, causing cysticercosis in both (Chapter 101.1). Infection was related to heavy contamination of the environment with human feces and was expedited by heavy rains with standing ground water. Many people were heavily infected with multiple cerebral cysticerci (Fig. 101–3), and they and others frequently had multiple subcutaneous cysticercus nodules. Epileptic seizures occurring at night while sleeping near open fires caused the epidemic of severe burns. Those having seizures would roll into the fires and, being unconscious, would not be able to move out of the flames.

This is an example of a disease that caused a severe epidemic when first brought into a community. (Intestinal capillariasis [Chapter 82.3] appeared in a similar manner in the Ilocos Norte district of the Philippines in the late 1960s.) The epilepsy caused by cysticercosis in New Guinea occurred during the acute invasive phase of infection, unlike the epilepsy of chronic cysticercosis, common in Mexico, with which patients frequently have calcified cerebral cysts.

In the Arctic. Trichinosis has been reported frequently in the Eskimo populations of Canada, the United States, and Greenland. Infection is acquired by eating raw or undercooked polar bears or walruses. The arctic form of *Trichinella* is referred to as *T. nativa* (Chapter 90). It has some different biologic characteristics from *Trichinella* in more southern climates and it is more enteropathogenic and less muscle invasive. Prolonged diarrhea is the most important clinical manifestation.

In Temperate Climates. Prior to the middle of the twentieth century, the helminthiases were a significant cause of morbidity in the United States. Infections with the intestinal nematodes were particularly common in the Southeast.

In Natives

Intestinal Nematode Infections. Pinworm is still common in the United States (Chapter 82.1). Infections with other intestinal nematodes are unusual, except in such populations as poor rural people in the South, inhabitants of Indian reservations, those in institutions for the mentally retarded, recent immigrants and migrant laborers from developing countries, and long-term residents (e.g., missionaries and Peace Corps volunteers) in developing countries.

The principal exception to the association of infection with residence in the tropics during the past few years is *Strongyloides stercoralis* (Chapter 84.2). This intestinal nematode can replicate in humans (i.e., has the potential to cause autoinfection). Therefore, infections can persist for many years. Strongyloidiasis continues to be diagnosed in the United States and Great Britain in former Far Eastern prisoners of war. In addition, the strongyloidiasis hyperinfection syndrome can occur in immunosuppressed and malnourished individuals, including those with acquired immunodeficiency syndrome (AIDS). All patients infected with this helminth should be treated.

Trichinosis. This infection is becoming less common than previously in domestic pigs, but epidemics associated with eating undercooked bear and wild boar have been reported during the past few years (Chapter 90). Certain ethnic groups, e.g., Vietnamese and Central Europeans, often prefer cured but undercooked pork sausage. Several epidemics have followed consumption of sausage prepared in this manner from infected pigs. The increasing use of microwave ovens, which do not always heat meat evenly throughout, may cause an increase in the incidence of trichinosis.

Fish-Transmitted Helminthiases.

Diphyllobothriasis (Chapter 100.1) and anisakiasis (Chapter 95) are being recognized with increasing frequency in the United States. Fluke infections occur in people who ingest raw, inadequately cooked, or improperly salted or pickled freshwater or brackish-water fish: heterophyasis and metagonimiasis (Chapter 97.3), clonorchiasis (Chapter 98.2), and opisthorchiasis (Chapter 98.1).

A digenetic trematode, *Nanophyetus salmincola*, has recently been reported to infect people in the Pacific Northwest of the United States who ingested incompletely cooked or home-smoked salmon or steelhead trout. About half of the patients with nanophyetiasis had abdominal pain or discomfort, loose stools or diarrhea and excessive bloating and gas, and/or eosinophilia. Clinical manifestations in other patients from Siberia with nanophyetiasis were dose related, i.e., those with heavier infection had greater symptoms. Praziquantel, 60 mg/kg body weight given in 3 divided doses in a single day, was curative. The life cycle of this parasite is similar to that of the other intestinal trematodes, *Heterophyes* and *Metagonimus*, and involves a mollusk, fish, and fish-eating definitive host. This newly described zoonosis must be added to the list of potential infections associated with the habit of eating raw fish.

In Immigrants and Travelers.

Many helminths are commonly found in immigrants to the more developed countries from the tropics (Chapter 120) and in those who have lived for prolonged periods in less developed countries. The usual intestinal nematodes as well as the liver flukes (*Clonorchis sinensis* and *Opisthorchis viverrini*), the lung fluke *(Paragonimus westermani)*, and *Schistosoma mekongi* (Chapter 96.2) and *S. japonicum* (Chapter 96) are often found in emigrants from Southeast Asia. Those from the Caribbean may have intestinal nematode and *S. mansoni* (Chapter 96) infections. Those from Mexico and Central America may have intestinal nematodes. Epilepsy can be caused by cerebral cysticercosis, which is particularly common in Mexico (Chapter 101.1). Emigrants and visitors from Africa can have a multitude of helminth infections, including those with the intestinal nematodes, *S. mansoni* and *S. haematobium, Taenia saginata* (Chapter 100.2), *W. bancrofti* (Chapter 85.1), and *O. volvulus* (Chapter 87).

Acquired Immunodeficiency Syndrome. Because helminths, with rare exceptions, do not multiply within the human host, they do not cause opportunistic infections in patients with AIDS. The exception could be *Strongyloides,* which has the capability to autoinfect, causing long-lasting infections (Chapter 84.2). In the normal host it produces chronic gastrointestinal disease, which is often undetected. In immunocompromised individuals, e.g., those receiving corticosteroids and/or chemotherapy for malignancies, *Strongyloides* can produce a hyperinfection syndrome with rampant multiplication and dissemination of larvae throughout the lungs and other organs. Although *Strongyloides* infection can be transmitted between homosexuals, the hyperinfection syndrome does not appear to occur with increased frequency in patients infected with human immunodeficiency virus (HIV).

Other helminths, including schistosomes, ascarides, hookworms, flukes, and tapeworms, are not more frequent or more pathogenic in those with HIV infections.

CHEMOTHERAPY

Praziquantel. The introduction of effective and safe drugs to treat schistosomiasis has been a major achievement in the past 10 or 15 years: metrifonate (for treating *Schistosoma haematobium*); oxamniquine (for *S. mansoni*); and praziquantel (for treating all *Schistosoma* species) (Chapter 96.1). Praziquantel gives high cure rates and usually only requires a single dose. Fortunately, the cost of this important drug has been decreasing as countrywide control programs are obtaining it in bulk.

Praziquantel is also effective in treating other fluke infections, with the exception of *Fasciola hepatica* (Chapters 97 to 99) and the tapeworms (Chapter 100). Most importantly, it has provided, for the first time, a specific agent to treat cerebral cysticercosis (Chapter 101.1).

Broad-Spectrum Anthelmintics. There are several newer, excellent broad-spectrum anthelmintics available for treating intestinal nematode infections (Table VI A–2). Thiabendazole is still the drug of choice for strongyloidiasis, although some recent investigations have shown that ivermectin can also cure this infection (Chapter 84.2).

Levamisole, an excellent broad-spectrum anthelmintic that was never approved in the United States for that purpose, is now being shown to be an immunomodulator in the treatment of various malignancies.

Mebendazole, in prolonged and high doses, was the first effective chemotherapeutic agent for treating hydatid disease (Chapters 101.2 to 101.4). Albendazole, which is better absorbed following oral ingestion, is proving useful against *Echinococcus granulosis* in ongoing clinical trials.

Ivermectin. This drug, under the careful guidance of the late Dr. Mohamed Aziz of Merck Sharpe and Dohme Research Laboratories, has been extensively evaluated for the treatment and control of onchocerciasis during the past 6 to 8 years (Chapter 87). It is effective and safe following single-dose treatment. The drug company, with the assistance of the World Health Organization, is providing ivermectin to the countries where onchocerciasis is a major health problem. It is being used in large control programs to reduce clinical disease and transmission. Ivermectin has also been evaluated for treating filariasis. As in treating *Onchocerca volvulus*, it kills microfilariae, but not the adult worms. Cure rates are better and toxicity is less than with the use of diethylcarbamazine, and it can be given as a single dose (Chapter 85). Ivermectin is also used in veterinary practice for treating and preventing canine heartworm and onchocerciasis in cattle. This drug appears to have some therapeutic benefit against most nematodes, including intestinal parasites in humans.

BIBLIOGRAPHY

Abdel-Wahab MF, Esmat G, Milad M, et al: Characteristic sonographic pattern of schistosomal hepatic fibrosis. Am J Trop Med Hyg 40:72, 1989.

Abdel-Wahab MF, Esmat G, Narooz SI, et al: Sonographic studies of schoolchildren in a village endemic for *Schistosoma mansoni*. Trans R Soc Trop Med Hyg 84:69, 1990.

Drugs for parasitic infection. Med Lett Drugs Ther 30:15, 1988.

Freedman DO, Zierdt WS, Lujan A, Nun TB: The efficacy of ivermectin in the chemotherapy of gastrointestinal helminthiasis in humans. J Infect Dis 159:1151, 1989.

Frische TR, Eastburn RL, Wiggins LH, Terhune CA Jr: Praziquantel for treatment of human *Nanophyetus salmincola (Troglotrema salmincola)* infection. J Infect Dis 160:896, 1989.

Gajdusek DC: Introduction of *Taenia solium* into West New Guinea with a note on an epidemic of burns from cysticercus epilepsy in the Ekari people of the Wissel Lakes areas. Papua New Guinea Med J 21:329, 1978.

Greene BM, Taylor HR, Cupp EW, et al: Comparison of ivermectin and diethylcarbamazine in the treatment of onchocerciasis. N Engl J Med 313:133, 1985.

Kumaraswami V, Ottesen EA, Vijayasekaran V, et al: Ivermectin for the treatment of *Wuchereria bancrofti* filariasis. Efficacy and adverse reactions. JAMA 259:3150, 1988.

McKerrow JH, Deardorff TL: Anisakiasis: Revenge of the sushi parasite. N Engl J Med 319:1228, 1988.

McLean JD, Viallet J, Law C, Staudt M: Trichinosis in the Canadian Arctic: Report of five outbreaks and a new clinical syndrome. J Infect Dis 160:513, 1989.

Naquira C, Jimenez G, Guerra JG, et al: Ivermectin for human strongyloidiasis and other intestinal helminths. Am J Trop Med Hyg 40:304, 1989.

Ruttenber AJ, Weniger BG, Sorvillo F, et al: Diphyllobothriasis associated with salmon consumption in Pacific coast states. Am J Trop Med Hyg 33:455, 1984.

—

SECTION A

INTESTINAL NEMATODE INFECTIONS*

GENERAL PRINCIPLES

Richard L. Guerrant
Joseph D. Schwartzman
and Richard D. Pearson

MAGNITUDE OF THE PROBLEM. Intestinal nematode infections constitute by far the most common parasitic infections in humans, with one or more species infecting the intestinal tracts of well over one-fourth of the world's population. *Ascaris* and *Enterobius* (pinworm) infect 1 billion people each; *Trichuris* and hookworm infect a half billion each; and including numerous transient pinworm infections, there are estimated to be over 50 million helminthic infections in the United States. In endemic areas where indiscriminate defecation is common, as in recently studied Somalia communities, the prevalence of intestinal nematodes and protozoa may reach 85%, often with individuals being infected with more than 1 intestinal parasite.

Few enteric nematodes multiply in their human hosts. Infections thus tend to be self-limited over weeks or months to a few years if the individual is no longer subjected to repeated exposure from the environment. However, important exceptions exist, as with *Strongyloides stercoralis,* which may persist by autoinfection for more than 40 years. *Strongyloides* is also the only nematode infecting humans that has a free-living, as well as parasitic, generation in its life cycle. *Capillaria philippinesis* is the other nematode that may cause progressive "autoinfection." Like *Strongyloides, Trichuris* may rarely cause overwhelming superinfection in immunocompromised hosts. Systemic tissue migration is

---

*This section and Chapters 82 to 84 were modified from the Sixth Edition of *Hunter's Tropical Medicine* and chapters published in *Clinical Medicine,* J. B. Lippincott Company, Philadelphia, 1985.

often associated with eosinophilia, another characteristic of nematode infections.

GENERAL MORPHOLOGY. The general structure of nematodes is diagrammed in Figure VI A–1. Intestinal nematodes range in size from microscopic *(Trichinella, Strongyloides,* and *Capillaria)* to 30 to 35 cm or more *(Ascaris).* The elongated, cylindrical, unsegmented bodies are covered with a secreted, non-nucleated glistening *cuticula* with cephalic or caudal sensory papillae (amphids and phasmids). A muscular layer with the excretory system and longitudinal nerve trunks lies beneath the subcuticular secretory cells. The simple tubular alimentary canal includes an anterior buccal cavity (sometimes with teeth or cutting plates), a muscular esophagus, valve, midgut, rectum, and ventral cloaca. The smaller male has a single tubular reproductive system with testis, vas deferens, seminal vesicle and ejaculatory duct with copulatory spicules, gubernaculum, and extremity. The larger female has a threadlike, tubular ovary, oviduct, seminal receptacle, uterus, and vaginal opening that may be single *(Trichuris),* double (pinworm), or multiple (others). Ova have a vitelline membrane in a chitinous shell with yolk granules and fertilized cell that may embryonate or have larval development when passed, as in hookworm and pinworm ova (Fig. VI A–2).

TYPES OF INTESTINAL NEMATODE INFECTIONS. Intestinal nematode infections are best approached according to their types of life cycles in the human host and environment (Table VI A–1).

Nematodes Limited to the Intestinal Tract (Chapter 82). Those nematodes that have life cycles that are limited to the gastrointestinal tract include pinworm *(Enterobius vermicularis)* (Chapter 82.1) and whipworm *(Trichuris trichiura)* (Chapter 82.2) (Fig. 82–3), as well as *Trichostrongylus* sp. and *Capillaria philippinensis.* Pinworms and whipworms require no intermediate host and development from larvae to adult worms is completed in the human gut. Embryonated pinworm eggs become infective as early as a few hours after deposition at 37C, whereas whipworm eggs require a few days for the development of infective larvae within the shell. Although less well understood, *C. philippinensis* (Chapter 82.3) and *Trichostrongylus orientalis* (Chapter 82.4) are ingested as larvae (in raw fish or plants, respectively) that mature and remain localized in the human small bowel. Like *Strongyloides,* adult female *Capillaria* produce infectious larvae that may cause progressive, life-threatening autoinfections.

Unlike the other common intestinal nematodes, this group of nematodes do not migrate through the lung or the liver. Instead, eggs or larvae are ingested, usually from fecally contaminated soil or water, and the larvae mature to adults in the intestinal tract. The adults then reside in the upper small bowel *(C. philippinensis),* cecum *(E. vermicularis),* or colon *(T. trichiura)* for 2 to 4 weeks *(E. vermicularis)* up to 20 years *(T. trichiura).* Adults measure from 2 mm to 5 cm and lay up to 10,000 eggs per day, which are usually shed in the stool *(E. vermicularis* are shed as adult worms) to complete the life cycle. With only rare exceptions, the adult worms remain in the intestinal lumen or wall and cause disease by local mucosal or perianal irritation and inflammation.

Nematodes That Migrate Through Lungs (Chapter 83). These have a more complex life cycle. Humans ingest embryonated *Ascaris* eggs that have matured for 1 to 2 weeks in the environment; these hatch in the small intestine (Chapter 83.1). The larvae penetrate the bowel wall and migrate via the venous blood stream through the heart to the lungs, muscle, or meninges (Fig. 83–1). In the lungs, *Ascaris* larvae break into alveoli and move or are coughed up the trachea to be swallowed and mature into adult worms in the intestine. Adult female worms measuring up to 30 to 35 cm may then lay up to 200,000 eggs per day. This entire cycle takes approximately 3 months. Adult worms live about 1 year. *A. lumbricoides* may infect one-fourth of the world's population. Symptoms are caused by allergic reactions to the systemically migrating parasite, by mechanical obstruction, or by irritation from adult worms in the intestine.

The related ascarids, *Toxocara* and *Anisakis,* primarily cause infections in domestic animals (dogs and cats) and marine mammals (seals, dolphins, whales), which are the definitive hosts. Only the larval stages cause limited disease in humans, in whom the life cycle is not completed. Visceral larva migrans results from infection of children with larval dog or cat ascarids (Chapter 91), whereas superficial intestinal irritation or ulceration may follow ingestion of *Anisakis* larvae in raw fish (Chapter 95).

Nematodes That Migrate Through Skin and Lungs (Chapter 84). This cycle is the most complex: penetra-

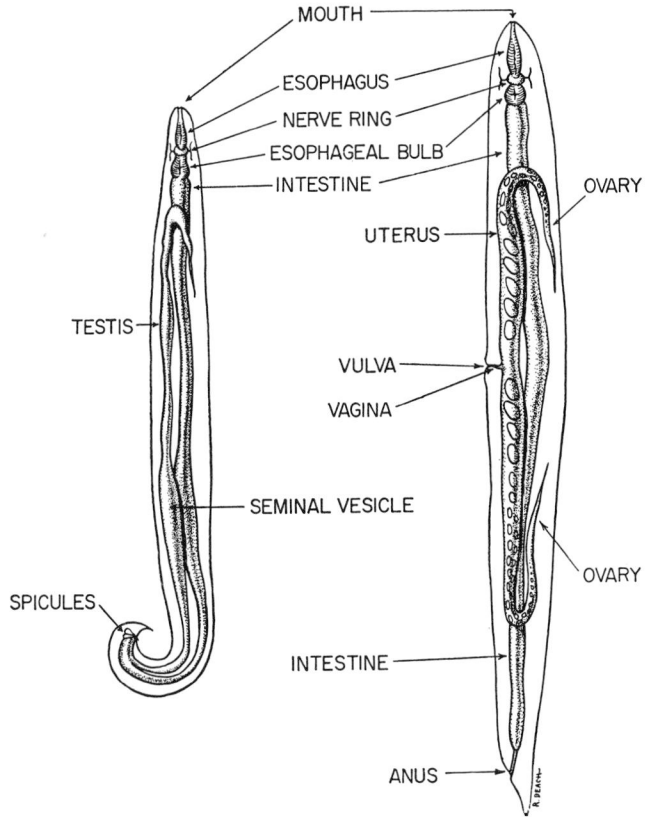

FIGURE VI A–1. Morphology of a typical nematode.

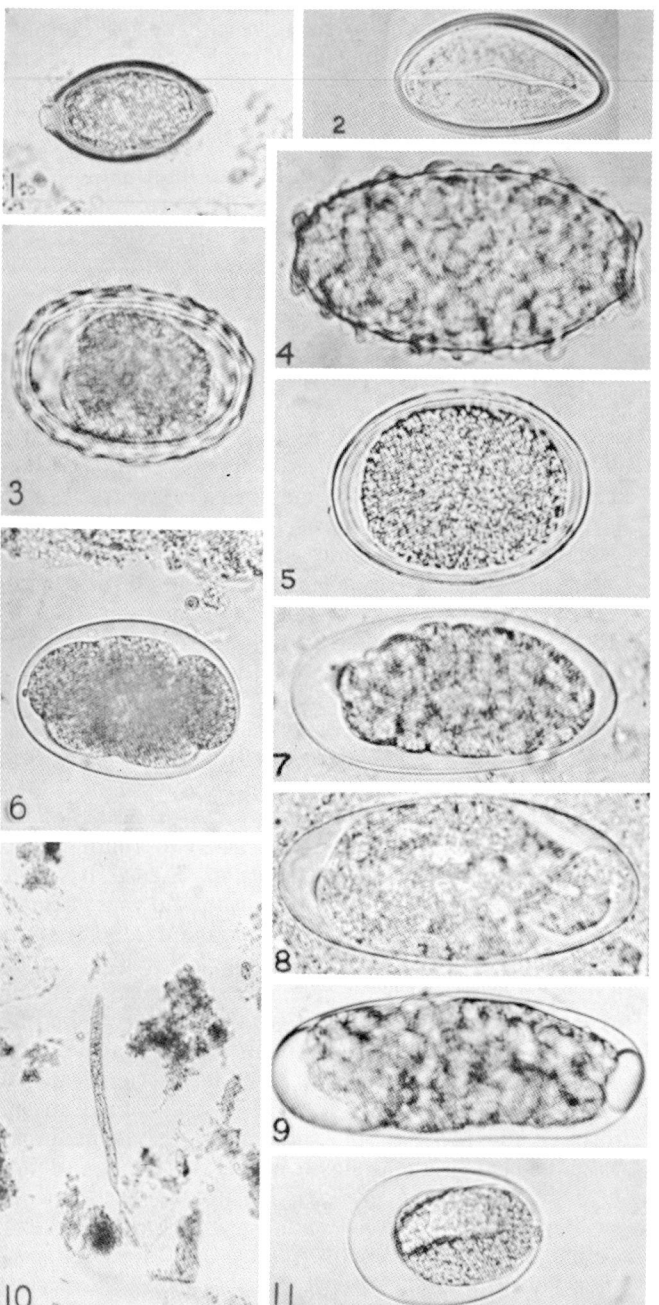

FIGURE VI A–2. Some common nematode eggs; *(1)* whipworm, *Trichuris trichiura; (2)* pinworm, *Enterobius vermicularis; (3)* large roundworm, *Ascaris lumbricoides,* fertilized egg; *(4) A. lumbricoides,* unfertilized egg; *(5) A. lumbricoides,* decorticated egg; *(6)* hookworm egg; *(7)* immature egg of *Trichostrongylus orientalis; (8)* embryonated egg of *T. orientalis; (9)* egg of *Meloidogne javanica,* a plant nematode, which sometimes is found in stools; *(10)* rhabditiform larva of *Strongyloides stercoralis,* the stage usually found in the stool; *(11)* egg of *S. stercoralis,* rarely seen in the stool. All figures × 500 except *(10)* × 75.

tion of the skin by larvae that migrate through the venous blood to the lungs, into alveoli, and up the trachea and are swallowed. Adults develop in the intestine and produce eggs that are shed in the stool or hatch in the bowel (Figs. 84–2 and 84–4). Intestinal nematodes transmitted in this manner probably cause greater morbidity and mortality than the others. Hookworm, particularly *Ancylostoma duodenale,* is the greatest cause of potentially severe anemia on a global scale (Chapter 84.1). Hookworm infections are usually limited to within 2 to 5 years after the last exposure. In contrast, *Strongyloides stercoralis* is capable of completing its life cycle in the same human host and can persist by "autoinfection" for 40 to 45 years (Chapter 84.2). In immunocompromised individuals, *S. stercoralis* may produce a life-threatening clinical syndrome of "hyperinfection."

The canine hookworms that cause cutaneous larva migrans in humans remain in the skin and fail to complete their life cycle in humans (Chapter 94). The curious "false hookworm" *Ternidens* is found localized primarily to Zimbabwe (Chapter 84).

CONTROL. General control measures include community-based education (about hygienic practices), socioeconomic development (with improved sanitary facilities, water supplies, and food handling), and individual or selected mass chemotherapy. Although many nematodes are eradicated by broad-spectrum agents such as mebendazole, most clinicians would reserve therapy in endemic areas to a targeted population with heavy or symptomatic infections, especially after the characteristic peak transmission season for that area. Soil dysinfection as by acidic lemongrass (to reduce hookworm and

TABLE VI A-1. Types of Life Cycles of Enteric Nematodes

Host Tissue Involved	Infective Stage	Mode of Transmission	Parasites*	
			Common Name	*Scientific Name*
Intestine only	Eggs	Direct oral	Pinworm	*Enterobius vermicularis*
			Whipworm	*Trichuris trichiura*
	Larvae		*Capillaria*	*Capillaria philippinensis*
	Larvae		*Trichostrongylus*	*Trichostrongylus orientalis*
	Larvae		Roundworm	(*Anisakis* sp)
			Anisakis	
Intestine and lung	Mature egg	Direct oral	Visceral larva migrans	*Ascaris lumbricoides* (*Toxocara canis* and *T. cati*)
			Trichinosis	*Trichinella spiralis*
			Eosinophilic meningitis	(*Angiostrongylus contonensis*)
			Eosinophilic gastroenteritis	(*Angiostrongylus costaricensis*)
Skin, lung, and intestine	Larvae	Skin	Hookworm	*Ancylostoma duodenale* and *Necator americanus*
			Cutaneous larva migrans	(*Ancylostoma braziliense*)
			Threadworm	*Strongyloides stercoralis*
		?Arthropod	Pseudohookworm	*Ternidens deminutus*

*In parentheses are related parasites that complete their life cycles in animal hosts; *Toxocara* (dog and cat ascarids that cause visceral larva migrans in children) and *Ancylostoma braziliense* (dog hookworms that cause cutaneous larva migrans) are discussed in detail in separate chapters, as is trichinosis and *Anisakis*.

Strongyloides) or ovicidal soil fungi may play accessory, limited roles in conjunction with other control measures.

TREATMENT. A number of relatively safe, effective drugs are available for the treatment of the intestinal nematodes (Table VI A-2). Mebendazole and albendazole (not yet licensed for use in the United States) have broad ranges of activity and are effective against hookworms, *Ascaris lumbricoides*, *Trichuris trichiura*, and *Enterobius vermicularis*. Pyrantel pamoate has activity against all of these common intestinal nematodes except for *T. trichiura*. Other drugs such as bephenium hydroxynaphthoate, pyrvinium pamoate, piperazine, and levamisole have more restricted spectrums of activity and, in several instances, are more toxic but less expensive than mebendazole, albendazole, or pyrantel pamoate. Thiabendazole is the treatment of choice for *S. stercoralis*. The pharmacology and untoward effects of these drugs are reviewed below. Specific details of therapy are covered separately in the sections on individual nematodes.

Mebendazole (Vermox). Mebendazole, a benzimidazole, is highly effective for the treatment of disease due to *A. lumbricoides*, hookworms, *T. trichiura*, and *E. vermicularis*. It is also used for the treatment of *Capillaria philippinensis*, *Angiostrongylus cantonensis*, and *Trichinella spiralis* infections and for other conditions such as inoperable echinococcal cysts and *Mansonella perstans* infection.

Mebendazole inhibits microtubule assembly and blocks glucose uptake by nematodes. Immobilization and death of susceptible nematodes follow, but it can take several days for nematodes to be cleared from the gastrointestinal tract. Mebendazole also inhibits the development of the ova of hookworms and *T. trichiura*.

Mebendazole is available in 100-mg chewable tablets. It is poorly absorbed orally and extremely well tolerated at the dosages used to treat intestinal nematode infections. Transient abdominal pain and diarrhea occur in some persons. Occasionally, *A. lumbricoides* will migrate to the pharynx during mebendazole therapy, but this is not a contraindication to its use. Embryotoxicity and teratogenicity have been observed in pregnant rats

treated with mebendazole, and mebendazole should not be administered during pregnancy. Rarely, mebendazole causes leukopenia, agranulocytosis, or hypospermia. These untoward effects are more likely when prolonged, high-dose therapy is used, as in the case of inoperable echinococcosis.

Albendazole (Zentel) and Flubendazole. Albendazole has a spectrum of anthelmintic activity similar to that of mebendazole, but albendazole has the advantage of being effective when administered as a single dose for the treatment of *T. trichiura*, *A. lumbricoides*, and the hookworms. Albendazole is consequently better suited for mass treatment programs. Albendazole is also better absorbed than mebendazole from the gastrointestinal tract, and its primary metabolite, albendazole sulfoxide, is scolicidal for echinococcal cysts. Albendazole has replaced mebendazole for the treatment of inoperable echinococcal cysts, and preliminary studies indicate that albendazole may be effective for the treatment of neurocysticercosis.

Albendazole is formulated in 200-mg tablets and as a 2% oral solution. It is usually well tolerated when administered as a single dose for the treatment of intestinal nematode infections. High-dose, prolonged therapy for echinococcal disease has been complicated by hepatitis and obstructive jaundice in a few patients.

Flubendazole, the parafluoro analogue of mebendazole, also has a range of activity similar to that of mebendazole. Although initially thought to lack terato-

TABLE VI A-2. Efficacy of Broad-Spectrum Anthelminthics

Infection	Mebendazole	Albendazole	Pyrantel Pamoate	Pyrvinium Pamoate
Enterobiasis	+++	+++	+++	+++
Ascariasis	+++	+++	+++	−
Hookworm	+++	+++	++	−
Trichuriasis	++	++	−	−

−	Less than 30% cured.
+	30 to 60% cured.
++	60 to 85% cured.
+++	Greater than 85% cured.

genicity, recent animal studies have shown that fluben-dazole is teratogenic when administered by gavage.

Thiabendazole (Mintezol). Thiabendazole, also a benzimidazole, is one of the most potent anthelmintic drugs, but a high frequency of untoward effects has limited its use primarily to infections with *Strongyloides stercoralis* and *S. fuelleborni, Trichostrongylus* species, *Angiostrongylus costaricensis;* cutaneous larva migrans; visceral larvae migrans; and trichinosis. It has been used as an alternative drug for *Capillaria philippinensis* and *Dracunculus medinensis.*

Thiabendazole is available in 500-mg tablets and as an oral suspension of 500 mg/5 ml. It is rapidly absorbed after oral administration. No parenteral preparation is available. This is a potentially important limitation in patients with disseminated *S. stercoralis* infection. The precise mechanism of action is unknown. Initial studies indicated that thiabendazole could inhibit fumarate reductase in helminths. More recent work suggests that thiabendazole, like mebendazole, interferes with microtubule assembly. This may be the primary mechanism of action.

Side effects are experienced by approximately half of the persons treated with thiabendazole. The most frequent are nausea, vomiting, anorexia, and dizziness. Less common are diarrhea, epigastric pain, pruritus, drowsiness, giddiness, headache, hallucinations, leukopenia, crystalluria, olfactory disturbances, and allergic manifestations, including rash, pruritus, erythema multiforme, and Stevens-Johnson syndrome. The release of helminthic antigens probably is responsible for some of the allergic reactions. Rare side effects include tinnitus, numbness, hypotension, and elevated liver enzyme levels. Activities requiring alertness should be avoided during therapy. Thiabendazole should be given with caution to persons with hepatic disease or dysfunction, and it is relatively contraindicated in pregnancy.

Pyrantel Pamoate (Antiminth). Pyrantel pamoate is effective for the treatment of *Enterobius vermicularis, Ascaris lumbricoides,* and hookworms, but not *Trichuris trichuria.* The m-oxyphenol derivative, which is not licensed in the United States, has activity against *T. trichiura.*

Pyrantel pamoate is available in tablets with 125 mg of pyrantel base and as a suspension with 50 mg of base/ml. Pyrantel and its analogues are depolarizing neuromuscular blocking agents in susceptible helminths. They result in nicotinic activation and spastic paralysis of worms. Pyrantel also inhibits acetylcholinesterases.

Pyrantel has minimal toxicity at the dosages used to treat intestinal helminths. Mild gastrointestinal side effects, including anorexia, nausea, vomiting, and abdominal discomfort, are experienced by some persons. Headache, dizziness, rash, or fever occur on occasion. The nitrosylated metabolites of pyrantel are mutagenic for bacteria. Consequently, pyrantel is not recommended for use during pregnancy. Finally, pyrantel should not be used with piperazine, which produces hyperpolarization in helminths. The two appear to be mutually antagonistic.

Bephenium hydroxynaphthoate (Alcopar). This is used for the treatment of hookworm infections in some areas. It is more effective against *Ancylostoma duodenale* than against *Necator americanus;* a single dose of 5 gm of the salt (2.5 gm of base) is effective for the former, whereas 5 daily 5-gm doses are needed for the latter. Bephenium hydroxynaphthoate also has some activity against *Ascaris lumbricoides,* and it has been used to treat persons with mixed hookworm and *Ascaris* infections. The drug is dispensed in small granules and is administered with water on an empty stomach, usually before breakfast. Bephenium is generally well tolerated, but nausea and vomiting occur on occasion.

Pyrvinium pamoate (Povan, Vanquin). A cyanide dye, this is effective against *Enterobius vermicularis,* but it has largely been replaced by mebendazole or pyrantel pamoate. Pyrvinium pamoate is no longer marketed in the United States. It is a deep-red solid, which is formulated in tablets containing 50 mg of pyrvinium base or as a suspension containing 10 mg of pyrvinium base/ml. Pyrvinium is thought to inhibit the respiration of aerobic organisms and to interfere with the absorption of glucose by intestinal helminths.

Pyrvinium is generally well tolerated. Side effects, which are not common, include nausea, vomiting, and abdominal cramps. Emesis has been associated with the suspension. Pyrvinium makes stools bright red, and the suspension can stain if spilled or vomited on clothing.

Piperazine (Piperazine Citrate). Piperazine is effective for the treatment of *Ascaris lumbricoides* and *Enterobius vermicularis,* but it has largely been replaced by mebendazole or pyrantel pamoate, which are less toxic. In a few developing areas, piperazine is still used because it is inexpensive.

Piperazine salts are available as 500-mg tablets and as syrups or suspensions containing 100 mg/ml. The drug is well absorbed orally and is usually well tolerated. On occasion, there are gastrointestinal disturbances, transient neurologic side effects, or urticarial reactions. Visual disturbances, ataxia, and hypotonia occur rarely. Epileptic activity may be exaggerated, and piperazine should not be given to persons with a history of seizures. Neurotoxicity has also been observed in persons with impaired renal function.

Levamisole (Ketrex). Levamisole can be used for the treatment of *Ascaris* and hookworm infections. It is given by mouth as a single dose of 2.5 mg/kg body weight. Adverse effects are observed in a small minority of patients and include nausea, vomiting, anorexia, abdominal discomfort, headache, and dizziness. These side effects are usually mild and transient. The drug is not licensed for use in the United States. Levamisole is also capable of stimulating cell-mediated immune responses in an antigen-independent manner.

BIBLIOGRAPHY

Beaver PC, Jung RC, Cupp EW: Clinical Parasitology, 9th ed. Philadelphia, Lea & Febiger, 1984.

Ilardi I, Shiddo SC, Mohamed HH, et al: The prevalence and intensity of intestinal parasites in two Somalian communities. Trans R Soc Trop Med Hyg 81:336, 1987.

Pawlowski ZS (ed): Intestinal helminthic infections. Clin Trop Med Comm Dis 2:489, 1987.

Pearson RD: Recent advances in helminthic infections. Curr Opin Infect Dis 1:238, 1988.

Schultz MG: The changing face of parasitic disease in developed countries. *In* Mettrick DF, Desser SS (eds): Parasites—Their World and Ours. Amsterdam, Elsevier Biomedical Press, 1982, pp 412–421.

Warren KS: Helminthic diseases endemic in the United States. Am J Trop Med Hyg 23:723, 1974.

82. NEMATODES LIMITED TO THE INTESTINAL TRACT (*ENTEROBIUS VERMICULARIS, TRICHURIS TRICHIURA, AND CAPILLARIA PHILIPPINENSIS*)

Richard D. Pearson
and Joseph D. Schwartzman

82.1. ENTERIOBIASIS

DEFINITION. Enterobiasis is due to the intestinal nematode, *Enterobius vermicularis*, the pinworm. *E. vermicularis* is an ancient parasite of humans; eggs of *E. vermicularis* in a coprolite from western Utah have been radiocarbon dated to 7837 B.C.

DISTRIBUTION. *E. vermicularis* is found worldwide in both temperate and tropical areas. It is the most common helminthic infection in the United States and Western Europe. The prevalence is greatest among young school-aged children living under conditions of high population density and indoor conditions.

ETIOLOGY. *E. vermicularis* was discovered by Lin-naeus in 1758 and originally named *Oxyuris vermicularis*. The disease was referred to as oxyuriasis for many years. *E. vermicularis* only infects humans, although related pinworm species infect animals.

Morphology. Adult females are 8 to 13 mm in length and up to 0.5 mm in width. The anterior extremity lacks a true buccal capsule. It is characterized by 3 labia and, laterally, by a pair of cephalic, winglike alae. The muscular esophagus terminates in a distinct bulb (Figs. 82–1*B* and 82–2*B*). The posterior tip of the female is distinctly attenuated and constitutes the posterior third of the worm (Fig. 82–1*A*). The reproductive system is T shaped. The vulva opens at the base of the T near the junction of the anterior and middle thirds of the body. The long, clear, pointed end of the female, the clear cephalic alae, and typical eggs within the uteri are demonstrated in Fig. 82–1. In cross-section, adult females are characterized by their bilateral crests and characteristic eggs within (Fig. 82–2*A*). Males have a ventrally curved tail with caudal alae and a single large copulatory spicule. They are smaller than the females, with a length of 2 to 5 mm.

Life Cycle. Approximately 11,000 eggs are produced by each gravid female. The eggs are ovoid, 50 to 60 mm by 20 to 30 mm, and asymmetrically flattened on one side (Fig. XI A-2[2]). The shell consists of a thick, outer, albuminous layer, which plays a role in adherence to objects in the environment; a thin inner hyaline layer; and the embryonic membrane.

At the time of oviposition, eggs contain larvae, which must undergo further maturation before they become infective. Atmospheric oxygen acts as a stimulus to development. At body temperature, eggs can become infective within 6 hours. They begin to lose infectivity after 1 or 2 days under warm, dry environmental conditions. Egg survival is greatest under conditions of

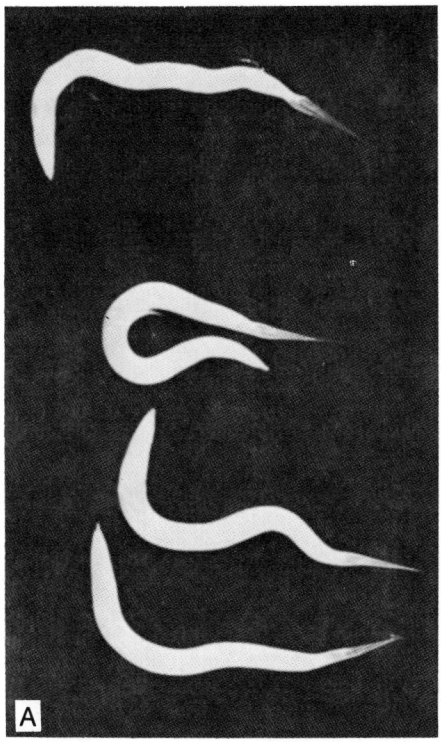
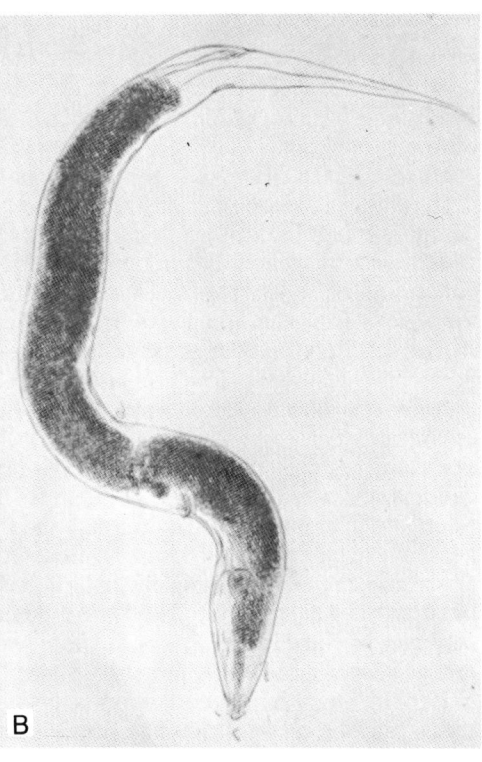

FIGURE 82–1. *Enterobius vermicularis* adult female worms. *A*, Note shapes and the clear, attenuated and pointed posterior end. *B*, Note cephalic alae, bulb behind esophagus, vulva, egg mass, anus, and pointed posterior end. (Courtesy of the Louisiana State University School of Medicine, New Orleans.)

A

B

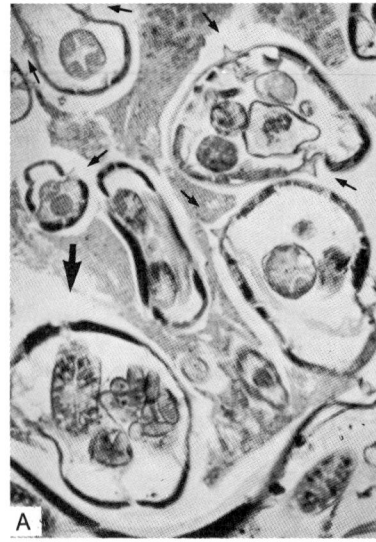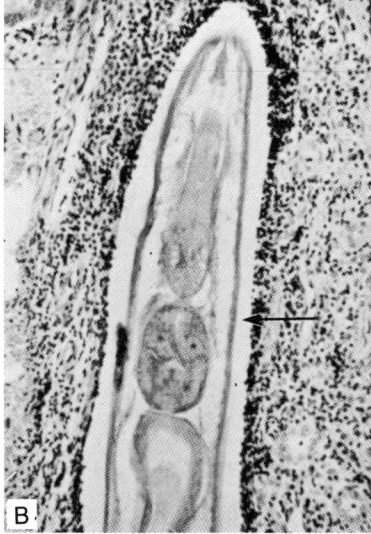

FIGURE 82–2. *E. vermicularis* in appendix. *A*, Cross-section of adult pinworms in lumen shows bilateral crests *(narrow arrows)*; 1 worm contains eggs *(wide arrow)*. *B*, Longitudinal section of adult worm in lymphatic nodule shows prominent esophageal bulb *(arrow)*. (Courtesy of the Louisiana State University School of Medicine, New Orleans.)

lower temperature and higher humidity. Eggs usually remain viable for less than 2 weeks; the maximum length of survival is reportedly 19 weeks.

After being ingested, eggs hatch in the upper small intestine, liberating larvae, which are 140 to 150 μm in length. The larvae migrate to the region of the ileum, molting twice along the way to become adults. Copulation takes place in the lower small intestine. Adult females finally settle in the cecum, appendix, or adjacent areas of the ascending colon. Adult females live up to 13 weeks and males for approximately 7 weeks. The earliest that oviposition is observed is 5 weeks. In most instances, there are a few to several hundred adult worms per patient.

At the time of oviposition, the gravid female leaves the colon and migrates out through the anus to lay her eggs while transversing the perianal or perineal skin. Female worms have been observed to move 2.5 inches in 30 minutes. Eggs are expelled by uterine contraction, death and disintegration of the worm, or disruption during scratching.

EPIDEMIOLOGY. *E. vermicularis* is found in children of all socioeconomic classes; males and females are equally susceptible. Infestation follows ingestion of eggs, which usually reach the mouth on soiled hands or contaminated food. The mechanical stimulation of migrating worms and the local irritation caused by the worms or deposited eggs often produce pruritus ani. Scratching results in contamination of the fingers and thereby contributes to autoinfection and spread to the environment.

Enterobiasis is most prevalent among school-aged children between the ages of 5 and 10 years; it is relatively uncommon in children less than 2 years. Poor personal hygiene and exposure to infected peers in the classroom are contributing factors. It has been postulated that as many as 20 to 30% of elementary school students in the United States are infected, although a recent report based on laboratory surveillance in New York City suggests that the number of cases of enterobiasis may be decreasing. The prevalence among children living in crowded conditions such as summer camps or institutions has been as high as 80 to 90% in some reports. Transmission of *E. vermicularis* is also common within families of infected children. Anyone who handles children's clothing or bedding is at increased risk. Enterobiasis has also been reported among male homosexuals, who likely become infected through the practice of anilingus.

PATHOLOGY. The most important consequence of *E. vermicularis* is cutaneous irritation in the perianal region. The associated pruritus results in scratching and self-induced trauma to the skin. Perianal eczematous dermatitis with secondary bacterial infection results in some children. Folliculitis has been reported with enterobiasis in adults. The eosinophil count in persons with *E. vermicularis* infection is usually normal.

Vulvovaginitis occurs in some girls when worms migrate to the vagina. An association between *E. vermicularis* infestation and urinary tract infection in young girls has also been suggested. It has been postulated that perineal irritation due to *E. vermicularis* with associated scratching results in introital colonization with coliforms and thereby predisposes to urinary tract infection.

E. vermicularis does not appear to produce any significant intestinal pathologic changes. Worms are occasionally found in the appendix after surgical excision, (Fig. 82–2*A*), but they do not cause acute appendicitis. On rare occasions, adult worms reach the peritoneum by traversing the female genital tract or migrating through a perforation in the bowel caused by appendicitis, diverticulitis, or intestinal malignancy. Granulomatous reactions to dead worms or eggs have been found in the vaginal wall, cervix, endometrium, salpinx, ovary, and peritoneum. On gross examination of the peritoneum, these appear as white or yellowish nodules, which may be confused with tuberculosis or metastatic neoplasms. Microscopically, there are granulomas with eosinophils and giant cells. Ova often remain well preserved even after worms are no longer identifiable.

E. vermicularis has on rare occasions been found in

other ectopic sites such as the conjunctival sac and the external auditory canal. Presumably eggs were delivered there by soiled fingers. Eggs are rarely found in the urine or vaginal smears.

CLINICAL CHARACTERISTICS. *E. vermicularis* infestation can result in perianal or perineal pruritus, but the majority of those infected never come to clinical attention. In 1 large study from New England, anal pruritus and perianal skin lesions were only slightly more common among those infected than in controls, and the differences were not statistically significant. Nonetheless, there are certainly instances in which intense perianal or perineal pruritus are associated with *E. vermicularis* and respond to appropriate anthelmintic chemotherapy. On some occasions, enterobiasis is complicated by secondary bacterial dermatitis or folliculitis.

Local symptoms vary from a mild, tickling sensation to acute pain. Symptoms tend to be most troublesome at night and may produce sleep disturbances, restlessness, and insomnia. There is no evidence that enterobiasis is responsible for abdominal pain, nail biting, or thumb sucking. The psychologic impact on parents who learn that their child has "worms" can not be totally disregarded.

E. vermicularis is a well recognized cause of vulvovaginitis in prepubertal girls. It has also been incriminated as a potential cause of secondary enuresis and urinary tract infection. In a few cases, peritoneal granulomas secondary to migrating *E. vermicularis* have been associated with abdominal pain in adult women. More commonly, peritoneal nodules are found incidently at the time of laparotomy (Fig. 82–2*B*).

DIAGNOSIS. The diagnosis of enterobiasis depends on the identification of adult worms or ova. Adult female worms are small, whitish, and pin shaped (Fig. 82–1*A*). They are occasionally seen in the perianal area or vagina of infected persons. The most successful diagnostic approach, however, makes use of a strip of transparent tape, which is held with adhesive side out affixed to a tongue depressor. Before the person defecates or bathes on arising in the morning, the buttocks are spread and the tape is pressed against the anal or perianal skin several times. The strip is then transferred to a microscope slide with adhesive side down. Debris can be cleared by adding a drop of toluene. Eggs are prominent at low power. Examination of 1 smear will detect approximately 50% of infections. Six consecutive negative swabs on separate days are necessary to exclude the diagnosis, but 90% of infections can be detected with 3 swabs. Parents can be taught the adhesive tape technique to obtain samples early in the morning. Other swab systems using glass or wooden applicators or cellophane have been used with similar efficacy.

Some physicians advocate a digital rectal examination to obtain anal material for analysis when the adhesive tape technique fails. Fecal material from the gloved finger is mixed with normal saline and examined under a coverslip. In contrast, routine stool examination for ova and parasites is positive in only 10 to 15% of infected persons. On rare occasions, *E. vermicularis* eggs are found incidentally in Papanicolaou-stained vaginal smears or in the urine sediment.

TREATMENT. *E. vermicularis* is susceptible to a number of anthelmintic drugs, with cure rates exceeding 90%. Pyrantel pamoate (Antiminth), mebendazole (Vermox), or pyrvinium pamoate (Povan) are effective and well tolerated, but pyrvinium pamoate is no longer marketed in the United States. Pyrantel pamoate is given as dose of 11 mg of base/kg body weight (maximum 1 gm) orally and repeated after 2 weeks. Piperazine (Vermizine), 65 mg/kg body weight (maximal dose of 2 gm) for 6 days, is also effective, but it is more likely to be associated with important untoward effects. Because multiple members of a family are usually infected, treatment for the entire family is often recommended. When there are no other children in the household, treatment of only the infected child should be adequate. Asymptomatic individuals who are unlikely to reinfect themselves or others do not need to be treated. In addition to chemotherapy, parents should be instructed in measures to reduce the risk of reinfection, and they should be reassured that enterobiasis is not a serious disease.

Mebendazole is administered in a dose of 100 mg orally. Some physicians recommend repeating the dose 2 weeks later. Pyrvinium pamoate is used in a single dose of 5 mg/kg (maximum dose 250 mg). Mebendazole inhibits the worm's microtubule function and causes glycogen depletion. It is poorly absorbed and, apart from occasional reports of abdominal pain or diarrhea, remarkably free of side effects at this dose. However, mebendazole has been associated with teratogenicity in animal studies and should not be given during pregnancy.

PREVENTION AND CONTROL. General and specific hygienic measures, including hand washing, particularly after bowel movements, are important. Simple laundering of clothes and linen is adequate to disinfect them. Linen and clothing should not be shaken because this can disseminate infective eggs. Extensive house cleaning is not necessary, but frequent vacuuming around beds, curtains, and other potentially contaminated areas is advised. Food should be covered to limit exposure to dust-borne eggs. Anthelmintic treatment of the entire household may be necessary to interrupt transmission in families with several small children.

BIBLIOGRAPHY

Cram EB: Studies on oxyuriasis. XXVIII. Studies and conclusions. Am J Dis Child 65:46, 1943.
Jones JJ: Pinworms. Am Fam Physician 38:159, 1988.
Symmers E St C: Pathology of oxyuriasis. Arch Pathol Lab Med [Chicago] 50:475, 1950.
Van Reken DE, Pearson RD: Antiparasitic agents. *In* Mandell GL, Douglas RG Jr, Bennett JE (eds): Principles and Practice of Infectious Diseases, 3rd ed. New York, Churchill Livingstone, 1990.

82.2. TRICHURIASIS

DEFINITION. *Trichuris trichiura* (the whipworm) is one of the most prevalent helminths of the world. It is basically a parasite of humans, known from antiquity and transmitted by eggs from fecally contaminated soil. The long association of this nematode with humans has allowed the parasite to adapt in such a way that it rarely compromises the health or reproductive fitness of the host; most infected persons are asymptomatic. Heavy infections or infections in those with other intestinal parasitoses and malnutrition may have a serious clinical outcome.

ETIOLOGY. *T. trichiura* infects humans as its primary host, but numerous members of the genus *Trichuris* infect domestic animals. *T. suis* is a morphologically identical parasite, which rarely and abortively infects humans. It can only be distinguished from *T. trichiura* by its biologic properties and its chromosome count. *T. vulpis* of dogs has also been reported occasionally from humans, based on the larger size of its eggs, although this may not always be a reliable criterion. The name whipworm derives from the morphology of the 3 to 5 cm adult. The anterior three-fifths of the worm is threadlike and the posterior two-fifths is more substantial, containing the reproductive organs.

Life Cycle. The life cycle of the parasite (Fig. 82–3) begins with ingestion of the embryonated egg. The larva penetrates the intestinal mucosa by its whiplike anterior end, molts, matures, and reattaches to the cecum of colon wall. The mature female produces 2000 to 6000 eggs per day. The eggs are passed in feces, where they must mature in soil for a period that varies with temperature, but is at least 10 to 14 days. About 3 months is required for a patent infection to be produced from the ingestion of eggs. Adult worms may persist for years.

EPIDEMIOLOGY AND DISTRIBUTION. *Trichuris* is distributed worldwide. It is prevalent generally in the same distribution as *Ascaris,* wherever fecal contamination of moist soils allows maturation of eggs. The egg is less resistant to low temperatures and drying than the eggs of *Ascaris,* and so trichuriasis is relatively more common in areas where warm, moist soil and shade prevail. In many areas of the developing world, where latrines have been installed, the incidence of soil-transmitted nematodes is still high because of the practice of using untreated fecal matter as fertilizer (night soil). *Trichuris* eggs are commonly found on vegetables that have been fertilized with night soil. The distribution of numbers of worms per host is uneven throughout communities; some persons harbor much higher numbers of parasites than others, but persons with a heavy infection with 1 nematode may not be heavily infected with others. Such "wormy persons" may represent an important target in public health campaigns designed to decrease the incidence of soil-transmitted nematodes. This phenomenon does not appear to be a genetic predilection to infection. In a study of infected children in Jamaica, heavily infected children cured by chemotherapy were not more likely than their less heavily infected peers to be reinfected with large numbers of *T. trichiura.*

PATHOLOGY AND CLINICAL MANIFESTATIONS. The adult worms buried by their anterior ends

LIFE CYCLE of—

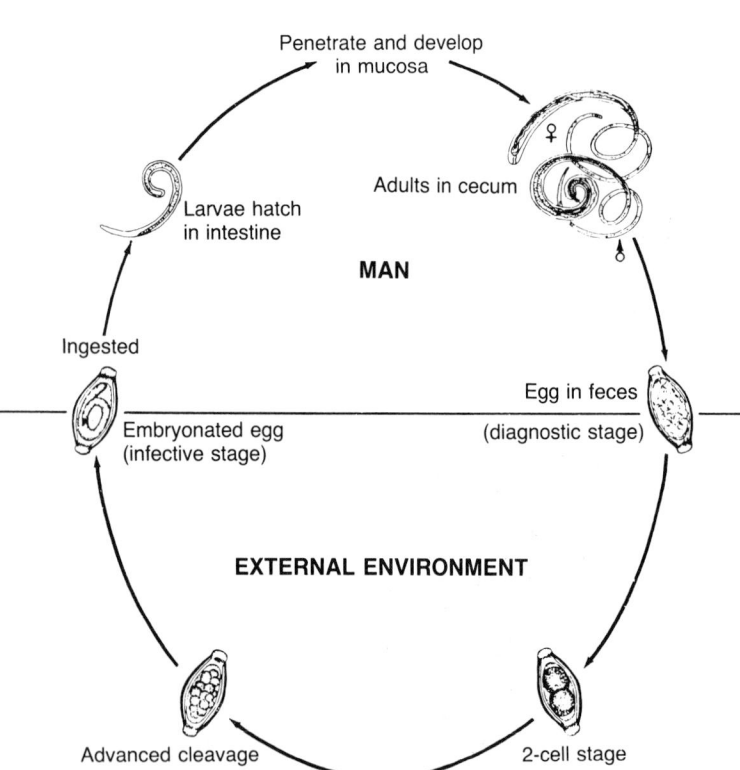

Trichuris trichiura

FIGURE 82–3. Life cycle of *Trichuris trichiura.* (From Melvin DM, Brooke MM, Sadun EH: Common Intestinal Helminths of Man. Atlanta, Centers for Disease Control. DHEW Publication No. [CDC] 75–8286, 1964.)

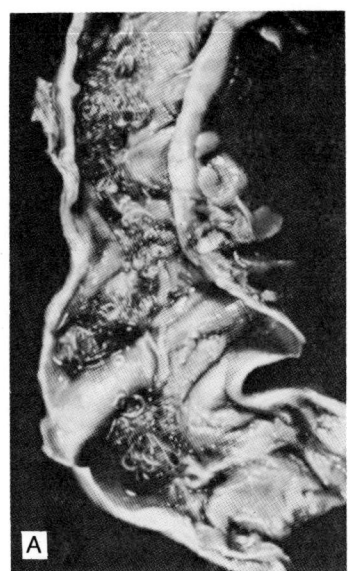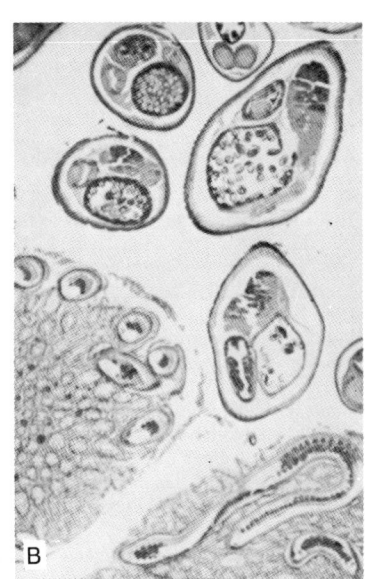

FIGURE 82–4. *A*, Masses of *T. trichiura* (whipworms) in colon of a child. *B*, Section of large intestine showing adult whipworms (natural infection of *T. vulpis* in dog). Thin anterior portions of worms are imbedded and threaded in the mucosa; broader posterior parts of worms, containing eggs, are in lumen. (Courtesy of the Louisiana State University School of Medicine, New Orleans.)

in the colonic mucosa cause only minor local inflammation in light to moderate infections. Local eosinophilic infiltration may be seen in the submucosa, and in heavy infection the bowel wall may be edematous and friable. Under these circumstances, the mucosa may bleed easily, but the worms do not actively suck blood. Blood loss from inflamed mucosa may be important in persons with marginal iron intake. Heavy infection (Fig. 82–4) may be manifest by abdominal pain and chronic diarrhea, but most infections are asymptomatic. Rectal prolapse (Fig. 82–5) is described in patients with heavy infection, but the relative frequency of this complication is unknown.

DIAGNOSIS, TREATMENT, AND PREVENTION. The diagnosis is made by finding the characteristic barrel-shaped eggs with their polar hyaline plugs in a stool specimen (Figs. VI A-2[1] and 82–7). The eggs are usually about 50 × 20 μm, but may be larger or abnormal in shape when the patient has been treated. Charcot-Leyden crystals are often present in stool, and eosinophilia (up to 15%) may be seen in peripheral blood. A light infection with *T. trichiura* may explain an asymptomatic eosinophilia.

Therapy of trichuriasis is somewhat more difficult than that of infection with other soil-transmitted nematodes, perhaps because immature worms are not affected by the chemotherapeutic agents; mebendazole, 100 mg twice a day for 3 days, is usually recommended. Other benzimidazole derivatives may be as effective as mebendazole, but they are not readily available in the United States. Flubendazole given in single doses of 200 to 600 mg was effective in reducing egg counts by more than 90%, but total cure was achieved in 65% or less of treated patients with this regimen. A single 500 mg dose of mebendazole in patients weighing more than 10 kg has been used in a mass chemotherapy trial, with about 75% efficacy in clearing trichuriasis. Albendazole administered as a 600 mg single dose cured 60% of patients, but none of the single-dose regimens appears to be as reliable as the recommended 3 day regimen of mebendazole for the treatment of individual patients. The single-dose regimens may be effective in endemic areas when the object is to reduce the worm burden in the community.

In residents of endemic areas, infection is largely unavoidable, but travelers may prevent infection by

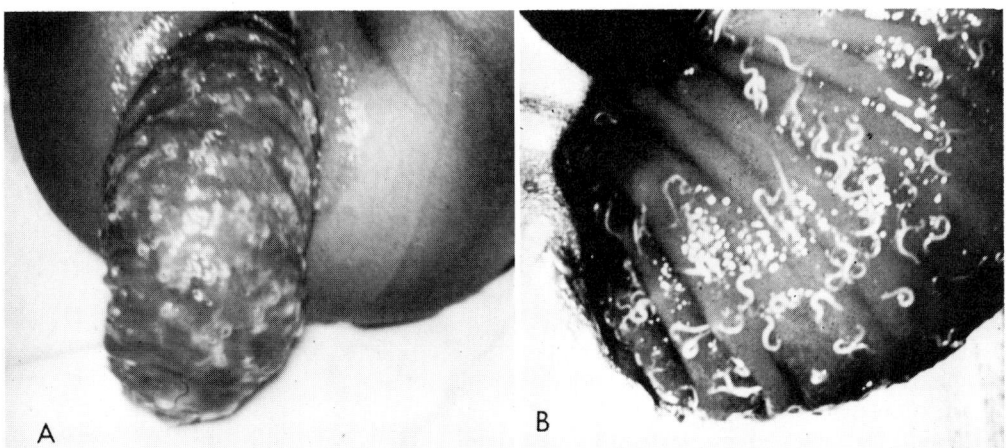

FIGURE 82–5. *A*, Prolapse of rectum in a heavy infection with *T. trichiura*. *B*, Adult *T. trichiura* attached to prolapsed bowel. (Both figures courtesy of Drs. P. C. Beaver and R. V. Platou, Tulane University School of Medicine, New Orleans.)

eating only cooked food or by rinsing vegetables in hot water (65C) or a 200 ppm iodine solution.

BIBLIOGRAPHY

Abadi K: Single dose mebendazole therapy for soil-transmitted nematodes. Am J Trop Med Hyg 34:129, 1985.

Arfaa F: Selective primary health care: Strategies for control of disease in the developing world. XII. Ascariasis and trichuriasis. Rev Infect Dis 6:364, 1984.

Bundy DA, Thompson DE, Golden MHN, et al: Population distribution of *Trichuris trichiura* is a community of Jamaican children. Trans R Soc Trop Med Hyg 79:232, 1985.

Bundy DA: Epidemiological aspects of *Trichuris* and trichuriasis in Caribbean communities. Trans R Soc Trop Med Hyg, 80:706, 1986.

Bundy DA, Cooper ES, Thompson DE, et al: Age-related prevalence and intensity of *Trichuris trichiura* infection in a St Lucian community. Trans R Soc Trop Med Hyg 81:85, 1987.

Bundy DA, Cooper ES, Thompson DE, et al: Epidemiology and population dynamics of *Ascaris lumbricoides* and *Trichuris trichiura* infection in the same community. Trans R Soc Trop Med Hyg, 81:987, 1987.

Bundy DA, Cooper ES, Thompson DE, et al: Predisposition to *Trichuris trichiura* infection in humans. Epidemiol Infect 98:65, 1987.

Croll NA, Ghadirian E: Wormy persons: Contributions to the nature and patterns of overdispersion with *Ascaris lumbricoides, Ancylostoma duodenale, Necator americanus* and *Trichuris trichiura.* Trop Geogr Med 33:241, 1981.

de Silva DG, Lionel ND, Jayatilleka SM: Flubendazole in the treatment of *Ascaris lumbricoides* and *Trichuris trichiura:* A comparison of two different regimens with single-dose. Ceylon Med J 29:199, 1984.

Fishman JA, Perrone TL: Colonic obstruction and perforation due to *Trichuris trichiura.* Am J Med 77:154, 1984.

Forrester JE, Scott ME, Bundy DA, Golden MH: Clustering of *Ascaris lumbricoides* and *Trichuris trichiura* infections within households. Trans R Soc Trop Med Hyg 82:282, 1988.

Gilman RH, Chong YH, David C, et al: The adverse consequences of heavy *Trichuris* infection. Trans R Soc Trop Med Hyg, 77:432, 1983.

Kan SP: Efficacy of single doses of mebendazole in the treatment of *Trichuris trichiura* infection. Am J Trop Med Hyg 32:118, 1983.

Kan SP: The anthelmintic effects of flubendazole on *Trichuris trichiura* and *Ascaris lumbricoides.* Trans R Soc Trop Med Hyg 77:668, 1983.

Ramalingam S, Sinniah B, Krishnan U: Albendazole, an effective single dose broad spectrum anthelmintic drug. Am J Trop Med Hyg 32:984, 1983.

Wolfe S: Oxyuris, trichostongylus and trichuris. Clin Gastroenterol 7:210, 1978.

82.3. INTESTINAL CAPILLARIASIS

DEFINITION. A small intestinal nematode related to *Trichuris trichiura* causes serious infections in areas of the Philippines and Thailand. *Capillaria philippinensis,* in the order Enoplida, superfamily Trichuroidea, is capable of autoinfection and therefore may cause extensive pathologic change of the small intestine following a relatively light exposure.

ETIOLOGY. The 2 to 4 mm adults are threadlike; the female has an esophagus in the anterior half of the body and reproductive organs in the posterior half, which may contain both eggs and the free larvae that are responsible for autoinfection and multiplication. The adults are in the mucosa of the small bowel and cause a syndrome of chronic diarrhea and wasting that may

be fatal if untreated. The infection is spread by the ingestion of several species of freshwater fish that have infectious larvae within muscle. The natural reservoir host has not been identified but fish-eating water birds are probable. Monkeys can be experimentally infected but have not been found to be infected in the wild. The custom of eating raw fish probably determines the transmission of infection. Outbreaks have occurred when fecal contamination of freshwater lagoons has allowed eggs from infected patients to be disseminated in large numbers to a local source of fish.

EPIDEMIOLOGY AND GEOGRAPHIC DISTRIBUTION. Most cases have been recognized in the Philippines, where the infection was first noted in the 1960s. Endemic areas are recognized in several provinces; both sporadic cases and outbreaks are seen. A few cases have been reported from Thailand and may be expected in other areas of Southeast Asia where freshwater fish are eaten without cooking. There have been 2 case reports from Egypt.

PATHOLOGY, CLINICAL MANIFESTATIONS, AND DIAGNOSIS. Larvae from infected fish can invade the small bowel on ingestion and cause a chronic malabsorption-diarrhea syndrome characterized by induration and villous atrophy, which is most prominent in the jejunum (Fig. 82–6). The adults invade the mucosa and lamina propria. Inflammation is not prominent around parasites, but chronic inflammation is noted within the lamina propria. The small intestine may contain thousands of parasites because of the ability of the adult females to produce infectious larvae. The chronic diarrhea, which is usually watery, leads to electrolyte and protein abnormalities. Muscle wasting and myocardial degeneration are seen terminally. Death has been attributed to hypokalemic or metabolic cardiomyopathy or to secondary infection of debilitated patients.

The diagnosis is made by finding the characteristic eggs in the stool (Fig. 82–7); larvae may also be seen. Multiple examinations may have to be made because shedding of diagnostic stages may be infrequent or sporadic.

TREATMENT AND PREVENTION. Because autoinfection may lead to multiplication and clinical dete-

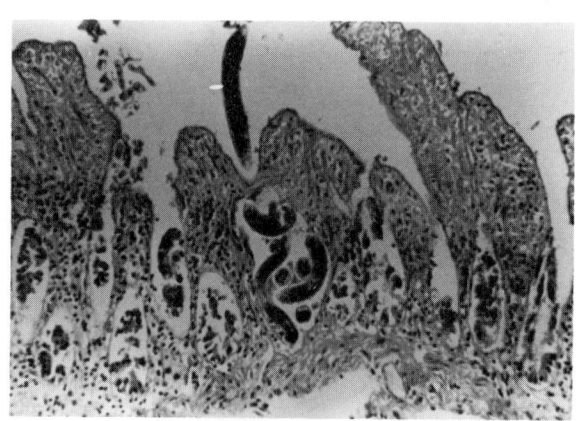

FIGURE 82–6. *Capillaria philippinensis.* Three transverse sections of larval *C. philippinensis* embedded in intestinal glands (× 100). (Courtesy of Armed Forces Institute of Pathology, Photograph Neg No 69–1065.)

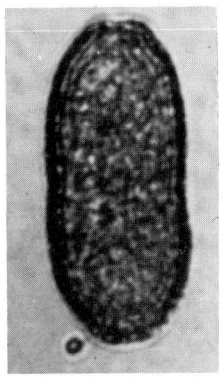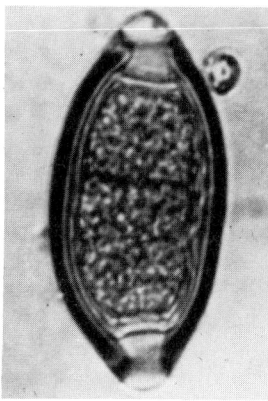

CAPILLARIA PHILIPPINENSIS	TRICHURIS TRICHIURA
Size: 45 X 21 μm	52 X 26 μm
Shape: peanut	ellipse
Plugs: bipolar not protuberant	bipolar protuberant
Shell: pitted	smooth

FIGURE 82–7. Comparison of *C. philippinensis* and *T. trichiura* eggs. (From Whalen GE, et al.: Lancet 1:13, 1969.)

rioration, infection with *Capillaria* should be promptly treated with mebendazole, 200 mg twice daily for 20 days. Albendazole is also effective. Supportive fluid, electrolyte, and nutritional therapy may also be necessary. Cooking of fish prevents infection.

BIBLIOGRAPHY

Alcantara AK, Uylangco CV, Cross JH: An obstinate case of intestinal capillariasis. Southeast Asian J Trop Med Public Health 16:410, 1985.
Cross JH, Basaca-Sevilla V: Albendazole in the treatment of intestinal capillariasis. Southeast Asian J Trop Med Public Health 18:507, 1987.

82.4. TRICHOSTRONGYLIASIS

Richard D. Pearson and Joseph D. Schwartzman

DEFINITION. Trichostrongyliasis is an infection caused by any of several *Trichostrongylus* species. These nematodes are primarily parasites of herbivorous animals, e.g., sheep or cattle. Humans become infected when they ingest food or water contaminated by the feces of infected animals or humans. *Trichostrongylus* adults reside in the duodenum or the upper jejunum with their heads embedded in the mucosa.

DISTRIBUTION. *Trichostrongylus* species have been reported with variable frequencies from many areas of the world. Human infections appear to be most prevalent in the Middle East and Asia. The most thorough investigations have been carried out in Iran, where 9 *Trichostrongylus* species have been identified from humans. In general, *T. colubriformis* is the species most frequently encountered in the Near and Middle East, whereas *T. orientalis* is the principal species in Asia.

ETIOLOGY

Morphology. *Trichostrongylus* adults are small, hairlike, reddish-brown roundworms. The males measure 4 to 6 mm in length, and the females, 5 to 8 mm. The head, which is unarmed, lies embedded in the mucosa of the small intestine. A distinct buccal capsule is absent, but there is a definite notch where the excretory pore opens. The males are characterized by a copulatory bursa with rays and spicules that are diagnostic for each species. In the female, the paired reproductive system opens through a common vulva. The eggs are elongated and oval, possess a transparent hyaline shell, and resemble those of hookworms, except that they are larger (85 to 115 μm) and slightly more pointed at one or both ends. When found in the feces, trichostrongylus eggs are usually in the morula stage (Fig. VI A–2 [7,8]). *Trichostrongylus* species can not be differentiated from one another on the basis of the morphologic characteristics of their ova.

Life Cycle. Under favorable conditions of humidity and temperature, ova hatch within 24 to 36 hours. They are remarkably resistant to long periods of cold and desiccation. The hatched larvae pass through 3 free-living stages, reaching the infective stage in 60 hours or more. Eggs and larvae flourish in areas with shade, high humidity, and grass or carpet vegetation. Infection usually follows ingestion of larvae in contaminated food or water, although larvae can enter through unbroken skin. Unlike *Strongyloides stercoralis* and the hookworms, migration of *Trichostrongylus* species through the lungs is not necessary for completion of the life cycle.

EPIDEMIOLOGY. *Trichostrongylus* species and related genera are common parasites of herbivorous animals, including cattle, sheep, donkeys, goats, deer, and rabbits. The use of sheep or cow manure as fertilizer contributes to the spread of infection in farming communities. Humans are often incidental hosts and vary in their susceptibility to various *Trichostrongylus* species. The prevalence of human infection may be as high as 1 or 2% in endemic areas. The use of night soil in the Orient creates conditions favorable to the spread of *T. orientalis*, which appears to be spread primarily from humans to humans.

PATHOLOGY AND CLINICAL MANIFESTATIONS. Little is known about the pathology of human trichostrongyliasis. The usual site of infection is the duodenum or the upper jejunum. Adult worms are thought to suck blood at times and to damage the mucosa of the small intestine at or near their sites of attachment. Shortened villi have been observed in the small intestine of experimentally infected rabbits.

Most human infections are mild and asymptomatic, but epigastric pain, diarrhea, and flatulence have been observed in some. Rarely, anemia and emaciation have been associated with heavy infections. Eosinophilia is present in a minority of those infected, and on rare occasions, the percentage of eosinophils may exceed 25%.

DIAGNOSIS. The diagnosis of trichostrongyliasis depends on the identification of ova in the stool. Concentration techniques are often necessary to find the rare ova in the usual, light infection. Care should be taken to differentiate *Trichostrongylus* eggs, which are larger and more pointed on one or both ends, from those of the hookworms (Fig. VI A-2). The diagnosis is occasionally made by finding *Trichostrongylus* larvae in duodenal aspirates. Identification of infecting *Trichostrongylus* species requires examination of adult worms, especially males.

TREATMENT. Thiabendazole, 25 mg/kg twice a day (maximal daily dose of 3 gm) for 2 days, is recommended, but thiabendazole-resistant *Trichostrongylus* strains have been identified and thiabendazole is frequently associated with side effects. Pyrantel pamoate, 11 mg/kg once (maximal dose 1 gm), has been used as an alternative, with better results reported from Japan and Korea than from Iran.

PROPHYLAXIS. Effective prophylaxis against trichostrongylus involves the sanitary disposal of human excreta and the prevention of fecal contamination of the topsoil by infected animals. The treatment of infected herd animals, such as cattle or sheep, may also reduce the risk to humans. Potentially contaminated vegetables should be thoroughly cooked and water boiled before ingestion.

BIBLIOGRAPHY

Ghadirian E: Human infection with *Trichostrongylus lerouxi* (Biocca, Chabaud, and Ghadirian, 1974) in Iran. Am J Trop Med Hyg 26:1212, 1977.

Hoste H, Kerboeuf D, Parodi AL: *Trichostrongylus colubriformis*: Effects on villi and crypts along the whole small intestine in infected rabbits. Exp Parasitol 67:39, 1988.

Markell EK: Pseudohookworm infection—trichostrongyliasis. N Engl J Med 278:831, 1968.

Wolfe MS: Oxyuris, trichostongylus and trichuris. Clin Gastroenterol 7:201, 1978.

83. INTESTINAL NEMATODES THAT MIGRATE THROUGH LUNGS (ASCARIASIS)

Joseph D. Schwartzman

DEFINITION. Infection by *Ascaris lumbricoides*, the largest of the intestinal nematodes, is more prevalent worldwide than infection with any other helminth. This is because the female worm produces a prodigious number of eggs that are relatively resistant to drying or to extremes of temperatures. *Ascaris* eggs in the soil are available to infect enormous numbers of people. The adult worms usually remain in the small intestine, while passage of the larvae through the lungs is accompanied by pneumonitis, which is usually subclinical.

ETIOLOGY

Adult Worms and Ova. The cylindrical, pink or cream-colored adult worm tapers at both ends. The male is smaller (120 to 250 mm × 3 to 4 mm) than the female (200 to 400 mm × 5 to 6 mm), and the male's posterior end is frequently slightly coiled or recurved. Females produce up to 200,000 fertilized or unfertilized eggs per day, which they deposit in the intestinal lumen. The 40 × 60 μm eggs have a characteristic mamillated outer coat and thick hyaline shell (Fig. VI A–2, [3–5]). *A. lumbricoides* has no important animal reservoir, although the morphologically similar *A. suum* may occasionally infect humans and *A. lumbricoides* may infect pigs. The 2 species may be difficult to distinguish but appear to be antigenically distinct. Genetic and immunologic analysis may soon clarify toxonomic relationships and may show the existence of strains with varying biologic behavior and pathogenic potential. Dog and cat ascarids of the genus *Toxocara* may infect humans but do not develop to sexual maturity in humans. The tissue-invasive larvae of these ascarids are responsible for the syndrome of visceral larva migrans.

Development. The life cycle of *Ascaris* begins with the production of eggs by adult female worms in the human distal small intestine; these are excreted in feces (Fig. 83–1). The mamillated outer coat of the egg may be important in survival, in that it may cause soil particles to adhere to the egg providing protection against complete desiccation. Under advantageous conditions of warm, moist, shaded soils the embryo molts within the eggshell; the infectious stage is a second-stage larva. The period of development in the soil is temperature dependent and may range from 2 weeks to several months. The eggs are infectious by ingestion, or possibly by inhalation of contaminated dust, but larvae do not hatch in soil and do not invade the skin. The larvae hatch in the jejunum, penetrate the intestinal wall, and migrate by way of the hepatic venules to the right side of the heart and the pulmonary circulation, where they break into the alveolar spaces and undergo 2 further molts. Most larvae will have reached the lung by 2 weeks following ingestion of eggs. From the alveoli, the 1.5 mm long larvae ascend to the trachea and are swallowed, undergo a last molt in the intestine, and develop to adults. Development from ingestion of eggs to the production of eggs may take from 10 to 12 weeks (Fig. 83–1). The number of adult worms per infected person may vary widely in an infected population; egg production per female worm decreases as the worm burden increases so that egg counts may not linearly reflect intensity of infection. Infections consisting only of female worms will produce infertile eggs, which will not develop to the infectious stage. Occasional male-only infections will result in no eggs in stool. Adults live for approximately a year.

EPIDEMIOLOGY. *A. lumbricoides* is distributed worldwide; an estimated 1.3 billion persons are infected. The infectious eggs are found in soil, where they remain viable for years. In the tropics, where moist shaded soils afford perfect conditions, the transmission of *Ascaris* is continuous. In regions where periods of aridity or temperature fluctuations may temporarily decrease the number of infectious eggs in soil, transmission of *Ascaris* may be seasonal. Clay soils favor *Ascaris* egg survival by retaining water around coated eggs and allowing

LIFE CYCLE of—

Ascaris lumbricoides

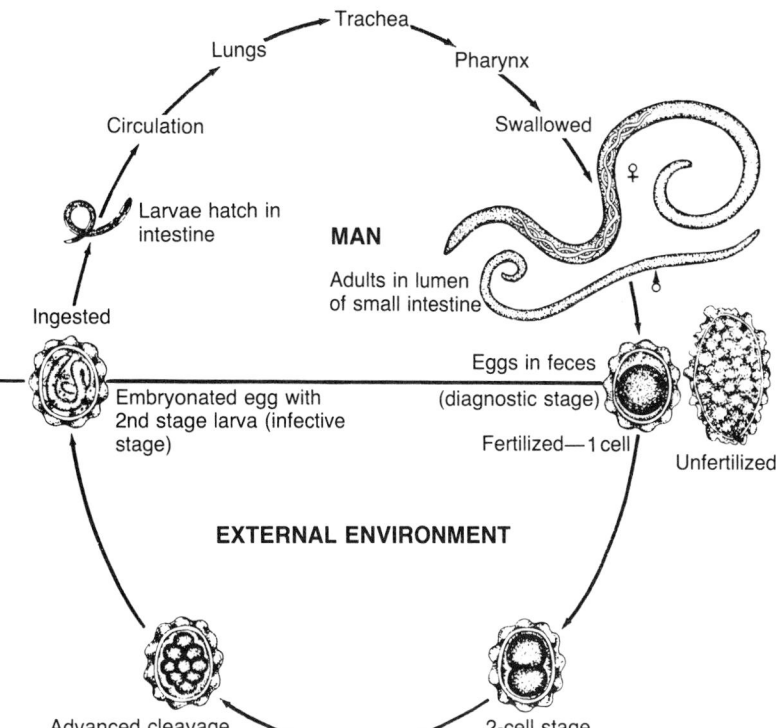

FIGURE 83–1. Life cycle of *Ascaris lumbricoides*. (From Melvin DM, Brooke MM, Sadun EH: Common Intestinal Helminths of Man. Atlanta, Centers for Disease Control, DHEW Publication No. [CDC] 75–8286, 1964.)

them to withstand desiccation. Eggs may also be more efficiently spread from clay soil; rain may spatter them onto vegetables, and eggs mixed with clay may adhere to persons and clothing, increasing the chances for ingestion or inhalation. *Ascaris* eggs can withstand freezing, and therefore, the infection is common even in northern temperate zones. Pawlowski has estimated that 9×10^{14} eggs per day contaminate the world's soil, which is a tribute to the enormous egg production of the worm and the general inadequacy of sanitation.

The prevalence of infection varies geographically, with approximately 73% of cases found in Asia, (including India and Southeast Asia), 12% in Africa, and 8% in Latin America. In areas of sporadic transmission, there may be small localized areas of high transmission. Only cold arid climates appear to be free of infection. Even in areas of high prevalence, the intensity of infection in the population is not uniform. A small proportion of the population usually harbors the majority of worms, and this subset of heavily infected persons is concentrated in children younger than 10 years, especially girls, who appear to have the highest infection rate.

PATHOLOGY. Most infected persons are asymptomatic. However, because there are so many individuals with infections, the overall morbidity caused by ascariasis is considerable.

Pulmonary Phase. Larvae migrating through the lungs may induce pulmonary hypersensitivity or inflammation in sensitized hosts, which can be manifest as asthma. This is especially likely to occur in localities where

transmission is seasonal or sporadic, such as in Saudi Arabia. The reaction to migration of larvae in tissue may be severe. Eosinophilic inflammation and granulomatous reaction may be seen in the lung, and local hypersensitivity may cause hypersecretion of mucus, bronchiolar inflammation, and serous exudate. In severe instances, vasculitis with perivascular granulomatous reactions may occur in conjunction with degenerating larvae. This spectrum of eosinophilic inflammation fits into the clinical entity referred to as Löffler's syndrome. Sputum containing eosinophils or Charcot-Leyden crystals may be produced, and larvae can sometimes be recovered from the sputum or gastric aspirate.

Other allergic manifestations to migrating larvae are also seen, including episodes of urticaria, which are more common at the end of the pulmonary phase.

Intestinal Phase. The intestinal phase of the disease is generally asymptomatic, and there is debate as to whether it is always harmful to the host. Although *Ascaris* infection can be shown to produce abnormalities of intestinal absorption (especially lactose malabsorption), malnutrition can usually not be attributed to this infection without involving other contributing factors such as inadequate diet or coexisting infections. In young children with the highest worm burdens, ascariasis may contribute to growth retardation.

Intestinal worms can cause serious complications; most frequently reported is intestinal obstruction at the terminal ileum (Fig. 83–2). This may be caused by a bolus of entangled worms, but a direct irritation caused

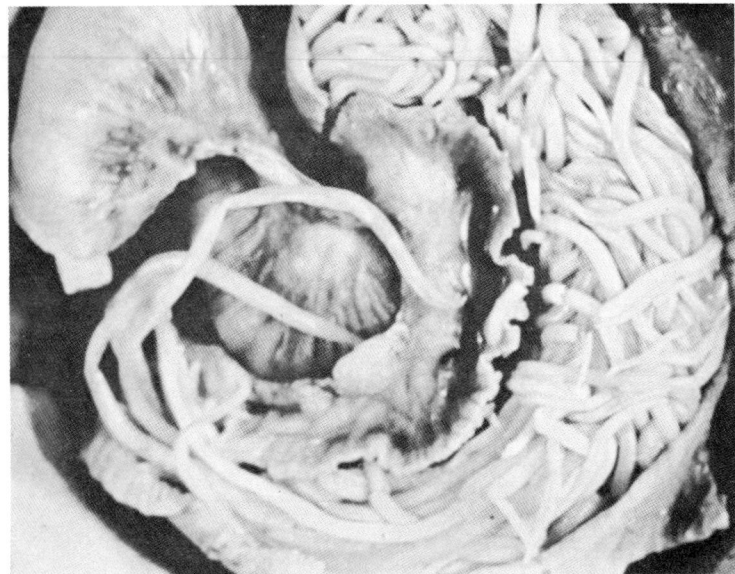

FIGURE 83–2. Terminal part of ileum opened, showing obstructing bolus of ascarids. (Courtesy of Drs. D. W. Aiken and F. N. Dickman. From JAMA 164:1317, 1957.)

by the worm, leading to spasm of the affected segment, has also been suggested. Ileocecal intussusception has been reported, and there have been less frequent reports of volvulus.

Migrating Adult Worms. Other complications of ascariasis result from the tendency of the adult worms to migrate. Numerous stimuli have been held responsible for worm migration, including fever, medication, anesthesia, and diet. Some drugs used to treat other parasitic infections (for instance, bephenium, which has been used to treat hookworm infections), may not kill *Ascaris* and may stimulate migration. Male worms are thought to be more prone to migrate and be expelled, which may explain the frequency of female-only infections. Worms migrate up or sometimes down the gastrointestinal tract and may cause bile duct obstruction (Fig. 83–3) or bile duct perforation with bile peritonitis or liver abscess. Pancreatic duct obstruction with pancreatitis is more rarely reported. Appendicitis (Fig. 83–4) and intestinal perforation have also been reported. Considering the prevalence of infections, all of the reported complications are infrequent, but the possibility of *Ascaris* infection is worth keeping in mind before treating patients with medicines or anesthetics that may induce migration and increase the chance of obstruction or perforation.

CLINICAL MANIFESTATIONS AND COMPLICATIONS

Pulmonary Migration. *Ascaris* larvae usually cause few symptoms along their migratory path, but in sensitized hosts, pulmonary manifestations may be noted starting within 1 week following the ingestion of eggs of either *A. lumbricoides* or *A. suum.* Fever, cough, wheezing, and dyspnea can be accompanied by sputum production, sometimes with small amounts of blood; chest pain and cyanosis are noted in the most severe cases. Chest film examination may show a variety of unilateral or bilateral abnormalities, ranging from nodular densities to diffuse interstitial patterns. The illness may persist as long as larvae continue to pass through the lungs but

usually is limited to several weeks. Leukocytosis is frequently associated and there may be marked eosinophilia, fulfilling the picture of Löffler's syndrome. Severe pulmonary inflammation associated with ascariasis has progressed to death, but this is rare.

Intestinal Infections. Adult worms probably cause few symptoms, except in heavy infections and unusual circumstances. It is difficult to know how frequently abdominal discomfort, nausea, anorexia, and diarrhea are attributable to ascariasis, although these symptoms are commonly seen in patients who are harboring *Ascaris.*

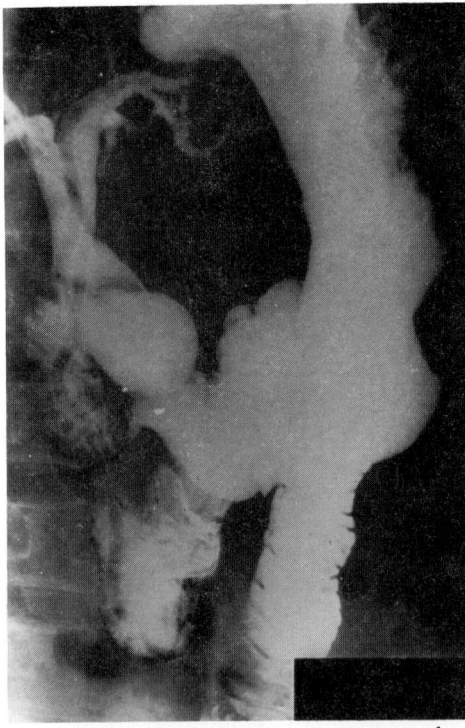

FIGURE 83–3. Ascariasis. Adult worms (linear lucencies) enter the bile ducts through the ampulla of Vater as well as through a surgically created choledochoduodenostomy. Barium was given orally.

The more serious complications of ascariasis, resulting from the migration of the adult worms, are unquestionably associated with symptoms. Migrating worms may reach the upper gastrointestinal tract and be vomited or may be passed per rectum. A number of worms may intertwine and form a bolus, which can cause partial or complete intestinal obstruction, with abdominal pain, vomiting, and occasionally a palpable abdominal mass (Fig. 83–2). Such a mass of worms may rarely cause intussusception with the attendant findings. Even less frequently, volvulus of a loop of small bowel has been attributed to a mass of entangled *Ascaris*. More frequently the migrating worms enter ducts or diverticuli, where they may perforate or cause obstruction. The common bile duct is perhaps the most often obstructed, causing biliary colic or cholangitis (Fig. 83–3). A worm that ascends higher in the biliary tree may result in liver abscess or may penetrate the bile duct and lead to bile peritonitis. The pancreatic duct may also be obstructed and lead to pancreatitis of various degrees of severity. Appendicitis may be triggered by *Ascaris* obstructing the appendix (Fig. 83–4). Perforation of the bowel has been reported, usually with a history of acute abdominal pain followed by symptoms of peritonitis or localized abscess, but the role of *Ascaris* in causing the perforation is unclear. Intestinal obstruction is occasionally caused by adhesions attributable to extraintestinal *Ascaris*.

DIAGNOSIS. The diagnosis of ascariasis is usually easily made by stool examination. Characteristic eggs (55 to 75 μm × 35 to 50 μm) may be seen on direct

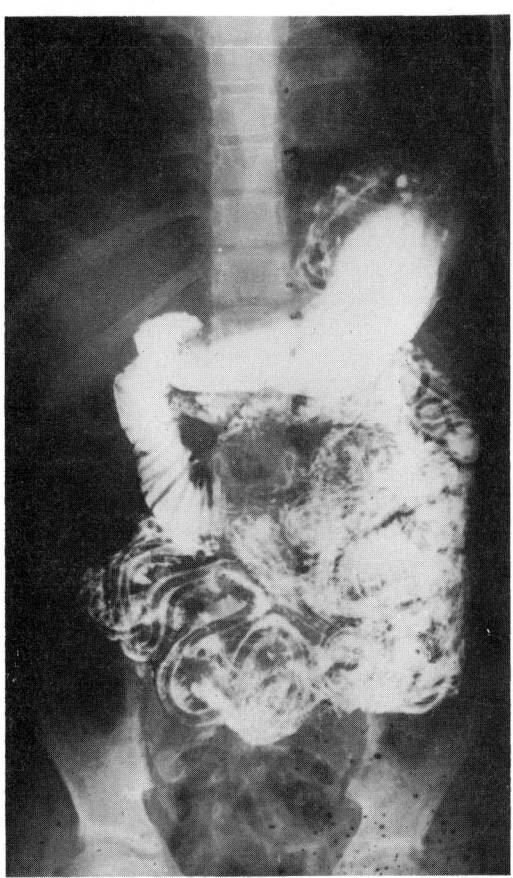

FIGURE 83–5. Adult *A. lumbricoides* visualized in small intestine by x-ray following barium. Ascarids may be detected at times without barium, by air contrast, but are less distinct. (Courtesy of Louisiana State University School of Medicine and the Charity Hospital of New Orleans.)

examination or may be concentrated by centrifugation techniques (Fig. VI A–2[3]). Unfertilized eggs may be somewhat more difficult to recognize because of their atypical size and appearance (Fig. VI A–2[4]). Decorticate eggs lacking the outer mamillated covering are sometimes produced (Fig. VI A–2[5]) and these may be confused with the eggs of other nematodes; the thick hyaline shell is typical of *Ascaris*. Infections consisting of only male worms will produce no eggs; if such infections are symptomatic, the worms may sometimes be detected radiologically as linear filling defects outlined by contrast media (Fig. 83–5). Intestinal worms may sometimes ingest barium and be seen as thin, curved linear densities after the barium meal has passed the portion of the intestine in which the worm resides.

TREATMENT

Chemotherapy. The treatment of ascariasis can be accomplished by several effective drugs. Pyrantel pamoate (11 mg/kg up to a maximum of 1 gm) can be given as a single dose. Adverse effects include occasional gastrointestinal disturbances, headaches, dizziness, rash, and fever. Mebendazole, 100 mg twice daily, should be given over 3 days. Occasional diarrhea, abdominal pain, and rare instances of leukopenia have been associated with mebendazole therapy. Mebendazole is contraindicated during pregnancy. Piperazine citrate, 75 mg/kg

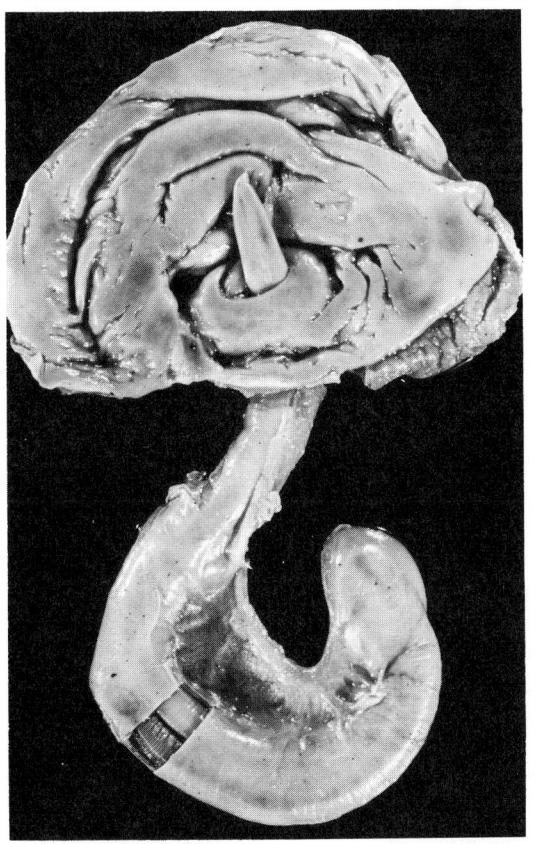

FIGURE 83–4. Adult *A. lumbricoides* in appendix. (Courtesy of the Louisiana State University School of Medicine, New Orleans.)

(maximum 3.5 gm daily), should be given for 2 days. Piperazine has occasionally caused urticarial reactions, gastrointestinal disturbances, and dizziness. On rare occasions, it may exacerbate epilepsy or cause ataxia, muscle weakness, and visual disturbances. Several regimens have been devised for effective single-dose therapy using benzimidazole derivatives. In 1 study, a single 500 mg dose of mebendazole was given to patients 10 kg and larger (excepting pregnant women and those with generalized neurologic disease) and was about 90% effective in eradicating *Ascaris*. Albendazole given in a single dose of 400 mg has cured 100% of *Ascaris* infections. Neither flubendazole nor albendazole is licensed for use in the United States.

Supportive Therapy. The therapy of complications of ascariasis depends on the presentation. Intestinal obstruction may necessitate surgery, although patients who are clinically stable and well hydrated have been successfully treated with diatrizoate meglumine and diatrizoate sodium solution, which induces an osmotic diarrhea. Obstruction of the bile or pancreatic ducts must be surgically relieved, but conservative therapy with nasogastric suction, intravenous hydration, antispasmodics, and anthelmintics (given by nasogastric tube) may be appropriate in simple biliary colic.

PREVENTION. Uncomplicated ascariasis in individual patients is relatively easy to treat. The more difficult problem is preventing reinfections, because the eggs may be stable in the environment for years. Soil treatments have been tried but are generally impractical, and sanitation must be adequate to prevent all untreated human waste from reaching the soil. Community-based mass chemotherapy must be repeated periodically to eradicate the infection. The problem is formidable, and, therefore, ascariasis is likely to persist as a common infection for the foreseeable future.

BIBLIOGRAPHY

Arfaa F: Selective primary health care: Strategies for control of disease in the developing world: XII. Ascariasis and trichuriasis. Rev Infect Dis 6:364, 1984.

Bar-Maor JA, de Carvalho JLAP, Chappell J: Gastrografin treatment of intestinal obstruction due to *Ascaris lumbricoides*. J Pediatr Surg 19:174, 1984.

Carrera E, Nesheim MC, Crompton DWT: Lactose maldigestion in *Ascaris*-infected preschool children. Am J Clin Nutr 39:255, 1983.

Croll NA, Ghadirian E: Wormy persons. Contributions to the nature and patterns of overdispersion with *Ascaris lumbricoides, Ancylostoma duodenale, Necator americanus* and *Trichuris trichiura*. Trop Geogr Med 33:241, 1981.

Crompton DWT, Nesheim NC, Pawlowski ZA: Ascariasis and its public health significance. London, Taylor & Francis, 1984.

Drugs for parasitic infections. Med Lett Drugs Ther 30:15, 1988.

Efem SEE: *Ascaris lumbricoides* and intestinal perforation. Br J Surg 74:643, 1987.

Elkins DB, Haswell-Elkins M, Anderson RM: The epidemiology and control of intestinal helminths in the Pulicat Lake region of Southern India. I. Study design and pre- and post-treatment observations on *Ascaris lumbricoides* infection. Trans R Soc Trop Med Hyg 80:774, 1986.

Elkins DB, Haswell-Elkins M, Anderson RM: The importance of host age and sex to patterns of reinfection with *Ascaris lumbricoides* following mass anthelmintic treatment in a South Indian fishing community. Parasitology 96:171, 1988.

El-Masry NA, Trabolsi B, Bassily S, Farid Z: Albendazole in the treatment of *Ancylostoma duodenale* and *Ascaris lumbriocoides* infections. Trans R Soc Trop Med Hyg 77:160, 1983.

Kan SP: The anthelmintic effects of flubendazole on *Trichuris trichiura* and *Ascaris lumbricoides*. Trans R Soc Trop Med Hyg 77:668, 1983.

Lord WD, Bullock WL: Swine ascaris in humans. N Engl J Med 306:113, 1982.

Martin J, Keymer A, Isherwood RJ, Wainwright SM: The prevalence and intensity of *Ascaris lumbricoides* infections in Moslem children from northern Bangladesh. Trans R Soc Trop Med Hyg 77:702, 1983.

Pawlowski ZS: Ascariasis: Host-pathogen biology. Rev Infect Dis 4:806, 1982.

Pawlowski ZS: Ascariasis. Clin Trop Med Comm Dis 2:595, 1987.

Ramalingam S, Sinniah B, Krishnan U: Albendazole, an effective single dose, broad spectrum anthelmintic drug. Am J Trop Med Hyg 32:984, 1983.

Schultz MG: Ascariasis: Nutritional implications. Rev Infect Dis 4:815, 1982.

Stephenson LS, Holland C: The impact of helminth infections on human nutrition: Schistosomes and soil-transmitted helminths. London, Taylor & Francis, 1987.

84.   INTESTINAL NEMATODES THAT MIGRATE THROUGH SKIN AND LUNG

Richard D. Pearson and Richard L. Guerrant

84.1.   HOOKWORM INFECTIONS

DEFINITION. Human hookworm disease (ancylostomiasis) is caused by *Necator americanus* and *Ancylostoma duodenale*. In addition, *Ancylostoma ceylonicum*, which infects a number of animals, is occasionally found in humans in restricted geographic areas. Hookworms have a complex life cycle of entering the skin, migrating through the lungs, and residing in the small intestine. The hallmark of hookworm disease is iron deficiency anemia due to chronic blood loss.

DISTRIBUTION. The hookworms are among the most important helminthic pathogens of humans. Both *A. duodenale* and *N. americanus* are widely distributed in tropical and subtropical Asia and Africa, but *A. duodenale* occurs in the Middle East, North Africa, and southern Europe. *N. americanus* is the predominant species in the New World, but there are focal sites of *A. duodenale* in the Caribbean islands and in Central and South America. *N. americanus* is found sporadically in the southeastern United States. Human infection with *A. ceylonicum* has been reported in the Philippines and in Calcutta, India.

ETIOLOGY

Morphology

Adults. Adult hookworms are small, cylindrical, creamy-white nematodes. Males measure 5 to 11 mm in length and 0.3 to 0.45 mm in width. The females are 9 to 13 mm in length and 0.35 to 0.6 mm in width. Males and females of *A. duodenale* are slightly larger than those of *N. americanus*. The anterior end of *N. americanus* is sharply curved in a direction opposite to the curve of the rest of the body, giving the worm a hooklike appearance. The head of *A. duodenale* continues in the same direction as the curvature of the body.

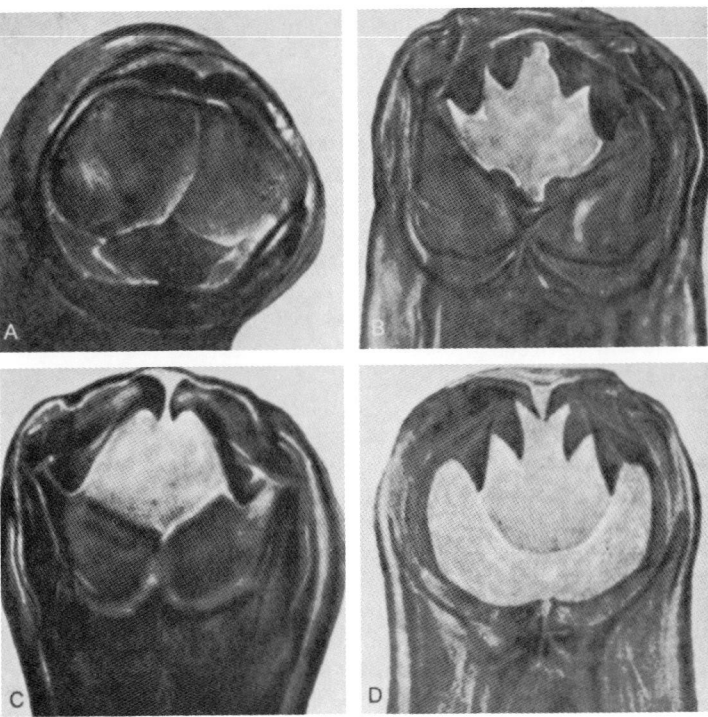

FIGURE 84–1. *A*, Mouthparts of *Necator americanus*. Note two pairs of chitinized cutting plates characteristic of this species. *B*, Mouthparts of *Ancylostoma duodenale*. Note two large pairs of teeth, each of the medial pair bearing a small accessory process. *C*, Mouthparts of *A. braziliense*. Note two pairs of teeth, a large outer pair and a small inner pair without accessory processes. *D*, Mouthparts of *A. caninum*. Note three well-developed pairs of teeth.

Identification of hookworm species is based on the length, the number and arrangement of the teeth or cutting plates (Fig. 84–1), the length of the esophagus, the morphology of the bursa of the male, the position of the vulva in the female, and the size of the eggs. These points are summarized in tabular form for *A. duodenale* and *N. americanus* and for 2 closely related hookworm species in Table 84–1.

The posterior tip of male hookworms is expanded to form a typical copulatory bursa supported by fleshy rays with a pattern that is characteristic of the species. The alimentary canal and genital ducts open into this bursa.

A pair of long copulatory spicules is regulated by an accessory copulatory device, the gubernaculum.

The females have a subterminal ventrally located anus on the conical posterior extremity. The reproductive system is double, the tubules of the ovary being coiled intricately over the alimentary canal and confined to the posterior two thirds of the body. The vulva is located ventrally at the junction of the anterior third and the middle of the body of *N. americanus* and at the beginning of the posterior third of the body of *A. duodenale*. During copulation, the copulatory bursa of the male surrounds the vulva, thus giving the spermatozoa access

TABLE 84–1. Differential Characteristics of Common Hookworms*

	Necator americanus	*Ancylostoma duodenale*	*Ancylostoma braziliense*	*Ancylostoma caninum*
Shape	Head curved opposite to curvature of body, giving a hooked appearance to anterior end	Head continues in same direction as curvature of body	Similar to *A. duodenale*	Similar to *A. duodenale*
Length				
Female (mm)	9–11 × 0.35	10–13 × 0.60	9–10.5 × 0.38	14 × 0.6
Male (mm)	5–9 × 0.30	8–11 × 0.45	7.8–8.5 × 0.35	10 × 0.4
Buccal capsule	A pair of dorsal and ventral semilunar cutting plates	2 pairs of curved ventral teeth of nearly the same size, rudimentary inner pair	2 pairs of ventral teeth, inner smaller	3 pairs of ventral teeth, inner smallest
Length of esophagus	0.5–0.8 mm in length. Opening small, oval, long axis dorsoventral	1.3 mm in length. Opening oval, long axis transverse	Opening very small, long axis dorsoventral	Opening large, oval, long axis dorsoventral
Bursa of male	Long, wide and rounded, dorsal ray small, bipartite	Broader than long, dorsal ray tripartite	Small, almost as broad as long, with short stubby rays	Large and flaring, with long slender rays
Caudal spine in female	Absent	Present	Present	Present
Vulva	Anterior third to middle of body	Posterior to middle of body	Posterior to middle of body	Posterior to middle of body
Size of eggs (μm)	64–76 × 35–40	50–60 × 35–40	55–60 × 34–40	60–75 × 38–45

*Adapted from Belding DL: Textbook of Parasitology, 3rd ed. New York, Appleton-Century-Crofts, 1965, p 426.

to the reproductive system of the female. After mating, the male becomes detached. Fertilization takes place in the upper portion of the uterus or in the seminal receptacle.

Ova. *N. americanus* produces an estimated 10,000 to 20,000 eggs per female per day, and *A. duodenale,* 10,000 to 25,000. The eggs of the 2 species are almost indistinguishable, differing only in size. *N. americanus* is 64 to 76 μm × 36 to 40 μm, and *A. duodenale* is 56 to 60 μm × 36 to 40 μm. The eggs are eliminated in feces in 2- to 8-celled stages of cleavage. A clear space is present between the cells and the shell (Fig. VI A–2*[6]*).

Development

Soil Stage. Hookworm ova are passed in the feces and develop in the soil (Fig. 84–2). Under optimal conditions of moisture and temperature (23 to 33C), eggs hatch in 1 to 2 days. Each one liberates a rhabditiform larva, which is 250 to 300 μm long. The anterior end is bluntly rounded and characterized by a long, narrow buccal cavity. The larvae feed actively on bacteria and organic debris, gradually double in size, and molt twice to become slender, nonfeeding, infectious third-stage or filariform larvae. Development from eggs to filariform larvae requires 5 to 10 days under favorable conditions.

Filariform larvae live in the top one-half inch of soil, with their ends projecting upward from the surface. They spend their lives within a few inches of where eggs were deposited. Larvae survive best in light soil that is protected from drying or excessive water. Under tropical conditions of high temperature and periodic rainfall, they can survive for 3 to 4 weeks.

Host Stage. Filariform larvae can migrate vertically through the soil to a potential host in response to contact (thigmotropism), carbon dioxide, or warmth. When contact is made with human skin, the larvae use discontinuities in the epidermis of the host, such as fissures or hair follicles, to penetrate the skin. They exsheath as they enter the host. The usual site of entrance is the dorsum of bare feet or between the toes. Miners and farmers may acquire infection through the interdigital spaces of the hand.

The larvae gain access to the venous circulation and are carried to the lungs, where they break out into the alveoli and move through the respiratory tree to the pharynx. They are swallowed, pass through the esophagus and stomach, and arrive in the small intestine before molting to become adults.

Although infection is principally acquired through the skin, *A. duodenale* can enter by the oral route when larvae are present on vegetables grown in soil contaminated with feces. Maturation then occurs entirely in the intestine without tissue invasion. *A. duodenale* has been

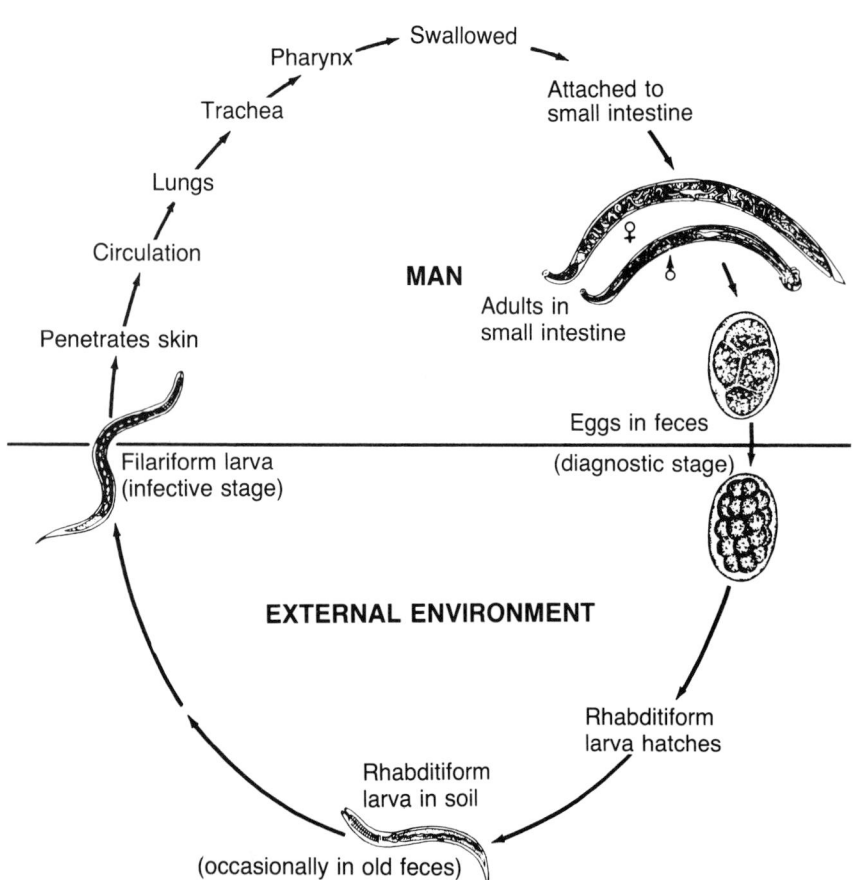

FIGURE 84–2. Life cycle of hookworm. (From Melvin DM, Brooke MM, Sadun EH: Common Intestinal Helminths of Man. Atlanta, Centers for Disease Control, DHEW Publication No. [CDC] 75–8286, 1964.)

shown to migrate to and remain dormant within the muscle of pigs, calves, rabbits, and other animals. Experimental models suggest that infection may result if meat of such a paratenic host is eaten uncooked, but whether this results in human infection is uncertain. Finally, transmammary transmission of hookworms is well documented in animals but has not been demonstrated in humans.

Eggs first appear in the stool 5 weeks or more after invasion of the skin by filariform larvae. Maximal egg production occurs at 12 to 18 months. *A. duodenale* adults can live up to 6 to 7 years. *N. americanus* usually live 5 to 6 years, but in 1 case, persisted for as long as 15 years. In general, the worm burden begins to fall within 1 to 3 years in the absence of reinfection.

EPIDEMIOLOGY. Several factors favor the spread of hookworm infection: poor sanitary practices in which infected individuals defecate in areas frequented by others; shaded sandy or loam soil; a warm, moist climate; and a population that does not wear shoes. Special habits or customs of a region are often important factors in transmission. In some regions, there are certain defecation areas that adults use. These spots often provide the proper environment for the development of infective hookworm larvae. Adults revisit these sites daily thus exposing themselves to infection and reinfection. Young children often defecate close to their houses in areas in which they play.

Cultural differences in attitude toward human excrement also contribute to the prevalence and intensity of infection. For example, the heavy infections attributable to the use of night soil as fertilizer in China contrast to the generally light infections found in India where Hindu culture limits the use of human feces as manure.

Temperatures ranging between 26.7 and 32.2C (80 and 90F) are optimal for larval development. Larvae are readily killed by desiccation or freezing. Hookworm infection is also limited to those tropical and subtropical areas where the rainfall averages 50 inches or more per year.

Sex-associated differences in the prevalence or severity of infection have been observed in some populations, but are probably due to occupational activities that result in different degrees of exposure. In the past, hookworm infection was common among underground workers who were exposed in mines or tunnels that lacked sanitary facilities. In hyperendemic areas, the prevalence of infection increases with age during childhood, but plateaus during the second to fifth decade, suggesting that there may be development of partial immunity.

Hookworm infections were once common in the southern United States. A large survey commissioned by the Rockefeller Foundation in 1910 revealed a prevalence of 42% in some areas of the South. The treatment and control measures that followed led to a dramatic reduction in the disease. For example, in eastern counties of Kentucky, the prevalence dropped from 37% in 1914 to 4% in 1963. As the prevalence diminished, so did the intensity of infections and the frequency of symptomatic disease. Severe anemia due to hookworm disease is now extremely rare in the United States.

PATHOLOGY

Larvae. The penetration of the skin by infectious filariform larvae of *N. americanus* often causes local dermatitis, which is associated with edema, erythema, and a vesicular or papular eruption. These changes subside spontaneously in approximately 2 weeks unless secondary bacterial infections occur. Cutaneous reactions seem to be less common with *A. duodenale*.

As the migrating larvae leave the capillaries of the lungs and penetrate into the alveoli, minute hemorrhagic lesions are produced. These are numerous in heavy infection and may be accompanied by an infiltrate with eosinophils and mononuclear cells. In general, the pulmonary reaction is mild.

Adults. Adult hookworms inhabit the upper half of the small intestine, where they attach and suck blood (Fig. 84–3). Transient injury to the intestinal mucosa results from the mechanical and lytic destruction of tissue at the point of attachment. Blood loss is due to bleeding at the site of attachment as well as to the blood removed by the worms. Less than half of the erythrocytes sucked into the worm are destroyed during passage through the worm's gut; the remainder enter the host's intestinal tract.

N. americanus seems to be more benign then *A. duodenale*. Blood loss is on the order of 0.03 ml/day per *N. americanus* adult and from 0.15 to 0.26 ml/day per *A. duodenale* adult. Hypoproteinemia frequently accompanies hookworm disease, but there is no evidence that hookworms themselves cause malabsorption or result in permanent damage to the intestinal mucosa.

CLINICAL MANIFESTATIONS. The clinical features of hookworm infection correspond to the life cycle of the organism and the intensity of infection.

Dermatitis. Penetration of the skin by filariform larvae can produce intense pruritus. In some instances, erythematous, pruritic papules develop at the entry site. Vesiculation and local edema may follow. This has been termed "ground itch" or "dew itch" and persists for up to 2 weeks. Secondary bacterial infections occur in some persons.

Pulmonary Manifestations. As larvae pass through the lungs, patients may complain of cough and wheezing. In a small percentage of patients, infiltrates may appear on the chest film in conjunction with eosinophilia. This can lead to the diagnosis of Löffler's syndrome, but in general, the pulmonary manifestations are relatively mild.

Gastrointestinal Manifestations. Epigastric pain, flatulence, and tenderness occur early in the intestinal phase of infection. In experimentally induced human *N. americanus* infections, abdominal pain and flatulence appeared 35 to 40 days after exposure to filariform larvae; eosinophilia (1350 to 3828/mm^3) peaked between 38 and 64 days; and eggs first appeared in the stool during the sixth week. The abdominal pain with hookworm infection may be severe enough to suggest peptic ulcer disease. On occasion, it is accompanied by diarrhea with blood and mucus. Rarely, massive exposure to filariform larvae results in acute gastrointestinal hemorrhage with uncompensated blood loss, a condition that is severe and potentially life threatening. This is most likely to occur in young children with heavy primary infections.

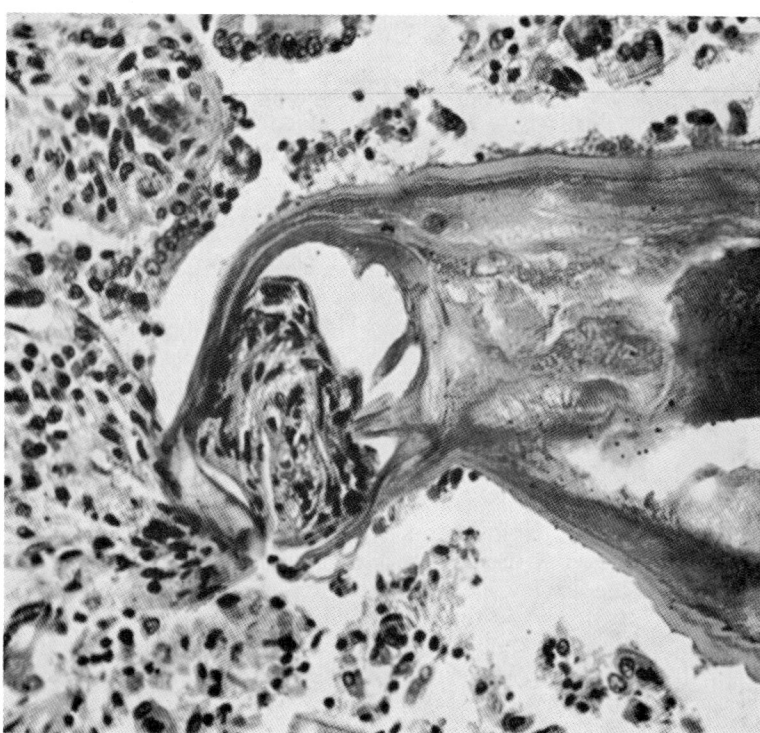

FIGURE 84–3. Longitudinal section through hookworm attached to intestinal mucosa. (Courtesy of Dr. Pedro Morera, Facultad de Microbiologia, Universidad de Costa Rica.)

Anemia. The hallmark of chronic hookworm disease is iron deficiency anemia, the development of which is dependent on the number and species of infecting hookworm, the iron reserves and requirements of the host, and the availability of iron in the diet. Iron loss is due to bleeding at the site of hookworm attachment as well as to blood sucked into the worm. In areas where iron intake is high, even relatively heavy hookworm infections may not cause anemia. However, if the iron content of the diet is low, even moderate worm burdens can result in severe iron deficiency (Chapter 108.1).

Clinical Findings. The anemia of hookworm disease is usually chronic and may be severe, with hemoglobin levels in the range of 3 to 8 gm/dl (Chapter 5). Lassitude, weakness, apathy, and depression are characteristic of anemia. On physical examination, the mucous membranes, conjuctivae, and skin appear pale. Iron deficiency has also been associated with koilonychia and angular stomatitis. In blacks, the skin may appear depigmented. A yellowish-green hue (chlorosis) was once commonly observed in Caucasians with severe hookworm disease, but is now extremely rare.

Complications. Severe cases of anemia and hypoalbuminemia are accompanied by cardiovascular changes. Dyspnea, palpitations, and sinus tachycardia are common. The physical findings may suggest a high-output state with widened pulse pressure, peripheral arterial bruits, a systolic flow murmur usually best heard in the pulmonic area, elevated jugular venous pressure, and cardiomegaly. Peripheral edema may be a manifestation of congestive heart failure and/or hypoalbuminemia. Cardiomegaly may be observed on the chest radiograph, and nonspecific ST-T wave changes may be present on the electrocardiogram. The effects of hookworm disease can be particularly severe in growing children and during pregnancy. Severe anemia is thought to stunt physical and intellectual growth and to contribute to increased maternal and neonatal mortality.

Laboratory Findings. Erythrocytes are hypochromic and microcytic in patients with hookworm disease, and the reticulocyte count is low. The serum ferritin and iron levels are low, and the iron-binding capacity (transferrin) is elevated. The bone marrow iron stores are depleted. Eosinophilia is common, but the total white blood cell count is usually normal. Of note, hookworm infection was the most common explanation for eosinophilia among Southeast Asian refugees referred for evaluation of eosinophilia at one center. Low levels of parasite-specific IgG and IgE can be detected in serum. Hookworms do not produce malabsorption, but in some areas, iron deficiency due to hookworms may be present concurrently with folic acid deficiency due to other causes, such as tropical sprue. The effects of folic acid deficiency may become overt only after iron repletion.

Hypoalbuminemia often accompanies hookworm infection and generally correlates with the degree of anemia. The relative contributions of worm-induced intestinal protein loss, diminished protein intake, and decreased albumin synthesis in malnourished persons have not been determined, but in general, hookworm patients are no more malnourished than uninfected subjects living in the same geographic area.

DIAGNOSIS. Hookworm disease should be considered in any patient from an endemic area who presents with anemia. The diagnosis is confirmed by identifying hookworm ova in the stool (Fig. VI A–2[6]). It is not easy or necessary to differentiate between eggs of *N. americanus* and those of *A. duodenale*. Direct fecal examination in saline or an iodine solution is suitable for detection of clinically significant infections. This technique will identify persons with more than 1200 eggs/gm of stool. Zinc sulfate flotation or formalin-ether concentration techniques can be used to identify persons with lighter infections.

In stool specimens that have not been examined for several days, it may be necessary to distinguish between the rhabditiform larvae of hookworms and those of *Strongyloides stercoralis* (Fig. 84–5; Table 84–2). In contrast to *S. stercoralis*, a rhabditiform hookworm larva has a long buccal tube extending from its mouth to its esophagus. The presence of embryonated eggs and rhabditiform larvae in the same stool is suggestive of hookworm infection or a mixed infection with hookworm and *S. stercoralis*. If only rhabditiform larvae are present, *S. stercoralis* should be suspected, but it must be borne in mind that mixed infections are common, especially in the tropics. On rare occasion, it may be necessary to differentiate hookworm larvae from those of *Trichostrongylus* species, which are larger and more pointed at 1 end (Fig. 84–5).

TREATMENT

Infection Therapy. The therapy of hookworm disease consists of iron repletion and anthelmintic medications. The benzimidazoles, albendazole and mebendazole; pyrantel pamoate; and bephenium hydroxynaphthoate are effective against hookworms and generally well tolerated. Tetrachloroethylene has also been used and is the least expensive, but it is more toxic.

Unless there are mitigating circumstances, treatment of light, asymptomatic infections is not necessary in endemic areas where reinfection is likely. Persons with heavy infections or iron deficiency should be treated. Discretion should be used in the treatment of light, asymptomatic infections in travelers returning to the United States or Europe who will not have further exposure. Only rarely will they develop anemia, but most are treated because safe, effective medications are available.

Mebendazole and Albendazole. Mebendazole is effective against both hookworm species; the standard dosage is 100 mg twice a day for 3 days. This regimen results in a cure rate of 76 to 95% and in reduction of mean egg counts by 83.7 to 99.9%. Mebendazole is also effective against *Ascaris lumbricoides* and *Trichuris trichiura* and is the drug of choice for persons concurrently infected with hookworm and these intestinal nematodes. Mebendazole is usually well tolerated, but it should not be used during pregnancy, because there has been evidence of teratogenicity in animal studies (VI A, General Principles). Albendazole is a newer benzimidazole. It has a spectrum of activity and toxicity similar to those of mebendazole but, in studies to date, has been effective when given as a single dose. Albendazole

thus holds promise for mass treatment programs. It is not licensed for use in the United States.

Pyrantel pamoate. This drug is more active against *A. duodenale* than against *N. americanus*. It is given as a single dose of 11 mg of pyrantel base/kg body weight (maximal dose 1 gm) orally. Pyrantel is usually well tolerated but, on occasion, causes mild gastrointestinal side effects, headache, dizziness, or drowsiness. Transient elevations of liver enzymes have also been reported (VI A, General Principles).

Bephenium hydroxynaphthoate. This drug is also more active against *A. duodenale* than against *N. americanus*. The standard treatment regimen for *A. duodenale* is a single dose of 5 gm of the salt (2.5 gm of base). For *N. americanus* infections, 3 single daily doses of 5 gm are needed to ensure a high cure rate. The drug is dispensed in small granules and is usually given with water on an empty stomach before breakfast. Bephenium can excite *Ascaris lumbricoides* and cause its migration; mebendazole and albendazole are better choices when persons are concurrently infected with hookworm and *A. lumbricoides* (VI A, General Principles).

Anemia Therapy. Rapid correction of anemia is best accomplished by the administration of ferrous sulfate. Iron replacement is continued for 3 months after normal hemoglobin values are achieved to replete iron stores. Anemia can be corrected even without anthelmintic therapy. During pregnancy, anemia is treated with ferrous sulfate alone and anthelmintic treatment is delayed until after delivery because of the potential teratogenicity of the anthelmintic drugs.

Chronic anemia due to hookworm infection is usually well tolerated, even if severe, and blood transfusion is seldom indicated. If required, blood should be given carefully because it may lead to hypervolemia and precipitate congestive heart failure. The use of packed red blood cells, administration of diuretics, and monitoring of central venous pressure have been recommended when transfusions are given to minimize these risks. The potential for human immunodeficiency virus (HIV) infection is another reason to limit transfusions.

CONTROL. Transmission of hookworm infection can theoretically be interrupted by sanitary disposal of human feces, use of footwear, or treatment of infected persons. In developing areas, local habits and customs may be obstacles to the use of latrines or to discontinuation of the use of night soil as fertilizer. In the southern United States, control was rendered cost effective by targeting for treatment those subpopulations with a high prevalence of clinical disease, but mass chemotherapy in holoendemic areas is often impractical because of the cost of drugs and high rates of reinfection. Immunity during natural infections is acquired slowly if at all, and no vaccine against human hookworms is available.

Some physicians have taken an alternative approach to the control of hookworm disease and advocated the use of iron supplements in food staples such as sugar or flour. However, a note of caution is necessary because, in the case of some malnourished populations, iron supplementation has been associated with an apparent increased risk of bacterial and protozoal infections.

TABLE 84–2. Rhabditiform Larvae

Characteristics	*Strongyloides*	Hookworm
Size, average	225 × 16 μm	275 × 17 μm
Posterior tip	Blunter	Sharper
Buccal chamber	Short or absent	Long
Genital primordia	Larger	Smaller

BIBLIOGRAPHY

Botero D, Castano A: Comparative study of pyrantel pamoate, bephenium hydroxynaphthoate, and tetrachloroethylene in the treatment of *Necator americanus* infections. Am J Trop Med Hyg 22:45, 1973.

Crosby WH: The deadly hookworm: Why did the Puerto Ricans die? Arch Intern Med 147:577, 1987.

Farid Z, Nichols JH, Bassily S, Schulert AR: Blood loss in pure *Ancylostoma duodenale* infection in Egyptian farmers. Am J Trop Med Hyg 14:375, 1965.

Fulmer HS, Huempfner HR: Intestinal helminths in eastern Kentucky: A survey in three rural counties. Am J Trop Med Hyg 14:269, 1965.

Gilles HM, Williams EJW, Ball PAJ: Hookworm infection and anaemia: An epidemiological, clinical, and laboratory study. Quart J Med 33:1, 1964.

Gilman RH: Hookworm disease: Host-pathogen biology. Rev Infect Dis 4:824, 1982.

Holzer BR, Frey FJ: Differential efficacy of mebendazole and albendazole against *Necator americanus* but not for *Trichuris trichiura* infestations. Eur J Clin Pharmacol 32:635, 1987.

Hotez PJ, Cerami A: Secretion of a proteolytic anticoagulant by *Ancylostoma* hookworms. J Exp Med 157:1594, 1983.

Little MD, Halsey NA, Cline BL, Katz SP: *Ancylostoma* larva in a muscle fiber of man following cutaneous larva migrans. Am J Trop Med Hyg 32:1285, 1983.

Martinez-Torres C, Ojeda A, Roche M, Layrisse M: Hookworm infection and intestinal blood loss. Trans R Soc Trop Med Hyg 61:373, 1967.

Maxwell C, Hussain R, Nutman TB, et al: The clinical and immunologic responses of normal human volunteers to low dose hookworm *(Necator americanus)* infection. Am J Trop Med Hyg 37:126, 1987.

Migasena S, Gilles HM: Hookworm infection. Clin Trop Med Comm Dis 2:617, 1987.

Miller TA: Hookworm infection in man. Adv Parasitol 17:315, 1979.

Nutman TB, Ottesen EA, Ieng S, et al: Eosinophilia in Southeast Asian refugees: Evaluation at a referral center. J Infect Dis 155:309, 1987.

Pugh RNH, Teesdale CH, Burnham GM: Albendazole in children with hookworm infection. Ann Trop Med Hyg Parastiol 80:565, 1986.

Ray DK, Shrivastava VB: The infectivity of ingested adult hookworm. Trans R Soc Trop Med Hyg 75:566, 1981.

de la Riva H, Escamilla DG, Frati AC: Acute massive intestinal bleeding caused by hookworm. JAMA 246:68, 1981.

Roche M, Layrisse M: The nature and causes of "hookworm anemia." Am J Trop Med Hyg 15:1030, 1966.

Schad GA, Chowdhury AB, Dean CG, et al: Arrested development in human hookworm infections: An adaptation to a seasonally unfavorable external environment. Science 180:502, 1973.

Variyam EP, Banwell JG: Hookworm disease: Nutritional implications. Rev Infect Dis 4:830, 1982.

84.2.   STRONGYLOIDES INFECTIONS

DEFINITION. Strongyloidiasis, sometimes called threadworm infection, results from infection by *Strongyloides stercoralis,* the female of which is usually embedded in the mucosa of the small intestine. *S. stercoralis* is less common than hookworm but may cause more severe, life-threatening illness. It is nearly unique among helminths in its ability to autoinfect and maintain persisting infection for many years. Recognized since 1876 when Normand described the larvae in stools of French soldiers in Southeast Asia with "Cochin-China diarrhea," *S. stercoralis* has a complex life cycle of entering the skin, migrating through the lungs, and residing in the small bowel (Fig. 84–4). Symptoms of chronic infection, which may persist for many years after

exposure, are primarily episodic, creeping urticaria (larva currens), epigastric or cramping abdominal pain, and diarrhea. The capacity of *S. stercoralis* to mature and multiply indirectly outside the host (heterogonic development) and its ability to overwhelm the immunocompromised host with autoinfection are well recognized.

Although the vast majority of *Strongyloides* infections are with *S. stercoralis*, the primate parasite *S. fulleborni* is recognized in humans in Africa and in Papua New Guinea.

ETIOLOGY AND DEVELOPMENT. As illustrated in Figure 84–4, the life cycle of *S. stercoralis* is complex. Like other intestinal nematodes, it may involve both host and soil stages. However, unlike most other helminths, the complete life cycle can also occur over prolonged periods completely in the soil (free-living cycle) or completely in the host (internal or external autoinfection). The free-living cycle enables the parasite to maintain itself and multiply in the external environment, thus improving its chances of infecting a new definitive host. Conversely, the autoinfection cycle is the basis of both persistence of infections for many years and the overwhelming hyperinfection syndrome. These 3 types of cycles thus involve (1) host and soil, (2) soil only (free-living or indirect cycle), and (3) internal or external autoinfection.

Host Stage. Human infection begins with exposure of the skin to filariform (third-stage) larvae that reside in fecally contaminated, moist soil for days to weeks (Fig. 84–4). These larvae measure 400 to 500 μm in length by 15 μm in width and have slender bodies, straight intestinal tracts, notched tails, and no visible genital primordium. Filariform larvae migrate through the venous blood stream to the lungs, where they penetrate into the alveoli and ascend the airways to the trachea and glottis before being swallowed to complete their life cycle in the small intestine. There, after 2 molts, adult females emerge that penetrate and reside in the superficial mucosa of the duodenum and jejunum, where mating is believed to occur. Adult females measure 2.2 mm long by 0.04 mm wide and have a delicate striated cuticula, elongated esophagus (less than one third of the body length), and paired ovaries, oviducts, and uteri. Nearly 1 month after initial infection, the adult female, after fertilization or by parthenogenesis (the latter analogous to the situation for *S. ratti* in rats), begins to lay oval, thin-shelled, embryonated eggs (32 × 55 μm) that closely resemble hookworm eggs but are usually not seen because they rapidly hatch in the intestinal mucosa to produce first-stage, noninfectious rhabditiform larvae (Figs. VI A–2[10] and 84–5). It is this rhabditiform larval stage that is characteristically found in the stool or the upper small bowel. The time from infection to the shedding of the larvae is usually 3 to 5 weeks. Rhabditiform larvae are shorter (200 to 250 μm) and wider (15 to 30 μm) than the infective filariform larvae and have a shorter buccal chamber and more prominent genital primordium when compared with the closely similar rhabditiform larvae of hookworm (Table 84–2). Under favorable soil conditions, rhabditiform larvae can transform into infected filariform larvae within 24 hours

LIFE CYCLE of—

Strongyloides stercoralis

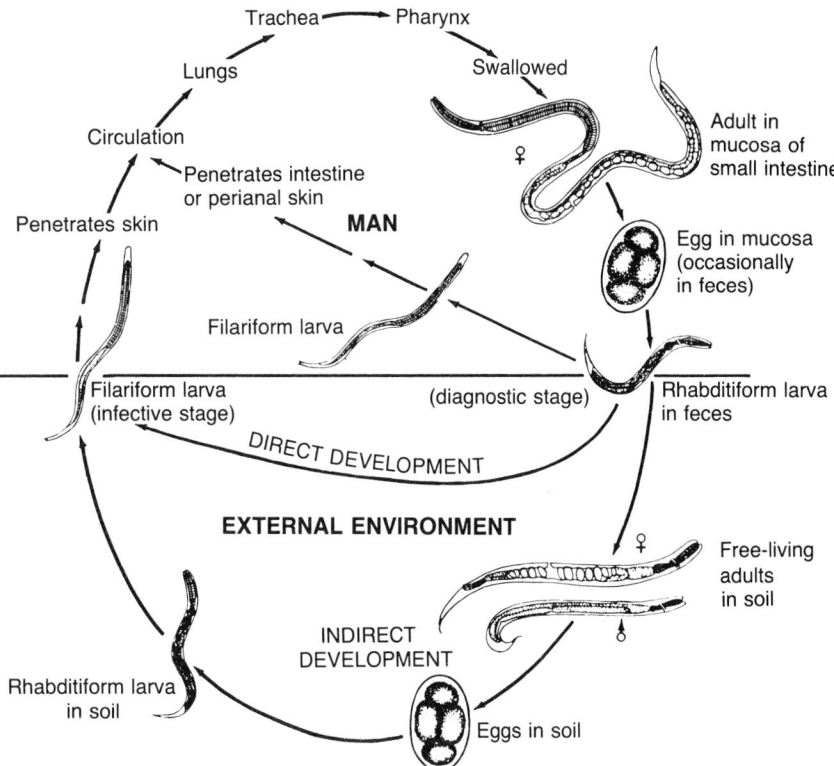

FIGURE 84–4. Life cycle of *Strongyloides stercoralis*. (From Melvin DM, Brooke MM, Sadun EH: Common Intestinal Helminths of Man. Atlanta, Centers for Disease Control, DHEW Publication No. [CDC] 75–8286, 1964.)

after fecal passage, a process that may also occur in the perianal region after defecation.

Soil Stage. Once passed into the soil, rhabditiform larvae may undergo 2 molts and mature over several days into infective filariform larvae (direct, homogonic cycle) that may survive for several weeks under moist conditions (Fig. 84–4). Alternatively, if conditions of light, warmth, oxygen, and moisture are optimal, non-infective rhabditiform larvae may develop into worms that are usually about half the size of the adults seen in the intestine (females about 1-mm and males about 0.75-mm long). By this latter process (indirect or heterogonic development), the parasite can multiply outside the host for several generations.

Autoinfection. Autoinfection may occur by the rapid transformation of rhabditiform larvae to infectious dwarf filariform larvae in the gut lumen, where they penetrate the intestinal mucosa ("intestinal" or "internal" autoinfection) to proceed via the lung to maintain infection in humans (Fig. 84–4). Alternatively, the filariform larvae may develop in the colorectal area and penetrate the perianal skin (with resultant pruritic creeping eruption or "larva currens" and "external autoinfection") before migrating through the lung back to the small intestine.

EPIDEMIOLOGY

Distribution. Although diagnostic methods are imperfect and precise prevalence data are not available, strongyloidiasis has a patchy, widespread distribution through warm, wet tropical and subtropical areas and is

often seen in regions or in institutions where sanitary facilities are poor or in moist conditions such as mines or tunnels under construction in temperate climates. Some have conservatively estimated that 50 to 100 million people are infected. *Strongyloides* infections are endemic in tropical Asia, Africa, and Latin America as well as in the southern United States, and southern and eastern Europe, including Hungary, Romania, Poland, and southern areas of the Soviet Union, with a recently reported autochthonous case from Nottingham, England. Prevalence rates of 3 to 21% are reported for Nigeria and of 2.5% in eastern Kentucky. Immigrants, travelers, or veterans from endemic areas such as southern Asia may have prolonged infections. The latter are primarily older males, veterans with prior histories of having lived in endemic tropical areas, and those with underlying malignant, metabolic, pulmonary, or renal disease who may be chronically infected and have mild to moderate, relapsing symptoms. A prospective study in rural Tennessee revealed *S. stercoralis* in 6.1% of 229 hospitalized patients and 2.6% of 346 domiciliary patients at the Johnson City Veterans Administration Hospital, one third of whom had never traveled abroad. Although *S. stercoralis* and other species may be found in dogs, cats, or monkeys (with apparent geographic preferences such as for dogs or cats with human *S. stercoralis* from Indochina or Calcutta, respectively), humans are the principal reservoir for *S. stercoralis*. Because infection can be maintained for 40 years or

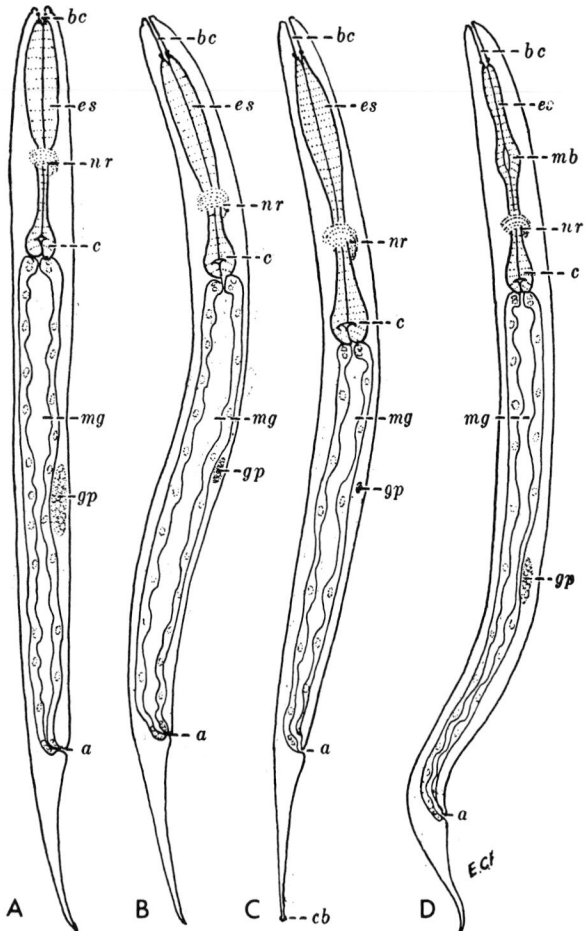

FIGURE 84–5. Figures of typical rhabditiform larval stages of: *A, Strongyloides; B,* hookworm; *C. Trichostrongylus;* and *D, Rhabditis* (ca. × 400). Explanation of labels: *a,* anus; *bc,* buccal chamber; *c,* cardiac bulb of esophagus; *cb,* beadlike swelling of caudal tip; *es,* esophagus; *gp,* genital primordia; *mb,* midesophageal bulb; *mg,* midgut; *nr,* nerve ring. (Drawing by E.C. Faust. From Beaver PC. Jung RC, Cupp EW: Clinical Parasitology, 9th ed. Philadelphia, Lea & Febiger, 1984.)

more, and because effective therapy (thiabendazole) has only been available since 1967, many persons, such as military personnel who were in the South Pacific in World War II, the Korean War, or the Vietnam War, may remain infected and at risk for episodic symptoms of chronic infection or overwhelming hyperinfection if they become immunosuppressed.

Transmission. The free-living cycle of *S. stercoralis* in the environment ensures the maintenance of the parasite in the appropriate conditions of moisture and temperature, even if the suitable mammalian host is not immediately available. Although transmission by direct contact may occur in institutions, transmission usually occurs via skin contact with the filariform larvae in moist soil. A *Strongyloides* sp. has also been reported in human breast milk in Africa; however, the importance of transmammary passage in the epidemiology of strongyloidiasis remains unclear.

There are no ideal experimental animal models of *S. stercoralis* infection. Besides highly variable infections (including autoinfection cycles) with *S. stercoralis* in dogs, animal models have been limited to the suboptimal *S. ratti* infection in rats that usually do not exhibit autoinfection.

PATHOGENESIS AND PATHOLOGY. Although the specific host and parasite factors that are responsible in the pathogenesis of strongyloidiasis are poorly understood, the capacity of *S. stercoralis* to persist despite normal host defenses characterizes the delicate balance of chronic infection. Intact cellular immunity appears to keep the tissue migration, as well as the development of the parasite in the intestine, under control with only intermittent symptoms. Any illness that results in loss of cellular immunity or corticosteroid therapy may lead to uncontrolled parasite multiplication and dissemination in the patient and the "hyperinfection" syndrome. The role of prior infection and the development of protective immunity remain unclear.

Migration Phase. The characteristic pruritic urticarial skin eruption and occasional eosinophilic pulmonary infiltrates or wheezing (Löffler's syndrome) appear to be related to immediate hypersensitivity reactions to the migrating larvae. In the lungs one can see alveolar hemorrhage and cellular reaction, and peripheral eosinophilia and increased IgE levels are often noticed.

Intestinal Phase. In the intestine, adult female worms, eggs, and larvae are found in the superficial submucosa and in the mucosal crypts, causing mechanical trauma, mucous discharge, and microscopic ulceration, but usually minimal inflammation. Increased epithelial cell turnover from the small bowel has been described in heavy infection and may cause malnutrition and hypoproteinemia. Occasionally, granulomas may form. Progressive involvement may lead to edema, flattened villi, malabsorption, and even ulceration, enteritis, and secondary bacterial invasion. Rarely, larvae are seen in the biliary or pancreatic ducts, liver, urine, or inflammatory exudates. Particularly in the hyperinfection syndrome, both direct filariform larval damage, as well as secondary polymicrobial infection, may be seen in virtually any organ. The usual sites of larval reinvasion are the ileum, appendix, and colon, where a granulomatous colitis may be seen along with steatorrhea, hypocalcemia, and hypoproteinemia. Although the pathophysiology of intestinal functional alteration remains poorly understood, decreased maltase and alkaline phosphatase levels have been seen with *Nippostrongylus brasiliensis* infections in a rat model.

CLINICAL MANIFESTATIONS. The clinical manifestations of *S. stercoralis* infection are acute infection, chronic persisting infection, and the disseminated hyperinfection syndrome in immunosuppressed hosts. The latter 2 syndromes are the best characterized.

Acute Infection. Clinical manifestations of acute strongyloidiasis reflect the intensity of the infection and are likely related to the 3 stages of infection, with: (1) skin penetration by filariform larvae, (2) pulmonary migration of larvae, and (3) intestinal penetration by adult worms. Although an estimated one third of individuals may remain asymptomatic, an initial pruritic, maculopapular rash or rapidly migrating linear urticaria called larva currens, which may move 10 cm/day, is well described at the site of skin penetration by the infectious filariform larvae. Larva currens is usually seen on the buttocks area with external autoinfection. Although infrequent, cough, shortness of breath, wheezing, fever, transient pulmonary infiltrates, and eosinophilia (Löffler's syndrome) may be seen with the migration of larvae through the lungs. Finally, when adult worms develop and penetrate the mucosa in the small bowel, nonspecific aching or epigastric abdominal pain and diarrhea may develop. With heavy infections in the upper small bowel, vomiting, malabsorption (of iron and other nutrients), steatorrhea, weight loss, edema, or even small bowel obstruction may occur. Obstruction may be due to paralytic ileus with edema in the small bowel wall.

Chronic, Persisting Infection. Best described in veterans or in former prisoners of war who have returned from endemic, tropical areas in Asia or in the South Pacific following World War I, World War II, or the Vietnam War, a syndrome of chronic strongyloidiasis with intermittent cutaneous and enteric symptoms extending for 40 years or more has been documented. Rates of infection determined by careful laboratory examinations of fecal specimens among former British, Australian, and American prisoners of war who had worked on the Burma-Thailand railroad during World War II were found 30 to 40 years later to be 21 to 37%. Although one third of documented infections were asymptomatic, two thirds of the patients had recurring episodic symptoms referable to the involved skin, lungs, or intestinal tract. The classically recognized triad of symptoms is urticaria, abdominal pain, and diarrhea. By far the most common was episodic, rapidly moving, creeping urticarial skin eruptions, most often on the buttocks or perianal area (at irregular intervals lasting 1 to 2 days), in 85 to 100% of symptomatic, infected individuals. Second in frequency were abdominal symptoms, led by intermittent epigastric pain, indigestion, or heartburn (65 to 67%), and watery diarrhea or cramping abdominal pain (42 to 67%). These symptoms were significantly reduced after treatment with thiabendazole, 25 mg/kg twice daily for 2 days, a course that was repeated once after 1 week. Symptoms of shortness of breath, wheezing, chest pain, and cough (35 to 52%) suggested pulmonary involvement, and eosinophilia and elevated serum IgE concentrations were common, but not universal. Immune complexes may rarely be associated with a reactive arthritis.

Further studies of chronic endemic infections in the United States have come from southeastern Kentucky, where infection with S. stercoralis is the most commonly diagnosed parasitic infection (in 2.5% of fecal specimens examined) at the University of Kentucky Medical Center. These endemic cases most commonly involved white male adults older than 50 years of age from lower socioeconomic backgrounds who often had a chronic or debilitating illness. The characteristic syndrome was one of mild to moderate chronic relapsing diarrhea, nausea, vomiting, and abdominal pain and tenderness, often with eosinophilia (in the range of 7 to 82% eosinophils) (in 85% of cases) and occasional hypoalbuminemia (in 20% of cases). In the prospective rural Tennessee study, Strongyloides infection was associated with abdominal bloating, eosinophilia, and guaiac-positive stools, as well

as with taking steroids, cimetidine, or antacid medications. S. stercoralis was also found in 3% of schoolchildren in a prospective survey conducted in Clay County, Kentucky, an area where 24% of children harbored intestinal parasites (Ascaris 14%; Trichuris 13%; Giardia 3%).

Hyperinfection Syndrome. When the critical host-parasite balance is upset in an individual chronically infected with Strongyloides by any drug or illness that compromises the host's immune status, a severe, life-threatening hyperinfection syndrome may result. Widely recognized since 1966, 103 reported cases of disseminated strongyloidiasis were recently reviewed, of which 89 were patients immunocompromised by recognized malignancies (especially lymphoma or leukemia) and/or corticosteroid therapy (for asthma, malignancy, lymphoma, leukemia, systemic lupus erythematosus, renal transplantation, ulcerative colitis, etc.). Severe strongyloidiasis has also been reported in at least 30 cases following renal transplantation as well as with cimetidine therapy. In a review of autopsies from Zaire and Washington, DC, in addition to the association with hematologic malignancies and corticosteroid therapy, several cases of disseminated strongyloidiasis were described in persons with protein-calorie malnutrition, lepromatous leprosy, and other severe infections such as tuberculosis and syphilis. It is apparent that loss of intact cellular immunity is associated with conversion of rhabditiform larvae to filariform larvae followed by uncontrolled, widespread dissemination of the filariform larvae via the blood stream to involve virtually any organ. Most often, extraintestinal infections involve the lung, with associated bronchospasm, focal or diffuse infiltrates, and even cavitation. In addition, abdominal lymph nodes, liver, spleen, pancreas, thyroid, endocardium, kidney, brain, and meninges may be involved. Intestinal symptoms with hyperinfection include profound diarrhea, malabsorption, and electrolyte abnormalities. Remarkably absent are cellular immune responses to migrating larvae. Thymic T-lymphocyte depletion and loss of the eosinophilia typify disseminated hyperinfection in immunocompromised hosts. Of special concern is the 86% mortality associated with the hyperinfection syndrome, often with bacterial infection secondary to extensive larval spread from the intestine. Sepsis, meningitis, peritonitis, or endocarditis was documented in 45% of cases studied. It is somewhat surprising that, despite the severity of cryptosporidial and Isospora infections in patients with the acquired immunodeficiency syndrome (AIDS), extraintestinal strongyloidiasis has not yet been associated with AIDS in areas of Africa highly endemic for S. stercoralis (Chapter 15.1).

DIAGNOSIS. As suggested throughout the previous discussion, the important aspects of diagnosing Strongyloides infections include a high index of clinical suspicion in patients with histories of exposure and characteristic skin and intestinal symptoms. Second, an experienced person may have to search extremely diligently (some report for up to 5 hours) in fecal specimens, even with formalin-ether concentration, to find the characteristic rhabditiform larvae (Fig. VI A–2[10]). It is important to recognize that Strongyloides larvae do not typically float in hypertonic saline solutions, which are often used to concentrate other parasites. Several authors have described the distinct advantages, particularly in endemic areas, of the Baermann funnel gauze method of concentrating *Strongyloides* larvae in fecal specimens, using warm water and larval sedimentation in the neck of the funnel (Chapter 122). Substantially improved yields of greater than fourfold have been described over other traditional methods, and some investigators have reported that this technique is superior even to duodenal aspiration. Our personal experience confirms the superiority of a Baermann funnel gauze method over simple, direct examinations and formalin-ether concentrations. Others have described a simple string capsule method (Enterotest) for obtaining duodenal fluid (Chapter 122).

Although previous serologic tests were complicated by lack of sensitivity and specificity, an improved immunofluorescence antibody assay using *Strongyloides* antigen has been described and may be helpful, but it is not yet widely available (Chapter 125). Neither total IgE nor *Strongyloides*-specific IgE or IgG levels are correlated with the severity of clinical disease during strongyloidiasis.

Great diagnostic problems may arise in persons who have traveled to endemic areas (even many years before) and then become immunocompromised by an underlying disease or are given corticosteroids for any reason. A careful search for larvae is required in stool or small bowel aspirates. Rarely, filariform larvae may be seen in the sputum, spinal fluid, or urine. In immunosuppressed patients, the clue of peripheral eosinophilia is lost, and indeed, less than 7% eosinophils was noted in three fourths of the 58 patients reviewed by Igra-Siegman and coworkers; these 43 patients had an 84% mortality (in contrast to the 27% mortality if greater than 8% eosinophils were present).

TREATMENT. Because of the potential for chronic symptomatic infection, autoinfection over many years, and the hyperinfection syndrome, all individuals who are infected with *S. stercoralis* should be treated. The safest and most effective form of treatment is thiabendazole, 25 mg/kg orally twice daily for 2 or 3 days. Because of the difficulty in confirming eradication of the infection, many experts prefer to repeat a 2-day course of therapy 1 week after the initial course, with careful follow-up for persisting symptoms or infection. Fifteen percent of patients relapsed after therapy in a prospective rural Tennessee study. Immunocompromised patients suspected of having a life-threatening, hyperinfection syndrome warrant this daily dosage for a longer period, probably 5 to 14 days. Because a parenteral preparation of thiabendazole is not available, intermittent administration via a nasogastric tube may be required in patients with intestinal obstruction. Schumaker and coworkers have described the administration of thiabendazole in patients undergoing hemodialysis.

Toxicity of thiabendazole, even in lower dosages, includes nausea, vomiting, malaise, dizziness, and smelly urine (VI A, General Principles). Although other related drugs, such as mebendazole and cambendazole, have been studied experimentally (cambendazole appears more effective in murine strongyloidiasis), they are not recommended for use in treating patients with strongyloidiasis at this time.

PREVENTION. As with most other enteric infections, critical to the prevention of strongyloidiasis is an improved standard of living, with particular reference to personal hygiene and improved sanitary and waste disposal facilities. Where sewage facilities are not available or where night soil is used for fertilization, adequate composting with vegetable refuse may provide high enough temperatures to kill the larvae.

Regarding the prevention of the hyperinfection syndrome, most important is an adequate awareness of the symptoms of chronic *Strongyloides* infection so that it can be treated with thiabendazole. This is particularly important in any immunocompromised patient or person given corticosteroids, especially when there is a history of exposure to an endemic area.

***STRONGYLOIDES FULLEBORNI* INFECTION.** Throughout several areas of equatorial Africa, widespread infection with *S. fulleborni* has been described in several species of "Old World" monkeys and other primates. Similar to *S. stercoralis* in morphology and life cycle, *S. fulleborni* may also cause cutaneous, pulmonary, and intestinal symptoms, as well as eosinophilia in humans in central and eastern Africa, in Zambia, and along the Fly River in the Kuringa region of Papua New Guinea, where nonhuman primates have not been found to be infected as in Africa. Although *S. fulleborni* has been associated with abdominal distention, respiratory distress, generalized edema, and a fatal outcome in infants, the capacity of *S. fulleborni* to cause prolonged autoinfection or the hyperinfection syndrome is not established. Also in contrast to *S. stercoralis*, *S. fulleborni* is diagnosed by finding characteristic 55×35 μm thin-shelled ovoid, embryonated eggs, rather than rhabditiform larvae, in the stool.

BIBLIOGRAPHY

Ashford RW, Barnish G: Strongyloidiasis in Papua New Guinea. Clin Trop Med Comm Dis 2:765, 1987.

Badaro R, Carvalho EM, Santos RB, et al: Parasite-specific humoral responses in different clinical forms of strongyloidiasis. Trans R Soc Trop Med Hyg 81:149, 1987.

Bartholomew C, Butler AK, Bhaskar AG, Jankey N: Pseudo-obstruction, and a sprue-like syndrome from strongyloidiasis. Postgrad Med J 53:139, 1977.

Beal CB, Viens P, Grant RGL, Hughes JM: A new technique for sampling duodenal contents: Demonstration of upper small-bowel pathogens. Am J Trop Med Hyg 19:349, 1970.

Berk SL, Verghese A, Alvarez S, et al: Clinical and epidemiologic features of strongyloidiasis: A prospective study in rural Tennessee. Arch Intern Med 147:1257, 1987.

Berry AJ, Long EG, Smith JH, et al: Chronic relapsing colitis due to *Strongyloides stercoralis*. Am J Trop Med Hyg 32:1289, 1983.

Brown RC, Girardeau MHF: Transmammary passage of *Strongyloides* sp. larvae in the human host. Am J Trop Med Hyg 26:215, 1977.

Cadranel JF, Eugene C: Another example of *Strongyloides stercoralis* infection associated with cimetidine in an immunosuppressed patient. Gut 27:1229, 1986.

Carvalho EM, Andrade TM, Andrade JA, Rocha H: Immunological features in different clinical forms of strongyloidiasis. Trans R Soc Trop Med Hyg 77:346, 1983.

Cruz T, Reboucas G, Rocha H: Fatal strongyloidiasis in patients receiving corticosteroids. N Engl J Med 275:1093, 1966.

Da Costa LR: Small-intestinal cell turnover in patients with parasitic infections. Br Med J 3:281, 1971.

Faust EC, De Groat A: Internal autoinfection in human strongyloidiasis. Am J Trop Med 20:359, 1940.

Genta RM: Strongyloidiasis. Clin Trop Med Comm Dis 2:645, 1987.

Gill GV, Bell DR: *Strongyloides stercoralis* infection in former Far East prisoners of war. Br Med J 2:572, 1979.

Grove DI: Strongyloidiasis in Allied ex-prisoners of war in Southeast Asia. Br Med J 280:598, 1980.

Grove DI: Treatment of strongyloidiasis with thiabendazole: An analysis of toxicity and effectiveness. Trans R Soc Trop Med Hyg 76:114, 1982.

Grove DI, Blair AJ: Diagnosis of human strongyloidiasis by immunofluorescence using *Strongyloides ratti* and *S. stercoralis* larvae. Am J Trop Hyg 30:344, 1981.

Hira PR, Patel BG: Human strongyloidiasis due to the primate species *Strongyloides fulleborni*. Trop Geogr Med 32:23, 1980.

Igra-Siegman Y, Kapila R, Sen P, et al: Syndrome of hyperinfection with *Strongyloides stercoralis*. Rev Infect Dis 3:397, 1981.

Lima JP, Delgado PG: Diagnosis of strongyloidiasis: Importance of Baermann's method. Am J Dig Dis 6:899, 1961.

Milder JE, Walzer PD, Kilgore G, et al: Clinical features of *Strongyloides stercoralis* infection in an endemic area of the United States. Gastroenterology 80:1481, 1981.

Milner PF, Irvine RA, Barton CJ, et al: Intestinal malabsorption in *Strongyloides stercoralis* infestation. Gut 6:574, 1965.

Morgan JS, Schaffner W, Stone WJ: Opportunistic strongyloidiasis in renal transplant recipients. Transplantation 42:518, 1986.

Pampiglione S, Ricciardi ML: Experimental infection with human strain *Strongyloides fülleborni* in man. Lancet 1:663, 1972.

Pelletier LL Jr: Chronic strongyloidiasis in World War II Far East ex-prisoners of war. Am J Trop Med Hyg 33:55, 1984.

Pelletier LL Jr, Gabre-Kidan T: Chronic strongyloidiasis in Vietnam veterans. Am J Med 78:139, 1985.

Petithory JC, Derouin F: AIDS and strongyloidiasis in Africa. Lancet 1:921, 1987.

Purtilo DT, Meyers WM, Connor DH: Fatal strongyloidiasis in immunosuppressed patients. Am J Med 56:488, 1974.

Sampson IA, Grove DI: Strongyloidiasis is endemic in another Australian population group: Indochinese immigrants. Med J Aust 146:580, 1987.

Schumaker JD, Band JD, Lensmeyer GL, et al: Thiabendazole treatment of severe strongyloidiasis in a hemodialyzed patient. Ann Intern Med 89:644, 1978.

Scowden EB, Schaffner W, Stone WJ: Overwhelming strongyloidiasis: An unappreciated opportunistic infection. Medicine 57:527, 1978.

Smith JD, Goette DK, Odom RB: Larva currens: Cutaneous strongyloidiasis. Arch Dermatol 112:1161, 1976.

Sprott V, Selby CD, Ispahani P, Toghill PJ: Indigenous strongyloidiasis in Nottingham. Br Med J 294:741, 1987.

Stemmermann GN: Strongyloidiasis in migrants: Pathological and clinical considerations. Gastroenterology 53:59, 1967.

Vince JD, Ashford RW, Gratten MJ, et al: *Strongyloides* species infestation in young infants at Papua New Guinea: Association with generalized oedema. Papua New Guinea Med J 22:120, 1979.

Walzer PD, Milder JE, Banwell JG, et al: Epidemiologic features of *Strongyloides stercoralis* infection in an endemic area of the United States. Am J Trop Med Hyg 31:313, 1982.

Willis AJP, Nwokolo C: Steroid therapy and strongyloidiasis. Lancet 1:1396, 1966.

■

SECTION B

FILARIAL INFECTIONS

GENERAL PRINCIPLES

Alfred A. Buck

BIOLOGY. The filarial parasites are long threadlike tissue-dwelling round worms that live for many years, continuously producing enormous numbers of microfilariae. The microfilariae are immature larvae that are found in either the blood or the skin and are the infective stages for the insect host. The filarial parasites infecting humans are not uniform species; each species has developed local forms that are adapted by means of the remarkable phenomenon of periodicity, i.e., the spatial distribution of microfilariae in the skin for transmission by particular vectors. For example, throughout most of its distribution *Wuchereria bancrofti* produces microfilariae with a distinct nocturnal periodicity and peak appearance in the blood at night as an adaptation to night-biting culicine and anopheline mosquitoes. However, in the Eastern Pacific Islands, where these night-biting mosquitoes are absent, the parasite has developed a diurnal periodicity as an adaptation to day-biting *Aedes* mosquitoes. In the same way, the skin-dwelling microfilariae of *Onchocerca volvulus* in Africa adapt for transmission by low-biting *Simulium damnosum*, i.e., the highest concentrations of microfilariae are in the lower part of the body. In Guatemala the maximum concentrations of parasites are in the skin of the upper part of the body, as an adaptation to transmission by the high-biting *Simulium ochraceum*. These variations in the behavior of the filarial parasites are also reflected in differences in other epidemiologic features; marked differences in the pathogenicity of the same species may occur in different regions of the same country. For example, the strain of *O. volvulus* that is transmitted by savanna simuliids is much more likely to be associated with severe eye lesions in humans and experimental animals than is the *O. volvulus* transmitted by rain forest simuliids. These differences in parasite-vector relationships in different areas indicate the need for detailed local studies of epidemiology before control measures can be introduced.

LIFE CYCLES. All the human filarial parasites have the same basic life cycle, with 5 larval stages of development: 3 in an intermediate insect host and 2 in humans. Each stage is represented by growth and then shedding of the nematode cuticle to allow further growth of the parasite, in much the same way as a growing snake periodically sheds its skin (Fig. VI B–1). Following copulation and fertilization, the female produces as many as 50,000 microfilariae per day. In some cases the egg membrane is retained around the microfilariae; this constitutes the sheath, which is a useful characteristic for distinguishing the different species. When the microfilariae are ingested by a susceptible insect host, they rapidly penetrate the wall of the midgut and migrate through the insect's tissues until they find an appropriate and specific type of "nurse" cell, where they undergo development. For example, *W. bancrofti* will develop

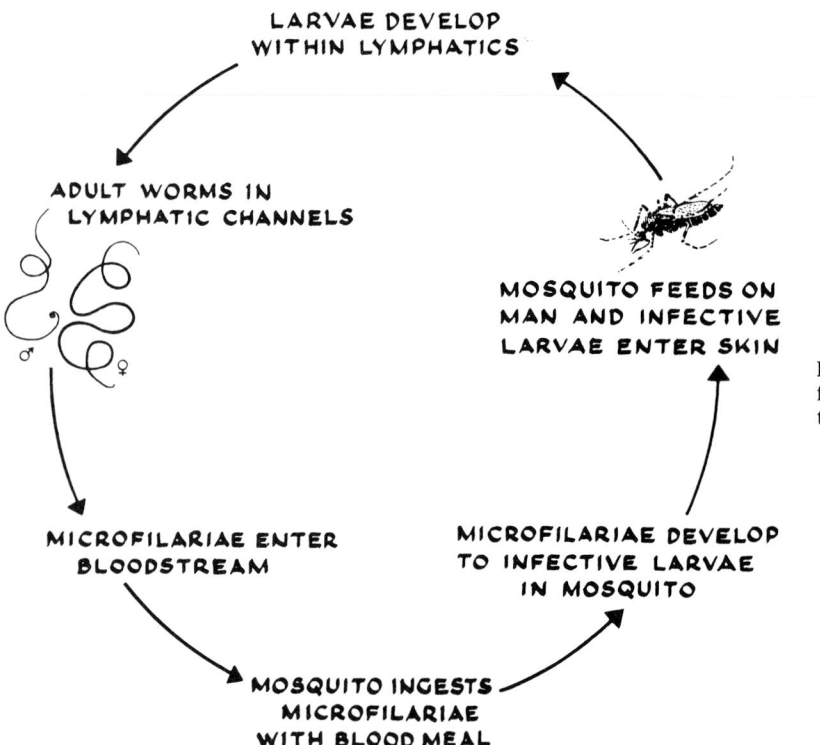

FIGURE VI B–1. Life cycle of lymphatic-dwelling filariae of humans. In addition to the elements illustrated, subperiodic *Brugia malayi* has a zoonotic cycle.

only in the flight muscle of genetically susceptible mosquitoes. Here, during a period of 12 days, the delicate microfilariae, which are 250 μm long, will be transformed into robust third-stage infective larvae 1500 μm long. The mosquito is now infective, and when it bites a human, the larvae will penetrate the skin at the site of the bite and then rapidly enter the nearest lymphatic vessel, where during the next few months they will undergo 2 further molts before reaching the adult stage. There is no multiplication of the filarial worms in humans, so that the worm load and the severity of the disease are proportional to the number of infective larvae acquired. This usually occurs over a long period, so the chronic and dreaded complications of elephantiasis in lymphatic filariasis and blindness in onchocerciasis are seen only in long-term residents in endemic areas.

SPECIES INFECTING HUMANS

Human Pathogens. Of the 8 species of filarial worms that develop normally in humans, only 6 are generally recognized as pathogens: those that live in the lymphatics, i.e., *W. bancrofti*, *Brugia malayi*, and *Brugia timori*, which produce elephantiasis and numerous lymphopathic complications; *Loa loa*, which causes Calabar swelling and other allergic manifestations; *O. volvulus*, the blinding filaria, which is also responsible for a disfiguring dermatitis; and *Mansonella streptocerca*, which causes skin lesions but not blindness. The other 2 parasites are *Mansonella perstans* and *Mansonella ozzardi*. Humans have developed a remarkable tolerance to these 2 parasites. In some areas, individuals have a high prevalence of these worms, often with millions of microfilariae, in their blood but have no symptoms.

Animal Reservoirs. In most areas the filarial parasites affecting humans are maintained by interhuman transmission, but 1 strain of *B. malayi* has a reservoir of infection in leaf-eating monkeys, and in parts of Malaysia the disease is a definite zoonosis. Under these circumstances reinfection is likely, even in areas where there are well-organized mass chemotherapy campaigns. A subspecies of *L. loa* is found in monkeys, and *M. perstans* and *M. streptocerca* have been reported from chimpanzees. *O. volvulus* has also been recorded from the gorilla, but it is unlikely that the animal reservoirs are of significance in the epidemiology of these infections.

Animal Pathogens Infecting Humans. There are hundreds of other species of filarial worms in wild and domestic animals, and if the vectors of these parasites bite humans, they can produce aberrant infections together with immunologic reactions that might affect the interpretation of serologic tests. One of the most prevalent filarial infections in animals is *Dirofilaria immitis*, the heartworm of the dog. This parasite is transmitted by mosquitoes that frequently bite humans, and cases of pulmonary nodules have been caused by the worm.

INCIDENCE AND DISTRIBUTION.
Although Manson first observed the development of filarial worms in mosquitoes as long ago as 1877, filariasis remains a major public health problem. More than 300 million people, mostly in India and Southeast Asia, are constantly exposed to lymphatic filariasis, and at least 30 million people live in areas where onchocerciasis is endemic. Bancroftian filariasis is increasing, mainly because of the resistance of the insect vectors to insecticides but also, paradoxically, because of the increase in mosquito breeding sites as a result of the provision of new water supplies in urban and rural areas. Together with the uncontrolled, large-scale population move-

ments from rural areas to the fringes of large cities, these developments have created conditions favorable to the transmission of *W. bancrofti* by mosquitoes of the genus *Culex*, which breeds in highly polluted water. Urban filariasis has become a new and difficult public health problem in many countries of Southeast Asia and Africa.

Following the discovery of diethylcarbamazine, it was hoped that mass chemotherapy might replace vector control. There has been some success with chemotherapeutic control in a few countries in Southeast Asia and the Pacific where *Wuchereria* and *Brugia* are endemic, but it has proved too difficult to apply on a mass scale in the major endemic areas of India and Africa. Because of the serious side reactions associated with treatment with diethylcarbamazine, the drug could not be used for mass treatment of onchocerciasis. In 1984, ivermectin, a new drug registered for animal health, was found to be highly effective against microfilariae of *O. volvulus*. Since then, large scale clinical trials have confirmed its safety and efficacy as a microfilaricide for single-dose treatment of onchocerciasis in endemic areas of Africa and Latin America. Ivermectin has become available to clinical investigators under the trade name of Mectizan. The drug is also effective against the microfilariae of *W. bancrofti*, *B. malayi*, and *L. loa*, but not against those of *M. perstans*. So far, the control of onchocerciasis has depended on the logistically difficult and expensive method of dosing rivers with insecticides to kill the larvae of *Simulium* vectors. The introduction of ivermectin for mass treatment in the onchocerciasis control programs in 11 West African countries has shown that a single dose of this powerful microfilaricide is well tolerated and that mass administration of this drug offers a new tool for disease control of endemic filariasis.

BIBLIOGRAPHY

Hawking F: Diethylcarbamazine and new compounds for the treatment of filariasis. Adv Pharmacol Chemother 16:129, 1979.
Nelson GS: The pathology of filarial infections. Helminth Abst 35:(Part 4), 311, 1966.
Sasa M: Human Filariasis. A Global Survey of Epidemiology and Control. Baltimore, University Park Press, 1976.
WHO Expert Committee on Filariasis: Lymphatic Filariasis. Fourth Report. WHO Tech Rep Ser 702, 1984.

85. FILARIASIS

Alfred A. Buck

85.1. BANCROFTIAN FILARIASIS

DEFINITION. Bancroftian filariasis is caused by the mosquito-borne nematode *Wuchereria bancrofti*. The adult worms, males and females, live in lymphatic vessels and nodes of humans, whereas the embryos, or microfilariae, are found mostly in the blood, where they reach peak densities at night. The infection may be clinically inapparent or manifest by a wide range of symptoms, of which most are due to inflammation and destruction of lymphatics. Humans are the only natural host for *W. bancrofti*. The lack of an experimental laboratory animal has hampered biomedical research of bancroftian filariasis, especially studies of the immunologic, biochemical, and genetic determinants of its pathogenesis.

HISTORY. Elephantiasis, surely one of the most bizarre of tropical diseases, was described in early Indian and Persian writings and drew the attention of medical observers in Africa and the South Pacific in the seventeenth and eighteenth centuries. It was common among Africans and their descendants in the West Indies colonies, where the term "Barbados foot" arose. The worldwide distribution of elephantiasis in tropical and subtropical areas and the epidemiologic association of elephantiasis with hydrocele, chylocele, and chyluria were established by the middle of the nineteenth century. Their common etiology, however, remained a mystery until discoveries were made of microfilariae in hydrocele fluid (Demarquay, 1863), chylous urine (Wucherer, 1868), and blood (Lewis, 1872) and of the adult worm in a lymphatic abscess (Bancroft, 1877). Manson's great contribution in Amoy, China, between 1875 and 1879, was his recognition of (1) the association of endemic microfilaremia with elephantiasis and other obstructive manifestations, (2) the uptake of microfilariae by *Culex* mosquitoes, promoted by the swarming of the parasites in the blood during the peak mosquito-feeding period around midnight, and (3) the critical role of the mosquito in "nursing" the parasite during its development to an infective form.

Despite the early advances, filariasis has remained one of the least understood of the major parasitic diseases. The need to develop new, effective methods of disease control through biomedical research has been recognized by the inclusion of filariasis as 1 of the 6 target diseases of the Special Program for Research and Training in Tropical Diseases (TDR) of the World Health Organization, the United Nations Development Fund, and the World Bank.

ETIOLOGY

Morphology. *W. bancrofti* (Cobbold, 1877; Seurat, 1921) reaches sexual maturity in lymphatic vessels and nodes of humans. The adults are white, threadlike worms that are usually much convoluted in situ. The female, which is about twice the size of the male, measures between 80 and 100 mm in length and 0.2 to 0.3 mm in width. Thousands of developing embryos may be found within the gravid paired uteri of the female, enclosed within translucent hyaline membranes that elongate to become the sheaths of the released microfilariae. Diagnosis is established by examining microfilariae in stained blood films. When treated in the standard manner with Giemsa's or Field's stain, the microfilaria has a body length of 250 to 300 μm and a width of 7 to 9 μm and is covered loosely by a translucent or pinkish-staining sheath. It usually assumes a gracefully curved position and has a short cephalic space followed by a column of discrete, loosely spaced, and dark-staining nuclei that do not reach the tip of the tail (Fig. 85–1). Differential characteristics are listed in Table 85–1.

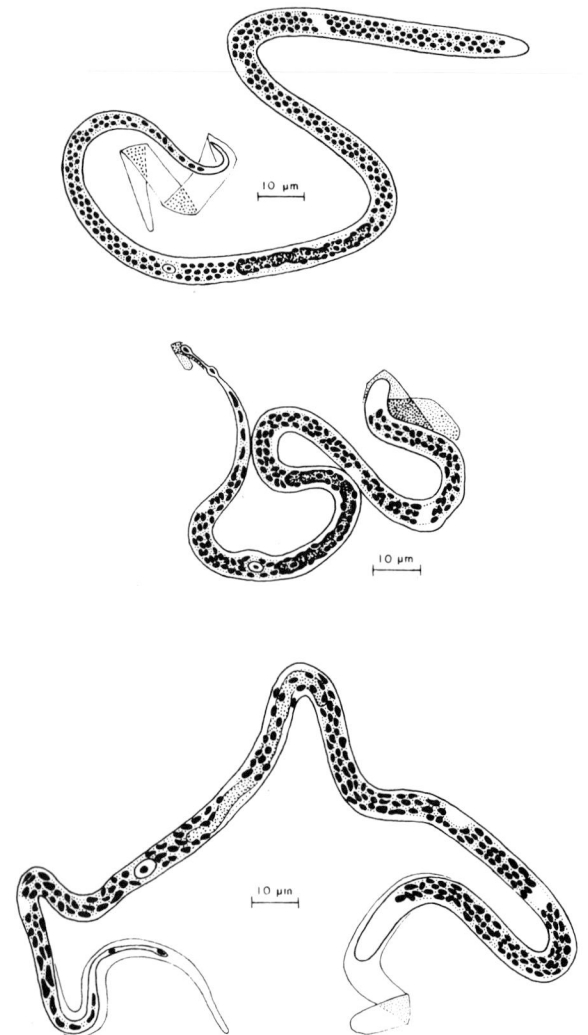

FIGURE 85–1. Microfilariae of (from top to bottom) *Wuchereria bancrofti,* *Brugia malayi,* and *Brugia timori,* as seen in Giemsa-stained blood films.

Development and Life Cycle (Fig. VI B–1). The infective (third-stage) larvae escape from the proboscis sheath (labella) of the mosquito at the time of feeding and penetrate the skin at the puncture wound. They then migrate within lymphatics to a suitable site within or adjacent to a lymph node, whereupon they grow to maturity and mate. Microfilariae first appear in the peripheral blood 6 months to 1 year later, and even in the absence of reinfection, microfilaremia may persist over a 5- to 10-year period. In completing the life cycle, microfilariae are taken up in the blood meal of mosquitoes, and within hours of arrival in the midgut of an appropriate host, these microfilariae cast their sheaths, penetrate the wall of the gut, and find their way to the muscles of the thorax. In the thorax, over a period of 10 to 14 days, the filariae pass through 2 ecdyses and develop into infective (third-stage) larvae.

EPIDEMIOLOGY

Distribution (Fig. 85–2). *W. bancrofti* is the most widespread of the filariae infecting humans and is focally distributed throughout much of the tropics and subtropics between latitudes 40 degrees north and 30 degrees

south. It has been estimated that 250 million persons are affected, mostly in South Asia and tropical sub-Saharan Africa. In Asia, the parasite is endemic in both urban and rural areas in the Indian subcontinent, the island of Sri Lanka, and Burma; in scattered rural foci in Thailand and Indochina; extensively in the south and the eastern alluvial plains of China; among aboriginal and proto-Malay peoples in the hill forests of the Malayan peninsula and northern Borneo; and in varied forest and agricultural ecotypes in the Philippine Islands. *W. bancrofti* has been nearly eliminated from Taiwan and from southern Japan. In Indonesia the parasite is focally endemic in low prevalence in low-lying hill forests of Sumatra, Kalimantan, and Sulawesi and more intensely along coastal fringes of small islands east of Lombok. The urban form is found in the northern Javanese cities of Jakarta and Semarang. In the South Pacific the parasite is highly endemic in low-lying areas of the island of New Guinea, and although considerable progress has been made in control, filariasis continues to be an important problem in many islands of Melanesia, Micronesia, and Polynesia. The parasite is diurnally subperiodic throughout Polynesia, New Caledonia, and the Loyalty Islands.

Infections with the nocturnally periodic, anopheline-borne rural strain of *W. bancrofti* are found in patchy distribution throughout a wide belt across tropical sub-Saharan Africa from 25 degrees north to 20 degrees south. The parasite in East Africa is adapted to *Culex* species, as well as anophelines, and occurs along the Indian Ocean coasts of Tanzania and Kenya, in Madagascar, and in other offshore islands, where transmission occurs in urban as well as rural areas. Bancroftian filariasis is endemic in many West African countries from Senegal to Zaire and in the southern Sudan and the low-lying western areas of Ethiopia. In Egypt, the parasite is mostly confined to the Nile Delta. In many of the old endemic foci in the Nile Delta the prevalence of *Culex*-transmitted filariasis has increased during the past decade. Moreover, the infection has now spread to urban areas. The scattered endemic foci reported previously along the north coast of Africa and the Mediterranean littoral of southern Europe have apparently disappeared. The infection is not found in the Middle East.

Bancroftian filariasis was introduced to the Western Hemisphere from Africa with the slave trade. It became endemic in most of the major islands of the Caribbean south of the Bahamas and on the eastern coastal plains of South America, especially those of the Guianas and of Brazil. Isolated foci of infection were reported in the past from the eastern coastal areas of Central America, Mexico, and, in the early part of the twentieth century, from Charleston, South Carolina. The disease has been greatly reduced in the Americas. Bancroftian filariasis is now a focal public health problem only in Haiti and the Dominican Republic, in the Guianas, and in some semiurban and urban areas of coastal Brazil.

Determining Factors. Differences in human, parasite, intermediate host (vector), and environmental factors are responsible for considerable variation in patterns of bancroftian filariasis from 1 locality to another. The

TABLE 85–1. Some Differential Characteristics of the Lymphatic-Dwelling Filariae of Humans

| Features | Wuchereria bancrofti | | Brugia malayi | | Brugia timori |
	Nocturnal	Diurnal	Periodic	Subperiodic	
Distribution	Asia, Africa, Americas, West Pacific	South Pacific beyond 165° E	South and East Asia	Southeast Asia	Southeast Indonesia
Ecotype	Urban, rural coastal fringes, tropical forests, open woodland, savanna, flood plains	Rural, coastal fringes, forest	Rural, open swamp and irrigated rice fields, hill forests	Rural, riverine, freshwater swamp forests	Rural, lowland riverine rice fields, coastal fringes
Vectors	Anophelines, *Culex* species, *Aedes* species	*Aedes* species	*Mansonia* species, anophelines, *Aedes togoi*	*Mansonia* species	*Anopheles barbirostris*
Microfilaria morphology (Giemsa stain)	Graceful; discrete nuclei that do not reach tip of tail; translucent sheath; total length: 275–325 μm	Same	Kinked; crowded nuclei with indistinct margins that reach tip of tail; dark-pink sheaths, many cast; total length: 225–275 μm	As for periodic, but less than 10% of sheaths cast, shorter innenkörper; total length: 200–250 μm	Sinuous; long cephalic space, and nuclei more distinct than *B. malayi;* sheath translucent and less than 50% cast; nuclei to tip of tail; total length: 290–325 μm
Reservoir hosts	Humans	Humans	Humans	Humans, monkeys, domestic cats, forest carnivores	Humans

prevalence of infection and the frequency and severity of signs and symptoms in communities are mostly related to the intensity of transmission. The dynamics of transmission within populations is based on the following major variables: (1) the rates and densities of microfilaremia in the human reservoir; (2) the potential of the vector population for acquiring, nurturing, and transmitting the parasite; and (3) the ability of the parasite to enter into a satisfactory relationship with the human host in order to mature, mate, and produce patent microfilaremia. All strains of *W. bancrofti* are thought to be maintained by interhuman transmission, and there is as yet no evidence of a natural animal reservoir. However, monkeys of the genus *Presbytis* can be infected in the laboratory, and they are the natural hosts of a closely related species, *W. kalamantani*, found in Indonesia.

The Vector. Foremost in determining the geographic distribution of bancroftian filariasis is the adaptability of the parasite to local vectors. Several dominant patterns of adaptation have emerged. The most primitive association is perhaps that found in tropical hill forest ecotypes of Southeast Asia, in which infection is transmitted by sylvatic anophelines of the *Anopheles umbrosus* group. The distribution is patchy, microfilaremia rates are usually low, and the disease in affected communities is described as mild. It may be hypothesized that the parasite next adapted to mosquito species breeding in alluvial valleys and plains, such as members of the *A. hyrcanus* group, and to coastal brackish-water

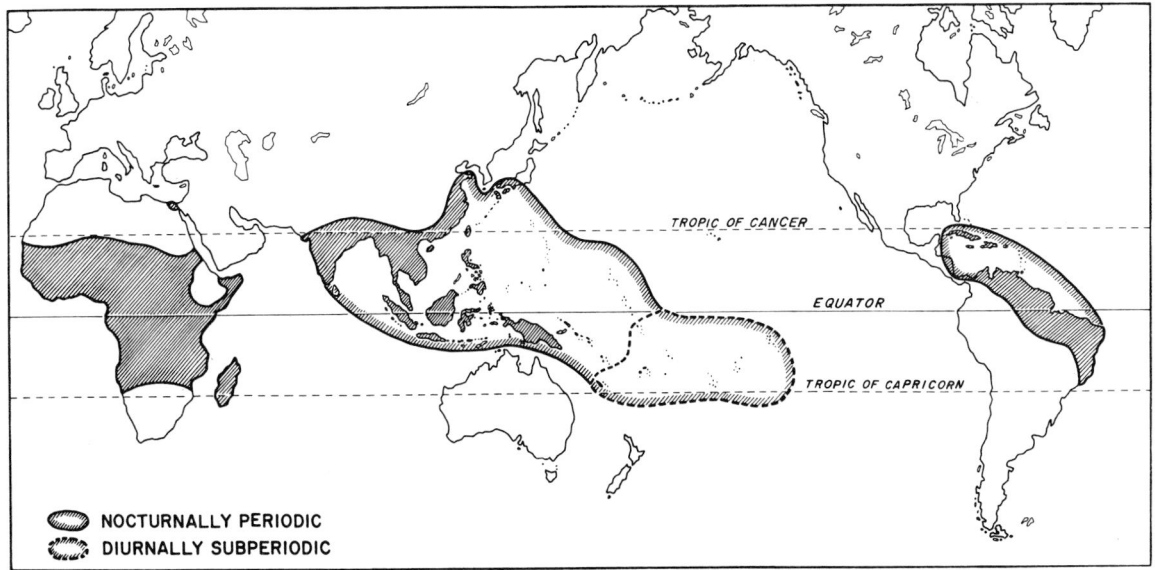

FIGURE 85–2. Worldwide distribution of *W. bancrofti*, with the interrupted line demarcating the limits of the diurnally subperiodic strain in the South Pacific region east of longitude 170° (Buxton's line).

breeders. From coastal Southeast Asia the parasite may have spread via trade and migration routes to India and the African coast to the west, to China, and to Japan and the South Pacific to the east by adjusting to local anopheline and culicine mosquitoes. Adaptation to the day-biting *Aedes* mosquitoes of the Pacific has depended on the evolution of a strain of *W. bancrofti* that has diurnal periodicity. Transmission by sewage-breeding *Culex* species allowed the establishment of infection within urban and semiurban populations.

The human-biting density and the proportion of feeds obtained from humans (human-biting index) are important measures in determining the vectorial capacity of a susceptible mosquito species. Other factors include the amount of blood ingested, the degree of concentration of parasites in the blood meal, the timing of feeding as related to the rhythms of circulating microfilariae within the human host, and the survivability of the vector and its efficiency in supporting development of the microfilariae to the infective stage and in delivering these larvae to humans. This is summarized in the annual transmission potential (ATP), the estimated number of infective larvae to which a person is exposed during 1 year.

The Parasite. A large number of parasite factors operate to ensure the maintenance and spread of infection within the human population. These include (1) the number of infective larvae gaining access to lymphatics and the proportion of those reaching fecundity, (2) the duration of patent infection, (3) the density of microfilariae in peripheral blood at times of vector feeding, and (4) the success with which microfilariae develop to infective larvae, taking into account rates of maturation and effects of the parasite on survivability of the vector. The quantitation of these variables is difficult, but some idea of the bionomics of transmission can be obtained from calculations made in Samoa, where the mean duration of patency of a single worm pair has been estimated to be 2 to 4 years, producing a theoretical maximum density of circulating microfilariae of 70/60 μl of peripheral blood. The mortality rate of mated females was calculated to be 0.02 to 0.05 per month, with an average load of fecund pairs in microfilaremic persons of about 7 pairs for men, 6 for women, and 3 for children.

Inefficiency of urban transmission is exemplified by studies in Rangoon indicating that some persons living there received about 83,000 *Culex* bites a year, 300 by infective mosquitoes. The proportion of parasites completing the phases of the cycle from third-stage larvae to microfilariae was so low that nearly 16,000 bites by infective mosquitoes resulted in 1 new patent infection in a person. Transmission in rural areas is considerably more efficient, and studies in Tanzania suggest that less than 200 infective bites a year per person maintain transmission at endemic levels.

Host Factors. Indicators of the level of endemicity in the human population are the microfilaremia rate, the density of microfilariae in peripheral blood, the immunopositivity rate, and the prevalence and severity of clinical manifestations. These indicators are not evenly distributed among the populace at risk but are selective for certain host attributes and variables. Infections may

be acquired at an early age, with recorded instances of patent microfilaremia occurring in children younger than 1 year of age. Usually, however, there is a low rate of microfilaremia in early childhood, a fairly rapid rise between the ages of 5 and 20 years, and a gradual increase or plateau thereafter. Overall microfilaremia rates in communities generally do not exceed 40%. When the exposure to bites of infective mosquitoes is more or less even throughout the population, age differences in microfilaremia rates perhaps reflect differences in cumulative infection and in the host's immune response. A slow periodic rise and fall of microfilarial density in individuals extends over a period of years. Thus, densities are not a useful indication of intensity of infection or severity of disease in an individual. Within a community, however, the collective microfilaremia rate and log median microfilarial density reflect the intensity of transmission and the disease impact.

Age is likewise important in determining clinical illness. In the usual endemic situation, the infection is fairly silent within the first decade, with recurrent episodes of adenolymphangitis and fever being the earliest manifestations, followed by the gradual appearance of genital lesions and lymphedema of extremities in some persons during the latter part of the second decade. These signs generally show a steady increase in frequency and severity thereafter, with a plateau or reduction after the fourth decade of life.

The role of gender, per se, is less well understood. Even in areas in which occupational and other behavioral factors do not apparently place men and women at differing levels of exposure, men often have higher rates of microfilaremia and of clinical signs. *W. bancrofti* tends to reside within lymphatics of the testis, epididymis, and spermatic cord, and hydrocele is a hallmark of infection in endemic communities.

Exposure. Occupation may be an important risk factor in infection, especially in rural areas. Well-known examples include work in abaca plantations in the Philippines and in coconut plantations in Polynesia, as breeding of the *Aedes* vectors occurs in axils of the abaca plant and within discarded coconut husks and tree holes. Filariasis primarily affects persons of the lowest socioeconomic level, owing to inadequate protection from mosquitoes and to unhygienic environmental conditions favorable to breeding of vectors. Ethnicity has not been shown to be a determining factor in infection and disease, although immigrant populations, newly exposed as adults, may show a more rapidly developing and severe disease than that of indigenous populations. Examples of translocated populations at high risk of infection include military groups, rural inhabitants moving to urban slums and urban fringe settlements and from mountainous to lowland areas, and settlers of new frontiers.

Immune Response. Recent studies of human immunologic responses to filarial infection have greatly increased the understanding of the host-parasite relationship. Complex cellular and humoral immune mechanisms actively participate in modulating host responses. Immunosuppression against specific stages of the parasite has been shown in various phases of manifest infections.

Lymphocytes from microfilaremic individuals are not activated by microfilarial antigens. On the other hand, a high prevalence of cellular and humoral immune reactivity is found in persons living in endemic communities who do not have other evidence of infection. Persons with filariasis without microfilaremia have specific antibodies directed against the microfilarial sheath, whereas those with microfilaremia do not. The diverse clinical and pathologic signs of filariasis are believed to reflect immune responses initiated by antigenic components of various stages of the parasites and their products. This is most clearly defined for tropical eosinophilia, which appears to be a disease of hyperreactivity to microfilariae.

PATHOLOGY AND PATHOGENESIS. Adult worms reside within lymphatic channels, most frequently within dilated vessels of the parenchyma or capsule of inguinal, epitrochlear, and axillary nodes; within major lymphatics distal to these nodes; and within the lymphatics of the testis, epididymis, and spermatic cord. They are also found in the abdominal cavity, from the thoracic duct downward (Fig. 85–3) and in the abdominal retroperitoneal regions. The basic lesion in bancroftian and Malayan filariasis is inflammation in and around lymphatic nodes and vessels at the site of developing and adult worms. In the typical attack of adenolymphangitis, retrograde spread of this inflammation occurs within afferent lymphatic tributaries. Histologic studies reveal a sequential pathologic pattern, as follows: The earliest change is dilatation of the affected vessel. The endothelial lining thickens and a chronic infiltrate of lymphocytes, histiocytes, plasma cells, and eosinophils accumulates around the parasite and in adjacent tissues. Thickening of the vessel proceeds along with further proliferation of endothelial and connective tissue cells, which may lead to obliterative lymphangitis with scarred, cordlike vessels. The most severe inflammation surrounds dead or dying adult worms and includes acute reactions with necrosis and infiltrates of polymorphonuclear cells and histiocytes. Granulomatous changes may supervene, characterized by the presence of epithelioid and giant cells, and the parasites may be enveloped by coagulated lymph or caseous material. Dead worms lyse or become calcified and surrounded by concentric fibrosis (Fig. 85–4).

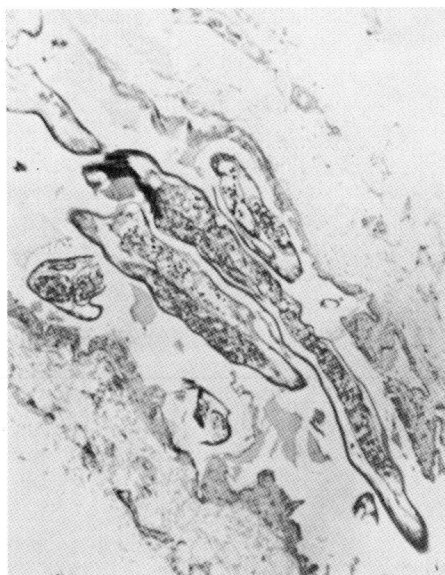

A

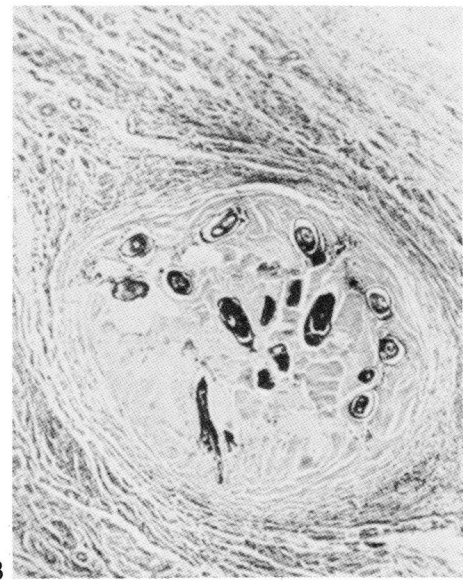

B

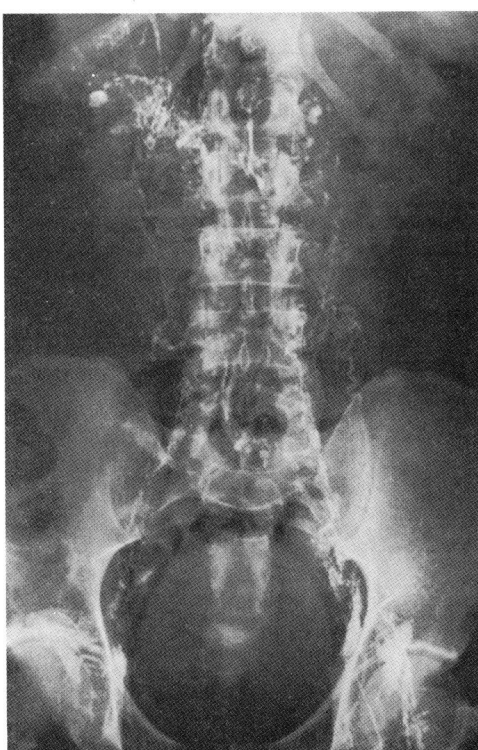

FIGURE 85–3. Filariasis. Bilateral lower extremity lymphangiogram of a patient infected with *W. bancrofti* demonstrates dilated and tortuous varicosed lymphatics and distended and distorted femoral, inguinal, and retroperitoneal lymph nodes. Obstruction to cephalad flow of lymph produced retrograde filling of the renal pericaliceal lymphatics and rapid excretion of the contrast material in the urine. (Note the faintly opacified distended bladder in the pelvis.) This explains the pathophysiology of chyluria in filariasis.

FIGURE 85–4. *A*, Longitudinal section of intact filarial worm in a lymph vessel. *B*, Granuloma containing a partially calcified filarial worm. (From Galindo L, von Lichtenberg F, Baldizón C: Am J Trop Med Hyg 11:739, 1962.)

Living microfilariae do not generally produce lesions. Dead microfilariae, however, are efficiently cleared by reticuloendothelial tissue in which an inflammatory reaction occurs that is characterized by capillary congestion, edema, and collections of lymphocytes, plasma cells, and eosinophils.

Lymphatic abscesses may form at sites of dead or degenerating adult worms, with the accumulation of considerable pus and marked edema of surrounding tissues.

The pathologic sequelae of repeated inflammatory reactions include obstruction to normal flow of lymph, with dilatation and valvular incompetence of afferent lymphatic channels, stasis, and dermal backflow of lymph. Lymphatic obstruction results in lymph varices, lymph scrotum, and hydrocele and in elephantiasis, most usually of the legs, scrotum, arms, and breasts. The penis and labia are less commonly affected. Rupture of abdominal lymphatics is responsible for chyluria (Fig. 85–3), chylous ascites, and rarely, the discharge of lymph into the intestine.

In acute lymphedema, inflammation of the corium and subcutaneous tissue develops. As the condition progresses to elephantiasis, there is increased hyperplasia of the connective tissue; diffuse infiltrations of eosinophils, plasma cells, and macrophages; and the accumulation of mucoid edema. The skin may be greatly thickened and may become verrucous or nodular in long-standing cases.

CLINICAL MANIFESTATIONS. Not all persons exposed to the parasite or known to be infected develop signs and symptoms of illness. Furthermore, there is considerable variation in the clinical manifestations among affected individuals in the same community and in patterns of disease between populations in different geographic areas. Basically, however, the signs and symptoms predictably follow the pathologic processes described earlier and may be grouped as inflammatory, chronic obstructive, or atypically hypersensitive in character.

Inflammatory Signs. The acute attack of localized pain, tenderness, swelling, and erythema is the hallmark of lymphatic filariasis. In United States servicemen acquiring a first infection in the South Pacific during World War II, the initial sign of filariasis was almost always an acute, unifocal inflammatory lesion. Time between first exposure and the development of illness, "the incubation period," was generally from 3½ to 12 months, with increasing frequency of symptoms after the sixth month. The first signs in this nonindigenous population were localized to the genitalia (42%), arms (25%), and legs (11%). In other geographic locations, attacks are more frequent in the lower extremities.

Filarial Adenolymphangitis. Lymphadenitis and lymphangitis of the arms and legs are characteristic of both bancroftian and Malayan filariasis. There is typically an acute onset of pain and tenderness in a single node or small group of adjacent nodes at a single inguinal, axillary, cervical, or epitrochlear site. This is rapidly accompanied by fever, sweats, sometimes chills, headache, lethargy, weakness, generalized mild aches and pains in the muscles and joints, and anorexia. Within 4 to 8 hours of onset, a retrograde lymphangitis of major afferent vessels frequently begins. The affected nodes and lymphatics become swollen, and the overlying skin is indurated and erythematous, producing a red streak 1 to 2 cm wide running down the medial aspect of the leg or the volar surface of the arm. The inflammation increases over the first 24 hours, and acute lymphedema may accumulate in the distal extremity. In endemic areas, uncomplicated attacks are generally mild and persist for a few days only. The distal edema, however, may take one to several weeks to resolve. Filarial adenolymphangitis commonly recurs, often with several attacks a year. Some persons may experience only one or a few attacks during their lifetime; others may have one or more attacks a month during periods of greatest activity of their disease. Episodes are most frequent during adolescence and early adulthood, with a tapering off of acute symptoms in later life. Affected persons frequently associate acute inflammatory episodes with periods of hard physical labor, such as planting crops.

Filarial Orchitis. Onset is sudden, with pain, swelling, and tenderness in the testicle and fever. The pain may be severe and frequently radiates up the spermatic cord and, less commonly, to the inguinal region. In other cases the inflammation may radiate downward to the testis. The testis frequently swells to twice its usual size and has a boggy, edematous consistency. Epididymitis, funiculitis, and varicoceles are common, as are edema and erythema of the scrotal skin. Small accumulations of fluid in the tunica vaginalis are also common during the acute attack. Fever (to 40C) and sometimes chills, malaise, anorexia, and lethargy are usual. The acute symptoms generally last for 3 to 5 days, but may persist for 1 to 2 weeks, and recur at irregular intervals.

Funiculitis and Epididymitis. Inflammation of the lymphatics of the epididymis and spermatic cord occurs alone or along with filarial orchitis. Repeated attacks result in thickening of these structures, which, together with hydroceles, may be the most common physical signs of filarial disease encountered in community surveys of endemic foci (Fig. 85–5). The effects of these lesions on fertility have not been established.

"Filarial" and "Elephantoid" Fever. Adenolymphangitis is almost always accompanied by fever. In endemic communities attacks of irregularly recurring fever without demonstrable lymphadenitis or lymphangitis, or other assignable causes such as malaria, may be due to inflammation of deep-seated lymphatics. These episodes have been termed "elephantoid fever" in cases of elephantiasis.

Filarial Abscess. Two forms of abscess occur in association with lymphatic filariasis. In the South Pacific, especially in Samoa, some abscesses occur deep within fascial spaces of muscle groups of the extremities, especially the arms and thighs. In general, however, they develop within superficially placed lymphatics draining into the inguinal and axillary regions and less frequently occur in the distal portions of the extremities, the breasts, and the pectoral areas. The onset of these abscesses is similar to a typical attack of adenolymphangitis, but progressive pain and swelling occur over the affected vessel for a period of one to several weeks prior

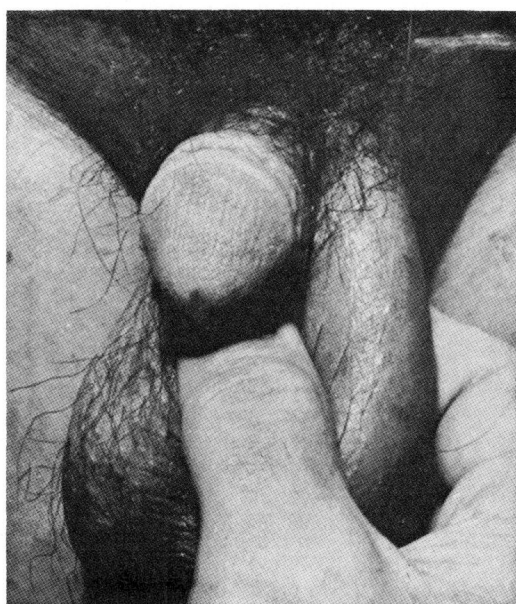

FIGURE 85–5. Filariasis, thickened spermatic cord.

to rupture. Considerable edema accumulates at the site, and there is often distal lymphedema. The expression of pus, sterile or containing streptococcal or staphylococcal bacteria, is followed by the leakage of lymph as the local and constitutional signs rapidly abate. The clean-based ulcer heals by granulation quickly and without complications, leaving a characteristic scar overlying a cordlike sclerotic vessel.

Chronic Obstructive Signs. Inflammation of lymphatic vessels and nodes causes constriction and obliteration of vascular spaces proximally and dilatation and valvular incompetence distally. This results in stasis with accumulations of lymphedema in the skin and subcutaneous tissues and of serous fluid within the potential space created by the folding of the tunica vaginalis. Chronic obstructive disease usually follows repeated acute inflammatory attacks and is rarely manifest until 10 or more years following first exposure. In the inhabitants of a typical endemic community, chronic lymphedema and hydroceles first appear late in the second decade, with peak incidence in the third and fourth decades. Once established, the obstructive sequelae are often slowly progressive, with greatest deformities occurring in the oldest age group. Despite repeated exposure to infection, in some patients hydrocele and unremitting edema never progress beyond the earliest stages, whereas in others severe disease develops rapidly at an early age. Disease signs generally appear earlier, and in greater frequency and severity, in foci of intense transmission.

Lymph Varices. Varicose lymphatic nodes are most commonly found among the superficial inguinal and axillary groups, where they form soft and lobular protuberances, sometimes associated with varicosity of afferent lymphatic vessels.

Lymph Scrotum. Varicosity of the lymphatics of the skin of the scrotum may result in a soft, sometimes vesiculated thickening of the affected part, which can be a prelude to elephantiasis.

Hydrocele (Fig. 85–6). Hydrocele, or chylocele, depending on whether the exudate is straw-colored and lymphous (hydrocele) or milky and chylous (chylocele), is often associated with orchitis. It is the hallmark of chronic bancroftian filariasis in most endemic areas and may be found in 25% or more of the adult male population in rural foci. Microfilariae are more often present in the blood of persons with hydrocele than in those with elephantiasis and can also commonly be recovered from the hydrocele fluid aspirate. As much as 500 ml of fluid may be drawn from the tunica, but relief is usually short-lasting. Large hydroceles cause considerable discomfort and restriction of normal activity.

Lymphedema and Elephantiasis. Swelling of the distal body parts typically first appears during an acute attack of adenolymphangitis, especially when there is retrograde spread of the inflammation. In early episodes, the swelling is slight and resolves completely. With subsequent attacks, however, the swelling increases and resolves more slowly, until finally it remains between episodes. The edema in the early stages is soft and pitting; when it persists for more than 6 months, it may be classified as elephantiasis, with or without the chronic thickening of the skin frequently associated with the term. In the natural history of lymphatic filariasis, elephantiasis is the most slowly developing manifestation. In endemic situations, there is usually a slow and steady rise in prevalence beyond age 20, with a peak occurrence of new cases between the ages of 25 and 40. Although elephantiasis usually follows repeated episodes of adenolymphangitis and remitting edema, in some patients

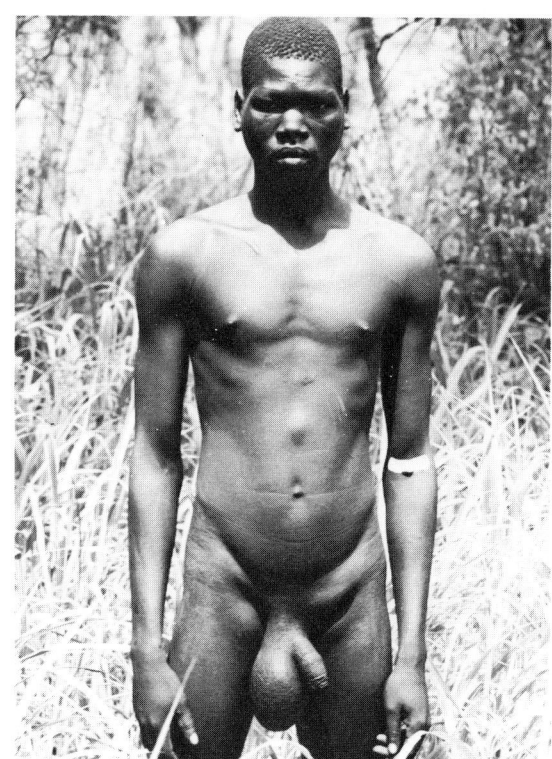

FIGURE 85–6. Nilotic tribesman of lowland western Ethiopia with bilateral filarial hydrocele and inguinal lymphatic varices progressing toward "hanging-groin."

the condition develops insidiously without acute symptoms. The legs and scrotum are most commonly affected, followed in frequency by the arms. The breasts, penis, and labia are less frequently involved. The condition is painless, but the affected parts are subject to attacks of inflammation. Fissures, maceration, and a susceptibility to trauma, coupled with poor healing and impaired defenses against bacteria, dispose to ulceration and infection. Although at first confined to the dorsum of the foot and the ankle or to the hand, the swelling may progress proximally to involve the entire extremity. Elephantiasis of the extremities is often bilateral, and a high proportion of persons with elephantiasis have swelling of more than 1 part. As the condition progresses, the swelling assumes a nonpitting solid firmness owing to extensive hypertrophy and fibrous hyperplasia of the skin and subcutaneous tissues. The skin may remain smooth or become verrucous or nodular (Fig. 85–7). The swelling may reach great proportions and be incapacitating because of its size and weight alone, and there are obvious psychosocial problems associated with the condition.

Chyluria. The passage of chylous urine from the rupture of abdominal lymphatics into the urinary tract (Fig. 85–3) comes on abruptly. It is often accompanied by pain in the back and lower abdomen and sometimes by fever. Difficulty in passing urine may arise from coagula. The fluid may be milky in appearance, or pinkish if mixed with blood. If passed into a glass container, the fluid quickly coagulates into an upper white fatty layer, a cloudy middle layer of gray lymphuria, and a thin pink or reddish sediment at the bottom. Attacks of chyluria and lymphuria usually last for a few days, but may persist for weeks and tend to recur. Serious complications include obstruction of the renal pelvis or ureters from coagula and hypoproteinemia from chronic loss of albumin.

DIAGNOSIS. The clinical diagnosis is made by associating the pattern of inflammatory and obstructive signs with a history of travel to or residence in an endemic area. Recurring attacks of lymphangitis or inflammation of scrotal contents should alert the practitioner to the possibility of early lymphatic filariasis.

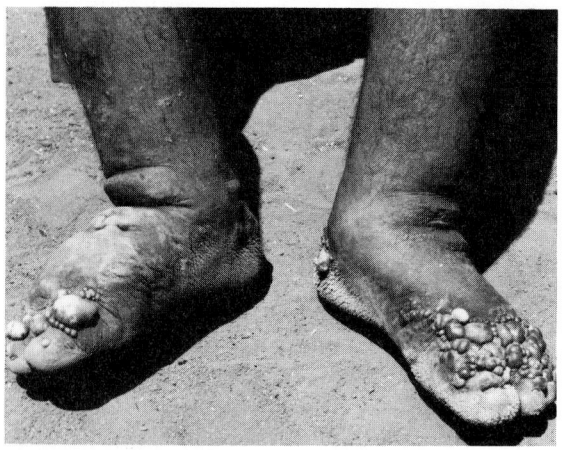

FIGURE 85–7. Filarial elephantiasis showing nodular and verrucous changes of the skin. Note the characteristic skin folds at the junction of the foot and ankle.

These acute-phase symptoms are often accompanied by a moderate eosinophilia.

Parasitemia. The diagnosis is best established by identifying the microfilariae in peripheral blood. If stained films of 60 μl of blood obtained during the day are negative, subsequent films should be made from blood taken at night or larger amounts of blood should be examined by concentration techniques. The most sensitive method of concentration is to collect 3 to 5 ml of heparinized venous blood within a 10-ml syringe and pass it directly through a Nuclepore membrane filter having pores with a diameter of 3 or 5 μm. The membrane is held in a standard Swinney-25 adapter. After the blood has been passed through the membrane, the syringe is disconnected and used to pass 10 ml of distilled water through the filter to clear it of debris. The membrane is removed from the adapter, placed on a glass microscope slide, and allowed to dry prior to staining in the usual manner with Giemsa or Field's stain. A drop of clear mounting medium is placed on the filter, followed by a coverslip, and the preparation examined with a compound microscope. This method is so efficient that, in many cases, the examination of day blood is satisfactory for detecting nocturnally periodic parasites.

Another useful procedure is that of Knott, in which 1 ml of blood is mixed with 9 ml of distilled water to which 1 ml of 40% formalin has been added. The mixture is shaken to ensure lysis of erythrocytes and centrifuged in a conical tube, and the sediment examined in a wet or stained preparation on a microscope slide.

A third method is to administer a single dose of 100 mg of diethylcarbamazine (DEC) and take blood specimens for routine examination 45 minutes to 1 hour later. The DEC causes sequestered microfilariae to emerge in the blood. This method avoids taking blood specimens at night, but is not as sensitive or reliable as a properly obtained night blood film. It is contraindicated in areas endemic for onchocerciasis or loiasis, because it may precipitate dangerous reactions in persons infected with these parasites.

Microfilariae may also be found in aspirates of hydrocele fluid and in chylous urine. Lymph node or vessel biopsy to search for parasites should be avoided, as removal of tissue may further compromise the return of lymph to the circulation.

Serology. Not all patients with filariasis will have circulating microfilariae, and diagnosis in these persons is limited to the use of immunologic techniques. The best results at present are obtained with tests that detect specific circulating antigens of microfilariae and adults. Antibody detection tests are sensitive but lack species specificity. This is of particular importance in rural areas where concomitant infections with other helminths can cause cross-reactions in the diagnostic antibody tests. In a few research laboratories diagnostic tests (usually enzyme-linked immunosorbent assay [ELISA]) have considerable sensitivity and specificity.

Differential Diagnosis. Diseases to be considered in the differential diagnosis of the individual case of adenolymphangitis include (1) acute bacterial lymphangitis that spreads proximally, often from an open lesion of the foot, lower leg, or hand; (2) phlebitis; and (3) unusual conditions, e.g., bubonic plague, anthrax, tuberculous adenitis, and lymphogranuloma inguinale. Recurrent filarial fever is often mistaken for malaria and may be confused with tuberculosis, urinary tract infection, and osteomyelitis. Filarial orchitis, epididymitis, and funiculitis have to be distinguished from gonococcal disease, tuberculous epididymitis, strangulated hernia, torsion, mumps orchitis, and trauma. Filarial hydrocele, without chyle or microfilariae in the aspirate, may have to be distinguished on epidemiologic grounds. Nonfilarial causes of chyluria, lymphedema, and elephantiasis include (1) infiltrative and granulomatous processes such as tumor, fungal infection, tuberculosis, and leprosy; (2) chronic venostasis and phlebitis; (3) cardiac insufficiency; (4) nutritional deficiencies; and (5) hereditary forms of lymphostasis such as Milroy's disease. Endemic "bigfoot" disease of highland areas of Africa, especially Ethiopia, is most probably caused by lateritious soils gaining entrance to lymphatics from fissures of the feet. It may be clinically indistinguishable from filarial elephantiasis, but occurs at altitudes above the limits for filarial transmission and is not associated with hydrocele.

TREATMENT

Chemotherapy. Diethylcarbamazine, a piperazine derivative, is the current chemotherapeutic agent of choice against lymphatic-dwelling filaria. DEC (Hetrazan, Banocide, Notézine, Filarizan) is a rapid and efficient microfilaricide for *Wuchereria* and *Brugia*, and in one or more treatment courses kills most adult parasites. It is inactive against the parasite in vitro, and the drug presumably works with the host's immune response, perhaps by unmasking the parasite as foreign or by removing immune suppressive factors. The usual dosage is 4 to 6 mg/kg body weight daily in single or spaced doses given after meals for 14 to 21 days. Most infections will be cured with this regimen, although in some persons low levels of microfilaremia may persist. Reexamination of the blood is recommended to detect a persisting infection. The drug is rapidly excreted and relatively nontoxic; repeat treatment may be safely given 1 month following completion of a previous course. Furthermore, a single treatment usually reduces or eliminates episodes of acute lymphatic inflammation, and obstructive lesions may become static and in some instances regress. No improvement can be expected in the advanced lesions in which fibrosis is prominent.

Recently, a new microfilaricidal drug, ivermectin (Mectizan) was introduced for treatment of onchocerciasis. In several clinical trials, ivermectin was also found effective against infections with *W. bancrofti*. The new drug can be given in a single dose. Untoward side reactions appear to be less severe than those observed from treatment with DEC. Ivermectin is still under clinical investigation but is promising as a chemotherapeutic agent for lymphatic filariasis, although it appears to be only microfilaricidal.

DEC Reactions. Untoward effects of DEC are of two types: those arising directly from toxicity of the drug itself and those resulting from destruction of the parasite. Symptoms of toxicity, including dizziness, weakness, and nausea, are unusual in children but common among adults, especially at single doses of 8 mg/kg of body weight or greater. These symptoms are mild and last for a few hours only. Reactions to the death of parasites, however, may be considerably more severe and take 2 forms. The rapid destruction of microfilariae may precipitate variable acute generalized symptoms of fever up to 41C (Fig. 85-8), headache, pains in muscles and joints (especially of the back), abdominal pain, nausea and vomiting, weakness, dizziness, lethargy, and asthma. These symptoms develop within the first 2 days of treatment, often within 12 hours, and persist for the first 2 to 4 days of treatment. Presumed damage to or death of adult worms may result in acute attacks of adenolymphangitis and sometimes abscesses. These local signs may arise at any time during treatment, and even for several weeks following therapy. Atypical bullous reactions of the skin may occur during treatment.

Reactions are usually most severe in infections with *Brugia malayi* and *Brugia timori*, and their incidence and severity are directly related to the microfilarial density and adult worm burden. Reactions are less common and less severe with repeat drug doses. Treatment seldom needs to be interrupted, but patients should be told about the reactions in advance. DEC is contraindicated during pregnancy and in persons with cardiac and renal disease. Special care should be exercised in treating the elderly and patients in areas where onchocerciasis and loiasis are prevalent. Reactions may be lessened somewhat by starting treatment with low doses and are almost always relieved by analgesic-antipyretic preparations such as salicylic acid and phenacetin.

Other Treatment. Filarial abscesses seen in the field are best managed conservatively with antibiotics, but may require incision and drainage. Hydroceles are temporarily relieved by aspiration and may be treated by more definitive procedures such as obliteration of the tunica sac. Lymphedema and elephantiasis are managed by reducing periods of dependency of the affected part and by firm bandaging. Excision of redundant tissue of scrotal elephantiasis may afford relief, but operations on extremities should be performed with caution (Chapter 12).

CONTROL AND PREVENTION. Control of lymphatic filariasis depends on mass and selective treatment

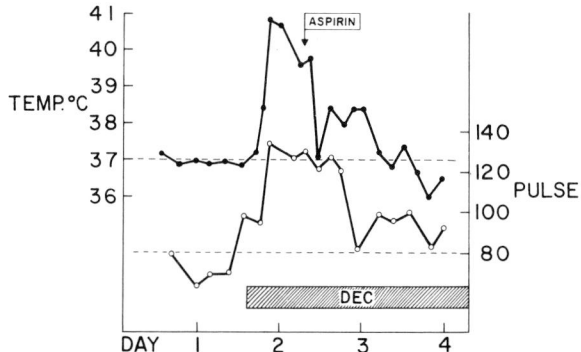

FIGURE 85-8. Fever course of a patient with *B. timori* infection who is experiencing a generalized reaction to treatment with diethylcarbamazine (DEC). This reaction is presumably due to massive destruction of microfilariae and is rapidly ameliorated by aspirin.

with DEC or (probably by 1991) with ivermectin, vector suppression, and improved personal protection from mosquitoes. Mass treatment results in a rapid reduction in microfilaremia rates and densities and in acute symptoms. Success depends on the skill and persistence of treatment teams in obtaining a complete course of treatment for everyone in the area by means of cooperation and health education. Follow-up "selective" treatment of persons with continuing microfilaremia or acute symptoms is often conducted at 3 to 6 months following a mass campaign and at one to several years later if the residual infection rate is brought below 5%. When the rate is 5% or greater at protracted follow-up, it is probably best to repeat treatment of the entire population to eliminate any subpatent infections. DEC is administered in a dose of 4 to 6 mg/kg of body weight at variable intervals of days to weeks or even months, for a total dosage of 30 to 75 mg/kg. Differing schedules are used to obtain the greatest coverage with the fewest and mildest reactions.

Significant reductions have been achieved wherever a serious program has been undertaken. Reluctance of patients to cooperate for fear of incurring reactions has been a major problem in some locales, especially in areas with *Brugia* infection. Treatment of communities with very low doses of DEC over prolonged periods, using medicated salt, has produced some notable successes, especially in China.

Control by vector suppression is useful in areas in which indoor residual insecticide spraying is effective and where mosquito breeding sites can be reduced. Personal protection includes complete clothing, improved housing and community hygiene, and use of repellents, insecticides, and bed nets. The value of DEC in prophylaxis is unknown.

BIBLIOGRAPHY

Freedman DO, Nutman TB, Ottesen EA: Protective immunity in bancroftian filariasis. J Clin Invest 83:14, 1989.
Goodwin LG, Ottesen EA, Southgate BA: Recent advances in research on filariasis. Trans R Soc Trop Med Hyg 78 (Suppl):1, 1984.
Kumaraswami V, Ottesen EA, Vijayasekaran V, et al: Ivermectin for the treatment of *Wuchereria bancrofti* filariasis. JAMA 259:3150, 1988.
Mahoney LE, Kessel JF: Treatment failure in filariasis mass treatment programs. BULL WHO 45:35, 1971.
Nutman TB, Kumaraswami V, Ottesen EA: Parasite-specific anergy in human filariasis. J Clin Invest 79:1516, 1987.
Weil GJ, Jain DC, Santhanam S, et al: A monoclonal antibody–based immunoassay for detecting parasite antigenemia in bancroftian filariasis. J Infect Dis 156:350, 1987.
Witte CL, Foldin M (eds): Lymphedema. Lymphology 18:143, 1985.
WHO Expert Committee on Filariasis: Lymphatic filariasis. Fourth Report. WHO Tech Rep Ser 702, 1984.

85.2. MALAYAN FILARIASIS

DEFINITION. Malayan filariasis denotes infection with *Brugia malayi*. Although this parasite is closely related to *Wuchereria bancrofti*, there are important differences in their biology, epidemiology, and clinico-pathologic characteristics of infection. Malayan filariasis is limited in distribution to South and East Asia, where it is a disease of rural communities. Two major forms of the parasite are distinguished: the nocturnally periodic and the nocturnally subperiodic. The subperiodic form, which is transmitted by *Mansonia* species of riverine swamp forest ecotypes, is zoonotic with an important reservoir in monkeys. The periodic type is transmitted by *Mansonia* and *Anopheles* species of open swamp and wet rice cultivation areas and by anophelines in hill forest locales; there is no known animal reservoir. As in bancroftian filariasis, the parasite in humans resides in lymphatic vessels, where it causes inflammatory and chronic obstructive disease. Adenolymphangitis of the extremities is, however, the most prominent feature. In contrast to the case with *W. bancrofti*, there is no evidence that *Brugia* cause genital lesions.

ETIOLOGY

Morphology. *B. malayi* (Brug, 1927; Rao and Maplestone, 1940) is similar to *W. bancrofti* in life cycle (Fig. VI B–1) and morphology. The adult worms are about half the size of those of *W. bancrofti* and have distinguishing characteristics of male genitalia and adjacent papillae. The sheathed microfilariae are readily distinguished from those of *W. bancrofti* in properly stained blood films (Fig. 85–1 and Table 85–1). They are 200 to 275 μm in length and 4 to 7 μm in width and have an ungraceful and kinked appearance, a long cephalic space with a length:width ratio of about 2:1, a packed nuclear column in which the cells are overlapping and indistinct in margin, a prominent innenkörper, and 2 discrete terminal nuclei that reach the tip of the tail. The sheath stains bright pink when treated with Giemsa or Field's preparations. Although there is overlap, periodic microfilariae have a greater total length and a longer innenkörper than the subperiodic microfilariae. In routine blood film preparations, at least 50% of periodic microfilariae are unsheathed, whereas only about 5% of the subperiodic form are unsheathed.

Development and Life Cycle. The development and life cycle of the parasite are essentially the same as that of *W. bancrofti* (Fig. VI B–1). However, *Brugia* has a more rapid development in infective forms in some mosquitoes, a generally shorter prepatent period in humans, and an animal reservoir of the subperiodic form.

EPIDEMIOLOGY

Distribution (Fig. 85–9). *Brugia malayi* is found throughout the Oriental biogeographic zone in a focal ecotype-dependent distribution, from India in the west to Korea in the northeast. The parasite probably originated in the tropical rain forests of Southeast Asia, perhaps in the once great land mass of Sundaland, which comprised present-day Sumatra, Java, Borneo, and Peninsular Malaysia and the intervening seas. Nowhere else is there such a rich diversity of parasite forms, vector

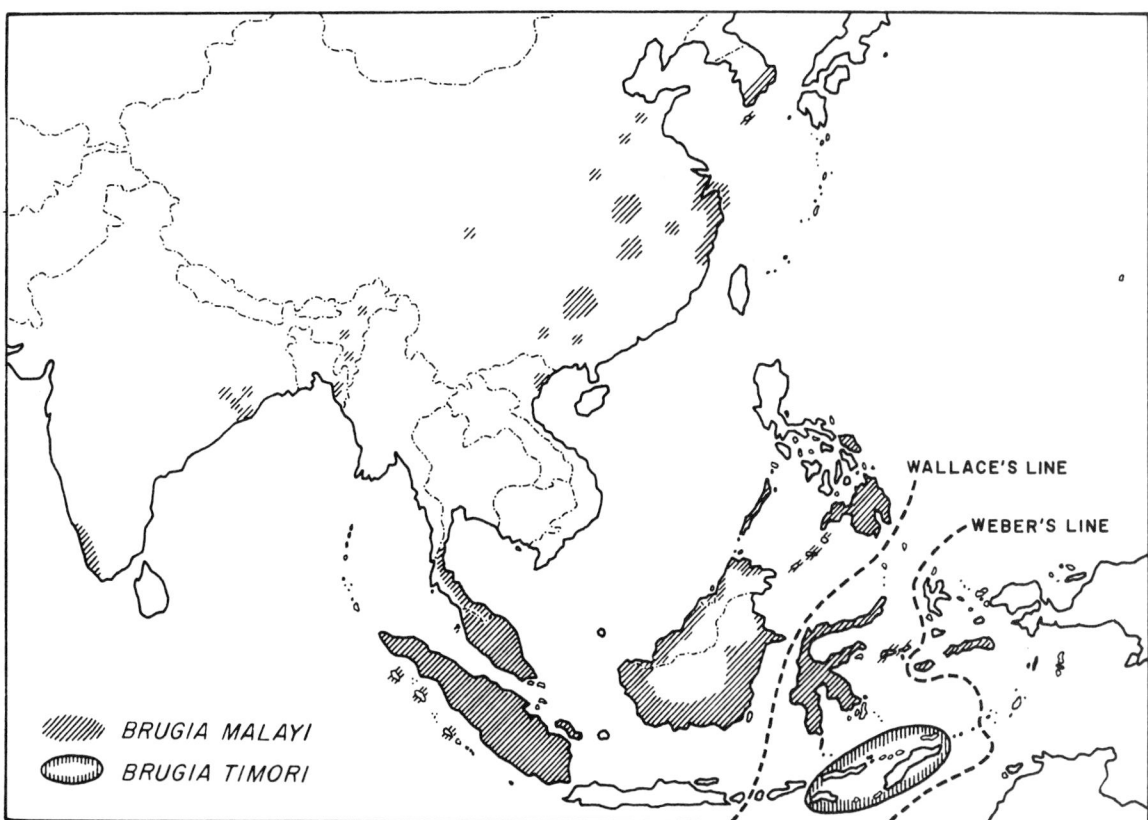

FIGURE 85–9. Distribution of filariasis due to *B. malayi* and *B. timori*. The subperiodic, as well as the periodic, strain of *B. malayi* occurs in Malaysia, Indonesia, and the Philippines. *B. timori* is found only on the islands of southeastern Indonesia.

species, and animal hosts. The parasite spreads by adapting itself to locally available vectors as diverse as *Aedes togoi* in coastal China and Korea and *Anopheles barbirostris* in eastern Indonesia. It is not found east of Weber's line, which divides the Oriental mosquito fauna from the Australian at the interface of the Moluccas and New Guinea.

Only the nocturnally periodic form is found in India, especially in the coastal belt of Kerala and in several other limited rural foci where there are water plants suitable for the breeding of *Mansonia uniformis* and related mosquitoes. The parasite has practically disappeared from Sri Lanka.

The periodic and subperiodic forms are both found in the southern peninsular section of Thailand in ecotypes similar to those described in Malaysia. In Malaysia, where the most thorough studies of the parasite have been conducted, the periodic strain occurs in the open coastal rice field areas and to a limited extent among aboriginal peoples living in hill forests, whereas the subperiodic strain is endemic in rural villages and plantations along the lower reaches of major rivers, in swamp forest ecotypes associated with a zoonotic reservoir. The periodic form is transmitted by anophelines and mosquitoes of the *Mansonia uniformis* group, whereas the subperiodic form is transmitted mostly by *M. bonneae* and *M. dives*.

The parasite is widespread in Indonesia, with perhaps 5 to 10 million persons at risk of infection. The subperiodic form occurs in Sumatra; throughout Borneo Island, including the eastern Malaysian state of Sabah; and in

the nearby southern islands of the Philippine archipelago. Periodic forms are endemic in Sumatra and Sulawesi; 3 isolated foci in Java have died out. Strains with both periodic and subperiodic characteristics have been reported as far east as Ceram, in the Moluccas. The parasite is apparently absent in those islands of southeastern Indonesia endemic for *Brugia timori*.

Malayan filariasis is endemic in the Red River delta of Vietnam, and is more widely distributed in China than previously believed, mostly in eastern lowland rice-growing areas, where *Anopheles sinensis* is the vector. The parasite is found in the southern Korean peninsula and in offshore islands. *Aedes togoi* transmits infection in some coastal foci of Korea and China.

Host, Parasite, and Environmental Factors. In the more highly endemic areas, microfilaremias and acute lymphatic symptoms develop at an early age, reaching a plateau in the third decade. Elephantiasis follows a time course similar to that of bancroftian filariasis. Beyond adolescence, infection and disease rates are generally higher in men than in women. No ethnic difference in susceptibility is evident, although exposure patterns differ greatly; e.g., in Malaysia, rubber tappers of Indian origin and rural Malay farmers are most affected.

Leaf monkeys of the *Presbytis* group are important zoonotic reservoirs of the subperiodic form in Malaysia and Indonesia; the reservoir role of less suitable natural hosts, such as domestic cats, is dubious. The relatively limited success of filariasis control efforts in forest and forest fringe areas, including rubber and palm estates, is most likely due to continued spillover from monkeys to humans. Domestic cats and dogs, leaf monkeys, and other forest animals are infected with *Brugia pahangi*. No natural infections with *B. pahangi* have yet been reported in humans, although this parasite has been transmitted to humans experimentally.

CLINICAL MANIFESTATIONS. Recurring lymphadenitis and lymphangitis of the extremities, with fever, are the major signs of Malayan filariasis. These episodes occur with a greater frequency than in bancroftian filariasis. The inguinal and axillary nodes and their afferent lymphatics are most often affected. Lymphatic abscesses and consequent scarring are common features in areas where the intensity of transmission is high. Lymphedema appears during the course of acute lymphangitis and progresses to elephantiasis in a small proportion of cases. The swelling in Malayan filariasis is most frequently limited to a mild, soft, pitting edema of the distal extremities, producing a "water-bag" deformity in the more advanced cases (Fig. 85–10). The edema does not usually extend above the elbows or knees and is infrequently accompanied by nodular or verrucous changes of the skin. The prevalence rates of adenolymphangitis may exceed 50% in some endemic communities, but the elephantiasis rate does not often exceed 3 to 5%. *B. malayi* has not been documented as

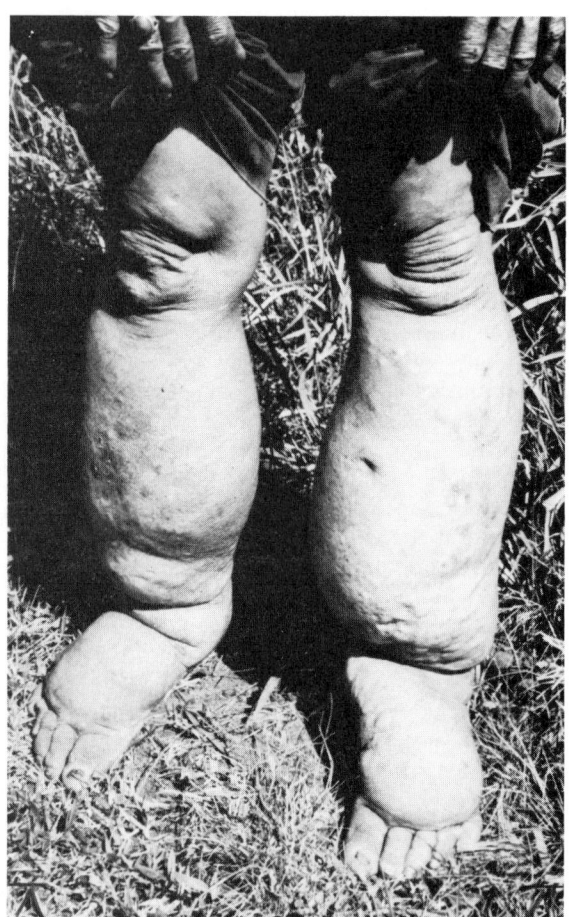

FIGURE 85–10. The so-called water-bag deformity of elephantiasis due to *Brugia* infection. The swelling does not often extend above the knee.

a cause of urogenital disease. The findings of sclerotic, cordlike lymphatics and enlarged firm nodes of the arms and legs are usual.

DIAGNOSIS. See Chapter 85.1.

TREATMENT AND CONTROL. See Chapter 85.1.

BIBLIOGRAPHY

Denham DA, McGreevy PB: Brugian filariasis: Epidemiological and experimental studies. Adv Parasitol 16:243, 1977.

Dissanaike AS: Zoonotic aspects of filarial infections in man. Bull WHO 57:349, 1979.

Mak JW: Filariasis in Southeast Asia. Ann Acad Med Singapore 10:112, 1981.

Mak JW, Cheong WH, Yen P, et al: Studies on the epidemiology of subperiodic *Brugia malayi* in Malaysia. Acta Trop 39:237, 1982.

Piessens WF, Ratiwayanto S, Tuti S, et al: Antigen-specific suppressor cells and suppressor factors in human filariasis with *Brugia malayi*. N Engl J Med 302:833, 1980.

Wilson T: Filariasis in Malaya—A general review. Trans R Soc Trop Med Hyg 55:107, 1961.

85.3. TIMORIAN FILARIASIS

DEFINITION. In 1965, microfilariae of a new parasite were identified in the blood of persons living on the island of Timor, southeastern Indonesia. Adult worms and larval forms were subsequently described from the nearby island of Flores, and the parasite was designated *Brugia timori*. Disease caused by the parasite is similar to that of *B. malayi*, but manifestations are unusually severe in the more heavily endemic communities. The microfilariae are nocturnally periodic. *Anopheles barbirostris*, a malaria carrier, is the only known vector. Infections in animals have not yet been found, although cats and gerbils have been infected in the laboratory.

ETIOLOGY. *B. timori* (Partono et al., 1977) has a life cycle similar to that of *B. malayi* (Fig. VI B–1). The microfilaria of *B. timori* is distinguished by a mean body length of 310 μm, a sheath that does not stain in Giemsa preparations, a long cephalic space with a length:width ratio of about 3:1, a compact nuclear column, and small terminal nuclei that reach the tip of the tail. It is a long and gracefully sinuous parasite with clear cellular features in stained blood films (Fig. 85–1 and Table 85–1).

EPIDEMIOLOGY. The parasite is limited in distribution to the small volcanic islands of southeastern Indonesia that surround the Savu Sea, including Timor, Alor, Flores, Sumba, Roti, and Savu (Fig. 85–9). It is especially endemic in low-lying riverine valleys of foothills and in coastal aprons, where the vector breeds in irrigated rice fields and along the banks and feeder streams of shallow perennial rivers. The vector feeds mostly indoors at night, and inhabitants of endemic communities are evenly exposed to infection. Microfilaremia and attacks of adenolymphangitis rapidly increase in prevalence from the ages of 5 to 15 years, and more slowly thereafter. Microfilaremia rates in areas of high transmission are in the range of 20 to 30%. In some foci, 50% of the population may experience acute recurring symptoms, usually inguinal adenitis and retrograde lymphangitis. Lymphatic abscesses are com-

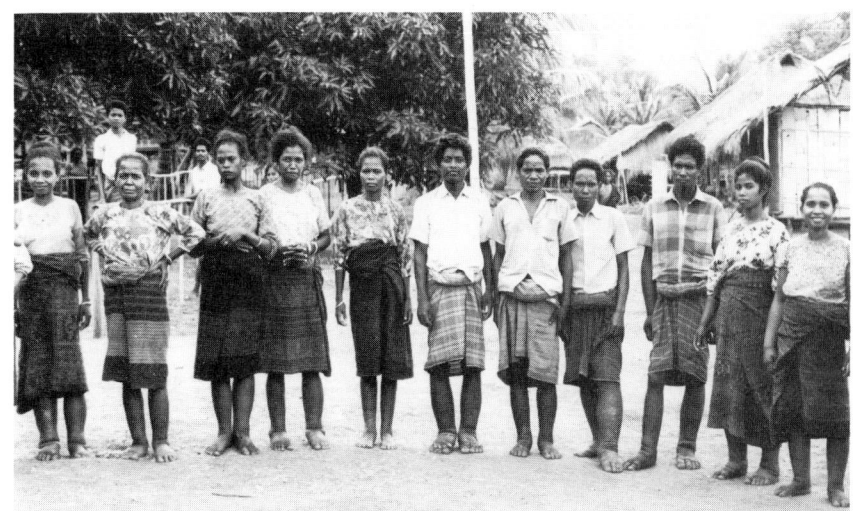

FIGURE 85–11. Elephantiasis of legs and arms (the 3 persons on the far right) due to *B. timori*. The elephantiasis is mostly bilateral.

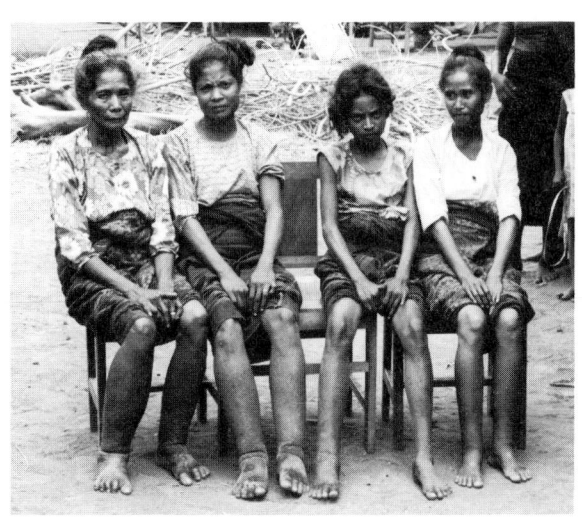

FIGURE 85–12. Elephantiasis in timorian filariasis showing the "water-bag" deformity and fissuring at ankles.

FIGURE 85–13. Filarial abscesses developing in the lower leg with acute lymphedema distally. The abscesses are covered by a locally prepared poultice.

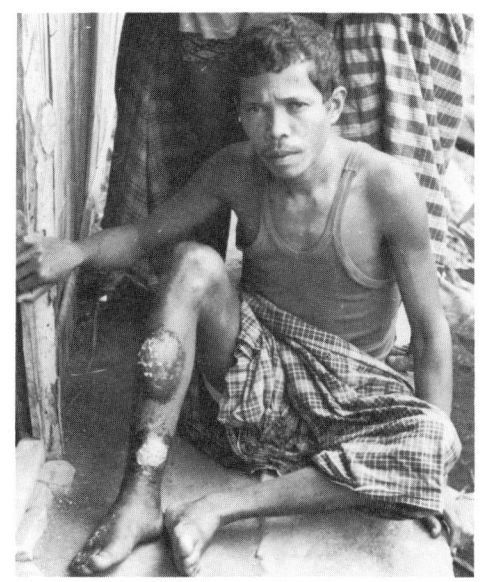

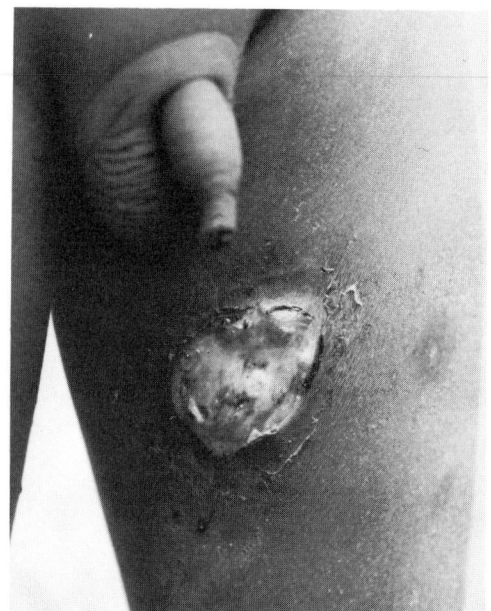

FIGURE 85–14. Clean-based ulcer resulting from the rupture of a filarial abscess.

mon, especially in the saphenous and brachial drainage sites; and the prevalence of scarring is a useful epidemiologic index. Elephantiasis is found in most endemic communities at rates of 5% or less, but in some unusual situations, 35% of the adult population may be affected (Fig. 85–11). Disease rates are slightly greater in males than in females.

CLINICOPATHOLOGIC DESCRIPTION. The clinical pattern is the same as that described for Malayan filariasis. Acute recurrent attacks of inguinal and axillary lymphadenitis with retrograde lymphangitis and fever, lasting 3 to 7 days, are the characteristic signs of the disease. Lymphedema of the legs, and less frequently of

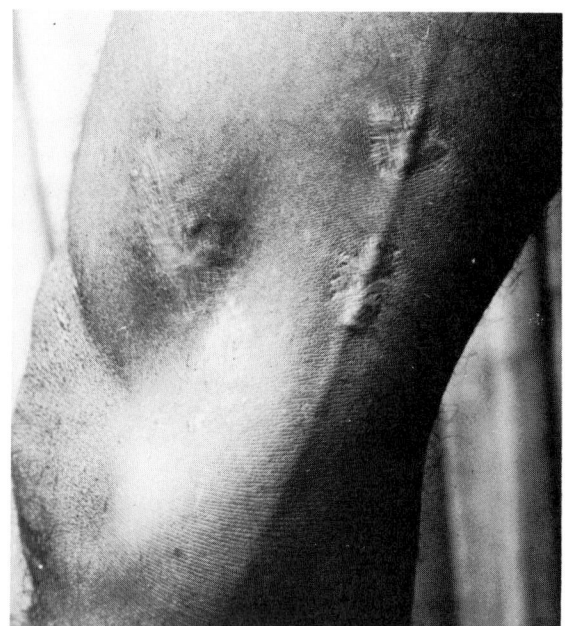

FIGURE 85–15. Filarial scars overlying a cordlike sclerotic lymphatic vessel.

the arms, often progresses to elephantiasis with minimal thickening and deformity of the skin (Figs. 85–11 and 85–12). Lymphatic abscesses account for considerable incapacitation in endemic communities (Fig. 85–13). Fever, lethargy, weakness, and pain and limitation of motion of the affected extremity may persist for the 3 to 5 weeks during the development and localization of the abscess prior to its rupture (Fig. 85–14). Single and multiple scars may be found over the pathways of the greater saphenous and brachial lymphatics (Fig. 85–15) and less commonly at other sites such as the distal extremities, breasts, and pectoral and cervical regions. Genital lesions are not seen, and there have been no reports of chyluria.

Human pathologic studies have not been done, although disease manifestations point to a pathogenesis similar to *B. malayi*, with localization of adult worms in glands and vessels of the proximal extremities. Occasional cases of severe abdominal pain during treatment with diethylcarbamazine (DEC) suggest that some worms lodge in abdominal lymphatics.

DIAGNOSIS. See Chapter 85.1.

TREATMENT AND CONTROL. The parasite is sensitive to DEC, with a rapid clearance of microfilariae following total doses of 60 mg/kg body weight. It should be possible to eliminate this disease by a combined program of mass chemotherapy and vector control with indoor residual insecticides (Chapter 85.1).

BIBLIOGRAPHY

Dennis DT, Partono F, Purnomo, et al: Timor filariasis: Epidemiologic and clinical features in a defined community. Am J Trop Med Hyg 25:797, 1976.
Partono F, Purnomo, Dennis DT, et al: *Brugia timori* sp. n. (nematoda: filarioidea) from Flores Island, Indonesia. J Parasitol 63:540, 1977.
Partono F, Purnomo, Pribadi W, et al: Epidemiological and clinical features of *Brugia timori* in a newly established village, Karakuak, West Flores, Indonesia. Am J Trop Med Hyg 27:910, 1978.

85.4. FILARIAL HYPEREOSINOPHILIA

DEFINITION. Hypereosinophilia of filarial origin (tropical pulmonary eosinophilia [TPE]) describes a complex of symptoms arising from an atypical sensitivity of the lungs and the reticuloendothelial system (especially the lymph nodes and spleen) to microfilariae. This term was first used to describe hypereosinophilia with prominent pulmonary symptoms (i.e., paroxysmal nocturnal cough and wheezing, scanty sputum production, and diffuse fine pulmonary markings) in amicrofilaremic persons from areas of India endemic for filariasis. Meyers and Kouwenaar had earlier described a condition in several persons in Indonesia characterized by marked eosinophilia, with or without asthma, in which microfilariae were absent from the peripheral blood but were present in hyperplastic lymph nodes and the spleen. These syndromes were combined under a common term, "occult filariasis," by Lie in 1962.

PATHOLOGY. Lungs, spleen, lymph nodes, and liver are the organs most affected. As determined by biopsy, infiltrates of eosinophils, histiocytes, and lymphocytes organize in small foci that, with time, become more histiocytic and granulomatous. These are the small yellowish-gray Meyers-Kouwenaar bodies or nodules, within which microfilariae may be surrounded by acidophilic hyaline material and foreign body giant cells. In the lymph nodes, the lesions are less granulomatous and contain more eosinophils than elsewhere.

CLINICAL MANIFESTATIONS. Some criteria useful in diagnosing filarial hypereosinophilia are recent residence in an area endemic for filariasis, especially South and Southeast Asia; strikingly elevated eosinophilia, usually greater than 3000 cells/mm³; isolated or generalized lymph node enlargement; pulmonary symptoms of paroxysmal cough, most frequently nocturnal, with little or no sputum production, but with dyspnea, a coarse rhonchi, and rales or wheezing; increased bronchovascular markings and diffuse miliary mottling in chest roentgenograms; absence of circulating microfilariae; elevated levels of IgE; high titers of antifilarial antibodies; and a favorable and rapid response to treatment with diethylcarbamazine (DEC).

Microfilariae of *Wuchereria bancrofti*, *Brugia malayi*, and unidentified species have been recovered from lungs and lymph nodes. Acute focal lymphadenitic forms of the disease were caused by *W. bancrofti* in American servicemen in the South Pacific and by *B. malayi* in French troops serving in Vietnam. The syndrome has resulted from experimental infection in humans with both *B. malayi* and the animal parasite *Brugia pahangi*.

DIAGNOSIS. The most straightforward approach to the diagnosis of filarial hypereosinophilia in a person with suggestive symptoms from an area endemic for filariasis is to rule out major differential diagnostic possibilities, determine whether antifilarial antibodies are present, and begin presumptive treatment with DEC.

Differential diagnoses include Löffler's syndrome, chronic eosinophilic pneumonia, allergic aspergillosis, autoimmune vasculitis, drug allergies, and infections with other parasites, e.g., trichinellosis and strongyloidiasis and seasonal pneumonitis due to *Ascaris*. Tissue biopsies, if warranted, may be specific.

TREATMENT. DEC, 4 to 6 mg/kg body weight daily for 14 to 21 days, is the treatment of choice, and is usually followed by rapid improvement. Steroids should be avoided if the diagnosis is uncertain, as they may mask the true etiology and may be harmful in some conditions, e.g., strongyloidiasis.

BIBLIOGRAPHY

Beaver PC: Filariasis without microfilaremia. Am J Trop Med Hyg 19:181, 1970.
Danaraj TJ, Pacheco G, Shanmugaratnam K, Beaver PC: The etiology and pathology of eosinophilic lung (tropical eosinophilia). Am J Trop Med Hyg 15:183, 1976.
Geddes DM: Pulmonary eosinophilia. J R Coll Physicians Lond 20:139, 1986.
Lie KJ: Occult filariasis: Its relationship with tropical eosinophilia. Am J Trop Med Hyg 11:646, 1962.
Meyers FM, Kouwenaar W: Over hypereosinophilie en over een markvaardigen vorm van filariosis. Geneesk Tijdschr Ned-Ind 79:853, 1939.
Neva FA, Ottesen EA: Current concepts in parasitology. Tropical (filarial) eosinophilia. N Engl J Med 298:1129, 1978.

86. LOIASIS

Brian O.L. Duke

DEFINITION. Loiasis is caused by infection with the filarial nematode *Loa loa*. The adult worms migrate through the subcutaneous tissues causing fugitive "Calabar swellings" and sometimes migrate beneath the conjunctiva (hence, the popular name "eye worm"). Microfilariae are found in the peripheral blood during the day. Vectors are tabanid flies belonging to the genus *Chrysops*.

DISTRIBUTION. Loiasis is endemic to the rain forest areas of Central and West Africa, including Zaire, Northwest Angola, Congo, Gabon, Central African Republic, Cameroon, Nigeria, Chad, Southwest Sudan, and Equatorial Guinea; and perhaps also Uganda.

TRANSMISSION

Adult Worms. Adult *Loa* in the subcutaneous connective tissues are thin, transparent worms; the females measure 50 to 70 × 0.5 mm, the males, 30 to 35 × 0.3 to 0.4 mm. The cuticle of the middle region in both sexes has numerous, small bosses that aid in identifying portions of worms removed at biopsy. The head has a ring of 6 small papillae behind the mouth. The posterior end of the female has a pair of terminal papillae; that of the male is curved ventrally with 5 pairs of large pedunculated papillae, 3 pairs of small sessile papillae, and 2 unequal spicules.

Microfilariae. The microfilariae in the peripheral blood stream show a diurnal periodicity, being most plentiful between 8:00 AM and 5:00 PM. They are sheathed and measure 230 to 300 × 6 to 8 μm.

Vectors. The vectors are large tabanid flies of the genus *Chrysops*, known in Africa as red flies. The species *C. silacea* and *C. dimidiata* are the most important. The day-biting female flies pick up the microfilariae of *Loa* in their blood meals. The ingested microfilariae lose their sheaths, penetrate the gut wall, and migrate to the cells of the fat body, where they molt twice. The infective filariform larvae develop in 10 to 12 days and move to the proboscis. Many larvae (up to 100) can develop in a single fly. When the fly bites a new host, larvae enter through the puncture wound, and males and females develop in the subcutaneous connective tissues. Fertilization occurs by 90 days, and microfilariae appear in the peripheral blood stream in 6 to 12 months. The adult worms may survive for 4 to 17 years.

Epidemiology. The distribution of the disease is determined by that of the vectors, which breed in wet mud on the edge of shaded streams beneath the high-canopied rain forest in which the adult *Chrysops* live. Flies descend to ground level to bite humans and are attracted by the movement of people or vehicles or by rising wood smoke. Particularly favorable vector-host conditions are created by rubber plantations, which form a dense canopy 30 to 50 feet above ground level. Infection

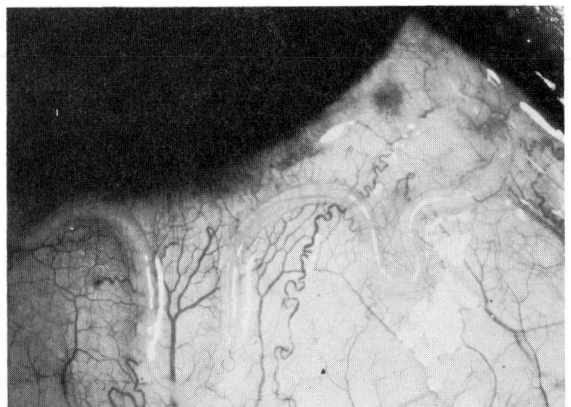

FIGURE 86–1. Adult *Loa* worm migrating beneath conjunctiva. (Courtsey of Dr. J. Anderson.)

rates are usually higher in adults, particularly males, than in children, probably because of an increased exposure to biting flies. Flies are most common during the rainy season and will enter houses only if they are well lit inside.

Reservoirs. Monkeys, especially the drill (*Mandrillus leucophaeus*), harbor a form of *Loa*, but the microfilariae of this form are nocturnally periodic and the vectors are night-biting *C. langi* and *C. centurionis*. Although the 2 strains have been hybridized experimentally, it is unlikely that monkeys act as reservoir hosts because the nocturnal vector species *Chrysops* do not usually bite humans.

CLINICAL MANIFESTATIONS

Calabar Swellings. The first definite signs are usually the formation of recurrent subcutaneous swellings, most commonly in the region of the wrists and forearms and often following use of the part. These are known as Calabar swellings and are a hypersensitivity response to antigenic material released by a migrating, developing, or adult worm. The overlying skin becomes erythematous, edematous (nonpitting), and itchy. The swelling lasts a few hours or days and is usually painless but, if near a joint, may cause difficulty in flexion. It may also

be accompanied by fever, irritability, urticaria, and pruritus.

Other Symptoms and Signs. Not infrequently, adults or migrating larvae cross the eye, beneath the conjunctiva (Fig. 86–1) or in the skin, and cause swelling of the lids (Fig. 86–2) with itching and pain. Dying worms under the skin may cause a granulomatous reaction and fibrosis (Fig. 86–3); worms have been excised from the subcutaneous tissues of many parts of the body.

Many patients have no clearly defined signs or symptoms for years before infection is diagnosed, but there may have been undetected symptoms of fatigue, recurrent fever, and perhaps arthritic pains. In most cases loiasis is a relatively benign disease with a good prognosis.

Eosinophilia is common and may exceed 70% (or 20,000 cells/mm³).

Complications. Various visceral lesions have been attributed to loiasis, but the most serious complication is meningoencephalitis, which is sometimes fatal. It is accompanied by retinal hemorrhages and appears to be associated with diethylcarbamazine (DEC) treatment in patients with a high microfilaremia. Occasionally, microfilariae are found in the cerebrospinal fluid of such patients, and encephalitis is presumably caused either by an allergic reaction to dead and dying microfilariae that obstruct the capillaries of the brain or by the

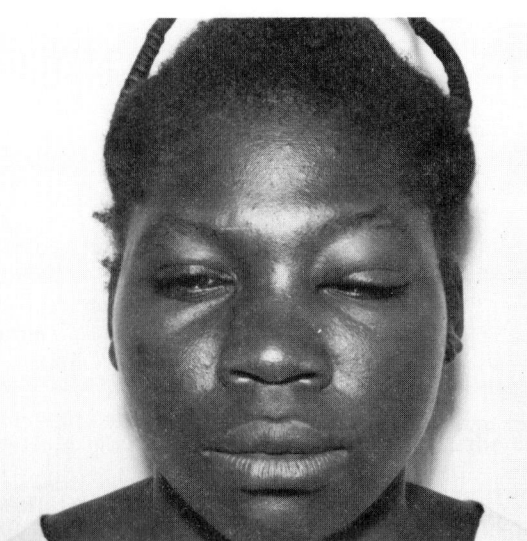

FIGURE 86–2. Zairian woman with Calabar swelling around left eye. (Courtesy of the Armed Forces Institute of Pathology. Photograph Neg. No. 68–7638–15.)

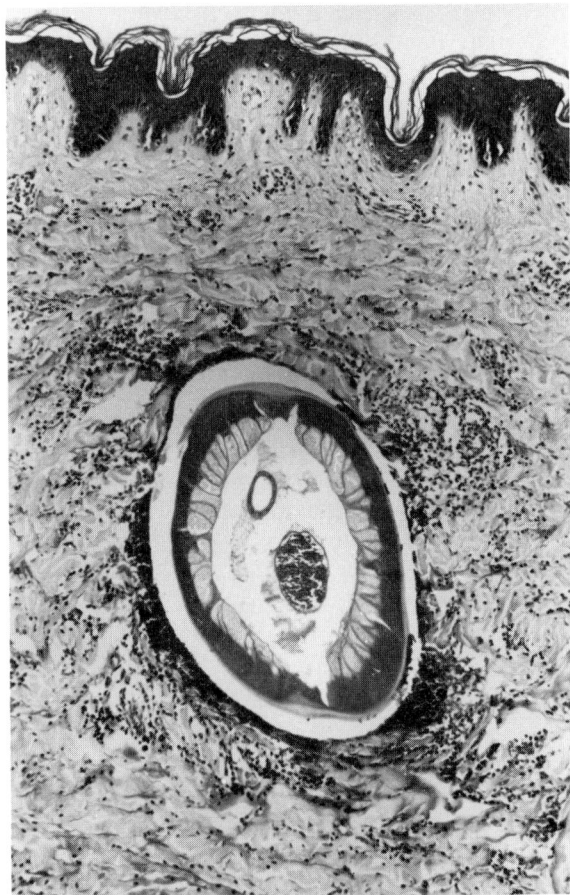

FIGURE 86–3. Section of dying adult male *Loa* worm in subdermis surrounded by intense tissue reaction. Biopsy specimen of Calabar swelling.

neurotoxic effect of their death. In a few cases neurologic manifestations may be severe and even fatal.

A proportion of patients, particularly chronic sufferers, are amicrofilaremic, and it is probable either that these are unisexual infections or that microfilariae are being destroyed by immune responses in these hypersensitized individuals. Endomyocardial fibrosis and nephrotic syndrome, which are sometimes reported from such patients, are considered autoimmune disorders.

DIAGNOSIS

Microfilariae in Blood. The routine method is to identify microfilariae in a peripheral thick blood film (20 to 60 mm³) taken during the day. The sheathed microfilariae have a kinked appearance in stained blood films, with nuclei extending to the tip of the tail; the sheath does not stain with Giemsa stain. Concentration techniques can be tried in patients with few circulating microfilariae. One of the best methods is to pass about 5 ml of hemolyzed blood through a 3-μm Nuclepore membrane filter and then stain this after fixation in methyl alcohol.

Clinical Observations. In many cases diagnosis is not made until the characteristic Calabar swellings appear or until adult worms are seen migrating across the eye or under the skin. Sometimes dead calcified worms are seen on a roentgenogram.

Serology. Immunodiagnostic tests are confined to academic institutions and are rather nonspecific. The indirect fluorescent antibody (IFA) and enzyme-linked immunosorbent assay (ELISA) tests are helpful in amicrofilaremic patients and can be useful for diagnosis in travelers from endemic areas of Africa who are suffering from general malaise accompanied by a high eosinophilia.

TREATMENT

Diethylcarbamazine. This drug has been used since 1951 and is effective in killing microfilariae. It also has a much slower action against adult worms, and higher doses may be necessary. The drug does not have a straightforward lethal effect but works in conjunction with the body's cellular defense responses, in some way enabling the host to recognize the parasite as foreign.

In cases of loiasis with no or few circulating microfilariae, 50 mg of DEC can be given to an adult on the first day of treatment and the dose doubled each day for 4 days. The final dosage of 400 mg/day should be continued for 7 to 21 days and may have to be repeated after 1 to 3 months. However, in patients with a high microfilaremia, e.g., 500 microfilariae/20 mm³ of blood, 25 mg should be given the first day and 50 mg the next, and then, if there are no untoward side effects, the regular dosage schedule can be followed. Otherwise, the DEC may be given under corticosteroid coverage, or in extreme cases, it may be necessary to perform plasmapheresis to remove most of the microfilariae from the peripheral blood before treating with DEC. This is to avoid the possibility of meningoencephalitis, which can follow treatment. With any dosage regimen, mild side effects may occur at the beginning of treatment, e.g., urticaria, fever, and nausea; these can be treated with an antihistamine preparation. Care should be taken to ascertain whether the patient also has onchocerciasis, since DEC can cause severe cutaneous reactions in these patients.

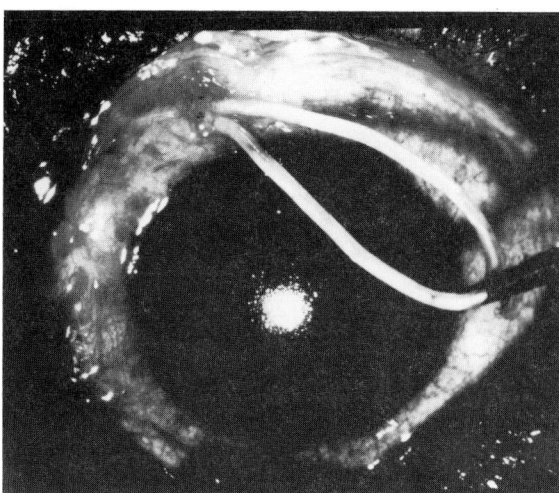

FIGURE 86–4. Surgical removal of *Loa* worm from eye. (Courtesy of the Armed Forces Institute of Pathology. Photograph Neg. No. 75–1789–4.)

Recently, mebendazole, in dosages of 100 to 500 mg 3 times a day for 28 days, has been shown to reduce microfilaremia over 4 to 6 weeks without complications. It is not known whether it affects the adult worms, but it could be used to reduce the high microfilaremia before giving DEC.

Prophylaxis. A prophylactic daily dose of DEC, 5 mg/kg body weight for 3 days every month, has been suggested.

Surgery. Adult worms not infrequently wander across the eye beneath the conjunctiva at a speed of about 1 cm/minute. They can then be anesthetized with a few drops of 10% cocaine and removed after cutting the conjunctiva with a surgical needle (Fig. 86–4).

CONTROL. Elimination of the insect vectors by larval insecticides is feasible but is not usually a cost-effective proposition. The clearance of forest around dwellings, screening of houses for mosquitoes, and wearing long trousers and long-sleeved shirts can effectively reduce personal exposure to *Chrysops* in endemic areas.

BIBLIOGRAPHY

Duke BOL: Behavioural aspects of the life cycle of *Loa*. *In* Canning EU, Wright CA (eds): Behavioural Aspects of Parasite Transmission. London and New York, Academic Press, 1972, pp 97–108.
Fain A: Les problèmes actuels de la loase. Bull WHO 56:155, 1978.

87. ONCHOCERCIASIS

Brian O.L. Duke
and Hugh R. Taylor

DEFINITION. Onchocerciasis is infection of humans by the filarial nematode *Onchocerca volvulus*. The parasite is transmitted by blackflies of the genus *Simulium*. In many individuals the infection produces little or no disease, but those with heavy infections usually have 3 cardinal manifestations: dermatitis, eye lesions, and subcutaneous nodules. The clinical pattern varies from patient to patient and also from one geographic region to another. There are many regional and local names for onchocerciasis, a few of which reflect particular features of the disease, e.g., river blindness, blinding filarial disease, enfermedad de Robles, erisípela de la costa, mal morado, craw-craw, gâle filarienne, and ceguera de los rios.

ETIOLOGY AND MORPHOLOGY OF ADULT WORMS AND MICROFILARIAE. Female worms are 23 to 50 cm long and 250 to 450 μm wide; male worms are 16 to 42 mm long and 125 to 200 μm wide. A helpful diagnostic feature is the regularly spaced cuticular annulations of the adult female. These are circular ridges about 8 μm wide and spaced about 50 μm apart at midbody. Typical transverse sections of the female at midbody reveal 2 thin-walled uteri and an intestine. The cuticular annulations of the male worm are between 5 and 10 μm wide and are adjacent to each other. Longitudinal and transverse sections of adult worms usually reveal hypodermis, lateral cords, and somatic muscle, any of which may be prominent or barely perceptible.

Microfilariae vary from 220 to 360 μm by 5 to 9 μm (Fig. 87–1*A*). They are unsheathed and have a cephalic space 7 to 13 μm long and anterior nuclei that are side by side (Fig. 87–1*B*). The caudal space is 9 to 15 μm, the terminal nuclei are elongated, and the tail is tapered to a fine point (Fig. 87–1*C*). These features distinguish the microfilariae of *O. volvulus* from those of *Mansonella streptocerca*, which also live extravascularly in the dermis, and from those of *Mansonella ozzardi*, which live in the superficial capillaries. The presence of either *M. streptocerca* or *M. ozzardi* may result in a false-positive diagnosis of onchocerciasis unless care is taken to examine the microfilariae.

PREVALENCE AND DISTRIBUTION. Onchocerciasis occurs in regions of the tropics where there are abundant human-biting *Simulium* vectors, i.e., near rivers where these blackflies breed. As of 1985 the estimated global total of persons infected with *O. volvulus* was 17.75 million, of whom 340,000 were blind and a like number had severely impaired vision.

Onchocerciasis is most prevalent in Africa and is a major public health problem along the main rivers of the northern Sudano-Guinean savanna: from Senegal, Guinea, Sierra Leone, and Liberia in the west through the World Bank/World Health Organization Onchocerciasis Control Programme area (which includes parts of Mali, Ivory Coast, Upper Volta, Ghana, Togo, Benin,

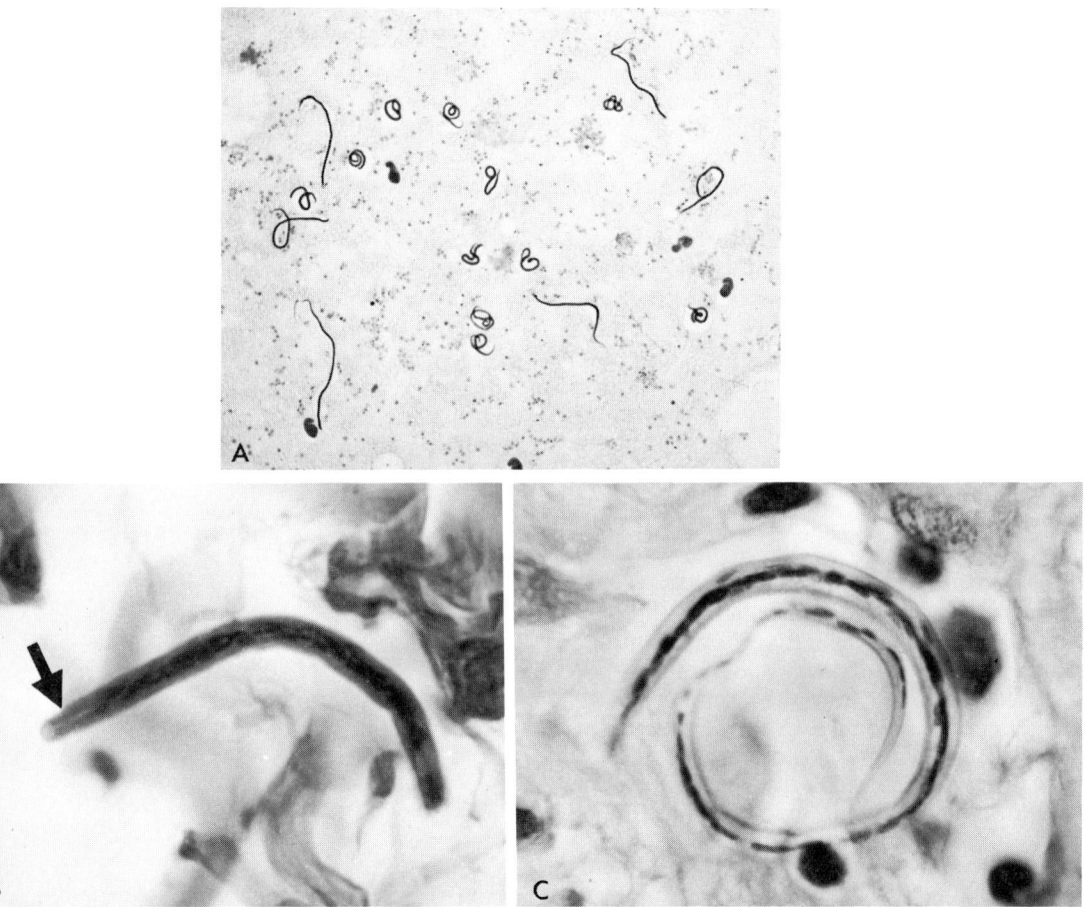

FIGURE 87–1. Microfilariae of *Onchocerca volvulus*. *A,* Touch smear preparation from dissected onchocercal nodule on iliac crest of patient in Zaire. Coiled and extended microfilariae at different stages of development were released from the uteri of gravid female worms during dissection (Giemsa stain, × 100). (Courtesy of the Armed Forces Institute of Pathology, Photograph Neg. No. 72–507.) *B,* Anterior end of a microfilaria of *O. volvulus* in skin. There is a characteristic cephalic clear space of about 9 μm before the first nucleus (*arrow*) (hematoxylin & eosin stain, × 1080). (Courtesy of the Armed Forces Institute of Pathology, Photograph Neg. No. 72–3238.) *C,* Posterior end of a microfilaria of *O. volvulus* in dermal collagen. There is a caudal clear space of about 12 μm from the elongated terminal nucleus to the tip (hematoxylin & eosin stain, × 1080). (Courtesy of the Armed Forces Institute of Pathology, Photograph Neg. No. 71–100072.)

and Niger) and then into Nigeria, Chad, Cameroon, the Central African Republic, Zaire, and the Sudan to reach as far east as the Ethiopian highlands and Uganda (Fig. 87–2). A less severe but equally widespread form of onchocerciasis occurs throughout most of the rain forest regions of West Africa and the Congo River basin, with an extension into the southern savanna regions of Angola, Tanzania, and Malawi. Onchocerciasis was at one time prevalent in western Kenya, but this focus has been eliminated. There is an extension into Arabia in South Yemen, North Yemen, and north along the mountain ridge stretching into Asir Province in Saudi Arabia (Fig. 87–2).

In Latin America there are foci of onchocerciasis in Guatemala, Mexico, Venezuela, Colombia, Ecuador, and Brazil (Fig. 87–2). The discoveries of isolated foci in forest areas and of differences in the biologic properties and pathogenicity of the parasites in Central and South America, as compared with the African parasites, suggest that the parasite may have existed in the former region for a long period and also suggests the possibility of an animal reservoir in South America. In Africa there are many different species of *Onchocerca* in wild and domestic animals, but *O. volvulus* has been detected only in the gorilla. With the exception of the chimpanzee, which is susceptible to some strains of the parasite, attempts to transmit the infection to animals have failed.

THE VECTOR. The species of blackfly that transmit *O. volvulus* vary from one endemic region to another. In West Africa the common vectors are related sibling species referred to as the *Simulium damnosum* complex (Fig. 87–3). They are hard to distinguish on morphologic grounds, but they have different banding patterns on the polytene chromosomes of the larval salivary glands and they occupy different niches in the environment. The most important vectors in the Western Hemisphere are *S. ochraceum* in Guatemala and Mexico, *S. metallicum* in Venezuela, *S. exiguum* and *S. quadrivittatum* in Colombia and Ecuador, and *S. oyapockense* and *S. guianense* on the Brazil-Venezuela border. All of the *Simulium* vectors breed in fast-flowing streams and rivers (Fig. 87–4). Although both healthy and infected blackflies may travel great distances (up to 400 km for *S. damnosum*) on the wind, transmission is most intense along the banks of the turbulent streams and rivers in which these flies multiply. Humans who develop severe infections frequent these streams regularly, where they are bitten repeatedly while wading, washing, fishing, bathing, or collecting water.

TRANSMISSION AND LIFE CYCLE. Onchocerciasis is spread from person to person by the bite of *Simulium* species, known popularly as blackflies. Blackflies have short, coarse mouth parts that rasp and tear through the keratin and dermis, where they produce a pool of cells, debris, and tissue fluids into which the microfilariae of *O. volvulus* are attracted. The saliva of the fly acts as an anticoagulant and an attractant that enables the *Simulium* vector to ingest large numbers of the tissue-dwelling microfilariae. The microfilariae then migrate into the flight muscles; after a period of 7 to 9 days, the infective larvae emerge. They move into the proboscis and are transmitted when the fly next bites a person (Fig. 87–5). It is assumed that the infective larvae remain in the subcutaneous tissue undergoing 2 further molts before they become mature worms. In experimentally infected chimpanzees, development to patency, i.e., when the microfilariae can be found in the skin, may take 10 months to 2 years; in humans the prepatent interval appears to be of the same order.

In Africa adult worms are predominantly found in the dermis and subcutaneous tissues around the pelvis. In heavy infections they are found over many other bony prominences and in deeper sites. In Guatemala and Mexico a greater proportion of adult worms are found in the upper part of the body, especially the head. After the male and female adult worms copulate, the gravid female produces millions of microfilariae, which tend to concentrate in skin, eyes, and lymph nodes. Adult worms survive for up to 15 years after cessation of transmission, as was noted following the elimination of the vector in Kenya. The microfilariae may persist for up to 2 years after the death of the adult worms.

PATHOLOGY. The adult worms are usually innocuous, apart from the production of unsightly nodules. By contrast, the microfilariae migrate through many tissues of the body and cause damaging and progressive lesions. After several months of active life the microfilariae degenerate and provoke the inflammatory lesions and subsequent scar tissue that characterize the disease.

Nodules. Most adult worms eventually become encapsulated and form discrete nodules in the deep dermis and subcutaneous tissue, especially over bony prominences (Figs. 87–6 and 87–7), or in deeper sites near joints, muscles, and bones. The triggering mechanism for encapsulation is unknown. Adult worms may release antigens, causing inflammation that leads to encapsulation, or they may be traumatized while migrating over bony prominences, provoking inflammation and eventual encapsulation. This might explain the anatomic location of nodules over bony prominences. The inflammatory reaction to adult worms includes (1) suppuration with neutrophils and fibrin; (2) a granulomatous component characterized by foamy histiocytes, epithelioid cells, and foreign body giant cells; and (3) granulation tissue that gradually matures to form a hyalinized "capsule." The female worms within this capsule are tightly coiled and "incarcerated" (Fig. 87–8*A* and *B*). The male worms tend to be found on the outer surface of the nodules and may migrate from one nodule to another.

Cutaneous Lesions. The gravid female worms produce microfilariae for many years. Degenerating microfilariae provoke 2 distinct types of reaction. The first is an accumulation of eosinophils around microfilariae. This also occurs within minutes after taking diethylcarbamazine (DEC). Associated changes are local edema, deposits of fibrin and inflammatory mucins, and hyperemia (Fig. 87–9). The second type of reaction is formation of a granuloma; the degenerating microfilaria is surrounded by histiocytes, epithelioid cells, and giant cells. The inflammatory changes take place in the upper dermis and include edema, fibrosis, dilated lymphatics, and tortuosity of blood vessels, with the inflammatory cells concentrated around vessels and appendages. The mi-

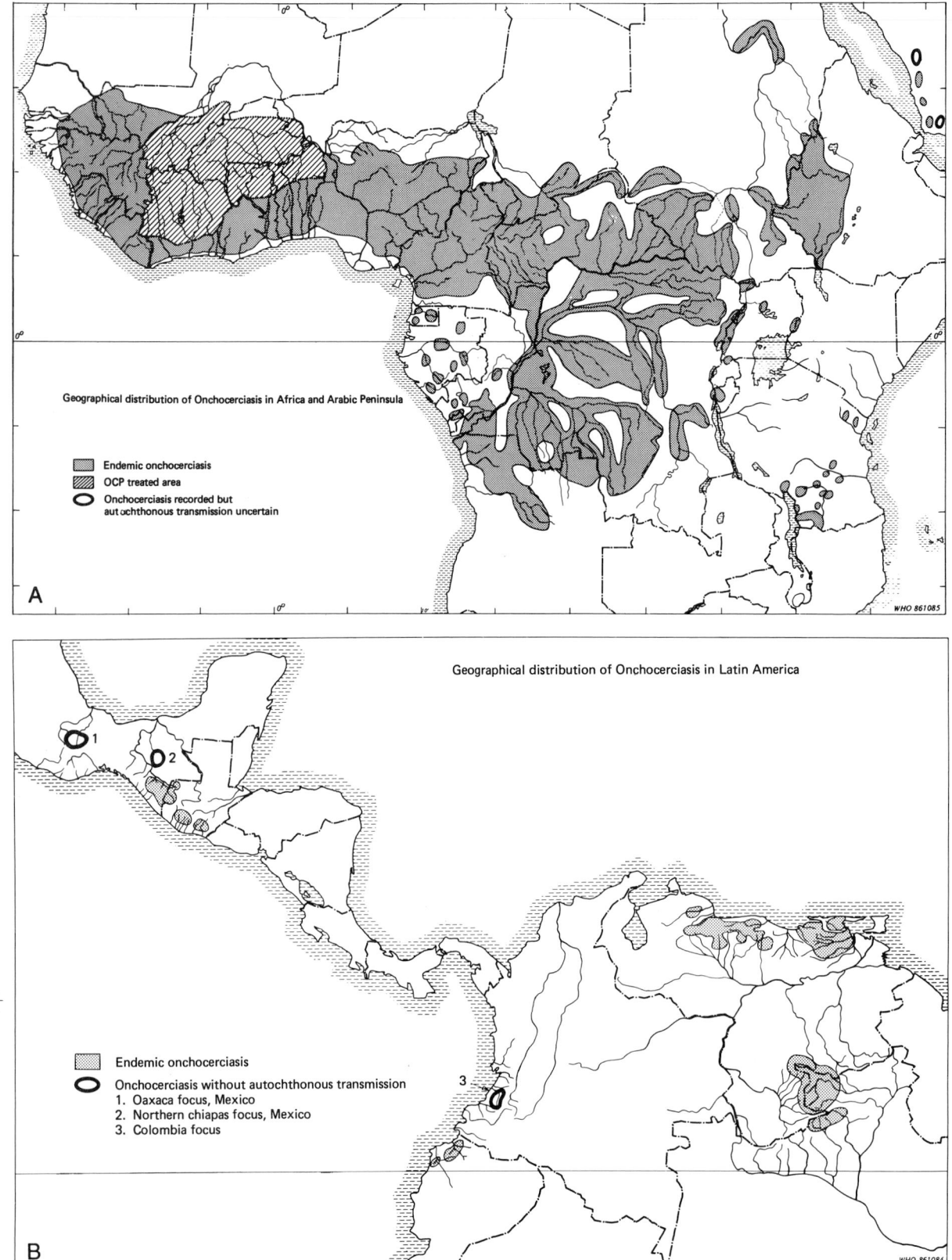

FIGURE 87–2. Maps showing the distribution of onchocerciasis: Africa, Arabia, and Central and South America. (By permission of the World Health Organization.)

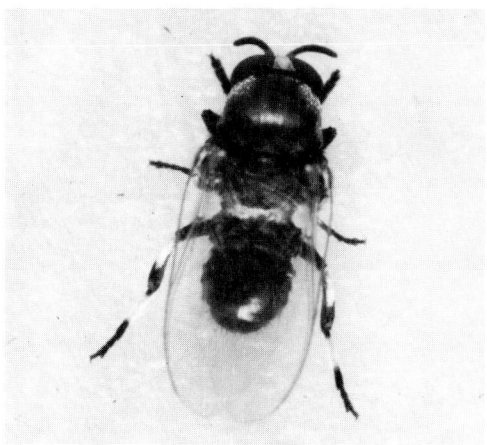

FIGURE 87–3. One of the blackflies in the *Simulium damnosum* complex, feeding on a person. The length of the fly is about 3.5 mm (× 14.8). (Courtesy of the Armed Forces Institute of Pathology, Photograph Neg. No. 72–4519E.)

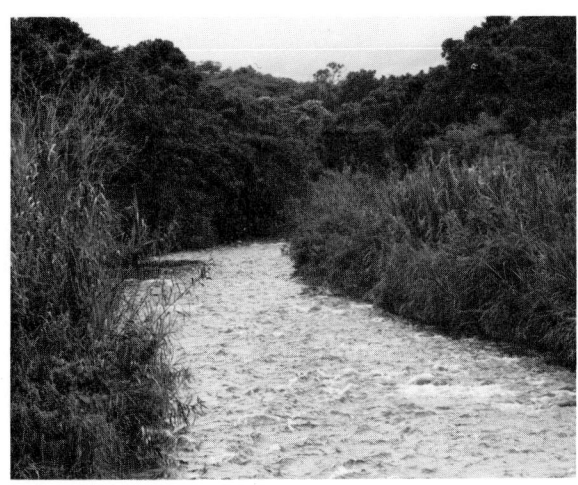

FIGURE 87–4. A turbulent river in Uganda with overhanging vegetation—characteristic features of breeding sites of the *S. damnosum* complex. (Courtesy of the Armed Forces Institute of Pathology, Photograph Neg. No. 68–2392.)

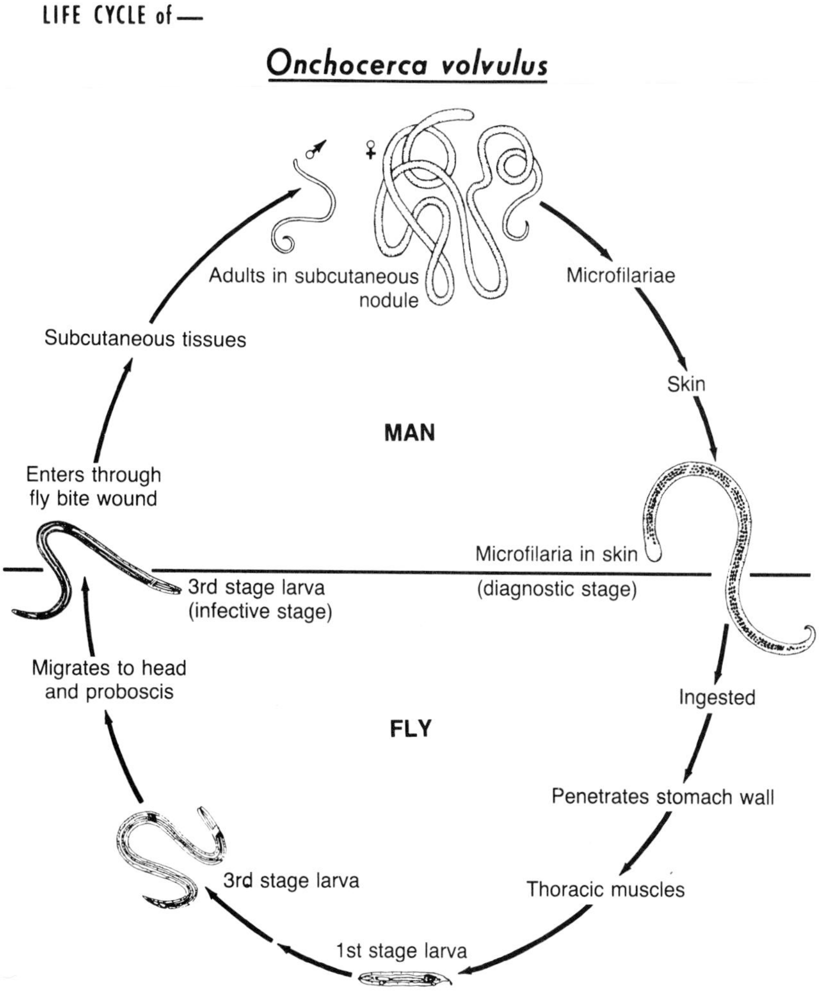

crofilariae are outside the vessels between dermal collagen fibers; they may be numerous or few but tend to be concentrated in the upper dermis and the dermal papillae.

There is often an associated enlargement of lymph nodes, especially with "sowda," the Arabian form of the disease, which is characterized by a hyper-reactive

inflammatory cell infiltrate of the dermis with sclerosis and edema, often affecting only 1 limb. Phagocytosed melanin is prominent in the epidermis, the number of elastic fibers is reduced, and there are few microfilariae. However, with the more usual form of the disease, the skin changes are more diffuse. The elastic fibers are

LIFE CYCLE of—

Onchocerca volvulus

FIGURE 87–5. Life cycle of *O. volvulus*. (From Melvin DM, Brooke MM, Healy GR, et al: Common Blood and Tissue Parasites. Life Cycle Charts. Atlanta, Centers for Disease Control, 1961.)

Adults in subcutaneous nodule

Microfilariae

Subcutaneous tissues

Skin

MAN

Enters through fly bite wound

Microfilaria in skin (diagnostic stage)

3rd stage larva (infective stage)

Migrates to head and proboscis

Ingested

FLY

3rd stage larva

Penetrates stomach wall

Thoracic muscles

1st stage larva

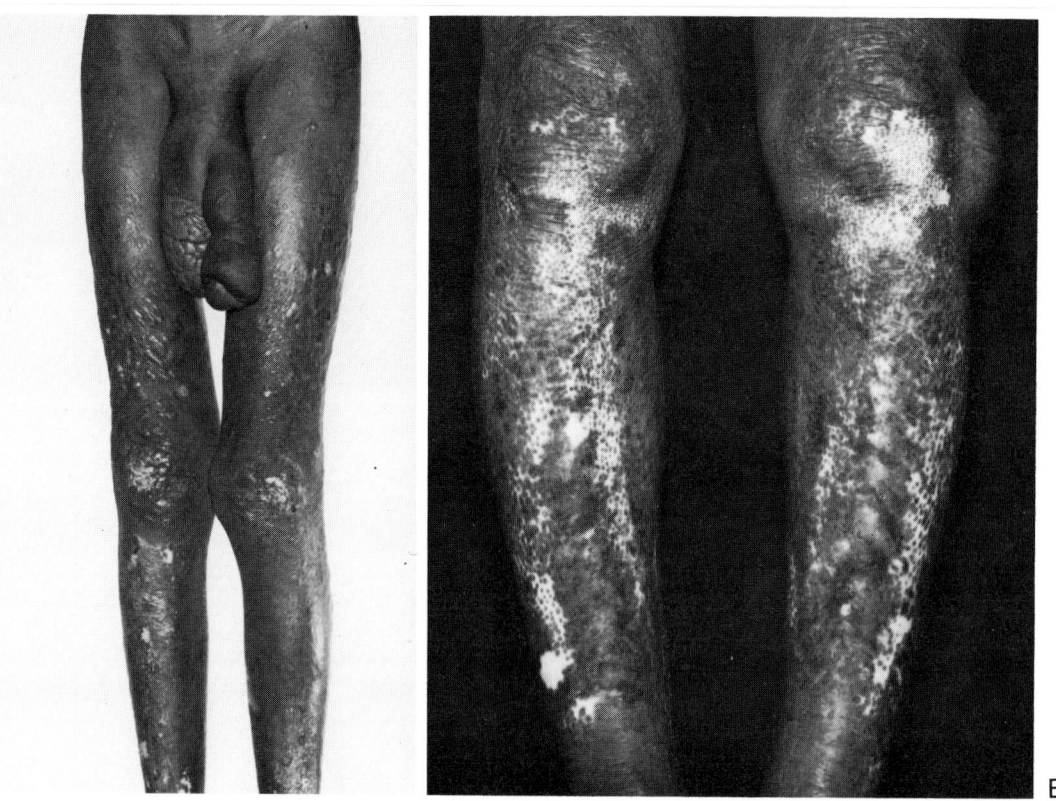

A

B

FIGURE 87–6. *A,* This 11-year-old boy in the Ubangi Territory of northern Zaire has onchocercal nodules over the knees and ribs; severe dermatitis with depigmentation, papules, wrinkling, and thickening; and inguinal lymphadenopathy with elephantoid changes of the penis and scrotum. (Courtesy of the Armed Forces Institute of Pathology, Photograph Neg. No. 68–7912-1.) *B,* This 48-year-old man in the rain forest of Cameroon has a cluster of onchocercal nodules over the left knee and "leopard skin" of the knees and shins. (Courtesy of the Armed Forces Institute of Pathology, Photograph Neg. No. 72–17223.)

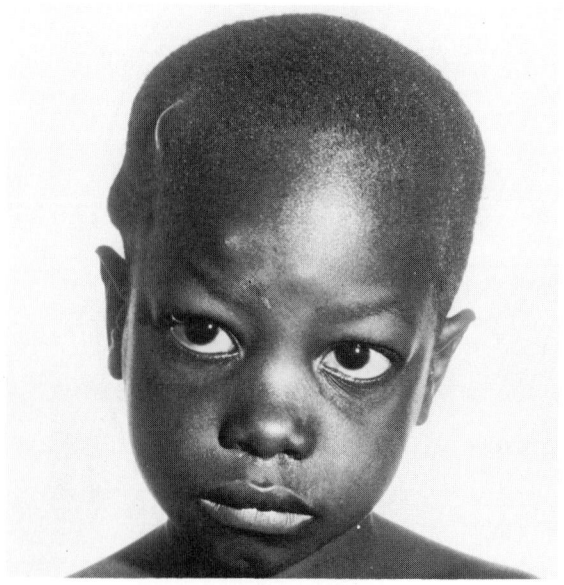

FIGURE 87–7. Young boy in Ubangi Territory of Zaire, who has 3 onchocercal nodules on the forehead and skull. (Courtesy of the Armed Forces Institute of Pathology, Photograph Neg. No. 69-3619.)

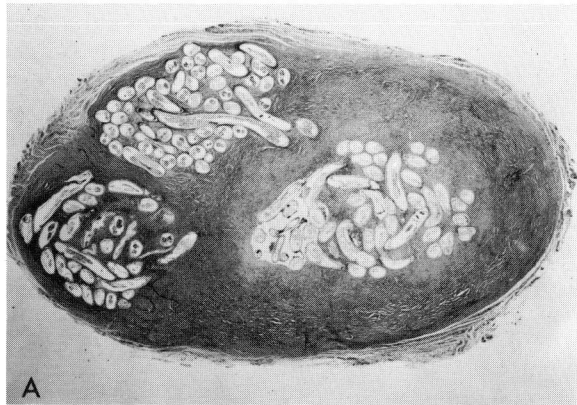

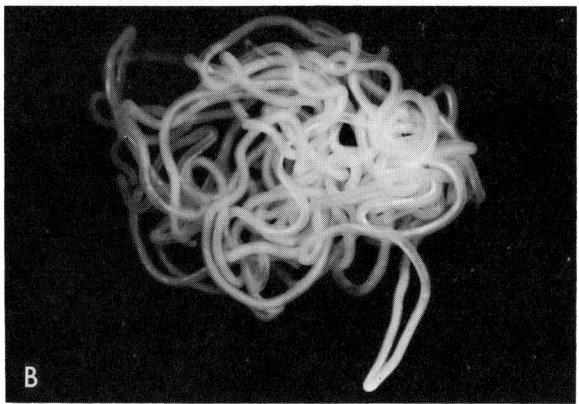

FIGURE 87–8. Adult worms of *O. volvulus*. *A*, Microscopic section through an onchocercal nodule (1.3 × 0.7 cm), showing several coiled adult worms (mostly gravid females). The worms are surrounded and incarcerated by hyalinized scar (Russell-Movat, × 8.2). (Courtesy of the Armed Forces Institute of Pathology, Photograph Neg. No. 69-3639.) *B*, Entangled adult worms, after collagenase digestion of an onchocercal nodule. The cluster measures about 1.1 × 0.9 cm. The individual worms are up to 0.5 mm across and 50 cm long (× 6.9). (Courtesy of the Armed Forces Institute of Pathology, Photograph Neg. No. 80-12068.)

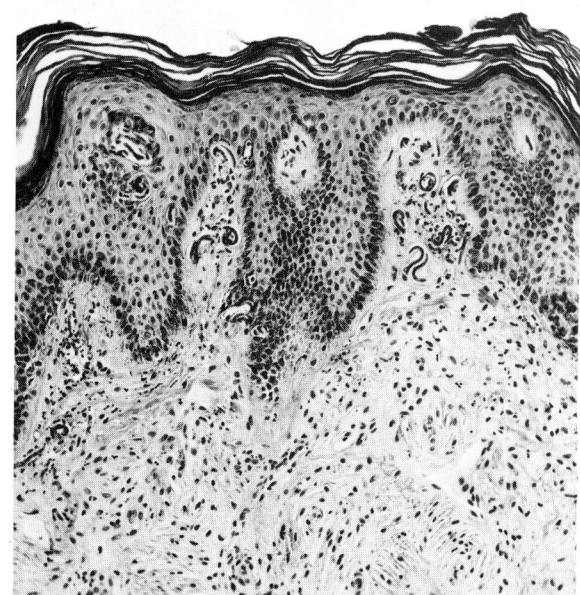

FIGURE 87–9. Post-treatment skin of buttocks of patient in Cameroon, after 2 oral doses of diethylcarbamazine (DEC). There are many microfilariae in the dermal papillae, with some migrating into the epidermis as a result of the treatment. Other features characteristic of onchocercal dermatitis include edema, dilated lymphatics, hyperkeratosis, and acanthosis with elongation of rete ridges (hematoxylin & eosin stain, × 125). (Courtesy of the Armed Forces Institute of Pathology, Photograph Neg. No. 73-5681.)

destroyed and the dermal collagen is replaced by scar tissue, resulting in an aged appearance (presbydermia). Scarring in lymph nodes may eventually obstruct the flow of lymph and cause regional lymphedema with "hanging groin" (Fig. 87–10) or sometimes elephantiasis (Fig. 87–6 *A*).

IMMUNOPATHOLOGY. The immune system of individuals infected with *O. volvulus* clearly recognizes the presence of the parasite, as is shown by the occurrence of specific antibodies and primed lymphocytes, and the presence in infected tissues of various cells associated with the immune system. Despite this recognition, the way in which the immune system actually responds varies considerably from patient to patient, and a clinical spectrum paralleling an immunologic spectrum appears to be present in this disease, as it does in other tropical diseases such as leprosy. This spectrum is best demonstrated in the cell-mediated immune (CMI) responses, in which patients with active skin disease—who in all probability are actively killing a majority of their resident microfilariae—also have a strong CMI response to *O. volvulus* antigens. Patients with quiescent skin disease, and often with high numbers of microfilariae, do not have an active CMI response; it is probable

that a specific immunosuppression exists in these individuals.

As with other helminths, in vitro studies have implicated eosinophils as the cells central to immunologically mediated damage to microfilariae, and probably to other

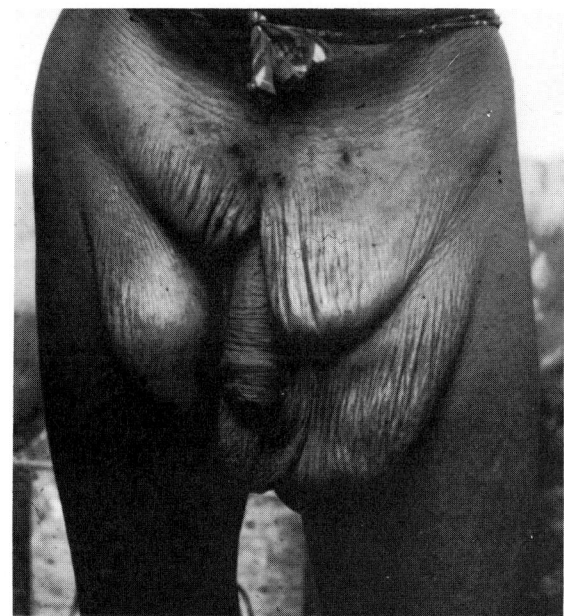

FIGURE 87–10. This 45-year-old man in Cameroon has bilateral inguinal and femoral hanging groins (adenolymphoceles). Inguinal and femoral lymph nodes beneath hanging groins are fibrotic and contain microfilariae of *O. volvulus*. (Courtesy of the Armed Forces Institute of Pathology, Photograph Neg. No. 73-6655; contributed by Dr. John Anderson, Helminthiasis Research Unit, Kumba, Cameroon.)

stages of *O. volvulus* as well. These findings support the observations of eosinophils and eosinophil-derived products at the in vivo sites of dying microfilariae. The function of eosinophil in vitro requires the presence of a surface antigen–specific IgG antibody and is greatly enhanced by the presence of complement. The sera most effective in this in vitro phenomenon are those taken from patients who are actively killing most of their microfilariae. For example, patients whose corneal-residing microfilariae are involved in detectable host reactions (i.e., punctate fluffy opacities) also commonly have serum that mediates eosinophil damage to microfilariae in vitro. Eosinophils also adhere to and damage infective larvae in vitro, provided suitable serum is present. The mechanisms involved in the destruction of adult worms are not understood. Adult worms within nodules often have host serum proteins, including specific anti–*O. volvulus* IgG, present on their epicuticle, and similar proteins are present within degenerating worms. Cells known to be involved in immune-mediated damage, particularly eosinophils and macrophages, are also commonly associated with the surface of adult worms and are likely to be involved in their destruction.

The involvement of the immune system in the development of pathologic lesions is perhaps most clearly seen in those patients with concurrent active CMI and active dermatitis, typified by the condition known as sowda. The consequences of the active immune killing of the microfilariae in these individuals are highly undesirable. Although there is some evidence that patients with active CMI have more severe corneal lesions, in general few data are available on the role of the immune system in the ocular lesions. This is particularly so with regard to the important fundal lesions. It has long been suggested, in the absence of any evidence of a direct role for microfilariae, that the fundal lesions are caused by soluble factors, including antigens and immune complexes. Levels of immune complex in patients with onchocerciasis vary greatly, as is to be expected in persons who concurrently have a number of other complex-stimulating diseases (e.g., malaria). Specific immune complexes and circulating antigens of *O. volvulus* can be isolated from sera, and serum antiretinal antibodies can be found in patients with chorioretinal disease. However, to date no clear correlation between these findings and clinical features has been determined. Nevertheless, aspects of onchocerciasis do involve vascular changes, and immunopathologic phenomena may be occurring in or around vessels, possibly involving immune complexes.

Changes in an individual's immune status occur during the adverse reactions following DEC therapy. Both nonspecific and specific immune complex levels increase, and there is an infiltration of eosinophils into the tissues (where the cells degranulate around microfilariae), together with degranulation of mast cells and basophils. DEC also promotes the microfilaria-damaging function of eosinophils, probably via a drug receptor on the surface of these cells. Specific antibody levels rise following DEC therapy, and there is some increase in lymphocyte sensitivity to *O. volvulus*; however, the significance of these findings is unclear, and they may simply occur in response to the death of microfilariae.

One of the main goals for the immunologic studies of onchocerciasis, other than aiding the characterization of the clinicopathologic spectrum, is in immunodiagnosis. The development of a less invasive and more sensitive test than skin snips is most likely to involve an immunoassay. Tests using stage-specific antigens of *O. volvulus* to detect circulating antigen in serum are being developed. Several microassays and skin tests using *O. volvulus* antigens, as well as antigens of other filariae, have been employed with varying success; delayed hypersensitivity to *O. volvulus*, however, is useful in the diagnosis of patients with severe dermatitis and low microfilarial loads.

The important question of whether the immune system affords any protection to infected individuals has not been answered. Heavily infected patients cleared of *O. volvulus* by chemotherapy do not appear to be substantially protected against reinfection. Nevertheless, active killing of microfilariae in certain patients suggests that immunoprotection can occur, at least to this stage. Immunomodulation of the disease remains a distant promise. This is emphasized by the fact that uncontrolled immunostimulation may lead to worsening of the pathologic lesions, rather than to their reduction. Despite these facts, immunoprotection against infective larvae may be achievable.

OCULAR LESIONS. Lesions of the eye are directly or indirectly related to invasion and local death of microfilariae. Relatively few eyes have been examined histopathologically, and most have had end-stage disease that obscured the earlier changes. Live microfilariae may be found in many parts of the eye, including the conjunctiva, cornea, posterior sclera, anterior and posterior chambers, vitreous, uveal tract, inner retina, and the optic nerve and its sheath. Live microfilariae in these sites cause little reaction; their death produces lesions.

Corneal Lesions. There are two types of corneal opacity: (1) "Fluffy" or "snowflake" punctate opacities (Fig. 87–11) clear without residual change and are focal collections of lymphocytes and eosinophils, with some interstitial edema, which form around dead or dying microfilariae. (2) Sclerosing keratitis (Fig. 87–12) is a progressive fibrovascular pannus and inflammatory infiltrate composed mainly of lymphocytes and eosinophils and starting at the level of Bowman's membrane.

Uveitis (Fig. 87–12). Mild, chronic, nongranulomatous uveitis is common with heavy microfilarial invasion. More severe uveitis occurs less often but may lead to anterior and posterior synechiae, seclusio- or occlusio-pupillae, secondary cataract, and secondary glaucoma.

Chorioretinal Lesions (Fig. 87–13). The severity and extent of chorioretinal changes vary. The retinal pigment epithelium may show areas of migration, clumping, atrophy, or focal hyperplasia. Chronic nongranulomatous chorioretinitis consists of an infiltrate of lymphocytes, plasma cells, and eosinophils with secondary degenerative changes in the overlying retinal pigment epithelium and neuroretina. Profound chorioretinal atrophy may develop, with loss of almost all the retina and choroid, so that the internal limiting membrane of the retina lies on the large choroid vessels. Optic atrophy is common in the more advanced stages of ocular

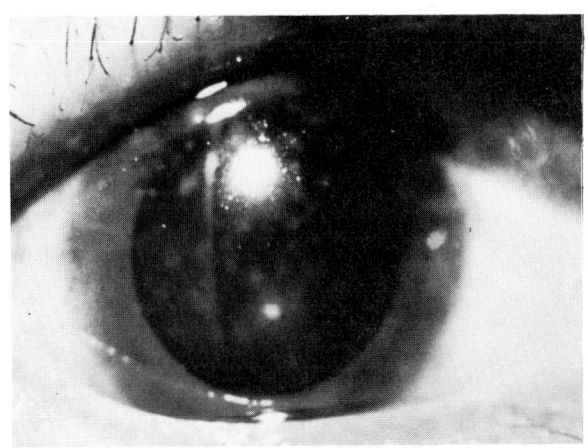

FIGURE 87–11. Ocular onchocerciasis with snowflake opacities (punctate keratitis), which usually occur in the peripheral cornea. Although a few opacities are common in people who have microfilariae in the cornea, they are seen especially during treatment with suramin or with DEC, as was the case in this patient.

onchocerciasis and may be associated with a large glaucomatous cup.

CLINICAL MANIFESTATIONS AND COMPLICATIONS. In heavily affected areas onchocerciasis causes severe morbidity, not only from blindness, which may affect 15% of a community, but also from severe itching and unsightly skin involvement. Entire communities have been disrupted and fertile valleys deserted. Onchocerciasis is often an "end of the road" disease in rural areas, where the skin lesions may be misdiagnosed and treated as scabies and where there are no ophthalmologists to recognize the characteristic eye lesions. Extensive new foci are often discovered by chance, either because a "nodule" thought to be a fibroma has been removed and sent for sectioning or because an ophthalmologist in an urban area has seen something wriggling in the eye. Onchocerciasis is not a uniform disease; there are major differences in different geographic regions. For example, the sclerosing keratitis that causes a high rate of blindness in the Sudano-Guinean savanna of Africa is an uncommon complication in the rain forest areas, even though the parasite densities may be higher in people in the forest areas (Fig. 87–14). Hanging groins, which are a feature of focal lymphatic obstruction and loss of elasticity in the skin, are common only in Africa. In Central America, the parasites are more concentrated in the upper part of the body, occasionally producing a leonine facies. Another geographic variant of the disease is called sowda—after the black hyperpigmented skin lesion first associated with the disease in Yemen and later recognized as a hyper-reactive form in Africa.

The differences in the clinical manifestations also depend on the worm load. Individuals with light infections, such as many expatriates or temporary visitors to endemic areas, usually have an unsightly skin rash affecting one part of the body but do not usually have eye lesions or palpable nodules. In these cases microfilariae are difficult to find, and a definite diagnosis is rarely established unless a typical Mazzotti reaction occurs following a test dose of DEC. Skin and eye lesions and nodules may not be present, even in infected individuals who have lived all their lives in the endemic area. In general, the worm load increases with age, and the severity of the disease is proportional to the intensity of transmission and the duration of exposure to the infection.

Dermatitis. The earliest manifestation of onchocercal dermatitis is itching, usually most severe over the lower trunk, pelvis, buttocks, and thighs. Itching and scratching may be the only manifestation of mild infections, but there is often a papular rash, usually involving the buttocks and legs. Altered pigmentation of the skin, i.e., distinct macules or poorly defined areas of hyper- and hypopigmentation, is an early sign. Scratching may produce ulcers, bleeding, and secondary infection. Later, papules, scaling, edema, and depigmentation may all develop (Fig. 87–6). The intradermal edema produces a "peau d'orange" effect with pitting around the hair follicles and sebaceous glands. This is usually followed by loss of elasticity and extensive scarring of the dermis and overlying atrophy of the epidermis, producing presbydermia, i.e., a characteristic feature of long-standing severe onchocercal dermatitis in which the skin of relatively young men and women has an aged appearance.

The wrinkled skin is usually extremely thin with little subcutaneous tissue. In some cases there is persistence of hypertrophy of the epidermis with lichenification, resulting in elephantoid or "lizard" skin. A characteristic feature of the disease in the rain forests of West Africa is the "leopard spot" depigmentation over the shins, which can extend to other areas of the body (Fig. 87–6B). This complication has been mistaken for leprosy, although there are no sensory changes.

In Guatemala, Mexico, and South America, the chronic skin lesions of onchocerciasis are not present to the same extent as in Africa. A variety of more acute manifestations occur in Central America, including "erisípela de la costa," with a macular rash and edema of the face, and "mal morado," with reddish-mauve discoloration, especially on the trunk and upper limbs.

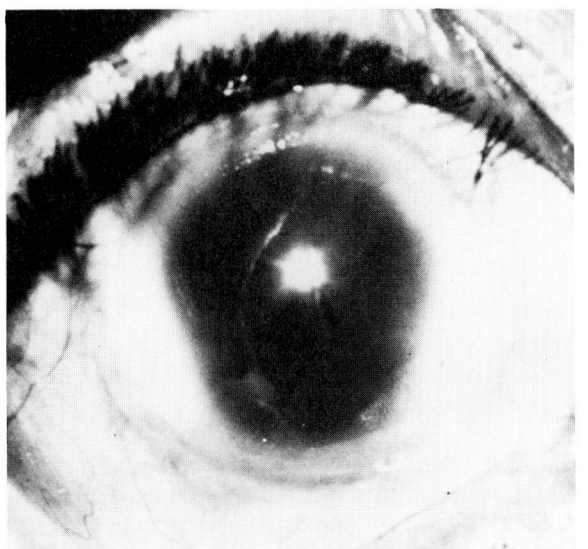

FIGURE 87–12. Ocular onchocerciasis with sclerosing keratitis, which usually begins at the nasal and temporal periphery and slowly progresses centrally. This Guatemalan man also has a pear-shaped distortion of his pupil, which is characteristic of onchocercal uveitis.

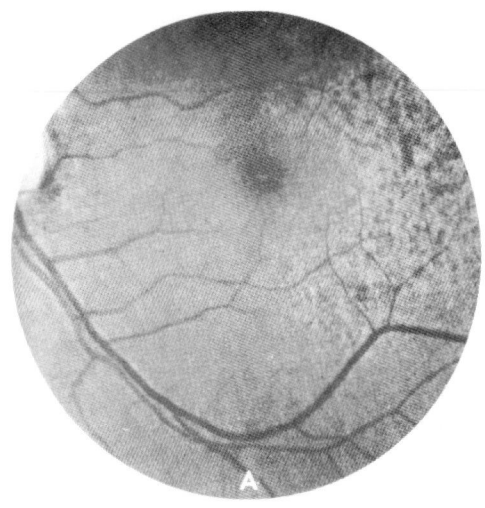

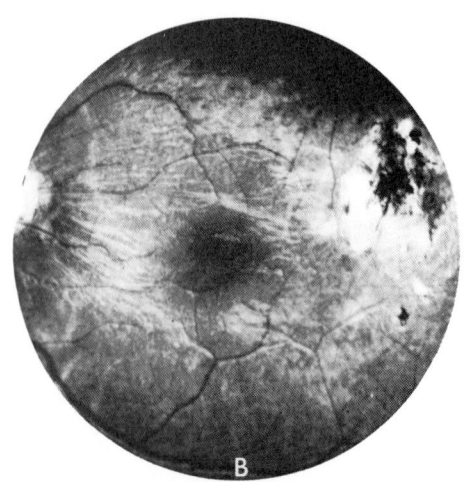

FIGURE 87–13. *A,* Ocular onchocerciasis with atrophy of the retinal pigment epithelium, temporal to the macula. (Courtesy of the Armed Forces Institute of Pathology, Photograph Neg. No. 75-1628.) *B,* Ocular onchocerciasis with a patch of chorioretinal atrophy with scarring superotemporally to the macula. (Courtesy of the Armed Forces Institute of Pathology, Photograph Neg. No. 75–1629.) *C,* Ocular onchocerciasis with extensive Ridley-type chorioretinal degeneration, with sparing of the macula and optic atrophy. (Courtesy of the Armed Forces Institute of Pathology, Photograph Neg. No. 75-1632; contributed by Dr. J. Anderson, Kumba, Cameroon.)

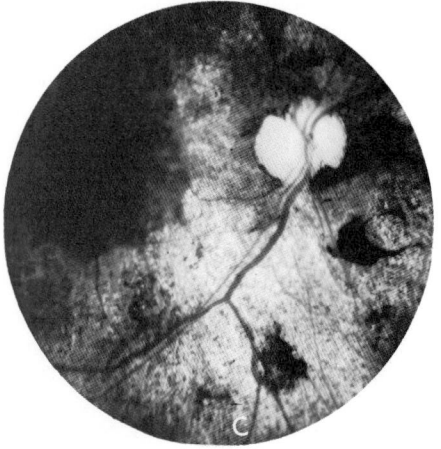

"Sowda" the feminine form of the Arabic word "as-wad," meaning black, is the name given to one of the manifestations of onchocerciasis in South and North Yemen and neighboring Saudi Arabia (with similar cases reported from the Sudan and from West Africa). The changes are usually limited to 1 limb and include edema, hyperpigmented papules, and regional lymphadenopathy. Few microfilariae can be found in patients with sowda, but other members of the community may be heavily infected with more typical lesions. It is thought that this syndrome is due to a hyper-reactive immunologic response.

Nodules. The onchocercal nodule, or onchocercoma, contains adult worms (see Fig. 87–8). These nodules are in the dermis or subcutaneous tissue and are characteristically located over bony prominences. In Africa, the

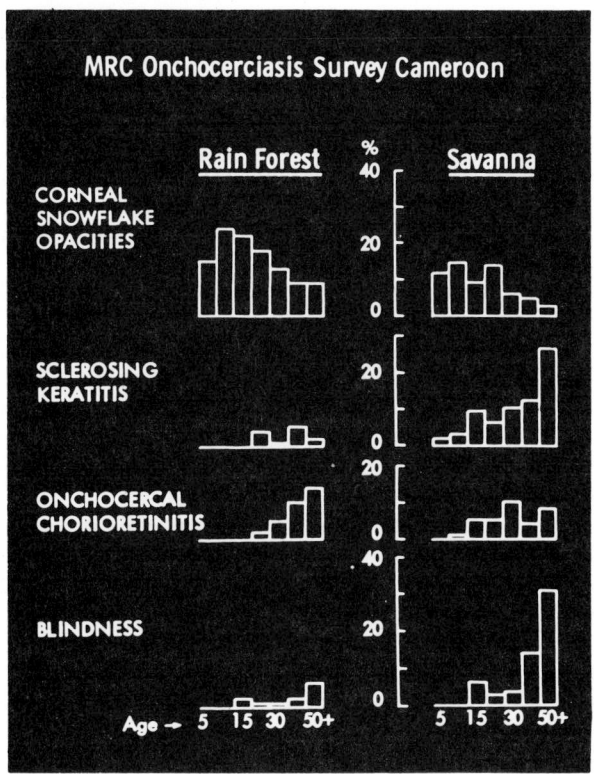

FIGURE 87–14. Geographic differences between the savanna and rain forest regions of Cameroon in frequencies of various lesions of ocular onchocerciasis. (Contributed by Dr. G. Nelson, Liverpool School of Tropical Medicine, with data from studies by Drs. J. Anderson and H. Fuglsang, Kumba, Cameroon.)

most common location is around the pelvis, over the anterior superior iliac spine, the trochanter of the femur, the iliac crest, the sacrum, and the coccyx. In heavy infections, nodules are commonly present over the ribs and around the knee joint (Fig. 87–6). They may also be found in the upper part of the body, near the scapula, near the elbow, and on the head (Fig. 87–7). In Guatemala and Mexico, a greater percentage of nodules are found around the head and upper part of the body.

Some nodules are too small or too deep to be felt. A typical nodule containing viable worms is firm, round or ovoid, nontender, "slippery" to the touch, movable, and well defined. Some nodules are discrete and isolated, but in long-standing infections they may present as conglomerate masses with an irregular outline and be firmly attached to the underlying fascia. Lesions vary from about 5 mm to clusters of nodules 10 cm or more across.

Lymphadenitis. Many patients with onchocerciasis have changes in inguinal or femoral lymph nodes (Fig. 87–6A). These are the nodes that drain areas of onchocercal dermatitis. Usually they are only slightly enlarged, firm, movable, discrete, and not tender. In some African patients, onchocercal lymphadenitis leads to a unique manifestation, i.e., "hanging groin," also called "adenolymphocele" (Fig. 87–10). This is a pouch of lymphedematous tissue hanging from a cluster of inguinal or femoral nodes. It occurs predominantly in males, and in some areas it predisposes to hernia. In the female the hanging groin may be represented by a "Hottentot

apron," a pathologic hanging down of the labia resembling the cosmetic apron produced in some communities by attaching weights to the labia. Involvement of deeper nodes may lead to elephantiasis of the limbs or genitalia (Fig. 87–6A).

Ocular Changes

Intraocular Microfilariae. The earliest sign of ocular involvement is the invasion of the eye by microfilariae. Intraocular microfilariae can be detected by slit-lamp examination, although they may be difficult to see. Microfilariae in the anterior chamber are seen as small wriggling white worms. Live microfilariae in the cornea are transparent and coiled up, whereas dead microfilariae are more opaque and straight and are thus easier to see. Less commonly, microfilariae may be found in the anterior vitreous and at times may even be attached to the lens capsule or to Descemet's membrane. With careful biomicroscopic examination, live microfilariae can be seen in the retina.

Punctate Keratitis. In the cornea, dead microfilariae are usually surrounded by an ill-defined fluffy opacity of inflammatory infiltrate, about 0.5 mm in diameter, called "snowflake" opacities or punctate keratitis (Fig. 87–11). Although these opacities can occur spontaneously, they are especially frequent following treatment with the microfilaricidal drug DEC.

Sclerosing Keratitis. Sclerosing keratitis may progress until the entire cornea is opaque and vascularized. The earliest change is an increased translucency, or haze, in the peripheral cornea. This limbal haze opacifies, extending from the limbus toward the central cornea (Fig. 87–12). This opacification advances in an arc, being most marked at each side and below, and progresses to cover the central cornea. Eventually the entire cornea may become opaque. Sclerosing keratitis occurs more commonly and is more severe in the savanna areas of Africa than in the rain forest regions.

Anterior Uveitis. The presence and severity of anterior uveitis are extremely variable; mild uveitis is common. At times, the eye may remain noninflamed despite heavy infiltration by microfilariae. In some patients severe anterior uveitis occurs, leading to posterior synechiae and pear-shaped deformity of the pupil (Fig. 87–12). Mild uveitis has been related to microfilarial invasion of the iris and the more severe granulomatous uveitis to invasion of the ciliary body. Extensive synechiae may cause seclusio- and occlusio-pupillae, secondary cataracts, and secondary glaucoma. Sequelae of anterior uveitis are probably the main causes of onchocerciasis-related blindness in Central America.

Chorioretinitis. A variety of changes are seen in the fundus. The most common is retinal pigment epithelial atrophy (Fig. 87–13A), seen as small, round white dots in the fundus. Mild forms may be revealed only by fluorescein angiography. Focal areas of hypertrophy and clumping of pigment may also be present. Larger areas of chorioretinal atrophy are common, and the choroidal vessels can be seen through the atrophic layers. Subretinal fibrosis appears as well-defined plaque-like white areas (Fig. 87–13B). New vessels may develop in areas of subretinal fibrosis. Active inflammation can be seen as areas of posterior retinal edema or as pale, ill-defined areas of swelling in the choroid.

Although all of these chorioretinal changes may occur together, one may predominate. The variation in prominence and distribution of each type of change leads to differences in the fundal appearance. Fundal changes are usually symmetrical; they may be localized or widespread. The extent of the fundal involvement is not necessarily related to the severity of the morphologic change or of the infection. The most common distribution of changes is temporal rather than macular. However, even when there is extensive involvement of the posterior pole, the macula may remain as a relatively intact island (Fig. 87–13C).

Optic Neuritis and Optic Atrophy. These are frequent complications of onchocerciasis. Microfilariae can be found within the optic nerve and its sheaths, and the death of these microfilariae could initiate an inflammatory response with later atrophic changes. Consecutive optic atrophy also occurs after the loss of ganglion cells in areas of retinal atrophy (Fig. 87–13C). Secondary glaucoma can also cause optic atrophy. However, optic atrophy can occur in patients treated with either DEC or suramin, and it may be a complication of treatment rather than due to the infection itself.

Glaucoma. The association between onchocerciasis and glaucoma is variable. Intraocular pressure can be elevated during the onchocerciasis-induced anterior uveitis, and severe secondary glaucoma occurs from extensive synechiae formation. However, there is no direct relationship between onchocerciasis and chronic open-angle glaucoma.

Geographic Differences in Eye Lesions in Africa. African Sudano-Guinean savanna and rain forest regions show differences in the frequencies of the various eye lesions associated with onchocerciasis (Fig. 87–14). In particular, sclerosing keratitis and the resulting blindness are common in the savanna regions but rare in the rain forest.

Other Complications. At one time the "Nakalanga dwarfs" of the Mabira Forest in Uganda were thought to have been stunted by onchocerciasis. They lived in areas where onchocerciasis prevailed and generally showed evidence of heavy infection with *O. volvulus*. It was suspected that the condition might be caused by parasitic involvement of the pituitary gland. This requires further study to see if dwarfism has persisted following control of blackflies, which has interrupted transmission of *O. volvulus* in the Mabira Forest.

There have been several reports from Central America of erosion of the skull by onchocercal nodules, with associated epilepsy. Seizures have also been reported as a complication of the disease in the Sudan. Acute arthritis and tenosynovitis are sometimes seen as complications of treatment. It has been suggested that the presence of adult worms around the hip and other joints may be responsible for some of the chronic arthritic conditions seen in the endemic areas.

DIAGNOSIS. Everyone in endemic regions is at risk; the longer one remains in these areas, the greater the chance of infection.

Skin Snip. This is the most commonly used procedure for diagnosis. The traditional method is to pick up the skin with a dermal hook or needle, then snip the minute tip off with a razor or scalpel. A simpler technique of snipping is to use an ophthalmologic instrument, the scleral-corneal punch. This is more convenient because it quickly bites out snips that are approximately uniform in size. The snip should include tips of the dermal papillae. The snip itself should be bloodless, but blood will well up into the bed of the wound after it is removed. The snip is put into normal saline or tissue culture medium in the well of a microtiter plate and examined at least 1 hour later (preferably at least 3 hours later). Microfilariae emerge progressively over the first hour or so, at which time 80 to 90% have emerged. Some workers leave the skin snips in tissue culture medium for 24 hours before counting the emerged microfilariae.

If 1- to 3-hour waiting periods are not convenient, the snips can be left longer in the saline, where the emerged microfilariae can be killed and preserved in situ by adding a drop of formol-saline. The specimens can then be kept for subsequent examination. Snips are usually taken from one or more standard sites, e.g., buttock, iliac crest, scapula, or lower calf, depending on where the clinical manifestations are most severe and on the biting habits of the local flies. In epidemiologic studies or in chemotherapy trials, the necessary quantitative data on parasite densities are best obtained by weighing the snips and calculating the number per milligram of skin.

Microfilariae emerging from the skin snip confirm the diagnosis. These are identified by their size and configuration and by their rapid wriggling. If in doubt or in areas where there is possible confusion with *M. streptocerca* or *M. ozzardi*, slides should be prepared and stained. In lightly infected individuals, only one or a few microfilariae will emerge; however, in heavily infected patients, there may be hundreds of microfilariae.

In many heavily infected individuals small numbers of microfilariae can be found in the urine or peripheral blood using the Nuclepore filter technique (Chapter 85.1). After treatment with DEC, the microfilariae can often be seen in large numbers in the blood, urine, sputum, lacrimal fluid, and cerebrospinal fluid.

Nodulectomy. Diagnosis may also be confirmed by the identification of adult *O. volvulus* worms in a surgically excised nodule (Fig. 87–8) or, less commonly, by the identification of fragments of the adult worms in aspirates of the nodules.

Slit-Lamp Examination. A noninvasive technique for confirming the diagnosis is the identification of microfilariae in the cornea and/or anterior chamber of the eye with a slit lamp. Prior to examination, the patient should sit with his or her head between the knees for at least 2 minutes. When the patient sits up, the microfilariae are concentrated behind the central cornea and thus are easier to see and count. This simple maneuver increases the absolute counts of microfilariae in the anterior chamber.

The patient is examined with a slit lamp, using an intense oblique beam similar to that used when looking for flare and cells in the anterior chamber. Microfilariae in the anterior chamber may at times be seen with a direct ophthalmoscope set at +20 diopters by looking against the red fundal reflex. Microfilariae in the cornea are more difficult to see. They can be found by using retroillumination produced by an oblique beam oriented to give a red reflex through the dilated pupil. The cornea is then examined carefully with the slit lamp, using high magnification ($\times$ 25).

The Mazzotti Test. An indirect technique for diagnosis is the Mazzotti test; this should be used only after skin snips reveal no microfilariae. The patient is given a single dose of 50 mg of DEC by mouth. Infected individuals develop intense pruritus within a few hours. The itching is maximal in areas of the most numerous microfilariae and may be accompanied by erythema, edema, and papules. The itching subsides in 2 to 3 days.

More heavily infected patients may have severe systemic manifestations following a test dose of DEC, including fever, malaise, swollen and tender lymph nodes, facial and periorbital edema, eosinophilia, and arthralgias. Patients with numerous microfilariae in the eye can develop serious ocular complications following treatment with DEC, and rarely death may follow. Therefore, heavily infected or debilitated persons should be excluded before using the Mazzotti test for diagnosis. Many experts believe that the test is dangerous and should not be used for diagnostic purposes.

Serology. A characteristic feature of onchocerciasis is eosinophilia. Immunologic diagnostic tests are of minimal value in individual patients. If no microfilariae are detected in the skin and eyes and if the Mazzotti test is negative, it is unlikely that the patient is infected with *O. volvulus*; in such cases, immunologic tests can be both misleading and unnecessary. There are no commonly available serologic test kits, and the antigens used in the tests are usually from related animal species. A wide variety of tests has been developed, including a skin test, complement fixation, hemagglutination, indirect fluorescent antibody test, immunoelectrophoresis, enzyme-linked immunosorbent assay (ELISA), and tests for the presence of circulating antigens (Chapter 125). The results are often misleading owing to the high rate of false-positive reactions caused by infections with other helminths such as *Strongyloides* species or to heterologous reactions from exposure to filarial infections of animal origin. However, prospects for better tests are good because of the development of species-specific diagnostic tests based on the isolation of pure antigens of *O. volvulus*.

Differential Diagnosis. The dermatitis of onchocerciasis is rarely diagnosed in early cases unless there is a history of exposure to infection in an endemic area and a positive skin snip or Mazzotti reaction. In expatriates, the dermatitis may be confused with food allergies, contact dermatitis, insect bite reactions, prickly heat, and the pruritus of scabies. The chronic skin lesion may be mistaken for eczema, tertiary yaws, malnutrition, and, in older patients, the presbydermic changes that develop at an earlier age in some inhabitants of the tropics. The leopard skin spots must be distinguished from other forms of vitiligo, leprosy, and streptocerciasis—the last of which is often a concomitant infection in many of the rain forest areas of Africa.

TREATMENT AND PROGNOSIS. The advent of ivermectin, registered in France under the name of Mectizan by Merck Sharp & Dohme (MSD), for the treatment of human onchocerciasis bids fair to change many of the views previously held on treatment when the only available drugs with activity against *O. volvulus* were DEC, suramin, and mebendazole. The indications for treatment with the older drugs had become more stringent as more was learned about the serious side effects of chemotherapy. In many patients, who lived in endemic areas and were virtually symptom free, specific chemotherapy with the older drugs was often unnecessary and even unethical because of its associated hazards where medical facilities were inadequate. The major indication for treatment is sight-threatening disease, as judged by the presence of more than 20 microfilariae in the anterior chamber, more than 50 in the cornea, severe anterior uveitis, or early sclerosing keratitis. Because advanced chorioretinal changes will not improve with treatment, their presence alone is not an indication for therapy. Other advocated indications for treatment include decreased night vision, visual field constriction, the presence of more than 10 microfilariae/mg of skin snips from the outer canthus, and nodules on the head. Patients with severe acute skin lesions and pruritus also benefit from treatment aimed at reducing the numbers of microfilariae and adult worms; and it is advisable to treat patients with "sowda." Treatment can alleviate the acute lesions, but it does not reduce scarring from longstanding inflammation of the skin, eyes, or lymphoid tissue. With the development of ivermectin, the community-based treatment of populations living in endemic areas is being considered.

Nodulectomy. A less hazardous and useful adjunct to chemotherapy is the removal of palpable nodules. This has been popular in Guatemala and Mexico, where nodules on the head are common. In Guatemala, in particular, prolonged nodulectomy campaigns may have reduced the incidence of ocular onchocerciasis; whereas in Ecuador removal of all palpable nodules reduces the load of microfilariae and improves clinical manifestations. In Africa, however, nodulectomy has never been widely practiced, as the nodules tend to be deeper, lying against bones and joints or between layers of muscle, and are thus more difficult to remove. Also, a smaller proportion of the nodules are found on the head. A field trial of mass nodulectomies in West Africans with the danger signs of visual impairment was abandoned when it proved too difficult and expensive. In 2 other trials in West Africa, nodulectomy failed to reduce microfilarial counts over 2 years of observation.

Chemotherapy

Ivermectin. Ivermectin, a widely used veterinary gastrointestinal anthelmintic and ectoparasiticide, must now be regarded as the microfilaricidal treatment of choice for onchocerciasis, thereby replacing DEC. The drug is a macrocyclic lactone produced by a fermentation process. In *O. volvulus* infection it is a rapidly effective, single-dose microfilaricide, which excites relatively little or no Mazzotti reaction. It also prevents the escape of microfilariae from the uteri of the female worm; the trapped microfilariae degenerate and prevent further microfilarial production for a period of 6 to 12 months; the drug thus acts as a microfilarial suppressant.

After treatment, microfilariae usually disappear from the eye within 2 to 3 months and the development of ocular and dermal lesions is arrested. However, the drug has no macrofilaricidal action nor is it a causal prophylactic for *O. volvulus*.

The optimal dosage of ivermectin is 150 µg/kg (usually 2 tablets of 6 mg for an adult) and this microfilaricidal suppressant treatment can be repeated every 6 to 12 months. The drug should not be given to children younger than 5 years, to pregnant women, to mothers in the first 3 months of lactation, or to those who are otherwise severely ill, or during outbreaks of cerebrospinal meningitis. If a significant Mazzotti reaction occurs, palliative symptomatic treatment with antipyretics, antihistamines, oral fluids, and possibly corticosteroids may be necessary.

Mectizan tablets can be purchased through normal channels in some developed countries for the treatment of individuals with onchocerciasis. It is also supplied free of charge by MSD for the large-scale treatment of infected persons in developing countries where the disease is endemic. To obtain this free supply, application has to be made to the Mectizan Expert Committee at the Carter Center, Atlanta, GA. Applications have to satisfy certain criteria laid down by the committee as to the means by which the drug will be distributed so as to avoid overdosage, etc., and it requires the written endorsement of the Ministry of Health of the country concerned.

Ivermectin is in effect the first filaricide effective against *O. volvulus* that appears to be safe for large-scale use. As of May 1988, it had been used to treat some 50,000 onchocerciasis patients in endemic areas without serious mishap. Furthermore, there is a strong likelihood that, provided adequate treatment coverage can be achieved in infected populations, the drug may be effective in reducing the human microfilarial reservoir sufficiently to control transmission by the *Simulium* vector. Already there is some experimental evidence indicating that this is possible.

Ivermectin has many advantages over DEC and should replace it as the microfilaricide of choice. It seems likely that it could satisfactorily precede treatment with suramin and effect a radical cure of *O. volvulus* infection.

Diethylcarbamazine. DEC (Banocide, Hetrazan, Notézine) kills microfilariae but has no effect on adult worms, and the microfilariae recur 3 to 12 months after treatment. In 30 minutes to 24 hours after the first dose of DEC, the patient usually develops itching and sometimes papular eruptions, swollen and tender lymph nodes, joint pain, headache, malaise, and edema of the head, neck, and eyelids. There may be an accentuation of the eye lesion. The heavier the infection, the more severe this Mazzotti reaction tends to be. Some patients may have an immediate collapse with hypotension and shortness of breath. Therefore, cautiously starting with small doses is recommended. It is advisable to give all heavily infected patients oral corticosteroids when starting DEC treatment and continue steroids until the most severe reactions have subsided.

The following course has been suggested: A single 50-mg tablet of DEC is usually given on the first day of treatment. Two 50-mg tablets are given (morning and evening) for the next 7 to 10 days. Frequently, aspirin is needed, especially for fever and pain of arthralgia and lymphadenitis. The routine use of systemic steroids is sometimes advocated, beginning with dexamethasone, 4 mg/day, 1 to 2 days before the start of DEC. The severe hypotensive reactions following treatment with DEC are usually relieved by corticosteroids, but neither these nor antihistamines completely relieve severe pruritus. Some workers, however, use steroids more sparingly and only in those patients who have the more severe reactions to DEC therapy.

DEC does not kill microfilariae in vitro, but instead alters them in some way that causes 2 immediate, almost simultaneous events: degeneration of microfilariae and an inflammatory reaction to them. In experimental animals with other filarial infections, the efficacy of the drug is dependent on a T-cell response. Patients given repeated doses of DEC continue to relapse, because the adult worms remain viable for several years. It is therefore necessary to give a macrofilaricidal drug (i.e., suramin) if the aim is to relieve all symptoms (see section below on combined microfilaricide and suramin treatment).

Suramin. Suramin (Bayer 205, Germanin, Moranyl, Antrypol) is both a macrofilaricide and a microfilaricide. It is a complex water-soluble urea derivative and must be given cautiously. A fresh 10% solution is injected intravenously, starting with a test dose of 100 mg given slowly over 2 minutes to test for hypersensitivity. Treatment with the full dose may then be continued. The high-dosage regimen of 1 gm/week has been abandoned. The following weekly doses are now recommended: 0.2 gm, 0.4 gm, 0.6 gm, 0.8 gm, 1.0 gm, and 1.0 gm, with a proportional reduction for patients under 60 kg in weight.

This dosage minimizes the risk of toxic reactions and kills nearly all adult worms and microfilariae in the skin and eyes. However, there are still the dangers of rare fatalities and of the eye lesion's becoming worse. Direct toxicity includes tenderness of the palms and soles, polyuria and increased thirst with albuminuria and granular casts in the urine, fatigue, anorexia, malaise, and sometimes ulceration of the mouth, diarrhea, and prostration. Reactions to dying adult worms include urticaria and swelling around dying worms, tenderness and swelling around nodules, extrusion of adult worms from the skin, abscesses of the deep fascia or the muscle around degenerating adult worms, painful and immobilized hip joints (usually semiflexed) from reaction around dying worms that lie against the capsule of the hip joint, and pain above the knee joint from reaction around nodules. Reactions may also be a consequence of the death of microfilariae and resemble a delayed Mazzotti reaction with itching of infected skin, fever with cough, iritis, and pain, swelling, and limitation of joints, especially the fingers, wrists, elbows, toes, and knees. The most serious complications are exfoliative dermatitis and usually fatal progressive wasting with diarrhea. Some of the complications may be prevented if the patient is given concomitant corticosteroids and if the main load of microfilariae is first removed by careful treatment with a microfilaricide, preferably ivermectin.

Combined Microfilaricide and Suramin. In the past many workers had recommended a combined treatment regimen with both DEC (microfilaricidal) and suramin (macrofilaricidal). When the DEC treatment course is completed (see above), 6 weekly intravenous injections of suramin are given, starting with 0.2 gm and then 0.4 gm, 0.4 gm, 0.8 gm, 1.0 gm, and 1.0 gm for a total dose of 3.8 gm. In all probability ivermectin should now be used as the pre-suramin microfilaricide, instead of DEC.

New Drugs. The World Health Organization (WHO) is conducting an active program of drug screening and development for drugs with a macrofilaricidal activity or a prolonged sterilizing or microfilarial suppressant action against *O. volvulus*. This program has assisted with the development of ivermectin and is currently concentrated on a series of derivatives of amoscanate developed by Ciba-Geigy Ltd, of which the leading compound now in clinical trials (1988–1989) is coded as CGP 6140.

PREVENTION. There are no effective prophylactic drugs or vaccines. All *Simulium* species vectors are day-biting insects that rarely enter houses. Their highest biting intensity is near their breeding sites along the rivers. The most effective method of prevention, therefore, is to avoid areas where the vectors are biting and, if this is not possible, to wear protective clothing. Long trousers with socks and shoes are of value against the low-biting vectors in Africa and Venezuela; in Guatemala and Mexico a hat and veil will be necessary to protect against the voracious high-biting vector, *S. ochraceum*. Insect repellents temporarily reduce fly exposure. The worm load in affected communities can be greatly reduced by providing alternative water supplies and locating houses and villages away from the rivers.

CONTROL. As with all vector-borne parasitic diseases, there are 3 principal methods of control: (1) reduce transmission by attacking the vector, (2) reduce the parasite reservoir in the community by mass chemotherapy, and (3) change human behavior to reduce exposure to the vector. Since the previously available drugs were unsuited for mass chemotherapy, control campaigns hitherto relied almost entirely on reducing the vector population. This can be achieved by treating the aquatic breeding sites with rapidly biodegradable insecticides; the natural flow carries the chemical downstream to kill the larvae that are usually attached to stones and vegetation (or to crabs, in the case of *S. neavei*) in the highly oxygenated water near waterfalls and rapids.

The success of any control campaign depends on the flight range or dispersal of the vector and the degree of isolation of the endemic area. In Kenya where the flight range of *S neavei* was only a few miles, the vector and parasite were totally eliminated by treating the rivers with DDT. Continual vigilance was necessary because it took 15 years for the parasite to die off.

The foci in West Africa are much more extensive, and complete eradication of the vector, members of the *S. damnosum* complex, has not been attempted, since reinvasion occurs with flies that are transferred on wind currents as far as 400 km from their breeding sites.

However, a multimillion dollar program, the Onchocerciasis Control Program (OCP), has been established by the World Bank, with WHO as the executive agent, to attempt to reduce the severity of the disease in the West African savanna. Helicopters and fixed-wing aircraft spray the rivers with the biodegradable insecticides Abate and *Bacillus thuringiensis* H14, while epidemiologic and entomologic teams monitor transmission and clinical manifestations. The objective is to reduce the number of flies to an "annual transmission potential" of less than 200 infective larvae per person per year. This has been achieved in more than 90% of the original OCP area; there are now no further cases of blindness and the disease is disappearing.

Unfortunately, there is already evidence of insecticide resistance by some of the vectors. This has resulted in accelerating the search for more effective and less toxic drugs to supplement control measures. Reduction of the parasite reservoir by periodic treatment of the infected human population with ivermectin is currently being evaluated and looks very promising.

BIBLIOGRAPHY

Anderson J, Fuglsang H: Ocular onchocerciasis. Trop Dis Bull 74:257, 1977.

Awadzi K, Dadzie KY, Schulz-Key H, et al: The chemotherapy of onchocerciasis. X. An assessment of four single-dose treatment regimens of MK-933 (ivermectin) in human onchocerciasis. Ann Trop Med Parasit 79:63, 1985.

Buck AA (ed): Onchocerciasis: Symptomatology, Pathology, Diagnosis. Geneva, World Health Organization, 1974.

Connor DH, Gibson DW, Neafie RC, et al: Sowda–onchocerciasis in North Yemen: A clinicopathologic study of 18 patients. Am J Trop Med Hyg 32:123, 1983.

Connor DH, Morrison NE, Kerdal-Vegas F, et al: Onchocerciasis: Onchocercal dermatitis, lymphadenitis, and elephantiasis in the Ubangi Territory. Hum Pathol 2:553, 1970.

Cupp EW, Bernado MJ, Kiszewski AE, et al: The effects of ivermectin in transmission of *Onchocerca volvulus*. Science 231:740, 1986.

Gibson DW, Connor DH: Onchocercal lymphadenitis: Clinicopathologic study of 34 patients: Trans R Soc Trop Med Hyg 72:137, 1978.

Gibson DW, Duke BOL, Connor DH: Onchocerciasis: A review of clinical, pathologic and chemotherapeutic aspects, and vector control program. Prog Clin Parasitol 1:57, 1988.

Greene BM, Taylor HR, Cupp EW, et al: Comparison of ivermectin and diethylcarbamazine in the treatment of human onchocerciasis. N Engl J Med 313:133, 1985.

Martins da Silva M (ed): Research and Control of Onchocerciasis in the Western Hemisphere. Pan American Health Organization Scientific Publication No. 298, Washington, DC, 1974.

Meyers WM, Neafie RC, Connor DH: Onchocerciasis: Invasion of deep organs by *Onchocerca volvulus*. Am J Trop Med Hyg 26:650, 1977.

Nelson GS: "Hanging groin" and hernia, complications of onchocerciasis. Trans R Soc Trop Med Hyg 52:272, 1958.

Paul EV, Zimmerman LE: Some observations on the ocular pathology of onchocerciasis. Hum Pathol 1:581, 1970.

Piessens WF, Mackenzie CD: Immunology of lymphatic filariasis and onchocerciasis. *In* Cohen S, Warren KS (eds): Immunology of Parasitic Infections, 2nd ed. London, Blackwell, 1982, pp 622–653.

Raper AR, Ladkin RGL: Endemic dwarfism in Uganda. Onchocerciasis. East Afr Med J 25:357, 1950.

Rodger FC: The pathogenesis and pathology of ocular onchocerciasis: I–V. Am J Ophthalmol 49:104, 110, 127, 327, 560, 1960.

Sasa M: Human Filariasis—A Global Survey of Epidemiology and Control. London, University Park Press, 1976.

Taylor HR, Greene BM: Ocular changes with oral and transepidermal diethylcarbamazine therapy of onchocerciasis. Br J Ophthalmol 65:494, 1981.

White AT, Newland HS, Taylor HR, et al: Controlled trial and dose-finding study of ivermectin for treatment of onchocerciasis. J Infect Dis 156:463, 1987.

World Health Organization: Third report of the WHO Expert Committee on Onchocerciasis. WHO Tech Rep Ser 752, 1987.

88. MISCELLANEOUS FILARIAL INFECTIONS

GENERAL PRINCIPLES

George S. Nelson

Other filariae infecting humans include the following: (1) *Mansonella ozzardi* is a parasite that has a high prevalence in parts of Central and South America and the Caribbean, but is usually nonpathogenic with no clearly defined disease syndrome. (2) *Mansonella perstans* (previously called *Dipetalonema perstans*) is a common infection of humans in tropical Africa and also in some parts of South America. Although this parasite may produce minor allergic manifestations, it cannot be identified as the cause of a particular disease. (3) *Mansonella streptocerca* (previously called *Dipetalonema streptocerca*) for many years was thought to be nonpathogenic, but it is now associated with clearly recognizable skin lesions. (4) *Dirofilaria* and other zoonotic filarial parasites rarely reach maturity as adult worms in humans and never produce patent infections.

88.1 *Mansonella ozzardi* INFECTION

George S. Nelson

DEFINITION. Infection with the filarial nematode *Mansonella ozzardi* (Manson, 1897) has been associated with an ill-defined syndrome referred to as mansonellosis.

ETIOLOGY AND HISTORY. The parasite was first described by Manson in 1897 from specimens obtained by Ozzard from the blood of Amerindians in Guyana. Also in Guyana, Daniels obtained fragments of adult worms from the peritoneal cavity, which led Faust in 1929 to define the new genus *Mansonella*. The parasite has been transmitted to patas monkeys *(Erythrocebus patas),* and as a result of taxonomic studies, Orihel and Eberhard suggested that the genus *Mansonella* should also include *Dipetalonema perstans* and *Dipetalonema streptocerca*.

The worms are small and slender; females measure about 49 mm in length and 0.15 mm in diameter, and males measure 26 mm in length and 0.07 mm in diameter. The microfilariae are quite distinct; they are delicate unsheathed parasites 220 μm long by 3 to 4 μm wide, with a clear cephalic space and a long thin tail without nuclei (Fig. 88–1). Although most of the microfilariae are in the peripheral blood and are readily seen on routine blood slides, they may be found also in skin snips, causing confusion with onchocerciasis, especially in the Amazon region of Brazil.

DISTRIBUTION AND EPIDEMIOLOGY. The parasite has been reported only in the Western Hemi-

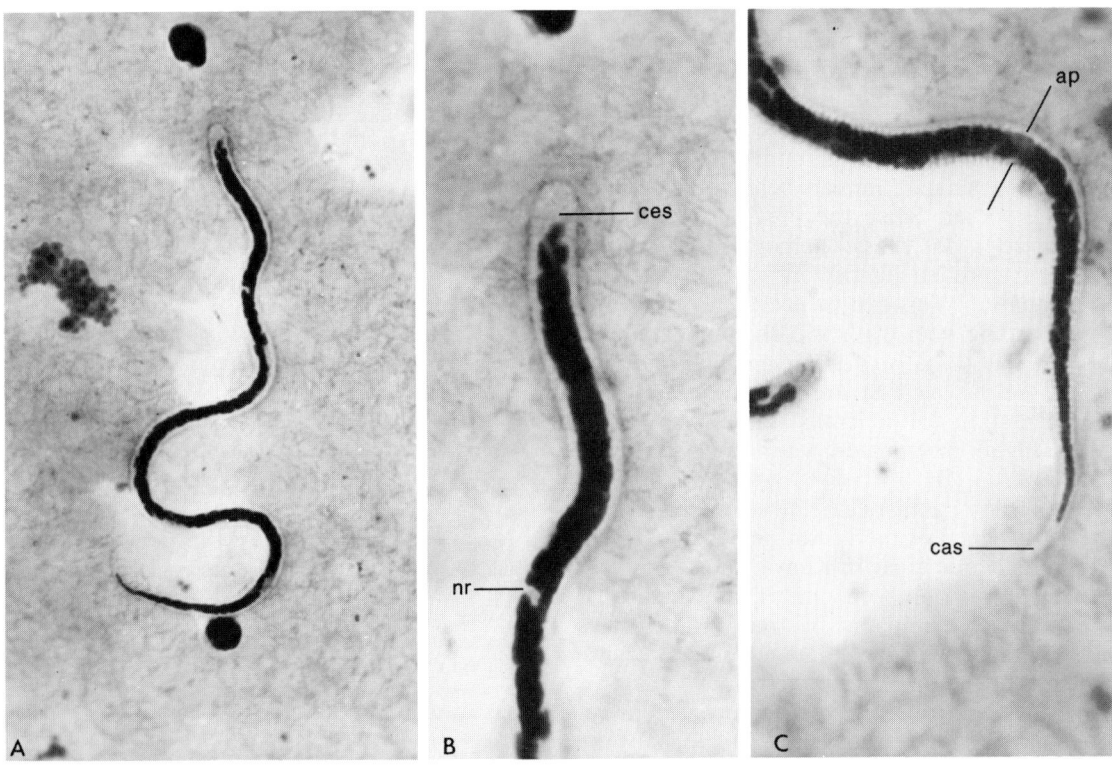

FIGURE 88–1. Thick blood film, *Mansonella ozzardi* microfilaria (Giemsa stain). *A,* × 820 (Courtesy of the Armed Forces Institute of Pathology, Photograph Neg. No. 74-19692.) *B,* Anterior end, cephalic space (ces), nerve ring (nr), × 1620. *C,* Posterior end, anal pore (ap), caudal space (cas), × 1620.

sphere, in Central and South America, and the Caribbean region. The northern focus in Yucatan seems to have disappeared, but there is active transmission in Haiti and several other Caribbean islands. While working on one of these islands (St. Vincent), Buckley in 1933 found that the nuisance "sandfly" *Culicoides furens* was an important vector. More recent studies have shown transmission by *Culicoides* in Trinidad. However, in Brazil and Guyana, the vectors are blackflies of the *Simulium amazonicum* group. A similar, if not identical, parasite has been recorded as far south as Argentina.

Humans are the only definitive host. There is increasing prevalence with age, the rate often reaching more than 70% in parts of Colombia and Brazil. Both sexes are affected, but the parasite is seen rarely in children.

PATHOGENESIS AND CLINICAL MANIFESTATIONS. Studies in Brazil and Colombia have suggested that *Mansonella* infections are associated with miscellaneous symptoms, including headaches, coldness of the legs, pruritus, and articular swellings. An epidemiologic study in Trinidad has confirmed that infection is associated with chronic arthritis, but nothing is known about the pathogenesis of the lesions, and there have been no autopsy studies. The microfilariae typically inhabit the subcutaneous tissues, and those seen in skin biopsy specimens are associated with perivascular cell infiltrates.

DIAGNOSIS. The characteristic nonperiodic unsheathed "sharp tailed" microfilariae (Fig. 88–1) are found in peripheral blood films and sometimes in skin snips taken during onchocerciasis surveys. If the Nuclepore filtration technique is used, the membranes must have a pore size of 3 μm, as the microfilariae can pass through the 5-μm filter used for *Wuchereria bancrofti*.

TREATMENT. There have been claims from Mexico that diethylcarbamazine can kill the parasites, but studies in Trinidad have shown that in this area there is no response to treatment.

BIBLIOGRAPHY

Buckley JJ: On the development, in *Culicoides furens* Poey, of *Filaria* (= *Mansonella*) *ozzardi* Manson, 1897. J Helminthol 12:99–118, 1934.
Marinkelle CJ, German E: Mansonelliasis in the Comisaria del Vaupes of Colombia. Trop Geogr Med 22:101–111, 1970.
Nelson GS, Davies JB. Observations on *Mansonella ozzardi* in Trinidad. Trans R Soc Trop Med Hyg 70:16, 1976.
Orihel TC, Eberhard ML: *Mansonella ozzardi:* A redescription with comments on its taxonomic relationships. Am J Trop Med Hyg 31:1142–1147, 1982.

88.2 *Mansonella perstans* INFECTION

George S. Nelson

DEFINITION. An ill-defined group of allergic symptoms has been associated with *Mansonella perstans* (Manson, 1891) infections together with an eosinophilia. However, most patients are asymptomatic. Until recently, this parasite was called *Dipetalonema perstans*.

ETIOLOGY AND EPIDEMIOLOGY. The adult worms are rarely seen in humans, but they occur in the serous cavities in the abdomen and chest of chimpanzees. The female worms are 60 to 80 mm by 100 to 150 μm and the males are 35 to 45 mm by 50 to 70 μm. The small nonperiodic unsheathed microfilariae average 200 μm in length by 4 to 5 μm in width; the tail is blunt and has a large nucleus at the tip (Fig. 88–2). The parasite is transmitted by midges or "noseeums" of the genus *Culicoides,* which are often found in the rotting stems of old banana plants.

M. perstans is widely distributed in tropical Africa, particularly in the rain forest areas of West and Central Africa. It is found also in sylvatic foci as far south as Zimbabwe. In Central and South America, there are limited foci among Amerindian communities in the rain forests. Infection rates of more than 50% occur without any detectable disease.

PATHOGENIC AND CLINICAL FEATURES. There have been no autopsy studies in humans to find the significance of *M. perstans* infections. The most commonly reported manifestation has been an eosinophilia with vague allergic signs observed in expatriates from Africa studied in Europe and America. In these cases, there is always the possibility of coexisting but unrecognized nonpatent nematode infections of *Loa, Onchocerca,* and *Strongyloides*. Microfilariae are frequently seen in the cerebrospinal fluid (and at one time were thought to be the etiologic agent of sleeping sickness).

Neurologic complications have been reported from Zimbabwe, but it has been suggested that the parasite involved is not *M. perstans* but *Meningonema peruzzi,* a common filarial parasite inhabiting the meninges of monkeys in Africa.

DIAGNOSIS AND TREATMENT. Diagnosis depends on finding the characteristic microfilariae in the peripheral blood (Fig. 88–2). Serologic tests are nonspecific and of little value. Treatment is not recommended in asymptomatic patients, but if there is a suspicion that the parasite is responsible for ill effects, a course of up

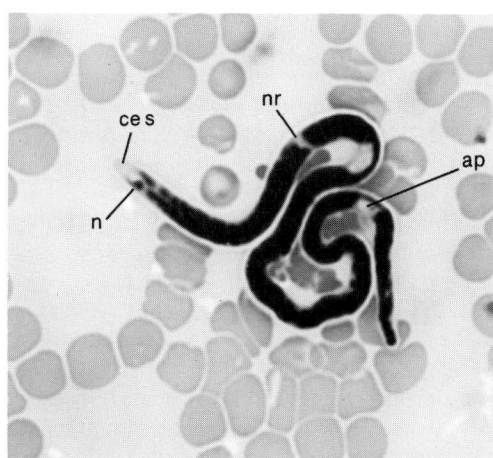

FIGURE 88–2. Thin blood film. *Mansonella perstans* microfilaria (Giemsa stain, × 890); cephalic space (ces), nucleus (n), nerve ring (nr), anal pore (ap). (Courtesy of the Armed Forces Institute of Pathology, Photograph Neg. No. 74-5605.)

to 75 mg/kg of diethylcarbamazine can be administered, following the same precautions and dose schedule as are used in treating filariasis (Chapter 85). This might provoke an inflammatory reaction around the adult worms, as was seen in the hernial sac of a patient treated in Zaire. Mebendazole has shown some promise as an alternative therapy.

BIBLIOGRAPHY

Adolphi PE, Kagan IG, McQuay RM: Diagnosis and treatment of *Acanthocheilonema perstans* filariasis. Am J Trop Med Hyg 11:76–88, 1962.
Maertens K, Wery M: Effect of mebendazole and levamisole on *Onchocerca volvulus* and *Dipetalonema perstans*. Trans R Soc Trop Med Hyg 69:355–360, 1975.
Orihel TC: "Cerebral filariasis" in Rhodesia—a zoonotic infection? Am J Trop Med Hyg 22:596, 1973.

88.3   STREPTOCERCIASIS

Wayne M. Meyers
and Ronald C. Neafie

DEFINITION. Streptocerciasis is an infection caused by the filarial nematode *Mansonella streptocerca* (Macfie and Corson, 1922), which was called *Dipetalonema streptocerca* until recently.

ETIOLOGY AND HISTORY. In the course of their studies on onchocerciasis in the Gold Coast (Ghana), Macfie and Corson in 1922 found microfilariae in skin snips that they recognized to be distinct from other known microfilariae that infect humans. Adult filariae presumed to be *M. streptocerca* were first seen in the chimpanzee in 1946 and in the tissues of humans in 1972. Adult female *M. streptocerca* are approximately 27 mm by 0.075 mm, and the adult male is 17 mm by 0.05 mm. The cuticle is thin and smooth, and the lateral chords are inconspicuous. The microfilariae are 180 to 240 μm by 2.5 to 5.0 μm and are unsheathed; sharp curving of the posterior end frequently gives them a characteristic "shepherd's crook" configuration (Fig. 88–3). In fresh mounts they swim less actively than do microfilariae of *Onchocerca volvulus*. The cephalic clear space is 3 to 5 μm long, and the first 4 nuclei are oval, occur in single file, and are followed by 7 to 10 smaller, more rounded nuclei (Fig. 88–4*A*). The terminal nucleus is oval or round, and the caudal clear space is 1 μm long (Fig. 88–4*B*).

EPIDEMIOLOGY AND DISTRIBUTION. Streptocerciasis is limited to western and central Africa and is most abundant in the tropical rain forest, where it is transmitted by the biting midge *Culicoides grahami*. Prevalence rates vary widely. In Zaire, up to 90% of the inhabitants of limited geographic areas are infected. Whether or not streptocerciasis is a zoonosis has not been established, but morphologically identical parasites found in chimpanzees suggest this possibility.

PATHOGENESIS AND PATHOLOGY. All adult filariae thus far observed (in approximately 100 patients) have been found in the dermis of long-term residents of

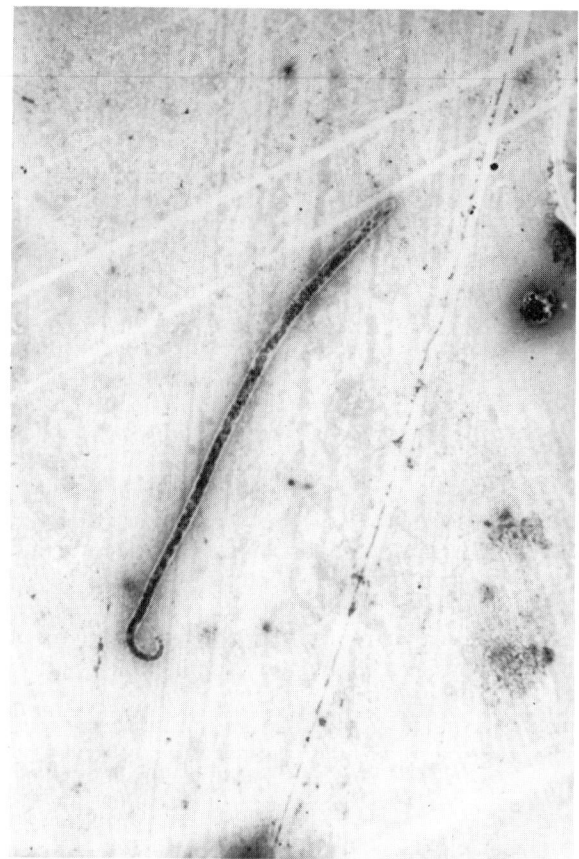

FIGURE 88–3. Whole microfilaria of *Mansonella streptocerca* obtained from skin snip. Note the "shepherd's crook" configuration (Giemsa stain, × 350). (Courtesy of the Armed Forces Institute of Pathology, Photograph Neg. No. 70-7193.)

endemic areas; thus, the length of the incubation period is unknown. Most worms inhabit the skin of the upper trunk and shoulder girdle. Live worms appear to glide readily between the dermal collagen bundles, provoking no reaction, but when worms die, an intense cellular response develops. Microfilariae are extravascular and have been observed between collagen fibers in the dermis and, rarely, in lymph nodes. Microscopic changes in the skin resemble those of onchocerciasis, but are less intense. There is as yet no evidence that the eye is affected by *M. streptocerca*. With diethylcarbamazine (DEC) therapy, a marked increase in the cellular exudates and edema occurs, especially around microfilariae. DEC kills adult worms, and papules then form around the coiled dead worms (Fig. 88–5). Lymph nodes are diffusely fibrotic, and the lymphatics are dilated. Whether or not these changes can cause elephantiasis is unknown.

CLINICAL MANIFESTATIONS. Many patients are asymptomatic, but the most consistent complaint is a chronic itching dermatitis, most pronounced over the thorax and shoulder girdle. The skin is thickened, hypopigmented macules develop, and one or a few papules are sometimes present. Axillary and inguinal lymphadenopathy is common. The macules in the skin are confused frequently with lesions of leprosy, and many patients with streptocerciasis are misdiagnosed and treated for leprosy for long periods. Macules of strep-

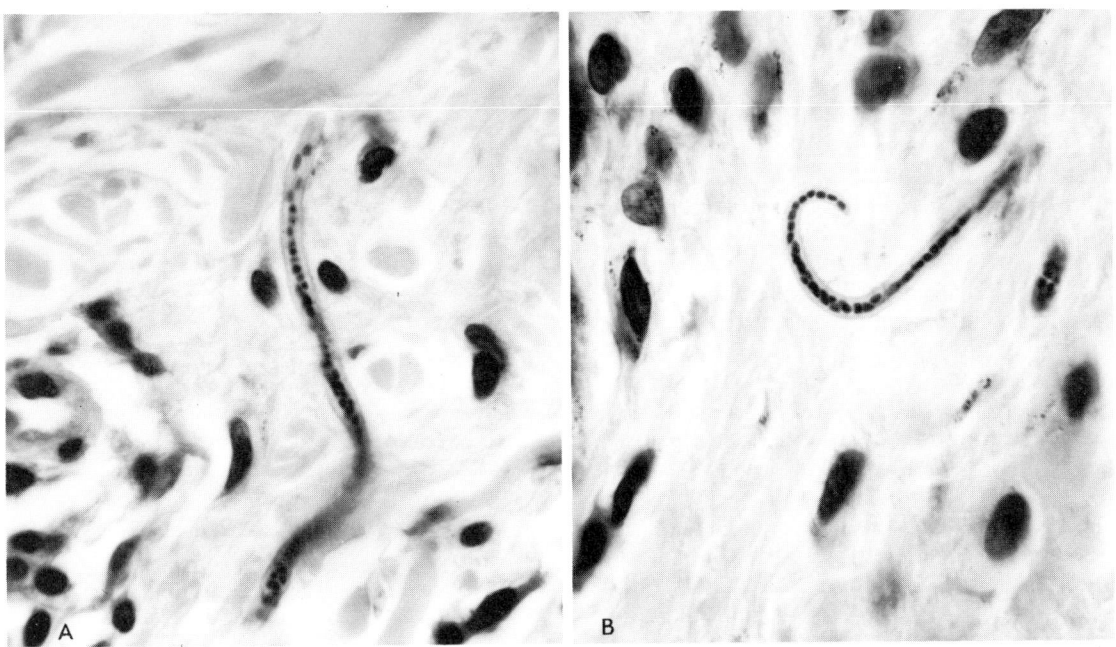

FIGURE 88–4. Diagnostic features of microfilariae of *Mansonella streptocerca* in sections of skin. The microfilariae are extravascular in the dermal collagen. *A,* Anterior end, showing cephalic space and nuclei (× 1080). (Courtesy of the Armed Forces Institute of Pathology, Photograph Neg. No. 71-10075.) *B,* Posterior end with "shepherd's crook" configuration and nuclei that reach nearly to the tip (× 1080). (Courtesy of the Armed Forces Institute of Pathology, Photograph Neg. No. 71-10074.)

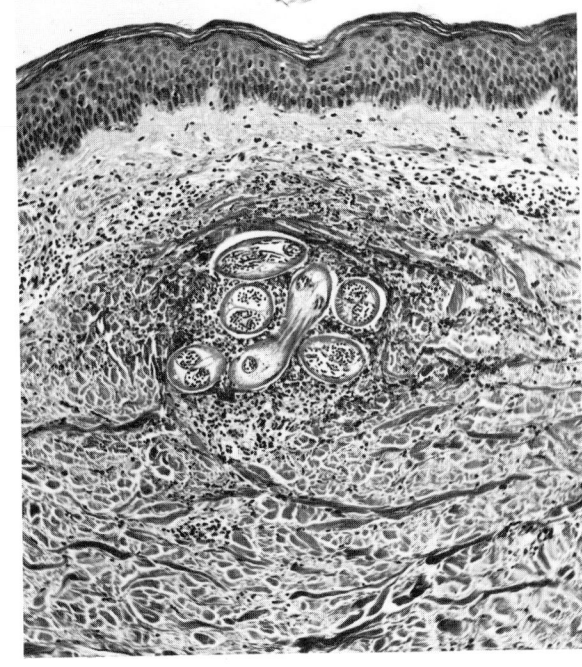

FIGURE 88–5. Section of skin containing multiple cross sections of adult *Mansonella streptocerca.* Biopsy specimen was from a papule that formed within 18 hours after ingestion of diethylcarbamazine. Note cellular exudate surrounding the coiled worm (× 110). (Courtesy of the Armed Forces Institute of Pathology, Photograph Neg. No. 73-1230.)

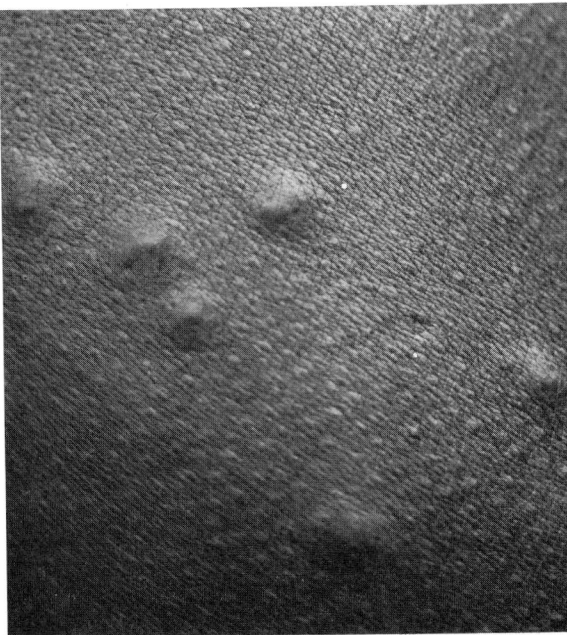

FIGURE 88–6. Multiple papules on the chest of a Zairian man with streptocerciasis. Papules developed within 18 hours after ingestion of 50 mg of diethylcarbamazine. (Courtesy of the Armed Forces Institute of Pathology, Photograph Neg. No. 77-5005.)

tocerciasis are not hyperesthetic, but many clinicians prefer to rely on the results of histopathologic studies for diagnosis, because sensory changes in early leprosy are often difficult to detect.

DEC at an initial dose of as little as 50 mg provokes a response analogous to the Mazzotti reaction. There is exacerbation of itching with cutaneous edema and the formation of papules around killed adult worms (Fig. 88–6). Occasionally the severity of this reaction requires the interruption of therapy and the administration of antihistamines.

DIAGNOSIS. Rapid diagnosis in most patients is made by demonstrating microfilariae in wet mounts of skin snips, usually obtained from skin over the scapulae (Fig. 88–3). In contrast with those of *O. volvulus*, the microfilariae of *M. streptocerca* are sluggish and when immobile assume the "shepherd's crook" configuration (Figs. 88–3 and 88–4*B*). Diagnosis is frequently made by the histopathologic identification of microfilariae of *M. streptocerca* (Fig. 88–4).

TREATMENT. Diethylcarbamazine kills the microfilariae and adults of *M. streptocerca*. Optimal dosages have not been established, but the drug is usually given at the same dosage as for onchocerciasis. Because DEC kills the adult worms, repeated courses of therapy may be curative for patients who do not dwell in endemic areas. Prognosis is excellent.

BIBLIOGRAPHY

Meyers WM, Connor DH, Harman LE, et al.: Human streptocerciasis. A clinicopathologic study of 40 Africans (Zairians) including identification of the adult filaria. Am J Trop Med Hyg 21:528–545, 1972.
Meyers WM, Moris R, Neafie RC, et al.: Streptocerciasis: Degeneration of adult *Dipetalonema streptocerca* in man following diethylcarbamazine therapy. Am J Trop Med Hyg 27:1137–1147, 1978.

88.4 DIROFILARIASIS

Ronald C. Neafie
and Wayne M. Meyers

DEFINITION. Dirofilariasis is an infection caused by filarial nematodes of the genus *Dirofilaria*. There are two forms of dirofilariasis: (1) pulmonary dirofilariasis caused by *Dirofilaria immitis*, the dog heartworm, and (2) subcutaneous dirofilariasis caused by *D. tenuis* (*Dirofilaria conjunctivae*), *D. repens*, and *D. ursi*-like worms.

PULMONARY DIROFILARIASIS

Morphology. Only immature *D. immitis* have been found in the lungs of humans. The worms are 100 to 350 μm in diameter. The cuticle is thick and multilayered and projects inward at the lateral chords to form prominent internal longitudinal ridges (Fig. 88–7). Lateral chords are usually poorly preserved, whereas somatic musculature is usually abundant. Internal organs consist of an intestine and 2 reproductive tubes in the female and an intestine and a single reproductive tube in the male.

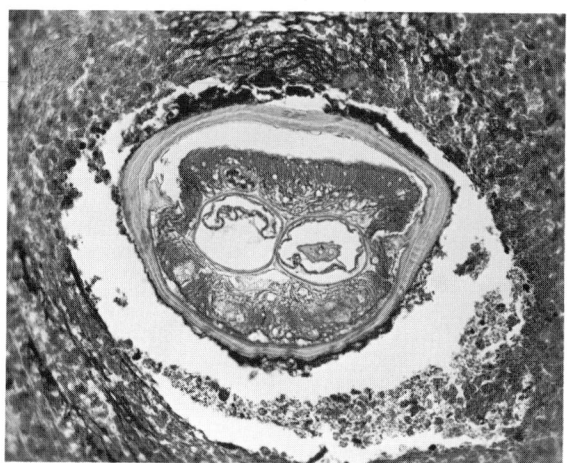

FIGURE 88–7. Transverse section of immature female *Dirofilaria immitis* in lung (Movat stain, × 275). (Courtesy of the Armed Forces Institute of Pathology, Photograph Neg. No. 71-1045.)

Epidemiology

Distribution. Pulmonary dirofilariasis has been reported from Japan, Australia, and the United States (especially the southern and eastern states, where approximately 50 cases have been reported). Human infection is largely determined by the prevalence of canine dirofilariasis and the extent to which humans are exposed to bites from the mosquito vectors.

Life Cycle. Although *D. immitis* infection occurs in the cat, fox, wolf, coyote, sea lion, and other mammals, the dog is by far the most important reservoir host. Coiled masses of adult worms inhabit the right ventricle of the definitive host, and their microfilariae circulate in the peripheral blood. The parasite is transmitted by many species of mosquitoes, which probably also transmit the parasite to humans, a dead-end host. Parasites probably develop partially in the right ventricle before

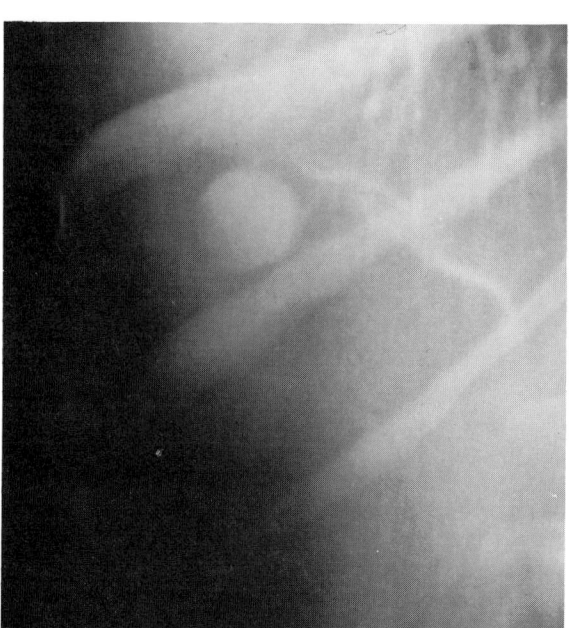

FIGURE 88–8. Roentgenogram of "coin lesion," 2.5 by 2.0 cm, in right lung. (Courtesy of the Armed Forces Institute of Pathology, Photograph Neg. No. 72-10156.)

dying and being swept into small pulmonary arteries. Neither mature worms nor microfilariae have been found in humans.

Pathology. Lesions are usually limited to the periphery of the lung and are sharply defined. They have a central area of necrosis surrounded by a zone of granulomatous inflammation and a fibrous wall. A single, coiled, usually necrotic, and occasionally calcified worm is found in the lumen of an artery within the area of necrosis. Multiple lesions are rare.

Clinical Manifestations. Most patients are asymptomatic; "coin lesions" detected during routine x-ray examinations of the chest are the most common presentation (Fig. 88–8). These lesions are 1 to 3 cm in diameter and well circumscribed. Clinical symptoms, when present, include chest pain, cough, hemoptysis, fever, chills, and malaise.

Diagnosis. Diagnosis is made by identifying the worm in biopsy or autopsy specimens.

Treatment. There are no chemotherapeutic agents. The lesions are removed frequently because the "coin lesion" is mistaken for cancer.

SUBCUTANEOUS DIROFILARIASIS

Etiology, Epidemiology, and Life Cycle. In 1957, Faust reviewed 37 known cases of dirofilariasis in humans. Most patients had worms in the skin and lived in the southern United States. Most infections previously attributed to *D. conjunctivae* are probably due to *D. tenuis,* a parasite of the subcutaneous tissue of the raccoon. *D. repens,* a parasite of the subcutaneous tissue of dogs and cats in Europe, Africa, and Asia, has also occasionally caused lesions in humans. Mosquitoes transmit both *D. tenuis* and *D. repens* to natural hosts and probably transmit the parasite from animals to humans. Subcutaneous dirofilariasis has been reported from the United States, Africa, Asia, Europe, and South America.

Morphology. *D. tenuis* females are 80 to 130 mm by 260 to 360 μm, and males are 40 to 48 mm by 190 to 260 μm. The cuticle is thick and multilayered and contains external and internal longitudinal ridges. Other morphologic characteristics are the same as for *D. immitis. D. repens* is greater in diameter than *D. tenuis.*

Pathology. Humans are an abnormal host, and although the parasites may reach maturity in humans, no microfilariae are seen in the circulation. Early lesions consist of a coiled, degenerating worm in an abscess in subcutaneous tissue. Chronic lesions are granulomatous

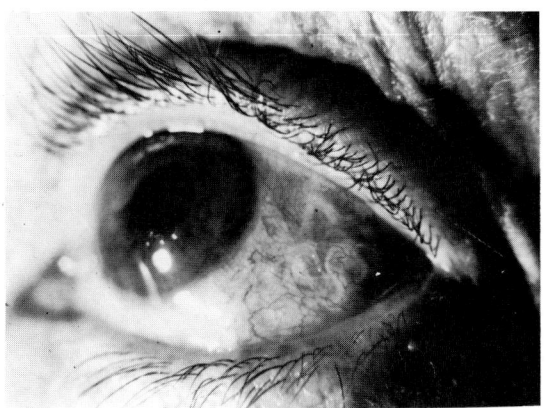

FIGURE 88–9. Female *Dirofilaria tenuis* in conjunctiva of left eye. (Courtesy of the Armed Forces Institute of Pathology, Photograph Neg. No. 74-6351-2.)

and contain epithelioid cells, foreign body giant cells, histiocytes, and eosinophils.

Clinical Manifestations. Lesions caused by *D. tenuis* and *D. repens* occur in many parts of the body but most commonly are found in the conjunctiva (Fig. 88–9), eyelid, scrotum, breast, arm, and leg. The lesion develops over a period of several weeks into a subcutaneous nodule that may be tender, painful, erythematous, and occasionally migratory.

Diagnosis. Diagnosis is usually made by identifying the worm in the biopsy specimen. Occasionally worms are extracted from the lesion and identified by gross examination.

Treatment. The only known treatment is surgical removal of the worm.

BIBLIOGRAPHY

Beaver PC, Orihel TC: Human infection with filariae of animals in the United States. Am J Trop Med Hyg 14:1010, 1965.

Beaver PC, Wolfson JS, Waldron MA, et al.: *Dirofilaria ursi*-like parasites acquired by humans in the northern United States and Canada: Report of two cases and brief review. Am J Trop Med Hyg 37:357–362, 1987.

Dayal Y, Neafie RC: Human pulmonary dirofilariasis: a case report and review of the literature. Am Rev Res Dis 112:437, 1975.

Font RL, Neafie RC, Perry HD: Subcutaneous dirofilariasis of the eyelid and ocular adnexa; report of six cases. Arch Ophthalmol 98:1079, 1980.

SECTION C

OTHER TISSUE NEMATODE INFECTIONS

89. DRACUNCULIASIS

Harrison C. Spencer

DEFINITION. Dracunculiasis (dracontiasis, guinea worm disease) is a painful, incapacitating disease caused by the parasite *Dracunculus medinensis* and transmitted by ingestion of drinking water containing cyclopoid copepods, fresh water microcrustaceans that harbor infective larvae. This nematode lives in the connective and subcutaneous tissues of humans until the female worm emerges through the skin to discharge its larvae into water. The clinical course is characterized by allergic prodromal symptoms, cutaneous ulceration, and secondary infection, and severe disability frequently results. Dracunculiasis is the only disease that can be eliminated completely by the provision of safe drinking water.

HISTORY. Guinea worm disease has been recognized since antiquity. Some believe it to be the "fiery serpent" referred to by Moses. Galen coined the term dracontiasis, and famous Roman and Greek physicians such as Plutarch and Pliny described the parasite in recognizable terms. Dracunculiasis was known to Persian and Arabic physicians including Avicenna who first described its clinical symptoms and called the disease "Medina sickness" because it was common in Medina. The contemporary term guinea worm disease derives from a European explorer who named the disease he found along the West African coast for the geographic region. The staff of Aesculapius, Roman god of medicine, may have originated from the ancient, still valid practice of removing the adult guinea worm by slowly winding it around a stick.

The role of the copepod intermediate host was first described by Aleksei Fedchenko in the early 1870s. It was the first recognition that the life cycle of a human parasite required an arthropod as an intermediate host. Linnaeus gave the parasite its modern scientific name of *Dracunculus medinensis* in his *Systema Naturae,* published in 1758.

ETIOLOGY. The family Dracunculoidea includes parasites of birds and mammals. Dracunculoidea are nematodes characterized by extreme sexual dimorphism and complete atrophy of the anus in the adult female. Only 1 species, *Dracunculus medinensis,* is found in humans.

Morphology and Physiology. The adult female worm appears as a creamy white, thin, translucent cord and is one of the longest nematodes known. It measures 60 to 80 cm (2 to 2–½ feet), and worms 120 cm have been recorded. It is slender also, approximately 1.7- to 2.0-mm wide. The uterus, which occupies most of the body cavity, contains millions of eggs, embryos, and first-stage larvae. The adult male is seen rarely and measures only 12- to 29-mm long and 0.4-mm wide. Little is known of how the worms subsist in the body.

Life Cycle (Fig. 89–1). After an incubation period of 10 to 14 months, the female worm migrates to the subcutaneous tissue, usually at the feet or legs, where a painful blister appears. When the affected part is immersed in water, the blister bursts, and the female worm protrudes through the skin and expels thousands of larvae into the water by contracting its uterus. The uterus may contain as many as 3 million larvae. On first immersion approximately 500,000 to 600,000 larvae are released. The adult female continues to release larvae upon subsequent contact with water, but the number decreases substantially.

Intermediate host. Larvae are actively motile until they are ingested by the copepod intermediate host, a species of *Cyclops* (Fig. 89–2). These carnivorous microcrustaceans, barely visible to the naked eye, measure 1 to 3 mm in length. On reaching the midintestine of the copepod, the larvae break through the soft wall and enter the hemocoel where they remain. Larvae remain active in pond water for 4 to 7 days, but the ability to infect Cyclops decreases after 3 days.

The development time of *D. medinensis* larvae in the copepod is temperature-dependent and species-specific but at optimal temperatures (25 to 30C) is approximately 2 to 3 weeks. The larvae molt twice. Third-stage larvae measure 240- to 608-μm long and 12- to 23-μm wide. Naturally infected adult copepods usually harbor only 1 infective larva; multiple infections are rare and may kill the copepod.

Definitive host. Humans become infected with guinea worm by drinking water containing cyclops infected with third-stage larvae. The copepods are killed by gastric juices. The liberated larvae penetrate the intestinal tract wall and migrate into the abdominal or thoracic cavity where they develop into mature adults. Mating occurs at about 3 months. The female worm continues to mature until its body consists almost entirely of a coiled distended uterus containing millions of rhabditoid larvae. Sometime during maturation the female begins an extensive migration that ends at the site of emergence. The worm begins to emerge from the body after an incubation period of 10 to 14 months.

EPIDEMIOLOGY

Distribution. More than 120 million poor, rural people in Africa and 20 million in Asia (Fig. 89–3) are considered at risk of infection with guinea worm. The annual incidence of infection is estimated at between 10 to 15 million. In Asia the disease is known to be present in parts of India and Pakistan. Residual disease may be present also in Yemen and Saudi Arabia. Dracunculiasis does not occur south of the equator in Africa. In West and Central Africa, known endemic countries include

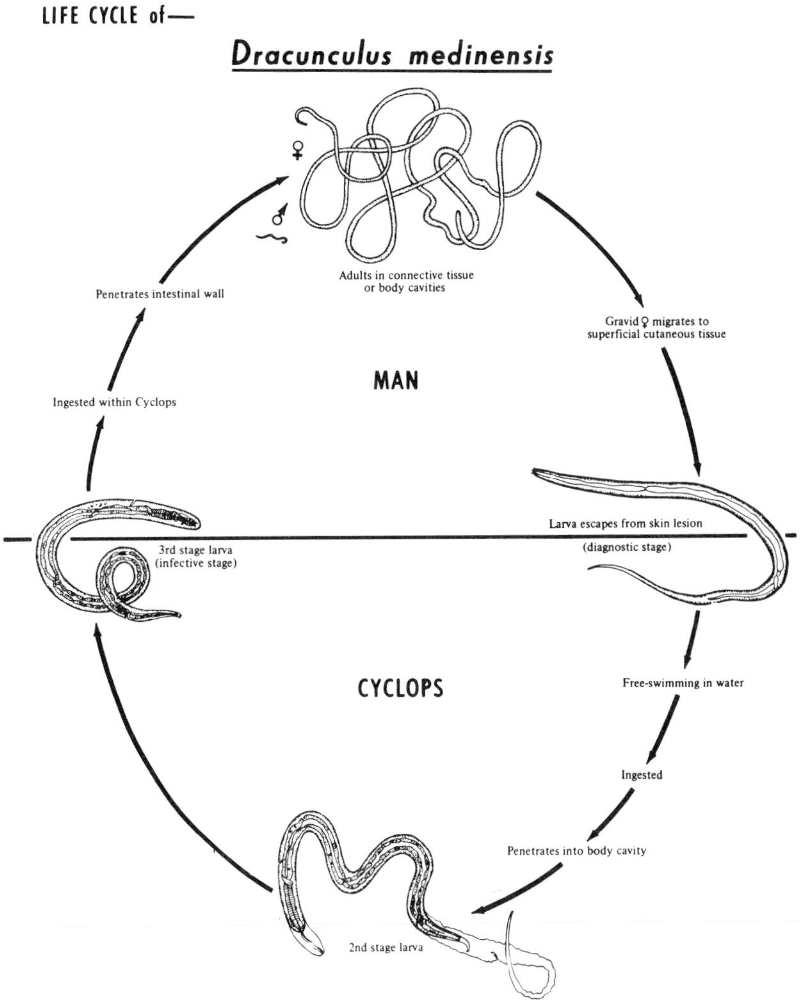

LIFE CYCLE of—

Dracunculus medinensis

FIGURE 89–1. Life cycle of *Dracunculus medinensis*. (From Melvin DM, Brooke MM, Healy GR, et al.: Common Blood and Tissue Parasites of Man. Life Cycle Charts. Atlanta, Georgia, Centers for Disease Control, 1979.)

Adults in connective tissue or body cavities

Penetrates intestinal wall

Gravid ♀ migrates to superficial cutaneous tissue

MAN

Ingested within Cyclops

Larva escapes from skin lesion (diagnostic stage)

3rd stage larva (infective stage)

CYCLOPS

Free-swimming in water

Ingested

Penetrates into body cavity

2nd stage larva

Benin, Burkina Faso, Cameroon, Central African Republic, Chad, Ghana, Cote d' Ivoire, Mali, Mauritania, Niger, Nigeria, Senegal, and Togo. In East Africa dracunculiasis is endemic in Ethiopia, Sudan, and northern Uganda. There is a small focus of the disease in northwest Kenya. Two African countries, Gambia and Guinea, may have eradicated the infection, but documentation is lacking.

Accurate estimates of prevalence and morbidity of guinea worm disease are not readily available. Dracunculiasis is typically a disease of rural communities that may be far from health centers and therefore from normal case-finding mechanisms. Few patients seek medical help, because there is no effective treatment. Furthermore, dracunculiasis is a disabling disease; those infected cannot travel long distances without help. In rural endemic areas, infected persons often remain at home while recuperating.

Transmission. Dracunculiasis is a focal disease that occurs seasonally. There are 2 general seasonal patterns. In semiarid areas such as the Sahel of West Africa and parts of India and Pakistan, contaminated surface sources of drinking water are present only during the brief rainy season, and transmission coincides with the rains. In endemic areas with surface sources of water throughout the year but distinct rainy and dry seasons, transmission occurs usually during the dry season when surface water sources are scanty and polluted. Severe drought, if sustained in semiarid areas, may interrupt transmission of the parasite, because people are forced to use drinking water from sources other than surface sources and because infection does not persist for more

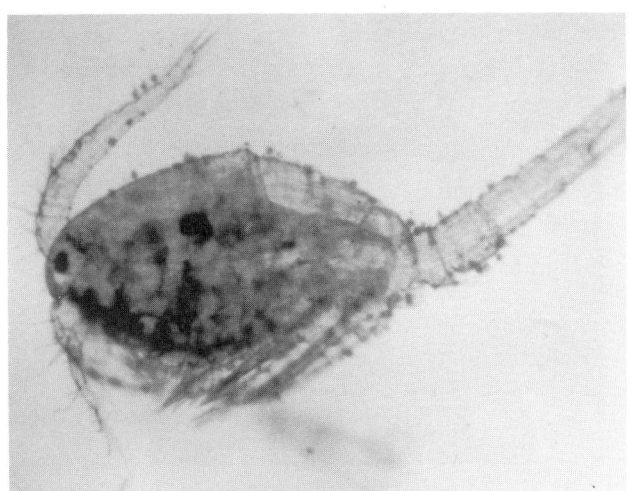

FIGURE 89–2. Lateral view of a cyclopoid copepod, the microcrustaceans that serve as the intermediate host of the guinea worm.

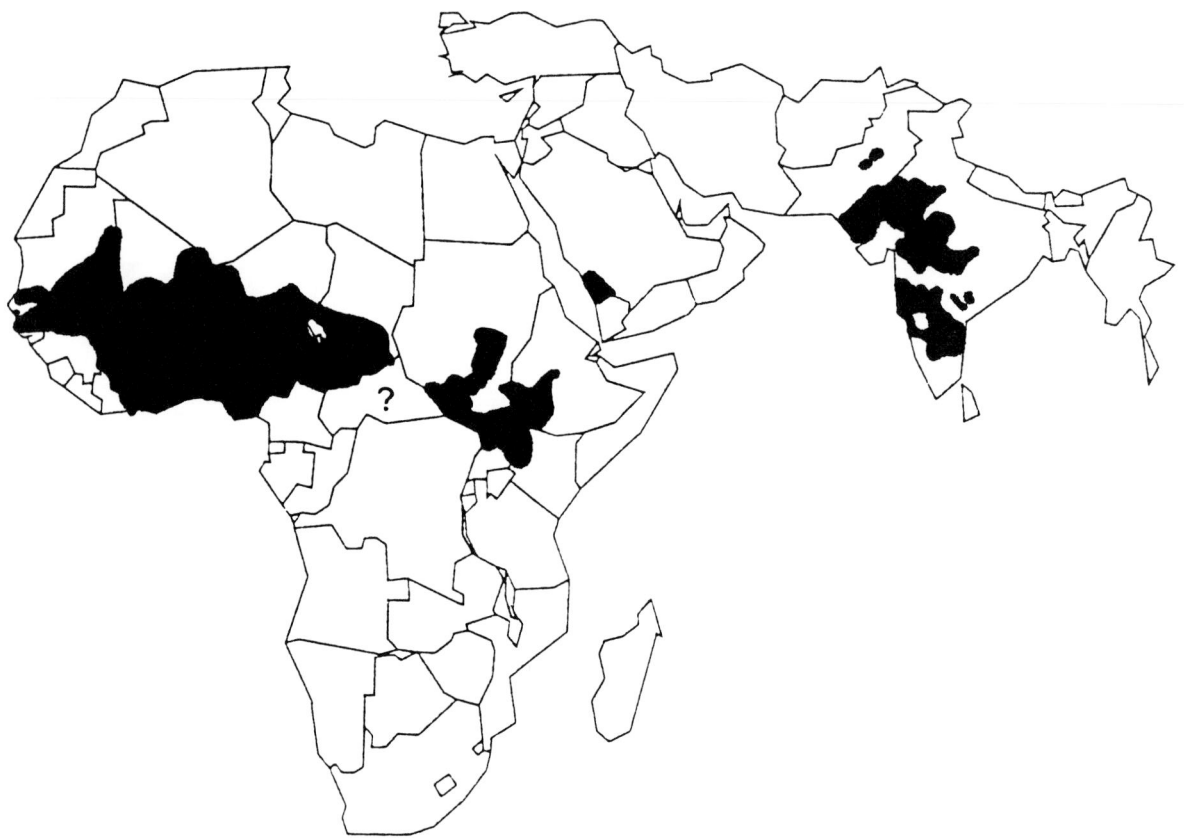

FIGURE 89–3. Distribution of *Dracunculus medinensis*. Endemic areas are in black. Guinea worm is not present in the New World.

than 1 to 2 years. These conditions applied to the Sind region of Pakistan in the 1930s and the Nara region of Mali in the 1970s.

A temperature of at least 15C is required for complete development of the larvae in the copepod and optimal temperatures are 25 to 30C. *D. medinensis* larvae cannot penetrate cyclops; therefore, only predatory cyclops species that ingest larvae serve as intermediate hosts (vectors). The copepod intermediate host flourishes only in standing, surface water as is found in ponds and large open wells, such as the step wells of India and Pakistan (Fig. 89–4). Guinea worm disease is uncommon in communities where people obtain their drinking water from flowing rivers or streams.

Humans are the only known host of *D. medinensis*. A wide range of mammals from many parts of the world have been reported to be infected, but the species of *Dracunculus* has not always been clear. The occasional cases of dracunculiasis reported in animals (usually from dogs) are probably isolated accidental infections with *D. medinensis* from humans. The apparent absence of zoonotic transmission is evidenced by failure of the disease to reappear in areas such as southern Russia where it has been eradicated from humans.

Socioeconomic Factors. The epidemiologic pattern of infection in a community is related to exposure as influenced by occupation and water consumption habits. There is no evidence for the development of acquired immunity nor for resistance to infection due to sex or age. Although the presence of developing or mature worms probably prevents new infections, some people

experience recurrent infections. A proportion of a population at risk never becomes infected; this has been attributed to the killing of larvae by high gastric acidity. However, x-rays show calcified worms in some supposedly uninfected people.

Unlike many other infectious diseases, dracunculiasis affects adults more frequently than children (Fig. 89–5). The highest infection rates usually occur in the 15- to 45-year age group, the most economically productive segment of society. Rural farmers are at particular risk because they may drink comparatively large amounts of water from ponds or other contaminated water sources

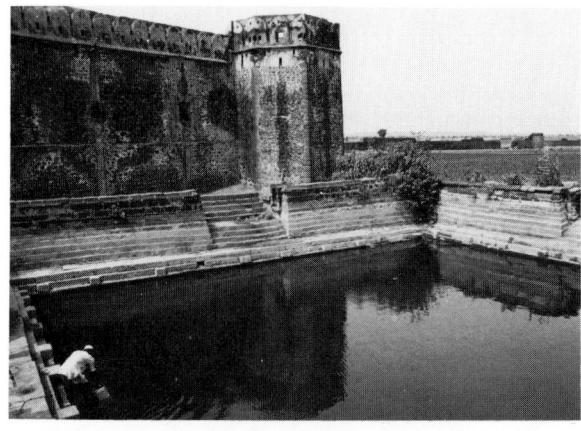

FIGURE 89–4. A step well in Maharashtra State, India. These large open wells, which also collect rainwater, provide ideal conditions for breeding of *Cyclops* and for contamination of the water by larvae.

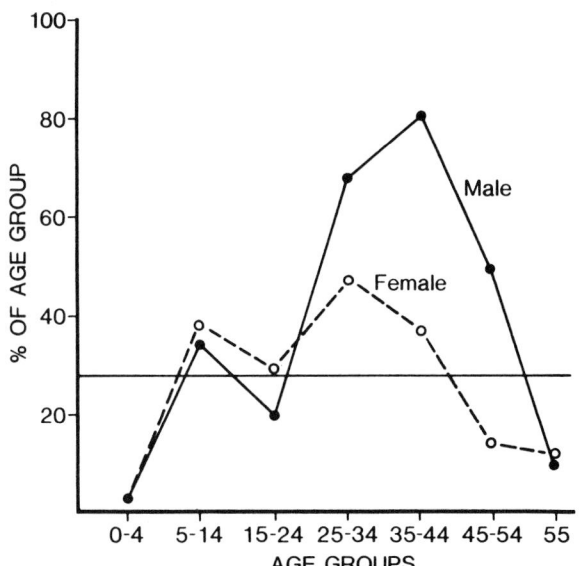

FIGURE 89–5. Guinea worm attack rate by age and sex in Ghana. (From Belcher DW, et al.: Am J Trop Med Hyg 24:246, 1975. Reprinted by permission.)

near their work. Children under 5 and adults over 55 are rarely infected. The male to female infection rates are inconstant and relate to the degree of exposure to *D. medinensis* as determined by occupation and water consumption habits.

Guinea worm is a disabling and economically crippling disease. Worms take an average of 3 to 8 weeks to fully emerge; the reported period of incapacitation averages 3 months and may be as long as 9 months or more. During this time infected persons may be unable to walk or move about easily. It has been reported that rarely victims are permanently crippled by dracunculiasis. Because guinea worm infection is not usually fatal, its true impact on communities has been underestimated. The disease is a major economic burden because of agricultural work loss; peak case rates coincide often with major agricultural activities of clearing land, planting, or harvesting. In one fertile area of 1.6 million inhabitants in Nigeria, estimated losses in rice production alone due to high dracunculiasis infection rates were $20 million a year. Dracunculiasis has also been shown to have an adverse effect on the ability of mothers to care for themselves and their children and to contribute to family income. School absenteeism increases during the guinea worm season (Fig. 89–6). Absenteeism is for 2 reasons: some children are infected themselves; whereas others must remain at home to carry out critical agricultural activities that infected adults are unable to perform. In areas where prevalence rates are high and onset of disease coincides with farming activity, substitute agricultural labor cannot always be obtained.

CLINICAL MANIFESTATIONS. Infected persons are asymptomatic during most of the 10- to 14-month incubation period. Symptoms begin just before a worm emerges. About one third of patients detect the serpiginous form of the worm or can palpate it just beneath the skin, usually a few days but occasionally up to a month before the worm emerges.

Allergic Manifestations. A few hours before the development of the local cutaneous lesion, there are pronounced systemic symptoms (e.g., erythema, urticarial rash, intense pruritis, nausea, vomiting, diarrhea, giddiness, syncope, and occasional fever) in 30 to 80% of patients. Suborbital edema may be present. Urticaria may appear up to 8 days before the worm begins to emerge.

Local Lesion. In most patients, the first physical sign is the formation of a reddish papule 2 to 7 cm in diameter with a vesicular center and an indurated margin. This is due to the cephalic end of the worm approaching the skin. The papule may at first be unnoticed. Within 1 to 3 days, however, the papule changes into a blister, probably due to either the production of some necrotizing secretion by the adult worm or by the release of larvae into the tissues. Formation of the blister is accompanied by local pruritis and an intense burning pain that induces the patient to immerse the affected body part in water for relief. The blister fluid is bacteriologically sterile and at first contains predominantly polymorphonuclear leukocytes, followed by increasing numbers of lymphocytes, eosinophils, and macrophages. Larvae are always present and usually white cells adhere to them. Lesions are most common (95%) on the lower extremities, particularly on the feet and ankles, but may be found anywhere on the body, including the hand, arm, trunk, buttocks, scrotum, knee joints, calf, thigh, shoulders, or even the angle of the jaw.

After 3 to 5 days the blister ruptures and discloses a small, superficial ulcer, 1.2 to 1.8 cm in diameter. At the center of the erosion, which sometimes heals quickly and spontaneously, is a minute hole large enough to admit a probe. Occasionally, the head of the worm

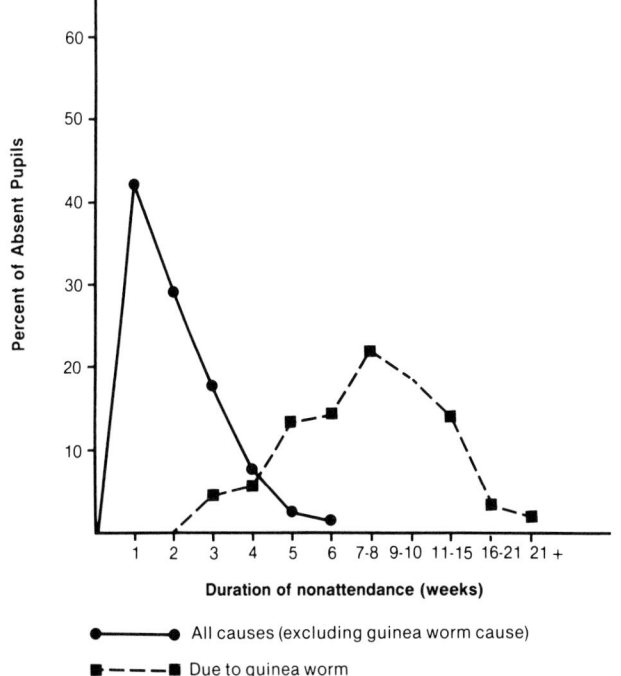

FIGURE 89–6. Comparison of percent duration school absenteeism from all causes excluding guinea worm (●–●) and from guinea worm (■ – – – ■) in Idere, Nigeria. (From Ilegbodu VA, et al.: Am J Trop Med Hyg 35:963, 1986. Reprinted by permission.)

protrudes through the hole, but usually the worm is not visible (Fig. 89–7). In response to contact with fresh water, a loop of uterus prolapsed through a ruptured anterior part of the body or through the mouth of the worm is projected through the hole. When the uterus has projected about 2.5 cm, it suddenly bursts and discharges an opaque, whitish material containing motile, first-stage, rhabditoid larvae. The process is repeated on subsequent exposure to water until the entire uterus is freed and all the larvae discharged. The act of prolapsing the uterus and releasing the larvae results in the death of the worm.

In general, only 1 to 2 worms emerge per year. However, massive infections have been reported; in one instance 56 adult worms emerged from one person in the same year. Severe local reactions may occur if the worm becomes injured or lacerated while lying in the subcutaneous tissues. The extremity may become extremely painful, inflamed, and edematous. The patient may be unable to walk.

Complications. Worms that fail to emerge usually die, become calcified, and cause no symptoms. They may be detected by x-ray (Fig. 89–8) or felt as hard, convoluted cords under the skin. However, nonemergent or aberrant worms may cause abscesses. Worms have been found in an abscess cavity in the pericardium of a 35-year-old male with constrictive pericarditis, in the subconjunctival space, and in extradural abscesses.

The principal complication of guinea worm disease is secondary bacterial infection. Depending on the site of emergence, there may be acute abscesses, cellulitis, arthritis, synovitis, epididymo-orchitis, bubo, chronic ulcerations, fibrous ankylosis of joints, and contractures of tendons. Approximately 40% of patients are totally incapacitated for about 6 weeks. Worms may rupture in the tissues leading to the formation of large abscesses. Intra-articular infections with acute arthritis, usually of the knee or ankle joints, may occur. Tetanus is a potentially lethal complication.

DIAGNOSIS. Diagnosis of guinea worm disease requires demonstration of or a documented history of worm emergence. Guinea worm is distinctive (Fig. 89–7). Once the blister has broken, the diagnosis can be confirmed by placing cold water on the ulcer or ethyl chloride near it. This results in release of actively mobile larvae that can be viewed through a microscope under low power.

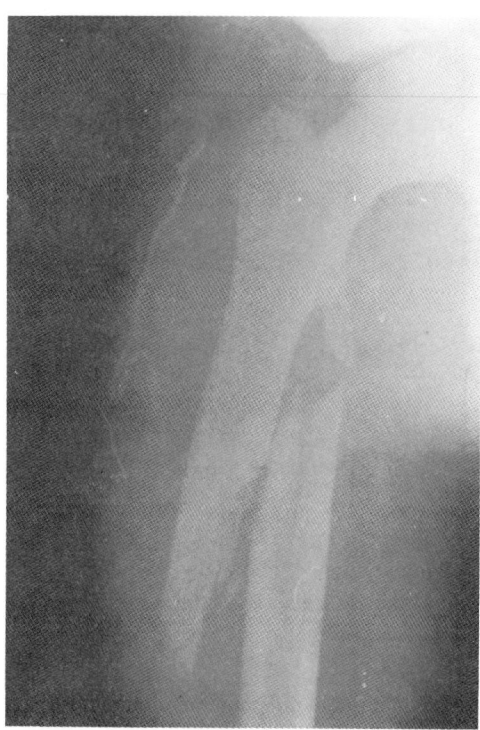

FIGURE 89–8. Dracunculiasis. Radiograph of a fractured femur demonstrates a calcified guinea worm in the subcutaneous tissues of this African.

On occasion a worm can be palpated in the subcutaneous tissues or its outline seen by reflected light. In doubtful cases, cold water placed over the site may cause the worm to emerge or to move. Worms that fail to emerge may become calcified and produce a characteristic radiologic picture (Fig. 89–8). Cutaneous larvae migrans may be confused with a serpiginous guinea worm beneath the skin. However, cutaneous larvae migrans is caused by abortive infections with dog or cat hookworms that are much shorter than guinea worm. Eosinophilia has been documented frequently during worm emergence. Levels vary usually between 13 to 18%, although values more than 30% have been recorded. Although eosinophilia occurs before worm emergence and in cryptic infections, its presence is not useful for diagnosis.

Immunodiagnostic tests are not useful in routine diagnosis. Several tests have been developed; however, none have proven sufficiently sensitive and specific.

TREATMENT. Winding each emerging worm onto a small stick a few centimeters a day as has been done for centuries is useful provided that it begins when the worm just emerges and precautions, such as sterile dressings and antiseptics, are used to prevent secondary infection (Fig. 89–9). The process can be facilitated by plunging the affected body part into cold water. This causes the worm's uterus to contract and expel larvae; then, the anterior portion of the worm becomes flaccid.

Drugs. Four benzimidazole compounds have been reported to have an effect on the emerging adult female worms: metronidazole (400 mg for an adult, given daily for 10 to 20 days), niridazole (25 mg/kg of body weight given daily for 10 days), thiabendazole (50 mg/kg of

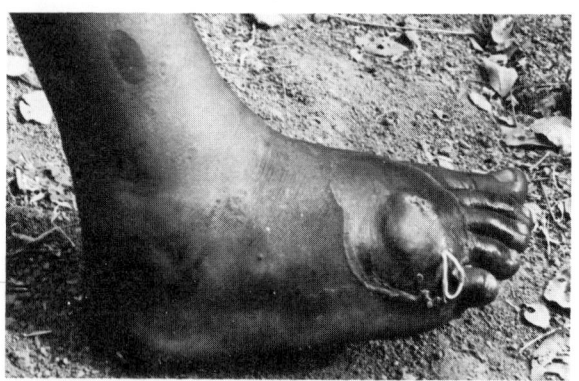

FIGURE 89–7. Large suppurating blister on the foot of a 6-year-old girl. A portion of a female *Dracunculus* is being extruded.

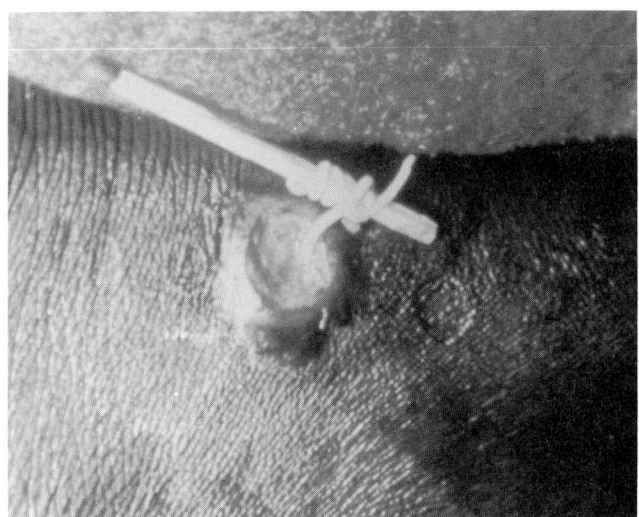

FIGURE 89–9. Traditional method of winding emerging guinea worm onto a small stick a few centimeters each day.

body weight given daily for 3 days), and mebendazole (400 to 800 mg for an adult, given daily for 6 days). All appear to act similarly; they provide symptomatic relief and facilitate removal of worms. These compounds have marked anti-inflammatory properties and thus reduce the intense tissue reaction that develops around the worm once it begins to emerge from the skin. However, they have no effect on pre-emergent worms or on the larvae.

Surgery. Surgical removal of pre-emergent female worms, after administration of a local anesthetic, is sometimes practiced in India. If the outline of the worm can be seen or palpated, the whole parasite can be easily extracted intact after making a small incision. However, complete removal is difficult if the worm is in the deep fascia or wound around tendons or if the surface has been damaged and there is adherence to the surrounding tissue.

PREVENTION AND CONTROL. Guinea worm disease is acquired only by drinking water contaminated with infected copepods. Therefore, it is the only communicable disease that could be eradicated completely if populations living in endemic areas were provided with and used safe drinking water. In Kwara State, Nigeria, the provision of protected water supplies in the form of boreholes reduced the prevalence of dracunculiasis in affected communities from 50% or more to near zero within 3 years of intervention. The epidemiology of guinea worm disease suggests that it can be eradicated, and a global effort to eradicate dracunculiasis is currently underway. The disease is focal, and its geographical range is limited. Infection is obvious, and there is low infectivity. Humans are the only host for *D. medinensis*. The fragility of the guinea worm transmission cycle is attested to by the eradication of the disease from areas once endemic for dracunculiasis in Asia, the Middle East, parts of Africa, and a small focus in the Americas.

There is no effective vaccine or treatment for dracunculiasis. However, health education alone or with the provision of new or improved sources of drinking water,

filtration of drinking water, and/or chemical treatment of drinking water sources can significantly reduce incidence of the disease.

Improvement of Water Supplies. Introduction and use of safe water supplies virtually eliminate guinea worm disease in a community within 1 to 2 years. Piped water supplies are ideal. When cases continue to occur in urban centers with piped water, it is because patients are infected elsewhere. For example, guinea worm disease persisted in Ibadan, Nigeria, after piped water was installed because many inhabitants had land in the surrounding areas that they farmed about 1 month each year. During that time they would often drink contaminated pond water. When technically and economically feasible, boreholes and tube wells can provide safe water.

Much can be done even without economic resources to develop sophisticated methods of water supply. The disease has been eliminated in areas of India and Russia by filling in step wells and replacing them with protected bore holes and tube wells. Raised edges and concrete barriers for draw wells can help to prevent infected persons from contaminating water.

Filtering household or individual drinking water is also an effective way to prevent guinea worm infection. A cloth filter is placed over the neck of a vessel from which drinking water is poured. Cheap, durable, efficient nylon filters have been developed. A pore size of 100 μm removes all copepod stages capable of ingesting and nurturing larvae but allows free flow of water. A 100 μm filter may clog; a mesh of 200 μm allows freer flow of water and retains large copepodid stages, including virtually all infected ones. When synthetic filters are too costly, water can be filtered effectively through locally available cotton cloth double- or triple-folded.

Chemical Treatment of Ponds and Wells. A number of chemical disinfectants and pesticides have been shown under field conditions to control cyclops when applied to sources of drinking water. However, temephos (Abate) is considered the compound of choice because of its efficacy, low toxicity, and safety for the environment. The World Health Organization Expert Committee on Pesticides has declared temephos to be safe for use in drinking water at a target dose of 1 mg/L. That concentration eliminates copepods from a water source for 4 to 7 weeks.

There are many considerations for the use of temephos. Chemical treatment is expensive and less permanent than provision of safe water. Depending on the formulation used, temephos may give an unpleasant odor and taste to water. Repeated applications are necessary. The cost greatly escalates if there are multiple, large water sources. Timing of application to coincide with transmission is crucial. Temephos is best applied when there are a few, well-defined water sources and when transmission is highly seasonal.

Health Education. There is widespread local ignorance of the etiology and mode of transmission of guinea worm. Health education is vital to acceptance and use of control measures, such as filters. In Burkina Faso, health education to promote filtration of drinking water through a nylon cloth reduced prevalence rates from as high as 54% to zero in only 2 transmission seasons. Health education may be critical to whether people choose safe drinking water when multiple sources of water are available. Health education also can change behavior so that persons with emerging worms do not place the affected part in water. This simple change in behavior would result in eradication.

BIBLIOGRAPHY

Adamson PB: Dracontiasis in antiquity. Med Hist 32:204–209, 1988.
Belcher DW, Wurapa FK, Wand WB, et al.: Guinea worm in Southern Ghana: Its epidemiology and impact on agricultural productivity. Am J Trop Med Hyg 24:243–249, 1975.
DeRooy C: Guinea worm control as a major contributor to self-sufficiency in rice production in Nigeria. Lagos: UNICEF, Nigeria, 1987.
Edungbola LD: Babana Parasitic Diseases Project II. Prevalence and impact of dracontiasis in Babana District, Kwara State, Nigeria. Trans R Soc Trop Med Hyg 77:310–315, 1983.
Edungbola LD, Watts SJ: Epidemiological assessment of the distribution and endemicity of guinea worm infection Asa, Kwara State, Nigeria. Trop Geogr Med 37:22–28, 1985.
Edungbola LD, Watts SJ, Alabi TO, et al.: The impact of a UNICEF-assisted rural water project on the prevalence of guinea worm disease in Asa, Kwara State, Nigeria. Am J Trop Med Hyg 39:79–85, 1988.
Hoeppli R: Parasites and Parasitic Infections in Early Medicine and Science. Kuala Lumpur, Malaysia, University of Malaya Press, 1959.
Ilegbodu VA, Kale OO, Wise, RA, et al.: Impact of guinea worm disease on children in Nigeria. Am J Trop Med Hyg 35:962–964, 1986.
Muller R: Guinea worm disease: Epidemiology, control and treatment. Bull WHO 57:683–689, 1979.
Nowasu ABC, Ifezulike EO, Anya AO: Endemic dracontiasis in Anambra State of Nigeria: Geographical distribution, clinical features, epidemiology and socioeconomic impact of the diseases. Ann Trop Med Parasitol 76:187–200, 1982.
Reddy CRRM, Devi CS, Reddy M, et al.: Dracontiasis. Review of surgical problems and treatment. Int Surg 52:481–488, 1969.
Reddy CRRM, Narasaiah IL, Parvath G: Epidemiological studies on guinea worm infection. Bull WHO 40:521–529, 1969.
Sullivan JJ, Long EG: Synthetic-fibre filters for preventing dracunculiasis. 100 vs 200 micrometres pore size. Trans R Soc Trop Med Hyg 82:465–466, 1988.
U.S. National Research Council: Opportunities for control of dracunculiasis. Washington, D.C., National Academy Press, 1985.
World Health Organization: Dracunculiasis: Global surveillance summary—1986. Wkly Epid Rev 62:337–339, 1987.

90.   TRICHINOSIS

K. Darwin Murrell

DEFINITION. Trichinosis is a disease caused by parasites of the genus *Trichinella* (Owen, 1835) that humans acquire from eating the muscles of wild animals or domestic pigs. The severity is usually proportional to the number of larvae ingested, and the disease is characterized by fever, gastrointestinal symptoms, myositis, swollen eyelids, and eosinophilia.

HISTORY. Some authorities believe the disease syndrome was recognized in Biblical times and was responsible for the Mosaic proscription of pork. This is questioned by Old Testament scholars, however, who believe the admonition was against beasts of prey and animals

with obnoxious habits. The encysted larval stage of *Trichinella spiralis* was first examined microscopically in 1835 by James Paget, a British medical student who was studying muscle tissue from a cadaver. Sir Richard Owen confirmed Paget's findings and published the first description and scientific designation for this parasite. Joseph Leidy of Philadelphia demonstrated the parasite in swine muscle in 1844, and Zenker related human trichinosis to the ingestion of infected pork in 1860. The essentials of the life cycle of *T. spiralis* were clarified during the 1850s by Leuckhart and Virchow. By the early twentieth century, trichinosis was recognized as an important public health problem. Despite improvements in many countries, notably in Europe, it remains a problem in the United States, Mexico, Chile, and other South American countries and is increasing in significance in several tropical regions, including Thailand, Kenya, Tanzania, and Senegal. Recent studies on isolates of *Trichinella* indicate that there are major differences in the genetic and biologic properties of parasites of arctic, temperate, and tropical regions.

ETIOLOGY. Infection occurs by the ingestion of meat containing infective, encysted larvae. The severest manifestations of the disease or infection are due to the larval offspring of the viviparous female worms rather than to the adult worms. Extensive invasion of the striated muscles and the epithelial lining of the small intestine stimulates a pronounced inflammatory response to the worm and its released antigens; it is this defensive response of the host that produces illness and sometimes death.

Biology. *T. spiralis* is nearly unique among helminthic parasites in that all stages of development occur within a single host; over 100 species of mammals have been reported to be susceptible to infection. The infective encysted larvae may remain viable in the host's musculature for many years; they may also survive long periods in decaying and putrefying muscle. These attributes confer a high probability of successful transmission.

Morphology. The adult worms are small and slender, with slightly tapered anterior ends, a common feature of the superfamily Trichuroidea (Fig. 90–1A). The males measure 1.4 to 1.6 mm in length by 40 to 60 μm in transverse diameter. The male has 2 pseudobursal flaps at the posterior end, with 2 pairs of papillae between the flaps; the pseudobursae aid in embracing the female during coitus. The female is a little more than twice as long as the male, 2.2 to 3.6 mm, and about one and a half times as broad. The vulva is situated near the middle of the esophageal region. A column of cells called stichocytes are associated with the capillary-like esophagus; the secretions of these cells contain potent antigens that are important in the host's response to the parasite.

LIFE CYCLE. When humans consume raw or rare flesh infected with cysts of *Trichinella* (Fig. 90–2), the cysts are digested out of the muscle in the stomach; the larvae (L_1 or first stage) are resistant to gastric juice. After passage to the small intestine, the larvae burrow beneath the columnar epithelium and lie just above the lamina propria, completely enveloped by tissue. There they undergo 4 molts within about 36 hours and develop

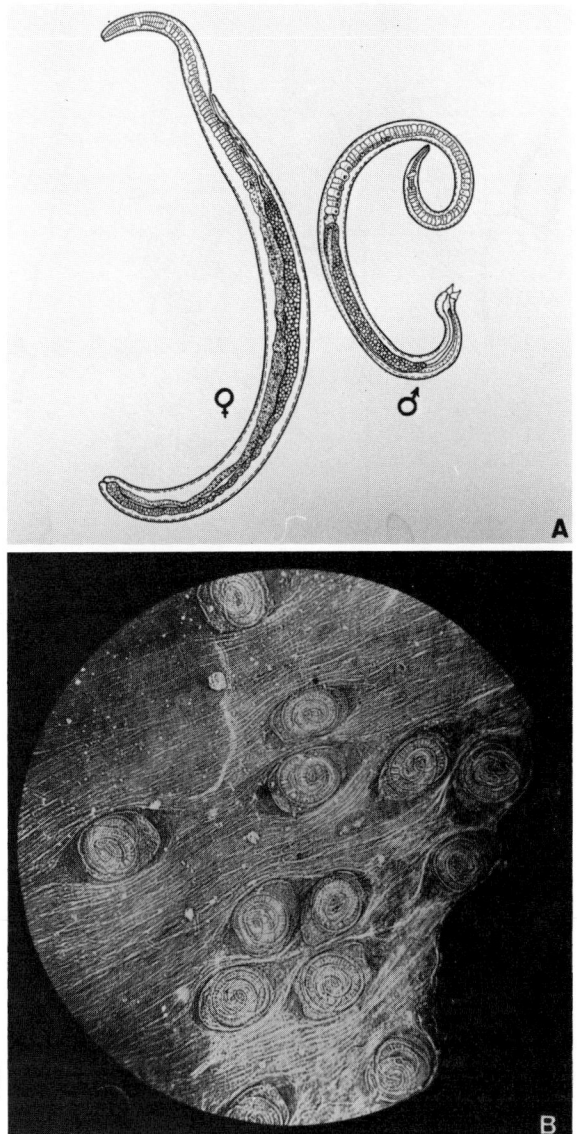

FIGURE 90–1. *A,* Morphology of adult male and female *Trichinella spiralis. B,* Compression of hog diaphragm muscle showing encysted trichinae.

humans averages 400 by 260 μm; the encysted larvae have grown to 800 to 1000 μm in length and are now fully infective. Unusual for nematodes of this group, these larvae can be typed as to sex after artificial excystation. In humans, calcification of the cyst may begin within 6 months to a year, a process that eventually leads to death of the encysted larvae.

EPIDEMIOLOGY AND DISTRIBUTION. *Trichinella* is widespread among wild mammals, especially carnivores, wild pigs, and other species that are cannibalistic or eat carrion. Formerly, infected pork was considered the only important source of infection for humans, who infected their domestic pigs through the practice of feeding them garbage containing meat scraps. However, on a worldwide basis, pork is decreasing in importance as a source of trichinosis, whereas wild animal meat is increasing in importance. For instance, in 1986, infected bear meat accounted for 38% of traceable human cases in the United States. In the Soviet Union, over 90% of trichinosis cases are attributed to eating bear and wild boar meat. In tropical Africa, trichinosis is primarily sylvatic, and humans are infected through the ingestion of improperly cooked bush pigs and wart hogs. Trichinosis also occurs in Egypt and Lebanon, where pork appears to be the main source of infection. Sylvatic infections in wild animals are also reported from Asia, although direct transmission to humans rarely occurs except in Thailand and China. Most human infections in Central and South America have been traced to domesticated pigs, but too few wild animals have been examined to be certain that there is no indigenous cycle in wild animals in this region.

Species and Strains of *Trichinella*. The natural maintenance cycle of *Trichinella* is among carrion-feeding or cannibalistic carnivores. Domestic pigs and rats are secondary hosts, although domestic pigs have been the main source of human infections in most developed and agricultural societies (Fig. 90–3). The relative importance of both domestic pigs (synanthropic) and wild animals (sylvatic) as potential sources of human infection must be considered carefully in designing control programs. Not all wild animal infections are directly transmissible to swine; the pig is more resistant to sylvatic *Trichinella* than humans are.

Isolates from different hosts of geographic localities should not be considered identical; *T. spiralis* is a species complex with at least 3 subspecies: *T. s. spiralis*, a parasite mainly of temperature regions, with domestic pigs as the main host for man; *T. s. nativa*, common to carrion-feeding carnivores in northern temperate regions, especially in such Arctic species as polar bears and walruses (both are chief sources of infection to humans); and *T. s. nelsoni*, a parasite maintained in nature in equatorial Africa. These subspecies may be raised to specific rank when more details are known. *Trichinella pseudospiralis* appears to be most distinctive. It is characterized by the absence of a cyst around the muscle larvae and has not been reported from humans. *T. s. nelsoni* from hyenas in Kenya and *T. s. nativa* from polar bears in the Arctic have low infectivity for domestic pigs and rats. Recent studies have demonstrated, however, that the domestic pig subspecies, *T. s. spiralis*,

into adult worms. Still within the tissue, the male and female worms mate. After fertilization, the females begin to discharge live larvae (as early as 4 to 7 days after infection). Production of larvae may continue for 4 to 16 weeks or more, depending on host species, until the worms are finally expelled from the intestine; the longevity of adult worms in the human intestine is not known with certainty.

Each newborn larva (about 100 μm long by 6 μm in diameter) makes its way into the lamina propria, where it enters a draining lymph node or blood vessel and is carried to the arterial circulation via the thoracic duct. The newborn larva is capable of invading nearly any tissue but can survive only in a striated skeletal muscle cell. Invasion of the muscle cell induces changes that culminate in a new host unit termed the "nurse cell." The larva begins to coil, and the nurse cell completes the formation of the cyst around the larva by 17 to 21 days after infection (Fig. 90–1*B*). The cyst size in

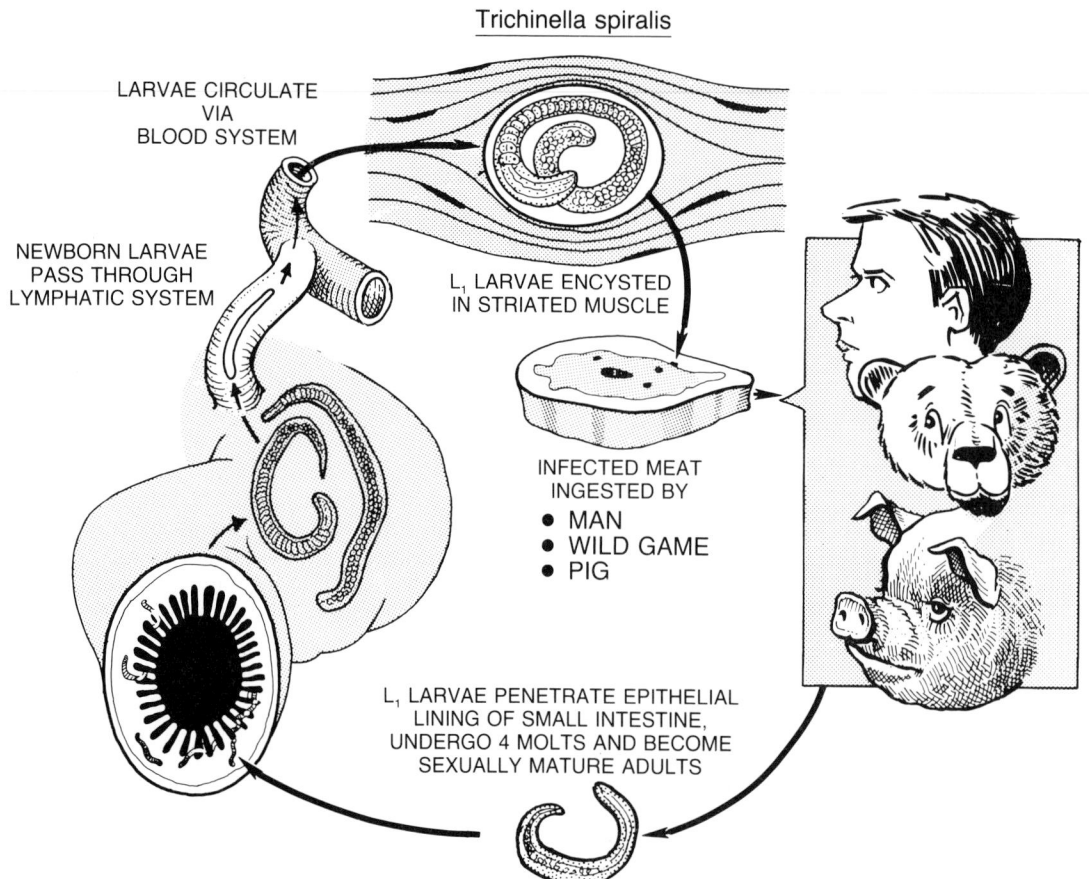

FIGURE 90–2. Life cycle of *Trichinella spiralis* showing stages and locations of development.

has been introduced into wild animal populations, increasing the importance of a sylvatic reservoir of *Trichinella* to the domestic cycle. An important difference between the Arctic parasites and those from domestic pigs is the remarkable resistance to freezing shown by the former.

Swine. The high incidence of human trichinosis previously reported in the United States and Europe was caused primarily by failure to control the disease in swine. A strong association between garbage feeding and swine trichinosis was apparent from prevalence data obtained on market hogs; in the United States in the 1950s, the prevalence rate of trichinosis in garbage-fed hogs was about 11%, whereas only 1% of grain-fed hogs were found to be infected. With the introduction of garbage-cooking laws to prevent the transmission of vesicular exanthema and hog cholera in swine, the rates for garbage-fed hogs fell to about 0.5 to 1% by the 1980s. The use of frozen foods undoubtedly also played an important role in this decrease. In Europe, a major factor in reducing the incidence of swine trichinosis has been the adaptation of routine inspection procedures at the slaughter plants. In Germany, for example, the reported prevalence of swine trichinosis is less than 0.00003%. It is 0.0008% in the USSR and 0.0% in Denmark.

Rats have traditionally been assigned an important role in the transmission of *T. spiralis* to hogs. Rats obtain their infections from the same source as hogs and

represent only one of several important sources of infection. The fact remains, though, that hogs will eat rats when they are available; thus, the opportunity for direct transmission of *T. spiralis* to hogs by infected rats must be considered significant in any epidemiologic investigation.

Ethnic Eating Habits. Certain eating customs play an important role in perpetuating human trichinosis. For example, ethnic groups of central European and Southeast Asian origin prefer the taste of raw pork; others may be infected by tasting raw sausages to check the flavor of seasonings. Thus, in the United States, persons of German and Italian extraction have an infection rate at autopsy of nearly 2½ times the national average because of their affinity for cured but uncooked sausage products. Recently, 2 large outbreaks of trichinosis among Indochinese refugees were reported. Investigation revealed they had cooked locally purchased pigs for community celebrations according to their practice in their homeland, an area with apparently low or nonexistent incidence of swine infections. The widespread adoption of fast cooking methods using microwave ovens may become an increasing problem; the reported difficulty of these ovens in achieving uniform heat distribution requires more care to ensure thoroughness of the cooking.

PATHOGENESIS AND CLINICAL MANIFESTATIONS. The level of infection generally determines the symptomatology of trichinosis, although the patient's

LIFE CYCLES IN VARIOUS PARTS OF THE WORLD

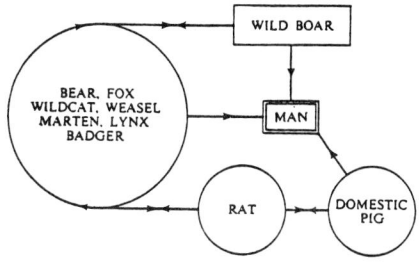

TEMPERATE **T.s.spiralis**

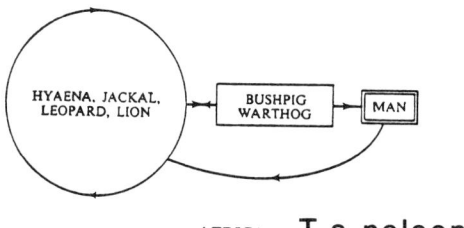

AFRICA **T.s.nelsoni**

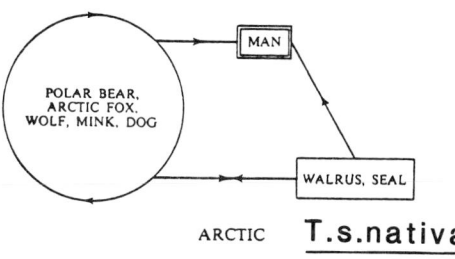

ARCTIC **T.s.nativa**

FIGURE 90–3. Major transmission pattern of *T. s. spiralis*, *T. s. nelsoni,* and *T. s. nativa* in endemic regions.

TABLE 90–1. Pathogenesis of Trichinosis

Days After Infection	Developmental Phase	Symptoms and Signs (Heavy Infections)
1 to 7	Intestinal	Gastrointestinal signs, i.e., nausea, abdominal pain; headache
9 to 28	Muscle	Muscular pain, facial edema, fever, chills, eosinophilia, tachycardia, coma, respiratory difficulties
14+	Encystment or chronic	Mental apathy, neurotoxic symptoms, possible myocarditis, anemia, muscular swelling

reflect chronic exposure and the development of intestinal immunity.

Muscle Invasion Phase. This stage, beginning about 7 to 9 days after exposure, is associated with penetration of the newborn larvae into muscle cells, initiating a strong inflammatory response, especially in the extraocular muscles, masseters, muscles of the larynx, tongue, diaphragm, and neck, intercostals, and muscular attachments to tendons and joints. The fibers become edematous and enlarged. Inflammation is attended by an infiltration of neutrophils, eosinophils, lymphocytes, and tissue histiocytes; this process reaches its peak at about 5 to 6 weeks of infection and diminishes when the encapsulation process ends. Early symptoms of this stage are swelling of the eyelids and facial edema. Following this, muscle swelling, tenderness, pain on movement, and fever usually develop. Headache, fainting, urticaria, "splinter" hemorrhages beneath the fingernails and toenails, conjunctivitis, loss of appetite, hoarseness, dysphagia, dyspnea, and edema of the legs may also occur. Fever can be delayed until several weeks after infection but may eventually reach 104°F for a week or more in heavy infections. Pain is noticed at about the time facial edema appears. It is most severe between the second and fourth weeks of infection but may persist for a longer period and can be so intense as to make chewing, talking, and swallowing difficult. Respiratory symptoms, including dyspnea, result from involvement of respiratory muscles, and myocarditis may also be apparent resulting from unsuccessful attempts by the larvae to invade the heart.

Neurologic Complications. Neurologic symptoms may accompany migration of the larvae through central nervous system tissue; the resulting intracerebral hemorrhage and marked meningeal irritation may simulate meningitis. Patients may exhibit dizziness, ataxia, hysteria, and psychotic disturbances. Seizures, monoparesis, and, eventually, coma can accompany severe infections. Larvae cannot successfully encyst in the nervous system.

Myocardial Complications. Myocarditis is a frequent serious complication of trichinosis and may lead to acute congestive heart failure, usually 4 to 8 weeks after infection. Larvae migrate through the myocardium between the second and fifth weeks, producing at least 2 clinical patterns: (1) sudden death, presumably from dysrhythmia, or (2) in the majority of patients, a prolonged illness associated with tachycardia, hypotension, elevated venous pressure, and peripheral edema. Pericardial effusion is common in the absence of echocar-

resistance, size, age, and general health are important variables. Usually, the degree of illness is related to the number of larvae/gm of muscle: light infection, probably subclinical, up to 10 larvae; moderate infection, 50 to 500 larvae; and severe, life-threatening infection, 1000 or more larvae. Strains of *T. spiralis* may be an important variable also because infections with the Kenyan and the southern European types appear to be less clinically severe.

Intestinal Phase. The initial consequences of infection occur within the first week after ingestion of infected meat, during the intestinal phase (Table 90–1); this period is associated with the development of worms to the adult stage within the small intestine. The symptoms reflect mucosal irritation and include nausea, abdominal aches or cramps, loss of appetite, vomiting, mild fever, and either mild diarrhea or constipation. The patient may complain of frontal headaches, dizziness, and weakness. These symptoms are easily confused with flu, especially in light to moderate infections. Severe diarrhea, persisting for weeks, sometimes occurs in patients with heavy infections. Infected Innuit Indians in North America experienced an unusually high frequency of diarrhea and a low frequency of myalgia. This may diographic evidence of ventricular dilation or impaired systolic function. Although most patients who survive trichinosis recover completely, a few continue to have chronic cardiac manifestations. Focal granulomas are eventually replaced by interstitial fibrosis. Larvae cannot successfully encyst in heart muscle.

Convalescent Phase. The third, or chronic, period, the convalescent phase, is associated with a decrease in muscular symptoms beginning in the second month after infection. Fever and itching subside also. At this time, evidence of congestive heart failure may appear, especially if the patient is allowed up too soon. Larvae remain alive in the cysts for many years, even after the cyst wall becomes calcified. These larvae release antigens that cause a continuing low to moderate eosinophilia, circulating antibody, and immediate and delayed hypersensitivity responses to skin-test antigens.

Fatal outcome is infrequent in trichinosis, normally occurring only in massive infections, and is most frequently associated with myocarditis, encephalitis, and pneumonitis. About 2% of cases in the United States end in death.

DIAGNOSIS. Guidelines for the diagnosis of infection have been recommended by the International Commission on Trichinellosis. Diagnosis may be made by either a direct or an indirect demonstration of infection.

Direct Demonstration

Enteral Phase. Adult *Trichinella* can sometimes be recovered from the intestinal mucosa at postmortem examination and could theoretically, but not practicably, be recovered from a living patient by duodenal aspiration or biopsy.

Parenteral Phase. (1) Dissemination Stage: Newborn larvae are transported via the blood stream and are disseminated to various parts of the body. Experimentally, they can be filtered from the blood by means of a 3-μm-pore filter, but it is unlikely that this method will be useful in routine diagnosis because of the relatively small number of newborn larvae in the blood at any given time.

(2) Muscle Stage: This stage offers the best chance for direct demonstration of the organism. The larvae may be found by examination of a biopsy specimen taken from a superficial skeletal muscle. The procedure should not be undertaken if a firm diagnosis can be made by other means. A specimen measuring approximately 1 cm^3 should be taken, preferably from either the deltoid or gastrocnemius muscles. A portion of the specimen is fixed and examined histologically. The remainder is handled in either one or both of the following ways: (a) compression between glass slides, followed by microscopic examination (Fig. 90–1*B*), and/or (b) digestion in 1% pepsin and 1% hydrochloric acid, with agitation, followed by microscopic examination of a filtrate or washed sediment of the digested specimen. The digestion time required for liberation of any larvae depends on the size of the muscle fragments and the volume of digestive fluid, but under most circumstances, digestion for a few hours is sufficient for the detection of any larvae that may be present. Larvae that have reached the musculature within the first 3 weeks of infection are more readily detected by the compression

and histologic techniques; otherwise, digestion of muscle tissue is the preferred method.

Indirect Demonstration. A negative biopsy does not exclude the possibility of infection, however. Circulating antibody can be detected even in lightly infected patients 3 to 4 weeks after infection and as early as 2 weeks in heavily infected individuals. A variety of serologic tests can be used, but the bentonite flocculation test (BFT), fluorescent antibody test (FAT), and the enzyme-linked immunosorbent assay (ELISA) have proved most useful. With the BFT, titers of 1:5 are considered positive; titers generally fall markedly after 1 or 2 years, so that a rise and fall in titer generally indicates recent infection. The ELISA is more sensitive and can also detect a rise and fall in titer. However, some problems in specificity have been observed when these tests are used with crude antigen extracts. Considerable effort has been made recently to produce more refined antigens. Stichosome antigens derived either from the larva's excretions and secretions during in vitro culture, or by somatic extraction, have proved superior to crude extracts. Skin tests can be performed also, but these lack specificity and are further handicapped by the persistence of reactivity in patients as long as 10 years after initial infection.

Differential Diagnosis. Trichinosis can mimic a wide variety of diseases. Most mild cases are misdiagnosed as influenza or other viral fevers unless the clinician recognizes a history of recent ingestion of pork or game, febrile myalgia, periorbital edema, and rising eosinophilia (to 50% or higher) and takes steps to confirm the diagnosis by either serologic tests or muscle biopsy. Similar symptoms among others who dined on the same occasion reflect a common source of infection and further substantiate the diagnosis.

TREATMENT. The efficacy of treatment of human trichinosis depends on the intensity and duration of the infection and on the character and intensity of the host's response. Guidelines for treatment have also recently been issued by the International Commission on Trichinellosis.

Intestinal Stage. Removal of adult worms from the intestine is necessary to stop the production of newborn larvae. This can be accomplished by several anthelmintics, e.g., thiabendazole (50 mg/kg for 5 days), pyrantel (10 mg/kg for 4 days), or mebendazole (200 mg/day for 4 days); mebendazole should not be given in the first trimester of pregnancy.

Muscle Stage. Corticosteroids are the drugs of choice in acute trichinosis because of their anti-inflammatory and antiallergic action. The usual dose is 40 to 60 mg of prednisone/day, taken until the fever and allergic signs subside. In life-threatening infections, higher doses may be required. Bed rest is always necessary, and any cardiac, circulatory, neurologic, or pulmonary complications may need specific treatment.

Thiabendazole has been used in severe infections but with controversial effects. By destroying muscle larvae and liberating antigenic substances, thiabendazole may provoke a systemic hypersensitivity response and be a potential hazard to patients already suffering an allergic response. Mebendazole (5 mg/kg/day) has commonly replaced thiabendazole. Mebendazole and corticosteroids have been reported also to be highly effective in severe trichinosis caused by sylvatic or polar strains of *Trichinella*.

Moderate or Mild Infection. Because corticosteroids may suppress the intestinal inflammatory response to the adult worms, immune expulsion may not occur, thereby prolonging the period of production of newborn larvae and muscle invasion. Therefore, the use of corticosteroids should be restricted to patients with fever, allergic symptoms, high leukocytosis, and eosinophilia; antipyretic and analgesic treatment alone may produce a satisfactory result.

Chronic Infection. Trichinosis is a self-limiting disease in both intestinal and muscular phases, and recovery usually occurs within a few months. In sporadic cases, myalgia and weakness persist for several years. In these cases an active process demonstrated by examination of a muscle biopsy specimen may justify the use of larvicidal drugs, e.g., mebendazole or thiabendazole. Usually, symptomatic treatment and proper mental and physical rehabilitation are effective; the patient should be convinced that the presence of *T. spiralis* larvae encapsulated in the muscles is not unique and is often well tolerated.

PREVENTION AND CONTROL. Because infection in humans is by the consumption of meat containing encysted larvae, direct prevention should be directed at preparing pork or game so that any larvae present are uninfective. In contrast to some countries in Europe, government inspection of pork is not practiced in the United States or in most of Asia, Africa, and South and Central America. The consumer should cook all pork to at least 170F (76.6C) to allow for a safety margin, because the thermal death point for *T. spiralis* in pork is 135F (57.2C) if the meat is kept at that temperature for about 4 minutes. Pork less than 6 inches thick can also be rendered safe if frozen to 5F (− 15C) for 20 days, − 10F (− 23C) for 10 days, or − 20F (− 29C) for 6 days. However, *T. s. nativa* larvae in bear meat are reported to survive freezing for a year or longer.

In those areas where pork is the primary source of infection, it is important to prevent infection of pigs. The requirement that garbage used for feeding swine be thoroughly cooked (boiled for 30 minutes) is an important control procedure. Vigorous efforts to control rodent populations and to prevent hog cannibalism are required. Furthermore, the education of farmers, meat processors, hunters, and trappers about the potential dangers of feeding wild game to swine should be promoted. The identification and elimination of infected hogs would have the effect of reducing transmission of *T. spiralis* to other swine and would eventually lower the transmission level below the threshold required to maintain the domestic pig-human cycle. Some countries may soon require that hogs be tested serologically for trichinosis at slaughter by an automated ELISA test. The effectiveness and practicality of whole hog carcass gamma irradiation to kill larvae have been demonstrated; 30 krads have been shown to be completely effective in sterilizing the encysted larvae. Research is also in progress to develop a vaccine for swine that could be administered to baby pigs.

Meanwhile, the control of trichinosis acquired from eating the flesh of wild animal hosts, e.g., polar bears in the Arctic, black bears in the United States, wild boars in Europe, or wart hogs in Africa, can be achieved only if the meat is properly cooked.

BIBLIOGRAPHY

Bessoudo R, Marrie TJ, Smith ER: Cardiac involvement in trichinosis. Chest 79:698, 1981.

Campbell WC: History of trichinosis: Paget, Owen and the discovery of *Trichinella spiralis*. Bull Hist Med 53:520, 1979.

Campbell WC, Denham DA: Chemotherapy. *In* Campbell WC (ed.): *Trichinella* and Trichinosis. New York, Plenum Press, 1983, pp. 335–366.

Dame J, Murrell KD, Stringfellow F, et al.: Genetic evidence for the presence of *Trichenella spiralis spiralis* in wildlife from DNA hybridization analysis. Exp Parasitol 64:195–203, 1987.

Forrester ATT, Nelson GS, Sander G: The first record of an outbreak of trichinosis in Africa south of the Sahara. Trans R Soc Trop Med Hyg 55:503, 1961.

Gamble WR, Anderson WA, Graham CE, et al.: Diagnosis of swine trichinosis by Elisa using an excretory-secreting antigen. Vet Parasitol 13:349–356, 1983.

Gould SE: Anatomic pathology. *In* Gould SE (ed): Trichinosis in Man and Animals. Springfield, Illinois, Charles C. Thomas, 1970, pp. 147–189.

Kim CW, Ruitenberg EJ, Treppema S: Trichinellosis. Proceedings of the 5th International Conference on Trichinellosis. September 1980. Survey, Reedbooks Ltd, 1981.

Kociecka W: Intestinal trichinellosis. Clin Trop Med Comm Dis 2:755–764, 1987.

Madsen H: The distribution of *Trichinella spiralis* in sledge dogs and wild mammals in Greenland. Medd Grnland 159:52, 1961.

Murrell KD: Strategies for the control of human trichinosis transmitted by pork. Food Technology 39:65–68, 1985.

Nelson GS: Carrion-feeding cannibalistic carnivores and human disease in Africa with special reference to trichinosis and hydatid disease in Kenya. Symp Zool Soc Lond 50:181, 1982.

Pawlowski ZS: Clinical aspects in man. *In* Campbell WC (ed.): *Trichinella* and Trichinosis. New York, Plenum Press, 1983, pp. 367–401.

Schad GA, Kellog M, Lieby D, et al.: Swine trichinosis in mid-Atlantic slaughterhouses: Possible relationship to hog marketing systems. Prev Vet Med 3:391–399, 1985.

91. TOXOCARIASIS

Michael E. Kilpatrick

DEFINITION. Toxocariasis in humans is a result of infection with embryonated eggs of dog and cat ascarids, *Toxocara canis* and *T. cati,* or possibly other *Toxocara* species. This roundworm is not able to complete its life cycle in humans and causes a spectrum of diseases ranging from no symptoms to eosinophilia, visceral larvae migrans (VLM), or ocular larva migrans (OLM).

ETIOLOGY AND EPIDEMIOLOGY

Life Cycle. Adult *T. canis* and *T. cati* live in the intestines of dogs and cats, respectively. Eggs are shed in the feces and require 2 to 3 weeks in moist soil at temperatures at or above 27C to embryonate and become infective. Puppies are commonly infected vertically and shed eggs by 3 weeks of age; egg shedding is less after dogs reach 6 months of age. Transmission of this parasite to humans occurs through ingestion of embryonated eggs from the soil or from contaminated hands (Fig. 91–1). The eggs hatch and release larvae in the proximal small intestine where they penetrate the mucosa and are carried to the liver by the portal circulation. Some larvae remain in the liver causing granuloma to form; others are carried to the lungs and some then enter the systemic circulation and are carried to various parts of the body until they reach a vessel too small for passage. There the larvae penetrate the vessel and migrate into the surrounding tissue.

Transmission. Humans are infected only through ingestion of embryonated eggs (Fig. 91–1). Studies of soil samples where dogs have access in most areas of the world have shown embryonated eggs of *Toxocara* species. Putting fingers, toys, or other objects into the mouth after they were in contact with contaminated soil is an obvious means of infection, which explains the predominance of toxocariasis in childhood. Serological surveys show a higher prevalence of antibody titers in children up to 10 years of age than in other groups. Most infections are asymptomatic or are unrecognized. VLM is more common in younger children (mean age of 3), whereas OLM is more likely to occur in older children (mean age of 8).

HISTORY. Werner described *T. canis* as a parasite of dogs in 1782. It was not until 1952 that the first infections in humans with the larvae of the parasite were reported by Beaver and associates. Only sporadic cases were reported until Woodruff and colleagues developed a standardized skin test in 1964 and a fluorescent antibody test in 1968 and conducted surveys that indicated a 2% prevalence rate of present or past infection in the population of Great Britain. Glickman and coworkers and DeSavigny and associates developed highly specific enzyme-linked immunosorbent assay (ELISA) techniques for diagnosing this infection. The use of a *T. canis* exoantigen in the ELISA diagnostic test has improved the sensitivity, particularly for OLM.

DISTRIBUTION. *T. canis* in dogs and infection of humans with its larvae have a worldwide distribution. Many studies performed in the United States, Great Britain, Canada, Brazil, Africa, and the Middle East have revealed the prevalence of infection in dogs to vary from 2 to 90%.

The prevalence of eggs in soil has not been widely investigated, but 17% of soil samples in Montreal parks contained eggs, which remained infective over winter, and up to 32% of soil samples taken in the Sudan and the Middle East contain eggs.

PATHOGENESIS AND PATHOLOGY. In humans the infective process begins when embryonated eggs are swallowed; in the intestine, the shell is digested partially, and the contained larva escapes. The 16 to 20 mm larvae enter the vascular system, and those that pass through the liver and the lungs into the systemic circulation eventually reach capillaries and are arrested. They may

LIFE CYCLE of—

Toxocara canis

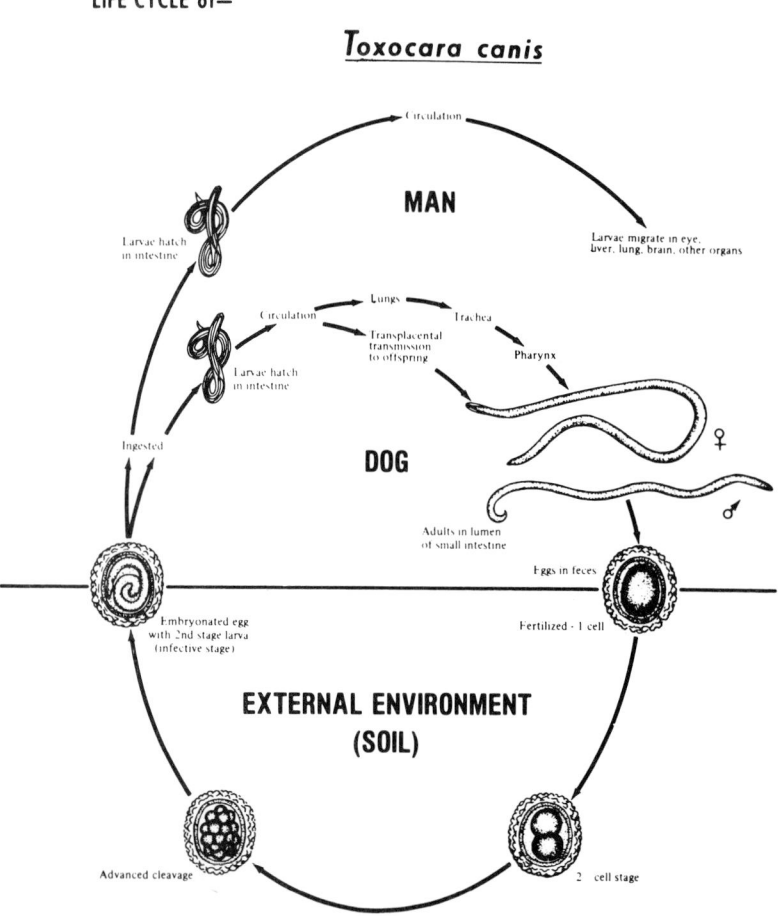

FIGURE 91–1. Life cycle of *Toxocara canis*. (From Melvin DM, Brooke MM, Healey GR, et al.: Common Blood and Tissue Parasites of Man. Life Cycle Charts. Atlanta, Georgia, Centers for Disease Control, 1961.)

burrow then into the tissue, causing hemorrhage, necrosis, and secondary inflammation. Some larvae die and some become dormant for years before again becoming active. Granuloma, 1 to 2 mm in diameter, usually form. These have a preponderance of eosinophils (Fig. 91–2). Later, fibrosis and possible calcification occur.

CLINICAL MANIFESTATIONS. The clinical manifestations depend on the number of invading larvae and the part(s) of the body affected. In many cases, infection is asymptomatic; in all cases, however, infection is potentially capable of causing severe disease. Initial infections in children sometimes cause abdominal pain, hepatomegaly, anorexia, nausea, vomiting, lethargy, sleep and behavior disturbances, pneumonia, cough, wheeze, pharyngitis, cervical adenitis, headache, limb pains, fever, skin rash, and/or eosinophilia. The more symptoms present, the more likely the diagnosis.

Ophthalmic Lesions. Ocular involvement is more common in older children and adults. It is believed that with fewer infecting larvae the immune response is less and the eye is invaded randomly several months after infection. Loss of vision in one eye in a child may not be recognized immediately. Disuse of the affected eye commonly leads to strabismus, and the parents may note that a squint has developed. In other individuals, routine examination may reveal poor or absent sight in one eye, and ophthalmoscopy will demonstrate a retinal scar or, if invasion of the eye has been recent, a tumor formed by the granuloma. There is often some vitreous haze; sometimes a cataract develops. Prior scar formation with consequent flattening, a tumor-like lesion of the fundus of one eye, and eosinophilia are highly suspicious signs of the presence of ophthalmic toxocariasis. Rarely, the patient has periorbital swelling caused by a subcutaneous granuloma containing toxocaral larva. They seldom have the VLM syndrome. At one time it was thought that there was a special predilection for toxocaral larvae to invade the eye, but ophthalmic lesions are found in a minority of patients with toxocaral infection. However, larvae in the eye usually cause symptoms and are detected more readily than are those in other organs.

Hepatic and Pulmonary Lesions. In heavy infections, larval invasion of the liver may cause slight to moderate hepatomegaly with tenderness and eosinophilia. Their presence in the lungs may give rise to patchy areas of pneumonitis, and in some persons, asthma may be provoked. Evidence of past or present toxocaral infection is increased significantly in asthmatics. Pulmonary nodules from granulomas surrounding dead larvae are sometimes detected on a chest radiograph.

Cerebral Lesions. Encephalitis with convulsions and chronic epilepsy have been associated with toxocaral involvement of the brain. Older lesions may be a cause of cerebral calcifications.

Laboratory Findings. Eosinophilia is common in active infections, but its duration is inconsistent and is probably related to the quantity of the infecting dose and the frequency of reinfection. In OLM, peripheral eosinophilia may be absent and evaluation of aqueous humor will reveal eosinophils and normal levels of lactic dehydrogenase and phosphoglucose isomerase.

DIAGNOSIS. The definitive diagnosis of VLM and OLM is identification of the larva in tissue (Fig. 91–2). Patients with hepatomegaly, epilepsy, a patchy pneumonitis, and/or a chorioretinal eye lesion with eosinophilia should be suspected of having toxocariasis, particularly if they are children and if there is a history of ingestion of possibly contaminated soil.

Serologic Tests. A presumptive diagnosis of *Toxocara* infection can be made with the ELISA. Two antigens are used to detect antibodies to *T. canis—T. canis* embryonated egg (TEE) antigen and *T. canis* exoantigen (TEX). TEE requires preabsorption of serum with ascaris antigens to decrease false positive; TEX does not. TEX has a greater sensitivity and specificity than does TEE, which has an 80 to 90% sensitivity and a 90% specificity.

Differential Diagnosis. In OLM the most important differential diagnosis is retinoblastoma. Testing of serum and aqueous humor can assist in the diagnosis, but it is possible that a patient with a retinoblastoma could have had exposure to *T. canis*.

Hepatic capillariasis can be confused with toxocariasis involving the liver. Patients have hepatomegaly, eosinophilia, and abnormal liver function tests. A liver biopsy may demonstrate eggs of *Capillaria* species within a hepatic granuloma (Fig. 91–3).

TREATMENT AND PROGNOSIS

Chemotherapy. There is no evidence of benefit from treatment for asymptomatic individuals with toxocariasis. There is improvement of symptoms with treatment, but there are no well-controlled studies. Both experimentally and clinically, diethylcarbamazine (DEC) gives good results when administered orally in doses of 3 mg/kg of body weight 3 times daily for 21 days. Preliminary doses of 1 mg/kg, increased according to tolerance to 3 mg/kg, are advisable because of occasional allergic reactions to dying parasites. DEC is generally superior to thiabendazole, which is also given orally but in 3 divided doses of 50 mg/kg daily for 5 days. Treatment causes a burst of eosinophilia, which then returns to baseline, and there is a slow decrease in the ELISA titers. DEC and thiabendazole will kill living

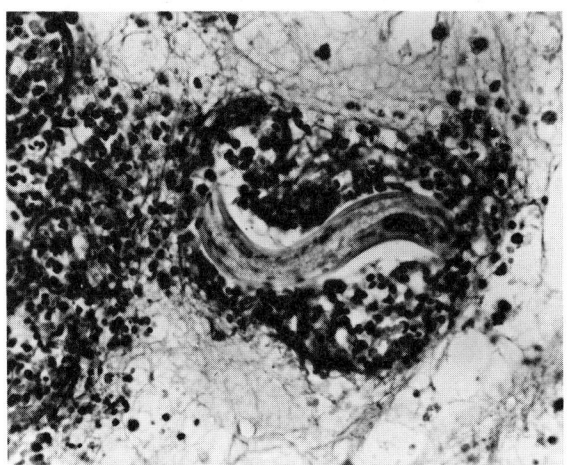

FIGURE 91–2. A portion of a *T. canis* larva is surrounded by inflammatory cells in a preretinal mass (× 220). (Courtesy of the Armed Forces Institute of Pathology, Photograph Neg. No. 298563-29081.)

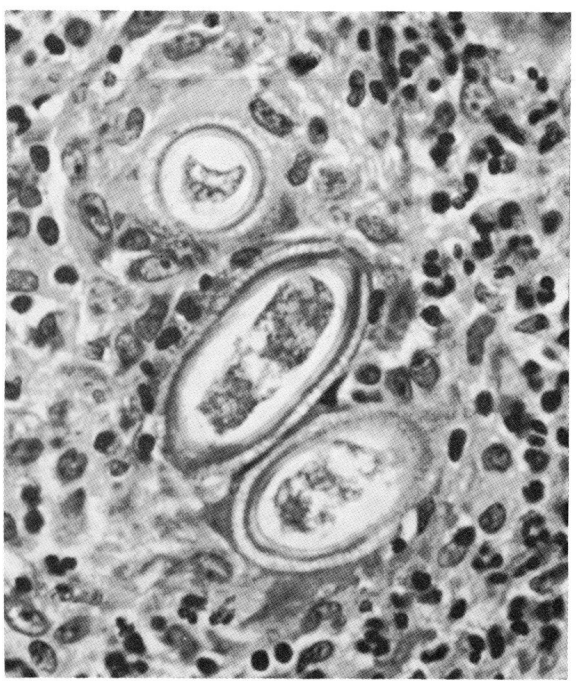

FIGURE 91–3. Focus of granulomatous reaction around 3 eggs of *Capillaria* species (H & E stain, × 450). (Courtesy of Dr. V.M. Areán, University of Florida College of Medicine.)

larvae, thus preventing further migration and additional damage, but will not reverse lesions already present. For ophthalmic toxocariasis, coincidental administration of corticosteroids locally and/or systematically reduces inflammation around larvae. In most internal organs, larvae-induced damage is usually not critical, but there is always the potential for serious damage in all toxocaral infections.

PROGNOSIS. The prognosis following treatment is good in limiting further damage. For OLM with severe symptoms, subtotal pars planus vitrectomy has produced good therapeutic results.

PREVENTION. Dogs are the reservoir of *T. canis*, the primary cause of toxocariasis. Prevention can be achieved only when pets are identified as infected and treated and when exposure to contaminated soil is eliminated. Prompt disposal of dog feces, which are not infectious because the *T. canis* eggs have not embryonated yet, is imperative.

Toxocariasis is a disease of major public health importance, particularly for children. Simple preventive measures can eradicate this disease.

BIBLIOGRAPHY

Bass JL, Mehta KA, Glickman LT, et al.: Asymptomatic toxocariasis in children. Clin Pediatr 26:441, 1987.
Belmont JB, Irvine A, Benson W, et al.: Vitrectomy in ocular toxocariasis. Arch Ophthalmol 100:1912, 1982.
Cypress RH, Karol MH, Zidian JL, et al.: Larva-specific antibody in patients with visceral larva migrans. J Infect Dis 135:633, 1977.
Glickman LT, Grieve RB, Fauria SS, et al.: Serodiagnosis of ocular toxocariasis: A comparison of two antigens. J Clin Pathol 38:103, 1985.
Glickman LT, Schantz PM, Dombroske RL, et al.: Evaluation of serodiagnostic tests for visceral larva migrans. Am J Trop Med Hyg 27:492, 1978.
Morris PD, Katerndahl DA: Human toxocariasis. Postgrad Med 81:263, 1987.
Pollard ZF: Long-term follow-up in patients with ocular toxocariasis as measured by ELISA titers. Ann Ophthalmol 19:167, 1987.
Roth RM, Gleckman RA: Human infections derived from dogs. Postgrad Med 77:169, 1985.
Schantz PM, Glickman LT: Toxocaral visceral larva migrans. N Engl J Med 298:436, 1978.
Schantz PM, Meyer D, Glickman LT: Clinical, serologic, and epidemiologic characteristics of ocular toxocariasis. Am J Trop Med Hyg 28:24, 1979.
Schantz PM, Weis PE, Pollard ZF, et al.: Risk factors for toxocaral ocular larva migrans: A case-control study. Am J Public Health 70:1269, 1980.
Taylor MRH, Keave CT, O'Connor P, et al.: The expanded spectrum of toxocaral disease. Lancet 1:692, 1988.

92. GNATHOSTOMIASIS
Thanongsak Bunnag

DEFINITION. Gnathostomiasis, also called eosinophilic myeloencephalitis, Tau-cheed (Thailand), Yangtze edema (China), and Chokofishi (Japan), is a sporadic infection caused by *Gnathostoma spinigerum* (Owen, 1836), a tissue nematode. Typically, the disease is manifested by intermittent subcutaneous migratory swelling, less commonly involving internal organs. Often, an immature adult worm has been recovered from the subcutaneous tissues, internal organs, or the central nervous system.

ETIOLOGY
Morphology. The adult worm is a reddish-colored, slightly transparent nematode with a globular cephalic bulb. The cuticle of the head bulb is armed with 8 to 11 transverse rows of minute hooklets; only the anterior half of the body below the cervical region constriction is spinous (Fig. 92–1). Males are 10 mm to 25 mm long and females 25 mm to 54 mm long. The 65 μm to 70 μm by 38 μm to 40 μm eggs are ovoid, unsegmented, and greenish-tinged and have a mucoid plug at one end.

Life Cycle. The adult worms lie coiled in a tumor mass in the stomach wall of the definitive host—domestic and wild cats and dogs, and several wild carnivorous animals (Fig. 92–2). Eggs are extruded from the lesions and evacuated in the feces. They hatch 10 to 12 days after reaching water, releasing cylindrical, ensheathed first-stage rhabditiform larvae that, following ingestion by a freshwater copepod (*Cyclops*), undergo development to second-stage larvae in the body cavity within 2 weeks (Fig. 92–3). When the infected copepod is eaten by any of many second intermediate or transport hosts, including fish, amphibians, reptiles, birds, and mammals, encystation of the third-stage larvae occurs in the flesh of the host. On ingestion by the definitive host, the parasites become localized in the stomach wall, where they mature in 3 to 12 months.

EPIDEMIOLOGY
Geographic Distribution. Ten species of the genus have been reported from different kinds of animals in various localities. *Gnathostoma spinigerum* is the species causing almost all cases of human gnathostomiasis; *G. hispidum* (Fedchenko, 1872), a nematode of the wild

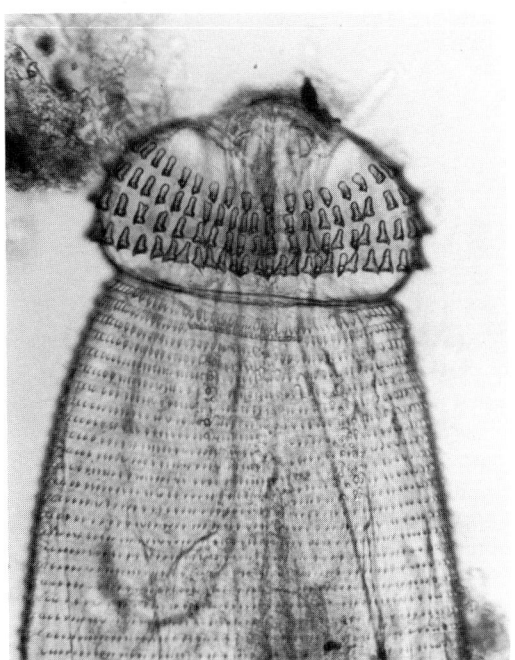

FIGURE 92–1. Anterior end of adult *Gnathostoma spinigerum* showing the globular cephalic bulb and the transverse rows of hooklets.

and domestic pig, has been found recently in Japan to infect humans who consumed infected loaches imported from China.

Gnathostomiasis has been reported mainly from Asia. Thailand and Japan are the endemic countries with the highest incidence, both in humans and in reservoir hosts. Sporadic human gnathostomiasis has occurred in Australia, Burma, China, India, Indonesia, Laos, Mexico, the Philippines, and Vietnam. A wide variety of animal infections occurs also in Bangladesh, Palestine, the United States, USSR, and Zimbabwe. The prevalence

of infection in cats and dogs in rural endemic areas of Thailand was 26 to 30%.

Transmission. *G. spinigerum* shows low host specificity; 44 species of vertebrates (including 16 species of freshwater fish, 2 of frog, 11 of reptiles, 11 of birds, and 4 species of mammals) serve as the natural second intermediate hosts.

Humans acquire infection usually through consumption of the raw or undercooked flesh of second and transport hosts having encysted third-stage infective larvae. The common sources of infection are the salted fermented freshwater fish locally called *Somfuk* in Thailand, and raw freshwater fish eaten with rice (sasemi) in Japan. Infection from drinking water contaminated with infected copepods is less common. In Thailand and Japan, the disease occurs throughout the year with a variable monthly incidence. All age groups are susceptible to infection, and there is no sex preference.

PATHOGENESIS AND PATHOLOGY. Humans are abnormal hosts in whom the worm is unable to complete the normal life cycle. Pathology is caused by mechanical injury to the tissues by the migrating worm and the immunologic response and the toxic products of the parasites. The lesions occur along the worm's migratory routes: track-like necrosis and/or varying degree of hemorrhage. Acute inflammation with diffuse eosinophilic infiltration, together with peripheral hypereosinophilia, is prominent in edematous skin lesions. Unilateral ocular invasion occurs occasionally, with subconjunctival edema, hemorrhage, and occasionally retinal damage (Fig. 92–4). The neuropathology of cerebral gnathostomiasis consists of large, multiple areas and tracks of hematoma and/or necrosis (Fig. 92–5), with immature or morphologically mature *G. spinigerum* recovered from the brain, spinal cord, and choroid plexus.

CLINICAL MANIFESTATIONS. The incubation

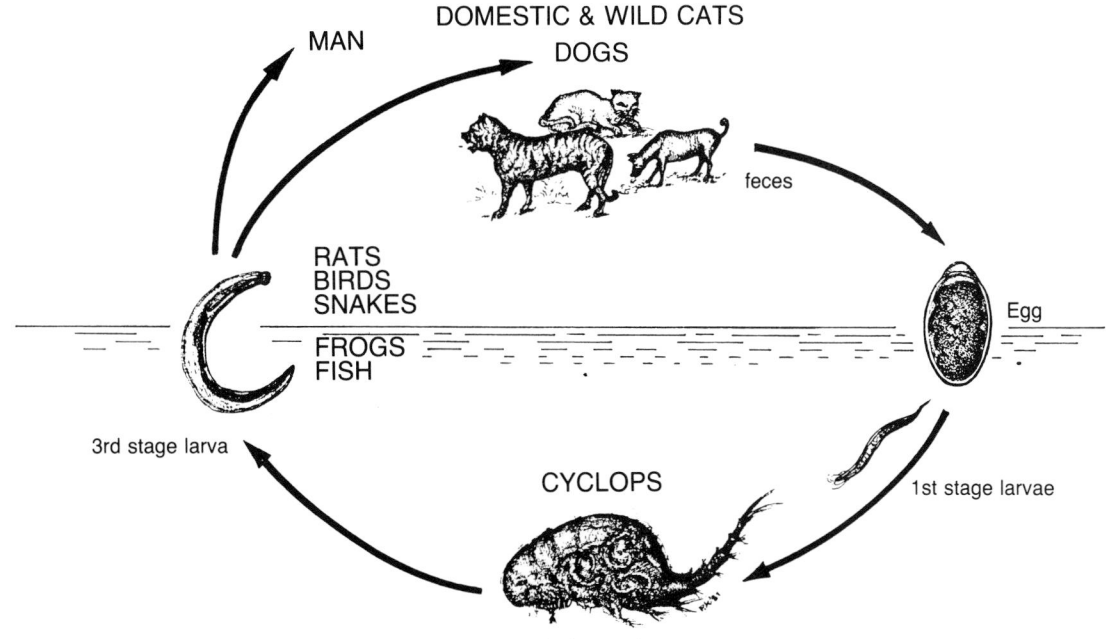

FIGURE 92–2. Life cycle of *Gnathostoma spinigerum*.

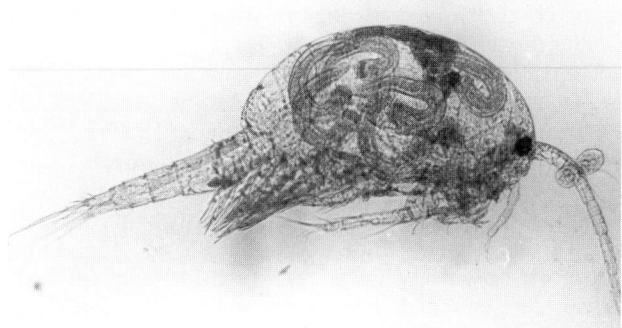

FIGURE 92–3. An intermediate host, *Cyclops,* which has ingested second-stage *G. spinigerum* larvae.

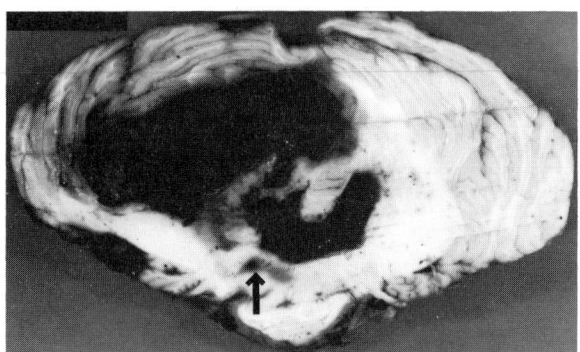

FIGURE 92–5. Section of cerebellum showing massive hemorrhage, necrosis, and small track *(arrow).*

period is unknown in most cases. Patients present usually with either of 2 distinct clinical forms: larval gnathostomiasis or eosinophilic myeloencephalitis.

Larval Gnathostomiasis. An early manifestation of abdominopulmonary hypereosinophilic syndrome consists of low-grade fever, abdominal pain in the right upper quadrant, an enlarged and tender liver, pleuritis or pneumonitis, malaise, and hypereosinophilia. This form of gnathostomiasis may be mild and unrecognised or may be severe and last for more than 6 weeks. Creeping eruption, the serpentine track similar to, but bigger than, those produced by animal hookworm larva, is rare (Fig. 92–6). Intermittent subcutaneous swellings are due to the migration of an immature adult worm. It usually is a painless swelling with local inflammatory reaction, edema, intense pruritis, and leukocytosis with a relatively high eosinophilia. Often, the swelling occurs in the eyelid. Chemosis, conjunctival edema, and/or hemorrhage may be observed in ocular gnathostomiasis (Fig. 92–4), and in a few cases a nematode worm can be found in the anterior chamber, the vitreous humor, or the retina (Fig. 92–7). Visual impairment is due to inflammation, hemorrhage, and sometimes, retinal detachment. Blindness due to larval gnathostomiasis has been reported in Thailand.

Rapidly occurring subcutaneous swelling without a regional lymphadenitis or fever may recur near or distant to the original site and lasts about 1 week. The interval between episodes of swelling varies from days to months. Other symptoms depend on the internal organs involved, imitating an acute abdomen or an abdominal

tumor, or causing spontaneous pneumothorax, hemoptysis, pneumonitis, or hematuria.

Eosinophilic Myeloencephalitis. The neurologic manifestations of gnathostomiasis are a unique symptom-complex called eosinophilic myeloencephalitis. The worm migrates along a large nerve trunk into the central nervous system, commonly producing agonizing nerve root pain, followed by paralysis of the extremities with urinary retention and, rarely, quadriplegia. Sudden severe headache and sensorial impairment, followed by coma, occurs in a few cases, suggesting a cerebrovascular accident. In rare instances, neurologic episodes occur in association with cutaneous migratory swelling. In endemic areas, cerebral gnathostomiasis should be considered a cause of cerebral hemorrhage, especially in younger individuals (Fig. 92–5).

Laboratory Findings. A peripheral blood leukocytosis with relatively hypereosinophilia always occurs in acute cases. The degree of eosinophilia, sometimes as high as 90%, does not correlate with clinical severity. In cerebral gnathostomiasis the cerebrospinal fluid is usually bloody or xanthochromic and has a pleocytosis. The CSF cell count is below 500 cells/cu mm. The predominant cells may be either lymphocytes or neutrophils; an

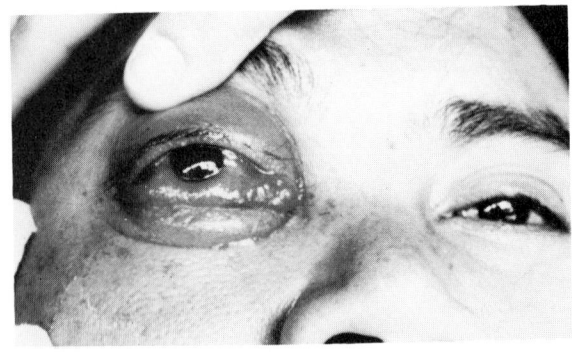

FIGURE 92–4. Subconjunctival edema and hemorrhage caused by *Gnathostoma spinigerum.*

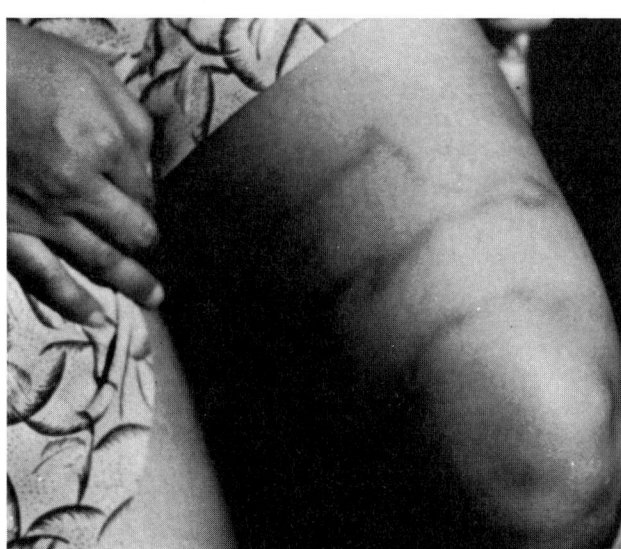

FIGURE 92–6. Gnathostomal creeping eruption is large, serpiginous, and has a transient pruritic track. (Courtesy of Professor Manoon Bhaibulaya.)

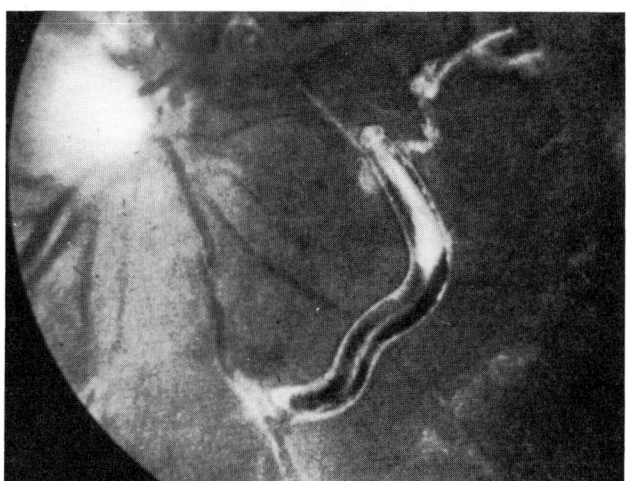

FIGURE 92–7. *Gnathostoma spinigerum* larva in the vitreous humor of a Thai patient. It causes hemorrhage, retinal detachment, and later, blindness.

eosinophilia of greater than 20% is present in most cases. Other investigations (e.g., electroencephalograms, cerebral angiography, computerized tomography) are usually not diagnostically helpful.

Up until now, an intradermal skin test and an immunoenzyme test (ELISA) for IgG antibody against aqueous extract of the third-stage larvae have not been clinically useful.

DIAGNOSIS. The diagnosis of larval gnathostomiasis is frequently difficult. It is presumptively suggested by a positive dietary history in endemic areas and by the clinical characteristics of the disease. Other eosinophilic syndromes, including tropical pulmonary eosinophilia and visceral toxocariasis, are misdiagnosed sometimes. Painless, recurrent migratory subcutaneous swellings and eosinophilic leukocytosis must be differentiated from other larval helminthic infections, such as ectopic fascioliasis, paragonimiasis, and sparganosis. Calabar swellings (caused by *Loa loa*) found associated with microfilariae in the blood in Central Africa and bilateral eye edema in acute stage of trichinosis can be differentiated usually by epidemiologic and clinical findings. Gnathostomal creeping eruptions are most likely to be confused with those caused by dog and cat hookworms. The former is rather large, serpiginous, and has a transient pruritic, sometimes hemorrhagic, track (Fig. 92–6). Eosinophilic myeloencephalitis differs clinically from eosinophilic meningitis caused by *Angiostrongylus cantonensis*. It should be suspected if the patient develops paralysis of the extremities following severe nerve root pain of the involved extremities or impairment of sensorium with hemorrhagic or xanthochromic cerebrospinal fluid and eosinophilic pleocytosis. The definitive diagnosis of gnathostomiasis depends mainly on the identification of the worms in surgical specimens and secretions such as expectorated sputum, urine, or vaginal discharge.

TREATMENT. Surgical removal of the worm is the only specific and effective treatment for gnathostomiasis. A combination of supportive, symptomatic, and anti-inflammatory treatments are preferable, however.

Broad spectrum anthelmintic drugs (e.g., thiabendazole, mebendazole, albendazole, and praziquantel) have been tried without convincing effects. Ultrasound may be useful in cutaneous gnathostomiasis. Intensive neurologic care is important in critical cases. High potency analgesics, such as morphine hydrochloride, are required to relieve pain in severe radiculitis.

PROGNOSIS. The recurrence of subcutaneous swelling, migratory or stationary, occurs intermittently for months or years without apparent damage. Blindness and impaired vision of varying degrees are usual in ocular gnathostomiasis. Permanent neurologic sequelae, such as paraplegia, are the most prominent morbidity. The fatality rate in cerebral gnathostomiasis is estimated to be as high as 40% in Thailand but is much lower because many milder cases are either not diagnosed or medical advice is not sought.

PREVENTION. In endemic areas, the disease can be prevented by the adequate cooking of freshwater fish, chicken, frogs, snakes, eels, and other intermediate or transport hosts. Untreated ground water is potentially infectious, because it can contain infected copepods.

BIBLIOGRAPHY

Bunnag T, Comer DS, Punyagupta S: Eosinophilic myeloencephalitis caused by *Gnathostoma spinigerum:* Neuropathology of nine cases. J Neurol Sci 10:419–434, 1970.
Chitanondh H, Rosen L: Fatal eosinophilic encephalomyelitis caused by *Gnathostoma spinigerum.* Am J Trop Med Hyg 16:638–645, 1967.
Miyazaki I: On the genus *Gnathostoma* and human gnathostomiasis, with special reference to Japan. Exp Parasitol 9:338, 1960.
Punyagupta S: Recent knowledge on clinical gnathostomiasis. J Med Assoc Thai 50:686, 1967.
Punyagupta S, Juttijudata P, Bunnag T, et al.: Two fatal cases of eosinophilic myeloencephalitis. A newly recognized disease caused by *Gnathostoma spinigerum.* Trans R Soc Trop Med Hyg 62:801–809, 1968.
Punyagupta S, Limtrakul C, Vichitpanthu P, et al.: Nine cases of radiculomyeloencephalitis associated with eosinophilic pleocytosis. Am J Trop Med Hyg 17:551–560, 1968.
Punyagupta S, Bunnag T, Juttijudata P: Eosinophilic meningitis in Thailand. Clinical and epidemiological characteristics of 162 patients with myeloencephalitis probably caused by *Gnathostoma spinigerum.* J Neurol Sci 96:241, 1990.
Suntharasamai P, Desakorn V, Migasena S, et al.: ELISA for immunodiagnosis of human gnathostomiasis. Southeast Asian J Trop Med Public Health 16:274–279, 1985.

93. ANGIOSTRONGYLIASIS

93.1 *ANGIOSTRONGYLUS* MENINGITIS

Thanongsak Bunnag

DEFINITION. Eosinophilic meningitis (eosinophilic meningoencephalitis, cerebral angiostrongyliasis) is a clinical zoonotic disease characterized by central nervous system involvement associated with an eosinophilic pleocytosis. *Angiostrongylus cantonensis,* a rat lungworm, has been recognized as the causative agent, and immature parasites have been recovered from the eye chamber, brain, and cerebrospinal fluid (CSF) of humans.

ETIOLOGY

Morphology. *A. cantonensis* was described by Chen (1933) in the lungs of rats, and the life cycle was elucidated by Mackerras and Sanders (1955). Both male and female adult parasites are delicate filiform and taper slightly at both ends. The cephalic tip is simple, and the cuticle is smooth and bears transverse striae; it is transparent when alive. Fully mature females average about 25 mm in length. The milky white uterine tubules are wound spirally around the blood-filled intestine, giving a "barber's pole" appearance. Fully developed males average 18 mm in length and possess well-developed caudal bursa copulatrix. Third-stage infective larvae are about 500 μm in length.

Life Cycle. *A. cantonensis* is a neurotropic parasite that requires a period of development in the central nervous system of its definitive vertebrate hosts. Mature adult *A. cantonensis* inhabits the pulmonary arteries of a wide variety of rodents of the genus *Rattus* and *Bandicota* (Fig. 93–1). Eggs laid by the female lodge in the pulmonary arteries, where they hatch. The first-stage larvae enter the alveolar space, migrate up the trachea and down the alimentary tract, and are excreted in the rodent's feces. Terrestrial snails, slugs, and aquatic snails serve as intermediate hosts either by being penetrated by the first-stage larvae or by ingesting rodent feces containing the larvae. Two further stages of development take place in the mollusk, where the parasites reach the third-stage larvae in about 2 weeks. When ingested by the rat, infective third-stage larvae migrate via the circulation to the rodent's brain, where they undergo 2 further stages of development, becoming young adult worms within 4 weeks. Then, they migrate to the surface of the brain, enter the venous system, and go to the pulmonary arteries where, after 2 more weeks, sexual maturity is attained. In humans, an accidental host, survival of the fifth-stage larvae is not certain: some die in the brain and spinal cord, some reach the eye chamber, and only a few reach the lungs.

The nematode parasite *A. cantonensis* shows little host specificity; a wide variety of terrestrial slugs and snails as well as freshwater species can transmit infection. Some of the major host species are the slugs—*Veronicella alte* and *V. siamensis;* the terrestrial snails—*Achatina fulica* and *Bradybaena similaris;* and the freshwater snails—*Pila ampulacea, P. polita, P. scutata,* and *Viviparus* species. *Pila* species and *Achatina fulica* are important sources of human infection in Thailand and Taiwan. Suitable paratenic hosts of *A. cantonensis* include fish, amphibians, reptiles, crustaceans, land planarians, and possibly vegetables contaminated with these larvae.

EPIDEMIOLOGY

Geographic Distribution. *Eosinophilic meningitis* occurs widely in the tropics from 23 degrees north to 23 degrees south, where there is a warm climate, moderate to heavy rainfall, and abundant vegetation suitable for the propagation of both the rodent vertebrate hosts and the mollusk intermediate hosts. The parasite was first recognized in the rat in Canton and in humans in Taiwan in 1933 and 1944, respectively. Cerebral angiostrongyliasis is more common in Southeast Asia and its archipelagoes than in the Pacific islands. It occurs in the Cook Islands, the Caroline Islands, Hawaii, Tahiti, New Hebrides, New Caledonia, American Samoa, the Philippines, Indonesia, Malaysia, Thailand, Vietnam, Taiwan, Hong Kong, Okinawa, Papua New Guinea, and Australia. It has been reported also from Cuba, Egypt, and the Ivory coast. In addition, the parasite has been found in the Malagasy Republic, Sri Lanka, India, mainland China, and all Southeast Asian countries, where the giant African snail *Achatina fulica* has been imported.

Distribution of cases in Southeast Asia correlates with

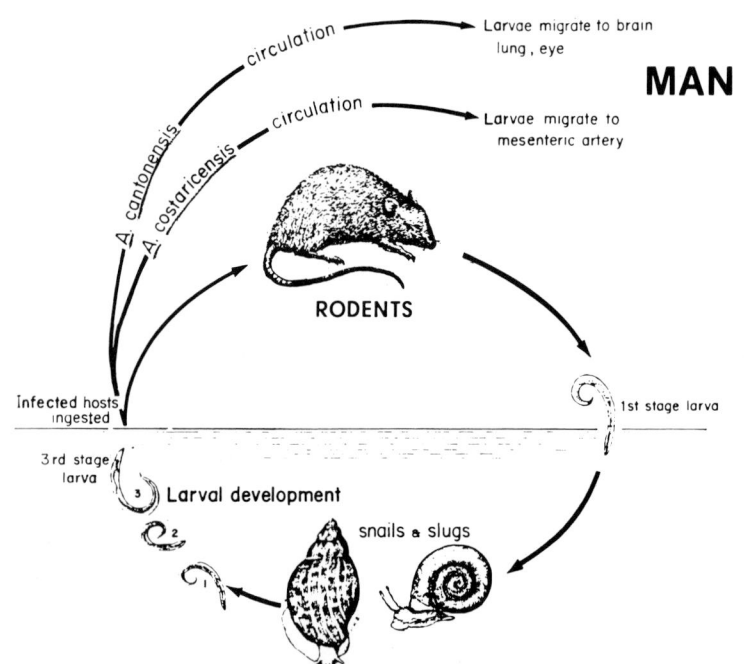

FIGURE 93–1. Life cycle of *Angiostrongylus cantonensis* and *A. costaricensis.*

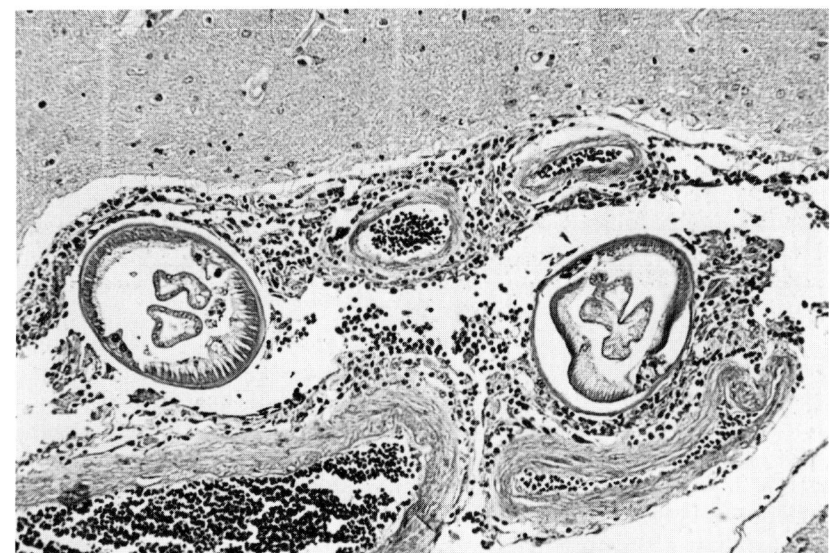

FIGURE 93–2. Cross section of *Angiostrongylus cantonensis* larvae in the meninges with lymphocytes and eosinophils.

the rainy season, when the invertebrate hosts are active. Elsewhere the disease is sporadic, varying with local customs. There have been dozens of parasitologically proven cases and thousands of clinically diagnosed cases, with occasional fatalities reported.

Transmission. Humans accidentally acquire infection by ingesting the tissues of infected mollusks, either by ingesting improperly cooked intermediate hosts (snails and slugs), or raw paratenic hosts (e.g., freshwater shrimp, *Macrobrachium lar*) or by eating food (e.g., salad greens) contaminated by slugs or snails. Drinking water containing third-stage larvae liberated from dead mollusks is difficult to validate as a source of infection. The disease is prevalent in adults in Thailand and the Pacific islands, whereas it is more common among children in Taiwan. Twice as many males are infected as females in Thailand, but a sex preference is not observed in other areas.

PATHOLOGY AND PATHOGENESIS. The neuropathology of human angiostrongyliasis has been well described. There is brain congestion and inflammation of the leptomeninges. Gross hemorrhage is unusual, and living larvae of *A. cantonensis* are seen often on the surface of the brain and spinal cord. The development and movement of the living parasites as well as dead and/or degenerating worms in the brain tissue and subarachnoidal space provoke the inflammatory reaction.

Microscopically, the pathologic changes are characterized by marked cellular infiltration of lymphocytes, plasma cells, macrophages, and eosinophils in the meninges and granulomas surrounding the dead worm. Invariably noted are numerous tracks or microcavities representing the passage of migrating worms in the brain and spinal cord. Older tracks contain debris, glitter cells, and Charcot-Leyden crystals; newer tracks show disruption of brain tissue with and without evidence of microscopic hemorrhage. Venous engorgement with necrosis of vessel walls and perivascular hemorrhage has been noted. Sections of *A. cantonensis* larvae are easily

recognized in the brain, in the meninges and sometimes in the blood vessels (Fig. 93–2). The lungs are the only other organ involved; in a few instances mature worms, alive or dead, have been found in the pulmonary artery. Living worms have been removed frequently from human eyes without apparent eye pathology.

CLINICAL MANIFESTATIONS. The disease is generally benign and self-limiting, and recovery is uneventful. However, patients may have a severe illness with lasting neurologic sequelae or even fatality, depending on the number of infecting larvae, which may range from a few to hundreds.

Symptoms and Signs. The usual incubation period is about 2 weeks (range of 3 to 36 days). Nausea, vomiting, and abdominal discomfort are seen in some cases soon after ingestion of the suspected food. Severe headache of insidious onset is the chief complaint in 96% of cases in Thailand; but in Taiwan 78% have an abrupt onset of headache. The headache is intermittent, intractable, bitemporal or occipital, and continues throughout the clinical illness. Nausea, vomiting, and moderate stiffness of the neck and/or back are frequent during the early stage. Paresthesia of the trunk and extremities commonly consists of exaggerated sensitivity to touch, which may persist for a few weeks or months. Sensorial impairment of varying degrees, characterized by somnolence to lethargy that may progress to coma, has been reported from 5% of clinical cases in Thailand and 82% of those in Taiwan. Generalized weakness to flaccid paralysis of the extremities associated with coma occurs in a few severe cases. Low-grade pyrexia or an absence of fever is usual, except in those with severe symptoms and in children.

Cranial nerves are involved sometimes, particularly the optic, facial, and abducens nerves. Visual impairment is observed; 12% have an abnormal fundus examination. Diplopia, abnormal visual fields, optic atrophy, and periorbital edema are present occasionally. Living young adult parasites have been recovered from the eye chambers in a dozen cases, and the CSF in these cases showed concomitant eosinophilic meningitis. Retinal hemorrhage and detachment are serious complications of ocular angiostrongyliasis. Unilateral facial paralysis of the lower motor neuron type and lateral abducens paralysis occur in less than 5% of patients (Fig. 93–3).

Definitive pulmonary symptoms, such as productive cough, audible rales, and confirmed chest roentgenographic abnormalities, have been recognized in some severe cases, and *A. cantonensis* adults have been seen histologically in the pulmonary arteries.

Laboratory Findings. Elevation of the initial CSF pressure above 200 mm of water (in some cases over 500 mm of water) with grossly opalescent or turbid, but not purulent, fluid occurs in 88% of cases in Thailand. Most cases have a characteristic pleocytosis consisting of a leukocyte count of 500 to 2000/mm^3 with a relatively high percentage of eosinophils, typically 25 to 75%. Eosinophilic pleocytosis reaches a peak around the 12th day of illness and gradually disappears over a few months. In a few cases, the pleocytosis may recur together with the symptoms after 2 or 3 months. The protein content is elevated in approximately two thirds of patients, but reduced glucose levels are rare.

An increased number of eosinophils (15 to 50%) is observed also in the peripheral blood and persists for about 3 months. There is no correlation between the degree of eosinophilia in the peripheral blood and the percentage of eosinophils in the CSF.

Other investigations, including serum biochemical tests, electroencephalography, and cerebral angiography, are usually normal.

DIAGNOSIS. In endemic areas, cerebral angiostrongyliasis is diagnosed usually on the basis of epidemiologic, clinical, and CSF findings. Computed axial tomographs (CAT scan) of the brain may be abnormal. The enzyme-linked immunosorbent assay (ELISA) with an-

tigen prepared from fourth-stage larvae has been positive at titers of 1:64 or greater in some patients believed to have *A. cantonensis* infection, but this test is not readily available. A definitive diagnosis can be made only by recovering *A. cantonensis* larvae from the CSF, ocular chambers, or at autopsy (Fig. 93–2). However, this is rare.

Differential Diagnosis. In endemic areas, eosinophilic pleocytosis associated with neurologic involvement has been found in other helminthic diseases, including infections with *Gnathosoma spinigerum*, *Paragonimus westermani*, *P. heterotremus*, *Schistosoma japonicum*, and *Taenia solium* cysticerca. Of these, cerebral gnathostomiasis is encountered most frequently, and should be suspected if a patient with hemorrhagic or xanthochromic spinal fluid and eosinophilic pleocytosis develops paralysis of the extremities following severe radiculitis or sensorium impairment.

TREATMENT. In mild and moderately severe cases, analgesics and sedatives give only minimal relief. Headache usually subsides dramatically, but temporarily, following the spinal tap. Therefore, careful removal of CSF at intervals of 3 to 7 days should be performed until there is a definite clinical as well as laboratory improvement. In more critical cases, corticosteroids may be employed to reduce cerebral pressure, or to treat those with cranial nerve involvement. No benefit has been obtained in milder cases.

Although effective broad spectrum anthelmintics (e.g., thiabendazole, mebendazole) are available, they should not be used, because clinical deterioration or death can follow the reaction to the dead or dying worms in the brain. In ocular involvement, emergency surgical removal of *Angiostrongylus* larva is required, but complications are inevitable if the worm gets into the posterior chamber.

PROGNOSIS. The disease is self-limiting. Clinical symptoms persist usually for only 2 to 4 weeks and generally become normal within a few days after initial treatment. In about 40% of cases, headache persists longer than 1 month; the neurologic deficit may last longer. The fatality rate is low: 3% in Taiwan; 0.5% in Thailand; and no deaths reported in Tahiti. Those who die do so in coma between 2 and 4 weeks after infection.

PREVENTION. Health education advising the nature and source of the disease, proper cooking of mollusks or paratenic hosts (such as edible snails, prawns, and crabs), and proper washing of salad vegetables is beneficial. Freezing of mollusks and crustaceans at −15C for 12 hours will destroy infective larvae of *A. cantonensis*. Community control measures consist of the control of mollusks and land planarians, but the most effective measure is rodent eradication.

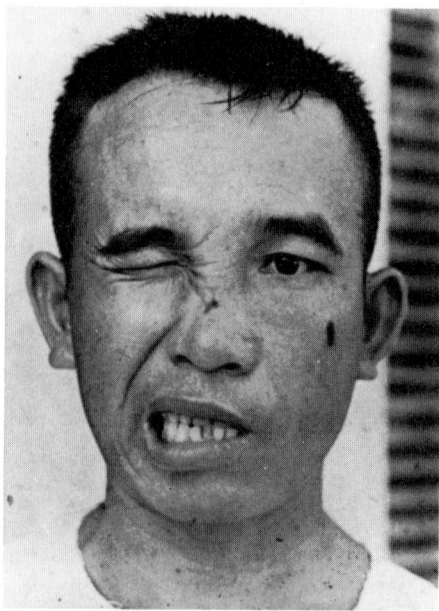

FIGURE 93–3. Unilateral facial paralysis of the lower motor neuron type in a patient with *Angiostrongylus* meningitis.

BIBLIOGRAPHY

Bunnag T, Benjapong W, Noeypatimanond S, et al.: The recovery of *Angiostrongylus cantonensis* in the cerebrospinal fluid in a case of eosinophilic meningitis. J Med Assoc Thai 52:665–672, 1969.

Prommindaroj K, Leelawongs N, Pradatsundarasar A: Human angiostrongyliasis of the eye in Bangkok. Am J Trop Med Hyg 11:759–761, 1962.

Punyagupta S, Bunnag T, Juttijudata P, et al.: Eosinophilic meningitis in Thailand: Epidemiologic studies of 484 typical cases and the etiologic role of *Angiostrongylus cantonensis.* Am J Trop Med Hyg 19:950–958, 1970.

Punyagupta S, Juttijudata P, Bunnag T, et al.: Eosinophilic meningitis in Thailand: Clinical studies of 484 typical cases probably caused by *Angiostrongylus cantonensis.* Am J Trop Med Hyg 24:921–931, 1975.

Rosen L, Loison G, Laigret J, et al.: Studies on eosinophilic meningitis: III. Epidemiologic and clinical observations on Pacific islands and the possible etiologic role of *Angiostrongylus cantonensis.* Am J Epidemiol 85:17–44, 1967.

Scrimgeour EM: Distribution of *Angiostrongylus cantonensis* in Papua New Guinea. Trans R Soc Trop Med Hyg 78:776–779, 1984.

Sonakul DS: Pathological findings in four cases of human angiostrongyliasis. Southeast Asian J Trop Med Public Health 9:220–227, 1978.

Yii CY: Clinical observations on eosinophilic meningitis and meningoencephalitis caused by *Angiostrongylus cantonensis* in Taiwan. Am J Trop Med Hyg 25:233–249, 1976.

93.2 ABDOMINAL ANGIOSTRONGYLIASIS

Pedro Morera

DEFINITION. Abdominal angiostrongyliasis is a granulomatous inflammatory reaction with heavy eosinophilic infiltration of the intestinal wall, especially of the ileocecal region, caused by *Angiostrongylus costaricensis* Morera and Céspedes, 1971 (= *Morerastrongylus costaricensis* Chabaud, 1972).

HISTORY. This disease has been observed in Costa Rican children since 1952. In 1971, the parasite was described. Subsequently, the definitive and intermediate hosts were identified, and the life cycle was elucidated. Since then, human cases of the disease have been reported from Central and South America, from Mexico to Argentina. In addition, naturally infected cotton rats have been found in the United States.

ETIOLOGY

Morphology. *A. costaricensis* is a filiform nematode normally living within the mesenteric arteries of the definitive host. The female is 33 mm long, and the vulva and anus are located near the caudal end. The male is 20 mm long, with a copulatory bursa and two spicules approximately 300 μm in length.

Development. Eggs are oviposited within the mesenteric arteries and carried by the blood into the intestinal wall, where they embryonate (Fig. 93–1). First-stage larvae hatch, migrate through the intestinal wall, and by excretion in the rat feces reach the soil, where they are eaten by the intermediate host, usually slugs. Two molts take place in the mollusk, and after 18 days the infective third-stage larva matures. The definitive host, a rodent, usually the cotton rat, becomes infected by eating the mollusk. The prepatent period lasts 24 days.

DISTRIBUTION AND INCIDENCE. The disease has been reported from Mexico to Argentina. Although it has been observed in the Continental United States, we do not know whether the cases are autochthonous or not. In addition, the first African human case has been reported. In Costa Rica, 20 to 60 cases were reported yearly since its first recognition; however, since the mid 1980s a better understanding of the disease by medical personnel has increased the annual incidence to 300 cases per year (11 per 100,000 inhabitants). In that country, its distribution is universal, from sea level to an altitude of 2000 m.

TRANSMISSION AND EPIDEMIOLOGY. Studies in Costa Rica demonstrated that the cotton rat *Sigmodon hispidus* is the most important definitive host, and at least 12 different species of rats and one coati *(Nasua narica)* have been found naturally infected with the parasite. Also, marmosets *(Saguinus mystax)* from Iquitos (Peru) have been found naturally infected with *A. costaricensis.*

Although several mollusks are naturally infected with *A. costaricensis,* veronicellid slugs are considered the main intermediate hosts. There is no evidence that persons intentionally eat slugs; however, small ones deeply hidden in salad greens could be finely chopped and inadvertently eaten raw. In addition, several cases are known of ingestion of these mollusks by infants. Nevertheless, most human infections are probably caused by ingestion of the infective larvae shed in the secretion of the mollusks. Slugs have been found in ripe fruits that have fallen to the ground. The characteristic mucous trails left by the mollusks can be observed throughout the endemic areas. The propensity for small children to put things in their mouths could explain why they have the highest infection rates (Fig. 93–1).

At least 2 species of veronicellid slugs in Costa Rica, 1 in Ecuador and 1 in Brazil, are naturally infected with *A. costaricensis;* 50% of 6025 slugs from 20 Costa Rican localities, from sea level to an altitude of 2000 m, were found to be infected; more than 14,000 infective larvae were counted in a single specimen.

PATHOLOGY. In most cases, the lesions are located in the ileocecal region. They have been observed also in the hepatic flexure, descending colon, regional lymph nodes, liver, and testicles.

Two major pathogenetic mechanisms are clearly distinguishable in the infections caused by *A. costaricensis:* (1) the adult worms living within the mesenteric arteries

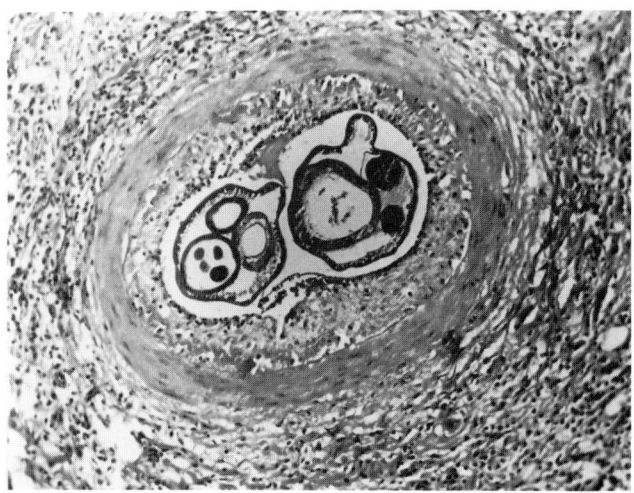

FIGURE 93–4. Adults of *Angiostrongylus costaricensis* within a mesenteric artery. The intima is swollen, and the endothelium is damaged.

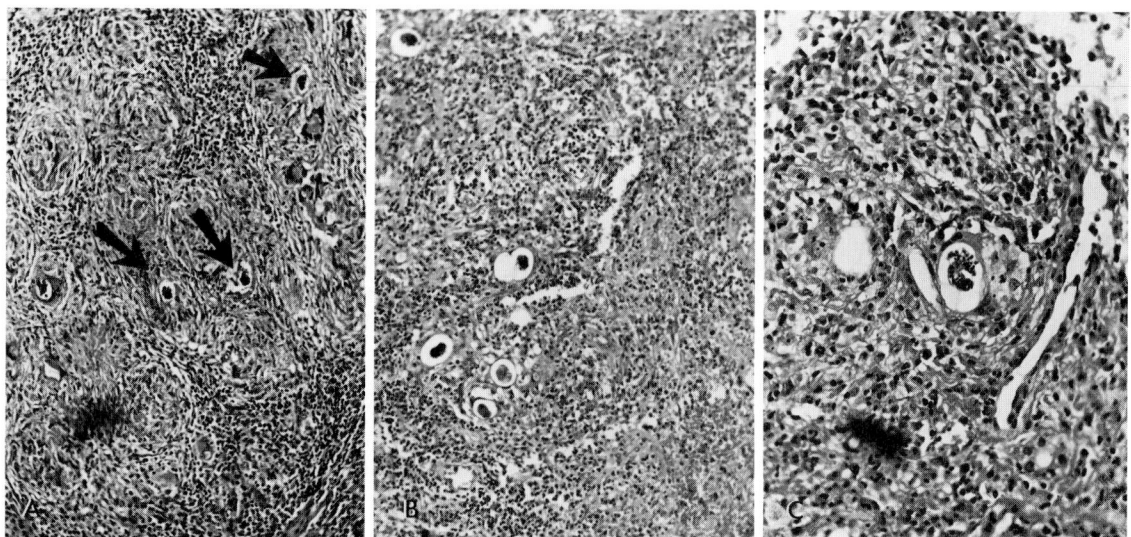

FIGURE 93-5. *Angiostrongylus costaricensis* ova in tissues. *A,* Section of intestine showing several granulomas and giant cells: eggs *(arrows)* are scattered in the tissue. *B,* Eggs in the cecum wall surrounded by inflammatory cells (eosinophils). *C,* Embryonated egg in the liver.

(Fig. 93–4) damage the endothelium, inducing thrombosis and, consequently, necrosis of the tissues formerly irrigated by the vessel; and (2) eggs, embryos, and larvae, as well as excretion/secretion products, cause inflammatory reaction. Combinations of these phenomena, as well as the patient's susceptibility and the number and localization of parasites, determine clinicopathologic differences, ranging from cases in which only the appendix is damaged to those in which major surgery is required.

The gross examination shows a hardened and thickened intestinal wall with yellowish foci on the serosal surface and in the mesentery. The intestinal lumen is reduced, sometimes causing partial or complete obstruction. Necrotic areas can perforate. In many cases, the surgeon observes lesions of the cecum during an appendectomy.

Histopathology demonstrates granulomatous inflammatory reactions (Fig. 93–5A) with heavy eosinophilic infiltration, especially in the mucosa and submucosa; often the serosa and muscular layers are involved to a lesser degree. Eggs (Fig. 93–5B), embryos, and larvae appear in small cavities lined by endothelium. Unfertilized eggs usually degenerate and are difficult to recognize. These structures, as well as the excretion/secretion antigens, are identified easily by immunochemical techniques. Large areas of necrosis are caused by arterial thrombosis. Eggs and embryos are present in the mesenteric lymph nodes, which also show reticuloendothelial hyperplasia and eosinophilic infiltration.

Hepatic lesions caused by *A. costaricensis* are similar to those caused by *Toxocara canis.* However, the finding of eggs (Fig. 93–5C), embryos, and even adult worms in the hepatic parenchyma establishes the diagnosis. In excised necrotic testicles histologically showing extensive parenchymal hemorrhagic necrosis, worms have been observed obstructing the arteries of the spermatic cord.

CLINICAL MANIFESTATIONS. Abdominal angiostrongyliasis affects children predominantly. From 116 patients studied in a pediatric hospital, 53% were

of school age, 37% were of preschool age, and 10% were infants. Of these patients, 64% were male and 34% female. When the worms are located in the ileocecal region, most patients complain of pain in the right iliac fossa and the right flank. Palpation in this area often causes pain. Rectal examination is also painful in about one half of the cases, and most patients present with fever ranging from 38C to 38.5C (100.4F to 101.3F), but rarely accompanied by chills. In chronic cases, a mild fever may persist for several weeks. Anorexia, vomiting, and constipation are also present in about one half of the patients. An important finding is a tumor-like mass that, if present, can be palpated in the lower right quadrant and may be confused with a malignancy.

Although a few patients have no hematologic abnor-

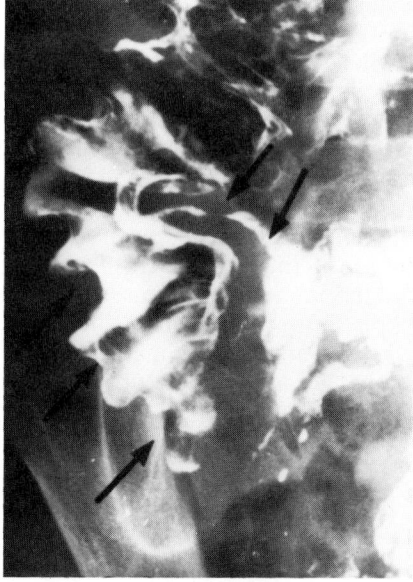

FIGURE 93-6. Radiograph after barium enema showing filling defect of the ileocecal region and ascending colon. The external wall of the colon shows festooned aspect of the mucosa.

malities, leukocytosis and eosinophilia are usually present. White blood cell counts usually range between 15,000 and 50,000/mm^3 and eosinophilia from 20 to 50%. The leukocytosis has been as high as 169,000/mm^3, with a 91% eosinophilia. A roentgenographic examination is often helpful in making the clinical diagnosis. Radiologic changes are localized in the terminal ileum, cecum appendix, and ascending colon. The contrast medium shows incomplete filling and irritability of the involved areas. The lumen is reduced by the thickening of the intestinal wall (Fig. 93–6).

Sometimes the patient complains of pain in the upper right quadrant; in these cases, the liver is almost always enlarged and tender to palpation. At laparoscopy, small yellowish spots are seen on the surface of the liver. Most patients have hepatic involvement along with intestinal angiostrongyliasis.

When the testicle is involved, the most remarkable finding is acute pain, accompanied by redness that later changes to purple. Eosinophilia and leukocytosis are also conspicuous. All patients with testicular necrosis have been misdiagnosed as having testicular torsion, and the correct diagnosis was only made following surgery.

DIAGNOSIS. The clinical diagnosis is based on the aforementioned features. The symptoms and findings can be confused with appendicitis, and the appendix is involved frequently in the process. The diagnosis is often made at surgery. Barium enema examination can show filling defects in the colon (Fig. 93–6) that often resemble carcinoma of colon. A latex test and enzyme-linked immunosorbent assay (ELISA) are used in the serodiagnosis. Eggs and larvae do not appear in the stool.

TREATMENT. When necessary, surgery is the treatment of choice for abdominal angiostrongyliasis. However, as knowledge of this often self-limiting disease increases, more nonsurgical cases have been followed. Two drugs, diethylcarbamazine and thiabendazole, have been used, with remission of symptoms reported. However, there has been no objective evidence to prove that cure was attributable to the drugs. In fact, in vitro and in vivo trials in experimentally infected rats demonstrate that the parasites are excited by the drugs instead of killed, causing erratic migrations and worsening of the lesions. Thus, chemotherapy is not recommended until experimental studies demonstrate a more efficacious drug.

BIBLIOGRAPHY

Loría-Cortes R, Lobo-Sanahuja HF: Clinical abdominal angiostrongyliasis. A study of 116 children with intestinal eosinophilic granuloma caused by *Angiostrongylus costaricensis*. Am J Trop Med Hyg 29:538, 1980.

Morera P: Abdominal angiostrongyliasis. Clin Trop Med Comm Dis 2:747–754, 1987.

Morera P: Life history and redescription of *Angiostrongylus costaricensis* (Morera and Céspedes, 1971). Am J Trop Med Hyg 22:613, 1973.

Morera P, Céspedes R: *Angiostrongylus costaricensis* n. sp. (Nematoda: Metastrongyloidea), a new lungworm occurring in man in Costa Rica. Rev Biol Trop 18:173, 1971.

Morera P, Pérez F, Mora F, et al.: Visceral larva migrans-like syndrome caused by *Angiostrongylus costaricensis*. Am J Trop Med Hyg 31:67, 1982.

94. CUTANEOUS LARVA MIGRANS

Ronald C. Neafie
and Wayne M. Meyers

DEFINITION. Cutaneous larva migrans is the dermatitis caused by invasion of the skin by larval nematodes. The filariform larvae of the dog and cat hookworm, *Ancylostoma braziliense,* account for most infections, but several other larval nematodes can cause the disease also (Table 94–1). The major emphasis of this chapter, however, will be on hookworm larvae that cannot or rarely complete their life cycle in man. Synonymous terms include creeping eruption, sandworm, plumber's itch, duckhunter's itch, and epidermitis linearis migrans.

ETIOLOGY

Morphology. Infective filariform larvae (third stage) of *Ancylostoma braziliense* measure 850 μm long and 35 μm in diameter. In processed tissue sections they are

TABLE 94–1. Causes of Cutaneous Larva Migrans

	Common Name	Incidence	Clinical Characteristics
Ancylostoma braziliense	Cat, dog hookworm	Most common	Thread-like, linear burrows, highly pruritic, moves 1–2 cm/day, may persist for months.
Ancylostoma caninum	Dog hookworm	Common	Papular, rarely linear burrows, clears spontaneously in 1–3 weeks.
Ancylostoma duodenale	Human hookworm	Common	Papulovesicular, pruritic, minimal migration in the skin, clears within 2 weeks.
Necator americanus	Human hookworm	Common	Same as for *A. duodenale.*
Uncinaria stenocephala	European dog hookworm	Rare	Thread-like, linear burrows, pruritic, moves 1–2 cm/day, may persist for months.
Gnathostoma spinigerum	Cat, dog nematode	Rare	Deep, wide burrows, furunculoid, may persist for years.
Bunostomum phlebotomum	Cattle hookworm	Rare	Papular lesion, minimal migration, clears within 2 weeks.
Strongyloides stercoralis (larva currens)	Human threadworm	Rare	Perianal band of urticaria and pruritic induration extends up to several cm/day around anus, may persist for weeks, recurrent owing to autoinfection.
Strongyloides myopotami	Nutria strongylid	Rare	Papular or linear, thread-like, serpiginous, pruritic lesion.

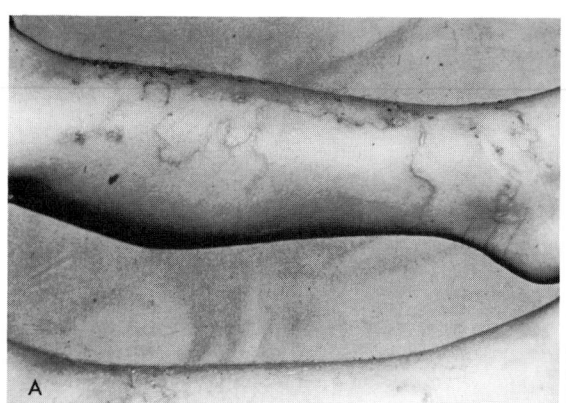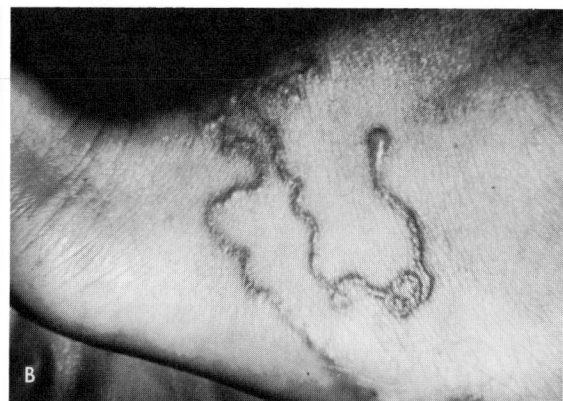

FIGURE 94–1. *A* and *B*, Creeping eruption caused by the larva of *Ancylostoma braziliense*.

only about 20 μm in diameter. They have double lateral alae that extend most of the length of the larva. All hookworm larvae that cause cutaneous larva migrans in humans and those of *Strongyloides stercoralis* are similar morphologically. In contrast, the larvae of *Gnathostoma spinigerum* are several hundred μm in diameter and can be readily identified by their numerous cuticular spines.

Life Cycle. The general life cycles of hookworms, threadworms, and *Gnanthostoma* have been described in Chapters 84.1, 84.2, and 92. Adult *A. braziliense* and *A. caninum* inhabit the intestines of dogs and cats. Embryonated eggs passed in the stool, under appropriate conditions of temperature and humidity, hatch and release rhabditiform larvae within 1 or 2 days. After feeding, growing, and undergoing 1 molt, they become infective filariform larvae, usually in about a week. Humans are an aberrant host of these hookworms; thus, these larvae invade the skin of humans but ordinarily penetrate no deeper than the epidermis.

GEOGRAPHIC DISTRIBUTION AND EPIDEMIOLOGY. Cutaneous larva migrans occurs wherever bare skin contacts contaminated soil containing the infective larvae of dog or cat hookworms. Thus, the disease is most common in warmer tropical or subtropical regions. It is especially prevalent in southeastern United States and is most frequent during the warm and rainy seasons. Children are more likely to acquire the infection because of their frequent contact with contaminated soil, such as in sandpiles. People who frequent beaches (hence, the synonym "sandworm") are at increased risk. "Plumber's itch" came into use because the disease is acquired often while repairing plumbing underneath houses.

PATHOLOGY. The larvae are limited to the epidermis, where they wander about producing serpiginous tunnels or tracks (Fig. 94–1). They are located in burrows in the deeper layers of the epidermis (Fig. 94–2) and are found most likely in biopsy specimens taken just ahead of the clinically evident track. Usually the specimen does not contain the larva but reveals only an infiltration of lymphocytes and eosinophils in the upper dermis. Often, the exact identification of the larva is impossible. It is not known why the larvae are unable to complete the life cycle. Some believe the larvae lack the specific collagenase needed for penetration of human dermis.

CLINICAL MANIFESTATIONS. Within a few hours after penetration of the skin by a larva, an itching red papule develops. A serpiginous track arises from the papule as the worm wanders aimlessly, creating tunnels within the epidermis. The surrounding tissues are edematous and acutely inflamed, and the unoccupied portion of the track dries and becomes encrusted and scarred. The larva may migrate several centimeters a day. This migration is associated with a severe pruritus that leads to scratching and frequently to secondary infection. In severe infections itching may be so intense that the patient suffers intolerably, cannot sleep, and may even become psychotic. The larvae can live for several months if untreated.

DIAGNOSIS. Diagnosis is usually made on the basis of the clinical history and the appearance of the characteristic serpiginous track. Biopsy is not recommended,

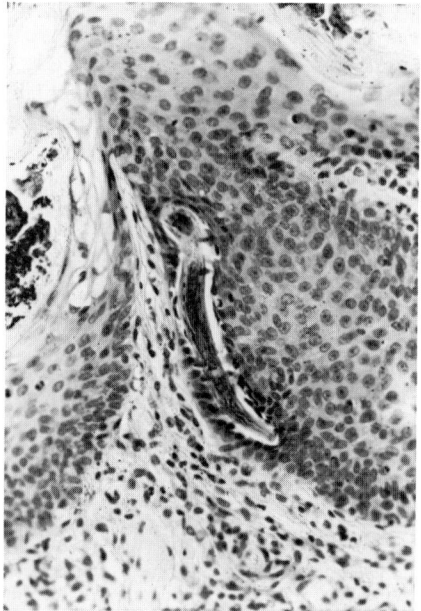

FIGURE 94–2. Longitudinal section of a larva of *Ancylostoma* species in epidermis. (H & E stain, ×175.) (Courtesy of the Armed Forces Institute of Pathology, Photograph Neg. No. 76-888.)

because the larva is usually beyond the obvious lesion and is rarely seen in the specimen.

PREVENTION AND TREATMENT. Avoiding contact of exposed skin with contaminated soil, e.g., wearing shoes and using a beach towel when lying on the sand, is the most appropriate preventive measure. Periodic deworming of domestic cats and dogs reduces soil contamination. Sandboxes and other similar facilities where children play frequently should be protected from dogs and cats, especially cats that may use them as defecation sites.

Thiabendazole taken orally or applied topically in an ointment or cream is effective and has generally replaced local freezing with ethyl chloride or carbon dioxide. Thiabendazole can be administered in a dosage of 25 mg/kg twice a day for 2 or 3 days. If lesions persist, this regimen should be repeated in 3 to 7 days. Topical thiabendazole should be given as a 10% suspension overlaid with 0.1% dexamethasone cream for 3 days. Mebendazole, 100 mg, 3 times a day for 7 days, is effective. Penicillin or other appropriate antibiotics should be given for secondary bacterial infections.

BIBLIOGRAPHY

Davis CM, Israel RM: Treatment of creeping eruption with topical thiabendazole. Arch Dermatol 97:325, 1968.
Edelglass JW, Douglass MC, Stiefler R, et al.: Cutaneous larva migrans in northern climates. A souvenir of your dream vacation. Am Acad Dermatol 7:353, 1982.
Katz R, Ziegler J, Blank H: Natural course of creeping eruption and treatment with thiabendazole. Arch Dermatol 91:420, 1965.
Stone OJ, Mullins JF: Thiabendazole therapy for creeping eruption. Arch Dermatol 89:557, 1964.

95. ANISAKIASIS

Tomoo Oshima

DEFINITION. Anisakiasis is the disease caused by the larval nematodes belonging to the subfamily Anisakinae through the consumption of raw or inadequately cooked marine fish or squid. It is commonly called herring worm disease or codworm disease.

ETIOLOGY. The disease is usually caused by infection with the third-stage larvae of *Anisakis simplex* and *Pseudoterranova decipiens;* occasionally other *Anisakis* larvae are involved. *Anisakis simplex* larvae are 19 to 36 mm in length and 0.3 to 0.6 mm in width and white or milky in color with a long stomach, an intestine with no cecum, and a blunt tail with mucron (type I larva). Rarely, another type of *Anisakis* larvae with a shorter stomach and attenuated tails (type II larva) causes human infection. *Pseudoterranova decipiens* larvae are 25 to 50 mm in length and 0.3 to 1.2 mm in width and yellowish or brownish in color; they have an anteriorly projected cecum.

DISTRIBUTION AND TRANSMISSION. Anisakiasis occurs mainly in Japan, and less frequently in the Hawaiian Islands and coastal areas of North America and Northern Europe, where people consume raw or inadequately cooked saltwater fish or squid. Humans are usually infected by eating raw herring, salmon, cod, mackerel, flat fish, greenling, red snapper, and squid in which the infectious larvae are present.

Life Cycle. The primary hosts of *Anisakis* are dolphin, porpoise, and whale; those of *Pseudoterranova* are seal, fur seal, walrus, and sea lion. Adult worms attach to the stomach wall and discharge eggs into the sea. Eggs develop and hatch in the cold water of the polar seas. Swimming second-stage larvae are ingested by small marine crustacea, such as krills, and develop to the third stage in their haemocoels. The third-stage larvae are transferred from krills to squid or fish and further from squid to fish or fish to fish by the predatory food chain. More than 150 species of fish become transport hosts of the third-stage larvae; when sea mammals ingest these transport hosts, the larvae develop to adults in their stomachs (Fig. 95–1). In general, the third-stage larvae are concentrated in the fish viscera; relatively few fish harbor larvae in their muscle. Among numerous transport hosts only the fish that have larvae in their flesh (Fig. 95–2) are important infectious sources for human anisakiasis. Herring, salmon, common mackerel, cod, and squid can transmit *Anisakis* infection, while cod, halibut, flatfish, greenling, and red snapper can transmit *Pseudoterranova* infection.

PATHOGENESIS AND PATHOLOGY. When humans consume raw or inadequately cooked infectious fish or squid, the larvae invade the submucosa of the stomach or intestine. The site of invasion is swollen and becomes hemorrhagic; larvae in the submucosa are surrounded by inflammatory cells, mostly eosinophils (Fig. 95–3). Occasionally, ecdysis occurs; however, the larvae die within 10 days and the exudative inflammation gradually subsides. An eosinophilic granuloma develops around the dead worm. Intestinal lesions are much more exudative and acute than stomach lesions.

CLINICAL MANIFESTATIONS

Stomach Anisakiasis. This usually begins 1 to 7 hours after eating the fish or squid. Most patients complain of severe epigastric pain that recurs every 5 to 10 minutes with nausea and vomiting. After a few days, the acute symptoms subside and a vague epigastric pain remains with intermittent nausea and vomiting for several weeks or months.

Intestinal Anisakiasis. This is caused by *Anisakis simplex* larvae or (rarely) by *Pseudoterranova* larvae. They usually invade the distal ileum. Usually 1 to 5 days after the infecting meal the patient has the sudden onset of abdominal pain with nausea and vomiting. Slight or no fever and a mild leukocytosis with eosinophilia of less than 10% are observed. Peritoneal fluid may be recognized; however, muscle guarding of the abdominal wall is frequently absent, occurring in only 20% of patients with intestinal anisakiasis. Usually, inflammation is limited to the intestine, and the parietal peritoneum is not involved. In some cases the larvae escape from the stomach or intestinal walls and migrate into the peritoneal or pleural cavity, causing peritonitis or pleurisy.

DIAGNOSIS. A history of consumption of raw or

inadequately prepared fish or squid shortly before the onset of the disease is an important clue. In the case of stomach anisakiasis, fiber optic endoscopy is the most useful method for diagnosis. Larvae invading the stomach wall are recognized easily and can be removed for morphologic identification of the worm (Fig. 95–4). If only a tumor is seen, biopsy should be made for detection of an eosinophilic granuloma. When endoscopy is not feasible, double contrast x-ray shadowing or ultrasonic echo analysis of the stomach is helpful.

Generally, intestinal anisakiasis is difficult to diagnose. Symptoms of an acute abdomen following consumption of raw fish strongly suggest intestinal anisakiasis. However, it mimics appendicitis, ileus, and regional enteritis, and patients often undergo laparotomy. Experienced physicians can differentiate intestinal anisakiasis when the characteristic history and findings, e.g., no or slight fever, mild leukocytosis with eosinophilia, peritoneal fluid, and no abdominal spasms, are present. Radiology is helpful when it shows luminal narrowing of the terminal ileum with proximal dilatation. Serological diagnosis, if available, is helpful. Antibodies to *Anisakis simplex* have been detected in some patients and appear to be sensitive and specific.

TREATMENT. The patient may regurgitate the worm, thereby terminating the illness. Endoscopic removal of the larvae is the best treatment for stomach anisakiasis. Larvae invading the stomach wall are removed easily by the forceps of a fiberoptic endoscope (Fig. 95–4). Eosinophilic granuloma present in chronic stomach anisakiasis requires no surgery; only symptomatic conservative treatment is recommended. Intestinal anisakiasis, if correctly diagnosed, also needs no surgery and should be treated conservatively with fluid and nutritional therapy. Effective drugs are not yet established. However, mebendazole (200 mg twice daily for 3 days) is worth trying for the expulsion of worms.

PREVENTION. Distribution of anisakid worms

among sea mammals is worldwide, and the contamination of marine fish and squid with anisakid larvae is widespread. It is necessary to know the hazardous species of fish that have anisakid larvae in their edible meat. Notorious species are cited above. The best prevention is not to consume raw or inadequately cooked, smoked, salted, or marinated fish or squid. They should be consumed only after thorough cooking or freezing below −20C for 60 hours. However, sushi served in professional sushi bars are rarely responsible for *Anisakis* infection. Professional chefs do not usually use fish, e.g., salmon, cod, mackerel, herring, whiting, haddock, which are infected with anisakid larvae, for preparation of sushi. Never order salmon sushi in a sushi bar.

INFECTION BY LARVAL EUSTRONGYLIDS

Three fishermen in Baltimore, Maryland, developed severe abdominal pain after swallowing live freshwater minnows. Laparotomy demonstrated roundworms penetrating the cecum and ecchymosis of the transverse colon in 1 patient and perforation of the cecum in a second. The third patient, who developed similar symptoms, recovered 4 days later without surgery. Roundworms were found in the abdominal cavity of both patients who had surgery. Minnows collected in East Baltimore waters were infected with roundworms identical to those recovered from the 2 patients at surgery. These worms were identified as fourth-stage larval nematodes of the genus *Eustrongylides*. They were 80 to 120 mm long and 1 to 2 mm in diameter.

A 24-year-old man from New York City developed eustrongylidiasis from eating sushi. He had right lower abdominal pain with exquisite tenderness, guarding,

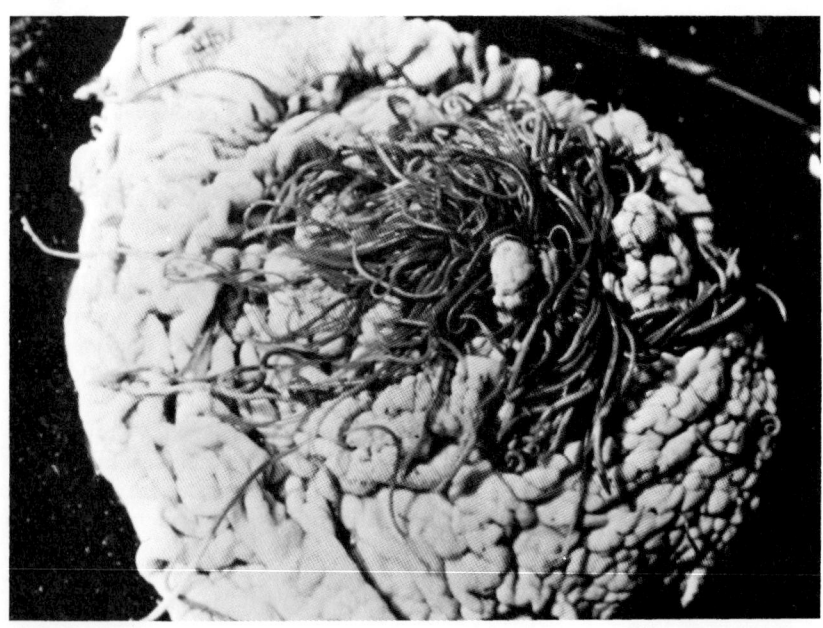

FIGURE 95–1. *Anisakis simplex* adult worms attached to the first stomach of a blue-white dolphin. (Courtesy of the Armed Forces Institute of Pathology. Photograph Neg. No. 76-2114.)

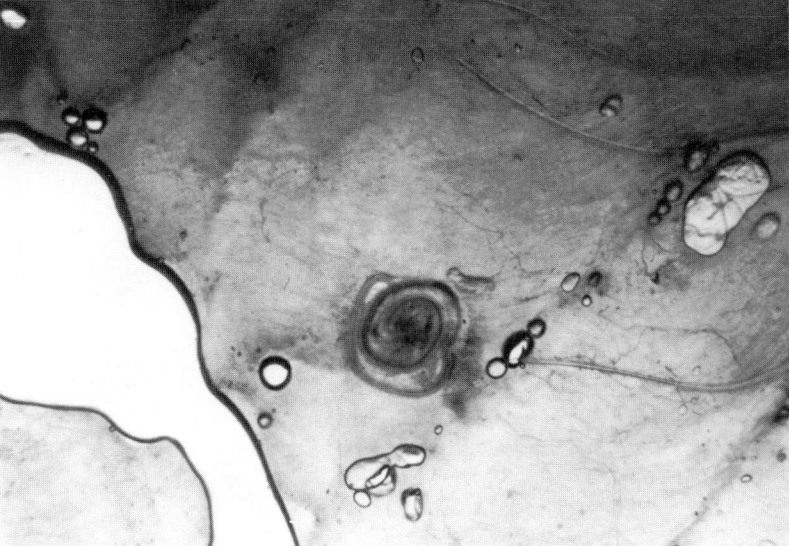

FIGURE 95–2. *Anisakis simplex* third-stage larva in salmon fillet.

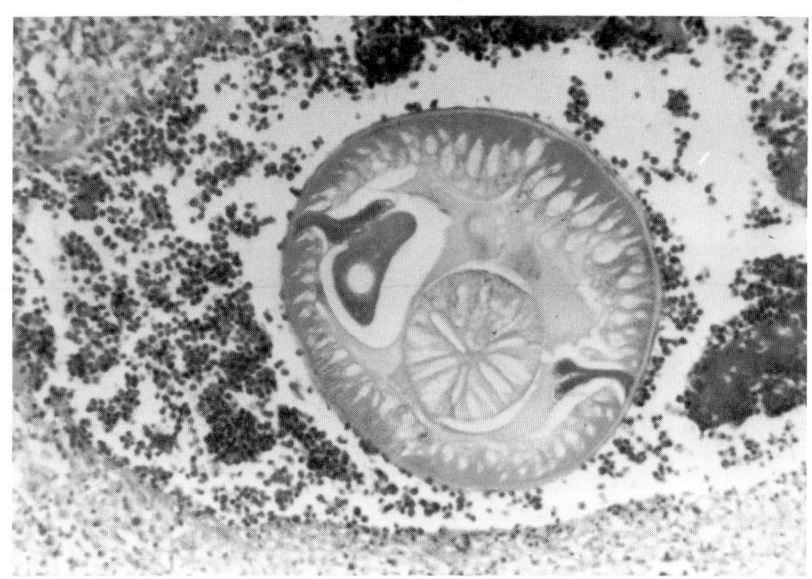

FIGURE 95–3. Intestinal anisakiasis with extensive infiltration of eosinophils surrounding an intact larva.

FIGURE 95–4. *Anisakis* larva caught by the biopsy forcep of the endoscope.

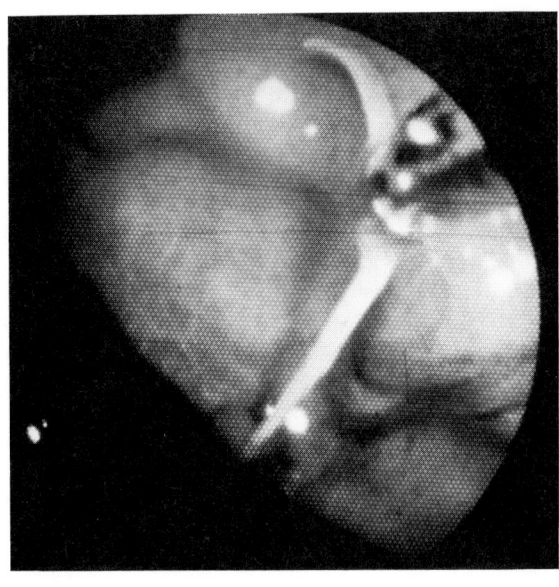

and rebound tenderness. An appendectomy was performed. The appendix and distal ileum appeared normal, but a 4.2 cm pinkish-red fourth-stage larva of the genus *Eustrongylides* was detected moving on the surgical drapes.

Nematodes of the genus *Eustrongylides* lack phasmids and belong to the subclass Adenophorea, order Enoplida, and superfamily Dioctophymatoidea. Adult eustrongylids are parasites of the gastrointestinal tract of fish-eating birds, and their larvae are found in the connective tissue or body cavity of freshwater fish. Amphibians, reptiles, and, rarely, mammals may become infected with larval eustrongylids and may be paratenic hosts.

BIBLIOGRAPHY

Centers for Disease Control: Intestinal perforation by larval *Eustrongylides*—Maryland. MMWR 31:383–384, 1982.
Kliks MM: Anisakis in the western United States: Four new case reports from California. Am J Trop Med Hyg 32:526–532, 1983.
Margolis L: Public health aspects of "Codworm" infection: A review. J Fish Res Board Can 34:887–898, 1977.
Oshima T: Anisakiasis—Is sushi bar guilty? Parasitol Today 3:44–48, 1987.
Oshima T, Kliks M: Effect of marine mammal parasites on human health. Int J Parasitol 17:415–421, 1987.
Smith JW, Wooten R: Anisakis and anisakiasis. Adv Parasitol 16:93–163, 1978.
Wittner M, Turner JW, Jacquette G, et al: Eustrongylidiasis—a parasitic infection acquired by eating sushi. N Engl J Med 320:1124–1126, 1989.

SECTION D

TREMATODE INFECTIONS

GENERAL PRINCIPLES

Robert Goldsmith

The phylum Platyhelminthes (flatworms) contains 3 classes of animals: the classes Trematoda and Cestoidea contain only parasitic forms, whereas the class Turbellaria contains chiefly free-living species. Animals belonging to the Platyhelminthes characteristically have a flattened, bilaterally symmetric body, without body cavity or coelom. Generally, flatworms are hermaphroditic and most are symbionts, living on or in the body of their hosts.

Most trematode (fluke) species are parasites of vertebrates and undergo initial development in snails through a series of multiplying larval stages. The trematodes display marked host specificity toward their snail host but less so toward the vertebrate host. Many flukes that primarily infect other animals are found sporadically as human parasites, whereas those considered to be primary human parasites may have either domestic or wild animals as important reservoir hosts (Tables VI D–1 to VI D–3).

TREMATODES OF HUMANS EXCLUSIVE OF THE SCHISTOSOMES. The trematodes of humans, exclusive of the schistosomes, are hermaphroditic, generally flat and leaf-shaped as adults, and range in length from a few millimeters to several centimeters. A representative life cycle, that of the lung fluke *Paragonimus*, is shown in Figure VI D–1. Adult worms have both oral and ventral suckers, a digestive tract that bifurcates a short distance below the oral sucker and ends blindly, and complete sets of male and female organs. Two testes are located usually in the posterior part of the body. A single ovary anterior to the testes connects with a system of laterally placed glands that produce the eggshell materials and also with a uterus that coils to a genital pore located near the ventral sucker (Fig. VI D–1). Eggs are usually passed in host feces (Fig. VI D–2). In all species, the eggs possess an operculum (a lid-like covering or "escape hatch") at one end of the shell through which the larva escapes. Generally, free-swimming ciliated miracidia are released, which penetrate the first intermediate host, a freshwater snail. In some species, however, the egg must be ingested by an appropriate snail host before emergence of the miracidium. Within the snail, a complex developmental cycle results in liberation, after several weeks, of large numbers of the free-swimming larval stage, the cercariae. After a brief period of independent existence, the larvae encyst in or on a second intermediate host, which (depending on the trematode species involved) may be another mollusk, a fish, a crab or other crustacean, or a plant. The encysted metacercaria (actually an immature adult worm) cannot undergo further development until ingested by humans or another suitable definitive (vertebrate) host. In such a host, after excystation is facilitated by the digestive process, the worms develop in a relatively simple way to adulthood, although some worms that do not parasitize the intestinal tract may migrate through the body.

SCHISTOSOMES OF HUMANS. The schistosome species that infect humans differ in several ways from other trematodes. They are diecious organisms (separate

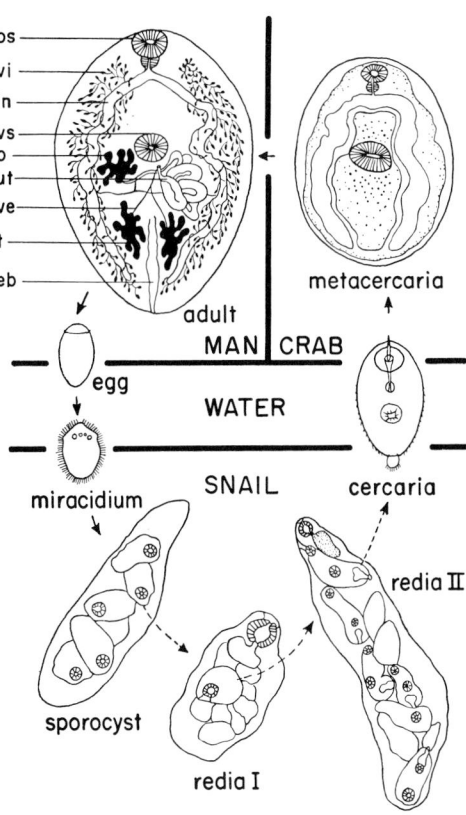

FIGURE VI D–1. *Paragonimus*, an example of a trematode life cycle: *eb*, excretory bladder; *in*, intestinal caeca; *o*, ovary; *os*, oral sucker; *t*, testis; *ut*, uterus; *ve*, vas efferens; *vi*, vitellaria; *vs*, ventral sucker. (From Markell EK, Voge M: Medical Parasitology, 5th ed. Philadelphia, WB Saunders Company, 1981.)

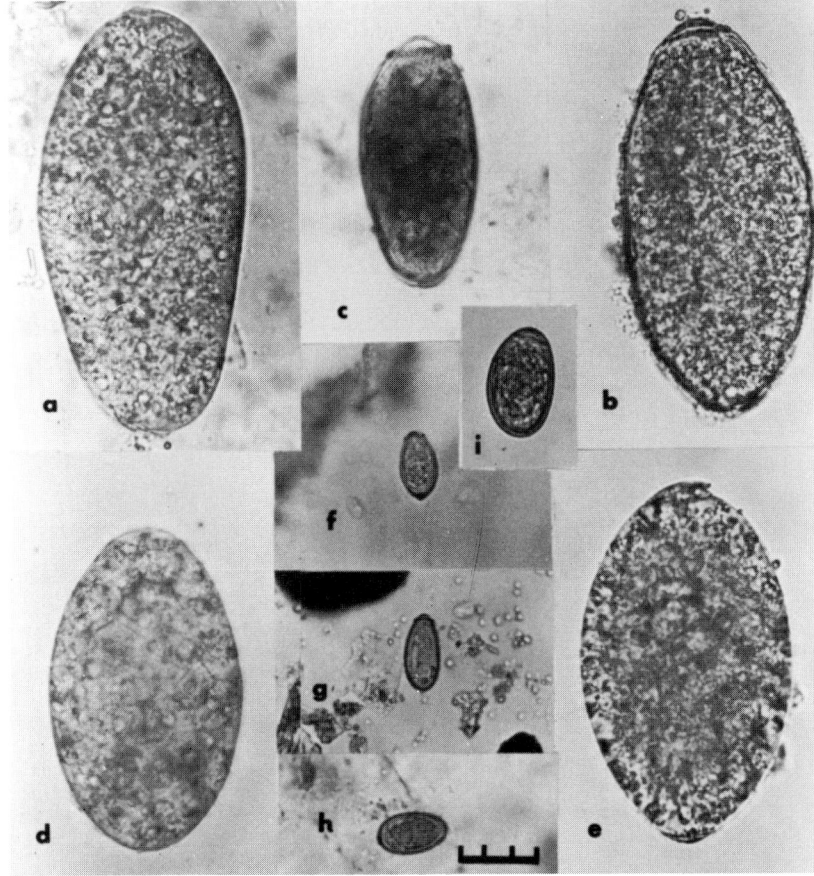

FIGURE VI D–2. Some trematode eggs. *a, Fasciola gigantica; b, Fasciola hepatica; c, Paragonimus westermani; d, Fasciolopsis buski; e, Echinostoma* species; *f, Opisthorchis viverrini; g, Clonorchis sinensis; h, Metagonimus yokogawai; i, Dicrocoelium dendriticum.* (Eggs of *O. viverrini, M. yokogawai* and *D. dendriticum* kindly supplied by Dr. Lawrence Ash.) All eggs photographed at same magnification: whole scale equals 30 μm.

TABLE VI D–1. Reservoirs of Some Intestinal Flukes

Species of Trematode	Host	Typical Location in Host
Fasciolopsis buski	Pigs, occasionally dogs, rabbits, and humans	Duodenum, jejunum
Echinostoma ilocanum	Dogs, rats, mice, and humans	Small intestine
Echinochasmus perfoliatus	Dogs, cats, pigs, foxes, and humans	Small intestine
Heterophyes heterophyes	Cats, dogs, foxes, other piscivorous mammals, and humans	Small intestine
Metagonimus yokogawai	Piscivorous mammals, mice (experimental infection), pelicans, and humans	Small intestine
Gastrodiscoides hominis	Pigs, "mouse deer" *(Tragulus napu)*, rats *(Rattus brevicaudatus)*, and humans	Cecum, colon

TABLE VI D–3. Reservoirs of Some Lung Flukes

Species of Trematode	Host	Typical Location in Host
Paragonimus westermani	Tigers, cattle, many crab- or crayfish-eating mammals, and humans	Lungs
Paragonimus kellicotti	Mink, many other crayfish-eating mammals, and humans	Lungs
Paragonimus africanus	Mongooses (two species), civet cats, dogs, and humans	Lungs
Paragonimus miyazakii	Weasels, yellow martens, dogs, wild boars, and experimentally in white and brown rats, cats, dogs, rabbits, and humans	Lungs

sexes) that live in the mesenteric or vesicular veins; infection results from skin invasion by free-swimming cercariae in fresh water. The schistosome species differ from each other in internal and external morphology of the adults (Fig. 96–2), in shape of their eggs (especially the form and location of the single spine on the shell) (Fig. 96–3), in the snails that serve as intermediate hosts (Fig. 96–5), and in the range of mammalian hosts they parasitize.

The body of the male has a short, preacetabular portion and a wide, flattened postacetabular portion, whereas the female (up to 2.6 × 0.03 cm) is filiform, round in transverse section, with a thinner but longer

TABLE VI D–2. Reservoirs of Some Liver Flukes

Species of Trematode	Host	Typical Location in Host
Clonorchis sinensis	Dogs, cats, and humans	Biliary passages
Opisthorchis felineus	Dogs, cats, foxes, pigs, rats, martens, wolverines, beavers, rabbits, seals, and humans	Biliary and pancreatic passages
Opisthorchis viverrini	Dogs, cats, civet cats, piscivorous mammals, and humans	Biliary passages
Fasciola hepatica	Sheep, cattle, wild rabbits, hares, other herbivorous and omnivorous mammals, and humans	Liver and biliary passages
Fasciola gigantica	Cattle, water buffalo, other herbivorous mammals, and humans	Biliary passages
Dicrocoelium dendriticum	Sheep, goats, deer, other herbivorous and omnivorous mammals, and humans	Biliary passages

body. Adults have a glandular anterior end and a ventral sucker (acetabulum) on the ventral surface. The alimentary system is an oral cavity that leads to the esophagus and then to the gut, which bifurcates into 2 ceca that reunite posteriorly to form a single posterior stem that ends blindly. The male reproductive system includes a number of testes dorsal and posterior to the ventral sucker, the number and arrangement varying by species. Females have an elongated ovary in their posterior half, the location of which also varies by species. The male worm possesses a ventral, longitudinal cleft, the gynecophoric canal, in which a female is enclosed. Nonoperculated eggs are passed in host feces, except for one species, *Schistosoma haematobium,* in which they are passed in host urine. On reaching fresh water, the eggs hatch by rupture, releasing miracidia (Fig. 96–4) that swim in search of an appropriate snail host. After penetrating the snail, the miracidia undergo polyembryonic multiplication that gives rise to and release of large numbers of infective cercariae. The life cycle is completed when the free-swimming cercariae penetrate the skin of the human or animal definitive host and complete their development in the liver and then in the mesenteric or vesicular blood vessels (Fig. 96–6).

BIBLIOGRAPHY

Beaver PC, Jung RC, Cupp EW (eds.): Clinical Parasitology, ed 9. Philadelphia, Lea & Febiger, 1984.

Binford CH, Connor DH (eds.): Pathology of Tropical and Extraordinary Diseases. An Atlas. Washington, DC, Armed Forces Institute of Pathology, 1976.

Hillyer GV, Hopla CE (vol eds.): Section C: Parasitic Zoonoses, Trematode Zoonoses, vol 3, pp. 3–210. *In* Steele JH (ed): Handbook Series in Zoonoses. Boca Raton, Florida, CRC Press, 1982.

Malek EA (ed.): Snail-transmitted Parasitic Diseases. Boca Raton, Florida, CRC Press, 1980, vols 1 & 2.

Rollinson D, Simpson AJG (eds.): The Biology of Schistosomes. From Genes to Latrines. San Diego, Academic Press, 1987.

Soulsby EJL (ed.): Immune Responses in Parasitic Infections: Immunology, Immunopathology, and Immunoprophylaxis. Trematodes and Cestodes, vol 2. Boca Raton, Florida, CRC Press, 1987.

96. SCHISTOSOMIASIS

G. Thomas Strickland
and M. Farid Abdel-Wahab

DEFINITION. Schistosomiasis is a parasitic disease with a wide range of clinical manifestations and affects more than 200 million people in 75 countries. Infection with any of 3 species (*Schistosoma japonicum, S. mansoni,* or *S. haematobium*) of the digenetic trematode *Schistosoma* commonly results in human disease. Infection takes place when cercariae, shed into fresh water by snail intermediate hosts, penetrate the skin of an individual exposed to contaminated water. After multiorgan migration, adult worms abide in intestinal and bladder venules. Human disease is most associated with the host's granulomatous response to eggs retained in the tissues.

HISTORY. The probable biologic origin of *S. japonicum* was the Yangtze River Valley; that of *S. mansoni* was the upper Nile River basin; and that of *S. haematobium* was the lake plateau of Africa. Ancient Egyptian papyri refer to hematuria in males, and nineteenth dynasty pharonic temple murals depict men with probable ascites and scrotal edema, commonly thought to be the result of hepatosplenic schistosomiasis (Fig. 96–1). This dates the African clinical disease as early as 1500 B.C. Other clinical descriptions have been found in Babylonian inscriptions, medieval Arabic literature, and Napoleonic remembrances of the "menstruating males of Egypt." Furthermore, calcified *Schistosoma* eggs have been identified in Egyptian mummy tissue from the twentieth dynasty (1200 to 1090 B.C.). In China, there are records of schistosomiasis of comparable antiquity. *Schistosoma* infections in the New World are more recent in origin, probably beginning with African slave trade to the Americas during the sixteenth and seventeenth centuries.

In 1851, Theodore Bilharz, whose name became synonymous with the clinical human disease (bilharziasis), first identified the etiologic agent of Egyptian endemic hematuria as the worm *Distomum haematobium* (later

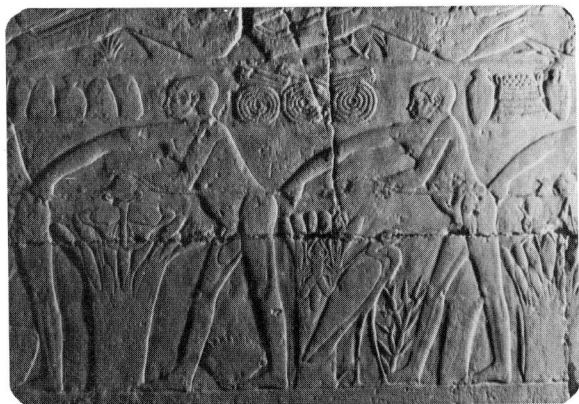

FIGURE 96–1. Photograph of nineteenth dynasty Egyptian pharaonic temple mural showing a boatman with ascites and scrotal edema said to be the result of hepatosplenic schistosomiasis. (Courtesy of Mr. Abdel Aziz Salah, U.S. Naval Medical Research Unit No. 3. Cairo, Egypt.)

Schistosoma haematobium). The differentiation of the 3 major disease-causing species was not noted until the early twentieth century by Sir Patrick Manson. The role of the snail intermediate host was defined in 1913 by Miyairi and was confirmed experimentally by the splendid work of Leiper in 1915. The first effective chemotherapy, tartar emetic, was introduced by McDonough in 1918. Interest in schistosomiasis remained somewhat circumscribed until the 1960s, when the immunologic complexities of the host's granulomatous response to the schistosome egg and the mechanisms of concomitant protective immunity began to be defined. Along with this renewed interest in schistosomiasis have come successful focal biologic control programs, particularly in Japan and Puerto Rico, as well as a new generation of less toxic and more effective antischistosomal drugs.

ETIOLOGY

Parasite Species. *Schistosoma,* the only bisexual genus of the class Trematoda, constitutes a rather large group of helminth parasites that differ from other human flukes by (1) living in blood vessels, (2) having nonoperculated eggs, and (3) lacking an encysted metacercarial stage. The human is a definitive host for 3 species of *Schistosoma: S. japonicum, S. mansoni,* and *S. haematobium,* each requiring a snail intermediate host. *S. mekongi* is a separate disease-causing schistosome similar to *S. japonicum. S. intercalatum* and *S. mattheei* are associated with human infections and pathology, whereas *S. bovis, S. rodhaini, S. margrebowiei, S. spindale,* and *S. incognitum* eggs or worms have been found in humans without evidence of significant pathophysiology. The cercariae of approximately 20 species of nonhuman schistosomes, mostly of birds or small mammals, are known to penetrate human skin, die without migration or maturation, and produce a dermatitis.

Biology of Parasite Stages

Adult Worms. Adult worms are just visible without using magnification, being from 12 to 26 mm in length and from 0.3 to 0.6 mm in width. The adult male worm is shorter and thicker than the longer, slender female. The male has a longitudinal body cleft, the gynecophoral canal or schist, in which the female lies in a folded fashion most of her life (Fig. 96–2). Both sexes have rudimentary attachment structures, the oral and ventral suckers. The former surrounds the mouth. The alimentary canal passes from the oral cavity into an esophagus, dividing just anterior to the ventral sucker and forming 2 intestinal canals that fuse near the middle of the worm to form a single trunk. This tubular structure ends in a blind terminus near the posterior end of the worm. The male tegumental surface may be tuberculated or smooth, depending on the species; the surface of the female worm is smooth in all species.

The reproductive organs vary slightly in number and location among the major schistosome species. In general, those in male worms consist of several testes, a number of vasa deferentia joining to form a vesicula seminalis, an ejaculatory duct, and a genital pore situated posterior to the ventral sucker. The female reproductive system is composed of a single elongate ovary, an oviduct, vitelline glands, shell glands, and an ootype

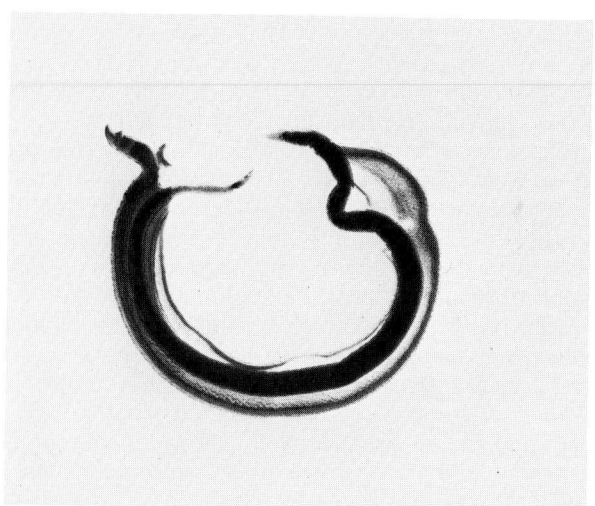

FIGURE 96–2. *Schistosoma mansoni.* Adult male with female in gynecophoral canal (× 10). The black color in the female is due to pigment in ingested erythrocytes. (Courtesy of the Armed Forces Institute of Pathology, Photograph Neg. No. 56-3334.)

in the central canal that passes forward to the uterus. The straight or slightly sinuous tubule-shaped uterus leads to the genital pore just behind the ventral sucker. The rudimentary excretory system consists of a few special function cells joined to a series of collecting tubules.

The worms take up nutrients by way of their intestine and integument. The energy metabolism of the adult worm is nearly totally dependent on energy-inefficient anaerobic glycolysis. Only egg production requires oxygen and aerobic metabolism. The adult schistosome utilizes one fifth of its dry body weight of glucose per hour, converting 80% to lactic acid. Adult worms contain a proteolytic enzyme, hemoglobulin protease, which breaks down hemoglobin, and the ingestion of red blood cells is thought to be important to their nutrition. As the gut terminates blindly, the insoluble hematin-like pigment is regurgitated. This pigment is phagocytized by the nearby hepatic reticuloendothelial cells and results in pigmentation of the liver. The high metabolic rate of the schistosome is probably related to the female worm's continuous high output of eggs.

Adult worms mate in the small vasculature of the liver and make a paired migration against the flow of venous blood to the predestined venous plexus. When the vessel caliber impedes further paired migration, the female progresses further alone and lays her eggs. The favored eventual location of the adult worm and, consequently, egg deposition varies according to species; *S. haematobium* is concentrated near the bladder, *S. mansoni* in the inferior mesenteric vessels of the large intestine, and *S. japonicum* in the superior mesenteric vessels of the large and small intestine. The life span of the adult worm is not precisely known, but studies of transmigrated populations suggest a usual longevity of 3 to 7 years and up to 30 years in exceptional cases.

Ova. Schistosome eggs are round or oval with one spiny appendage (Fig. 96–3). Size and shape vary according to species. Each fertilized female worm releases many eggs each day (Table 96–1). The eggs of *S.*

mansoni are released singly, whereas those of *S. japonicum* and *S. haematobium* are deposited in groups. Clusters of *S. japonicum* eggs have a greater predilection for calcification. Each egg contains a single miracidium, a ciliated larval stage, which matures over 6 to 10 days and may remain alive up to 3 weeks after oviposition. Most eggs desiccate and die if they do not come into contact with fresh water soon after leaving the host; however, mature *S. japonicum* eggs may survive outside the body for up to 80 days under moist winter conditions, e.g., in China and Japan, where they will hatch and

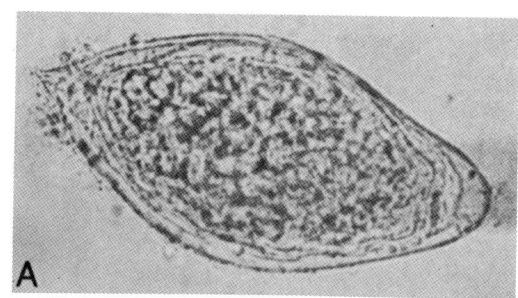

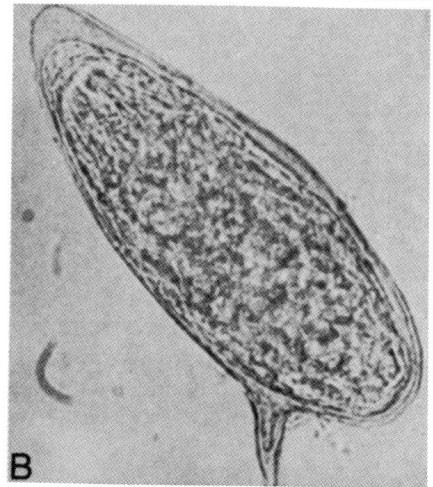

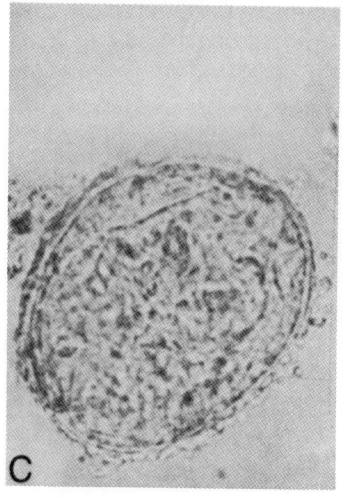

FIGURE 96–3. Ova of schistosomes commonly infecting humans. *A, S. haematobium* with terminal spine, taken from urine (× 500). *B, S. mansoni* with prominent lateral spine, taken from feces (× 500). *C. S. japonicum* taken from feces (× 500). (Courtesy of Dr. R. L. Roudabush. Ward's Natural Science Establishment, Rochester, New York.)

TABLE 96–1. Characteristics of Schistosomal Eggs

Species	Shape	Dimensions (μm)	Intrauterine Eggs	Eggs Produced/ Female Worm/Day
S. japonicum	Round, small lateral hook	70–100 × 50–65	30–50	500–3500
S. mansoni	Oval, prominent lateral spine	115–175 × 45–70	1–5	100–300
S. haematobium	Oval, terminal spine	110–170 × 40–70	20–100	20–200

infect snails the following spring. It is likely that the spiny appendage of the egg serves as an anchor against blood flow. All schistosome eggs absorb nutrients and secrete histiolytic enzymes, which facilitate their teleologic passage through tissue into the environment. Approximately 50% of released schistosome eggs are excreted into the environment in a viable state.

Miracidia. Human schistosome eggs, housing the miracidia, are viable only in fresh water. The hatching and survival of the miracidia are dependent on freshwater contact at a temperature between 20 and 30C. Miracidia are ovoid and about 160 μm long and are propelled by flagellating cilia on 4 rows of epidermal plates. Miracidia of all schistosome species are similar in appearance, containing a bilobate nonfunctional gut and 4 flame cells that function as the excretory system (Fig. 96–4). Miracidia demonstrate negative geotaxis and positive phototaxis. At a rate of about 700 cm/minute, miracidia swim to and attach to the soft part of the appropriate snail intermediate host. Penetration is aided by lytic substances secreted from miracidial glands.

Sporocysts. After snail penetration, the miracidium loses its cilia and becomes a nonmotile sac, the mother sporocyst. Over the next 10 to 15 days, germinal cells in the mother sporocyst differentiate into motile daughter sporocysts. The daughter sporocysts migrate to and grow in the hepatic and gonadal tissue of the snail. Cercariae metamorphose from germinal cells in the daughter sporocysts, migrate through the vascular sinuses, and exit from the edge of the snail's mantle. Sporocysts may regenerate and produce more cercariae. During this 4- to 6-week asexual stage in the snail, as many as 100,000 cercariae may be produced by each snail. Snail life expectancy is reduced by schistosome infection because of damage to hepatic and gonadal tissue.

Cercariae. The infective larva emerges from the snail

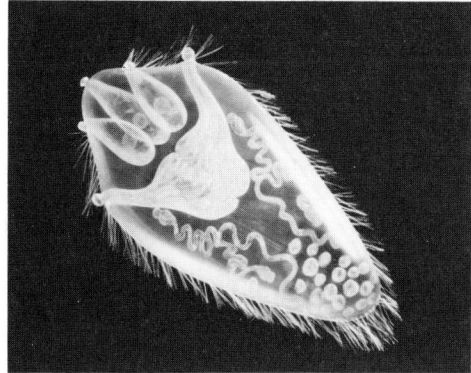

FIGURE 96–4. Miracidium of *S. japonicum* (darkfield, × 1000). (Courtesy of the Armed Forces Institute of Pathology, Photograph Neg. No. 218934-42.)

intermediate host under specific conditions of light and temperature. Maximum stimulants for shedding of *S. mansoni* and *S. haematobium* cercariae are provided by bright, direct sunlight and water temperatures of 25 to 30C, leading to higher rates of transmission during the summer months in the subtropics. *S. japonicum* cercariae are shed at night. Snails may be infected by multiple miracidia, but the mean daily output of a snail singly infected with *S. mansoni* or *S. haematobium* is 500 to 2000 cercariae/day. Snails infected with *S. japonicum* will yield only 2 to 20 cercariae/day.

Cercariae are unisexual fish-like organisms with a pear-shaped head and a forked tail, measuring 400 to 600 μm in length. The head contains oral and ventral suckers, flame cells, a primitive nervous system, and a nonfunctional gut. Cercariae may survive in fresh water up to 72 hours but gradually begin to lose infectivity after 12 hours. Although all species of cercariae are similar in appearance, their activity in water varies with the species: *S. mansoni* and *S. haematobium* cercariae move vertically, alternating between active movement toward the surface and slow sinking; *S. japonicum* cercariae attach themselves to the water surface film, where they tend to remain at rest unless disturbed. In contrast to schistosomula and adult worms, cercariae utilize aerobic metabolism. Cercariae attach themselves to the skin of the definitive host by their ventral or oral suckers, assisted by mucoid secretions from the unicellular posterior postacetabular glands. Penetration of the skin, usually complete within 3 to 5 minutes, is accomplished by vertical, vibratory movements of the cercarial body and lytic secretions from the cephalic preacetabular penetration glands. Only about 40% of cercariae that penetrate the skin eventually become viable adult worms. Survival is inversely related to the host's acquired immunity to schistosomiasis.

Schistosomula. The schistosomulum is the tail-less cercarial body that has undergone dramatic outer membrane modification. The trilaminar cercarial membrane becomes heptalaminar and is now tolerant to a saline environment. Metabolism shifts from an efficient tricarboxylic acid cycle to the less efficient anaerobic glycolysis. The schistosomulum remains in the subcutaneous tissue for approximately 48 hours before beginning the 3- to 6-day migration to the lungs.

Transition of the schistosomulum into an adult worm occurs between 1 and 4 weeks after skin penetration and is marked by the previously described anatomic developments. However, its most striking change is the development of an immunologically tolerant tegumental membrane.

Intermediate Host

Morphology and Biology. The snail intermediate hosts of *S. mansoni* and *S. haematobium* belong to the same family, Planorbidae, class Gastropoda (Table 111–

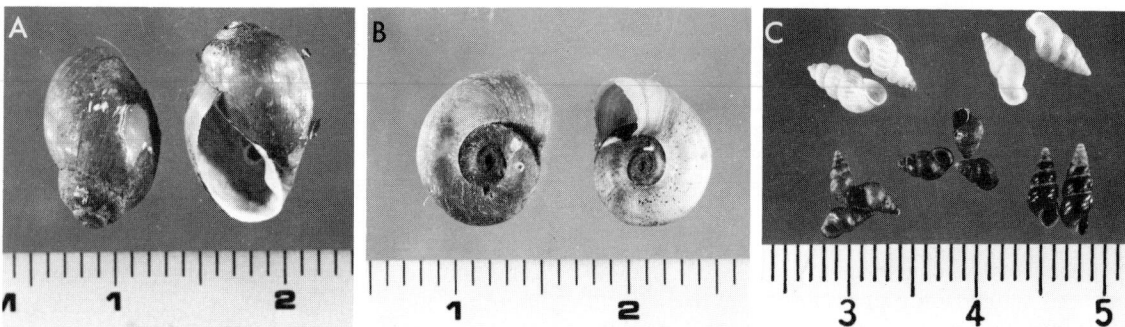

FIGURE 96–5. *A.* Both sides of an empty shell of a typical *Bulinus* species, the intermediate hosts of *S. haematobium* (× 5.7). (Courtesy of the Armed Forces Institute of Pathology, Photograph Neg. No. 70-11816-22.) *B.* Both sides of an empty shell of a typical *Biomphalaria* species, the intermediate hosts of *S. mansoni* (× 6.1). (Courtesy of the Armed Forces Institute of Pathology, Photograph Neg. No. 70-11816-21.) *C.* Empty shells of species of the genus *Oncomelania*, the intermediate hosts of *S. japonicum* (× 5). (Courtesy of Col. Myron Radke, MSC, USA, and the Armed Forces Institute of Pathology, Photograph Neg. No. 70-11816-18.)

1). These freshwater, nonoperculate, hermaphroditic snails have lungs and have hemoglobin in their blood, which gives them a characteristic pink or red color. The subfamily Bulininae are the major intermediate hosts for *S. haematobium* and *S. intercalatum* and are distinguishable by their ovate shells (Figs. 96–5*A* and 111–2); the genus *Biomphalaria* serves as the intermediate host for *S. mansoni* and is characterized by its disk- or lens-shaped shells (Figs. 96–5*B* and 111–2).

The amphibious snail intermediate hosts of *S. japonicum* are members of *Oncomelania hupensis* species; they are unisexual, have gills instead of lungs, and are operculate freshwater snails with conical or turriculate shells that are adapted to live on land and tend to be confined to stable marshy habitats with constant high humidity (Table 111–1 and Figs. 96–5*C* and 111–1).

The freshwater mollusks that serve as intermediate hosts for incomplete avian schistosome infections (cercarial dermatitis) include species of *Lymnaea*, *Physa*, *Polypylis*, *Gyraulus*, *Segmentina*, *Stagnicola*, and *Chilina* (Table 111–1). Some of the saltwater molluscan hosts include representatives of *Nassarius*, *Littorina*, *Haminoea*, *Cerithidea*, and *Batillaria*.

Life Cycle. The life cycle of the schistosome is complex and alternates between sexual (vertebrate host) and asexual (invertebrate host) generations. However, as seen by the survival of the schistosome from antiquity, the life cycle is obviously functional (Fig. 96–6).

Vertebrate Host. In the mesenteric venous plexus of the human host, the shorter, thicker male worm mates with the longer, thinner female worm in the male gynecophoral canal (Figs. 96–2 and 96–7). The female leaves the male after successful mating and migrates against the flow of blood to the small venules of the intestine or bladder, depending on the species. Incompletely embryonated eggs are laid, with approximately 50% being swept upstream, where they become lodged in the microvasculature of the liver and other organs, and 50% becoming attached to and embedded in the mesenteric venule wall. By a process not completely understood, but that probably includes the release of lytic enzymes from the egg and is assisted by host muscular contractions, the egg penetrates the lumen of the host organ, e.g., the intestine or bladder. The

penetration process takes approximately 8 to 12 days, coincident with egg maturation. The process of penetration is arrested in a certain percentage of eggs, whereupon a granuloma is formed and the egg dies, calcifies, and is eventually absorbed by the host. Eggs that reach the lumen of the intestine or bladder are passed out in the stool or urine.

Invertebrate Host. With satisfactory environmental conditions, each mature egg that reaches fresh water hatches a single ciliated miracidium, which then seeks out its own regionally specific freshwater intermediate snail host. Fortunate miracidia penetrate the snail, lose their cilia, and metamorphose into 2 generations of sporocysts, which migrate to the digestive gland of the snail and mature into hundreds of fork-tailed cercariae. The intermediate host phase takes 3 to 5 weeks.

At full maturity, cercariae emerge from the snail and swim tail first near the water surface in a teleologic search for a human host. Without successful host contact, the cercariae will die within 48 to 72 hours.

Vertebrate Host. Following cercarial contact with skin for as little as 5 minutes, penetration takes place. The now tail-less schistosomula find their way into the microcirculation, to the heart, then to the lungs, and eventually (e.g., 5 to 10 days after skin contact) to the small vessels of the liver. Histologic studies show that schistosomula are able to stretch the capillaries between the arterioles and venules of the lungs and thus remain within the circulation during this most hazardous stage of their migration. Those schistosomula not reaching the hepatic portal system on the first pass may return to the heart-lung circulation to restart the circuit. It is unlikely that any schistosomula running this gauntlet 3 times and not reaching the portal system survive. Over the next 2 to 3 weeks, following settling in the liver, schistosomula become mature adult unisexual worms, which, if they mate, begin laying eggs about 4 to 6 weeks after initial cercarial skin penetration.

EPIDEMIOLOGY

Distribution. Schistosomiasis is increasing in prevalence, largely because of increased exposure to contaminated water associated with (1) greater use of irrigation for agricultural development; (2) increase and redistribution of world population (from hunter/nomad to

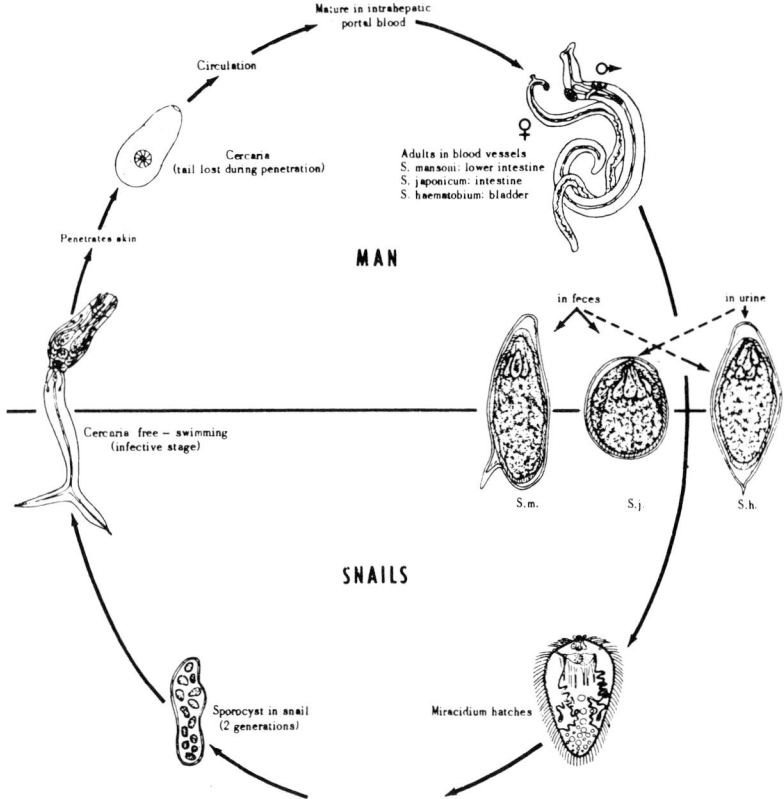

FIGURE 96–6. Life cycle of schistosomes in human infection. (From Melvin DM, Brooke MM, Sadun EH: Common Intestinal Helminths of Man. Life Cycle Charts. Atlanta, Georgia, Centers for Disease Control, 1964.)

farmer); and (3) inadequate control measures. An estimated 500 to 600 million people in 75 countries are exposed to infection and about 200 million are believed to be infected. The geographic distribution of schistosomiasis is confined to an area between 36 degrees north

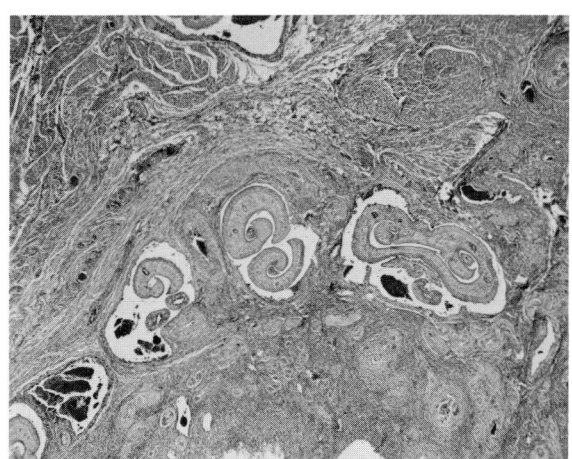

FIGURE 96–7. Biopsy sample from bladder wall showing worm pair(s) of *Schistosoma mansoni* within veins. The dark material is schistosomal pigment within the female. Note also the multiple granulomas and ulceration in the bladder mucosa and submucosa that is caused by the parasite ova. (× 25.) (Courtesy of Ron Neafie and the Armed Forces Institute of Pathology, Photograph Neg. No. 83-5186.)

and 34 degrees south latitude, where freshwater temperatures average 25 to 30C. In general, this includes: (1) *S. japonicum,* which is transmitted only in China, Indonesia, and the Philippines by *Oncomelania hupensis* (Fig. 96–8). A parasite resembling *S. japonicum* and transmitted by *Robertsiella kaporensis* in Malaysia has been found infecting humans; (2) *S. mansoni,* which is transmitted by members of the *Biomphalaria* genus in 53 countries from the Arabian peninsula, much of Africa, Brazil, Suriname, Venezuela, and some Caribbean islands (Fig. 96–9); and (3) *S. haematobium,* which is transmitted by members of the *Bulinus africanus* group in 52 countries in subSaharan Africa, by tetraploid members of the *B. tropicus/truncatus* complex in the Mediterranean region and Southwest Asia, by members of *B. forskalii* group in Arabia and Mauritius, and by all 3 snail groups in West Africa (Fig. 96–8). Incomplete infections with avian schistosomes, causing cercarial dermatitis, occur in fresh water throughout the Americas (particularly around the Great Lakes of the United States), Europe, Africa, Japan, and Malaysia.

Endemic Infection

Prevalence. Endemic populations show human infection beginning as early as 6 months of age. The peak intensity and prevalence of infection, as measured by egg excretion, usually occur between 8 and 12 years of age in heavily infected communities and somewhat later

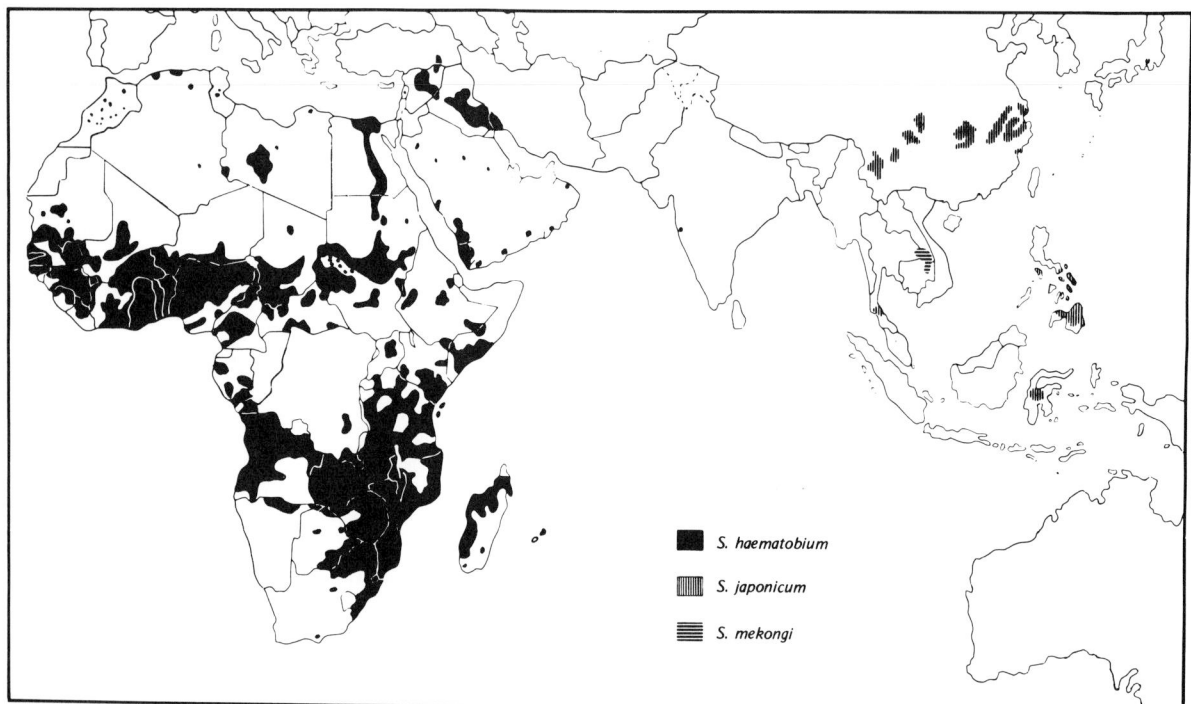

FIGURE 96–8. Global distribution of schistosomiasis due to *Schistosoma haematobium, S. japonicum,* and S. mekongi. (From The control of schistosomiasis: Report of a WHO Expert Committee. Geneva, World Health Organization, 1985 (WHO Technical Report Series, No. 728, 1985, pp. 17–18. Reprinted by permission.)

in lightly infected areas. In most communities, both the intensity and prevalence of ova excretion decrease after the preadolescent/adolescent peak. Infants first become infected while being bathed in the local irrigation canal, river, or lake. People, particularly children, in tropical and subtropical regions frequently use the same water source for defecation and urination, swimming, and

bathing. The greatest cercarial exposure usually occurs in boys aged 5 to 10 years. Adolescents usually have less recreational time in the water but have more potential exposure during vocational activities, e.g., agricultural activities for males and some females and washing dishes and clothes and bathing younger siblings for females. Adults also have considerable exposure to

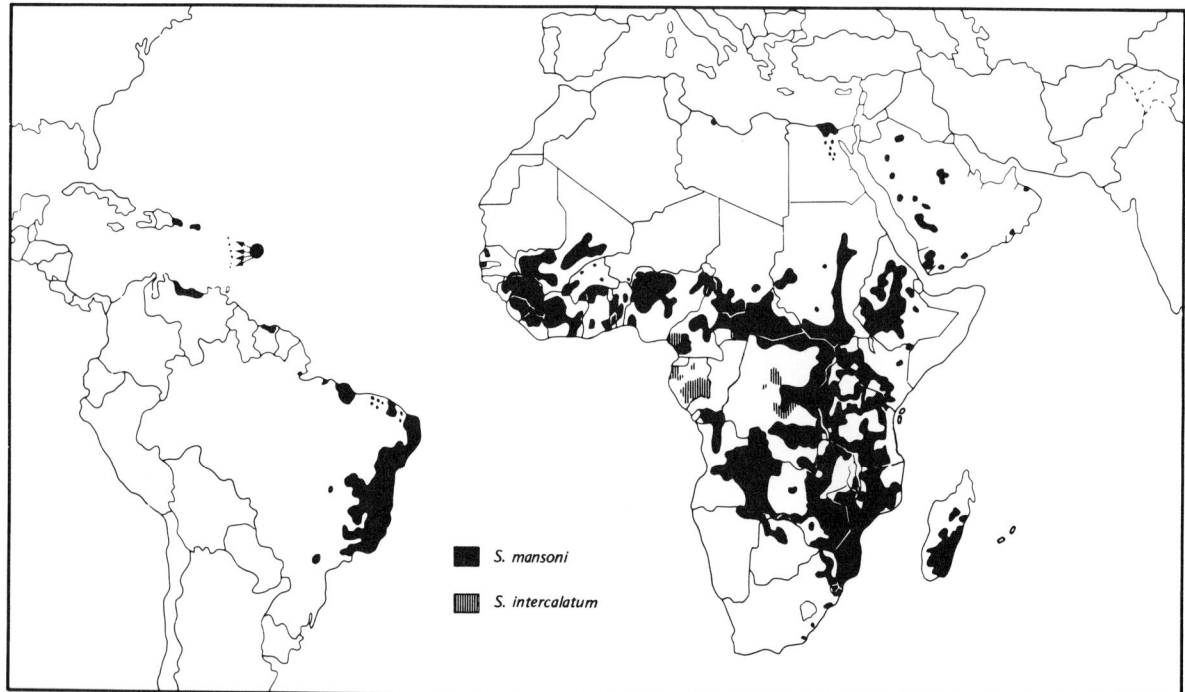

FIGURE 96–9. Global distribution of schistosomiasis due to *Schistosoma mansoni* and *S. intercalatum.* (From The control of schistosomiasis: Report of a WHO Expert Committee. Geneva, World Health Organization, 1985 (WHO Technical Report Series, No. 728, 1985, pp. 17–18. Reprinted by permission.)

cercariae-infested waters; however, the slightly lower prevalence and significantly lower intensity of infection among them probably reflects a partial acquired immunity, as well as less recreational exposure to the water. Most endemic rural populations will have a 40 to 60% prevalence rate of schistosome egg excretion at any one time; but almost everyone (i.e., 95%) has had an infection sometime during his life. These estimates, superimposed on the 1.5 billion humans in schistosome endemic areas, easily qualify schistosomiasis as one of the major world public health problems.

Morbidity. The distribution of infection intensity within a population is best described by a negative binomial curve, with a majority of the infected community members harboring a small number of worms and only a small proportion having heavy worm burdens. Because the morbidity of schistosomiasis correlates with the worm burden, as determined by fecal and urinary egg counts, a large proportion of the infected community will be asymptomatic during a single cross-sectional observation.

The precise morbidity of a schistosome infection is difficult to quantitate. The toll taken by hepatosplenic disease with incapacitating ascites or fatal hematemesis or renal failure from chronic urinary obstruction and pyelonephritis is dramatic and important but undoubtedly reflects only a fraction of the schistosome burden in an endemic community. More difficult to measure is the impact of chronic mild diarrhea, anemia, hypoproteinemia, hematuria, bacteriuria, or other more subtle schistosome-associated symptoms and secondary diseases on the socioeconomic output of a population.

Schistosomiasis in Nonendemic Countries. Owing to the absence of an appropriate snail population and the presence of more sophisticated sanitation systems, schistosomiasis is not transmitted in North America and Europe. However, because of a large immigrant population from endemic areas, physicians in California, England, and France (large Middle East and Far East immigrant populations) and in New York and Florida (large Caribbean immigrant populations) as well as university physicians (foreign students) throughout the developed world are increasingly being called upon to diagnose and treat schistosomiasis.

Ecology

Snails. Endemic human schistosomiasis is ecologically most dependent on the presence of the snail intermediate host and the deposition of human and reservoir host excreta into its warm freshwater habitat. These snails are *Schistosoma* species-specific and frequently geographically specific (Table 111–1). For instance, *Oncomelania hupensis*, the snail hosts for *S. japonicum,* are not compatible with the similar species, *S. mekongi,* and the snail host for the latter, *Tricula aperta,* cannot be infected by *S. japonicum.*

The aquatic snails important to the transmission of *S. mansoni* and *S. haematobium* live in lightly shaded, slow-flowing (15 meters/minute), shallow (<2 meters) water, whereas the amphibious intermediate host of *S. japonicum* spends much of its time out of water, preferring moist soil at the edge of slow-flowing streams or irrigation canals. The infective dynamics of the inter-

mediate host are such that low percentages of snails (e.g., 0.2 to 2%) are infected at any one time in an area highly endemic for schistosomiasis; even though a single snail may shed thousands of cercariae, the numbers detectable in an infested body of water are vanishingly small. Furthermore, snail cercarial shedding is seasonal in many areas.

Reservoir Hosts. There has been no identified functional reservoir host for *S. mansoni* and *S. haematobium.* However, *S. mansoni* infections have been found in rodents, baboons, and insectivores in Africa and South America. *S. haematobium* has been found in animals but rarely. In marked contrast, reservoir hosts play a significant role in the transmission of *S. japonicum* infections. Natural infections have been demonstrated in 31 mammalian species, including dogs, cats, cattle, water buffaloes, pigs, horses, sheep, and goats. A few wild rodents have been found to be heavily infected. On the island of Taiwan, a strain of *S. japonicum* is infectious to water buffaloes and other animals but not to humans.

PATHOGENESIS AND PATHOLOGY. The pathogenesis and pathology of schistosomiasis are largely ones of host reaction to a foreign body, e.g., the different stages of the schistosome parasite. During the migratory larval stage, mild transient foreign body reactions are seen. However, most pathology results from the granulomatous response to the schistosome egg and is directly related to the intensity of infection. In chronic schistosomiasis increased collagen synthesis occurs in the granuloma. Schistosomal fibrosis is caused by an imbalance between collagen synthesis and degradation.

Migratory Phase

Dermatitis. Cercariae penetrate the skin by opening the epidermis with lytic enzymes and wiggling into the epidermis (Fig. 96–10). Careful examination will reveal mild erythema at the point of entry, but this usually goes unnoticed. However, with prior cercarial humoral and cell-mediated immune sensitization, schistosome dermatitis, a pruritic papular rash, may result. Pathologically, each focal lesion demonstrates edema and heavy dermal and epidermal eosinophil and mononuclear cell infiltrates. The greatest pathologic responses are seen with avian schistosomes, probably because of subcutaneous cercarial death. Lesser pathology is seen with *S. mansoni* and *S. haematobium,* and cercarial dermatitis is unusual with *S. japonicum.* Cercarial dermatitis resolves in 7 to 10 days without permanent tissue damage or scarring.

Pulmonary Lesions. The metamorphosed cercariae, the schistosomula, migrate via the hemolymphatic system through the heart to the lungs, usually without recognizable pathology. In heavy infections, schistosomula may produce a pneumonitis akin to hookworm pneumonitis. This pathogenic state is histologically undocumented but is logically one of eosinophil-dominated acute inflammatory response to a helminthic foreign body.

Hepatic Stage. The schistosomula next appear in the liver, by way of the vascular system, where they develop into adult worms without causing overt hepatic pathology. Adult worms migrate to the mesenteric and vesic-

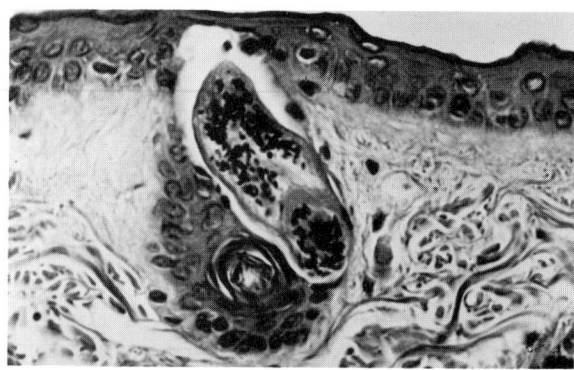

FIGURE 96–10. *S. mansoni* schistosomulum in dermis immediately after skin penetration in biopsy sample taken from a primate with experimental infection (× 255). (Courtesy of the Armed Forces Institute of Pathology, Photograph Neg. No. 74-9470.)

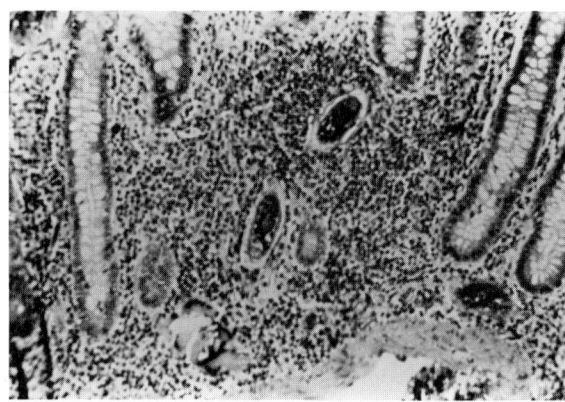

FIGURE 96–11. *S. mansoni* ova in the colon causing a heavy mononuclear cellular infiltrate in the submucosa. (Courtesy of U.S. Naval Medical Research Unit No. 3, Cairo, Egypt.)

ular microvasculature, also without host damage. While living in the mesenteric vessels the adult worm is nonpathogenic.

Acute Schistosomiasis

Katayama Fever. Approximately 4 to 6 weeks after initial infection, at the time of first egg release, acute systemic schistosomiasis, also called Katayama fever, may occur. It is more common in *S. japonicum* infections but has been reported in infections with *S. mansoni* as well. Circumstantial evidence suggests that this sometimes fatal serum sickness–like disease results from the release of large numbers of schistosome eggs that antigenically cross-react with a high level of antibody to a shared cercariae-schistosomula-adult worm antigen. This results in an antigen:antibody ratio that leads to large-sized immune complexes that must be cleared by reticuloendothelial cells, causing hypertrophy of lymphoreticular tissue. Antigen-antibody complexes have been detected in other stages of schistosomal infection, and stage-common antigens are suspected, but firm causal documentation of this pathogenic mechanism is absent. The prototypic Katayama syndrome has been rarely seen in recent years, and thus, the pathology remains incompletely defined.

Chronic Schistosomiasis. The pathogenesis of chronic schistosomiasis is almost exclusively explained by the host's granulomatous response to schistosome eggs deposited in tissues.

Egg Granuloma. Eggs trapped in tissues release enzymes and other antigenic substances that sensitize local host lymphocytes. These lymphocytes secrete lymphokines, which recruit other immune cells (Fig. 96–11). Eventually, macrophages, lymphocytes, eosinophils, and fibroblasts make up a compact cellular infiltrate, the egg granuloma (Fig. 96–12). Schistosome egg granulomas are similar for all species, although in *S. japonicum* infections granulomas usually show a greater amount of necrosis, perhaps owing to egg clustering at the site of inflammation. Early, acute granulomas are usually composed of eosinophils and neutrophils as well as mononuclear cells. The chronic granuloma is dominated by macrophages, lymphocytes, fibroblasts, and multinucleated giant cells. The acute granuloma is large and diffuse, whereas the more chronic granuloma is smaller and better circumscribed. The dynamics of the

evolving egg granuloma are based on the concept of immune modulation and are discussed in the Immunology section. Collagen deposition and fibrosis are integral features of the chronic granuloma and account for most of the irreversible pathology in all forms of schistosomiasis.

The egg granuloma is protective as well as pathologic. Animal studies using athymic or otherwise lymphocyte-depleted mice incapable of generating a granulomatous response show hepatocellular necrosis in the area surrounding the schistosome egg. The same is true in other tissues, e.g., intestine, spleen, brain, and spinal cord. Most authors agree that the granuloma reduces or confines this tissue necrosis.

Hepatosplenic Schistosomiasis

Hepatomegaly. In *S. mansoni* and *S. japonicum* infections, the major hepatic pathology of egg granulomas results from simple physical obstruction and tissue compression. Portal presinusoidal egg granulomas of the liver (Fig. 96–12) result in hepatomegaly and portal fibrosis with little primary hepatocellular damage. Portal hypertension follows with the shifting of hepatic blood flow from mainly portal to arterial sources. A disproportionate enlargement of the left lobe of the liver, frequently seen in early hepatosplenic disease, may reflect a preferential egg flow distribution.

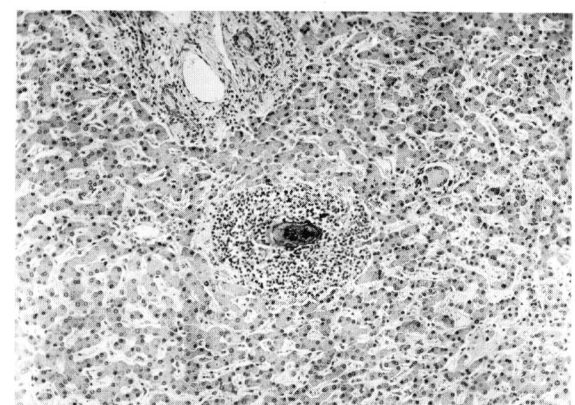

FIGURE 96–12. Egg of *S. mansoni* within hepatic lobule. Mixed leukocytic infiltrate around eggs may occur anywhere in the hepatic substance. (× 175.) (Courtesy of the Armed Forces Institute of Pathology, Photograph Neg. No. N-7661.)

Splenomegaly. Increased hepatic presinusoidal venous pressures lead to increased splenic vein pressures and vessel tortuosity. Intrasplenic venous pressures are also increased, with resultant congestive splenomegaly.

A second factor contributing to splenomegaly is splenic hyperplasia. Cell proliferation in the red pulp and germinal centers of lymphoid follicles occurs early in infection. Later, at a time when serum immunoglobulins are elevated, basophil proliferation may be seen. Histologic sections of the spleen show distended venous sinuses and dense splenic cords, reflecting changes from both portal hypertension and hypercellularity. Giant follicular lymphoma has been reported in association with schistosome hypersplenism.

Varices and Ascites. Severe long-standing hepatosplenic schistosomiasis leads to esophageal varices and ascites. This "collateralization" of the abdominal venous system may enable schistosome eggs to bypass the liver and reach areas of the body not normally accessible, e.g., the lungs and spinal cord.

Symmers' Pipe-Stem Fibrosis. This is a periportal fibrosis without bridging, nodular formation, or significant hepatocellular destruction and is undoubtedly a result of egg-induced chronic presinusoidal inflammation leading to the deposition of fibrous material. These fibrotic changes cause a broadening and lengthening of the portal areas so that they are seen prominently on anatomic cross section to resemble a "pipe stem" (Fig. 96–13). This is most often a part of the later stages of the portal hypertensive syndrome and is seen in all human schistosome infections; in *S. japonicum* disease, however, the onset may be more rapid and the prevalence greater.

More information is known about liver fibrosis in schistosomiasis than in any other liver disease. Products of schistosome eggs, inflammatory cells, and stimulating factors from these cells all promote fibroblast activity. This leads to a proliferation of collagen-synthesizing cells, increased peptide synthesis, and increased turnover of collagen. The balance between collagen formation and degradation is critical for determining whether the schistosome-infected liver returns to normal structure or becomes fibrotic. Tissue collagenases, mainly of macrophage origin, are greatly increased in the schistosome-infected liver. A predominance of collagenolysis over collagen synthesis explains the reversal of fibrosis that occurs clinically and has been demonstrated in experimental animals infected with *Schistosoma*.

Intestinal Schistosomiasis. As egg-laying worms may be found in the microvasculature of both the superior (*S. japonicum*) and inferior (*S. mansoni*) mesenteric venous distribution, all areas of the small and large intestine may be involved. Small intestinal biopsies have shown schistosome eggs and their attendant inflammatory response, and autopsy studies have demonstrated the "sandy patches" of long-standing schistosome granulomatous lesions throughout the small intestine. The protein-losing enteropathies and malabsorption-type anemias of schistosomiasis are likely the result of this phenomenon.

Intestinal Polyposis. The large intestine usually demonstrates the most severe pathology. Multiple focal

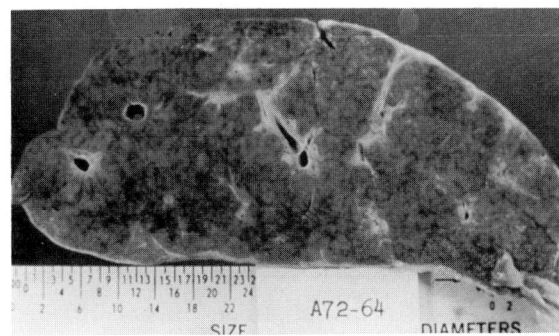

FIGURE 96–13. Cut surface of the liver showing Symmers' clay pipe-stem fibrosis in a patient infected with *Schistosoma mansoni*. (Courtesy of U.S. Naval Medical Research Unit No. 3, Cairo, Egypt.)

granulomatous lesions can be extensive and, in severe cases, coalesce to form a large hemorrhagic granuloma, denuded of all normal mucosa. In some cases, the granulomatous lesions become polypoid. The polyps are usually friable and on biopsy show acute and chronic inflammatory reaction and large numbers of schistosome eggs. Polyp formation results from deposition of ova in the superficial layers of the submucosa where the connective tissue is loose, thus permitting greater accumulations of granulation tissue. Subsequently, the muscularis mucosa becomes involved, and the overlying mucosa undergoes hyperplastic changes. This same process is the most likely explanation of rectal prolapse, which is also seen in severe intestinal schistosomiasis.

Other Complications. Severe and long-standing large bowel granulomatous lesions may become fibrotic and constrict the normal bowel caliber. These large granulomatous and later fibrotic lesions begin usually as microperforations of extensive bowel wall granulomas. Frank bowel perforation is rarely found.

Urinary Tract Schistosomiasis. The pathogenesis of urinary schistosomiasis (*S. haematobium*) relates to the mucosal and submucosal granulomatous lesions of the ureters and bladder. As in the intestine, granulomatous lesions may be seen throughout the urinary tract and are prone to the same hemorrhagic, polypoid, and fibrotic complications.

Obstructive Uropathy. Obstructive uropathy occurs when egg granulomas are located in the ureteral mucosa or in the bladder mucosa near the ureteral inlet or when massive bladder granulomatous and/or polypoid lesions obstruct the ureteral inlet. The pathogenesis of chronic bacteriuria relates in part to bladder and ureteral obstructive phenomena with resultant urine stasis and probably in part to the disruption of the normal bacteriostatic mechanisms of the intact bladder mucosa.

Bladder Cancer. Bladder carcinoma is associated with chronic heavy urinary schistosomiasis. The cell type is usually squamous, and the early in situ stages are found near bladder granulomas. It usually spreads laterally and from the mucosa through the bladder wall and into contiguous tissues. Lymphatic spread to the para-aortic lymph nodes is common.

Epidemiologic studies comparing populations highly endemic for heavy urinary schistosomiasis and those without *S. haematobium* infection show (1) a dramatic, multifold rate increase in bladder cancer; (2) an abnormal age distribution of bladder cancer, following the pattern of heaviest endemic urinary schistosomiasis; and (3) a predominance of an unusual cancer cell type, squamous cell, suspected in other circumstances (e.g., lung cancer, cervical cancer) to be a result of chronic irritative lesions.

Three pathogenic mechanisms have been suggested to explain the association of bladder cancer and urinary schistosomiasis:

1. Prolonged irritation of bladder epithelium resulting from long-standing egg granulomas leads to a constant reparative process that progresses to hyperplasia and then to malignancy.

2. A localized bladder obstructive state leads to urine stasis, local sepsis, and consequent alkalinity of an inflamed schistosomal bladder, which induces malignancy. This mechanism is supported by the autopsy observation of schistosomal fibrotic stenosis below the site of the neoplasm.

3. Carcinogens have been found in the urine of patients with schistosomal bladder cancer. Large amounts of the enzyme glucuronidase are found regularly. In the presence of urinary stasis, secondary bacterial infection, and alkaline urine, this enzyme may release carcinogenic substances from the harmless conjugated forms. Furthermore, carcinogenic metabolites of tryptophan have been found in high levels in patients with schistosomal bladder cancer. These metabolites are reduced by the administration of vitamin B_6, which is needed for the growth, maturation, and oviposition of schistosomes. Perhaps a schistosome-induced vitamin B_6 deficiency results in carcinogenic tryptophan metabolites.

Renal Schistosomiasis

Glomerulonephritis. Although common in schistosomiasis mansoni, glomerulonephritis is usually asymptomatic and clinically insignificant. A renal biopsy study of patients with *S. mansoni* infection without clinical renal disease showed a high prevalence of histopathologic glomerulonephritis with schistosome antigen-antibody immune complex deposits in the glomeruli. This finding is not unexpected, because circulating schistosome immune complexes are found frequently in *S. mansoni* infections, and an immune complex syndrome, e.g., Katayama fever, occurs.

Nephrotic Syndrome. This is seen occasionally in patients with *S. mansoni* and/or *S. haematobium* infections. There remains some controversy as to the precise infectious cause of nephrotic syndrome in this setting, as many reported cases also have had associated chronic *Salmonella* bacteremia and/or *Salmonella* bacteriuria. The few renal biopsy specimens available from such patients have shown minimal-change disease and only schistosome immune complex deposits.

Amyloid. Deposits of amyloid have been detected also in renal biopsy samples from patients with chronic schistosomiasis haematobia and mansoni who have no other long-standing infection. The pathogenic mechanism is undefined but is presumed to be the same as that of other chronic infection states and is hypothesized to be the result of an aberrant immunoregulatory condition.

Cardiopulmonary Schistosomiasis

Pneumonitis. The pathogenesis of larval pneumonitis, seen shortly after heavy schistosome infection, and the Loeffler-like pneumonitis, seen soon after antischistosome chemotherapy for heavy infections, is undoubtedly based on a local allergic reaction, although specimens for pathologic study are rarely available. In the case of larval pneumonitis, there is an allergic reaction to the migratory schistosome larvae as they congregate in the pulmonary microvasculature on their way to the liver. The posttreatment pneumonitis is hypothesized to be the allergic response to the abrupt release of common antigen(s) from the dying adult worms. The pulmonary focus of this response may be due to sensitization of local immune cells by larvae or perhaps to the fact that the lungs happen to be the most visible organ of a systemic immune complex phenomenon (although generalized lymphadenopathy is not found). Peripheral eosinophilia, a marker of a reaginic allergic response, is much more prominent in larval pneumonitis than in the Loeffler-like syndrome.

Schistosomal Cor Pulmonale. Cor pulmonale, seen infrequently in the 3 human schistosome infections, manifests pathologically as 3 groups of vascular changes: (1) organic changes produced by multiple schistosome egg tubercules; (2) toxic-allergic changes leading to arteritis; (3) medial hypertrophy, diffuse intimal arteriolar proliferation, and premature atheroma of the pulmonary artery.

These changes occur after prolonged deposition of large numbers of schistosome eggs in the prearteriolar pulmonary circulation. The resulting obliterative arteritis leads to pulmonary hypertension, increased right heart pressures, pulmonary artery and right atrial dilatation, and right ventricular hypertrophy (Figs. 2–6 and 2–7). Histologic sections of the lung demonstrate rather characteristic dumbbell-shaped interarterial and paraarterial granulomas. Cor pulmonale is more common in schistosomiasis mansoni and is closely associated with the presence and severity of portal hypertension and the resulting propensity for ova to bypass the portal venous system and reach the systemic venous system, from which they are trapped as they pass through the lungs.

Central Nervous System (CNS) Schistosomiasis.
CNS schistosomiasis is usually the result of embolic egg deposition within the cranial or spinal cord vasculature, resulting in infarctions and/or granulomatous lesions. All 3 species can produce such lesions, although *S. japonicum* is responsible for 60% of all CNS infections and virtually all brain lesions, and *S. mansoni* infection is the most common cause of spinal cord lesions (i.e., transverse myelitis). The smaller, more numerous *S. japonicum* eggs would seem more likely to range farthest from the hepatosplenic vasculature. In rare cases, the aberrant location of an adult worm can cause focal deposition of ova or can obstruct the anterior spinal artery and cause local spinal cord necrosis.

Association of Schistosomiasis and Other Infections

Chronic Salmonella Infections. Chronic persistent *Salmonella* bacteremia occurs with increased frequency in patients infected with the 3 major human schistosomes. Among intracellular bacteria, only *Salmonella* has been found to be associated with greater frequency with schistosomiasis. Likewise, other nonintracellular gram-negative or gram-positive bacteria, commonly causing bacteremia in other groups with hepatic abnormalities, are not frequent causes of infection in chronic schistosomiasis. *Salmonella* species specificity is a prominent feature of this syndrome, as is the absence of mortality from this gram-negative bacteremia.

The pathogenesis of chronic *Salmonella* infections in schistosomiasis has followed 2 major hypotheses: (1) an immunologic tolerance caused by schistosomiasis that allows *Salmonella* organisms to survive and persist and (2) the physical attachment and proliferation of *Salmonella* bacteria on the integumentum or in the intestinal tract of the adult schistosome worm with persistent release of bacteria into the blood stream.

The latter (physical attachment) hypothesis began with the in vitro observations that both gram-positive and gram-negative bacteria could colonize the intestine of the adult schistosome worm. Later, it was shown that *Salmonella paratyphi A* would firmly attach to *S. mansoni* adult worms taken from a schistosome-infected patient. The integumental attachment was randomly distributed over the surface of the worm and was probably related to somatic antigen and the bacterial pili.

The immunologic tolerance hypothesis is based on shared schistosome adult worm/*Salmonella* bacteria immune tolerance. Shared antigens have been demonstrated between the schistosome adult worm and *Salmonella*. By using large numbers of adult schistosome worms, *Salmonella* antibody may be adsorbed out of serum from patients with typhoid fever, turning their serum from Widal positive 1/640 to negative. Conversely, it could be further demonstrated that rabbit serum became Widal positive after immunizing the rabbit with the insoluble fraction of macerated adult schistosome worms.

More recently, work using in vitro spleen cell cultures has shown a reduced antibody response to *Salmonella* lipopolysaccharide antigen in mice with chronic schistosomiasis but a normal response to other gram-negative lipopolysaccharide antigens. Further dissection of this specific immune defect indicated a B-lymphocyte origin, independent of macrophages and T lymphocytes. These data suggest that the previously described antigenic associations between the schistosome and *Salmonella* may provide partial immune tolerance for *Salmonella* bacteria along with the immunologic tolerance to the adult worm.

Hepatitis B Infections. Hepatitis B infections are usually common in populations with endemic schistosomiasis. Patients with hepatosplenic schistosomiasis have hepatitis B surface antigen (HB$_s$Ag) rates significantly greater than those of noninfected controls, as well as schistosome-infected patients with less evidence of hepatic involvement. Patients with chronic schistosomiasis mansoni when infected with hepatitis B virus are prone to have clinically more severe infections, to develop persistent hepatosplenomegaly, and to be chronic carriers of HB$_s$Ag. In addition, a history of prior parenteral treatment for schistosomiasis has been associated with serologic evidence for hepatitis B virus infection, sug-

gesting that this has been a cause of transmission of the virus in the past. Many patients with decompensated liver disease have evidence of active infections with both agents. It appears that in many cases chronic active hepatitis and/or cirrhosis caused by hepatitis B virus leads to hepatic decompensation with ascites, portal hypertension, and bleeding esophageal varices in a patient with chronic schistosomiasis mansoni.

IMMUNOLOGY. The host's acute and chronic immunologic response to the different parasite stages (i.e., cercaria, schistosomulum, adult worm, and schistosome egg) is extremely complex and has been studied extensively in both human and animal models over the past 20 years. Much of the recent work in humans has, by necessity, been performed in vitro and therefore risks incomplete translation to the in vivo circumstance. Drawing from this wide range of experimental evidence, the immunologic response may be divided into 2 categories: (1) mechanisms of resistance to reinfection or protective immunity (e.g., antibody production and cell cytotoxicity), and (2) immune responses resulting from schistosome infection, which can affect the host in a negative manner (e.g., granuloma formation and fibrosis leading to bladder lesions and obstructive uropathy, or hepatosplenomegaly and portal hypertension), or morbid immunity.

Protective Immunity. In nature, protective immunity seems limited to a reduction in the rate of survival of reinfecting schistosomula, without effect on the worms that have reached the adult stage. This protective response is maintained while a living adult worm remains in the host and, consequently, has been called concomitant immunity. Recent studies in the mouse model indicate that there are 2 distinct mechanisms: (1) an early elimination phase, while schistosomula are still in the skin, and (2) a later fatality of schistosomula as they pass from the lung to the liver.

Immunity During Skin Penetration. The mechanism of protective immunity during the early skin-penetration stage involves 2 separate and probably complementary mechanisms:

Eosinophils and IgG. First, in in vitro studies, eosinophils have been shown to play an important role in protective immunity. Many workers have shown subsequently that this is mediated by an antibody-dependent cell-mediated cytotoxicity. The Fc portions of IgG antischistosome antibodies attach to the Fc receptors of eosinophils to bring the schistosomula and the eosinophils together, whereupon degranulation with the release of eosinophil major basic protein leads to irreversible binding of the eosinophils to the schistosomula. This is followed by (1) eosinophil release of lytic agents, (2) schistosomula membrane damage, and (3) parasite death. Activated eosinophils, irrespective of the specificity of the activation stimulus, were more efficient at killing schistosomula than nonactivated eosinophils. Some authors suggest that the mast cell is important in this eosinophilic antibody-dependent cell-mediated cytotoxicity, functioning in the arming of the effector eosinophil.

Macrophages and IgE Immune Complexes. The second cytotoxic system involved in the early skin-penetration stage of reinfection immunity involves IgE immune complexes and is mediated by the macrophage. Specifically, antischistosomal IgE, in aggregate form, binds to a receptor site on the surface of the schistosomulum-attached macrophage. This triggers the release of lysosomal enzymes, resulting in the death of the schistosomulum.

Immunity During Migration. Schistosomula are killed also during passage from the lung to the liver. The mechanism is unknown, but it has been associated with the advent of mature egg laying during primary infection.

Schistosomule Immune Evasion. Schistosomula are attacked by immunologic processes triggered by adult worms. They attempt to evade immunologic destruction by at least 2 mechanisms. There is a continuous turnover of surface membranes that leads to a loss of antigenic components that could be recognized by antibodies. Also, as the young schistosomula mature, their surfaces become covered with or converted to host-like antigen such that by day 4 to 5, the aforementioned antischistosome antibody-mediated protective immune responses are no longer functional.

Immunity to Adult Worms. There appears to be no effective protective immunologic response against the adult schistosome worm, although specific adult worm antibodies and lymphocyte responses can be detected and have been modestly useful as a diagnostic assay. Conversely, the adult worm is responsible for no significant immunopathology.

Morbid Immunity. The immunopathology of schistosomiasis can be divided into early and late disorders.

Schistosome Dermatitis. The first early immunopathology seen is the allergic dermatitis occurring after heavy exposure to skin-penetrating cercariae and is probably more protective than morbid. Both humoral and cell-mediated immune responses to cercarial antigens have been demonstrated in infected humans and experimental animals.

Katayama Fever. This is probably the first significant morbid immunologic phenomenon and manifests as a serum sickness–like disease, which is seen usually in a nonendemic populace about 6 weeks after heavy initial schistosome infection (see the section on Katayama Fever). It has been associated with 2 immunologic abnormalities: (1) depression in cell-mediated immunity to nonschistosome antigens and (2) demonstrable circulating large immune complex formation. Both of these occur at a time when a high schistosome egg antigen load is being presented to the host.

In heavy schistosomal infections in mice, an acute humoral and cellular immunodepression to nonschistosome antigens has been demonstrated, and immune complex formation is easily detected, both being found at the time of first egg deposition. Some considered this to represent an animal model of Katayama fever. However, as mortality and morbidity are high in mice heavily infected with schistosomes, the depressed immune response may reflect only their moribund state.

The suggested immune mechanism of Katayama fever is one of an antibody-excess immune complex phenomenon, as seen in serum sickness, in which excess antibody in relation to antigen forms lattice structures. It is well known that larger immune complexes, when cleared by the reticuloendothelial system, activate the complement scheme, generating chemotactic factors that produce an inflammatory response at the site of complex entrapment.

Immune Complex Lesions. Other more chronic immune complex lesions in schistosomiasis have been demonstrated; however, their clinical and pathologic significance is uncertain. For example, biopsy of subclinical glomerulonephritis has shown schistosome immune complex deposits on the glomerular basement membrane, and circulating immune complexes of schistosome origin have been demonstrated regularly in the serum of experimental animals and humans. However, circulating antigens and antigen-antibody complexes may play a beneficial role in the immune regulation of concomitant immunity and in the protective modulation of the granuloma formation.

Egg Granuloma Formation. During the chronic stages of infection, egg granuloma formation, with the accompanying immune modulation, is the dominant immunologic phenomenon. Cell-mediated immune responses are almost exclusively the cause of granuloma formation around *S. mansoni* and *S. haematobium* eggs. Humoral immune responses appear to play a more important role in the granulomas around *S. japonicum* ova.

Immunologic Modulation. The importance of immune modulation is derived from its teleologic necessity (i.e., granulomas are protective but must be modulated or they cause host mortality and loss of parasite perpetuation) and because the chronic egg granuloma stage is the most prevalent form of human schistosomiasis. The acute florid granulomatous response to the schistosome egg results in a large-volume granuloma that causes a severe obstructive state in the affected organ. Only in the immune modulated state, as in chronic schistosomiasis, when the granulomas are smaller but still protective, does the host's immunologic response and the disease state maintain an acceptable balance.

The cause of the immune modulation of the granulomatous response to the schistosoma egg is complicated. The most complete information collected about this important immune response has been gathered using the *S. mansoni*–infected mouse model, in which immune modulation begins around the twelfth week after cercarial penetration and reaches its maximum stage 16 to 24 weeks after infection. During this time, the schistosome egg granuloma decreases in volume and changes in cellular composition. With the reduction in granuloma volume comes some relief of the vascular obstruction, resulting in reduced organ size and pathology. Associated with the downward modulation of granuloma size is an inversely proportional increase in humoral responses to schistosome antigens. With immune modulation comes a marked increase in serum antibody levels to the schistosome major serologic antigen (MSA), soluble egg antigen (SEA), and soluble worm antigen preparation (SWAP). In the spleens of mice with chronic schistosome infection, this parallels the relative decrease in the T-lymphocyte population and the relative and absolute increase in B-lymphocyte populations. Examination with direct fluorescent antibody techniques of liver biopsy specimens and colon biopsy specimens of polyps from patients has shown that the lymphocytes surrounding *S. mansoni* ova granulomas secrete considerable antibody. Studies with *S. mansoni*–infected mice have shown, as expected, that IgM is predominant during the first few weeks. After about 8 to 12 weeks, IgG becomes predominant. The role of localized antibody or immune complexes in this immunologic modulation is intriguing.

This unique and protective granulomatous immune modulation response can be transferred adoptively by spleen or lymph node cells from mice with chronic schistosome infection only, not from those with acute infection. Nor can it be transferred with immune serum. The reduction in granuloma size after spleen cell transfer is specific for schistosome egg granulomas and does not affect the granulomatous response to nonschistosomal agents such as MeBSA-coupled sepharose beads. Granulomatous modulation is abrogated after T-lymphocyte depletion of transferred spleen cells by anti-Thy 1.2 serum but is maintained in macrophage-depleted, B-lymphocyte–depleted, or unfractionated transferred spleen cells. Schistosome immune modulation does not take place in athymic, genetically T-lymphocyte–deficient or otherwise T-cell–depleted mice. Splenic suppressor T lymphocytes have been implicated as being responsible for immune modulation.

Cell-Mediated Immunity. Concurrent with granulomatous immune modulation, mice with chronic schistosome infection demonstrated a depressed lymphocyte proliferation response to SEA, MSA, and SWAP. This same immunosuppression to specific schistosome antigens is also seen in chronic human schistosomiasis.

Other T-lymphocyte–dependent responses such as footpad swelling, production of macrophage migration inhibitory factor, mitogenic responses to PHA and Con A, cytotoxic responses to foreign histocompatibility antigens, and production of eosinophil stimulation promoter were found to be depressed in chronic murine schistosomiasis. In addition, a progressive loss of T-helper cell activity directed at TNP-schistosomula has been demonstrated.

In humans, where controlled schistosome infections are not possible, the picture is less clear. For instance, serum and adherent peripheral blood mononuclear cells, in addition to the T lymphocyte, have been implicated as suppressive agents. Several investigators have shown evidence of a suppressive serum factor in chronic human schistosomiasis. Schistosome immune complexes are suspected as the suppressor factor in the serum, although their exact mechanism of action is open to speculation. Adherent peripheral blood mononuclear cells have been found responsible also for a depressed response to schistosome-specific antigens in patients with chronic but not acute schistosomiasis.

Summary. Protective immunity in schistosomiasis is effective against skin stages of the schistosomulum by means of antibody-dependent cell-mediated cytotoxicity and, later, during the lung-to-liver schistosomulum stage, by a mechanism as yet undefined. Adult worms

are protected from any effective host immune response, probably through a camouflage mechanism. The morbid immunology of schistosomiasis centers around the host's granulomatous response to ova trapped in the tissues. The host's granulomatous response may protect host tissue from toxic egg excretions but is frequently obstructive to the local microcirculation, resulting in host organ pathology. Uniquely and to the host's benefit, this granulomatous response to the schistosome egg is reduced or modulated during the chronic stages of the disease. The immune modulation is mediated by an antigen-specific suppressor T-lymphocyte response and perhaps also by adherent cells and serum factors, including localized antibodies and/or immune complexes.

CLINICAL MANIFESTATIONS AND MANAGEMENT

Schistosome Cercarial Dermatitis. Cercarial dermatitis results from incomplete infection by small mammal or avian schistosomes and occurs in immune populations from endemic areas following heavy re-exposure to *S. mansoni* and *S. haematobium; S. japonicum* rarely causes dermatitis. Depending on the circumstances under which the disease is acquired, it has been variously designated as "swimmer's itch," "schistosome dermatitis," "clam digger's itch," "sawah itch," or "koganbyo." In all cases, it involves the association of humans and cercariae-shedding intermediate snail hosts.

Unsensitized and sensitized individuals respond with marked differences to the penetration of the skin by cercariae. Initial exposures to these cercariae produce only mild, transient reactions that often pass unnoticed or cause a prickling sensation as the water evaporates and the parasites penetrate the skin. Macules usually appear within 12 hours and, in nonsensitized individuals, soon disappear. However, in persons sensitized by previous exposures to these cercariae, the macules will be followed by papules, possibly accompanied by erythema, vesicle formation, edema, and pruritus, which may persist for 7 to 10 days (Fig. 96–14). Reactions vary markedly, not only because of differences in host susceptibility but also because human and nonhuman schistosome cercariae differ in their ability to produce a response in the human host.

Treatment is usually not needed. Palliative topical agents, e.g., corticosteroid creams, can be applied, and in severe cases, oral or parenteral antihistamines can be administered.

Katayama Fever. This distinct syndrome has been reported after initial heavy infection with the 3 common human schistosome species. However, the name is derived from an area endemic for *S. japonicum,* and the disease is seen most often in those infected with that species. It also occurs following infection of nonimmune individuals with *S. mansoni.* In Egypt, where the syndrome is being reported more frequently, acute schistosomiasis is rarely occurring in those with chronic schistosomiasis haematobia who are being infected with *S. mansoni* for the first time.

Katayama fever became known after nineteenth-century reports from the Katayama River Valley in Japan (an area hyperendemic for schistosomiasis japonica) detailed a clinical syndrome of abrupt onset of fever,

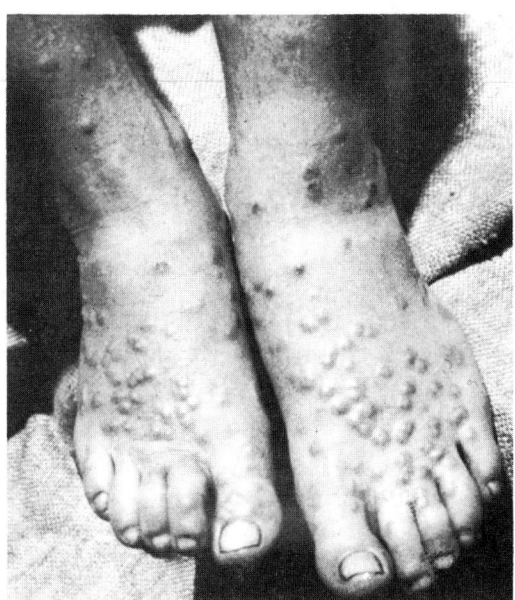

FIGURE 96–14. Marked reaction in sensitized amateur fisherman about 4 days after fishing in a brackish-water lagoon near Sydney, Australia. The infection was caused by cercariae of *Austrobilharzia terrigalensis*. (Courtesy of Dr. A.J. Bearup, School of Public Health and Tropical Medicine, University of Sydney, N.S.W., Australia.)

chills, abdominal pain, diarrhea, nausea, vomiting, cough, headache, urticaria, hepatosplenomegaly, and lymphadenopathy. There is marked eosinophilia and usually marked elevations in levels of IgE and IgG. This illness may last from several days to weeks and may cause significant mortality. It was seen most often in immigrants to the Katayama River Valley and was said to have led to the prohibition of marriage between people of this area and outsiders because of illness and deaths among new spouses. With the advent of schistosomal chemotherapy and control and the reduction in the intensity of infections, Katayama fever has become less common in recent decades. The clinical syndrome most resembles serum sickness and usually occurs 4 to 6 weeks after heavy initial infection—when the first schistosome egg production and release would be expected.

In nonendemic countries, it would most likely be seen in tourists who had wandered into heavily cercariae-infested waters and returned home within a month of exposure. Thus, a history of water contact in a schistosome-endemic area, perhaps with a history of mild swimmer's itch, in a patient with a serum sickness–like disease would provide the clues necessary to search for schistosomal eggs. Treatment has not been established, but anti-inflammatory therapy with salicylates or corticosteroids would seem rational. In life-threatening disease, corticosteroids are recommended.

Chronic Schistosomiasis. Chronic schistosomiasis is the most prevalent form of this disease; most clinicians and laymen refer to this when they indicate that a patient "has schistosomiasis." All forms of chronic schistosomiasis share the basic pathogenic mechanism of long-standing egg granuloma formation in an organ or organ system. This form of disease is rarely brought to the physician's attention before 6 months after the initial

infection. Because of the different selective places of egg laying among schistosome species dwelling in the venous circulation of the abdomen, 2 basic patterns of disease are easily distinguishable: gastrointestinal (*S. mansoni* and *S. japonicum*) and urinary (*S. haematobium*). However, the clinician must be aware of significant overlap between these 2 categories.

Most individuals with *Schistosoma* infections are asymptomatic, and owing to the sociocultural milieu of most endemic populations who readily endure general poor health, only those with severe disease usually seek medical attention.

In North America and Europe, patients would likely first present with lethargy, chronic mild mucohemorrhagic diarrhea with mild cramping abdominal pain, and minimal hepatomegaly (gastrointestinal) or with lethargy, dysuria, and perhaps terminal hematuria (urinary). The differential diagnoses of these insidious and nonspecific signs and symptoms are myriad, and unless the physician takes a travel history and is clinically alert, schistosomiasis is unlikely to even be considered.

Endemic populations usually accept these early signs and symptoms as normal. Only as the heavier infections progress does schistosomiasis become a specifically recognizable clinical disease, and even then, the differential diagnosis can be confused by other complicating factors, e.g., concomitant viral hepatitis infection. Therefore, the clinician's awareness of the epidemiology and pathogenesis of schistosome disease is essential for proper diagnosis and management.

Hepatosplenic Schistosomiasis. This is the most well-known form of chronic disease and usually results from chronic heavy *S. mansoni* or *S. japonicum* infections. The heavy infection and consequent egg burden are thought to be largely responsible for this manifestation of schistosomiasis, although limited studies of HLA typing have suggested a genetic predisposition to the hepatosplenic syndrome. On clinical examination, patients have grossly enlarged livers, with the left lobe often disproportionately enlarged (Fig. 96–15). The liver is firm, finely nodular, and nontender. Jaundice is characteristically absent, and liver cell function is usually normal until the terminal stages.

Hypersplenism. The spleen is invariably palpable and, in many cases, massively enlarged. On examination, the spleen is firm, without sharp edges, and nontender. Usually, splenomegaly is moderate and tolerable to the patient, although resultant clinicolaboratory hypersplenism with mild hemolytic anemia and increased red cell destruction has definitely been documented. A small group of patients with massive hypersplenism (Hackett size 5) complain of severe abdominal discomfort and have on occasion undergone splenectomy without obvious ill effects on the underlying schistosomal disease.

Portal Hypertension. The major clinical findings beyond hepatosplenomegaly are a direct result of portal hypertension. Esophageal varices occur frequently, and fatal hemorrhage is not uncommon. However, patients with schistosomiasis tolerate variceal bleeding episodes better than patients with alcoholic or hepatitic causes of hepatic portal hypertension, because the parenchymal cells and the resulting hepatic function remain intact.

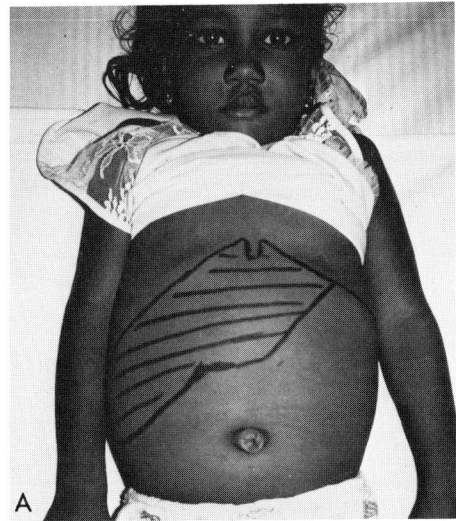

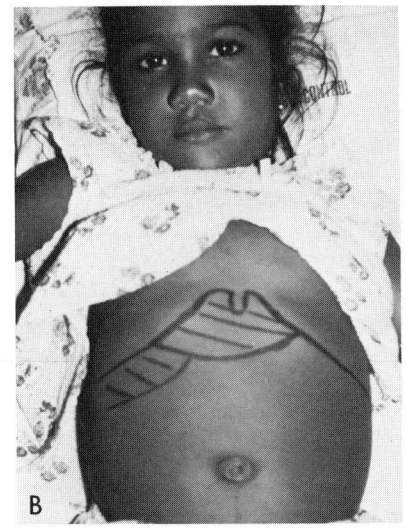

FIGURE 96–15. *Schistosoma mansoni* infection. Four-year-old girl with a distended abdomen with hepatomegaly. *A,* Before therapy. *B,* Two months after therapy. (Courtesy of Dr. Joseph Cook.)

End-stage hepatosplenic schistosomiasis is heralded by massive ascites. Although ascites may predate death by years, it is generally refractory to medical treatment and pathologically irreversible.

Sigmoidoscopy will show mild to moderate focal granulomatous bowel disease. Radiographs taken after a barium swallow frequently demonstrate esophageal varices, but studies after a barium enema and upper gastrointestinal radiographs are usually normal. Sonography of the liver is an excellent noninvasive technique to demonstrate the pathognomonic periportal fibrosis (Figs. 4–1 and 96–16) and can estimate the degree of portal hypertension by measuring the distention of the portal vein.

Chemotherapy for *Schistosoma* infection is warranted even in severe disease if an active infection can be demonstrated, with the rationale that the irreversible disease state might be arrested.

Intestinal Schistosomiasis. This is common in *S. mansoni* and *S. japonicum* infections but is much less common in *S. haematobium* infection. The entire intestinal tract may be diseased; however, the large intestine is usually involved more often and more severely.

Mild to moderate infections result in colonic irritative bowel habits, manifested as malaise, mild mucohemorrhagic diarrhea, and frequent cramping abdominal pains. Physical examination may be normal or may show moderate abdominal distention, diffuse mild abdominal tenderness, and hyperactive bowel sounds. In general, the signs and symptoms are those of focal granulomatous large bowel disease. Sigmoidoscopy may show areas of granular inflammation with hyperemic pinpoint elevations, shallow ulcerations, or small hemorrhages. Patients rarely present with both severe bowel disease and severe hepatosplenomegaly; in nearly all cases, one or the other syndrome is dominant.

Intestinal Granulomatosis and/or Polyposis. This is

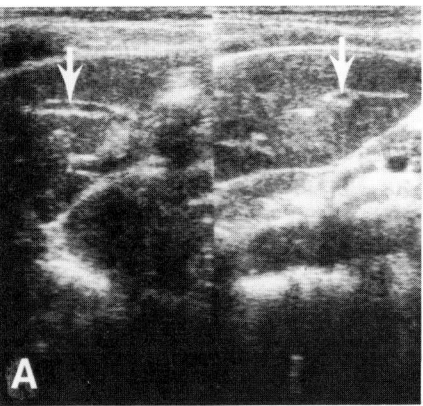

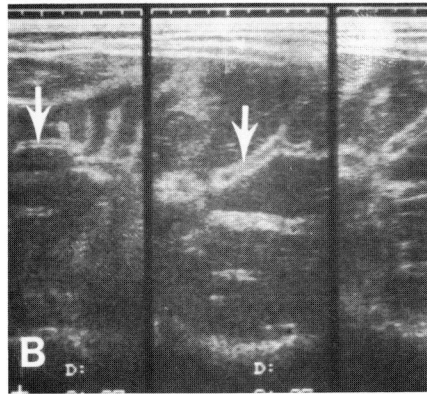

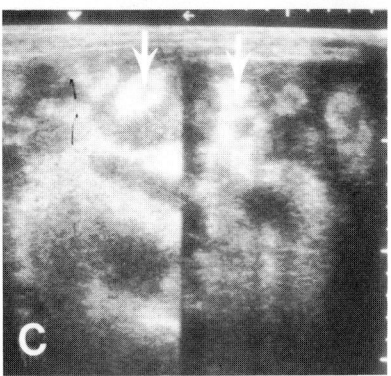

FIGURE 96–16. Examples of minimal *(A)*, moderate *(B)*, and extensive *(C)* periportal fibrosis of the liver demonstrated by ultrasonography. The arrows point to typical lesions.

found in up to 20% of some Middle Eastern symptomatic *S. mansoni*–infected populations requiring hospitalization and is usually accompanied by a protein-losing enteropathy manifesting as chronic severe mucohemorrhagic diarrhea with weight loss and anemia. Physical examination reveals a distended abdomen with diffuse tenderness or localized tenderness in the area of the transverse and descending colon. Lesions in the descending colon are recognized most frequently, and this area is usually most heavily involved. Barium enema, sigmoidoscopy, and colonoscopy have demonstrated over 100 pedunculated and sessile polyps in some cases (Fig. 96–17). Some large, severe, long-standing granulomatous or polypous lesions may result in partial or complete lower bowel obstruction. These patients frequently have a palpable, tender, sausage-like mass in an area corresponding to one of the colonic segments. Overt large bowel perforation rarely occurs. Usually, the obstructive lesions are at least partially reversible with chemotherapy, particularly with niridazole. However, residual fi-

brotic scarring may lead to permanent partial bowel obstruction or bowel wall deformation.

Complications. Localized bowel granulomas may also serve as the focal point for intussusception. Reduction of this lesion by barium enema must be undertaken with extreme care to avoid perforation. Rectal prolapse occurs rarely in intestinal disease of this extent and is usually slowly reversible with chemotherapy. Anorectal fistulas and perianal abscess formation are common. An increased incidence of colonic carcinoma in association with severe intestinal schistosomiasis has never been documented.

Many of the manifestations and complications of schistosomal intestinal granulomas and/or polyp disease are the same as those of some of the noninfectious causes of inflammatory bowel disease (e.g., Crohn's disease and ulcerative colitis). Disastrous errors in medical management have occurred when this form of schistosomiasis was mistaken for other granulomatous bowel diseases or mass lesions with resultant surgical and/or corticosteroid therapy.

Hypertrophic Osteoarthropathy. This clinical complex occurs in a few patients with severe schistosomal bowel disease. Patients present usually with mucohemorrhagic diarrhea, arthritis in several large joints, and clubbing of the digits. Periosteal inflammation with new bone formation is seen on the radiograph. This syndrome is associated most often with severe intestinal polyposis and heavy *S. mansoni* infection. However, the expected pulmonary symptoms or findings on the chest radiographs that are usually seen with other forms of hypertrophic osteoarthropathy are absent. It is reversible with treatment of the underlying schistosome infection, although symptomatic treatment with corticosteroid anti-inflammatory agents may bring more immediate relief to the patient.

Urinary Tract Schistosomiasis. *S. haematobium* has a predilection for the urinary tract venous plexus. Most infections are mild and asymptomatic. However, more complications are seen in light and moderate *S. haematobium* infections than in light or moderate *S. mansoni* and *S. japonicum* infections because of the small caliber of the ureter and its high risk for obstruction. Most symptomatic disease begins months after the initial cercarial penetration. Dysuria, urinary frequency, and terminal hematuria of an insidious onset are the earliest symptoms and signs and often go unnoticed in endemic populations. Physical examination is usually normal, but urinalysis reveals many red blood cells and a few white blood cells on microscopic examination and hematuria and proteinuria by chemical reagent strips. Symptoms and laboratory findings are related directly to intensity of infection and are often reversible with appropriate chemotherapy.

Chronic infection may lead to 4 major disease manifestations: obstructive uropathy, chronic bacteriuria, carcinoma of the bladder, and bladder calcification.

Obstructive Uropathy. This complication is usually silent clinically but can be demonstrated by intravenous pyelogram (Fig. 96–18), by ultrasonography, or by renogram function testing in up to 20% of symptomatic patients and in many asymptomatic patients with *S.*

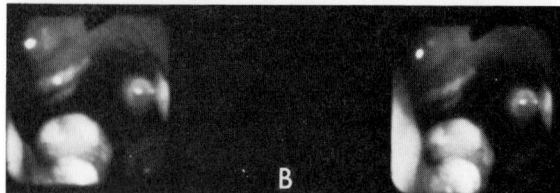

FIGURE 96–17. Colonic polyposis. *A,* Radiograph after air contrast barium enema demonstrates multiple rectosigmoid polyps in a patient heavily infected with *S. mansoni. B,* Colonoscopic view of polyps. (Courtesy of U.S. Naval Medical Research Unit No. 3, Cairo, Egypt.)

haematobium infection. The expected clinical pathologic syndromes are seen, e.g., hydronephrosis, hydroureter, pyelonephritis, and renal failure (Figs. 96–18 and 96–19). Most lesions occur in the lower third of the ureter or in the bladder (Figs. 96–19 and 96–20) and are reversible with early chemotherapy (Fig. 96–24). However, as noted previously, chronic granulomas do become fibrotic in time, and reversibility diminishes.

Pyelonephritis. Pyelonephritis secondary to obstruction and leading to gram-negative septicemia is not uncommon and may be the presenting manifestation as well as a leading cause of mortality in urinary schistosomiasis.

Renal Failure. Renal failure secondary to any of the complications of schistosomal obstructive uropathy is also a common cause of fatal schistosomiasis. Unfortunately, because obstructive disease is associated with heavy and extensive infection, bilateral ureteral obstruction occurs more commonly than would be predicted. Therefore, the bilaterality of the human urinary tract offers little protection in this disease. Renal failure may be the direct result of prolonged ureteral obstruction, chronic pyelonephritis, or severe ureterovesicular urinary reflux, each a complication of severe urinary schistosomiasis. Because of the clinically silent nature of many of these early obstructive lesions, all patients with documented urinary schistosomiasis should have an intravenous pyelogram or ultrasonography.

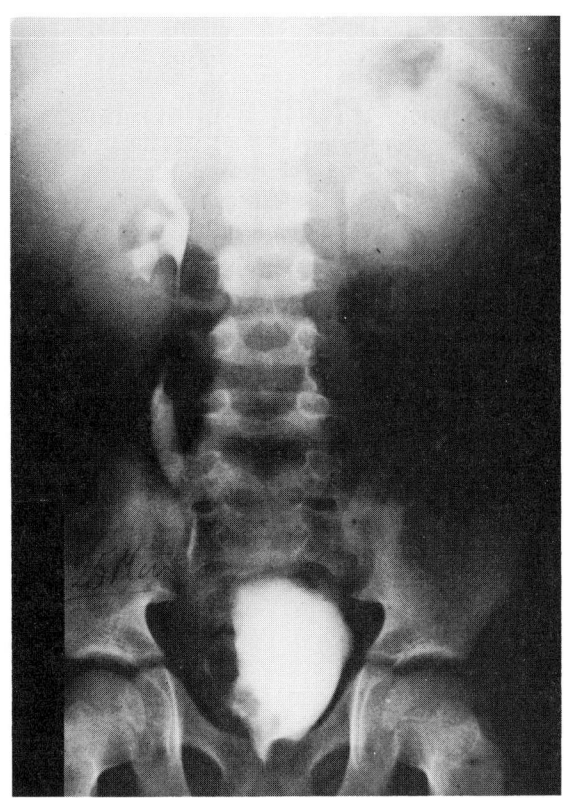

FIGURE 96–19. Intravenous pyelogram showing a large bladder filling defect caused by granulomatous polyp formation in a patient infected with *S. haematobium.* Early right hydronephrosis and hydroureter may also be seen. (Courtesy of U.S. Naval Medical Research Unit No. 3, Cairo, Egypt.)

Chronic Bacteriuria. Epidemiologic surveys in endemic populations have demonstrated bacteriuria rates of up to 5% in school boys with asymptomatic *S. haematobium* infection, and bacteriuria rates in symptomatic patients are higher. Several species of coliform bacteria have been identified as the causative organism, although a *Salmonella* species was the most frequent cause. The clinical importance of this bacteriuria lies in (1) the inherent morbidity of chronic bacteriuria; (2) the ready source or direct cause of pyelonephritis in obstructive and nonobstructive disease; and (3) the suggested chemical carcinogenic agents, either as direct

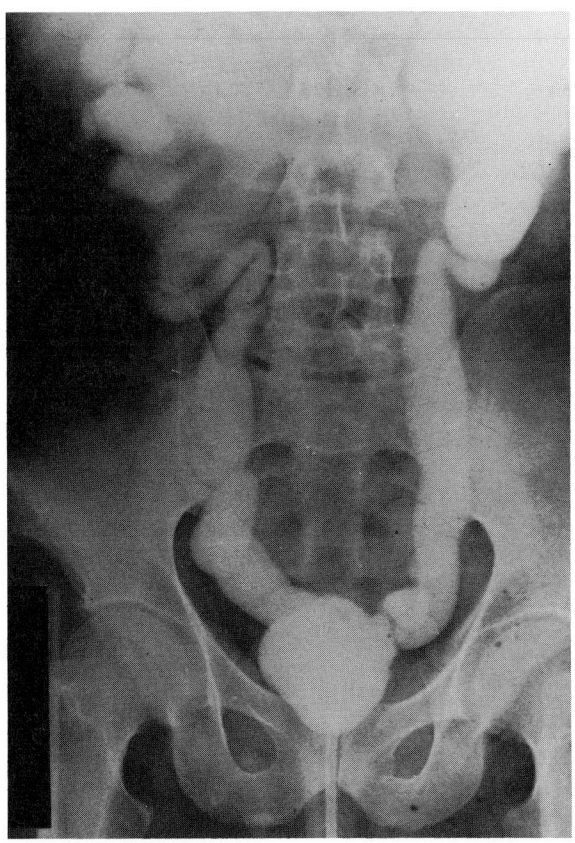

FIGURE 96–18. Severe obstructive uropathy with severe bilateral hydronephrosis and hydroureter in a patient with chronic *S. haematobium* infection. (Courtesy of U.S. Naval Medical Research Unit No. 3, Cairo, Egypt.)

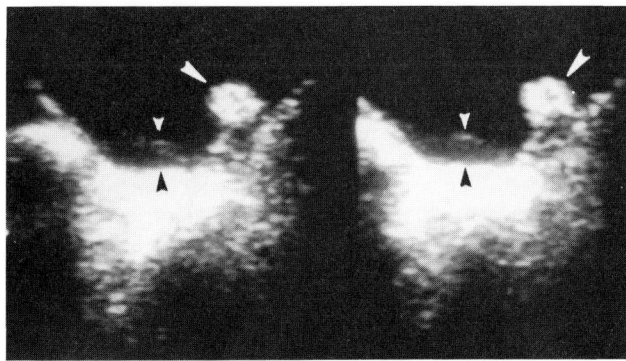

FIGURE 96–20. Ultrasonographic view of bladder of patient with schistosomiasis caused by *S. haematobium.* Thickening and irregularity of the bladder wall *(small arrows)* and a large polyp *(large arrow)* are present.

bacterial products or as other chemicals converted to carcinogens by bacteria, hypothesized to be important in the etiology of schistosomal bladder carcinoma. Antibiotic treatment of bacteriuria is usually incomplete unless it follows antischistosomal treatment and elimination of the underlying schistosomal mucosal lesions.

Bladder Carcinoma. Bladder carcinoma is an epidemiologically important complication of chronic *S. haematobium* infection. The presenting signs and symptoms of bladder irritation, gross hematuria, weight loss, and metastasis (particularly to inguinal, femoral, and retroperitoneal lymph nodes) usually lag 10 to 20 years behind the peak *S. haematobium* infection age. Most bladder cancer is diagnosed in the third and fourth decades of life. Diagnosis is by biopsy, although urine LDH levels and urinary cytologic studies are sometimes helpful.

Bladder Calcification. The "fetal head" sign (Fig. 96–21) is seen in abdominal radiographs and reflects calcium deposits around myriads of schistosome eggs in bladder and ureteral walls. Sonography can also demonstrate the calcification in the bladder wall. Although the *S. haematobium*–infected bladder frequently loses distensibility and contractibility because of thickened fibrotic walls, it does not become as rigid as it would appear on the radiograph. Bladder calcification accounts for no specific pathology or clinical symptoms, but it may be useful as a diagnostic marker of heavy chronic infection. Schistosome bladder calcification will resolve over years if the patient remains free of schistosome infection.

Renal Disease. Nephrotic syndrome is occasionally related to *S. mansoni* infections. In Egypt, schistosome nephrotic syndrome is accompanied often by *Salmonella* bacteriuria and/or bacteremia. The characteristic findings of edema, hypoalbuminemia, massive proteinuria, and hyperlipidemia are evident. As with other forms of infection associated with nephrotic syndrome, management is relatively easy, and fatal renal disease is rare. Resolution, although slow, is nearly 100% after treatment with antischistosomal and antibacterial agents.

Amyloid deposits have been found in renal biopsy material from patients with long-standing schistosomiasis, usually *S. mansoni* infection, although clinical amyloid renal disease is rare.

Cardiopulmonary Schistosomiasis. This is a complex of primary pulmonary pathologic conditions, some of which secondarily affect the heart after exposure to chronic abnormal pressure gradients. All 3 human schistosomes participate in these disease states.

Larval Pneumonitis. Larval pneumonitis, similar to other helminth larval migrations (e.g., hookworm), occurs days to weeks after heavy cercarial exposure and is marked by low-grade fever of gradual onset and mild cough. Basilar crepitations and scattered wheezing may be heard on examining the chest, and radiographs reveal basilar mottling. These symptoms last 2 to 4 weeks and are associated with marked eosinophilia and spontaneous resolution. Embolic worms are thought to cause a similar, more localized disease and may develop into mass lesions of the lung.

Reactionary Pneumonitis. This Loeffler-like syn-

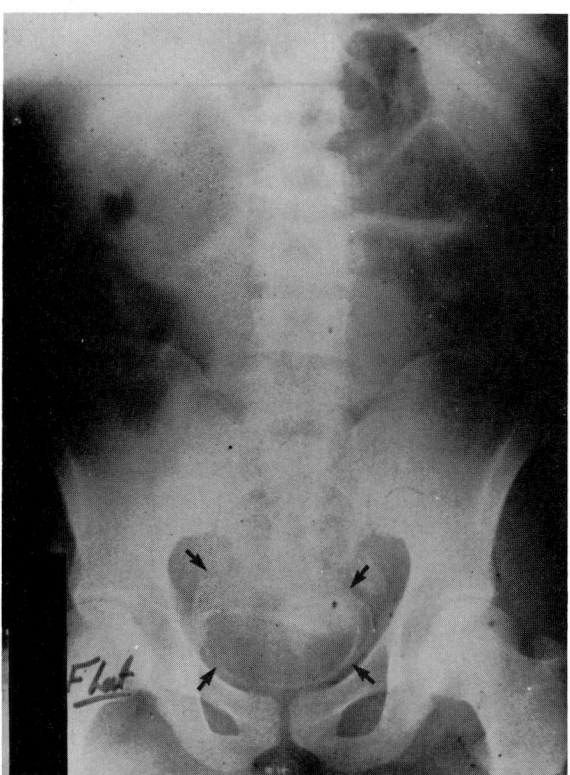

FIGURE 96–21. "Fetal head" bladder calcification may be seen *(arrows)* in this plain radiograph of the abdomen of a patient with chronic *S. haematobium* infection. (Courtesy of U.S. Naval Medical Research Unit No. 3, Cairo, Egypt.)

drome is commonly seen in patients carefully observed during chemotherapy of heavy infections. The clinical and laboratory findings are similar to those of larval pneumonitis, except that spontaneous resolution is usually more rapid and eosinophilia less striking. Marked reactionary pneumonitis is an indication to temporarily discontinue chemotherapy.

Schistosomal Cor Pulmonale. This uncommon presentation of chronic schistosomiasis is seen in all schistosome endemic areas of the world, although most often reported in *S. mansoni* infections from Egypt and Brazil. It is seen most frequently in patients having hepatosplenic schistosomiasis mansoni with portal hypertension, which allows shunting of eggs through portosystemic collaterals to the lungs.

Hallmarks of this disease are easy fatigability, palpitations, dyspnea on exertion, cough with occasional hemoptysis, right ventricular hypertrophy, and dilation of the pulmonary artery (Fig. 2–7). The electrocardiogram may show right ventricular hypertrophy and strain (Fig. 2–6), and occasional patients develop large aneurysms of the pulmonary arteries. Lesser degrees of these features are seen more commonly. Antischistosomal therapy usually has no effect, but it is given to prevent further progression of disease.

Central Nervous System (CNS) Schistosomiasis. Clinical presentation relates to the location of egg granulomas. Clinical diagnosis of all nervous system schistosomiasis is invariably presumptive. Only occasional autopsy or surgical findings firmly support the diagnosis.

Cerebral Schistosomiasis. Focal and generalized seizures are the most common presenting symptom of cerebral schistosomiasis, with headache, optic field defects, and speech abnormalities also being reported. Diagnosis is difficult and may be heralded only by focal encephalographic changes or a cerebrospinal fluid examination showing slightly increased pressure, a mild increase in protein, and the presence of a few lymphocytes. Isotopic brain scans and CT scans can localize the lesions. The vast majority of cases of cerebral schistosomiasis are seen in *S. japonicum* infections and occur in 2 to 4% of diagnosed cases.

Spinal Schistosomiasis. Most often seen in *S. mansoni* infections, spinal schistosomiasis usually presents as a transverse myelitis of variable degrees with attendant localizing neurologic signs (i.e., paraplegia and loss of bladder and anal control). Antischistosomal chemotherapy will presumably reduce the likelihood of future lesions but would be unlikely to reduce the manifestations of the offending egg granuloma. As with other space-occupying lesions in the CNS, corticosteroid anti-inflammatory therapy must be considered along with specific antischistosomal therapy.

Other Schistosome Lesions. Ectopic lesions in schistosomiasis, the result of the aberrant location of either worm or egg, are not common, are frequently asymptomatic or undiagnosed, and may span all organ systems and tissues of the body. *S. haematobium* egg granulomas have occurred in extraocular spaces and on the globe, resulting in proptosis, reduction of extraocular movements, and visual disturbances. Perigenital subcutaneous egg granulomas have been reported, as have granulomas in the spermatic cord, epididymis, testes, prostate, seminal vesicle, uterine cervix, ovary, and urethra, causing local clinical disease. Pancreatic, gallbladder, omental, peritoneal, and stomach egg granulomas have also been documented and are thought to be responsible for local pathology. Egg granulomas have also been found incidentally in the heart, kidney, and adrenal glands at postmortem examination without recognized clinical manifestations.

Association of Schistosomiasis and Other Infections
Salmonella-Schistosome Syndrome. Chronic persistent *Salmonella* bacteremia has been described in association with *S. mansoni*, *S. haematobium,* and *S. japonicum* infections in patients from many endemic areas of the world. The most common characteristics of the clinical syndrome are (1) a long history (from several weeks to 1 year) of an indolent febrile disease; (2) a frequent, sometimes daily, bacteremia with one of many species of the genus *Salmonella;* and (3) chronic active schistosomiasis. Patients complain of fatigue, malaise, weight loss, and fever. Some authors have described the clinical features as being "more like kala-azar than typhoid fever." The clinical disease bears no resemblance to clinical typhoid fever. Prostration and delirium never occur, and only rarely are salmonella isolated from the stool. A petechial rash on the lower extremities is common, but the classic abdominal rose spots are rarely seen. Localized infections, as are found in the osteomyelitis of sickle cell disease, chronic cholecystitis, or abscess formation, do not occur. In the Egyptian delta region, where *S. mansoni* and the urinary tract–associated *S. haematobium* are both endemic, chronic *Salmonella* bacteriuria is a common clinical problem.

Chronic persistent *Salmonella* bacteremia is not the result of end-stage or moribund schistosomiasis. It occurs most commonly in males between the ages of 15 and 30 years. Mortality is rare, and the response to antibiotic therapy is dramatic. However, recurrent *Salmonella* bacteremia is common if the underlying schistosome disease is not treated.

Hepatitis B Infection. Recent clinical studies have demonstrated an association between hepatosplenic schistosomiasis and hepatitis B infection. The greatest clinical relevance lies in the knowledge that in severe hepatosplenic disease the clinician may be dealing with 2 infections. Patients with this dual infection more often develop jaundice, intractable ascites, and hepatic failure. Mild to moderate elevations in hepatocellular liver function test results occur commonly, as does the demonstration of HB_sAg. Proper precautions for dealing with potentially infected blood products should be taken. The clinical management is more complicated and the prognosis more guarded than for chronic hepatosplenic schistosomiasis alone.

DIAGNOSIS. Because the epidemiology of schistosomiasis is well known, residence or travel history is of utmost importance. History and physical examination may also supply one of the rare specific features, "swimmer's itch" (Fig. 96–14). Other aspects of clinical history and findings on physical examination, although important and supportive, are usually nonspecific and of minimal assistance in the diagnosis of schistosome infections. X-ray examinations, such as barium enema (Fig. 96–17A), barium swallow, and intravenous pyelogram (Figs. 96–18, 96–19, and 96–24) frequently document pathology but are not diagnostic, the one exception being the "fetal head" bladder calcification (Fig. 96–21) seen in chronic urinary schistosomiasis. Sonography will also document hydronephrosis, hydroureter, bladder polyps, and calcification (Fig. 96–20). It can demonstrate the thickened fibrosed portal tracts, which are characteristic of Symmers' pipe-stem fibrosis (Figs. 4–1 and 96–16), and the enlargement of the portal vein, which correlates with portal venous pressure. Computed tomography is likely to demonstrate pathologic hepatic findings but is largely untested. Esophagoscopy will document esophageal varices but does not establish their etiology. Sigmoidoscopy, colonoscopy (Fig. 96–17B), and cystoscopy will document granulomatous or polyp disease but are of greatest value in providing access to biopsy specimens for tissue egg identification.

Laboratory Findings
Schistosome Egg Identification. Egg identification is the appropriate method of establishing the diagnosis (Fig. 96–3). Egg quantitation is also important in the assessment of clinical disease and its epidemiologic impact, as is egg viability. The Kato thick smear technique is described. Other methods are described in detail elsewhere (Chapter 122).

Kato Thick Smear. A 50-mg sample of feces (an amount about the size of a garden pea) is pressed through a 105-mesh steel sieve onto a glass slide. This sample is covered with a cellophane coverslip impregnated with glycerin and is then inverted and pressed onto a bed of filter paper. The slide is turned so that the coverslip is facing up and is left for 24 to 48 hours while the fecal matter clears. Then, all eggs on the slide are counted using 100 magnification. Multiplying by 20 gives the number of ova/gm of stool. The daily ova excretion can be calculated if the day's stool weight is known.

The Kato thick smear (Fig. 96–22) involves no equipment beyond a simple microscope, but results are not available for 24 to 48 hours. The Kato thick smear is quantitative and useful for special clinically and epidemiologically based studies. However, because of the small volume of stool examined, it has a low sensitivity and will not detect most light infections.

Rectal Biopsy or Bladder Mucosal Biopsy. These are valuable when stool samples are difficult to obtain or are negative, as is often the case in light or partially treated infections. These biopsies may be performed easily during proctoscopy, sigmoidoscopy, or cystoscopy by taking 1 to 3 small mucosal samples from inflamed or granulomatous lesions or from random areas of normal mucosa. The mucosal sample is pressed between a coverslip and a glass slide, where it becomes transparent, and any eggs may be seen with low-power microscopy (Fig. 96–23). Schistosome eggs are seen sometimes in biopsy samples from the small bowel in patients with *S. mansoni* and *S. japonicum* infections, but this is not advocated as a primary diagnostic procedure. A portion of the biopsy sample should be fixed in formalin and processed for histologic examination.

Urine Specimens. Eggs in the urine may be detected by simple centrifuge sedimentation or micropore urine filtrates and microscopic examination (Chapter 123). The excretion of schistosome eggs into the urine is not uniform over a 24-hour period, and samples collected between 10 AM and 2 PM are more likely to be positive.

Egg Quantitation. This clinically important examination is usually measured over 24 hours by collecting an entire day's urine or stool sample, homogenizing the entire sample, and then counting the eggs in a measured aliquot (see preceding sections and Chapter 122). Twenty-four-hour stool and urine egg counts < 100 are

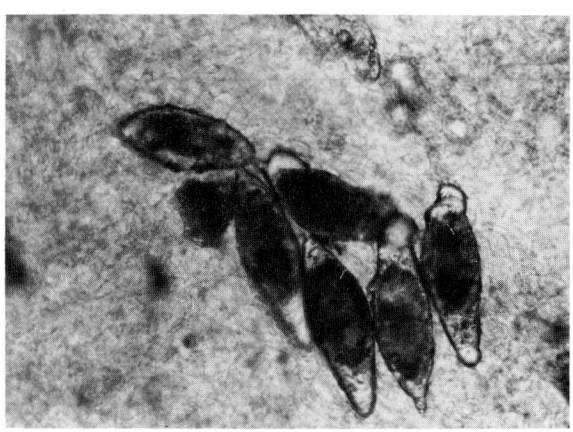

FIGURE 96–23. Calcified *S. haematobium* eggs in a crushed piece of bladder mucosa from an Egyptian patient (unstained, × 316). (Courtesy of the Armed Forces Institute of Pathology, Photograph Neg. No. 76-2408.)

considered light infection; counts of 100 to 400 are considered moderate infection; and those > 400 are considered heavy infection.

Egg Viability. Egg viability is also important in determining the activity of schistosome infections, especially in areas where antischistosomal drugs are available locally. Schistosome eggs are excreted in the urine and stool long (e.g., months to years) after a patient has been treated successfully. Eggs passed more than 1 week after treatment are usually not viable. Egg viability testing is accomplished by 2 methods: (1) Careful examination of single viable eggs will show a living ovum as clear and transparent. Under high magnification, living ova may show the moving organelles (flame cells) of the miracidium. (2) A more reliable but more difficult method is induced egg hatching. It is performed by diluting a small amount of urine or stool sediment in distilled water at room temperature and exposing it to light for 15 to 20 minutes. Examination with a hand lens will reveal swimming miracidia (Chapter 122).

Serologic Tests. These are abundant but, at present, are of little practical use (Table 96–2). Most serologic tests are not helpful because they (1) become positive too late after infection; (2) become negative too long after cure; or (3) cross-react with other helminths (Chapter 125).

The circumoval precipitin test (COPT), the cercaria-Hullen reaction, the miracidia immobilization test, and the cercarial fluorescent antibody test are reasonably accurate but rarely practical because of the need for viable schistosome eggs, viable cercariae, and viable miracidia, respectively. The hemagglutination test will detect high levels of antischistosome antibody, but the sensitivity and specificity are highly variable because of the wide range of type and purity of schistosome antigens used. Enzyme-linked immunosorbent assays (ELISA) are becoming available for detecting both schistosomal antibodies and antigens. With the advent of hybridoma technology, allowing for antigen purification and standardization, the sensitive ELISA methodology has produced useful serologic tests for schistosomiasis. However, only a few specialized laboratories can provide clinically useful serologic assays at this time.

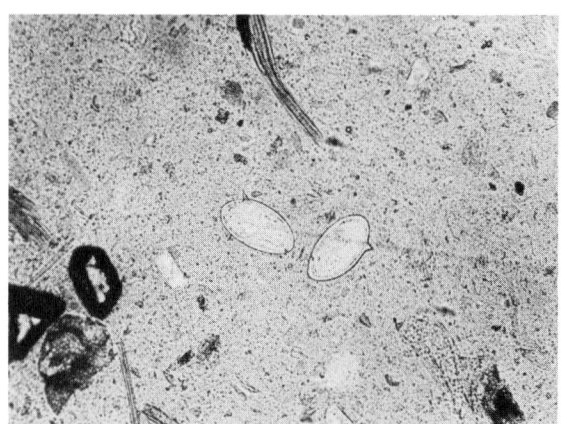

FIGURE 96–22. *S. mansoni* eggs in feces (Kato preparation, × 125). (Courtesy of the Armed Forces Institute of Pathology, Photograph Neg. No. 76-2406.)

TABLE 96–2. Immunologic Diagnostic Tests in Schistosomiasis

Test	Comment
Intradermal test (IDT)	Becomes positive 4 to 8 weeks after infection; immediate type reaction read 15 to 20 minutes after 0.05 ml ID injection of adult worm antigen; need Merthiolate control for wheal response; positive for years after successful treatment.
Circumoval precipitin test (COPT)	Detects presence of antibodies against ova; negative shortly after cure; semiquantitative; procedure—incubate patient serum with viable egg, giving oval precipitate at 24 hours.
Cercaria-Hullen reaction (CHR)	Positive early after infection and negative 3 weeks after cure; cercariae incubated with patient's serum; membrane forms around cercariae.
Miracidia immobilization test (MIT)	Positive in acute stage; heat-inactivated patient's serum immobilizes miracidia.
Hemagglutination test (HA)	Variable sensitivity and specificity according to antigen type adsorbed to red cell; sensitivity and specificity may be high in laboratories with experienced personnel.
Fluorescent antibody test (IFA)	Cercariae or adult worm sections attached to slide coated with patient's serum, then labeled with antihuman globulin; positive serum shows fluorescence of schistosomal material.
Enzyme-linked immunosorbent assay (ELISA)	Sensitivity and specificity vary with antigen type used and the skill and experience of the laboratory personnel.
Antigen detection ELISA	Sensitivity and specificity depend upon reagents used; becomes negative shortly after cure.

As with other infectious diseases, serologic tests are most useful in epidemiologic studies of endemic populations, in specific diagnoses in nonendemic populations, and in the assessment of individual response to treatment.

Associated Clinical Laboratory Findings. Mild anemia is a common finding associated with schistosomiasis. It has several etiologies resulting from the malabsorptive complications of intestinal disease, the iron loss of chronic mucohemorrhagic diarrhea or gross hematuria, the hemolysis of hypersplenism, or any combination of these. Hypoalbuminemia is common and may be caused by intestinal malabsorption or chronic infection. Normal liver function tests are the rule, except for an elevation in alkaline phosphatase. Hypergammaglobulinemia is common. Mild albuminuria and red cells in the urine sediment are consistent findings in *S. haematobium* infections.

BIBLIOGRAPHY

Abdel-Wahab MF: Schistosomiasis in Egypt. Boca Raton, Florida, CRC Press, 1982.

Abdel-Wahab MF: Schistosomiasis mansoni in Egypt. Clin Trop Comm Dis 2:371–395, 1987.

Abdel-Wahab MF, Esmat G, Milad M, et al.: Characteristic sonographic pattern of schistosomal hepatic fibrosis. Am J Trop Med Hyg 40:72–76, 1989.

Abdel-Wahab MF, Esmat G, Narooz SI, et al.: Sonographic studies of school children in a village endemic for *Schistosoma mansoni.* Trans R Soc Trop Med Hyg 84:69–73, 1990.

Anderson RM: Determinants of infection in human schistosomiasis. Clin Trop Med Comm Dis 2:279–300, 1987.

Andrade ZA, Andrade SG: Pathogenesis of pulmonary arteritis. Am J Trop Med Hyg 19:305, 1970.

Andrade ZA, Cheever AW: Alterations of intrahepatic vasculature in hepatosplenic schistosomiasis mansoni. Am J Trop Med Hyg 20:425, 1971.

Ariizum M: Cerebral schistosomiasis japonica: Report of one operated case and fifty clinical cases. Am J Trop Med Hyg 12:40, 1963.

Barral-Netto W, Hoffstetter M, Cheever AW, et al.: Specificity of antibody and cellular immune responses in human schistosomiasis. Am J Trop Med Hyg 32:106, 1983.

Bassily S, Farid Z, Baroum RS, et al.: Renal biopsy of Schistosoma-Salmonella associated nephrotic syndrome. J Trop Med Hyg 79:256, 1976.

Biempica L, Dunn MA, Kamel IA, et al.: Liver collagen-type characterization in human schistosomiasis. Am J Trop Med Hyg 32:316, 1983.

Browning MD, Narooz SI, Strickland GT, et al.: Clinical characteristics and response to therapy in Egyptian children infected with *Schistosoma haematobium.* J Infect Dis 149:998–1004, 1984.

Capron A, Dessaint JP, Capron M, et al.: Immunity to schistosomes: Progress towards vaccine. Science 238:1065–1072, 1987.

Carvalho EM, Andrews BS, Martinelli R, et al.: Circulating immune complexes and rheumatoid factor in schistosomiasis and visceral leishmaniasis. Am J Trop Med Hyg 32:61, 1983.

Cheever AW, Kamel IA, Elwi AM, et al.: *Schistosoma mansoni* and *S. haematobium* infections in Egypt IV. Hepatic lesions. Am J Trop Med Hyg 27:939–943, 1978.

Colley DG: Dynamics of the human immune response to schistosomes. Clin Trop Med Comm Dis 2:315–332, 1987.

Colley DG, Lewis FA, Goodgame RW: Immune responses during human schistosomiasis mansoni. IV. Induction of suppressor cell activity by schistosome antigen preparations and concanavalin A. J Immunol 120:1225, 1978.

David JR, Butterworth AE, Vadas MA: Mechanism of the interaction mediating killing of *Schistosoma mansoni* by human eosinophils. Am J Trop Med Hyg 29:842, 1980.

Dunn MA, Kamel R: Hepatic schistosomiasis. Hepatology 1:653, 1981.

Ellner JS, Olds GC, Kamel R, et al.: Suppressor splenic T-lymphocytes in human hepatosplenic schistosomiasis mansoni. J Immunol 125:308, 1980.

Hillyer GV, Ruiz-Tiben E, Knight WB, et al.: Immunodiagnosis of infection with *Schistosoma mansoni:* Comparison of ELISA, radioimmunoassay, and precipitation tests performed with antigens from eggs. Am J Trop Med Hyg 28:661, 1979.

Hoeffler DF: Cercarial dermatitis. Its etiology, epidemiology and clinical aspects. Arch Environ Health 29:225, 1974.

Laughlin LW, Farid Z, Manzour N, et al.: Bacteriuria in urinary schistosomiasis in Egypt. A prevalence study. Am J Trop Med Hyg 27:916, 1978.

Lehman JS, Farid Z, Bassily S, et al.: Intestinal protein loss in schistosomal polyposis of the colon. Gastroenterology 59:433, 1970.

Lehman JS, Farid Z, Smith JH, et al.: Urinary schistosomiasis in Egypt. Clinical, radiological, bacteriological and parasitological correlations. Trans R Soc Trop Med Hyg 67:384, 1973.

LoVerde PT, Amento C, Higashi GI: Parasite-parasite interaction of *Salmonella typhimurium* and *Schistosoma.* J Infect Dis 141:177, 1980.

Lyra LD, Rebouca G, Andrade ZA: Hepatitis B surface antigen carrier state in hepatosplenic schistosomiasis. Gastroenterology 71:641, 1976.

Madwar MA, El Tahawy M, Strickland GT: The relationship between uncomplicated schistosomiasis and hepatitis B infection. Trans R Soc Trop Med Hyg 83:233–236, 1989.

Nebel OT, El Massry NA, Castell DO, et al.: Schistosomiasis disease of the colon: A reversible form of polyposis. Gastroenterology 67:939, 1974.

Olveda RM, Domingo EO: Schistosomiasis japonica. Clin Trop Med Comm Dis 2:397–417, 1987.

Ottesen EA: Modulation of the host response in human schistosomiasis. I. Adherent suppressor cells that inhibit lymphocyte proliferative responses to parasite antigens. J Immunol 123:1639, 1979.

Peters PAS, Kazura JW: Update on diagnostic methods for schistosomiasis. Clin Trop Med Comm Dis 2:419–433, 1987.

Prata A: Schistosomiasis mansoni in Brazil. Clin Trop Med Comm Dis 2:349–369, 1987.

Queiroz FP, Brito E, Martinelli R, et al.: Nephrotic syndrome in patients with *Schistosoma mansoni* infection. Am J Trop Med Hyg 22:622, 1973.

Rocha H, Cruz T, Brito E, et al.: Renal involvement in patients with hepatosplenic schistosomiasis mansoni. Am J Trop Med Hyg 25:108, 1976.

Rocklin RE, Brown AP, Warren KS, et al.: Factors that modify the cellular-immunity response in patients infected by *Schistosoma mansoni.* J Immunol 125:1916, 1980.

Sadigursky M, Andrade ZA: Pulmonary changes in schistosomal cor pulmonale. Am J Trop Med Hyg 31:779, 1982.

Schwartz DA: Helminths in the induction of cancer. II. *Schistosoma haematobium* and bladder cancer. Trop Geogr Med 33:1, 1981.

Scrimgeour EM, Gajdusek DC: Involvement of the central nervous system in *Schistosoma haematobium* infection. A review. Brain 108:1023–1038, 1985.

Shaw AFB, Ghareeb AA: The pathogenesis of pulmonary schistosomiasis in Egypt with special reference to Ayerga's disease. J Path Bact 46:401, 1938.

Smith JH, Kamel TA, Elwi A, et al.: A quantitative post mortem analysis of urinary schistosomiasis in Egypt. I. Pathology and pathogenesis. Am J Trop Med Hyg 23:1054, 1974.

Smithers SR, Miller KL: Protective immunity in murine schistosomiasis mansoni: Evidence for two distinct mechanisms. Am J Trop Med Hyg 29:832, 1980.

Strickland GT: The prevention and control of schistosomiasis. Rev Infect Dis 4:951, 1982.

Strickland GT, Merritt W, El-Sahly A, et al.: Clinical characteristics and response to therapy in Egyptian children heavily infected with *Schistosoma mansoni.* J Infect Dis 146:20–29, 1982.

Sturrock RF: Biology and ecology of human schistosomes. Clin Trop Med Comm Dis 2:249–266, 1987.

Warren KS: Determinants of disease in human schistosomes. Clin Trop Med Comm Dis 2:301–313, 1987.

Wilkins A, Gilles H: Schistosomiasis haematobia. Clin Trop Med Comm Dis 2:333–348, 1987.

World Health Organization: Atlas of the global distribution of schistosomiasis. Parasitic Diseases Programme. Geneva, World Health Organization, 1987.

World Health Organization: Progress in assessment of morbidity due to *Schistosoma haematobium* infection: A review of recent literature. WHO/Schisto/87.91, World Health Organization, 1987.

96.1   TREATMENT AND CONTROL OF SCHISTOSOMIASIS

CHEMOTHERAPY. After active infection is confirmed by the demonstration of viable egg excretion, chemotherapy should be considered. Over the past 10 years, there has been a marked improvement in the management of patients with schistosomiasis. Three new nontoxic and efficacious drugs are now available, and 2 others are in the developmental phase (Table 96–3). All sporadically infected patients currently living in nonendemic areas as well as all symptomatic and moderately and heavily infected asymptomatic patients living in endemic areas should be treated. However, treatment in endemic areas is frequently modulated by overriding social, cultural, and economic factors.

Chemotherapeutic Agents

Oxamniquine. This tetrahydroquinoline compound is effective against *S. mansoni,* especially the strains in the Americas and West Africa. It is well absorbed from the gastrointestinal tract, and its metabolites are excreted in the urine. The site of metabolism and the mechanism of action are unknown.

Dosage and Toxicity. Oxamniquine is effective in a single oral dose of 15 mg/kg in strains from the Caribbean and South America. A dose of 20 mg/kg has been more efficacious in children in several studies. North and East African strains of *S. mansoni* are less sensitive to this compound, and doses of up to 60 mg/kg given over 2 or 3 days have been required to achieve the same results as 15 mg/kg with strains in the Western Hemisphere. Side effects, usually mild, are decreased by the administration of the single dose after a meal and late in the day. Drowsiness and dizziness are the most commonly reported side effects (7 to 15%). Fever on day 3 or 4 after initiation of therapy has been noted in carefully monitored patients and appears to be related to worm death and shift to the liver but is of little clinical importance. Oxamniquine is uniquely useful in the treatment of decompensated hepatosplenic schistosomiasis and severe colonic polyposis caused by *S. mansoni* infection, in which all prior drugs induced unacceptable toxic side effects for safe use. This drug has been used successfully in Africa and in Brazil, where a countrywide control effort was based on community chemotherapy with oxamniquine.

The drug is relatively expensive, making it difficult to use in control programs in which the higher dosage is needed (i.e., in Egypt, Sudan, and Kenya).

Metrifonate. This organophosphate compound is metabolized slowly to dichlorvos. It is an anticholinesterase and presumably acts by blocking the worm's acetylcholinesterase, thereby causing paralysis of the worm. It is active only against *S. haematobium,* and there is some evidence to suggest that the worm paralysis may be only temporary. Other worms (e.g., *S. japonicum* and *S. mansoni*) in the mesenteric plexus are only swept into the portal vein, where they survive and later migrate back to their usual habitat. (The same may happen to *S. haematobium* worm pairs in the mesenteric plexus.) Egg laying may be temporarily interrupted, but the disease state is not affected in this case. However, *S. haematobium* worms, when temporarily paralyzed, are swept from the vesicular plexus into the vena cava and onto the pulmonary vasculature where they are unable to return to their habitat and are destroyed by the immune response.

Dosage and Toxicity. Clinical tolerance to this drug is generally good. Nausea, vomiting, and bronchospasm have been reported but are rare. Plasma cholinesterase activity drops to less than 5% of pretreatment levels within 6 hours of dosage but quickly returns to normal, whereas erythrocyte cholinesterase is inhibited to 50% of pretreatment values and takes 8 to 10 weeks to resume normal levels. The usual dose is 7.5 to 10 mg/kg of body weight, but it is necessary to give 3 doses at biweekly intervals. Cure rates have been 40 to 50% after 2 doses and 70 to 80% following the full course. There are no contraindications to re-treatment.

Praziquantel. This is the most important drug for treating schistosomiasis. It is effective orally in a single dose against all species of schistosomes infecting humans. Praziquantel is a mixture of stereoisomers of

TABLE 96–3. Antischistosomal Drugs Currently Used

Drug	Dosage (Route)	Schistosome Treated	Side Effects	Comments
Oxamniquine (Mansil, Vansil)	15 mg/kg in a single dose (60 mg/kg in 3 or 4 doses over 2 or 3 days in North and East Africa) (PO)	*S. mansoni*	Drowsiness and dizziness (10%); fever; dark urine	Children may need 20 mg/kg; 80–90% cure rate; expensive
Metrifonate (Bilarcil, Trichlofon)	7.5–10 mg/kg per dose to be given 3 times at 2 weekly intervals (PO)	*S. haematobium*	Mild nausea and vomiting; bronchospasm (rare)	Anticholinesterase drug; paralysis of worm; 70–80% cure rate; inexpensive
Praziquantel (Biltricide)	40 mg/kg in a single dose (60 mg/kg in 2 or 3 doses for *S. japonicum*) (PO)	*S. mansoni* *S. haematobium* *S. japonicum* *S. mekongi* *S. intercalatum*	Nausea and vomiting; abdominal pain (mild to moderate)	Effective against other cestodes and flukes; 70–90% cure rate; expensive

pyrazinoisoquinoline ring structures. It is active not only against the digenetic trematodes but against many cestodes (e.g., *Diphyllobothrium latum*, *Taenia saginata*, and *Hymenolepis nana*) and other flukes (e.g., *Clonorchis sinensis* and *Paragonimus westermani*). Although the mode of action is unknown, a strong tetanic contraction of the helminth's musculature occurs within a few minutes of administration of the drug. It has been shown to uncover a specific antigen on the worm's surface that can then be attacked by the host's immune response.

Dosage and Toxicity. Single doses of 40 mg/kg of body weight have resulted in 70 to 95% cure rates in both *S. mansoni* and *S. haematobium* infections. Side effects (e.g., nausea, abdominal pain, and vomiting), usually of short duration, beginning a few hours after treatment, and disappearing spontaneously within 48 hours, have been reported. The drug has been well tolerated in community control efforts. Treatment of *S. japonicum* has generally required a higher dose, the most efficacious being a total dose of 60 mg/kg (i.e., 3 doses of 20 mg/kg of body weight given within 24 hours). This higher dose can be used in infections with *S. mekongi,* a relatively rare species of schistosome that is transmitted in Southeast Asia. Praziquantel is currently (1990) approved in the United States only for the treatment of schistosomiasis.

Amoscanate. This lipophilic compound with a reactive isothiocyanate group has shown efficacy in treating *S. haematobium, S. mansoni,* and *S. japonicum.* A smaller particle formulation has caused less toxicity than earlier large particle size formulations that produced erratic therapeutic results and liver and central nervous system reactions. Amoscanate induces a rapid hepatic shift of *S. mansoni* in rodents and causes damage to the tegument and female reproductive organs of schistosomes. It is uncertain if this drug will undergo field testing at this time. As long as praziquantel remains as effective, amoscanate's history of toxicity could prevent further development.

Oltipraz. This 1.2-dithiole chemically synthesized antischistosomal compound has efficacy against human *S. mansoni, S. haematobium,* and *S. intercalatum.* Clinical evaluation was suspended in 1984 because of late-onset toxicity. It has a slow onset of antischistosomal

action that is believed to be related to the parasite's glutathione metabolism. Its activity is greater against mature worms than against immature forms. Primate studies show that more than 40% of an oral dose is absorbed; the plasma half-life is 4.5 hours. Female worms concentrate the drug to a greater extent than male worms. About 40% of the drug and its metabolites are excreted in the urine, with the other 60% being passed in the feces.

Dosage and Toxicity. In small groups of patients, oltipraz has produced cure rates of 86 to 92% with *S. haematobium* infection, and 96 to 100% with *S. mansoni* infection. However, this promising new drug may be too toxic for clinical use.

General Side Effects. In addition to the chemical side effects of the chemotherapeutic agents, worm death, relocation, and degeneration may also result in pathology. Most drugs cause worm paralysis or mechanical dysfunction, which results in release from attachment to the venule wall. Worms are then swept away by blood flow, usually lodging in the liver, lungs, or, in rare cases, the central nervous system. This results in large focal granuloma formation with the expected complications. Beyond this local response to a large foreign body, the degeneration of the adult worm undoubtedly releases large amounts of soluble or small particulate antigens over a relatively short period of time. It is speculated that this antigenic release is responsible for the fever and the Loeffler-like pneumonitis commonly seen 2 or 3 days after the initiation of chemotherapy. Usually, these generalized side effects are mildly symptomatic or subclinical, but in heavy infections, they may be severe. It is common practice to interrupt chemotherapy if the patient becomes symptomatic, although the damage has doubtlessly already been done. Severe generalized side effects of this type usually have an immunologic basis and may be treated with a short course of corticosteroids.

Evaluation of Therapy. Definitive parasitologic cure of schistosomal infections is considered to have occurred only when there is total disappearance of viable eggs from the excreta for at least 6 months after treatment, in the absence of exposure to reinfection. Not infrequently, adult worms are incapacitated only temporarily by chemotherapy. In this case, egg release is interrupted only to begin again a few weeks later. Final laboratory examination should include examination of excreta on 3 consecutive days and, if negative for viable eggs, is followed frequently by a similar examination of a rectal mucosa biopsy in cases of *S. mansoni* and *S. japonicum* infections.

In epidemiologic studies and antischistosomal drug trials in endemic areas, these rigid criteria for cure are impractical and not pertinent. Therefore, study results are reported as cure rates after 6 weeks, with the rationalization that reinfection has yet to become patent. Percentage of egg reduction is another way of assessing the incomplete early effects of chemotherapy. The early cure rates and egg reduction measurements are undoubtedly representative of the positive impact of the drug on the infection, but they must not be confused with complete cure.

Management of the Individual Patient. Because of the wide range of clinical disease presentation, the multiorgan involvement of complications, and the variation in antischistosomal chemotherapy according to infecting species and strain, a simplified standard management regimen for schistosomiasis cannot be devised. In many circumstances, patient care must be individualized. Table 96–4 offers broad guidelines for the management of the more common presentations of schistosomiasis.

Prognosis. The long-term prognosis for heavy untreated schistosomiasis or heavy recurrent infection is guarded. Heavy urinary schistosomiasis often leads to obstructive uropathy and/or pyelonephritis with gram-negative bacteremia and resultant renal failure. Bladder cancer is a long-term potential consequence of chronic heavy *S. haematobium* infection. If untreated, long-standing hepatosplenic schistosomiasis may eventually result in intractable portal hypertension with recurrent esophageal variceal bleeding and ascites. Hepatic failure with associated hepatitis B infection can be a terminal event also. Some patients develop cor pulmonale from pulmonary hypertension and are markedly limited in their physical activities.

Certain local fibrotic changes of schistosomal granulomatosis (e.g., of the ureter, intestine, or liver) may remain after complete eradication of infection and may cause permanent and potentially fatal disease if not surgically repaired. However, with the advent of the newer efficacious and less toxic chemotherapeutic agents, the prognosis in most schistosomal infections is excellent, providing reinfection can be prevented and end-stage irreversible disease has not yet been established (Fig. 96–24).

PREVENTION AND CONTROL. The complicated and seemingly fragile life cycle of the schistosome seems easily interrupted and difficult to sustain unmolested. However, the antiquity of the disease and recent unsuccessful attempts at eradication indicate otherwise. Most scientists agree that schistosomiasis cannot be eradicated on a worldwide scale at present, although certain foci have been cleared successfully. To date, all successful focal eradication programs have been multifaceted in approach, and this undoubtedly is the direction for future attempts at worldwide eradication of schistosomiasis.

Schistosomiasis control is the realistic goal of the present and near future. Control logically falls into 2 parallel interdependent strategies: control of population morbidity and control of transmission, which incorporate 5 general methods (Table 96–5).

Chemotherapy. This is the most cost-effective form of control and the only one that reduces both the transmission of the biologic cycle (by reducing the number of ova in the excreta) and the disease morbidity (by reducing the number of ova released within the body). Both effects can be obtained by lowering the body burden of parasites; complete cure is not essential. Until recently, the drugs available for treating schistosomiasis were not sufficiently efficacious and were too toxic for routine use in control programs. However, a new generation of antischistosomal drugs are available that can be given in the field safely in single (or only a few) doses, that cure at least 75% of those infected, and that reduce ova excretion by 90% to 95% in those not cured: oxamniquine (for *S. mansoni* infections), metrifonate (for *S. haematobium* infections), and praziquantel (for *S. mansoni, S. haematobium,* and *S. japonicum* infections). These drugs may be applied in 2 ways—mass chemotherapy or targeted population chemotherapy.

Mass Chemotherapy. This is most appropriate in a defined, medically manageable population with high prevalence rates approaching or exceeding 40%. It is performed by giving all members of the population drug treatment with no attempt at individual diagnosis or evaluation of cure. The rationale is that the savings in time, effort, and money to diagnose and to evaluate cure in individual patients outweigh the cost and relatively small risk of a safe drug being administered to noninfected community members. Overall population morbidity should be reduced, and with the addition of other control methods, the reduction of eggs excreted into the environment might break the transmission cycle.

Targeted Population Chemotherapy. This approach relies on the identification of individual moderate to heavy egg excretors followed by specific treatment and evaluation of cure. This method is more medically esthetic (e.g., noninfected persons are not given an unnecessary drug), and drug costs may be reduced considerably. However, it requires more time, technology, and equipment. A cost-effective method to detect those in a community who may be infected with *S. haematobium* is to screen for hematuria and proteinuria using chemical reagent strips. Many community-based studies have shown that both hematuria and proteinuria correlate with *S. haematobium* infection. When both are positive, the sensitivity and specificity are both usually greater than 90%.

Chemotherapy, either mass or targeted, is the linchpin of control and should be an integral part of every program.

Snail Control. Although snail control is a rapid and effective means of reducing transmission, it requires a prolonged effort (Chapter 111). The snails almost always return in significant numbers, and, if they are infected by schistosome miracidia, the biologic cycle is resumed. Therefore, snail control should be used in combination with other approaches.

TABLE 96–4. Management of Schistosomiasis

Schistosome dermatitis	Self-limited and usually not diagnosed.
	Topical corticosteroids and parenteral antihistamines will reduce symptoms in severe cases.
Katayama fever	Anti-inflammatory therapy (salicylates) for mild or moderate disease.
	Corticosteroids for life-threatening disease.
	Antischistosome therapy according to species.
Gastrointestinal schistosomiasis	
S. mansoni	Oxamniquine, 15 mg/kg in a single dose for adults (20 mg/kg for children), except in North and East Africa, where the dose is 60 mg/kg over 2 or 3 days, given in 3 or 4 equally divided doses; or
	Praziquantel, 40 mg/kg in a single dose.
S. japonicum	Praziquantel, 60 mg/kg in 2 or 3 doses given in one day.
Hepatosplenic disease	
S. mansoni	Oxamniquine or praziquantel.
	Ultrasonography to establish extent of disease.
S. japonicum	Praziquantel. Ultrasonography to establish extent of disease.
Ascites	Low-salt diet and diuretics.
Bleeding esophageal varices	Barium swallow and/or esophagoscopy to establish diagnosis. Usually can be managed conservatively with transfusion and esophageal sclerotherapy.
	Surgical shunt procedures for portal hypertension may be considered in severe cases (after repeated hemorrhage). A selective shunt operation that decompresses the splenic venous compartment without interfering with portal venous perfusion of the liver gives best long-term results.
Colonic polyposis	Barium enema and colonoscopy to establish extent of disease.
	Chemotherapy usually shrinks polyps; pedunculated polyps may be removed at colonoscopy; surgical bowel resection if permanent fibrotic obstructive bowel lesion.
	For intussusception, barium enema treatment must be performed with great care to avoid perforation.
	For rectal prolapse, chemotherapy only.
	For anorectal fistulas and abscess, surgical drainage and antibiotic therapy.
Hypertrophic osteoarthropathy	Chest radiograph and barium enema to document extent of disease.
	Steroid therapy for 2 to 4 weeks for symptomatic relief of severe bone and joint pain.
Urinary schistosomiasis	Metrifonate, 7.5–10 mg/kg biweekly × 3 or praziquantel.
Uncomplicated	Intravenous pyelogram or ultrasonography in all patients to detect silent obstructive disease.
Obstructive uropathy	Often responds to chemotherapy; may require surgery if permanent obstructive fibrotic lesion is present.
Urinary tract infection	Bacteriuria will not be eradicated with antibiotic unless accompanied by antischistosomal therapy.
	Pyelonephritis may be life-threatening and requires parenteral antibiotics.
Renal failure	Hemodialysis or renal transplant.
Bladder cancer	Radical surgery and cancer chemotherapy are usually only palliative.
Cardiopulmonary schistosomiasis	
Larval pneumonitis	Self-limited disease.
	Short-course steroid therapy if there is respiratory distress.
Reactionary pneumonitis	Interrupt antischistosomal chemotherapy until resolution.
	Short-course steroid therapy if respiratory distress is present.
Cor pulmonale	Antischistosomal therapy to arrest further progression of disease; symptomatic therapy.
CNS schistosomiasis	Antischistosomal therapy according to species.
	Steroid therapy is recommended to reduce inflammation and size of space-occupying lesions.
Other	
Salmonella-schistosome syndrome	Simultaneous antischistosomal and antibiotic therapy.
	Re-treatment with both may be necessary.
Hepatitis B/schistosome disease	Antischistosomal therapy.
	Precautions to prevent transmission of hepatitis B to hospital and laboratory staff.

Mollusciciding. This is the usual method of snail control. Niclosamide is the most frequently used chemical and is most cost-effective when a small body of water is to be treated. It is well suited to arid areas where transmission is seasonal and confined to relatively small habitats. It also can be targeted to focal areas to kill infected snails, as has been done in the Cul-de-Sac Valley and elsewhere in St. Lucia and areas in Puerto Rico. These projects show that routine focal control of snails is as effective as areawide control and is less expensive.

Biologic Control. This is an alternate method of snail control. Potential competitors or predators (including ducks, fish, turtles, fungi, and parasites) are introduced into the environment. In Puerto Rico, a competitive species of snail, *Marisa cornuarietis,* has been effective in reducing the transmission of *S. mansoni* by *Biomphalaria glabrata* in some habitats.

Environmental Modification. The burying of snails by digging out irrigation ditches was an effective but labor-intensive method of *Oncomelania* snail control in China. Other methods of environmental modification, e.g., cementing over or enclosing irrigation ditches, not only reduced the snail habitat but reduced human exposure to water.

Reduction of Water Contact and Contamination. The provision of clean water supplies to infected populations not only reduces exposure to cercariae but also reduces other water-borne infections. However, sociocultural habits are difficult to modify, and frequently the population continues to use the nearby contaminated stream or irrigation canal. Likewise, the provision of indoor or outdoor latrines has not always reduced the transmission of schistosomiasis. A successful program requires that the provision of clean water and sanitary excreta disposal be combined with health education and the other meth-

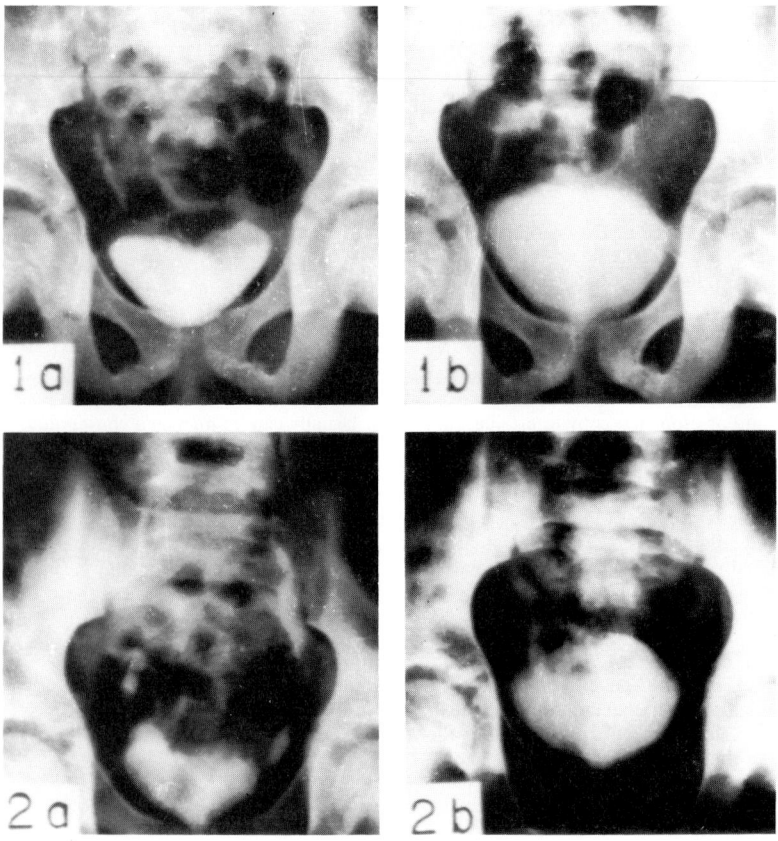

FIGURE 96–24. Intravenous pyelograms demonstrating bladder masses due to *S. haematobium* infection in 2 Egyptian patients (*1a* and *2a*). These abnormalities were reversible following praziquantel therapy (*1b* and *2b*).

ods of control. Those living in endemic areas must understand how to prevent the biologic transmission of schistosomiasis and must have the incentive and the tools to participate in its control.

Vaccination. A vaccine to prevent or attenuate infection with schistosomes would be the single most important control method and would provide a tool for eradication of schistosomiasis. With the recent renewed interest in vaccine development using modern immunologic and molecular biology techniques it is hoped that a vaccine will be available for extensive field-testing by the year 2000. It is not necessary that a vaccine provide total protection to be effective. One with 50% efficacy would prevent almost all disease, and its use in combination with chemotherapy and focal molluscicid-ing should interrupt transmission.

Improved Living Standards. As living standards improve, e.g., in Puerto Rico and Japan, it becomes much easier to control and, eventually, eradicate schistoso-

miasis. A more educated population, supplied with indoor water and toilets and working in offices or factories or farming with tools and equipment that reduce water contact, is less likely to be infected with schistosomes. Communities with improved living standards are also more likely to have satisfactory diagnostic and therapeutic facilities available for detecting and treating schistosomiasis.

BIBLIOGRAPHY

Bella H, Rahim AGA, Mustafa MD, et al.: Oltipraz—antischistosomal efficacy in Sudanese infected with *Schistosoma mansoni*. Am J Trop Med Hyg 31:775, 1982.

Butterworth AE: Potential for vaccines against human schistosomes. Clin Trop Med Comm Dis 2:465–483, 1987.

Cook JA: Strategies for control of human schistosomiasis. Clin Trop Med Comm Dis 2:449–463, 1987.

Davis A, Biles JE, Urlich AM: Initial experiences with praziquantel in the treatment of human infections due to *Schistosoma haematobium*. Bull WHO 57:773, 1979.

Jolles G: Oltipraz: Metabolism, pharmacokinetics and mechanism of action. WHO Scientific Working Group on the Biochemistry and Chemotherapy of Schistosomiasis. Geneva, WHO, 1987, pp. 1–19.

Jordan P, Bartholomew RK, Grist E, et al.: Evaluation of chemotherapy in the control of *Schistosoma mansoni* in Marquis Valley, Saint Lucia. I. Results in humans. Am Trop Med Hyg 31:103, 1982.

Jordan P, Cook JA, Bartholomew RK, et al.: Schistosomiasis mansoni control in Cul de Sac Valley, Saint Lucia. II. Chemotherapy as a supplement to a focal molluscicing programme. Trans R Soc Trop Med Hyg 74:493, 1980.

Katz N, Rocha RS, Chaves A: Preliminary trials with praziquantel in human infections due to *Schistosoma mansoni*. Bull WHO 57:781, 1979.

Kilpatrick ME, Farid Z, Bassily S, et al.: Treatment of schistosomiasis

TABLE 96–5. Schistosomiasis Control Methods

1. Chemotherapy
   a. Mass
   b. Targeted population
2. Snail control
   a. Molluscicing
   b. Biologic control
   c. Environmental modification
3. Reduction of water contact and contamination
   a. Provision of domestic water supplies
   b. Provision for sanitary disposal of excreta
4. Vaccination
5. Improved living standards

mansoni with oxamniquine—five years' experience. Am J Trop Med Hyg 30:1219, 1981.

McMahon JE, Kolstrup N: Praziquantel: A new schistosomicide against *Schistosoma haematobium*. Br Med J 2:1369, 1979.

Nash TE, Hofstetter M, Cheever AW, et al.: Treatment of *Schistosoma mekongi* with praziquantel: A double-blind study. Am J Trop Med Hyg 31:977, 1982.

Omer AHS: Oxamniquine for treating *Schistosoma mansoni* infection in Sudan. Br Med J 2:163, 1978.

Omer AHS, Teesdale CH: Metrifonate trial in treatment of various presentations of *Schistosoma haematobium* and *S. mansoni* infections in the Sudan. Ann Trop Med Parasitol 72:145, 1978.

Prentice MA, Jordan P, Bartholomew RK, et al.: Reduction in transmission of *Schistosoma mansoni* by a four-year focal mollusciciding programme against *Biomphalaria glabrata* in Saint Lucia. Trans R Soc Trop Med Hyg 75:789, 1981.

Santos AT, Blas BL, Nosenas JS, et al.: Preliminary clinical trials with praziquantel in *Schistosoma japonicum* infections in the Philippines. Bull WHO 57:793, 1979.

Sleigh AC, Hoff R, Mott KE, et al.: Manson's schistosomiasis in Brazil: 11-year evaluation of successful disease control with oxamniquine. Lancet 1:635–637, 1986.

World Health Organization: The control of schistosomiasis. WHO Tech Rep Ser 728, 1985, p. 113.

96.2. OTHER HUMAN SCHISTOSOMAL INFECTIONS

Schistosomiasis Intercalatum

DEFINITION. Schistosomiasis intercalatum is an endemic intestinal disease with abdominal pain, diarrhea, and other symptoms that is caused by the blood fluke *Schistosoma intercalatum*.

ETIOLOGY

Adult Morphology. The dimensions of the adult parasites may vary with the host and may be confused with other species of schistosomes. The males range in length from 115 to 145 mm and in breadth (with the gynecophoral canal folded) from 3 to 5 mm. The testes vary in number from 2 to 7, but most of these parasites have 4. The ventral, lateral, and dorsal surfaces of the male are spinose, and from the testes posteriorly, the cuticula is tuberculate. Adult female worms range from 130 to 240 mm in length by 3 mm in breadth. The ovary lies between the intestinal ceca and, in many specimens, is spirally twisted.

Ova. The intrauterine eggs measure 140 to 180 μm in length by 30 to 50 μm in breadth. After 80 days, the number of eggs that are passed from an experimental host averages between 25 and 60 per worm. Eggs that occur in the feces are characterized by a terminal spine that is usually slightly bent. The eggshells are Ziehl-Neelsen–positive, i.e., acid-fast, when fixed in Bouin's solution; frequently, the contained miracidium appears to be hourglass-shaped.

Intermediate Hosts. The proven intermediate hosts consist of *Bulinus forskalii* in Cameroon and Gabon and *B. africanus* group in parts of Zaire.

UNIQUE BIOLOGIC CHARACTERISTICS. The best criteria for considering *S. intercalatum* as a separate species and distinguishing it from other schistosomes lie in a number of biologic characteristics. The most distinctive features are (1) the Ziehl-Neelsen–positive staining reaction of the eggshell in histologic sections; (2)

the behavioral pattern of the cercariae, which tend to congregate near or at the water surface (as do those of *S. japonicum*); (3) the tendency of the cercariae to adhere to objects; (4) the cercarial glandular secretions that take the form of granular strings; and (5) it is the sole species that is found in most of the known transmission foci (in a few places *S. intercalatum* coexists with *S. mansoni;* it coexists with *S. haematobium* only in the Cameroons).

Natural hybrids between *S. haematobium* and *S. intercalatum* are found in Loum, Cameroon. Over a 10-year period the number of cases of intestinal schistosomiasis caused by *S. intercalatum* has markedly decreased, while the cases of urinary schistosomiasis caused by *S. haematobium* and the hybrid parasite have increased. *S. haematobium* and *S. intercalatum* hybrids raised in the laboratory exhibit heterosis by their enhanced infectivity to both snail hosts and experimental animals as well as by an increased growth rate and reproductive potential.

EPIDEMIOLOGY. The epidemiology of *S. intercalatum* is essentially similar to that of *S. mansoni*, and the ranges of the 2 parasites overlap in a few areas.

Distribution and Incidence. This distinctly African disease is endemic in parts of Cameroon, Gabon, and north and east Zaire, and possibly other parts of Central and West Africa (Fig. 96–9). The disease is spread to new foci by migrant African laborers as well as by the regular seasonal migration of nomads between the southern and northern Cameroons, especially because potential snail vector species are widely disseminated throughout Central Africa. Surveys made in endemic regions reveal a prevalence rate for *S. intercalatum* of between 5 and 25%.

Animal Reservoirs. Two natural infections have been found in *Hybomys univittatus,* the one-striped mouse. However, more potential hosts need to be examined in endemic foci. Laboratory infections have been produced in hamsters, gerbils, rats, mice, guinea pigs, rabbits, goats, sheep, and rhesus monkeys. Other species of monkeys and the American opossum have also been infected.

PATHOLOGY. Lesions occur when the often bent, terminal-spined eggs of *S. intercalatum* are deposited in the mesenteric venules and break through to the lumen of the intestine, where they are passed in the feces. The infection causes less tissue reaction than do the other human schistosomes, for undefined reasons. Hepatomegaly may occur frequently and may be severe; liver biopsies reveal perioval granulomas.

CLINICAL MANIFESTATIONS. The clinical symptomatology may include episodes of pain in the left iliac fossa with tenesmus. Anorexia, nausea, abdominal pain, and diarrhea occur frequently, and blood and mucus may be present in the stool. Proctoscopy may reveal hyperplasia of the mucosa near the rectal valves, inflammation of the wall, and sometimes polyposis. These conditions are usually relieved following adequate treatment. There may be alterations in the results of liver function tests.

DIAGNOSIS. The diagnosis rests on the demonstration of the characteristic bent, terminal-spined eggs.

These may be demonstrated in the feces or in mucosal snips from the rectum. The eggs are Ziehl-Neelsen–positive, i.e., acid-fast, whereas those of the other species with terminal-spined eggs, *S. haematobium,* are not. The contained miracidium is often narrowed in the middle, giving it something of an hourglass shape.

TREATMENT. The treatment of choice is praziquantel, which gives high cure rates when used in a single dosage of 40 mg/kg.

Schistosomiasis Mekongi

DEFINITION. Schistosomiasis mekongi occurs in the lower Mekong River Basin of Southeast Asia and is caused by an *S. japonicum*–like schistosome, *S. mekongi.* Clinical disease has gastrointestinal manifestations and may be severe.

ETIOLOGY
Adult Worm. The morphologic characteristics of the adult worm are similar to those of *S. japonicum,* although some morphologists believe that *S. mekongi* adult worms are slightly larger and have more testes and larger ovaries and other more subtle anatomic differences.

Ova. The eggs are round, with a mean diameter of 57 to 66 μm, and have a small knob-like appendage. They are similar in appearance to *S. japonicum* ova but are more rounded and slightly smaller.

Intermediate Host. The strongest evidence for separate speciation of *S. mekongi* rests with its intermediate host. The miracidium of the Mekong schistosome will develop only in the aquatic *Tricula aperta. Oncomelania* snails, the intermediate host of *S. japonicum,* cannot be infected by *S. mekongi* miracidia.

EPIDEMIOLOGY
Distribution and Incidence. *S. mekongi* infection was first described on Khong Island, the largest island in the Mekong River, and in the Lower Mekong Basin region in Cambodia, Laos, and Thailand (Fig. 96–8). Population studies indicate a prevalence rate of 15 to 50%, with school children to age 15 years being most heavily and most frequently infected.

Reservoir Hosts. Dogs are the only known reservoir host for *S. mekongi,* and their role in the maintenance of the disease cycle is yet to be determined.

PATHOGENESIS AND PATHOLOGY. Because of the small population infected with *S. mekongi* and the few clinical or pathologic studies, little information is available about the pathogenesis and pathology. However, most observers agree that the disease most resembles schistosomiasis japonica. Animal model experiments indicate that the pathology is identical to that of the Philippine strain of *S. japonicum.* Pathogenesis is likewise similar, except for delayed oviposition in mice and the inability to infect rabbits.

CLINICAL MANIFESTATIONS. Clinically, schistosomiasis mekongi mirrors *S. japonicum* infection. Presenting complaints include generalized weakness, mild diarrhea, and "thong darn," or abdominal distress. A single clinical study found hepatomegaly in 44% and splenomegaly in 18% of infected patients. Two of 25 patients with hepatosplenomegaly had portal hypertension with ascites. Central nervous system or cardiopulmonary complications have not been reported.

DIAGNOSIS. Demonstration of eggs in the stool establishes the diagnosis. Other clinical laboratory findings are normal or unhelpful; however, as noted in other forms of schistosomiasis, alkaline phosphatase levels are markedly elevated.

TREATMENT. Praziquantel (60 mg/kg) is the treatment of choice for schistosomiasis mekongi, based on clinical trials.

Schistosomiasis Mattheei

DEFINITION. Schistosomiasis mattheei is a natural schistosome infection of sheep, cattle, and horses that

TABLE 96–6. Geographic Distribution and Hosts of the Zoonotic Mammalian Schistosomes

Schistosome	Geographic Distribution	Snail Intermediate Hosts	Natural Definitive Hosts
Schistosomatium douthitti	Northern United States (including Alaska), Canada	*Stagnicola pabistris* *Lymnaea stagnalis*	Muskrats, meadow mice
Heterobilharzia americana	United States: Florida, Georgia, Texas, Louisiana, North Carolina and South Carolina	*Lymnaea cubensis* *Pseudosuccinea columella*	Bobcats, raccoons, dogs, nutria, white-tailed deer, rabbits, opossums
Schistosoma spindale	Malaya, Sumatra, and India South Africa, Zambia, and Rhodesia	*Indoplanorbis exustus* *Bulinus tropicus*	Cattle, buffalos, goats Cattle, reedbucks, other antelopes
Schistosoma bovis	Southern Europe Northern Africa and southwestern Asia East Africa West Africa South Africa Central Africa	*Planorbarius metidjensis* *Bulinus (Bulinus) truncatus* *B. forskalii* *B. senegalensis* *B. (Ph.) africanus* *B. ugandae*	Sheep, goats, cattle, equines, camels, humans
Schistosoma mattheei	South Africa, Zaire	*B. (Ph.) globosus*	Cattle, sheep, goats, zebras, impalas, humans
Schistosoma margrebowiei	Zambia, South Africa		Equines, cattle, sheep, antelopes, humans
Schistosoma rodhaini	Zaire, Uganda	*Biomphalaria sudanica* *B. pfeifferi*	Rodents, dogs, humans
Schistosoma incognitum	Indonesia	*Radix rubiginosa*	Rodents

also infects humans in South Africa, causing mild gastrointestinal disease.

ETIOLOGY

Adult Worm. Adult worms most resemble *S. intercalatum*. The female worm is able to produce eggs parthenogenetically and is perhaps carried by excess males of other species. It was once thought that *S. intercalatum* was a hybrid of *S. mattheei* and *S. haematobium*.

Ova. *S. mattheei* eggs may be found in urine or feces, measure 120 to 280 μm in length, have a terminal spine, and resemble *S. intercalatum* eggs in general configuration.

EPIDEMIOLOGY. Sheep, cattle, horses, and antelope are the natural hosts of *S. mattheei;* humans are only a secondary host. In humans, *S. mattheei* infection has invariably been found in association with *S. haematobium* or *S. mansoni* and has been seen in up to 30% of some populations in South Africa. Because of mild human disease and the limited distribution of disease, *S. mattheei* infection in humans does not constitute a serious public health problem; its veterinary importance is significant, however.

PATHOGENESIS AND PATHOLOGY. The pathogenesis and pathology of human *S. mattheei* infection are thought to be similar to those of other human intestinal schistosome infections. Typical egg granulomas have been found in the large intestine and liver and are responsible for mild hepatosplenomegaly and granulomatous bowel disease. Because of the invariable coinfection with *S. mansoni* or *S. haematobium*, the overall pathologic impact of *S. mattheei* is difficult to assess.

CLINICAL MANIFESTATIONS. Human *S. mattheei* infections are associated with schistosomal bowel disease. Patients most often present with mild blood-containing mucoid diarrhea, diffuse intermittent cramping abdominal pain, and general malaise. However, as in other schistosome infections, the majority of infected patients are asymptomatic. Mild hepatosplenomegaly may be found on physical examination, and sigmoidoscopy will reveal mucosal granulomatous lesions. Severe gastrointestinal disease and cardiopulmonary or central nervous system complications have not been reported. However, because of its limited distribution and its mild clinical manifestations, detailed clinical studies have not been performed.

DIAGNOSIS. Clinical diagnosis rests with finding *S. mattheei* eggs in the stool or, occasionally, in the urine and is supported by the known epidemiologic distribution of disease.

TREATMENT. Clinical drug trials have not been performed in *S. mattheei* infections. Praziquantel should be efficacious.

Some Potential Human Schistosomes

Several other species of schistosomes, normally parasites of mammals, may occasionally infect humans. Experiments with monkeys suggest that nonpatent visceral schistosomiasis may be produced in humans as a result of infection with the cercariae of *Schistosomatium douthitti, Heterobilharzia americana,* and *Schistosoma spindale.* Young preadult worms were recovered from livers of rhesus monkeys exposed to these schistosomes, but later the worms were lost. However, in South American monkeys, cebus, and squirrel, *Heterobilharzia americana* produces a patent infection with the deposition of large numbers of eggs in the tissues and their excretion in the feces. Other zoonotic species of *Schistosoma* include *S. bovis, S. margrebowiei,* and *S. rodhaini.* These produce a patent infection in humans, with passage of viable eggs in the stools or urine. *S. incognitum,* commonly found in rodents in Indonesia, is suspected to occasionally infect humans. The geographic distribution and hosts of these mammalian schistosomes are indicated in Table 96–6.

BIBLIOGRAPHY

Hofstetter M, Nash TE, Cheever AW, et al.: Schistosomiasis due to *Schistosoma mekongi* in Southeast Asian refugees. J Infect Dis 144:420, 1981.
Sornmani S, Vivatanasesth P, Thirachantra S: Schistosomiasis due to *Schistosoma mekongi* in Southeast Asian refugees. J Infect Dis 144:420, 1981.

97. INTESTINAL FLUKE INFECTIONS

Thanongsak Bunnag,
Danai Bunnag,
and Robert Goldsmith

Intestinal trematode (fluke) infections have been reported from Southeast Asia, the Far East, the Middle East, and North Africa. More than 50 species infect an estimated 50 million persons, but only a few cause disease. These species include the families Fasciolidae, Echinostomatidae, Heterophyidae and, to a lesser extent, the Gastrodiscidae, Lecithodendriidae, Plagiorchiidae, Microphallidae, and Diplostomatidae. In recent years, many species have been identified after anthelminthic treatment and recovery of the adult worms, but the full distribution of fluke infections and their public health importance is not known.

BIBLIOGRAPHY

Harinasuta T, Bunnag D, Radomyos P: Intestinal fluke infections. Clin Trop Med Comm Dis 2:695, 1987.
Radomyos P, Bunnag D, Harinasuta T: Worms recovered in stools following praziquantel treatment. Arzneimittelforsch/Drug Res 34:1186, 1984.

97.1. FASCIOLOPSIASIS

DEFINITION. Fasciolopsiasis buski is an infection by the giant intestinal fluke, *Fasciolopsis buski.* In general, it causes only mild or no symptoms, but in individuals with heavy worm loads, there may be intestinal symptoms, toxemic and allergic manifestations, malabsorption, and rarely, death.

GEOGRAPHIC DISTRIBUTION. *F. buski* is a common intestinal parasite of humans and pigs in Central and South China, Taiwan, Vietnam, Thailand, Laos, Kampuchea, Bangladesh, India, and Indonesia. The distribution of infection within these countries is limited, and prevalence rates are low. Recently, human infections have been reported also from Japan, Malaysia, the Philippines, a number of western countries, and in some instances, in immigrants from endemic areas.

ETIOLOGY

Morphology. *F. buski* is the largest of the intestinal trematodes and attaches to the duodenal and jejunal walls. It has a fleshy, reddish beef color, is generally elongate-ovoid, has no cephalic cone, and measures 20 to 75 mm in length, 8 to 20 mm in width, and 0.5 to 3 mm in thickness (Fig. 97–1*A*). Its large egg is hen egg-

shaped, yellowish-brown, has a clear thin shell with a small operculum at one end, measures 130 to 140 μm by 80 to 85 μm, and is unembryonated when laid (Fig. 97–1*B*). In appearance, the egg is nearly identical to those of *F. hepatica* and *F. gigantica* (Fig. VI D–2).

Life Cycle. The adult flukes live in the small intestine of pigs and humans. Eggs are passed with feces. On reaching fresh water, miracidia develop in 3 to 7 weeks at warm temperatures, hatch, and enter the snail, the first intermediate host; they then form sporocysts, rediae, and then cercariae. The cercariae swim about and encyst on various water plants where they develop into metacercariae in approximately 4 weeks. When pigs or humans ingest freshwater plants, the metacercariae excyst in the duodenum, attach to the mucosa, and develop into adult worms in about 3 months. The life span of the fluke is about 1 year (Fig. 97–2).

F. buski is distributed widely among several planorbid snail hosts. In mainland China, Vietnam, and Taiwan

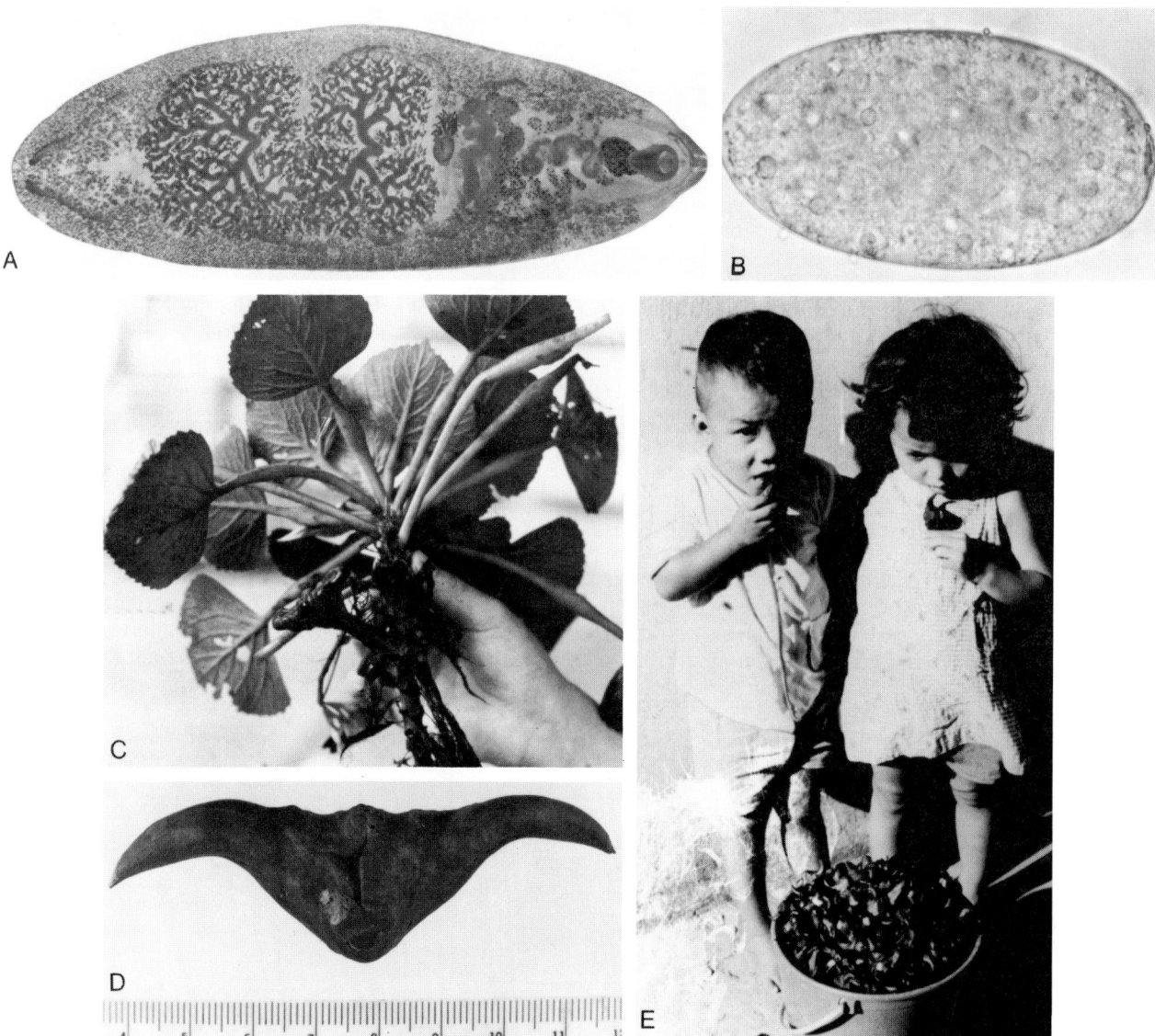

FIGURE 97–1. *A*, Adult *Fasciolopsis buski* (7 cm). *B*, Egg with a relatively small operculum (130 to 140 μm × 80 to 85 μm). *C* and *D*, Water caltrop *Trapa bicornis* with fruit seed. *E*, Children get infected by peeling with their teeth the outer layers of the fruit seed, where the metacercariae are encysted. (Courtesy of Associate Professor Prayong Radomyos, Faculty of Tropical Medicine, Mahidol University, Bangkok, Thailand.)

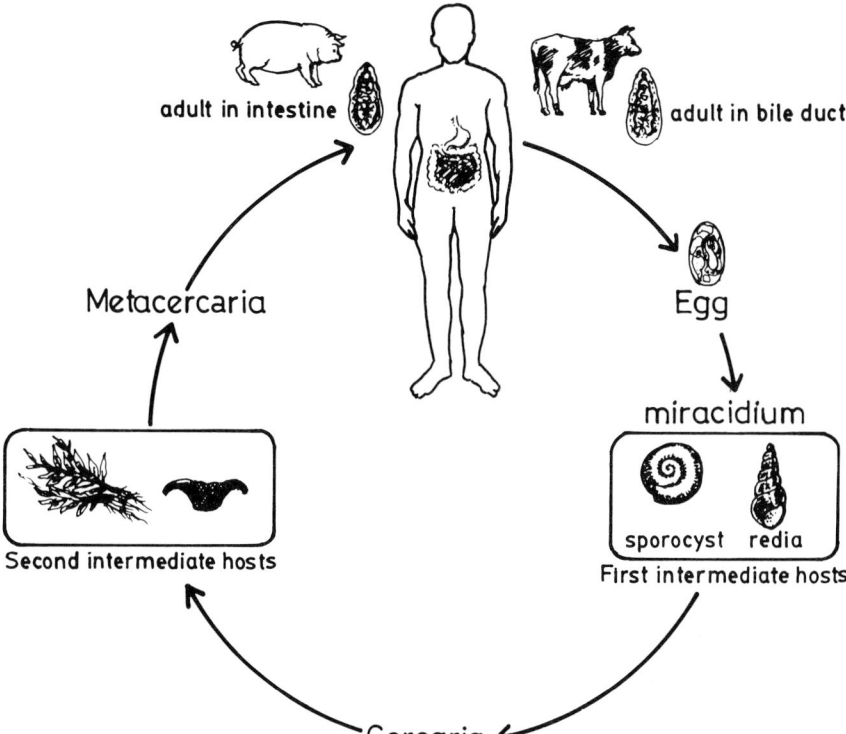

FIGURE 97–2. Life cycle of the Fasciolidae: *Fasciolopsis buski* and *Fasciola hepatica* and *gigantica*.

the snail hosts include *Segmentina hemisphaerula, Hippeutis cantori,* and *Gyraulus* species. In India (Assam), Bangladesh, and Thailand, *Segmentina (Trochorbis) trochoideus* is a host. The metacercariae encyst on the seed pods of the water caltrop (*Trapa natans* in China and *T. bicornis* in Thailand and Bengal) (Figs. 97–1*C, D*), the bulb of the water chestnut (*Eliocharis tuberosa*) and water lily shoots in Bangladesh, and other edible aquatic vegetation, including water morning glory (*Ipomoea aquatica*), water bamboo (*Zizania aquatica*), and watercress (*Neptunia Oleracea*).

EPIDEMIOLOGY. Information on the distribution of fasciolopsiasis is limited. It is distributed focally in endemic areas, with reported prevalence rates that range from 5% in parts of China to 50% in Assam, Bangladesh, and Thailand. The infection seems restricted to areas where people raise pigs and water plants, and to populations that commonly eat freshwater plants. On many farms, pigs are kept near the ponds where water plants are grown. Pig excreta are washed into the ponds that have abundant snail intermediate hosts. The cycle is continued when water plants are fed to pigs.

Humans are infected by consuming raw edible water plants, the stems, bulbs, tubers, and seed pods of which are often peeled with the teeth. In central Thailand and rural Bangladesh, where water caltrop and water lilies are cultivated in canals along the roadside, there is a high prevalence of fasciolopsiasis in children 5 to 14 years old. On their way to school they pick water caltrop and eat it fresh (Fig. 97–1*E*). Over age 7, females are infected more often than males.

PATHOGENESIS AND PATHOLOGY. The flukes normally attach to the duodenal and jejunal mucosa, but in heavy infections they may be found in the pylorus, ileum, and colon. Localized inflammation, mucous secretion, and ulceration occur at attachment sites, which may be followed by deep erosions and hemorrhage. Heavy worm burdens may result in intestinal obstruction. In severe cases in children, there is profound intoxication and sensitization from absorption of fluke metabolites. Hypoalbuminemia secondary to malabsorption or protein-losing enteropathy may result in edema of the face and extremities. Impaired vitamin B_{12} absorption and reduced serum vitamin B_{12} levels are occasional findings.

CLINICAL MANIFESTATIONS. Most infections are light and asymptomatic. In heavy infections, diarrhea occurs accompanied by hunger pain that may simulate a peptic ulcer. Initially, the diarrhea alternates with constipation but later may be persistent. The stool is greenish-yellow, foul-smelling, and contains undigested food. The appetite is usually normal or even excessive, but some patients are anorexic, nauseated, and vomit. In severe cases, anasarca and ascites develop, and the skin becomes dry and rough. Death is rare, associated with extreme cachexia and prostration.

DIAGNOSIS. Specific diagnosis is by demonstrating the characteristic eggs (Fig. 97–1*B*) or adult flukes in feces and vomitus. The eggs must be distinguished from those of various echinostomes and *Fasciola* species. Leukocytosis with relative eosinophilia is common.

The symptoms associated with heavy infections may be confused with those of giardiasis or peptic ulcer, or with other causes of bowel obstruction. Generalized edema may mimic nephrotic syndrome and other causes of hypoproteinemia.

TREATMENT. Three drugs are recommended in treatment. *Praziquantel* is the drug of choice, as a single

15 mg/kg dose given after the evening meal or before retiring to bed. The flukes are expelled the following day, and 100% cure rates are achieved. Side effects, which include headache, dizziness, abdominal pain, drowsiness, nausea, pruritus, and myalgia, are minimal and generally disappear within 48 hours.

Niclosamide, 40 mg/kg/day (up to a maximum of 4 gm), is given for 1 or 2 days. *Tetrachloroethylene*, 0.1 ml/kg (up to a maximum of 5 ml) given once only, is less effective.

PREVENTION. In endemic areas, water plants should be cooked before being eaten. Health education, prohibition of use of night soil and pig excreta as pond fertilizer, mass treatment of infected humans and pigs, modern methods of pig husbandry (i.e., pigs fed on commercial feeds rather than water plants), snail destruction when practical, and ecologic modification through urbanization and industrialization have resulted in reduced prevalence rates in some endemic areas in Thailand and Taiwan, and eradication of some foci of infection.

BIBLIOGRAPHY

Bunnag D, Radomyos P, Harinasuta T: Field trial of the treatment of fasciolopsiasis with praziquantel. SE Asian J Trop Med Public Health 14:216, 1983.
Gilman RH, Mondal G, Maksud M, et al: Endemic focus of *Fasciolopsis buski* infection in Bangladesh. Am J Trop Med Hyg 31:796, 1982.

97.2. ECHINOSTOMIASIS

DEFINITION. Echinostomiasis is an infection by trematodes of the genus *Echinostoma* and related genera.

ETIOLOGY. There are as many as 30 genera in the family Echinostomatidae, mostly parasites of birds, dogs, cats, and other mammals. Of 12 species reported in humans, the most common are *E. ilocanum, E. malayanum, E. revolutum,* and *Hypoderaeum conoideum.* Less common are *E. lindoense, E. recurvatum, E. jassyense (E. melis), E. macrorchis, E. cinetorchis, Echinochasmus perfoliatus, Paraphostomum sufrartyfex,* and *Himasthla muehlensi* (Table 97–1).

Morphology. In general, the echinostome flukes have either a characteristic horseshoe-shaped collar or 1 or 2 rows of straight spines that surround the dorsal and lateral sides of the oral sucker (Fig. 97–3I). The flukes are elongated and small, measuring 5 to 15 mm in length and 1 to 2 mm in width, with slightly tapering rounded ends (Fig. 97–3A, C, F). The cuticle of the anterior portion of the body is covered by minute scalelike spines that vary by species.

The eggs are large, yellow to yellowish-brown, thin-shelled, operculated, ovoid, and unembryonated when laid. They vary in size from 83 to 154 μm by 53 to 95 μm (Fig. 97–3B, D, E).

Life Cycle. The adult worms live attached to the intestinal wall of birds, mammals, and sometimes humans. Eggs are passed in the feces. On reaching water, miracidia develop, hatch, and penetrate snails (the first intermediate host); then, over 6 to 7 weeks, they develop into sporocysts, mother rediae, daughter rediae, and cercariae. The cercariae escape from the snails to encyst either in freshwater snails (e.g., *Pila, Viviparus, Lymnaea*), fish, tadpoles, or possibly in vegetation. Humans and definitive hosts become infected if they ingest the raw or undercooked second intermediate host.

EPIDEMIOLOGY. Human echinostomiasis is common in Indonesia, the Philippines, Taiwan, and Thailand. In some endemic areas in northeast Thailand, the prevalence rate is about 50%. A few cases have been reported also in Malaysia, Japan, and some western countries (Table 97–1).

High prevalence of infection in reservoir hosts, wide range of definitive and intermediate hosts, lack of sanitary facilities, nonhygienic health practices, and the custom of eating raw or undercooked freshwater animals are all important in transmission of the infection to humans.

Echinostoma (Euparyphium) ilocanum (Fig. 97–3C, D) is highly endemic in Luzon, Mindanao, and Leyte in the Philippines, where local prevalence rates have ranged from 1 to 44%. Human infections have been reported also from Indonesia, and a new endemic area was discovered in 1982 in northeast Thailand. In China, only enzootic foci have been found (14% in dogs).

The collar of the *E. ilocanum* has 49 to 51 spines. The planorbid snails, *Gyraulus convexiusculus* (Philippines, Indonesia), *Hippeutis umbilicus* (Philippines), and *G. prashdi* (India) are first intermediate hosts. Any

TABLE 97–1. Distribution, Hosts and Size of Ova of Some Less Common Echinostomids

Species	Definitive Hosts (Excluding Humans)	Source of Infection	Size of Ova (μm)	Locality
Echinostoma melis (E. jassyense)	Unknown	Tadpole	132–154 × 75–85	Romania, China
E. cinetorchis	Rat	Tadpole, frog	96–100 × 61–70	Japan, Taiwan, Korea, Indonesia
E. macrorchis	Rat	Tadpole, frog, snail	81–89 × 54–58	Japan, Taiwan, Indonesia
E. japonicus	Cat, dog, rat, mouse, chick	Fish	77–90 × 51–57	China, Korea
E. recurvatum	Bird, mammals, wild rat	Tadpole, frog	88–111 × 54–75	Taiwan, Indonesia, Egypt
E. lindoense	Rat, bird	Clam	92–124 × 65–76	Indonesia, Brazil
Echinochasmus perfoliatus	Cat, dog, hog, fox, rat, wild boar	Fish	90–135 × 55–95	Japan, Italy, Romania, Russia, northern Asia, Egypt, Taiwan
Episthmium caninum	Dog	Fish	84 × 50–60	Thailand
Paraphostomum sufrartylex	Hog, dog, rat	Digoniostoma pulchella	90–125 × 60–75	India (Assam)

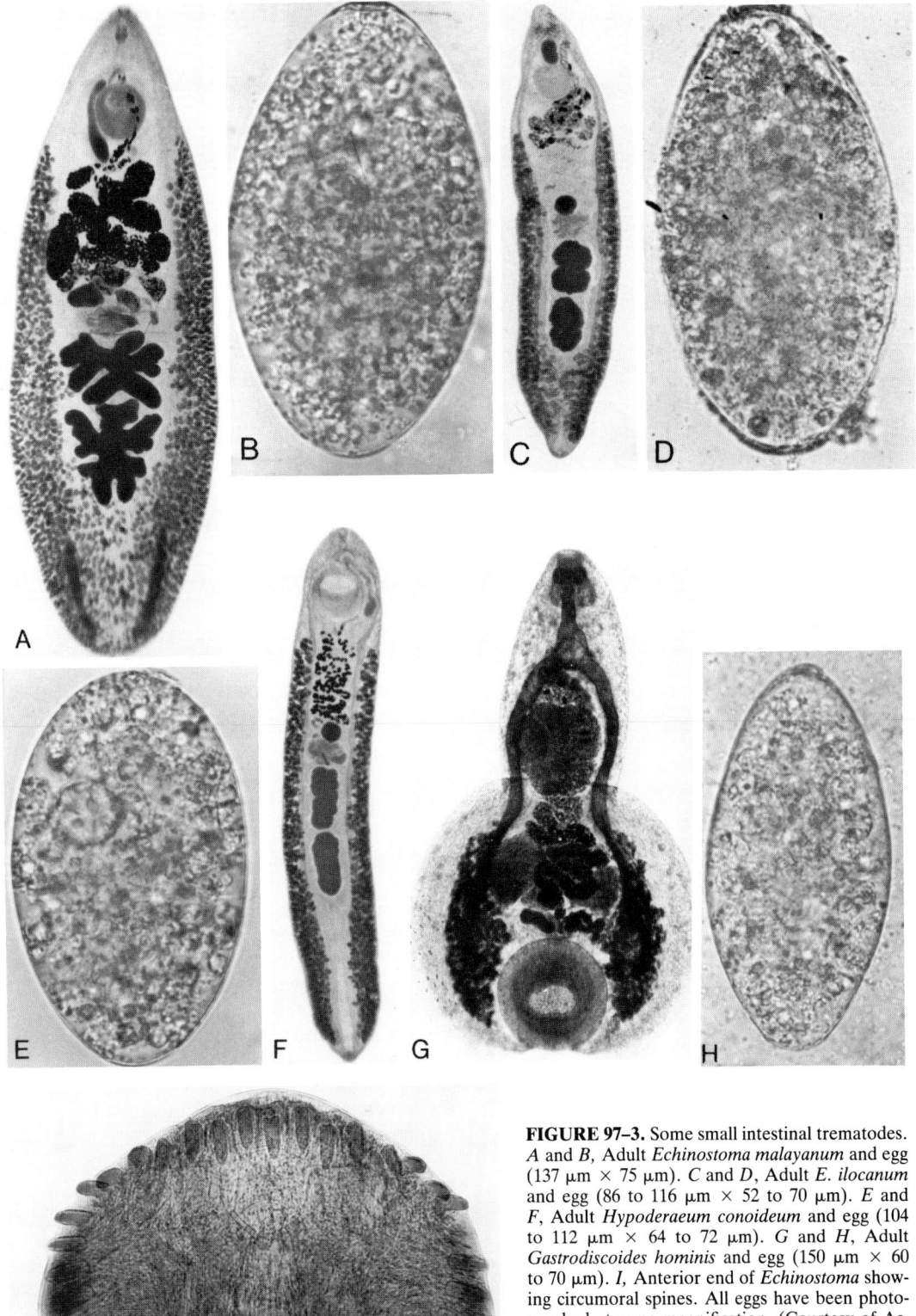

FIGURE 97–3. Some small intestinal trematodes. *A* and *B,* Adult *Echinostoma malayanum* and egg (137 μm × 75 μm). *C* and *D,* Adult *E. ilocanum* and egg (86 to 116 μm × 52 to 70 μm). *E* and *F,* Adult *Hypoderaeum conoideum* and egg (104 to 112 μm × 64 to 72 μm). *G* and *H,* Adult *Gastrodiscoides hominis* and egg (150 μm × 60 to 70 μm). *I,* Anterior end of *Echinostoma* showing circumoral spines. All eggs have been photographed at same magnification. (Courtesy of Associate Professor Prayong Radomyos, Faculty of Tropical Medicine, Mahidol University, Bangkok, Thailand.)

freshwater snail, such as *Pila conica* (Philippines) and *Viviparus javanicus* (Indonesia), is a source of infection.

Echinostoma malayanum (Fig. 97–3A, B) is enzootic-endemic in northeast and northern Thailand. In Malaysia and Indonesia, human infection is rare, because freshwater snails are usually well cooked before eaten. The adult worms possess 43 crown spines and inhabit the small intestine of reservoir hosts (e.g., rats, dogs). A variety of freshwater snails, such as *Indoplanorbis exustus* (Thailand) and *Lymnaea leuteola* (India), are first intermediate hosts. Metacercariae are found in *I. exustus, L. (Radix) rubiginosa, G. convexiusculus* and in tadpoles in Thailand and *Vivaparus javanicus* and *Pila scutata* in Malaysia and Indonesia.

Echinostoma revolutum is normally a parasite of ducks, geese, and rats. The worm has 37 circumoval spines. The worm was first recognized in Taiwan, where human infection is estimated at 3 to 7%. The northeast provinces of Thailand are also endemic-enzootic areas, but the prevalence is unknown. A few cases have been recorded in Indonesia also. In addition to the first intermediate snail hosts, *I. exustus* and *L. (Radix) rubiginosa* in Thailand and *Physa* species (*Segmentina* species and *Helisoma* species) in Taiwan, a second mollusk host or tadpole in Thailand and clams (*Corbicula producta*) in Taiwan are required for encystment of the metacercariae.

Hypoderaeum conoideum is a common intestinal parasite (Fig. 97–3E, F) of ducks, other fowl, rats, and humans in northeast Thailand, where a 55% prevalence rate was found in 1965. The body of the fluke is elongated and tapered posteriorly; the head collar has 2 rows of 45 to 53 spines. Intermediate hosts are freshwater snails, including *I. exustus, L. (Radix) rubiginosa,* and tadpoles.

Echinostoma lindoense was highly endemic a few decades ago among humans and animals in the remote Lindu Valley in Central Sulawesi, Indonesia. The infection has since disappeared, probably as a result of biological competition between the snail hosts in Lindu lake and *Tilapia mossambica* fish, introduced in 1951.

PATHOLOGY AND CLINICAL MANIFESTATIONS. The pathology and clinical manifestations of echinostomiasis have not been well studied. The flukes attach to the small intestine mucosa and produce shallow ulcers and a mild inflammatory response with cellular infiltration. Heavy infections may result in local necrosis.

Apparently, mild infections produce little morbidity. With heavy infections, there is diarrhea and vague abdominal complaints of flatulence and intestinal colic. In children, symptoms similar to those of *Fasciolopsiasis buski*, including diarrhea, abdominal pain, anemia, and edema, have been reported.

DIAGNOSIS. Diagnosis is by recovery of eggs (Fig. 97–3B, D, E) in the feces; the eggs must be differentiated from those of other trematodes such as *Fasciola hepatica, F. gigantica,* and *Fasciolopsis buski* (Fig. VI D–2). Definitive identification depends upon the morphology of adult worms (Fig. 97–3A, C, F, I) recovered in feces after anthelmintic therapy or at autopsy.

TREATMENT. Praziquantel in a single dose of 40 mg/kg at bed time, or albendazole 400 mg twice daily for 3 days, is effective.

PREVENTION. Echinostomiasis can be prevented by ensuring that snails or other aquatic animals are cooked adequately before eaten.

BIBLIOGRAPHY

Bhaibulaya M, Charoenlarp P, Harinasuta C: Report of cases of *Echinostoma malayanum* and *Hypoderaeum concideum* in Thailand. J Med Assoc Thai 47:720, 1964.
Carney WP, Sodoma M, Purnomo: Echinostomiasis. A disease that disappeared. Trop Geogr Med 32:101, 1980.

97.3. HETEROPHYIASIS

DEFINITION. Heterophyiasis is an infection by the minute intestinal flukes of the genus *Heterophyes* or related members of the family Heterophyidae, which sometimes cause abdominal colic and mucous diarrhea.

HETEROPHYIASIS DUE TO HETEROPHYES HETEROPHYES

GEOGRAPHIC DISTRIBUTION. More than 10 heterophyid species have been found in humans, of which *Heterophyes heterophyes* and *Metagonimus yokogawai* are the most important. Human infection is common in the Nile delta of Egypt and in Iran, Tunisia, and Turkey. In Asia, foci have been reported in Japan, Korea, Taiwan, mainland China, the Philippines, and Indonesia. Possibly the infection occurs throughout Southeast Asia. In India, infection is found in dogs.

ETIOLOGY

Morphology. *H. heterophyes* is a pyriform, grey, minute fluke measuring 1.0 to 1.8 mm by 0.3 to 0.7 mm with a broadly rounded posterior end. Its tegument scales are closely set and most numerous in the anterior portion of the body. The oral sucker is subterminal and one third the size of the ventral sucker. The eggs are ovoid, light brown, operculated, and measure 28 to 30 μm by 15 to 17 μm. They are the same size as other heterophyid and opisthorchid eggs but differ from *M. yokogawai* in having a thicker shell.

Life Cycle. Adult *H. heterophyes* attach to the intestinal mucosa of the jejunum and upper ileum of fish-eating mammals. Eggs are passed in feces but hatch only after ingestion by brackish or freshwater snails, the first intermediate hosts, in which they undergo development through 1 or 2 generations of sporocysts. Resulting cercariae emerge from the snails and encyst in brackish or freshwater fish, the second intermediate host, in which they become infective metacercaria.

Proven snail hosts are *Perinella conica* in Egypt and *Cerithedea cingulata* (Syn. *Tymphonotonus microptera*) in Japan. Fish hosts in Egypt are mullet species *Mugil cephalus* and *M. capito, Tilapia nilotica,* and *Aphanius fasciatus;* hosts in Japan are the minnow *Gambusia affinis* and *Acanthogobius* species.

Dog, cat, fox, bird, and other fish-eating mammals are reservoir hosts.

EPIDEMIOLOGY. Humans become infected when parasitized fish are eaten raw, cooked inadequately, or pickled or salted improperly. Metacercariae are capable of living up to 7 days in salted fish. The brackish-water fish, *Mugil capito*, caught off the coast of Israel, have been found heavily infected, some with 2300 to 6000 metacercariae/gm of fish.

PATHOLOGY. The flukes attach to the small bowel mucosa and may cause shallow ulcers, mild inflammation, or superficial necrosis. Ova and sometimes adult flukes may enter blood vessels and embolize to the heart and central nervous system.

CLINICAL MANIFESTATIONS. Following ingestion of infective metacercariae and a prepatent period (average, 9 days), clinical findings may include mild and intermittent mucous diarrhea, dyspepsia, and abdominal colic. Eosinophilia may be present. Eggs that filter through the mesenteric lymphatics may result in (1) a myocarditis that can lead to chronic congestive cardiac failure or death, or (2) embolisms to the brain with findings similar to cerebral hemorrhage. In the Philippines, severe cardiac damage has been described due to vessel occlusion by the ova.

DIAGNOSIS. Diagnosis is generally based on recovery of characteristic eggs in feces. They may be difficult to differentiate, however, from those of other *Heterophyes* or from *Clonorchis* or *Opisthorchis* (Fig. VI D–2). The specific diagnosis can be made only by morphologic identification of adult worms recovered after anthelmintic therapy or at autopsy. Geographic and epidemiologic information may aid in diagnosis. *Heterophyes* and *Metagonimus* infection can be excluded in persons who have not eaten potentially infectious fish for 1 year, because both flukes have relatively short lives. This is not true for *Opisthorchis*, however, which have a longer lifespan.

TREATMENT. The drug of choice is praziquantel as a single 15 to 25 mg/kg dose.

PREVENTION AND CONTROL. Efforts must focus on health education to inform about the danger of eating raw, undercooked, or improperly salted or pickled fish, and on reduction of infection in the reservoir hosts.

METAGONIMIASIS

DEFINITION. Metagonimiasis is infection by the minute trematode, *Metagonimus yokogawai*, a species closely related to *H. heterophyes*.

ETIOLOGY

Morphology. *M. yokogawai*, which resembles *H. heterophyes* in size and shape, measures 1.0 to 2.5 mm by 0.4 to 0.75 mm and is wider posteriorly than anteriorly. The ventral sucker is located to the right of the midline. The eggs are 26 to 28 μm by 15 to 17 μm, fully mature when laid, and difficult to distinguish from those of *H. heterophyes* (Figs. VI D–2 and 97–4F).

Life Cycle. The life cycle is similar to *H. heterophyes*. The first intermediate host is the snail *Semisulcospira libertina* and related species. The second intermediate hosts are several species of freshwater fish, particularly Cyprinidae: trout (*Plectoglossus altivelis* and *Odontobulis obscurus*) and salmon (*Salmo perryi* and *Tribolodon hakonensis*). The cercariae encyst under the scales or in the tissue of the gills, fins, and tail.

Dogs, cats, pigs, and pelicans are important reservoirs.

GEOGRAPHIC DISTRIBUTION AND EPIDEMIOLOGY. The parasite is probably the most common intestinal fluke infection in the Far East. It is endemic in parts of China, Japan, Korea, Taiwan, the Philippines, and Indonesia. Prevalence is particularly high in Japan, Korea, and Taiwan, with rates of 2 to 50% reported from Japan. Infections have been reported also from Siberia, the Balkans, Spain, and Israel.

Humans are infected by eating raw or undercooked fish. The prevalence rate of metagonimiasis is difficult to estimate in endemic areas where clonorchids and other heterophyids are also present, because the eggs are similar (Fig. VI D–2).

PATHOLOGY. The flukes invade the mucosa of the small intestine, duodenum, or jejunum causing inflammation, granulomatous infiltration, and ulcerations. They ultimately become encapsulated. On rare occasions, eggs deposited in the tissue are carried by the blood stream and embolized in other organs, as in heterophyiasis.

CLINICAL MANIFESTATIONS. The disease caused by *M. yokogawai* is similar to that by *H. heterophyes*. Mucous diarrhea is the usual finding, but serious manifestations may result from massive embolization of eggs to vessels in the heart or brain.

DIAGNOSIS. Diagnosis is by demonstrating eggs in the feces (Figs. VI D–2h and 97–4F) or finding adult flukes after an anthelmintic or at autopsy. The eggs resemble those of *H. heterophyes*.

TREATMENT. Treatment is as for heterophyiasis.

PROGNOSIS. The prognosis is good except when there are ectopic lesions in the brain or heart.

PREVENTION. Abstinence from eating raw or inadequately cooked freshwater fish will prevent infection.

OTHER HETEROPHYID INFECTIONS IN HUMANS

Infections by other Heterophyidae species occur in areas of Asia where people eat raw or partially cooked freshwater fish. The flukes are minute, usually less than 1 mm long. The reservoir hosts are fish-eating birds and mammals. The following species have been reported from humans: *Centrocestus formosanus* from Taiwan and mainland China; *Haplorchis pumilio* (Fig. 97–4G), *H. yokogawai*, and *H. taichui* (Fig. 97–4C, H) from Taiwan, the Philippines, Indonesia, and Thailand; *Metagonimus minutus*, *Diorchitrema formosanum*, and *D. amplicaecale* from Taiwan; *Procerovum calderoni* from the Philippines and China; *Stellantchasmus falcatus* from Hawaii (from eating raw mullet), Japan, the Philippines, and Thailand; and *Pygidiopsis summa* from Korea (up to 4,000 worms have been recovered from individuals).

The intestinal lesions produced by these flukes are similar to those described for *H. heterophyes* and *M. yokogawai*. At autopsy, eggs of *Haplorchis yokogawai*,

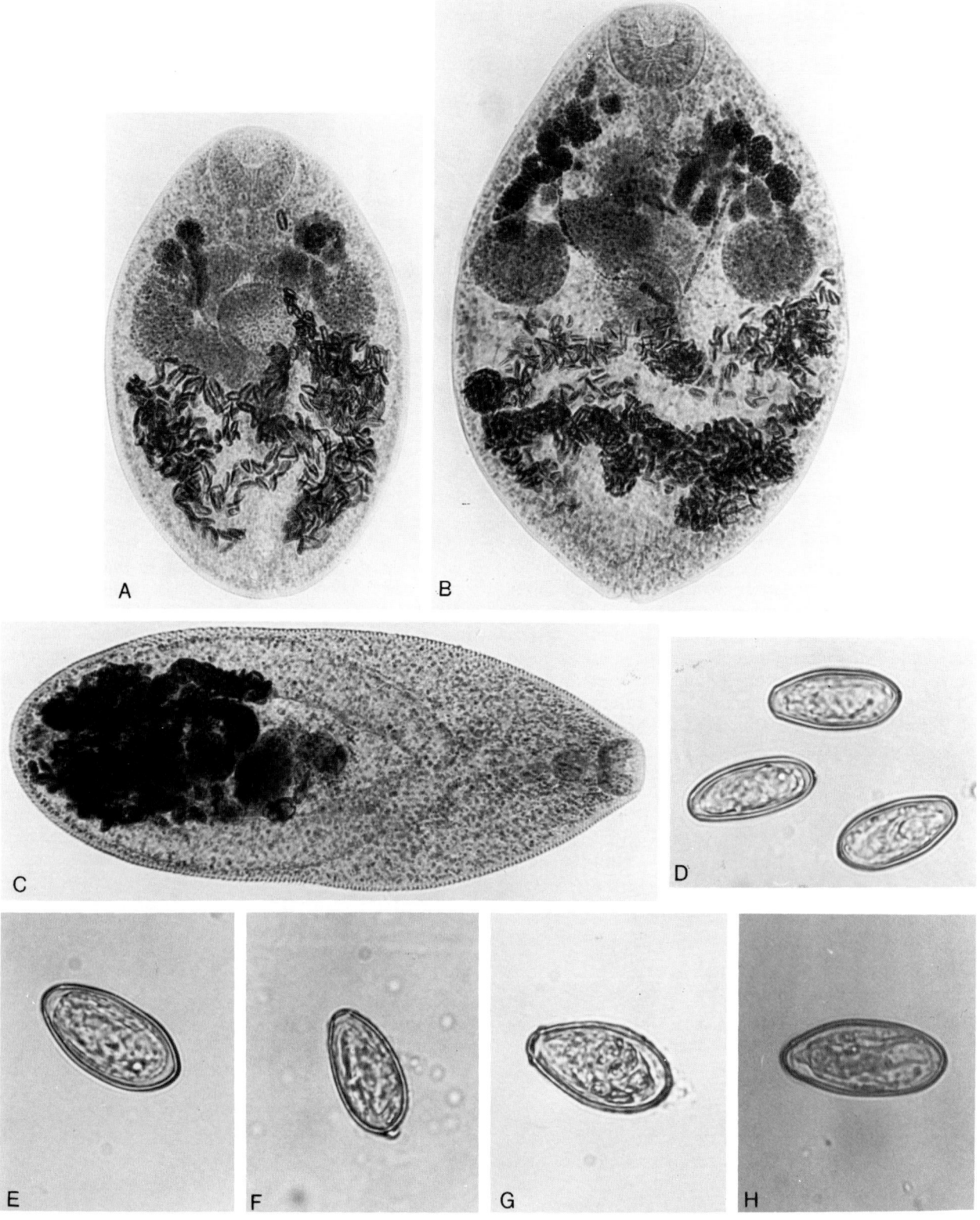

FIGURE 97–4. Some minute intestinal trematodes. *A* Adult *Phaneropsolus bonnei. B*, Adult *Prosthodendrium molenkempi. C,*Adult *Haplorchis taichui. D*, Eggs of *P. molenkempi. E, P. bonnei. F, Metagonimus yokogawai. G, Haplorchis pumillo. H, H. taichui.* All eggs were photographed at the same magnification. (Courtesy of Associate Professor Prayong Radomyos, Faculty of Tropical Medicine, Mahidol University, Bangkok, Thailand.)

H. pumilio, and *H. taichui* have been found in cardiac lesions but rarely cause vascular occlusion. Treatment with a single dose of 15 to 25 mg/kg of praziquantel is effective.

BIBLIOGRAPHY

Sheir Z, El-Shabrawy A–EM: Demographic, clinical and therapeutic appraisal of heterophyiasis. J Trop Med Hyg 73:148, 1970.

97.4. GASTRODISCIASIS

DEFINITION. Gastrodisciasis is an infection by the small amphistome trematode *Gastrodiscoides hominis*, which inhabits the cecum and ascending colon.

ETIOLOGY

Morphology. The adult worm, 5 to 14 mm long by 4 to 6 mm wide, is bright pink and pyriform in shape with a conical anterior. The ventral surface of the discoidal posterior portion has a large acetabulum that bears a characteristic notch (Fig. 97–3*G*). The eggs are greenish-brown, operculated, immature when laid, and measure 150 μm by 60 to 70 μm (Fig. 97–3*H*); they resemble those of *F. buski* but are slightly narrower.

Life Cycle. The complete life cycle is unknown but is probably similar to that of the amphistomes.

EPIDEMIOLOGY. *G. hominis* is a relatively common human parasite in Asia. It has been reported from Assam, Bihar, and Orissa in India; Vietnam, Burma, China, the Philippines, and Thailand; Kazakstan in the Soviet Union; and British Guiana. In India, a 41% prevalence was found in one survey in which pigs were the reservoir host. Other known reservoirs are the mouse deer (*Tragulus napu*) in Malaysia and rats in Indonesia, Japan, and Thailand.

PATHOLOGY. Adult *G. hominis* attach to the mucosa of the cecum and ascending colon, where they may produce lesions similar to those described in pigs. At the attachment site, papular lesions with minute surface desquamation may progress to necrosis. Lymphocytes, plasma cells, and eosinophils infiltrate the mucosa and submucosa.

CLINICAL MANIFESTATIONS. The flukes live in the cecum and ascending colon but usually produce no symptoms. However, mucous diarrhea has been reported.

DIAGNOSIS. Diagnosis is by finding characteristic eggs or the adult fluke after an anthelmintic. The eggs resemble those of *F. buski* but are narrower and have a greenish-brown color (Fig. 97–3*H*).

TREATMENT. Praziquantel at the same dosage used in fasciolopsiasis may be effective.

BIBLIOGRAPHY

Ahluwalia SS: *Gastrodiscoides hominis* (Lewis and McConnell) Leiper, 1913. The amphistome parasite of man and pigs. Indian J Med Res 48:315, 1960.
Surinthrangkul B, Gonthian S, Pradatsundarasar A: *Gastrodiscoides hominis* from man in Thailand. J Med Assoc Thai 48:96, 1965.

97.5. MISCELLANEOUS INTESTINAL FLUKE INFECTIONS

LECITHODENDRIIDAE FLUKE INFECTIONS

DEFINITION. *Phaneropsolus bonnei* and *Prosthodendrium molenkempi* are 2 minute trematodes in the Lecithodendriidae that infect humans.

ETIOLOGY

Morphology. *P. bonnei* is small, ovoid, and 0.48 to 0.78 mm long by 0.22 to 0.35 mm wide (Fig. 97–4*A*). Its cuticular spines are long at the posterior end. The eggs are small, 23 to 33 μm by 13 to 18 μm, oval, thin-shelled with indistinct operculum, dark-colored, and unembryonated when laid (Fig. 97–4*E*).

P. molenkempi is small, 0.4 to 0.8 mm long by 0.4 to 0.6 mm wide (Fig. 97–4*B*). The body is round and covered with cuticular spines. The subterminal oral sucker and the acetabulum are in the middle third of the body. The eggs are 24 to 26 μm by 8 to 10 μm, operculated, oval, dark brown, and unembryonated when laid (Fig. 97–4*D*). Eggs of both species are similar to those of *O. viverrini* and can be differentiated only with great difficulty (Fig. VI D–2).

Life Cycle. The life cycles of *P. bonnei* and *P. molenkempi* are not completely understood. Natural infections in reservoir hosts have been found in monkeys (*Macaca iris* and *Nycticebus coucang* in Malaysia, *Macaca mulatta* in India, and *Macaca fuscicularis* in Thailand), in insectivorous bats (*Scotophilus kuhlii* and *Taphozons melanopogon*), and in rats (*Rattus rattus*) in Thailand. It is highly probably that *Bithynia goniomphalus* is the snail intermediate host and that dragon and damselflies (*Crocothemis servilia, Orthetrum sabina, Trithemis pallidinervis, Brachythemis contaminata*) act as the second intermediate hosts.

GEOGRAPHY AND EPIDEMIOLOGY. Both flukes were recognized initially at autopsy in Indonesia and subsequently following anthelmintic treatment and during surveys. Both flukes are endemic among rural populations of northeast Thailand and adjacent Laos, and in some areas prevalence rates vary from 10 to 40%. Infections with both species have sometimes been found in the same individuals. Infection for both flukes results from consumption of raw or inadequately cooked small fish contaminated with infected naiads (water nymphs of dragonflies). Manning has suggested, however, that *P. bonnei* and *P. molenkempi* are present in a sylvatic cycle throughout Southeast Asia, but that humans are only accidentally infected when they eat infected naiads collected with freshwater fish.

PATHOLOGY AND CLINICAL MANIFESTATIONS. Although large numbers of flukes (4356 *P. bonnei* and 1339 *P. molenkempi*) have been recovered following treatment, there are no established intestinal pathologic or clinical findings. It has been difficult to separate clinical symptoms caused by the lecithodendriids from those caused by other parasites in northeast Thailand and Laos, where polyparasitism is common.

DIAGNOSIS. The diagnosis is based on finding the characteristic eggs and adult worms in feces or at autopsy. It is difficult to differentiate the eggs of *P. bonnei* and *P. molenkempi* from each other and from *Opisthorchis viverrini* and other heterophyid eggs (Figs. VI D–2 and 97–4D–H).

TREATMENT AND PREVENTION. A single dose of 40 mg/kg of praziquantel is effective. Prevention is by not eating raw freshwater fish or naiads.

MICROPHALLIDAE FLUKE INFECTION

The members of this trematode group are minute intestinal parasites of a wide range of vertebrates. Morphologically they resemble the Heterophyidae; their life cycle resembles that of the Plagiorchiidae.

Spelotrema brevicaeca has been reported on several occasions in humans in the Philippines. The eggs are suspected of causing lesions in the heart, brain, and spinal cord of patients dying of acute cardiac dilation. The complete life cycle is unknown. The encysted metacercarial stage has been found in the crab, *Cararius maenas*, which is the source of infection for Filipinos. The adult worms are small, pyriform, and measure 0.5 to 0.7 mm by 0.3 to 0.4 mm wide, and have a spinose cuticle. The eggs are operculated, yellowish, and 15 to 16 μm by 9 to 10 μm in size. Diagnosis is based on finding the eggs in stools or in tissue, or recovery of adult worms after treatment.

PLAGIORCHIIDAE FLUKE INFECTION

Three species of *Plagiorchis* infect humans in the Philippines, Indonesia, Japan, and Thailand.

P. philippinensis was recovered at autopsy in Ilocanos, Philippines. The infection is acquired by eating larvae of certain insects, the second intermediate host. *P. javensis* was found once in an Indonesian, and *P. muris* once in Japan.

Human infections by these species may be misdiagnosed, because the fluke eggs are small and similar to those of *Opisthorchis viverrini* and *Clonorchis sinensis*.

DIPLOSTOMATIDAE FLUKE INFECTION

Flukes in this family are intestinal parasites of birds and mammals. In humans, the disease results from eating raw or inadequately cooked flesh of frogs or snakes that contain the larval stage "mesocercariae."

ALARIASIS

In North America, the adult stage of various species of *Alaria* inhabit the intestine of wild carnivores (e.g., wolves, foxes, raccoons, bobcats, and skunks). Eggs in feces hatch in water and invade freshwater snails of the genus *Helisoma* from which cercariae emerge and infect frog tadpoles. A fatal case of *Alaria americana* infection reported from Ontario, Canada is assumed to have resulted from eating inadequately cooked frogs' legs.

Autopsy revealed numerous mesocercariae in ascitic fluid, lungs, liver, heart, kidneys, pancreas, spleen, brain, and spinal cord. Another patient had an eye infection that probably resulted from direct penetration of the tissues by the infective mesocercarial stage while frogs were being prepared for the table.

FIBRICOLIASIS

Fibricola seoulensis is the only diplostomatid fluke known to infect humans in Korea, and has been reported among snake eaters. The parasite is enzootic among house rats, frogs and their tadpoles, and several terrestrial snakes. Epigastric discomfort or pain, diarrhea, fever, and eosinophilia have been seen in humans. Eggs from the feces are readily differentiated from those of *Paragonimus*, *Echinostoma*, or *Fasciola*. They measure 81 to 102 μm long by 51 to 63 μm wide, and are golden brown, bilaterally asymmetric with an oblique opercular margin, and immature when laid.

Almost 100% of persons treated with praziquantel (20 mg/kg in a single dose) have been cured. Bithionol is less effective.

BIBLIOGRAPHY

Freeman RS, Stuart PF, Cullen JB, et al: Fatal human infection with mesocercariae of the trematode *Alaria americana*. Am J Trop Med Hyg 25:803, 1976.

Hong ST, Cho TK, Hong SJ, et al: Fifteen human cases of *Fibricola seoulensis*. Korean J Parasitol 22:61, 1984.

Manning GS, Lertprasert P: Studies on the life cycle of *Planeropsolus bonnei* and *Prosthodendrium molenkempi* in Thailand. Ann Trop Med Parasitol 67:361, 1973.

98. LIVER FLUKE INFECTIONS

Danai Bunnag,
Thanongsak Bunnag,
and Robert Goldsmith

Seven species of flukes in 3 distomate families—Opisthorchiidae, Fasciolidae, and Dicrocoelidae—infect the liver, more specifically, the biliary tract of humans. Some are found worldwide, whereas others are limited in geographic distribution. The major liver flukes that cause disease in humans are *Opisthorchis viverrini*, *O. felineus*, and *Clonorchis sinensis*. Of less importance and with sporadic occurrence are *Fasciola hepatica*, *F. gigantica*, *Dicrocoelium dendriticum*, and *Eurytrema pancreaticum*.

98.1. OPISTHORCHIASIS

DEFINITION. Opisthorchiasis is infection of the intrahepatic biliary tract by *Opisthorchis viverrini* and *O. felineus* (the cat liver fluke). Most infections in humans are asymptomatic. Clinical manifestations include abdominal discomfort or pain, hepatomegaly, an enlarged gallbladder, and relapsing cholangitis. Occasional complications are gallstones and obstructive jaundice; cholangiocarcinoma is associated with opisthorchiasis.

GEOGRAPHIC DISTRIBUTION. *O. viverrini* in humans is endemic in north and northeast Thailand and in Laos and Kampuchea. Up to 7 million persons may be infected; the overall prevalence rate is 35% but in some areas is over 90%. *O. felineus* has been reported from central, eastern, and southern Europe, particularly Poland, Germany, and European USSR and western Siberia, with scattered reports from other parts of Asia. A few million persons may be infected with *O. felineus*; prevalence rates up to 85% have been reported in areas of the USSR. Reports of finding *O. felineus* in Southeast Asia may have been in error.

ETIOLOGY

Morphology. Living *O. viverrini* and *O. felineus* are transparent, have a leaf-like shape, and are 8 to 12 mm in length (Fig. 98–1*B*). The length to width ratio of *O. viverrini* is approximately 2:1 and thus resembles *Clonorchis sinensis* (Fig. 98–1*A*), whereas that of *O. felineus* is about 3:1. Their eggs are yellowish-brown, oval, and have an operculum that rests on shoulders with or without a tubercle-like knob at the abopercular end (Figs. VI D–2*F* and 98–1*B*). The eggs average 28 μm by 16 μm in size and contain a miracidium when laid.

TRANSMISSION AND EPIDEMIOLOGY

Life Cycle. The life cycles of *Opisthorchis* and *Clonorchis* are similar (Fig. 98–2). The adult worms live in the distal biliary ducts and sometimes in the gallbladder. Eggs are released into the bile and pass to the feces. On reaching water, the eggs are eaten by appropriate species of snails, the first intermediate host. Within the snails, the miracidia hatch and develop sequentially as sporocysts, rediae, and cercariae. In 4 to 6 weeks, mature cercariae are released into the water and penetrate the muscle of susceptible freshwater scally fish to develop into metacercariae. The metacercariae mature and become infective in 6 weeks. Consumption of infected fish is the source of infection for the definitive hosts, humans or other fish-eating mammals. The metacercariae excyst in the duodenum or jejunum and migrate through the ampulla of Vater and the common bile duct to the bile ducts, where they mature within 4 weeks and begin to produce eggs. The life span of the flukes is over 20 years. This natural cycle continues almost year round; snail infection rates are generally less than 0.1% and cercarial output averages 280 per snail.

INTERMEDIATE HOSTS. The snail intermediate hosts for *O. viverrini* are *Bithynia siamensis goniomphalos*, *B. (Digoniostoma) funiculata*, and *B. siamensis siamensis*; hosts for *O. felineus* are *Bithynia leachi* and *B. infata*. Second intermediate hosts for *O. viverrini* are many species of cyprinoid fish or carp: *Cyclocheilicthys apogon* (*Pla Kua Na*), *Puntius leiacanthys* (*Pla Tapein Sai*), and *Hampala dispar* (*Pla Suud*); infection rates in the fish are commonly over 95%. In central, eastern, and southern Europe and in Siberia, the metacercariae of *O. felineus* are found in several freshwater fish (e.g., *Leuciscus rutilus*, *Blicca bjorkna*, *Tinca tinca*, and *Barbus barbus*).

In hyperendemic-enzootic areas, domestic cats, dogs, and many fish-eating mammals are definitive hosts. Infection rates of 22.6% have been found in cats compared to 1.9% in dogs.

***O. viverrini* Infection.** The high prevalence in northeast Thailand is explained by lack of hygienic knowledge and facilities, increasing development of water reservoirs and irrigation systems, flourishing snail and fish intermediate host populations, and the popular practice of consuming raw fish, e.g., in *Koi Pla*, a dish prepared from chopped, raw cyprinoid fish. Prevalence of infection in some villages is over 90%. Intensity of infection increases generally with age owing to continuing new infections, lack of protective immunity, and the long life span of the flukes. In older age groups, the worm burden in males is twice that in females.

***O. felineus* Infection.** In western Siberia, people consume raw freshwater fish and 1-day-old salted fish. Newly arrived immigrants acquire the infection during their first year of residence.

PATHOLOGY AND PATHOGENESIS. The pathologic changes induced by the worms are apparently the result of mechanical irritation caused by the worm suckers, toxic metabolic substances, immunologic response of the host, and secondary bacterial infection. These effects increase with intensity and duration of infection; as many as 20,000 worms have been found at autopsy. Early changes are mild, with excessive mucin production, desquamation, and adenomatous hyperplasia of duct epithelium. With progression, glandular proliferations project into the lumen. In heavy and severe infections, there is biliary obstruction, bile retention, periductal infiltration with eosinophils and round cells, fibrosis, and necrosis and atrophy of surrounding hepatic cells (Fig. 98–3). Dilatation of the intrahepatic bile ducts is uniform, accompanied by distal clubbing or cyst formation. The gallbladder is frequently nonfunctional, contains white or muddy bile, and enlarges to 10 to 20 cm in length.

Severe opisthorchiasis has been associated with cirrhosis, obstructive jaundice, pancreatitis, cholangitis, and cholangiocarcinoma.

CLINICAL MANIFESTATIONS. The signs and symptoms are similar for the 3 liver fluke infections: opisthorchiasis viverrini, opisthorchiasis felineus, and clonorchiasis sinensis. In endemic areas, although infection begins early in life, most patients are asymptomatic, have a benign infection, and are diagnosed only on routine stool examination. If symptoms occur, they usually start in the third decade of life or later.

Acute symptoms starting shortly after exposure have been reported only for *C. sinensis* and *O. felineus* infections. They may resemble serum sickness or Katayama fever; following a 2- to 3-week prepatent period, there is irregular high fever, lymph node enlargement, myalgia, arthralgia, rash, and eosinophilia. Facial edema occurs occasionally; an allergic hepatitis has been observed in severe cases.

An early symptom is dull pain or discomfort in the right upper abdominal quadrant that may radiate to the epigastrium and left hypochondrium; typically, it appears in the late afternoon and lasts 1 to 3 hours. The

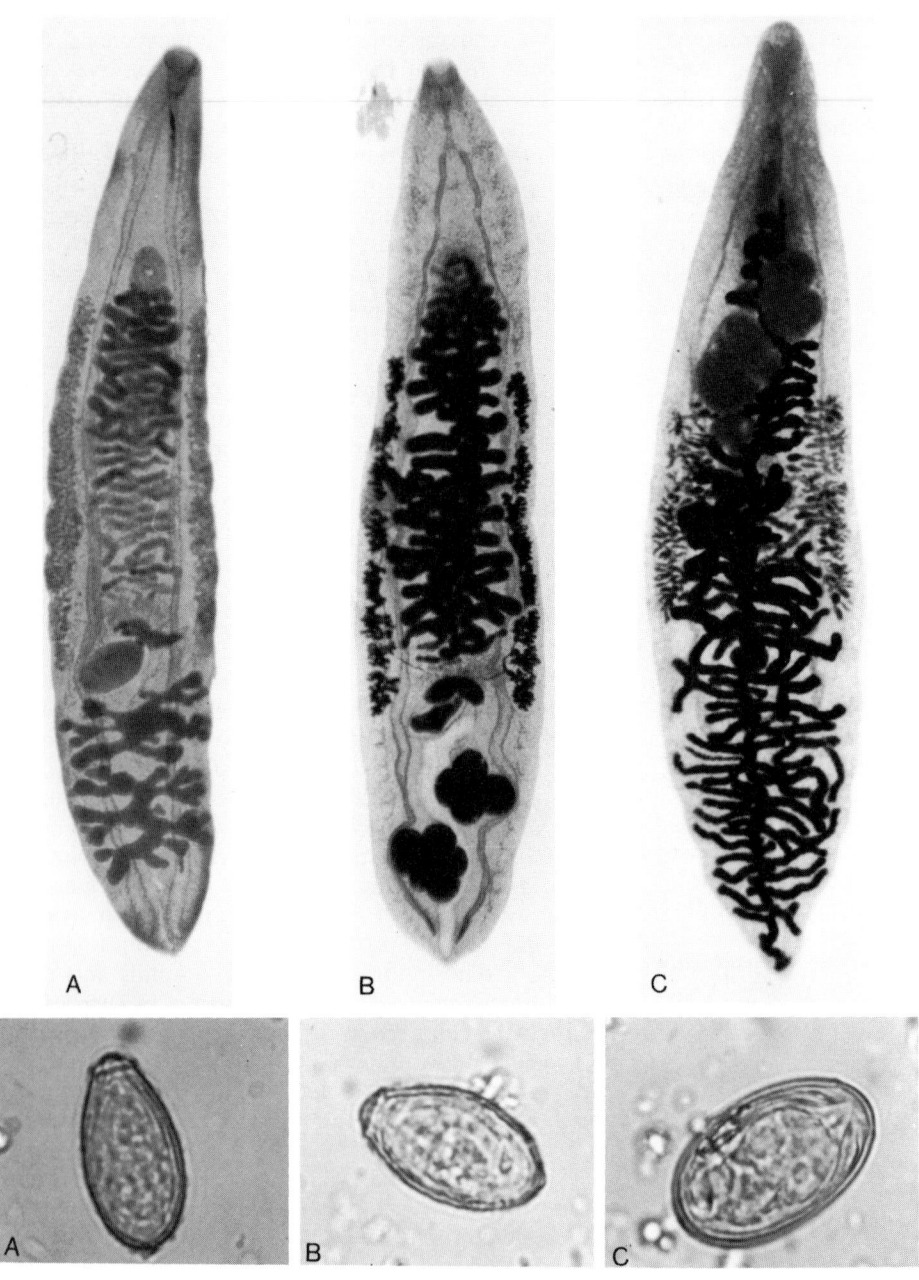

FIGURE 98–1. Small liver flukes. *A*, Adult *Clonorchis sinensis* and egg. *B*, Adult *Opisthorchis viverrini* and egg. *C*, Adult *Dicrocoelium dendriticum* and egg. All eggs photographed at same magnification. (Courtesy of Associate Professor Prayong Radomyos, Faculty of Tropical Medicine, Mahidol University, Bangkok, Thailand.)

pain may return in days or weeks, or there may be intermittent remissions for months or years. With progression, the pain may limit the patient's physical activities. Other symptoms are lassitude, anorexia, flatulence, occasional loose stools, poor appetite, low-grade fever, and hepatomegaly. With associated malnutrition, weight loss and slight pedal edema are common. A peculiar "hot cutaneous sensation," felt over the upper abdomen or the back, is characteristic of opisthorchiasis. It bears no anatomical relation to somatic nerves.

Complications. In the advanced stage of infection, the liver is enlarged, and the gallbladder is palpable and functions poorly. Some patients develop intermittent fever and jaundice from relapsing cholangitis or pyogenic cholangitis.

Cholangiocarcinoma is commonly observed in association with opisthorchiasis. Deterioration is rapid and the outcome fatal.

DIAGNOSIS AND DIFFERENTIAL DIAGNOSIS. Diagnosis is by finding *Opisthorchis* eggs in feces (Figs. VI D–2*F* and 98–1*B*); in patients with biliary obstruction, however, the eggs can be recovered only in bile by needle aspiration or at surgery or autopsy. The eggs are difficult to differentiate from those of the small intestinal flukes, *Metagonimus yokogawai, Heterophyes heterophyes, Phaneropsolus bonnei, Prosthodendrium molenkampi,* and *Haplorchis taichui* (Figs. VI D–2 and 97–4*D–H*). Geographic distribution of the parasites may assist in diagnosis. Definitive diagnosis is by identification of adult worms recovered after anthelminthic treatment, at operation, or at autopsy (Fig. 98–2*B*).

In patients with biliary obstruction, the condition must be differentiated from other causes and from enlarged gallbladder, cholangitis with jaundice, carcinoma of the liver, and cholangiocarcinoma. Often, ultrasonography and liver scanning can show lesions compatible with the

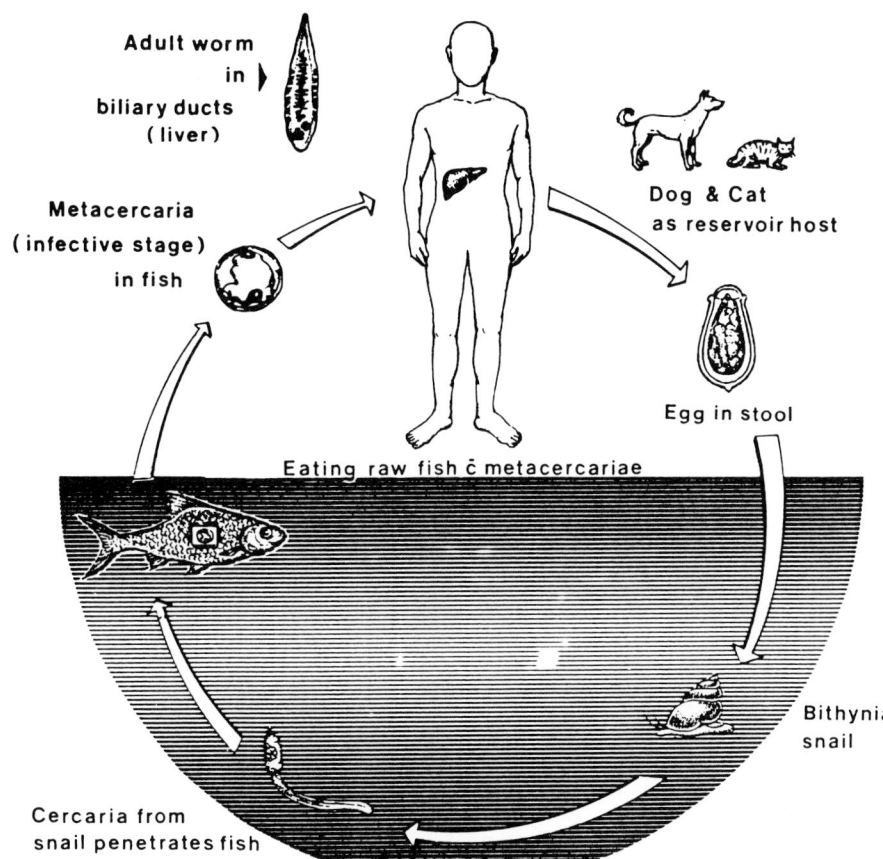

FIGURE 98–2. Life cycle of *Opisthorchis viverrini*.

Adult worm in biliary ducts (liver)

Metacercaria (infective stage) in fish

Dog & Cat as reservoir host

Egg in stool

Eating raw fish c̄ metacercariae

Bithynia snail

Cercaria from snail penetrates fish

infection. Immunodiagnosis by ELISA using crude somatic extracts of *O. viverrini* is available in a few laboratories and may assist in establishing the diagnosis.

TREATMENT AND PROGNOSIS. Praziquantel is highly effective and safe. In asymptomatic and mild to moderate cases, a one-day regimen of 25 mg/kg 3 times after meals, or a single dose of 40 mg/kg yielded 100 and 90% cure rates, respectively. In heavy infection, a single dose of 50 mg/kg gave a cure rate of 97%. Eggs disappear from the feces in 1 week; clinical symptoms

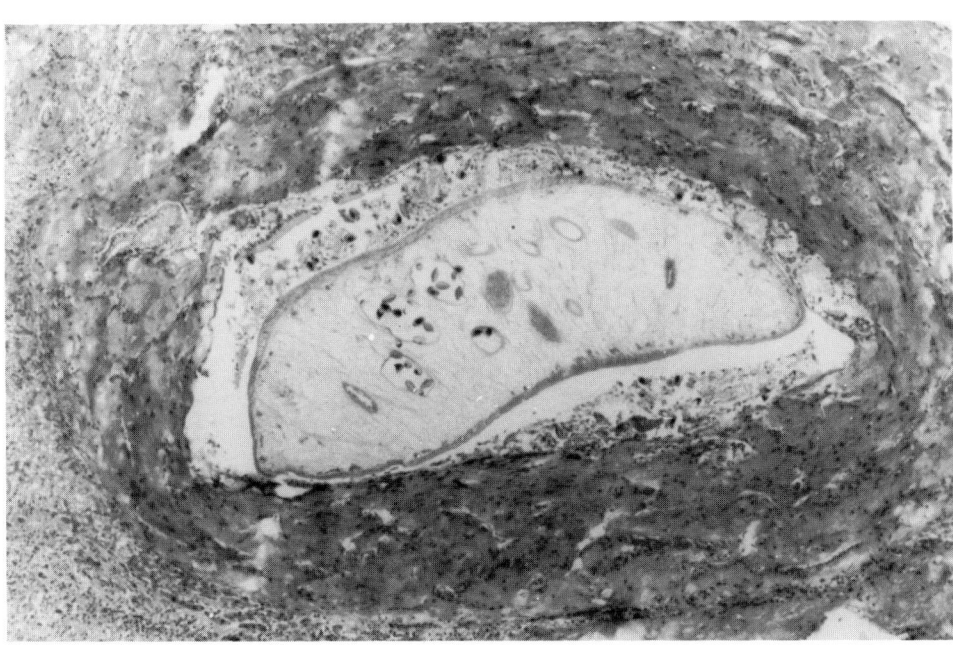

FIGURE 98–3. The bile duct shows marked dilation and glandular hyperplasia of duct epithelium, and a cross-section of *Opisthorchis viverrini* in the lumen. (Courtesy of Dr. M. Riganti, Faculty of Tropical Medicine, Mahidol University, Bangkok, Thailand.)

and a dysfunctioning enlarged gallbladder take several months to return to normal (Fig. 98–4). Drug side effects are mild and transient; they include headache, dizziness, sleepiness, nausea, and vomiting. Administration of the drug at bedtime, if the single dose regimen is used, will minimize side effects.

Mebendazole, 30 mg/kg/day for 3- and 4-week periods gave cure rates of 89 and 94%, respectively. No flukes were recovered post-treatment.

Albendazole at a dosage of 400 mg twice daily for 3 and 7 days gave cure rates of 40 and 63%, and egg excretion was reduced by 92% after each regimen. Most of the flukes were expelled within 3 days of treatment.

Relapsing cholangitis and obstructive jaundice should be treated with antimicrobials also because only 5 to 10% of cases are relieved with praziquantel alone. Palliative surgery may be required in complicated cases with obstructive jaundice.

The prognosis is good in persons with light infections. Death is rare in patients with heavy, long-standing infections that progress to cholangitis and septic shock. Cholangiocarcinoma associated with opisthorchiasis has a poor prognosis.

PREVENTION AND CONTROL. In endemic areas, infection can be prevented by cooking freshwater fish. Extensive health education in concert with local primary health care programs can successfully change local eating habits, improve sanitation, and stop the use of night soil as fertilizer in fish ponds. Mass treatment of infected populations is recommended with praziquantel as a single 40 to 50 mg/kg dose at bedtime; however, at the present time the drug is too expensive for large scale programs in endemic countries. Currently, molluscicide application is impractical and expensive.

BIBLIOGRAPHY

Bunnag D, Harinasuta T: Studies of the chemotherapy of human opisthorchiasis in Thailand: I. Clinical trial of praziquantel. Southeast Asian J Trop Med Public Health 11:528, 1980.
Bunnag D, Harinasuta T: Studies of the chemotherapy of human opisthorchiasis in Thailand: III. Minimum effective dose of praziquantel. Southeast Asian J Trop Med Public Health 12:413, 1981.
Jaroonvesama N, Chareonlarp K, Cross JH: Treatment of *Opisthorchis viverrini* with mebendazole. Southeast Asian J Trop Med Public Health 12:595, 1981.
Pungpark S, Bunnag D, Harinasuta T: Albendazole in treatment of opisthorchiasis and concomitant intestinal helminthic infections. Southeast Asian J Trop Med Public Health 15:44, 1984.

98.2 CLONORCHIASIS

DEFINITION. Clonorchiasis is an infection of the biliary tract by *Clonorchis sinensis*, the Chinese liver fluke. The scientific name of the species is *Opisthorchis sinensis*, but because the genus *Clonorchis* is well established, the name is retained.

ETIOLOGY

Morphology. *C. sinensis*, 10 to 25 mm long and 3 to 5 mm wide, is larger than *O. felineus* and *O. viverrini* (Fig. 98–1A). The eggs are small, 20 to 30 μm long and 15 to 17 μm wide; they resemble those of *O. viverrini* but are broader than those of *O. felineus* (Figs. VI D–2G and 98–1A).

Life Cycle. The life cycle of *C. sinensis* is similar to that of *Opisthorchis* (Fig. 98–2). The first intermediate hosts for *C. sinensis* are hydrobiid snails: *Parafossarulus manchouricus, Bithynia fuchsianus, Alocinma longicornis* in most endemic areas; and *Thiara granifera, Semisulcospira libertina,* and *Melanoid tuberculata* in some areas. The snails live in fish-culturing ponds, lakes, and slow-moving waters. Infection rates in the snails are usually low. The fish second intermediate host is carp of the families Cyprinidae and Anabantidae, among which at least 49 species have been found infected in China, 29 in Korea, 27 in Japan, and 15 in Taiwan. Reservoir (definitive) hosts include dogs, cats, pigs, mink, rats, and other fish-eating mammals.

EPIDEMIOLOGY. Human clonorchiasis is mainly endemic in Japan, Korea, China, Taiwan, and Vietnam, where the first and second intermediate hosts are found and where the populations are accustomed to consuming raw fish, such as sashimi and pickled fish in vinegar (sunomono) in Japan, fish covered with pounded chili paste in Korea, and raw fish congee (*Yu shun chuk*) in Hong Kong. In most endemic areas, fish are raised in ponds fertilized with night soil from human or animal feces. However, the many cases reported from Hong Kong (where neither the snail nor fish intermediate hosts are indigenous) are due to importation of infected fish from China.

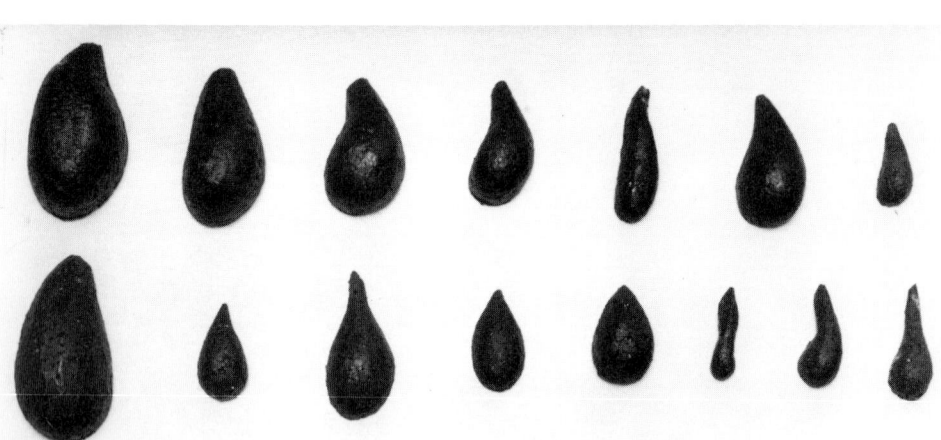

FIGURE 98–4. Models of cholecystography in patients with opisthorchiasis treated with praziquantel and showing pre- and post-fatty meals at intervals of 0, 14, 30, and 180 days. After treatment, function improved gradually, size decreased, and normal state was reached within 6 months.

Over 20 million people in China and 4.5 million in Korea are estimated to be infected. Some reduction in prevalence has occurred among those under age 40 in Japan and Taiwan; this is attributed to industrialization, insecticide pollution of water, land reclamation, and health education, all of which have contributed to a decrease in the snail population. In recent years, clonorchiasis has been reported frequently in the United States, Canada, France, Australia, and other countries, all in refugee immigants from endemic areas.

PATHOLOGY AND PATHOGENESIS. The pathogenesis and pathologic changes in clonorchiasis are similar to those seen in opisthorchiasis (Chapter 98.1).

CLINICAL MANIFESTATIONS. Clinical manifestations are similar to findings in opisthorchiasis (Chapter 98.1). On rare occasions, acute symptoms have been noted in visitors to endemic areas: anorexia, epigastric pain, diarrhea, and leukocytosis with eosinophilia. These findings start 10 to 26 days after consumption of inadequately cooked, massively infected fish and last 2 to 4 weeks. Cholangitis, cholelithiasis, pancreatitis, and cholangiocarcinoma are common complications of chronic infection and can be fatal.

DIAGNOSIS. Diagnosis of clonorchiasis is as for opisthorchiasis (Chapter 98.1).

TREATMENT. The drug of choice is praziquantel, 25 mg/kg after meals 3 times for 1 or 2 days. These regimens yielded cure rates of 85 and 100%, respectively.

PROGNOSIS. The majority of patients do well except those who suffer from pyogenic cholangitis, obstructive jaundice (Fig. 98–5), or associated cholangiocarcinoma.

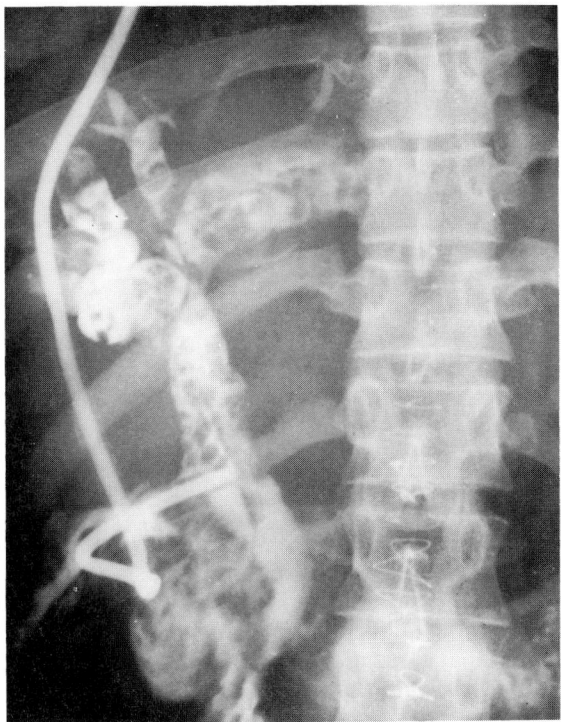

FIGURE 98–5. Clonorchiasis, T-tube cholangiogram demonstrating dilated bile ducts filled with flukes. (Courtesy of the Armed Forces Institute of Pathology, Photograph Neg. No. 69-5522-3.)

PREVENTION AND CONTROL. Prevention is by thorough cooking or freezing of freshwater fish. Educational efforts should be directed toward changing eating habits and improving sanitation. The use of night soil or feces from reservoir hosts for fertilizing fish ponds should be prevented; alternatively, storage of night soil is recommended, for eggs of *C. sinensis* will die within 2 days at 26°C.

BIBLIOGRAPHY

Rim HJ, Lyu K–S: Chemotherapeutic effect of praziquantel (EMBAY 8440) in the treatment of clonorchiasis sinensis. Korea Univ Med J 16:459, 1979.

Xu Z, Zhong H, Cao W: Acute clonorchiasis: Report of 2 cases. Chin Med J 92:423, 1970.

98.3. FASCIOLIASIS

DEFINITION. Fascioliasis (sheep liver fluke disease) is infection by 1 of 2 species: *Fasciola hepatica* or *F. gigantica*. The former occurs principally in temperate climates, the latter in the tropics. They are both common hepatic flukes of sheep and other domestic livestock. In humans, both occasionally infect the bile ducts, the gallbladder, or extrahepatic sites.

FASCIOLA HEPATICA INFECTION

ETIOLOGY

Morphology. *F. hepatica* is relatively flat and leaf-like, fleshy, measures 20 to 30 mm in length by 8 to 13 mm in width, and its broader, anterior portion is covered with scale-like spines. A distinct cephalic cone gives a characteristic shouldered appearance (Fig. 98–6*A*). The eggs are large, ovoid with an inconspicuous operculum, light yellowish-brown, measure 130 to 150 μm by 60 to 90 μm, and are unsegmented when laid (Figs. VI D–2*B* and 98–6*A*).

Life Cycle. The adult parasites live in the large biliary ducts. Eggs passed in host feces require 9 to 15 days for the miracidia to develop and hatch in water of optimal temperatures of 22° to 26°C. The miracidia penetrate various lymnaeid snails, the first intermediate hosts, and develop (within 4 to 7 weeks) from sporocysts, rediae, and daughter rediae to cercariae. The mature cercariae emerge from the snail and encyst within hours as minute white spherules on various kinds of aquatic vegetation; a few sink to the bottom, where they develop into metacercariae.

When metacercariae are ingested, they excyst in the duodenum, migrate through the intestinal wall into the peritoneal cavity, subsequently leave through Glisson's capsule, and then traverse the liver parenchyma into the bile ducts, where they grow to maturity. The prepatent period in humans may take 3 to 4 months. Although the life span of the flukes in humans is not known, it is about 3 years in rabbits and at least 5 in sheep.

Numerous species of amphibious snails of the genus

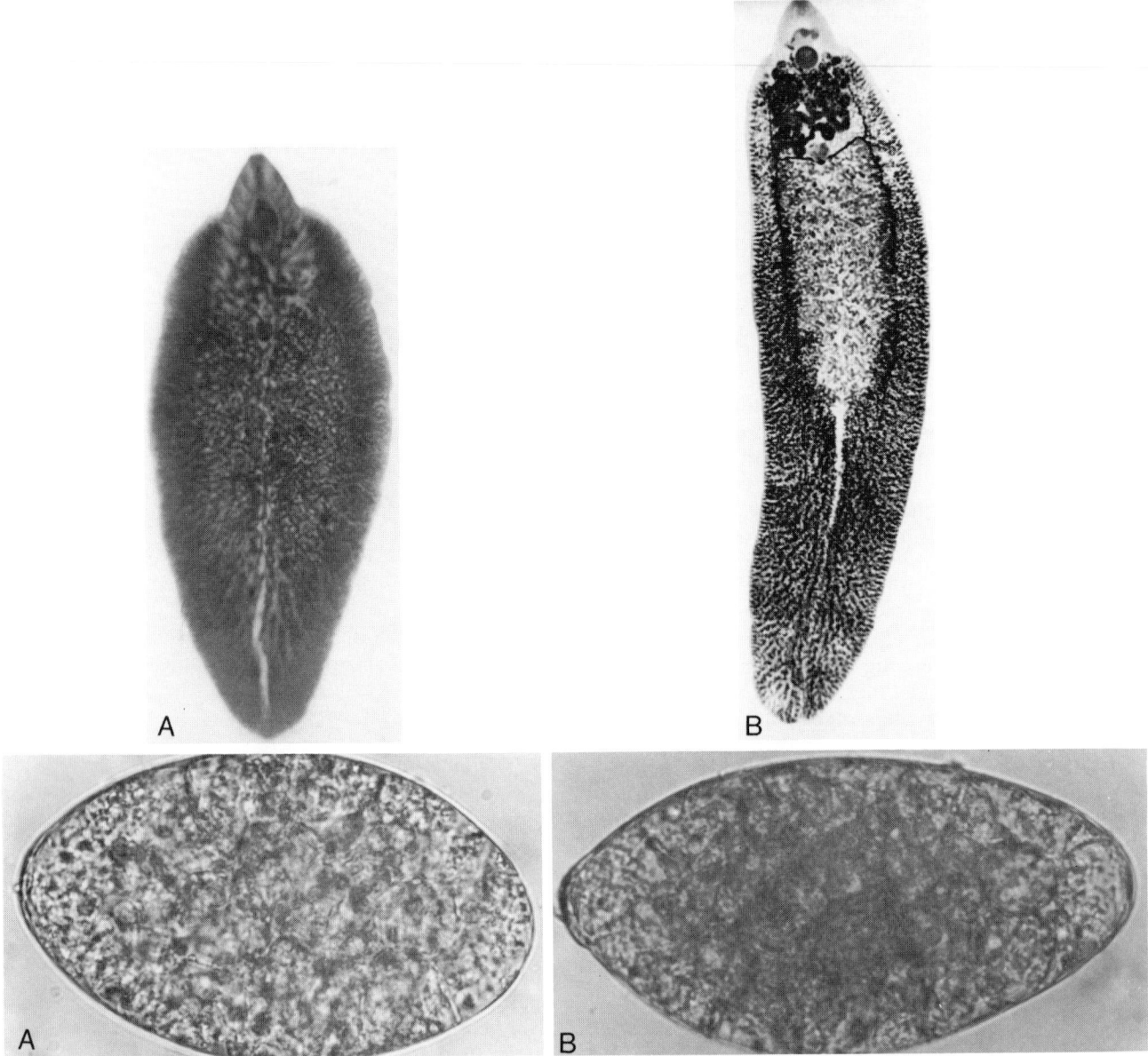

FIGURE 98–6. Large liver flukes. *A,* Adult *Fasciola hepatica* (3 cm) and egg (130 to 150 μm × 60 to 90 μm). *B,* Adult *Fasciola gigantica* (7 cm) and egg (160 to 190 μm × 70 to 90 μm). (Courtesy of Associate Professor Prayong Radomyos, Faculty of Tropical Medicine, Mahidol University, Bangkok, Thailand.)

Lymnaea serve as intermediate hosts. *L. truncatula* is the most important and widespread host in Europe, Africa, and north Asia; *L. bulimoides* is the principal host in North America and *L. tomentosa* in Australia.

The most important definitive hosts are sheep, but other herbivores, including goats, cattle, horses, camels, hogs, vicuna, rabbits, and deer, are commonly infected.

EPIDEMIOLOGY. *F. hepatica* has a cosmopolitan distribution, being prevalent in most sheep-raising areas. Sporadic human fascioliasis hepatica has been reported from mainland United States and Hawaii, South America (Venezuela, Uruguay, Argentina, Chile, Colombia, Mexico, Cuba, Puerto Rico, Costa Rica, Brazil), Europe (France, England, Poland, the USSR, Italy, Corsica, Spain, Hungary, Romania, Turkey), Africa (Egypt, Somaliland, Algeria, South Africa), and Asia and the Middle East (Japan, China, Iran, Syria).

Human infection is usually acquired by eating watercress grown in sheep-raising areas.

PATHOGENESIS AND PATHOLOGY. Experimental animal studies indicate that migrating metacercariae cause local hepatic parenchymal destruction, necrosis, and abscess formation. Adult flukes may cause hyperplasia, desquamation, thickening, and dilatation of the bile ducts. Sheep heavily infected with *F. hepatica* develop "liver rot"; the amount of tissue damage is correlated with the worm load; 600 flukes will cause death. Although infection in humans is usually mild, rarely, in heavy infections there is extensive liver parenchymal necrosis that sometimes results in internal hemorrhage. Ectopic fascioliasis is common.

The fluke's antigens provoke various types of complement fixing, precipitating, and hemagglutinating antibodies.

CLINICAL MANIFESTATIONS. Clinical findings relate to the phase of infection.

Acute Phase. Acute symptoms may persist for several weeks to months. They occur during the period in which the larval flukes migrate through the liver and stop when the larvae penetrate the bile ducts. Patients may develop acute dyspepsia, anorexia, nausea, vomiting, prolonged high fever, abdominal pain in the right hypochondrium and, sometimes, hepatomegaly, hepatic tenderness, and urticaria with marked eosinophilia. Severe illness with prostration and jaundice is unusual. Asymptomatic acute infection has been reported and seems to be common in Peru.

Chronic Phase. Most will have few or no symptoms after the flukes have lodged in the biliary passages. However, some patients have pain in the epigastrium and right hypochondrium, diarrhea, nausea, vomiting, hepatomegaly, and jaundice. If the flukes lodge in the extrahepatic biliary ducts, symptoms may be those of cholelithiasis. Abnormal liver function and eosinophilia are common.

Ectopic Infection Sites. Aberrant sites (e.g., lungs, intestinal wall, heart, brain, skin) are observed frequently. Manifestations are visceral larval migrans-like, including vague abdominal migratory pain to severe colic when the biliary tract is involved. Exploratory abdominal surgery may be needed to make the diagnosis.

Halzoun. In endemic areas, acute nasopharyngitis known as "halzoun" in Lebanon or "marrara" in Sudan is caused by eating raw infected liver of sheep or goats. Young flukes emerge from the ingested liver and attach to mucosa in the laryngopharyngeal region, where they induce irritation and edema that results in discomfort, dysphagia, and dyspnea.

Laboratory Findings. These may include leukocytosis with relative hypereosinophilia, anemia, increased erythrocyte sedimentation rate, hypergammaglobulinemia, abnormal liver function tests, and eosinophilic hyperplasia of the bone marrow.

DIAGNOSIS. In enzootic areas, fascioliasis is suspected in patients suffering from fever, hepatomegaly, and eosinophilia who have a history of consuming raw freshwater plants. Serologic tests (indirect hemagglutination, complement fixation, counterimmunoelectrophoresis, ELISA) are particularly useful for diagnosing ectopic disease and in the early acute phase when the flukes are young and eggs have not appeared yet in the feces. Liver biopsy sometimes demonstrates the flukes or compatible lesions.

Definitive diagnosis is by finding the eggs in feces or sometimes by duodenal aspiration. Spurious infection must be ruled out. As the eggs of *F. hepatica* (Fig. 98–6*A*), *F. gigantica* (Fig. 98–6*B*), and *F. buski* (97–1*B*) are similar and difficult to distinguish from each other (Fig. VI D–2), recovery of adult flukes at surgery, autopsy (Fig. 98–6*A*), or after anthelminthics confirms the diagnosis.

TREATMENT. Bithionol given orally at a dose of 1 gm 3 times a day on alternate days to a total dosage of 45 gm is the preferred drug and has little toxicity. In biliary infection, praziquantel is sometimes effective at a dosage of 25 mg/kg 3 times daily after meals for 2 days. In Egypt, praziquantel has not been effective. Treatment with potentially toxic drugs, such as emetine hydrochloride, or extended treatment with chloroquine has been of little value.

PREVENTION AND CONTROL. Prevention is by not eating watercress salad in endemic areas and by thoroughly cooking sheep and goat livers. In endemic-enzootic areas, control measures are elimination of snail intermediate hosts by adequate drainage of pastures, application of effective molluscicides (e.g., copper sulfate and frescon), and by adequate therapy of definitive herbivorous animal hosts (e.g., with Niclofolan).

FASCIOLA GIGANTICA INFECTION

Fasciola gigantica is a species closely related to *F. hepatica*; it infects domestic livestock in tropical and subtropical areas and sometimes infects humans.

GEOGRAPHIC DISTRIBUTION. *F. gigantica* is the common liver fluke of herbivorous mammals, particularly cattle in Africa, southern Europe, southern United States and Hawaii, USSR, the Middle East, and Southest Asia. Mixed *F. gigantica* and *F. hepatica* infections have been reported from highland areas of Pakistan.

ETIOLOGY

Morphology. *F. gigantica* resembles *F. hepatica* and may attain a length of 7.5 cm; it is more lanceolate, however, and has a less distinct cephalic cone (Fig. 98–6*B*). Its eggs are larger, measuring 160 to 190 μm by 70 to 90 μm (Figs. VI D–2*A* and 98–6*B*).

The snail hosts of *F. gigantica* belong to the *Lymnaea* (*Radix*) *auricularia* complex: *L. auricularia rufescens* in the Indian subcontinent, *L. auricularia rubiginosa* in Malaysia and Thailand, and *L. natalensis* in Africa.

EPIDEMIOLOGY. Infection develops in a wide range of susceptible mammals, the definitive hosts, when they ingest infected aquatic vegetation or water containing encysted metacercariae (white spherules). Infection rates in herbivorous mammals may be high in endemic areas: in China, cattle (50%), goats (45%), and water buffalo (33%); in Iraq, water buffalo (71%) and cattle (27%); and in northeast Thailand, cattle (60%). Human fascioliasis gigantica has been reported occasionally from Zimbabwe, Uganda, Tashkent in the USSR, Iraq, Vietnam, Hawaii, and Thailand, areas in which infection in animals is not common.

The prepatent period in the definitive host, from infection until the worms complete liver migration and reach the bile ducts, is 9 to 12 weeks.

CLINICAL MANIFESTATIONS, DIAGNOSIS, AND TREATMENT. The life cycle, pathology, and clinical manifestations of *F. gigantica* are similar to those of *F. hepatica*. Patients may have fever, abdominal pain, nausea, vomiting, hepatomegaly, hepatic tenderness, and eosinophilia; unrecognized milder manifestations undoubtedly exist. *F. gigantica* has been observed frequently in ectopic locations. In some cases, *F. gigantica* has induced an abscess or tumor-like reaction either in subcutaneous tissue or in the liver (Fig. 98–7).

Eggs are often absent from the stool. Serodiagnosis

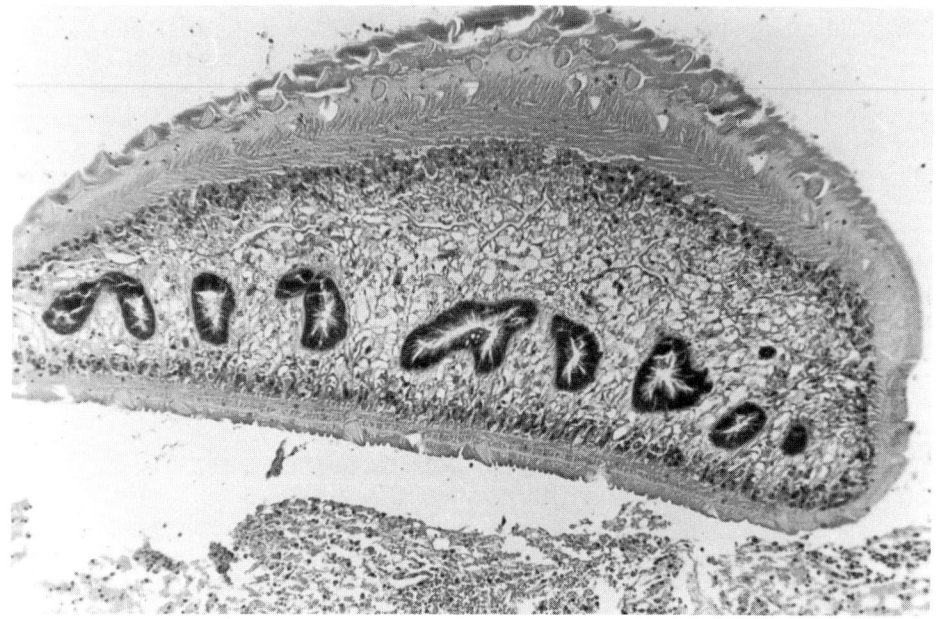

FIGURE 98–7. Histologic section of *Fasciola gigantica* from a Thai patient, showing necrotic and hemorrhagic areas of liver parenchyma.

is inconclusive, but fascioliasis gigantica can sometimes be excluded on geographic grounds. Recovery of adult flukes by surgical exploration confirms the diagnosis.

Treatment and preventive measures are similar to those for *F. hepatica*.

BIBLIOGRPAHY

Hillyer GV: Fascioliasis in Puerto Rico: A review. Bol Asoc Med PR 73:94, 1981.
Jones EA, Kay JM, Milligan HP, et al: Massive infection with *Fasciola hepatica* in man. Am J Med 63:836, 1977.
Parichatikanond P, Sarasas A: Human biliary fascioliasis: Report of the first case in Thailand. Siriraj Hosp Gaz 36:131, 1984.
Stork MG, Venables GS, Jennings SMF, et al: An investigation of endemic fascioliasis in Peruvian village children. J Trop Med Hyg 76:231, 1973.

98.4. DICROCOELIASIS AND EURYTREMIASIS

DEFINITION. Dicrocoeliasis and eurytremiasis are infections of the bile ducts and pancreatic ducts of herbivorous animals by trematodes of the genus *Dicrocoelium dendriticum* and *Eurytrema pancreaticum*. The parasites rarely infect humans; when they do, however, they are more commonly spurious infections due to ingestion of infected animal livers.

ETIOLOGY

Morphology. The dicrocoeliid fluke is transparent, flat and lanceolate, and measures 5 to 15 mm long by 1.5 to 2.5 mm wide (Fig. 98–1*C*). Its eggs are dark-brown, 38 to 45 μm by 22 to 30 μm, operculated, thick-shelled, and fully embryonated when laid (Figs. VI D–2*I* and 98–1*C*). *E. pancreaticum* (8 to 16 mm by 5 to 9 mm) is more ovate and broader than *D. dendriticum*. Eggs of the 2 species are indistinguishable.

Life Cycle. The life cycles of the 2 trematodes are similar and require 2 intermediate hosts, a snail and an insect. The adult flukes live in the biliary and pancreatic passages of the herbivore. Eggs are passed in the feces and ingested by land snails, which are the first intermediate host. The snail hosts of *D. denriticum* are *Zebrina detrita* and *Helicella candidula* in Europe, *Cionella lubrica* in North America, and *Bradybaena similaris* in Malaysia. Two generations of sporocysts develop in the snail. Cercariae are released in slime balls shed by the snail on vegetation as it crawls along. The cercariae develop into infective metacercariae only if ingested by ants, the second intermediate hosts: *Formica fusca* in the United States and Germany, *F. gigantis* or *F. rufibarbis* in the Middle East, and *F. cinerea* and *F. picea* in the central USSR. Snail hosts for *E. pancreaticum* in China are *Ganesella* species. For second intermediate hosts, *E. pancreaticum* uses grasshoppers (*Conocephalus maculatus*) in Malaysia and tree crickets (*Oecanthus longicaudus*) in the USSR. The life cycle is completed when the infected insects are eaten by grazing herbivores. The metacercariae excyst and migrate to the biliary passage for *D. dendriticum* and to the pancreatic ducts for *E. pancreaticum* where they develop to adults.

Humans become infected when they accidentally eat infected ants or grasshoppers.

GEOGRAPHIC DISTRIBUTION AND EPIDEMIOLOGY. *D. dendriticum* is a common parasite in the bile ducts of sheep, deer, water buffalo, and cattle. Its enzootic distribution is reported from Europe, Turkey, northern Africa, and parts of the Far East. Most reported human cases were spurious infections; a few genuine human cases have rarely been reported from Europe, Egypt, Iran, Nigeria, Ivory Coast, and China.

E. pancreaticum is a common parasite of pancreatic ducts and rarely of the bile ducts of herbivorous mammals (cattle, sheep, goats, monkeys, and camels). Eurytremiasis has been reported in humans in Hong Kong, Kiang-Su Province in China, and at least 6 times in Japan, twice at autopsy.

CLINICAL MANIFESTATIONS. Dicrocoeliasis and eurytremiasis usually cause mild symptoms. In heavy infections, however, there may be vague biliary and gastrointestinal disturbances, including abdominal distress, flatulence, biliary colic, vomiting, and diarrhea or constipation. Jaundice, an enlarged liver, and systemic symptoms are reported occasionally. Eosinophilia is rare.

DIAGNOSIS. Diagnosis is made by finding the characteristic eggs in feces, bile, or duodenal fluid (Fig. 98–1C). Spurious infection must be ruled out by repeated fecal examination. Definitive diagnosis is by recovery of adult flukes at surgery or autopsy (Fig. 98–1C).

TREATMENT. Praziquantel is recommended at the same dose as for opisthorchiasis. Bithionol may be effective also.

PREVENTION AND CONTROL. As infection in humans is generally accidental, no preventive measures are effective.

BIBLIOGRAPHY

Ishii Y, Koga M, Fujino T, et al: Human infection with the pancreas fluke *Eurytrema pancreaticum.* Am J Trop Med Hyg 32:1019, 1983.

99. LUNG FLUKE INFECTIONS: PARAGONIMIASIS

Robert Goldsmith, Danai Bunnag, and Thanongsak Bunnag

DEFINITION. Paragonimiasis is infection by lung flukes of the genus *Paragonimus,* the most common of which is the oriental lung fluke, *P. westermani.* The adult worms usually live encapsulated in pockets in the lung, but may be found also in extrapulmonary locations.

ETIOLOGY. About 48 species and subspecies of *Paragonimus* have been described, some of which may not be valid. In animal hosts, they appear to be widely distributed; in humans, 7 species are known to cause disease.

Paragonimus species are distinguishable by their cuticular spines, ovarian shape, relative size of oral and ventral suckers, ova characteristics, chromosomes, and migration route in tissues.

Morphology. The living adult parasites are reddish-brown, ovoid, and have a broad anterior end. They measure 7 to 16 mm in length, 4 to 8 mm in width, and 2 to 5 mm in thickness. The tegument is covered with cuticular spines (Fig. 99–1A). The eggs are golden brown, asymmetrically ovoid with a thick shell, have a relatively flattened operculum, measure 80 to 120 μm by 50 to 65 μm, and are immature when deposited (Fig. 99–1B).

Life Cycle. The adult flukes live in and lay eggs within a pulmonary cyst (Fig. 99–2). The eggs are passed along a tunnel that connects to a large bronchus and are expectorated with sputum or swallowed and passed in feces. On reaching water, they embryonate and hatch

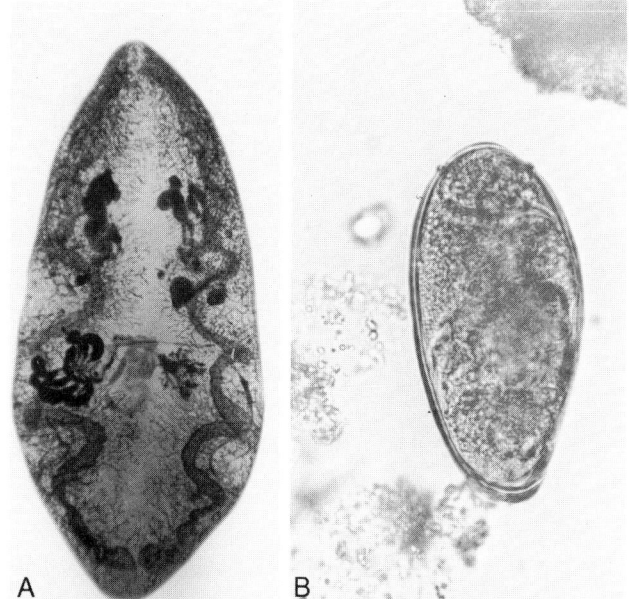

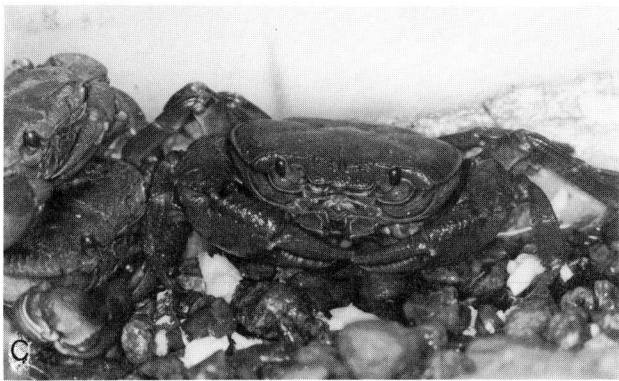

FIGURE 99–1. Adult *Paragonimus heterotremus* (A) and egg (B). Mountainous stream crab *Larnaudia beusekomae* (Tawaripotamon) (C) is an important second intermediate host of paragonimiasis in Thailand. (Courtesy of Associate Professor Prayong Radomyos, Faculty of Tropical Medicine, Mahidol University, Bangkok, Thailand.)

in about 3 weeks into miracidia that invade the tissues of appropriate snails (the first intermediate host), in which they undergo asexual transformation into sporocysts, rediae, and daughter rediae. Cercariae emerge from the snails in 3 to 5 months and penetrate crustaceans (crabs or crayfish) (the second intermediate host), in which they develop to become infective-stage metacercariae in 6 to 8 weeks. However, some crabs acquire infection by eating infected snails. When infected crustaceans are eaten raw by a mammalian host (the definitive host), the metacercariae excyst in the duodenum, penetrate the intestinal wall into the abdominal cavity, and then migrate through the abdominal wall into the liver, where, after about a week, they grow to young flukes. The flukes reappear in the abdominal cavity and then penetrate the diaphragm to enter the lung tissue, where, enclosed in a pseudocapsule, they grow to adult worms in 5 to 6 weeks. Eggs are produced and appear in the sputum or feces as early as 8 to 10 weeks after infection. In humans, flukes have been known to live for over 20 years.

INTERMEDIATE HOSTS. About 20 species of

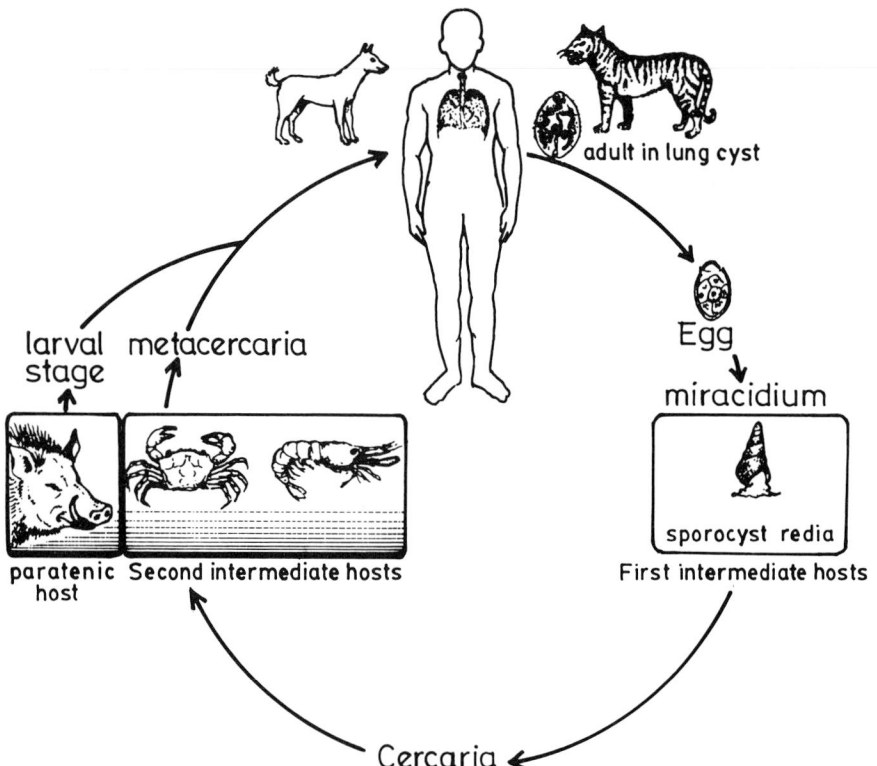

FIGURE 99–2. Life cycle of *Paragonimus heterotremus*.

freshwater snails serve as hosts, mainly members of the families Thiaridae, Pleuroceridae, and Pomatiopsidae. Important snail hosts in China, Japan, Korea, and Taiwan are the pleurocerid *Semisulcospira (Melania) libertina* and *Tricula gregoriana*, and the thiarid *Thiara (Tarebia) granifera*; in the Philippines, *Brotia asperata*; in Malaysia, *B. costula episcopalis* and other melanoid-allied species. Crustacean intermediate hosts are several kinds of freshwater crabs: in China, Japan, and Taiwan, they are *Eriocheir japonicus, Potamon dehaani,* and *P. rathburni*; in Thailand, *Larnaudia (Tawaripotamon) buesekomae* (Fig. 99–1C); in the Philippines, *Sundathelphusa philippina*; and in Korea, the crayfish *Cambaroides similis*. The freshwater shrimp, *Macrobrachium nipponensis* and *Caridina* species, are of less importance as secondary intermediate hosts in Japan, Korea, and China; other crustacean species are hosts elsewhere in the world. In endemic areas of Japan, some mammals (e.g., rat, mouse, pig, and wild boar) serve as paratenic hosts and as sources of human infection when they carry the immature fluke in their muscles (Fig. 99–2).

EPIDEMIOLOGY. Paragonimiasis is essentially a zoonotic disease among carnivorous animals throughout the world, but there are 3 main endemic foci of human paragonimiasis: Asia, Africa, and Central and South America (Table 99–1).

Geographic Distribution. In Asia, several million people are infected; the infection is prevalent particularly in Korea, China, Japan, and Taiwan but also occurs in India, Sri Lanka, Malaysia, Papua New Guinea, Thailand, Laos, Vietnam, and the Philippines. Of the approximately 25 zoonotic species of *Paragonimus* in Asia and Oceania, 4 cause infections of humans: *P. wester-*

mani, P. (szechuanensis) skrjabini, P. miyazakii, and *P. (tuanshanensis) heterotremus.*

In Africa, where *P. africanus* and *P. uterobilateralis* have been identified in humans and animals, paragonimiasis is endemic in eastern Nigeria, Cameroon, Liberia, Guinea, and The Gambia. In Central and South America, where *P. mexicanus* is the principal species in humans and animals, human infections have been reported in Mexico, Guatemala, Panama, Colombia, Peru, Ecuador, Costa Rica, Honduras, Venezuela, El Salvador, and Nicaragua.

TABLE 99–1. Geographic Distribution of Confirmed Lung Flukes in Humans

Species	Country
Paragonimus westermani (Kerbert, 1818)	China, Japan, Korea, Taiwan, India, Sri Lanka, Thailand, Laos, Indonesia, Philippines, USSR, Solomon Islands, Western and American Samoa
Paragonimus heterotremus (Chen and Hsia, 1964; Syn. *P. tuanshanensis*)	Thailand, Laos, China
Paragonimus skrjabini (Chen, 1959; Syn. *P. szechuanensis*)	China
Paragonimus miyazakii (Kamo et al., 1961)	Japan
Paragonimus africanus (Voelker and Vogel, 1965)	Cameroon, Nigeria
Paragonimus uterobilateralis (Voelker and Vogel, 1965)	Cameroon, Nigeria, Liberia, Congo, Guinea
Paragonimus mexicanus (Miyazaki and Ishii, 1968; Syn. *P. peruvianus* and *P. ecuadoriensis*	Mexico, Guatemala, Panama, Colombia, Peru, Ecuador, Costa Rica, Honduras, Venezuela, El Salvador, Nicaragua, Canada

Transmission. Contributing factors responsible for transmission of infection to humans include presence of a large number of reservoir hosts (human and animals), abundance of first and second intermediate hosts, and social customs among certain Asian populations of eating raw or inadequately cooked crabs, crayfish, or shrimp. Infection results from such dishes as "Drunken-crab" (immersion of live crabs in wine for 12 hours), raw crab sauce or jam, and crayfish-curd in China; in Thailand, *Kung Ten* (raw shrimp salad) and *Nam Prik Poo* (crab sauce); in the Philippines, *Sinugba* (roasted crab) and *Kinilao* (raw crab); and in Korea, *Ke Jang* (crab immersed in soy sauce). In Korea and Japan, raw juice of crabs or crayfish is used in traditional medicine in treatment of measles, diarrhea, and urticaria. Another source of infection is contamination of utensils, chopping blocks, and cloths used during food preparation. In Africa, some women have the local custom of eating raw crustaceans to increase fertility. In Kyushu in Japan, humans have been infected by eating raw infected wild boar meat, a paratenic host.

The prevalence of paragonimiasis, as assessed by intradermal test in 21 provinces of China, ranged from 15 to 45%, and in South Korea from 0.3 to 78%.

PATHOLOGY AND PATHOGENESIS. The wide variation in pathologic findings depends on the number of infecting worms, duration of infection, and tissues affected. Toxic and allergic factors may be involved also.

Pulmonary Lesions. Migrating larval flukes in the lung (and frequently in other tissues) induce local necrosis, hemorrhage, and inflammatory exudate, which are followed by fibrous encapsulation into a "worm cyst" (Fig. 99–3). In the lungs, initial lesions are located usually a few centimeters beneath the pleural surface, near bronchioles or bronchi. Pathology includes bronchopneumonia, interstitial pneumonia, bronchitis, bronchiectasis, atelectasis, fibrosis, pleural thickening, angiitis obliterans, and periphlebitis.

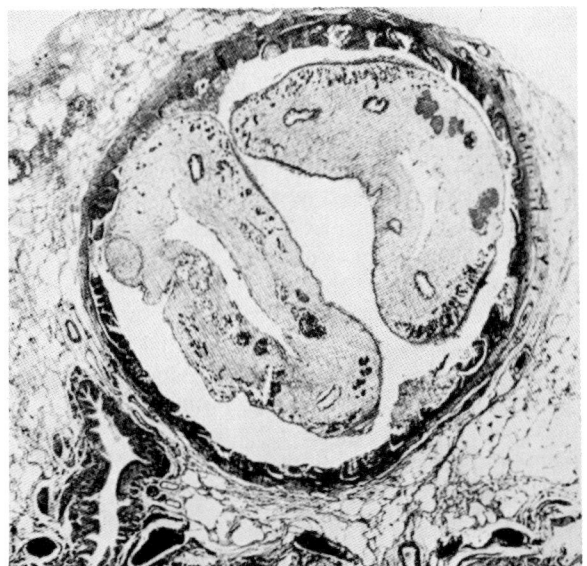

FIGURE 99–3. *Paragonimus westermani* in the lung of a Bengal tiger. (Courtesy of Dr. T. W. M. Cameron, Macdonald College of McGill University.)

Macroscopically, the worm cysts are generally 1 to 4 cm, distended, grayish-white nodules. In cross-section, they have irregular outlines and cavities; within are generally 1 to 2 worms, uncommonly 3 to 4 or none. The total number of cysts in the lungs is usually less than 20, with the larger proportion located in the right lung.

Microscopically, the cyst wall consists of granulation tissue with fibroblasts, lymphoid cells, mononuclear cells, plasma cells, and eosinophils. Within the cavity are numerous Charcot-Leyden crystals, *Paragonimus* eggs, and necrotic material. In the vicinity of the cysts are tunnels, burrows, egg tubercles, and calcified eggs.

Ectopic Lesions. Though uncommon, young or even mature flukes may migrate from the lungs and reach almost any organ, including the psoas muscle, testes, scrotum, spermatic cord, liver, gut wall, other abdominal viscera, uterine and vaginal wall, and spinal cord. In the ectopic site, the flukes reach sexual maturity. Cysts, granulomas, or abscess may then form around the flukes or their eggs. Some immature flukes migrate from the lungs through the jugular or carotid foramen at the base of the skull to reach the temporal and occipital lobes of the brain, where they produce necrosis and eosinophilic granulomatous reactions. In China, migratory subcutaneous swellings are particularly common with *P. skrjabini* infection, and ova have been found at the centers of small eosinophilic granulomas in such aberrant sites as the pericardium, meninges, and liver.

CLINICAL MANIFESTATIONS. In light infections, the majority of patients are asymptomatic. In heavy infections, patients may have few symptoms and appear well despite severe pathology.

Acute Stage. This stage corresponds to the period of invasion and migration of the young flukes. Although this stage often passes undiagnosed, findings may include diarrhea, abdominal pain, urticaria, and eosinophilia, followed by fever, chest pain, cough, dyspnea, malaise, and night sweats.

Pulmonary Paragonimiasis. The incubation period is about 6 months (range, 1 to 27 months). Cough, sputum, and chest discomfort increase gradually, and are similar to those seen in chronic bronchitis. The cough is spasmodic, usually occurs on walking or after exertion, and is productive of a characteristic gelatinous, tenacious, rusty-brown or golden-flake sputum. About half of the patients complain of breathlessness on exertion and some of wheezing. Mild fever may be present. Episodic pleuritic pain and frank hemoptysis are common; the latter is induced usually by heavy work, and rarely is severe and life-threatening. Physical signs in the chest are not distinct; digital clubbing may be seen. Pulmonary tuberculosis may coexist; secondary bronchopneumonia and lung abscess are complications.

Laboratory tests show normal hemoglobin with relative eosinophilic leukocytosis. Chest radiographs in the early stage show ill-defined opacities (Fig. 99–4). Later radiographic findings include cysts (that may have a ring shadow with a crescent-shaped opacity along one side) (Fig. 99–5), extensive infiltration (nodular, exudative, or linear), calcified foci, pleural thickening, loculated

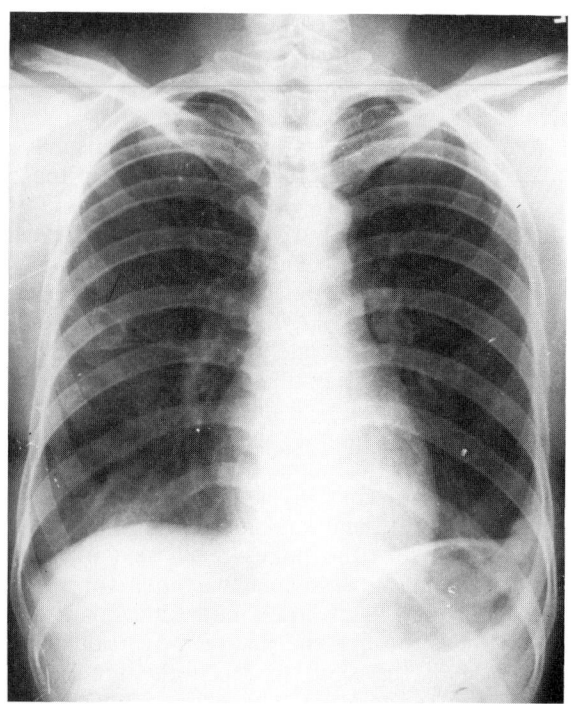

FIGURE 99–4. Pulmonary paragonimiasis. Chest roentgenogram shows thick-walled cystic lesion in the right upper lobe with pericystic fibrosis and thickening of the interlobular septum on both lower lobes. (Courtesy of Associate Professor Sirivan Vanijanonda, Faculty of Tropical Medicine, Mahidol University, Bangkok, Thailand.)

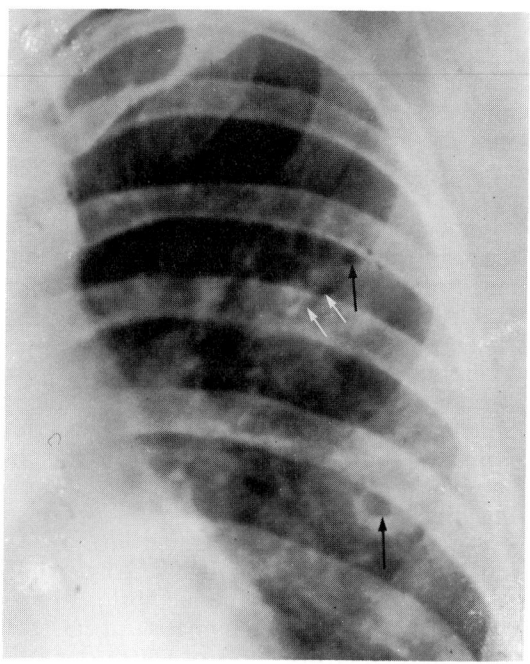

FIGURE 99–5. Pulmonary paragonimiasis with ring shadows (black arrows) and linear lucency (white arrows) representing burrow tract. (Courtesy of R. Suwanik Dhonburi, Thailand.) (From Markell EK, Voge M, John DT: Medical Parasitology. 6th ed. Philadelphia, W.B. Saunders Company, 1986.)

pleural effusions, multilocular cavities, and hilar enlargement.

Cerebral and Spinal Paragonimiasis. In endemic areas of Asia, 25% of hospitalized cases are due to brain invasion. Eighty percent of these patients are under age 10 and most are males. Cerebral disease is particularly prevalent in rural South Korea, where it is the most common cause of cerebral tumor. Up to 10 round or oval cysts, a few mm to 10 cm in diameter, are found in the temporal and occipital lobes, near the jugular foramen.

In the acute phase, manifestations may resemble meningoencephalitis. There is headache, vomiting, fever, and visual disturbances. With progression, patients may have papilledema, bitemporal hemianopsia, facial palsy, hemiplegia, paraplegia, Jacksonian seizures, and coma. Death during the acute attack is not uncommon. In nonfatal cases there is spontaneous remission in 1 to 2 months, but recurrence may occur within 2 years.

Pleocytosis of the cerebrospinal fluid with a high eosinophil count is common. Plain skull radiographs show signs of increased intracranial pressure or cerebral calcification. Cysts can be demonstrated by computerized axial tomography or angiography.

Rarely, spinal cord involvement presents as paraplegia or monoplegia, with weakness of the extremities and disturbance in sensation.

Abdominal Paragonimiasis. Findings may include abdominal pain and tenderness, bloody diarrhea, nausea, vomiting, palpable nodules, and abscess formation in the liver, spleen, or abdominal cavity that may simulate a bacterial infection. In some instances, cyst rupture

into the intestinal lumen releases *Paragonimus* eggs that can be recovered in the feces.

Migratory Subcutaneous Paragonimiasis. Migratory subcutaneous nodules occur in 20 to 60% of patients with *P. skrjabini* and 10% of those with *P. westermani* infections. They are firm, slightly mobile, tender, a few mm to 10 cm in diameter, and often are mildly irritating. The most common sites are the lower abdomen, inguinal region, and thigh; nodules up to 6 cm in diameter have also been seen behind the ear lobe.

In China, *P. westermani* var *szechuanensis* (*P. huei-tungensis*) is unable to develop to maturity in the lungs. Instead of findings of hemoptysis and ova in the sputum, the striking feature is "trematode larva migrans," associated with migratory subcutaneous nodules accompanied by marked eosinophilic leukocytosis. In many cases, the nodules contain juvenile flukes. Brain involvement with subarachnoid hemorrhage is common.

DIAGNOSIS. A presumptive diagnosis can be made in a patient with a history of chronic bronchitis, blood-streaked sputum, and occasional hemoptysis who lives in an endemic area and has eaten raw crustaceans. Confirmation is by finding characteristic eggs in sputum, stool, pleural effusion, or cerebral spinal fluid (Fig. 99–1B), or adult flukes in subcutaneous nodules, in other surgical specimens, or rarely in sputum (Fig. 99–1A).

Immunodiagnosis by complement fixation, counter-current immunoelectrophoresis, and ELISA, especially in extrapulmonary disease, can help establish the diagnosis. Most treated cases become seronegative after about 6 months. Intradermal tests have been used in screening in epidemiologic surveys.

Differential diagnosis of pulmonary paragonimiasis includes pulmonary tuberculosis, lung abscess, chronic pulmonary infection of other causes, and primary and metastatic pulmonary carcinoma. Cerebral and spinal paragonimiasis must be differentiated from abscess, tuberculoma, and othe₁ helminthic infections, including fascioliasis, schistosomiasis japonica, cysticercosis, hydatid disease, angiostrongyliasis, and gnathostomiasis.

Abdominal symptoms mimic many acute conditions, including appendicitis and amebic liver abscess. Subcutaneous paragonimiasis may be confused with gnathostomiasis, sparganosis, and onchocerciasis.

TREATMENT. The drug of choice is praziquantel at 25 mg/kg 3 times at 4 hour intervals after meals for 3 days. The cure rate is almost 100%; only a few cases with heavy infections need a second course of treatment. Symptoms improve rapidly and disappear within a few months. Eggs clear from the sputum in a few weeks, whereas the radiologic pulmonary lesions take some months to clear, depending on duration and severity of the disease. Drug side effects, including drowsiness and headaches, are mild and transient. The dosage in cerebral paragonimiasis is often higher and must be adjusted according to the clinical response. As convulsions and coma have been observed, treatment should proceed with caution in the hospital and corticosteroids should be given as in certain cases of cerebral cysticercosis treated with praziquantel (Chapter 101.1).

Bithionol (Bitin, Actamer), 2,2'-thiobis (4,6-dichlorophenol), is another effective drug; 30 to 50 mg/kg given orally on alternate days for 10 to 15 doses has given cure rates of 80 to 100% in pulmonary paragonimiasis in Asia and Africa.

PROGNOSIS. Pulmonary paragonimiasis is rarely fatal; even without treatment, flukes die or disappear within 10 to 20 years. In most cases of cerebral disease, there is chronic morbidity from epilepsy, dementia, and other neurologic sequelae; 5% of the patients die owing to hemorrhage, and usually in the first 2 years of the disease.

PREVENTION AND CONTROL. Health education, especially for young school children, is needed to change the dietary customs of eating raw or undercooked crab or crayfish. Mass treatment with bithionol in some endemic areas in Korea proved effective in reducing the prevalence of paragonimiasis, but the drug is too costly to be used in large-scale programs. Mollusciciding is at present impractical.

BIBLIOGRAPHY

Bunnag D, Harinasuta T: Trematode infections excluding schistosomiasis. In Gilles HE (ed.): Recent Advances in Tropical Medicine No. 1. Edinburgh, Churchill Livingstone, 1984, pp. 223–227.

Chung HL, Ho LY, Hsu CP, et al.: Recent progress in studies of *Paragonimus* and paragonimiasis control in China. Chin Med J 94:483, 1981.

Chung PR: Review and problem on *Paragonimus* and paragonimiasis with special reference to its intermediate and natural final hosts. Yonsei Rep Trop Med 14:44, 1983.

Miyazaki M: Lung flukes in the world: Morphology and life history. *In* Sasa M (ed.): A Symposium on Epidemiology of Parasitic Diseases. Tokyo International Medical Foundation of Japan, 1984.

Sachs, R, Voelker J: Human paragonimiasis caused by *Paragonimus uterobilateralis* in Liberia and Guinea, West Africa. Tropenmed Parasitol 33:15, 1982.

Vanijanonda S, Bunnag D, Harinasuta T: Radiological findings in pulmonary paragonimiasis heterotremus. Southeast Asian J Trop Med Public Health 15:122, 1984.

Yokogawa M: Paragonimiasis: Current concepts, laboratory diagnosis and chemotherapy. *In* Kan SPl (ed.): Asian J Clin Sci Monograph No. 7: Parasites and Parasitic Infections. Singapore, Melirwin Enterprises, 1986, pp. 79–92.

SECTION E

CESTODE INFECTIONS

GENERAL PRINCIPLES

Herbert B. Tanowitz
and Murray Wittner

Infection with tapeworms is one of the oldest recognized afflictions of humankind. Their huge size and, at times, untimely egress from the body, could hardly go unnoticed. The Cestoda, or tapeworms, are a class of the phylum Platyhelminthes and are exclusively parasitic. In addition to the Cestoda, other classes of Platyhelminthes are the Turbellaria, almost all of which are free living, and the Trematoda, or flukes, which are exclusively parasitic (Section VI D, General Principles, Chapters 96–99). Tapeworms are flattened, and do not possess a body cavity. They infect members of all vertebrate classes, whereas their larvae may infect both vertebrates and invertebrates.

CLASSIFICATION. Of the 4 main groups of cestodes, only 2 are important as parasites of humans and domestic animals. The order Pseudophyllidea is characterized by the presence of a scolex, or attachment organ, containing 2 sucking grooves. Examples of this group are members of the genus *Diphyllobothrium* and include *Diphyllobothrium latum* (the broad or fish tapeworm) (Chapter 100.1) and worms that infect humans only at the larval stage, such as the sparganum (Chapter 101.5). The order Cyclophyllidea, to which all other tapeworms that parasitize humans belong, is characterized by a scolex with 4 suckers. This group includes those belonging to the genus *Taenia*, examples of which are the beef and pork tapeworms (Chapter 100.2). The life cycles of the Pseudophyllidea involve a minimum of 3 hosts. Those of the Cyclophyllidea generally require 2, although in some cases the definitive host can serve also as the intermediate host. Adult tapeworms that are medically important range in size from the minute *Echinococcus* (Chapter 101.2, 101.3, and 101.4), which has a scolex and 3 segments, to *Taenia saginata*, reported at times to reach 25 to 30 m in length.

MORPHOLOGY

Adult. Adult tapeworms typically possess a scolex or head that may be modified or adorned with structures or organelles that serve as holdfast organs for attachment to the small intestinal mucosa. In the Pseudophyllidea, the structures that function for attachment are termed bothria, which are 2 shallow sucking grooves on the sides of a spatulate scolex (Fig. VI E–1A). Some species of Cyclophyllidea, in addition to having 4 sucking cups or acetabula (Fig. VI E–1B), possess hooklets that may form a ring at the top of the scolex or be mounted on a protrusion known as the rostellum (Fig. VI E–1C). The distal portion of the scolex is termed the "neck," an area of intense metabolic activity, which in most groups of tapeworms is the zone from which new segments or proglottids proliferate and form the strobila. Clinically, the scolex is highly significant, because therapy is aimed at its destruction or elimination, inasmuch as failure to do so will result in regrowth of the entire tapeworm. Usually the most proximal proglottids are immature. When stained they will contain only the earliest rudiments of the organs that develop in mature proglottids in the middle of the strobila. Those further distal become mature proglottids and contain 1 set, and in some species 2 complete sets, of male and female sex organs, i.e., they are hermaphroditic. The distal-most segments are filled with eggs and are termed "gravid proglottids." In cyclophyllidean cestodes the sex organs have atrophied, leaving the segment occupied largely by a uterus filled with eggs.

The surface epithelium or tegument is actually a syncytium composed of an anucleate ectocytoplasm that covers the body of the tapeworm and an underlying layer containing nucleated cell bodies or perikarya. The ectocytoplasm has a prominent brush border composed of modified microvilli or microtriches. These structures are cytoplasmic extensions supported by a microfilamentous core. This cestode tegumental brush border increases the absorptive surface and, in addition, may assist in motility and anchoring. Because cestodes lack a digestive system or alimentary canal, all of their nutriment is obtained by absorption across this highly organized surface tegument, which also serves to protect the worm from its environment, i.e., host digestive enzymes. Small molecules and carbohydrates are absorbed directly from the lumen of the small intestine, but there is evidence that amino acids are transported directly from the host's mucosal cells to the proglottids, which are thought to lie in close apposition to one another.

The nervous system present in the scolex consists of ganglia with connecting commissures. Lateral nerve trunks extend distally and serve to coordinate movement of the chain of proglottids or strobila. The excretory system is developed primitively.

Eggs. The eggs of the tapeworms are characteristic (Fig. VI E–2). In members of the genus *Diphyllobothrium*, eggs are discharged through a muscular uterine pore, and therefore, they are found regularly in the feces. However, in many Cyclophyllidea the gravid proglottids split, and the eggs are released through the rents in the proglottids. The eggs of the smaller tapeworms, such as *Hymenolepis nana* and *H. diminuta*, are found in the stool after the disintegration of the gravid proglottids, whereas often those of the genus *Taenia* are not found in the stool because they are passed out in intact segments. In fact, a "scotch tape" preparation similar to that used for the diagnosis of pinworm infection is more reliable in finding *Taenia* eggs. Eggs of the diphyllobothriid tapeworms are operculate (Fig. VI E–

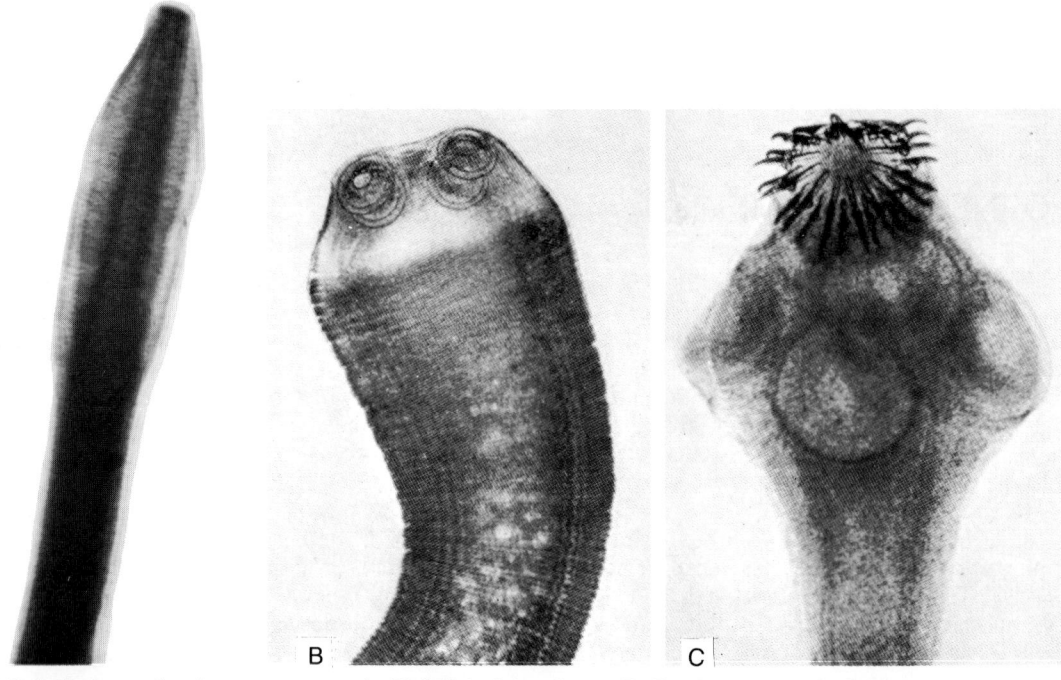

FIGURE VI E–1. Scoleces of various tapeworms. *A, Diphyllobothrium latum. B, Taenia saginata. C, Taenia solium.* (Photomicrographs by Zane Price.) (From Markell EK, Voge M, John DT: Medical Parasitology. 6th ed. Philadelphia, W.B. Saunders Company, 1986.)

FIGURE VI E–2. Cestode eggs. *a, Hymenolepis nana; b, Hymenolepis diminuta; c, d, Taenia* species; *e, Diphyllobothrium latum.* All eggs photographed at same magnification; scale equals 50 μm. (From Markell EK, Voge M, John DT: Medical Parasitology. 6th ed. Philadelphia, W.B. Saunders Company, 1986.)

2E), resembling that of many trematodes, and hatch in water to release a free-swimming larva, the coracidium. Cyclophyllidean tapeworm eggs all contain a fully developed hexacanth (6-hooked) embryo, the oncosphere. The embryonic envelope that surrounds this oncosphere constitutes what is generally referred to as the egg shell, and its morphology is often diagnostic of the species (Fig. VI E–2).

LIFE CYCLE. With the single exception of *Hymenolepis nana*, tapeworms that infect humans require 1 or more intermediate hosts to complete their life histories. The life cycle of diphyllobothriid cestodes involves 2 or more intermediate hosts. Coracidia, ingested by water flies or copepods, develop in the body cavity of these hosts into procercoid larvae, which, while retaining the embryonic 6 hooklets, show evidence of developing bothria. When infected copepods are ingested by the appropriate piscine hosts, the procercoid larva enters the musculature of the fish, where it becomes a plerocercoid or sparganum larva (Fig. 100–1).

Interestingly, the latter may have a number of transfer or paratenic hosts. Thus, a plerocercoid that has developed in a minnow may next parasitize a somewhat larger fish, and may even pass through a series of such transitory domiciliary relationships until its final piscine host is ingested by a suitable mammal, in which it will develop to the adult stage.

Some cestodes only infect humans in the larval stage, e.g., the plerocercoid (sparganum) of *Spirometra mansonoides* (Chapter 101.5), whereas others infect humans in both the adult and larval stages, e.g., *Taenia solium*, (Chapters 100.2 and 101.1). In the genera *Multiceps* (Chapter 101.6) and *Echinococcus* (Chapters 101.2–101.4), larval development results in considerable multiplication. Therefore, when ingested by a suitable host, there may be large numbers of adult worms produced.

CLINICAL MANIFESTATIONS. The clinical manifestations of tapeworm infection may be due to infection with the adult or larval stage. Adult tapeworm infection may persist for many years or even for the life of the host. During this period, it may be relatively asymptomatic or cause persistent symptoms and deprive the host of important and/or essential nutriment. In general, however, these infections are well tolerated. In contrast to infection with adult stage, the infection with the larval stage of a tapeworm often causes serious or fatal disease and can be of great economic consequences.

TREATMENT. Several drugs are used in the treatment of tapeworm infections. Niclosamide is a chlorinated salicylanilide that is poorly absorbed from the gastrointestinal tract and rapidly kills both the segments and the scolex of *D. latum*, and *Taenia* species. For the treatment of *Hymenolepis* infection it requires a prolonged treatment schedule (Chapter 100.3). Because it is absorbed minimally from the gastrointestinal tract, few side effects are reported, although mild nausea, vomiting, and colicky abdominal pain are seen occasionally. Taken in the morning on an empty stomach, niclosamide tablets should be chewed thoroughly and then swallowed with water. For small children it may be pulverized and mixed with water. The patient may eat 2 hours later.

Praziquantel is an acylated isoquinoline-pyrazine that presumably acts by altering calcium fluxes resulting in tetanic contractions of the worm. In addition, there is rapid killing of the scolex and segments. It is absorbed rapidly and metabolized; 70% is excreted by the kidneys within 24 hours. Side effects may occur within hours of ingestion and may include headache, dizziness, drowsiness, nausea, abdominal pain, pruritus, urticaria, arthralgia, and myalgia. However, when they do occur they are mild and disappear by 48 hours. Recently, this drug has been reported to be efficacious in the killing of protoscoleces of *Echinococcus* within cysts.

BIBLIOGRAPHY

Campbell WC, Rew RS: Chemotherapy of Parasitic Diseases. New York, Plenum Press, 1986.
Groll E: Praziquantel for cestode infections in man. Acta Trop 37:293, 1980.
Harnett W: The anthelminthic action of praziquantel. Parasitology Today 4:144–146, 1988.
Kociecka W: Intestinal cestodiasis. Clin Trop Med Comm Dis 2:677–694, 1987.

100. TAPEWORM INFECTIONS

Herbert B. Tanowitz and Murray Wittner

100.1. DIPHYLLOBOTHRIASIS

ETIOLOGY AND LIFE CYCLE. The life cycle of *Diphyllobothrium latum* requires 3 hosts: the definitive hosts are humans and fish-eating carnivores; the first intermediate hosts are a large number of Copepoda (crustaceans); and the second intermediate hosts are freshwater fish (Fig. 100–1).

The fish or broad tapeworm, *D. latum*, is a frequent human intestinal parasite in many areas where uncooked freshwater fish is consumed. *D. latum* is a large tapeworm often consisting of 3000 to 4000 segments or proglottids measuring from 3 to 12 m that inhabits the ileum and jejunum. It possesses a scolex that is characteristically elongate or spoon-shaped with a ventral and dorsal sucking groove or bothrium (Fig. VI E–1*A*). Most of this tapeworm is made up of mature or maturing proglottids. Egg production usually takes place in many proglottids simultaneously over a relatively extended period. The mature proglottid is broader than it is long and contains both male and female reproductive organs. In the center of the mature proglottid is a characteristic dark rosette, i.e., the egg-filled uterus (Fig. 100–2), that aids in its recognition. The uterus leads to a uterine pore on the ventral surface of the segment through which the eggs pass into the feces. Typically, proglottids do not break off and migrate out of the body as occurs in taeniasis (Chapter 100.2), but upwards of a million eggs per day are extruded into the small intestinal lumen by contractions of the muscular uterine pore. Spent proglottids disintegrate eventually and pass out of the body. Occasionally, a long chain of proglottids is passed with the stool.

The characteristic light yellow eggs are 42 to 50 μm by 59 to 75 μm. They possess an operculum or lid at one end; at the abopercular end there is often a characteristic tiny knob (Fig. VI E–2*E*). In fresh water, at a temperature between 15 and 25C, the eggs take about 10 days to 2 weeks to mature, whereupon the operculum opens and a ciliated hexacanth, i.e., 6-hooked embryo, or coracidium, emerges swimming; within 6 to 12 hours

it must be ingested by one of several crustacean species of copepods or perish (*Cyclops* species; *Diaptomus* species). The larva penetrates the midgut and enters the hemocoel of the copepoda and in 10 to 21 days transforms into an elongated procercoid larva, about 0.5 mm in length, where it remains until ingested by one of many species of freshwater plankton-eating fish (second intermediate host). The procercoid larva next makes its way through the tissues of the fish and settles between the muscle fibers of the fish where, within a month, it transforms into a plerocercoid or sparganum larva. The latter has the characteristic rudiments of a scolex but is unsegmented. Next, these fish are eaten by larger carnivorous fish, such as rainbow trout, wall-eyed pike, or the burbot (paratenic or transport hosts). The plerocercoid larvae reinvade the muscles of these fish and if consumed raw or inadequately cooked by a suitable host, i.e., humans, the larva attaches to the wall of the small intestine and becomes a mature tapeworm in about 5 to 6 weeks (Fig. 100–1).

Other adult diphyllobothriid species, normally parasites of fish-eating mammals, have been found occasionally in humans, dogs, and cats in China; *Diplogonoporus grandis*, a whale parasite found on rare occasions in humans in Japan; *Diphyllobothrium dendriticum*, found commonly in piscivorous birds and mammals in the northern hemisphere; and *Diphyllobothrium pacificum*, found in seals (its natural host) and marine fish (its intermediate host) in Peru and Chile.

DISTRIBUTION AND EPIDEMIOLOGY. *D. latum* biotypes are mostly shallow freshwater littorals with vegetation favoring the development of copepods and fish. Infection with this parasite is most prevalent in parts of the northern temperate and sub-arctic zones where freshwater fish is commonly consumed.

During recent years the prevalence has decreased in many areas of the world. The estimated worldwide prevalence of human infection is about 9 to 10 million. In North America, highly endemic foci have been found among Eskimos in Alaska and Canada and in the smaller lakes of the the Great Lakes region. Fish from the lakes of the north central region of the United States, especially in Minnesota, Michigan, Florida, and California, have been found to be infected. In the highly endemic regions of Finnish and Soviet Karelia, the proportion of infected fish has ranged from 25 to 100%. In addition, areas of Sweden, France, Switzerland, northwestern Russia, the Danube and lower Volga basins, and the lake regions of northern Italy and Switzerland contain infected fish. Freshwater lakes in many parts of Africa, including the island of Madagascar, China, Taiwan, Japan, Turkey, Ireland, Israel, Papua-New Guinea, Australia, the Philippines, Argentina, and southern Chile contain infected fish. However, some of these records may be the result of misidentification.

Humans are the primary definitive host and most important reservoir of infection. Other definitive and reservoir hosts are fish-eating mammals, e.g., fox, mink, bear, domestic and wild cat, dog, pig, walrus, and seal. Secondary intermediate hosts are many species of brackish and freshwater fish, including fish that spawn in fresh water, e.g., salmonids. Salmon has been the cause of

LIFE CYCLE of —

Diphyllobothrium latum

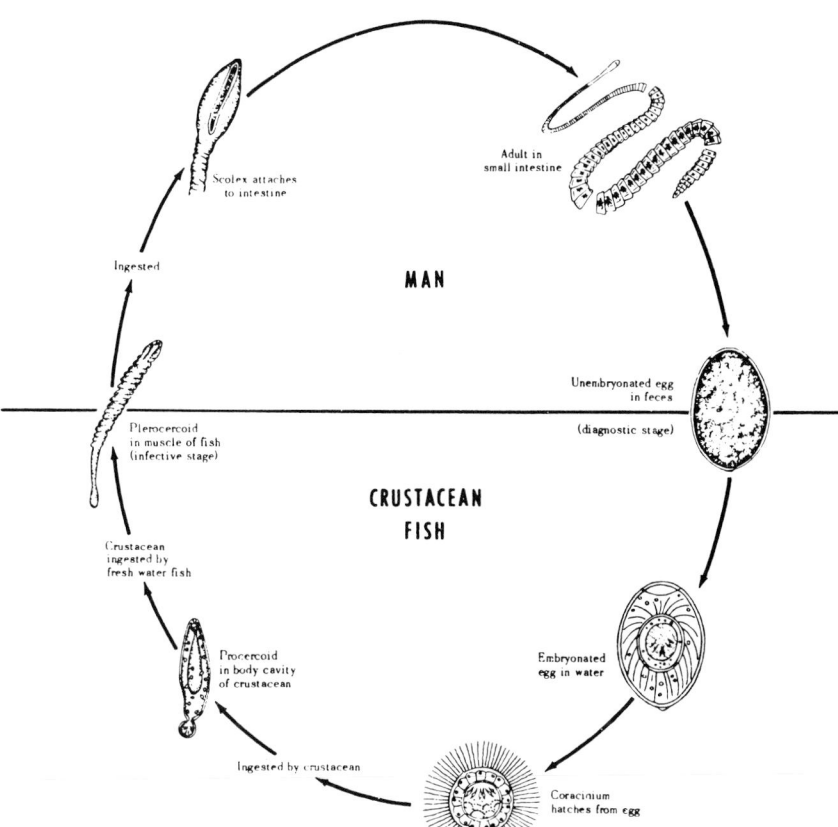

FIGURE 100–1. Life cycle of *Diphyllobothrium latum*. (From Melvin DM, Brooke MM, Sadun EH: Common Intestinal Helminths of Man. Atlanta, Centers for Disease Control, DHEW Publication No. [CDC] 75–8286, 1964.)

the transmission of this parasite in Japan and the West coast of the United States where sushi has been prepared with fresh salmon. Important factors contributing to the spread of infection have been the emigration of infected populations, the construction of dams and other water projects, and the practice of allowing untreated sewage to enter freshwater lakes. Cases of diphyllobothriasis sometimes occur outside of endemic areas as a result of infected fish being shipped under refrigeration.

Eating raw, insufficiently cooked, or lightly pickled fish or fresh roe is common among many ethnic groups where it is considered a delicacy. For example, for many

years in New York City, infected fresh fish, transported on ice, was the main source of this tapeworm infection among Jewish housewives who made gefüllte fish. Typically, small amounts of raw fish are sampled in order to season this ethnic delicacy to taste. In northern Minnesota and Michigan where large numbers of individuals of Scandinavian background live, raw and/or pickled fish are still eaten, and infection with *D. latum* is not uncommon. There are other diphyllobothriids that cause disease. *D. pacificum* has been reported from Japan and is endemic in coastal areas of Peru. Unlike *D. latum*, infection with this parasite is acquired from eating marine fish that have been prepared in lime juice. *Diplogonoporus grandis*, another member of this group, is found in Japan and thought to be acquired by consumption of raw anchovies and sardines.

CLINICAL MANIFESTATIONS AND PATHOLOGY. Harboring this large tapeworm is often associated with surprisingly few symptoms or pathologic changes in the intestinal mucosa. Often the infection is recognized first in an asymptomatic patient as a result of a stool examination carried out for other reasons. However, some individuals complain of vague abdominal pain and some patients describe the sensation that "something is moving inside." Others describe bloating, sore tongue, sore gums, allergic symptoms, headache,

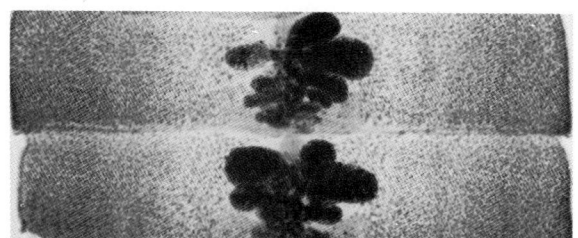

FIGURE 100–2. Gravid proglottids of *Diphyllobothrium latum*. (Photomicrograph by Zane Price from material furnished by Dr. Justus F. Mueller.) (From Markell EK, Voge M, John DT: Medical Parasitology, 6th ed. Philadelphia, W.B. Saunders Company, 1986.)

hunger pains, loss of appetite, and/or increased appetite. On rare occasions, mechanical intestinal obstruction may occur as a result of several worms becoming entangled. Diarrhea may occur also. Almost all patients become aware of the infection when spontaneously passing a large section of the spent proglottids; most often this startling event brings the patient to the office or clinic. Unlike the proglottids of *Taenia saginata*, those of *D. latum* do not crawl spontaneously through the anus.

Megaloblastic Anemia. In a small number of patients, megaloblastic and pernicious anemia have been shown to be caused by infection with *D. latum* ("bothriocephalus anemia"). When fully manifest, this anemia is a hyperchromic, macrocytic, megaloblastic anemia with thrombocytopenia and mild leukopenia.

Clinical and experimental studies suggest that worms situated in the ileum or jejunum successfully compete with the host for vitamin B_{12}. Tracer studies have shown that the parasite absorbs more than 80% of administered vitamin B_{12}. However, the precise mechanism of the anemia is poorly understood. Folate absorption by the host may be diminished also, and decreased levels of ascorbic acid, thiamine, and riboflavin have been described. For unknown reasons, anemia associated with diphyllobothriasis is found primarily in the Scandinavian countries.

Approximately 40% of persons harboring the worm have reduced serum vitamin B_{12} levels, but less than 2% develop anemia. The anemia is usually moderate, but can become severe, with pallor, glossitis, dyspnea, and tachycardia. Neurologic findings, which include weakness, numbness, paresthesias, disturbances of motility and coordination, and impairment of deep sensations, can occur in the absence of hematologic abnormalities. The basic pathologic lesion is subacute combined spinal and peripheral nerve degeneration.

In the spinal cord, the posterior and lateral columns are involved. Central scotoma, secondary to optic atrophy, has been described. The anemia and neurological manifestations respond to vitamin B_{12} and do not recur after the worm has been expelled.

DIAGNOSIS. The infection can be diagnosed readily by finding characteristic ova in the feces (Fig. VI E–2E). Concentration methods are usually unnecessary, because the numbers of eggs present are often so great that direct examination of a small amount of the patient's feces in a drop of saline is usually sufficient. In addition, a strobila may be expelled in the feces and on rare occasions portions of worm may be vomited. Tapeworm-induced anemia may be associated with free hydrochloric acid in the gastric juice; in contrast, pernicious anemia is associated with achlorhydria. There is no reliable serologic test to aid in diagnosis. It is not uncommon to find an eosinophilia of 5 to 10% in patients with *D. latum* infection accompanied by a minimal leukocytosis.

TREATMENT. The treatment of choice for adults is niclosamide or praziquantel. Niclosamide is given as a single dose of 4 tablets (2 gm) chewed thoroughly. A single dose of 1 gm (2 tablets) is recommended for children weighing 11 to 34 kg and a single dose of 1.5

gm (3 tablets) for those children weighing more than 34 kg. Praziquantel is given as a single dose of 10 to 20 mg/kg for both adults and children. It cures virtually all infections.

PREVENTION. Careful cooking of freshwater fish would eliminate all possibility of human infection. The sale of fish originating in heavily infected lakes should be regulated. Freezing at −10C for 24 hours kills the plerocercoid larva. In the United States smoked salmon is usually brined before smoking and is not considered a source of infection. Other control measures include the education of cooks regarding the sampling of raw fish during preparation. In addition, the discontinuation of dumping raw sewage into freshwater lakes would prevent viable eggs from contaminating various intermediate hosts. In highly endemic areas, human infection should be detected by survey and treated; pet dogs should be dewormed several times a year.

BIBLIOGRAPHY

Centers for Disease Control: Diphyllobothriasis associated with salmon—United States. MMWR 30:331–338, 1981.
Von Bondsorff B: Diphyllobothriasis in Man. London, Academic Press, 1977.
Von Bondsorff B, Bylund G: The ecology of *Diphyllobothrium latum*. Ecol Dis 1: 21–26, 1982.

100.2. TAENIASIS

ETIOLOGY AND LIFE CYCLE. The pork tapeworm, *Taenia solium*, and the beef tapeworm, *Taenia saginata*, are the common tapeworm parasites of humans. These infections have been known since ancient times and occur whenever infected insufficiently cooked beef or pork is consumed.

Several other species of this genus infect animals, and some, e.g., the cat tapeworm *Taenia taeniaeformis*, have been reported rarely as a human parasite. Human infection caused by larvae of *T. solium*, known as cysticercosis, is discussed in Chapter 101.1.

Adult *T. saginata* vary in size from 4 to 12 m and may be composed of 1000 to 2000 proglottids. In multiple infections with either *T. saginata* or *T. solium*, however, a "crowding effect" is noted so that each worm is usually smaller. As proglottids mature and become gravid, the testes and other reproductive organs first appear and finally disappear, giving place to the enlarging uterus. The proglottids have no uterine pore; instead, eggs are released into the feces or onto the perineum through a longitudinal ventral split in the distended gravid segments (Fig. 100–3). The scolex of *T. saginata* is distinctive, being about 1.5 to 2 mm wide and possessing 4 sucking discs. It lacks a crown or rostellum with hooks and is said to be an "unarmed" scolex (Fig. VI E–1B).

T. solium is somewhat smaller, varying from 2 to 8 m with a total of about 1000 proglottids. The characteristic scolex is about 1 mm and possesses a well-developed crown or rostellum upon which are a double row of 22 to 32 large and small hooklets, i.e., an "armed" scolex (Fig. VI E–1C).

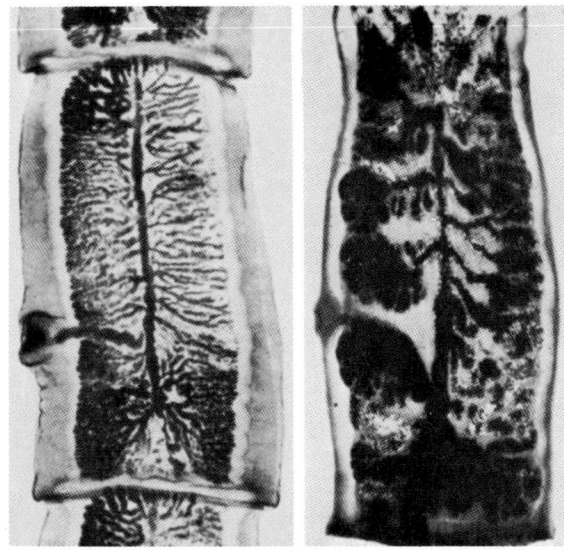

FIGURE 100–3. Gravid proglottids of *Taenia saginata (A)* and *Taenia solium (B)*. (Photomicrographs by Zane Price.) (From Markell EK, Voge M, John DT: Medical Parasitology. 6th ed. Philadelphia, W.B. Saunders Company, 1986.)

Adult taenia are found only in humans and generally are attached 40 to 50 cm below the ligament of Treitz, i.e., in the jejunum. The worm is not fixed in position but moves frequently even against the peristaltic stream. Gravid proglottids hold tens of thousands of eggs. The spherical, thick-walled egg is striated radially and contains a mature 6-hooked (hexacanth) embryo, termed an oncosphere. The eggs are 30 to 40 μm in diameter and are similar in all members of the genus (Fig. VI E– 2C and D).

Cattle or hogs become infected by ingesting mature eggs, contaminating low-lying pastures or barn yards. The action by gastric juice, intestinal enzymes, and bile has been shown necessary to stimulate hatching. Embryos that then penetrate the intestinal mucosa of cattle or hogs enter the circulation and are transported throughout the body. Encystment usually occurs in striated muscle, and within 10 to 11 weeks the larvae, termed *Cysticercus cellulosae* in hogs or *Cysticercus bovis* in cattle, are infectious. Cysticerci measure 4 to 6 mm by 7.5 to 10 mm. They are ellipsoidal, white, translucent bladder-like cysts into which an inverted scolex has developed. Upon consumption of infected raw or inadequately cooked beef or pork, the cysticercus is activated by gastric juices, and surface active agents, e.g., bile salts, stimulate evagination of the scolex. Then, it attaches to the jejunal wall, becoming a mature tapeworm in 10 to 12 weeks in the case of *T. saginata* and in 5 to 12 weeks with *T. solium*. The adult tapeworm may live as long as 25 years (Figs. 100–4 and 100–5).

EPIDEMIOLOGY AND DISTRIBUTION. Both infections have a worldwide distribution, but there are no reliable statistics as to their prevalence. In 1973 it was estimated that 3 million people were infected with *T. solium* and 45 million people infected with *T. saginata*. *T. saginata* is commonly found in the United States, Western and Eastern Europe, South America, and East and West Africa. *Taenia solium* infection is common in

Mexico, Central and South America, Czechoslovakia, Yugoslavia, Northern China, focally in East Africa, and India.

Humans are the definitive host for both *T. saginata* and *T. solium*. Human infection with the pork tapeworm has become rather uncommon in the United States, although cysticercosis of hogs still occurs. In many areas of the world, especially Mexico and parts of South and Central America, *T. solium* infection is relatively common. Human infection with *Cysticercus cellulosae*, or cysticercosis, is found wherever adult *T. solium* infection is common (Chapter 101.1). Thus, human cysticercosis is often encountered in Mexico, South and Central America, southeastern Europe, Africa, India, and parts of China. *T. saginata* infection occurs among those who prefer to eat raw or insufficiently cooked beef. In the United States it is common to find raw beef included on menus as "steak tartare" at "chic" metropolitan restaurants, indicating the extent of the popularity of this food. Moreover, rare beef is served commonly at home and is preferred by many individuals. Throughout the world beef consumption has increased; thus, combined with various ethnic factors, it has favored increased transmission of *T. saginata* infection. Fortunately, human infection with larval *T. saginata* almost never occurs. *T. saginata* infection is an anthrozoonosis in which humans are the mandatory definitive host that disseminates the infection to bovine intermediate hosts. While direct transmission from humans to cows is unusual, it may occur if contaminated hands are used to feed calves. More commonly, however, it is believed that transmission occurs through feces-contaminated grazing lands, cattle feed, and is spread by birds and flies. Intrauterine infection of calves has been reported.

CLINICAL MANIFESTATIONS AND PATHOLOGY. The scolex lodges generally in the upper jejunum. Usually only 1 worm is present, but multiple infections can occur, and concurrent infections with both species of *Taenia* have been described. Adult tapeworms cause minimal pathologic changes. However, intestinal mucosal biopsies in patients harboring *T. saginata* have shown minimal inflammatory reactions, suggesting that the worms can have an irritative effect resulting in symptoms.

Most individuals who harbor *T. solium* or *T. saginata* infection are either asymptomatic or have mild to moderate complaints. Occasionally the infection can cause serious, life-threatening disease from intestinal, appendiceal, biliary or pancreatic obstruction resulting in an acute surgical abdomen. Rarely an individual may regurgitate and aspirate a proglottid. Among the most frequently reported signs or symptoms of adult *Taenia* infection are spontaneous discharge of proglottids from the rectum, abdominal pain, nausea, weakness, loss of appetite, increased appetite, headache, constipation, dizziness, diarrhea, pruritus ani, and hyperexcitability. Abdominal pain and nausea are reported to be more common in the morning and characteristically relieved by food. Children are more frequently symptomatic than adults. Worms are immunogenic, and allergic symptoms, e.g., urticaria, pruritus, and other skin disorders, have been reported. Eosinophilia is often present; it is usually from 5 to 15%. Serum IgE levels may be increased.

LIFE CYCLE of—

Taenia saginata

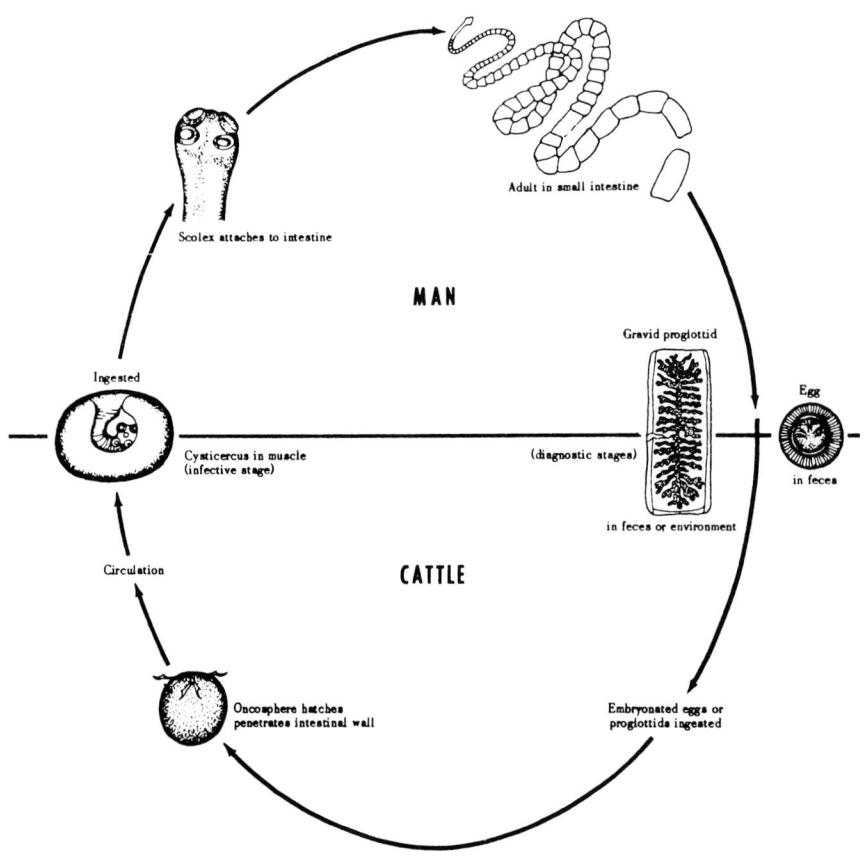

FIGURE 100–4. Life cycle of *Taenia saginata*. (From Melvin DM, Brooke MM, Sadun EH: Common Intestinal Helminths of Man. Atlanta, Centers for Disease Control, DHEW Publication No. [CDC] 72–8286, 1964.)

LIFE CYCLE of—

Taenia solium

FIGURE 100–5. Life cycle of *Taenia solium*. (From Melvin DM, Brooke MM, Sadun EH: Common Intestinal Helminths of Man. Atlanta, Centers for Disease Control, DHEW Publication No. [CDC] 72–8286, 1964.)

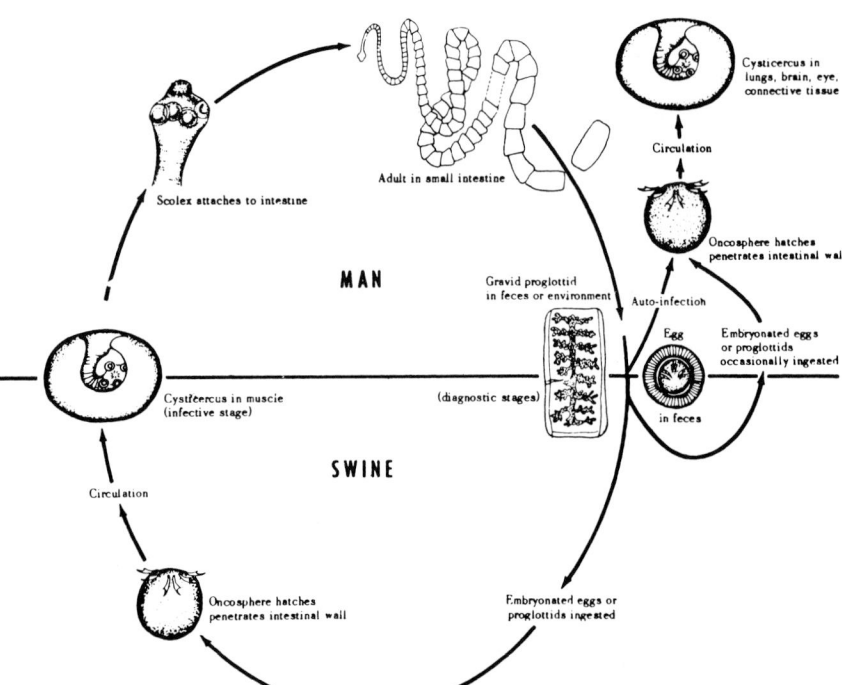

Human cysticercosis with the larvae of *T. solium* is an important and sometimes fatal disease. Cysticerci have been found in almost every tissue and organ of the body (Chapter 101.1).

DIAGNOSIS. Because the finding of *Taenia* eggs in the stool is not sufficient to make a specific diagnosis, a gravid proglottid must be obtained. This is not difficult, because proglottids are passed in the stool or emerge on the perianal or perineal region frequently and spontaneously at irregular intervals.

Identification of proglottids is done by pressing the segment between 2 glass microscope slides and counting the main lateral branches of the uterus. *T. solium* has fewer primary branches, usually 7 to 13 on each side; *T. saginata* usually has greater than 15 lateral primary branches per side, i.e. 15 to 20 (Fig. 100–3). Fecal examination, especially in the case of *T. saginata*, is often unrewarding inasmuch as gravid proglottids tend to be eliminated or "crawl" out on the perianal area prior to ovipositing. Thus, anal swabs, e.g., the "scotch tape" method as is usually done for the diagnosis of pinworm, is recommended for detecting the ova. In addition, the embryophore of *T. saginata* can be stained with the Ziehl-Neelsen stain, whereas that of *T. solium* is acid-fast negative. There are no serologic tests for the diagnosis of *Taenia* infections. However, serologic tests are useful in making the diagnosis of cysticercosis (Chapter 101.1).

TREATMENT. The treatment of both tapeworm infections is similar. Niclosamide or praziquantel in the same dosage schedule as for *D. latum* is given (Chapter 100.1). Since the advent of praziquantel, paromomycin and dichlorophen are rarely prescribed. In the treatment of *T. solium* infections, precautions should be taken to prevent autoinfection or dissemination. Drugs that induce vomiting should be avoided, because retrograde peristalsis might bring gravid proglottids into the gastroduodenal area, resulting in their subsequent digestion followed by egg hatching, penetration, and cysticercosis. In addition, since niclosamide and praziquantel kill the worm but not the eggs released from the disintegrating gravid segments, cysticercosis is theoretically possible following treatment. It is also unknown whether larvae released from eggs in the colon are capable of penetrating the intestinal wall. However, no cases of cysticercosis have been reported by this mechanism. As a precaution, however, some clinicians advise that a purge be given 2 hours after treatment of *T. solium* infections to eliminate all mature segments before eggs can be released. The patient should be followed to ensure prompt evacuation. Post-treatment follow-up stool examination should be performed after approximately 5 weeks and 3 months. The treatment of human cysticercosis is discussed in Chapter 101.1.

PREVENTION. The prevention of beef and pork tapeworm infection can be accomplished by adequate cooking or freezing of these meats. *Cysticercus cellulosae* are killed by moderate temperatures of 65C or if the pork is frozen at −20C for at least 12 hours. Pickling in brine and salting are not always adequate. *Cysticercus bovis* is killed by thorough cooking at 56C or freezing at −10C for 5 days. Pickling of beef in 25% brine for 5 to 6 days is said to render the beef safe. Meat inspection would help reduce transmission to humans who fail to properly prepare meat. Treatment of all infected individuals would eliminate the source of soil and sewage pollution with *Taenia* eggs.

BIBLIOGRAPHY

Pawlowski Z, Schultz MG: Taeniasis and cysticercosis (*Taenia saginata*). Adv Parasitol 10:269–310, 1972.

100.3. HYMENOLEPIASIS

Two species of small tapeworms of the genus *Hymenolepis* infect humans. The dwarf tapeworm, *Hymenolepis nana*, is a common infection, especially of children, throughout the world and can be passed from human to human. In moderate to heavy infections it may cause a variety of abdominal and neurologic symptoms. *Hymenolepis diminuta* is primarily a parasite of rodents and also, infrequently, of humans.

HYMENOLEPIS NANA INFECTION

ETIOLOGY AND LIFE CYCLE. *H. nana* is the smallest adult tapeworm to infect humans regularly, measuring about 25 to 30 mm long by about 0.8 to 1.0 mm wide (Fig. 100–6). The entire chain of proglottids from the anterior immature to the distal gravid segments often consists of no more than 175 to 220 segments. However, there may be considerably fewer proglottids per worm if many worms are present at one time, i.e., the "crowding effect." The minute rounded scolex (3 mm in diameter) possesses 4 sucking disks and a short-armed retractable rostellum. The infective eggs (Fig. VI E–2a), liberated when the distalmost proglottids disintegrate, are most characteristic, measuring 35 to 52 µm in diameter; they contain a hexacanth embryo or oncosphere that resides within an inner membrane. The latter possesses 2 polar thickenings from which there arise typically 4 to 8 polar filaments. These eggs are released by the gradual disintegration of the terminal gravid proglottids and are infective immediately when passed in the feces. Unlike most other tapeworms that infect humans, no intermediate host is required. Therefore, if the egg is ingested by another or the same host, the oncosphere is liberated in the small intestine and penetrates the villi, where it becomes a cysticercoid larva (a small larva that has a single scolex but does not have a bladder characteristic of a cysticercus) (Fig. 100–7). In about 96 hours, the larva re-enters the lumen and attaches to a small intestinal villus by its scolex, usually at a more distal location. In about 10 to 20 days, it matures, and eggs may be found in the feces.

There is evidence that hyper- or autoinfection occurs when ova liberated in the small intestine spontaneously hatch and immediately penetrate a villus to undergo a new cycle. Individual worms live about a year. However,

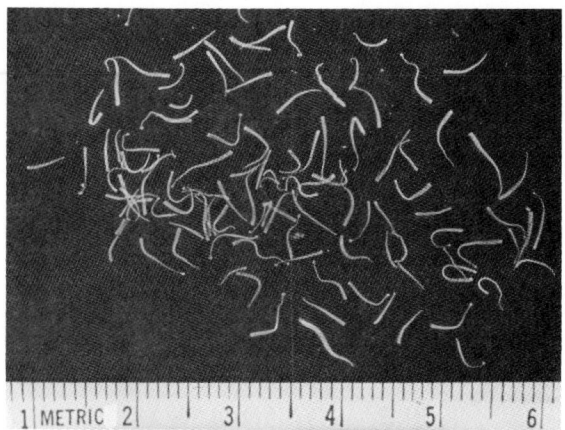

FIGURE 100–6. *Hymenolepis nana,* dwarf tapeworm, adults. (Courtesy of Dr. Francisco J. Aguilar, Guatemala.)

as a result of hyperinfection, individuals may have a large worm burden for many years. In experimental animals, the worm burden is limited by the development of immunity, and immunosuppression can cause hyperinfection. In addition, experimental evidence suggests that certain strains of *H. nana* undergo larval or cysticercoid development in various fleas and meal worms. Subsequently, the larvae have been found to develop to adult tapeworms in mice. At the present time, human infection with these murine strains is regarded as most unusual.

EPIDEMIOLOGY AND DISTRIBUTION. Infection with this parasite is worldwide in distribution; millions of people are infected. It is commonly regarded as a hand to mouth infection and, as a result, is encountered most frequently in children and in inhabitants of institutions for the mentally retarded and chronic care psychiatric hospitals.

H. nana infection is most common in rural communities in the southeastern portion of the United States, where it is has been reported to infect almost 1% of young school children. Higher infection rates are reported in South and Central American countries, Puerto Rico, and Mexico, where conditions of overcrowding and poor personal and environmental hygiene are pres-

ent. Families from Latin America who have emigrated recently to urban areas are often heavily parasitized. The infection is also common throughout southern Europe, the Middle East, the Soviet Union, and the Indian subcontinent.

Humans are the natural resevoir for the parasite, and transmission is generally direct from human to human by ingestion of eggs from feces of infected individuals. Although transmission may occur by fomites, water, and food, this is less common, because the eggs succumb quickly outside the host. Larvae of fleas and grain beetles can become infected after ingesting *H. nana* eggs and develop cysticercoids in their hemocoeles. However, probably these insects are seldom of importance as intermediate hosts in human infection. Some murine strains are infectious for humans. Thus, pet mice, rats, and hamsters are sometimes the source of infection.

CLINICAL MANIFESTATIONS, PATHOLOGY, AND DIAGNOSIS. Necrosis and desquamation of intestinal epithelial cells have been observed at the site of attachment of the mature worm. Light infections generally cause no significant mucosal damage and are either asymptomatic or cause vague abdominal complaints. Even heavy parasitism is usually well tolerated. It is believed that many of the clinical symptoms are immunologically mediated. Young children are particularly troubled with this infection, especially when they are infected with many worms. Commonly, these patients have loose bowel movements or occasionally frank diarrhea with mucus. Bloody diarrhea is rare. Diffuse, persistent, abdominal pain is the most common complaint. Pruritus ani and nasi and urticaria are encountered occasionally. Many children have headaches, dizziness, and sleep and behavioral disturbances, which clear after successful therapy. Serious neurologic disturbances, such as seizures, have been reported. Many patients with hymenolepiasis have a moderate eosinophilia of 5 to 10%. Internal auto- or hyperinfection has been reported in immunosuppressed mice.

The diagnosis is made by identifying the characteristic ova in a fecal specimen (Fig. VI E–2*a*). Proglottids are usually not found because they degenerate before passage.

TREATMENT. Successful therapy depends upon understanding the life history of this infection and, therefore, one should recall that the larval stage or cysticercoid is buried in the intestinal mucosa (Fig. 100–7) and presumably is not killed by the drugs as ordinarily employed for treating other tapeworm infections. The treatment of choice is praziquantel inasmuch as it is lethal to the cysticercoid stage within the tissue as well as the worm in the lumen. The recommended dose for adults and children is 25 mg/kg in a single dose. Niclosamide, which is not absorbed, is an alternative drug that may be given to adults as a single dose of 2 gm (4 tablets) followed by 2 tablets daily for 6 additional days. The drug should be chewed thoroughly. The pediatric dose schedule is: for 11 to 34 kg, a single dose of 2 tablets (1 gm) followed by 1 tablet daily for 6 days; for greater than 34 kg, a single dose of 3 tablets followed by 2 tablets daily for 6 days.

PREVENTION. Control depends on improved per-

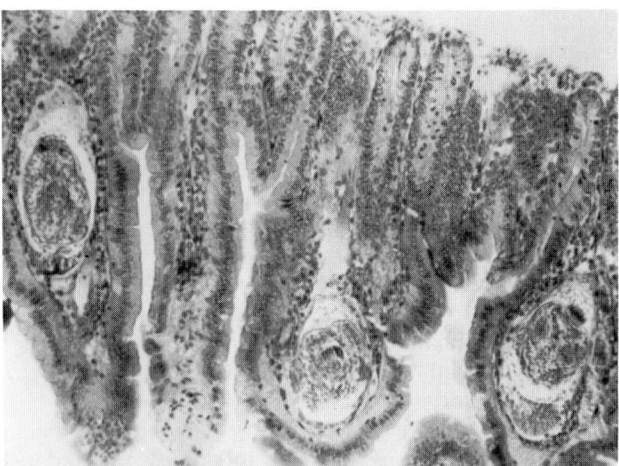

FIGURE 100–7. *Hymenolepis nana* cysticercoid larvae in the small intestinal villi. (Courtesy of Herman Zaiman, M.D.)

LIFE CYCLE of—

Hymenolepis diminuta

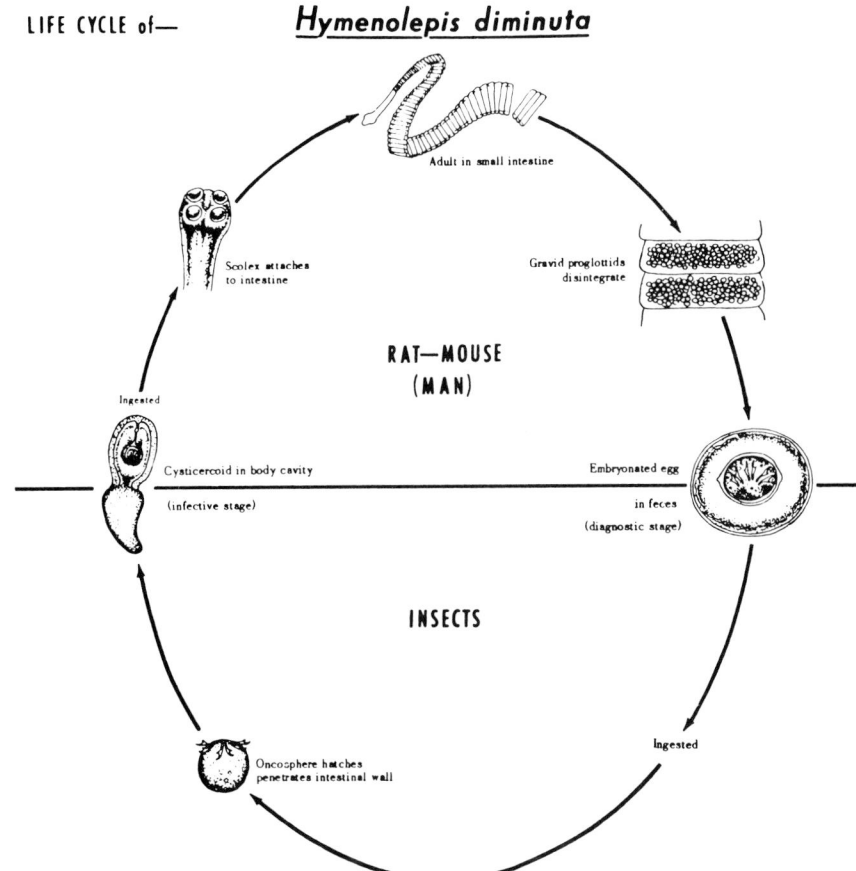

Adult in small intestine

Scolex attaches to intestine

Gravid proglottids disintegrate

RAT—MOUSE
(MAN)

Ingested

Cysticercoid in body cavity

(infective stage)

Embryonated egg

in feces

(diagnostic stage)

INSECTS

Oncosphere hatches penetrates intestinal wall

ingested

FIGURE 100–8. Life cycle of *Hymenolepis diminuta*. (From Melvin DM, Brooke MM, Sadun EH: Common Intestinal Helminths of Man. Atlanta, Centers for Disease Control, DHEW Publication No. [CDC] 75–8286, 1964.)

sonal and environmental hygiene. In institutions, mass chemotherapy may be necessary. Although rodents have not been proven to be an important source of infection to humans, the possibility of murine infection should be considered when rodents, pets, or laboratory animals are present.

HYMENOLEPIS DIMINUTA INFECTION

The definitive hosts for this tapeworm are primarily rats, mice, and other murine species. It is closely related to *H. nana* and infrequently infects humans. Over 200 human cases have been reported and most frequently occur in children under 3 years of age. The adult worm is 10 to 60 cm by 3 to 5 mm; larger than *H. nana*, it has 800 to 1000 proglottids. The scolex is club-shaped and has a rudimentary apical unarmed rostellum and 4 small suckers. The mature proglottids resemble *H. nana*. The

eggs are spherical and 60 to 86 μm in diameter; their thin, yellowish outer membrane is separated from the inner embryonic envelope by a clear area that, in contrast to the eggs of *H. nana*, contains no polar filaments (Fig. VI E–2b). Development of this tapeworm requires an intermediate host. Presumably, rat fleas (*Nosopsyllus, Xenopsyllus*) and meal worms infected with larvae are ingested accidentally, and mature adults develop in about 3 weeks. Cockroaches may serve as intermediate hosts also. These insects become infected by ingesting eggs passed in rodent feces. The eggs develop into cysticercoids in the hemacoele of the insect; when ingested, the cysticercoids are infectious to rodents or humans (Fig. 100–8). Human infection probably occurs by accidental ingestion of mealworms or grain beetles found in dry grains, cereals, flour, and dried fruits.

The adult tapeworms attach to duodenal or jejunal mucosa (Fig. 100–9). Human infections are light, and the life span in humans is short. The diagnosis is made by finding ova in the stool (Fig. VI E–2b). Treatment is the same as for *H. nana*.

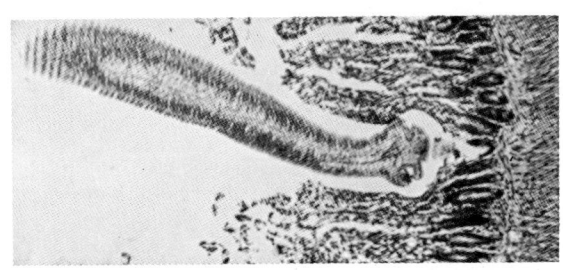

FIGURE 100–9. *Hymenolepis diminuta* attached to intestinal mucosa of rat.

BIBLIOGRAPHY

Arai HP (ed): Biology of the tapeworm *Hymenolepis diminuta*. New York, Academic Press, 1980.

Biswash H, Arora RR, Sehgal S: Epidemiology of *Hymenolepis nana* infections in a selected rural community. J Commun Dis 10:170–174, 1978.

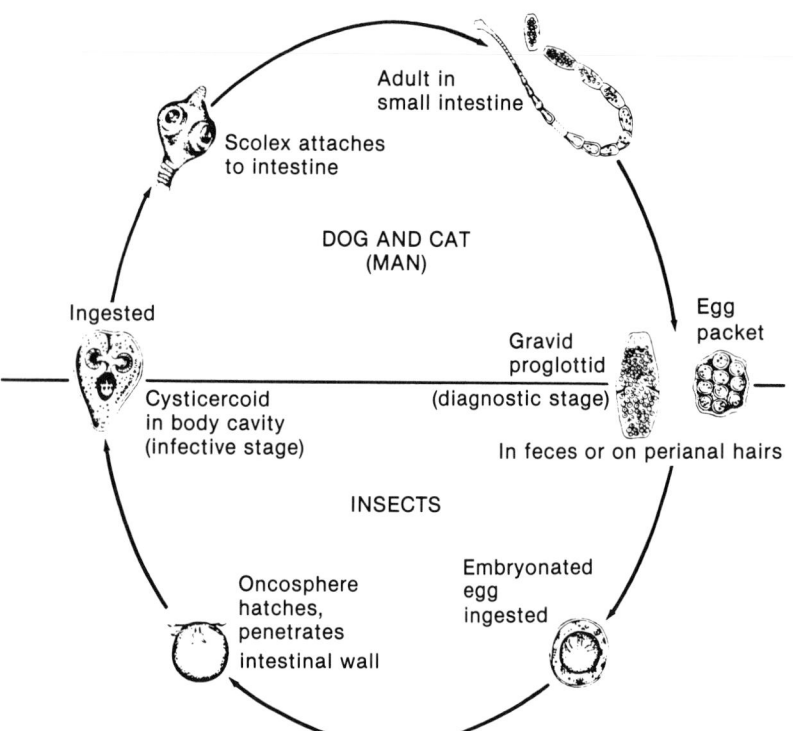

Adult in
small intestine

Scolex attaches
to intestine

DOG AND CAT
(MAN)

Ingested

Egg
packet

Gravid
proglottid

(diagnostic stage)

Cysticercoid
in body cavity
(infective stage)

In feces or on perianal hairs

INSECTS

Oncosphere
hatches,
penetrates
intestinal wall

Embryonated
egg
ingested

FIGURE 100–10. Life cycle of *Dipylidium caninum*. (From Melvin DM, Brooke MM, Sadun EH: Common Intestinal Helminths of Man. Atlanta, Centers for Disease Control, DHEW Publication No. [CDC] 75–8286, 1964.)

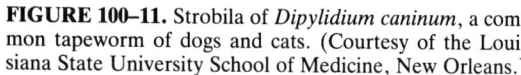
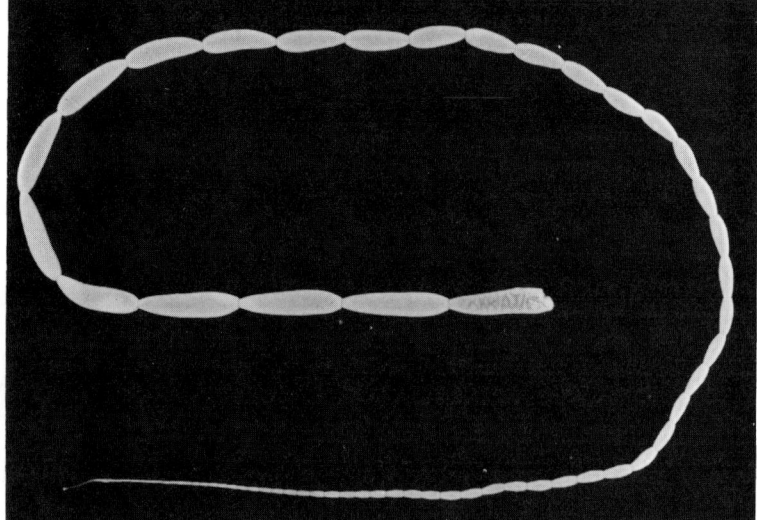

FIGURE 100–11. Strobila of *Dipylidium caninum*, a common tapeworm of dogs and cats. (Courtesy of the Louisiana State University School of Medicine, New Orleans.)

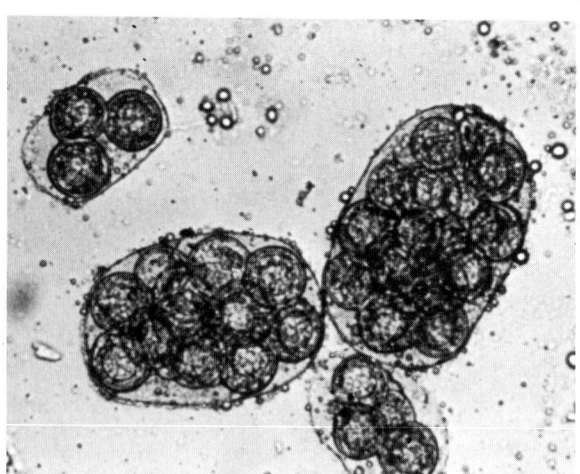

FIGURE 100–12. Egg capsules of *Dipylidium caninum*. (Photograph by H.J. Griffiths. From Zaiman H (ed.): A Pictorial Presentation of Parasites.)

100.4. DIPYLIDIASIS

ETIOLOGY AND LIFE CYCLE (Fig. 100–10). *Dipylidium caninum* is a cestode of dogs, cats, and wild Carnivora that occasionally infects humans. Adult tapeworms inhabit the small intestine and measure 15 to 20 cm in length. The worm usually contains 60 to 175 proglottids (Fig. 100–11). *D. caninum* has a characteristic rhomboidal scolex with 4 oval suckers and an armed retractible conical rostellum containing 30 to 150 thorn-shaped hooks arranged in transverse rows. The vase-shaped proglottids possess a double set of reproductive organs with genital pores midway on each lateral margin. The gravid proglottids are usually packed with 15 to 25 eggs. Each egg is 35 to 60 μm in diameter and contains an onchosphere with 6 hooklets (Fig. 100–12).

Strobila (Fig. 100–11) are capable of moving several inches per hour and pass out of the anus or are passed in the feces. Eggs are expelled by contraction of the proglottids or disintegration of the proglottid outside of the intestine on the perianal region.

The intermediate hosts of *Dipylidium* are larval dog, cat, and human fleas. Those cysticercoid larvae that survive metamorphosis of the larval flea are ingested by the definitive host. The larvae are liberated in the small intestine and become adults in about 20 days (Fig. 100–10).

EPIDEMIOLOGY. Most of the infections have occurred in children under 8 years of age, with one third occurring in infants under 6 months. Transmission is thought to be due to accidental swallowing of infected adult fleas, most likely due to the close association between children and dogs and cats. In addition, transmission may occur as a result of hand to mouth contamination.

CLINICAL MANIFESTATIONS AND DIAGNOSIS. Most patients are asymptomatic, but clinical findings attributed to *D. caninum* include abdominal pain, diarrhea, urticaria, and pruritus ani. Multiple infections are not uncommon. Definitive diagnosis is made by finding typical eggs or proglottids in stool (Fig. 100–12). However, examination for eggs may be unreliable, because proglottids usually do not release eggs within the intestines. There may be moderate eosinophilia.

TREATMENT. Treatment is the same as for *D. latum* infections. Children should not be allowed to fondle infected dogs or cats. Household pets should be treated with antihelmintics, and insecticides should be used to remove pet ectoparasites and to disinfect their sleeping areas.

BIBLIOGRAPHY

Jones WE: Niclosamide as a treatment for *Hymenolepis diminuta* and *Dipylidium caninum* infection in man. Am J Trop Med Hyg 28:300–302, 1979.
Wijesundera M de S: The use of praziquantel in human infection with *Dipylidium*. Trans R Soc Trop Med Hyg 83:383, 1989.

101. LARVAL CESTODE INFECTIONS

Patrick B. McGreevy
and George S. Nelson

GENERAL PRINCIPLES

In 1850, Von Siebold suggested that "bladder worms," which were found frequently in animals and occasionally in humans, were the larval stages of adult tapeworms. He confirmed this in 1852 by feeding hydatid cysts to dogs and recovering adult *Echinococcus*. The most dramatic demonstration of this alternation of generations was provided by Friedrick Kuchenmeister in 1853 when he fed bladder worms from a pig to a convict who was "scheduled to be dispatched from this life to death by the Guillotine." At autopsy, the adult tapeworm *Taenia solium* was recovered from the intestine. Although the biology of most larval tapeworms infecting humans is now described in considerable detail, several new species have been discovered in recent years, and the fundamental details of their life cycles are largely unknown.

The classification and life cycles of the larval tapeworms commonly found in humans are listed in Table 101–1. There are 2 orders of larval tapeworms found in humans: (1) in the order Pseudophyllidea, there is the genus *Spirometra*, and (2) in the order Cyclophyllidea, there are the genera *Hymenolepis*, *Taenia*, and *Echinococcus*.

There is often confusion with cestode terminology because the names given to the cystic larval stages before the life cycles were delineated are still in common use by meat hygienists, e.g., *Cysticercus bovis* for the intermediate stage of *Taenia saginata* in the cow, and *Cysticercus cellulosae* for the cystic stage of *T. solium* in the pig.

MORPHOLOGY. The morphologic characteristics of larval tapeworms vary widely among species, but there are 3 features shared by all cestode larvae: (1) a scolex, (2) an external brush border, and (3) calcareous corpuscles. The scolex is usually visible to the naked eye, and the holdfast organs, suckers and hooks, can be distinguished under the compound microscope (Figs. 101–1*A* and *B*, 101–2*A*, and 101–14). The brush border consists of millions of microvilli called microtrichs that increase the absorptive area of the larval surface (Fig. 101–1*C*). The microtrichs are visible in tissue sections magnified 1000 times. The calcareous corpuscles are thin, oval, mineral concretions that are found in the parenchyma (Fig. 101–1*D*). Their size is variable, but the average is usually 5 × 10 μm. It is unlikely that all of these features will be found in a single tissue section, and a series of sections must be studied to make an identification. Furthermore, a particular cyst may not have all of these features. Some cysts are sterile and have no scoleces, whereas others may lack both microtrichs and calcareous corpuscles. However, the recognition of any one of these structures is all that is required to establish a diagnosis of larval cestode infection.

TABLE 101–1. Tapeworms with Larval Stages Infecting Humans

Scientific Name	Larval Stage	Disease	Type of Life Cycle	Definitive Hosts	Intermediate Hosts
Spirometra species	Sparganum (Plerocercoid)	Sparganosis	Aquatic	Carnivores	Copepods, fish, amphibians, reptiles, mammals
Taenia solium	*Cysticercus* (*C. cellulosae*)	Cysticercosis	Domestic	Humans	Pig
Taenia (Multiceps) species	*Coenurus* (*C. cerebralis, C. serialis*)	Coenuriasis	Domestic Wild	Dog Fox, jackal, genet	Sheep Rodents, lagomorphs
Echinococcus granulosus	Unilocular hydatid cyst	Cystic hydatid disease	Domestic	Dog	Sheep, goat, camel, buffalo, reindeer
			Wild	Fox, wolf, coyote, dingo, jackal, wild dog	Moose, deer, reindeer, wallaby, antelope, wild pig
Echinococcus multilocularis	Multilocular hydatid cyst	Alveolar hydatid disease	Domestic	Dog, cat	House mouse
			Wild	Fox, coyote, wolf	Field mouse, mole, lemming, shrew
Echinococcus vogeli	Polycystic hydatid cyst	Polycystic hydatid disease	Wild	Bush dog, feral dog	Paca, spiny rat

ORDER PSEUDOPHYLLIDEA. The life cycles of pseudophyllidean tapeworms are discussed in Chapter 100. Pseudophyllidean larvae found in vertebrates are called plerocercoids or spargana (see Fig. 101–13). These larvae are vermiform in shape and have an undifferentiated head that is identified by a deep invag-ination of the tegument (Fig. 101–13*C* and *D*). Internally, the body of the sparganum is solid parenchyma containing scattered longitudinal muscle bands. The only cavities in the sparganum are the central excretory channels that are lined with an epithelium. Usually, spargana infecting humans do not reproduce in the larval

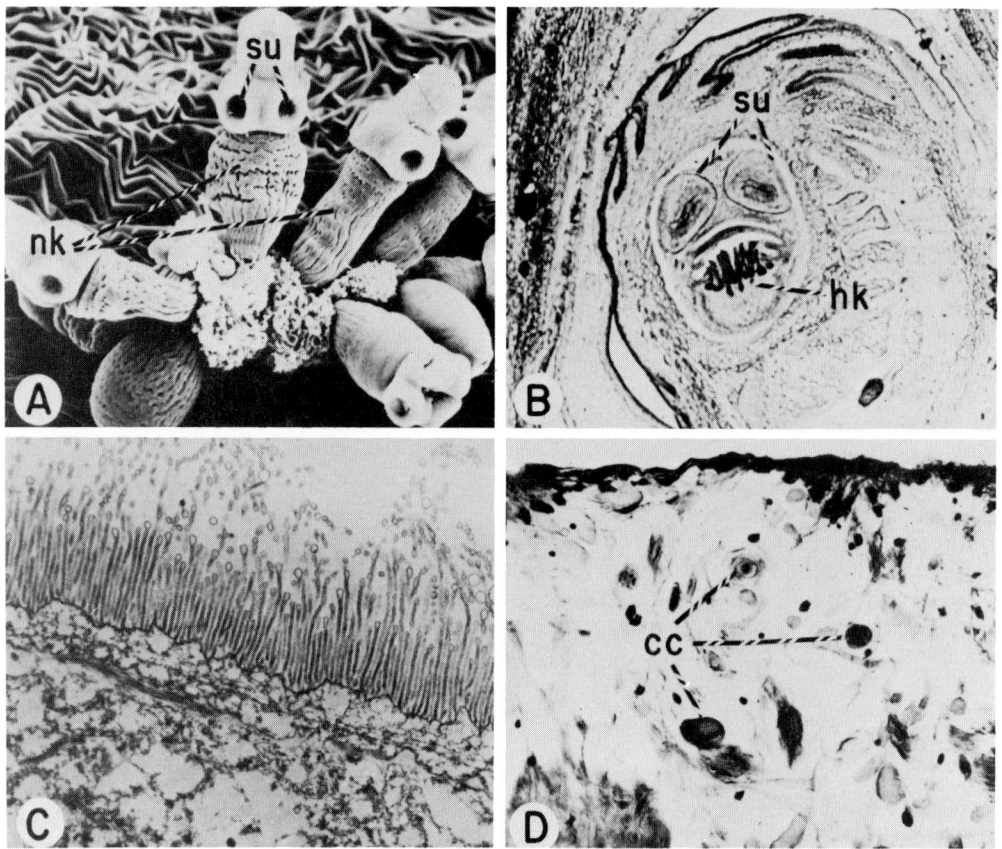

FIGURE 101–1. Morphologic features unique to tapeworms. *A,* Scanning electron micrograph of *Echinococcus multilocularis* showing cyst interior. Scoleces with prominent suckers (su) are supported by wrinkled necks (nk) that connect with the germinal membrane in the background. (Courtesy of A.A. Marchiondo, University of Notre Dame.) *B,* Histologic section of a cysticercus of *Taenia solium* from a human eye showing invaginated scolex with suckers (su) and hooks (hk). (Courtesy of P.M. Schantz, Centers for Disease Control.) *C,* Electron micrograph showing tegumental microvilli. The villi are visible under oil immersion. (Courtesy of the Armed Forces Institute of Pathology, Photograph Neg. No. 74-19368). *D,* Histologic section showing calcareous corpuscles (cc) in the parenchyma under high power. Their number varies, and they may be absent in some sections. (Courtesy of the Armed Forces Institute of Pathology, Photograph Neg. No. 70-6406.)

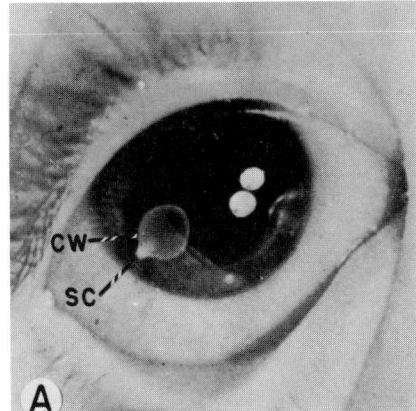

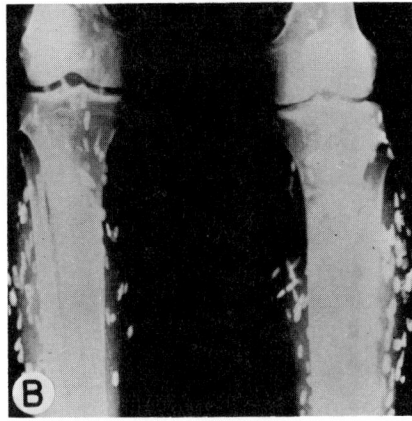

FIGURE 101–2. Cysticercosis. *A,* Viable cysticercus of *Taenia solium* in human eye showing scolex (sc) and cyst wall (cw). (Courtesy of Dr. A. Trejos, Costa Rica.) *B,* Radiograph of legs showing calcified cysticerci. (Courtesy of Dr. M. Campagna.)

stage, but proliferating larvae have been found on rare occasions.

ORDER CYCLOPHYLLIDEA. The life cycles of cyclophyllidean tapeworms are discussed in Chapter 100. Cyclophyllidean larvae are usually cystic, with a cavity or bladder lined with parenchyma rather than an epithelium (see Figs. 101–1*B* and 101–2*A*). The muscle bands are limited to the body wall, where they separate the cortical tegument from the medullary germinal membrane. The scolex and neck develop from the germinal membrane. The scoleces are invaginated and have suckers and hooks similar to those found on the adult tapeworms (see Fig. 101–1*A* and *B*). When ingested by the definitive host, the cyst wall digests away, the scolex attaches to the intestinal epithelium, and the neck generates new segments to form the strobila.

The larval Cyclophyllidea most frequently found in humans are the cysticercoid of *Hymenolepis,* cysticercus of *T. solium,* coenurus of *Taenia (Multiceps)* species, unilocular hydatid cyst of *Echinococcus granulosus,* polycystic hydatid cyst of *Echinococcus vogeli,* and multilocular hydatid cyst of *Echinococcus multilocularis* (Table 101–1). *Hymenolepis nana* was discussed in Chapter 100 and will not be considered here.

Cysticercus. From a reproductive viewpoint the simplest larva is the cysticercus of *T. solium* (Figs. 101–1*B* and 101–2*A*). When ingested by the intermediate host, pig or human, each egg develops into a fluid-filled cyst

containing a single scolex that produces a single adult worm when eaten by the definitive host.

Coenurus. When *Taenia (Multiceps)* eggs are ingested by the intermediate host, sheep or humans, each egg develops into a fluid-filled spherical coenurus that contains several scoleces (Fig. 101–14), each capable of growing into an adult tapeworm. Thus, a single coenurus produces multiple tapeworms in the intestine of the definitive host, the dog.

Hydatid Cysts. Hydatid cysts of the genus *Echinococcus* are the most prolific tapeworm larvae. Like the coenurus, one egg of *Echinococcus* grows into a single spherical cyst, and many scoleces develop from the germinal membrane. In contrast to the coenurus, the germinal membrane of the hydatid cyst proliferates endogenously and/or exogenously to increase its surface area and to facilitate the development of large numbers of scoleces.

Unilocular Hydatid Cyst. The unilocular hydatid cyst of *E. granulosus* appears as a fluid-filled sphere (Figs. 101–7 and 101–9*C*). The germinal membrane secretes a thick, laminated membrane, which is usually covered by a thick pericyst of fibrous tissue of host origin. The germinal membrane proliferates endogenously to form brood capsules within the cyst cavity. The brood capsules frequently detach from the germinal membrane to form what is commonly called hydatid sand. Each scolex is infective to the dog or other definitive hosts, and hundreds of adult tapeworms can develop after the ingestion of a single cyst.

Polycystic Hydatid Cyst. The polycystic hydatid cyst of *E. vogeli* is unique because the germinal membrane proliferates exogenously to form new cysts and endogenously to form septa that divide the hydatid cavity into numerous microcysts (Fig. 101–12). Brood capsules develop from the septate germinal membranes, and scoleces develop from the walls of the brood capsules.

Multilocular Hydatid Cyst. The hydatid cyst of *E. multilocularis* is unique because it only buds exogenously to form a multilocular cyst (Fig. 101–11). The external laminated membrane and the fibrous pericyst of the host are typically thin, and the parasite infiltrates host tissue like a malignancy by external proliferation of the germinal membrane to form new cysts. Humans are an abnormal host for *E. multilocularis,* and the slow-growing multilocular cysts rarely produce brood capsules, scoleces, or calcareous corpuscles.

BIBLIOGRAPHY

Beaver PC, Rolon FA: Proliferating larval cestode in a man in Paraguay. A case report and review. Am J Trop Med Hyg 30:625–637, 1981.

Muller R: Worms and Disease. A Manual of Medical Helminthology. London, William Heinemann Medical Books, 1975, p 161.

Rausch RL: Taeniidae. *In* Hubbert WT, McCulloch WF, Schnurrenberger PR (eds.): Diseases Transmitted from Animals to Man. 6th ed. Springfield, IL, Charles C Thomas, 1975, pp 678–707.

Rickard MD, Williams JF: Hydatidosis/cysticercosis: Immune mechanisms and immunization against infection. *In* Baker JR, Muller R (eds.): Advances in Parasitology, Vol. 21. New York, Academic Press, 1982, pp 230–296.

Schmidt GD, Roberts LS: Foundations of Parasitology. 2d ed. St Louis, C. V. Mosby, 1981.

Thompson RCA (ed.): The Biology of Echinococcus and Hydatid Disease. London, George Allen & Unwin, 1986.

Turner JA: Other cestode infections. *In* Hubbert WT, McCulloch WF, Schnurrenberger PR (eds.): Diseases Transmitted from Animals to Man. 6th ed. Springfield, IL, Charles C Thomas, 1975, pp 708–744.

101.1. CYSTICERCOSIS

DEFINITION. Cysticercosis is caused by infections with the larval stage (cysticercus) of *Taenia solium.*

ETIOLOGY

Definitive Host. The adult tapeworm is host-specific to humans (Chapter 100.2 and 100.5). The scolex is anchored into the jejunum, and the strobila extends throughout the ileum. Gravid segments break from the posterior of the strobila and may pass intact in feces, where they are often described as melon seeds by the distressed patient. Alternatively, the gravid segments disintegrate in the lower intestine to free the eggs, which pass individually in the feces.

Intermediate Host. The only normal intermediate host of significance is the domestic pig, and infected pig meat is called "measly pork." Humans are an incidental intermediate host and could play a role in the life cycle only in areas where cannibalism is prevalent. Ingested eggs begin to hatch in the stomach, where gastric secretions dissolve the embryophore blocks that form the egg shell. Hatching is completed in the duodenum, where the activated oncospheres use their hooks to break out of the egg shell and penetrate the intestinal epithelium to the lymphatic and vascular systems, where they are carried to a variety of tissues. Within 2 to 3 months, the oncospheres lose their hooks and develop into fluid-filled bladder worms or cysticerci (Fig. 101–2A).

T. solium is the most common helminth found in the central nervous system of humans (Figs. 101–3 to 101–

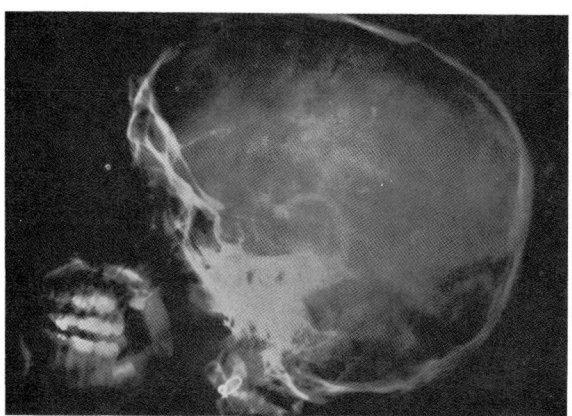

FIGURE 101–4. Cysticercosis. Skull film showing multiple target-like calcifications in the brain of a child infected with the cysticerci of *Taenia solium.*

5). Cysticerci are also found in the eye (Figs. 101–1B and 101–2A), skeletal muscle (Fig. 101–2B), oral cavity, and internal organs.

Humans acquire cysticercosis by ingesting the eggs of *T. solium.* Person-to-person transmission occurs when eggs defecated by an individual with adult tapeworms contaminate the food or beverages consumed by a second individual. A person with the adult tapeworm may infect himself also by external autoinfection via the fecal-oral route. Theoretically, internal autoinfection could result from reverse peristalsis of gravid proglottids to the stomach where egg hatching commences. Although massive cysticercosis from internal autoinfection has never been reported, it has inhibited clinicians from treating patients for infection by the adult tapeworm. Internal autoinfection is not thought to be a complication with the newer anthelmintics (Chapter 100.2).

DISTRIBUTION AND PREVALENCE. Cysticercosis is endemic on all continents except Australasia. In the Americas, cysticercosis is endemic throughout Latin America from Mexico to Chile. Simple, inexpensive

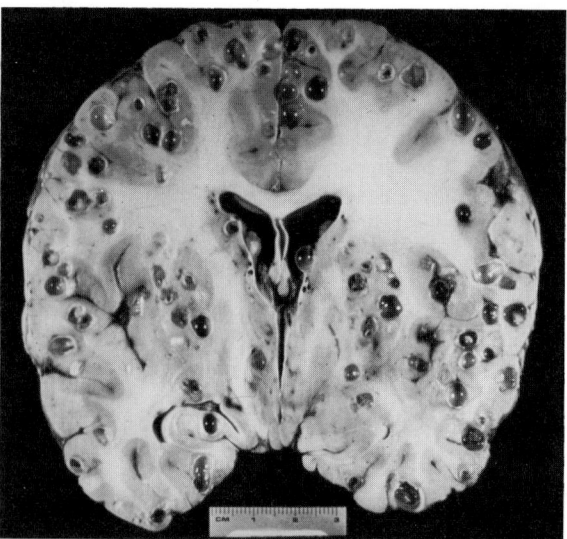

FIGURE 101–3. Sagittal section of brain of a 13-year-old Ekari girl who died from a massive infection with cerebral cysticercosis. (Courtesy of Dr. D.C. Gajdusek of the National Institute of Health and Dr. S.C. Bauserman of the Armed Forces Institute of Pathology; Papua New Guinea Med J 21:329, 1978.)

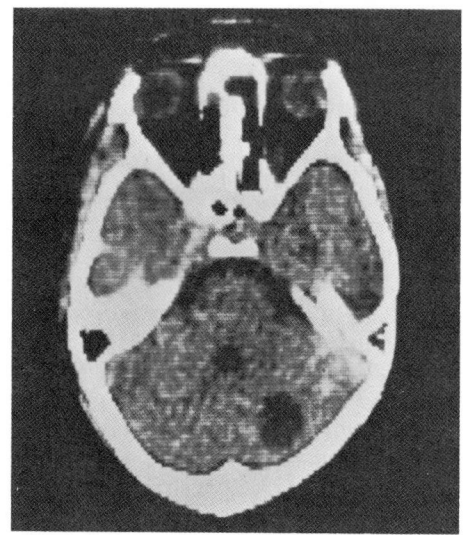

FIGURE 101–5. Cysticercosis. Cerebral lesion in the brain demonstrated by CT scan. The lesion was not seen on the radiograph because it was not calcified.

diagnostic tests with acceptable sensitivity and specificity are not available, and accurate prevalence rates in endemic areas remain to be determined. However, the significance of cysticercosis in Latin America is emphasized in data from Mexico City, where *T. solium* accounts for 10% of all hospital admissions for neurologic conditions and up to one third of all craniotomies for brain tumors. Autopsy data from Mexico City show that the prevalence rate of neurocysticercosis ranges from 1.4 to 3.6% in the general population, and it is likely that similar rates exist elsewhere. *T. solium* is not endemic in the United States, but cysticercosis is prevalent in immigrants from Latin America and Southeast Asia. At the University of Southern California School of Medicine, cysticercosis accounts for 1% of all hospital admissions for neurologic and neurosurgical conditions.

Cysticercosis is uncommon in Europe except in Spain and eastern Europe. In Asia, it has a focal distribution in Russia, China, India, Pakistan, the Philippines, and Indonesia. Cysticercosis occurs sporadically throughout the African continent.

EPIDEMIOLOGY. *T. solium* is prevalent in communities where there is close contact between pigs and people, hygienic standards are low, and meat is eaten undercooked. Because humans are the only host for adult tapeworms, they are the sole source of tapeworm eggs. The transmission of eggs largely depends on promiscuous defecation. In communities without sewage disposal or latrines, adults, and particularly children, defecate in the environment around the house. The concentration of tapeworm eggs is therefore highest in the yard and garden, where humans spend much of their time. In contrast to the pig, humans are not coprophagic, and transmission to humans via the soil-to-mouth route depends on the disintegration of feces and dispersion of eggs throughout the environment. Taeniid eggs (Fig. VI E–2c,d) may disperse up to 80 m in a radial pattern in 10 days. Alternatively, taeniid eggs may be dispersed from feces to food via coprophagic flies. Up to 50% of filth flies feeding on infested feces ingest taeniid eggs, and 5000 eggs have been recorded in a single blowfly. Viable eggs are voided from these flies 48 hours after ingestion.

In addition to defecation habits, other cultural practices may facilitate the transmission of *T. solium* to humans. In southern Africa, there are cases of cysticercosis attributed to the use of *T. solium* proglottids by witch doctors. Humans may also acquire cysticercosis from aberrant sexual practices that facilitate the ingestion of whole proglottids.

The focus in Irian Jaya is of particular interest because it occurred after a gift of pigs from endemic Bali to people in western New Guinea. This resulted in an epidemic of severe burns that was eventually linked to neurocysticercosis with epilepsy. During seizures, infected individuals fell into fires that are used for heat at night in this highland area.

CLINICAL MANIFESTATIONS AND PATHOLOGY. The clinical manifestations of cysticercosis are most variable and depend on the number, age, and location of the cysts. Cysticerci are reported in the brain in 60% of the patients (Figs. 101–3 to 101–5), in the eye in 3% (Fig. 101–2A), and in the muscles in 5% (Fig. 101–2B). Intramuscular cysts are probably more prevalent, but they usually escape clinical attention. Viable cysts stimulate a chronic lymphocytic and granulomatous inflammation, and these space-occupying lesions may persist for 20 years. Dying cysts provoke acute inflammation, which is associated with tissue damage. Dead cysts may resolve or calcify and remain in situ for years (Figs. 101–2B and 101–4). As calcification occurs, symptoms subside, and the patient may become asymptomatic.

Cerebral Features. Cysticerci may localize in any area of the brain, and clinical manifestations are expressed in only half of the infected people. Neurocysticercosis can be grouped into 4 patterns. *Parenchymal cysts* are found in the majority of patients, and they cause seizures, focal deficits, and increased intracranial hypertension (Figs. 101–3 and 101–5). *Meningeal cysts* are found frequently in the basal meninges and occur in about one half of the patients. They cause intense inflammation manifested by obstructive hydrocephalus, arterial thrombosis, and stroke. *Ventricular cysts* are found in 15% of the patients. They may be free-floating or attached and occur most frequently in the fourth ventricle. Ventricular cysts are asymptomatic unless they block the flow of cerebrospinal fluid to cause intracranial hypertension. *Spinal cord cysts* are found in 3% of the patients, and they cause arachnoiditis or signs of compression. More than half of the patients have multiple cysts, and they may express a mixture of these basic patterns of disease.

Ocular Features. Cysticerci infect the eye, where they float freely in the anterior and vitreous chambers or adhere to the subretinal tissue (Figs. 101–1B and 101–2A). Subretinal larvae cause retinal edema, hemorrhage, and vasculitis of the disk. Larvae in the vitreous cavity cause clouding, chorioretinitis, and detachment of the retina. Cystercerci have been found also in the lacrimal gland and eyelid.

Muscular Features. Cysticerci are found in muscles throughout the body, including the buccal mucosa, tongue, and subcutaneous tissues, and may cause severe myositis during acute illness. In addition to inflammation around the cysts, inflammatory cells invade neighboring tissues, where the muscle fibers swell, undergo atrophy, and become fibrosed. The cysticerci often calcify (Fig. 101–2B).

DIAGNOSIS. Cysticercosis occurs most frequently in people between 20 and 50 years old. A suspicion of neurocysticercosis should prompt efforts to establish whether the patient has been exposed to the eggs of *T. solium*. It is important to know if the patient has resided in an endemic area, keeping in mind that the onset of symptoms occurs from a few months to 30 years after infection. Family and friends, as well as the patient himself, may serve as a source of infection, and stool examinations for adult tapeworms should be conducted. Finally, the patient should be examined for muscular cysticercosis by palpating the entire body for pea-sized nodules that can be excised for parasite identification.

Differential Diagnoses. Signs and symptoms vary greatly because cysticerci produce single or multiple space-occupying lesions in any part of the brain, eye, and musculature. The most common manifestations of neurocysticercosis are seizures, acute or progressive focal neurologic deficits, chronic meningitis, and increased intracranial pressure. To establish a diagnosis of neurocysticercosis, other diseases with similar manifestations must be excluded, including tuberculosis, coccidioidomycosis, cryptococcosis, neurosyphilis, sarcoidosis, and primary and metastatic malignancy.

Biopsy. The definitive diagnosis of cysticercosis by parasite identification depends on direct observation of cysts in the eye or on the availability of the cysts for excisional biopsy (Fig. 101–2A). The gross specimen is a fluid-filled opaque bladder measuring 1 to 70 mm in diameter that contains a single, solid, white sphere, the scolex. In live specimens, movement may be seen in the bladder wall and the scolex. Carefully prepared wet mounts viewed under the microscope will reveal the 4 suckers and the double row of hooks on the rostellum. The short hooks measure 130 μm in length, and the long hooks measure 170 μm. In tissue sections, the diagnostic features include the surface microtrichs, calcareous corpuscles, the wrinkled neck, and the scolex (Fig. 101–1B).

Radiography. The hallmark of cysticercosis revealed by plain radiography is multiple elliptiform calcifications (Figs. 101–2B and 101–4). Pathognomonic features are the central calcified scolex and the surrounding calcified cyst wall. Computerized tomography is more sensitive than plain radiography and reveals noncalcified and calcified cysts (Fig. 101–5). Because cysticerci may have the same absorption values as cerebrospinal fluid, contrast enhancement might be required to visualize cysts in the ventricles.

Cerebrospinal Fluid and Blood. Examinations of cerebrospinal fluid and blood may show nonspecific changes that are helpful in diagnosing cysticercosis in combination with the aforementioned parameters. Changes in the cerebrospinal fluid associated with neurocysticercosis are the presence of eosinophils, an increase in total protein and IgG concentrations, and the presence of antibody to *T. solium.* Changes in the blood include leukocytosis, eosinophilia, and the presence of specific antibody. Most of the generally available tests for antibody lack sensitivity and specificity and cross react with antigens from hydatid cysts, coenuri, and other tapeworms (Chapter 125), but recent developments in Mexico and South Africa suggest that ELISA tests can become much more reliable.

TREATMENT. The management of neurocysticercosis varies with clinical manifestations and includes no intervention, symptomatic treatment, surgery, or chemotherapy. Asymptomatic neurocysticerci do not always warrant treatment. In one study, 90% of the patients with hemispheric lesions present on CT scans had a nonprogressive course during a 1-year observation period. Ventricular cysts have been found also at autopsy in patients who died of other causes.

Symptomatic Treatment. When infection of the brain is accompanied by clinical manifestations, symptomatic treatment should precede surgery. Epilepsy may be controlled with anticonvulsants, and meningitis and cerebral edema may be controlled with corticosteroids.

Surgery. Cystectomy may eradicate central nervous system (CNS) disease in operable cases involving a single cyst. Patients with hydrocephalus, in whom extirpation of cysts should be avoided, might obtain symptomatic relief by ventricular shunting.

Chemotherapy. Praziquantel does not affect disease caused by calcified cysts or unrepairable tissue damage, but it does cross the blood-brain barrier and the cyst wall to kill cysticerci. Apparently most of the dead cysts are resorbed, but a few calcify. In one preliminary trial, intracranial hypertension was cured in 90% of the patients, and the remainder improved. Post-treatment epilepsy was controlled with anticonvulsants in 75% of the patients, and the frequency of seizures was reduced in the remainder. In anticipation of allergic reactions, patients were given prednisone to dampen the inflammatory response to disintegrating larvae. About 15% of the patients experienced headache, nausea, and vomiting that required no treatment. An additional 15% had severe side effects such as increased intracranial hypertension, which was managed with parenteral steroids and mannitol.

Praziquantel is also effective against muscular cysticercosis, and most of the nodules disappear 2 to 3 months after treatment. In one study, 38% of the patients with muscular larvae had seizures, indicating that they had neurocysticercosis as well.

The following recommendations should be considered for the treatment of neurocysticercosis: (1) praziquantel, 50 mg/kg/day in 3 divided doses for 10 to 14 days, or albendazole as for treatment of hydatid cysts (Chapter 101.2), repeating the treatment if symptoms persist; (2) dexamethasone to suppress inflammation around degenerating cysts; (3) surgical removal of some cysticerci, such as those in the fourth ventricle and the eye; and (4) hospitalization with neurosurgical consultation in case complications arise.

CONTROL. Because humans are the only definitive host, control should focus on education in health and hygiene. Cysticerci can be killed by freezing pork, the usual source of the adult tapeworm, at −20C for 12 hours or by cooking it at 50C. Although cysticerci can be found in live pigs by examination of the tongue or in carcasses by examination of the intercostal and cervical muscles, meat inspection is an insensitive method for detecting measly pork. To prevent the infection of pigs, indiscriminate human defecation should be discouraged, and sewage should be treated to kill tapeworm eggs. Poor husbandry practices must be corrected, because pigs wander everywhere and eat anything, including human feces.

RACEMOSE CYSTICERCUS. This larval cestode is found on rare occasion in the central nervous system, particularly at the base of the brain. This cyst is acephalic and multiplies by exogenous budding to form multilocular cystic cavities. Grossly, the racemose cysticercus may appear as a mass of thin-walled cysts resembling a bunch of grapes, with the larger cysts measuring up to 10 cm in diameter. This larva is classified as a cestode because it has surface microtrichs. It belongs to the Cyclophyllidea because it has characteristic muscle bands that separate the tissue of the worm into cortical and medullary zones and a cysticercus lacuna, a large cavity lined with parenchyma rather than an epithelium. Because generic classification is based on the number, distribution, and morphologic features of the scoleces, the exact taxonomic status of these acephalic larvae is unknown. The racemose cysticercus is believed to be an aberrant larva of *T. solium* or *Taenia (Multiceps)* species.

BIBLIOGRAPHY

Botero D, Castano S: Treatment of cysticercosis with praziquantel in Colombia. Am J Trop Med Hyg 31:811, 1982.

Brown JW, Voge M: Neuropathology of Parasitic Infections. Oxford, Oxford University Press, 1982.

Dixon HBF, Lipscomb FM: Cysticercosis: An analysis and follow-up of 450 cases. Medical Research Council Special Report Series No. 299. London, Medical Research Council, 1961.

Escobedo J, Penagos P, Rodriguez J, et al.: Albendazole therapy for neurocysticercosis. Arch Intern Med 147:738–741, 1987.

Flisser A, Willms K, Laclette JP, et al.: Cysticercosis. Present State of Knowledge and Perspectives. New York, Academic Press, 1982, p 700.

Gemmel M, Matyas Z, Pawlowski Z, et al. (eds.): WHO Guidelines for Surveillance, Prevention and Control of Taeniasis/Cysticercosis. Geneva, WHO, VPH/83.49.

McCormick GF, Zee CS, Heiden J: Cysticercosis cerebri. Review of 127 cases. Arch Neurol 39:534, 1982.

Pammenter MD, Rossouw EJ: The value of an antigenic fraction of *Cysticercus cellulosae* in the serodiagnosis of cysticercosis. Ann Trop Med Parasitol 81:117–123, 1900.

Spina-França A, Nobrega JPS, Livramento JA, et al.: Administration of praziquantel in neurocysticercosis. Tropenmed Parasitol 33:1, 1982.

101.2. CYSTIC HYDATID DISEASE

DEFINITION. Cystic hydatid disease is a zoonotic disease of humans caused by infection with the larval stage (unilocular hydatid cyst) of *Echinococcus granulosus.*

ETIOLOGY. Humans acquire cystic hydatid disease by ingesting the eggs of *E. granulosus* (Fig. 101–6). The eggs hatch in the intestine, and the liberated oncospheres penetrate the mucosa to the blood and lymphatic systems for transport to the liver, lungs, and other organs. The larvae grow slowly into hydatid cysts and produce chronic, space-occupying lesions.

DISTRIBUTION AND PREVALENCE. Cystic hydatid disease is prevalent in most parts of the world where dogs are kept as pets or used as guards or for herding livestock. It is distributed throughout the Americas, but most of the human cases come from southern Brazil, Uruguay, Argentina, Chile, and Peru. The disease is widespread in the Old World, particularly in Yugoslavia, Bulgaria, Cyprus, Sardinia, Lebanon, Turkey, Iraq, southern USSR, Mongolia, Tibet, and China. Cystic hydatid disease is a problem throughout Australasia. It is distributed widely in North and East Africa with a high prevalence in Libya, northern Kenya, southern Sudan, and southern Ethiopia.

In some areas, cystic hydatid disease is an important cause of human morbidity and necessitates major expenditures for diagnosis and surgical treatment. The economic loss to the livestock industry can be substantial also in terms of the decreased production of meat, milk, and wool and the condemnation of organs at slaughter.

EPIDEMIOLOGY. The life cycle of *E. granulosus* requires 2 hosts and is dependent on the food chain (Fig. 101–6) and the high biotic potential of the hydatid cyst. The adult is found in the small intestine of dogs or other canids. It is one of the smallest cestodes, with only 2 to 5 segments and a length of 3 to 8 mm, but it compensates for its small size by occurring in large numbers. Eggs are eliminated in feces, contaminate herbage, and remain viable for long periods in cool, damp places. When viable eggs are ingested by susceptible herbivores, they develop into unilocular cysts in the viscera, particularly the liver and lungs. Enormous numbers of scoleces are produced from endogenous budding of the germinal membrane, and 60,000 to 70,000 adult tapeworms have been recovered from dogs that were fed individual cysts.

The adult stage of *E. granulosus* has been recorded from more than 12 species of carnivores throughout the world, and the larval stage has been recorded from over 50 species of herbivores. Taxonomic studies have detected morphologic, developmental, biochemical, and physiologic differences among geographic strains, and these differences have been linked to local patterns of transmission. For example, *Echinococcus* from horses and sheep in Britain are distinct, and it is unlikely that the horse strain infects humans. In Australia, there are 3 strains of *Echinococcus:* the sheep-dog and macropod-dingo strains on mainland Australia and another sheep-dog strain in Tasmania.

Wild Cycles. Both taxonomic and epidemiologic studies have delineated wild and domestic cycles of *E. granulosus.* The wild cycles exist throughout much of the distribution of *E. granulosus.* In the Arctic, this cycle involves the wolf as the final host and the moose, caribou, and reindeer as intermediate hosts. In California, there is a coyote-deer cycle. In Sri Lanka, there is a jackal-deer cycle. In Africa, adult tapeworms have been found in hunting dogs, hyenas, jackals, and lions, with cysts occurring in antelopes and wild pigs. In Australia, there is a dingo-macropod cycle.

Domestic Cycle. The domestic cycle of *E. granulosus* is essentially the same in all endemic areas of the world. The dog is always the definitive host, and sheep are by far the most important intermediate hosts, but goats, horses, cows, camels, yaks, and pigs may also serve as hosts.

Transmission between the wild and domestic cycles depends on the infectivity of the *Echinococcus* strains to the wild and domestic hosts. The intensity and direction of this transmission are related to the behavior of the wild and domestic animals. Transmission from wild herbivores to domestic dogs is usually of minor importance. However, wild carnivores often contaminate pastures with *Echinococcus* eggs, which infect domestic herbivores and humans. Transmission from wild carnivores to domestic herbivores could jeopardize the success of control schemes.

Animal Husbandry. With few exceptions, cystic hy-

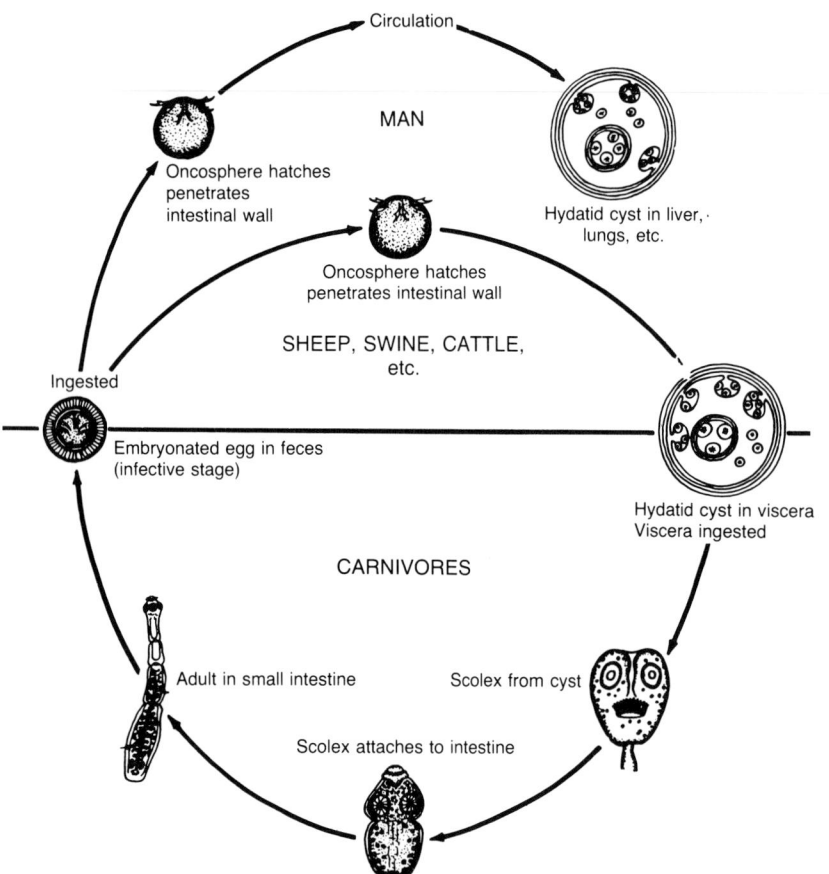

FIGURE 101–6. Life cycle of *Echinococcus granulosus*. (Modified from Melvin DM, et al.: Common Blood and Tissue Parasites of Man. Life Cycle Charts. Atlanta, Georgia, Centers for Disease Control, 1979.)

FIGURE 101–7. Cystic hydatid disease. *A,* Abdominal distention from hydatid cysts in Turkana, Kenya. (From Muller R: Worms and Disease. London, William Heinemann Medical Books, 1975.) *B,* Unilocular hydatid cyst in human liver containing hydatid sand consisting of daughter cysts and free scoleces in the cyst fluid. (Courtesy of the Armed Forces Institute of Pathology, Photograph Neg. No. N-31977.) *C,* Histologic section showing external laminated membrane (lm), internal germinal membrane (gm), and scoleces (SC). (Courtesy of the Armed Forces Institute of Pathology, Photograph Neg. No. 706612.) *D,* Histologic section showing brood capsules (bc) attached to the germinal membrane (gm). Fibrous wall of the host (fw) and laminated membrane of the parasite (lm) are also shown. (Courtesy of the Armed Forces Institute of Pathology, Photograph Neg. No. N-74378.)

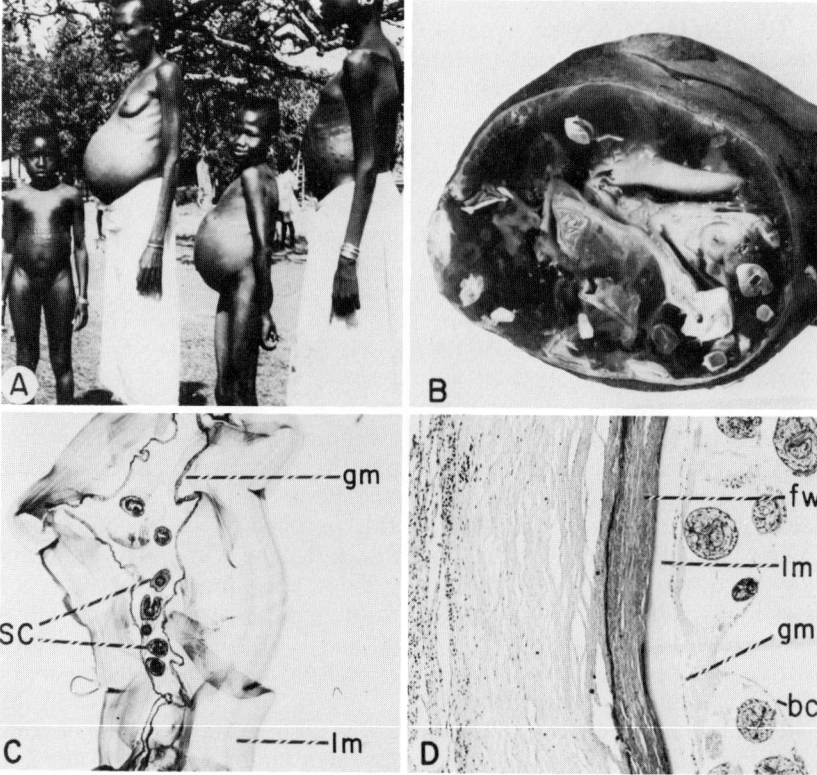

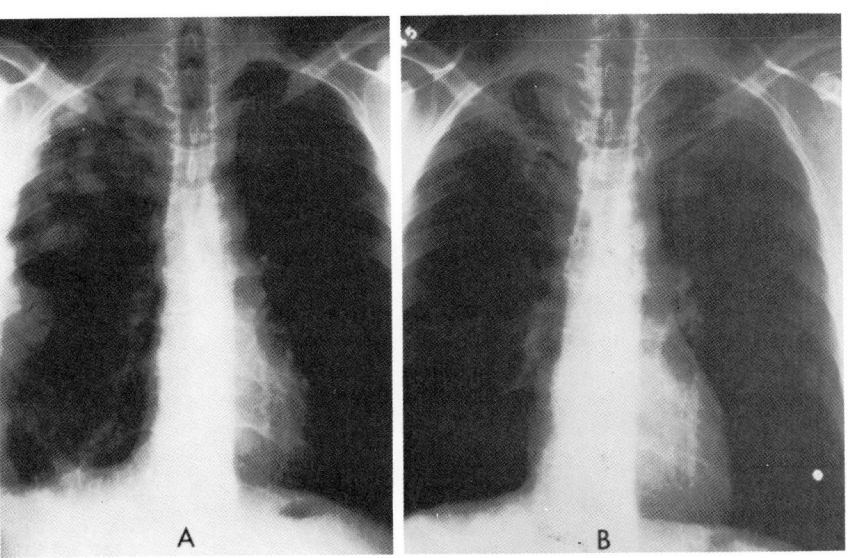

FIGURE 101–8. Echinococcosis. *A*, Chest radiograph of a young Italian carpenter with multiple cysts in the right upper lung fields and a large cyst on the right lateral chest wall. *B*, Chest radiograph almost 4 years later following a prolonged course of mebendazole therapy. No lesions are present on the radiograph.

datid disease in humans is a rural disease; the communities at highest risk of infection are those where working dogs are used to manage the flocks and where they have access to sheep carcasses. In the United States, vast areas are used to raise sheep, but hydatid disease is prevalent only in small groups of ranchers who feed their dogs the entrails of slaughtered animals—the Basques in the Central Valley of California, some Mormon ranchers in Utah, and the Navajo and Zuni Indians of Arizona and New Mexico.

In addition to husbandry practices, cultural, occupational, and religious practices affect the transmission of *Echinococcus* eggs from the feces, paws, and fur of dogs to humans. The risk of infection is often linked with poor hygiene combined with frequent and intimate contact with dogs. Despite the fact that eggs are killed by exposure to temperatures above 40C, cystic hydatid disease is hyperendemic in the desert-dwelling Turkana tribe of Kenya because they value dogs highly and maintain intimate contact with them. In this arid region where water is scarce, the women, among whom there is an unusually high prevalence of hydatid disease, are always accompanied by dogs and even use them to clean up their menses and to lick vomit from the faces and diarrhea from the anal regions of their children (Fig. 101–7A). In Lebanon, the prevalence was high in shoemakers, who used dog feces to cure leather. The use of dog feces in traditional medicine may be a factor also in transmission in some primitive regions.

CLINICAL MANIFESTATIONS. The majority of cases of cystic hydatid disease are probably asymptomatic and are discovered by sonography and chest radiography or at autopsy. Signs and symptoms vary according to the number and size of cysts and the organ involved. Single cysts are found in 80% of the patients and have the following distribution: liver, 63% (Fig. 101–7B); lungs, 25%; muscle, 5%; bones, 3%; kidney, 2%; spleen and brain, 1%; and other organs, 1%. Signs and symptoms largely result from pressure exerted by the growing cyst and mimic those of an expanding tumor, but in many cases the cysts are relatively benign.

Because the initial oncosphere is only 20 μm in diameter and the larger cysts grow at a variable rate, averaging 1 to 5 cm in diameter per year, the symptoms of hydatid infection are usually manifested in the middle and older age groups. However, cysts in the eye and brain may produce earlier symptoms in children.

Signs and Symptoms. The chronic signs of hepatic hydatid disease include hepatomegaly and obstructive jaundice accompanied by symptoms such as mild epigastric pain, bloating, indigestion, and nausea. A hydatid cyst may also become secondarily infected with bacteria and present as an hepatic abscess. Features of lung involvement include coughing, hemoptysis, dyspnea, and, sometimes, fever. Brain cysts produce increasing intracranial pressure, epilepsy, and blindness; vertebral cysts compress the spinal cord and cause paraplegia; renal cysts produce hematuria, albuminuria, and loin pain; and bone cysts produce spontaneous fractures and deformity.

Cyst Rupture. Acute signs and symptoms of hydatid disease are associated with the traumatic and surgical rupture of the cysts. Rupture of cysts in the abdominal organs may cause peritonitis, and rupture in the lungs may cause pneumothorax and empyema. In addition to these local signs and symptoms of acute hydatid disease, rupture of a cyst also causes allergic manifestations, including pruritus, urticaria, edema, dyspnea, asthma, vomiting, diarrhea, colicky pain, anaphylactic shock, and even death.

DIAGNOSIS. Signs and symptoms indicating a space-occupying lesion should warrant the inclusion of cystic hydatid disease in the differential diagnosis. The space-occupying lesions can be further defined with roentgenography (Fig. 101–8A), CT scanning (Fig. 101–9A), and sonography (Fig. 101–9B). Sometimes the cyst may be calcified, and it will be demonstrated by a plain x-ray (Fig. 101–10). For hydatid disease to be included in the differential diagnosis, the patient must have lived in or traveled to endemic areas.

Serology. Antibody may not be detected in all patients. The indirect hemagglutination and latex aggluti-

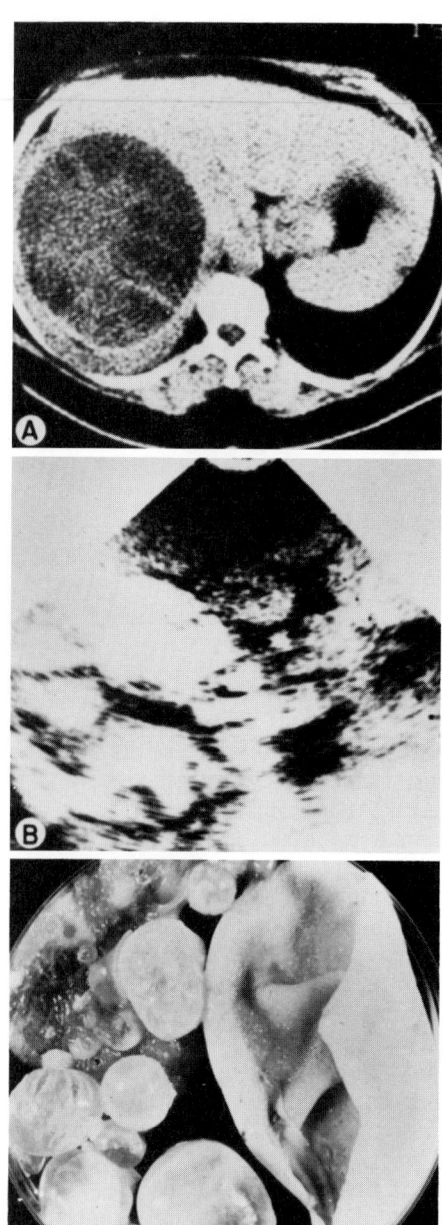

FIGURE 101–9. Cystic hydatid disease. *A,* CT scan showing septate densities within the 12-cm cyst. *B,* Sonogram of the same cyst showing the septate densities. *C,* Daughter cysts removed from the same cyst. (Courtesy of the Armed Forces Institute of Pathology.)

nation tests are used often for initial screening, because they are simple procedures with adequate sensitivity (Chapter 125). These tests lack specificity, however. When cross-reactions are suspected, the diagnosis can be narrowed by using double diffusion, immunoelectrophoresis, or counterimmunoelectrophoresis tests to detect antibody against "Arc-5"—a genus-specific antigen isolated from unilocular hydatid cyst fluid. Antibody tests may be negative in patients with large active cysts. In these cases the sera can be examined for immune complexes and circulating antigens. The Casoni skin test is nonspecific and of little value in diagnosis.

Sputum Samples. Lung cysts sometimes rupture, and the diagnosis might be confirmed by examination of

sputum. The hooks of *Echinococcus* stain well with the Ziehl-Neelsen technique used for *Mycobacterium tuberculosis,* and the laminated membrane stains with the periodic acid-Schiff technique.

Parasitology. The gross specimen will have one fluid-filled cavity covered by a translucent white membrane with underlying, opaque dots representing scoleces, brood capsules, and hydatid sand (Fig. 101–9C). Parasite identification can be made in wet-mount preparations. The scolex has 4 spherical suckers and a rostellum with 2 rows of hooks. The large hooks are 30 to 40 μm in length, and the small hooks measure 22 to 34 μm. In hematoxylin-eosin-stained sections, the brush border and calcareous corpuscles (see Fig. 101–1) are characteristics unique to cestodes, whereas brood capsules, hydatid sand, and the acellular, multilayered, laminated membrane are characteristics unique to the genus *Echinococcus* (Fig. 101–7C and D).

TREATMENT. Between 1 and 4% of the diagnosed cases of cystic hydatid disease are fatal. In uncomplicated cases, surgical resection remains the treatment of choice, but patients with multiple cysts or cysts in the brain or bone should be treated with albendazole.

Surgery. During surgery, special care must be taken to remove the cyst intact. Leakage of cyst fluid may cause general toxicity and anaphylaxis. In addition, scoleces or microscopic fragments of the germinal epithelium can generate entirely new cysts, and their dissemination may cause secondary disease. This can be prevented by treatment with albendazole from 2 weeks before until 2 weeks after surgery.

To minimize leakage of hydatid fluid, the resection

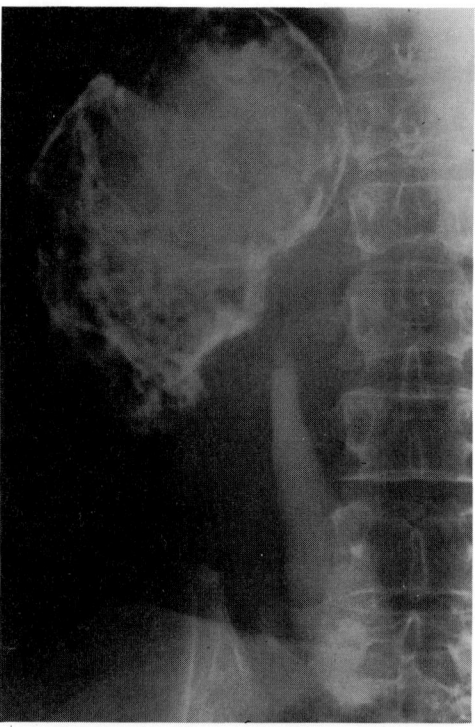

FIGURE 101–10. Echinococcosis. Plain film of the abdomen demonstrating a calcified mass in the liver. Serologic testing was positive for *Echinococcus.* The patient, being elderly and asymptomatic, was not treated.

can be conducted inside a metal cone that is frozen to the cyst. Prior to resection, the area of the cyst is swabbed with a scolecidal chemical such as 0.1% Cetrimide (cetyltrimethylammonium bromide) or hypertonic saline solution. The cyst contents are then aspirated and replaced with the scolecide. After a 5-minute incubation period, the procedure is repeated. Finally, the laminated membrane of the cyst is separated from the fibrous host pericyst, and the cavity is irrigated with more scolecide. Formalin should not be used as a scolecide because it may cause an adverse shock reaction and fix host tissue.

With liver cysts, the fibrous tissue should be left to prevent bleeding. If the liver cyst is too large for closure of the cavity, marsupialization may be necessary. Pulmonary cysts should be removed intact by making an incision through the adventitia, aided by increasing the intrapulmonary pressure with an inflated cuff tube in the trachea.

Chemotherapy. Preliminary studies on the efficacy of mebendazole for the treatment of cystic hydatid disease produced conflicting results (Fig. 101–8*B*). This drug has now been replaced by albendazole, which is much better absorbed from the intestine and much more effective. In some areas, for example in Kenya, albendazole has replaced surgery as the first treatment and it has been dramatically successful in the treatment of cysts in the liver, abdomen, lungs, bones, and eye. This is particularly the case with young, actively growing cysts. Albendazole was administered at a dose of 10 to 15 mg/kg/day over 8 weeks, and good results have been obtained with 2 28-day courses separated by 2 weeks at a dose of 800 mg/day.

The mixed results obtained with chemotherapy relate to difficulties in measuring the success of treatment. Because cyst material is difficult to obtain, parasitologic criteria for parasite viability, including the motility of scoleces, in vitro culture, and growth in gerbils, are rarely used. Changes in cyst volume and density can be monitored by radiography (Fig. 101–8), sonography, and CT scanning (Figs. 101–9 and 101–10), but the relationship between these parameters and cyst viability is ill defined. Of the serologic parameters, a decrease in the titer of specific IgE is the most reliable indication of cure, but this test is complicated and is not always available.

CONTROL. The control of hydatid disease rests on mass chemotherapy of dogs, the destruction of stray dogs, and an active health education program. Mass chemotherapy using praziquantel (see Chapter 100.4) focuses on the elimination of adult worms from dogs to reduce environmental contamination with *Echinococcus* eggs and their transmission to herbivores and humans. Because the prepatent period is 45 to 50 days, treatment should be given at monthly intervals, but this is usually not feasible. The success of mass chemotherapy depends on the proportion of dogs that are successfully treated and the frequency of transmission from wild canids to domestic herbivores and humans.

Health education on hydatid control focuses on the management of the domestic dog population, animal husbandry, and personal hygiene. Domestic dogs are infected because humans feed them viscera with hydatid cysts; therefore proper disposal of infected organs by commercial and home butchers is essential. Behavioral patterns that encourage human-dog contact and foster transmission of *Echinococcus* eggs from dogs to humans must be corrected.

These control measures have been successful in Iceland, where strict regulations precluding dogs from human habitations probably led to the elimination of *Echinococcus*. In Cyprus, Tasmania, and New Zealand, where there is no wild cycle, mass treatment of dogs and health education have greatly limited transmission to humans.

101.3. ALVEOLAR HYDATID DISEASE

DEFINITION. Alveolar hydatid disease is a zoonotic disease of humans caused by infection with the larval stage (multilocular hydatid cyst) of *Echinococcus multilocularis*.

HISTORY. It was known for many years that some hydatid cysts in the liver of humans failed to develop a restricting laminated membrane and spread through the tissue to produce the so-called alveolar or malignant hydatid cyst. It was not until the 1950s that Vogel in Germany, Rausch and colleagues in Alaska, and Lukashenko in the USSR clearly recognized *E. multilocularis* as a distinct species with a life cycle that differs from that of *E. granulosus*.

ETIOLOGY. Humans acquire alveolar hydatid disease by ingesting the eggs of *E. multilocularis*. The oncospheres hatch from the eggs in the intestine, penetrate the mucosa to the portal circulation, and are carried to the liver, where they develop into multilocular hydatid cysts. These cysts grow slowly by exogenous proliferation and spread throughout the entire liver (Fig. 101–11) and contiguous organs to produce chronic, space-occupying lesions. The cysts occasionally metastasize to the lungs and brain.

DISTRIBUTION AND PREVALENCE. *E. multilocularis* is enzootic in the Northern Hemisphere. In North America, it is distributed throughout the northern tundra and in a large focus along the central portion of the United States–Canadian border that includes 3 provinces and 6 states. Human disease in North America is rare, with records of 33 autochthonous cases from Alaska and 1 from Minnesota.

E. multilocularis is found in central Europe, including Switzerland, where 122 cases of alveolar hydatid disease were reported from 1950 to 1969. In Asia, it is distributed throughout much of the Soviet Union and in some parts of Siberia, where the prevalence reaches 9 per 1000 inhabitants. It is also found in the northern islands of Japan, and there is an extensive focus in western China.

EPIDEMIOLOGY. The fox is the primary definitive host of *E. multilocularis*, but wolves, coyotes, dogs, and cats have been found infected. The adult tapeworm lives in the small intestine, and eggs are voided in feces. The intermediate hosts include voles, lemmings, shrews, and mice.

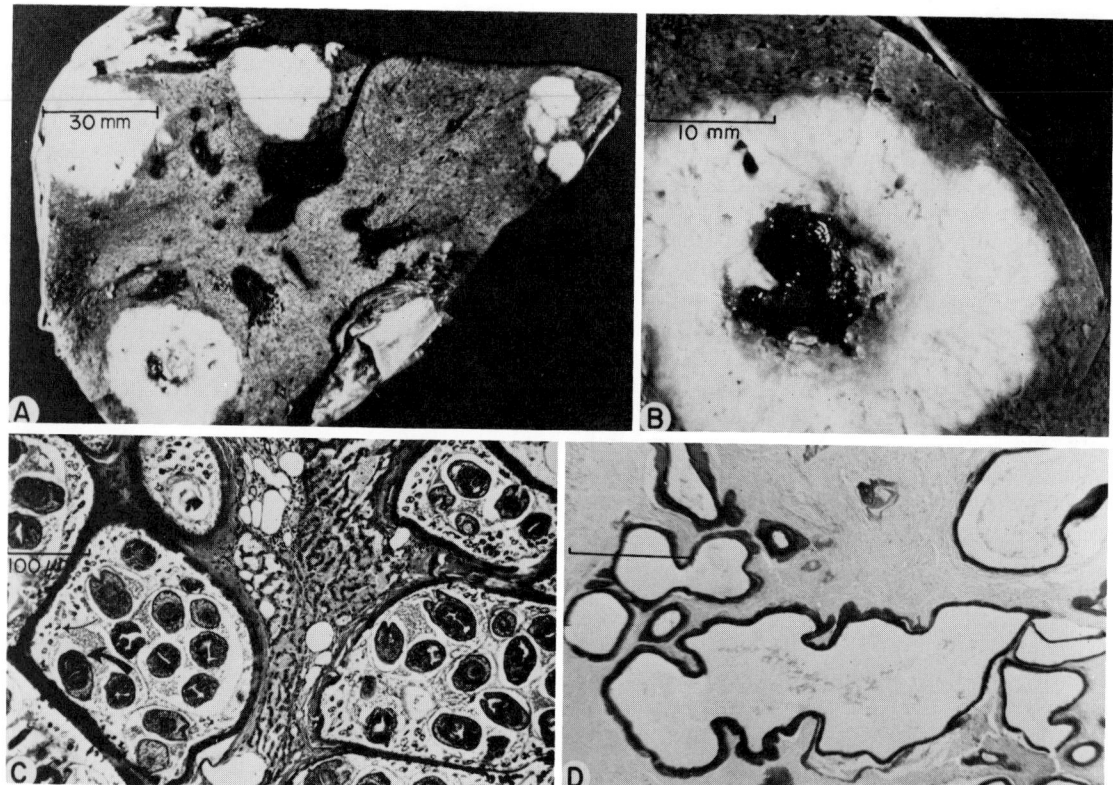

FIGURE 101–11. Multilocular hydatid disease. *A,* Multiple primary lesions in human liver. *B,* Enlargement of one of the lesions seen in *A* showing central necrosis. *C,* Histologic section of cyst from a vole, the normal host, stained with hematoxylin and eosin showing abundant scoleces (large arrow) and calcareous corpuscles (small arrow). *D,* Histologic section of a cyst from man, an abnormal host, stained by the periodic acid–Schiff technique showing the intensely stained laminated membrane surrounding vesicles void of scoleces and calcareous corpuscles. (From Wilson JF, Rausch RL: Am J Trop Med Hyg 29:1340, 1980.)

Throughout most of its range, *E. multilocularis* is an arctic or alpine parasite, and special adaptations have evolved to facilitate its transmission in these harsh environments. The adult tapeworm survives the winter in the intestines of canids, and the cyst survives in hibernating rodents with low body temperatures. The parasite eggs also resist cold climate and accumulate in the environment for transmission to rodents at the spring thaw.

The arctic and alpine summers are short, and the multilocular cysts grow quickly in the natural rodent hosts, with scoleces developing in 2 to 4 months. The biotic potential of the cysts is high, because there are 100 to 200 scoleces per mg of tissue (Fig. 101–11*C*). The cysts produce massive infections in canids, and the intensity of infection can range from 100,000 to 160,000 worms per dog. Eggs develop 30 to 35 days after infection. Each gravid segment contains about 100 eggs, so that environmental contamination is high.

E. multilocularis is a zoonotic parasite that is maintained in a fox-rodent cycle. The role of foxes in terms of transmission to humans is important to hunters and fur traders. However, domestic cycles may become established within rural communities, where dogs and cats can serve as definitive hosts, with wild rodents serving as intermediate hosts. The intensity of transmission in arctic villages is high because populations of sled dogs are large and there are no precautions to prevent contamination of the environment and food stores with

their feces. It is in this setting that humans are most frequently exposed to infection from the eggs of *E. multilocularis.*

PATHOLOGY. The hepatic lesions appear as one or more firm, yellow-gray masses that may occupy any area of the liver, including the surface (Fig. 101–11*A* and *B*). In advanced cases, the liver lesion includes extensive hepatic degeneration, with central necrosis presenting as a large, pus-filled cavity with a firm wall several millimeters thick that may occupy half the organ. The outer layer of the cyst has an ill-defined margin and diffuses inconspicuously into the host tissue.

Microscopically, there are multiple convoluted vesicles of varying sizes lined with the external laminated membrane of the parasite (Fig. 101–11*D*). This hyaline membrane is much thinner than that in the cyst of *E. granulosus,* and it is best visualized by the periodic acid-Schiff technique. Because humans are an abnormal host, brood capsules, scoleces, and calcareous corpuscles rarely develop. The large vesicles represent older portions of the cyst that give rise to the smaller microcysts by exogenous proliferation of the germinal membrane. The vesicles are usually surrounded by a dense layer of scar tissue that may be 3 to 15 mm thick. Inflammatory cells consisting of histiocytes and eosinophils have a focal distribution around the proliferating vesicles at the periphery of the cyst.

CLINICAL MANIFESTATIONS. The multilocular cyst grows slowly in humans (an abnormal host), and a person may be infected for 30 years before symptoms appear. The primary lesion in alveolar hydatid disease is always in the liver (Fig. 101–11*A* and *B*). These lesions involve the right lobe in 30% of patients, the left lobe in 10%, and both lobes in 60%. There is spread to contiguous organs in 15% of patients to infect the inferior vena cava, portal vein, and common bile duct. Pieces of the germinal membrane metastasize to distant organs in 2% of patients to infect the brain, lungs, and mediastinum. The signs and symptoms identified in retrospective studies show palpable livers in 80% of patients, right upper quadrant pain in 60%, an abdominal mass arising from the liver in 50%, jaundice in 20%, and shortness of breath in 10%. The rate of cyst growth varies among individuals, and there may be some self-cures, but without treatment, proliferation usually continues and ultimately leads to the death of the patient.

DIAGNOSIS. Alveolar hydatid disease is usually diagnosed in people who are 50 years of age or older and have a history of living in an endemic area. Radiographs will reveal diffuse space-occupying lesions that permeate the liver. Diffuse mineralization of dead cyst material can also be visualized.

Serology. Serologic tests are helpful in supporting the diagnosis if the history, signs, and symptoms are compatible with alveolar hydatid disease (Chapter 125). The indirect hemagglutination test using fluid from the cyst of *E. granulosus* is positive in 90% of patients with alveolar hydatid disease, and the titers are much higher than those found in patients with cystic hydatid disease. Antibodies to the genus-specific *Echinococcus* antigen called "Arc-5" are detected by gel diffusion techniques in 70% of patients with alveolar hydatid disease. This test can be used to check the specificity of a positive hemagglutination test (Chapter 101.2).

The extent of the disease is usually determined at laparotomy, and confirmation of the diagnosis is established histologically by demonstrating the multilaminar cyst membrane using the periodic acid-Schiff technique (Fig. 101–11*D*).

TREATMENT

Surgical Resection. Surgical resection of the primary cyst is the traditional treatment for alveolar hydatid disease. In contrast to the unilocular cyst of *E. granulosus*, which is a well-defined sphere contained in a fibrotic pericyst, the multilocular cyst is pleomorphic and infiltrates the organ in all directions. It is impossible to separate the cyst from host tissue, and resection must include the cyst, diseased tissue, and surrounding normal tissue. There is little risk of toxic and anaphylactic reactions, as the cyst does not contain free fluid. When partial hepatectomy is feasible, the cure rate of cyst resection is excellent. Success is indicated by the permanent decrease in antibody titer.

Chemotherapy. Mebendazole has been used for treatment of inoperable patients with encouraging results. Several patients have been given continuous high doses (40 mg/kg/day) for as long as 5 years. Cyst growth usually stops, and some cysts even regress. Many patients feel better while receiving therapy, and their survival is prolonged. Unfortunately, post-treatment antibody titers remain high, suggesting that the cysts are not killed. The side effects of long-term, high-dose treatment with mebendazole are rare and include febrile reactions, reversible leukopenias, and reversible alopecia. Better results are being reported now with the much less toxic drug albendazole at similar dose levels as used for *E. granulosus* but given for longer periods (Chapter 101.2).

CONTROL. Until recently, control rested solely on education to improve hygienic practices and to encourage the elimination of surplus dogs in enzootic areas. There is now hope that transmission of *E. multilocularis* might be reduced by mass treatment of village dogs with praziquantel to eliminate the adult tapeworm population and reduce environmental contamination with eggs (Chapter 101.2).

101.4. POLYCYSTIC HYDATID DISEASE

DEFINITION. Polycystic hydatid disease is a zoonotic disease of humans caused by infection with the larval stage (polycystic hydatid cyst) of *Echinococcus vogeli.*

ETIOLOGY AND EPIDEMIOLOGY. The etiologic agent of polycystic hydatid disease of humans was originally assumed to be *Echinococcus oligarthrus*, a tapeworm of wild felids with polycystic larvae in the agouti. Recent evidence does not exclude *E. oligarthrus* as a human pathogen but indicates that *E. vogeli* is the more likely cause of human disease. This conclusion is based on 2 observations: (1) The morphology and size of the hooks recovered from human cysts correspond to those of *E. vogeli*, and (2) adult *E. vogeli* have been recovered from dogs that were fed cysts resected from humans.

E. vogeli is a zoonotic parasite maintained in a wild life cycle. The adult tapeworm is found in the intestine of the bush dog and the polycystic larva in pacas and spiny rats. Domestic dogs have been infected experimentally, and 1 hunting dog from Colombia was found infected naturally. Humans are probably infected with eggs from their domestic dogs. Polycystic hydatid cysts have been recovered from a number of human organs, including the liver, lungs, stomach, heart (Fig. 101–12*A*), diaphragm, omentum, mesenteries, and intercostal muscles.

DISTRIBUTION AND PREVALENCE. About 20 human cases of polycystic hydatid disease have been recorded from Panama, Colombia, and Ecuador. The natural hosts of *E. vogeli* range throughout Central and South America, and the distribution of this parasite is probably more extensive than is currently recognized. Because polycystic hydatid disease of humans is found in rural communities where diagnostic expertise and technology are unavailable, its morbidity and mortality are probably higher than now believed.

CLINICAL MANIFESTATIONS, PATHOLOGY, AND DIAGNOSIS. The general lack of knowledge about polycystic hydatid disease is reflected by the high frequency of misdiagnosis. For example, the clinical and surgical diagnoses were incorrect in all 9 Colombian

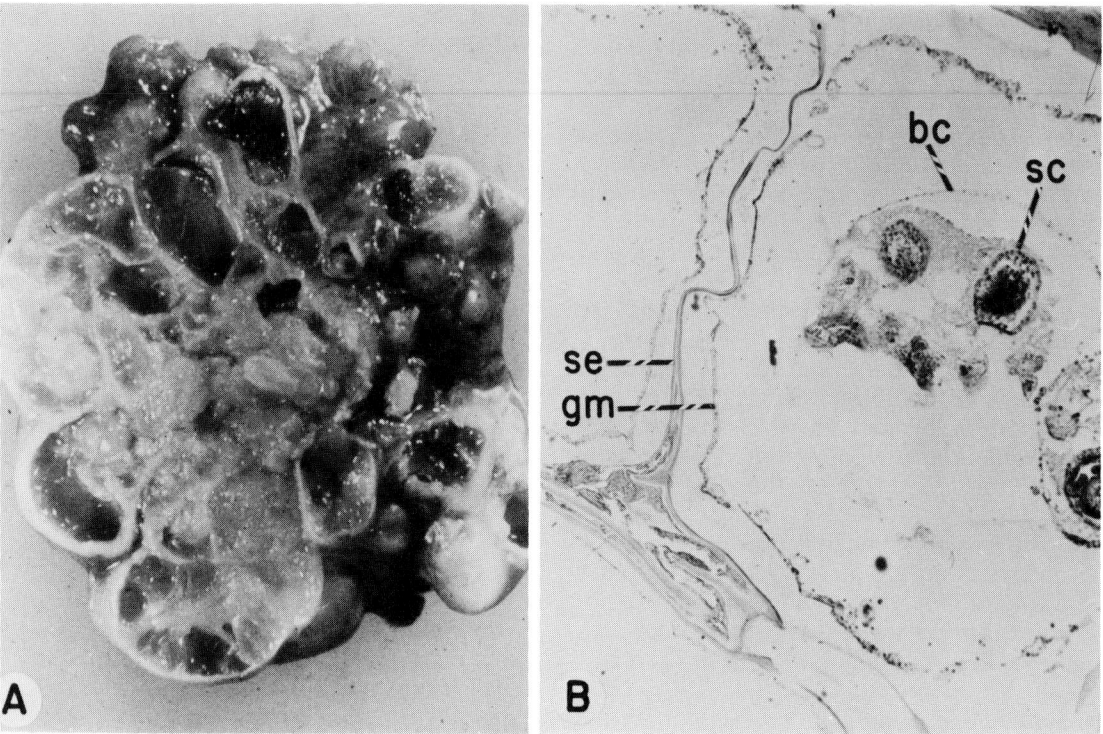

FIGURE 101–12. Polycystic hydatid disease. *A,* Frontal section of a human heart showing a polycystic hydatid cyst of *Echinococcus vogeli. B,* Histologic section of a portion of a cyst showing internal septa (se), germinal membrane (gm), brood capsules (bc), and necrotic scoleces (sc). (From D'Alessandro A, et al.: Am J Trop Med Hyg 28:303, 1979.)

cases that were later confirmed as *E. vogeli* infection by the pathologist. The clinical diagnoses included hepatic tumor, hepatic abscess, cirrhosis, gastric tumor, and chondrosarcoma of a rib.

The median age at diagnosis is 43 years, and the most common signs are hepatomegaly, palpable peritoneal masses, and jaundice. Preliminary observations indicate that the indirect hemagglutination and "Arc-5" gel diffusion tests using antigen from unilocular hydatid cysts are useful diagnostic tools. Radiographs may demonstrate polycystic structures in the peritoneal cavity and diffuse mineralization.

At laparotomy, the larva of *E. vogeli* appears as a whitish-gray polycystic structure that contains a yellow fluid or gel (Fig. 101–12*A*). The entire cyst may measure only 10 mm in diameter or may form vesicular aggregates that replace most of the liver. The scolex with its 4 circular suckers and rostellum with hooks can be seen in wet-mount preparations and tissue sections. The large hooks are 38 to 46 μm in length, and the small hooks measure 30 to 37 μm.

Microscopically, there are multiple vesicles, varying in size from a few millimeters to centimeters (Fig. 101–12*B*). The vesicles are partitioned by septa formed from the hyaline laminated membrane that is 8 to 65 μm thick and stains intensely by the periodic acid-Schiff technique. The internal surface of the septa is lined with a germinal membrane that is 3 to 13 μm thick and contains calcareous corpuscles. The brood capsules bud internally from the germinal epithelium. Externally, the cyst is surrounded by fibrous tissue, with only slight cellular infiltration. Portions of these cysts are frequently ne-

crotic and mineralized, and the only remains of *Echinococcus* are the hooks and calcareous corpuscles.

TREATMENT. Surgical resection of the cysts is the only proven therapy for polycystic hydatid disease, but mebendazole and albendazole are likely to be of some value, as with *E. multilocularis* infections (see Chapter 101.4).

BIBLIOGRAPHY

Amir-Jahed AK, Fardin R, Farzad A, et al.: Clinical echinococcosis. Ann Surg 182:541, 1975.

Craig PS, Nelson GS: The detection of circulating antigen in human hydatid disease. Ann Trop Med Parasitol 78:219–227, 1984.

Craig PS, Macpherson CNL, Watson-Jones DL, et al.: Immunodetection of *Echinococcus* eggs from naturally infected dogs and from environmental contamination sites in settlements in Turkana, Kenya. Trans R Soc Trop Med Hyg 82:268–274, 1988.

Craig PS, Zeyhle E, Comig T: Hydatid disease: Research and control in Turkana. II. The role of immunological techniques for the diagnosis of hydatid disease. Trans R Soc Trop Med Hyg 80:183–192, 1986.

D'Alessandro A, Rausch RL, Cuello C, et al.: *Echinococcus vogeli* in man, with a review of polycystic hydatid disease in Colombia and neighboring countries. Am J Trop Med Hyg 28:303, 1979.

Eckert J, Gemmel MA, Soulsby EJL (eds.): FAO/UNEP/WHO Guidelines for Surveillance, Prevention and Control of Echinococcosis/Hydatidosis. VPH/81.28. Geneva, WHO, 1981.

Little JM: Hydatid disease at Royal Prince Alfred Hospital, 1964 to 1974. Med J Aust 1:903, 1976.

Morris DL, Smith PG: Albendazole in hydatid disease—hepatocellular toxicity. Trans R Soc Trop Med Hyg 81:343–344, 1987.

Nelson GS: Hydatid disease: Research and control in Turkana, Kenya. I. Epidemiological observations. Trans R Soc Trop Med Hyg 80:177–182, 1986.

Okelo GBA: Hydatid disease: Research and control in Turkana. III. Albendazole in the treatment of inoperable hydatid disease in Kenya—a report on 12 cases. Trans R Soc Trop Med Hyg 80:193–195, 1986.

Schantz PM: Echinococcosis. *In* Steele JH, Arambulo P (eds.): Handbook of Zoonoses, Section C, Vol 3. Parasitic Zoonoses. Boca Raton, Florida, CRC Press, 1982, p. 231.

Schantz PM, Van den Bossche H, Eckert J: Chemotherapy for larval echinococcosis in animals and humans: Report of a workshop. Z Parasitenkd 67:5, 1982.

Smyth JD, Barrett NJ: Procedures for testing the viability of human hydatid cysts following surgical removal, especially after chemotherapy. Trans R Soc Trop Med Hyg 74:649, 1980.

Thompson RCA (ed.): The Biology of Echinococcus and Hydatid Disease. London, George Allen and Unwin, 1986.

Thompson RCA, Lymbery AJ: The nature, extent and significance of variation within the genus Echinococcus. Adv Parasitol 27:210–263, 1988.

Todorov T, Vutova K, Petkov D, et al.: Albendazole treatment of human cystic echinococcosis. Trans R Soc Trop Med Hyg 82:453–459, 1988.

Wilson JF, Rausch RL: Alveolar hydatid disease: A review of clinical features of 33 indigenous cases of *Echinococcus multilocularis* infection in Alaskan Eskimos. Am J Trop Med Hyg 29:1340, 1980.

101.5. SPARGANOSIS

DEFINITION. Sparganosis is caused by infection with spargana, which are second-stage larvae (plerocer-coids) of diphyllobothrid tapeworms of the genus *Spirometra*.

ETIOLOGY. Many species of *Spirometra* have been described, but they are morphologically similar and taxonomically confusing. It is usual to refer to the parasite in Southeast Asia as *Spirometra mansoni* and that in North America as *Spirometra mansonoides*. The adult tapeworms occur in domestic and wild carnivores and are similar to *Diphyllobothrium* (Chapter 100.1). They are distinguished by the characteristic compact uterine coils and mature proglottids. The life cycles also differ, as *Spirometra* usually use amphibians, reptiles, and mammals as second intermediate hosts, whereas *Diphyllobothrium* use fish (Fig. 100–3). The adult parasite does not develop in humans, but humans can be infected with the larval stages by ingesting the procercoid in the first intermediate host, *Cyclops,* when drinking contaminated water. Humans may also act as a paratenic host by ingesting the plerocercoid in second intermediate hosts such as frogs or mammals. Another route of infection in Southeast Asia is from poultices prepared from frogs infected with plerocercoids that are applied directly to ulcers, sores, and inflamed eyes.

DISTRIBUTION AND PREVALENCE. Humans are a rare incidental host of these zoonotic parasites that are prevalent in cats, dogs, and wild carnivores in many parts of the world. Human infections are seen

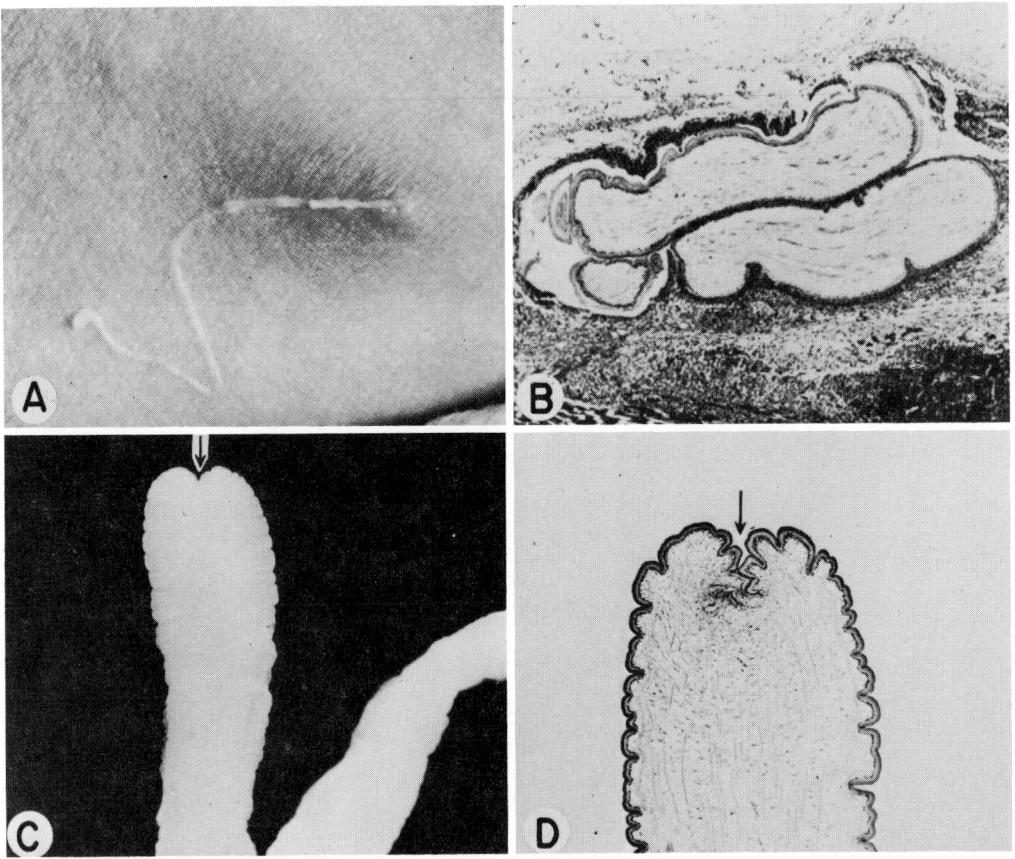

FIGURE 101–13. Sparganosis. *A,* Sparganum of *Spirometra* species from incised lesion on the chest. (Courtesy of Drs. J.H. Miller and S.H. Abadie, Louisiana State University School of Medicine.) *B,* Histologic section of sparganum showing inflammation. (Courtesy of Dr. J.F. Mueller, State University of New York Medical Center, Syracuse.) *C,* Flattened anterior end of a sparganum demonstrating the invaginated slit of the head (arrow) and pseudosegmentation. (Courtesy of the Armed Forces Institute of Pathology, Photograph Neg. No. 70-7390.) *D,* Histologic section showing head and pseudosegmentation. (Courtesy of the Armed Forces Institute of Pathology, Photograph Neg. No. 70-7310.)

most commonly in Southeast Asia, but infections have been recorded in East Africa and North America.

CLINICAL MANIFESTATIONS AND PATHOLOGY. Spargana cause little reaction in the normal host, but in humans they usually migrate to the subcutaneous tissues, where they become encapsulated in inflammatory nodules that may develop into abscesses. Under these circumstances, the parasite is discharged, and it may be mistaken for a guinea worm unless the specimen is carefully examined (Fig. 101–13*A*). In the subconjunctival tissues, the larvae provoke a more acute inflammation with conjunctivitis and periorbital edema. Spargana have also been reported as causing brain abscesses.

The inflammation consists of lymphocytes, histiocytes, plasma cells, and neutrophils; eosinophils may be abundant or absent (Fig. 101–13*B*). The parasites can usually be extracted alive, and they may be several centimeters in length. They are glistening white, opaque worms with a typical undulating cestode movement (Fig. 101–13*A* and *C*).

DIAGNOSIS. If the intact parasite is extracted, it can be recognized by the head with the characteristic deep invagination (Fig. 101–13*C* and *D*). Histologic sections of the worm show the typical features of cestode larvae (Fig. 101–13*D*). The worm-like appearance and the solid body of the spargana along with the absence of suckers and hooks usually distinguish them from the cystic stages of other cestodes that occur in subcutaneous tissues.

TREATMENT AND CONTROL. Surgical excision is usually possible, but in patients with multiple infections, supplementary treatment with praziquantel might be advisable (Chapter 101.1). In endemic areas, the local population should be discouraged from drinking "raw" water from natural ponds. The archaic use of frog poultices should be discouraged.

SPARGANUM PROLIFERUM. This is a rare larval cestode found in the skin, muscles, viscera, and brain of humans. These larvae are cylindric or slightly flattened and can measure 20 cm long and 2 mm wide; they proliferate by lateral budding to produce massive infections.

BIBLIOGRAPHY

Daly JJ: Sparganosis. *In* Steele JH, Arambulo P (eds.): Handbook of Zoonoses, Section C, Vol 3. Parasitic Zoonoses. Boca Raton, Florida, CRC Press, 1982, p. 293.
Nelson GS, Pester FRN, Rickman R: The significance of wild animals in the transmission of cestodes of medical importance in Kenya. Trans R Soc Trop Med Hyg 59:507–524, 1900.
Norman SH, Kreutner A Jr: Sparganosis: Clinical and pathologic observations in ten cases. South Med J 73:297, 1980.

101.6.   COENURIASIS

DEFINITION. Coenuriasis is a zoonotic disease of humans caused by infection with the larval stage (coenurus) of *Taenia (Multiceps)* species.

ETIOLOGY, DISTRIBUTION, AND EPIDEMIOLOGY. Adult tapeworms are found in the small intestine of canids, usually dogs. Gravid proglottids are passed at defecation. The proglottids eventually disintegrate to free the eggs, which disperse over the environment. When ingested by susceptible herbivores or humans, the eggs develop into coenuri in the subcutaneous muscles and central nervous system.

The taxonomy of coenuri is confusing, but the anatomical location of the coenuri may relate to the species. *Taenia (Multiceps) multiceps* has a wide distribution in temperate areas, where it usually circulates in a domestic cycle between dogs and herbivorous mammals, including sheep, goats, cattle, and horses. The coenurus infects the brain and spinal cord of the intermediate host and causes a common disease of sheep known as gid or staggers. Human neurocoenuriasis is rare but has been reported from the United States, England, France, Africa, and Brazil.

Taenia (Multiceps) serialis is also a parasite of temperate areas with wide distribution. Coenuri are usually

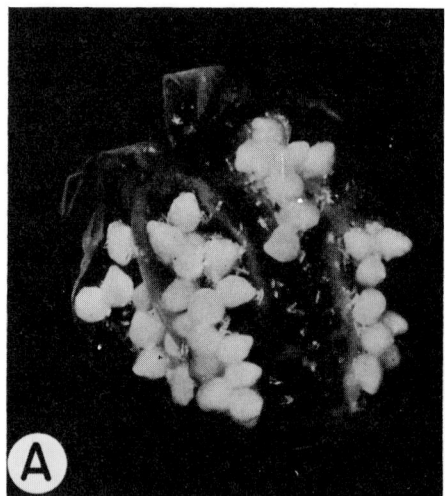
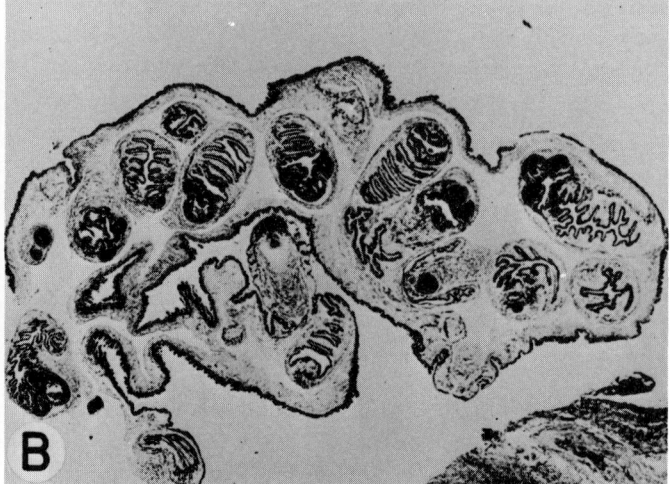

FIGURE 101–14. Coenuriasis. *A,* Coenurus from subcutaneous tissue of man showing scoleces attached to cyst wall. (Courtesy of the Armed Forces Institute of Pathology, Photograph Neg. No. 70-4295.) *B,* Section of coenurus showing thin cyst wall and numerous scoleces developing from the germinal membrane. (Courtesy of the Armed Forces Institute of Pathology, Photograph Neg. No. 69-4736.)

found in intermuscular connective tissue of lagomorphs and rodents, including the rabbit, squirrel, and nutria. *T. serialis* is rare in humans and has been found in Canada, the United States, France, and Africa.

Taenia (Multiceps) brauni is a tropical tapeworm of eastern Africa with a sylvatic life cycle, including the dog, fox, jackal, and genet as definitive hosts and rodents such as the swamp rat, porcupine, and gerbil as intermediate hosts. The coenuri infect subcutaneous tissue of the intermediate hosts. There are less than 100 reports of *T. brauni* in humans.

Taenia (Multiceps) glomeratus has been found in subcutaneous tissue of humans in Nigeria.

CLINICAL MANIFESTATIONS AND PATHOLOGY. Patients with coenuriasis usually have a space-occupying lesion caused by a single cyst measuring 2 to 6 cm in diameter. Neural coenuri have been found in the cerebrum, ventricles, posterior horn of the lateral ventricle, brain stem, and spinal cord and among the cranial nerves. The clinical manifestations of neurocoenuriasis are similar to those of neurocysticercosis (Chapter 101.1). Subcutaneous coenuri are commonly found in the intercostal region and anterior abdominal wall. These cysts may be confused with a lipoma, ganglion, and neurofibroma. Ocular coenuri have been recorded from the vitreous, anterior chamber, and conjunctiva.

DIAGNOSIS. Space-occupying lesions in the deep organs are visualized with radiographic techniques, e.g., x-rays, radioisotopic scans, CT scans, and sonograms. Subcutaneous coenuri may be palpated, and ocular coenuri may be observed directly by endoscopic examination. Definitive diagnosis rests on surgical excision and parasitologic identification. The coenurus has a thin wall surrounding a single cavity that contains a clear fluid (Fig. 101–14*A* and *B*). Numerous scoleces measuring 3 mm in diameter attach to the cyst wall, and there are no brood capsules as found in the unilocular hydatid cyst of *E. granulosus*. Each scolex has 4 circular suckers and 2 rows of hooks on a rostellum. There are large and small hooks. The hook lengths for *T. multiceps* are 150 to 170 μm and 90 to 130 μm; those for *T. serialis* are 135 to 175 μm and 68 to 120 μm; those for *T. brauni* are 95 to 140 μm and 70 to 90 μm; and those for *T. glomeratus* are 90 to 100 μm and 65 to 70 μm.

TREATMENT AND CONTROL. Surgical excision is the usual treatment, although both praziquantel and albendazole are likely to be as effective as in the treatment of cysticercosis. Preventive measures include hygienic practices to reduce contact with dogs and to break the transmission of eggs from dog feces to humans. Elimination of adult worms with praziquantel or niclosamide will reduce environmental contamination with eggs.

BIBLIOGRAPHY

Benger A, Rennie RP, Roberts JT, et al.: A human coenurus infection in Canada. Am J Trop Med Hyg 30:638–644, 1981.
Templeton AC: Anatomical and geographical location of human coenurus infection. Trop Geogr Med 23:105–108, 1971.

PART VII

POISONOUS AND TOXIC PLANTS AND ANIMALS

102. POISONOUS PLANTS AND FISH

William A. Sodeman, Jr.

Toxic and poisonous plants and animals exist in all environments. The numerical richness of tropical flora and fauna increases the relative number of toxic species. Poisonings are increasing in frequency. This increase is related directly to increased exposure. Several factors are involved in this increase. Indigenous populations receive some protection from the tradition and folklore that serve as a repository for prior experience concerning foodstuffs that are toxic at any given time. Development of natural resources in the tropics has opened vast areas to immigration, which exposes a naive population to new toxins and poisons. This same development, coupled with technological progress in processing and transportation of foodstuffs, permits wide dissemination of occasionally toxic foods, usually fish or shellfish. Distribution occurs often before their toxicity can be recognized. Finally, the ease of travel has opened previously remote areas to tourism. The resultant increase in population at risk is followed by an increase in numbers of poisonings.

102.1. SHELLFISH POISONING

Clinically, 3 types of shellfish poisoning may be recognized.

GASTROINTESTINAL SHELLFISH POISONING. The onset of symptoms, i.e., nausea, vomiting, diarrhea, and abdominal pain, is 8 to 12 hours after ingestion. Bacterial contamination of the shellfish is believed to be the cause.

ALLERGIC SHELLFISH POISONING. The onset of symptoms occurs 30 minutes to 6 hours after ingestion. In this type, symptoms include skin rash and itching, nasal congestion, dryness of the throat, and edema of the tongue, causing potentially fatal respiratory distress. It is thought to be due to individual sensitivity to the shellfish.

PARALYTIC SHELLFISH POISONING. This is also called dinoflagellate poisoning and saxitoxin poisoning.

Etiology and Pathophysiology. This is an acute poisoning due to saxitoxin, a powerful curare-like neuro-

toxin that is produced by toxic species of planktonic dinoflagellates and concentrated in filter-feeding mollusks (clams, oysters, scallops, mussels). The principal action of the toxin occurs centrally on the respiratory and vasomotor centers and peripherally at the neuromuscular junctions and the sensory nerve endings. The toxin is absorbed through the gastrointestinal tract and excreted by the kidneys.

Clinical Manifestations and Prognosis. The onset of symptoms, which are usually neuromotor in nature, is usually 30 minutes following ingestion of the shellfish. Paresthesia starts in the lips and tip of the tongue and spreads to involve the face, scalp, neck, and extremities. This may be accompanied by weakness of the limbs, ataxia, incoherent speech, aphonia, tightness of the throat and chest, and increased salivation. The pulse is thready; superficial reflexes may be lost, whereas deep reflexes are depressed. If the patient survives the first 12 hours, the prognosis is good. However, the mortality rate is 1 to 7%, with death usually occurring from respiratory paralysis within 24 hours.

TREATMENT. As no specific antidote is known, treatment is symptomatic and supportive. In the gastrointestinal type of shellfish poisoning, reports indicate that in most cases the signs and symptoms responded to the administration of a broad-spectrum antibiotic, diphenoxylate hydrochloride with atropine sulfate (Lomotil), and rehydration (intravenously when indicated). Antihistamines, epinephrine, and corticosteroids have been used to good effect in the allergic type of shellfish poisoning. The paralytic type of poisoning, however, often requires treatment of respiratory and circulatory collapse by means of intravenous infusions and cardiotonic drugs, as well as drugs to control the arrhythmias. In some cases, assisted ventilation is needed.

102.2. FISH POISONING

There are 500 species of known toxic fish; most are reef fish. Some are toxic at all times; others are toxic only during certain seasons. In some fish, all the tissues are toxic; in others, only the tissues of certain organs are toxic.

CIGUATERA POISONING. Etiology. From the medical and economic standpoints, this is the most important type of poisoning. Three hundred species of fish have been incriminated in a wide geographic distribution from the West Indies to the Pacific. The ciguatoxic fish cannot be recognized by external appearance. Species that are toxic in one locality may be nontoxic in another. Evidence suggests that the origin of the toxin is the dinoflagellate *Gamberdiscus toxicus* and possibly others. It is thought to be transferred by transvection via the food chain through herbivorous reef fish to carnivorous tropical reef fish (groupers, snappers, dolphins, barracuda) where it is concentrated. It is harmless to the fish themselves.

Clinical Manifestations and Prognosis. In the United States, the disease occurs most frequently during the late spring and summer. The onset of clinical manifestations of poisoning occurs 4 to 30 hours after ingestion. In the main, the manifestations are gastrointestinal and neurologic, with nausea (and, on occasion, a metallic taste in the mouth), vomiting and diarrhea, abdominal pain and cramps, paresthesia around the mouth (and in some cases the fingers and toes), cold-to-hot sensory reversal dysesthesia, increased salivation, dilatation of the pupils, strabismus, ptosis, weakness, myalgia of the legs, incoordination, and even paralysis. Pruritus of the soles of the feet and palms of the hands may be present. The mortality rate is as high as 10%. Usually, death occurs from respiratory failure or hypovolemic shock.

Treatment. Treatment is supportive and symptomatic. A wide variety of pharmacologic agents have been used both experimentally and clinically. Emesis should be induced, a cathartic given, 10% calcium gluconate given intravenously (to relieve neurologic symptoms), sedation for convulsions, e.g., diazepam or paraldehyde, and nikethamide for respiratory depression. Atropine sulfate has been used in patients in whom there is excessive production of mucus, but it tends to make aspiration of secretions more difficult. Intravenous administration of fluids with supplements of vitamin B and C has been advocated and used with some success. Patients with laryngeal obstruction will require intubation or tracheostomy. In patients severely affected, the myalgia, paresthesia of the hands and feet, and pruritus may recur intermittently for as long as 6 months to a year after the initial attack.

TETRAODON POISONING. Etiology. Tetraodontoxin, a neurotoxin, is widely distributed among the order Tetraodontoidea (Plectognathi). This includes puffers (blowfish, toadfish, fugu), ocean sunfish, and porcupine fish. They are characterized by having very small scales. The toxin concentrates mainly in the liver, ovaries, intestine, and skin of the fish. Puffer musculature is generally considered nonpoisonous. Toxicity is related to the reproductive cycle, being highest just before spawning in late spring or early summer.

Clinical Manifestations and Prognosis. The clinical features of tetraodon poisoning are characterized by the rapid onset, within 5 to 30 minutes, of weakness; dizziness; paresthesia of the lips, tongue, throat, and, later, the limbs; nausea (but often not vomiting or diarrhea), and abdominal pain. Pallor, sweating, and increased salivation may be present. There is a tachycardia, hypotension, and increasing difficulty with breathing, which may be complicated by a general flaccid ascending paralysis, leading to respiratory failure, convulsions, and death in 6 to 24 hours. Usually, consciousness is retained throughout. The mortality rate was as high as 60% in Japanese outbreaks.

Treatment. Treatment is symptomatic and supportive because there is no specific therapy or antidote. It should include induced emesis (but in patients in whom there is evidence of increasing paralysis only when there is a cuffed endotracheal tube in place), administration of a cathartic, and administration of 10% intravenous calcium gluconate to combat neurologic symptoms. Respiratory and cardiac stimulants and assisted respiration are indicated in many cases.

SCOMBROID POISONING

Etiology. Scombrotoxic poisoning follows ingestion of contaminated fish (which have been imperfectly refrigerated) of the tuna and mackerel families and, occasionally, sprats and pilchards. Bacterial contaminants (*Proteus, Salmonella, Clostridium,* and *Escherichia coli*) break down the histidine of fish muscles to saurine, a histamine-like substance. Victims often complain that the fish has a peppery taste.

Clinical Manifestations and Treatment. Signs and symptoms resemble those of a histamine poisoning. The onset occurs about 3 hours after ingestion of the fish, and the findings are of an acute allergic or histamine-like reaction, with headache; flushing of the head and upper trunk; generalized urticaria; swelling of the eyelids, periorbital tissue, lips, tongue, and throat; muscular weakness; myalgia; and diarrhea. Recovery usually takes place in about 3 to 16 hours, although occasional deaths have been reported. Antihistamines are effective with or without emesis or gastric lavage.

OTHER FISH POISONING

Elasmobranch Poisoning. This occurs after ingestion of the liver or skeletal muscles of sharks and rays. The onset of symptoms usually occurs after 30 minutes. These are usually mild following ingestion of the musculature and include some abdominal pain but mainly diarrhea. Symptoms are more severe after ingestion of the liver and include, in addition to diarrhea and abdominal pain, nausea, vomiting, headache, tingling around the mouth, and a burning sensation of the tongue. In severe cases, this may progress to ataxia, visual disturbances, difficulty with breathing, coma, and death. Most patients, however, recover completely in 5 to 20 days.

Hallucinatory Fish Poisoning. This may occur after ingestion of certain species of mullet. Signs and symptoms begin about 2 hours after ingestion of the fish and are all neurologic, e.g., incoordination, nightmares, ataxia, and hallucinations. No fatalities have been recorded, and cathartics are recommended in treatment.

Miscellaneous. Other intoxications have been described, e.g., fish roe poisoning, fish blood poisoning, and fish liver poisoning. Treatment is symptomatic.

The contamination of the sea and its fauna by metallic wastes, particularly mercury, has been described in Japan, i.e., Minamata disease.

BIBLIOGRAPHY

Banner AH: Hazardous marine animals. *In* Tedeschi CG, Eckert WG, Tedeschi LG (eds.): Forensic Medicine. Vol. 3, Environmental Hazards, Philadelphia, W.B. Saunders Company, 1977.

Lawrence DN: Ciguatera fish poisoning in Miami. JAMA 244:254,1980.
Russel FE: Poisonous Marine Animals. London, T.F.H. Publications, Inc., and Academic Press, Inc. (London) Ltd., 1971.
Southcott RV: The neurologic effects of noxious marine creatures. *In* Hornabrook RW (ed.): Topics of Tropical Neurology. Philadelphia, F.A. Davis, 1975.

102.3.   MUSHROOM POISONING

DEFINITION AND ETIOLOGY. Hundreds of toxin-containing mushroom species are known worldwide. A small but significant percentage can produce fatal poisoning. Most poisonings are accidental, as a result of either culinary error or ingestion by small children. Mushrooms of certain species are abused as hallucinogens, and there are suicide attempts by mushroom ingestion.

Mushroom toxicity is highly variable. Toxin content may vary with season, geographic origin, maturity of the fungus, and method of preparation. Some mushrooms are toxic when raw but not when cooked. Individual human sensitivity to some toxins is variable.

CLINICAL MANIFESTATIONS AND MANAGEMENT. Manifestations of toxicity may be immediate or may be delayed for up to 17 days. Outcome in any individual case is heavily dependent on the dose of toxin.

Identification of the suspect mushroom in a case of poisoning is often not possible. Species abound, toxic effects may be delayed long after ingestion, and mistaken identification as an edible mushroom is often the problem in the first place. The recognition of a characteristic syndrome plus a history of recent ingestion of wild mushrooms should prompt clinical intervention, especially when the syndrome has lethal implications.

Mushroom intoxications may be classified by the species involved, by the toxin involved, or by the clinical presentation. For the nonmycologist physician it is the clinical presentation that proves most useful. There are 3 basic patterns of clinical presentation: gastrointestinal symptoms, renal symptoms, and neuropsychiatric symptoms. These in turn may be subdivided into more specific presentations.

Gastrointestinal Symptoms. The key criterion that separates the various gastrointestinal syndromes is the duration of the latent period between ingestion of the mushroom and the onset of the signs and symptoms.

Rapid Onset. Many different genera and species have toxins that affect the gastrointestinal tract and have a rapid, almost immediate, onset of action. These tend not to be fatal intoxications. Generally, the toxins induce nausea, vomiting, and/or diarrhea. Symptoms can persist for days and become clinically significant largely as a result of dehydration and acid-base imbalance. In patients with limited tolerance for dehydration and electrolyte abnormality, such as patients on cardioactive drugs, the very old or very young, or patients with other intercurrent diseases such as diabetes, special attention must be paid to early intervention and management.

The mechanism of toxin action is not well understood. One exception is the ingestion of *Coprinus atramentar-*

ius, the Inky Cap. This mushroom produces coprine, which after metabolic conversion to cyclopropanone hydrate, inhibits acetaldehyde dehydrogenase. This causes a disulfiram-like effect following the ingestion of alcohol. The mushroom is not toxic in the nonalcohol drinker. Alcohol ingestion produces headache, nausea, and vomiting. Diarrhea does not occur. The sensitization to alcohol may last up to 72 hours. Several other species of *Coprinus* in Europe and Africa have been implicated in causing this syndrome. *Clitocybe clavipes* in Japan has been reported to cause this syndrome also.

Delayed Onset—6 Hours. Ingestion of *Gyromitra esculenta* produces gastrointestinal symptoms after a latent interval of about 6 hours. The toxin involved is gyromitrin or monomethylhydrazine. This can be found in other species of *Gyromitra* as well. The toxin causes vomiting, headache, abdominal cramping, diarrhea and, when severe, neurologic symptoms and evidence of liver damage. The most prominent sign is the emesis, which may be persistent enough to cause acidosis. The demonstration of methemoglobin in the circulation is evidence of ingestion of *Gyromitra*. The management is largely that of treating the dehydration and electrolyte abnormalities. Pyridoxine will reverse some of the toxicity. It should be administered IV in a dose of 25 mg/kg, adjusting the dose to the patient's symptoms. Severe intoxication requires the management of the liver damage and coma.

The toxin is water soluble and volatile. It can be leached out of the mushroom by parboiling or volatilized by drying. Detoxifying is common practice in Europe. Toxin-containing vapor from cooking fresh mushrooms can itself be toxic if inhaled.

Delayed Onset—12 Hours. *Amanita phalloides* and other amatoxin-containing mushrooms (in at least 4 genera) can cause fatal intoxication, which occurs with delayed onset of symptoms. Amatoxins act directly on the intestine to produce acute gastroenteritis. The usual latent interval is 12 hours. The gastrointestinal response is nausea and vomiting, cramping abdominal pain, and diarrhea. This runs a short course of about 8 hours, and then the patient experiences a symptom-free interval of 3 to 5 days. Following this interval, the character of the illness changes, and there is the development of hepatic insufficiency. Clinically the picture is that of severe viral hepatitis. There is elevation of hepatocellular enzymes, falling levels of liver-produced coagulation factors, and finally hypoglycemia. Amatoxins also have an affinity for the proximal convoluted tubule of the kidney and can produce acute tubular necrosis with renal failure.

Amatoxins are cyclic octapeptides that are hepatoselective. They interfere with the activity of RNA polymerase and eventuate in cell death. They are not destroyed by drying or leached by parboiling. Treatment is a complex process that varies with the stage of development of the intoxication. If the ingestion is recognized early (within 6 hours) as in a culinary error, a suicide attempt, or inadvertent ingestion by a child, the stomach should be evacuated by induced emesis or lavage. The fatal dose for an adult is 5 to 10 mg of toxin, an amount that could be found in a single large cap. Vigorous attempts to lower the dose are proper.

Amatoxin binds strongly with activated charcoal, and once the stomach has been cleaned, administration of a slurry of activated charcoal in water may bind some of the toxin in the intestinal lumen.

The acute gastroenteritis is treated symptomatically with fluid and electrolyte replacement. Even if recognition of toxin ingestion is delayed, administration of activated charcoal may help break the enterohepatic cycle of the toxin by binding it in the lumen. A forced diuresis may speed the excretion of the toxin and lessen its stay within the kidney. Once liver or renal failure supervenes, these are managed by standard approaches.

Renal Syndromes. In addition to the amatoxin-containing mushrooms described above, which can cause acute tubular necrosis, some species of *Cortinarius* can cause renal failure also. Several toxins are known in this genus, but the one responsible for the renal failure and its mechanism of action is not known. This mushroom species has great variability in toxicity. Some species seem safe if eaten raw but toxic if cooked. The latent interval may be long, 3 to 17 days.

The initial manifestation of the renal toxicity is the appearance of polydipsia and polyuria. There may be associated chills, headache, and muscular pain. In some patients there are gastrointestinal symptoms. The renal failure develops as a result of acute tubular necrosis. Fatalities do occur. The management is that of acute renal failure. Dialysis over XAD-4 Amberlite may remove toxin.

Neuropsychiatric Syndromes. Several distinct neuropsychiatric syndromes occur following toxic mushroom ingestion. These may present as muscarine toxicity, coma, or hallucinations.

Muscarine Toxicity. Mushrooms of the genera *Clitocybe* and *Inocybe* contain muscarine. This compound, even in small doses, acts as a parasympathetic stimulant and can produce sweating, abdominal pain, and miosis. The effect is temporary, and atropine in full doses can reverse most of the symptoms.

Coma Producers. *Amanita muscaria* and *A. pantherina* contain ibotenic acid. This is metabolized to muscimol, which is a GABA agonist in the CNS. Patients become drowsy and then comatose, but this is interrupted by periods of delirium and excitement. It is fatal in heavy doses.

Hallucinogens. Many mushrooms are known and abused for their effect as hallucinogens. The active toxin is psilocybin. Mushrooms of many genera (Table 102–1) have been implicated. The effect is that of alcohol intoxication with hallucinations. Responses vary with chronic use. In children, particularly with high doses,

TABLE 102–1. Genera with Psilocybin- and/or Psilocin-Containing Species

Amanita	Naematoloma
Boletus	Panaeolus
Clitocybe	Pluteus
Conocybe	Psathyrella
Copelandia	Psilocybe
Gymnopilus	Russula
Lycoperdon	Stropharia

Compiled from Lincoff and Mitchel, 1977; Lampe and McCann, 1985.

severe reactions occur with hyperthermia and convulsions. Treatment is symptomatic for mild intoxications. In the long-term abuser specific management for substance abuse may be in order. Severe intoxication requires specific management of the hyperthermia and the seizures.

BIBLIOGRAPHY

Campbell GR: An Illustrated Guide to Some Poisonous Plants and Animals of Florida. Englewood, Pineapple Press Inc., 1983.
Hardin JW, Arena JM: Human Poisoning from Native and Cultivated Plants. Durham, Duke University Press, 1974.
Lampe KF, McCann MA: Handbook of Poisonous and Injurious Plants. Chicago, American Medical Association, 1985.
Lincoff G, Mitchel DH: Toxic and Hallucinogenic Mushroom Poisoning. New York, Van Nostrand Reinhold Co., 1977.

102.4. PLANT POISONING

DEFINITION AND ETIOLOGY. Many plants have responded to the challenge for survival by evolving chemical toxins and irritants to fend off browsing animals. Many of these compounds are extracted and purified for use as drugs in combating human disease, e.g., digitalis, belladonna, and curare. Many of these compounds also cause disease as a result of inadvertent ingestion or contact. The numbers are so large that only the most common can be listed (Table 102–2) and these with limited detail. Generally plant toxins pose the greatest hazard for young children and visitors new to an environment. Most native residents have absorbed a body of folklore that identifies hazardous plants.

The outcome of most plant poisonings is dose related. Toxin concentrations vary with season, the maturity of the plant, and geographic origin. Not all parts of a plant need be toxic. In many areas methods of food preparation have been evolved to detoxify the plant material. The processing of bitter manioc, *Manihot utilissima*, is one example. Rapid, inexpensive transportation of fresh foodstuffs, coupled with a keen interest in culinary experimentation, has greatly enhanced the possible exposure to toxic plants.

In addition to plant toxins, mycotoxins and external and internal environmental contaminants can cause disease. Pesticide residues pose the most common hazard, but other adulterants are known.

CLINICAL MANAGEMENT. There is a great individual variability in response to some plant toxins. Also, some reactions are allergic and depend on individual development of hypersensitivity. Hayfever and *Rhus* dermatitis, poison ivy sensitivity, are perhaps the most common examples. This too, has changed with the sophistication of food delivery systems and the palate. A new generation of grocery store check-out clerks has discovered mango sensitivity dermatitis.

The range of toxins present in various plants is so great that there are no really useful general rules concerning the management of plant poisonings except that prevention is always more effective than treatment.

The most useful clinical separations of plant poison-

Text continued on page 869

TABLE 102–2. Table of Common Toxic Plants

Toxic Plants	Clinical Manifestations	Guidelines for Therapy
DERMATITIS PRODUCING PLANTS— **examples include**:		
Mechanical Injury		
Yucca (Spanish bayonet)		
Zygophyllaceae		
Tribulus terrestris (puncture vine)		
IRRITANTS AND ALLERGENS— **examples include:**		
Anacardaceae		
Anacardium occidentale (cashew nut) Nut shell oil contains cardol, cardanol, anacardic acid	Irritation and vesiculation as well as purgative effect if ingested.	Corticosteroid creams and lotions.
Mangifera indica (mango) Foliage, sap, and skin of the unripe fruit contain cardanol-like compound	Irritant and allergic—*mango dermatitis*.	Corticosteroid creams and lotions.
Rhus (Toxicodendron) radicans (poison ivy) Leaves and stem contain substance similar to cardanol	Irritation and vesiculation.	Corticosteroid creams and lotions.
Other *Rhus* species		
Araceae		
Dieffenbachia species All parts except fruit contain calcium oxalate and other toxic principles	Irritation of the skin. If ingested, burning of the mouth and swelling of the tongue. In severe poisoning, convulsions, coma, and death in uremia.	If ingested, gastric lavage or emesis and symptomatic treatment.
Related genera that may cause less severe injury: *Philodendron* species *Alocasia* (elephant ear) species *Monstera* (Swiss cheese) species		Corticosteroid creams and lotions; antihistamines orally.
Euphorbiaceae		
Euphorbia species, e.g., *Euphorbia pulcherrima* (poinsettia) Latex in all parts	Dermatitis and blistering, swelling of the face, rash, and burning eyes (if rubbed into the eye, may cause keratoconjunctivitis or uveitis).	Corticosteroid creams and lotions; antihistamines orally.
Hippomane mancinella (manchineel) All parts containing latex	Similar to above.	
Hura polyandra (devil tree) All parts containing sap	Dermatitis, keratoconjunctivitis.	
Ricinus communis (castor bean) Entire plant is poisonous (Fig. 102–1)	Dermatitis (in sensitive individuals), in addition to other toxic effects if ingested.	
Photosensitization (inflammation of any exposed, highly vascularized area of the skin)		
Verbenaceae		
Lantana camara (wild sage)	Photosensitization, in addition to clinical features of atropine-like poisoning if ingested (see Neuromuscular Poisons).	
NARCOTIC POISONS—examples include:		
Amaryllidaceae		
Boophone disticha (gifbol) Bulb contains alkaloid buphanine (like hyoscine)	*Buphanine poisoning*. This presents as acute drunkenness. There is rapid onset of ataxia, giddiness, and mydriasis. Patient is initially talkative and later subdued, becoming stuporose, and coma supervenes. Death occurs from respiratory failure.	Gastric lavage with activated charcoal added to the water. Symptomatic treatment.
Celastraceae		
Catha edulis (khat, wild tea) Leaves contain cathine, cathinine, and cathidine	*Khat poisoning*. Leaves are chewed or infused and are an inebriant narcotic. Effects are initially stimulative and later depressive. Subject is often excessively polite but later becomes divorced from reality and deteriorates mentally.	Treatment of drug addiction.
Cannabaceae		
Cannabis sativa (cannabinol, cannabidol) Leaves at top of plant	Causes cerebral stimulation, later depression, and in some cases, delirious rages. Intoxication may cause death from cardiac failure.	Treatment of drug addiction.
Solanaceae		
Datura stramonium (jimsonweed, thorn apple) Unripe seed pods contain alkaloids hyoscyamine and scopolamine	Mydriasis, thirst, dry mouth, headache, rapid pulse, high blood pressure, hallucinations, delirium, coma, and death.	Gastric lavage with activated charcoal, emesis, pilocarpine, and sedation.

TABLE 102–2. Table of Common Toxic Plants *Continued*

Toxic Plants	Clinical Manifestations	Guidelines for Therapy
Nicotiana species (tobacco) Nicotine	Poisoning has occurred through use of nicotine-containing insecticide. Manifestations include vomiting, diarrhea, muscular weakness, irregular pulse, palpitations, and death from respiratory paralysis.	Gastric lavage with potassium permanganate added. Tannin (which binds nicotine by forming nicotine tannate).
Solanum species (including potato skin not covered by earth and immature sprouting) Potatoes contain solanine	Manifestations of intoxication are nausea and vomiting, ataxia, hallucinations, drowsiness, and dilation of the pupils.	Gastric lavage with addition of activated charcoal. Symptomatic treatment.

NEUROMUSCULAR POISONS—examples include:

Leguminosae

Lathyrus sativus (pea) Seeds contain alkaloid	*Lathyrism.* Onset is slow, suggesting that the toxin is cumulative. Outbreaks have been described in India and elsewhere. Larger-than-usual amounts of the pea consumed over a period of 6 months lead to abrupt or insidious onset of spastic paralysis in the lower limbs of (usually) young males. Signs are thought to be due to damage to pyramidal tracts and motor nerves.	Cumulative poison—neurologic changes are irreversible.

Loganiaceae

Gelsemium sempervirens (yellow jessamine) All parts, especially root and nectar, contain alkaloids that depress and paralyze motor nerve endings	Mydriasis, sweating, weakness, impaired speech, ataxia, asphyxia, and death.	Gastric lavage, atropine, and supportive treatment.
Strychnos nux-vomica All parts contain alkaloids	Signs of strychnine poisoning; constriction of the throat, chest, and abdomen; involuntary muscle spasms; miosis; convulsions; asphyxia; and death.	Gastric lavage with activated charcoal and symptomatic treatment.

Meliaceae

Melia azedarach (chinaberry or syringa) Alkaloids in fruit and bark	Vomiting and diarrhea, excitement, sweating, mydriasis, paralysis, and asphyxiation.	Gastric lavage and symptomatic treatment.

Ranunculaceae

Aconitum napellus (monkshood) All parts (especially roots and seeds)	Nausea and vomiting, burning of the mouth and pharynx, numbness, paralysis, difficulty with breathing, convulsions, and death.	Atropine and symptomatic treatment.

Verbenaceae

Lantana camara (wild sage) All parts, especially unripe beans	Produce symptoms of atropine-like poisoning, vomiting and diarrhea, dilatation (later constriction) of pupils, muscular weakness, coma, and death; photosensitization dermatitis.	Gastric lavage (or emesis) and symptomatic and supportive treatment.

TOXINS PRODUCING PURGATION AND LATER SYSTEMIC EFFECTS

Ericaceae

Rhododendron (azaleas) species All parts toxic; andromedotoxin	Salivation, lacrimation, vomiting, hypotension, slowing of pulse, paralysis, and convulsions.	Gastric lavage with activated charcoal, atropine, and antihypotensive drugs.

Euphorbiaceae

Euphorbia species All parts contain latex euphorbon	Dermatitis and, if ingested, diarrhea, vomiting, coma, and death.	Gastric lavage and symptomatic treatment.
Hippomane mancinella (manchineel) All parts are toxic, especially fruit; toxic principle resembles alkaloid physostigmine	Abdominal pain, vomiting, diarrhea, and reportedly death.	Gastric lavage with activated charcoal; symptomatic and supportive treatment.
Hura polyandra (devil tree) All parts, particularly seeds and sap, contain hitrine, crepitine, and hurin	Ingested seeds produce nausea, vomiting, abdominal pain, bloody diarrhea, coma, convulsions, and death.	Same as above.
Jatropha curcas (Barbados nut) Contains curcin and oil	Nausea, vomiting, abdominal pain, bloody diarrhea, coma, convulsions, and even death.	Same as above.
Ricinus communis (castor bean) Whole plant toxic, ricin (highest in seeds), an allergen, and purgative oil (seeds)	Allergic dermatitis. Ingested seeds, if chewed, produce nausea, vomiting, diarrhea (bloody), mydriasis, convulsions, and death in uremia and/or jaundice in 3 to 7 days.	Same as above.

Leguminosae

Abrus precatorius (rosary pea, black-eyed Susan) (Fig. 102–2) Seeds contain abrin, abrine, hemagglutinin, and abralin (a glycoside)	If bitten or drilled (as in necklaces), seeds, when ingested, may after a latent period produce nausea, vomiting, diarrhea, weakness, abdominal pain, rapid pulse, and rectal bleeding or other evidence of a bleeding diathesis, as well as hemolytic anemia, oliguria, and uremia.	Gastric lavage with activated charcoal, symptomatic and supportive treatment. Blood transfusion and dialysis when indicated.

Table continued on following page

TABLE 102–2. Table of Common Toxic Plants *Continued*

Toxic Plants	Clinical Manifestations	Guidelines for Therapy
Laburnum species All parts, particularly seeds and bark, contain alkaloid cytisine	Abdominal pain, diarrhea and vomiting, excitement, mydriasis, incoordination, convulsions, respiratory depression, and death.	Gastric lavage with activated charcoal or emesis.
Wisteria sinensis (wisteria) Pods contain resin and glycoside wisterin	Severe diarrhea, vomiting, and collapse.	Gastric lavage or emesis, and symptomatic treatment.
Liliaceae *Colchicum autumnale* (autumn crocus) Whole plant contains alkaloid colchicine	Thirst, mydriasis, nausea and vomiting, diarrhea (bloody), oliguria, weakness, difficulty with breathing, and death.	Gastric lavage with activated charcoal; symptomatic and supportive treatment (assisted respiration and dialysis when indicated).
Phytolaccaceae *Phytolacca americana* (pokeweed) Mature leaves, stems, roots, and seeds contain alkaloid and saponin	Vomiting and diarrhea, abdominal pain, salivation, respiratory paralysis, and death.	Gastric lavage with activated charcoal; symptomatic treatment.
Umbelliferae *Cicuta maculata* (water hemlock) Often mistaken for parsnips; roots contain resin and cicutoxins	Abdominal pain, vomiting, convulsions, respiratory paralysis, and death.	Gastric lavage or emesis, and symptomatic treatment.
Conium maculatum (poison parsley) All parts contain alkaloid coniine	Abdominal pain, vomiting, diarrhea, muscular weakness, respiratory depression, convulsions, and death.	Gastric lavage or emesis, and symptomatic treatment.
TOXINS PRODUCING SYSTEMIC EFFECTS **Cardiac** Apocyanaceae *Nerium oleander* (oleander) All parts contain glycosides resembling digitalis, oleandrin, and neriin	Dermatitis and, if ingested, dilated pupils, nausea, vomiting, bloody diarrhea, cardiac irregularity, labored respiration, coma, paralysis, and death.	Gastric lavage; emesis; in the main, symptomatic and supportive treatment with drugs to combat irregularity of cardiac rhythm.
Thevetia peruviana (yellow oleander) All parts, particularly the seed, contain cardiac glycosides thevetin, thevetoxin, neriifolin, peruvoside, and ruvoside	Clinical manifestations are similar to those with *Nerium*.	Same as above.
Papaveraceae *Argemone mexicana* Seeds contain a glycoside sanguinarine	*Epidemic dropsy.* This is seen in India (Bengal) and also in Mauritius, Fiji, and South Africa. Seeds may contaminate mustard seed oil. Toxin causes dilatation and increased permeability of capillaries and interferes with pyruvic acid oxidation. Characteristics of the disease are edema; dilatation of vessels in skin, subcutaneous tissues, and uveal tract (glaucoma); cardiac insufficiency; and liver abnormalities. Mortality rate may be 5 to 44%.	Bed rest, high-protein diet, vitamin supplements, and digitalis (but its action is variable); glaucoma may require surgical intervention.
Scrophulariaceae *Digitalis purpurea* Leaves, stem, and flowers contain glycoside	*Digitalis poisoning.* Leaves used medicinally, also in herbal tea. Manifestations of toxicity include nausea, psychiatric disturbances, cardiac arrhythmias, paresthesia, sometimes facial neuralgia, and death from cardiac arrhythmias and refractory hyperkalemia.	Gastric lavage or emesis, treatment of arrhythmias, and supportive treatment.
Liver and Pancreas Compositae *Senecio burchelli* (ragwort) All parts contain pyrrolizidine alkaloids	Seeds often contaminate wheat. Manifestations of toxicity may produce *veno-occlusive disease of the liver,* which has been described in Jamaica, Israel, Egypt, India, and South Africa. The acute stage of the disease is characterized by the sudden onset of abdominal distention with slight tenderness over the liver, which is smooth and slightly enlarged, acute ascites, and ankle edema. In the later stages, there is progressive liver failure, hematemesis (portal hypertension), and death. At autopsy, the liver shows centrilobular thrombosis, congestion, and nonportal fibrosis.	Admission to hospital for evaluation; "treatment" is prevention.

TABLE 102–2 *Continued.* **Table of Common Toxic Plants**

Toxic Plants	Clinical Manifestations	Guidelines for Therapy
Euphorbiaceae *Manihot esculenta* (bitter cassava, manihot, tapioca) Root contains cyanogenic glucosides (normally leached out by boiling the root)	Possibly pancreatic calcification and goiter. *Manihot* is a pest-resistant high-yield crop that forms the staple diet for 10% of global caloric needs. It is in the areas where this plant forms the staple diet that the incidence of pancreatic calcification is highest. It has been incriminated as a cause of goiter and tropical ataxic neuropathy. Manifestations of acute toxicity (which might occur if cooking water is ingested) include convulsions, respiratory difficulty, and death from depression of cardiac and respiratory centers.	"Treatment" is prevention—adequate processing of food. In acute cases, gastric lavage with potassium permanganate (to neutralize hydrocyanic acid) and glucose (to retard the liberation of further acid).
Leguminosae *Crotalaria fulva* All parts contain alkaloid	Veno-occlusive disease of liver and lungs.	
Sapindaceae *Blighia sapida* (akee) Unripe fruit contains hypoglycine and hypoglycine A (Fig. 102–3)	*Vomiting sickness of Jamaica.* Six to 48 hours after ingestion, there is vomiting, followed by a period of drowsiness or sleep, after which the vomiting recurs. There is hypoglycemia (due to blocking of gluconeogenesis), often with coma and death. It is particularly severe in young children, in whom the speed of recognition and treatment often determines the outcome.	Emetic and intravenous glucose.
ABORTIFACIENTS **Euphorbiaceae** *Euphorbia* species *Jatropha curcas* (purging nut)	May be inserted into the vagina. Nut is ingested.	Treatment of acute poisoning, as indicated above.
Leguminosae *Abrus precatorius* (rosary pea, black-eyed Susan)	A paste is made of the seeds, applied to a stick, and inserted into the vagina. (Subcutaneous administration can kill an animal or human in a few hours.)	Complications of an abortion and/or intoxication (e.g., renal shutdown) will require appropriate medical and gynecologic treatment.

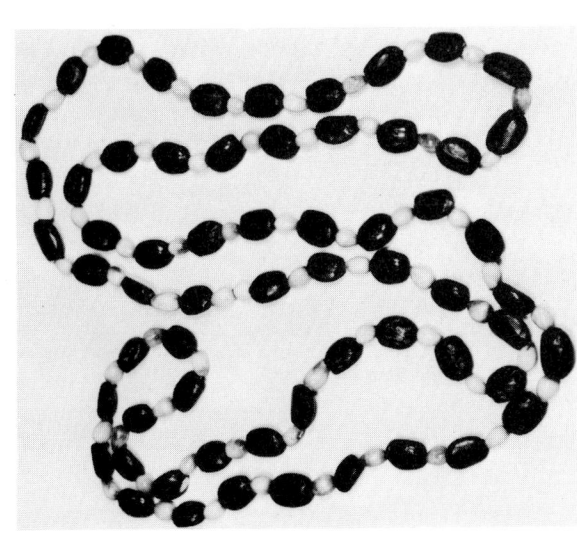

FIGURE 102–1. Necklace made from the toxic castor bean *(Ricinus communis)* (small, light-colored bean) and Job's tears *(Coix lacryma-jobi)* seeds, which are nontoxic. (Courtesy of Julia Morton.)

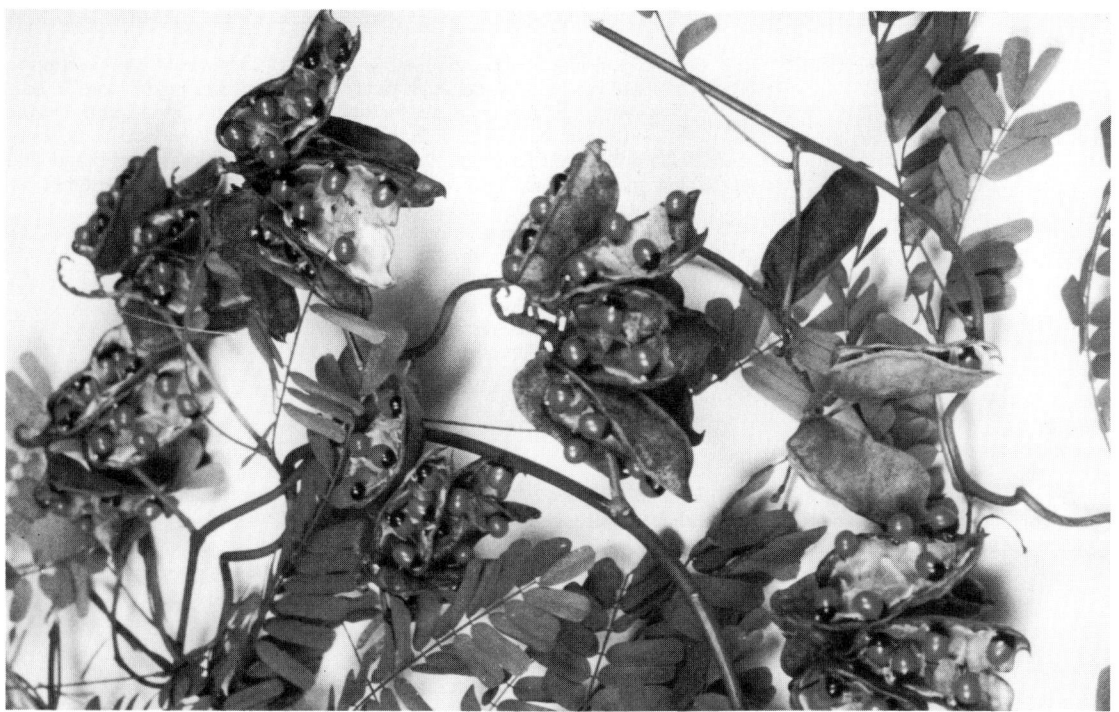

FIGURE 102–2. Rosary pea *(Abrus precatorius)* is toxic when ingested. (Courtesy of Julia Morton.)

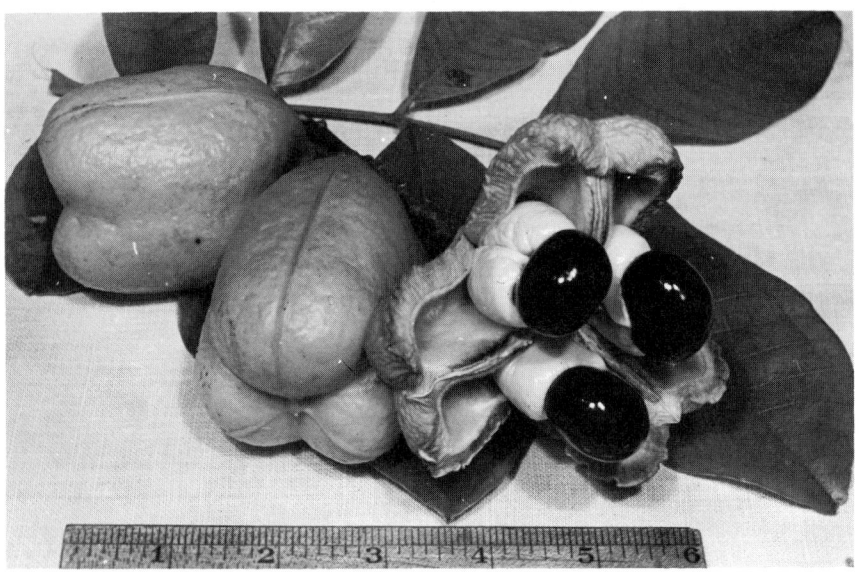

FIGURE 102–3. Akee *(Blighia sapida)*. (From Morton K, Morton J: Fifty Tropical Fruits of Nassau. Text House, Florida, 1946. By permission.)

ings are those due to plant toxins causing contact dermatitis, those causing allergic sensitivity, and those responsible for internal or systemic poisoning.

MYCOTOXINS. *Aspergillus flavus.* Aflatoxins resulting from contamination of peanuts with this fungus are believed to be a cause of the high incidence of primary cancer of the liver in the indigenous inhabitants of Africa and the Orient. Prevention of ingestion of this toxin is the only "treatment" available.

Claviceps purpurea. This fungus, which infects rye, wheat, and other grains, produces ergotism. Its LSD-like fraction may produce hallucinogenic visions, whereas other alkaloids produce contraction of smooth muscle. Symptoms of toxicity include vomiting, diarrhea, abdominal pain, cold extremities, claudication, ischemic peripheral gangrene, hypotension, compensatory bradycardia, headache, convulsions, and coma. Treatment is largely symptomatic and includes the use of analgesics and vasodilators.

Fusarium Species. These grow on grain stored in open fields in winter and produce the toxins responsible for toxic alimentary aleukia. The disease is characterized by necrotic rashes on the skin, leukopenia, agranulocytosis, necrosis, hemorrhages, and, ultimately, death.

BIBLIOGRAPHY

Morton JF: Poisonous and injurious higher plants and fungi. *In* Tedeschi CG, Eckert WB, Tedeschi LG (eds.): Forensic Medicine. Vol. 3, Environmental Hazards, Philadelphia, W. B. Saunders Company, 1977.

Mushroom poisoning. (Editorial.) Lancet 2:351, 1980.

North P: Poisonous Plants and Fungi. London, Blandford Press, 1967.

Short ALK, et al.: Poisoning by *Cortinarius speciosissimus.* Lancet 2:942, 1980.

Watt JM, Breyer-Brandwijk MG: The Medicinal and Poisonous Plants of Southern and Eastern Africa. Edinburgh, Churchill Livingstone, 1962.

103. ANIMALS HAZARDOUS TO HUMANS

GENERAL PRINCIPLES

William A. Sodeman, Jr.

Humans' interaction with the rest of the animal kingdom has always been fraught with the possibilities of injury from either direct trauma or by venoms. The process of urbanization and cultivation had for many years reduced the opportunities for untoward interaction between humans and animals. Two circumstances led to a resurgence of injury related to animals. The first, erratic in occurrence but not uncommon, is the temporary stress caused by natural cataclysm. Natural catastrophes, floods, storms, droughts, tend to press humans and animals into uncommon juxtaposition. The second feature is the popularity of recreational visits to the diminishing natural environments. The numbers of people who engage in caving, diving, wilderness hiking, bird watching, photo safaris, and the like have undergone remarkable increase, and with this comes increased exposure and increased numbers of untoward incidents. Previously uncommon or rare hazards have emerged as significant health problems.

103.1. VENOMOUS MARINE ANIMALS

William A. Sodeman, Jr.

Venomous marine animals range worldwide. Relative numbers and varieties are greater in the warm waters of tropical and subtropical seas. Their clinical importance has undergone a recent and rather unexpected escalation. In the past, human exposure was limited by geography, because many venomous marine animals are abundant only in less populated areas. The predominant exposure had been occupational, usually among fishermen and professional divers. There was a relatively limited recreational exposure. Currently professional and recreational diving has undergone a greater than geometric expansion in popularity, vastly increasing the exposure.

Much of the recreational diving focuses on marine reef environments rich in venomous species. A second feature is the change in access with easy travel opportunities to previously remote areas also rich in venomous marine species. The consequence is a greatly increased incidence of injury and fatality from venomous marine animals.

Toxin-containing marine protozoans abound, but because their expression is as a food chain poisoning they are discussed in Chapter 102 under shellfish poisoning, ciguatera poisoning, and other poisonings.

INVERTEBRATES. Venomous invertebrates are found in 5 phyla: the Porifera, the Coelenterata, the Mollusca, the Annelida, and the Echinodermata. Relatively few of the many thousands of species in these 5 phyla pose a hazard to humans.

Sponges, Porifera. Sponges produce a number of toxins that may be retained on the surface of the sponge or released into the water. These prove an effective defense, and few sponges are eaten by higher forms. Toxic sponges are widespread and not necessarily tropical. The most common toxic sponges and their distribution are listed in Table 103–1. Human exposure is a result of handling or otherwise contacting the sponge with abraded skin. Russell reports a case with both local and systemic symptoms after handling sponges. Local symptoms include pain, pruritus, and swelling of the skin. The papules may go on to vesiculate. Left untreated, the dermatitis may be unusually persistent. Systemic complaints include malaise, weakness, and syncope. Nausea and paresthesia are described also.

Sponge fisherman's disease, an occupational problem among Mediterranean fishermen, is associated with a coelenterate living in close association with the sponges rather than a Porifera toxin.

Coelenterates, Coelenterata. Three classes, the Hydrozoa (fire coral, the Portuguese man-of-war, and the stinging hydroids), Scyphozoa (true jellyfish), and An-

TABLE 103–1. Toxic Marine Sponges

Name	Common Name	Distribution
Fibulia nolitangere (Duchassaing and Michelotti)	Do-Not-Touch-Me sponge	West Indies
Microciona prolifera (Ellis and Solander)	Red moss, Oyster sponge	Cape Cod to North Florida
Haliclona viridis (Duchassaing and Michelotti)	Green sponge	West Indies
Tedania ignis (Duchassaing and Michelotti)	Fire sponge	West Indies
Tedania nigrescens (Schmidt)		West Indies
Neofibularia mordens Hartman	Australia stinging sponge	Australia

Compiled from Russell, 1971; Campbell, 1983; Halstead, 1988.

thozoa (the true corals and sea anemones) all have venomous forms. Injuries are produced by nematocysts, individual stinging units, which when triggered inject minute quantities of venom into the skin of an intruder. The severity and the consequences of coelenterate stings depends primarily on the species involved in the sting but also varies with the site of the sting, the total number of nematocysts involved, and the duration of contact. Nematocysts are located frequently on the tentacles, and 1 measure of the exposure is the length of the tentacles involved.

Hydrozoa. *Aglaophenia cupresina* Lamouroux, *Lytocarpus philippinus* (Kirchenpauer) and *Rhizophysa eysenhardti* Gegenbaur are seaweed-like organisms with, collectively, a worldwide distribution (Table 103–2). Skin contact produces a painful papulovesicular dermatitis that may last for days.

Millepora alcornis (Linnaeus), *M. dichotoma* (Forskål), and *M. complanata* (Lamarck) are referred to commonly as fire corals. The various species are found in tropical waters worldwide (Table 103–2). They produce primarily skin irritation with painful pruritic papules.

Physalia physalis (Linnaeus), the Portuguese man-of-war, is a colonial hydroid often mistaken for a true jellyfish. It has a wide geographic distribution in the Atlantic Ocean and the Mediterranean Sea, and a related species, *Physalia utriculus* (La Martinière), has an equally wide Indo-Pacific distribution (Table 103–2). They are more plentiful in the tropics, but they can be found as far north as Canada, the Hebrides, and Japan. *Gonionemus vertens* (Agassiz) and *Olindioides formosa* Goto (Table 103–2) are toxic jellyfish-like hydroids. Envenomation causes painful cutaneous lesions and in some cases systemic reactions. Contact with the tentacles produces lines of papules, which are extremely painful. These may vesiculate and heal with pigmentation. Muscle spasms and pain may appear in the involved extremity.

With extensive exposure, systemic reactions may occur. Nausea, vomiting, headaches, vertigo, and weakness are all described. Pain and muscle spasm, particularly in the back, occur but are less frequent. Lacrimation, rhinorrhea, pain on respiration, and ar-

TABLE 103–2. Venomous Coelenterates (Representative List)

Name	Common Name	Distribution
HYDROIDS		
Aglaophenia cupressinia Lamouroux	Stinging hydroid	Indian Ocean
Lytocarpus philippinus (Kirchenpauer)	Feather hydroid	Tropical Pacific, Indian, and Atlantic Oceans, Mediterranean Sea
Rhizophysa eysenhardti		Tropical oceans
Millepora alcornis Linnaeus	Fire coral	Caribbean Sea
Millepora dichotoma Forskål	Fire coral	Red Sea, Indo-Pacific
Millepora complanata Lamarck	Fire coral	West Indies
Physalia physalis (Linnaeus)	Portuguese man-of-war	Tropical Atlantic Ocean, Mediterranean Sea
Physalia utriculus (La Martinière)	Portuguese man-of-war	Indo-Pacific
Gonionemus vertens (Agassiz)	Orange-striped jellyfish	Temperate Pacific and Atlantic Oceans, Mediterranean Sea
Olindioides formosa Goto	Stinging medusa	Japan
JELLYFISH		
Chironex fleckeri Southcott	Deadly sea wasp	Northeastern Australia
Chiropsalmus quadrigatus Haeckel	Sea wasp	Northern Australia, Indian Ocean, Philippine Islands
Chiropsalmus quadrumanus (Müller)	Sea wasp	North Australia, Indian Ocean, Atlantic Coast—Carolina to Brazil
Carukia barnesi Southcott		Australia—Queensland coast
Carybdea rastoni Haacke	Sea wasp	Tropical Pacific Ocean—Southern Japan to Australia
Carybdea alata Reynaud	Sea wasp	Tropical Indian, Pacific, and Atlantic Oceans
Cyanea capillata (Linnaeus)	Giant jellyfish	Atlantic and Pacific basins—arctic to tropics
Cassiopea xamachana Bigelow	Upside down jellyfish	Caribbean Basin, Gulf of Mexico
ANTHOZOA		
Acropora palmata (Lamarck)	Elk horn coral	Florida, Bahamas, West Indies

Various sea anemones in the families:
ACTINIIDAE
ACTINODENDRONIDAE
ACTINODISCIDAE
ALICIIDAE
HORMATHIIDAE
RENILLIDAE
SAGARTIIDAE
STOICHACTIIDAE
ZOANTHIDAE

Compiled from Russell, 1971; Campbell, 1983; Halstead, 1988.

rhythmia may occur. Neurotoxins are suspected to be involved.

Treatment of stings involves 3 separate steps. The first goal is to arrest the envenomation by inactivation and/or removal of the nematocysts. Next is to treat the local reaction, pain, and swelling. The third step, when necessary, is the treatment of systemic reactions. Prompt removal of any adhering tentacles will reduce envenomation. These should be lifted away rather than brushed across the skin, with care that the rescuing finger does not get stung. A sea water rinse, not a scrub, may wash away loose nematocysts. Prompt application of vinegar or dilute (3 to 10%) acetic acid will inactivate the nematocysts. Methyl alcohol or ethyl alcohol, which in the past has been the recommended treatment, should be avoided. Alcohol has now been shown to stimulate nematocyst discharge. Fresh water is also a stimulant for nematocyst discharge. Removal of adherent nematocysts is a problem with a number of possible solutions that often have to be adapted to available resources. Rubbing the affected area with wet sand, a cloth, or vigorous washing is likely to cause further discharge of nematocysts and, thus, should be avoided. Dusting the area with fine sand, baking soda, powder, or flour and then scraping the caked powder off with the dull back edge of a knife has proven effective and safe. Application of aerosol shaving cream, then shaving the nematocysts off with a safety razor, is a handy alternative method of removal. A host of other agents are part of the folklore of treatment, including papain, ammonia, lime juice, and boric acid. None have had any systematic study.

Relief of pain and swelling may be facilitated with topical application of steroid cream and/or anesthetic creams or aerosols. Antihistamines in some cases will reduce the swelling. Occasionally the pain will be severe enough to require narcotic analgesics. Secondary infection may follow vesiculation, particularly if the sting has occurred in a grossly contaminated environment. Topical or systemic antibiotics may be in order. Muscle spasms can be alleviated with intravenous calcium gluconate, 10 ml of a 10% solution. Evidence of toxicity affecting the cardiovascular system or the pulmonary system may require the use of epinephrine or intervention with CPR.

Scyphozoa. Several of the true jellyfish are distinguished as lethal for humans. Many others, although not lethal, cause painful skin lesions and disturbing systemic reactions. *Chironex fleckeri* Southcott, the deadly sea wasp (Fig. 103–1), is distributed on the Australian coastline. Other sea wasps, *Carybdea rastoni* Haacke and several species of *Chiropsalmus,* are found in all tropical oceans. *Cassiopea* species are found in the Caribbean Sea and the Gulf of Mexico. *Cyanea capillata* (Linnaeus), which grows to giant proportions, may be found in arctic as well as tropical waters in both ocean basins. A number of other stinging species are known (Table 103–2).

Chironex fleckeri Southcott is a small, up to 5 inches in length, undistinguished jellyfish with lethal potential (Fig. 103–1). *Chiropsalmus quadrigatus* Haeckel and *Chiropsalmus quadrumanus* (Müller) are only slightly less dangerous and far more widespread in distribution. The sting is followed by almost immediate pain, then swelling, which proceeds to vesiculation and then to necrosis with further breakdown. The pain is agonizing. There can be rapid progression through muscle spasm, pulmonary edema, vascular collapse, and respiratory

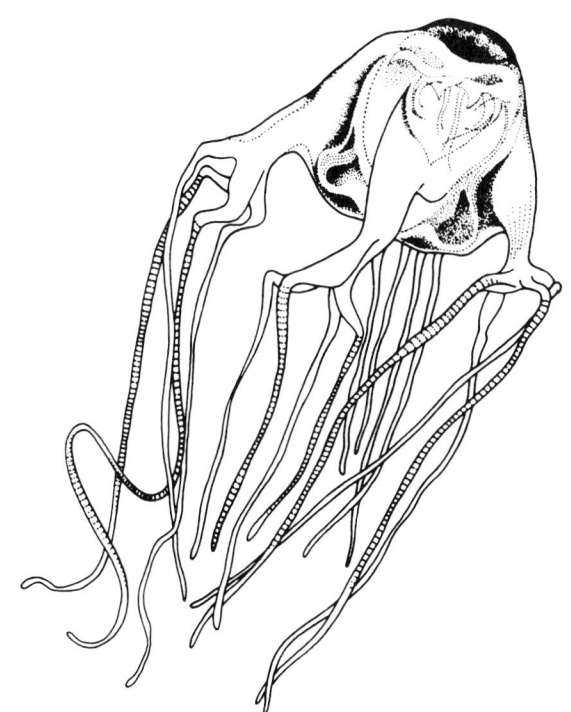

FIGURE 103–1. *Chironex fleckeri,* although usually associated with the north coast of Australia, can be found in the Atlantic Ocean, the Gulf of Mexico, and Caribbean Sea as well. (Courtesy of A. A. Fischer, M.D.: Atlas of Aquatic Dermatology. Copyright 1978 American Cyanamid Company, Lederle Laboratories Division. Reproduced by permission.)

failure with death. Although patients may survive as long as 2 to 3 hours, death can be rapid—1 minute or less. An antivenin is manufactured in Australia and, if available, can be lifesaving. Otherwise, treatment follows that outlined above.

Carukia barnesi Southcott is responsible for the Irukandji syndrome, a severe but not fatal envenomation, that is reported from Australia. The sting appears as an erythematous patch with localized pain that increases in severity and spreads to involve the back and extremities. There may be systemic symptoms with fever and tachycardia. Respiratory symptoms with cough, tightness, mucoid sputum, and hemoptysis are distinguishing features.

Many jellyfish stings remain unidentified as to causative organism. Repeated stings can give rise to hypersensitivity with the possibility of anaphylaxis.

Anthozoa. This class includes the true corals, sea anemones, and sea pansies. Many species are toxic, and the geographic distribution collectively spares no marine environment (Table 103–2).

The toxicity associated with coral cuts is poorly characterized. Cuts are associated frequently with a stinging sensation. These cuts break down frequently to form painful ulcerations that are slow to heal and tend to recur. Treatment is scrupulous care of the sort that would be applied to any laceration.

Sea anemones and sea pansies are highly variable in their toxicity, and many cause only mild stinging. Severe reactions do occur, with local edema and necrosis that results in slow-healing ulcers. Relatively nonspecific systemic symptoms are reported. Treatment is careful cleansing, protection of the affected area, and specific treatment of secondary infection.

Echinoderms, Echinodermata. Venomous echinoderms are found among the Asteroidea (starfishes), Echinoidea (sea urchins), and Holothuroidea (sea cucumbers). Whereas many creatures in this phylum have proven toxic on ingestion, relatively few are venomous for humans.

Asteroidea. Only one starfish, *Acanthaster planci* (Linnaeus) (Table 103–3) has proven venomous, although several other species have produced dermatitis on contact. This starfish, commonly known as the crown of thorns, grows to a large size. It is covered with large spines that in turn are covered by an integument containing venom-producing glands. Envenomation is a result of wounding by contact with the spines. Wounds are painful with associated swelling and erythema. Systemic reactions include nausea, vomiting, numbness, and paralysis. There is no specific antidote, and treatment is first aid and supportive care.

Echinoidea. Many sea urchins are known for their venomous stings (Table 103–3). There are 2 venom delivery systems. The first involves the long needle-like spines of the families Diadematidea, Echinidea, and Echinothuridae. These spines can contain venom that is released after the spine penetrates the integument. The second method of venom delivery involves pedicellariae. These are seizing organs found scattered among the spines on the surface of the urchin. They come in many varieties and are utilized in taxonomic classification of urchins. The jaws of the pedicellariae clamp onto prey and maintain their hold even if broken free from the urchin. Venomous pedicellariae continue envenomation even when broken off and must be removed promptly. Penetration of spines is associated with the release of a colored fluid (violet-purple) that stains the wound and is a good clinical marker of possible envenomation. With an envenomating sting, another diagnostic sign is pain, which develops quickly, and is out of proportion to the trauma of the sting. Pain is followed by the development of edematous swelling and redness. In addition to local reactions, partial paralysis of an involved extremity, facial edema, and arrhythmia have been reported. Generally the pain will subside after several hours, although the staining of the wound may persist for days. Secondary infection does occur and may require attention.

Pedicellarial stings have been associated with local complaints of pain and somewhat more frightening systemic reactions, including paralysis, aphonia, respiratory distress, and occasionally death. The pain will subside in about 1 hour, but paralysis persists often for several hours longer.

Treatment is largely symptomatic. There are no specific antidotes. Two therapeutic features specific to sea urchins are the need to inspect the bite carefully and promptly remove any adherent pedicellariae to terminate the envenomation. Spines may break off in the wound also. There is much folklore concerning the need or lack of need for their removal. Unlike pedicellariae, there is no apparent need for urgent extraction of spines, but they may require surgical removal at a later date.

Holothuroidea. Sea cucumbers are spineless echinoderms that are wormlike in appearance. Several species (Table 103–3) are equipped for defense with organs of Cuvier. These tubules, derived from the respiratory tree, are filled with the toxin holothurin. The organs can be extruded from the body of the sea cucumber to cause release of holothurin into the water. Skin contact with this venom has caused dermatitis, and corneal contact has caused blindness in humans. The treatment is symptomatic.

Mollusca. Of the 5 classes of Mollusca only the gastropods and cephalopods harbor species venomous for humans. Shellfish are a common food item, and many more are poisonous than venomous. Some families, particularly the Muricidae, have well-developed poison glands but lack a mechanism for delivery of the venom. A number of species of the family Aplysiidae, nudibranchs or sea hares, feed on coelenterates and carry undischarged nematocysts, which they use for defense and predation. Contact with these animals can produce the coelenterate stings discussed above.

Conidae. Cone shells are much sought after gastropod mollusks. More than 400 species are described, and they are found worldwide in warm water oceans and seas. They are carnivorous predators with highly developed venom delivery systems used in hunting and defense. Eight species are lethal for humans (Table 103–4). Many of the remaining species are capable of inflicting painful stings.

Venom is delivered by injection through a modified radular tooth, which is hollow, barbed, and carries an attached venom sac (Fig. 103–2). The cone shell is a desirable collector's item, and stings are associated usually with handling during collection. The best characterized component of venom is a neurotoxin that has an

TABLE 103–3. Venomous Echinoderms (Representative List)

Name	Common Name	Distribution
STARFISH		
Acanthaster planci (Linnaeus)	Crown of thorns starfish	Indo-Pacific
SEA URCHINS		
Diadema antillarum Philippi	Black urchin	West Indies
Diadema setosum (Leske)	Black sea urchin	Indo-Pacific, China, Japan
Paracentrotus lividus Lamarck	Sea urchin	Atlantic coast of Europe and West Africa
Araeosoma thetidis (Clark)	Tam o'shanter urchin	Australia, New Zealand
Toxopneustes pileolus (Lamarck)	Sea urchin	Indo-Pacific, Japan
Tripneustes ventricosus (Lamarck)	White sea urchin	West Indies, Tropical South Atlantic
SEA CUCUMBERS		
Cucumaria echinata Von Marenzeller		Japan
Holothuria argus (Jaeger)	Tiger fish	Indo-Pacific
Euapta lappa (Müller)		West Indies

Compiled from Russell, 1971; Campbell, 1983; Halstead, 1988.

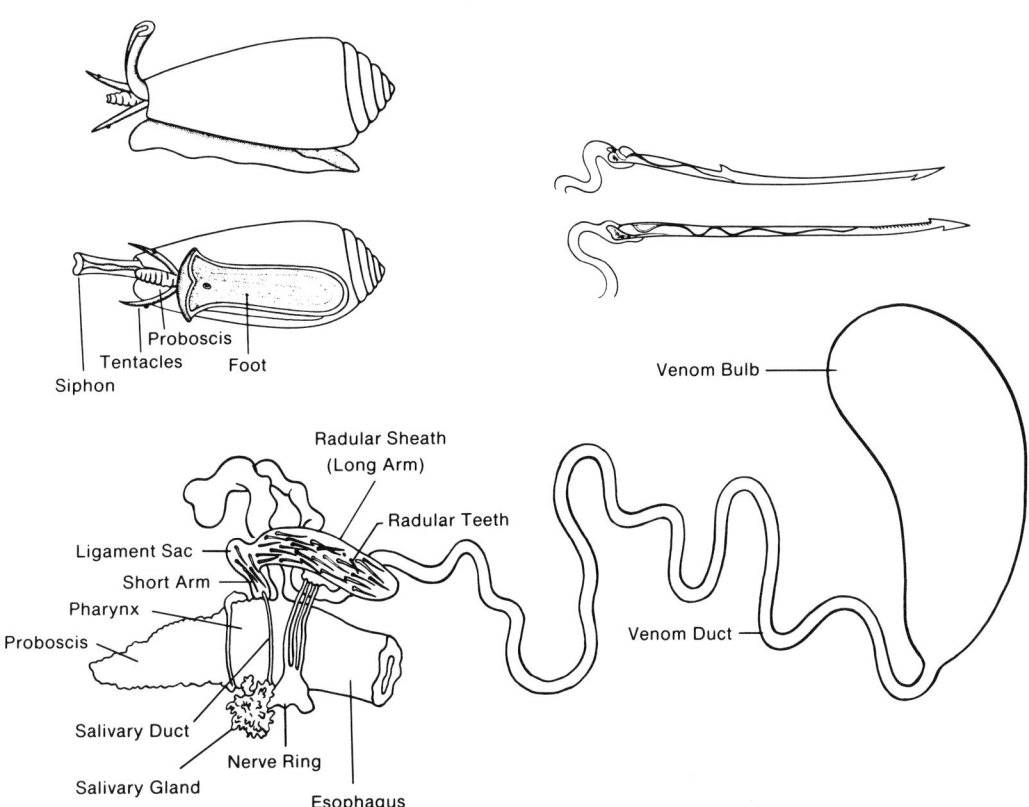

FIGURE 103–2. This general representation of the venom apparatus of *Conidae* is applicable to all species, whether or not toxic for humans. The armed, barbed tooth is held in the proboscis and thrust into the integument of prey or an attacker. (Courtesy of Bruce W. Halstead, M.D.: Poisonous and Venomous Marine Animals of the World, 2nd ed.)

effect on the neuromuscular junction and causes paralysis of skeletal muscle. There are other venom components that vary from species to species.

The sting results in prompt pain at the site of puncture. There is associated swelling and erythema. The perception of the pain is highly variable from person to person. Neurologic symptoms appear promptly. Sensory symptoms include numbness and paresthesias. Motor symptoms include incoordination and muscular paralysis. In mild envenomation only weakness may be manifest as a motor change. In the case of severe envenomation paralysis will progress to become generalized. Deep tendon reflexes will disappear. Aphonia, dysphagia, diplopia, and blurred vision all may occur. Fatal cases proceed to coma and death from cardiac or respiratory failure. Nausea is an early complaint, but there is little else in the way of smooth muscle dysfunction. Recovery is slow and in the cases of serious envenomation may take weeks before the return of full muscular function.

Whereas most of the attention has focused on the 8 cones that are lethal for humans, *Conus aulicus* Linnaeus, *C. geographus* Linnaeus, *C. gloriamaris* Hwass, *C. magus* Linnaeus, *C. marmoreus* Linnaeus, *C. striatus* Linnaeus, *C. textile* Linnaeus, and *C. tulipa* Linnaeus, the other cones are capable of producing a limited systemic reaction with nausea, weakness, and limited paralysis. Should these reactions occur while diving to collect shells, they can cause fatality by drowning. All live cone shells should be treated with care and respect as venomous animals.

Treatment is largely symptomatic. The curare-like effect of the neurotoxin may respond to the use of neostigmine. Maintenance of airway and provision of artificial ventilation may be required.

Pteropoda. The pteropod *Creseis acicula* Rang (Table 103–4) is a gastropod commonly called a sea butterfly. Contact with its needle-like shell has caused stings associated with a self-limited maculopapular dermatitis.

TABLE 103–4. Venomous Mollusks

Name	Common Name	Distribution
CONE SHELLS		
Conus aulicus Linnaeus	Court cone	Polynesia
Conus geographus Linnaeus	Geographer cone	Indo-Pacific
Conus gloriamaris Hwass	Glory-of-the-Sea	Philippines, Malaysia
Conus magus Linnaeus		Indo-Pacific
Conus marmoreus Linnaeus	Marbled cone	Polynesia
Conus striatus Linnaeus	Striated cone	Indo-Pacific
Conus textile Linnaeus	Textile cone	Indo-Pacific
Conus tulipa Linnaeus	Tulip cone	Indo-Pacific
PTEROPOD		
Creseis acicula Rang	Sea butterfly	Atlantic and Pacific Oceans
CEPHALOPODS		
Octopus maculosus Hoyle	Blue-ringed octopus	Indo-Pacific, Japan

Compiled from Russell, 1971; Campbell, 1983; Halstead, 1988.

Little is known concerning possible toxins in this organism. Treatment is symptomatic.

Cephalopoda. The cephalopods include cuttlefish, squid, and octopi, all of which utilize venom in the predation for food. Only the octopus is associated with envenomation in humans (Table 103–4). Fatalities and near fatal serious envenomations have been associated only with *Octopus maculosus* Hoyle, the Australian blue-ringed octopus, in Australian waters. There is some taxonomic confusion, and several other spotted octopi may be implicated also. There are a few reports of envenomation by other octopi, but none have been well studied.

Envenomation in humans is associated with a bite. The jaws of the octopus are beak-like and produce 2 puncture wounds. These bites bleed freely. Envenomation is associated with a rapidly spreading burning sensation. The wound site becomes edematous and erythematous. If the envenomation is severe, neurologic symptoms may occur. These may be both motor and sensory. Paralysis, difficulty with swallowing, and loss of equilibrium are described. In a well-documented fatality reported by Mabbet, the patient developed respiratory distress and was placed in a respirator, but died despite the treatment.

Treatment is symptomatic. Mild envenomations are self-limited. CPR measures may be lifesaving to permit severely bitten patients to reach medical facilities. Most envenomations are a result of handling the octopus, and caution is advised.

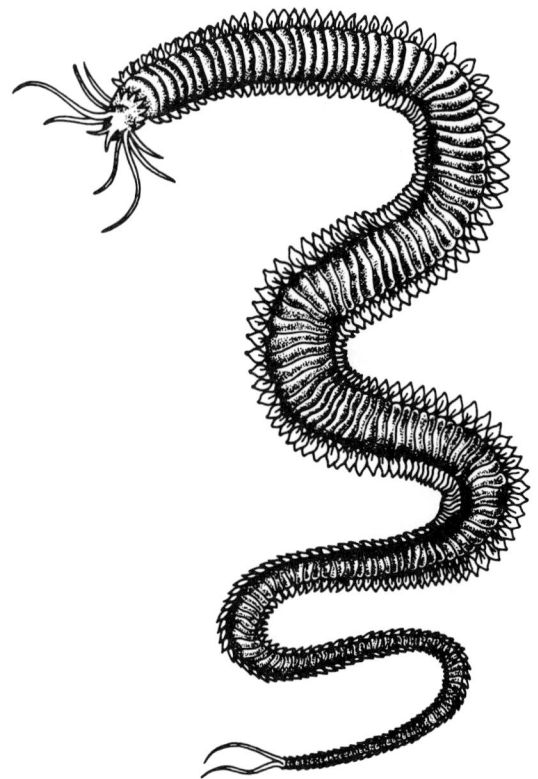

FIGURE 103–3. The bristle worm can cause cutaneous envenomation, with the development of dermatitis, as a result of contact with the bristles. (Courtesy of A.A. Fischer, M.D.: Atlas of Aquatic Dermatology. Copyright, 1978 American Cyanamid Company, Lederle Laboratories Division. Reproduced by permission.)

TABLE 103–5. Venomous Roundworms

Name	Common Name	Distribution
BRISTLE WORMS		
Chloeia flava (Pallas)	Sea-mouse	Indo-Pacific, Japan
Chloeia viridis Schmarda	Red-tipped bristle worm	Both coasts of tropical America
Eurythoë complanata (Pallas)	Orange bristle worm	Tropical worldwide
Glycera dibranchiata Ehlers	Blood worm	Canada to Carolina
Hermodice carunculata (Pallas)	Green bristle worm	West Indies, Florida

Compiled from Russell, 1971; Campbell, 1983; Halstead, 1988.

Flatworms, Platyhelminthes. The nemertean *Amphiporus lactifloreus* (Johnston), the ribbon worm, has a true venom apparatus, but human envenomation has not been described.

Roundworms, Annelida. Several polychaetes of the family Amphinomidea, the bristle worms, (Table 103–5), have venom-containing setae, bristles, which can extend and contract and are capable of penetrating skin (Fig. 103–3). The resulting painful dermatitis may be associated with secondary infection and gangrene. Treatment is symptomatic but must include the removal of any retained setae.

Several species of the family Glyceridae have biting jaws associated with venom glands. The bite of *Glycera dibranchiata* Ehlers produces pain, swelling, and erythema. The wound heals over several days with gradual subsidence of symptoms.

VERTEBRATES

Fishes. There are over 200 species of marine fish known to be venomous, mainly shallow-water reef fish or inshore fish (Table 103–6). Many species are found off the coasts of California and Florida and in the Gulf of Mexico and the Caribbean. They include stingrays, scorpion fish, zebra fish, stonefish, weevers, toadfish, stargazers, certain sharks, catfish, and surgeon-fish. Ill effects result from puncture of the skin by spines and

TABLE 103–6. Venomous Fish Families

Families	Common Name	Distribution
DASYATIDAE	Stingrays	Collectively worldwide in temperate and tropical waters
GYMNURIDAE	Butterflyrays	Same as stingrays
MYLIOBATIDAE	Bat stingrays	Same as stingrays
UROLOPHIDAE	Round stingrays	Pacific and Indian Oceans
RAJIDAE	Skates	North and South Atlantic
TORPEDINIDAE	Electric rays	Atlantic and Indian Oceans, Mediterranean Sea
CHIMAERIDAE	Catfish	North Atlantic, North Pacific, Australia
HETERODONTIDAE	Hornshark	California coast
SQUALIDAE	Dogfish	Atlantic and Pacific Oceans
ARIIDAE	Marine catfish	Worldwide
TRACHINIDAE	Weever fish	European coast
SCORPAENIDAE	Scorpion fish	Indo-Pacific
BATRACHOIDIDAE	Toadfish	Worldwide
ACANTHURIDAE	Surgeon fish	Indo-Pacific
URANOSCOPIDAE	Stargazers	Indo-Pacific

Compiled from Russell, 1971; Campbell, 1983; Halstead, 1988.

inoculation of venom, as occurs in the case of stingrays, scorpion fish, stonefish, stargazers, and various sharks, or from eating fish eggs or blood of certain fish (the toxic substance in this case being intrinsic, i.e., originating in a gland or other structure).

Rajiformes, Stingrays, and Skates. These are bottom feeders (Table 103–6). When stepped on, the muscular tail with its barb is wielded vigorously and may cause extensive wounds, and even death from hemorrhage. The venom affects the cardiovascular system, causing peripheral vasoconstriction or dilatation and cardiac arrythmias (including asystole). It can cause depression of respiration (mediated by the medullary centers) and convulsions as well. Other symptoms include nausea, vomiting, diarrhea, and weakness. Pain at the site of injury is immediate and intense, spreading and intensifying over a period of 30 to 90 minutes and then gradually diminishing over the next 6 to 48 hours.

Treatment is common to all wounds inflicted by venomous fish. It should be directed at (1) relief of pain, (2) neutralization of the effects of the venom, and (3) prevention of secondary infection. The pain results from the inoculation of the venom, the traumatization by the spine, and probably the introduction of other foreign bodies. Wounds should be irrigated, therefore, with saline solution. If the puncture wound is small, it should be excised and then irrigated. Opinions vary on the use of tourniquets. Heat treatment, i.e., soaking the limb in hot water (120°F) for 30 minutes to 1 hour, is efficacious. Stingray venom is destroyed by heat. Intravenous administration of calcium gluconate (to relieve muscle spasms) and local infiltration of 0.5 to 2% procaine give some relief of pain. Occasionally, however, meperidine hydrochloride may be necessary. Débridement and suturing (with or without a drain) are usually necessary. Tetanus toxoid and an antibiotic to combat secondary infection should be given. Secondary shock may occur as a result of the direct action of the venom on the cardiovascular system and requires prompt and vigorous therapy. Cardiovascular and respiratory stimulants, as well as assisted ventilation, may be indicated.

Electric rays, members of the family Torpedinidae, can produce a discharge of up to 220 volts, which can temporarily disable a swimmer.

Scorpion Fish and Zebra Fish (Table 103–6). These are becoming popular with tropical marine aquaria enthusiasts. They have venomous spines that, on penetration, produce immediate and intense local pain that radiates along the course of lymphatics. This pain may last 16 to 24 hours. The surrounding tissues become swollen, discolored, and even gangrenous. General symptoms include shock, nausea, vomiting, diarrhea, hypotension, respiratory distress, convulsions, and, occasionally, death. Treatment is supportive and symptomatic, similar to that used to treat stingray wounds.

Stonefish (Table 103–6). These are found only in the tropical Indo-Pacific and are the most dangerous of the venomous fish, particularly because of their camouflaged appearance. Injury causes immediate pain, which is moderately severe to excruciating in intensity, with the victim often rapidly losing consciousness. The pain may

last for hours or days. At the site of the injury, there is swelling and, in many instances, ischemia, which leads to subsequent necrosis and sloughing. General signs and symptoms include shock, respiratory distress, and, sometimes, death, probably as a result of direct action of the toxin on the heart. Treatment is symptomatic and supportive, although procaine and morphine are said to do little to alleviate the intense pain. Heat treatment reportedly produces some relief. Antivenom should be used if available.

Weever Fish. These perch-like marine fish are distributed on the Atlantic and Mediterranean coasts of Europe and North Africa (Table 103–6). The venom of these fish has effects similar to those of stingray venom. Victims are usually fishermen (fish being caught in nets) or bathers (fish being stepped on in the sand). Pain in the immediate area is instantaneous, spreading in the first half hour and then gradually subsiding and disappearing over the next 2 to 24 hours. Rarely, envenomation has been fatal. Swelling, which involves the wound and the regional lymph glands, may last for days. Treatment should include opening of the wound with a knife and suction and irrigation with cold water or sterile saline solution to remove as much poison as possible. It is of interest to note that weevers can cause wounds even when dead.

Catfish. Both freshwater (North American) and marine catfish can cause injuries. The marine variety is a shore fish and is commonly found in muddy waters around boat slips. On envenomation, the victim experiences sharp pain. This lasts 30 minutes to 48 hours. The area surrounding the wound (and possibly the entire limb) becomes ischemic; later, it becomes cyanotic and edematous. Numbness and localized gangrene occur in some cases, and the complications of shock and respiratory distress may occur also in severe injuries. Treatment is symptomatic and supportive and follows the general principles indicated previously for the treatment of other venomous fish stings.

103.2. LEECHES

William A. Sodeman, Jr.

Leeches belong to the phylum Annelida of the class Hirudinea. They occur mainly in Southeast Asia, India, tropical Australia, and parts of South America. The blood-sucking species of medical importance are either terrestrial or live in fresh water.

Leeches have 2 suckers, 1 anteriorly (containing the mouth and cutting parts) and 1 posteriorly. The leech attaches to the skin of animals, including humans, by means of the cutting plate, rapidly perforates the skin, and secretes an anticoagulant, hirudin, into the wound. With the sucker, it then draws blood from the victim. If present in large numbers, leeches may cause considerable blood loss, as well as psychological trauma. If ingested, they may become attached to the buccal mucosa, pharynx, or larynx, producing hemorrhage and signs of obstruction. Leeches attached to the skin may be fairly easily detached by rubbing them with salt or by burning them with a match. Those attached internally have been removed endoscopically with a snare, but some may require surgical removal. All wounds should be irrigated and dressed. Antibiotics may be indicated in the event of secondary infection. Prophylaxis includes the use of protective clothing and repellent creams (particularly those containing diethyltoluamide).

103.3. FISH

William A. Sodeman, Jr.

SHARKS. Only about 30 of 350 species of sharks have been identified in attacks on humans. Sharks tend to inhabit waters between latitude 47 degrees south and 46 degrees north, with a slight preponderance in the Southern Hemisphere and where water temperature is above 68F. Attacks usually occur in the late afternoon and night, when sharks normally feed, or whenever there is food or blood in the water.

Sharks use vision as the primary sensory organ at distances of 50 feet or less; their visual acuity for color and moving objects is better than previously thought. At distances greater than 50 feet, other sensory organs are used. These include (in some species) visual adaptations for sight under low light conditions, a highly developed olfactory sense, chemoreceptors in the skin that detect water movement and changes in salinity, and "hearing" sense. Sharks have the ability to detect low-frequency vibrations at great distances in the water (bathers and other fish), as well as electrical fields of infinitesimal energy, by means of electroreceptors located in the head.

Sharks are unpredictable, and there does not appear to be any uniform attack approach. Attacks may be provoked or unprovoked. Bright colors or patterns may attract sharks. The fatality rate of shark attacks based on records of a series of 1165 attacks was 35%.

Attack prevention is not absolute, but a few precautionary measures should be observed. Swim in groups; if water is shark-infested, stay out; do not enter or remain in water with a bleeding wound; avoid turbid or polluted water; and wear dark protective clothing. Shark repellents and nets in beach areas have been used effectively.

The bites of sharks will generally produce severe, ragged wounds. Initial first aid is of the greatest importance. A pressure bandage or tourniquet should be used to control hemorrhage; analgesics should be given and transfusions started to combat shock. Some advocate that these measures should be instituted on the beach and that undue haste in removing the patient to a hospital decreases his chances of survival. In any event, when conditions permit, the patient should be hospitalized for more complete evaluation and definitive treatment.

GIANT DEVILFISH OR MANTA RAY. The manta ray is not aggressive but is dangerous because of its large size, measuring up to 5 m across. The coarse dermal tentacles may cause skin abrasions and may interfere with divers' air lines.

BARRACUDA. There are about 20 species of barracuda, which vary in aggressiveness. The great barracuda can be exceedingly pugnacious. It can measure up to 8 feet in length and is usually found in the Caribbean, off the coast of Brazil, and in the Indo-Pacific.

The barracuda relies almost entirely on sight and is attracted to bright colors, shiny reflections, or injured fish. It will follow divers without attacking. If it does attack, it usually does so only once, but this may be fatal. Bites (which are straight cuts as opposed to the curved cuts of shark bites) should be treated similarly to shark bites.

MORAY EELS. These eels are notoriously powerful biters, but attacks are usually provoked by poking into crevices between rocks. Wounds produced by the bite are ragged, and treatment of victims should follow the same principles as for treatment of shark bites.

NEEDLEFISH. Needlefish are found in tropical waters, bays, and inshore areas. They are attracted by light and may leap out of the water toward the light, impaling anyone in the way, especially if the victim happens to be light fishing at night. Puncture wounds may be severe, even fatal if vital organs are penetrated. Wounds require prompt surgical attention.

GIANT GROUPERS OR SEA BASS. These fish may bite or cause injury by their very size (up to 3.6 m in length and weighing up to 360 kg).

BIBLIOGRAPHY

Banner AM: Hazardous marine animals. *In* Tedeschi CG, Eckert WG, Tedeschi LG (eds.): Forensic Medicine. Vol 3, Environmental Hazards. Philadelphia, W.B. Saunders Company, 1977.

Campbell GR: An Illustrated Guide to some Poisonous Plants and Animals of Florida. Englewood, Pineapple Press, 1983.

Clark E: Sharks: Magnificent and misunderstood. National Geographic 160:138, 1981.

Halstead BW: Dangerous Marine Animals That Bite, Sting, Shock and Are Nonedible. Centerville, Maryland, Cornell Maritime Press, 1980.

Halstead BW: Poisonous and Venomous Marine Animals of the World, ed 2. Princeton, The Darwin Press, 1988.

Iverson ES, Skinner RH: How to Cope with Dangerous Sea Life. Miami, Windward Publishing, 1977.

Mabbet H: Death of a skin diver. Australia Skin Diving and Spear-Fishing Digest. December:13, 1954.

Russel FE: Poisonous Marine Animals. London, T.F.H. Publications, Inc. and Academic Press, Inc. (London) Ltd., 1971.

Southcott RV: The neurologic effects of noxious marine creatures. *In* Hornabrook RW (ed.): Topics of Tropical Neurology. Philadelphia, F.A. Davis, 1975.

103.4. LIZARDS

William A. Sodeman, Jr.

There is one genus of poisonous lizards, *Heloderma*, which has two species: *H. suspectum* (Gila monsters) and *H. horridum* (Mexican beaded lizards). They inhabit the desert areas of Mexico and Arizona and are easily recognizable, being heavy and yellow or pink in color.

The actual venom of the Gila monster is as poisonous as that of the rattlesnake, but the mechanism for venom transfer is poorly developed. Submaxillary glands secrete poison that is passed along ducts to grooved teeth, and the victim is envenomated by the chewing action of the powerful jaws. The venom has its effect on the central nervous system, causing paralysis, dyspnea, and convulsions. Treatment is symptomatic and supportive.

Some of the large lizards, turtles, and crocodiles are capable of producing severe injury by biting.

103.5. SNAKES

David A. Warrell

The 4 families of venomous snakes, Atractaspididae, Elapidae, Hydrophiidae, and Viperidae, contain some 500 species, whereas the fifth family, the Colubridae, once considered nonvenomous, contains at least 40 species venomous to humans. Less than 200 species have caused clinically severe envenoming, ending in death or permanent disability (Table 103–7).

DISTRIBUTION OF VENOMOUS SNAKES. Venomous species are widely distributed, except at altitudes above 5000 m, in polar regions, and in most islands of the western Mediterranean, Atlantic, Caribbean, and Pacific, and in Madagascar, New Caledonia, New Zealand, Hawaii, Ireland, Iceland, and Chile. The range of *Vipera berus* extends into the Arctic Circle. Sea snakes exist in the Indian and Pacific Oceans and in estuaries, rivers (New Guinea), and freshwater lakes (Philippines, Cambodia).

CLASSIFICATION. Medically important snakes always possess 1 or more pairs of enlarged teeth in the upper jaw, the fangs, which penetrate the skin of their victim and conduct venom into the tissues along a groove or through a lumen.

Colubridae. The fangs of colubrids are relatively short, are situated at the posterior end of the maxilla, and are capable of only restricted movement. Three species found in Africa, the boomslang (*Dispholidus typus*) and the vine, twig, or bird snake (*Thelotornis kirtlandi* and *T. capensis*), have been responsible for the deaths of a few people who handled them injudiciously. Over the last 55 years, the Japanese yamakagashi (*Rhabdophis tigrinus*) has caused at least 20 cases of coagulopathy with 2 deaths, whereas the related Southeast Asian red-necked keelback (*R. subminiatus*) has been responsible for cases of severe envenoming.

Atractaspididae. The burrowing asps, also known as burrowing or mole vipers or adders, have long front fangs and strike sideways.

Elapidae. This family includes cobras, kraits, mambas, coral snakes, and Australasian terrestrial venomous snakes (sometimes classified with Hydrophiidae). The relatively short anterior fangs of these snakes are permanently erect and capable of little movement (Fig. 103–4). In the ringhals, and 2 African and 2 Asian species of spitting cobras, the venom channel opens forward before it reaches the tip of the fang, allowing venom to be ejected as a fine spray for a distance of several meters into the eyes of an aggressor.

Hydrophiidae. The fangs of sea snakes are short,

TABLE 103–7. Glossary of English and Latin Names of Snakes Mentioned in This Chapter

Latin Name	English Name
Acanthophis	Death adders
Agkistrodon blomhoffi brevicaudus = A. halys	Pallas's viper, mamushi
Atractaspis engaddensis *A. irregularis*	Burrowing asps or mole adders or vipers
A. microlepidota	
Bitis arietans	Puff adder
B. atropos	Berg adder
B. gabonica	Gaboon viper
B. nasicornis	Rhinoceros viper or river Jack
Bothrops atrox	Fer-de-lance, barba amarilla, caissaca
B. jararaca	Jararaca
Bungarus caeruleus	Common Indian krait
B. candidus	Malayan krait
B. fasciatus	Banded krait
Calloselasma (Agkistrodon) rhodostoma	Malayan pit viper
Causus	Night adders
Crotalus adamanteus	Eastern diamondback rattlesnake
C. atrox	Western diamondback rattlesnake
C. durissus durissus	Central American rattlesnake
C. durissus terrificus	South American rattlesnake
C. horridus	Timber rattlesnake
C. scutulatus	Mojave rattlesnake
C. viridis	Western rattlesnake
C. viridis helleri	Southern Pacific rattlesnake
Dendroaspis polylepis	Black mamba
D. viridis	Western green mamba
Dispholidus typus	Boomslang
Echis carinatus *E. ocellatus*	Saw-scaled or carpet viper
Enhydrina schistosa	Beaked sea snake
Hemachatus haemachatus	Ringhals
Malpolon monspessulanus	Montpellier snake
Micruroides *Micrurus*	American coral snakes
Naja kaouthia	Monocellate cobra
N. melanoleuca	Black or forest cobra
N. mossambica	Mozambique cobra
N. naja	Asian cobra
N. nigricollis	Black-necked or spitting cobra
Notechis scutatus	Tiger snake
Ophiophagus hannah	King cobra
Oxyuranus scutellatus	Taipan
Pseudonaja textilis	Eastern brown snake
Rhabdophis subminiatus	Red-necked keelback
R. tigrinus	Japanese keelback or yamakagashi
Thelotornis capensis *Th. kirtlandi*	Bird, twig, or vine snake
Trimeresurus flavoviridis	Japanese habu
T. mucrosquamatus	Chinese habu
Vipera berus	European adder or viper
V. lebetina	Levantine viper
V. palaestinae	Palestine viper
V. russelli	Russell's viper
V. russelli pulchella	Sri Lankan Russell's viper

placed anteriorly, and have limited movement (Fig. 103–5).

Viperidae. The fangs are situated anteriorly, are long, curved, and capable of a wide range of movement (Fig. 103–6). Members of the subfamily Crotalinae—rattlesnakes, moccasins, South American lance-headed vipers, and Asian pit vipers—possess a heat-sensitive pit organ behind the nostril (Fig. 103–7). The Old World

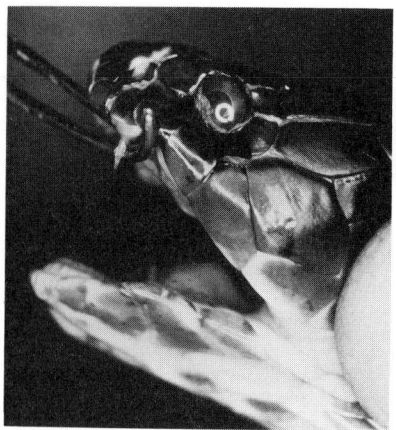
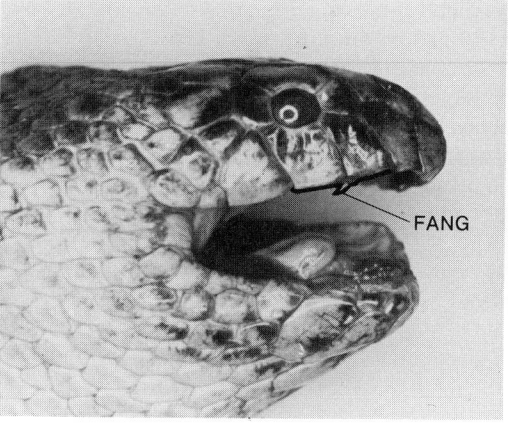
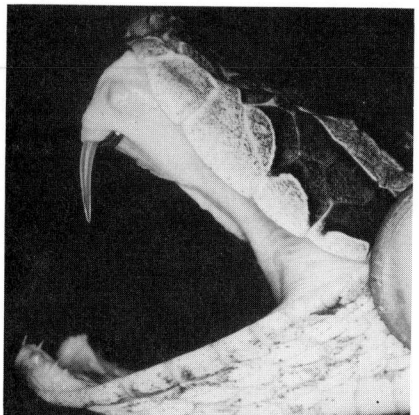

Fig. 103–4   Fig. 103–5   Fig. 103–6

FIGURE 103–4. Short fixed front fang of an elapid snake (Thai spitting cobra *Naja sputatrix*).
FIGURE 103–5. Small fixed front fang of sea snake *(Lapemis hardwicki)*.
FIGURE 103–6. Long hinged front fang of Malayan pit viper *(Calloselasma rhodostoma)*.

vipers, subfamily Viperinae, include the European adder and African and Asian vipers and adders.

MEDICALLY IMPORTANT VENOMOUS SPECIES. Table 103–8 lists some of those species that commonly cause human deaths and serious disability (usually resulting from local necrosis). Some species, such as the night adders (genus *Causus* of Africa) and green pit vipers (genus *Trimeresurus* of Asia), frequently bite, but the effects are usually trivial.

INCIDENCE AND IMPORTANCE OF SNAKEBITE. Snakebite is largely a problem of the rural tropics, and as a result, reliable data for incidence, morbidity, and mortality are scarce. The following examples probably represent underestimates of the true incidence of mortality resulting from snakebite. In India, the reported annual mortality has exceeded 20,000 during the last 100 years, and in Maharashtra State alone, there are more than 1000 deaths each year. In Myanmar (Burma), where Russell's viper is the most important species, snake bite has been the fifth most common

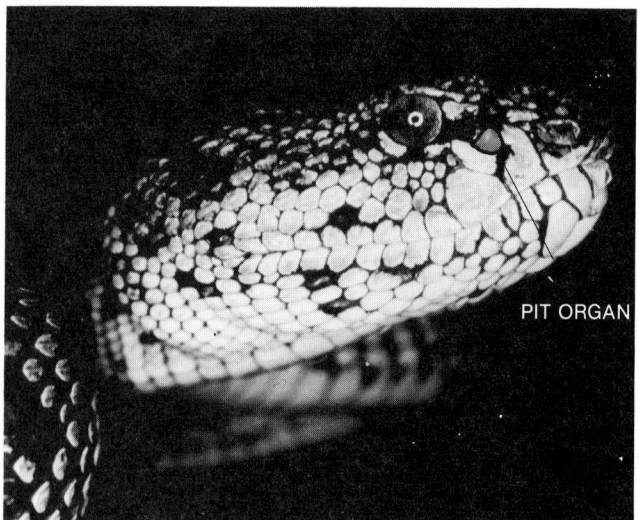

FIGURE 103–7. Heat-sensitive pit organ of mangrove pit viper *(Trimeresurus purpureomaculatus)*.

cause of death and is currently responsible for more than 1000 deaths each year (approximately 3.3/100,000 population). In Sri Lanka, the annual death rate exceeds 800 (6/100,000 population). In parts of West Africa (northeastern Nigeria, central Benin) the incidence of snake bites exceeds 400/100,000 population/year with a mortality of up to 12%. Snakebite is common in parts of Latin America. In Brazil there are an estimated 20,000 bites each year, but with less than 100 reported deaths.

The highest snakebite mortalities have been reported in certain hunter-gatherer tribes. Among the Yanomamo of Amazonian Venezuela, snakebite is responsible for 2% of adult deaths, and among the Waorani of Ecuador, for 5% of all deaths. The Phi Tong Luang of northeastern Thailand, the Hadza of Tanzania, some tribal groups in Papua New Guinea, and the aborigines of central Australia have suffered a high mortality from snakebite.

In the United States, there are approximately 45,000 bites/year, 7000 of which are caused by venomous species, with 9 to 14 deaths/year.

EPIDEMIOLOGY. Most snakebites occur on the lower limbs of farmers, herdsmen, and hunters in the rural tropics. The incidence of bites by a particular species in a particular geographic area depends on the size of human and snake populations, the snake's irritability (its inclination to bite when trodden on or disturbed) and diurnal rhythm, and the extent to which human activities encroach on its chosen habitat. There are few convincing reports of unprovoked aggression by snakes, and, in the tropics at least, snakebite is always the result of an inadvertent tread or touch. Many bites happen when the snake is trodden on in the dark. However, most cases of spitting cobra *(Naja nigricollis)* bite in West Africa and krait bite in Southern Asia *(Bungarus caeruleus, B. candidus)* occur while the victims are asleep in their homes. These commensal species enter houses in search of their prey—rodents, toads, lizards, and other snakes. In developed countries, snakes inspire curiosity and are popular pets, and most bites occur on the hands as a result of the snake's being

TABLE 103–8. Species Responsible for Most Deaths and Morbidity Resulting from Snakebite

Area of Distribution	Latin Name*	English Name
North America	Crotalus adamanteus	Eastern diamondback rattlesnake
	C. atrox	Western diamondback rattlesnake
	C. viridis	Western rattlesnake
Central America	C. durissus durissus	Central American rattlesnake
	Bothrops asper	Terciopelo, caissaca
South America	B. atrox	Fer-de-lance, barba amarilla
	B. jararaca	Jararaca
	C. durissus terrificus	South American rattlesnake
Europe	Vipera berus	Viper, adder
	V. ammodytes	Long-nosed viper
Africa	Echis species	Saw-scaled or carpet viper
	Bitis arietans	Puff adder
	Naja nigricollis, N. mossambica etc.	African spitting cobras
	N. haje	Egyptian cobra
	Dendroaspis species	Mambas
Asia, Middle East	E. carinatus	Saw-scaled or carpet viper
	Vipera lebetina	Levantine viper
	V. palaestinae	Palestine viper
Southeast Asia	Naja naja, N. kaouthia	Asian cobras
	Bungarus caeruleus	Indian krait
	V. russelli	Russell's viper
	E. carinatus	Saw-scaled or carpet viper
	Calloselasma (Agkistrodon) rhodostoma	Malayan pit viper
	Trimeresurus species	Green pit vipers
Far East	N. naja	Asian cobra
	Trimeresurus flavoviridis	Habu
	T. mucrosquamatus	Chinese habu
Australasia	Acanthophis antarcticus	Death adder
	Notechis scutatus	Tiger snake
	Oxyuranus scutellatus	Taipan
	Pseudonaja textilis	Eastern brown snake

*Scientific (Latin) names are important because they are used internationally to describe the range of specificity of antivenoms.

picked up. In the United States, 25% of bites result from snakes being attacked or handled. Irritable species that strike readily when disturbed include *E. carinatus,* the Malayan pit viper *(Calloselasma rhodostoma,* formerly known as *Agkistrodon rhodostoma),* and most species of rattlesnake *(Crotalus),* lance-headed vipers *(Bothrops),* and cobras *(Naja),* whereas the giant gaboon *(Bitis gabonica)* and rhinoceros *(B. nasicornis)* vipers and the banded krait *(Bungarus fasciatus)* seem relatively reluctant to bite. Serious bites by back-fanged (colubrid) snakes have been confined to professional and amateur herpetologists who were handling the snakes. Seasonal variation in the incidence of snakebite is attributed to farming activity in relation to rainfall and to the yearly reproductive cycle of the snake. Severe flooding, by flushing out and concentrating the snake population, has given rise to epidemics of snakebite in Colombia, Pakistan, and India. Development of jungle areas for highways and irrigation or hydroelectric schemes have resulted in an increased incidence of snakebite in Brazil and Sri Lanka. On rare occasions, snakebite or injection of snake venom has been used for suicide or murder.

VENOM APPARATUS. The venom glands are surrounded by compressor muscles and are situated behind or below the eye. The venom duct opens within a sheath at the base of the fang, and venom is conducted toward the tip in a partially or completely closed groove or fang canal (Fig. 103–8). Venomous snakes can inject doses of venom lethal to their natural prey at each of up to 10 or more consecutive strikes; the quantity of venom injected is highly variable, with no convincing evidence that it can be adjusted according to the size of the prey or the mood of the snake. The high proportion of bites without envenoming reported for species such as *C. rhodostoma* is more likely to be the result of mechanical inefficiency than to voluntary control by the snake, and the concept of a defensive bite may not be valid. Of a group of 824 patients bitten by venomous species, 53% showed only trivial or no evidence of envenoming. There is no support for the popular belief that snakes are less dangerous after they have eaten. It is most important to emphasize that the snake uses only a fraction of the content of its venom gland at each strike.

VENOM COMPOSITION. Snake venoms may contain 20 or more components, so their effects cannot be interpreted in terms of the activity of a single toxin. Dried venom is more than 90% protein, consisting of a rich variety of enzymes, nonenzymatic polypeptide toxins, and nontoxic proteins. Metals such as zinc are associated with some of the enzymes, such as ecarin, the procoagulant enzyme of *E. carinatus* venom, which activates prothrombin. Carbohydrate is present in glycoproteins, such as the serine protease ancrod (Arvin), the procoagulant of *C. rhodostoma* venom, which cleaves fibrinopeptide A from fibrinogen and has been used to treat thrombotic disorders. Biogenic amines such as histamine and 5-hydroxytryptamine may be partly responsible for the pain of snakebite; they are found in greater quantity and variety in venoms of Viperidae than in those of Elapidae or Hydrophiidae. Many snake venoms contain phospholipases A_2, which are responsible for presynaptic neurotoxic activity, rhabdomyolysis, vascular endothelial damage, and hemolysis. The bright yellow color of some Viperidae venoms is attributable to L-amino acid oxidase, which has a riboflavin prosthetic group. Other venom enzymes include phosphoesterases, monoesterases, diesterases, acetylcholinesterase, proteolytic enzymes, and hyaluronidase. The role of these enzymes in human envenoming is uncertain.

Polypeptide Toxins (Neurotoxins). These low molecular weight proteins are found in elapid, hydrophiid, and several viperid venoms. Postsynaptic (α-) neurotoxins, such as α-bungarotoxin and cobrotoxin, contain 60-62 "short chain" or 67-74 "long chain" amino acids and bind to acetylcholine receptors on the motor end-plate. Presynaptic (β-) neurotoxins, such as β-bungarotoxin, crotoxin, taipoxin, and notexin, are phospholipases A_2 consisting of approximately 120 amino acids; they prevent release of acetylcholine at the neuromuscular junction. Other neurotoxins of doubtful clinical significance

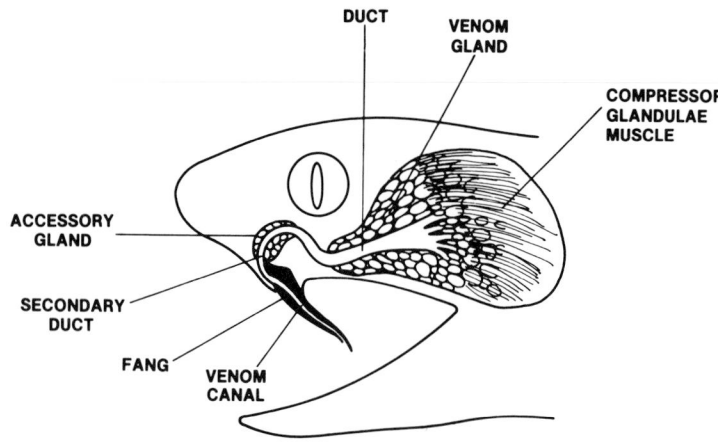

FIGURE 103–8. Venom apparatus of a viperine snake.

interfere with ionic fluxes and stimulate release of ace-tylcholine from nerve endings.

Hemorrhagin activity is found mainly in Viperidae venoms and is responsible for spontaneous hemorrhage by damaging vascular endothelium. Procoagulant venom factors (enzymes) act at various points of the clotting cascade (Fig. 103–9), while fibrinolytic factors may act directly or by activating plasminogen. Defibrination and associated platelet abnormalities result in persistent bleeding from vessels damaged by hemorrhagin, vene-puncture, or other trauma but do not cause spontaneous hemorrhage in the absence of hemorrhagin. Local swell-ing, blistering, and necrosis, prominent features of en-venoming by Viperidae and some cobras, are caused by primary effects of cytotoxic venom components and by the release of endogenous substances that increase cap-illary permeability. Autopharmacologic effects of ven-oms, mainly of Viperidae, include the release and potentiation of bradykinin, histamine, 5-hydroxytrypta-mine, and adenosine triphosphate from platelets and inhibition of angiotensinase. In humans, presynaptic neurotoxins of Hydrophiidae, several Australasian Elap-idae, and a few species of Viperidae (e.g. *Crotalus durissus terrificus* and *Vipera russelli pulchella*) produce systemic rhabdomyolysis. A number of other venoms cause myonecrosis at the site of local injection.

Variation in Venom Composition. The diversity of clinical manifestations of snakebite is explained by the variation of venom composition from species to species. There may be considerable variation also in venom composition within a single species throughout its geo-graphical range, at different seasons of the year, and as a result of aging.

Pharmacology. The toxic polypeptides of Elapidae and Hydrophiidae venoms are relatively small molecules that are absorbed rapidly into the blood stream, whereas the much larger molecules of Viperidae venoms are taken up more slowly through lymphatics. The distri-bution of venoms from the site of inoculation is affected also by their binding to tissues, the production of local thrombosis and vasoconstriction, and the presence of spreading factors such as hyaluronidase. Some venoms, notably of the Viperidae, break down permeability barriers leading to extravasation and edema. Most ven-oms are concentrated and bound in the kidney, and some components are eliminated in the urine, whereas crotaline venoms are selectively bound in the lungs, concentrated in the liver, and excreted in bile.

CLINICAL MANIFESTATIONS. The patient who has been bitten by a snake may present with symptoms resulting from fear, from prehospital treatment, and from effects of the venom itself. A snakebite is a terrifying experience, especially for those who believe that all bites are rapidly fatal. Physiologic manifestations of anxiety, and even frank hysteria, may confuse the clinical picture. Thus, patients who are bitten but not envenomed may feel flushed, dizzy, and breathless, with constriction of the chest, and may notice a thumping pulse, palpitations, sweating, and effects of hyperventi-lation. Such symptoms dominate many accounts of snak-ebites written by the victims and are falsely attributed to neurotoxicity. Misguided prehospital treatment can result in congestion and ischemia of a limb whose circulation is occluded by a tourniquet, bleeding or sensory loss resulting from local incisions, and vomiting and other side effects caused by herbal remedies. Rarely, the terror of snakebite may precipitate angina pectoris, myocardial infarction, or cardiac arrhythmia.

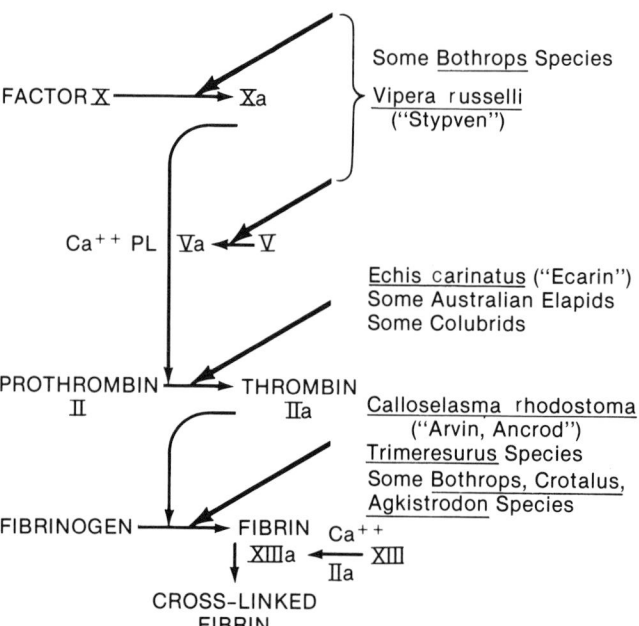

FIGURE 103–9. Sites of action of some snake venom procoagulants on the clotting cascade.

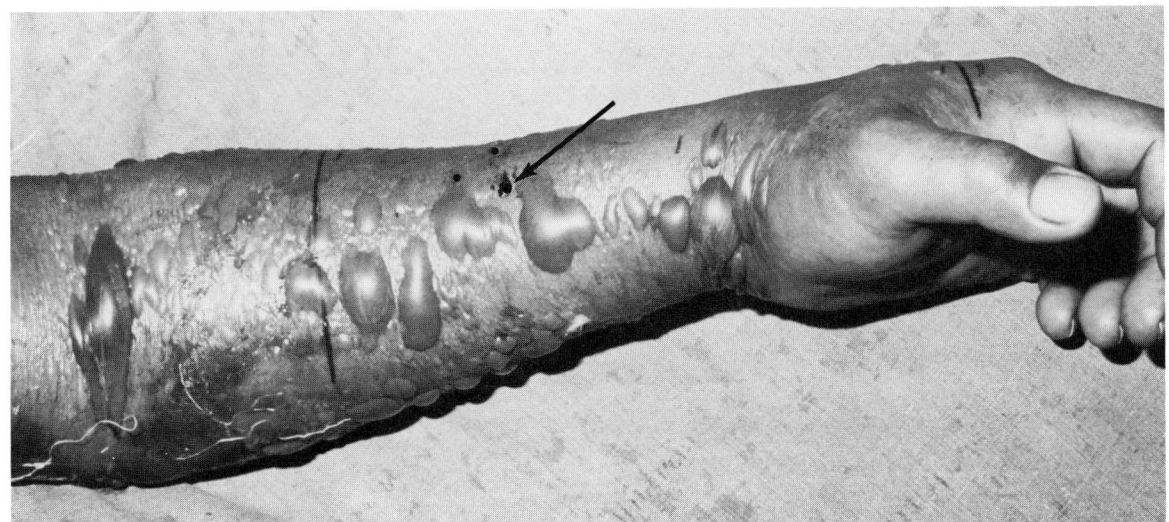

FIGURE 103–10. Intense edema, bruising, and formation of bullae 24 hours after a bite on the forearm *(arrow)* by a Malayan pit viper *(Calloselasma rhodostoma).*

General Symptoms and Signs. The evolution of symptoms and signs of envenoming depends on the nature of the venom, the dose, and the site of injection.

The earliest symptom is pain, which is usually felt immediately. Local swelling may start within minutes, and total defibrination can develop in half an hour *(C. rhodostoma* and *E. carinatus).* Rarely, death may occur as soon as 15 minutes after an elapid (e.g., *N. naja* or *Dendroaspis* species) or viper (e.g., *V. russelli)* bite. Usually, however, death comes hours after an elapid or sea snake bite and days after a viper bite.

Clinical Snakebite

Local Effects. This is characteristic of bites by the Viperidae, including the pit vipers of the subfamily Crotalinae, African spitting cobras (e.g., *N. mossambica, N. nigricollis)* and Asian cobras (e.g., *N. naja* and *N. kaouthia).* Tender swelling spreads from the site of the bite, and there is early tender enlargement of lymph nodes draining the bitten area. Within a few hours, serosanguineous bullae may appear under the epidermis (Fig. 103–10). With elapid bites, blistering is nearly always followed by tissue necrosis, usually superficial, which may extend up the fascial planes of the limb (Fig. 103–11). Bullae caused by Viperidae bites frequently dry up and slough without the development of necrosis. A pale, anesthetic, demarcated area of skin with a characteristic odor of putrefaction signals the appearance of necrosis. This is an effect of the venom, but the necrotic tissue is at risk from secondary infection by bacteria, including anaerobes.

An important result of massive swelling of the bitten limb is loss of circulating volume; a swollen limb can accommodate several liters of blood. The result may be hypotension due to hypovolemia. Envenomating by rattlesnakes *(Crotalus)* produces local pain with swelling that appears within 15 minutes of the bite and may spread rapidly. Bruising along the path of lymphatics, bullae, and local necrosis may develop. Paresthesia of the tongue and lips and an abnormal metallic taste are common early symptoms following bites by western *(C. viridis),* eastern diamondback *(C. adamanteus),* western

diamondback *(C. atrox),* and timber *(C. horridus)* rattlesnakes. Other symptoms include weakness, rigors, sweating, fasciculation, spontaneous bleeding, and neurotoxic effects *(C. adamanteus, C. scutulatus).* Bites by the Mojave rattlesnake *(C. scutulatus)* and *C. durissus terrificus* may produce little or no local swelling but severe systemic signs.

Bleeding and Clotting Disturbances. This combination is characteristic of vipers such as *V. russelli* and *E. carinatus,* pit vipers such as *C. rhodostoma, C. viridis, Trimeresurus* and *Bothrops* species, and some Australian snakes such as the eastern brown snake *(Pseudonaja textilis),* tiger snake *(Notechis scutatus)* and taipan *(Oxyuranus scutellatus).* Spontaneous bleeding is most frequently detected in the gingival sulci (Fig. 103–12). The most dangerous forms of hemorrhage are intracerebral, gastrointestinal, and retroperitoneal. Incoagulable blood is suggested by oozing from venipuncture sites or other sites of recent trauma.

Hypotension and Shock. Early syncope can occur as part of the autopharmacologic syndrome after bites by

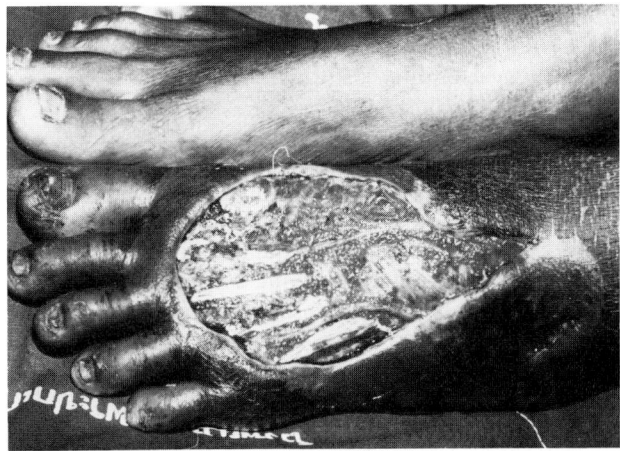

FIGURE 103–11. Necrosis of skin and subcutaneous tissue 1 week after a bite on the dorsum of the foot by a Thai monocellate cobra *(Naja kaouthia).*

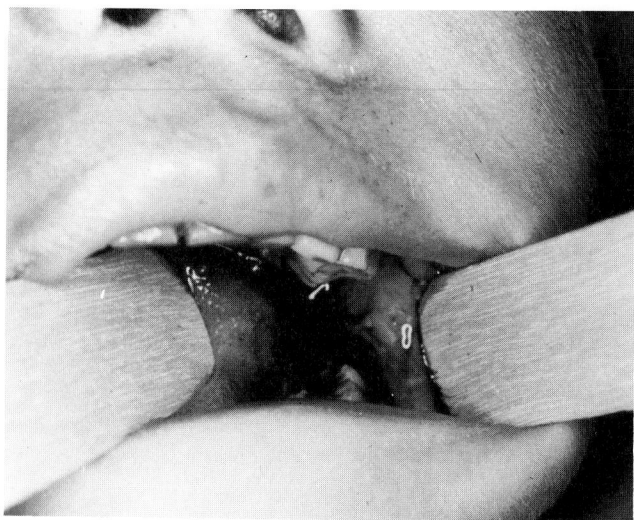

FIGURE 103–12. Extensive spontaneous bleeding from gingival sulci 1 hour after a bite by a Malayan pit viper *(Calloselasma rhodostoma).*

Vipera, Australasian elapids, and *Atractaspis.* More common causes of hypotension are hypovolemia resulting from massive hemorrhage or local or systemic leakage from the vascular compartment (Fig. 103–13), vasodilatation, and a direct action on the myocardium. Acute pituitary adrenal insufficiency may cause shock within the first 10 days of bites by *Vipera russelli* and *Bothrops* species.

Neurotoxicity. This is a feature of envenoming by elapids, Australian snakes, and sea snakes. A few species of Viperidae also produce neurotoxic effects. These include *C. d. terrificus,* Pallas's pit viper *(Agkistrodon blomhoffi brevicaudus), B. atropos,* and *V. russelli* (apparently only in Sri Lanka). Typically, neurotoxic symptoms develop early, but after krait bite there may be a delay of 10 or more hours. Symptoms include vomiting, headache, paresthesia, drowsiness, apathy or euphoria, hyperacusis, diplopia, blurred vision, heaviness of the eyelids, and difficulty in speaking.

The levator palpebrae superioris and extraocular muscles are the most sensitive to neuromuscular blockade, and in some patients, the only feature of envenoming is ptosis and ophthalmoplegia (Fig. 103–14). More serious effects are paralysis of the palate, jaws, tongue, vocal cords, neck muscles, and muscles of deglutition and respiration. The intercostal muscles are affected before the diaphragm and limbs. The patient appears to be curarized. Objective sensory impairment is unusual. It is unlikely that neurotoxic venoms have any effect on the central nervous system in humans. Coma and convulsions could result from hypoxemia caused by respiratory paralysis or circulatory failure. Ptosis and fatigue may be misinterpreted as coma. Neurotoxicity is completely reversible; in some cases there is a rapid response to specific antivenom or anticholinesterase, and in others there is slow, spontaneous resolution. With no specific antivenom, patients supported by artificial ventilation recover sufficient diaphragmatic movement to breathe adequately in 1 to 4 days. The ocular muscles recover in 2 to 4 days, and there is usually full recovery of motor function in 3 to 7 days. Upper airway obstruction by the

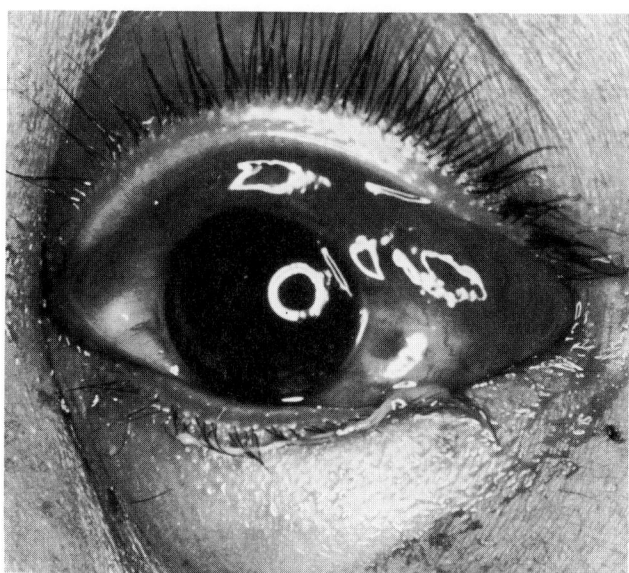

FIGURE 103–13. Clinical evidence of increased systemic vascular permeability: chemosis (edema of the conjunctiva) 48 hours after a bite by Russell's viper *(Vipera russelli siamensis)* in Burma (copyright, D. A. Warrell).

tongue or inhaled vomitus may precipitate respiratory arrest.

Rhabdomyolysis. This must be distinguished from local muscle necrosis caused by cytotoxic venoms. The neurotoxins of sea snakes, Australasian elapids, *C. d. terrificus* and *V. russelli* in Sri Lanka produce systemic rhabdomyolysis. The symptoms are muscle pain and stiffness, with trismus and respiratory muscle paralysis. Myoglobinemia, myoglobinuria, hyperkalemia, and renal failure may result.

Renal Failure. Renal failure can complicate almost any severe case of snakebite, but it is the major cause of death in victims of *V. russelli* and *C. d. terrificus.* Mechanisms of renal damage include ischemia (from hypotension, renal vasoconstriction, or disseminated intravascular coagulation), hemorrhage, direct nephrotoxicity or pigment nephropathy associated with massive

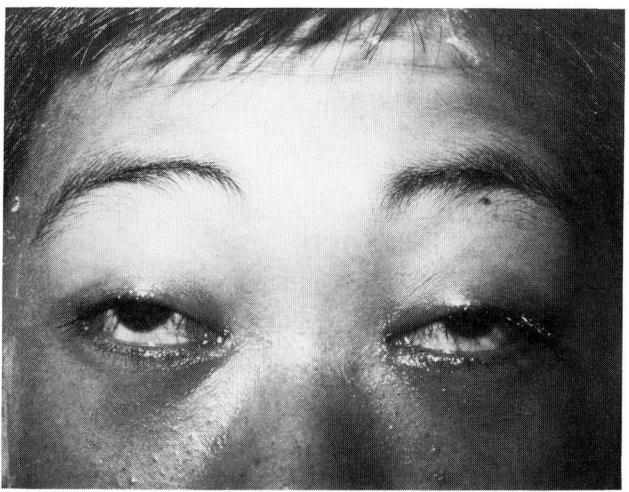

FIGURE 103–14. The earliest clinical evidence of neurotoxic envenoming: bilateral ptosis and external ophthalmoplegia after a bite by a Malayan krait *(Bungarus candidus)* (copyright, D. A. Warrell).

intravascular hemolysis, generalized rhabdomyolysis, and their attendant electrolyte disturbances. Antivenom may cause immune complex nephritis as part of the late reactions occurring 7 days or more after treatment.

Autopharmacologic Effects and Venom Hypersensitivity Reactions. Patients bitten by the Palestine viper *(V. palaestinae)* commonly develop abdominal colic, persistent diarrhea, sweating, hypotension, and angioneurotic edema of the tongue and lips and may collapse within minutes of the bite. Similar symptoms have been described, less commonly, in patients bitten by *V. berus* and other European vipers, the Israeli burrowing viper *(Atractaspis engaddensis)*, and some Australasian snakes, and strongly suggest release by the venom of endogenous amines such as histamine, a known property of many snake venoms. Another possible explanation, in those previously exposed to the same venom, is hypersensitivity. Laboratory workers who habitually handle venoms are prone to become sensitized. They may develop conjunctivitis, rhinitis, asthma, and dermatitis on re-exposure.

Venomous Ophthalmia Caused by Spitting Cobras. The ringhals *(Hemachatus haemachatus)* and spitting cobras *(N. nigricollis)* of Africa, and some populations of the Asian cobra *N. naja* in Thailand, Indochina, Malaysia, Indonesia, and the Philippines, can eject venom in a fine stream from the tips of the fangs for a distance of a few meters. If venom enters the eye, there is intense local pain, leukorrhea, blepharospasm, and palpebral edema. Because most patients make an uneventful recovery, these injuries used to be thought trivial, but slit lamp examination reveals corneal erosions in more than half of the cases. There is the same risk of secondary infection as with other corneal injuries (Fig. 103–15), leading to permanent blindness in some cases. The venom may be absorbed also into the anterior chamber, resulting in anterior uveitis with hypopyon.

PATHOLOGY. Patients who died from predominantly neurotoxic envenomation show no postmortem abnormalities except those attributable to terminal hypoxia. Those who died from the action of venoms with predominant hemorrhagin and procoagulant activity may show extensive hemorrhages in the bitten limb, body cavities, gastrointestinal tract, retroperitoneal tissues, renal tract, and brain. Hemorrhagic infarction of the anterior pituitary may complicate bites by *V. russelli* in Burma and southern India (Fig. 103–16). Sea snake

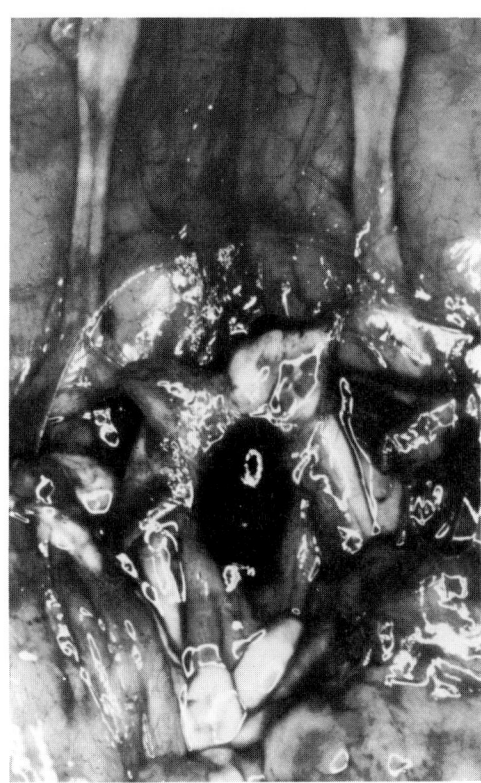

FIGURE 103–16. Hemorrhagic anterior pituitary stump in a patient who died 36 hours after a bite by Russell's viper *(Vipera russelli siamensis)* in Burma.

venom causes scattered and discrete death of skeletal muscle fibers, clogging of the renal tubules with myoglobin, and myoglobinuria. The commonest renal lesion in patients dying with acute renal failure is tubular necrosis. Fibrin thrombi may be found in renal arterioles (Fig. 103–17). A variety of histologic changes have been described in survivors. In some cases these may be attributable to pre-existing renal disease and in others to serum sickness induced by antivenom. In patients dying of an unknown cause, the discovery of fang marks with or without local changes should raise the possibility of snakebite, which can be confirmed by immunodiagnostic and other tests (see Detection of Venoms in Snakebite Victims).

LABORATORY INVESTIGATIONS. The peripheral white blood cell count is raised in patients severely envenomed by many species of snakes. Anemia is the result of bleeding or, much more rarely, hemolysis. Venoms of *Vipera russelli* in India and Sri Lanka and some colubrids cause intravascular hemolysis. Venoms containing procoagulant often produce thrombocytopenia; this is common following bites by *V. russelli, Trimeresurus, Bothrops, C. rhodostoma,* and the Pacific rattlesnake *(Cr. viridis helleri)* but is relatively rare after an *E. carinatus* bite. Important simple tests for venom-induced defibrination are the simple whole blood clotting test and clot quality test. A few milliliters of blood are placed in a clean, dry glass test tube, left undisturbed for 20 minutes, and then tipped to check for clotting. The tube is examined again after 12 hours to assess clot size. Serum potassium is elevated by the generalized

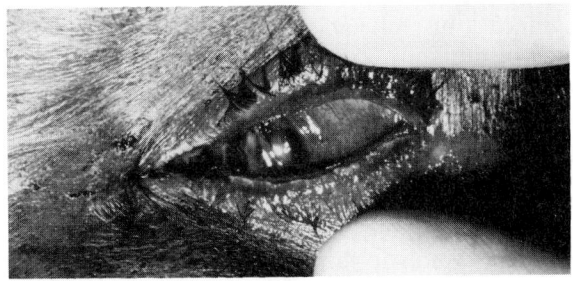

FIGURE 103–15. Severe venom ophthalmia that led to blindness in a patient "spat at" by the cobra *Naja nigricollis* in Nigeria. Failure to treat with a local antimicrobial agent may allow secondary infection of corneal abrasions with these disastrous results.

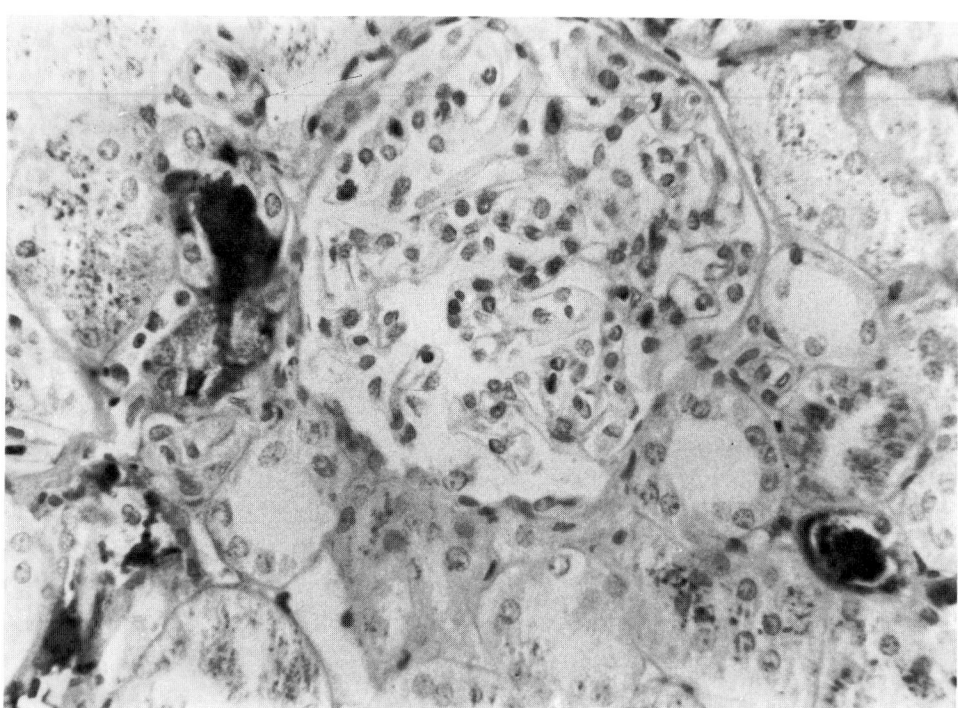

FIGURE 103–17. Kidney of a patient who died 15 hours after being bitten by Russell's viper *(Vipera russelli siamensis)* in Burma. The glomerulus is congested, and there is granular material in the tubules. Arterioles contain fibrin (dark staining). (Anti-human fibrinogen PAP method × 512.) (Courtesy of Dr. Nicholas Francis.)

rhabdomyolysis of sea snake envenoming. Serum enzymes, such as aspartate and alanine aminotransferases and creatine phosphokinase, are mildly elevated in patients with local tissue damage but are grossly raised in victims of sea snake bite. Electrocardiographic changes, such as inverted T waves, raised ST segments, prolonged Q-T$_c$ intervals, and arrhythmias, have been reported in patients bitten by vipers and pit vipers. The urine of snakebite victims commonly contains red and white blood cells and granular casts. Dark urine should be tested for hemoglobin and myoglobin.

DETECTION OF VENOMS IN SNAKEBITE VICTIMS; IMMUNODIAGNOSIS. Specific snake venom antigens have been detected in wound aspirate, blood, urine, cerebrospinal fluid, and other body fluids by a variety of techniques, including immunodiffusion, countercurrent immunoelectrophoresis (CIE), passive hemagglutination, radioimmunoassay, and enzyme immunoassay (EIA). The latter appears to be the simplest and most sensitive technique. The Commonwealth Serum Laboratories (CSL) in Australia have issued venom detection kits based on this principle. In some cases, the EIA and CIE may give results in time to guide clinical management, but their main value is in the investigation of the pathophysiology and epidemiology of snakebite and, for forensic purposes, in confirming the cause of deaths suspected to have been caused by snakebite. Venom antibody is also detectable by EIA and may persist for many years after the bite.

MANAGEMENT OF SNAKEBITE. Snakebite is a rare emergency in most parts of the world, and because its management is thought to require specialized knowledge, many clinicians close their minds to the simple therapeutic principles that could prevent morbidity and mortality. Management starts with first aid by relatives, friends, or fellow workers of the snakebite victim who happen to be present when the bite occurs. Therefore,

first aid principles should be a priority subject for community health education in schools, at clinics, and via the media.

First Aid Treatment. Most snakebite victims are terrified and require reassurance. The bitten limb should be immobilized, if possible, with a splint or sling and the patient quickly moved to the nearest treatment facility. Pain can be treated with oral acetaminophen or intravenous meperidine. Aspirin should not be used, as it may lead to persistent gastric bleeding in patients with incoagulable blood. Local incisions and suction are more likely to introduce infection and cause persistent bleeding than to remove significant amounts of venom from the wound. In one study of viper bites in Jammu, India, 94% of patients who had received incisions developed local infection, compared with none in the group without incisions. Potassium permanganate and ice packs can cause local necrosis. Electric shock treatment is potentially dangerous and of unproven value.

Tourniquets. The value of tourniquets has not been adequately investigated in human patients. A broad, firm (but not tight), constricting band may temporarily delay the spread of viper venoms along lymphatics and superficial veins, but this effect has not been proved to be clinically useful and may lead to congestion and edema of the limb—confusing signs that suggest envenoming where there may be none. A tight (arterial-occlusive) tourniquet is effective in preventing venous return from the occluded limb and delays death in animals given elapid and Australasian snake venoms. However, such tourniquets have also been responsible for gangrenous limbs; peripheral nerve damage; and increased fibrinolytic activity, bleeding, and local effects of venom. Recent studies in restrained monkeys have shown that crepe bandaging and splinting of the injected limb are effective in delaying the spread of snake and spider venoms. The use of a tight crepe bandage (with splint) or arterial tourniquet is justified only in the case of bites by dangerously neurotoxic elapids, sea snakes, and Australasian snakes when the delay in reaching medical care is likely to be more than 30 minutes but less than 2 hours. In these particular circumstances, the tourniquet may delay the development of respiratory paralysis or cardiovascular collapse until medical help is available. The arterial tourniquet must be released for 15 seconds every 30 minutes and should not be applied for more than 2 hours.

Early Complications. Problems that may arise on the way to a medical facility include the following: (1) Vomiting may occur; therefore, patients should lie on their side to avoid aspiration. Persistent vomiting can be treated with chlorpromazine (25 mg for adults, 1 mg/kg for children), by intravenous injection. (2) Anaphylactic shock with angioneurotic edema and diarrhea can be treated with antihistamines, such as chlorpheniramine maleate (10 mg for adults, 0.2 mg/kg for children) by intravenous injection. (3) Respiratory or cardiac arrest should be treated by mouth-to-mouth respiration and external cardiac massage. (4) Airway obstruction due to paralysis of the jaw and tongue should be treated by laying the patient on his or her side, inserting an oropharyngeal airway, and raising the jaw. (5) Intramuscular injections can lead to large hematomas in patients with defibrinated blood; therefore, oral or intravenous routes should be used whenever possible. A pressure pad should be applied to venipuncture sites.

Patients should bring the dead snake to the hospital, provided no risk of further bites is involved. Snakes, even those that appear dead, and severed heads should not be handled but should be carried on a stick or maneuvered into a container.

Treatment by Medically Trained Personnel in Hospital or Dispensary. Because of the uncertainties about the type, quantity, and quality of venom injected and the variable time course for development of signs of envenoming, all victims of snakebite should be hospitalized and observed for at least 24 hours. Frequent observations of the level of consciousness, blood pressure, pulse rate, and respiration should be made. Any ligatures should be released, preferably after starting administration of antivenom (see Antivenom Treatment). Physical examination should include assessment of local swelling, almost invariably present within 15 minutes of significant pit viper envenoming and within 2 hours of viper envenoming but absent in patients bitten by some neurotoxic species (especially kraits, sea snakes, and coral snakes). Tender enlargement of regional lymph nodes draining the bitten area is an early sign of envenoming by Viperidae and Australasian snakes. Spontaneous bleeding is most often detected in the gingival sulci (Fig. 103–12), at venepuncture sites, from partially healed wounds, and from the nose, gastrointestinal tract, and genitourinary tract. Hypotension is an important sign of hypovolemia or cardiotoxicity in patients bitten by vipers, pit vipers, and cobras. Ptosis is the earliest sign of neurotoxic envenoming (Fig. 103–14). Respiratory muscle power should be assessed objectively, e.g., by measuring vital capacity. If a procoagulant venom is suspected, hemostasis should be checked at the bedside by the simple whole blood clotting test.

Antivenom Treatment. The only specific treatment for snake venom poisoning is antivenom, also known as antivenin and antisnakebite serum, which is usually raised in horses. Most commercial antivenoms are now purified immunoglobulins but still carry a risk of serum reactions. Unfortunately, the clinical testing of antivenoms has been neglected, and consequently, the indications, dosage, and assessment of the activity of most antivenoms in patients remain uncertain. The WHO Publication "Progress in the Characterisation of Venoms and Standardisation of Antivenoms" (1981), Chippaux and Goyffon (1983), and various other directories list the antivenoms available worldwide and their range of activity.

Indications. Because of their high cost and the inherent danger of reactions, antivenoms should not be used indiscriminately. Antivenom is indicated if there is severe systemic envenoming evidenced by hypotension or other signs of cardiovascular toxicity, signs of neurotoxicity or generalized myotoxicity, impaired consciousness, spontaneous systemic bleeding, and incoagulable blood. Supporting evidence of severe envenoming is provided by a peripheral leukocytosis of more than 20,000/mm³, electrocardiographic abnormalities, elevated serum enzymes, hemoglobinuria, myoglobinuria, severe anemia or hemoconcentration, uremia, and oliguria. In the absence of systemic envenoming, massive local swelling (involving more than half of the bitten limb) following bites by species known to cause necrosis is an indication for antivenom.

Special Indications. In the case of rattlesnake envenoming, especially by the most dangerous species (*C. atrox, C. adamanteus, C. durissus* subspecies, *C. scutulatus, C. viridis* subspecies, and *C. horridus*), it is recommended that antivenom be given early, before systemic envenoming has become obvious. In this case, the rapid spread of local swelling is considered an indication for antivenom. Similarly, with bites by several species of North American coral snake (genera *Micrurus* and *Micruroides*), antivenom is recommended following definite bites in which there is immediate pain and any other symptom or sign of envenoming. In Australia, the Commonwealth Serum Laboratories (CSL) recommend that antivenom be given for any proved or suspected snakebite if there are tender regional lymph nodes or other evidence of systemic spread of venom, as well as for any bite by an identified highly venomous snake.

Contraindications. There is no absolute contraindication to antivenom, but because of the increased danger of severe reactions, atopic individuals and those known to be hypersensitive to equine serum should be treated only if effects of envenomation are thought to be life-threatening and after pretreatment with epinephrine, hydrocortisone, and antihistamine.

Timing of Antivenom Treatment. Antivenom should be given as soon as indicated, but it is almost never too late. For example, sea snake envenoming has been reversed up to 2 days after the bite, and blood coagulability has been restored in victims of *E. carinatus* bite 10 days or more after the bite.

Administration of Antivenom. The most highly refined commercial antivenoms are now prepared by pepsin digestion, ammonium sulfate precipitation, dialysis,
and ultrafiltration. The expiration date stated on ampules of antivenom may be too rigid if storage has been
at 4C, but opaque solutions should always be rejected,
as precipitation of protein indicates loss of activity and
increased risk of antivenom reactions. Only specific
antivenom, i.e., antivenom whose range of specificity
includes the biting species, should be given. Some antivenoms raised against the venom of 1 or 2 species have
wide paraspecific activity. For example, the Australian
CSL "Tiger-Sea-Snake Antivenom" raised against the
venoms of *Notechis scutatus* and *Enhydrina schistosa*
appears to neutralize at least 12 different sea snake
venoms.

Ideally, antivenom should be diluted in an appropriate
volume of fluid and given by "push" injection over 10
to 15 minutes or by intravenous infusion over 30 minutes. The incidence and severity of reactions are the
same with both techniques, but where equipment and
supervision are available, administration is controlled
more easily by infusion. Epinephrine, 0.5 ml for adults
or 0.01 ml/kg for children of 0.1% solution, must be
ready for inoculation during the infusion. The patient
must be watched carefully while antivenom is being
given and for at least 1 hour afterward. At the first sign
of a reaction, administration of antivenom should be
stopped and epinephrine should be given by subcutaneous injection. In severe reactions, epinephrine may
be given intramuscularly, intravenously, or even by
intracardiac injection if there is cardiac arrest. In most
cases, however, the subcutaneous route is effective and
avoids the danger of inadvertent intravenous injection
that exists with intramuscular administration. Once the
symptoms of the reaction have subsided, antivenom
infusion can be continued slowly if the patient's condition still warrants it. Intravenous chlorpheniramine maleate (10 mg in adults, 0.2 mg/kg in children) can be
given later to prevent recurrent urticaria and to calm
the patient. Corticosteroids are not indicated, except for
the treatment of serum sickness-type reactions.

Antivenom reactions are not predicted reliably by
conjunctival or intradermal tests. In patients known to
be hypersensitive to equine serum, pretreatment with
epinephrine and antihistamine may be partially effective
in preventing reactions. "Rapid desensitization" is not
recommended.

The appropriate initial dose in humans has been
established for only a few antivenoms. Assessment of
antivenom dose will remain a matter of clinical judgment, but guidelines are needed to help judge the range
of doses commonly required by patients. Antivenom
potencies based on animal protection tests may be highly
misleading for calculating the dose required in human
victims. Approximate initial starting doses of a selected
group of antivenoms for bites by some of the most
important species are presented in Table 103–9. *The
dose for children should be the same or greater.*

Response to antivenom may be dramatic. Patients
often feel indefinably better soon after the infusion has
started. In patients with cardiotoxicity, the blood pres-

sure may rise to normal within a few minutes. Dramatic
recovery of consciousness or recovery from respiratory
paralysis in patients with neurotoxic envenomation is
rare but has occasionally been described, e.g., in bite
victims of the Australian and Papuan death adder (genus
Acanthophis). Spontaneous systemic bleeding usually
stops within 15 to 30 minutes of initiating antivenom
therapy in the case of *E. carinatus* and *C. rhodostoma*
bites, and blood clotting is usually restored within 1 to
6 hours if an adequate neutralizing dose of antivenom
has been given. Further antivenom should be given if
severe signs of envenomation persist after 1 to 2 hours
or if blood coagulability is not restored within about 6
hours. Some effects of envenoming, such as nephrotoxicity following Russell's viper bites, generalized rhabdomyolysis, and some types of neurotoxicity, are unlikely to be reversed by antivenom.

Antivenom Reactions. There are 3 types of antivenom
reaction.

Early (anaphylactic) reactions usually develop within
10 to 20 minutes of intravenous injection of antivenom
or within 30 minutes to 3 hours of starting intravenous
infusion of diluted antivenom. Premonitory symptoms
include restlessness, cough, itching of the scalp, nausea,
vomiting, a feeling of heat, or an increase in pulse rate.
Later, there is diffuse and confluent urticaria, generalized pruritus, fever, tachycardia, autonomic manifestations, and, in a few patients, dangerous hypotension,
airflow obstruction, and angioedema. The incidence of
early reactions is greatest when large doses of relatively
unrefined antivenom are given by intravenous injection.
The original assumption that all of these reactions resulted from immediate (IgE-mediated Type I) hypersensitivity to equine serum was not correct. The mechanism
is complement activation by IgG aggregates. Mortality
from antivenom reactions is low if appropriate treatment
is given.

Pyrogenic reactions, which may be nonspecific and
nonimmunologic, may occur within 1 or 2 hours of
antivenom treatment and can precipitate febrile convulsions in children.

Late reactions of the serum sickness type may develop
5 to 10 days after antivenom treatment. A high incidence
of these reactions, related to the dose of antivenom
given, has been reported in North America. Clinical
features include fever, urticaria, subcutaneous and periarticular swellings, polyarthritis, lymphadenopathy,
mononeuritis multiplex and other neurologic symptoms,
and proteinuria.

Supportive Treatment

Neurotoxic Envenoming. Many patients, unable to
swallow their secretions, aspirate, develop upper airway
obstruction,a nd die. Others die of respiratory paralysis.
As in tetanus, elective tracheostomy should be performed at an early stage, before obstruction or respiratory arrest has developed. Because most patients with
neurotoxic envenomation remain fully conscious, insertion of a cuffed tracheostomy tube under a local anesthetic is preferred to endotracheal intubation. If respiratory muscle power is inadequate, ventilation must be
assisted by mouth-to-tube respiration, Ambu-bag, or
respirator. Patients have recovered from respiratory

TABLE 103–9. A Guide to Initial Dosage of Selected Important Antivenoms

Species		Manufacturer, Antivenom	Approximate Initial Dose
Latin Name	*English Name*		
Acanthophis antarcticus	Death adder	CSL,* monospecific	3000–6000 units
Bitis arietans	Puff adder	Behringwerke, SAIMR,† polyspecific	80 ml
Bothrops atrox *B. jararaca*	Lance-headed vipers	South American Institutes, *Bothrops,* polyspecific	40 ml
Bungarus caeruleus	Indian krait	Haffkine, polyspecific	100 ml
Calloselasma (Agkistrodon) rhodostoma	Malayan pit viper	Thai Red Cross (Saovabha), Bangkok, monospecific	100 ml
		Thai Government Pharmaceutical Organization, monospecific	50 ml
		Twyford Pharmaceuticals	10 ml
Crotalus adamanteus	Eastern diamondback rattlesnakes		
C. atrox	Western diamondback rattlesnakes	Wyeth, Crotalidae polyspecific	30–100 ml
C. viridis subspecies	Western rattlesnakes		
Echis carinatus	Saw-scaled or carpet viper	SAIMR, *Echis,* monospecific	20 ml
		Behringwerke, *Bitis-Echis-Naja,* polyspecific	100 ml
Hydrophiidae	Sea snakes	CSL, *Enhydrina schistosa*	1000 units
Naja kaouthia	Monocellate Thai cobra	Thai Red Cross, monospecific	100 ml
N. naja	Indian cobra	Haffkine, Kasauli, polyspecific	100 ml
Notechis scutatus	Tiger snake	CSL, monospecific	3000–6000 units
Pseudonaja textilis	Eastern brown snake		
Trimeresurus albolabris	Green pit viper	Thai Red Cross, monospecific	100 ml
Vipera berus	European adder	Imunoloski Zavod-Zagreb Vipera polyspecific	10 ml
V. palaestinae	Palestine viper	Rogoff Medical Research Institute, Tel Aviv, Palestine viper monospecific	50–80 ml
V. russelli	Russell's viper	Burma Pharmaceutical Industry, monospecific	40 ml
		Haffkine, polyspecific	100 ml

*Commonwealth Serum Laboratories, Australia.
†South African Institute for Medical Research.

paralysis after being manually ventilated by relays of relatives or nurses for up to 30 days and after mechanical ventilation for up to 10 weeks. All effects of neurotoxic envenomation are fully reversible; therefore, artificial ventilation should always be attempted.

Circulatory Collapse. This may be a direct effect of the venom on the heart and vasculature, the result of hypovolemia or autopharmacologic effects of the venom. In all cases, antivenom, followed by plasma expanders, is indicated. Clinical observation of jugular venous pressure or measurement of central venous pressure or pulmonary wedge pressure (via a Swan-Ganz catheter) helps to prevent fluid overload and precipitation of pulmonary edema. If hypotension persists despite restoration of central venous pressure to +10–15 cm, an infusion of dopamine should be started at a dose of 2 µg/kg/minute through the central catheter.

Occlusion of Major Arteries. This usually occurs in tensely swollen limbs and could result from compression in fascial compartments or from high local concentrations of venom procoagulant. It may be difficult to diagnose vascular occlusion in an edematous limb that is cold and has impalpable pulses. Arteriography could be used in patients with no coagulation disturbance, or blood flow could be detected by the Doppler method.

Local Necrosis. Once definite signs of necrosis have appeared, surgical débridement, immediate split-skin grafting, and antibiotic prophylaxis, to include coverage for anaerobic organisms, are necessary. Occasionally, thrombosis of a major vessel or neglected local necrosis may necessitate amputation of a limb. This is usually the result of inadequate initial antivenom treatment,

prolonged application of a tight tourniquet, or inadvisable treatment such as cryotherapy. On rare occasions, increased pressure within tight fascial compartments, e.g., in the digits and anterior tibial compartment, may contribute to ischemic necrosis. In view of the great dangers of decompression by fasciotomy in patients with incoagulable blood, objective evidence of a high compartmental pressure or vascular occlusion should be obtained before surgery is considered. Fasciotomy is rarely, if ever, indicated in snakebite victims.

Renal Failure. Some snakebite victims admitted with oliguria and elevated blood urea nitrogen and creatinine levels are simply hypovolemic. Acute tubular necrosis resulting from hypotension is the most common cause of renal failure in snakebite. Urine output, specific gravity, and sodium concentration should be followed, and the patient should be treated conservatively by strict fluid balance or, if necessary, by peritoneal dialysis or hemodialysis. In patients bitten by sea snakes and the other species whose venoms cause generalized rhabdomyolysis, alkaline diuresis should be initiated with mannitol, sodium bicarbonate, and furosamide to prevent renal damage from myoglobin. Hyperkalemia should be corrected by the usual methods.

Other Drugs. Heparin, antifibrinolytic agents such as epsilon-aminocaproic acid, corticosteroids, antihistamines, and a large range of herbal and other remedies have been advocated for treatment of snakebite. There is no adequate evidence, based on controlled trials, that any of these agents is other than harmful. In particular, heparin has exaggerated bleeding and contributed to the death of snakebite victims.

Anticholinesterases appear to have a variable but sometimes useful effect in patients with neurotoxic envenoming. It is worth giving to any patient with severe neurotoxic envenoming a test dose of edrophonium chloride by intravenous injection (for adults 2 mg followed after 45 seconds by 8 mg if there is no response) as in the Tensilon test for myasthenia gravis. Atropine 0.6 mg should be given first by intravenous injection to block the unpleasant muscarinic effects of edrophonium. The effects should be assessed objectively, and if convincing, neostigmine methylsulfate and atropine should be given at least every 4 hours or by continuous infusion. The dose of neostigmine is 50 to 100 μg/kg every 4 hours. Anticholinesterases have proved most effective in cases of bites by Asian *N. naja,* but there are also reports of benefit after bites by green mamba *(Dendroaspis viridis),* forest cobra *(Naja melanoleuca),* and Malayan and Indian kraits *(Bungarus candidus* and *B. caeruleus).*

Management of Snake Venom Ophthalmia (Eye Injuries Caused by Spitting Cobras). First aid consists of immediate generous irrigation of the affected eye or mucous membrane with water or any other plentiful bland liquid. At the hospital or dispensary, the eye should be examined by fluorescein staining or with slit lamp. Unless the possibility of corneal abrasions can be excluded, topical antimicrobials should be applied and the eye closed with a dressing pad.

PREVENTION OF SNAKEBITE. To reduce the risk of bites, snakes should never be disturbed, attacked, or handled, even if they are said to be harmless species or appear to be dead. In snake-infested areas, boots, socks, and long trousers should be worn for walks in undergrowth or deep sand. A light should always be carried at night. Particularly dangerous activities are collecting firewood; dislodging logs and boulders with the bare hands; pushing sticks into burrows, holes, or crevices; and climbing rocks and trees covered with dense foliage. Unlit paths and roads are especially dangerous after heavy rains.

It is pointless and undesirable to attempt to exterminate of dangerous species of snakes.

BIBLIOGRAPHY

Bhat RN: Viperine snake bite poisoning in Jammu. J Indian Med Assoc 63:383, 1974.
Bücherl W, Buckley EE, Deulofeu V (eds.): Venomous Animals and Their Venoms, Volumes I and II. New York, Academic Press, 1971.
Campbell CH: Venomous snake bite in Papua and its treatment with tracheotomy, artificial respiration and antivenene. Trans R Soc Trop Med Hyg 58:263, 1964.
Efrati P, Reif L: Clinical and pathological observations on sixty-five cases of viper bite in Israel. Am J Trop Med Hyg 2:1085, 1953.
Gans C, Gans KA (eds.): Biology of the Reptilia. Vol. 8. London, Academic Press, 1978.
Ho M, Warrell MJ, Warrell DA, et al.: A critical reappraisal of the use of ELISA in the study of snake bite. Toxicon 24:211–221, 1986.
Lee CY: Snake Venoms. Handbook of Experimental Pharmacology. Vol. 52. New York, Springer-Verlag, 1979.
Malasit P, Warrell DA, Chanthavanich P, et al.: Prediction, prevention and mechanism of early (anaphylactic) antivenom reactions in victims of snake bites. Br Med J 292:17–20, 1986.
Myint-Lwin, Warrell DA, Phillips RE, et al.: Bites by Russell's viper *(Vipera russelli siamensis)* in Burma: Haemostatic, vascular and renal disturbances and response to treatment. Lancet 2:1259–1264, 1985.
Phillips RE, Theakston RDG, Warrell DA, et al.: Paralysis, rhabdomyolysis and haemolysis caused by bites of Russell's viper *(Vipera russelli pulchella)* in Sri Lanka: Failure of Indian (Haffkine) antivenom. Q J Med 68:691–715, 1988.
Reid HA, Thean PC, Chan KE, et al.: Clinical effects of bites by Malayan viper *(Ancistrodon rhodostoma).* Lancet 1:617, 1963.
Sutherland SK: Australian animal toxins. The creatures, their toxins and care of the poisoned patient. Melbourne, Oxford University Press, 1983.
Tun-Pe, Phillips RE, Warrell DA, et al.: Acute and chronic pituitary failure resembling Sheehan's syndrome following bites by Russell's viper in Burma. Lancet 2:763–767, 1987.
Warrell DA, Davidson NM, Greenwood BM, et al.: Poisoning by bites of the saw-scaled or carpet viper *(Echis carinatus)* in Nigeria. Q J Med 46:33, 1977.
Warrell DA, Greenwood BM, Davidson NM, et al.: Necrosis, haemorrhage and complement depletion following bites by the spitting cobra *(Naja nigricollis).* Q J Med 45:1, 1976.
Warrell DA, Looareesuwan S, Theakston RDG, et al.: Randomized comparative trial of three monospecific antivenoms for bites by the Malayan pit viper *(Calloselasma rhodostoma)* in southern Thailand: Clinical and laboratory correlations. Am J Trop Med Hyg 35:1235–1247, 1986.
Watt G, Theakston RDG, Hayes CG, et al.: Positive response to edrophonium in patients with neurotoxic envenoming by cobras *(Naja naja philippinensis).* A placebo-controlled study. N Engl J Med 315:1444–1448, 1986.
World Health Organization: Progress in the Characterisation of Venoms and Standardisation of Antivenoms. Geneva, World Health Organization, 1981, WHO Offset Publication No. 58.

103.6.   BATS

William A. Sodeman, Jr.

Bats are of medical importance because they transmit disease to humans and in some cases are direct agents of injury. In addition, bat roosts provide an environment highly suited to the transmission of some fungal diseases to humans. The role of bats in the direct transmission of diseases to humans has been characterized best for the viral infections, rabies, and Venezuelan equine encephalomyelitis. Many other viral, bacterial, fungal, and parasitic organisms have been described as associated with bats (Table 103–10) but the human risk is not well characterized. Vampire bats cause direct injury during feeding. Secondary infections or parasitization of these open lesions by fly larvae, particularly screwworm, can be serious health problems at times. *Histoplasma capsulatum* often contaminates guano deposits and has caused human infection. Several other fungi are associated with bats, but transmission to humans has not been established.

Almost all of the direct transmission and injury related to bats is in association with the New World vampire bats. The three species, *Desmodus rotundus* (Geoffroy), *Diphylla ecaudata* Spix, and *Diaemus youngi* (Jentinck) have a wide distribution in Central and South America. These bats have a great economic impact as a result of injury to, or transmission of, infection to livestock.

Vampire bats feed primarily on blood. These bats will prey on mammals, birds, and reptiles. Domesticated animals are the preferred target. The incisor and canine

TABLE 103–10. Viruses, Bacteria, Fungi, and Parasites Associated with Bats

Organism	Location
VEE	Mexico, Guatemala, Ecuador, Panama, USA, Colombia
Rabies	USA, Mexico, Colombia, Venezuela, Guyana, Brazil, Peru, Bolivia, El Salvador, Trinidad, Canada, Guatemala, Panama, Argentina, Germany, Turkey, Yugoslavia, India, Thailand, South Africa
Yellow Fever	Ethiopia
Rio Bravo virus	USA, Mexico, Trinidad, Guatemala
Tamana Bat virus	Trinidad
St. Louis encephalitis	USA, Guatemala
Tacaribe virus	Trinidad, Guatemala
Nepuyo virus	Honduras, Trinidad
Catu virus	Brazil
Bimiti virus	Trinidad
Guama virus	Trinidad
Japanese encephalitis virus	Japan
Leptospira	Brazil, Trinidad
Brucella	Brazil
Histoplasma capsulatum	Panama, Mexico, Colombia, Trinidad, USA
Scopulariopsis	Mexico, Colombia
Trypanosoma evansi	Mexico, Central and South America

teeth are modified to permit painless incision. The bat laps blood with its tongue. A plasminogen activator, Desmokinase, has been isolated from *Desmodus,* and a similar substance has been demonstrated in *Diaemus.* Saliva flows down a groove on the dorsal surface of the tongue, and blood returns up paired ventral grooves. The anticoagulant and the mechanical licking combine to maintain blood flow. Bats are nocturnal feeders.

RABIES. Most bat rabies in humans is transmitted by the vampire bats, but bat rabies does occur in many other genera of bats. There are occasional reports of transmission to humans by frugivorous or insectivorous bats, but these are rare. When this does occur the bats appear to be driven to attack by furious rabies. Rabies virus seems to undergo compartmentalization in bats. The strain associated with vampire bats produces paralytic rather than furious rabies.

Bats infected with rabies generally develop paralytic disease. Death is a result of inanition because of the paralysis. It is possible some bats survive, but a healthy carrier state does not seem to occur. The virus is transmitted in saliva. Several cases of apparent infection of humans exposed to aerosolized saliva, but not to bites, have been reported.

Bat rabies in humans has been reported from many countries in all continents except Australia (Table 103–10). Immunization against rabies offers the best protection. Sleeping in bat-proof lodgings affords protection also. Environmental control to eliminate bat roosts is difficult to implement. Bat rabies in livestock causes considerable economic loss in the tropics. The disease is called derriengue or limping illness, emphasizing its paralytic nature. Treatment of cattle with controlled doses of warfarin will cause death of a feeding vampire bat from hemorrhage.

VENEZUELAN EQUINE ENCEPHALOMYELITIS (VEE). Epidemic VEE in horses has been associated with the presence of virus-infected vampire bats. Bats may be responsible for mechanical transmission of the virus under such circumstances, but this would be a minor route of dissemination.

OTHER VIRUSES. Many other viruses have been shown to occur naturally in bats: yellow fever virus, Montana myotis leukoencephalitis virus, Rio Bravo virus, Tamana bat virus, Nepuyo, St. Louis encephalitis virus, Catu virus, Tacaribe virus, Mount Elgan virus, and Entebbe virus. The role of bats in the natural history and transmission of these viruses is not clear.

BACTERIAL INFECTIONS. *Leptospira* and *Brucella* have both been reported to occur naturally in bats. *Leptospira* infected bats are found in Asia and Europe as well as the Americas. *Brucella* infection has been found in vampire bats in Brazil. There is no evidence yet for transmission from bats to humans.

HISTOPLASMOSIS. Bat guano provides a rich medium for the growth of *Histoplasma capsulatum.* The environment in the bat roost fosters this growth. Humans exposed to dried guano have suffered massive infection and death by inhalation.

OTHER FUNGI. Many other fungi have been found in association with bat roosts, including *Candida* and *Scopulariopsis,* which can infect humans. The involvement of bats seems limited to the provision of a rich environment in the roost to foster the growth of these organisms.

PARASITES. *Trypanosoma evansi,* the causative agent of surra in domestic animals, has been demonstrated in vampire bats. These bats can mechanically transmit the trypanosome from host to host. *Trypanosoma cruzi* has been reported also, but evidence for transmission to humans is lacking.

BIBLIOGRAPHY

Baer GM (ed.): The Natural History of Rabies. Academic Press, New York, 1975.
Crespo RF, et al.: Intramuscular inoculation of cattle with warfarin; a new technique for control of vampire bats. Bull Pan Am Health Organ 13:147, 1979.
Greenhall AM, Schmidt U (eds.): Natural History of Vampire Bats. Boca Raton, CRC Press, 1988.
Meredith CD, Standing E: Lagos bat virus in South Africa. Lancet 1:832, 1981.
Price JL: Serological evidence of infection of Tacaribe virus and arboviruses in Trinidadian bats. Am J Trop Med Hyg 27:162–167, 1978.

104. PENTASTOMIASIS

Joseph J. Drabick

DEFINITION. Pentastomiasis is a parasitic zoonosis of humans caused by pentastomes, members of an unusual, exclusively parasitic phylum—Pentastomida—with characteristics of both annelids and arthropods. Synonymous terms are tongue worm infection, porocephalosis, and linguatuliasis.

ETIOLOGY. Adult pentastomes generally parasitize the respiratory tracts of reptiles or carnivorous mammals in whom they are well tolerated. Usual intermediate hosts are herbivorous mammals, but many classes of animals have been infected depending on the infecting pentastome. Upon infection humans can act as an intermediate host or a temporary definitive host. The disease was first described by Pruner in 1847, making it one of the earliest described parasitic zoonoses.

Classification. The phylum is old; it is speculated that pentastomes probably parasitized carnivorous dinosaurs in mesozoic times. The phylum Pentastomida comprises 2 orders: Porocephalida and Cephalobaenida, the latter being more primitive. Ninety-nine percent of human infection is caused by 2 species within the first order: *Armillifer armillatus* and *Linguatula serrata*. Infection has been ascribed anecdotally to *Armillifer moniliformis*, *Armillifer grandis*, *Leiperia cincinnalais*, and *Raillietiella hemidactyli*. Only the latter is a member of the order Cephalobaenida.

Morphology. Pentastomes range from a few millimeters to more than 15 cm in length, dependent upon the species. The sexes are separate; the males are much smaller than the females. They tend to be colorless and transparent and possess 2 pairs of hooks on either side of a projection that bears the true mouth. Because of this arrangement, the phylum was misnamed pentastome (5-mouthed). External pseudoannulation can give a corkscrew or string-of-beads appearance in some species (Fig. 104–3). Others (Linguatulidae) are flattened and resemble tongues. Superficially, adults resemble helminths and are frequently mistaken for them; however, the first larval stage superficially resembles a mite. In the past it was felt pentastomes may be degenerate arthropods of the mite line (Acarina).

EPIDEMIOLOGY

Life Cycle. Adult parasites exist in the respiratory tract of the definitine host, where they attach themselves by means of their hooks and suck epithelial cells, blood, lymph, and mucus into their digestive tract (Figs. 104–1 and 2). After internal fertilization, the embryonated eggs pass into the environment in nasal discharge, saliva, and feces where the eggs are well adapted to an aqueous environment; hence, water as well as wet vegetation may be the sources of infection for the intermediate host. Upon ingestion, the first stage larva hatches and tunnels through the tissues of the host until it finally encysts. After a series of molts, the third-stage larva may excyst and wander freely through the peritoneal cavity of the intermediate host. With ingestion of the tissues of the intermediate host by the carnivorous definitive host, the third stage larvae migrate up the esophagus to the lungs and/or nasopharynx. After several more molts they mature, mate, and lay eggs. Both encysted and migrating third-stage larvae are infectious for the definitive host.

Distribution. Pentastomes are cosmopolitan with a concentration in tropical and subtropical areas. Most cases of pentastomiasis have been reported from equatorial Africa, the Middle East, and Southeast Asia. Sporadic cases have been noted in the Americas and Southeastern Europe. Eating habits and lifestyles are the primary factors in determining the rates and severity of infection.

PATHOLOGY AND PATHOGENESIS. In humans there is a minimal to moderate immune response to the parasite. Most encysted larvae die eventually and leave fibrotic nodules that may calcify, appearing as radiopaque densities on radiographs. Lesions are found most commonly in the liver (Fig. 104–4), but can also involve the intestinal wall, mesentery, peritoneum, and lung. Eosinophilia is not a feature of pentastomiasis.

CLINICAL MANIFESTATIONS. An individual becomes a secondary host for *A. armillatus* by ingesting eggs in contaminated food or drink or by intimate contact with the definitive host reptile in the preparation of food or the harvesting of skins (Fig. 104–1). Likewise, an individual can be infected as a secondary host by *L. serrata* by exposure to canine nasal secretions or feces containing eggs (Fig. 104–2). Humans are highly tolerant of this form of pentastomiasis. The vast majority of cases are asymptomatic, manifested only as an incidental finding at autopsy or radiologic examination (Fig. 104–3). Problems can arise when the encysted larvae enlarge during molting, causing pressure on vital structures or when migrating larvae perforate organs. Hypersensitivity reactions probably occur also. Anecdotal cases of pneumonitis, atelectasis, intestinal obstruction, bile duct blockage, and pericarditis have been reported. Eye involvement has been reported, including some cases in the southern United States. Acute unilateral glaucoma as a complication has been described.

Halzoun. The other form of pentastomiasis is found in the Middle East and is caused by ingested third-stage larvae found in the raw liver or lymph nodes of sheep or goats. In this instance, humans are infected as temporary definitive hosts. The infection is called Halzoun and occurs when such foods are consumed. In Sudan the syndrome is called Marrara after the dish that causes it. The syndrome is characterized as an acute, self-limited nasopharyngitis associated with coughing, sneezing, dysphagia, hoarseness, and facial edema. Symptoms usually last 7 to 10 days, resolving spontaneously, but airway obstruction and pyogenic complications can occur. Third-stage larvae can be demonstrated in nasal discharge, sputum, and vomitus and are described as small living worms 5 to 10 mm in length. In extremely rare case reports, infection with adults in the nasopharynx has been described.

Subcutaneous Lesions. Cases of subcutaneous human infection with *R. hemidactyli*, called creeping disease, has been observed in Southeast Asia among tribes who swallow small live lizards as a folk remedy.

DIAGNOSIS AND TREATMENT. The diagnosis of pentastomiasis is usually made by demonstrating the presence of the parasite in tissues at autopsy, biopsy, or surgery (Figs. 104–3 and 4). The typical radiographic lesion is a C-shaped or "cashew nut" opacity less than 1 cm in diameter with lesions predominantly in the liver and hili of the lungs. A serologic test for *Armillifer* has been developed in France, but its role in diagnosis is unclear.

Treatment of larval pentastomiasis is unnecessary except in rare instances in which symptoms arise owing

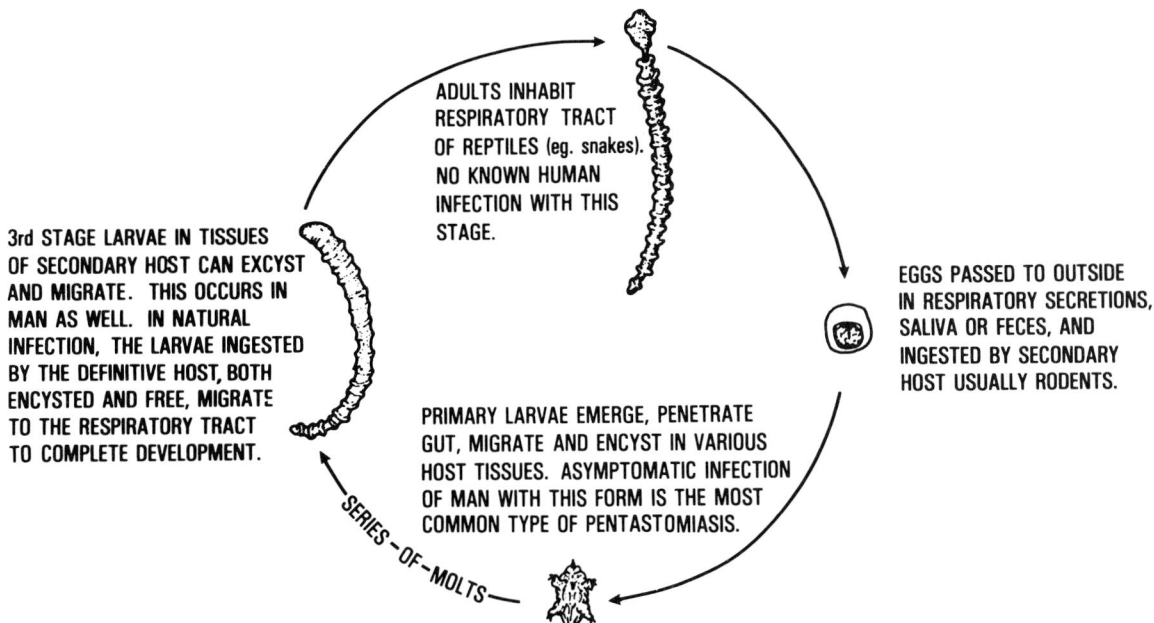

ADULTS INHABIT
RESPIRATORY TRACT
OF REPTILES (eg. snakes).
NO KNOWN HUMAN
INFECTION WITH THIS
STAGE.

EGGS PASSED TO OUTSIDE
IN RESPIRATORY SECRETIONS,
SALIVA OR FECES, AND
INGESTED BY SECONDARY
HOST USUALLY RODENTS.

3rd STAGE LARVAE IN TISSUES
OF SECONDARY HOST CAN EXCYST
AND MIGRATE. THIS OCCURS IN
MAN AS WELL. IN NATURAL
INFECTION, THE LARVAE INGESTED
BY THE DEFINITIVE HOST, BOTH
ENCYSTED AND FREE, MIGRATE
TO THE RESPIRATORY TRACT
TO COMPLETE DEVELOPMENT.

PRIMARY LARVAE EMERGE, PENETRATE
GUT, MIGRATE AND ENCYST IN VARIOUS
HOST TISSUES. ASYMPTOMATIC INFECTION
OF MAN WITH THIS FORM IS THE MOST
COMMON TYPE OF PENTASTOMIASIS.

SERIES–OF–MOLTS

FIGURE 104–1. Life cycle of *Armillifer*. (From Drabick JJ: Rev Infect Dis 9:1087, 1987. Reprinted by permission.)

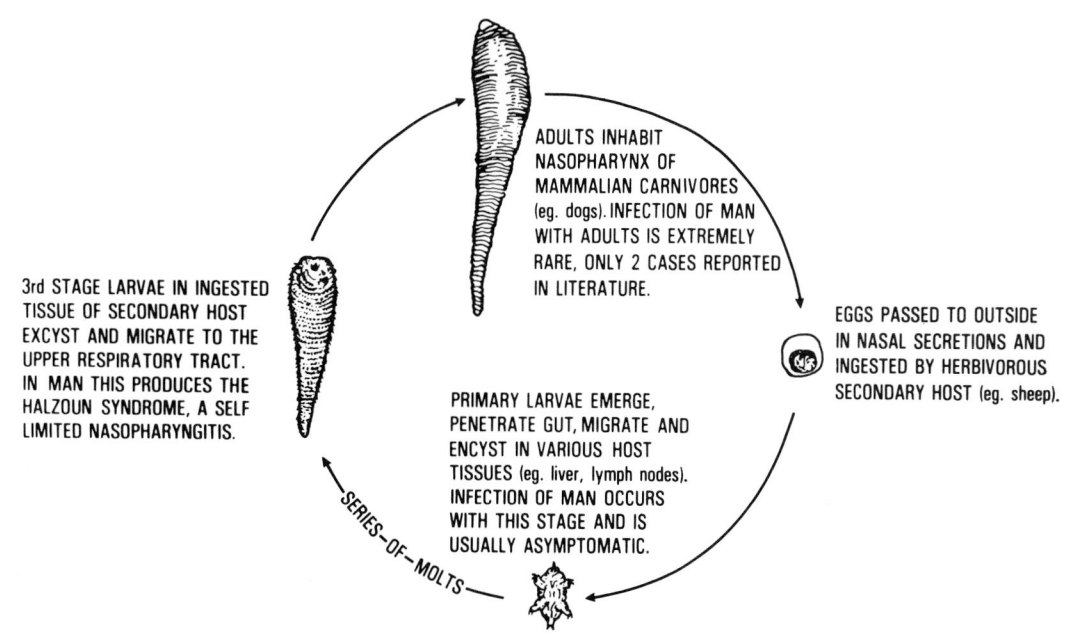

ADULTS INHABIT
NASOPHARYNX OF
MAMMALIAN CARNIVORES
(eg. dogs). INFECTION OF MAN
WITH ADULTS IS EXTREMELY
RARE, ONLY 2 CASES REPORTED
IN LITERATURE.

EGGS PASSED TO OUTSIDE
IN NASAL SECRETIONS AND
INGESTED BY HERBIVOROUS
SECONDARY HOST (eg. sheep).

3rd STAGE LARVAE IN INGESTED
TISSUE OF SECONDARY HOST
EXCYST AND MIGRATE TO THE
UPPER RESPIRATORY TRACT.
IN MAN THIS PRODUCES THE
HALZOUN SYNDROME, A SELF
LIMITED NASOPHARYNGITIS.

PRIMARY LARVAE EMERGE,
PENETRATE GUT, MIGRATE AND
ENCYST IN VARIOUS HOST
TISSUES (eg. liver, lymph nodes).
INFECTION OF MAN OCCURS
WITH THIS STAGE AND IS
USUALLY ASYMPTOMATIC.

SERIES–OF–MOLTS

FIGURE 104–2. Life cycle of *Linguatula*. (From Drabick JJ: Rev Infect Dis 9:1087, 1987. Reprinted by permission.)

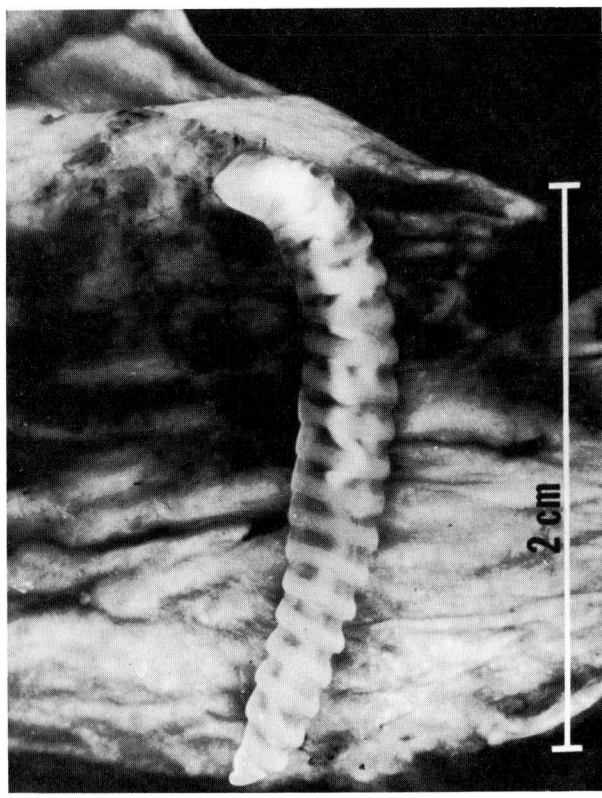

FIGURE 104–3. *Armillifer armillatus* excysted third-stage larva. This specimen had emerged from its cyst and was found crawling over the abdominal surface of the diaphragm of a Zairean man necropsied 18 hours after an accidental death. Several other specimens were found free and motile in the abdominal cavity. (Courtesy of Armed Forces Institute of Pathology, Photograph Neg. No. 72-4558.)

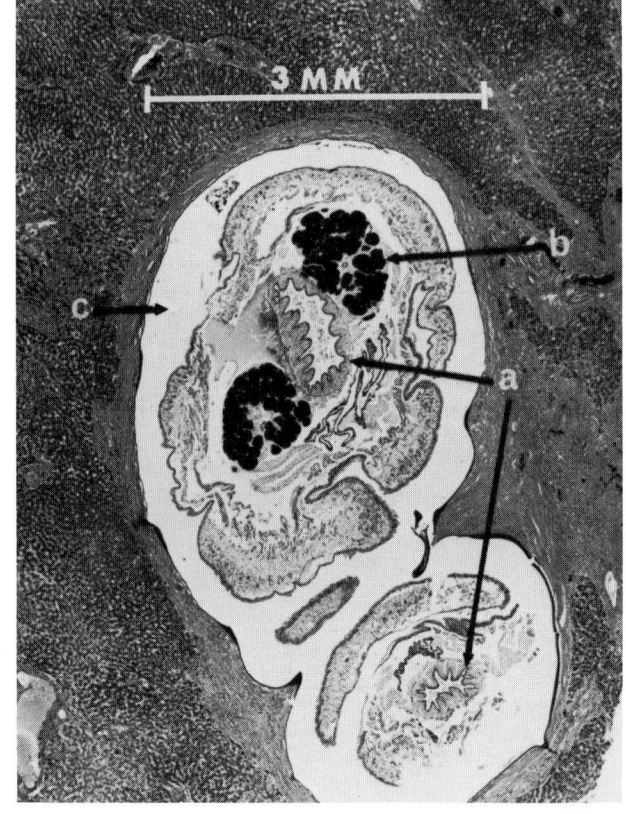

FIGURE 104–4. *Armillifer armillatus* larval pentastomid cyst in human liver. This viable larva can excyst and migrate. The intestine *(a)* and acidophilic glands *(b)* are apparent. There is a space *(c)* between the current cuticle and that of a former molt. The host reaction is predominantly fibrosis. (Courtesy of Armed Forces Institute of Pathology, Photograph Neg. No. 75-2703.)

to pressure effects, in which case surgery is indicated for removal. Halzoun is usually self-limited, but airway protection may be required in cases with severe laryngeal edema. Antibiotic and surgical therapy may be required for secondary pyogenic complications.

PREVENTION. As with so many tropical diseases, control of pentastomiasis would be best realized with more effective water and food sanitation. As in the case of other parasitic infections, the eating of uncooked exotic meats can cause infection.

BIBLIOGRAPHY

Drabick JJ: Pentastomiasis. Rev Infect Dis 9:1087–1094, 1987.
Haugerund RE: Human Pentastomiasis. Tidsskr Nor Laegeforen 108:28–31, 1988.
Lang Y, Garzozi H, Epstein Z, et al.: Intraocular pentastomiasis causing unilateral glaucoma. Br J Ophthalmol 71:391–395, 1987.
Riley J: The biology of Pentastomids. Adv Parasitol 25:45–128, 1986.
Self JT, Kuntz RE: Host-parasite relations in some Pentastomida. J Parasitol 53:202–206, 1967.

105. INJURIOUS ARTHROPODS

Robert A. Wirtz
and Abdu F. Azad

Contact with arthropods and their products can result in adverse reactions in humans that range from mild seasonal annoyance to anaphylactic shock and death. The severity of these reactions is dependent on the way in which the arthropod or its products is encountered, the type and composition of the allergen, and the prior history of exposure.

The most common modes of exposure are through arthropod bites or stings (envenomization) and direct contact, ingestion, or inhalation of venoms or allergens. Stinging arthropods (e.g., wasps, bees, ants, scorpions) actively inject venom mixtures through specialized structures. Biting arthropods (e.g., spiders, flies, bugs, mites, ticks) inject digestive or salivary secretions and venoms through piercing mouthparts or modified appendages (e.g., fangs). Biting arthropods can be grouped according to duration of host contact, i.e., transient versus prolonged (Fig. 105–1). Passive envenomation is the release of venom in or onto the surface of the skin; this includes defensive irritants and vesicants (e.g., blister beetles, millipedes, cockroaches) and venom-containing hollow spines (e.g., caterpillars). Some arthropods may forcibly release toxins from some distance (millimeters to over 1 meter). Potent allergens and toxic secretory products, such as defensive secretions, dried feces (frass), wing scales, other exoskeleton fragments, and whole arthropods (e.g., mites, thrips, aphids), are often ingested or inhaled.

Venoms and salivary secretions are also capable of eliciting an allergic reaction. These are usually mild; however, in sensitized individuals they can be life-threatening. Allergic reactions to stings cause more deaths than any other type of arthropod injury, and

hypersensitive individuals often die before supportive therapy can be given.

In general, important determinants of the envenomation effect of arthropod bites relate to the arthropod, its toxin, and the human host. The species of arthropod, the effectiveness of toxin delivery, and the number of arthropods making the attack will all influence the medical outcome. Likewise, the volume and nature of the toxin will be important. Finally, the status of the victim with regard to age, size, weight, and the nature of the immune response will be critical. Arthropod injury is one of the most common causes of lesions of the human integument. Although winter brings some relief from flying insects in temperate climates, the ectoparasites persist. In the tropics, the densities of biting insects can reach remarkable proportions. In developed countries, the widespread use of insecticides has reduced insect populations.

We have deliberately avoided the area of identification of arthropods. Biting and envenoming arthropods from many orders and families are commonly involved in producing similar dermatologic conditions. Different species within the same genus, however, can produce remarkably different effects. Furthermore, a given arthropod may produce different symptoms in different people.

Delusory parasitosis is an emotional disorder in which the individual has an unwarranted belief that he or she is infested with live organisms, usually mites or other small arthropods. Excoriation and gouging may be seen as a result of desperate scratching and cleansing. This disease can become intractable and induce a consuming anxiety in the patient and family. Victims can be well educated and appear rational and sensible about other matters not pertaining to their obsession. Delusory parasitosis has occasionally been misdiagnosed owing to the small size of many arthropods. An adequate search for parasites on the patient, pets, and in the immediate work and home environment should be made before symptoms are labeled as delusional. "Sick building syndrome" and "cable mite dermatitis" exemplify cases in which symptoms initially attributed to arthropod infestations or diagnosed as psychoneurotic were later associated with physical irritants found in the work or home environment.

Entomophobia (acarophobia), often used in referring to delusory parasitosis, is an unfounded fear of insects. Greater understanding of—and familiarity with—insects generally lessens this fear.

105.1. ALLERGY

Allergies to arthropods are recognized as a significant health threat worldwide. The tremendous diversity of arthropods and their products and the large biomass represented by this phylum present a continuing, complex array of potent allergens to the immune system.

Chronological exposure to arthropod allergens usually results in a sequence of reactions. Initially, there is no discernible response; this is followed by the appearance

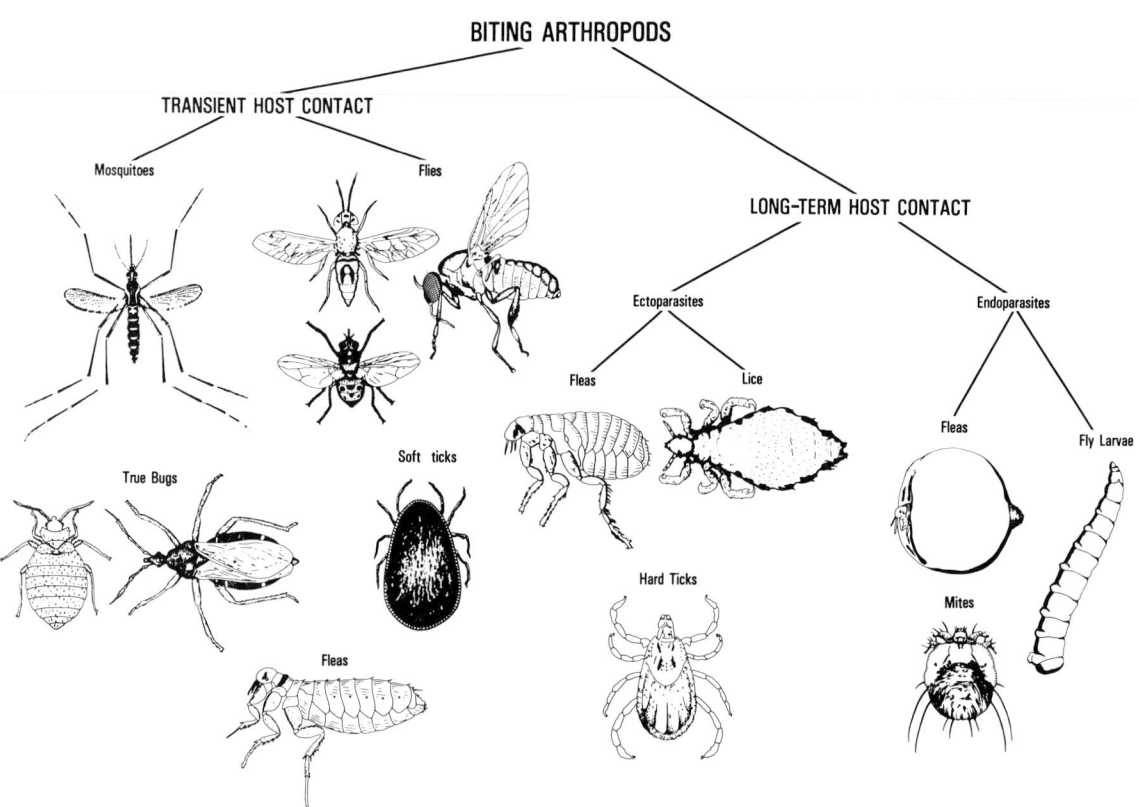

FIGURE 105–1. Biting arthropods can be broadly grouped into categories based on the length of contact with humans.

of only a delayed reaction. Both immediate and delayed reactions usually occur with further exposure. Many individuals remain at this stage, whereas others progress to only an immediate response, and finally to a point at which no reaction is observed with exposure. It may be difficult to determine when clinical symptoms are attributable to reaginic hypersensitivity and IgE antibodies and when the reactions are due to the nonallergenic components of arthropod products. Development of an arthropod allergy is dependent on the genetic predisposition of the individual, the species of arthropod and size of infestations, and the type of allergens as well as the duration of exposure. Cross-reactivity among different arthropod allergens exists, so that once sensitized, a subject may react to a variety of species. Potent arthropod allergens can promote two very different types of reaction—immediate and delayed. The immediate reaction may advance to a state of hypersensitivity in some individuals.

REAGINIC HYPERSENSITIVITY. In the immediate (within 6 hours) anaphylactic (type I) response, reaginic IgE antibodies formed on previous exposure to the allergen are fixed to tissue mast cells. When the antigen is reintroduced into the host, it binds with the antibody attached to the cell surface, triggering the release of histamine and other substances. Local anaphylaxis in the skin, an urticarial or bullous response, is the immediate reaction to an insect bite. In generalized anaphylaxis, such as that seen after a bee sting in a sensitized person, a massive release of histamine and other mediators results in life-threatening complications, e.g., cardiovascular shock or laryngeal edema.

DELAYED HYPERSENSITIVITY. Papular urticaria was the name applied to insect bites before their true origin was determined. These nodules represent the delayed reactions. They are common in children whose experience of exposure is limited. Because the skin is irritated by bites, scratching with subsequent secondary infection often modifies their appearance. Bites on the lower leg often show greater reaction owing to relative circulatory stasis. The bite marks of fleas, mosquitoes, black flies, midges, or assassin bugs frequently have the same appearance. Treatment is usually limited to calamine lotions and the prevention of secondary infection.

Delayed hypersensitivity reactions to insect bites are mainly the result of a type IV reaction, in which the allergen may be different from that responsible for type I reactions. In the type IV reaction, mononuclear cells respond to the allergen at the site of introduction, producing an intense cellular infiltration that results in a nodule. Histologic studies of insect bites show that immediate macular wheal reactions, which may be associated with an erythematous flare, have prominent eosinophilic infiltration. This is in contrast to a delayed response, in which lymphocytes and plasma cells predominate.

TESTS FOR HYPERSENSITIVITY. Hypersensitivity is an exaggerated type I immediate response. The division into local and systemic response is somewhat artificial because a sufficient stimulus will result in a generalized reaction.

Skin Tests. Skin testing is the initial method used to determine sensitivity. Within minutes of introduction of the allergen, histamine release from skin mast cells causes vasodilation (erythema), localized edema from increased vascular permeability (wheal), and itching. Many antigens are available commercially in cutaneous and intracutaneous skin test kits.

Blood Tests. Two more sensitive techniques are sometimes available in specialized laboratories. The histamine release assay is a technique that requires the incubation of a patient's leukocytes with the relevant allergen. If the basophils are coated with specific IgE, histamine release can be measured. The radioallergosorbent test (RAST) measures the amount of specific IgE antibody present in the serum and is sensitive to 0.0001 μg of antibody. Although these in vitro methods avoid the risk of sensitizing the patient, they are not as sensitive as skin testing, and their correlations with the clinical history are 85% and 70%, respectively. In addition, they are more time-consuming and more expensive than skin tests.

CONTACT, AIRBORNE, AND INGESTED ALLERGENS. Disorders resulting from inhalation or ingestion of arthropod parts and products, or from direct contact, are separated from those resulting from envenomization. The pathogenic mechanisms include hypersensitivity reactions (allergies) from arthropod allergens and irritant effects from the physical structure of spines, setae, and other materials. Inhalation and physical contact with airborne materials are the mechanisms most pertinent to these allergies. Whole arthropods, body parts, secretions, and excretions can become airborne. Symptoms are often seasonal, with the frequency of exposure increasing as arthropod populations burgeon, or are occupational in nature. Symptoms can range from mild dermal irritation to anaphylaxis.

House dust mites and cockroaches are the most prevalent sources of inhalation allergies in a domestic environment. Notable examples of seasonal variation in public health or occupational exposure include reactions to mayflies (Ephemeroptera), caddis flies (Trichoptera), midges (Diptera), larval and adult moths (Lepidoptera), dermestid and carpet beetle larvae, and adult staphylinid and blister beetles (Coleoptera) (Fig. 105–2).

Mite Allergies. House dust allergy, in which several species of *Dermatophagoides* mites and other arthropods are sources of the inhalation and contact allergens, is estimated to affect 4% of the United States population and is a significant public health problem worldwide. Mites breed best at relatively high temperatures and

humidity, and studies have shown enormous volumes of mites and mite products in living areas. Using extracts of mite cultures for skin testing, over 50% of asthmatic and nonasthmatic atopic individuals have exhibited positive tests. Most allergens in mite cultures are present in fecal particles, and potent glycoprotein fractions of low molecular weight have been isolated. Diagnosis and immunotherapy of the house dust mite allergy is currently based on crude mite preparations. Molecular cloning of mite allergens is being investigated to circumvent the limitations of the small and variable quantities present in these extracts.

Treatment of house dust mite allergies by hyposensitization with *Dermatophagoides* extracts has yielded variable results, possibly because of the use of relatively crude preparations and the possible involvement of other allergens. Reduction of exposure by using specially designed vacuum cleaners, laundering bed sheets, and enclosing mattresses in plastic covers may have some long-term effect. Recent studies indicate that treatment of living areas with tannic acid solutions can chemically alter dust mite allergens so that they no longer elicit allergic reactions; this may be of clinical benefit.

Most instances of mite-induced occupational dermatitis are observed in individuals whose work brings them in contact with infested materials. The majority of mites infesting stored and processed foods belong to the families Acaridae, Carpoglyphidae, Glyciphagidae, and Pyroglyphidae. A specific type of product usually harbors a given species; the common terms applied to mite-induced skin inflammations reflect the respective industries (e.g., baker's itch, grain itch, straw itch).

Cockroach Allergies. Hypersensitivity to cockroach allergens is worldwide. Only approximately 50 of the 4000 species of cockroaches are pestiferous, and fewer than a dozen substantially affect health and welfare. Individuals living in environments heavily infested with cockroaches have a higher prevalence of positive skin tests (59%) than do those in areas with lower infestation rates (5%). Over 50% of asthmatics have positive skin scratch tests, while the incidence among nonasthmatic atopics approaches 35%. Over 12% of individuals without a history of allergy also exhibit cockroach hypersensitivity. These data suggest that 10 million to 15 million North Americans are allergic to cockroaches; studies in Asia showed similar prevalences.

Other Arthropod Allergies. Lepidopterism is the general term for the ill effects that larval and adult moths and butterflies have on humans. Included are problems associated with inhalation, ingestion, dermal contact, and tissue penetration by products or structures from any life-cycle stage. The urticating hairs or nettling setae (macrotrichia) of caterpillars can be a source of contact dermatitis in an occupational environment and in some instances a significant public health problem. Barbed setae of some species can be difficult to extract. If these enter the eye, fragments may embed in the eyelid, scratching the conjunctiva or cornea, or even penetrate into the interior, resulting in loss of vision.

The barbed setae of adult female *Hylesia* spp. are responsible for serious outbreaks of urticating rashes and upper respiratory tract complications in South

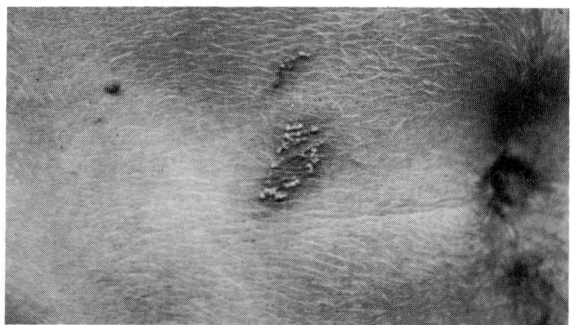

FIGURE 105–2. Contact dermatitis from staphylinid beetle (*Paederus* species) on the body of an adult in Ethiopia. (Courtesy of the Armed Forces Institute of Pathology, Photograph Neg. No. 75–5784.)

America, most notably in Brazil and Peru, where cases may number in the thousands. Symptoms usually occur seasonally, often when moths are attracted to lights in inhabited areas.

Periodic increases in the moth population have resulted in public health problems affecting thousands of individuals in the United States. Both the gypsy moth, *Lymantria dispar,* and the puss moth, *Megalopyge opercularis,* have been implicated. An estimated 500,000 individuals were affected by windblown hairs of the mulberry tussock moth, *Euproctis similis,* near Shanghai, China. Last-instars larvae carry over 2 million urticating setae per caterpillar. The Oriental tussock moth, *Euproctis flava,* also was associated with symptoms affecting an estimated 250,000 persons on Honshu Island, Japan, in 1956. Areas throughout the Far East are routinely affected by these moths.

The mass emergence of nonbiting midges (Diptera: Chironomidae) along the Nile in northern Sudan results in allergic symptoms, especially bronchial asthma and rhinitis. Low molecular weight hemoglobins appear to be the primary allergens. Larval populations can reach $100,000/M^2$, and the adult midges at times reach levels that hinder or prevent work and recreation for thousands of individuals. Palliative measures include the use of strong decoy lights to attract midges away from populated areas, which are illuminated by weak reddish lights.

DESENSITIZATION. The clearest indication for desensitization is a patient who has had a life-threatening anaphylactic episode and shows marked skin sensitivity to insect venom. Mixed venom preparations are available containing bee, wasp, and vespid (yellow jacket, yellow hornet, and white-faced hornet) components. Purified venom antigens are preferable to whole-body extracts, which promote many nonspecific immunoglobulins. Because systemic reactions may occur during the course of treatment, therapy is best given in special clinics. The duration of treatment necessary to achieve persistent blocking immunity to stings is unknown. Many allergists advise that treatment be discontinued after 5 years, or sooner if RAST or skin tests become negative. Both IgE and IgG levels may rise during immunotherapy, and modified forms of the type I reaction may be seen. A serum sickness syndrome has been reported with whole-body extract. There is some evidence that factors other than venom-specific IgE may contribute to clinical anaphylaxis. In desensitization to salivary allergens, whole-body extracts are used because salivary antigens are not usually available.

There are few studies on the immunotherapy of patients with allergic respiratory diseases due to inhalation of insect allergens. The recommended treatment follows methods used for patients with asthma caused by plant pollens and molds.

105.2. BITING ARTHROPODS

Transient Host Contact

Most arthropods that bite man have only transient host contact (Fig. 105–1). Hematophagous insects are frequently winged and highly mobile. This accounts for their ability to quickly attack and escape capture or detection. Some arthropods hide in structures close to the host and feed only when the host is nearby. Other arthropods that bite man may have no intention to attack, bites being stimulated by various conditions, i.e., defense, attractive odors, or erroneous food selection.

Penetration or irritation of skin can be caused by bites of some members of the phylum Arthropoda in the classes Chilopoda, Insecta, and Arachnida. Adults, larvae, or nymphs, both terrestrial and aquatic, of many different arthropods can bite humans. Biting mouth parts are generally classified into chewing (mandibulate) and sucking (haustellate). Mandibulate mouth parts are generally not structurally adapted for biting man, although various members of the orders Coleoptera (beetles), Neuroptera (aphis lions and dobson flies), Hymenoptera (wasps, bees, and ants), and Odonata (damselflies and dragonflies) may use their mouth parts for breaking the skin. Bites often become infected with bacteria, usually pathogenic cocci, present on the human skin or on contaminated arthropod mouth parts. Cockroaches (Dictyoptera) do not usually attack humans but will eat dried or fresh blood, skin, and fingernails of incapacitated individuals. This scavenger behavior suggests a source of direct injury and possible contamination.

HEMATOPHAGOUS ARTHROPODS. These arthropods normally feed on warm-blooded vertebrates (including man) for blood that is both life-supporting and necessary for growth and gonotropic development. Therefore, their mouth parts are designed for probing and sucking blood and tissue fluids. In general, the term "biting arthropod" implies piercing and sucking mechanisms. Hematophagous arthropods have to pierce the host's skin to obtain blood. Since injury to skin triggers a series of repair reactions in the host (e.g., blood clotting, platelet aggregation, increased vascular permeability, and leukocyte chemotaxis), to obtain blood, hematophagous arthropods must modify or antagonize some of these adverse reactions. Arthropod saliva contains vast amounts of pharmacologic substances (e.g., proteases, carbohydrases, anticoagulants, and antiplatelet, anticomplement, and vasodilatory prostaglandins) that counteract host hemostasis.

The arthropod mouth parts are highly variable in morphology. The adults of the order Diptera have the most diverse mouth part types. Only females of the lower Diptera (i.e., mosquitoes, black flies, biting midges, horse flies, and snipe flies) are hematophagous. Males and females of the higher muscid Diptera (i.e., tsetse flies, biting house flies, and stable flies) are blood feeders. Although the goal of acquiring blood is the same, the structure and function of mouth parts of these distinct groups differ. Consequently, the damage to human tissue caused by these mouth parts is different.

Diptera. Diptera (flies and mosquitoes and their relatives) is a large order, containing over 100 families. They develop by complete metamorphosis (egg-larva-pupa-adult).

Mosquitoes have mouth parts composed of 6 united stylets, which can be seen as only a single filament-like structure with the unaided eye. The major part of the food channel is formed by the labrum-epipharynx, the mandibles, and the hypopharynx; the last is also used for injection of salivary fluids. A pair of maxillae and mandibles serve to penetrate surface capillaries. Although mosquitoes are considered solenophageous (vessel blood feeders), some evidence suggests that they are telmophageous (pool blood feeders).

The mouth parts of horse flies (Tabanidae), black flies (Simuliidae), biting midges (Ceratopogonidae), phlebotomine sand flies (Psychodidae), and some snipe flies (Rhagionidae) have 6 short bladelike structures. Cutting and penetration are accomplished by a pair of mandibles that act as scissors and a pair of maxillae that may aid in piercing and thrusting into the tissues (some horse flies) or be used for anchoring mouth parts in the tissues (some black flies, biting flies, and sand flies). The labium, which ensheaths the blades, has a labellum that is used for sponging and lapping blood. Frequently, flies that feed in this manner leave spots or streams of blood (Fig. 105–3). These bites can be very painful and produce local lesions that persist for hours or days. Sensitized individuals develop allergic reactions. The very minute biting midges cause pain inverse to their size, and frequently, much larger insects, i.e., mosquitoes or black flies, are blamed for the discomfort.

Some mosquitoes and flies (i.e., some biting midges and sand flies) bite at various times of the day and night. Black flies, horse flies, snipe flies, some mosquitoes (especially those of the genus *Aedes*), some biting midges, and many sand flies are daytime feeders. On the eastern and southern coastal areas of the United States, the salt-marsh mosquito, *Aedes sollicitans,* attacks man and other animals at the rate of thousands per 15 minutes of exposure time. Similarly, synchronous emergence of black flies in large numbers, especially in temperate climates, renders certain areas uninhabitable for man, livestock, and even wild animals.

The mouth parts of stable flies (Muscidae) and tsetse flies (Glossinidae) have a labrum-epipharynx for the

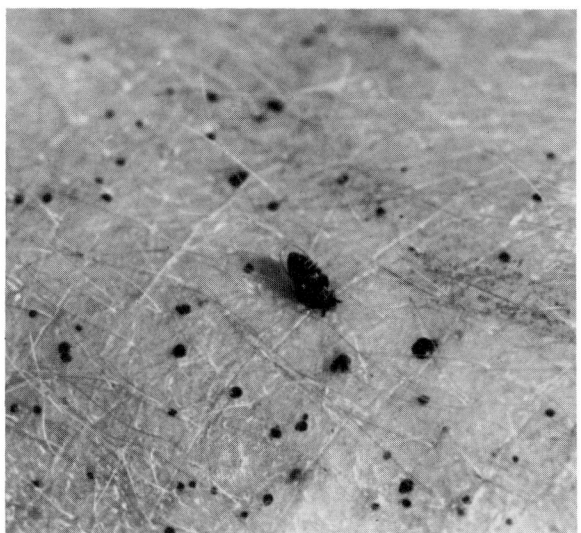

FIGURE 105–3. Blood-encrusted lesions following *Simulium* bites. A simulium is seen feeding. (Courtesy of Dr. Harold Trapido, Louisiana State University School of Medicine, New Orleans.)

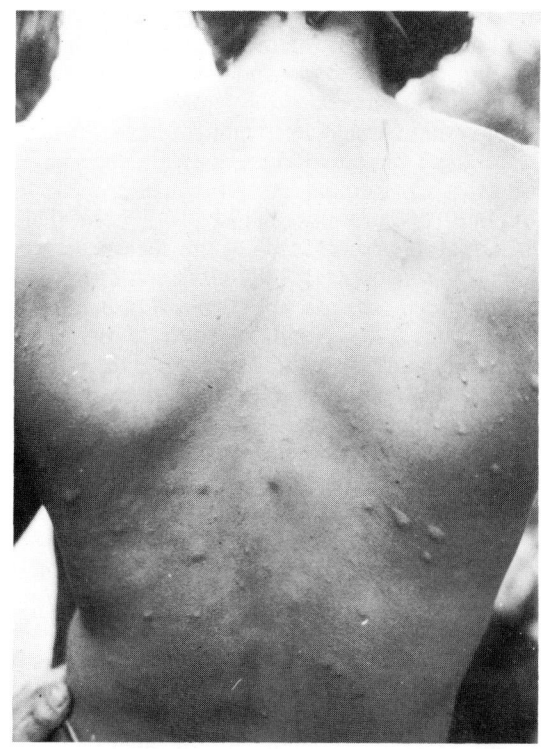

FIGURE 105–4. Tsetse fly *(Glossina fuscipes)* bites on the back of an adult male in Ethiopia. (Courtesy of the Armed Forces Institute of Pathology, Photograph Neg. No. 75–5783.)

food canal and a hypopharynx with the salivary duct. The haustellum has tissue-cutting denticles on the tip of the labellum. The tsetse fly has a thinner haustellum that can probe deep into the skin, whereas the stable fly has a thicker, shorter proboscis. The stable fly and tsetse fly are daytime blood feeders. They cut through tissues and capillaries while probing for blood. Salivary fluids are inoculated in the process of pooling blood for ingestion. The stable fly, *Stomoxys calcitrans,* is a serious biting pest; it resembles a house fly in general appearance, but the stable fly possesses a prominent proboscis, which both sexes use for sucking blood. When ready to feed, it quickly redirects the proboscis downward. The tsetse fly (*Glossina* species) has a similar proboscis. The fly may lower the mouth parts to probe a number of times before settling down to feed. Each time the fly probes, intense pain can be felt (Fig. 105–4).

Diptera Larvae. Mouth parts of Diptera larvae are neither used in the same way nor morphologically similar to the mouth parts of adults. In general, the larvae are found within special habitats. Mouth hooks of some maggots are attached to a cephalopharyngeal sclerite. The hooks act to lacerate tissue. A few larvae can bite man on a short-term basis. The bite of a predatory tabanid larva can be quite painful. A hole is punched in the dermis, and salivary toxins can be inoculated; blood can be drawn but is not usually ingested. In equatorial Africa, the Congo floor maggot, *Auchmeromyia luteola,* is a hematophagous larva that feeds at night and hides in the walls of houses during the day. In these respects, it resembles the South American *Triatoma* species. However, the Congo floor maggot does not transmit disease. It is restricted to feeding at floor level; thus, a bed or hammock solves the problem of bites in humans.

True Bugs. The piercing and sucking mouth parts of bloodsucking Hemiptera of the families Reduviidae (assassin bugs) and Cimicidae (bedbugs) have 4 fascicles to penetrate the skin and blood vessels. There are over 2500 species of Reduviidae, of which the subfamily Triatominae (or cone-nose bugs) (14 genera, 111 species) is hematophagous. Some of the species are vectors of Chagas' disease (i.e., *Triatoma infestans, T. dimidiata, Rhodnius prolixus, Panstrongylus megistus*). In cone-nose bugs, the maxillae penetrate the skin and blood vessels, and the mandibles anchor into the skin.

Of the 74 species of cimicids, only 2 have well-known associations with humans. The bedbugs are cosmopolitan in distribution. The common bedbug, *Cimex lectularius,* is widespread throughout the temperate and tropical regions, whereas the distribution of the Indian bedbug, *C. hemipterus,* is restricted to tropical and subtropical climates. Bedbugs use both mandibles and maxillae for feeding from blood vessels. Bites of males, females, and nymphs from both species occur at night or under subdued light on people in bed. Ingestion of blood and engorgement may require only a few minutes. Little pain may be associated with their bites. Reactions to bites are variable, depending on the allergic response. The insects hide in the cracks and crevices of walls and beds during the day. The foul odor of the feces of bedbugs is pungent in heavily infested houses.

Fleas. Adult fleas are obligate parasites of warm-blooded vertebrates. Bladelike structures called maxillary stylets and the epipharynx can quickly penetrate capillaries. The cat flea *(Ctenocephalides felis),* a very common pest of dogs, can cause severe bite reactions. The nonparasitic eggs, larvae, and pupae are found in pet resting areas, e.g., on rugs, in dog bedding, and under furniture in the home. Other species of fleas that attack man are the Oriental rat flea *(Xenopsylla cheopis)* and the human flea *(Pulex irritans).* Fleas readily bite man when they are starved and can prove very annoying.

Soft Ticks. Argasidae (order Acarina) can produce painful bites. Species of the genus *Ornithodoros* are found in both hemispheres. They are usually associated with wild animal resting areas. The mouth parts of soft ticks have teeth on the chelicerae for cutting tissues and a hypostome for collecting pooled blood and tissues. These ticks feed quickly and are different from the hard ticks that anchor into the dermis.

NONHEMATOPHAGOUS ARTHROPODS. Occasionally, bites by non-bloodsucking insects can be as painful or even more excruciating than those by bloodsucking insects. The rasping mouth parts of minute thrips (order Thysanoptera) can be surprisingly painful, but little reaction occurs except in sensitive individuals. Other plant-eating insects and predators of other insects have mouth parts just as capable of penetrating human skin as of entering the epidermis of a leaf or the chitinous membranes of insects. Blood can be ingested by some in this process. Many species of centipede (Chilopoda), and spiders (Araneida) do occasionally bite humans if they are touched. Such bites may include transitory pain, swelling, necrotic lesions, systemic reactions (vom-

iting, headache, cardiac arrhythmias, and convulsions), or even death. Predatory assassin bugs (e.g., Platymeris) inoculate enzyme-rich saliva with trypsin, hyaluronidase, and phospholipase, causing severe, persistent pain. Some arthropods that cannot inject salivary fluid may deposit the fluid on the skin surface and thus cause a reaction. Millipedes will not bite, and many of the known species are harmless. However, their exuded secretions may cause intense burning if they enter the eyes or may produce blisters on the skin.

Long-Term Host Contact

Some biting arthropods require considerable time on the host to complete a normal life cycle (Fig. 105–1). The continuous availability of food from one host reduces the necessity for these arthropods to seek another. Depending on the species, only one life stage may be found on the host for an extended time. If development and reproduction occur on the host, the extent of the damage to the host may be correlated with the length of stay and arthropod population size. In most cases, their sedentary parasitologic role allows more potential for secondary dermal infection.

ECTOPARASITES

Fleas. Fleas were mentioned earlier as transient biters of man. Hundreds of adult fleas can infest the body and head hairs, a problem that may have originated from an animal pet. For example, the sticktight flea, *Echidnophaga gallinacea,* and the cat flea, *Ctenocephalides felis,* may remain and feed on the same host for a long time, if undisturbed. The fleas, protected by the head hair and body warmth, have a continuous food supply. Pyrethrum soaps and shampoos are effective in control.

Hard Ticks. These maintain contact with the human host for several days while feeding on blood cells and tissue fluids. The bite of hard ticks is not usually detected during feeding. The discovery of a tick on the body or head may be well after the tick is fully engorged, even as large as 2 cm. The larvae, called seed ticks, may occur in large numbers, whereas usually fewer nymphs and adults are found on the body. Ticks that enter the ear canal can cause complications due to their engorged size, which makes it difficult to remove them intact.

Removal. Contact is rendered more certain by the depth of hypostomal (mouth part) penetration and the recurved denticles of the hypostome. In some genera that have shorter hypostomes, the secretion of a cementing substance aids in anchoring the tick, making removal more difficult. If the tick is forcibly pulled off, the mouth parts may remain in the tissues and promote a chronic granulomatous reaction. The accepted method for removing ticks is with forceps (lift the abdomen of the tick upward and forward over the front of the tick, grasping very near the point of attachment (not the skin), and pull outward and forward). Formamidine derivatives are effective in causing ticks to detach.

Tick Paralysis. Ticks can cause a more serious condition, paralysis, which occurs worldwide and resembles acute poliomyelitis. More than 40 species of soft and hard ticks secrete salivary toxins that are responsible for paralysis in man and some animals. In the United States, the Rocky Mountain wood tick, *Dermacentor andersoni,* and the American dog tick, *D. variabilis,* are implicated. Five or 6 days after attachment of the tick, the patient becomes restless and irritable and may have numbness or tingling of the extremities, lips, throat, and face. Difficulty in walking is followed by an inability to stand. Rapidly progressive ascending flaccid paralysis, which can reach the bulbar centers, causing dysphagia, slurred speech, and diplopia, may occur. Death may result from respiratory failure or aspiration pneumonia.

Ticks responsible for this condition, which is more common in children, are often concealed in long hair at the nape of the neck, particularly in girls. Provided that the paralysis is not too far advanced, rapid and complete recovery follows removal of the tick. Diagnosis depends upon the clinical history and recovery of the tick.

Lice. Sucking lice (Phthiraptera) closely associated with man are the head louse *(Pediculus humanus capitis),* the body louse *(P. humanus corporis),* and the crab louse *(Phthirus pubis).* The lice are flattened dorsoventrally and have legs adapted for clinging to hair. The bite is accomplished with 3 stylets that are pushed into the skin from within the head of the louse. The paired maxillae form a food duct, and the hypopharynx forms the salivary channel. The mouth is held in place by a circlet of teeth at the end of the proboscis. Nymphs and adults require blood for survival. Lice must feed daily in order to survive. The names of the lice give some indication as to where they might be found on humans.

Head and Body Lice. The head louse is about 3 mm long. Nymphs are difficult to see on the head because they blend in color and size with flakes of the scalp; hence, the name "mechanical dandruff" has been used. The lice move surprisingly fast in the hairy environment, but the eggs (nits) remain as telltale signs. The female louse lays individual eggs or nits (approximately 0.6 mm in length) and attaches them to hairs of the host. Nits are so strongly glued on the hairs that they remain long after the lice are controlled. Infestation of head lice occurs on other parts of the body. Morphologic characteristics for the identification and separation of body and head lice overlap.

Lice are found in all socioeconomic groups but occur more frequently among the poor because of infrequent washing and overcrowding. Infestations have been common in military troops during wartime. Epidemics occur in many schools. Head lice appear to be most common in tropical South America, whereas body lice occur mainly in colder areas (e.g., in the Andes), a difference probably related to the amount of clothing worn. Body lice are more apt to be found in areas where clothing comes into close contact with the body, with nits being laid in the seams of clothes and rarely attached to hairs.

Bites of the lice cause pinpoint macules and pigmentation of the skin. Intense itching is the usual characteristic of heavy infestation. Pediculosis is associated with itching and rash and may be followed by irritability and depression. On the head, enlarged postauricular lymph nodes and scalp infection may result from scratching. Hemorrhagic macules or papules develop at the sites of feeding lice, and vertical excoriations due to scratching

may be present. The condition of postinflammatory skin thickening and pigmentation in people continuously exposed to lice has been called vagabond's disease.

Crab Lice. The crab louse, as the French name *papillon d'amour* implies, is usually acquired by sexual contact or contact with infested objects, e.g., blankets or articles of clothing. The normal habitat of this louse is the pubic hair, which it scales by means of its crablike claws. It sometimes can be found on eyebrows and eyelashes or on the axillary hairs. These somewhat sedentary lice cause irritating papules in the groin. Pruritus occurs at the feeding sites, and with continued feeding, bluish macules mark the skin.

Treatment. Lotions or shampoos that incorporate insecticides, e.g., benzene hexachloride or pyrethrins, are used to control lice. The compound should be applied only to the infested areas. Reapplication 1 week later may be necessary to control those nymphs that emerge following treatment. Clothing and bedding of infested individuals should be laundered at 55°C for 20 minutes or dry-cleaned to destroy nits and lice.

ENDOPARASITES

Tungiasis. This is caused by the female *Tunga penetrans* (1 mm) (chigoe flea, jigger flea), a highly specialized flea that burrows into the skin, feeds on tissue fluids, and grows to about 1 cm within 2 weeks of infestation as eggs develop beneath the dermis. In the skin, the flea is oriented with its head farthest from the dermal surface. Close inspection reveals a black dot in the center of the lesion, locating the female's posterior end, from which she respires and discharges excrement and eggs. After the eggs are extruded, the carcass of the flea collapses and sloughs along with the covering keratin. The eggs hatch, and the larvae develop to become adult fleas in about 3 weeks. After copulation the female flea begins a pattern of jumping that persists until she dies or attaches and burrows into the skin of a warm-blooded animal. Infestations usually occur on the feet and legs; fleas tend to concentrate on the ankles, the instep, and between the toes but generally avoid the weight-bearing portion of the soles (Fig. 105–5). Fleas may attack any portion of the body, including the trunk, limbs, head, face and even eyelids, of individuals who lie on the ground. Fleas beneath the nails are especially painful and have given rise to the sailor's oath, "Well, I'll be jiggered." Patients with leprosy, who have reduced sensation in their feet, are especially prone to severe and recurrent infestation.

Although tungiasis is usually innocuous, secondary infections, including tetanus and gas gangrene, kill some patients in tropical Africa.

Pigs are natural hosts of these fleas, which prefer sandy soil; close contact with pigs predisposes to infestation. The flea evolved in the tropical and subtropical Americas, spread to Africa in the late 1800s, and has since expanded its range into the Indian subcontinent.

Treatment involves removal of the chigoe by widening the cavity with a sterile needle so that the flea can be extracted intact. The usual care should be taken to dress the cavities and prevent secondary infection.

Myiasis. Human myiasis is the invasion or infestation of man's body and tissues by Diptera larvae or maggots.

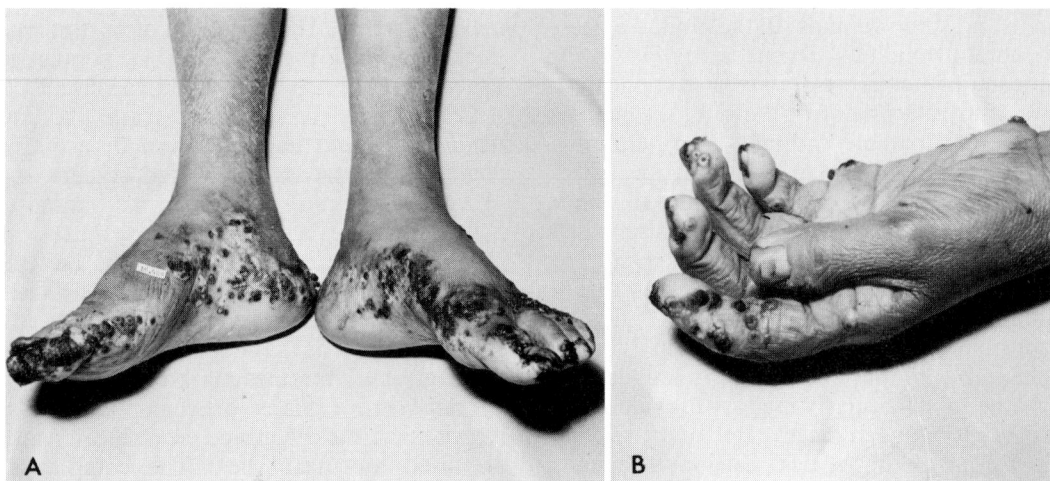

FIGURE 105–5. Tungiasis. Lesions due to *Tunga penetrans,* the chigoe or burrowing flea. (Courtesy of Dr. Rodolfo Cespedes. Hospital San Juan de Dios, San José, Costa Rica.)

The families of flies commonly involved are very diverse (i.e., Muscidae, Calliphoridae, Sarcophagidae, Piophilidae, Stratiomyidae, Syrphidae, Oestridae, Gasterophilidae, and Cuterebridae). Myiasis can be divided into primary and secondary types: Primary myiasis implies a breach in the skin made by the larva itself; in secondary myiasis, open devitalized tissues, i.e., wounds, infections, or burns, are parasitized. Although certain species of flies are obligate parasites and require living tissue for their development, some other species are facultative and require either live or dead tissues for their development. Some members of family Piophilidae (cheese skippers), Stratiomyidae (soldier fly larvae), and Syrphidae (rat-tailed larvae) can cause accidental gastrointestinal myiasis. The classification adopted by James (1947) is probably most useful to the clinician because it is based on the part of the body affected. Except for the various types of skin myiasis (i.e., furuncular, creeping dermal myiasis, and wound infection), myiasis (of the nose, mouth, ear, eye, gastrointestinal tract, anal or sexual orifices, and urinary passages) is treated on an individual basis.

Traumatic (Wound) Myiasis. Although the wounds through which the larvae enter are usually sizable, a minor injury can be the portal of entry. The female fly, often attracted by blood or pus, lays her eggs near the lesion. The quickly hatching maggots have easy access to the wound. Skin breaches due to disease, e.g., leprosy, treponematoses, leishmaniasis, or cancer, or to wounds can also be parasitized in this way. Often the maggots remain superficial, but they can penetrate deep, causing meningitis or even necessitating amputation of a limb. Female flesh flies (Sarcophagidae) deposit freshly hatched first-stage larvae directly in wounds, ulcers, or even unbroken skin.

The dominant fly species involved vary with the geographic location. In southern Europe, Russia, Africa, and the Middle East, *Wohlfahrtia magnifica* is the most common species. The Old World screwworm *(Chrysomyia bezziana)* is a major cause of myiasis in the Orient and sub-Saharan Africa. In the Americas, the primary screwworm, *Cochliomyia hominivorax,* is well known to livestock farmers as a serious pest. Eggs laid in batches of 10 to 300 hatch within 24 hours. The larvae penetrating the tissues in a head-down position are gregarious and form a pocket-like wound. The female fly prefers clean, fresh wounds for oviposition. Because she mates only once, an extensive program of sterile male release was effective in controlling the problem in livestock in the United States, and in eradicating it from Curaçao, although it has since started to return. Before this control program, in 1935 in Texas, 12 million livestock cases and 55 human cases of myiasis were recorded. In the northern part of the United States, *Wohlfahrtia vigil* is an important agent of myiasis.

Many other fly species may infest wounds but stay on the surface of the lesion. In the 1930s, before the advent of antibiotics, some species of blowfly maggots were used in medicine to debride suppurating wounds.

Furuncular Myiasis. In subcutaneous myiasis, the skin lesion can be mistaken for a staphylococcal boil—hence the name. Although the lesion is often complicated by a secondary bacterial infection, close inspection reveals a maggot with its posterior spiracles visible in the wound (Fig. 105–6). Two species of obligatory myiasis producers are responsible: *Dermatobia hominis* in South and Central America and *Cordylobia arthropophaga* in Africa. No previous skin lesion is necessary for the larva to effect penetration. *Dermatobia hominis* (berne, tórsalo) is named the human botfly, even though it principally infests cattle and other animals and is responsible for great economic losses in hides and milk and meat production. The mechanism of infection is unique because the fecund female fly catches mosquitoes or flies during flight. She glues her eggs to the undersurface of the captured insect and then releases it. When this insect comes into contact with a mammalian host, the eggs hatch with a spring-lid mechanism at the operculum, and the larvae burrow into the skin. Scalp infections are common in man, but lesions may occur on any exposed skin. The growing larvae assume a bottle shape, with the narrow posterior end juxtaposed

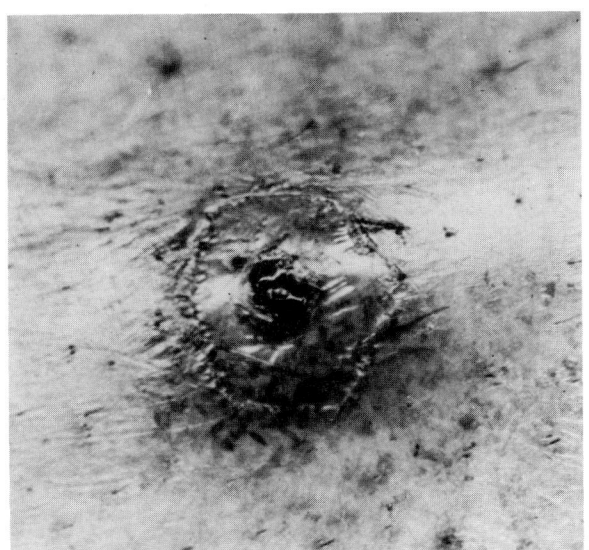

FIGURE 105–6. Myiasis. The posterior end of the warble *Dermatobia hominis* can be seen, with the shiny black spiracles in the center of the dermal lesion. (Courtesy of the Armed Forces Institute of Pathology, Photograph Neg. No. N–49503.)

to the skin surface, thus making removal more difficult. The larvae mature in about 4 weeks and then leave the host to pupate in the soil.

The adult female *Cordylobia anthropophaga* (Tumbu fly) deposits over 100 eggs, usually on urine- or feces-contaminated sand, soil, or clothing (e.g., clothes hung out to dry, soiled bedding). Within 2 days, larvae emerge; they can remain alive for 2 weeks without feeding, but on contact with skin, they penetrate. Because larvae mature within 9 days, skin tumors form rapidly. The erythema is more marked and secondary infection less common than in myiasis caused by the human botfly. The larva is easier to extract, but a large number of lesions may be present.

Creeping Dermal Myiasis. This is strictly a form of larva migrans and as such must be distinguished from subdermal migrating eruptions caused by helminths, e.g., *Ancylostoma braziliense, Strongyloides stercoralis,* and *Gnathostoma spinigerum* (Chapter 92). Creeping dermal myiasis involves man as an accidental host of botflies. *Gasterophilus intestinalis,* a natural parasite in horses, produces narrow, raised lines in the skin because the first-stage larva is incapable of developing beyond the first stage in man and migrates about in the dermis. Itching is the accompanying symptom. In contrast, the galleries of *Hypoderma lineatum,* the common cattle grub, are deeper and wider because *Hypoderma* larvae can complete development in man. Typical tumor-like warbles containing mature larvae may form, such as those seen in cattle. The deep tissue migration is accompanied by pain; severe complications may ensue.

Myiasis of the Nose, Mouth, Ear, and Accessory Sinuses. This is usually caused by the same species responsible for wound myiasis and may be a complication when the wound is on the head. Debilitated or comatose patients are especially at risk because oviposition is easier. Pain, edema, and purulent discharge are often associated with maggot growth in cases restricted

by bone and cartilage. Destruction and erosion of the nose or mouth can be caused by maggots (Fig. 105–7). Movement of maggots to the base of the brain can result in meningitis and death. In aural myiasis, pain and discomfort are accompanied by deafness and tinnitus. Infection and penetration of tympanum can ensue. Larvae of the obligatory myiasis producer flies, such as the old world screwfly *(Chrysomyia bezziana),* sheep nasal botfly *(Oestrus ovis),* and Russian gadfly *(Rhinoestrus purpureus),* are most commonly the cause of nasal myiasis.

Ocular Myiasis. Although some maggots may destroy the eye by spreading from a contiguous wound, there are other types of ocular myiasis. For example, external ophthalmomyiasis, an acute catarrhal or parasitic conjunctivitis, is caused by first-stage larvae of *Oestrus ovis,* the sheep botfly. Close inspection of the inflamed conjunctival area will reveal a wriggling mass of tiny larvae, a sequel to an opportunistic deposition of the larvae during a fly strike by the female *Oestrus.* This type of myiasis is most common among those working with sheep and goats. Internal ophthalmomyiasis is produced by deep migrating larvae of species such as *Hypoderma lineatum.* If the maggot is in the anterior chamber, it can be seen moving, and there is a chance of extraction. Posterior chamber involvement may cause retinal detachment or optic nerve invasion, with resultant blindness.

Myiasis of the Anal Region and Vagina. Secretions and excretions from these areas are highly attractive to many species of flies. Deposition of large numbers of eggs from filth flies and flesh flies can result in large numbers of larvae in as few as 8 to 12 hours. Poorly cared for and exposed children or adults can become victims. This is especially true in areas with high fly populations, such as the tropics.

Myiasis of the Bladder and Urinary Passages. The preceding explanation applies to this location as well.

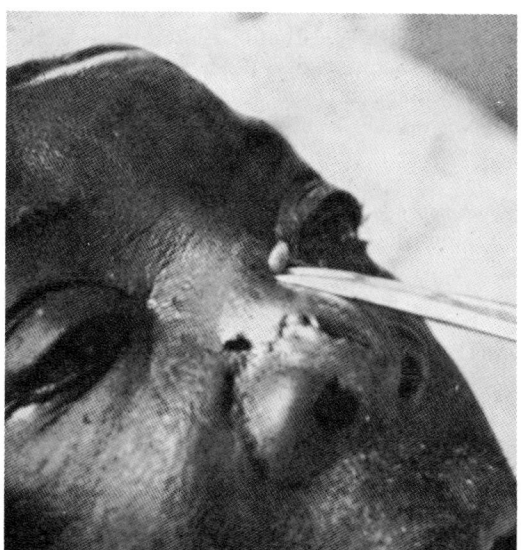

FIGURE 105–7. Infection with *Cochliomyia hominivorax.* Over 230 screwworm larvae were removed from this patient's nasal passages. (Courtest of Dr. W. E. Dove and associates, Bureau of Entomology and Plant Quarantine, U.S. Department of Agriculture.)

Newly hatched larvae at the urinary meatus migrate up the urethra only to be subsequently passed in the urine. Bladder and urethral pain may be associated with dysuria. Priapism may occur, but it is rare. Small flies of the genus *Fannia,* which resemble house flies, are most frequently implicated. Members of the genera *Psychoda, Musca, Calliphora,* and *Sarcophaga* are also implicated in urinary myiasis. Care must be taken to confirm that the urine specimen was not passed into a receptacle already containing contaminating maggots.

Enteric Myiasis. Pseudomyiasis due to maggot contamination of passed feces must be included in this discussion, even though it is still debated whether real development occurs in the human enteron. In most cases, ingested fly eggs or larvae that were deposited on foodstuff may pass intact through the intestinal tract. Acute enteritis has been described, and many cases have been documented. The ingestion of fly larvae in food is the obvious route of infection. Maggots from the genera *Musca, Fannia,* and *Sarcophaga* have been recovered. One species often recovered from stools is the aquatic rat-tailed maggot *Eristalis tenax.*

Treatment. Although species of many different genera and families are implicated in human myiasis, it is worthwhile attempting a specific identification of the maggot. The chitinous spiracular plates of mature larvae have different configurations that often allow identification of the genus. The maggots should be preserved in 70% alcohol and sent to a reference laboratory. If possible, live maggots should be furnished to a local medical entomologist; some maggots can be reared to adults for more precise identification.

Treatment entails extraction of the maggots. In furuncular myiasis, the application of petroleum jelly to the lesion suffocates the maggots, which may come wriggling out backwards, e.g., the African Tumbu fly. *Dermatobia hominis* is more difficult to remove, and incision under local anesthesia is usually necessary. Maggots in orifices, tissues, and organs are best removed individually, but if they are lodged in the nose, this may require endoscopy and even a general anesthetic. There are no medications that will dislodge maggots. When exposed to any chemical insult, maggots tend to retract, making it more difficult to find and remove them.

Acariasis

Scabies. Infestation of the epidermis by *Sarcoptes scabiei hominis* is responsible for one of the most common itching dermatoses in the world. It is usually associated with crowded conditions. Transmission is from person to person by close body contact and through sharing the same bed and clothing. Often transmission of scabies occurs during sexual encounters. The newly fertilized female mite burrows into the epidermis and lays 2 to 3 eggs a day for 30 days. The larvae hatch in 3 to 4 days and migrate to the skin surface. Maturation from eggs to adults takes about 10 to 14 days. The females feed on cells of the stratum corneum, and it is their secretions and excretions that sensitize the host and produce the familiar irritation. Typical infection usually involves less than 20 mites.

Clinical Manifestations. Newly infested persons may have large populations before the infestation is noticed.

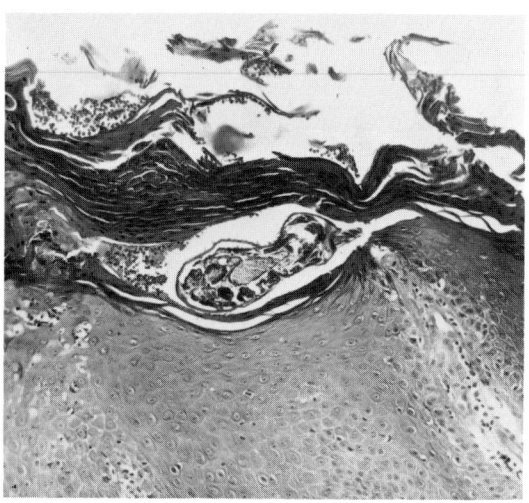

FIGURE 105–8. An adult *Sarcoptes scabiei hominis* in a burrow. Note the spinose walls. (Courtesy of the Louisiana State University School of Medicine. New Orleans.)

There is a period of about a month before sensitization and symptoms develop. Within 100 days from the arrival of a single fertilized female mite, several hundred females can develop; mite mortality is high, however, because scratching kills them. Although the mite may burrow anywhere on the skin (Fig. 105–8), there are certain sites that are more commonly affected, i.e., the hands and wrists (Fig. 105–9), the female breast, the penis, the natal cleft, and, in children, the feet. Scratching and secondary infection often cause puzzling skin lesions. The more classic sign of a run or burrow is seldom seen. This appears as a short, wavy, reddish line. A tiny blister at the distal extremity contains the female mite, which can be extracted with a pin and

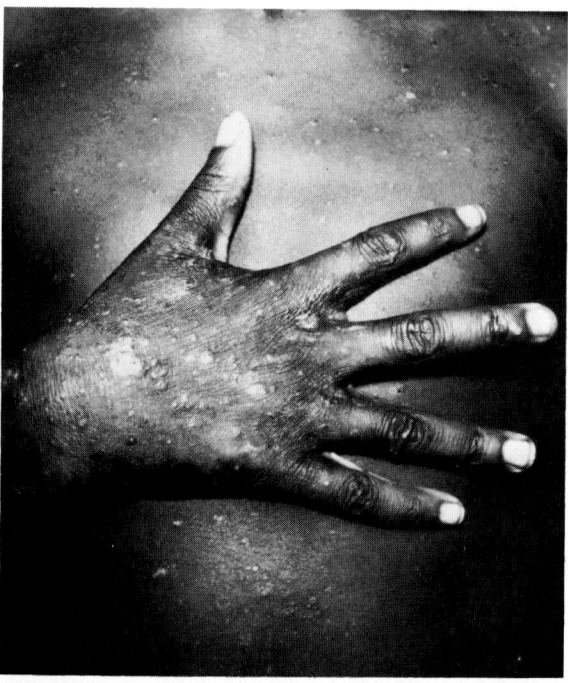

FIGURE 105–9. Advanced scabies infestation on the hand, thorax, and abdomen in a Zairean child. (Courtesy of the Armed Forces Institute of Pathology, Photograph Neg. No. 68–7834–20.)

TABLE 105–1. Example of Mites that are Implicated in Dermatitis and House Dust Allergies

Mite Species	Geographic Distribution	Hosts	Usual Habitat
*Ornithonyssus bacoti**	Worldwide	Mice, rats, chickens, wild rodents, carnivores, wild birds, humans	Nest-acquired mites, rodent burrows, cracks in buildings
*Ornithonyssus sylviarum**	Worldwide (temperate zones)	Mice, rats, chickens, pigeons, wild rodents, humans	Cracks and crevices in buildings; skin, feathers
Dermanyssus gallinae	Worldwide	Chickens, wild birds, pigeons, rats, rabbits, humans	Nests of chickens and other birds; rodent burrows
*Liponyssoides sanguineus**	Worldwide	Mice, rats, wild rodents, humans	Cracks and crevices in buildings; rodent burrows
*Pyemotes tritici**	Worldwide	Parasites of stored grain; insects, humans	Straw, grain, straw mattresses
*Cheyletiella yasguri**	Worldwide	Dog, humans	Skin, pelage, floors, furniture, mattresses
*Cheyletiella parasitovorax**	Worldwide	Rabbit, cat, humans	Skin, pelage
*Demodex folliculorum**	Worldwide	Humans	Sebaceous glands, hair follicles
*Eutrombicula alfreddugesi**	North and South America	Wide range of domestic animals, wild birds, humans	Grass, skin of host
Eutrombicula batatas	Central and South America, SW USA	Chicken, wild birds, rodents, domestic animals, humans*	Grass and weeds, skin of host
*Neotrombicula autumnalis**	Europe	Dog, horse, rabbit, various birds, humans	Grass, skin of host
*Sarcoptes scabiei**	Worldwide	Domestic animals, humans	Skin
Notoedres cati	Worldwide	Cats, rabbits, dogs, humans	Skin
Acarus siro	Worldwide	Pests of stored foods and vegetable products*†	Stored hay and grain, house dust
Tyrophagus putrescentiae	Worldwide	*†	House dust, pests of stored food products
Lepidoglyphus destructor	Worldwide	*†	Grain dust, barn dust, surface of mattresses, stored hay and grain
Dermatophagoides farinae	Worldwide	*†	House dust: surface of mattresses, blankets, pillows, floors, pets
Dermatophagoides pteronyssinus	Worldwide	*†	House dust: surface of mattresses, blankets, pillows, floors, pets, bedding and cages
Euroglyphus maynei	Worldwide	*†	House dust: surface of mattresses, blankets, pillows, floors, pets, bedding and cages

*Discussed in text.
†Free-living mites.

identified under the microscope. Erythematous itching papules are common lesions, and these may turn to pustules as a result of secondary staphylococcal infection. An eczematous reaction may occur, or, in long-standing infections, erythematous nodules may develop.

Complications. Epidemics of acute glomerulonephritis associated with pyoderma and scabies have been documented in Trinidad. Hyperinfestation of the epidermis with the skin honeycombed with mite burrows is sometimes referred to as Norwegian scabies. This situation results from hyperinfestation with thousands to a million mites. Clinically, this often appears as crusted psoriasiform lesions on the hands and feet and is highly contagious because of the large numbers of loosely attached, easily transferred mites present in the exfoliating skin. Itching is absent in many patients, suggesting that failure of the immune response has allowed the mites to multiply unchecked. Hyperinfection has been observed in patients immunosuppressed after renal transplant or in those using topical corticosteroids for a long period. In addition, this type of scabies occurs in demented and paralyzed patients who do not scratch.

Diagnosis and Treatment. Diagnosis, especially in the tropics, is based on the clinical appearance. Although ideally the identification of a mite is desirable, it is often impossible or too time-consuming. Treatment instructions should be precise. The patient should take a bath and discard his clothes, and bed linens should be laundered. The scabicide should be thinly applied with a swab over the entire body, sparing only the face. In children, the scalp may be affected. After donning fresh clothes, the patient should not bathe for 48 hours. A second successive treatment may be recommended. Worldwide, benzylbenzoate emulsion (20% to 35%) is the most common scabicide, but there are other effective preparations. Many are eye irritants, however. In the United States, gamma benzene hexachloride (lindane) in cream or lotion form is most frequently used. It is left on for only 12 hours to minimize percutaneous absorption. Secondary skin sepsis may be so marked as to require prior treatment with antibiotics. Simultaneous treatment of all affected family members is important. It is common to see a mother nursing a scratching child, and both have scabies.

Mite-Induced Dermatitis. Many species of mites that feed on humans actually do not burrow into the skin, but tissue swelling around them gives the appearance of dermal penetration. Most instances of mite-induced dermatitis are observed in individuals whose occupations bring them into contact with mite-infested materials. Several species of mesostigmatid, prostigmatid, and astigmatid mites can attack humans and cause irritating rashes (Table 105–1). Among mesostigmatid mites, members of the families Dermanyssidae, Macronyssidae, and Laelapidae are known to attack and bite humans. In rodent-infested buildings it is not uncommon for people to be bitten by the tropical rat mite *(Ornithonyssus bacoti)* and the house mite *(Liponyssoides sanguineus)*. Other species such as the chicken mite *(O. sylviarum)* frequently attack humans and their pets. The severity of dermatitis resulting from the bites of these mites varies with the sensitivity of the individual. The bite causes small urticarial wheals and papules that may be associated with pruritus. Many species of mites that commonly parasitize poultry, wild birds, commensal and wild rodents, and household pets may also cause dermatitis in humans and their pets. The family Sarcoptidae contains important parasitic species that cause scabies in humans and mange and other skin diseases in domestic and wild animals. *Sarcoptes scabiei canis* causes sarcoptic mange in dogs, and dog owners may become infested and develop sensitivity. This mite can penetrate the skin, but it does not multiply on the human host. Irritating papular lesions are similar to those with infestation by *S. scabiei hominis*. The families Acaridae, Glycyphagidae, and Pyroglyphidae contain many of the "stored product mites" that attack humans and occasionally cause the severe dermatitis known as grocer's itch *(Glycyphagus domesticus)*, baker's itch *(Acarus siro)*, and copra itch *(Tyrophagus putrescentiae)* (Table 105–1). Among prostigmatid mites, the straw itch mite *(Pymotes tritici)* and cheyletid mite *(Cheyletiella yasguri* and *C. blakei)* are common nuisances to humans, causing multiple lesions. Dermatitis associated with *P. tritici* is commonly known as straw, hay, or grain itch.

Chiggers. In many parts of the world, trombiculid mite larvae (chiggers) can cause severe skin irritation. In Europe *Trombicula autumnalis* (the harvester mite) and in the United States *T. alfreddugesi* and *T. splendens* are examples of the chiggers that cause much itching distress in man. Chiggers neither feed on blood nor burrow into the skin. The secretions of the mite and host reaction to the saliva and mouth parts combine to form a feeding tube (stylostome). At this stage, the mite

is strongly anchored to the skin, frequently in hair follicles and pores, for the ingestion of tissue fluids and predigested cells. Some blood cells are ingested. Red maculopapular lesions develop within 24 hours. A tiny dot in the center may be the larva, just barely visible. Again, welts and swelling around the mite may make it appear as though the chigger burrowed into the skin. After the mite is replete, it leaves the host, but itching may continue.

The natural environments of chiggers are grassy, rodent-infested areas. Persons walking through such areas should use insect repellent, e.g., diethyltoluamide, or should wear permethrin-treated clothing. Antiseptics applied to the welts will usually kill the chiggers. Temporary relief from itching is obtained with a combination of benzocaine (5%), methyl salicylate (2%), salicylic acid (0.5%), ethyl alcohol (73%), and water (19.5%).

105.3.   ENVENOMATION

The number of people seeking medical assistance because of bites is far fewer than those seeking attention because of stings of bees, wasps, hornets, and ants. A 1971 survey of physicians in Mississippi revealed that they were consulted about 2381 cases of bee, wasp, and ant stings, 499 spider bites, and 387 unidentified bites or stings. An earlier nationwide survey by Parrish showed that from 1950 to 1959, of 460 deaths due to venomous animals, 50% were caused by hymenopterans, 14% by spiders, 1.7% by scorpions, and 30% by snakes.

Active Envenomation

Envenomation by arthropods is commonly the result of the injection of a toxin used in defense or to subdue prey. (The main types of venomous arthropods are shown in Figure 105–10.) Active envenomation usually requires movement of the arthropod to inflict the injury. The mechanism of delivery of the toxin can be anteriorly stationed (i.e., mouth parts or modified front legs) or posteriorly stationed (i.e., stinging apparatus or venoms). Various mechanisms of muscular contraction serve to actively inoculate venom.

ANTERIORLY STATIONED VENOM

Spiders. The morbidity and mortality caused by spiders (class Arachnida) are usually rare, yet they are highly publicized. Fortunately, very few of the 100,000 species are considered dangerous to humans. Spiders have fangs on the end of the chelicerae, with venom stored in glands located in the cephalothorax or chelicerae. Almost all spiders have venom for the purpose of paralyzing or killing insects or small animals for food. Although man is not part of their diet, he can be victimized by some spiders that have fangs large enough to penetrate the dermis. Even the more toxic spiders, in the immature stages, may not be able to break the skin. Usually, they are not aggressive, but some will bite to defend themselves or their egg masses. Venoms

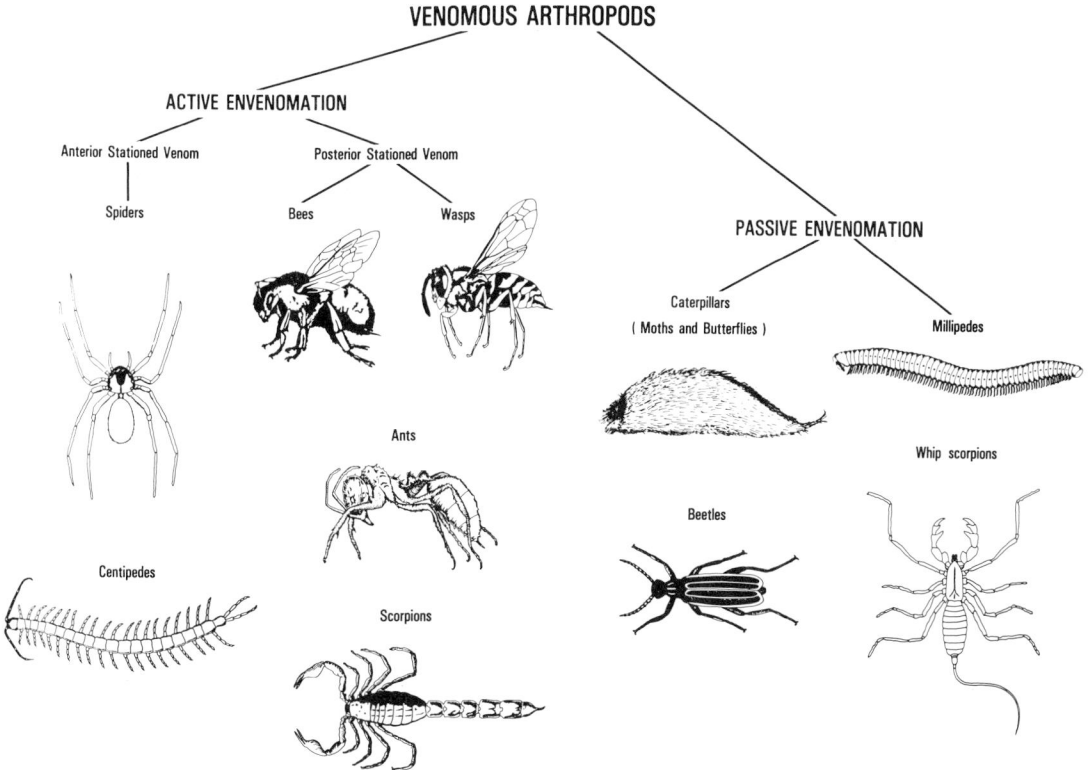

FIGURE 105–10. Venomous arthropods can be broadly categorized under active envenomation and passive envenomation.

of spiders can be very toxic, even in small quantities (0.2 to 5.0 mg of dry weight), with mouse LD_{50}, in mg/kg of body weight of 0.34 intravenously to 62.5 subcutaneously. Biochemicals found in spider venoms of several toxic species have been analyzed and have been found to be consistent intraspecifically but to vary between species. Amines, amino acids, proteins, and proteolytic enzymes are commonly pooled into potent complexes, causing variable medical abnormalities. Human fatalities have occurred after the bites of species from the genera *Latrodectus, Loxosceles, Phoneutria,* and *Atrax.*

***Latrodectus* Species.** Several species of *Latrodectus* are found worldwide, primarily in warmer climates. The female black widow, *L. mactans,* is well known by its large, glossy black abdomen with a red, hourglass-shaped marking on the ventral side. The mature female is about 30 mm long with legs extended. The spider spends her time in an irregularly patterned web, usually in the shadows of plants, woodpiles, and old buildings. Bites commonly occur on the hands. However, many people are bitten on the buttocks and genitals while using privies and outhouses.

The bite may pass unnoticed; two tiny red spots may be seen at the site, or a severe local reaction may occur. The neurotoxic fraction in the venom is a protein of low molecular weight that affects the spinal cord and nerve endings. Absorption is accompanied by pain and numbness in the affected part. In 15 minutes to a few hours, generalized agonizing muscular pains appear, together with symptoms of shock. The blood pressure falls, and there is marked sweating, a feeling of weakness and nausea, and labored respiration. The marked rigidity of the muscles of the abdominal wall may simulate tetanus or an acute abdomen. Rarely, if paralysis and coma ensue, they may be followed by cardiac or respiratory failure.

***Loxosceles* Spiders.** These spiders occur in the Americas. They are usually light brown with a darker violin-shaped mark on the cephalothorax. The body length of the adult is about 1 to 1.5 cm. They are commonly called fiddleback spiders or brown recluse spiders. The name "recluse" is appropriate, because they are secretive, shy spiders that hunt at night for silverfish and other insects. Their webs are not distinctive. In the central United States, *Loxosceles reclusa* can be collected in many homes. People are bitten indoors, often while sleeping or while donning clothing stored in closets or laid on the floor. *L. reclusa* can produce severe bites, but they are not as severe as those of *L. laeta* of South America.

The venom of *Loxosceles* is cytotoxic; it produces marked local necrosis that is slow to heal. The bite is associated with intense pain and local vasoconstriction and is followed by edema, erythema, blistering, and hemorrhage, with eventual frank necrosis and tissue loss (Fig. 105–11). Serious complications are acute hemolysis, pulmonary edema, and renal insufficiency.

***Phoneutria* Species.** The wandering spider or bird spider of South America, *Phoneutria nigriventer,* has one of the most pharmacologically active venoms of all spiders. The dose in mg/kg of body weight for killing 20 gm mice was 0.006 intravenously and 0.013 subcutaneously. The mean quantity of venom obtained by electric extraction was 1.25 mg of dry weight. In man, the venom is neurotoxic, affecting the central nervous sys-

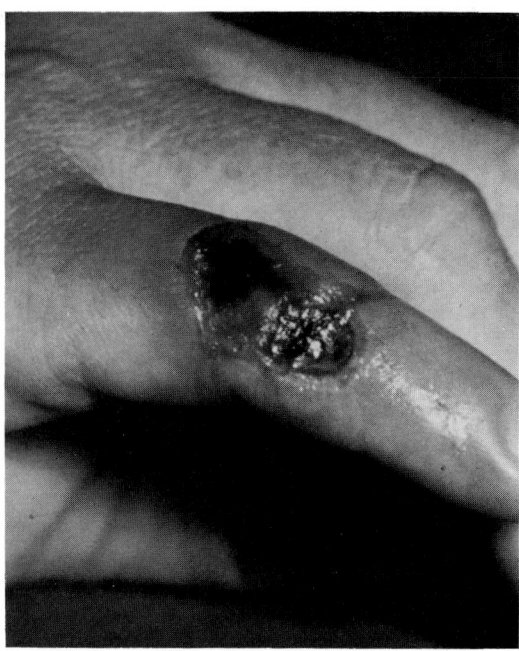

FIGURE 105–11. Local necrosis of a finger following the bite of the brown recluse spider *Loxosceles reclusa.* (From Dillaha CJ, Jansen GT, Honeycutt WM, et al: JAMA 188:33, 1964. Reprinted by permission.)

tem. There is intense local pain caused by the high serotonin content of the venom. In children, muscle spasms and convulsions may be followed by death in a matter of hours. *Phoneutria* spiders are hunting spiders with no apparent web for entrapping prey. They are large, having a body length of 3 cm, and very aggressive, usually hiding during the day and hunting between dusk and dawn. They are sometimes found in boxed fruit, particularly bananas. Other species of *Phoneutria* are also found in South and Central America.

Lycosidae Species. The venom of wolf spiders can cause marked local cytotoxic effects but little systemic illness. Local edema and necrosis are followed by crusting and scarring. There may be very little pain, although the resultant keloid scars are often painful. These spiders, which vary in size, are agile predators during the day and night. They usually run from man. Other members of this and other spider families have also been responsible for bites of varying degrees of severity.

Centipedes. Members of the class Chilopoda are also venomous because of a pair of strong hollow-tipped claws with venom glands located on the first body segment behind the head. Although centipedes are carnivorous, hunting prey at night, most species are harmless. Humans are not usually bitten. Centipedes can be quite large, measuring from 10 cm long in the southern United States to over 25 cm long in the tropics. Members of the genus *Scoloperdra* can cause severe local pain and occasional skin necrosis, but no human deaths have been reported as a result of their bites.

POSTERIORLY STATIONED VENOM

Bees, Wasps, and Hornets. The venoms of the insect order Hymenoptera are some of the most studied and characterized of all venoms. The venoms of bees and wasps have active toxic components that result in similar sting reactions.

Stings. A modified ovipositor, the stinging apparatus, penetrates the skin, and venom is injected by muscular action. The stinging apparatus is similar in structure in honeybees, wasps, hornets, and bumblebees. Honeybees, bumblebees, and vespids are social insects that use their venom for defense. Near a nest, multiple stings might be expected. The aggressiveness of bees usually increases near the hives, but there is some variability according to species. Stings from the varieties of honeybee, primarily *Apis mellifera mellifera, A. m. ligustica,* and *A. m. scutellata* (killer honeybee), are dangerous essentially for those individuals who are at risk. Systemic toxic reactions from stings may occur with multiple stings (≥ 50). Toxic reactions may include vomiting, diarrhea, shock, and renal failure. Most fatalities due to bee stings have followed the occurrence of more than 500 stings. Despite the dramatic reports about the so-called African killer bee *(A. m. scutellata)* stings, it has been shown that the killer bee venom is less lethal to animals than the European bee. Moreover, *A. m. scutellata* has considerably less venom in its venom reservoirs. The highly developed colony-defensive behaviors of *A. m. scutellata* makes it much more aggressive and unpredictable than the other subspecies.

Toxins. The polypeptide melittin, which constitutes 50% of honeybee venom, damages erythrocytes, leukocytes, and lysosomes, with the subsequent release of enzymes. Melittin stimulates the activity of endogenous phospholipase A, which then affects guanylate cyclase activity. Phospholipase A, 12% of honeybee venom, directly attacks phospholipids and tissue thromboplastin. Exogenous histamine (0.1% to 1.5% of bee venom) and melittin appear to be responsible for the pain associated with the inoculation, but the antigenicity of the bee venom appears to be primarily associated with phospholipase A. Hyaluronidase, composing 1% to 3% of bee venom, is a spreading factor that has some antigenicity. Apamin, composing about 2% of bee venom, has a neurotoxic effect. Mast cell peptide, composing 1% to 2% of bee venom, causes the destruction of mast cells (MCD).

Components of wasp and hornet venoms are histamine, hyaluronidase, serotonin, phospholipases A and B, kinins (one for wasps and another for hornets), and acetylcholine (hornets only). The kinins, apparently in the presence of trypsin, result in the formation of a kind of bradykinin. Interestingly, serotonin is part of wasp venom, and a secondarily derived compound from the hemolytic activity of melittin in bee venom. Acetylcholine is not often a common chemical in the venom of other stinging arthropods.

Ants. Ant stings are common in the southern United States. The imported fire ants, *Solenopsis richteri* and *S. invicta,* and the native United States fire ants, *S. geminata* and *S. xyloni,* cause stings that result in sharp pain similar to that of a bee sting, although less intense (Fig. 105–12).

Stings. The sting causes an immediate erythematous rash, followed by a wheal (up to 10 mm in diameter). After a few hours, a vesicle containing clear fluid forms. Within 24 hours, the vesicle becomes turgid and pustulated. The pustule will remain for several days to more

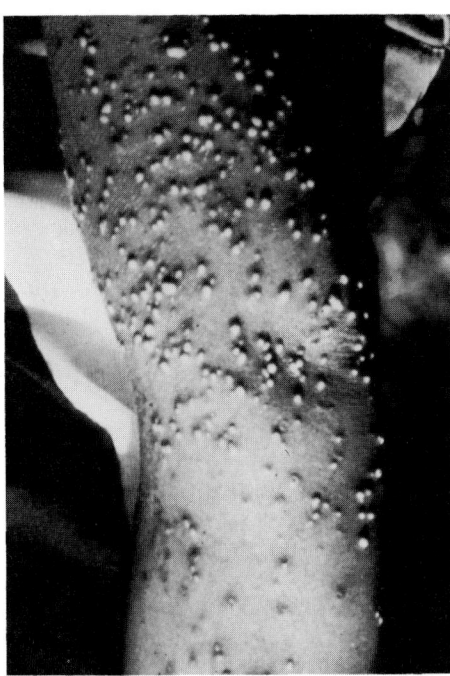

FIGURE 105-12. Fire ant stings. Severe reaction to multiple stings from *Solenopsis invicta* on the arm of a male in Mississippi. (Courtesy of the Armed Forces Institute of Pathology, Photograph Neg. No. 75-14977.)

than a week before rupturing or resolving to a scab formation. Inconspicuous, small fibrotic nodules or small pigmented areas can result.

Large numbers of stings on the extremities may occur in young children and in any unsuspecting person. Hundreds of fire ants can boil up the foot of a person who steps into the dirt mound nest. The stinging mechanism for some ants, e.g., fire ants and harvester ants, is to use the mandibles to hold onto the skin, to arch the back at the thread waist (peduncle), and to project the stinger from the posterior of the globular abdomen into the victim. Anaphylaxis can be caused by these and other species of ants, although much less frequently than with other Hymenoptera.

Toxins. Venoms of fire ants are primarily 2,6-dialkyl-piperidines (99%), which apparently cause the toxic effects. Only 0.1% of the venom is protein, containing three fractions with estimated molecular weights of 2000, 5000, and 10,000. Phospholipase A and hyaluronidase are also venom components.

More primitive ants, e.g., myrmecine and ponerine, have venoms that are more proteinaceous. Fractionation of these venoms resulted in isolation of histamines, hyaluronidase, kinin-like material, hemolytic proteins, and biochemicals that might resemble honeybee melittin.

The more advanced formicine ants have a reduced stinging apparatus and more developed anal glands for defensive and alarm secretions. Examples of compounds found in these glands are formic acid, terpenes, and ketones. Most of these seem to be used for communication between the ants themselves and other arthropods. However, the mandibles of some ants break the dermis and release a concentrated solution of formic acid into the wound. Formic acid, which is very cytotoxic, and a carrier compound, i.e., n-undecane, which aids penetration, are effective chemical combinations against human intruders.

Scorpions. These are nocturnally active arachnids; they can be easily recognized by having a pair of pincers in the front of a segmented body that ends in a 5-segment tail armed with a terminal stinger. They have 8 legs in addition to the pincers. Discovery of scorpions during the daytime is usually made by removing their protective shelter in the field (e.g., loose bark, piles of debris, rocks), in the house (e.g., in footwear, storage rooms and boxes, cabinets, clothing on the floor), and in other places somewhat protected from light. Usually, scorpions can be found immobile with the stinger laying flat or coiled next to the body. Although they may appear sluggish, the disturbance of removing their protection can cause a flurry of activity. The stinger or telson is raised above the abdomen in a defensive posture. Alternatively, they will run to other cover with the terminal segments flattened straight behind the body. The stinger is usually used to kill other arthropods. The method of striking its prey or victim (in attack or defense) is to thrust the telson over the back and head to the front. The pincers are used to hold the prey in attack, but in defense, the telson can be quickly thrust forward a number of times without the pincers being used. This is usually the case when a hand or bare foot finds the scorpion's hiding place. Unfortunately, children are often struck, possibly because of their exploratory nature.

Distribution. The distribution of dangerous scorpions is quite broad throughout the world. There are about 650 species. The most dangerous family of scorpions is Buthidae. In South America, there are 4 species of the genus *Tityus* (*T. serrulatus, T. bahensis, T. trinitatis,* and *T. trivittatus*) that are highly toxic to man. The genus *Centruroides* has about 25 species found in Mexico, Central America, and the southern United States that are considered important. In the Old World, the family Buthidae includes dangerous species in the genera *Androctonus, Buthacus, Leiurus, Buthus, Parabuthus,* and *Butheolus*. In the same region, the family Scorpionidae has perilous species in the genera *Heterometrus, Pandinus, Scorpio, Opisthophthalmus,* and *Hadogenes*.

Venom. A pair of venom glands found within the bulbous telson synthesize and store venoms of varying toxicity, depending on the species of scorpion. Consequently, information about the potentially hazardous species in a given geographic area is important. The biochemical components of the venoms of scorpions of some species are currently being studied, but little information is available as yet. In general, scorpions produce two types of venoms, hemolytic and neurotoxic. Proteins and enzyme toxins of some species cause only local reactions, whereas those of others may be highly toxic.

The local pain of some scorpion stings is sometimes caused by the presence of 5-hydroxytryptamine (serotonin). Hyaluronidase has also been found in the venoms of some scorpions.

Clinical Manifestations. The effects of envenomation

vary with the species. No severe reactions are produced by some scorpions; high mortality rates in children are caused by others. In addition to species differences, toxicity is probably based on a dose/weight relationship. Severe pain may occur at the site of the sting, with radiation into the affected limbs. Chills with abundant cold sweats may be associated with severe thirst and vomiting. Venoms may have neurotoxic effects with paralysis and convulsions or cardiovascular effects with myocarditis and tachycardia or may cause intravascular hemolysis. Death is often due to respiratory paralysis. Pancreatitis and defibrination syndromes have recently been described, with widespread hemorrhages present in most organs at autopsy. Stings by scorpions with neurotoxic venom may produce little local reaction.

TREATMENT OF ACTIVE ENVENOMATION

Anaphylaxis. Anaphylactic shock in people sensitized to venom components requires urgent treatment. The release of histamine and other mediators causes vasodilation and increased capillary permeability, with a sudden fall in blood pressure, edema of entire extremities, and bronchospasm. A fall in cardiac output may produce secondary myocardial and tissue hypoxia, arrhythmias, and metabolic acidosis. Intramuscular administration of epinephrine (Adrenalin) is immediately indicated in a dose of 0.5 ml of 1:1000. This dose should be repeated every 15 minutes until improvement occurs. Adrenalin causes constriction of the peripheral vasculature and bronchodilation. It may also inhibit further histamine release. Another treatment scheme, presented in Table 105–2, combines epinephrine with an intravenous antihistamine. Antihistamines are effective in the management of angioedema, pruritus, and urticaria (Table 105–3). Intravenous hydrocortisone sodium succinate may have a long-term beneficial effect. Circulatory collapse may require fluid replacements. In bronchospasm resistant to Adrenalin, intravenous aminophylline, oxygen, and assisted respiration may be indicated. Acute laryngeal edema may require an emergency tracheostomy.

Symptoms occur so rapidly in sensitized persons that they should carry an emergency kit of two syringes containing epinephrine and an antihistamine. Approximately 100 deaths a year occur in the United States as a result of bee or wasp stings.

Local Reactions. Large local reactions of the skin, i.e., urticaria, may be IgE-mediated. If the stinger is present (which frequently occurs in honeybee stings), it should be removed. Cold compresses are a useful first aid measure in hymenopteran sting treatment. Although antihistamines are invariably prescribed, there is no good evidence that they are beneficial. Superimposed

TABLE 105–2. Treatment of Anaphylaxis

Reaction	Immediate Treatment	Mild Reaction Treatment	Severe Reaction Treatment
Conjunctivitis Rhinitis Urticaria/angioedema Pruritus Erythema	Epinephrine hydrochloride (1:1000) 0.3–0.5 ml sc (adults) 0.15–0.3 ml sc (children) Diphenhydramine hydrochloride 25–50 mg po or terfenadine 60 mg po	Terfenadine 60 mg po every 8–12 hours	
Laryngeal edema	Epinephrine hydrochloride (1:1000) 0.3–0.5 ml sc Epinephrine (racemic) via nebulizer 0.5–0.75 ml in 3.0 ml total volume Diphenhydramine hydrochloride, 50 mg IV or IM	Epinephrine hydrochloride (1:1000) 0.3–0.5 ml sc every 20–60 minutes Epinephrine (racemic) via inhalation every 20–60 minutes Terfenadine 60 mg po every 8–12 hours	Oxygen Monitor blood gases Hydrocortisone or methylprednisolone IV Neublized racemic epinephrine (0.5–0.75 ml in 3.0 ml) every 20–60 minutes Tracheostomy
Bronchospasm	Epinephrine hydrochloride (1:1000) 0.3–0.5 ml sc Diphenhydramine hydrochloride 50 mg IV Albuterol, isoetharine, or metaproterenol nebulizer solution 0.3–0.5 ml in 3.0 ml total volume	Albuterol (up to 0.5 ml) *or* Metaproterenol (up to 0.3 ml) *or* Isoetharine (up to 0.3 ml) diluted to 3.0 ml in saline and nebulized every 20–60 minutes	Oxygen Intravenous fluids Monitor blood gases Observe for respiratory failure Methyl prednisolone 60–125 mg IV every 4–6 hours Nebulized beta-agonists every 20–60 minutes Aminophylline 5–6 mg/kg IV over 30 minutes if not on theophylline
Hypotension	Epinephrine hydrochloride (1:1000) 0.3–0.5 ml sc Diphenhydramine hydrochloride 50 mg IV Cimetidine, 300 mg IV	Intravenous fluids Epinephrine (1:1000) 0.3–0.5 ml sc every 20–30 minutes Methyl prednisolone 60–125 mg IV	Oxygen MAST (Military antishock trousers) Hydrocortisone or methylprednisolone IV Cimetidine 300 mg, IV very 4–6 hours Diphenhydramine hydrochloride, 50 ml IV every 5–6 hours Metaraminol bitartrate, 100 mg in 500 ml D5W drip

Modified with the assistance of Dr. Gary B. Carpenter, Chief of Allergy and Immunology, Walter Reed Army Medical Center, from a table used in the sixth edition.

TABLE 105–3. Antihistamines

Group	Generic Name	Trade Name	Average Oral Dose Adult	Average Oral Dose Child	Sedation
H₁ Antagonists					
Ethanolamines	Diphenhydramine hydrochloride	Benadryl	25–50 mg every 4–6 hours	12.5–25 mg every 4–6 hours	+ + + +
	Dimenhydrinate	Dramamine	50 mg every 4 hours	25 mg every 4 hours	+ + + +
Ethylenediamines	Tripelennamine hydrochloride	Pyribenzamine, PBZ	50 mg every 4–6 hours	25 mg every 4–6 hours	+ + +
Alkylamines	Chlorpheniramine maleate	Chlor-trimeton, CTM	4 mg every 6 hours	2 mg every 6 hours	+ + +
	Brompheniramine maleate	Dimetane	8 mg every 6 hours	4 mg every 6 hours	+ +
	Triprolidine hydrochloride	Actidil	2.5 mg every 6 hours	1.25 mg every 6–12 hours	+ +
Cyclizines	Hydroxyzine hydrochloride	Atarax	25–100 mg every 6–12 hours	10–25 mg every 6–12 hours	+ +
Phenothiazines	Promethazine hydrochloride	Phenergan	25–50 mg every 6–8 hours	12.5–25 mg every 6–8 hours	+ + + +
Miscellaneous	Cyproheptadine hydrochloride	Peractin	4 mg every 6 hours	2 mg every 6 hours	+ + +
	Terfenadine	Seldane	60 mg every 12 hours	30 mg every 12 hours	0
	Astemizole	Hismanal	10 mg every 24 hours	5 mg every 24 hours	0
*H₂ Antagonists**					
	Cimetidine hydrochloride	Tagamet	300–400 mg every 6 hours	20–40 mg/kg/day	0
	Rantidine	Zantac	150 mg every 12 hours		0
	Famotidine	Pepcid	20 mg every 12 hours or 40 mg at bedtime		0

*Although primarily anti–peptic ulcer and reflux medications, H₂ antagonists may be used in conjunction with classic (anti-H₁) antihistamines for the treatment of chronic urticaria or severe systemic anaphylaxis with hypotension.

Modified, with the assistance of Dr. Gary B. Carpenter, Chief of Allergy and Immunology, Walter Reed Army Medical Center, from a table used in the sixth edition.

infections such as cellulitis or septicemia require antibiotic therapy.

Ant Stings. In ant stings, medical treatment does not alter pustule formation. In fire ant stings in rabbits, no benefit is shown from treatment with topical or systemic steroids, antihistamines, sympathomimetics, local abrasion, topical povidone-iodine solution, or pustule aspiration. Care should be taken to avoid secondary infection.

Spider Bites. Rest and immobilization of a bitten limb are necessary. A firm compression with a bandage on the bite may reduce toxin dissemination, and ice packs are recommended for treating bites from *Lactrodectus* species. If systemic signs occur following a bite by this species, an ampule of antivenom (Lyovac) can be given by slow intravenous injection in 50 ml of saline solution after skin testing for hypersensitivity. Pain requires analgesics and may be sufficiently intense to justify the administration of meperidine (Demerol) or morphine. For muscle spasms, 10 ml of 10% calcium gluconate every 4 hours can be used, as can other muscle relaxants, e.g., methocarbamol. There is no clear indication for corticosteroids or antihistamines. Necrotizing bites of South American *Loxosceles* spiders can be treated by locally available antivenom. In other areas, treatment of bites consists of supportive care and 40 mg of dexamethasone given every 6 hours for the first 48 hours. Application of local antiseptic to open ulcers is necessary. In the healing phase, skin grafting may be indicated.

Centipede Bites. The pain of a centipede bite can be relieved by infiltrating the affected area with 1% lidocaine (Xylocaine).

Scorpion Stings. Immediate treatment of a scorpion sting is directed toward delaying absorption of the venom. A constricting band is applied to the limb and is released every 20 to 30 minutes. If available, ice packs should be applied to the site, and the patient should be kept at rest. Specific antiserum is available in some countries, e.g., Mexico and Brazil, and should be given if signs occur that the central nervous system is being affected.

Passive Envenomation

Some stinging arthropods play a more passive role. Specialized cells and morphologic structures, i.e., setae and spines, synthesize toxins and irritating chemicals to repel an offending animal. Man himself often provides the force necessary to introduce the venom.

CATERPILLARS. Irritant hairs or spines present on caterpillars (order Lepidoptera) cause dermatitis on skin contact. In Brazil, five families of nocturnal moths and the Morphidae family of butterflies have larvae with such structures. The spines are of two general types, either a simple linear shaft of a spinous hair that may be branched with a detachable cap. Both types have a simple poison gland at their hollow base. These urticating hairs may be distributed over the entire body of the caterpillar. The venoms are poorly characterized, but symptoms of itching papules or urticaria, often associated with transient edema, are well known. The puss caterpillars (*Megalopyge* species) in the United States and elsewhere are very hairy, with hidden spines. They should be avoided but are frequently brushed against by accident. Sticky cellophane tape applied to the skin will often pick up the spines, which can be seen microscopically. Calamine lotion is often sufficient to relieve itching. Stinging and irritation can also have an allergic basis, resulting in other medical complications.

BEETLES. Two families of beetles (order Coleoptera) have urticating substances causing skin reaction in man. The Staphylinidae contain a genus of small beetles, *Paederus.* When accidentally crushed on the skin, a vesicant in the hemolymph of *Paederus* causes painful erythema and blistering (Fig. 105–2). In the Amazon region of Brazil, reactions to these beetles may persist for several weeks and leave a pigmented scar. Another species in Kenya causes the so-called Nairobi eye, conjunctival contamination by the beetle resulting in a unilateral conjunctivitis and orbital edema. The Meloidae (blister and oil beetles) are larger and often brightly colored and are attacted to artificial light at night. Hemolymph exuded through integumental membranes or expelled on crushing contains cantharidin, a vesicant that often causes large blisters. Topical treatment of the blisters with magnesium sulfate or methyl alcohol has been recommended.

MILLIPEDES AND OTHERS. Secretions from a number of other arthropods can also irritate the eyes, nose, and skin. Millipedes (class Diplopoda) are scavengers living on decayed vegetation; some species can forcibly release a defensive, odoriferous fluid from segmental glands. Dermatitis may be followed by bullae and, occasionally, necrosis. The giant whip scorpion or vinegarroon *(Mastigoproctus giganteus),* and night-hunting arachnid, can directionally eject secretions of acetic acid and caprylic acid. Some beetles (e.g., Carabidae and Tenebrionidae) and true bugs (e.g., Coreidae and Pentatomidae) can also release obnoxious secretions. These are usually gaseous and are repugnant to humans.

REFERENCES

Barriga OO: Immune reaction to arthropods. *In* Immunology of Parasitic Infections, Baltimore, University Park Press, 1981, pp. 283–317.

Beard RB: Insect toxins and insect venoms. Ann Rev Entomol 8:1, 1963.

Bellas TE: Insects as a cause of inhalation allergies. A bibliography. CSIRO Australian Division of Entomology, Reprint No. 25. Canberra City, CSIRO. 2nd ed., 1982.

Bettini S (ed.): Arthropod Venoms. Handbook of Experimental Pharmacology. Vol. 48. New York, Springer-Verlag, 1978.

Biery TS: Venomous Arthropod Handbook. Washington, D.C., U.S. Government Printing Office, 1977, AFP 191–243.

Blum MS: Biochemical defenses of insects. *In* Rockstein M (ed.): Biochemistry of Insects, New York, Academic Press, 1978, pp. 465–513.

Bousquet J, Müller UR, Dreborg S, et al: Immunotherapy with Hymenoptera venoms. Allergy 42:401, 1987.

Bücherl W, Buckley E (eds.): Venomous Animals and Their Venoms. Vol. III. Venomous Invertebrates. New York, Academic Press, 1971.

Delori P, Rietschoten JV, Rochat H: Scorpion venoms and neurotoxins: an immunological study. Toxicon 19:393, 1981.

Ebeling W: Urban Entomology. Davis, University of California, Division of Agricultural Sciences, 1978.

Feingold BF, Benjamini E, Michael D: The allergic responses to insect bites. Ann Rev Entomol. 13:137, 1968.

Frazier CA, Brown FK: Insects and Allergy and What To Do About Them. Norman, University of Oklahoma Press, 1980.

Habermann E: Bee and wasp venoms. Science 177:314, 1972.

Harwood RF, James MT: Entomology in Human and Animal Health. New York, Macmillan, 1979.

Hopla CE: Arthropodiasis. *In* Steele JH (ed.): CRC Handbook Series in Zoonoses, Section C: Parasitic Zoonoses, Vol. III. Boca Raton, CRC Press, 1982, pp. 215–247.

James MT: Flies That Cause Myiasis in Man. Washington, D.C., U.S. Department of Agriculture, 1947, Miscellaneous Publication 631.

Keegan HL: Venomous bites and stings in Mississippi. J Miss State Med Assoc 8:495, 1972.

Le Mao J, Dandeu JP, Rabillon J, et al.: Antigens and allergens in *Dermatophagoides farinae* mite. Immunology 44:239, 1981.

Levine MJ, Lockey RF: Monograph on Insect Allergy. American Academy of Allergy Publication. Hartland, Wisconsin, Parker Printing, 1981.

Minton SA: Venom Disease. Springfield, Illinois, Charles C Thomas, 1974.

Mueller HL, Schmid WH, Ribiniztain R: Stinging insect hypersensitivity: A 20 year study of immunological treatment. Pediatrics 55:530, 1975.

Nelson WA, Bell JF, Clifford CM, et al.: Interaction of ectoparasites and their hosts. J Med Entomol 13:389, 1977.

Ori M; Biology and poisonings by spiders. *In* Tu AT (ed.): Insect Poisons, Allergens, and Other Invertebrate Venoms. New York, Marcel Dekker, 1984, pp 397–440.

Orkin M, Maibach HI, Parish LC, et al.: Scabies and Pediculosis. Philadelphia, J. B. Lippincott, 1977.

Owen S, Morganstern M, Hepworth J, Woodcock A: Control of dust mite antigen in bedding. Lancet 335:396, 1990.

Parrish HM: Analysis of 460 fatalities from venomous animals in the United States. Am J Med Sci 245:129, 1963.

Reisman RE, Lazell M, Doerr J: Insect venom allergy: A prospective case study showing lack of correlation between immunologic reactivity and clinical sensitivity. J Allergy Clin Immunol 68:406, 1981.

Riebeiro JMC, Makoul GT, Levine J, et al.: Antihemostatic, antiinflamatory, and immunosuppressive properties of saliva of a tick, *Ixodes dammini.* J Exp Med 161:332, 1985.

Schmidt JO: Biochemistry of insect venoms. Ann Rev Entomol 27:339, 1982.

Schumacher MJ, Schmidt JO, Egen NB, Lowry JE: Quality, analysis, and lethality of European and Africanized honey bee venoms. Am J Trop Med Hyg 43:79, 1990.

Smith KGV (ed.): Insects and Other Arthropods of Medical Importance. London, British Museum, 1973, Publication No. 720.

Tovey ER, Chapman MD, Platts-Mills TAE: Mite feces are a major source of house dust allergens. Nature 289:592, 1981.

Treatment of anaphylactic shock. Br Med J 282:1011, 1981.

Van Bronswijk JEMH, Sinha RN: Pyroglyphid mites (Acari) and house dust allergy. J Allergy 47:31, 1971.

Wikel SK: Immune responses to arthropods and their products. Ann Rev Entomol 27:21, 1982.

Wirtz RA: Allergic and toxic reactions to non-stinging arthropods. Ann Rev Entomol 69:47, 1984.

Yunginger JW: Advances in the diagnosis and treatment of stinging insect allergy. Pediatrics 67:325, 1981.

PART VIII

NUTRITIONAL PROBLEMS AND DEFICIENCY DISEASES

GENERAL PRINCIPLES

Michael C. Latham

Tropical diseases are generally those that are more common and important in the tropics than in other geographic regions. They include some that are confined primarily to the tropics because the organism causing the disease, or the vector carrying it, can easily propagate only in warm climates (e.g., trypanosomiasis and schistosomiasis). However, the majority of so-called tropical diseases are illnesses that are currently more prevalent in the nonindustrialized countries in the tropics or subtropics. However, many formerly existed in Europe and the Americas. Many of the tropical diseases are related also to poverty, inequity, and their accompaniments, including poor sanitation, contaminated water supplies, lack of education, and poor knowledge about disease etiology and prevention. The major remaining nutritional deficiency diseases in tropical and nonindustrialized countries are also not "tropical" in the sense that they have not always been confined by climate and geography. In general, they are most prevalent in the poor nonindustrialized nations because of their relationship to poverty and to food conditions in these countries. But none of them have been totally eradicated from the nontropical countries.

DEFINITION OF TROPICAL NUTRITIONAL PROBLEMS. Tropical medicine as a subject, or a discipline, has not truly embraced nutrition and has not given sufficient or proper recognition to different forms of malnutrition as tropical diseases. Yet kwashiorkor, nutritional marasmus, xerophthalmia, iodine deficiency disorders, and pellagra are just as much tropical diseases as are, for example, malaria, cholera, yellow fever, and ascariasis. Tropical medicine has been almost totally dominated by tropical infections, particularly parasitic infections. Tropical deficiency diseases are inadequately covered in most congresses, courses, journals, and textbooks dealing with "Tropical Medicine." When they are included, often it is not to consider them as tropical diseases, but rather to give consideration to how nutrition impinges on infections and vice versa. For example, at the 1988 International Congress on Tropical Medicine and Malaria held in Amsterdam, there were 3 round table sessions on nutrition; however, each was on the relationship between nutrition and tropical infections. There were no sessions on protein-energy malnutrition, xerophthalmia, iodine deficiency disorders, or nutritional anemias.

The relationship of nutrition to infections is important (Chapter 109.1). Tropical infections and nutritional deficiencies occur commonly in the same populations. Poor nutritional status can reduce the person's resistance to infection and can make the body more vulnerable to infection; in many cases, the infectious disease is more severe and more often fatal in the malnourished patient. Infections also adversely affect nutritional status. They commonly worsen the nutritional status and precipitate malnutrition.

THE DIMENSIONS OF THE MAJOR NUTRITIONAL PROBLEMS. There are no accurate figures on the global prevalence of malnutrition, and good estimates are difficult to obtain. Many would argue that malnutrition is the single most important public health problem for children in tropical countries. Millions of adults suffer from deficiency diseases also. Malnutrition tends to be greatly under-reported in morbidity and particularly in mortality statistics. This is because many children whose cause of death was recorded, for example, as being due to diarrhea or measles may have survived had they not been malnourished.

In 1974 at the World Food Conference in Rome it was stated that 500 million people in the world were underfed. That was probably an underestimate. Today the numbers are undoubtedly larger, because almost 2 billion people have been added to the world's population in the last 15 years, and most of these live in poor developing countries. An attempt by the World Health Organization (WHO) to provide prevalence rates of WHO's "big four" deficiency diseases is given in Table VIII–1.

Protein-energy malnutrition, nutritional anemias, vitamin A deficiency leading to xerophthalmia, and iodine deficiency disorders are the four most important nutritional problems in tropical countries. Each disease is due to a deficient intake of 1 or more nutrients, but the underlying etiology is often not straightforward. There are many contributing causes, because food has to be available to the individual, he or she has to consume it, the nutrients need to be properly absorbed and utilized, and metabolism has to be normal. If any link in the chain is broken, or interfered with, malnutrition may ensue. Therefore, factors such as poverty, inappropriate bulky foods, anorexia, infections, conditions affecting absorption, and metabolic disorders may contribute to malnutrition. There are also diet-drug interactions that may importantly influence nutrition (Chapter 109.3).

TABLE VIII–1. Gross Worldwide Estimate of Total Number of Persons Affected by Currently Preventable Malnutrition

Deficiency	Morbidity due to Malnutrition	Prevalence[1]	Age (years)	Mortality per Year
Protein and energy	Stunted growth[2, 10]	500 million	0–6	
	Clinical cases of kwashiorkor and marasmus[4]	1 million	1–4	10 million[3, 5]
Iron	Anemia[6]	900 million	All ages	
Vitamin A	Blindness[7]	6 million	All ages	750,000
Iodine	Goiter[8]	150 million	All ages	
	Cretinism[9]	6 million	All ages	

[1] The estimates are gross and do not express the significant variations occurring not only from country to country but within countries.

[2] Stunted growth defined by weight below the 2.5th percentile of the WHO growth standards. This figure includes mild malnutrition and is therefore higher than the usual estimated 200 million of moderate to severe malnourished.

[3] Often due to diarrhea as proximate cause of death. Most cases of death by diarrhea (about 1.5% of 1 to 4 year olds or 4.6 million a year) are associated with stunting and wasting.

[4] About 1.5% of those with stunted growth are so malnourished that they will show the life-threatening symptoms of marasmus and kwashiorkor within the year, e.g., 7.5 million cases per year. The mean duration of kwashiorkor is about a month and of marasmus, about 3 months, for an average of 2 months. The prevalence at any given time is thus over 1 million.

[5] Of the 7.5 million cases per year of kwashiorkor and marasmus, most die, e.g., 7 million. Many of these die with diarrhea.

[6] 33% of women aged 18 to 45 years are anemic. Some anemia results from hookworm infections.

[7] This is an underestimation of persons affected, because it includes only those cases in Southeast Asia. This area has the highest prevalence in the world, but further cases should be added from Africa and the Americas. Of a million new cases of blindness per year, 25% survive that year, so there are 250,000 blind survivors each year. These probably have another 40 years of mean life span, resulting in a prevalence of 6 million.

[8] 200 million estimated in 1960. We estimate successful campaigns against goiter have reduced the prevalence, so that about 150 million suffer from goiter today.

[9] In goitrous populations 1.5% of the children born have severe mental and physical retardation (cretinism). 750 million people live in goitrous areas (overall prevalence of 20% goiter in such areas). Thus, about 250,000 cretins are born a year in these areas. Even if their life span is half that of noncretins, 6 million persons living today are mentally deficient because of maternal iodine deficiency.

[10] The first manifestations of stunting appear at birth, defined by low weight for gestational age. A rough estimate has been made of 22 million live-born low-birth-weight infants, equivalent to ⅙ of total number of births. If ⅓ of these cases are due to other factors, there are at least 14 million nutrition-related stunted babies born each year. Some evidence suggests a higher mortality for these babies than for bigger babies.

Table VIII–2 provides a summary of the manifestations of the more important nutrient deficiency diseases discussed in the following pages. It gives a short-hand summary of the clinical manifestations and of the more commonly used laboratory tests for each disease.

The deficiency diseases described in this section are generally those that are considerably more prevalent in poor nonindustrialized countries than in the affluent nations. There is 1 exception—dental caries—but with greatly increased numbers of persons in urban areas of northern countries now consuming fluoridated water supplies, the rates of dental caries are diminishing in these countries, while rising in many poorer countries. Nutritional anemia is another condition that remains moderately prevalent among affluent populations but is much more common in tropical countries.

This section does not discuss nutritional conditions related to affluence, or those that are more common in the northern industrialized countries. For example, in Europe and North America the major diseases in which nutrition plays an important role are arteriosclerosis, often leading to coronary heart disease; obesity; hypertension (sometimes related to high sodium intakes) and stroke; diabetes mellitus; and possibly some cancers. Tropical populations are not immune to these important diseases. Some cancers that may be influenced by dietary intake are in fact commoner in tropical areas. But the other conditions are more associated with overconsumption of certain nutrients or foodstuffs and with western diets and lifestyles. In many tropical countries the more affluent and more westernized part of the population is now increasingly experiencing these disease conditions. The causes and clinical aspects of, for example, arteriosclerotic heart disease, hypertension, diabetes, morbid obesity, and malignant disease are well covered in textbooks of medicine.

As diets improve and as undernutrition becomes less important in developing countries, it is rather easy for populations to pass rapidly through a phase where nutrition is relatively good to a situation where problems related to overnutrition or overconsumption of certain nutrients become common. Countries where there is more equity, both in incomes and food consumption, may enjoy less malnutrition and also less heart disease and obesity compared with nations that are poor or where wealth and food are inequitably distributed.

RECOMMENDED DAILY INTAKES OF NUTRIENTS. The requirements for certain nutrients are based on research in both animals and humans. The physiologic and biochemical bases for recommended allowances of specific nutrients are discussed in standard textbooks of nutrition. Many countries have established their own recommendations of daily intakes or allowances of nutrients. These are designed usually to afford a margin of sufficiency above average physiologic requirements to cover variations in the general population. (Table VIII–3). They are useful as guidelines for the evaluation of the adequacy of diets of groups of people and to make policy recommendations for improvements. Their use is often dependent on obtaining reasonably accurate information on the quantity of foods being consumed in the diets of a population and then on the use of tables of nutrient content of foods eaten by that population. Often such data are not easy to obtain in tropical and other countries. It must be recognized also that great variations exist in the quantities and types of food consumed by different communities and in ecological areas within countries. The use of mean figures of

TABLE VIII–2. Manifestations of Important Nutrient Deficiency Diseases

Disease	Nutrient	Prevalence	Clinical Manifestations	Laboratory Tests
Protein-energy malnutrition, kwashiorkor, nutritional marasmus (Chapter 106)	Protein and energy	Very high	Growth retardation and wasting; in kwashiorkor—edema, flaky paint dermatosis, hepatomegaly, hair changes, mental signs; in marasmus—loss of subcutaneous fat, extreme wasting	In kwashiorkor—low total serum protein and very low serum albumin levels; low levels of digestive enzymes; in marasmus—low urinary hydroxyproline
Xerophthalmia (Chapter 107.1)	Vitamin A	High	Night blindness; conjunctival xerosis; Bitot's spots; corneal xerosis and ulceration; keratomalacia; corneal scarring	Low serum vitamin A levels; altered relative dose response; changed cytology of conjunctival cells
Beriberi, Wernicke's encephalopathy (Chapter 107.2)	Thiamine (Vitamin B_1)	Moderate low	Weakness; peripheral neuropathy; loss of reflexes; ataxia; weight loss; edema; dyspnea; heart failure; in infants—tachycardia, aphonia, heart failure. In Wernicke's syndrome—ataxia, ocular signs, psychosis	Low whole blood or erythrocyte transketolase activity; low urinary thiamine in 24 hour urines or per gm of creatinine; low thiamine in whole blood
Ariboflavinosis (Chapter 107.6)	Riboflavin	High	Cheilosis of the lips; angular stomatitis; glossitis; seborrheic dermatitis, often of genitalia	Raised levels of erythrocyte glutathione reductase; low urinary riboflavin levels in 24 hour urines or per gm of creatinine
Pellagra (Chapter 107.5)	Niacin	Moderate low	Photosensitive dermatitis on light-exposed areas; diarrhea; stomatitis; mental confusion, depression, and psychosis	Low levels of urinary N^1-methyl-nicotinamide in 24 hour urines or per gm of creatinine; low niacin in whole blood
Scurvy (Chapter 107.3)	Ascorbic acid (vitamin C)	Low	Swollen fragile papillae between teeth; bleeding gums; petechial and other skin hemorrhages; depression; weakness; in infants—tender swellings of bones; pithed frog position	Low leukocyte vitamin C; low serum ascorbate levels
Megaloblastic anemia (Chapter 107.7)	Folate, vitamin B_{12}	Medium	Anorexia; tiredness; dyspnea; ankle edema; cheilitis	Low hemoglobin; hypersegmentation of polymorphonuclear leukocytes; megaloblastic red cells; macrocytic RBCs; low levels of serum folate; increased FIGLU
Rickets, osteomalacia (Chapter 107.4)	Vitamin D	Moderate low	In rickets—craniotabes, bony deformities, rickety rosary due to enlargement of costochondral junctions, bow legs, kyphosis, bossing of skull; in osteomalacia—bone tenderness and pain, kyphosis and bony deformities, waddling gait, tetany	Low plasma 25-hydroxychole-calciferol levels; increased plasma alkaline phosphatase
Microcytic anemia (Chapter 108.1)	Iron	Very high	Tiredness, weakness, dyspnea, pallor of tongue, nailbeds and conjunctiva; occasionally pica	Low hemoglobin; low serum ferritin; low transferrin saturation; raised free erythrocyte protoporphyrin; hypochromic macrocytic RBCs
Iodine deficiency disorders, goiter, cretinism (Chapter 108.2)	Iodine	Very high	Enlargement of thyroid gland; in children born of iodine-deficient mothers—cretinism, mental retardation, deaf mutism; strabismus	Low urinary iodine levels
Zinc deficiency (Chapter 108.4)	Zinc	Low	Acrodermatitis enteropathica with bullous dermatitis; dwarfing; hypogonadism	Decreased plasma zinc levels
Dental caries (Chapter 108.3)	Fluoride (other causes)	Very high	Tooth cavities; tooth decay; loss of teeth. Excess fluoride causes dental fluorosis with mottling of teeth and skeletal fluorosis	

TABLE VIII–3. Recommended Intakes of Nutrients, FAO/WHO*

Age (years)	Body Weight (kg)	Energy kcal	Energy MJ	Protein† (gm)	Vitamin A‡ (µg)	Vitamin D§ (µg)	Thiamine (mg)	Riboflavin (mg)	Niacin (mg)	Folic Acid (µg)	Vitamin B₁₂ (µg)	Ascorbic Acid (mg)	Calcium (gm)	Iron‖ (mg)
Children														
<1	7.3	820	3.4	14	300	10.0	0.3	0.5	5.4	60	0.3	20	0.5–0.6	5–10
1–3	13.4	1360	5.7	16	250	10.0	0.5	0.8	9.0	100	0.9	20	0.4–0.5	5–10
4–6	20.2	1830	7.6	20	300	10.0	0.7	1.1	12.1	100	1.5	20	0.4–0.5	5–10
7–9	28.1	2190	9.2	25	400	2.5	0.9	1.3	14.5	100	1.5	20	0.4–0.5	5–10
Male adolescents														
10–12	36.9	2600	10.9	30	575	2.5	1.0	1.6	17.2	100	2.0	20	0.6–0.7	5–10
13–15	51.3	2900	12.1	37	725	2.5	1.2	1.7	19.1	200	2.0	30	0.6–0.7	9–18
16–19	62.9	3070	12.8	38	750	2.5	1.2	1.8	20.3	200	2.0	30	0.5–0.6	5–19
Female adolescents														
10–12	38.0	2350	9.8	29	575	2.5	0.9	1.4	15.5	100	2.0	20	0.6–0.7	5–10
13–15	49.9	2490	10.4	31	725	2.5	1.0	1.5	16.4	200	2.0	30	0.6–0.7	12–24
16–19	54.4	2310	9.7	30	750	2.5	0.9	1.4	15.2	200	2.0	30	0.5–0.6	14–28
Adult man moderately active	65.0	3000	12.6	37	750	2.5	1.2	1.8	19.8	200	2.0	30	0.4–0.5	5–19
Adult woman moderately active	55.0	2200	9.2	29	750	2.5	0.9	1.3	14.5	200	2.0	30	0.4–0.5	14–28
Pregnancy latter half		+350	+1.5	38	750	10.0	+0.1	+0.2	+2.3	400	3.0	50	1.0–1.2	**
Lactation first 6 months		+550	+2.3	46	1200	10.0	+0.2	+0.4	+3.7	300	2.5	50	1.0–1.2	**

*From Food and Agriculture Organization: Handbook on Human Nutritional Requirements Rome, FAO/WHO, 1974.
†As milk or milk protein for infants.
‡As retinol
§As cholecalciferol
‖On each line, the lower value applies when over 25% of calories in the diet come from animal foods, and the higher value applies when animal foods represent less than 10% of calories.
**For women whose iron intake throughout life has been at the level recommended in this table, the daily intake of iron during pregnancy and lactation should be the same as that recommended for nonpregnant, nonlactating women of childbearing age. For women whose iron status is not satisfactory at the beginning of pregnancy, the requirement is increased, and in the extreme situation of women with no iron stores, the requirement can probably not be met without supplementation.

nutrient consumption for a population may mask major differences between the best and the worst fed. Caution is warranted in using such data.

BIBLIOGRAPHY

Grant JP: The State of the World's Children 1987. Oxford, UNICEF/ Oxford University Press, 1987, pp 1–148.
Latham MC: International nutrition problems and policies. *In* World Food Issues, 2nd ed. Ithaca, NY, Cornell University, 1984.
Latham MC: Human Nutrition in Tropical Africa. Rome, FAO, 1979, pp 1–286.
Present Knowledge in Nutrition. Nutrition Reviews. 1984, pp 1–900.
Passmore R, Eastwood MA: Human Nutrition and Dietetics, 8th ed. Edinburgh, Churchill Livingstone, 1986, pp 1–666.
Shils ME, Young VR (eds.): Modern Nutrition in Health and Disease, 7th ed. Philadelphia, Lea & Febiger, 1988, pp 1–168.
WHO: A Health and Nutrition Atlas. Geneva World Health Organization, May 1988, pp 1–31.

106. PROTEIN-ENERGY MALNUTRITION

Derrick B. Jelliffe and E. F. Patrice Jelliffe

The term "protein-energy malnutrition" (PEM) covers not only the severe clinical syndromes of kwashiorkor and marasmus but also the much more numerous mild to moderate cases, best envisaged in the PEM "iceberg" (Fig. 106–1). In addition, the term has the advantage of emphasizing the often underappreciated importance of energy (calories) both in infant feeding and in treatment.

PEM is mainly a problem in early childhood but can occur in all forms, including kwashiorkor, in older children and even in adults, e.g., in malnourished multiparous women as a form of maternal depletion syndrome, especially in famine circumstances. Severe degrees of PEM, however, are rare outside early childhood, except in famine conditions.

106.1. KWASHIORKOR

DEFINITION AND HISTORY. Kwashiorkor is 1 of the 2 severe syndromes of PEM of early childhood. Characteristically, it occurs mainly in the second year of life, but the age of onset depends principally on local infant feeding practices. Kwashiorkor is usually considered to be due to an unbalanced diet, one that is low in protein but contains carbohydrate calories, associated with a variable burden of microbial and parasitic infections, toxic, and psychosocial factors. The name "kwashiorkor," first used in the medical literature by Cicely

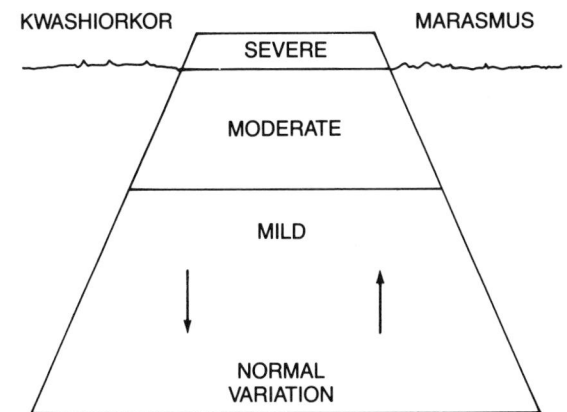

FIGURE 106–1. The protein-energy malnutrition (PEM) iceberg.

Williams in 1933, means "condition seen in the displaced child" in the Ga language of Ghana and reflected traditional recognition that the condition occurs commonly when the infant is weaned from the mother's breast.

ETIOLOGY. As with all forms of PEM, the detailed etiology of kwashiorkor varies from area to area, but it is always due to the cumulative effect of multiple factors—dietary, infective, and psychosocial.

Diet. As mentioned previously, the primary cause of kwashiorkor is an unbalanced diet, one that is low in protein but contains some carbohydrate calories, in the early years of life, when nutrient needs for growth are relatively much higher than in later childhood or adult life. Various other nutrient deficiencies will be present also, e.g., iron, riboflavin, and folic acid, varying with local dietary habits.

In many traditional communities, kwashiorkor is principally a disease of the second year of life. This can best be understood by examining the 4-stage weight curves seen commonly in these circumstances (Fig. 106–2). Despite an often low birth weight, for the first 6 months or so the breast-fed infant usually gains weight and is protected from infections by maternal antibodies acquired transplacentally and by the anti-infective properties of human milk. In the second 6 months of life, growth is often less, as the diet frequently comprises decreasing quantities of breast milk, together with a small amount of largely carbohydrate gruels or pastes. This inadequate and unbalanced nutrient intake is associated with waning passive immunity and increasing exposure to infections.

The third stage of growth occurs usually in the second year of life. Breast-feeding may have been stopped, or if lactation is continuing, the quantity of mother's milk is no longer adequate for the child's needs, and often other feedings will consist mainly of carbohydrate-rich foods of low nutritional value and "density." At the same time, the nonimmune child is exposed to a wide and cumulative burden of bacterial, viral, and parasitic infections of nutritional significance. During this dangerous phase, the weight curve may remain flat or may decline into moderate PEM. In severe instances, kwashiorkor develops, often precipitated by an added "contributory infection," such as measles or infectious diarrhea. In less affected children, the weight gradually starts to increase again in the third or fourth year of life, although the curve often remains below reference levels.

This type of inadequate diet may be due to poverty, lack of availability of food, lack of knowledge about and poor feeding practices (e.g., too few meals a day), "cultural blocks" (e.g., available foods being prohibited for infants because of cultural beliefs), or, very often, a combination of all of these.

Infections. The mechanisms leading to nutritional ill effects in infections include increased nutrient requirements, anorexia, vomiting, diminished absorption (in diarrhea), increased losses (e.g., protein loss in hookworm infection), or nutrient competition (e.g., large numbers of roundworms or the needs of literally millions of malarial parasites). This can sometimes be compounded further by ill-advised therapy, such as severe restriction of food or purgation.

Measles, whooping cough, diarrheal diseases, and tuberculosis are important as contributory infections. Heavy burdens of hookworm, roundworm, or whip-

FIGURE 106–2. Classic 4-stage weight curve characteristically seen in many traditional village circumstances. (Adapted from Jelliffe DB: Child Nutrition in Developing Countries. Washington, D.C., USAID, U.S. Government Printing Office, 1968, and Jelliffe DB: Protein-calorie malnutrition. *In* Woodruff AW [ed.]: Medicine in the Tropics. Edinburgh and New York, Churchill Livingstone, 1974.)

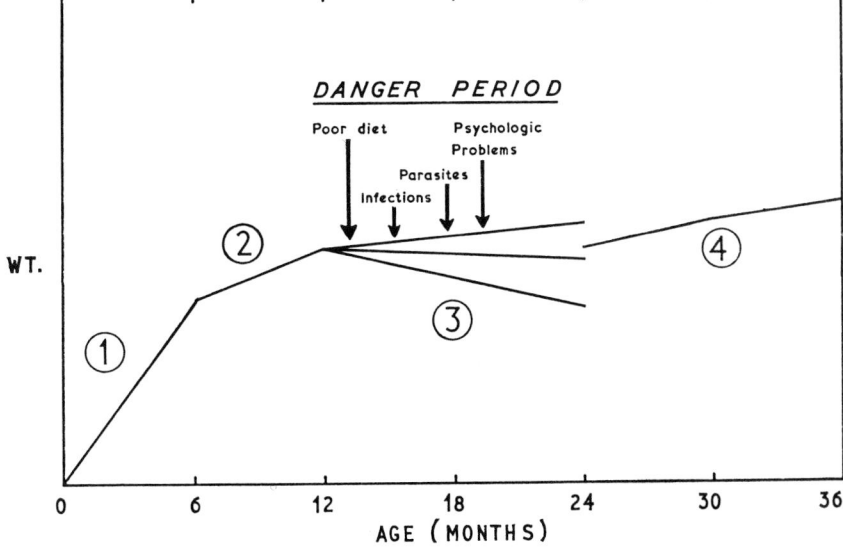

worm have considerable nutritional consequences also, as does the persistent heavy parasitemia found universally in young children in hyperendemic malarial areas.

Psychosocial Factors. Weaning, in the sense of separation from the breast, can have great nutritional and psychologic consequences. However, the process varies considerably in different cultures, and its effects depend on many factors, including its abruptness, the degree of preparation, whether the child is "compensated," whether there is actual geographic separation from the mother, and the age at which it occurs. Apart from the loss of the small but still significant quantity of breast milk, the psychologic trauma of the process may lead to a form of "maternal deprivation syndrome," long recognized in recently orphaned young children. This is characterized by depression, poor appetite, vomiting, and general lack of interest—all tending to produce nutritional deterioration.

Family instability, such as can occur with illegitimacy and paternal irresponsibility, may contribute to PEM both directly, as a result of lack of money to buy nutritious foods, and indirectly, because of defective child care by a sibling or low-paid caretaker when mothers leave home to work.

Toxins. Recent work has suggested that mycotoxins on moldy grain and legumes (especially aflatoxin) may play a part in the etiology of kwashiorkor, especially in producing liver damage. It has also been hypothesized that free radicals play a role in the etiology of kwashiorkor.

EPIDEMIOLOGY. Kwashiorkor occurs in areas with poverty, limited education, poor sanitation, insufficient food production, and inadequate health services, so that currently it is principally a public health problem in impoverished, less technically developed regions of the world, mostly situated in the tropics (Table 106–1). However, it has been reported occasionally in all parts of the world in disadvantaged families.

Kwashiorkor often has a seasonal incidence, related either to outbreaks of infectious diseases (e.g., measles or diarrhea) or to annual food shortages of the "hungry season," occurring in the early rains before the crops have been harvested. It has its main impact on young children in the early preschool group (1 to 4 years old), especially those in the second year of life.

Information on the incidence or prevalence of kwashiorkor is far from complete. Most statistics are derived from hospital or health centers and are therefore biased by many circumstances, including distances and local transportation problems, cultural beliefs about the condition, and hospital criteria for admission. Nevertheless, it is useful to gather information from health services as widely as possible by training medical and paramedical personnel and primary health care workers to recognize and record the condition as part of a nutritional surveillance system.

Field surveys performed in various developing countries in nonfamine circumstances often show a prevalence of 1 to 7% of this severe form of PEM in young children in the community at large, as opposed to a 10 to 20% admission rate to children's wards of hospitals.

PATHOLOGY. The major pathologic consequences of kwashiorkor are on the organs with the highest turnover rate of protein, although these are protected initially by depletion of the body's own basic protein reserves, e.g., muscle. The liver shows extreme fatty infiltration, and its dysfunction is reflected in low serum albumin levels. All enzyme systems are affected, including intestinal and pancreatic secretions, which further impairs digestion, exacerbating the nutritional status and interfering with treatment. Organs and tissues become smaller, and the gastrointestinal tract becomes thinner.

CLINICAL MANIFESTATIONS. These vary from one region of the world to another, depending on genetic background (e.g., normal hair color), age of onset, rapidity of development, chronicity, dietary details, and the types of conditioning infections present. Kwashiorkor is a variable syndrome, and it is unwise to generalize too widely from the picture seen in one area. Nevertheless, it is useful to divide the clinical features into 3 groups—constant, usual, and occasional (Fig. 106–3).

Constant. The 4 basic features of kwashiorkor are edema, growth failure, psychomotor change, and wasted muscles, with overlying subcutaneous fat.

Edema. Pitting edema is the cardinal diagnostic sign. It is first present over the feet, ankles, lower legs, and sacrum, but in severe cases, it may be generalized, involving the hands, forearms, and face. Impaired osmotic pressure associated with low serum albumin is partly responsible, but metabolic effects on the endocrine system, particularly the adrenal glands, lead to sodium retention.

Growth Failure. This is always present and is best detected by a failure to gain weight or a loss of weight on serial measurements. The extent of the depleted body weight is masked by the associated edema and is revealed only during treatment, when the edema subsides.

Psychomotor Change. This is characteristic but is impossible to measure objectively. It is typified by a whining, apathetic lethargy or by a miserable withdrawal.

Muscle Wasting. This is always present with some overlying subcutaneous fat. In the severely edematous child, muscle wasting is visible in the neck muscles and in those of the upper arms.

Usual

Anemia. Anemia of some degree is usual in kwashiorkor. This is basically due to lack of protein, together

TABLE 106–1. Total Numbers of Children Affected by Protein-Energy Malnutrition, WHO Estimates*

Area	Population Aged 0 to 5 Years (millions)†	Number of Children with Protein-Energy Malnutrition (millions)		
		Severe	Moderate	Total
Latin America	46	0.7	8.8	9.5
Africa	61	2.7	16.3	19.0
Asia‡	206	6.6	64.4	71.0
Total	313	10.0	89.5	99.5

*From De Maeyer E: Protein-energy malnutrition. *In* Beaton GH, Bengoa JM (eds.): Nutrition in Preventive Medicine. Geneva, World Health Organization, 1976.

†Averages for the years 1963 to 1973.

‡Excluding China and Japan.

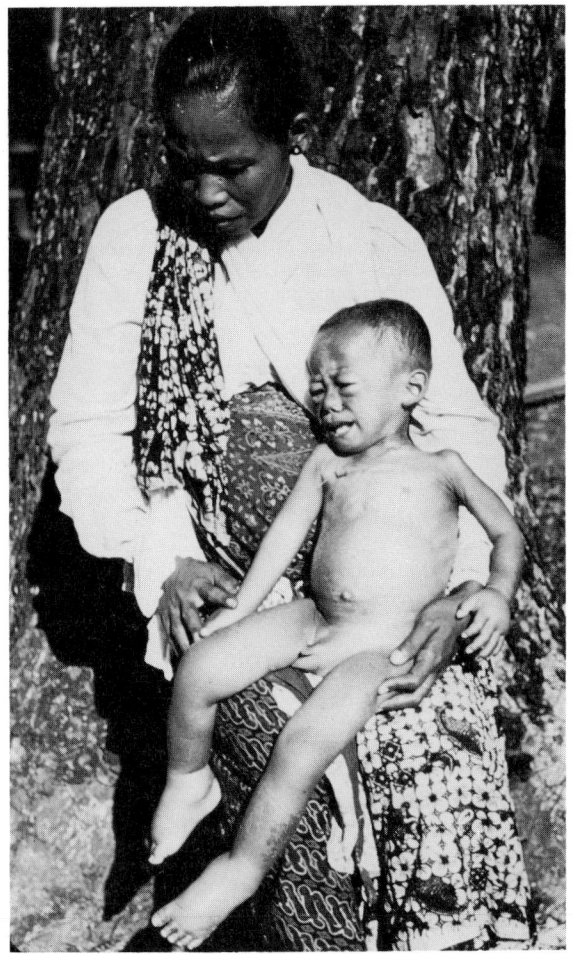

FIGURE 106–3. Kwashiorkor (Indonesia). Child in second year of life with edema, misery, growth retardation, and wasted muscles (with some subcutaneous fat present), together with "flaky paint" dermatosis (lower left leg), light, sparse hair, and hypopigmented skin (compared with mother). (Courtesy of the late Dr. H.A.P.C. Oomen.)

with an associated deficiency of iron or folic acid. The effects of malaria, the blood loss from such intestinal helminths as hookworm or whipworm, or the general effect of any bacterial infection may be contributory also.

Hair Changes. These are common in kwashiorkor, although neither universal nor necessary for diagnosis. For example, the hair may be normal in kwashiorkor of acute onset in the first year of life. Dyspigmentation of the hair can be striking. Various light shades may occur, including pale brown, red-brown, blonde, and grey. In kwashiorkor, the hair is also often sparse, easily pluckable, silky, and straight (in groups with naturally curly hair). Paralleling the dyspigmentation of the hair, there is often a lightening in color of the skin, especially that of the face (Fig. 106–3).

Loose Stools. Loose stools are caused by several factors, often interacting. Classic intestinal infectious pathogenic organisms, e.g., shigella, salmonella, or rotaviruses, may be present from a preceding diarrheal infection. In addition, PEM itself leads to loose stools from decreased secretion of pancreatic and intestinal enzymes, especially lactase, from altered microbial flora, and possibly from changes in gut motility.

Moon Face. This is partly due to subcutaneous fat but may be due also to adrenal dysfunction.

Occasional

Associated Vitamin Deficiencies. These may influence the clinical picture and treatment. They include avitaminosis A (xerophthalmia) and deficiency of riboflavin or folic acid.

Associated Infections. Other infections, e.g., tuberculosis, may also be present. However, these are usually difficult to detect clinically because of the malnourished child's lack of "textbook" response. For example, bronchopneumonia or tuberculosis can occur with no fever or obvious signs, and a tuberculin test may be negative. Dehydration can occur even in edematous children. There is abnormally decreased elasticity of the skin in severe PEM, so that a dry mouth and sunken eyeballs should be looked for carefully.

Liver Enlargement. As extreme fatty infiltration is a *constant* finding at autopsy, it is uncertain why hepatomegaly is only a variable feature. It is particularly marked when accentuated by malarial infection in hyperendemic areas, or perhaps where high intakes of sucrose (domestic sugar) are present (as in the "sugar babies" of the Caribbean of the 1940s to 1950s).

Skin Lesions. Skin changes include small indolent sores, groin rash, and the pathognomonic "flaky-paint" dermatosis, which characteristically presents as dark patches on the buttocks, backs of legs, and arms, later flaking off to leave thin, light-colored skin or superficial ulceration underneath (Fig. 106–3).

TREATMENT. See Chapter 106.3.

106.2. MARASMUS

DEFINITION. Marasmus is the other clinical syndrome of severe PEM. It is characterized by extreme growth failure (notably a weight of 60% or less than that expected for age) and wasted muscles and subcutaneous fat. It is mainly the result of a diet that is extremely low in both protein and calories and is often associated with infective diarrhea and sometimes with tuberculosis.

ETIOLOGY. There are 2 quite different forms of marasmus—early and late onset.

Early Marasmus (Figs. 106–4 and 109–2). This occurs in the first year of life and is usually due to ill-advised attempts to rear babies with dilute, contaminated bottle feedings. It is the result of an interacting deterioration due to starvation and infective diarrhea. Uncommonly, it can occur with inadequate breast milk production, as exemplified by lactating mothers during a famine or receiving oral contraceptives containing estrogens. In recent years, some infants with transplacentally acquired AIDS present with marasmus. This has been noted in parts of Africa.

Late Marasmus. This is seen characteristically in preschool-age children (Fig. 106–5). It is due to a diet that comprises inadequate quantities of local foods plus, in some cases, a small amount of breast milk. Diarrhea may be present also, as may tuberculosis. The cause

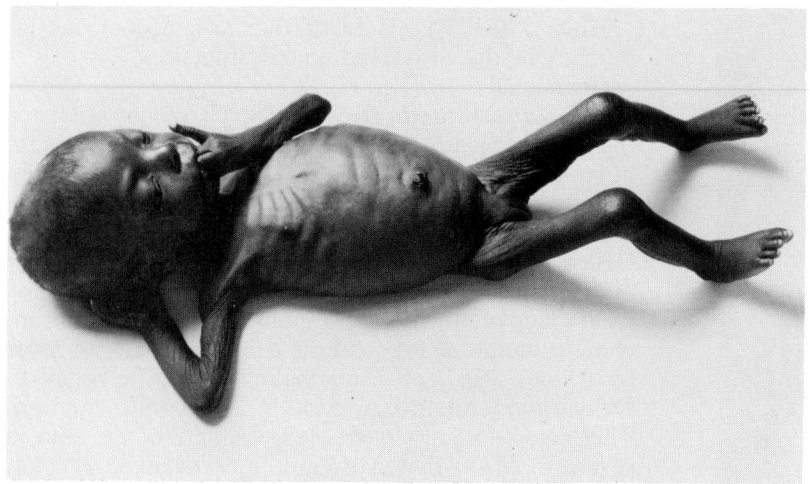

FIGURE 106–4. Early onset marasmus (West Indies). Inadequately bottle-fed 5-month-old baby with associated diarrhea and showing extreme growth retardation (weight < 60% of normal) and marked wasting of subcutaneous fat and muscles.

may be related to the cultural practice of delaying the introduction of semisolids. Today, late marasmus is occurring more commonly with the decreasing availability and increasing cost of foods and with natural and manmade disasters, such as famines and civil wars.

EPIDEMIOLOGY. Until recently, early marasmus had received inadequate attention compared with kwashiorkor, which has a more striking appearance and exotic name. In fact, marasmus is of worldwide distribution and is now increasing in many urbanized areas. This parallels a move to "mixed-milk" feeding or inadequate bottle-feeding, resulting from varying complex social and cultural pressures, especially the imitation of socioeconomic "superiors," the ill effects of pervasive advertising of costly and locally inappropriate formulas, the lack of emphasis given to breast-feeding by westernized health services, women going out of the home for salaried employment, or abandonment of unwanted babies (Chapter 109.2).

The universal advantage of breast-feeding is that human milk has an ideal species-specific composition and provides protection against numerous infections, especially those causing diarrhea. Other considerations include economy, ease of preparation, endocrinologic child spacing, and a close initial mother-child relationship, facilitating "bonding." For infants in less developed regions, breast-feeding is virtually essential for survival. For artificial feedings with cow's milk preparations, up to three fourths of the basic wage is often required to purchase enough formula for a 3-month-old infant. The water supply and the kitchen and storage facilities are such that a clean feeding is almost impossible to prepare. Under these circumstances, bottle-fed infants receive dilute doses of milk and a high concentration of bacteria, with resultant mutually reinforcing marasmus and infective diarrhea.

PATHOLOGY. The liver shows only slight fatty infiltration, and the serum albumin and enzyme levels are much less reduced than in kwashiorkor.

CLINICAL MANIFESTATIONS. The main clinical changes seen are in the muscles and subcutaneous fat—both of which are markedly wasted. Signs of dehydration and associated infections, e.g., tuberculosis or oral moniliasis, may be present. Apathy and hair changes are slight, at most, in contrast with kwashiorkor (Figs. 106–5 and 106–6).

TREATMENT (Chapter 106.3). Marasmus is treated similarly to kwashiorkor. However, although the marasmic baby usually has a better appetite and is less apathetic than is the child with kwashiorkor, the patient is often a young infant unable to assist in feeding himself. The need is great for "compact calories" in the form of vegetable oil to speed recovery, with amounts based on "ideal" weight rather than present weight.

PREVENTION. Breast-feeding is the key to the prevention of early marasmus, with attention focused on (a) avoidance of traditional and modern medical

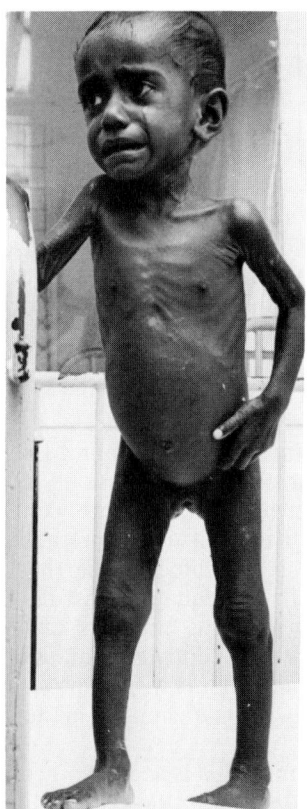

FIGURE 106–5. Late onset marasmus (Fiji) in a girl of preschool age (due to a generally inadequate diet that was especially low in calories and to multiple infections) (weight < 60% of reference level).

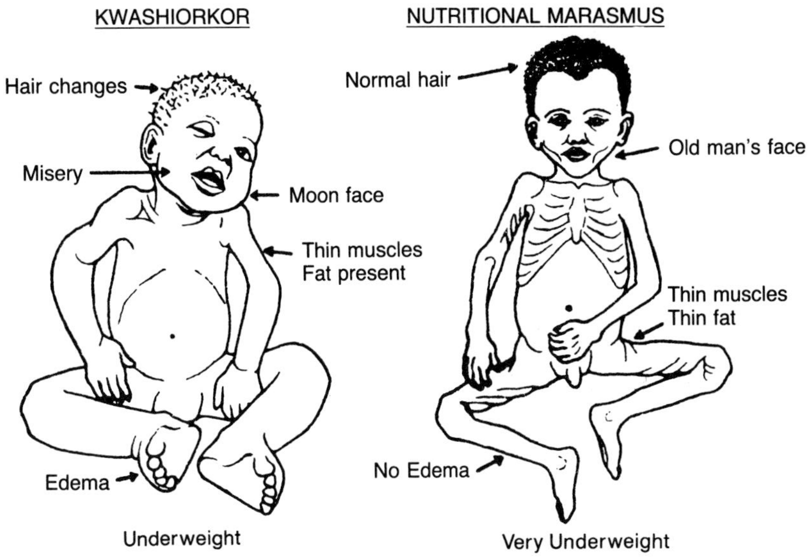

FIGURE 106–6. Some contrasting clinical signs in kwashiorkor and marasmus. (From Jelliffe DB: Child Nutrition in Developing Countries. Washington, D.C., USAID, U.S. Government Printing Office, 1968.)

practices, including maternity wards, that may interfere with the key maternal reflexes, i.e., diminished sucking stimulus and the prolactin reflex, and anxiety and the let-down reflex, (b) ensuring correct "management" (learned practical procedures, especially in urban conditions), (c) maternal health and nutrition in pregnancy and lactation, and (d) avoidance of estrogen-containing oral contraceptives. Late marasmus is prevented by the introduction before or by 6 months of age of locally prepared "multimixes," with special attention to compact calories, combined with continued breast-feeding (which then becomes an important nutritional supplement).

PROGNOSIS. Early marasmus has a mortality rate of 25% or more. It responds slowly to treatment, probably with a greater chance of brain damage than with kwashiorkor. In contrast, late marasmus usually responds to therapy more easily and relatively promptly, because such children accept an improved diet avidly.

106.3. MODERATE PROTEIN-ENERGY MALNUTRITION

Lesser degrees of PEM are far more common in the community than are the severe syndromes of kwashiorkor and marasmus (Table 106–1). More recent figures than those given indicate a deterioration in some areas related to economics, overpopulation, and political events.

CLINICAL MANIFESTATIONS. Moderate PEM is diagnosed by growth failure, as judged by a flattening weight curve in clinical circumstances or, in community surveys, by subnormal anthropometric measurements in young children.

ETIOLOGY. This is identical to that of severe PEM. In fact, children with moderate PEM represent those who are passing through the difficult transitional or weaning period with minimum immediate consequences but who can easily be precipitated into severe PEM by an additional infection, a family social catastrophe, or a national disaster, such as a drought or civil strife.

EPIDEMIOLOGY. Adequate information is not available, as most data on the incidence of PEM are derived from hospitals or health centers and are therefore primarily concerned with severe syndromes.

Community Surveys. One way in which community assessment can be undertaken is by longitudinal surveys, which are difficult to organize, expensive, and time-consuming but give detailed understanding of the interplay of the different factors at work in the syndrome. Alternatively, cross-sectional point-prevalence surveys can be made. These are relatively economical with regard to time, staff, and money but show the situation only at a certain season of that particular year.

Data for the assessment of the status of PEM in the community may be obtained from the following approaches:

1. *Direct assessment of human groups:* Clinical signs, biochemical tests, and anthropometric measurements.

2. *Indirect assessment of human groups:* Mortality and morbidity data in key age groups.

3. *Assessment of ecologic factors:* Conditioning infections, food consumption, cultural influences, socioeconomic circumstances, food production, and medical and educational services for major risk factors.

Criteria for PEM in Surveys. In community surveys, the presence of edema in young children should be noted as probably indicative of kwashiorkor, but anthropometric measurements are undoubtedly the best general method of assessing the prevalence of moderate PEM (Fig. 106–7). Measurements used most frequently include weight, length, circumference of the mid-upper arm, and triceps skinfold. The following levels of weight-for-age have been used often: $\leq 80\%$—moderate, and $\leq 60\%$—severe. Details have been much debated, but similar principles apply.

However, children with a low weight-for-age represent a mixture of the more acutely malnourished ("wasted") and more chronically affected ("stunted"). The limiting levels in this Waterlow classification are weight-for-height $\leq 80\%$ ($-2SD$) and height-for-age $\leq 90\%$ ($-2SD$). This classification has the advantage of sorting out children at greatest risk and with the highest need for attention, i.e., the "wasted." It has the

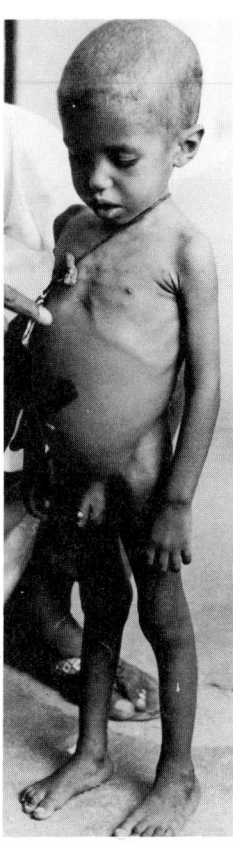

FIGURE 106–7. Moderate protein-energy malnutrition (West Africa). "Wasted" child of preschool age (Waterlow classification), with low weight for height (< 80%), relatively normal height (> 90%), and diminished muscle and subcutaneous fat. (Courtesy UNICEF/6786.)

disadvantage of requiring 2 measurements and a reasonably exact knowledge of age, which is often not possible in many less technically developed countries.

However, assessment of age may be attempted by constructing a "local events" calendar. Alternatively, "precise age-independent" anthropometry may be used, employing the weight-for-height or the arm circumference.

For children under surveillance, e.g., those attending Young Child or Under Five Clinics, serial recording of weight graphically, using a growth chart such as that devised by Morley (Fig. 106–8), is the best method for the early detection of lesser degrees of PEM. It can be useful as practical nutrition education for mothers (and fathers) who retain the chart. However, recent work has indicated that the understanding and practical usefulness of weight charts varies, particularly with the effectiveness of the training of community health workers.

TREATMENT. The treatment of all forms of PEM is similar and consists of (a) diet, (b) management of infections, and (c) emotional support. Details will vary in different countries and with health services of varying levels of sophistication.

Diet. In the initial therapy of severe PEM, the diet should be liquid or semisolid and high in calories, protein, and other nutrients.

Although cure can be obtained with vegetable-protein mixtures, therapeutic diets have been (and still are)

TABLE 106–2. Approximate Protein Content and Amino Acid Deficiency of Main Categories of Vegetable Food Used in Multimixes‡

Types of Food	Protein (approx. %)	Amino Acid Deficiency
Cereal grain	± 10	Lacking in lysine
Legumes*	± 20	Lacking in methionine
Dark-green leafy vegetables†	4–10	Lacking in methionine

*soy beans: <40%.
†Dried: 30%.
‡From Jelliffe DB: Infant Nutrition in the Subtropics and Tropics. WHO Monograph No. 29 (2nd ed.). Geneva, World Health Organization, 1968; and Jelliffe DB: Protein-calorie malnutrition. *In* Woodruff AW (ed.): Medicine in the Tropics. Edinburgh and New York, Churchill Livingstone, 1974.

characteristically based on reconstituted dried skimmed milk (DSM), with added calories in the form of sugar and/or vegetable oil. Details vary, but 3 to 4 gm of protein/kg and up to 150 kcal/kg are widely recommended, with supplements of potassium and magnesium, if feasible. Problems with anorexia are approached by employing small frequent feedings or gavage for a few days.

The routine administration of vitamins in early therapy is controversial, partly because vitamins greatly increase the cost of treatment. Ideally, a vitamin mixture covering recognized daily requirements should be added to the feedings. Also, if a particular deficiency, e.g., vitamin A, is well recognized, this nutrient should be given routinely in large amounts. Overt xerophthalmia, especially as keratomalacia, requires emergency treatment with large doses of oral vitamin A (Fig. 107–2).

As soon as possible, the diet should be widened to include local foods, given as "multimixes." These may be made from indigenous food mixtures (Tables 106–2 and 106–3) or from dried skimmed milk mixed with local staple porridge, or processed multimixes, e.g., wheat-soy blend, may be used. Hospital kitchens need to prepare such mixtures.

TABLE 106–3. Village-Level Multimixes*

Type of Multimix	Ingredients
Double mix	Staple† + legume
	or
	Staple + animal protein‡
	or
	Staple + dark-green leafy vegetable (DGLV)§
Triple mix	Staple + legume + animal protein
	or
	Staple + legume + DGLV
	or
	Staple + DGLV + animal protein
Quadrimix‖	Staple + legume + DGLV + animal protein

*From Jelliffe DB: Infant Nutrition in the Subtropics and Tropics. WHO Monograph No. 29 (2nd ed.). Geneva, World Health Organization, 1968; and Jelliffe DB: Protein-calorie malnutrition. *In* Woodruff AW (ed.): Medicine in the Tropics. Edinburgh and New York, Churchill Livingstone, 1974.
†Preferably a cereal.
‡Mixtures with animal protein preferable in all mixes.
§Source of minerals and vitamins.
‖**All mixes should have "compact calories" added when practical (e.g., oil, fat, sugar).**

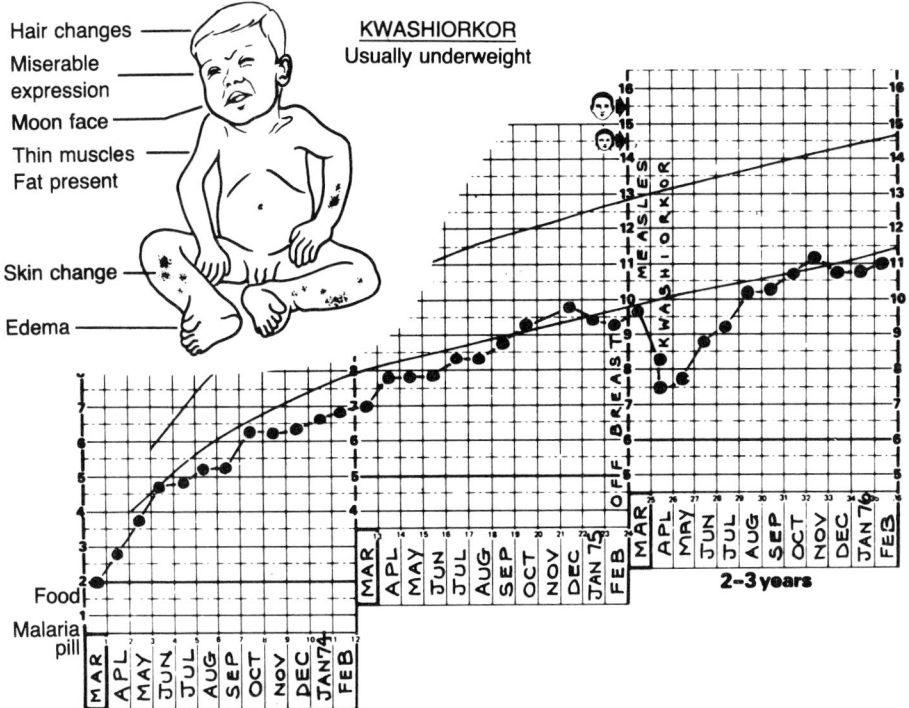

FIGURE 106–8. Growth charts used for surveillance for protein-energy malnutrition. This child developed kwashiorkor after 4 months of failing to gain weight following measles that precipitated the illness. Upper line: Fiftieth percentile boys. Lower line: Third percentile girls (International Children's Center Study, U.K. children). (From Morley D: Clinic Assessment. *In* Jelliffe DB, Jelliffe EFP [eds.]: Nutrition and Growth. New York, Plenum Press, 1979.)

Moderate PEM is best treated at a nutrition rehabilitation center but may be undertaken at home or in the village; in the latter situations, parents are supervised by home visiting. The present trend is toward village-level treatment with home-prepared multimixes either in the home or in village feeding centers, using primary health workers. The costs and risks of hospital treatment have also become increasingly clear—cross-infections from overcrowding, inadequate personnel for feeding, and, in some circumstances, removal from the mother.

Management of Infections. Overt conditioning infections, e.g., malaria, tuberculosis, and intestinal helminthic infections, should be treated as soon as the child can tolerate the chemotherapy.

Emotional Care. Children with severe PEM need emotional care in the form of attention, stimulation by play, and love (TLC), which is an additional reason for mothers to be admitted with their infants to overcrowded, understaffed children's wards.

Special Treatment. This may be indicated for continuing diarrhea (often caused by lactose intolerance), dehydration, severe anemia, convulsions, hypothermia, or cardiac failure.

PREVENTION. Preventive programs need to be based on knowledge of food customs, economics, and conditioning infections and to be undertaken collaboratively with extension workers in other fields, e.g., agriculture and education.

General public health measures with indirect nutritional benefits, e.g., improved water supply, environmental sanitation, and malaria control, are important. In addition, more specific activities may be undertaken by health personnel to prevent PEM.

Programs to Promote or Protect Breast-Feeding in the Community. These include (a) information and education; (b) modification of health services (e.g., maternity ward routines and training curricula); (c) monitoring of infant food industry activities; and (d) provision of facilities for working women who are breast-feeding.

Improved Feeding of Pregnant and Lactating Mothers and Young Children. This is accomplished by (a) nutrition education directed toward the best use of locally available food mixtures; and (b) supplementary feeding, if and when necessary and "targeted" (e.g., used for specified periods for agreed upon criteria).

Early Recognition of Moderate PEM. Children with

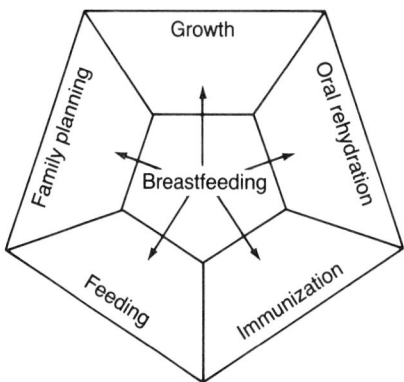

FIGURE 106–9. GOBI-FF. Main aspects of UNICEF programs and policy. Breast-feeding plays a role in most aspects. (G, growth and its monitoring; O, oral rehydration; B, breast-feeding; I, immunization; F, family planning: lactation, amenorrhea; F, feeding and weaning: breast-feeding with extra supplement in weaning period.)

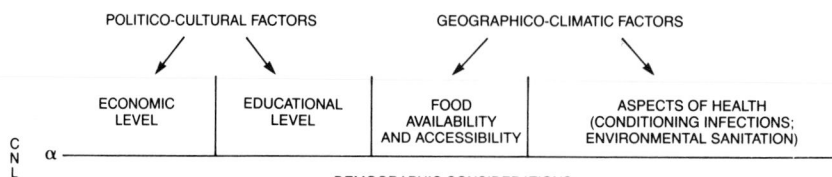

FIGURE 106–10. Factors affecting the community nutrition level (CNL).

PEM are detected by (a) serial weight and growth charts; and (b) screening by village health workers for low arm circumference.

Reduction of Conditioning Infections. These are reduced by (a) prevention and basic management (appropriate for main local health problems); and (b) immunization, malarial chemoprophylaxis, "deworming" for ascariasis, and oral rehydration for diarrhea.

Child Spacing. This is best approached by (a) encouragement of breast-feeding and lactation amenorrhea; and (b) information about and/or availability of contraceptives that do not interfere with lactation and are acceptable in local culture.

The main features of what has been termed by UNICEF and WHO as the "Child Survival Revolution" are covered by the acronym GOBI-FF (Fig. 106–9) and are the key aspects of prevention.

CONCLUSIONS. Moderate and severe forms of PEM with conditioning infections affect up to two thirds of young children in many developing tropical countries. PEM is responsible for millions of deaths not directly, but in combination with multiple microbial, viral, and parasitic infections. This is illustrated by the fact that the 1- to 4-year mortality rate may be 30 to 50 times as great in developing regions as in North America and Western Europe, with a particularly high death rate among 2-year-old children.

The economic cost is considerable if curative services are to be introduced to treat such malnutrition. High death rates from PEM (and associated infections) act as a deterrent to family planning. The long-term consequences can lead to stunting of growth or failure to achieve full intellectual potential in substantial numbers of children.

Prevention is the only logical approach, ideally taking into consideration all factors that can influence the "community nutrition level" (Fig. 106–10), principally "resource reallocation" (e.g., income and land). At the same time, the activities of the health services can play a major role in an immediate preventive attack on PEM via rural outreach channelled through primary health care services.

BIBLIOGRAPHY

Alleyne GAO, Hay HW, Picou DI, et al.: Protein-Energy Malnutrition. London, Edward Arnold, 1977.

Cameron M, Hofvander Y: Feeding Young Children. New York, United Nations, 1978.

DeMaeyer E: Protein-energy malnutrition. *In* Beaton GH, Bengoa JM (eds.): Nutrition in Preventive Medicine. Geneva, World Health Organization, 1976, p. 23.

Grant J: State of the World's Children 1988. New York, UNICEF, 1988.

Hendrickse RG: The influence of aflatoxins on child health in the tropics with particular reference to kwashiorkor. Trans R Soc Trop Med Hyg 78:427, 1988.

Jelliffe DB: Child Nutrition in Developing Countries. Washington, D.C., USAID, U.S. Government Printing Office, 1968.

Jelliffe DB: Cultural blocks and protein malnutrition in early childhood in rural West Bengal. Pediatrics 20:128, 1957.

Jelliffe DB: Infant Nutrition in the Subtropics and Tropics. WHO Monograph No. 29, 2nd ed. Geneva, World Health Organization, 1968.

Jelliffe DB: Protein-calorie malnutrition of early childhood—practical notes. J Trop Pediatr 5:96, 1959.

Jelliffe DB, Jelliffe EFP: Community Nutritional Assessment. Oxford, Oxford University Press, 1990.

Jelliffe DB, Jelliffe EFP (eds.): Growth Monitoring and Promotion in Young Children: Selection of Methods and Techniques of Training. New York, Oxford University Press, 1990.

Jelliffe DB, Jelliffe EFP: Human Milk in the Modern World, 2nd ed. Oxford, Oxford University Press, 1990.

Jelliffe DB, Jelliffe EFP: National policy and young child nutrition. Am J Clin Nutr 31:1421, 1978.

Jelliffe DB, Jelliffe EFP (eds.): Programmes to Promote Breastfeeding. Oxford, Oxford University Press, 1989.

Morley D: Clinic assessment. *In* Jelliffe DB, Jelliffe EFP (eds.): Nutrition and Growth. New York, Plenum Press, 1979.

Morley D: Nutritional surveillance of young children in developing countries. Int J Epidemiol 5:51, 1976.

Scrimshaw NS, Taylor CE, Gordon JE: Interactions of Nutrition and Infection. WHO Monograph No. 57. Geneva, World Health Organization, 1957.

Waterlow JC: Notes on the assessment and classification of protein-energy malnutrition in children. Lancet 2:87, 1973.

107. VITAMIN DEFICIENCIES

GENERAL PRINCIPLES

Michael C. Latham

Vitamins are organic substances present in small quantities in foods we consume that are necessary for metabolism. They are chemically unrelated and their physiological functions differ. They are grouped together because, as their name implies, they are vital factors in the diet, because of the way they were discovered, and because they do not fit into other nutrient categories—namely, carbohydrates, protein, and fats (all of which provide energy), and minerals or trace metals. Generally, vitamins are divided into those that are fat soluble (vitamins A, D, E, and K) and those that are water soluble (vitamin C and the B vitamins). In this section, those vitamins whose deficiencies result in serious clinical and public health problems are discussed.

107.1. VITAMIN A DEFICIENCY AND XEROPHTHALMIA

Michael C. Latham

DEFINITION. Vitamin A deficiency most commonly, and importantly, affects the eyes, although it may play a role in a variety of clinical conditions. Xerophthalmia is now the term used to cover all ocular manifestations of hypovitaminosis A. Xeros is the Greek word meaning dry, and xerophthalmia literally means a drying of the eyes. When vitamin A deficiency is at a level resulting in inadequate liver stores to satisfy the metabolic needs of the body, ocular signs may occur. First, there may be night blindness, then a drying of the conjunctiva and cornea, and eventually corneal destruction with resulting blindness. The advanced form is often termed "kerato-malacia." The serious eye manifestations are mainly seen in young children. Vitamin A deficiency may adversely affect other epithelial surfaces, may aggravate infections, and may be associated with an increased incidence of certain cancers.

ETIOLOGY. An inadequate intake of preformed vitamin A or of carotene, a poor absorption of the vitamin, or an increased metabolic demand can all lead to vitamin A deficiency. Of these 3, a dietary deficiency is by far the most important cause of xerophthalmia.

History. Vitamin A was discovered in 1913 when experiments showed that if the only fat present in diets of young animals was lard, their growth was retarded, and when butter was substituted the animals grew and thrived. A substance in butter, but not lard, was found also in egg yolk and cod liver oil. It was named vitamin A. It was later established that many products of vegetable origin had similar nutritional properties as the vitamin A in foods of animal origin; they contained a yellow pigment, carotene, that is converted to vitamin A in the body. Preformed vitamin A or retinol is a fat-soluble vitamin found only in animal products. Carotenes or carotenoids can act as a provitamin. There are many carotenoids in plants, but the most important for human nutrition is Beta-carotene. This can be converted to vitamin A by enzymatic action in the intestinal wall.

Dietary Sources and Requirements. In most nonindustrialized countries the majority of poorer people get most, often 80% or more, of their vitamin A from carotene present in foods of vegetable origin. The yellow color of carotene may be masked by chlorophyll in many dark green leafy vegetables.

Rich sources of retinol, or preformed vitamin A, are liver, fish liver oils, egg yolks, and dairy products. Carotenes are present in good quantities in a wide variety of green and yellow vegetables and fruits, and also in yellow corn or maize, and yellow root crops, e.g., sweet potatoes. A rich source is red palm oil eaten extensively in West Africa and widely grown but infrequently consumed in many areas, e.g., in Malaysia. In many tropical diets important sources are dark green leafy vegetables, e.g., amaranth, cassava, drumstick and other leaves, mangos and papayas, tomatoes, and sometimes, local yellow pumpkins, squash, and yellow maize. The wet tropics often abound in both cultivated and wild food sources of carotene. The poor often consume too little of these foods and young children often dislike green vegetables. Breast milk of mothers on a diet low in vitamin A will also contain relatively low levels of this vitamin.

The biologic activity of vitamin A is now usually expressed as retinol equivalents (RE) rather than in International Units (IU). One RE is equal to 1 μg of retinol or 6 μg of Beta-carotene. WHO has recommended an intake of 300 RE daily for infants and 750 RE for adults.

Metabolism. Vitamin A, either from preformed retinol or after conversion from carotene, is stored in the liver. For this reason the best criterion for judging vitamin A nutritional status is to obtain an estimate of levels of vitamin A in the liver. This can be performed easily only at autopsy. Retinol is transported from the liver to other sites in the body by retinol binding protein (RBP), a specific carrier protein. Protein deficiency may influence vitamin A status by reducing the synthesis of RBP.

A diet deficient in vitamin A results eventually in low hepatic stores; serum retinol levels often fall from normal levels of 30 to 50 μg/100 ml plasma to low or deficient levels below 20 μg/100 ml plasma. Ocular manifestations of xerophthalmia seldom occur until serum vitamin A levels are deficient.

PATHOPHYSIOLOGY. Prolonged intake of diets low in vitamin A and carotene is the most common cause of xerophthalmia. But the condition may be influenced by other factors, e.g., intestinal parasitic infections, gastroenteritis, or malabsorption. There may be seasons when the main sources of vitamin A are less available or more expensive. Measles often precipitates xerophthalmia because it leads to lower food intake (anorexia and stomatitis may be factors) and to increased metabolic demands for vitamin A, or the virus affects the eye and leads to lesions of vitamin A deficiency. Protein-energy malnutrition (PEM) is important also as a cause or as an accompaniment of xerophthalmia. Data from Indonesia and elsewhere suggest that serious corneal involvement of xerophthalmia seldom occurs except in children who have moderate or severe PEM.

EPIDEMIOLOGY

Distribution. Xerophthalmia is especially prevalent in children of poor rice-eating families in South and Southeast Asia (e.g., India, Bangladesh, Pakistan, Indonesia, and the Philippines). There is a high incidence in some African countries (e.g., Ethiopia, Burkina Faso, Zambia, and Mozambique) whereas other countries, especially in West Africa, are spared in part because of consumption of red palm oil, which is high in carotene. In the Western Hemisphere, Haiti and Northeast Brazil are areas where xerophthalmia is highly prevalent. It occurs also in many poorer areas of Central and South America. Vitamin A deficiency used to be a problem in the Middle East, but few recent data on its prevalence there are available. In Europe and North America, and in affluent people everywhere, vitamin A deficiency may occur in alcoholics, in those with malabsorption or anorexia nervosa, and in persons for any reason consuming diets low in carotene or vitamin A.

Prevalence. Although no truly accurate figures are available, it is believed that worldwide between 500,000 and 1 million children each year develop active xerophthalmia with some corneal involvement. Of these, perhaps half will become blind or have serious visual impairment, and a large proportion will die. Vitamin A deficiency, manifested by low liver stores of retinol,

TABLE 107–1. Classification of Xerophthalmia

Ocular Sign	Classification
Night blindness	XN
Conjunctival xerosis	X1A
Bitot's spots	X1B
Corneal xerosis	X2
Corneal ulceration/Keratomalacia <⅓ corneal surface	X3A
Corneal ulceration/Keratomalacia ≥⅓ corneal surface	X3B
Corneal scar	XS
Xerophthalmia fundus	XF

deficient serum vitamin A levels, or noncorneal eye involvement, affects many millions of people, particularly, but not confined to, children. Vitamin A deficiency is the most common cause of blindness in children in many endemic areas and is 1 of the 4 most important nutritional deficiency diseases in the world.

CLINICAL MANIFESTATIONS. WHO and others have accepted a classification of the ocular signs of xerophthalmia (Table 107–1). The shorthand code in the first column and this classification are now widely used in surveys. Prevalence criteria (in percentage of children 6 months to 6 years of age) for determining the public health significance of xerophthalmia and vitamin A deficiency in a population are given in Table 107–2.

Night Blindness. Night blindness (XN) often is the first evidence of vitamin A deficiency; the individual has a reduced ability to see in dim light. In many countries where xerophthalmia is endemic, there are local terms for night blindness, and it is well recognized even by uneducated persons. Night blindness occurs because vitamin A deficiency reduces the rhodopsin in the rods of the retina.

Early Eye Lesions. Then the conjunctiva becomes relatively dry and loses its shiny luster, and often becomes thickened, wrinkled, and sometimes pigmented. However, the cardinal sign is dryness, patches of xerosis giving the appearance of "sandbanks at receding tide." These changes are particularly common on the bulbar conjunctiva. This is known as conjunctival xerosis (X1A).

Sometimes accompanying the conjunctival xerosis are Bitot's spots (X1B), which are usually bilateral, triangular-shaped, raised whitish plaques. When examined closely they look like a fine foam with many tiny bubbles (Fig. 107–1). This foamy sticky material can be wiped away. Bitot's spots in the absence of xerosis may be due to a cause other than vitamin A deficiency.

Later Eye Lesions. The earliest corneal change is punctate keratopathy seen on slit lamp examination.

TABLE 107–2. Prevalence Criteria for Determining Public Health Significance of Vitamin A Deficiency

Criteria	Minimum Prevalence (%)
Bitot's spots	0.50
Corneal xerosis/Corneal ulceration/Keratomalacia (X2/X3A/X3B)	0.01
Corneal scar (XS)	0.05
Plasma vitamin A <10 μg/dL	5.00

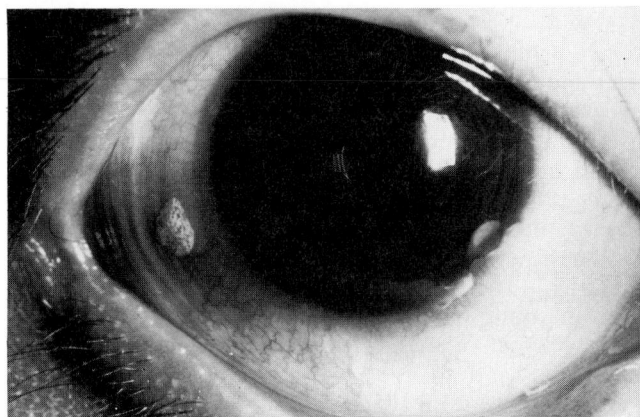

FIGURE 107–1. Temporal Bitot's spot (X1B). (From Sommer A: Field Guide to Detection and Control of Xerophthalmia. Geneva, World Health Organization, 1978.)

Corneal xerosis (X2) begins with drying of the corneal surface that first appears hazy and then granular on simple eye examination (Fig. 107–2). This is followed by a softening of the cornea, often with ulceration and areas of necrosis. Corneal ulcers (Fig. 107–3) are usually circular and punched out in appearance and often initially small (X3A) but may extend centrally to involve much of the cornea (X3B). This may lead to perforation of the cornea, prolapse of the iris, loss of ocular contents and, perhaps, destruction of the eye, a condition termed keratomalacia (X3B, Fig. 107–4). Although the lesions are usually bilateral, the corneal ulceration may be more advanced in 1 eye. With these severe manifestations the child is also usually seriously ill; sometimes with a high fever.

If treatment is instituted when only a small corneal ulcer is present, it will heal, forming a corneal scar (XS). The size of the scar and the limits it places on future vision will depend on how large or advanced the corneal ulceration was and its location.

Xerophthalmia of the fundus (XF) is sometimes seen early in the disease with an ophthalmoscope. The retina has white dots around the periphery of the fundus. They disappear following treatment.

Generalized Effects. Nonocular effects of vitamin A

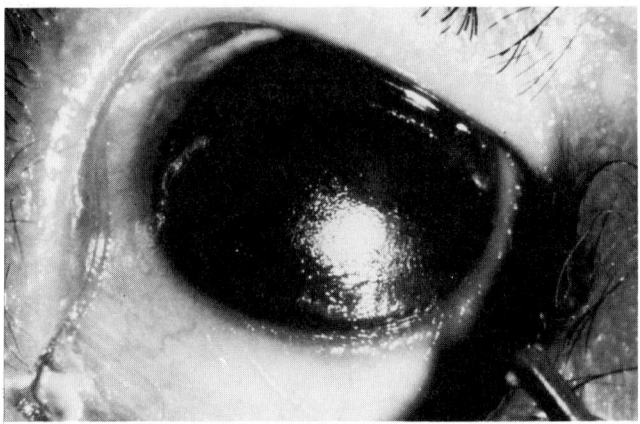

FIGURE 107–2. Advanced corneal xerosis (X2). (From Sommer A: Field Guide to Detection and Control of Xerophthalmia. Geneva, World Health Organization, 1978.)

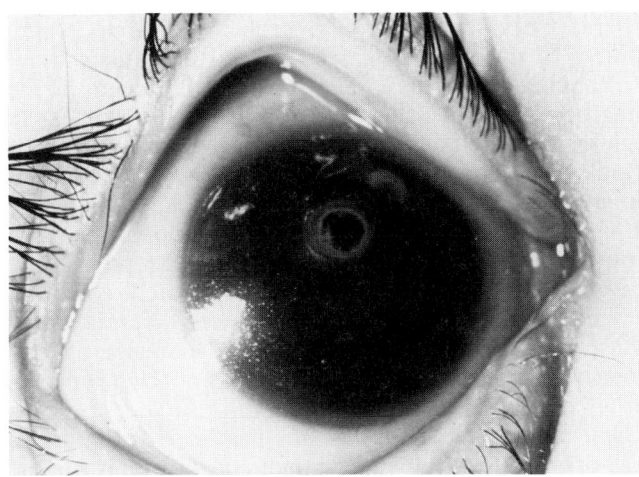

FIGURE 107–3. Typical xerophthalmic ulcer (X3A). (From Sommer A, Sugana T: Corneal xerophthalmia and keratomalacia. Arch Ophthalmol 100:404, 1982.)

deficiency are better described in experimental animals than in humans. In young animals growth retardation is marked. It is likely that vitamin A deficiency in children has similar consequences. In the young child xerophthalmia appears to depress the immune response and in this way makes infections more common and more serious. The association of common infections with xerophthalmia is well described. There is now experimental evidence from Indonesia to suggest that even in the absence of clinical signs of xerophthalmia, the provision of vitamin A may substantially reduce infant and child mortality in communities where vitamin A deficiency is prevalent. This work needs to be confirmed.

Further research may confirm that improved intakes of vitamin A or carotene both reduce the incidence and duration of common diseases such as diarrhea and respiratory infections, and also improve the growth of young children.

DIAGNOSIS

Clinical Exams. The ocular signs of xerophthalmia allow diagnosis on clinical grounds, especially when the condition is moderately advanced. Corneal xerosis and ulceration can be easily detected, and cannot be mistaken easily for trachoma, which usually begins on the conjunctival surface of the upper lid. A history of night blindness where vitamin A deficiency occurs provides strong evidence for vitamin A deficiency. The diagnosis is often missed because the sick child presents with serious PEM (kwashiorkor or nutritional marasmus), measles, tuberculosis, dehydration, or some other condition that occupies the attention of the medical attendant. The eyes of sick children must always be examined in good light.

Laboratory Tests. Determination of serum vitamin A levels is useful for community surveys. Children with xerophthalmia will usually have levels below 10 µg/100 ml. A technique known as the relative dose response is now favored but is more complex. It is said to give a better picture of liver vitamin A stores than does the simple measure of serum vitamin A levels. RBP levels may be low also. Conjunctival impression cytology is a new test that holds promise for early detection of vitamin A deficiency.

TREATMENT. Severe cases with corneal involvement should be treated as an emergency. Hours, and certainly days, may make the difference between reasonable vision and total blindness. Treatment for children 1 year or over should consist of providing 110 mg of retinol palmitate or 66 mg of retinol acetate (200,000 IU of vitamin A) orally or 100,000 IU of water-miscible vitamin A (retinol palmitate) by intramuscular injection. Vitamin A in oil should not be used for injection. The oral dose should be repeated on the second day and again on discharge from hospital or 7 to 30 days after the first dose. Half these doses are recommended for infants.

With corneal perforation or advanced keratomalacia, topical bacitracin or other antibiotics should be instilled into both eyes 6 times per day. Appropriate systemic antibiotics should be administered and bacteriologic studies performed to determine the etiology and antibiotic sensitivity of the causative bacteria.

Other diseases e.g., severe PEM, tuberculosis, and dehydration, need appropriate treatment. Night blindness and conjunctival xerosis are completely reversible and respond quickly to treatment using oral doses of vitamin A on an outpatient basis. Corneal ulceration is arrested by treatment and will heal within a week or 2 but will leave scars. There is often a high case fatality rate because of accompanying PEM and infections.

PREVENTION AND CONTROL. Xerophthalmia, in theory at least, is relatively easy to prevent and control. Commonly used strategies are listed:

1. Fortification with vitamin A of a suitable food. Sugar, MSG, rice, and other foods have all been successfully fortified.

2. Periodic large doses of vitamin A by mouth to all children or to children at risk. Usually 110 mg of retinol palmitate or 66 mg of retinol acetate (200,000 IU) with added vitamin E are provided every 6 months. However, every 4 months may be preferable.

3. Improved diets with more carotene or vitamin A-containing foods, nutrition education, and encouraging home gardening.

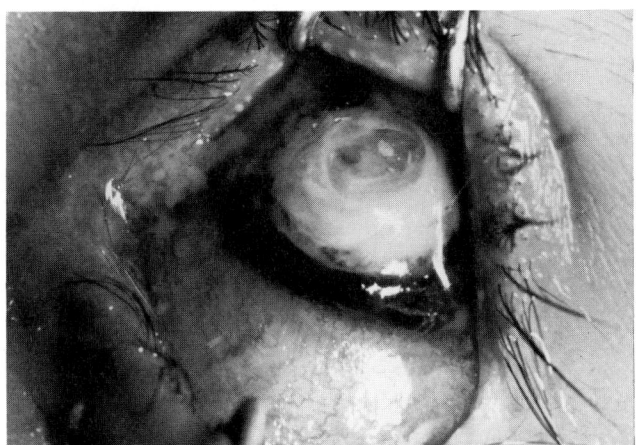

FIGURE 107–4. Total necrosis (keratomalacia) (X3B). (From Sommer A, Sugana T: Corneal xerophthalmia and keratomalacia. Arch Ophthalmol 100:404, 1982.)

4. Public health and medical measures, including early diagnosis and treatment at child health clinics or as part of growth monitoring; control of parasitic diseases and infections (including immunization); steps to reduce the extent of PEM.

5. Measures to reduce poverty and inequity that allow the purchase of adequate quantities of food.

The vitamin A content of breast milk is low in mothers consuming poor diets with inadequate carotene or retinol. Providing mothers at risk with 200,000 IU of vitamin A at delivery and at 4 monthly intervals will help ensure that breast-feeding infants obtain adequate vitamin A.

BIBLIOGRAPHY

Bauernfeind JC: Vitamin A Deficiency and Its Control. Orlando, Florida, Academic Press, 1986.
Control of vitamin A deficiency and xerophthalmia. Report of an International Meeting. WHO Tech Rep Ser, No. 672, 1982.
McLaren DS: Nutritional Ophthalmology. London, Academic Press, 1980.
Olson JA, Bridges CDB, Packer L, et al.: The function of vitamin A. Fed Proc 42: 2740–2746, 1983.
Solon F, Fernandez TL, Latham MC, et al.: An evaluation of strategies to control vitamin A deficiency in the Philippines. Am J Clin Nutr 32: 1445–1453, 1979.
Sommer A, Tarwotjo I, Djunaedi E, et al.: Impact of vitamin A supplementation on childhood mortality. Lancet 1: 1169–1173, 1986.

107.2.   BERIBERI

Daphne A. Roe

DEFINITION. Beriberi is a nutritional deficiency disease caused by a prolonged deficiency of thiamine (vitamin B_1), a water-soluble vitamin. The diagnostic term "beriberi" is applied to the 2 major forms of the disease that are characterized by peripheral neuritis and congestive heart failure. A third form of thiamine deficiency is seen in alcoholics; this bears the diagnostic term Wernicke's encephalopathy and is characterized by paralysis of ocular muscles and an acute confusional state.

ETIOLOGY. Beriberi can be caused by (1) intake of a monotonous diet of highly milled, refined cereal grains, particularly rice, which is low in thiamine; (2) intake of foods or beverages that contain thiamine antagonists; or (3) high intake of alcohol by people eating a cereal diet of low thiamine content.

Thiamine is one of the least stable of the B vitamins and readily loses activity during food storage, processing, and cooking. Cereals stored as whole grains lose thiamine if the moisture content is high. Thiamine is lost from rice when washed or boiled. Baking destroys thiamine in other cereal foods.

PREVALENCE AND DISTRIBUTION. Whereas beriberi was once a common nutritional disease and important public health problem in many Asian countries where polished rice was the cereal staple, its prevalence has declined because of social changes allowing the poor a more varied and nutritional diet and/or because of cereal enrichment programs adding thiamine

to rice. Beriberi was not a problem in areas where parboiled rice was the staple food, e.g., South India.

Populations at Risk. The disease still occurs in the neuropathic form and in the cardiac form in blacks in South Africa. It is present in urban populations who drink Bantu beer and subsist on diets prepared from unenriched, highly milled maize flour. The disease may be precipitated also in hospitalized alcoholics receiving intravenous glucose as a sole source of food energy. Subclinical thiamine deficiency is a prevalent condition in settled groups of previously hunter-gatherer San or Bushmen in Namibia who also show evidence of deficiency of other B vitamins. Thiamine deficiency occurs in elderly Thais who are heavy tea drinkers and who chew tea leaves. The deficiency has been attributed to the presence of polyphenolic thiamine antagonists in the tea. Breast-fed infants of women consuming a thiamine-deficient diet may develop infantile beriberi.

Cerebral thiamine deficiency, first described in its acute form in 1881 by Carl Wernicke, occurs in alcoholics, in pregnant women with hyperemesis gravidarum, and in prisoners in prison camps. Chronic effects of cerebral thiamine deficiency, Korsakoff's psychosis, is seen in alcoholics in psychiatric institutions.

CLINICAL MANIFESTATIONS

Dry or Neuropathic Beriberi. This is a slowly developing peripheral neuropathy. Onset is heralded by numbness of the feet and/or by paresthesias, including sensations of burning or pins and needles in the legs and feet. Loss of tendon reflexes in the lower limbs is common. Other frequent signs that usually involve the lower limbs include muscle weakness and atrophy. Paralysis of the phrenic nerves and retrobulbar neuritis are more rare. Cerebellar signs, e.g., ataxia, may be present also. The disease, if untreated, is progressive; the patient becomes weak, wasted, and bedridden, and dies of secondary infections.

Wet or Cardiac Beriberi. This is manifested by signs of congestive heart failure, i.e., massive dependent edema and increasing dyspnea. Patients with acute cardiac beriberi may have severe metabolic acidosis and circulatory collapse. Anorexia is profound in cardiac beriberi and is due in part to the acidosis. Untreated, the disease is frequently fatal.

Infantile Beriberi. This may have an acute onset in breast-fed infants of thiamine-deficient mothers. They have edema, dyspnea, cyanosis, aphonia, tachycardia, and oliguria.

Wernicke's Encephalopathy. This is a confusional state associated with paralysis of the ocular muscles, especially the external rectus muscle. The ophthalmoplegia is characterized by nystagmus and weakness of conjugate gaze. Frequently, hypothermia is present, which is fatal if untreated. The encephalopathy is considered a thiamine-dependent state because it is reversed only with pharmacologic doses of thiamine. If Wernicke's encephalopathy is untreated or undertreated, a chronic dementia, Korsakoff's psychosis, develops. These patients have a gross memory deficit and confabulation.

LABORATORY DIAGNOSIS

Erythrocyte Transketolase Measurement. Measurement of erythrocyte transketolase levels is the most acceptable biochemical method for assessing thiamine nutriture. This test determines the activity of a thiamine pyrophosphate-dependent enzyme in the pentose phosphate pathway. It compares the activity of the transketolase enzyme in 2 erythrocyte hemolysate samples, activity of the enzyme in 1 being stimulated by adding thiamine in vitro. If the individual is thiamine deficient, the activity of the stimulated hemolysate is greater than that of the unstimulated. Normal erythrocyte transketolase activity is 8 to 15 IU. When the cofactor, thiamine pyrophosphate, is added to the test mixture, there is less than 10% stimulation of enzyme activity. In thiamine deficiency, the erythrocyte transketolase activity values are less than 8 IU and there is more than 10% stimulation of the activity when the cofactor is added to the test mixture. A micromethod utilizes finger-prick blood and, because it requires no venipuncture, it would be useful in field surveys. However, the ease of collecting the blood sample is offset by the shortcomings of the simplified assay. Certain diseases, e.g., diabetes mellitus, interfere with transketolase assays and give low erythrocyte transketolase values, apparently because of reduced apoenzyme levels.

Thiamine Measurement. Plasma, serum, erythrocyte, red cell, and urinary thiamine levels have been used also to assess thiamine status. Measurement of thiamine in whole blood, using high-pressure liquid chromatography (HPLC), offers the most promise as an alternate to the erythrocyte transketolase method for diagnosis of beriberi. Both erythrocyte transketolase activity and whole blood thiamine are reduced significantly in patients with this vitamin deficiency. The thiamine content of urine varies directly with the level of intake of the vitamin.

TREATMENT AND PREVENTION. Dry beriberi is usually treated by administration of 10 mg of thiamine 3 times a day. This may be initiated with intramuscular thiamine at a dose of 25 mg twice daily for 2 or 3 days. Because many patients with dry beriberi are likely to also have severe protein-energy malnutrition, nutritional therapy must include provision of a diet of high food-energy content.

Cardiac beriberi is treated with 25 mg of thiamine intramuscularly twice daily for 3 or 4 days, followed by oral thiamine at a dose of 10 mg 3 times a day until all clinical signs have resolved and biochemical tests of thiamine metabolism normalize. Essential adjunct therapy for cardiac beriberi includes complete bed rest during the period of cardiac failure.

In infantile beriberi, the mother as well as the infant should receive 10 mg of thiamine twice daily by intramuscular injection for the first 2 to 3 days of treatment. Thereafter, they should both be given an oral thiamine supplement until the clinical and biochemical signs of the disease have resolved.

Wernicke's encephalopathy should be treated by 200 mg of thiamine IV, twice daily for 3 days. Korsakoff's psychosis does not respond to thiamine administration.

Large-scale prevention of beriberi has been achieved by fortifying the staple cereal. The most advocated intervention for prevention of beriberi in alcoholics is fortification of beer with thiamine. Those who are critical of this endeavor believe that the alcoholic would drink more, because this could be done with impunity.

BIBLIOGRAPHY

Campbell CH: The severe lactic acidosis of thiamine deficiency: Acute pernicious or fulminating beriberi. Lancet 2:446–449, 1984.

De Wardener HE, Lennox B: Cerebral beriberi (Wernicke's encephalopathy): Review of 52 cases in a Singapore prisoner of war hospital. Lancet 1:11–17, 1947.

Linder MC: Nutrition and metabolism of vitamins. In Linder MC (ed.): Nutritional Biochemistry and Metabolism with Clinical Applications. New York, Elsevier, 1985, pp. 69–74.

Naidoo DP: Beriberi heart disease in Durban: A retrospective study. South Afr Med J 72:241–245, 1987.

Passmore R, Eastwood MA (eds.): Davidson and Passmore's Human Nutrition and Dietetics. New York, Churchill Livingstone, 1986, pp. 311–317.

Roe DA: Nutrient deficiencies in naturally-occurring foods. In Jelliffe EFP, Jelliffe DB (eds.): Adverse Effects of Foods. New York, Plenum Press, 1982, pp. 407–426.

Sauberlich HE: Newer laboratory methods for assessing nutriture of selected B–complex vitamins. Ann Rev Nutr 4:377–407, 1984.

Somogyi JC, Hotzel D, Fujiwara M: Biological interactions and nutrition: A workshop report. In Taylor TG, Jenkins NK (eds.): Proc. XIII International Congress of Nutrition. London, John Libbey, 1986, pp. 480–481.

Truswell AS, Apeagyei F: Alcohol and cerebral thiamine deficiency. In Jelliffe EFP, Jelliffe DB (eds.): Adverse Effects of Foods. New York, Plenum Press, 1982, pp. 253–258.

van der Westhuyzen J, Davis RE, Icke GC, et al.: Thiamine status and biochemical indices of malnutrition and alcoholism in settled communities of Kung San. J Trop Med Hyg 90:283–289, 1987.

Wood B: Thiamine status in Australia. World Rev Nutr Diet 46:148–218, 1985.

Yellowlees PM: Thiamine deficiency and prevention of Wernicke–Korsakoff syndrome. Med J Aust 145:216–219, 1986.

107.3. SCURVY

Daphne A. Roe

DEFINITION. Scurvy is a nutritional deficiency disease caused by a severe lack of dietary vitamin C (ascorbic acid). It is characterized by capillary fragility and manifested in the skin by petechiae and large ecchymoses at the sites of trauma.

ETIOLOGY. In order to prevent vitamin C deficiency it is essential to consume foods containing the vitamin. Unlike most other mammals, humans cannot synthesize the vitamin endogenously. Vitamin C is necessary for collagen synthesis. In scurvy there is reduced hydroxylation of proline in a collagen component, tropocollagen. This reduces the stability of connective tissue and may explain the fragility of small blood vessels that occurs in scurvy. Vitamin C deficiency results also in reduced tissue carnitine levels. Lassitude and muscle fatigue that occur in scurvy are due to inadequate carnitine production. Reduced iron absorption in scorbutic infants, children, and adults is explained by the need for the vitamin to reduce ferric iron in the stomach and to keep iron soluble, expediting absorption from the duodenum.

Scurvy is caused most frequently by a prolonged dietary deficiency of vitamin C. Diets deficient in vitamin

C are those lacking in fruits and vegetables. Important food sources of vitamin C include citrus fruits and fruit juices, green peppers, tomatoes, and soft drinks that are fortified with the vitamin. Many tropical fruits, such as guavas and West Indian cherries, are even richer sources of vitamin C than citrus. Diets likely to induce scurvy in adults are those that are limited to breads or other cereal grains and canned meats. Alcoholics develop scurvy, not only because alcohol calories replace calories from food, but also because indigent alcoholics tend not to consume fruits and vegetables.

Approximately 10 mg of vitamin C is required daily to prevent scurvy. In the adult, clinical scurvy occurs after 60 to 90 days of a diet containing less than this. Because vitamin C is destroyed by prolonged cooking, it may be lost in overcooked foods.

The iron deficiency of scurvy is due not only to blood loss, linked to capillary fragility, but also to reduced absorption of nonheme iron. Absorption of this form of iron is promoted by dietary vitamin C. Because vitamin C enhances the absorption of iron from cow's milk formula and soy formula, its absence from the diets of infants fed such formulas may contribute to iron deficiency in a vulnerable age group.

PREVALENCE. Scurvy was prevalent in sailors in the days of sailing ships. The eighteenth century British naval surgeon, James Lind, recognized that it occurred on long voyages when sailors were deprived of fresh fruits. Lind showed that the condition could be prevented and treated by oranges or lemons consumed by sea men. In times past, scurvy has been a major health problem also in prisoners deprived of fruits and vegetables and in explorers who lived on canned meat and biscuits.

Infantile scurvy (Barlow's disease), first described in the nineteenth century, became a scourge when heat-treated milk products, including evaporated and condensed milk, and other breast-milk substitutes without added ascorbic acid increasingly replaced breast-feeding. The disease was prevalent in Europe and North America around the turn of the century, and has been seen in tropical countries also. Breast-fed infants rarely get infantile scurvy.

Today almost all infant formulas made by reputable manufacturers contain adequate ascorbic acid to prevent the disease. Scurvy no longer occurs as an endemic disease. It may be seen in infants suffering from child abuse. However, most recent reports of scurvy have been in men living alone and subsisting for long periods of time on diets totally lacking in fruits and vegetables. Scurvy has been recently reported also in children and adults who live on a strict macrobiotic diet for religious reasons, in which fruit and fruit juice consumption is proscribed and brown rice is the main diet.

There have been several reports of scurvy in patients with chronic gastrointestinal disease, including Crohn's disease and Whipple's disease. In Whipple's disease scurvy is believed to be due to malabsorption of the vitamin.

CLINICAL MANIFESTATIONS
Infantile Scurvy. Early signs of infantile scurvy include fretfulness and increasing pallor. As the disease pro-

gresses, the infant screams when the limbs are touched. Tenderness of the limbs and unwillingness to use the limbs for weight bearing become more evident as the child gets older. Often the legs are drawn up towards the trunk and held in a frog-like position, apparently in an attempt to limit pain. These symptoms are due to painful subperiosteal hemorrhages and hemorrhages within the muscles. Gum hemorrhages are found also when the teeth have started to erupt. Hemorrhages may be seen on the hard palate. Scorbutic beading of the ribs may occur due to hemorrhages at the costochondral junctions. Hematuria is a frequent sign, but bleeding from the rectum is rare. Bruises may occur with mild skin trauma; such bruising is often most evident on the scalp. Visceral hemorrhages are rare.

Anemia is a uniform sign of infantile scurvy and in these infants is due mainly to blood loss although it is also attributable to a diet with an extremely low iron content. Growth retardation occurs in scorbutic infants. Untreated, the disease may be fatal.

Adult Scurvy. Malaise is an early sign of adult scurvy. The earliest cutaneous sign of scurvy is follicular hyperkeratosis which is particularly evident on the thighs. The follicular hyperkeratosis is associated with a peculiar twisting of the hairs in the skin follicles (corkscrew hairs). These changes in the skin are followed rapidly by perifollicular, petechial hemorrhage. Later, skin changes include massive ecchymoses over sites of minor trauma.

In the adult who is not edentulous, early oral signs of scurvy include bleeding and swelling of the gums. Later signs of scurvy include loosening of the teeth. These signs may be overlooked as manifestations of a vitamin deficiency in individuals who have pre-existing periodontal disease. Hemorrhages from various sites may occur.

Severe scurvy in the adult is associated with prostration, hypotension, and massive edema of the feet and legs. When these signs are present, they herald a fatal outcome unless there is prompt intervention.

Other types of malnutrition that may be present in scorbutic patients include iron deficiency anemia and megaloblastic anemia due to folate deficiency. The occurrence of anemia is explained by bleeding caused by the scurvy, folate deficiency, and reduced iron absorption due to low intakes of fruits and vegetables that are rich food sources of folic acid and contain ascorbic acid, which enhances iron absorption.

DIAGNOSIS. In the infant, radiologic signs of scurvy include increased density of the epiphyseal lines and evidence of new bone formation around subperiosteal hemorrhages. Epiphyseal separation may be demonstrated also. Capillary fragility may be demonstrated by placing a sphygmomanometer cuff around the arm, inflating it to a point midway between the systolic and diastolic blood pressure for 5 minutes, and then examining the antecubital fossa for petechial hemorrhages. However, this test is not specific for scurvy and it may be positive for other conditions associated with capillary fragility. Biochemical evidence of vitamin C deficiency is by measurement of leukocyte levels of the vitamin. Deficient values for leukocyte ascorbic acid are less than

7 mg/dL; low values are more than 7 mg/dL but less than 15 mg/dL, and acceptable values for leukocyte ascorbic acid are more than 15 mg/dL.

PREVENTION AND TREATMENT. Infantile scurvy can be prevented by ensuring that all infant formula or breast–milk substitutes contain adequate amounts of vitamin C, and by assuring an adequate intake of vitamin C to pregnant women. Prenatal vitamin tablets are useful for this purpose. Administration of vitamin C is also necessary for all premature infants. For breast-fed, full-term infants of women who have had adequate intakes of vitamin C in pregnancy, there is no risk of scurvy. However, in both breast- and formula-fed infants, fruit juices or physiologic levels of vitamin C given in supplements are recommended from about 4 to 6 months of age to assure an adequate vitamin C status.

When scurvy is present, therapy should be with oral doses of 250 mg vitamin C, 4 times daily until all clinical and biochemical evidence of the deficiency has resolved.

BIBLIOGRAPHY

Berger ML, Siegel, DM, Lee EL: Scurvy as an initial manifestation of Whipple's disease. Ann Intern Med 101:58–59, 1984.

Carpenter KJ: The History of Scurvy and Vitamin C. Cambridge, Cambridge University Press, 1986.

Ellis CE, Vanderveen EE, Rasmussen JE: Scurvy. A case caused by peculiar dietary habits. Arch Dermatol 120:1212–1214, 1984.

Gerson CD, Fabry EM: Ascorbic acid deficiency and fistula formation in regional enteritis. Gastroenterology 67:428–433, 1974.

Hornig DH, Moser U, Glatthaar BE: Ascorbic acid. In Shils ME, Young VR (eds.): Modern Nutrition in Health and Disease, 7th ed. Philadelphia, Lea and Febiger, 1988, pp. 417–435.

Lonnerdal B: Vitamin–mineral interactions. In Bodwell CE, Erdman JW, Jr (eds.): Nutrient Interactions. New York, Marcel Dekker, 1988, pp. 163–186.

Reuler JB, Broudy VC, and Cooney TG: Adult scurvy. JAMA 253:805–807, 1985.

Robson JRK: Zen macrobiotic diets. In Jelliffe EFP, Jelliffe DB (eds.): Adverse Effects of Foods. New York, Plenum Press, 1982, pp. 473–480.

Roe DA: Current etiologies and cutaneous signs of vitamin deficiencies. In Roe DA (ed.): Nutrition and the Skin. New York, Alan R. Liss, 1986, pp. 81–98.

Stewart JS, Booth CC: Ascorbic acid absorption in malabsorption. Clin Sci 27:15–22, 1964.

107.4. RICKETS AND OSTEOMALACIA

Daphne A. Roe

DEFINITION. Rickets and osteomalacia are the manifestations of vitamin D deficiency in children and adults. Effects of the deficiency include primarily skeletal changes due to bone softening and dental abnormalities as well as hypocalcemia. These are caused by a lack of cutaneous synthesis, intake, or utilization of vitamin D that is required for calcium absorption.

ETIOLOGY. Rickets and osteomalacia are nutritional deficiency diseases of environmental origin, and are largely attributable to lack of exposure to ultraviolet (UV) light. However, it is increasingly recognized that many otherwise adequate diets do not satisfy normal requirements for vitamin D. Therefore, most people depend on skin exposure to obtain adequate amounts of vitamin D. Supplements or diets high in vitamin D play a role in prevention, but sunlight on the skin is more important. Both diseases are due to lack of vitamin D_3, a steroid hormone synthesized in a 2-stage process in the epidermis from the precursor substance, 7-dehydrocholesterol. Formation of the epidermal precursor of vitamin D_3, previtamin D, is an ultraviolet light-dependent synthetic step, requiring an action spectrum of UV light from 240–320 nm, with a maximum at 295–313 nm. The extent to which vitamin D_3 is synthesized in the skin is related to the time of day, the amount of cloud coverage, air pollution, and to the duration of exposure to UV light.

The capacity to synthesize vitamin D in the skin is unaffected by the degree of skin pigmentation, although synthesis is slower in blacks and Indians than in Caucasians.

Following its cutaneous synthesis, vitamin D is transported to the liver where hydroxylation forms the hepatic metabolite, 25-hydroxyvitamin D, which circulates in a protein-bound form. Seasonal variation in levels of 25-hydroxyvitamin D can be correlated with exposure to ultraviolet light.

The principal mediators of vitamin D-dependent functions are the renal metabolites of the vitamin, 1,25-dihydroxyvitamin D_3 and 24,25-dihydroxyvitamin D_3, which are formed from further hydroxylation of the hepatic metabolite. The important biologic target organs of this vitamin (or hormone) include the intestine, where absorption of dietary calcium is stimulated; the bone, where accretion and mobilization of calcium and phosphorus take place; and the kidney, where tubular reabsorption of calcium and phosphorus are promoted.

DISTRIBUTION
Rickets

Reduced UV Light Exposure. Rickets was first described by Glisson in the seventeenth century in well-to-do English infants and children, who were swaddled in early life and later overclothed and kept indoors. In the nineteenth and early twentieth centuries, it was largely seen in infants and children living in industrial slums, whose sunlight exposure was limited by air pollution and who were fed exclusively cereal diets. It is now seen in the children of Asian women who are immigrants to Great Britain. These women, who themselves are vitamin D depleted, breast-feed their infants for long periods and fail to give their children vitamin D supplements. Rickets is seen also in tropical and nontropical countries in infants and children who are kept indoors for cultural reasons, or who are the progeny of Rastafarians or other vegan sects who are unwilling to consume milk or milk products. Rickets has been identified as a particular risk in premature infants, especially if the mother is vitamin D deficient.

Drug-Induced. Drug-induced rickets occurs in children with seizure disorders who are on protracted maintenance therapy with the anticonvulsants, phenytoin and phenobarbital. Epileptic children at highest risk are on these drugs and confined indoors within institutions and provided with diets lacking in milk or other vitamin D-

fortified dairy products. The antituberculous drug isoniazid interferes also with the conversion of vitamin D_3
to its active metabolites, and imposes a potential risk if
other risk factors are also present and if drug administration is prolonged.

Inborn Errors of Metabolism. Rickets can rarely be
due to inborn errors of vitamin D metabolism, including
vitamin D-dependent rickets that is caused by defective
synthesis of the vitamin. Familial hypophosphatemic
rickets is caused by a renal tubular defect.

Complication of Malabsorption. Diseases associated
with the complication of rickets include malabsorption
syndromes, cholestatic liver disease, and chronic renal
disease. Common conditions associated with malabsorption in which rickets is prevalent include gluten-sensitive
enteropathy (celiac disease), cystic fibrosis, and chronic
giardiasis. In these conditions, risk of rickets is not only
associated with malabsorption of vitamin D and calcium
but also to the avoidance of milk due to lactose intolerance.

Osteomalacia. Osteomalacia, or adult rickets, is a
prevalent condition in India, where it has occurred in
women in purdah, and in middle eastern countries such
as North Yemen, where it occurs in veiled Moslem
women who cover all exposed skin areas with turmeric.

Reduced Skin Exposure to UV Light. Even in tropical
countries the elderly are at risk for osteomalacia because
of their reduced capacity to synthesize vitamin D within
the skin. Also, they stay indoors more than younger
people, they tend to wear heavy clothing, and they may
not consume milk because of custom, cost, or real or
perceived intolerance. Another risk factor identified
recently is the excessive use of sun screens that efficiently
block shorter wave ultraviolet light (UVB) required in
vitamin D synthesis. Elderly Caucasians, particularly
those living in a sunny climate, tend to use these
products more to protect themselves against skin cancer.

In the elderly, osteomalacia is associated frequently
with osteoporosis; this combination places them at highest risk of hip fracture. Institutionalized elderly in both
tropical and nontropical countries are at risk for hip
fractures due to osteomalacia and osteoporosis if they
are not taken outdoors.

A high prevalence of osteomalacia has been reported
in Bedouin women, with hypocalcemia and rickets being
reported in their infants. In a comparative study of
Bedouin and Jewish women, levels of 2 vitamin D
metabolites, 25-hydroxyvitamin D and 24,25-hydroxy-
vitamin D, were lower in Bedouin women at delivery.
In this same study, a high correlation was found between
25-hydroxyvitamin D in infants and in the maternal
blood.

Secondary Causes of Osteomalacia. Itai-itai disease,
associated with osteomalacia, has been reported in multiparous, postmenopausal Japanese women, and is believed to be due to cadmium exposure. Risk factors
include low intake of vitamin D and calcium.

Secondary drug-induced osteomalacia may be due to
abuse of aluminum-containing antacids, or laxatives,
including mineral oil, which impairs vitamin D absorption. It may be due also to phenobarbital and phenytoin,
prescribed to control seizure disorders.

CLINICAL MANIFESTATIONS

Rickets. Rickets is characterized by abnormal development of the skeleton and teeth. Clinical signs vary
with age of onset.

Bony Changes. When rickets develops in infants less
than 8 months of age, skeletal changes in the skull are
most marked. Ossification of the skull is slowed and
irregular. The anterior fontanelle remains unclosed for
a longer than normal period; i.e., instead of closing by
18 months of age, it remains open and membranous
until the second, third, or even fourth year of life. Other
changes in the skull of the infant include bone thickening
in the frontal and parietal regions to produce characteristic bosses of the skull known as "Parrot's nodes" (Fig.
107–5). This so-called bossing of the skull, separated by
the depressions formed by the skull suture lines, suggested to earlier observers that the head had the appearance of a hot cross bun. In certain areas of the
rickety skull, particularly along the occipitoparietal suture line, the bones are thin, and craniotabes is evident
when the skull can be indented and then snap back into
its usual configuration like a ping-pong ball.

Changes in the bony thoracic cage associated with
respiratory difficulties develop early (Figs. 107–5 and
107–6). There is combined bending of the lower ribs
along the attachment of the diaphragm, flaring of the
lower ribs, and a midsternal depression producing a
deformity known as "Harrison's sulcus." Additionally,
excess osteoid formation at the costochondral junctions
produces localized enlargements that in the thin child

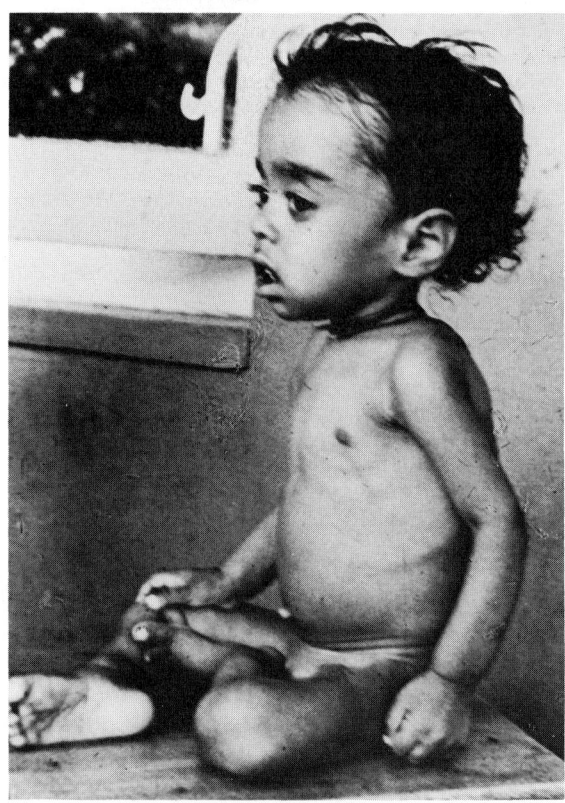

FIGURE 107–5. Child with active rickets showing bossing of the skull
bones and enlarged costochondral junctions (beading). (Courtesy of
the National Institute of Nutrition, Indian Council of Medical Research, Hyderabad, India.)

can be readily seen and palpated. The bony enlargements at the costochondral junctions are known as the "rickety rosary" (Figs. 107–5 and 107–6). Multiple rib fractures occur in severe cases.

Other skeletal changes that occur in rickets appear after the child has learned to sit up. During the first year of life, pelvic changes occur with forward projection of the sacrum and lateral bony narrowing. Kyphoscoliosis is present in severe cases. Bowing of the long bones of the arms is first manifested in the sitting infant; when the child begins to walk and weight bearing is transferred to the lower limbs, these too become bowed (Fig. 107–7). Although the extent of the bowing differs with the severity of the disease, a most constant skeletal change, attributable to rickets, is enlargement of the epiphyses, particularly found at the wrists and ankles (Fig. 107–8). Rickets may lead to pelvic deformities, which in females may in later years result in difficulties during childbirth, including obstructed labor. Eruption of the teeth of the primary dentition is delayed. When the teeth do erupt, they are small, pointed, and subject to early caries.

Complications. Infants and children with rickets have poor muscle tone and may find it difficult to sit up or stand. Tetany is a rarer complication. Infants and children with rickets often have frequent episodes of bronchitis that may lead to emphysema and chronic obstructive lung disease. The combined effects of the bone changes and repeated respiratory infections lead to marked growth retardation. Rickets was associated with high rates of infant and child mortality when it was endemic in Europe and North America.

Osteomalacia. Osteomalacia is characterized by bone pain and tenderness on pressure, loss of height, muscle weakness, which, when severe, leads to a waddling gait and difficulty in standing. Common skeletal changes lead to reduction in size of the pelvic cavity and kyphosis. Bowing of the femur and tibia may occur also. When osteomalacia develops in women in the reproductive

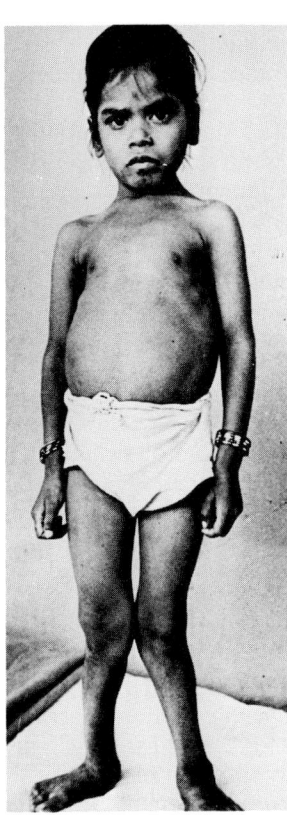

FIGURE 107–7. Girl with genu valgum due to rickets. (Courtesy of the National Institute of Nutrition, Indian Council of Medical Research, Hyderabad, India.)

period of life, the pelvic deformities impose a serious risk of obstructed labor leading to increased maternal and perinatal mortality. Tetany due to neuromuscular irritability secondary to hypocalcemia is relatively common and is associated with carpopedal spasm and facial twitching.

DIAGNOSTIC TESTS

X-ray Findings. Early radiographic changes in rickets include broadening of the lower end of the ulna and radius and rarefaction of the distal end of the shaft of these bones. Additionally, there is more intense rarefaction behind the epiphyses. As the disease advances, the widening of the distal ends of the long bones

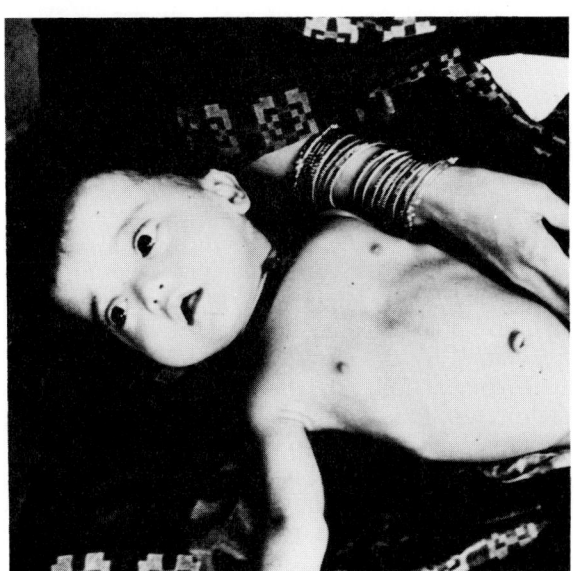

FIGURE 107–6. Infant with rickets showing rachitic beading. (Courtesy of the National Institute of Nutrition, Indian Council of Medical Research, Hyderabad, India.)

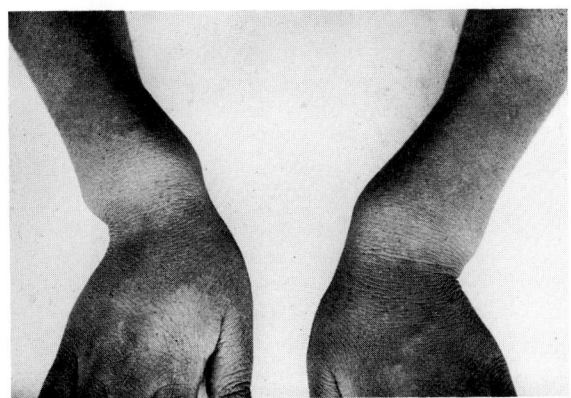

FIGURE 107–8. Widened epiphyses at the wrist in a child with active rickets. (Courtesy of the National Institute of Nutrition, Indian Council of Medical Research, Hyderabad, India.)

becomes more marked, and the ends of the shafts assume the appearance of an inverted cup (Fig. 107–9). There is delayed epiphyseal closure. Lamellated thickening of the cortex of long bones and subperiosteal bone formation are present also. Localized enlargements of the costochondral junctions ("rickety rosary") are evident on chest x-rays. Evidence of rickets can be obtained also by using photon absorptionometry to demonstrate decreased bone density. Radiographic changes in osteomalacia include generalized decalcification with incomplete fractures (Looser's zones) of the pubic rami, femoral neck, the medial border of the scapula or the upper end of the humerus.

Blood Tests

Biochemistry. Indicators of rickets and osteomalacia include combined hypocalcemia, hypophosphatemia, and elevated alkaline phosphatase activity. Whereas normally the product of serum calcium multiplied by serum phosphorus is about 50 mg/dL, in rickets this product is less than 40 and may be less than 30.

Radioimmunoassay of 25-hydroxycholecalciferol and 1,25-dihydroxycholecalciferol is measured. Deficiency levels of the vitamin D_3 metabolites are less than 10 ng/mL for 25-hydroxycholecalciferol (acceptable range 10 to 55 ng/mL), and for 1,25-dihydroxycholecalciferol, less than 20 pg/mL (acceptable range 20 to 76 pg/mL).

Bone Biopsy. A reliable method to diagnose osteomalacia is by iliac crest bone biopsy, which shows osteoid seams with absorption and atrophy of bone trabeculae.

TREATMENT. An oral dose of 25 to 125 μg (1000 to 5000 IU) of vitamin D will cure rickets or osteomalacia. A dose of greater than 125 μg vitamin D (calciferol) should be administered only in severe cases of rickets, because vitamin D toxicity can cause hypercalcemia, metastatic calcification, and renal failure.

PREVENTION. Rickets can be prevented by encouraging urban mothers to take their infants and children outdoors. Vitamin D supplements meeting the recommended nutritional requirements of the breast-fed infant need to be made available from prenatal clinics. Among Asian vegan populations, especially those who are immigrants to Great Britain, health education should include encouragement of regular use of vitamin supplements for infants and exhortation to get the children outdoors during fine weather, without excessive clothing. Prevention of osteomalacia in veiled Moslem women should be by explaining the need to expose some area of their skin, such as the hands, to sunlight. In institutionalized children and adults and in the homebound elderly, a prophylactic dose of vitamin D of 400-800 IU/day should be administered.

BIBLIOGRAPHY

Dunnigan MG, Robertson I: Residence in Britain as a risk factor for Asian rickets and osteomalacia. Lancet 1:770, 1980.

Dwyer JT, Dietz WH, Hass GH, et al.: Risk of nutritional rickets among vegetarian children. Am J Dis Child 133:134–140, 1979.

Frame B, Parfit AM: Osteomalacia: Current concepts. Ann Intern Med 89:966–982, 1978.

Henry HL, Norman AW: Vitamin D: Metabolism and biological actions. Annu Rev Nutr 4:493–520, 1984.

Holick MF: Vitamin D requirements of the elderly. Am J Clin Nutr 5:121–129, 1986.

Matsuoka LY, Wortsman J, Hanifan N, et al.: Chronic sunscreen use decreases circulating concentrations of 25-hydroxyvitamin D: A preliminary study. Arch Dermatol 124:1802–1804, 1988.

Roe DA: Drug-Induced Nutritional Deficiencies, 2nd ed. Westport, CT, AVI Publishing, 1985, pp. 32–42.

Shany S, Biale Y, Zuili I, et al.: Fetomaternal relationships between vitamin D metabolites in Israeli Bedouins and Jews. Am J Clin Nutr 40:1290–1294, 1984.

Sheldon W: Diseases of Infancy and Childhood, 5th ed. London, Churchill Ltd., 1943.

Spivey Fox MR: Nutrient interactions and the toxic elements aluminum, cadmium and lead. *In* Bodwell CE, Erdman JW, Jr (eds.): Nutrient Interactions. New York, Marcel Dekker, 1988, p. 313.

107.5. PELLAGRA

Daphne A. Roe

DEFINITION. Pellagra is a nutritional deficiency disease manifested by a rash on light-exposed areas of skin, diarrhea associated with malabsorption of nutrients, and a confusional state that is accompanied by depression. It is due to a severe deficiency of a vitamin of the B complex, niacin, which is mainly obtained from animal protein foods and vitamin-enriched cereals. The vitamin niacin denotes 2 compounds, niacin (also known as nicotinic acid) and niacinamide (also known as nicotinamide). The name of the disease, pellagra, is derived from the Italian words for rough skin, and it was so named in the eighteenth century because of the characteristic skin changes.

ETIOLOGY AND DISTRIBUTION. Pellagra used to be endemic in areas of the world where maize or

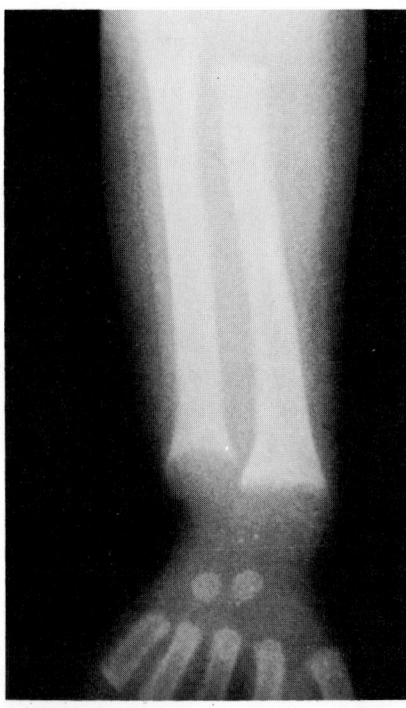

FIGURE 107–9. Radiograph of the wrist of a child with active rickets showing typical cupping and fraying of the epiphyses. (Courtesy of the National Institute of Nutrition, Indian Council of Medical Research, Hyderabad, India.)

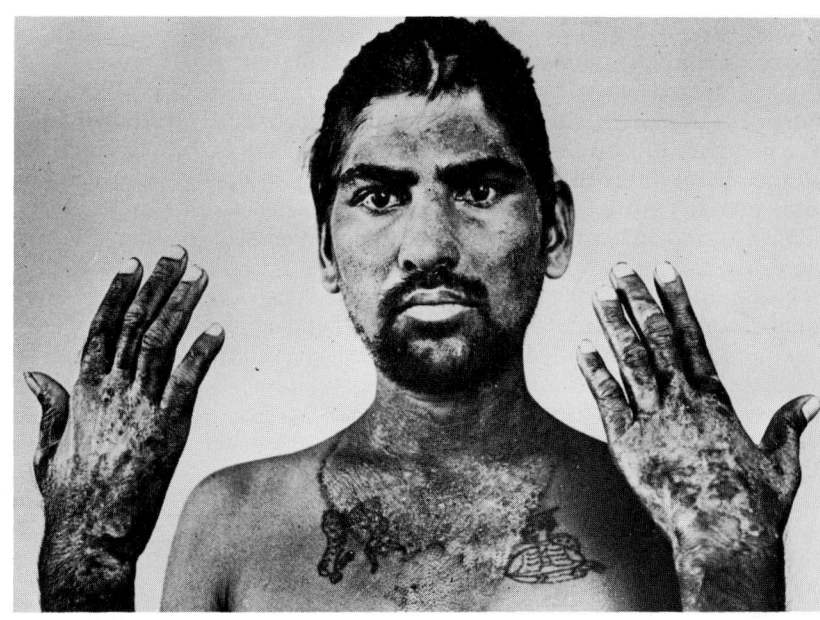

FIGURE 107–10. Pellagra showing the characteristic bilateral symmetric dermatitis on the dorsum of both hands and on the exposed part of the neck and chest. The patient has seborrheic dermatitis on the face. (Courtesy of the National Institute of Nutrition, Indian Council of Medical Research, Hyderabad, India.)

millet were the food staples and the poor could not obtain other foods. This was linked to sharecropping economies, such as those that existed in northern Italy, Egypt, and the southern United States. Pellagra is still endemic in rural blacks in South Africa who subsist on an unfortified maize meal porridge, and in India where it occurs among the poor who subsist on millet and where, as in other parts of the world, it occurs among alcoholics.

Inadequate dietary niacin is unlikely to cause pellagra if the diet contains sufficient tryptophan, an essential amino acid that can be converted to niacin in the body. Foods high in tryptophan are protein foods, particularly those of animal origin (which are also rich food sources of niacin). The niacin content of maize is not low, but much of the niacin in maize is present in a bound form. Release of the vitamin from its bound form can be achieved by treating the grain with alkali. This practice has been traditional in Mexico since early times. Poorer Mexicans who have subsisted on maize have not had endemic pellagra except during periods of severe famine.

Conditions that contribute to the risk of pellagra are improper infant feeding practices, alcoholism, tuberculosis, and diseases of genetic or acquired origin that cause malabsorption or malutilization of the vitamin. Feeding infants with corn starch rather than with breast milk and/or with infant formula of inadequate niacin content can cause infantile pellagra. Alcoholics develop pellagra not only because of inadequate intake of the vitamin, but also because of insufficient hepatic storage of the vitamin. Pellagra in persons with tuberculosis is linked to treatment with the antibacterial drug isoniazid, a vitamin B_6 antagonist. It inhibits the normal conversion of tryptophan to niacin.

CLINICAL MANIFESTATIONS. Pellagra is a chronic disease of infants, children, and adults. Four stages of the disease are identified, including an initial stage in which the individual feels unwell but has no definite symptoms. In the second stage, a confluent dermatitis of light exposed areas of the body appears. Distinctive features of the dermatitis are (a) its distribution is limited usually to areas exposed to the sun (Figs. 107–10 and 107–11) but may also include areas that are traumatized by friction or heat. A collarette of dermatitis around the neck, the so-called collar of Casal,

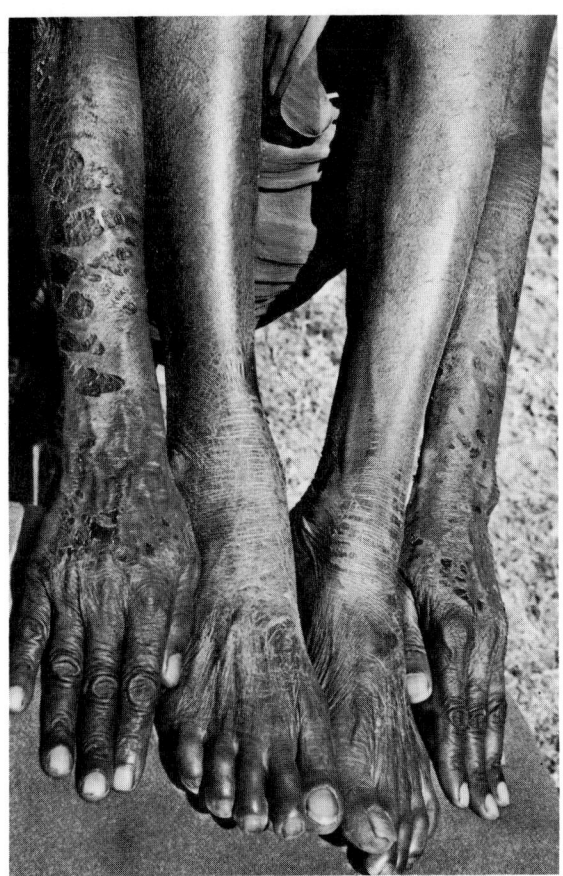

FIGURE 107–11. Pellagrous dermatitis on both arms and legs. (Courtesy of the National Institute of Nutrition, Indian Council of Medical Research, Hyderabad, India.)

is diagnostic (Fig. 107–10); (b) its progression from erythema and desquamation to hyperpigmentation of affected areas (hyperpigmentation may be followed by cutaneous atrophy); and (c) its seasonal appearance, which occurs during the time of maximal sunlight exposure. During this second stage gastrointestinal symptoms and signs (i.e., stomatitis, glossitis, gastritis and enteritis associated with malabsorption) are manifested also.

The third stage is when neuropsychiatric signs (i.e., mental confusion, irritability, delusions of sin, depression, and a suicidal tendency) appear. These psychiatric signs are associated occasionally with motor paresis and sensory neuropathy affecting the lower limbs.

The final stage in development of the disease is when protein-energy malnutrition becomes extreme. It is due to (a) the combined effects of refusal or inability to eat, (b) stomatitis, (c) psychosis in which there may be fear of eating, and (d) malabsorption. Death is either from inanition, secondary infection (e.g., tuberculosis), or suicide.

DIAGNOSIS

Clinical Diagnosis. Diagnosis is usually made clinically. The clinical signs long associated with pellagra are dermatitis, diarrhea, and dementia, but the clinician should be aware that these may develop one after the other as the disease progresses, and pellagra can be present when not all are present, e.g., before the dementia is manifested.

Laboratory Diagnosis. Preclinical diagnosis of niacin deficiency is from the levels of urinary excretion of N′-methyl-nicotinamide. For adult males and nonpregnant females, deficient values are less than 0.5 mg/gm creatinine; low values are 0.5 to 1.5 mg/gm creatinine; acceptable values are 1.6 to 4.9 mg/gm creatinine; and high values are more than 5.0 mg/gm creatinine. In pregnant women, deficient values are less than 0.5, 0.6, and 0.8 mg/gm creatinine for the first, second, and third trimesters of pregnancy, respectively.

An alternate method for diagnosis of niacin deficiency is measurement of the ratio of excretion of the urinary metabolites of niacin, e.g., 2-pyridone/N′-methylnicotinamide; a value of less than 2.0 indicates deficiency (acceptable values are more than 2.0). Another method to detect deficiency is by measuring the niacin in whole blood; a value of less than 24.4 μmol/l (3μg/mL) is considered deficient and values of 32.5 to 73.1 μmol/l (4 to 9 μg/mL) are acceptable values.

Differential Diagnosis. Phototoxic dermatoses (e.g., those due to drugs, or to ingestion of large quantities of chenopodium or other plant foods containing phototoxins) may be confused with pellagra. Another condition in the differential diagnosis is ariboflavinosis. In this condition the dermatitis is in skinfolds and flexures as well as on the genitalia; fissuring occurs at the corners of the mouth; glossitis is present as in pellagra; but the diarrhea and dementia of pellagra are absent. In infants and young children, the differential diagnosis is also from kwashiorkor with so-called "flaky paint" dermatitis of the limbs, particularly over areas of edema, but not specifically over areas exposed to the sun. In infants fed diets low in food energy and lacking both in protein and

in niacin, signs of kwashiorkor and pellagra can be present concurrently.

TREATMENT AND CONTROL. Niacin should be administered orally or by nasogastric tube when the oral and pharyngeal lesions make swallowing difficult. In all cases with overt clinical signs, 300 to 500 mg of niacin or niacinamide should be given in divided doses of 100 mg for the first 2 days. Thereafter, the dose can be reduced to 50 mg 2 to 3 times daily until all signs have disappeared and the laboratory tests have reached normal values. If it is impossible to give the niacin or niacinamide orally or by nasogastric tube due to the severity of mucositis of the mouth, pharynx, and esophagus, initial doses of 100 mg niacinamide may be given intramuscularly 3 times daily.

Prevention of pellagra is by providing a diet adequate in the vitamin, implying an adequate intake from animal protein as well as from enriched cereals. The adequacy of animal protein in the diet also assists in disease prevention by providing tryptophan. In all areas, the major public health measure found efficacious in preventing pellagra has been the enrichment of cereal grain with the vitamin. Such enrichment should be mandatory and should be at a level of 24 mg/lb of flour, whether it is wheat or corn or other cereal staple.

Isoniazid-related pellagra can be prevented by giving a vitamin B₆ supplement daily (25 mg) with the drug.

BIBLIOGRAPHY

Roe DA: A Plague of Corn: The Social History of Pellagra. Ithaca, New York, Cornell University Press, 1976, pp. 1–7.
Goldsmith GA: Curative nutrition—vitamins. In Schneider HA, Anderson CE, Coursin DB (eds.): Nutritional Support of Medical Practice, 2nd ed. Philadelphia, Harper & Row, 1983, pp. 168–170.
Bauernfeind JC: Nutrification of food. In Shils ME, Young VR (eds.): Modern Nutrition in Health and Disease, 7th ed. Philadelphia, Lea & Febiger, 1988, pp. 718–719.

107.6. ARIBOFLAVINOSIS

Daphne A. Roe

DEFINITION. Ariboflavinosis is a nutritional deficiency disease characterized by seborrheic dermatitis, angular stomatitis, and glossitis. It is due to a deficiency of the B vitamin, riboflavin, which is obtained mainly from dairy foods. It was first described in India in the 1930s but has since been seen as a widespread deficiency not only in India, but also in China, Taiwan, Iran, among the urban poor in Kenya, and Ecuador.

ETIOLOGY AND EPIDEMIOLOGY. Riboflavin occurs in food and in the body in three major forms: the free vitamin and the two active coenzyme forms, flavin 5′phosphate or flavin monophosphate (FMN) and flavin adenine dinucleotide (FAD). In its coenzyme forms, riboflavin is active in energy utilization and acts as an intermediary in the transfer of electrons in biological oxidation-reduction reactions.

Riboflavin is stable on heat processing and is not destroyed in high temperature treatment milks such as those recently made available in certain tropical countries. It is, however, unstable in light and is destroyed when sun drying of foods is undertaken or when milk is light-exposed in glass or plastic bottles.

Ariboflavinosis has a worldwide distribution, occurring among all populations and population subgroups subsisting on cereal-based diets. It may develop during the weaning period if the infant's diet does not contain milk. In older children and in adults, ariboflavinosis occurs in those who do not include milk in their diets, either because the milk is not available or because they are lactose intolerant. In urbanized communities, ariboflavinosis may occur even in those populations who traditionally drink milk, if milk is too expensive to buy or too difficult to obtain. Alcoholics are particularly at risk, not only because they do not drink milk and are often lactose intolerant, but also because their riboflavin absorption and utilization is impaired.

CLINICAL MANIFESTATIONS. Early symptoms of riboflavin deficiency include soreness and burning of the tongue. There may be discomfort in the mouth on eating highly seasoned food, such as curry. Signs of the disease include fissuring and peeling of the lips (cheilosis), cracks at the corners of the mouth (angular stomatitis) (Fig. 107–12), and a seborrheic dermatitis that occurs in the nasolabial folds (Fig. 107–13) around the eyes, in the umbilicus, on the genitalia, particularly on the scrotum, and in the flexures, including the inguinal areas.

Photophobia with lacrimation and burning of the eyes has been described and is associated with corneal vascularization. Normochromic anemia occurs in severe cases.

DIAGNOSIS
Differential Diagnosis

Pellagra. Differential diagnosis is from pellagra that may coexist (Chapter 107.5). The cutaneous manifestations of ariboflavinosis differ from pellagra in that the dermatosis of pellagra is predominantly on light exposed areas, whereas the skin changes in riboflavin deficiency are localized to skin creases and flexures that are not

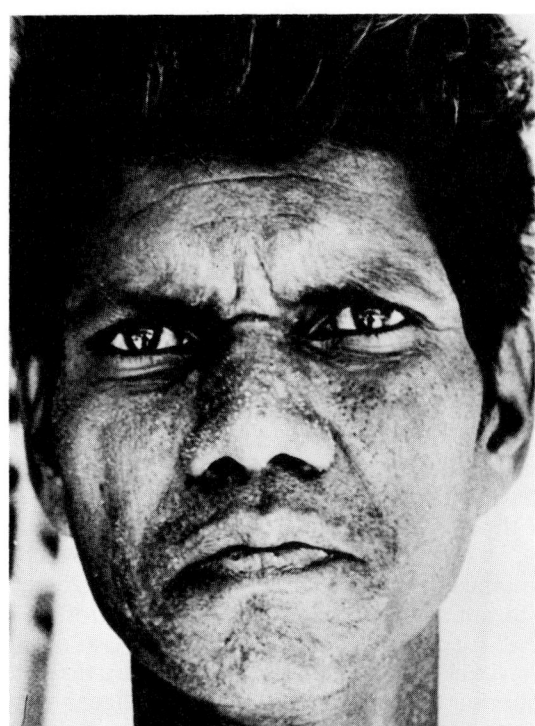

FIGURE 107–13. Seborrheic dermatitis due to riboflavin deficiency. Whitish sebaceous plugs can be seen on the nose. They have a characteristic fatty acid odor. (Courtesy of the National Institute of Nutrition, Indian Council of Medical Research, Hyderabad, India.)

usually exposed to light or are exposed to light less than unaffected areas of skin. Pellagra patients (pellagrins) also have more severe oral lesions than patients with riboflavin deficiency; pellagrins' oral lesions may interfere with chewing and swallowing, which rarely occurs in ariboflavinosis. Advanced cases of pellagra show psychiatric manifestations with profound depression and a confusional state; this does not occur in ariboflavinosis.

Zinc Deficiency. Zinc deficiency, like ariboflavinosis, is manifested by a red scaly dermatosis on the face (Chapter 108.4). However, in the former condition the dermatosis tends to be localized around the oral, perineal, and anal areas. It may be pustular and may extend to the trunk and limbs, where a mild erythema and desquamation occurs. The mucosal lesions in zinc deficiency are due to secondary candidiasis. Other manifestations of zinc deficiency not present in ariboflavinosis include loss of taste, severe impairment in cell-mediated immunity, and slow wound healing. Endemic zinc deficiency and ariboflavinosis occur in Middle Eastern countries in individuals subsisting on wheat-based cereal diets. Zinc deficiency and ariboflavinosis may both be present in alcoholics.

Stomatitis. The angular stomatitis of ariboflavinosis has to be differentiated from a simple monilial intertrigo, particularly in those who are edentulous; from herpetic infection of the commissures of the mouth; and from impetigo. These conditions do not heal when riboflavin is administered but do respond to anti-infective agents or, in the case of herpetic lesions, are self-limited in duration.

Biochemical Tests. The biochemical test for riboflavin

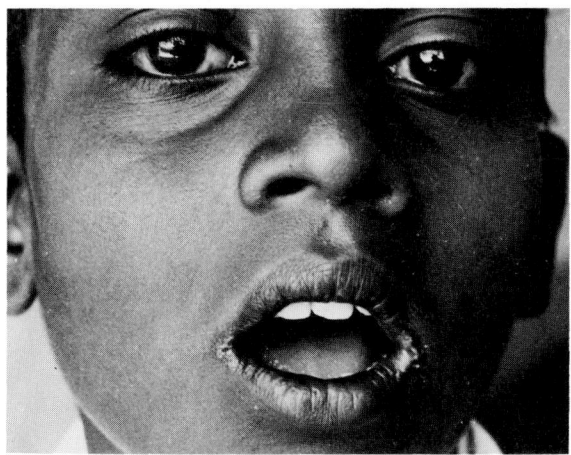

FIGURE 107–12. Angular stomatitis in a child caused by riboflavin deficiency. The lesion is an acute one. The sharp fissures at the angle of the mouth are evident. (Courtesy of the National Institute of Nutrition, Indian Council of Medical Research, Hyderabad, India.)

depletion or deficiency is the erythrocyte glutathione reductase assay (EGR). The test depends on the degree of stimulation of erythrocyte glutathione reductase activity by addition of FAD in vitro. Results are usually expressed as activity coefficients (EGRAC), as follows:

$$EGRAC = \frac{\text{Enzyme activity with added FAD}}{\text{Enzyme activity without added FAD}}$$

Acceptable normal EGRAC values are less than 1.2. In clinical riboflavin deficiency, the EGRAC is greater than 1.3. The test cannot be used in persons with glucose-6-phosphate dehydrogenase deficiency because of an increased avidity of the red cell enzyme for FAD in this disease. An alternate laboratory method of biochemical assessment of riboflavin status is to measure riboflavin excretion in 24-hour urine collections. However, the urinary excretion of the vitamin reflects intake of the vitamin rather than riboflavin status. When riboflavin intake is inadequate (e.g., less than 0.25 mg/1000 kcal for an adult or child), the urinary excretion is less than 30 μg/gm creatinine for an adult. Use of urinary riboflavin as a diagnostic test is limited by the problem of collecting 24-hour urine samples, the higher excretion of the vitamin by the riboflavin deficient, growing children, and the hyperexcretion of the vitamin by individuals of all ages who are catabolic.

TREATMENT. Treatment of riboflavin deficiency is by administration of a purified preparation of the vitamin at a dose of 5 mg twice daily until the clinical signs of deficiency have disappeared and biochemical status is normalized. Thereafter, the dietary intake of the vitamin needs to be adequate to prevent recurrence.

PREVENTION AND CONTROL. Riboflavin deficiency is prevented by including dairy products in the diet. An 8 fluid ounce glass of milk contains 0.4 mg of riboflavin. In areas where intake of dairy products is low, enrichment of cereal grains with the vitamin can prevent deficiency. In Great Britain, the recommended intake for an adult, nonpregnant nonlactating woman is 1.3 mg/day; for a man it is 1.7 mg/day; and the daily recommended intake of riboflavin in the United States for an adult is 0.6 mg/1000 kcal of food energy. Whereas these amounts may be inadequate to prevent riboflavin depletion in an individual undertaking heavy exercise or physical work, they are sufficient to prevent the appearance of clinical signs of riboflavin deficiency. Estimated requirements of riboflavin for physically active individuals range from 0.9 to 1.2 mg/day. Pregnant and lactating women (according to studies carried out in Gambia, West Africa) require at least 2.5 mg of riboflavin per day to achieve normal status as estimated by the red cell enzyme (EGR) test.

BIBLIOGRAPHY

Bates CJ, Prentice AM, Watkinson M, et al.: Riboflavin requirements of lactating Gambian women: A controlled supplementation trial. Am J Clin Nutr 36:902–909, 1982.

Belko AZ, Obarzanek E, Kalkwarf HJ, et al.: Effects of exercise on the riboflavin requirements of young women. Am J Clin Nutr 37:509–517, 1983.

Cooperman JM, Lopez R: Riboflavin. *In* Machlin LJ (ed.): Handbook of Vitamins: Nutritional, Biochemical and Clinical Aspects. New York, Marcel Dekker, 1984, pp. 299–327.

Goldsmith GA: Riboflavin deficiency. *In* Rivlin RS (ed.): Riboflavin. New York, Plenum Press, 1975, pp. 221–244.

Hunt SM: Nutritional intake of riboflavin. *In* Rivlin RS (ed.): Riboflavin. New York, Plenum Press, 1975, pp. 199–219.

Nicholalds GE: Riboflavin. *In* Labbe RF (ed.): Clin Lab Med 1:685–698, 1981.

Roe DA: Current etiologies and cutaneous signs of vitamin deficiencies. *In* Roe DA (ed.): Nutrition and the Skin. New York, Alan R. Liss, 1986, pp. 81–98.

Rosenthal WS, Adham NF, Lopez R, et al.: Riboflavin deficiency in complicated chronic alcoholism. Am J Clin Nutr 26:858–860, 1973.

Sebrell WH, Butler RE: Riboflavin deficiency in man. Preliminary note. Public Health Rep 53:2282–2284, 1938.

107.7   NUTRITIONAL MACROCYTIC (MEGALOBLASTIC) ANEMIA

Daphne A. Roe

DEFINITION AND HISTORY. Nutritional macrocytic (megaloblastic) anemia is a deficiency disease caused by inadequate intake and/or impaired absorption or utilization of the B vitamin, folic acid. It was first described in 1929 by Lucy Wills. She observed the anemia in pregnant Indian women and gave it the name "pernicious anaemia of pregnancy" because the blood picture resembled that of pernicious (Addisonian) anemia. Following her original observations of nutritional macrocytic anemia in pregnant women, she was able to show that the same disease occurred in nonpregnant women and in men, and she showed that the condition could be treated effectively with crude liver extracts as well as with preparations of yeast, which were identified as sources of a then unknown nutrient named for Dr. Wills, the "Wills factor" and from which folic acid was subsequently isolated.

ETIOLOGY AND EPIDEMIOLOGY. Folic acid deficiency has a worldwide distribution presently, but it differs greatly in severity. In its less severe form, no anemia is manifested.

Groups at Risk. Nutritional macrocytic anemia in its endemic form has greatest prevalence in pregnant women. Risk factors include multiple or frequent pregnancies and intake of diets that lack all types of dark green vegetables. It was described originally as a seasonal disease; the season of greatest occurrence being the time of lowest availability of green vegetables as sources of the vitamin. Other diet characteristics that have been shown to contribute to the risk of folate deficiency include cooking vegetables in large volumes of water, which is then discarded; the folate in the vegetables leaches into the cooking water. An observation, originally made by Dr. Wills, is that folate deficiency occurs most frequently in those subsisting on "white diets," i.e., diets based on white bread, polished rice, or white maize meal. This diet is lacking in both vegetables and animal protein, sources of the folate. In poverty areas, such as urban areas in South Africa, folate depletion is a problem of urban black school children.

Since its original description as a condition of pregnancy, nutritional macrocytic anemia has been found most commonly in alcoholics who eat diets low in vegetables, and who also are unable to absorb or metabolize folic acid normally.

Other groups at risk for folic acid deficiency include those with hemolytic anemias, e.g., sickle cell anemia, in whom folate deficiency develops following hemolytic episodes. Folic acid deficiency, with or without megaloblastic anemia, is common also in people with malabsorption syndromes, e.g., those having tropical sprue, chronic giardiasis, and gluten-sensitive enteropathy. It develops also in those who are taking drugs that are folate antagonists, including the protozoal drug, pyrimethamine, and the antibacterial drug, trimethoprim, as well as pentamidine, which is sometimes used in the treatment of trypanosomiasis, Kala-azar, and *Pneumocystis carinii* infection. Other drugs that induce folate depletion or deficiency include the anticonvulsant drugs, phenytoin and phenobarbital. Mild folate depletion may be found in women taking oral contraceptives. If women become pregnant within 6 months of taking these drugs, folate depletion may persist throughout the first trimester of pregnancy.

CLINICAL MANIFESTATIONS. Development of folic acid deficiency, by dietary deprivation, to a stage of anemia takes approximately 4 to 5 months if the individual's previous intake of the vitamin has been sufficient. However, in those who habitually consume diets low in the vitamin, the time required to become anemic is less.

Folic acid deficiency with severe anemia causes anorexia, fever, dyspnea due to hypoxia, ankle edema, and cheilitis associated with glossitis (Chapter 5).

Risks from folate deficiency include poor pregnancy outcome. In some groups of pregnant women, there has been a high prevalence of accidental hemorrhage and premature births. Birth defects are not associated with nutritional folate deficiency, though they are induced by drugs that are folate antagonists. There may be a risk of cancer developing at the site of folate deficiency megaloblastic changes in the cervix.

LABORATORY DIAGNOSIS
Hematologic Changes. The initial hematologic changes include hypersegmentation of the polymorphonuclear leukocytes (Chapter 5). This denotes an impairment in leukocyte maturation. Hypersegmentation of the granulocytes is associated with, or shortly followed by, the appearance of megaloblastic red cells in the peripheral blood, that is, red blood cells having an abnormally high corpuscular volume. Concurrently there is megaloblastic development of red and white cell precursors in the bone marrow and also of epithelial cells, including those lining the mouth, small intestine, vagina, and bladder. As the folate deficiency progresses, the red cell count markedly declines, and the fall in number of red blood cells is associated with a lowering of hemoglobin values.

Because folate deficiency is associated frequently with iron deficiency, the peripheral blood may contain both microcytic and macrocytic (megaloblastic) cells. This results in a dimorphic anemia; the average volume of red cells is not increased. It may mask the diagnosis

unless blood and/or bone marrow films are examined for megaloblasts or biochemical indicators of folate deficiency are obtained.

Biochemical Changes. Diagnosis of folate deficiency is made usually from combined hematologic and biochemical assessments. Hematologic changes per se are insufficient evidence for making a diagnosis of folate deficiency, because the same findings occur in vitamin B_{12} deficiency. Biochemical indicators of folate deficiency include low levels of plasma (serum) and red cell folate. Levels of folate in plasma and red cells that are considered deficient differ with the assay method. If the microbiologic assay technique is used, deficient levels of plasma folate are less than 3 ng/mL, and deficient levels of red cell folate are less than 140 ng/mL. If the patient has consumed aspirin or alcohol before the plasma folate assay, the values are lowered temporarily.

Other tests of folate deficiency include the urinary formiminoglutamic acid excretion (FIGLU) test, and the deoxyuridine (dU) suppression test. However, neither of these procedures is likely to be available except in a research unit or a tertiary care hospital.

Plasma or serum vitamin B_{12} levels less than 150 picograms/mL can differentiate vitamin B_{12} from folate deficiency. When the laboratory is unable to perform this measurement and the patient has megaloblastic anemia, it is appropriate to give 1000 µg of vitamin B_{12} by intramuscular injection and monitor the patient for a hematologic response. If reticulocytosis follows 1 or more vitamin B_{12} injections, the anemia is due to a deficiency of vitamin B_{12} and not of folate. In tropical countries, vitamin B_{12} deficiency is most likely due to prolonged subsistence on a vegan diet.

TREATMENT. Treatment of severe folate deficiency is with folic acid. It is usually given at a dose of 10 to 15 mg/day until the clinical signs disappear, the blood picture normalizes, and the plasma and red cell folate achieve acceptable levels. However, this high dose cannot be given if the patient is receiving phenytoin, because it interferes with seizure control. In such cases, the recommended dose is 1 mg/day, which is sufficient for most cases of folate deficiency.

Prior to giving folic acid in therapeutic doses it is important to differentiate folate deficiency from vitamin B_{12} deficiency. Failure to diagnose the latter condition imposes the risk of neuropathic complications.

PREVENTION AND CONTROL. Consumption of green leafy vegetables cooked in small volumes of water and the cooking liquid can prevent folate deficiency. Fortification of cereal grains has been carried out in certain countries, including South Africa, but only on a limited or experimental basis. The 1980 recommended dietary allowance for folate in the U.S. is 400 µg/day, which is more than enough to prevent deficiency.

In pregnancy, a common practice is to give folic acid supplements of 1 to 5 mg/day.

Programs to reduce alcohol abuse by improving social conditions and decreasing availability may reduce the prevalence of folate deficiency.

BIBLIOGRAPHY

Colman N: Laboratory assessment of folate status. *In* Labbe RF (ed.): Clin Lab Med 1:775–796, 1981.

Colman N, Green R, Metz J: Prevention of folate deficiency by food fortification. II. Absorption of folic acid from fortified staple foods. Am J Clin Nutr 28:459–464, 1975.

Halsted CH: Folate deficiency in alcoholism. Am J Clin Nutr 33:2736–2740, 1980.

Lamparelli RDV, van der Westhuyzen, Steyn NP, et al.: Nutritional anaemia in 11 year-old school children in the Western Cape. S Afr Med J 73:473–476, 1988.

Martinez O, Roe DA: Effect of oral contraceptives on blood folate levels in pregnancy. Am J Obstet Gynecol 128:255–257, 1977.

Roe DA: Diet and Drug Interactions. New York, Van Nostrand Reinhold, 1988, pp. 135–152.

Roe DA: Lucy Wills (1888–1964). A biographical sketch. J Nutr 108:1379, 1978.

Wagner C: Folic acid. In: Olson RE (ed.): Present Knowledge in Nutrition, 5th ed. New York, Nutrition Foundation, 1984, pp. 332–346.

Wills L, Mehta MM: Studies in pernicious anaemia of pregnancy: Part I. Preliminary Report. Indian J Med Res 17:777, 1929–1930.

Wills L, Talpade SN: Studies in pernicious anaemia of pregnancy: Part II. A survey of dietetic and hygienic conditions of women in Bombay. Indian J Med Res 18:307, 1930–1931.

108. MINERAL DEFICIENCIES

Many minerals are needed for normal health, some in small amounts ("trace elements"). Much is known about many of these micronutrients in veterinary medicine, and this field has begun to be explored in humans in recent years. The following sections deal only with 3 minerals about which there is considerable information—iron, iodine, and zinc.

108.1. IRON DEFICIENCY

Samuel G. Kahn

DEFINITION. Iron deficiency anemia results from a decrease in content of total body iron. The hemoglobin concentration is reduced to a level that is lower than an accepted standard value for a given population.

ETIOLOGY. Insufficient biologically available dietary iron is the most frequent cause of iron deficiency anemia. The availability of food iron is related to chemical properties of its iron salts, such as its association with other substances in the diet. Usually, other substances "bind" the iron molecule, making it less available for absorption. Thus, a food with a high iron content may be a relatively poor source of food iron. Overcoming this problem may involve (a) the addition of iron to a food at a level that exceeds that of the complexing substance, (b) the proper processing of the food, and/or (c) the addition of chemicals that favorably influence the increased absorption of iron.

Loss of blood promotes anemia when the dietary intake is insufficient to replace the iron lost. In the tropics, blood loss is often caused by parasitic infections, e.g., hookworm infection and schistosomiasis.

PREVALENCE AND DISTRIBUTION. Nutritional anemia has a worldwide distribution and is one of the most prevalent nutritional deficiencies. It is precipitated by an insufficiency of iron, vitamin B_{12}, or folic acid, or a combination of the three. The most common cause of nutritional anemia is an inadequacy of iron per se. Iron deficiency anemia occurs most frequently in infants, growing children, adolescents, and pregnant women. In the last group, a combined deficiency of iron and folic acid is often present.

In developing countries, iron deficiency anemia may affect half the population. In many of these countries, almost all pregnant women and 60% to 80% of women of childbearing age are anemic. This is especially true in rural areas. The prevalence of anemia in children 5 years old or younger is often 50 to 60% (Chapter 5).

IRON METABOLISM

Iron Distribution. Body iron is classified as either *functional* or *stored*.

Functional Iron. Functional compounds are *hemoglobin, myoglobin, heme* and *nonheme enzymes,* and *transferrin*. They are essential for many vital functions of the body. Approximately 85% of all functional iron serves as erythrocyte hemoglobin in the transport of oxygen. Another 14.5% resides in muscle as a component of myoglobin, which serves as a source of oxygen for muscle metabolism. The remaining 0.5% is part of a cofactor to enzymes that serve as either electron donors or acceptors in critical body reduction–oxidation reactions or is bound to transferrin, the iron transport protein. A healthy adult will have approximately 37 mg of functional iron per kg of body weight.

Stored Iron. Storage forms of iron are *ferritin* and *hemosiderin*. Ferritin is composed of a heterogeneous group of water-soluble proteins, approximately 20% iron by weight. The largest amounts of ferritin are found in liver parenchyma, but considerable quantities are also present in cells of the reticuloendothelial system (particularly in the spleen and bone marrow) and in skeletal muscle. Hemosiderin is water-insoluble and may contain up to 41% iron by weight. It is found chiefly in skeletal muscle, but smaller amounts may be found in parenchymal cells. The total amount of stored iron will vary because it reflects the adequacy of iron balance. A replete male may store as much as 1000 mg of iron, whereas a comparable female will store only 300 mg. This limited iron reserve and their greater physiologic requirement for iron explain why women are more vulnerable to developing iron deficiency anemia.

Iron Absorption. The amount of iron absorbed depends on several factors: (a) the total amount in the diet, (b) its absorbability, and (c) the regulation of its absorption through the intestinal mucosa. Conditions such as pregnancy and deficiency of iron stores increase absorption of iron by the small intestinal mucosa.

There are 2 categories of dietary iron: heme iron, which is readily absorbed irrespective of diet composition, and nonheme iron, which has a lower absorbability. Heme iron is found in meat, including poultry and fish, whereas nonheme iron is found in vegetable staples, e.g., cereals and legumes. The better absorption of animal tissue iron could be explained by the fact that heme iron is taken up directly by mucosal cells, and therefore, its iron is not vulnerable to substances and conditions that interfere with iron absorption. Most forms of nonheme iron enter a "common pool" during digestion and are similarly affected by dietary enhancers and inhibitors of iron absorption.

TABLE 108–1. Foods Rich in Ascorbic Acid

West Indian cherry	Cabbage
Guava	Akee
Papaya	Alfalfa shoots
Citrus fruit	Broccoli
Spinach	Cauliflower
Peas	Parsley
Sweet potato	Collard greens
White potato	Cashew (raw fruit pulp)
Beet greens	Lychee
Turnips and turnip tops	Mango
Amaranth leaves	Pineapple
Bean sprouts	Baobab (monkey bread)
Green and red peppers	Longan

TABLE 108–3. Foods with Relatively High Iron Content

Whole grain of oats, barley, canihua, millet, wheat, sorghum
Quinoa
Beans and peas
Soybeans and chickpeas
Seeds of pumpkin, sesame, sunflower, squash, almond
Blackstrap molasses
Red palm oil
Crickets, termites, grasshoppers
Peanuts
Betel nut
Dried dates and raisins
Jackfruit
Egg yolk

Insoluble iron compounds, e.g., ferric phosphates and ferric hydroxide, are poorly absorbed, and ferric oxide is not absorbed at all. Often, these iron compounds are present in the dirt that contaminates cereal, legume, and vegetable foodstuffs and contribute to relatively high iron content in the diet in areas where iron deficiency anemia is prevalent.

A number of foods contain substances that inhibit iron absorption by forming complexes with iron that are then poorly absorbed. Some examples are oxalates in spinach, phytates in cereal brans, tannates in tea and coffee, and phosphoprotein in egg yolk. In contrast, iron absorption can be significantly enhanced by ascorbic acid (vitamin C). Foods high in ascorbic acid are fruits and vegetables, examples of which are listed in Table 108–1. Foods with relatively high iron bioavailability are listed in Table 108–2, and those with relatively high iron content are listed in Table 108–3.

Meat, poultry, and fish are ideal for the treatment and prevention of iron deficiency; however, adequate amounts of animal proteins are beyond the economic means of the majority of those living in developing countries. A valid alternative is the use of vegetables and fruits that contain high amounts of ascorbic acid in conjunction with foods, e.g., cereals and legumes, that have adequate iron but of low bioavailability. Good iron nutriture is attainable, but often not obtained, on a vegetarian diet.

In more affluent populations, excessive food refinement, individual food idiosyncrasies, and, often, a decrease in meat consumption and food quantity in general have contributed to the prevalence of iron deficiency. A general rule of thumb for estimating the iron content of a "Western diet" is 6 mg of iron per 1000 kilocalories.

Iron Requirements. Individual iron requirements depend on age, sex, and special physiologic needs, e.g., pregnancy, lactation, and growth (Table 108–4).

Infants. At birth, the full-term infant is supplied with

TABLE 108–2. Foods with Relatively High Iron Bioavailability

Blood products
Beef, pork, chicken, animal muscle tissue, fish
Liver, kidney, spleen
Sausages
Oysters, clams, mussels
Spinach
Alfalfa shoots
Amaranth leaves

substantial amounts of stored iron—from fetal hepatic stores and from blood drained from the placenta ("placental transfusion"). The iron status of the mother does not appear to modify the iron stores of the full-term newborn, except in mothers with marked iron deficiency. Moreover, administration of supplements of either oral or parenteral iron to pregnant women does not influence the iron nutriture of the newborn. However, this fact should not minimize the importance of iron nutrition in the pregnant woman. During the first year after birth, the infant needs to double its body iron stores, making it necessary to replenish these stores with iron from its diet. The importance of breast-feeding in improving the bioavailability of iron present is well documented. The highest prevalence of iron deficiency anemia in children occurs between the ages of about 6 months and 3 years, when stores are likely to become depleted. As the growth rate subsides, the demand for iron lessens. Premature and small-for-date infants have reduced iron stores that are soon exhausted because of rapid postnatal growth. Consequently, they are in a more precarious situation with regard to iron stores and need exogenous iron earlier in life than the full-term infant does.

Children. Iron needs during childhood are not as demanding as those during infancy or adolescence. However, the child in the tropics is vulnerable to infections with hookworm and schistosomes, which can result in substantial blood loss and a concomitant greater iron need. During adolescence, children experience a rapid spurt in growth that requires increased iron. The need for iron in girls is soon increased by the start of menstruation.

Adults. The adult male has a relatively low iron requirement. Iron deficiency anemia in this group is usually due to blood loss from the gastrointestinal tract, e.g., chronic bleeding from a peptic ulcer or hookworm or schistosomal infections.

Women of childbearing age are the group at greatest risk of developing iron deficiency anemia. The cumulative frequency of daily iron requirements in normal women, as calculated from the sum of their basal obligatory iron losses plus menstruation, ranges from 1.3 to 2.1 mg of absorbed iron daily (Fig. 108–1). The estimated net iron cost of pregnancy is shown in Table 108–5. Onset of menopause diminishes a woman's requirement for iron to that of a man.

PATHOGENESIS. Conditions that precipitate iron

TABLE 108–4. Recommended Daily Intakes of Iron (mg/day)*†

	Age	USRDA (1974)	FAO/WHO (1970)		
			Percent Calories from Animal Foods		*Absorbed Iron*
			<10%	*>25%*	
	(Years)	*Iron (mg/day)*	*Iron (mg/day)*		*(mg/day)*
Infants	0.5–3	15	10	5	1.0
Children‡	4–10	10	10	5	1.0
Male	11–18	18	18	9	1.8
Female	11–18	18	24	12	2.4
Men	>19	10	9	5	0.9
Women	19–50	18	28	14	2.8
Women	>51	10	9	5	0.9

*From the International Nutritional Anemia Consultative Group (INACG): Iron Deficiency in Infancy and Childhood. September 1979.

†Recommended daily intakes are estimates of "upper limits" of requirements in normal individuals; they do not take into account any additional requirements imposed by unusual environmental stress, by disease, or by parasitic infection.

‡Age ranges for children are those of the USRDA: ranges in the FAO/WHO recommendations differ slightly as follows: 4–12, 3–16 yrs.

deficiency anemia are (1) insufficient iron intake, (2) blood loss, (3) malabsorption, and (4) repeated pregnancies.

Insufficient Intake. The inadequate consumption of dietary iron can be the result of the voluntary restriction of certain iron-rich foods because of economic or cultural constraints. This is especially true in developing countries, where vegetarian food habits or low income restricts the consumption of meat, poultry, and fish. These situations are further compounded by the fact that many cereal and legume diets contain ligands and other inhibitors of iron absorption. The problem can be further aggravated by tropical malabsorption syndromes (sprue), a problem widespread in countries such as India, Pakistan, Bangladesh, and Haiti.

Blood Loss. This results in anemia if the amount of blood lost depletes iron stores, a condition not uncommon in menorrhagia. The use of estrogen/progesterone contraceptive pills can reduce menstrual blood loss by 50%. However, the use of intrauterine devices tends to promote increased blood loss. One pregnancy causes an estimated loss of 500 mg of iron; consequently, repeated pregnancies frequently result in iron deficiency anemia, often of a serious nature.

In tropical areas, anemia due to blood loss, particularly in children, is frequently caused by hookworm, *Trichuris,* and schistosomal infections. Other causes of blood loss are bleeding peptic ulcers and hemorrhoids.

CLINICAL MANIFESTATIONS. Iron deficiency anemia often goes unrecognized, because the individual experiences no profound ill effect and/or has another disorder that is the focus of treatment. The clinical and public health significance of mild to moderate anemia varies from country to country (Chapter 5).

Mild anemia may be marked by weakness, fatigability, irritability, lightheadedness, headache, and shortness of breath. Paleness of the skin, conjunctivae, fingernails, and mucous membranes is observed.

Moderate iron deficiency anemia may be associated with papillary atrophy of the tongue and glossitis. Other symptoms may be anorexia, heartburn, flatulence, nausea, and constipation. Pica or bizarre food cravings have been associated with iron deficiency. There is evidence that anemia impairs work capacity and performance.

Severe anemia can lead to cardiac dilatation and congestive heart failure. Enlargement of the spleen has been reported in some individuals. In pregnant women,

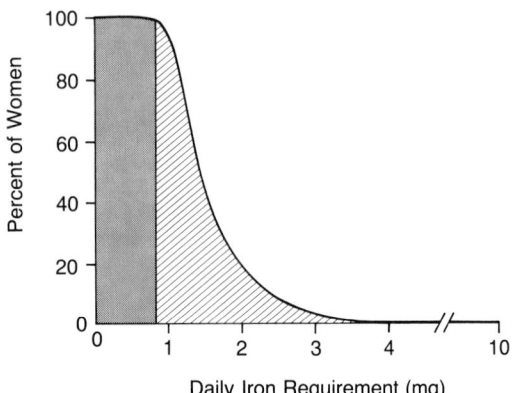

FIGURE 108–1. Cumulative frequency of daily iron requirements in normal women as calculated from the sum of their basal obligatory losses (dotted area) and loss due to menstruation (cross-hatched area). (From Iron Deficiency in Women. A Report of the International Nutritional Anemia Consultative Group [INACG], 1981. After Hallberg L, et al.: Variation in iron loss in women. *In* Occurrence, Causes, and Prevention of Nutritional Anemias, Symposia of the Swedish Nutrition Foundation VI, 1967. Stockholm, Almqvist and Wiksell, 1968.)

TABLE 108–5. Iron Losses During Pregnancy in a 55-kg Iron-Replete Woman*†

	Amount of Iron (mg)
Gross Losses	
Fetus	280
Umbilical cord and placenta	90
Maternal blood loss	150
Obligatory losses from gut, etc., during gestation	230
Expansion of maternal red cell mass	450
Gross Total	1200
Net Losses	
Contraction of maternal red cell mass after delivery	450
Net Total	750

*These represent average values. Considerable individual variations have been reported in different studies.

†From the International Nutritional Anemia Consultative Group (INACG): Iron Deficiency in Women. April 1981.

severe iron deficiency increases maternal morbidity and mortality and carries an increased risk to the fetus. The anemic child does not thrive, and death may result from other intercurrent diseases. There is increasing evidence that anemia and iron deficiency may contribute to the susceptibility of an individual to infection. In addition, studies suggest that iron deficiency anemia is causally associated with less than optimal behavior in infants and children, as demonstrated by lower scores on tests of development, learning, and school achievement.

DIAGNOSIS. Anemia is the result of iron deficiency and is reflected by a reduction in hemoglobin (Hb) and hematocrit (Hct). Table 5–1 lists the Hb concentrations that have been selected by the World Health Organization (WHO) to define normal and anemic values for populations by function of age and sex.

Other parameters, e.g., serum ferritin, transferrin, and free erythrocyte protoporphyrin, are more indicative of body iron depletion before anemia occurs. Figures 108–2 and 108–3 illustrate the changes occurring in body iron compartments and laboratory parameters of iron status precipitated by continuous negative iron balance. Each of these tests reflects a different aspect of iron deficiency; together they constitute an effective profile of iron nutrition.

A rise in the Hb concentration following the administration of iron will confirm that an anemia is due to iron deficiency. Nevertheless, one should be aware that factors other than iron deficiency, e.g., folate and protein deficiency, chronic infections, and hemoglobinopathy, may contribute to anemia, particularly in developing countries.

THERAPY. Treatment of iron deficiency anemia consists of oral iron therapy. It is usually given as 30 to 60 mg of elemental iron in its ferrous form 1 to 2 times a day. For example, 200 mg of exsiccated (1 H_2O) ferrous sulfate and 300 mg of hydrated (7 H_2O) ferrous sulfate both contain 60 mg of elemental iron. The recommended dose for young children is 3 mg/kg of body weight per day; iron elixirs are available for them. A divided dose facilitates greater absorption. Iron absorption is greatly improved when it is taken with vitamin C.

Acute iron poisoning can occur, predominantly in children from 1 to 5 years old who, out of curiosity, swallow sugar-coated iron tablets that are prescribed for their mothers. Therefore, great care must be taken to keep iron preparations inaccessible to young children.

If oral iron therapy is inappropriate, parenteral iron may be indicated. Because this is an iron-dextran complex, it is recommended that a small test dose be given initially to guard against the possibility of an anaphylactic reaction. In addition, care must be taken when treating individuals with protein deficiency, e.g., kwashiorkor, because parenteral preparations can make available large amounts of free iron, which, if not bound by serum transferrin and tissue ferritin, might lead to bacterial sepsis or cerebral malaria (Chapters 5 and 109).

Parenteral preparations can be administered either intramuscularly or intravenously at a daily dosage *not to exceed* 25 mg of iron for infants weighing less than 5 kg, 50 mg of iron for children weighing less than 10 kg, and 100 mg of iron for patients weighing more than 10 kg. Intravenous dextran should be administered slowly (1 minute or longer per ml [100 mg of iron]). Only in the most severe situations (when Hb is less than 3 gm/dl) may blood transfusion be necessary.

PREVENTION. Prevention of iron deficiency anemia is best achieved by the consumption of a diet adequate in bioavailable iron. Foods that should be included are meat, poultry, fish, whole cereals, legumes, certain dried fruits, and dark-green vegetables. The bioavailability of iron in nonmeat foods can be greatly enhanced if these foods are eaten with others rich in ascorbic acid, e.g., certain fruits and vegetables. (Tables 108–1 to 108–3).

Special attention must be given to women, particularly when pregnant, to infants and young children, and to others with symptoms and/or signs of iron deficiency. All pregnant women should receive ferrous sulfate tablets (or an equivalent iron supplement), and iron supplementation should continue during the first few months of lactation. Breast-fed babies usually need no additional iron for the first 6 months. All formula given to infants should be iron-fortified. Infants who are exclusively breast-fed for more than 1 year should be given an iron supplement. Although breast milk iron is bioavailable, the concentration is insufficient to provide adequate iron nutriture to growing children. In addition,

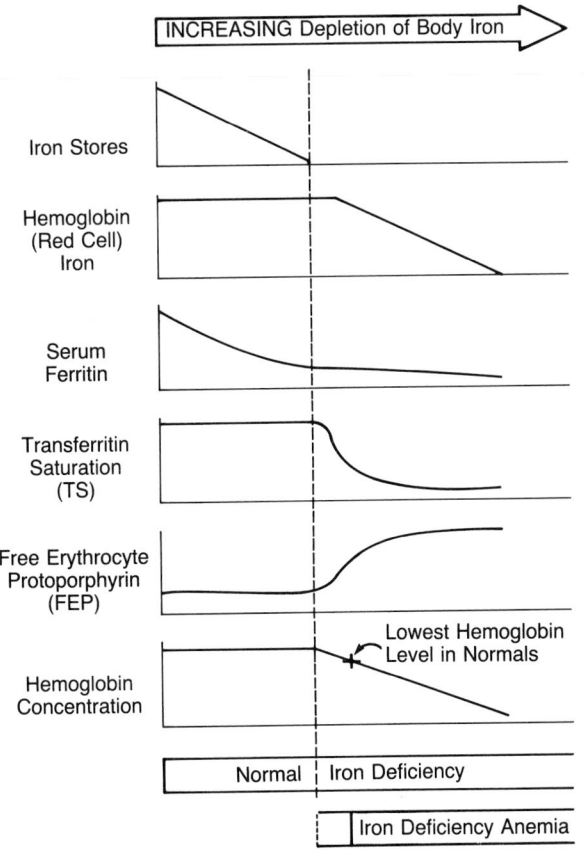

FIGURE 108–2. Changes in body iron compartments and laboratory parameters of iron status during development of iron deficiency due to a continuous negative iron balance. (From Guidelines for the Eradication of Iron Deficiency. A Report of the International Nutritional Anemia Consultative Group [INACG], 1977.)

Sequential Changes in the Development of Iron Deficiency

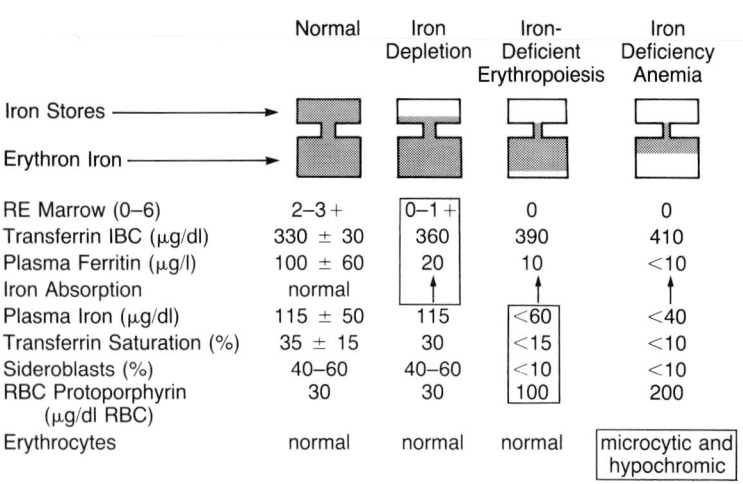

	Normal	Iron Depletion	Iron-Deficient Erythropoiesis	Iron Deficiency Anemia
RE Marrow (0–6)	2–3 +	0–1 +	0	0
Transferrin IBC (μg/dl)	330 ± 30	360	390	410
Plasma Ferritin (μg/l)	100 ± 60	20	10	<10
Iron Absorption	normal			
Plasma Iron (μg/dl)	115 ± 50	115	<60	<40
Transferrin Saturation (%)	35 ± 15	30	<15	<10
Sideroblasts (%)	40–60	40–60	<10	<10
RBC Protoporphyrin (μg/dl RBC)	30	30	100	200
Erythrocytes	normal	normal	normal	microcytic and hypochromic

FIGURE 108–3. The sequence of changes induced by gradual reduction in the iron content of the body. (From Bothwell TH, et al.: Iron Metabolism in Man. Oxford. Blackwell Scientific Publications, 1979.)

all premature or small-for-age infants should receive iron supplementation, because their iron store is much less than that of full-term infants.

When circumstances indicate that a diet is suboptimal in iron, an approach often used to prevent iron deficiency is the fortification of food staples that are consumed by the group most vulnerable to iron deficiency anemia. Currently, many countries fortify refined wheat flour and bread, rolls, or buns. Other products commercially fortified are corn flour, infant milk formulas, and soy products; currently under study are sugar, salt, fish sauce (used in the Far East) and whole wheat flour. The amounts of iron incorporated into foods by fortification are at levels sufficient to augment the daily iron intake but pose no danger to the target populations.

BIBLIOGRAPHY

Bothwell TH, Charlton RW, Cook JD, et al.: Iron Metabolism in Man. Oxford, Blackwell Scientific Publications, 1979.
Cook JD: Iron (Methods in Hematology, Vol 1). New York, Churchill Livingstone, 1980.
De Maeyer E, Adiels-Tegman M: The prevalence of anemia in the world. World Health Stat Q 38:302, 1985.
Hallberg L, Högdahl AM, Nilsson L, et al.: Variation in iron loss in women. *In* Occurrence, Causes, and Prevention of Nutritional Anemias, Symposia of the Swedish Nutrition Foundation VI, 1967. Stockholm, Almqvist and Wiksell, 1968, pp. 115–120.

108.2. GOITER AND THE IODINE DEFICIENCY DISORDERS

Frederick L. Trowbridge and John B. Stanbury

The iodine deficiency disorders, including endemic goiter, endemic cretinism, endemic deaf-mutism, and endemic neuromotor retardation, are extremely common in the developing countries. It is estimated that as many as 1 billion persons are currently at risk of these disorders.

REQUIREMENT FOR IODINE. The daily requirement for iodine based on balance studies in adults is estimated at 50 to 75 μg/day or approximately 1 μg/kg. In order to assure iodine sufficieny, an allowance of approximately 150 μg/day for adolescents and adults is recommended. Endemic goiter, reflecting iodine deficiency, is often seen in populations excreting less than 50 μg of iodine/gm of creatinine in the urine. Severe deficiency with a significant risk of endemic cretinism is encountered in populations excreting less than 25 μg of iodine/gm of creatinine.

SOURCES OF IODINE. Iodine is obtained principally from food, although drinking water may serve as a limited source. The iodine content of foods varies widely. Seafoods are generally a good source. Milk and dairy products may provide significant iodine intake, especially if animal feeds are supplemented with iodine or if iodine compounds are used as sanitizers in milk processing. Bread can provide significant iodine intake also if iodine compounds are used as dough conditioners. Iodized salt is an important source when available and utilized in food preparation and seasoning. The iodine content of plant foods depends on the level of iodine in the soil and on the methods of cooking or processing.

GEOGRAPHIC DISTRIBUTION OF DEFICIENCY. Iodine deficiency classically occurs in high mountainous areas, such as the Andes, the Himalayas, the Alps, central New Guinea, and Central Africa, but may occur also in less mountainous areas where erosion or glacial movements have stripped away the iodine-rich upper layers of soil. In developed countries, where diets are less dependent on local food production, where processed foods are widely consumed, and where iodized salt is commonly used, iodine deficiency has largely been eliminated, but it still is found in southern Germany, Central Europe, and in North and Central Italy. In less developed countries, and especially in more remote areas, where traditional diet and food preparation patterns persist, iodine deficiency remains an important public health concern.

ENDEMIC GOITER. Endemic goiter, the most obvious clinical manifestation associated with iodine deficiency, may be observed as iodine intake falls below approximately 50 μg/day. Goiter characteristically begins to develop in childhood or adolescence as a diffuse enlargement of the thyroid gland. Over time, a multinodular goiter develops that is histologically indistinguishable from the sporadic multinodular goiter found in areas not deficient in iodine. The incidence of endemic goiter is generally higher in women than in men, although in severe endemic areas 80 to 90% of adults of both sexes may have goiters.

Pathogenesis. Iodine deficiency is presumed to cause a mild underproduction of thyroid hormone, which in turn leads to an increase in thyroid-stimulating hormone (TSH), which produces thyroid enlargement. Chronic iodine deficiency with repeated severe iodine deficiency episodes leads, over time, to the development of a nodular goiter. It may be that the thyroid gland reacts heterogeneously to repeated stimuli, resulting in nodules rather than in a homogeneous, diffuse enlargement. There is considerable ability to adapt to low iodine intakes, because most individuals in goiter endemic areas are able to remain clinically euthyroid.

Although iodine deficiency is the most significant underlying factor in the etiology of endemic goiter and is the principal target of intervention efforts, studies in South America indicate that goiter may be observed in areas where iodine intake is considered adequate. These observations suggest that other factors may influence the development of goiters. Goitrogenic substances exhibiting antithyroid activity have been found in certain staple foods, such as cassava, and have been implicated in goiter in Africa. Protein-calorie malnutrition may be associated with decreased thyroid function and may contribute to the effects of iodine deficiency and other factors in goitrogenesis, but its importance is poorly defined.

Clinical Manifestations and Diagnosis. In endemic areas, goiter generally develops as a diffuse enlargement of the thyroid gland beginning in childhood or adolescence. In adulthood, goiters may become nodular. Individuals usually remain clinically euthyroid, without obvious signs or symptoms of hypothyroidism, but greatly enlarged thyroid glands can cause symptoms of tracheal compression and may be cosmetically undesirable (Fig. 108–4).

The diagnosis of endemic goiter is properly made on a population basis because sporadic goiter in individuals and endemic goiter in populations are not clinically distinguishable. Thus, the diagnosis is based on documenting an increased prevalence of goiter in a defined population. Examination of a representative sample of school children has been recommended as a first step because of their accessibility and their risk of developing goiter. A goiter prevalence of more than 10% among school children suggests the need to assess goiter in a sample of the total population. Although definitions are not precise, a goiter prevalence of 10% or greater in the general population suggests endemic goiter.

Standardization of goiter assessment is a critical issue in diagnosis. The use of a standardized classification permits comparison of goiter prevalence among surveys performed by different examiners in different areas. According to the widely used classification of Perez, goiter is considered to exist when either lobe of the

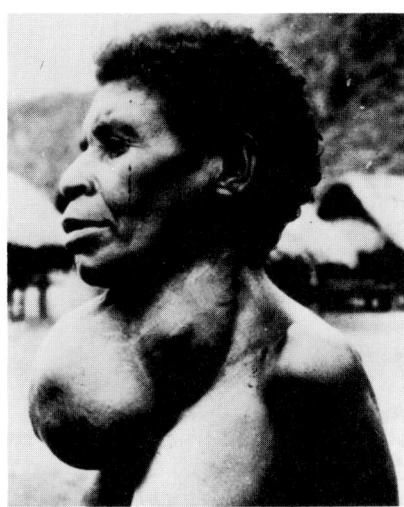

FIGURE 108–4. Native from New Guinea with a huge endemic goiter. (Courtesy of Dr. A. Querido, University Hospital, Leiden, The Netherlands.)

thyroid gland feels larger than the terminal phalanx of the thumb of the person being examined. Various classifications of goiter size have been proposed, but the following may be the most practical:

Grade O: No goiter (by Perez criterion).

Grade Ia: Goiter can be felt but not seen, even with the neck extended.

Grade Ib: Goiter can be felt but not seen with the neck in normal position, becoming visible when the neck is extended.

Grade II: Goiter is easily visible with neck in normal position.

Grade III: Goiter is large (visible at a considerable distance).

The diagnosis of endemic goiter should be based not only on the prevalence of goiter but also on the severity of iodine deficiency. A goiter prevalence of greater than 10% combined with an average urinary iodine excretion below 50 μg/gm or 5 μg/dL of creatinine suggests that goiter in the population is due to iodine deficiency. If urinary iodine excretion averages greater than 50 μg/gm of creatinine, other causes, such as goitrogenic substances in food or water, must be considered.

Treatment. The provision of adequate iodine intake to the population is the best therapy and means of prevention. Iodized salt has been widely used to increase iodine intake; it has been effective where the processing of salt can be adequately controlled and where the distribution of processed salt effectively reaches the populations at risk.

In more remote areas where iodized salt may not be effectively distributed, a more direct approach is to administer iodized oil by mouth or by intramuscular injection. The recommended dosage of iodized oil (Ethiodol) containing 475 mg of iodine/mL is 0.5 mL for infants 0 to 12 months of age and 1 mL for older children and adults to age 45 years. Rare complications consist principally of thyrotoxic symptoms in older subjects with nodular goiter, a reaction estimated to occur in approximately 1 in 300 of those treated who were over 40 years of age. There have been no reported allergic reactions to the high dose of organic iodine. Up to 70% of individuals with endemic goiter respond to iodized oil treatment with a significant reduction in thyroid size, although established goiters in older adults may not decrease in size.

Iodine supplementation is the only practical approach to the treatment of endemic goiter in developing countries with limited health facilities. Treatment of goiter with thyroid hormone preparations may be preferred when long-term follow-up can be assured, but standardized and stable thyroid hormone preparations often are unavailable or too expensive in developing countries, and patients may not cooperate reliably in a long-term therapeutic program. Surgical intervention may be indicated in rare instances when tracheal compression occurs, but such intervention can be dangerous except in well-equipped and well-staffed centers. These patients must receive 1-thyroxine or its equivalent indefinitely after surgery.

Prevention. Increased iodine intake is the most effective measure for the prevention of endemic goiter. The iodinization of salt has proved effective in many areas but depends on the central processing of the salt supply for a population, the enforcement of regulations requiring industry to add iodine in the proper quantity, the distribution of iodized salt at a competitive price to the population at risk and monitoring of the iodine content of the salt at the consumer level to assure that the iodine actually reaches the target population. Populations that are not effectively reached by iodized salt may require more direct intervention, such as the administration of iodized oil by injection or oral administration. A single dose of iodized oil intramuscularly should provide protection for up to 3 years, whereas oral administration is usually effective for about 1 year. Increased consumption of foods with a relatively high iodine content, e.g., fish and shellfish, may serve also to increase iodine intake if such foods are available and affordable to the population at risk.

ENDEMIC CRETINISM. Although endemic goiter is the most prevalent, the most striking health consequence of severe iodine deficiency is endemic cretinism, which may occur in over 5% of individuals in highly affected areas. Endemic cretinism lacks precise definition, but mental retardation is a characteristic feature, frequently combined with neurologic deficits, including a characteristic proximal spasticity and deaf-mutism. In other endemic areas, the most prominent features are mental retardation, hypothyroidism, and stunted growth. Thus, endemic cretinism is a syndrome with some common features but with a variable presentation, suggesting that etiologic factors other than iodine deficiency alone lead to a spectrum of clinical manifestations.

Pathogenesis. Endemic cretinism is thought to be related to maternal hypothyroidism combined with iodine deficiency during gestation and the early postnatal period, resulting in neurologic and developmental damage. Supplementation of iodine to the mother before conception appears to prevent this syndrome. In some areas, such as Central Africa, goitrogens from cassava may influence the predominant development of the hypothyroid form of cretinism.

Clinical Manifestations and Diagnosis. The neurologic and the hypothyroid types of endemic cretinism represent the extremes of a spectrum of abnormalities that constitute the syndrome.

Neurologic Type. The neurologic type of endemic cretinism, characterized by mental retardation associated with deaf-mutism and spastic diplegia but without clinically evident hypothyroidism, predominates in several South American, Asian, and South Pacific endemic areas. Cretins of this type may be relatively short in stature but are not severely dwarfed. Skin and hair may be course and dry, and the tongue may be protuberant. Abnormalities of locomotion are common, including a characteristic shuffling gait. Motor coordination is limited, and movements are generally slow. The bridge of the nose may be depressed and the hairline low. Facial expression is impassive but gives way, during amusement, to a vacuous smile, which is often noted as characteristic of the endemic cretin.

Hypothyroid Type. In the hypothyroid type of endemic cretinism, which predominates in some Central African countries, those affected display myxedematous thickening of the skin, are mentally retarded, and are severely dwarfed, with infantile body proportions. Delayed sexual development, dry skin, a protuberant abdomen, umbilical hernia, and lumbar lordosis are additional common features. Deaf-mutism is not usual, although hearing and speech in severely mentally retarded cretins are difficult to assess.

The neurologic and hypothyroid types of endemic cretinism may coexist, but one form usually predominates. The diagnosis of endemic cretinism rests on the observation of one of these clinically defined syndromes associated with endemic goiter and severe iodine deficiency.

Endemic Neuromotor Damage. The effects of iodine deficiency on the nervous system are undoubtedly the most important consequences of a chronic dietary lack of iodine. Damage to the nervous system is seen in its most florid form in the endemic cretin, as described above, but studies have shown more subtle damage manifested by retardation in neuromotor function, and later in school and social performance in persons whose mothers were iodine deficient during pregnancy. This damage may affect a much larger fraction of the population than cretinism, and is much more subtle. It may contribute substantially to retarded socioeconomic development in many parts of the globe where iodine deficiency occurs.

Prognosis and Prevention. The mental retardation and neurologic damage associated with endemic cretinism are irreversible. Efforts must therefore be aimed at prevention by iodine supplementation. The critical target group for iodine prophylaxis is women of childbearing age to prevent the occurrence of maternal iodine deficiency and hypothyroidism during pregnancy with its adverse effects on neural and statural growth.

BIBLIOGRAPHY

Dunn JT, Medeiros-Neto GA (eds.): Endemic Goiter and Cretinism: Continuing Threats to World Health. Washington, D.C., Pan American Health Organization, PAHO Scientific Publication No. 292, 1974.

Hetzel BS, Dunn JT, Stanbury JB (eds.): The Prevention and Control of Iodine Deficiency Disorders. New York, Elsevier, 1987.

Stanbury JB, Hetzel BH (eds.): Endemic Goiter. New York, John Wiley & Sons, 1980.

108.3 FLUORIDE, DENTAL CARIES, AND FLUOROSIS

Michael C. Latham

DEFINITION. Fluoride is a mineral nutrient present mainly in the teeth and skeleton, but the total amount found in the human body is small. An adequate level of fluoride intake, especially in childhood, helps protect the teeth against decay or dental caries. Excessive intakes of fluoride lead to dental fluorosis seen mainly as mottling of the teeth, and occasionally to skeletal fluorosis.

SOURCES OF FLUORIDE. Most foods contain traces of fluoride and a few, such as tea and seafoods, are rich sources. But, in general, humans get most of their fluoride from the water that they consume, or from beverages and foods containing water. If water contains about 1 part per million (ppm) of fluoride, then it will provide adequate amounts of the mineral to help protect the teeth from dental caries. Many waters contain considerably lower levels, and in the case of urban water supplies, the addition of fluoride (fluoridation) is feasible and an important public health measure. Water in some parts of the world contains excessive amounts ranging from 2 to 20 ppm or even higher. Regular drinking of water containing these amounts will lead to the development of dental fluorosis and sometimes skeletal fluorosis.

FLUORIDE AND DENTAL CARIES. A deficient intake of fluoride during infancy and childhood leaves the teeth less protected from dental caries. Research shows that the rates of dental caries in populations drinking water with fluoride concentrations of 0.8 to 1.2 ppm are much lower than communities consuming waters with 0.0 to 0.2 ppm (Fig. 108–5). Therefore, adequate intakes of fluoride significantly reduce tooth decay.

Dental caries is a major health problem worldwide, perhaps humans' most prevalent disease, and is costly to treat. Dental caries is caused by bacteria (most often *Streptococcus mutans*), which act on carbohydrate substrate adherent to the teeth or entrapped between them, producing an acid capable of eroding the teeth, particularly where the dental enamel is damaged or not adequately protective.

Optimal fluoride intakes during infancy and childhood make the enamel much more resistant to decay. A diet containing minimal reduced carbohydrates, such as sticky sweet foods and sugary sodas, will reduce caries. Dental flossing and tooth brushing to remove the carbohydrate substrate will help also. But having teeth strengthened by optimal intakes of fluoride in childhood is the most effective means of reducing caries. In tropical countries the increasing consumption of western diets,

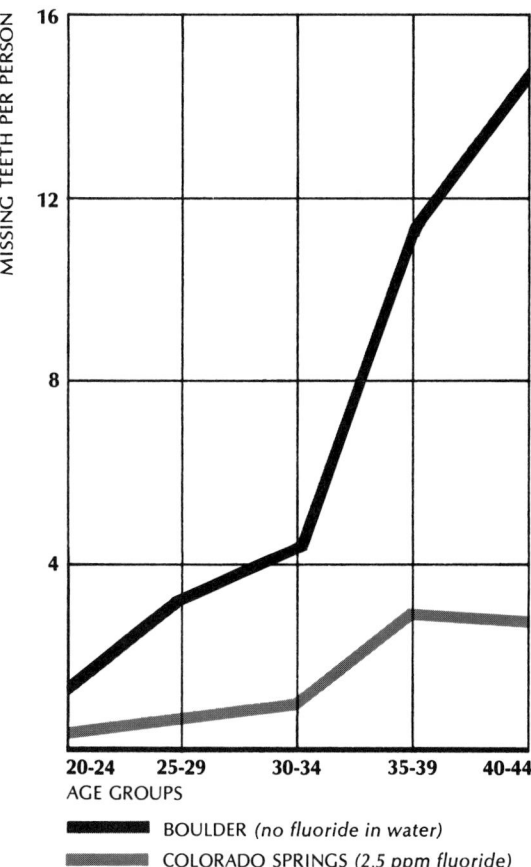

FIGURE 108–5. That the benefits of fluoride accrued during childhood are carried over into adulthood is shown by a comparison of missing teeth of adults in Boulder, Colorado (no fluoride in the drinking water) and Colorado Springs (2.5 ppm of fluoride in the drinking water). At age 40–44 the loss of teeth is less than 4 permanent teeth per person in Colorado Springs while it averages about 16 permanent teeth loss per person in Boulder, Colorado. The ratio of tooth loss is 4 to 5 times greater, at all times, in the non-fluoride area than in the fluoride area from age 20 to 44. (From Latham MC, et al.: SCOPE Manual of Nutrition. Kalamazoo, Upjohn, 1970.)

including sugary foods and beverages, is contributing to an increase in dental caries. In the past, dental caries rates were often low in children in most developing countries consuming traditional diets. However, rates are increasing rapidly. This is at a time when dental caries rates are declining in the industrialized countries, due mainly to fluoridation of water supplies and better attention to dental hygiene.

DENTAL AND SKELETAL FLUOROSIS. There are areas in tropical countries where the local water contains high levels of fluoride. If these are above 2 or 3 ppm, dental fluorosis will be seen; it may be extremely prevalent. With higher levels of fluoride consumption over long periods of time, skeletal fluorosis will occur, particularly in older persons.

Dental Fluorosis. The first change in dental fluorosis is a patchy white chalkiness, with areas of the tooth not glistening and possibly somewhat rough. These areas often become stained with brownish patches. It may be present in a large proportion of the population, and may be considered unsightly or aesthetically undesirable. This is the case in some highland areas of Kenya and in

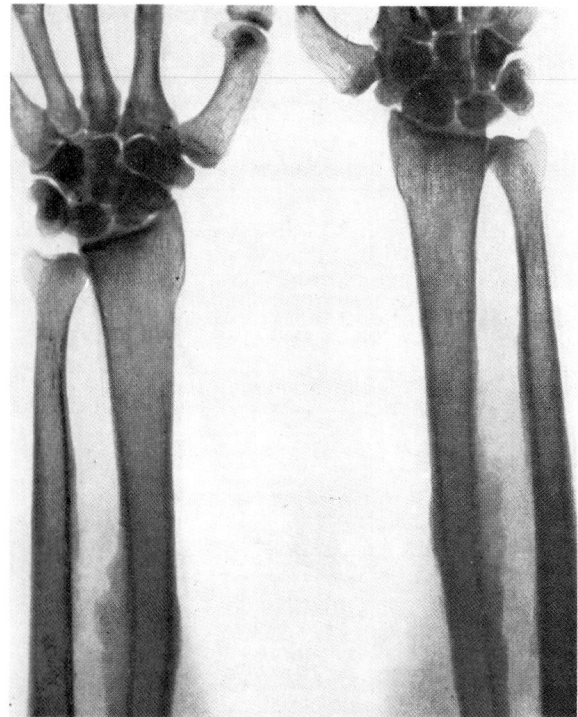

FIGURE 108–6. X-ray of forearm in fluorosis. Note the denseness of the bones and the calcification between them. (From Latham, MC: Human Nutrition in Tropical Africa. Rome, FAO, 1979.)

many other parts of the world. These fluorotic teeth apparently remain relatively resistant to dental caries.

Skeletal Fluorosis. Chronic consumption of water with high levels of fluoride over a period of years may lead to the development of skeletal fluorosis. This has been studied in Tanzania and India, and has been reported from many countries. The long-term ingestion of fluoride leads to excessive laying down of calcium in bones and in other tissues. This can be demonstrated radiologically; the x-rays show increased bone density (in long bones, skull, vertebrae, etc.) and calcification of adjacent tissues, such as in muscle insertions and in intervertebral tissue or between bones, such as the radius and ulna (Fig. 108–6). In older subjects these changes have been associated with pain, deformities, and in the case of vertebral involvement, reduced ability to flex the spine.

PREVENTION. The prevention of fluorosis can be achieved only by having communities consume water with lower levels of fluoride. Not infrequently, adjacent rivers or streams in the same geographic area may have different levels of fluoride. Rain water can be collected for drinking. City water supplies should not be allowed to have levels above 1.5 or 2 ppm of fluoride, although the "defluoridation" of water is an expensive undertaking.

BIBLIOGRAPHY

Jolly SS, Singh BM: Endemic fluorosis in Punjab (India). Am J Med 47:553, 1969.
Latham MC, Grech P: The effects of excessive fluoride intake. Am J Public Health 57:651, 1956.
Scherp HW: Dental caries: Prospects for prevention. Science 173:1199, 1971.
Singer L, Ophaug RH: Fluoride. *In* Present Knowledge in Nutrition, 5th ed. Nutrition Foundation, 1984, p. 538.
Sweeney EA, Shaw JH: Nutrition in relation to dental medicine. In Shils ME, Young VR (eds.): Modern Nutrition in Health and Disease, 7th ed. Philadelphia, Lea and Febiger, 1988, p.1069.
World Health Organization: Fluorides and human health. WHO Monograph Series No. 59, 1970.

108.4   ZINC AND OTHER TRACE ELEMENT DEFICIENCIES

Roger Shrimpton

The trace elements chromium, cobalt, copper, fluorine, iodine, iron, manganese, molybdenum, nickel, selenium, silicon, tin, vanadium, and zinc are all required by the body in quantities of less than a few milligrams a day. Characteristically they have low tissue concentrations, high chemical reactivity, and act primarily as catalysts in enzyme systems in cells. Iron (Chapter 108.1), iodine (Chapter 108.2), and fluoride (Chapter 108.3) deficiencies are well recognized in humans. Deficiencies of the other trace elements are still less clearly understood. Zinc is probably the best candidate for being a future trace element deficiency of public health significance.

ZINC DEFICIENCY. The importance of zinc in human nutrition has become evident only in the last 2 decades. Zinc-dependent enzymes exist in most metabolic pathways, and most critically that of the nucleic acids. Zinc deficiency, thus, stops cell division and protein synthesis. The daily requirement for zinc has not been fixed with certainty, but intakes of 3 to 5 mg/day for infants, 10 mg/day for children 1 to 10 years old, and 15 mg/day for older individuals have been recommended. A single unequivocal index of zinc status does not exist yet. Several indicators including a low zinc intake (<2 mg/1000 calorie), low serum zinc (<70 μg/dl), and low hair zinc (<110 μg/g) in combination can suggest zinc deficiency, but zinc supplementation studies are necessary for confirmation.

Etiology. Zinc deficiency may have a variety of causes, including insufficient intake, malabsorption, excessive excretion, or increased requirements. Food zinc content varies greatly, being greatest in the more protein-rich foods, such as meats, certain sea foods, eggs, milk, crustacea, whole grains, and nuts. Zinc-poor foods are fats, oils, sugar-rich foods such as jams and soft drinks, refined cereal products, tubers, plantains, and fish. Primary zinc deficiency has not been shown in free-living populations, except in the Amazon in association with fish and cassava diets. Primary zinc depletion is seen most commonly in patients on total parenteral nutrition, when insufficient care has been taken to supply adequate zinc intravenously.

A diet may contain sufficient total zinc, but it is not adequately absorbed. This may be for a variety of reasons including inhibitory factors such as phytates, oxalates, tannins, and fiber found in plant foods; excessive dietary iron or folate; or deficiency of the zinc binding factor in pancreatic secretions that occurs in the autosomal recessive disease acrodermatitis enteropathica.

Excessive excretion of zinc can occur owing to the intestinal hurry of diarrhea when the zinc excreted into the intestinal lumen with the pancreatic secretions is not reabsorbed. This occurs in Crohn's disease, coeliac disease, cystic fibrosis, and infectious diarrhea. Urinary zinc losses are high in diseases such as sickle cell anemia and chronic uremia, and when using the drugs isoniazid and tetracycline. Excessive sweating increases zinc losses, as does lactation.

Rapid creation of new tissue is the basis for increased zinc requirements. This process is seen in neoplastic diseases, during re-epithelialization after burns, and during rapid growth in infancy and adolescence.

Clinical Manifestations. The rare congenital disease acrodermatitis enteropathica is a manifestation of zinc deficiency and responds to treatment with the mineral. The condition is seen most frequently in infancy after weaning from the breast. It is characterized by a bullous dermatitis often beginning around the anus and mouth, chronic diarrhea, and growth failure, and it was invariably fatal in the past. The disease responds to treatment with zinc. Similar skin lesions, also responsive to zinc, have been reported in patients receiving parenteral nutrition therapy. In Iran and Egypt a condition seen in adolescent males characterized mainly by hypogonadism and dwarfing has been reported to respond to zinc therapy, but it is not certain that the cause is primarily dietary zinc deficiency. There is some evidence that increasing zinc intakes has improved growth of certain children with low serum or hair zinc in the United States and elsewhere. Zinc deficiency, as judged by low serum zinc levels, is sometimes seen in protein-energy malnutrition, in alcoholism, in certain malabsorption states, in some infections and in renal disease. But zinc deficiency is not the cause of these diseases.

Biochemical Changes. Experimental human zinc deficiency is characterized by decreased circulating zinc, carbonic anhydrase and alkaline phosphatase activity, elevated RNase activity, increased serum ammonia, and depressed testosterone levels. In energy inadequacy and other catabolic situations, zinc is liberated from catabolized muscle, maintaining circulating levels in the face of depletion. Infections cause circulating zinc to fall independent of zinc status.

Treatment and Prevention. Zinc deficiency is treated with 2 mg/kg, but not more than 40 mg a day, of oral zinc in the form of its sulfate, or gluconate. Public health measures to prevent zinc deficiency at the population level cannot yet be justified.

OTHER TRACE ELEMENT DEFICIENCIES. Copper deficiency leads to anemia and scorbutic bone changes in humans. The limited evidence that overt copper deficiency occurs in human populations is in children with Menkes' disease, or in the occasional patient maintained by total parenteral nutrition without copper, or during the rehabilitation of severely malnourished children. Selenium deficiency is manifested by a lack of reduced glutathione, leading to oxidant and free-radical damage. In low selenium areas of China, selenium deficiency in children is associated with Keshan disease, a cardiomyopathy. Evidence of deficiency of other trace elements is still lacking in humans.

BIBLIOGRAPHY

Chandra RK (ed.): Trace elements in nutrition of children. Nestle Nutrition Workshop Series, Vol. 8, New York, Raven Press, 1985.
Solomons NW: Zinc and copper. *In* Shils ME, Young VR (eds.): Modern Nutrition in Health and Disease, 7th ed. Philadelphia, Lea & Febiger, 1988.

109. OTHER NUTRITIONALLY RELATED PROBLEMS

109.1. INTERACTION OF NUTRITION AND INFECTION

Charlotte G. Neumann
and Lani S. Stephenson

The interaction of malnutrition and infection is the leading cause of morbidity and mortality in both developing countries and among the poorest populations of affluent nations. In tropical countries bacterial, viral, and parasitic infections all play an important role and have relationships to nutritional status. In many parts of the world, death rates in children 1 to 4 years old are 30- to 40-fold higher than those in industrialized nations, i.e., 50% die before their fifth birthday. Many observers in the health field have commented on the abundance, long duration, and complications of infections in malnourished individuals and on the severe course that ordinarily mild infections follow in the malnourished.

Because of their physiologic state and increased nutritional requirements, pregnant and lactating women, the developing fetus, the young child, and the adolescent, particularly if pregnant, are the most vulnerable to malnutrition and infection. There may be serious consequences not only in terms of immediate survival but also for the outcome of pregnancy and future physical and mental impairments of the children. Another vulnerable group are those with chronic debilitating disease, particularly AIDS.

INTRODUCTION. What is the nature of the interaction of nutrition and infection? What are the mechanisms and causative factors? What are the implications of the problem for intervention?

That there is a synergistic relationship between nutrition and infection has been well established in animal studies and in well-controlled human field studies. Infections adversely affect nutritional status, and malnutrition adversely affects the ability of the host to withstand infection.

Antagonism to infection, particularly to viral infection in animals, can occur when a nutritional deficiency or a metabolic disturbance produced by a deficiency has a greater effect on the agent than on the host. In humans, deficiencies severe enough to cause antagonism often result in an overall decreased resistance to infection. The Murrays' observations of suppression of infection by famine are most provocative, but these are not widespread observations, particularly among young children, and may refer specifically to the situation with unbound serum iron promoting sepsis. The observations, especially those on the refeeding of semistarved nomadic populations with promotion of sepsis, may represent interaction among a unique host, agent, and environment. However, the overwhelming interaction tends to be synergistic and harmful to human beings. In a vicious downward cycle, infection causes a worsening of malnutrition, thereby making the host more vulnerable to infections and to further deterioration of nutritional status.

THE EFFECTS OF INFECTION ON NUTRITIONAL STATUS. Almost all infections have a nutritional cost to the host. The obvious effects of infections are readily understandable through the signs and symptoms they cause. Fever increases the metabolic and the energy or caloric needs of the individual. Anorexia during an infection causes reduced food intake, as do cough, rapid breathing, and congested nasal passages, which also impair an infant or young child's ability to suckle or eat. Abnormal losses of nutrients accompany perspiration, diarrhea, and vomiting.

Infections of the gastrointestinal tract compromise nutritional status by interfering with absorption of foodstuffs because of rapid transit time and transient enzyme defects. Parasitic infections of the gastrointestinal tract are important owing to their ubiquitous nature in poverty-stricken and unsanitary environments. They contribute to malabsorption; they may result in loss of nutrients by the host, for example, loss of blood and iron in hookworm disease and vitamin B_{12} in infections with *Diphylobothrium latum;* and they may cause anorexia. Increased nitrogen losses occur in the urine even with mild infections and/or live virus immunizations. Such situations are catabolic with depletion of muscle tissue.

Interleukin-1 (IL-1), produced by infection-activated monocytes, has been identified as a potent mediator of the metabolic, immunologic, and nutritional alterations in animal models and humans. The acute phase reactants and lymphokines, whose production is activated by IL-1, promote recovery from the infection. Interleukin-1 also stimulates skeletal muscle catabolism to supply amino acids for the production of acute phase reactants. Presumably the anorexia and nutrient shifts, early in the illness, reduce the availability of nutrients essential to growth of the pathogens. Little is known about IL-1 production and activity in malnutrition. Among elderly adults endogenous pyrogen was significantly reduced with less fever produced than in controls. Also, infants and young children with protein-energy malnutrition (PEM) may not mount a febrile response to infection. Interferon is reduced in PEM as is cell-mediated immunity (CMI), both stimulated by IL-1, which is now thought to be depressed in malnutrition. The infection-induced stress reaction mediated through adrenal corticoids further depletes muscle tissue and depresses CMI;

thus, the net effect is diminished host ability to deal with infection.

The feeding of sick individuals, particularly during childhood and pregnancy, is often governed by cultural beliefs. Often certain foods or even all solid foods are withheld, and only thin watery fluids low in energy and protein are provided during acute illness. Purges may add to the nutritional difficulties. Therefore, it is common for a child already harboring intestinal parasites to have rather frequent acute viral and bacterial infections that together lower food consumption because of poor appetite or as a form of home treatment; decrease nutrient absorption; and increase nutrient loss, for example, nitrogen in the urine and blood in the stool. The net result is a deterioration in nutritional status including a slowing or cessation of growth, and perhaps development of anemia, xerophthalmia, or signs of other micronutrient deficiencies.

INFECTION IN THE MALNOURISHED INDIVIDUAL. Malnutrition adversely affects a wide range of nonspecific host factors.

Barriers to Infection. Among the body's mechanical barriers against infection that depend on good nutritional status are the connective tissue, the mucosal surfaces of the gums and oral cavity, and the epithelial coverings of the eye, respiratory tract, and gastrointestinal tract. Any break in the integrity of these tissues provides a portal of entry for disease-causing agents. Some of these cells have a specialized structure and function. For example, the respiratory epithelial cells secrete protective anti-infective substances, such as mucus, and have cilia that sweep away bacteria and other foreign materials. The eye and the respiratory and intestinal tracts are particularly vulnerable to infection. Vitamins A and C, the B vitamins, and protein play a major role in maintaining the integrity of these barriers.

Antibody. In undernourished individuals, antibody response to several pathogenic organisms may be reduced, e.g., those of typhoid, diphtheria, and yellow fever. Responses to measles and certain other infections appear to be normal.

White Blood Cells. As for the antibacterial activity of leukocytes in malnutrition, results are variable. Some studies show that leukocyte responses, e.g., the ability of leukocytes to phagocytize and kill infectious organisms, are diminished.

Cell-Mediated Immunity. Another important aspect of the immune response, CMI, is involved in the containment of tuberculosis and of many fungal, viral, bacterial, and parasitic infections. This immunity can become impaired in PEM as a consequence of depletion of the lymphoid tissue, which produces a variety of lymphocytes responsible for CMI and its many expressions. The degree of impairment is related directly to the degree of malnutrition and is readily reversed by nutritional rehabilitation. The depressed CMI prevents a good response to certain immunizations in the malnourished host, such as that of Calmette-Guérin bacillus (BCG) against tuberculosis. Infants malnourished in utero, a condition common in the developing areas of the world, may be born with impaired CMI, which is not readily reversible until at least 6 to 12 months of age and even longer. These young infants are especially vulnerable to infection.

Iron deficiency, globally prevalent, and zinc deficiency may depress CMI. Folic acid and pyridoxine deficiencies have also been associated with depressed CMI.

Secretory Antibody. Secretory IgA (sIgA) production by respiratory epithelium, in tears and saliva, and mucosal antibody responses may be decreased in subjects with moderate as well as severe PEM. The sIgA response to live attenuated measles and poliomyelitis immunizations was found to be greatly decreased or absent in malnourished children. This reduced secretory and mucosal immunity may permit penetration of and decreased mucosal binding of pathogens and increased shedding and colonization of pathogens in the malnourished host.

Serum Proteins. Some serum proteins that participate in combating infection are drastically reduced also in malnutrition. These include those that bind heavy metals, e.g., transferrin and lactoferrin. Free serum iron, unbound by protein, may actually promote bacterial growth, resulting in sepsis. The complement system, which enhances certain antibacterial and antiviral reactions of leukocytes, is depleted in PEM also.

Vitamin A and Infection Resistance. Several recent epidemiologic and clinical studies have shown that children with xerophthalmia also had higher mortality and morbidity rates. Respiratory, diarrheal, and other infections were more common in those with signs of vitamin A deficiency. Upon treatment with vitamin A the rates were reduced significantly. It is known that aside from the role of vitamin A in maintaining the integrity of mucosal and other mechanical barriers to infections, vitamin A deficiency may be associated also with decreased CMI. These may be the main mechanisms involved in increased infection with vitamin A deficiency and low carotene intakes.

EXAMPLES OF THE INTERACTION OF NUTRITION AND INFECTION

Measles. This is one of the most serious infectious diseases among children in developing areas (Chapter 16.1). Death rates from measles among children in developing countries exceed those in affluent industrialized nations by 200- to 400-fold. Case-fatality rates range from 20 to 40%, as compared with less than 1% in the United States. The complication rate is exceedingly high, particularly during the first year of life. Complications of measles in malnourished children include upper airway obstruction, pneumonia, mouth and eye infections, devastating ulcers of the face and extremities, and prolonged diarrhea. In Kenya, for example, complications developed in over 60% of poorly nourished children. Crowded living conditions, which increase the opportunity for droplet exposure, along with the lack of immunization programs, help to account for the early onset of this infection in Africa. However, the severity and high complication and mortality rates are due not to greater virulence of the virus, but to reduced host resistance caused by malnutrition and local food beliefs and practices.

Conversely, measles can have devastating effects on nutritional status. In populations in which protein and energy nutrition are only marginally adequate, measles may precipitate or be closely followed by full-blown kwashiorkor. Less dramatic effects may be prolonged weight loss and a fall in serum albumin.

"Weanling Diarrhea." The close relationship between nutritional status and frequency and severity of diarrhea is well established by numerous field studies. "Weanling diarrhea" refers to the bouts of diarrhea frequently seen at the time of weaning, when breast-feeding ends (Chapter 109.2). In marginally nourished children, this diarrhea may precipitate frank malnutrition because of nutrient losses and malabsorption. The diarrhea may be caused by a variety of viruses, bacteria and parasites.

Weaning is fraught with danger because the anti-infective protection from placentally transferred antibody has waned and the protective effects of breast milk are being lost. With weaning, the African child literally leaves the safety of the mother's back and is put down on the ground to toddle and crawl in an unsanitary environment. He or she is now deprived of the protection afforded by the many anti-infective substances and living phagocytic cells in breast milk. The suppression of pathogenic bacterial flora in the infant's intestine by bifidus factor in breast milk no longer occurs. In place of breast milk, the infant tends to be given low-protein and often contaminated and indigestible gruels. Formula feedings are often contaminated or diluted. Further damage occurs by the age-old custom of "starving" diarrheas by withholding food and liquids and by giving purges.

Concomitant with rapid urbanization in many developing nations, with mothers entering the labor force and no longer nursing their infants, diarrhea and malnutrition become evident much earlier in life. The use by families of oral rehydration fluids in the treatment of diarrhea at home is now widely credited with reducing deaths from acute gastroenteritis. Correcting dehydration must be combined with encouraging mothers to continue breast-feeding even when the child is ill with diarrhea (General Principles, III D).

Helminthic Infections. *Ascaris lumbricoides* infects perhaps 1,200 million persons in the world; hookworms about 800 million; *Trichuris trichuria* around 600 million; and schistosomiasis (including the 3 common human varieties) involves about 250 million people in Africa, Asia, and Latin America. All of these parasites have been shown to contribute to malnutrition. For many years it has been well documented that infections with *Necator americanus* and *Ancylostoma duodenale* cause significant blood loss from the mucosa of the intestines, and this results in increased iron loss in the feces (Chapter 84.1). In many populations where the prevalence of hookworm is high and where heavy loads are common, this parasite is a major cause of iron deficiency anemia, not only in children and women of child-bearing age, but also in adult males (Fig. 109–1). It may sap the health of people; it may reduce worker productivity; and it contributes to anemia, one of the most prevalent forms of malnutrition (Chapter 5).

Recent studies have illustrated that *Ascaris lumbricoides* (Chapter 83) and *Schistosoma* (Chapter 96) infections contribute to poor growth and therefore to PEM. Several studies in Kenya, Panama, India, and

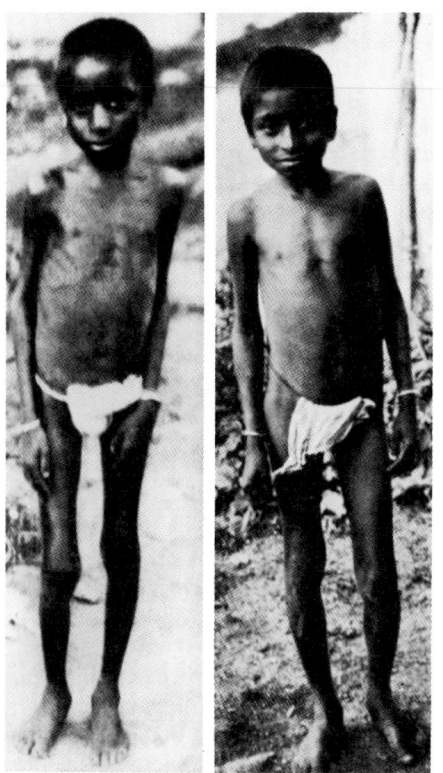

A   B

FIGURE 109–1. *A*, An Indian boy with malnutrition, severe wasting, and anemia. *B*, The same child 6 months after treatment for hookworm.

elsewhere have shown that children treated for *Ascaris* grew better than matched untreated controls. Treatment of Kenyan children with *S. haematobium* infections resulted in significantly improved growth, lower iron losses, increased physical fitness, and better appetite when compared with untreated children.

In many countries animals and farm livestock are dewormed routinely. Much evidence suggests that pigs grow better when they regularly receive anthelminthics. Now that highly effective, rather inexpensive, and safe broad-spectrum anthelminthics such as albendazole are available, it seems highly desirable that routine mass deworming be introduced in areas where parasitic infections are prevalent, and where PEM and anemia are common. Similarly, routine efforts to treat children with schistosomiasis using metrifonate or praziquantel seem highly desirable both to rid children of potential serious pathology but also to improve their nutritional status. More attention needs to be given to population-based chemotherapy for these infections while intensifying public health and other measures to reduce their transmission. Such efforts would improve the health and nutritional status of millions of the world's children.

Acquired Immunodeficiency Syndrome. A dramatic example of the interaction of nutrition and infection is exemplified by people with acquired immunodeficiency syndrome (AIDS). So devastating is the effect of AIDS on nutritional status of the individual that the disease was originally called Slim's disease in Uganda before the etiology was known (Chapter 15.1). There are relatively few studies that address the mechanisms of

action for the severe malnutrition in the infected host and fewer reports of attempts to improve nutritional status as an adjunct to therapy for HIV infection. Almost continuous bouts of malabsorption, severe diarrhea, and marked unrelenting weight loss occur secondary to opportunistic enteric and generalized infections (e.g., cytomegalovirus, tuberculous, *Pneumocytis carinii* mycoses). Loss of integrity of mucosal barriers, thinning of the villi, and infiltration of the mucosal layers by microorganisms are seen. The anorexia, malabsorption, negative nitrogen balance, and loss of skin and mucosal integrity collectively exert pronounced adverse effects on the host's nutritional condition. Selenium deficiency, with possible further deleterious effects on CMI, may be present. Upgrading the nutritional status of those with AIDS, particularly children, as a means of strengthening immune function, even in symptomatic patients, may improve the treatment outcome and the quality of life in their remaining years.

IMPLICATIONS. Comprehensive approaches for improving the nutritional status of a population include efforts directed toward environmental sanitation, immunization programs, and early treatment of infections. Conversely, to optimally control infections and obtain maximum responses from immunization, nutritional status must be improved simultaneously. Breast-feeding, with its excellent nutritional value and anti-infective properties, should be promoted agressively, and nutritious weaning foods should be demonstrated to mothers from locally produced and available foodstuffs.

Unfortunately, government agencies or services often deal with infectious diseases and with malnutrition in separate programs and campaigns. These services should be integrated and have sufficient outreach to peripheral populations. They must be simple, low-cost, and deliverable by health auxiliaries in the context of primary health care. Just as there is a synergism of malnutrition and infection, so must there be a "synergism of services."

BIBLIOGRAPHY

Beisel WR: Metabolic effect of infection. Prog Food Nutr Sci 8:43–75, 1984.

Bentler M, Stanish M: Nutritional support of the pediatric patient with AIDS. J Am Diet Assoc 87:488–491, 1987.

Chandra RK: Nutritional regulation of immunity and infection: From epidemiology to clinical practice. J Pediatr Gastroenterol Nutr 5:844–852, 1985.

Kauffman CA, Jones PG, Kluger MJ: Fever and malnutrition: Endogenous pyrogen/interleukin-1 in malnourished patients. Am J Clin Nutr 44:449–452, 1986.

Keusch GT, Farthing MJG: Nutrition and infection. Annu Rev Nutr 6:131–154, 1986.

Latham MC: Nutrition and infection in national development. Science 188:561–565, 1975.

McCarthy DO, Kleger MJ, Vander AJ: Suppression of food intake during infection: Is interleukin-1 involved? Am J Clin Nutr 42:1179–1182, 1985.

McLoughlin LC, Nord KS, Joshi VV, et al.: Severe gastrointestinal involvement in children with acquired immunodeficiency syndrome. J Pediatr Gastroenterol Nutr 6:517–524, 1987.

Moseson M: Nutrition and AIDS: Letter to the editor. Nutr Res 6:729–730, 1986.

Murray J, Murray A: Starvation suppression and refeeding activation of infection: An ecological necessity? Lancet 1:23–25, 1977.

Neumann CG, Lawlor GJ, Stiehm ER, et al.: Immunologic response in malnourished children. Am J Clin Nutr 28:89–104, 1975.

Serwadda D, Mugerwa RD, Sewankambo NK, et al.: Slim disease: A new disease in Uganda and its association with HTLV-III infection. Lancet 2:849–852, 1985.

Sommer A, Tarwotjo I, Hussaini G, et al: Increased mortality in children with mild vitamin A deficiency. Lancet 11:585, 1983.

Stephenson LS: The Impact of Helminth Infections on Human Nutrition. London, Taylor and Francis, 1987, p. 233.

Stephenson LS, Latham MC, Kurz KM, et al.: Relationships of *Schistosoma haematobium*, hookworm and malarial infections and metrifonate treatment to growth of Kenyan school children. Am J Trop Med Hyg 34:1109–1118, 1985.

109.2. INFANT FEEDING AND WEANING PROBLEMS

Michael C. Latham

DEFINITION. The proper feeding of the infant during the first 12 months of life is of great importance for the health, future development, and survival of the child. The term weaning is generally used for the process of accustoming the child to foods other than milk, and gradually moving from a milk diet to consumption of ordinary family foods. In the past weaning referred to weaning from the breast but now is also used for weaning from the bottle. The French use the term "sevrage" to indicate the age at which breast-feeding ceases, and because there is no exact English equivalent this term is increasingly entering the literature.

GENERAL PRINCIPLES. The benefits of breast-feeding for the young infant have been appreciated for many years. In the last decade there has been an avalanche of publications on the topic of lactation. The new studies have strengthened our view of the many advantages of breast-feeding over other methods of infant feeding, and especially for the infant brought up in a tropical environment where sanitation, education, and incomes are often poor.

It is now widely recommended that only breast milk be fed to infants for the first 4 to 6 months of life. In most instances breast milk will provide for all the nutritional needs of the infant up to this age, when other available local foods should be introduced gradually, whereas breast-feeding continues for as long as the mother feels able, and wishes, to do so. Breast milk during the period from 6 months to 18 months or beyond provides important nutrients and other benefits.

ADVANTAGES OF BREAST- OVER BOTTLE-FEEDING. There is now an appreciation that breast-feeding is the optimal form of infant feeding, and that the alternative, which is most commonly bottle-feeding using infant formula or animal milk, has major disadvantages. Nevertheless, there has been a major decline in breast-feeding. This has resulted in serious problems: in higher rates of infant and young child morbidity (including malnutrition), in higher mortality, in narrower spacing between births, and in other adverse consequences. The advantages of breast- over bottle-feeding include:

(1) breast milk provides a proper balance and quantity of nutrients ideal for the human infant;

(2) breast-feeding is convenient, the food is easily available for the infant, and no special preparations or equipment are needed;

(3) both colostrum and breast milk have anti-infective constituents that help limit infections;

(4) bottle-feeding enhances the risk of infections from contamination with pathogenic organisms in the milk, the formula, the water used in preparation, as well as bottles, teats, and other items used for infant feeding;

(5) economic benefits from breast-feeding when compared with the cost of purchasing infant formula or cows' milk, the bottles and teats, and the fuel necessary for sterilization;

(6) breast-feeding prolongs duration of postpartum anovulation, assisting mothers to space their children;

(7) enhanced bonding and relationship between mother and infant is fostered by breast-feeding; and

(8) an apparent lowered risk of allergies, obesity, and certain other health problems in breast-fed compared with artificially fed infants.

In terms of morbidity and mortality the increased risks of bottle- over breast-feeding are most apparent for poor families with little health knowledge living in homes with contaminated, inadequate water supplies, poor sanitation, inadequate facilities to prepare and store infant formula or cows' milk, and with insufficient income to afford to purchase adequate quantities of infant formula. These factors coupled with the loss of the anti-infective properties of breast milk contribute to high rates of gastroenteritis and other infections in bottle-fed compared with breast-fed babies. These infections may contribute to malnutrition (Chapter 109.1). Also, because of the high cost of breast-milk substitutes in relation to incomes of the poor, families often purchase too little, and try to stretch it, for example, by using less than the recommended amount of powdered formula per feed or per day. The correct number of feedings and the recommended volume of liquid may be given to the infant, but due to overdilution the contents of each bottle may be too low in calories, protein, energy, and other nutrients to sustain good growth and maintain good nutritional status. Often the result is first, growth faltering, and then perhaps, the development of marasmus and signs of other nutrient deficiencies (Fig. 109–2). These may be aggravated by infections, and the malnutrition may contribute to the seriousness of these infections.

FACTORS INFLUENCING FEEDING PRACTICES

Prevalence Changes. The prevalence and duration of breast-feeding varies widely between countries and within them. Among the more educated women in the industrialized western countries, where breast-feeding reached low levels in the 1950s, there has been a marked resurgence. In many tropical countries there is still a high prevalence and long duration of breast-feeding in traditional extended families, particularly in the rural areas, and a decline in breast-feeding in major urban centers. A recent study in 4 cities showed that at 6 months of age, 54% in Thailand, 56%

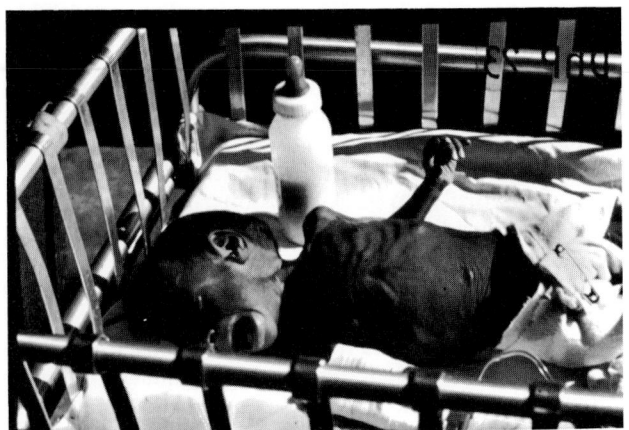

FIGURE 109–2. An example of the abundant evidence: "breast is best." (Photograph published with thanks to Professor David Morley, Institute of Child Health, London.)

in Colombia, and 86% of infants in both Indonesia and Kenya were still being breast-fed. It has been reported that in Chile the percentage of babies being breast-fed at 13 months of age dropped from over 90% in 1960 to less than 10% in 1968; that in Mexico the percentage being breast-fed at 6 months of age dropped from over 90% in 1960 to less than 40% in 1966; and at 3 months of age in Singapore from around 75% in 1951 to around 8% in 1971. These major declines were at a time when less than 20% of mothers leaving hospitals following delivery in the United States were breast-feeding their babies.

Factors Reducing Prevalence of Breast-feeding. Many factors influenced the decline in breast-feeding in tropical countries during the period from 1950 to 1980. The first was the aggressive promotion of infant formula by multinational corporations, hungry for new customers, new markets, and increased profits. The second was the failure of health professionals to appreciate the dangers of bottle-feeding, and to adequately advocate, protect, and support breast-feeding as the optimal means of nourishment for their young patients.

Manufacturers of Infant Formulas. The promotional activities of the infant formula companies have been limited to some extent by the passing at the World Health Assembly in 1981 of the WHO/UNICEF International Code of Marketing of Breastmilk Substitutes. The Code limits advertising to the public, but some undesirable corporation practices, such as the provision of free formula samples to mothers leaving maternity wards, still serve to undermine breast-feeding and to suggest that formula-feeding is superior and has the blessing of the medical profession.

Ignorance of Health Care Providers. The negative role played by the health profession is changing, but many physicians are relatively ignorant about breast-feeding. Often health services in tropical countries do not provide sensible and adequate advice about breast-feeding to women attending prenatal clinics, nor at the time of delivery, nor postnatally. Many maternity units do not encourage mothers to breast-feed their babies in the first minutes following delivery; many do not permit mothers to breast-feed on demand or allow their babies

to sleep with them; and others routinely feed newborn babies with glucose water, infant formula, or both while in the maternity ward or nursery. All of this should change.

Many obstetricians, pediatricians, and doctors wrongly believe that there are many medical contraindications to breast-feeding: prematurity or low weight for age at birth, Caesarian delivery, minor breast problems, and other maternal or infant health problems. Seldom are these valid reasons for not breast-feeding. A recent meeting of experts called by WHO and UNICEF concluded that contraindications to breast-feeding are few, certainly less than in 1% of births. Some extremely rare congenital metabolic diseases do preclude the provision of breast milk to an infant: galactosemia, maple syrup disease, and phenylketonuria.

Experience in many hospitals shows that most infants with low birth weight should receive breast milk; that congenital abnormalities such as cleft palate are not contraindications for breast-feeding; and that Caesarian delivery, mastitis, breast abscess, many infections (including pulmonary tuberculosis and leprosy) are not indications for denying breast-feeding to a newborn infant. Although there is evidence that a mother with acquired immune deficiency syndrome (AIDS) may transmit the virus in utero to her unborn child, at present few infants have been proved to have been infected with the AIDS virus as a result of breast-feeding. Even though HIV has been detected in breast milk, the risks of not breast-feeding the baby outweigh the risk of the infant acquiring AIDS in this manner.

THE INSUFFICIENT MILK SYNDROME. It is common for mothers to believe that they are not producing adequate milk for their baby. In many studies "insufficient milk" is cited as one of the more common reasons given for early termination of breast-feeding or for early supplementation with infant formula. The "insufficient milk syndrome" is not well understood either in research circles or by practicing doctors and pediatricians. Too often health professionals, when faced with a mother complaining of insufficient milk, simply advise her to supplement her breast milk with bottle feeds. Usually this is exactly the wrong advice to give. The maintenance of lactation is dependent on adequate nipple stimulation by the suckling infant, which leads to the release of the hormone prolactin. Therefore, the cause of "insufficient milk" may often be that alternative feeding has replaced breast-feeding to a variable degree. Advice to provide a supplement or more supplement, then, usually contributes to a reduction in breast-milk production. The most appropriate advice to a mother who wishes to breast-feed, but who believes she has insufficient milk, is to help her to breast-feed more, and not less, because this is likely to increase her milk production.

PROTECTION, SUPPORT, AND PROMOTION OF BREAST-FEEDING. In most developing countries mothers should be encouraged to provide breast milk as the only, or the main source of, food for the infant for the first 4 to 6 months of life. Breast-feeding should be continued as other foods are introduced into the diet of the baby. Three types of activities expediate this.

Protection of Breast-feeding. Policies and activities should shield women already breast-feeding or planning to breast-feed against forces that might influence them to do otherwise (e.g., curtailment of the promotion of breast-milk substitutes and measures that reduce the easy availability of infant formula—Papua New Guinea has placed infant formula on prescription as a means to protect breast-feeding).

Support of Breast-feeding. Activities, both formal and informal, that improve mothers' confidence in their ability to breast-feed should be encouraged. Employment away from home discourages breast-feeding. Legislation to provide women with maternity leave, and job security if they take a longer period of unpaid leave, would help. Advice by doctors and other health professionals before and after delivery can be helpful. Local breast-feeding support groups may play a useful role.

Promotion of Breast-feeding. This includes influencing women to breast-feed their infants. Education campaigns to make known the disadvantages of bottle-feeding and the advantages of breast-feeding are the usual approaches. It is important to know what led to the decline in breast-feeding in an area and to understand how women regard breast- and bottle-feeding. A lack of such understanding has led to failure of many promotional campaigns.

THE ECONOMICS OF BOTTLE-FEEDING

Impact upon Families. Manufactured breast-milk substitutes are extremely expensive in relation to the income of the majority of families in nonindustrialized countries. Figures from Kenya, Tanzania, and India show that it would take more than 60% of the total minimum wage of a father to buy adequate quantities of formula for his 3-month-old infant. The purchase of recommended quantities of breast-milk substitutes would divert scarce family resources away from other essential needs and increase poverty. Stretching the formula by overdiluting it will, as stated, lead to marasmus (Fig. 109–2).

Impact upon Nations. For many nations a decline in breast-feeding means an increase in the importation of breast-milk substitutes and of the paraphernalia needed for bottle-feeding. These contribute to already serious foreign exchange problems.

WEANING. Somewhere between 4 and 6 months of age foods other than breast milk need to be introduced into the diet of the infant. Prolonged use of breast milk alone will lead to an inadequate diet in terms of energy intake. This leads to growth faltering. The resulting low intake of other nutrients, e.g., iron, causes anemia and other deficiency states.

In some societies other beverages and foods are introduced unnecessarily early. Some Indian babies receive tea within hours of birth, and many Indonesian mothers introduce solid foods in the first few weeks, sometimes force-feeding foods previously masticated by the mother. The beginning of weaning introduces new hazards to the infant. These new foods and beverages may be contaminated with pathogenic organisms. Gastrointestinal infections occur frequently during this time, leading to the term "weanling diarrhea," which is prevalent worldwide.

In general, the first weaning foods should be soft and easily digestible, and should be introduced gradually while breast-feeding continues. Often gruels of the local staple food, be it rice or maize, cassava or plantain, are used as weaning foods. The addition of a little oil or fat will increase its caloric density. It is important that the food be cooked long enough to kill pathogenic organisms, and covered while it cools. Later, other family foods can be cut up or softened and added to the gruel or fed separately. Gradually the amount and frequency with which these supplementary foods are fed increases, and the percentage of nutrients received from breast milk becomes smaller, even though breast-feeding continues.

In general as the child gets older, multimixes including the staple food (usually a cereal or root crop), plus small amounts of foods rich in protein (often either a legume or meat, fish, or milk), fruits and vegetables (especially dark green leafy vegetables to provide carotene), and energy supplements (e.g. oils, fats, and/or sugar) are recommended. Recent work in Tanzania has shown that adding small amounts of pulverized sprouted seeds will serve to make a thick porridge thin, and thus increase energy density for a given viscosity.

As the child gets close to complete weaning, he or she should be increasingly eating normal family foods. However, it remains important that meals be frequent (4 to 6 per day) and that the food be relatively energy dense. A common contributory cause of childhood malnutrition is the feeding of 2-to 4-year-old children only 2 or 3 meals a day with most of the food in the form of a bulky staple (like ugali in East Africa, which is a thick maize product more solid than porridge, a bulky dish and heavy for a young child to eat in adequate quantities).

BIBLIOGRAPHY

American Academy of Pediatrics: Encouraging breastfeeding. Pediatrics 65:657, 1980.

Chandra RK: Prospective studies of the effect of breastfeeding on incidence of infection and allergy. Acta Paediatr 68: 691, 1979.

Cameron M, Hofvander Y: Manual on Feeding Infants and Young Children. Oxford, Oxford University Press, 1983.

Greiner T, Almroth S, Latham MC: The economic value of breast-feeding. Cornell International Nutrition Monograph Series No. 6. Ithaca, New York, Cornell University, 1979.

Jelliffe DB, Jelliffe EFP: Human Milk in the Modern World. London, Oxford University Press, 1978.

Jelliffe DB, Jelliffe EFP (eds.): Programmes to Promote Breastfeeding. Oxford, Oxford University Press, 1988.

Latham MC: Insufficient milk and the World Health Organization Code. East Afr Med J 58:87, 1982.

Latham MC: The relationship of breastfeeding to human fertility. *In* The Decline of the Breast. Cornell International Nutrition Monograph Series No. 10. Ithaca, New York, Cornell University, 1982.

Latham MC, Elliott TC, Winikoff B, et al.: Infant feeding in urban Kenya: A pattern of triple nipple feeding. J Trop Pediatr 32:276, 1986.

Minchin M: Breastfeeding Matters. Victoria, Australia, Allen and Unwin, 1985.

Potts M, Thapa S, Herbetson MA: Breast-feeding and fertility. J Biosoc Sci 9(Suppl):1, 1985.

WHO: The dynamics of breast-feeding. WHO Chron 37:6, 1983.

WHO: The prevalence and duration of breast-feeding: A critical review of available information. WHO Stat Quart 2:192, 1982.
Winikoff B, Castle MA, Laukaran VH: Feeding Infants in Four Societies. New York, Greenwood Press, 1988.

109.3. DRUG AND NUTRIENT INTERACTIONS

Daphne A. Roe

DEFINITION. Drug and nutrient interactions cover both beneficial and unwanted effects of drugs on the disposition of nutrients and on nutritional status as well as the effects of food or specific nutrient intake on the disposition of drugs.

ETIOLOGY AND PREVALENCE. In tropical countries, factors that influence the types of drug and nutrient interaction include the following:

(1) geography of disease, including both infectious and noninfectious disease;

(2) prevalence and types of malnutrition present in the population;

(3) local availablity of drugs and prescribing practices;

(4) prevalence of genetic diseases that alter the metabolism of drugs or modify responses to drugs;

(5) use of social drugs, including alcohol, that modify or alter the risk of interactions between therapeutic drugs and nutrients;

(6) consumption of foods containing natural food toxins that is influenced by the amount of the food consumed or the preparation of the food;

(7) promotion of breast-feeding during periods of drug administration.

ROLE OF DISEASE DISTRIBUTION, GENETIC VARIABLES, AND PRE-EXISTENT DIETARY DEFICIENCIES ON RISK OF DRUG-INDUCED MALNUTRITION. The prevalence of specific drug and nutrient interactions is influenced by disease distribution (Table 109–1). For example, the prevalence of drug and nutrient interactions relative to antimalarial drugs is determined not only by the local prevalence of malaria, but also by the types of malaria that are endemic, which defines the antimalarial drug prescribed. Thus, where *Plasmodium falciparum* is the parasite, and the drug combination prescribed is sulfadoxine with pyrimethamine (Fansidar), there is a higher prevalence of megaloblastic anemia and concurrent leukopenia. This is due to the antifolate effects of the pyrimethamine. Similarly, those taking pyrimethamine as a malaria prophylaxis are at increased risk of developing megaloblastic anemia (Chapter 107.7).

However, drug-induced hemolytic anemia due to antimalarial drugs is defined not only by specific drug usage, but also within these areas, and risk is limited to individuals who have glucose-6-phosphate dehydrogen-

ase deficiency (Chapter 5). Risk for hemolytic anemia is further linked to the local prescribing practices, which in turn may be influenced by whether or not chloroquine-resistant malaria is a problem.

The prevalence of drug-induced nutritional deficiencies is related not only to the prevalence of diseases for which drugs exerting an antinutrient effect are prescribed, but also is related to the nutritional status of those receiving the drug. For example, the common drug used in the treatment of tuberculosis is isoniazid. This drug is a vitamin B_6 antagonist, and as such, can induce the spectrum of clinical effects of vitamin B_6 deficiency, including neuropathy, sideroblastic anemia, and dermatitis (Chapter 107.5). Whether or not those on the drug are at risk for vitamin B_6 deficiency depends on whether or not local physicians routinely prescribe a prophylactic vitamin B_6 supplement with the isoniazid. In some clinics treating large numbers of cases of tuberculosis, vitamin B_6 is not routinely provided together with isoniazid because of its high cost. In this case early recognition and treatment of vitamin B_6 deficiency is important. When isoniazid-induced vitamin B_6 deficiency occurs in a population that is consuming a low niacin diet, pellagra may be a risk also. This secondary drug-induced vitamin deficiency is explained by the fact that in vitamin B_6 deficiency, the endogenous conversion of tryptophan to niacin is inhibited. This limits the total niacin available in the body. Because pulmonary tuberculosis is seen often in urban populations where alcoholism is common, it is within these populations that isoniazid-induced pellagra has been reported. Alcoholics often have low niacin intakes.

A pharmacogenetic determinant of vitamin B_6 deficiency in people under treatment with isoniazid for tuberculosis is their acetylator status. Isoniazid is acetylated prior to clearance, and those who are genetically slow acetylators are more at risk for vitamin B_6 deficiency, because the parent drug exerts its inhibitory effect on pyridoxal kinase longer and prevents conversion of the vitamin to its coenzyme forms.

Another factor influencing the risk of drug-induced vitamin B_6 deficiency in those under treatment for tuberculosis is whether other vitamin B_6 antagonists, such as cycloserine and pyrazinamide, are given concurrently with isoniazid.

DRUG DISPOSITION, NEEDS, AND TOXICITY IN MALNUTRITION. Whether the effects of protein-energy malnutrition (PEM) on the pharmacokinetic disposition of drugs and their toxicity is a clinical concern depends upon the extent PEM is a problem in a particular country or region. Pathophysiologic changes in PEM may alter drug pharmacokinetics. Decreased mucosal absorption and rapid intestinal transit can reduce the rate and amount of the drug absorbed. Edema, hypoalbuminemia, and increased extracellular and total

TABLE 109–1. Examples of Endemic Diseases as Determinants of Local Incidence of Drug-induced Nutritional Deficiencies

Endemic Disease	Location	Drug-Induced Deficiency	Clinical Manifestation
Malaria	Malawi	Folate deficiency due to the antimalarial, pyrimethamine	Megaloblastic anemia
Tuberculosis	Kenya	Vitamin B_6 deficiency due to the anti-TB drug, isoniazid	Neuropathy
Cerebral cysticercosis	South Africa	Folate deficiency due to the anticonvulsant, phenytoin	Megaloblastic anemia

water can alter drug disposition. Fatty infiltration of the liver can reduce the efficiency of drug metabolism. PEM can also reduce glomerular filtration and plasma blood flow, which can slow drug clearance (Chapter 106).

However, pharmacokinetic studies carried out in India in children with PEM and also in malnourished adults have shown the effects of the nutritional deficiency depend not only upon the type of PEM present (i.e., whether marasmus or kwashiorkor), but also on the drug prescribed. The latter variable is dependent on infections that are locally present and upon local prescribing habits. For drugs not protein bound, such as penicillin, excretion is slower before nutritional intervention, because the depressed renal function leads to slower renal clearance. The therapeutic dose would be lower than after successful nutritional rehabilitation. For certain protein-bound drugs, such as sulfamethoxazole and streptomycin, hypoalbuminemia is associated with more free drug in the plasma. Although the free drug concentration may be elevated, it is not clear whether this is associated with enhanced toxicity because more drug reaches the tissues. The risk of certain highly toxic drugs, such as chloramphenicol and gentamicin, is increased in PEM.

In women, during their reproductive years when iron deficiency is a risk from menstrual and pregnancy losses and low intake, nonsteroidal analgesics (e.g., aspirin and ibuprofen) add a further risk of iron deficiency anemia.

INCOMPATIBILITY REACTIONS DUE TO NON-NUTRIENTS IN FOOD AND ALCOHOLIC BEVERAGES. Acute drug-food incompatibility reactions occur when a food is consumed by an individual taking a drug that inhibits the metabolism of amines in the food. This causes either a direct reaction from the effects of amine, a flush reaction, or acute and severe hypertension from histamine or catecholamine release. Examples include the flush reaction from eating tuna, bonito, or other fish containing histamine by an individual receiving isoniazid, which inhibits histaminase; or from eating beans containing dopamine; or consuming wine, beer, or cheese containing tyramine by an individual who is receiving a drug that is a monoamine oxidase inhibitor (e.g., the antidepressant phenelzine).

The risk of these acute drug-food incompatibility reactions and of drug-induced nutritional deficiencies is influenced by social drug use and abuse. Alcohol abuse can modulate the outcomes and increase the risk of therapeutic drug interactions as well as potentiate the severity of malnutrition.

DRUGS IN BREAST MILK. A special risk where breast-feeding is practiced by women being treated for tuberculosis is the ingestion of isoniazid by the infant. The infant may develop hepatitis due to the drug. Other drugs taken by the mother may pass into the milk, but the risk to the infant from the drug is often smaller than the risk of abandoning breast-feeding.

NATURAL FOOD TOXINS: EFFECT OF FOOD PREPARATION AND MALNUTRITION ON RESPONSES. The unusual amino acid mimosine (beta-[N]-(3-hydroxypyridone-3)-alpha-aminopropionic acid) is present in the wild tamarind (*Leucaena glauca*). This plant has a wide distribution in South and Central America and the Far East. In Indonesia, where *L. glauca* is consumed, children and adults have developed edema of the scalp and extensive hair loss. However, this toxic response is not inevitable. Mimosine forms an iron complex that inactivates the amino acid. Therefore, if soups and stews containing *L. glauca* are cooked in iron pots, there is no adverse effect on the consumers' scalp or hair.

Famine. During famines, populations may rely on local wild plants containing a non-nutrient toxin, such as the wild tamarind, as a major food source. If this non-nutrient is harmless in small amounts, but toxic when consumed in large amounts, toxicity will be observed only under famine conditions. Alternate effects of famine on outcome are that the response to the toxin is affected by malnutrition or that when malnutrition is present, the dose required to exert a toxic effect is lower because of reduction in body mass, body composition, and hepatic or renal function. Phototoxins in wild spinach-like plants have been reported to produce a pellagra-like syndrome in times of famine. These different outcomes could be explained by differences in nutritional status, although they could also be linked to differences in the amounts of the plant consumed. Certain species of *Amaranthus* have been associated with acute photosensitivity when eaten by famine populations in China; the photosensitivity ceased after the famine was relieved.

CLINICAL MANIFESTATIONS. Problem diagnosis is necessary to identify unwanted outcomes of drug and nutrient interactions. From the clinical standpoint, there are 4 main types of problems (Table 109–2):

(1) disease that persists in spite of drug therapy because altered diet or nutritional status has altered the disposition of, and dose requirements for, a therapeutic drug;

TABLE 109–2. Examples of Clinical Problems Associated with Drug and Nutrient Interactions

Problem	Disease	Diet	Drug/Toxin	Mechanism
Persistence of lesions	Streptococcal impetigo	High kcal-protein	Penicillin	With nutritional rehabilitation more penicillin is excreted
Light sensitivity (pellagra-like syndrome)	Marasmus	Famine	Phototoxin in plant	Response to phototoxin altered by malnutrition
Flush reaction	Tuberculosis	Fish	Isoniazid	Histamine in fish not metabolized due to effect of drug on histaminase
Megaloblastic anemia	Malaria	Low folate	Pyrimethamine	Anti-folate effects of the antimalarial + effects of diet.

(2) drug or plant toxicity attributable to changes in eating or cooking practices or malnutrition;

(3) incompatibility reactions following consumption of food containing a non-nutrient substance that is only toxic if its metabolism is inhibited by a therapeutic drug;

(4) drug-induced nutritional deficiencies attributable to antivitamin effects of the drug, or to drug-induced malabsorption, or to drug-induced mineral depletion.

PREVENTION AND CONTROL. Outcomes of drug and nutrient interactions can be beneficial or adverse. Beneficial outcomes, which should clearly not be prevented, include improved nutritional status due to disease control by antibacterial or antiprotozoal agents. Inadequate treatment of infections due to too low a drug dose in children with malnutrition must be avoided. For example, streptococcal impetigo in children recovering from PEM requires higher doses of penicillin. Acute incompatibility reactions (e.g., flush reactions) can be avoided by warning patients who take drugs, such as isoniazid, to avoid intake of foods containing amines, such as histamine. Risk of hepatitis in breast-fed infants of women receiving isoniazid can be prevented by having the infant breast-fed by another lactating woman who is free of tuberculosis. Alternatively the mother can be treated with another antituberculosis drug if a suitable one exists.

Prevention of altered reactions to plant toxins during famine is by increasing local awareness of plants that can cause the reaction and by supplying food relief with cereal staples as well as other foods of high nutrient density.

Drug-induced nutritional deficiencies can be prevented by routinely giving a vitamin supplement with the drug. Examples include the administration of vitamin B_6 with isoniazid or folate with pyrimethamine. Megadoses of these vitamins are to be avoided, because they may interfere with the intended therapeutic action of the drug.

BIBLIOGRAPHY

Buchanan N: Effect of protein-energy malnutrition on drug metabolism in man. World Rev Nutr Diet 43:129–139, 1984.

Kirksey A, Groziak SM: Maternal drug use: Evaluation of risks to breast fed infants. World Rev Nutr Diet 43:60–79, 1984.

Krishnaswamy K: Effects of malnutrition on drug metabolism and toxicity in humans. *In* Hathcock JN (ed.): Nutritional Toxicology, Vol. 2. New York, Academic Press, 1987, pp. 105–128.

Price Evans DA, Clarke CA: Pharmacogenetics. Br Med Bull 17:234–240, 1961.

Roberts JMD: Malaria. *In* Vogel LC, Muller AS, Odingo RS, et al. (eds.): Health and Disease in Kenya. Nairobi, Kenya Lit. Bureau, 1974, pp. 305–330.

Roe DA: Diet and Drug Interactions. New York, Van Nostrand Reinhold, 1988.

Roe DA: Drug-Induced Nutritional Deficiencies, 2nd ed. Westport, CT, AVI Publishing, 1985, pp. 113–122, 193, 281–287.

Roe DA: A Plague of Corn: The Social History of Pellagra. Ithaca, New York, Cornell University Press, 1973, pp. 147–148, 156.

Seitz HK, Simanowski UA: Metabolic and nutritional effects of ethanol. *In* Hathcock JN (ed.): Nutritional Toxicology, Vol. 2. New York, Academic Press, 1987, pp. 63–103.

Shankar PS: Pellagra in Gulbarga. J Indian Med Assoc 54:273–275, 1970.

van Veen AG: Toxic properties of some unusual foods. *In* Toxicants Occurring Naturally in Foods. Washington, DC, Food Protection Committee, Food and Nutrition Board, NAS/NRC, 1966, pp. 174–182.

PART IX

VECTOR TRANSMISSION OF DISEASES

GENERAL PRINCIPLES

Trenton K. Ruebush II

Disease is produced by an interaction between a causative agent and a susceptible host. The basic principles of disease transmission apply equally well to diseases caused by infections, chemical and physical agents, and nutritional deficiencies or excesses.

In most cases of infectious disease, the causative agent, an infectious organism, is transmitted to the host from an external source *(exogenous infection)*. Less frequently, owing to a change in the host-agent relationship that favors the infective agent, disease is produced by an organism that is normally carried by the host without signs or symptoms of disease *(endogenous infection)*. The interrelationship among an infectious agent, its host, and the route by which the agent is transmitted from host to host has been termed the chain of infection. Environmental factors may affect all three links in the chain of infection.

INFECTIOUS AGENT

Pathogenicity and Virulence. The infectious agent may be a virus, chlamydia, rickettsia, bacterium, fungus, protozoan, or helminth. The ability of an infectious organism to cause disease in a susceptible host is termed *pathogenicity*. Rabies virus and smallpox virus are examples of highly pathogenic organisms; all infected persons develop clinically apparent illnesses. In contrast, *Staphylococcus epidermidis* rarely causes disease, although it is commonly found colonizing the skin.

The term *virulence* is used to characterize the severity of disease produced by an infectious organism. Rabies virus is highly virulent; only a few patients have ever recovered from such infections. In contrast, *Dientamoeba fragilis* rarely produces symptoms in infected patients. The virulence of most infectious agents varies, depending on the susceptibility of the host. Although *Toxoplasma gondii* usually causes asymptomatic or mild illnesses in normal hosts, infections during the first trimester of pregnancy may lead to severe birth defects, and in immunosuppressed patients, a fatal encephalitis may result.

Host Specificity. Several properties of an infectious agent may influence its pathogenicity and virulence. Host specificity refers to the preference of an infectious agent for a given host. Some organisms have very strict host specificities, e.g., *Treponema pallidum* and *Neisseria gonorrhoeae,* which are pathogenic only for man. In contrast, *Salmonella* species and *Trypanosoma cruzi* infect human beings as well as a wide variety of non-human animals. Different strains or developmental stages of an organism may also differ in their pathogenicity and virulence. The larval stages of most helminths are much less host-specific than the adult worms. Cutaneous and visceral larva migrans, for example, are usually caused by helminths that are incapable of developing into adults in man.

Invasiveness. The ability of an infectious agent to penetrate and spread through the host's tissues is referred to as invasiveness. *Vibrio cholerae* does not invade the intestinal mucosa. Instead, it produces its effects by the elaboration of a potent toxin. *Entamoeba histolytica,* however, may multiply within the intestinal lumen without causing disease, but when it does invade the mucosa, severe disease results, with occasional dissemination of organisms to other parts of the body via the blood stream. With most highly invasive organisms, such as *Streptococcus,* the production of lytic enzymes promotes the rapid spread of infection.

Infective Dose. The number of organisms necessary to cause infection also plays a role in the pathogenicity and virulence of infectious diseases. Neutralization of gastric acidity greatly reduces the number of enteric bacteria necessary to produce infection. A similar relationship between infective dose and severity of infection occurs in most helminthic infections. When the worm burden is low, patients usually have few or no symptoms, but heavy infections can result in severe disease.

Additional Factors. The longevity of an infectious agent, its resistance to antimicrobial agents, and the production of toxins are additional factors to be considered in the pathogenicity and virulence of an infectious agent.

Source and Reservoir. In considering programs for the control of infectious diseases, it is important that a distinction be made between the source of an infectious agent and its reservoir. The *source* of an infectious agent is the person, animal, object, or substance from which the organism passes directly to a susceptible host. The *reservoir* is the person, animal, arthropod, plant, or inanimate organic material in which an infectious agent normally lives and multiplies and on which it depends for its survival. The reservoir and source of an organism may be identical, as with *Salmonella typhi* infections. In contrast, with hepatitis virus, the reservoir is usually man, but the source may be contaminated food, water, or biologic products.

HOST

Site of Entrance of Infection. Infectious agents may enter a host via the skin, mucous membranes, respiratory tract, gastrointestinal tract, or genitourinary tract. *Schistosoma* and *Leptospira* are examples of organisms that can penetrate intact skin. Most other infectious agents require a break in the integrity of the skin due to trauma, surgical wounds or instrumentation, or the bite of an arthropod vector to invade a host and produce disease.

The site of entrance of infectious agents that are deposited in the respiratory tract depends primarily on the size of the organism. Particles smaller than 5 μm in diameter are usually carried to the terminal alveoli, where they may be transported across the alveolar membrane by macrophages. Larger particles are deposited in the bronchioles, bronchi, trachea, or nares.

Infection via the gastrointestinal tract in contaminated food or drink is the usual means of entrance of enteric bacteria and intestinal protozoa and helminths. Entrance to the genitourinary tract may occur during catheterization, instrumentation, or sexual intercourse. Infectious agents may also be transferred transplacentally to the developing fetus, as in the case of rubella and *Toxoplasma*.

Host Defenses. The response of a host to an infectious agent depends on the pathogenicity and virulence of the organism as well as on the host's susceptibility and defenses. The host response may range from inapparent or subclinical infection to severe or even fatal illness. Host factors that may influence susceptibility to an infectious agent and the severity of clinical manifestations include age, sex, race, ethnic group and other hereditary factors, nutritional and physiologic status, previous or concurrent diseases, and prior immunologic experience.

Carrier State. The carrier state, a form of inapparent infection in which a patient continues to harbor an infectious agent in the absence of clinical disease, is extremely important epidemiologically. Prolonged urinary or fecal excretors of *Salmonella typhi* and asymptomatic malaria gametocyte carriers play crucial roles in the transmission of these diseases and their maintenance during unfavorable periods.

Nonspecific and Specific Protection. Host defense mechanisms are of two types: nonspecific and specific. The barrier presented by the intact skin and mucous membranes, tears, saliva, and respiratory, gastrointestinal, and genitourinary secretions are examples of *nonspecific* defenses. The *specific* defense mechanisms of the host are natural and artificial immunity. *Natural immunity* develops following the natural occurrence of an infection. It may be short-lived, as with most viral respiratory illnesses, or essentially lifelong, as with rubella and poliomyelitis. Artificial immunity is of two kinds. *Active artificial immunity* results from vaccination with live, attenuated, or killed vaccines. *Passive artificial immunity* is produced by the administration of immunoglobulin or antitoxins or by the transplacental passage of antibody.

ROUTE OF INFECTION. There are four basic routes of transmission of infectious agents from a source to a susceptible host: contact, common-vehicle, airborne, and vector-borne. In many cases, infectious agents are transmitted by more than one of these routes; however, before specific control measures can be considered, the route of transmission must be identified.

Contact Transmission. Three types of contact transmission are recognized: *Direct-contact transmission* requires direct physical contact between an infected person or animal and a susceptible host, such as occurs with syphilis or gonorrhea. *Indirect-contact transmission* results from the contact between a susceptible host and a contaminated inanimate object, as in pinworm infections, which may be transmitted by clothing, bedding, and other articles contaminated with infective eggs. *Droplet spread* involves transmission of infection over short distances via large droplets that contain the infectious agent. The common cold and measles are examples of transmission by this route.

Common-Vehicle Transmission. In this situation, the infectious agent is spread to multiple hosts from a single inanimate source. The vehicle may be water (as in the case of giardiasis or typhoid fever), food (as with botulism and trichinosis), milk (as with brucellosis), or biologic substances such as blood, blood products, or intravenous fluids (as in the case of hepatitis and malaria).

Airborne Transmission. Dust particles or droplet nuclei that contain an infectious agent are responsible for disease transmission by the airborne route. These particles are much smaller than those involved in direct-contact transmission by droplets and may remain suspended in the air for considerable periods of time. Airborne infectious agents may arise from human, animal, or inanimate sources. Tuberculosis is an example of a disease transmitted by airborne spread from an infected patient. In ornithosis, airborne transmission results from infected birds, whereas Q fever may be transmitted by aerosols from inanimate sources.

Vector-borne Spread. Transmission of an infectious agent to a vertebrate host by an arthropod may be either mechanical or biologic. *Mechanical transmission* includes simple mechanical carriage of an infectious agent on the vector's body or within its intestinal tract, as in flies harboring *Salmonella* or *Shigella,* as well as the carriage of organisms on the mouth parts of biting insects, such as occurs with African trypanosomiasis. In *biologic transmission,* the infectious agent multiplies within the arthropod vector, and a finite period, known

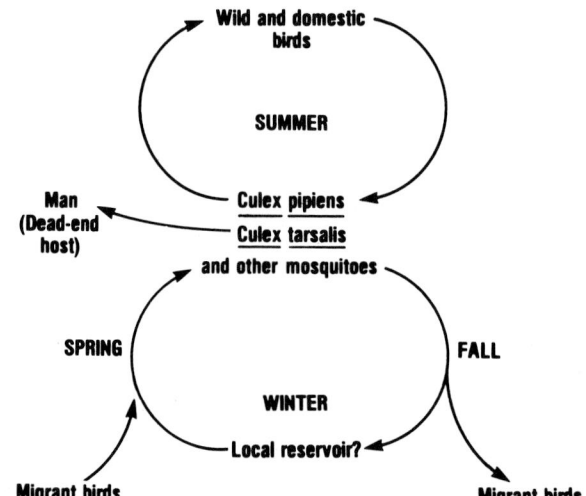

FIGURE IX–1. St. Louis encephalitis virus transmission cycle in the United States.

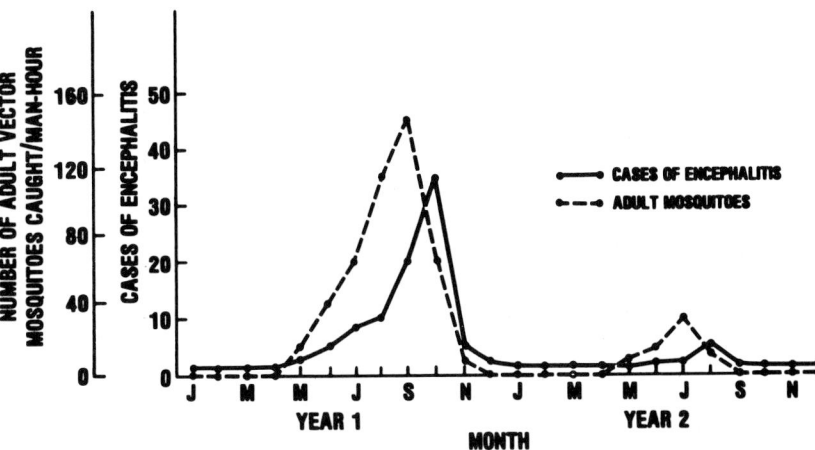

FIGURE IX–2. Mosquito-borne viral encephalitis. Outbreak in Year 1, before mosquito control program started, shows the occurrence of disease primarily during the summer months and the rise and peak of human cases following the rise in the mosquito population. Regular spraying with insecticide was initiated in Year 2, and no outbreak occurred.

as the extrinsic incubation period, is required before the arthropod becomes infective for another vertebrate host (Fig. IX–1).

Arthropod-borne infectious agents may enter the host by several routes. With malaria, dengue, and yellow fever, the infectious agent is injected directly into the subcutaneous tissues or the blood stream. With plague, the intestinal tract of the flea vector becomes blocked by large masses of bacilli, and when the flea attempts to feed, organisms are regurgitated into the bite wound. Infectious agents may also gain entrance to the host through contamination of the skin or mucous membranes. Rickettsiae of epidemic typhus and trypanosomes of Chagas' disease are discharged in the vector's feces and may be rubbed or scratched into the wound after the vector has fed. Relapsing fever spirochetes, present within the body fluids of infected body lice, may enter the bite wound when the lice are accidentally or purposely crushed.

A variety of factors influence the capability of an arthropod to serve as an efficient vector of human disease. These include the susceptibility of the vector to the infectious agent, the vector's ability to transmit the organism to man, the degree of association between the vector and man and its willingness to bite man, and the vector's population density and survival rate (Fig. IX–2).

Many infectious agents may be transmitted by several different routes. Rabies virus, for example, is most frequently transmitted by direct contact with an infected canine but also may be spread by the airborne route in caves inhabited by infected bats. Anthrax is usually spread by direct contact with contaminated tissues or products of infected animals, but it can also be transmitted by the airborne or common-vehicle route.

ENVIRONMENT. The environment, including its physical, biologic, and socioeconomic components, may influence any of the three major links in the chain of transmission so as to promote or limit the development of infection. *Physical factors* such as cold, heat, rainfall, humidity, and velocity of air currents may affect both the host's susceptibility to infection and the viability of the infectious agent. These physical factors are particularly important in the case of vector-borne diseases. *Biologic factors,* including human population density

and availability of food sources for vertebrate reservoir hosts and vectors, may also influence the transmission of infection. Finally, *socioeconomic and behavioral factors* such as occupation, sanitary conditions, hygienic habits, cultural and religious practices, and catastrophes such as wars, floods, and famines may affect the susceptibility of a host and the risk of acquiring infection.

BIBLIOGRAPHY

Benenson AS (ed): Control of Communicable Diseases in Man. 13th ed. Washington, DC, American Public Health Association, 1981.
Fox JP, Hall CE, Elveback LR: Epidemiology: Man and Disease. New York, Macmillan Company, 1970.
Lilienfeld AM: Foundations of Epidemiology. New York, Oxford University Press, 1976.

110.   ZOONOSES

Trenton K. Ruebush II

DEFINITION. Zoonoses are infections that are transmitted in nature between vertebrate animals and humans. They include those infections that man acquires from lower animals as well as infections that can be transmitted from man to lower animals. Also usually included are infestations with ectoparasites, such as scabies and myiasis, in which the arthropod burrows into or penetrates the body of the vertebrate host.

The economic cost of zoonotic diseases is very high. Not only are they a major cause of human disease throughout the world, but also they are responsible for serious economic losses to the livestock industry, thus indirectly affecting man's welfare.

HISTORY. Zoonotic diseases have been recognized for thousands of years. Perhaps the earliest reference to a zoonosis occurs in a Mesopotamian code from the twentieth century B.C. in which a fine was established for the owner of a dog that had bitten someone and was found to be rabid. Accurate clinical descriptions of anthrax appear in early Hebrew, Greek, Roman, and Hindu writings, and epidemics of plague have been recorded for more than 3000 years.

Zoonotic diseases have also played an important role

in history. The three major pandemics of bubonic plague that have been recorded since the beginning of the Christian era decimated populations and profoundly affected socioeconomic and cultural development. In Europe, for example, from the fourteenth to the late seventeenth century, it has been estimated that 25 million persons, or one fourth of the population, died as a result of the Black Death. During the eighteenth and nineteenth centuries, severe outbreaks of yellow fever spread via shipping routes to most major port cities in the Western Hemisphere. Yellow fever was also one of the major obstacles to the construction of the Panama Canal.

In recent years, with improvements in and more widespread application of clinical and laboratory diagnostic techniques, many "new" or previously unrecognized zoonotic diseases have been described. Because of their ability to adapt rapidly to changing ecologic conditions, the viruses offer a greater potential for these newly emerging zoonoses than do bacteria, protozoa, or helminths. Lassa fever and Marburg virus disease are just two examples of diseases that had not been recognized previously in either man or lower animals. Other organisms, such as *Babesia,* which have been known for many years but were thought to be restricted to lower animals, have been shown to be capable of infecting humans as well. As human and animal populations increase and man proceeds with the development of previously uninhabited areas, opportunities for contact between man and animals are constantly increasing. It seems likely, therefore, that additional zoonotic diseases will be recognized in the future and that these diseases will assume greater importance as the known diseases of man and animals are eradicated or brought under control.

EPIDEMIOLOGY. To understand the epidemiology of zoonotic diseases, it is first necessary to have a comprehensive understanding of the cycle of transmission of the organism in nature. As with any infectious disease, four factors must be considered in the transmission of zoonotic diseases: the infective agent, the host, the route of transmission, and the environment. However, as a group of diseases, the zoonoses tend to demonstrate much more complexity and variability in their epidemiology than do most infectious diseases. This is primarily due to the fact that a minimum of two hosts, the natural reservoir host and man, are involved in the transmission of all zoonotic diseases. As a result, a greater variety of host-infectious agent interactions may be established, and the epidemiology of the disease may vary with each host-agent combination.

Infective Agent and Reservoir Host. More than 150 different zoonotic diseases have been recorded. They may be caused by any family of infectious agents from the viruses to the helminths.

The natural or reservoir host of a zoonotic disease may be a wild animal, a domestic animal, or both. Human beings are not necessary for the transmission of zoonotic diseases in nature. They become infected when they accidentally come into contact with some part of the natural transmission cycle between the organism's animal reservoir hosts.

Arthropods may also act as a reservoir for certain infectious agents. The rickettsiae of Rocky Mountain spotted fever can be maintained for several years in the tick vector by transstadial and transovarial passage in the absence of infected vertebrate hosts. Transovarial transmission of some virus species also occurs in mosquitoes. *Babesia microti* apparently overwinters in the tick vector and then is transmitted to susceptible rodent hosts during the following spring.

Transmission. The transmission of an infectious agent from the reservoir host to man may take place by any of the four basic routes of disease transmission—by contact or by the airborne, vector-borne, or common-vehicle route. However, the route of transmission of an organism among the natural animal hosts and between the reservoir host and man is not necessarily identical. With tularemia, for example, tick transmission is the major route of spread among wild animals, but man generally acquires infection by direct contact with the tissues of infected animals.

With some zoonotic diseases, the route of transmission to man is quite complicated, and several different animal reservoir hosts are involved. In such cases, the different animal species may vary in their importance as reservoir hosts and in their role as a source of infection for man. Primary reservoir hosts are those that serve as permanent reservoirs of infection in the natural ecologic setting of the disease. Secondary reservoir hosts are animals that may be involved in the natural cycle of transmission and may play a very important role in the spread of infection to man but are not necessary for the survival of the infectious agent in nature. When the primary reservoir host of a zoonotic disease is a wild animal, secondary reservoir hosts may be domestic animals or other wild animals that come into closer contact with man. Plague is an example of a disease that is spread in such a way (Fig. 110–1). More than 200 different natural animal hosts have been identified for the plague bacillus. The primary reservoir hosts are wild rodents; the organism is transmitted between them by the bite of an infected flea. Sporadic human cases of plague arise when man enters a natural focus of the disease and is bitten by an infected flea or handles infected wild animals. The disease is spread from these sylvatic foci to urban areas when the secondary reservoir hosts, rats and mice living in close association with man, contract the infection from wild rodents. Transmission to man by the infected fleas of these peridomestic rodents may then result in severe outbreaks of human disease.

A similar situation occurs with Japanese B virus infections. Wild birds are the primary reservoir hosts, and a domestic animal, the pig, is the secondary reservoir host responsible for transmission of infection to man. The virus of yellow fever is maintained within the jungle between monkeys, the primary reservoir hosts, and various forest species of mosquitoes that rarely bite man (Fig. 110–2). Spread to urban areas may occur when infected monkeys carry the virus to areas adjacent to the forest and are bitten by mosquito species that live in close association with man and preferentially feed on human beings.

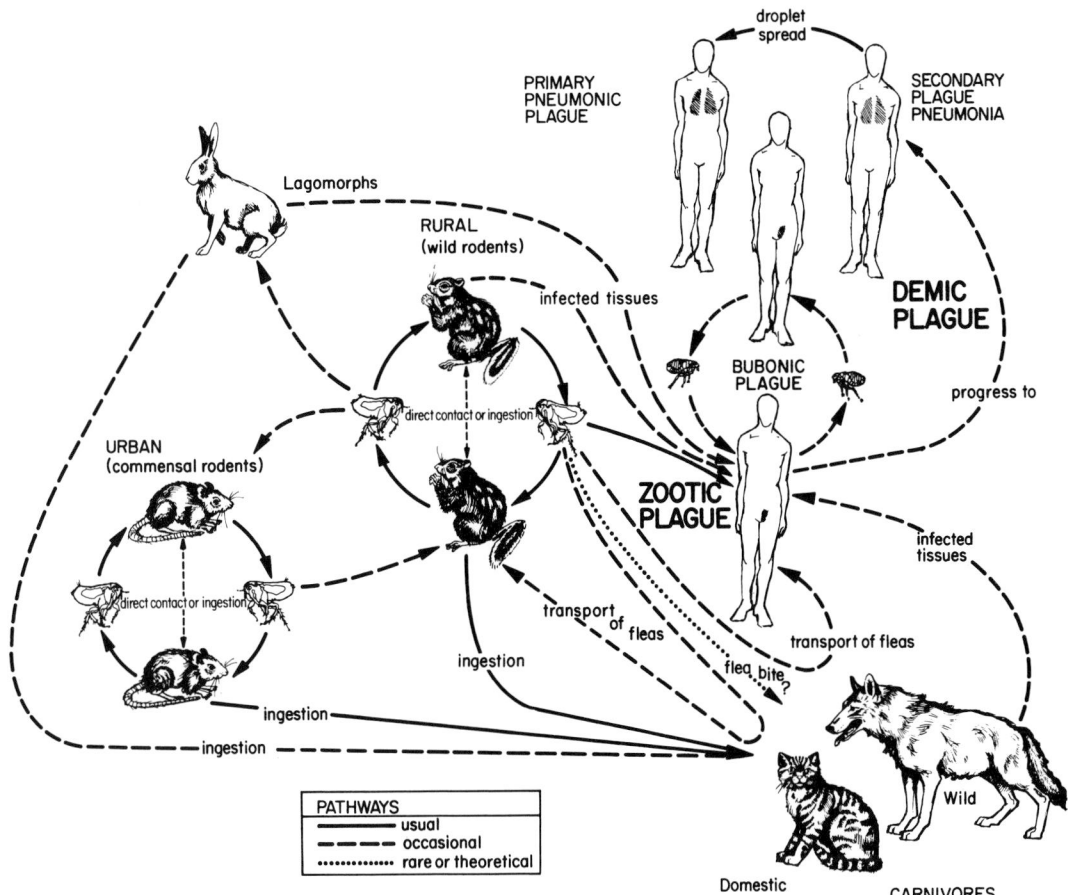

FIGURE 110–1. Transmission of plague. (From Hoeprich PD [ed]: Infectious Diseases. 3rd ed. Hagerstown, MD, Harper and Row, 1983.)

Reservoir hosts with inapparent or mild infections are usually more important epidemiologically to the transmission of zoonotic diseases than are animals with clinically apparent infections. Rabies is an exception, because most infected animals do not survive. In the case of this disease, however, a long and variable incubation period aids survival of the virus in nature.

Although human beings may serve as a reservoir for some zoonotic diseases, man is often a dead end in the chain of infection. With diseases such as leishmaniasis, trypanosomiasis, and the viral encephalitides, person-to-person transmission does occur but is uncommon and of little importance epidemiologically. In contrast, man's role as a reservoir for yellow fever virus and the plague bacillus is extremely important in promoting the rapid spread of these organisms within human communities. Without a human reservoir, fulminant outbreaks of yellow fever and pneumonic plague could not occur.

Environment. Environmental factors play an important role in the epidemiology of all zoonotic diseases

FIGURE 110–2. Transmission of yellow fever in Africa. (From Strode GK [ed]: Yellow Fever. New York, McGraw-Hill Book Company, 1951.)

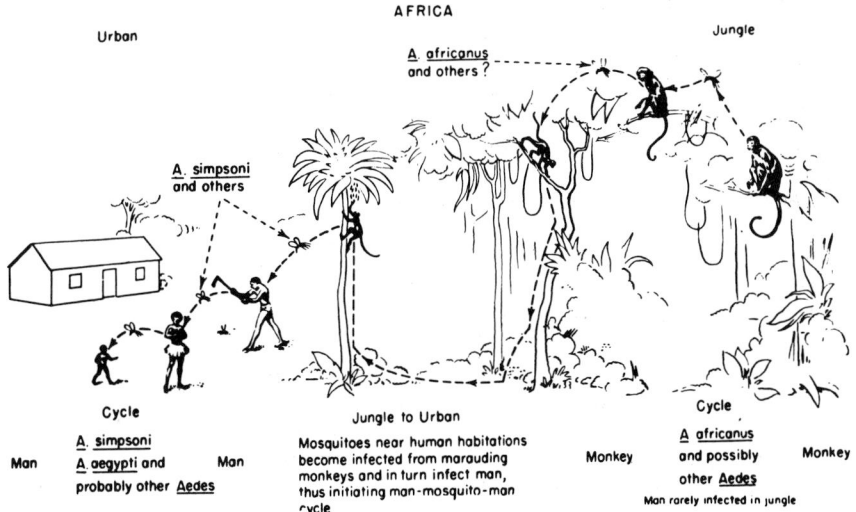

but particularly those with wild animal reservoirs. Study of these diseases in their natural settings has resulted in a concept known as the "focality" or "nidality" of infectious diseases. According to this concept, infectious diseases are not evenly distributed geographically. Just as animal species have defined habitats and associations with other species in a particular ecologic setting, so diseases tend to occur in foci in which the pathogenic organism circulates between its reservoir hosts and vectors. When man intrudes on one of these disease foci, he exposes himself to infection. The general term "landscape epidemiology" has been used to emphasize the epidemiologic importance of the environment in which a disease occurs and to indicate that the physical characteristics of a locality may suggest the likelihood of a given disease being present or not.

Tularemia provides an excellent example of disease focality. Eight different tularemia foci have been identified in the world, each one with its particular host-vector-infectious agent relationship. In the eastern North American continent, for example, the cycle is maintained between cottontail rabbits and hard ticks. In the western part of the continent, the jack rabbit is the major reservoir host, and either hard ticks or deer flies may serve as vectors. In Scandinavia, mosquitoes transmit the organism among lemmings, whereas in the area around the Black Sea, the water rat is the major reservoir host.

As environmental conditions change, changes may occur in the epidemiology of any zoonotic disease. Sporadic cases of American cutaneous leishmaniasis in hunters and woodsmen are common when the forest habitat of the rodent reservoir hosts and sandfly vectors is relatively undisturbed. Later, when communities are created within the forest, small outbreaks of the disease may occur among early settlers. As more and more of the forest is cleared, reservoir hosts and vectors are eliminated, and opportunities for exposure are reduced to a point at which human cases no longer occur. In such instances, it is conceivable that as man's contact with wild animals is reduced, domestic animals may come to be the most important reservoirs of many wild animal pathogens.

Introduction of control measures also may cause changes in the epidemiology of zoonotic diseases. Before the introduction of control programs, brucellosis was most frequently acquired by ingestion of contaminated milk or milk products. At present, the most common route of transmission is by direct contact with or inhalation of the organism.

In some cases, man may inadvertently create suitable environmental conditions for the spread of a zoonotic disease. Irrigation and hydroelectric projects in which large bodies of water are impounded greatly increase mosquito breeding sites and may result in severe outbreaks of mosquito-borne disease. Expansion of human communities into areas on the forest fringe or new settlements in previously uninhabited areas may expose a large number of residents to organisms normally limited to wild animals. Creation of wildlife and game preserves with the destruction of natural predators may result in high tick populations and may promote the spread of tick-borne pathogens to man.

Many zoonotic diseases are occupational hazards. Attack rates are much higher in workers engaged in activities that bring them into close contact with the natural transmission cycle of an organism than they are in the general population. Examples of such occupational diseases include leptospirosis in rice field workers, anthrax in carpet weavers, Q fever in abattoir workers, and cutaneous larva migrans in plumbers.

CONTROL. Zoonotic diseases present special problems in the planning of control and eradication programs. Control measures may be directed against any of the links in the chain of transmission—the infective agent, the natural host, or the route of transmission. Because of the variety of host animals involved in many zoonotic diseases, however, control of the infectious agent in one or two animal species alone is often not sufficient to eradicate the disease.

This is particularly true in the case of zoonotic diseases that have a wild animal reservoir, such as sylvatic plague, leishmaniasis, or yellow fever. Efforts directed against the reservoir of an infective agent offer a greater chance of success when the major reservoir host is a domestic animal. Control programs for bovine tuberculosis, anthrax, and brucellosis have been particularly successful. Even with these diseases, however, it is often not economically feasible to eliminate all infected reservoirs. As a result, the infection may persist at low levels in one or more reservoir hosts, and unless control measures are continued, further outbreaks will occur.

In the case of vector-borne zoonotic diseases, reduction of arthropod populations may be the most practical approach to control (Fig. IX–2). Urban yellow fever has been brought under control in many countries by reduction of breeding places and by regular insecticide use. Similarly, house spraying with residual insecticides for malaria has resulted in almost complete elimination of the sandfly vector of *Leishmania braziliensis peruviana,* which, unlike other vectors of American cutaneous leishmaniasis, lives in and around human dwellings.

Public health education and protection of food supplies are generally effective in controlling zoonotic diseases such as trichinosis, brucellosis, and salmonellosis, in which infection is acquired by ingestion of the causative agent. In the case of occupational diseases, measures directed toward reducing human exposure to the infectious agent through health education, improvement of working conditions, and vaccination of high-risk individuals may be the most satisfactory approach to disease control.

BIBLIOGRAPHY

Benenson AS (ed): Control of Communicable Diseases in Man. 13th ed. Washington, DC, American Public Health Association, 1981.

Hubbert WT, McCulloch WF, Schnurrenberger PR (eds): Disease Transmitted from Animals to Man. 6th ed. Springfield, IL, Charles C Thomas, 1975.

Steele JH (ed): CRC Handbook Series in Zoonoses, Vol 1. Boca Raton, FL, CRC Press, 1978.

111. MOLLUSKS INVOLVED IN DISEASE TRANSMISSION

William A. Sodeman, Jr.

Most mollusks have no relationship to man beyond their collection either as objects of beauty or as food. A few figure in the transmission of disease. Some mollusks transmit infection when eaten because of bacteria or viruses concentrated by filter feeding, such as the bivalves, oysters, mussels, and clams. Many parasites utilize the snail as a first and/or second intermediate host for their larval stages. Transmission to humans can occur with ingestion of raw or poorly cooked snails (Fig. 93–1), but most often the parasite leaves the snail and penetrates the skin of the host (Fig. 96–6) or encysts on another food item that is eaten raw (Figs. 97–1 and 97–2).

This chapter is designed to serve as a guide for the physician practicing in an area endemic for snail-transmitted diseases. Table 111–1 lists the principal snail-transmitted diseases, their mollusk intermediate host, and their geographic distribution. The list is long, but fortunately, in most areas the numbers of snails are limited, and once the species have been determined by expert identification, further field identification is feasible and practical.

Snail identification primarily depends upon morphology, including distinctive shells, radula (tooth) patterns, and soft-part anatomy, principally the anatomic variations of the genital apparatus. In a few cases, biochemical, immunologic, or cytogenetic characteristics must be ascertained to distinguish between morphologically similar, closely related species.

Shell morphology is often helpful in separating potential intermediate hosts from the many unsuitable mollusks. There are many areas where shell morphology alone can serve as an adequate guide to the presence or absence of suitable intermediate-host snails, but in some circumstances, the definitive species identification requires at least the study of soft-part anatomy and radular structure.

THE CLASSIFICATION OF MEDICALLY IMPORTANT GASTROPOD MOLLUSKS

The class Gastropoda is divided into two subclasses: Streptoneura, readily identifiable by the presence of an operculum, and the Euthyneura, of which the freshwater pulmonates are the primary concern.

SUBCLASS STREPTONEURA. Snails within the subclass Streptoneura are operculate, with the operculum, a trap door covering the aperture of the shell, fixed to the top of the foot behind the aperture. The operculum may be calcified, but in most freshwater families it is made of an organic noncalcified material. Soft-part anatomy shows a characteristic figure-eight twist to the visceral nerve and, in the aquatic forms, anterior gills. There are three orders, one of which, the Mesogastropoda, contains snails of medical importance.

Order Mesogastropoda. Snails of the order Mesogastropoda are responsible, as intermediate hosts, for the transmission of an extraordinary collection of trematodes that can produce disease in man. Eight families are of medical importance. These are the Ampullariidae (= Pilidae), Viviparidae, Pomatiopsidae, Bithyniidae, Thiaridae, Pleuroceridae, Potatimididae, and Littorinidae.

Family Viviparidae. The families Ampullariidae and Viviparidae can be distinguished by the appearance of the operculum, which grows with a concentric rather than a spiral pattern. Viviparidae are large, globular snails (Fig. 111–1) that are ovoviviparous (bear live young). They are widespread in lakes and rivers. A single species, *Viviparus javanicus,* serves as a second intermediate host for *Echinostoma ilocanum* in Java. Transmission is by ingestion of the raw snail. This snail can also serve as the intermediate host for the rat lungworm *Angiostrongylus cantonensis.*

Family Ampullariidae. Ampullariidae are also large, globular, egg-laying snails that have a worldwide distribution. Two of the many genera in this family are of medical significance. *Pila luzonica* and *P. conica* serve as second intermediate hosts for *E. ilocanum* on the Philippine Island of Luzon. *Marisa cornuarietis* (Linnaeus) (Fig. 111–1) is an aquatic carnivorous snail that has been utilized in the attempted biologic control of *Biomphalaria* species that can transmit *Schistosoma mansoni* in South America and the Antilles. It does not serve in the transmission of human infection. It is flat rather than globular in shape but differs from planorbids because of its small, red-brown operculum. Its shell is marked with reddish bands. It may be found in a broad range of freshwater habitats.

The remaining families of Mesogastropoda of medical importance all have an operculum with a spiral growth pattern.

Family Thiaridae. Although these snails have a worldwide distribution, their medical importance is principally in the Orient and Southeast Asia. One African genus is involved in the transmission of disease. The genus *Thiara* have tall, turreted shells measuring 2.5 to 5 cm as adults. There is a prominent axial beaded sculpture. *Thiara granifera* (Lamarck) (Fig. 111–1) in Taiwan and the islands of Southeast Asia and now introduced in Central America, the Antilles and the United States; *Melanoides tuberculata* (Muller) in both Africa and Asia; and *Brotia asperata* (Lamarck) in the Philippines all are reported to serve as first intermediate hosts for the lung fluke *Paragonimus westermani.* Subsequent evaluation suggests that *T. granifera* is not a first intermediate host for *P. westermani. T. granifera,* however, has served as an effective competitor in the biologic control of *Biomphalaria glabrata,* an intermediate host for *Schistosoma mansoni. T. granifera* is a first intermediate host of the intestinal fluke *Metagonimus yokogawai.*

In Africa, *Potadoma freethi* (Greer) (Fig. 111–1) has been identified as a first intermediate host of the lung fluke *Paragonimus africanus.* This snail is found in rivers and large streams. The snail intermediate host for *P. uterobilateralis,* another African lung fluke, has not been identified.

TABLE 111–1. Principal Mollusk-Transmitted Infections of Man

Disease	Pathogen	Mollusk (Genus and Species)	Geographic Range as Host
Clonorchiasis (Chapter 98.2)	*Clonorchis sinensis*	*Bithynia (Parafossarulus) manchourica*	China, Korea, Taiwan, Japan
		Bithynia fuchsiana	North China
		Bithynia chaperi	China
		Alocinma longicornis	China
		Semisulcospira amurensis	China
		Gabbia misella	Korea
Fascioliasis (Chapter 98.3)	*Fasciola hepatica*	*Lymnaea (Fossaria) truncatula*	Europe, Africa, Middle East, Asia
		Lymnaea viatrix	Argentina
		Lymnaea rubiginosa	Malaysia
		Lymnaea philippensis	Philippines
		Lymnaea swinhoe	Philippines
		Lymnaea tomentosa	Australia
		Lymnaea japonicum	Japan
		Lymnaea pervia	Japan
		Lymnaea columella	North and South America, Africa, Hawaiian Islands
		Fossaria bulimoides	United States
		Fossaria cubensis	United States
	Fasciola gigantica	*Lymnaea columella*	Africa
		Lymnaea rubiginosa	Malaysia
		Lymnaea acuminata	India
		Lymnaea auricularia	India
		Lymnaea natalensis	Africa
		Fossaria ollula	Hawaii
Fasciolopsiasis (Chapter 97.1)	*Fasciolopsis buski*	*Hippeutis umbilicalis*	India, Asia
		Hippeutis cantori	India, Asia
		Segmentina hemisphaerula	India, Asia
		Segmentina trochoideus	India, Asia
Gastrodisciasis (Chapter 97.4)	*Gastrodiscoides hominis*	*Helicorbis coenosus*	India, China
Heterophyiasis (Chapter 97.3)	*Heterophyes heterophyes*	*Cerithidea cingulata*	Japan
		Pirenella conica	Egypt, Oman
Metagonimiasis (Chapter 97.2)	*Metagonimus yokogawai*	*Thiara granifera*	Asia
		Semisulcospira libertina	Russia
		Semisulcospira laevigata	Russia
		Semisulcospira cancellata	Russia
Nanophyetiasis	*Nanophyetus salmincola schikhobalowi*	*Semisulcospira libertina*	Siberia
		Semisulcospira cancellata	Siberia
Opisthorchiasis (Chapter 98.1)	*Opisthorchis felineus*	*Bithynia leachii*	Europe, Siberia
	Opisthorchis viverrini	*Bithynia laevis*	Thailand, Laos, Malaysia
		Bithynia goniomphalus	Thailand, Laos, Malaysia
		Bithynia funiculata	Thailand, Laos, Malaysia
		Bithynia siamensis	Thailand, Laos, Malaysia
Paragonimiasis (Chapter 99)	*Paragonimus westermani*	*Semisulcospira libertina*	Japan, Taiwan, China, Korea
		Semisulcospira amurensis	North China, Korea
		Thiara tuberculata	Africa, Asia
		Brotia asperata	Philippines
	Paragonimus africanus	*Potadoma freethi*	Cameroon, Liberia, Nigeria, Zaire
	Paragonimus skrjabini	*Tricula microstoma*	China
		Tricula fujianesis	China
		Tricula minutoides	China
		Tricula humida	China
	Paragonimus heterotremus	*Tricula gregorina*	China
	Paragonimus caliensis	*Aroapyrgus columbiensis*	Central and South America
	Paragonimus mexicanus	*Aroapyrgus costaricensis*	Central and South America
Schistosomiasis (Chapter 96)	*Schistosoma japonicum*	*Oncomelania hupensis formosana*	Taiwan
		Oncomelania hupensis hupensis	China
		Oncomelania hupensis fausti	China
		Oncomelania hupensis tangi	China
		Oncomelania hupensis robertsoni	China
		Oncomelania hupensis guangxiensis	China
		Oncomelania hupensis lindoensis	Sulawesi
		Oncomelania hupensis nosophora	Japan
		Oncomelania hupensis quadrasi	Philippines
	Schistosoma mekongi	*Tricula aperta*	Thailand, Laos, Cambodia
	Schistosoma species	*Robertsiella* species	Malaysia
	Schistosoma haematobium	*Bulinus beccarii*	Southwestern Arabia
		Bulinus camerunensis	Cameroon
		Bulinus cernicus	Mauritius

TABLE 111–1. Principal Mollusk-Transmitted Infections of Man *Continued*

Disease	Pathogen	Mollusk (Genus and Species)	Geographic Range as Host
Schistosomiasis *continued*		*Bulinus senegalensis*	Gambia
		Bulinus wrighti	Saudi Arabia, Yemen, Oman
		Bulinus guernei	Gambia
		Bulinus rohlfsi	West Africa
		Bulinus truncatus	Eastern and western North Africa
		Bulinus abyssinicus	Ethiopia, Somalia
		Bulinus africanus	Eastern South Africa
		Bulinus jousseaumei	Gambia
		Bulinus obtusispira	Madagascar
		Bulinus globosus	Sub-Saharan Africa
		Bulinus nasutus	East Africa
		Planorbarius metidjensis	Portugal
		Ferrissia tenuis	India
	Schistosoma intercalatum	*Bulinus forskalii*	Cameroon, Gabon
	Schistosoma mattheei	*Bulinus globosus*	South Africa
	Schistosoma mansoni	*Biomphalaria glabrata*	Venezuela, Greater and Lesser Antilles, Guyana, Surinam, French Guiana, Brazil
		Biomphalaria tenagophila	Brazil, Argentina
		Biomphalaria straminea	Brazil, Martinique
		Biomphalaria pfeifferi	North Africa, Sub-Saharan Africa
		Biomphalaria choanomphala	Uganda, Tanzania
		Biomphalaria alexandrina	Egypt, Sudan
		Biomphalaria camerunensis	Zaire, Cameroon
		Biomphalaria sudanica	East Africa, Uganda, Sudan

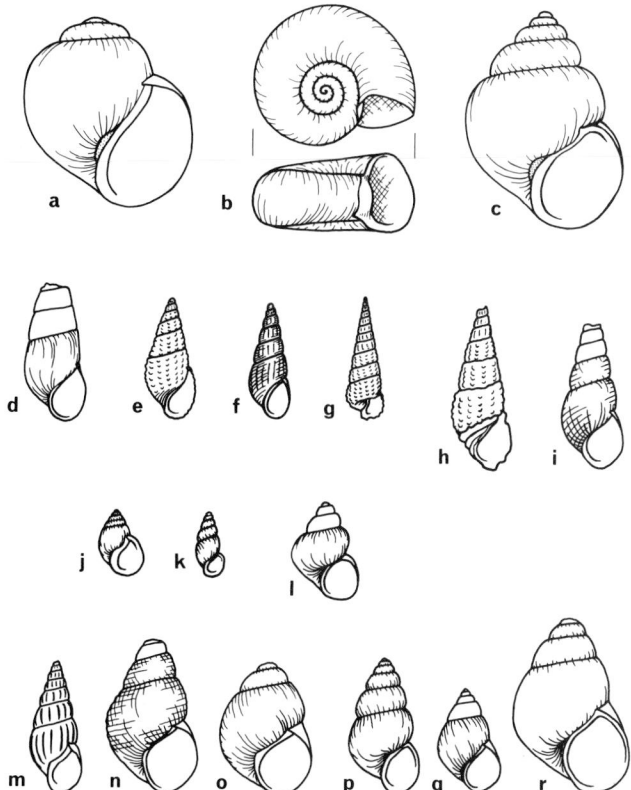

FIGURE 111–1. a, *Pila luzonica.* b, *Marisa cornuarietis.* c, Viviparidae: *Cipangopaludina chinensis.* d, *Potadoma freethii.* e, *Thiara granifera.* f, *Melanoides tuberculata.* g, *Pirenella conica.* h, *Semisulcospira amurensis.* i, *Semisulcospira libertina.* j, *Neotricula aperta.* k, *Robertsiella kaporensis.* l, *Bithynia leachii.* m, *Oncomelania hupensis.* n, *Parafossarulus manchouricus.* o, *Bithynia (Gabbia) longicornus.* p, *Pomatiopsis lapidaria.* q, *Bithynia fuchsiana.* r, *Bithynia goniomphalus.* (Scale line: a = 44 mm; a–i to scale; j = 4 mm; j–r to scale. Drawings by Susan Trammell. Produced by George M. Davis, using collections of the Academy of Natural Sciences of Philadelphia.)

Family Pleuroceridae. This family contains two genera of medical importance: *Oxytrema* in the United States (Table 111–2) and *Semisulcospira* in the Orient.

The genus *Semisulcospira* is widespread throughout the Orient, where various species serve as hosts for *Clonorchis sinensis, Metagonimus yokogawai, Paragonimus westermani,* and *Nanophyetus salmincola schikhobalowi. Semisulcospira libertina* (Gould) (Fig. 111–1) serves as a first intermediate host of *Metagonimus yokogawai* in Japan, while *S. laevigata* and *S. cancellata* (Benson) fill this role in Russia. Possible snail hosts in Spain and the Balkans have not been identified. *S. libertina* serves as the intermediate host for the lung fluke *Paragonimus westermani* in Japan, Taiwan, China, and Korea; *S. amurensis* (Gerstfeldt) is the host for this fluke in northern China and Korea. *S. amurensis* also serves as the first intermediate host for *Clonorchis sinensis* infection in China.

These snails are all large, measuring up to 5 cm in length, with high spires. *S. libertina* is found in the muddy bottoms of canals. *S. amurensis* frequents free-flowing streams. In the past, classifications have included many subgroups and races, with a resultant confusion in the literature.

Family Bithyniidae. This family contains three genera that can transmit disease, *Alocinma, Gabbia,* and *Bithynia.* These snails are 1.5 cm or less in length and ovate without a pointed spire. They are deeply sutured. The operculum is calcareous, with a small spiral nucleus that gives way to concentric development.

Genus Bithynia (= Bulimus). Bithynia leachii (Sheppard) is the first intermediate host of *Opisthorchis felineus* in Central and Eastern Europe and in Russia as far east as Siberia. This globular snail has wide distribution in ponds in northern Europe and the United States.

TABLE 111–2. Incidental or Rare Mollusk-Transmitted Infections of Man

Disease	Pathogen	Mollusk (Genus and Species)	Geographic Range as Host
Echinostomiasis (Chapter 97.2)	*Echinostoma ilocanum*	First intermediate host:	Philippines, Japan
		Gyraulus convexiusculus	Philippines
		Hippeutis umbilicalis	
		Second intermediate host:	
		Pila luzonica	Philippines
		Pila conica	Philippines
		Viviparus javanicus	Java
	Echinostoma malayanum	First intermediate host:	
		Lymnaea luteola	India
		Second Intermediate Host:	
		Indoplanorbis exustus	India
		Gyraulus convexiusculus	India
Salmon poisoning	*Nanophyetus salmincola*	*Oxytrema silicula*	Northwestern United States
Schistosomiasis (Chapter 96.2)	*Schistosoma bovis*	*Bulinus forskalii*	East Africa
		Bulinus senegalensis	Gambia
		Bulinus scalaris	Gambia
		Bulinus truncatus	Middle East
		Bulinus africanus	South Africa
		Bulinus ugandae	Sudan, Uganda
		Planorbarius metidjensis	Spain
	Schistosoma rodhaini	*Biomphalaria sudanica*	Zaire
		Biomphalaria pfeifferi	Uganda, Zaire
Swimmers' itch (cercarial dermatitis) (Chapter 96.2)	*Ornithobilharzia canaliculata*	*Batillaria minima*	Florida
	Gigantobilharzia gyrauli	*Gyraulus parvus*	United States
	Gigantobilharzia huronensis	*Physa gyrina*	United States
	Gigantobilharzia huttoni	*Haminoae antillarum*	Florida
	Gigantobilharzia sturniae	*Segmentina hemisphaerula*	Japan
	Austrobilharzia penneri	*Cerithidea scalariformis*	Florida
	Austrobilharzia varigalandis	*Littorina planaxis*	California
		Littorina pintado	Hawaii
	Trichobilharzia ocellata	*Lymnaea stagnalis*	United States and Europe
	Trichobilharzia physellae	*Physa parkeri*	United States
		Physa anatina	United States
	Trichobilharzia yokogawai	*Lymnaea swinhoe*	Japan

Four other species, *B. laevis* (Lea), *B. goniomphalus* (Morelet) (Fig. 111–1), *B. siamensis* (Lea), and *B. funiculata* (Walker), serve as first intermediate hosts of *O. viverrini* in Thailand, Laos, and Malaysia. These tiny snails favor muddy canals as habitats. *B. (Parafossarulus) manchourica* (Bourguignant) is widespread in the Orient, both on the mainland, including Korea, and on Taiwan and Japan. It is the host for *Echinochasmus perfoliatus,* an unusual and incidental parasite in man, and it is an important intermediate host for *Clonorchis sinensis* throughout its geographic range. This small snail is globular but has a spire and pronounced ridge sculpture. It is found in sluggish water, including swamps, canals, ponds, and rivers.

B. fuchsiana (Mollendorf) in northern China and *B. chaperi* act as first intermediate hosts in the transmission of *C. sinensis* in their respective distributions.

Genus Alocinma. The second genus of medical importance in this family includes one species, *Alocinma longicornis* (Benson) (Fig. 111–1), which also serves as a first intermediate host in the transmission of *C. sinensis* in China. The snail is small, measuring less than 10 mm, and globular, with a blunter spire than *Bithynia.* It, too, is prevalent in ponds and canal bottoms.

Genus Gabbia. *Gabbia misella* Gredler, a small globular snail with a pronounced spire, has been identified as an intermediate host of *C. sinensis* in Korea.

Family Hydrobiidae. There are two subfamilies.

Subfamily Triculinae. This subfamily contains 11 genera, of which two are hosts of human schistosomiasis;

one genus also harbors intermediate hosts of *Paragonimus heterotremus* and *P. skrjabini. Neotricula aperta* (Temcharoen) (Fig. 111–1), a tiny, globular, operculate snail found in Thailand, Laos, and Cambodia, is the only known host for *Schistosoma mekongi. Robertsiella kaporensis* (Davis and Greer) (Fig. 111–1) acts as an intermediate host for an as yet unnamed Malaysian *S. japonicum*—like schistosome species. Both these hosts are aquatic. *Tricula microstoma* Yue-ying, Wen-zhen, and Yao-xian; *T. fujianesis* Yue-ying, Wen-zhen, and Yao-xian; *T. minutoides* (Gredler); and *T. humida* (Heude) all serve as first intermediate hosts for *P. skrjabini* in China. *T. gregorina* serves as the first intermediate host for *P. heterotremus* in China and Thailand.

Subfamily Pomatiopsinae. This subfamily contains eight genera, one of which, *Oncomelania,* is of importance in human disease. One species, *Oncomelania hupensis* (Gredler) (Fig. 111–1), is responsible for the transmission of *S. japonicum* throughout Asia. There are a number of subspecies of *O. hupensis,* which are geographically isolated and include *O. h. chiui* (Habe and Miyazaki) and *O. h. formosana* (Pilsbry and Hirase) from Taiwan, *O. h. hupensis* (Gredler) *from China, O. h. fausti* (Bartsch), *O. h. tangi* (Bartsch), *O. h. robertsoni* (Bartsch), *O. h. guangxiensis* (Yue-ying, Tze-kong, Yao-xian, and Wen-zhen), *O. h. lindoensis* (Davis and Canby) from Sulawesi, *O. h. nosophora* (Robson) from Japan, and *O. h. quadrasi* (Mollendorf) from the Philippines. All of these except *O. h. chiui* will transmit human schistosomes. These various subspecies will hybridize. There are remarkable differences in cross-susceptibility to infection with *S. japonicum* from various geographic areas.

Oncomelania are tiny, high-spired operculates that are amphibious. They favor rotting vegetation along river banks, where the mud is moist, as well as rice paddies. The complex relationships among subspecies, races, and susceptibility to infection make specific identification difficult.

Family Potamididae (= Cerithiidae). These have brackish and sea water as well as freshwater representatives of minor medical importance. *Cerithidea cingulata* in Japan and *Pirenella conica* (Blaurville) (Fig. 111–1) in Egypt and Oman serve as hosts of the intestinal fluke *Heterophyes heterophyes*.

Genus Aroapyrgus. This neotropical hydrobiid genus contains several species that serve as first intermediate hosts for several species of American paragonimiases. *Aroapyrgus columbiensis* (Malek and Little) has been identified as first intermediate host for *P. caliensis*. *A. costaricensis* (Mörch) is the first intermediate host for *P. mexicanus*. Many other species of *Aroapyrgus* are suspected of serving as first intermediate hosts for *Paragonimus* species. Considerable controversy remains concerning the speciation of these parasites in the Americas.

SUBCLASS EUTHYNEURA. This subclass is separated into four orders, three of which—the Basommatophora, the Stylommatophora, and the Systellommatophora—have representatives of medical importance.

Order Basommatophora. This order has four families with genera of medical importance, all for their role as intermediate hosts of trematodes. These are the families Ancylidae, Lymnaeidae, Physidae, and Planorbidae.

Family Ancylidae. A single genus of the Ancylidae, *Ferrissia tenuis* (Bourguignant), has been implicated as the intermediate host for *Schistosoma haematobium* in India.

Family Lymnaeidae. This family is large and geographically widespread. The liver flukes *Fasciola hepatica* and *Fasciola gigantica* utilize genera of this family as intermediate hosts. Several species of *Trichobilharzia* that can cause schistosome dermatitis in man also use Lymnaeidae as hosts. Nine species of *Lymnaea* serve as intermediate hosts of *F. hepatica*. These include *Lymnaea (Fossaria) truncatula* (Müller) (Fig. 111–2) in Europe, Africa, the Middle East, and Asia; *L. viatrix* (Orbigny) in Argentina; *L. rubiginosa* (Mudrelin) in Malaysia; *L. philippensis* and *L. swinhoe* (Adams) in the Philippines; *L. tomentosa* (Pfeiffer) in Australia; and *L. japonica* and *L. pervia* in Japan. *L. columella* Say (Fig. 111–2) is now widespread in North and South America, Africa, and the Hawaiian Islands. Five species, *L. rubiginosa* in Malaysia, *L. acuminata* and *L. auricularia* (Linnaeus) in India, and *L. natalensis* (Krauss) (Fig. 111–2) and *L. columella* in Africa, are intermediate hosts for *F. gigantica*.

Two species of *Fossaria*, *F. bulimoides* (Lea) and *F. cubensis* (Pfeiffer), act as intermediate hosts for *F. hepatica* in the United States. *F. ollula* will transmit *F. gigantica* in Hawaii.

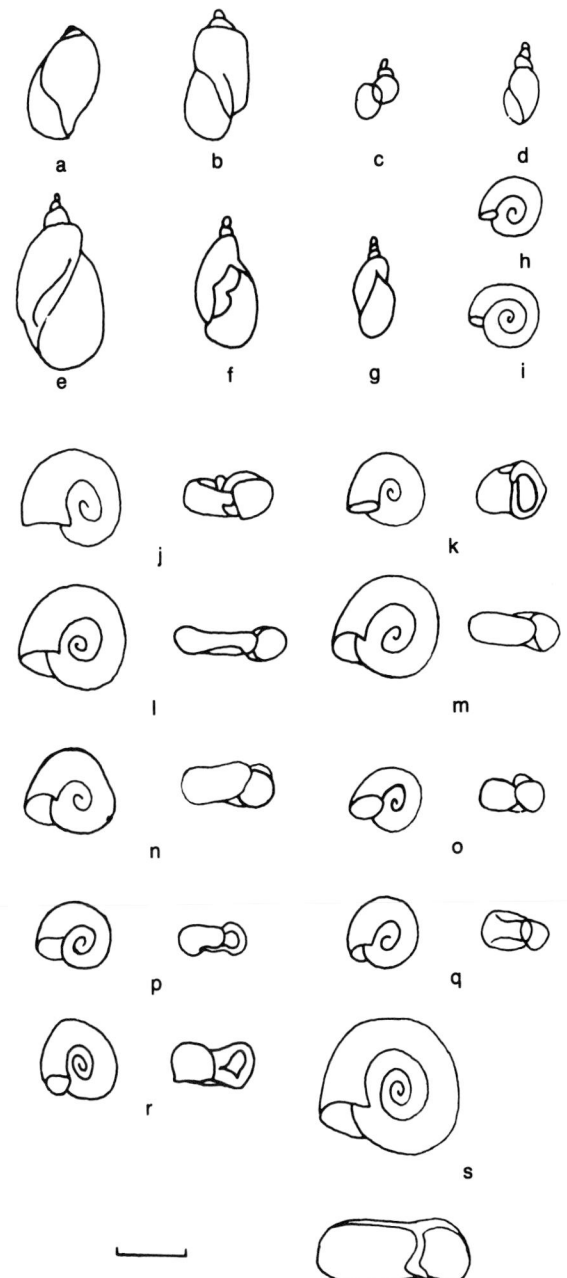

FIGURE 111–2. a, *Bulinus globosus.* b, *Bulinus truncatus.* c, *Bulinus wrighti.* d, *Bulinus senegalensis.* e, *Lymnaea natalensis.* f, *Lymnaea columella.* g, *Lymnaea truncatula.* h, *Hippeutis umbilicalis.* i, *Segmentina hemisphaerula.* j, *Planorbarius metidjensis.* k, *Indoplanorbis exustus.* l, *Biomphalaria sudanica.* m, *Biomphalaria camerunensis.* n, *Biomphalaria alexandrina.* o, *Biomphalaria pfeifferi.* p, *Biomphalaria choanomphala.* q, *Biomphalaria straminea.* r, *Biomphalaria tenagophila.* s, *Biomphalaria glabrata.* (Scale line = 1 cm.) (Redrawn in part with permission from Brown DS: Freshwater Snails of Africa and Their Medical Importance. London, Taylor & Francis, 1980.)

Family Planorbidae. Many species are medically important. The family is separated into two subfamilies, Planorbinae and Bulininae. Snails of the subfamily Planorbinae are discoidal and usually small, although some may reach as much as 4 cm in diameter.

Subfamily Planorbinae. *Gyraulus convexiusculus* (Hutton) acts as the first intermediate host of the intestinal trematode *Echinostoma ilocanum* in the Philippines and Java and as the second intermediate host of *Echinostoma malayanum* in India.

Hippeutis umbilicalis (Benson) (Fig. 111–2) also acts as a first intermediate host of *Echinostoma ilocanum* in the Philippines. This snail and *Hippeutis cantori* (Benson), *Segmentina trochoideus*, and *S. hemisphaerula* (Fig. 111–2) act as intermediate hosts of *Fasciolopsis buski* in India and the Orient. Infection is by ingestion of metacercarial cysts on plants such as water chestnuts.

The snail *Helicorbis coenosus* (Benson) is an intermediate host of the intestinal fluke *Gastrodiscoides hominis* in India and in China, and in India it acts as intermediate host of *Fasciolopsis buski*.

The genus *Biomphalaria* lies within the subfamily Planorbinae. This large genus contains all of the intermediate hosts of *Schistosoma mansoni* in Africa, Southwest Asia, and the Western Hemisphere. Eight of the 31 recognized species act as intermediate hosts of *S. mansoni*. In the Western Hemisphere, these include *Biomphalaria glabrata* (Say), *B. tenagophila* (Orbigny), and *B. straminea* (Dunker) (Fig. 111–2). *B. glabrata* serves as a host throughout its range in the islands of the Caribbean as well as the coastal strip from Venezuela to southern Brazil. *B. tenagophila* is a host in a much more restricted range in the southernmost part of Brazil and Argentina. *B. straminea* has a much broader geographic range through North, South, and Central America as well as the Antilles. It has been found infected only in Brazil and Martinique. Six of the 16 remaining species of Western Hemisphere *Biomphalaria* have proved to be susceptible to *Schistosoma mansoni* infection in the laboratory, but none serves as a host in nature.

There are five established intermediate hosts for *Schistosoma mansoni* in Africa and the Middle East. These are *B. pfeifferi* (Krauss), *B. choanomphala* (Martens), *B. alexandrina* (Ehrenberg), *B. camerunensis* (Boettger), and *B. sudanica* (Martens) (Fig. 111–2). Terminological complexity in the past concerning African *Biomphalaria* has now been greatly simplified. *B. pfeifferi* is the most widespread host, prevalent all over sub-Saharan Africa, with a few additional North African foci. Eight previously identified species and subspecies are now recognized as *B. pfeifferi*. In addition to *Schistosoma mansoni*, *B. pfeifferi* in Central Africa is the intermediate host for the rodent schistosome *S. rodhaini,* which rarely infects man.

Biomphalaria choanomphala (Martens) acts as the intermediate host for *S. mansoni* in Uganda and Tanzania. *B. alexandrina* is the intermediate host for *S. mansoni* in the highly endemic area of the Nile delta as well as in the Sudan. *B. camerunensis* serves as an intermediate host for *S. mansoni* in Zaire and the Cameroon. *B. sudanica* is the most important intermediate host of *S. mansoni* in East Africa as well as in Uganda and the southern Sudan. It also acts as an intermediate host for *S. rodhaini* in Zaire.

The relationships between many of the *Biomphalaria* are close, and species identification is often difficult. However, in many areas, only one species can be found, thus simplifying the problems of field identification for control purposes.

The remaining genus and species of medical importance in this subfamily is *Planorbarius metidjensis* (Forbes). This snail is found in Morocco and Algiers as well as in Spain and Portugal and has been the host for *S. haematobium* in Portugal and *S. bovis* in Spain.

Subfamily Bulininae. The genus *Bulinus* serves as the principal host for *Schistosoma haematobium* in Africa and the Middle East. This genus in turn is divided into two subgenera, *Bulinus* proper and *Physopsis*. There are 37 recognized species in these two subgenera, which are further divided into four groups. Fourteen of these serve as hosts for *S. haematobium* in nature (Table 111–1). The *Bulinus forskalii* group contains four susceptible snails: *Bulinus beccarii* (Paladike) in southwestern Arabia, *Bulinus camerunensis* (Mandahl-Barth) in Cameroon, *Bulinus cernicus* (Morelet) on Mauritius, and *Bulinus senegalensis* (Muller) (Fig. 111–2) in Gambia. In addition, *B. forskalii* (Ehrenberg) acts as the intermediate host for *Schistosoma intercalatum* in Cameroon and Gabon and for *Schistosoma bovis* in East Africa. *Bulinus senegalensis* and *B. scalaris* (Dunker) also serve as the intermediate hosts of *S. bovis* in Gambia. All of these snails are small, high-spired stream dwellers.

The Reticulatus group includes *Bulinus wrighti* (Mandahl-Barth) (Fig. 111–2), which serves as an intermediate host of *S. haematobium* in Saudia Arabia, Yemen, and Oman.

The Tropicus/Truncatus subgroup has three *S. haematobium* vectors: *Bulinus guernei* (Dantzenberg) in Gambia, *B. rohlfsi* (Clessin) in West Africa, and *B. truncatus* (Adouin) (Fig. 111–2) in both eastern and western North Africa. *B. truncatus* also functions as the principal host for *S. bovis* in the Middle East.

The Africanus subgroup comprises the subgenus *Physopsis*. *Bulinus abyssinicus* (Martens) serves as an intermediate host for *S. haematobium* in Ethiopia and Somalia, while *B. africanus* (Krauss) is a widespread intermediate host for both *S. haematobium* and *S. bovis* in eastern South Africa. *Bulinus jousseaumei* (Dantzenberg) is a host for *S. haematobium* in Gambia, and *Bulinus obtusispira* (Smith) plays the same role in Madagascar. *Bulinus globosus* (Morelet) (Fig. 111–2) is widespread in sub-Saharan Africa, where it is confined mainly to the lowland areas. It is a host for *S. haematobium* and *S. mattheei*. *Bulinus nasutus* (Martens) is an East African intermediate host for *S. haematobium*. *Bulinus ugandae* (Mandahl-Barth) is a natural host for *S. bovis* in the Sudan and Uganda.

Another genus in the subfamily is *Indoplanorbis*. *I. exustus* (Deshayes) is an intermediate host for *Echinostoma malayanum*, an intestinal fluke reportedly infecting man in Southeast Asia. This snail can also serve as an intermediate host for the nematode *Angiostrongylus cantonensis* in Malaysia.

Orders Stylommatophora and Systellommatophora. The former order contains terrestrial snails and some slugs, while the latter comprises only tropical slugs. Many terrestrial snails and slugs are involved as intermediate hosts in the transmission of four parasites that may infect man. Two are nematodes: the rat lungworm *Angiostrongylus cantonensis* (Chapter 93.1) and the related American parasite *Moreostrongylus costaricensis*

(Chapter 93.2). The other two parasites are the related liver flukes *Dicrocoelium dendriticum* and *Dicrocoelium hospes* that infect herbivores. Infections in man by all four of these parasites have been reported but are rare.

A. cantonensis does not seem to be terribly fastidious or, for that matter, very demanding concerning its intermediate host. It utilizes slugs of both orders as well as many terrestrial and aquatic snails. The parasite was originally identified in China and is now reported from the islands of the South Pacific, Cuba, Puerto Rico, and Louisiana. The intermediate host range in Cuba includes many terrestrial snails and slugs. Transmission is by accidental ingestion of a mollusk or by ingestion of poorly cooked snails and slugs.

M. costaricensis commonly utilizes veronicellid slugs as the intermediate host, but in Costa Rica, many terrestrial and aquatic mollusks have been shown to be naturally infected. These include *Helisoma trivolvus* (Say), *Succineidae* sp., and *Bulimus* sp. (personal communication from Dr. Pedro Morera). Again, transmission is by accidental ingestion of the slug or slug mucus containing larvae.

Dicrocoelium dendriticum is a fluke that normally parasitizes the biliary tree of sheep and other herbivores (Chapter 98.4). Its distribution includes both North and South America, Europe, the Middle East, India, and China. The fluke employs a variety of terrestrial snails as first intermediate hosts. Many genera of a number of families are involved. Infection may be quite localized in a given area despite widespread distribution of snails. Infection is acquired by accidental ingestion of infected ants, the second intermediate host. *D. hospes* has a much more limited distribution in Africa. It, too, is rare in man. The only identified host snails are in the genus *Limicolaria* (Schumacher) and include *Limicolaria aurora* as well as other species.

CONTROL

One obvious means of eliminating snail-related diseases is to control the intermediate host. The success of control measures is variable, and many factors affect their use. As a consequence, there is no simple protocol for control measures. Each attempt at control needs to consider the host, intermediate host, infecting agents, and physical setting, as well as the relationships among these four variables, if a workable approach is to be identified.

Control methods take the form of protection from exposure to the definitive host and the intermediate host, as well as antisnail measures.

EXPOSURE CONTROL. Logical approaches to controlling mollusk-transmitted diseases include restriction of human exposure to the mollusk and/or restriction of exposure of the mollusk to infecting organisms. Control of human contact with infected mollusks is largely accomplished by quarantine and posting of infected waters. This is effective, realistically, only in dealing with commercial food-processing operations. Regulation of shellfish beds is effective in the control of oyster- and clam-transmitted viral hepatitis as well as of transmission

of cholera and *Salmonella* infection. In cases in which water contact is an important feature of disease transmission, particularly the skin-penetrating trematodes, the wearing of boots and other protective aids can be effective. Most of these are voluntary measures and, for this reason, are only modestly effective. Continuing attention to public health education shows slow progress in this important control mechanism.

ANTISNAIL MEASURES. Four mechanisms for direct snail control may be employed. These include snail removal by mechanical or manual means, snail control by environmental manipulation, the use of molluscicides, and the use of biologic control.

Snail Removal by Mechanical Means. This is largely a measure of the past. No selective mechanisms currently exist to concentrate snails for removal.

Environmental Manipulation. This has proved to be a useful tool in snail control, but costs as well as local engineering problems severely limit its application. Where transmission of infection involves irrigation schemes or fish farms, it is often possible to plan for intervals of desiccation. Although some snails can estivate and survive dry periods by burrowing into moist, muddy bottoms, the snail population does tend to be held down by these measures.

Where desiccation is impossible, some control of snail population size is possible by the use of rapid flow in canals and channels. Many host snails are adapted only to slow-moving or stagnant habitats. There has been success, particularly in Japan, with cement lining of canals to create a habitat unsuitable for amphibious snails. Although these measures are effective, costs inhibit their extensive use.

Molluscicides. Four compounds are currently employed in the chemical control of mollusks. These compounds have been subjected to extensive trial and are commonly available in quantity.

Copper Sulfate. This compound has been used the longest and is effective only against aquatic snails. Its effect is considerably reduced by organic matter in the environment, and it currently has limited application.

Sodium Pentachlorophenate (NaPCP). This compound is available in many formulations, some of which have slow-release residual capability. NaPCP is absorbed by mud and is broken down by sunlight. It is a toxic substance and must be employed with attention to the safety of workers.

Niclosamide. Niclosamide (Bayluscid) is effective at a much lower concentration than NaPCP. It may be applied as a powder or an emulsion and is effective against amphibious snails.

N-Tritylmorpholine. N-Tritylmorpholine (Frescon) is available in many forms, including bait. It is less soluble than the other compounds mentioned. It has excellent stability in the environment and is effective in low concentration.

The use of all of the molluscicides is limited by the cost and the water dynamics, which control achievable concentrations of the compounds. There is concern that some of these compounds may damage the environment.

Molluscicides of Plant Origin. The only such molluscicide to receive extensive field trial is Euclod *(Phyto-*

lacca dodecundra) in Ethiopia. The ability to incorporate the use of such natural compounds into self-help programs offsets the comparative inefficiency of the compounds.

Biologic Control. Biologic control measures take two forms.

Competitive Species. The first is the introduction of competitive species that displace the snail intermediate hosts. The most successful has been the thiarid snail *Thiara granifera* in Puerto Rico, where, in some locations, it has displaced *B. glabrata,* the *S. mansoni* host. This snail has spread to Haiti, where it has displaced planorbids from a number of streams in the southern region.

Predator Species. The other approach to biologic control has been the use of predators or parasites to reduce snail populations. A number of parasites harmful to snails have been identified, but no extensive scientific evaluation of parasites has been performed.

Predators have been employed with variable success in snail control. The use of the predatory snails *Marisa cornuarietis* in Puerto Rico and *Pomacea haustrum* in Brazil has been partially successful in controlling *B. glabrata,* the host for *S. mansoni,* in these areas. The use of the sciomyzid fly, the larva of which attacks snails, has been field tested in Hawaii. There the fly *Sepeolon macropus* has been employed against *Lymnaea ollula,* the host for *Fasciola gigantica.* The difficulty of successful introduction of this fly into new environments limits the application of this measure.

A number of fish, including *Tilapia melanopleura* (Nile perch), as well as several species of chichlids that normally include snails in their diet, have proved useful, particularly in the control of snails in fish-farm tanks.

The combined problem of the introduction of new, potentially environment-damaging species, plus the difficulty of this introduction, markedly limits the use of this mechanism of control.

COLLECTION METHODS

The two most important aspects of snail collection are the collection site and the preservation of the snails. How the snails are picked up, whether by scoop, dredge, forceps, or spoon, is important only in quantitative studies. The method of collection should safeguard collectors from exposure to infectious material and should not damage the snail. There are quantitative collection methods useful in evaluations, particularly related to control programs, but these are not necessary for a casual survey.

SITE RECORD. This should include locations, preferably with reference points that can be identified on a map, the date and time, and a habitat description.

PRESERVED SPECIMENS. Ideally, both the shell and the soft parts should be preserved. Although the shell is useful to the taxonomist, soft parts are usually essential to complete species identification. Soft-part dissection as well as measurement is simplified if the snail is relaxed and extended when fixed. Two preservation protocols are recommended.

Alcohol Fixation. This is the simplest fixation method. Extended snails may be obtained as follows: A live snail is picked up with forceps and held until it is extended. With the aperture facing up, it is carefully lowered to the level of the aperture into water with a temperature of 65° to 70°C for 15 seconds. With care, the snail will remain extended and die, following which it can be plunged into the water for an additional 20 seconds. A temperature of 65° to 70°C will produce thermal death without cooking the snail or coagulating its hemolymph.

Obtaining extended specimens is somewhat easier if the snail is narcotized. Solutions of rapid-acting barbiturates, such as 0.2% Nembutal, will do this. The same effect can be achieved by placing the snail in a vial or dish with several menthol crystals added to the water. In either case, narcotization takes 4 to 6 hours. Slugs may be relaxed by overnight refrigeration.

After the relaxed snails are killed, large specimens can usually be removed from the shell by holding the snail in cool water and gently tugging the snail out of its shell by pulling on the foot with forceps. The snail is then placed in fixative and the shell dried. In this fashion, body and shell are preserved for study. Tiny snails or snails with internal lamellae in the shell usually cannot be withdrawn from the shell undamaged and must be dropped directly into a fixative.

Alcohol diluted to 70% is a suitable fixative for field work. The addition of glycerin 1:10 by volume also helps preservation. Alcohol fixation does produce some hardening and friability of tissues after long preservation.

Railliet-Henry Fixative. A better fixative for long-term preservation of dissectable material is Railliet-Henry fixative. This is made as follows:

Distilled water 930 ml
NaCl 6 gm
Formalin 50 ml
Glacial acetic acid 20 ml

These reagents are readily available in most clinical laboratories. Snails preserved in this fixative remain soft for many years. When shells are added to this acid fixative, CO_2 evolves, and care must be taken to prevent the tops from blowing off the vials.

With both fixation methods, a single change of fixative after 24 hours will improve preservation. Preserved specimens must be clearly marked with all identifying information.

BIBLIOGRAPHY

Ansari N: Epidemiology and Control of Schistosomiasis (Bilharziasis). Baltimore, University Park Press, 1973.

Boray JC: Studies on the relative susceptibility of some lymnaeids to infection with *Fasciola hepatica* and *F. gigantica* and on the adaptation of Fasciola spp. Ann Trop Med Parasitol 60:114, 1966.

Brown DS: Freshwater Snails of Africa and Their Medical Importance. London, Taylor & Francis, 1980.

Bruce JI, Sornmani S: The Mekong schistosome. Malacol Rev (Suppl 2), 1980.

Burch JB: A guide to freshwater snails of the Philippines. Malacol Rev 13:123, 1980.

Chung P: A comparative study of three species of Bithyniidae (Mollusca:Prosobranchia): *Parafossarulus manchouricus, Gabbia misella* and *Bithynia tentaculata.* Malacol Rev 17:1, 1984.

Davis GM: A taxonomic study of some species of *Semisulcospira* in Japan (Mesogastropoda: Pleuroceridae). Malacologia 7:211, 1969.

Davis GM: The Origin and Evolution of the Gastropod Family Pomatiopsidae, with Emphasis on the Mekong River Triculinae. Monograph 20. Philadelphia, Academy of Natural Sciences, 1979.

Davis GM, Ruff MD: *Oncomelania hupensis* (Gastropoda: Hydrobiidae): Hybridization, genetics and transmission of *Schistosoma japonicum.* Malacol Rev 6:181, 1974.

Frandsen F, McCullough F, Madsen H: A practical guide to the identification of African freshwater snails. Malacol Rev 13:95, 1980.

Grácio MA: Distribution and habitats of six species of freshwater pulmonate snails in Algarve, Southern Portugal. Malacol Rev 16:17, 1983.

Kendall SB: Relationships between species of Fasciola and their molluscan hosts. *In* Dawes B (ed): Advances in Parasitology, Vol 3. London, Academic Press, 1965, p 59.

Kitikoon V: Studies on *Tricula aperta* and related taxa, the snail intermediate hosts of *Schistosoma mekongi.* III. Susceptibility studies. Malacol Rev 14:37, 1981.

Kruatrachue M, Jantataeme S, Ratanatham S, et al: A culture method for *Bithynia* (Prosobranchia:Bithyniidae), snail hosts for the trematode *Opisthorchis viverrini.* Malacol Rev 15:63, 1982.

Malek EA: Studies on "tropicorbid" snails (Biomphalaria:Planorbidae) from the Caribbean and Gulf of Mexico areas, including the southern United States. Malacol Int J Malacol 7:183, 1969.

Malek EA: Snail-Transmitted Parasitic Diseases, Vols I and II. Boca Raton, FL, CRC Press, 1980.

Malek EA: Snail Hosts of Schistosomiasis and Other Snail-transmitted Diseases in Tropical America: A Manual. Scientific publication No. 478. Washington DC, Pan American Health Organization, 1985.

Mandahl-Barth G: Intermediate Hosts of Schistosoma African Biomphalaria and Bulinus. WHO Monograph Series No. 37. Geneva, World Health Organization, 1958.

Mandahl-Barth G: Revision of the African genera Potodoma Gran and Potodomoides Leloup, and description of a new species of Cleopatra. Rev Zool Bot Afr 76:110, 1967.

Morera P: Life history and redescription of *Angiostrongylus costaricensis* Morera and Cespedes. Am J Trop Med Hyg 22:613, 1973.

Pace GL: The freshwater snails of Taiwan (Formosa). Malacol Rev (Suppl 1), 1973.

Pan American Health Organization: A Guide for the Identification of the Snail Intermediate Hosts of Schistosomiasis in the Americas. Washington, DC, Pan American Health Organization, 1968.

Perera G, Yong M, Rodriguez J, Gálvez D: Cuban endemic molluscs infected with *Angiostrongylus cantonensis.* Malacol Rev 16:87, 1983.

Rosewater J: The family Littorinidae in the Indo-Pacific. Indo-Pacific Mollusca 2:417, 1970.

Saliba EK, Salameh E: A second finding of *Bulinus truncatus* in Jordan. Malacol Rev 14:65, 1981.

Tze-kong L, Yue-ying L, Wen-zhen Z, Yao-xian W: A discussion on the classification of *Oncomelania* (Mollusca). Sinozoologia 3:97, 1982.

Wallace GD, Rosen L: Studies on eosinophilic meningitis. I. Observations on the geographic distribution of *Angiostrongylus cantonensis* in the Pacific areas and its prevalence in wild rats. Am J Epidemiol 8:52, 1965.

Wright CA: The freshwater gastropod molluscs of Western Aden Protectorate. Bull Br Mus Nat Hist Zool 5:1, 1963.

Wright CA, Brown DS: The freshwater mollusca of Dhofar. *In* The Journal of Oman Studies Special Report No. 2. England, The Cray Press, 1975, pp 97–102.

Yokogawa M, Sodeman WA Jr: Current status of Paragonimus and paragonimiasis. Proceedings of the XI International Congress for Tropical Medicine and Malaria. Boca Raton, FL, CRC Press (in press).

Yue-Ying L, Tze-kong L, Yao-xian W, Wen-zhen Z: Subspecific deafferentation of Oncomelaniid snails. Acta Zootaxon Sinica, 6:253, 1981.

Yue-ying L, Wen-zhen Z, Yao-xian W: Studies on *Tricula* (Prosobranchia:Hydrobiidae) from China. Acta Zootaxon Sinica, 8:135, 1983.

112. TICKS AND MITES IN DISEASE TRANSMISSION

Daniel E. Sonenshine
and Abdu Fahrang Azad

GENERAL PRINCIPLES

Ticks and mites are members of the subclass Acari, one of the dominant subclasses of the Arachnida (chelicerate arthropods). Arachnids are believed to have appeared during the late Archeozoic or early Paleozoic eras, i.e., during the period of proliferation of bottom-feeding invertebrates (e.g., Trilobites). Adaptive radiation followed colonization of the terrestrial environment, with explosive multiplication of new life forms. Virtually all of the arachnid taxa, including the Acari, are believed to have evolved during this warm, moist period (Savory, 1977). Arachnids, including the ticks and mites, are distinguished from the insects by the lack of a clearly defined head, by chelicerae instead of mandibles, by the absence of antennae, and by the presence of 4 pairs of walking legs (except in larvae of the Acari). The body is subdivided into the anterior prosoma, bearing the appendages, and the posterior opisthosoma ("abdominal" region). The Acari are readily distinguished from other arachnids by the general absence of segmentation, so that the prosoma and opisthosoma are fused (in all but a few adult mites), and by the presence of the gnathosoma (i.e., capitulum in ticks), a unique structure at the anterior end of the body bearing the mouthparts. The gnathosoma is formed by the fusion of the pedipalp coxae to form a ring of cuticle that surrounds the chelicerae (i.e., basis capituli, or gnathosomal base). The remaining palpal segments lie lateral to instead of behind the chelicerae, allowing the 2 pairs of appendages to act collaboratively. An unpaired appendage, the hypostome, is located on the ventromedial surface between the palps. The remainder of the highly fused body is divided into 2 regions, the podosoma, bearing the walking legs, and the opisthosoma, or "abdominal" region, behind it. The opisthosoma is not a true abdomen, and no segmentation is evident to facilitate homology with the abdomen of other arachnid groups. The mite or tick body, exclusive of the mouthparts (gnathosoma), is termed the idiosoma. Thus, in the mites and ticks, tremendous fusion has taken place, and body segmentation is lost, except during embryonic development.

The Acari comprise a vast assemblage of species that have proliferated extensively throughout the many terrestrial and freshwater habitats available. Many are free living as herbivores, fungivores, and predators; others are parasitic, including both ectoparasitic and endoparasitic adaptations. These adaptations contribute to their harmful effects on human and animal health. In addition, mites and ticks are important as vectors of many pathogenic agents. Ticks transmit a greater variety of disease-causing pathogens than any other arthropod vector. As a result, the biology and disease relationships of the Acari are of intense interest to physicians, veterinarians, and public health officials, as well as to students and scientists.

112.1.   TICKS (Suborder Ixodida)

CHARACTERIZATION. All ticks are obligate bloodsucking parasites. Most ticks are relatively large, i.e., 5 to 10 mm long in adults, as compared with mites, which usually measure less than 1 mm in length. There is a single pair of respiratory pores, or spiracles (i.e., stigmata). The hypostome is prominent and covered with retrorse teeth for anchoring the tick to its host. This is the primary holdfast for attaching the tick to the host's body. In ixodids, copious quantities of cement, secreted during the first few hours of the attachment process, surround the hypostome and secure the tick to the host's skin. The hypostome bears the preoral canal, or food canal, that directs blood from the feeding site to the mouth, located at the hypostome base, and into the sucking pharynx. The chelicerae of ticks bear prominent cutting denticles, oriented laterally, that rip and tear tissue, facilitating the entry of the mouthparts into the skin and forming the feeding site. The dorsal surface of the tarsus of the first pair of legs (i.e., tarsus I) bears a distinctive sensory organ, the Haller's organ.

CLASSIFICATION. The subclass Acari is subdivided into 2 major orders, the order Parasitiformes, and the order Acariformes (Krantz, 1978). Ticks constitute the suborder Ixodida (i.e., Metastigmata of some authors), a suborder of the Parasitiformes. This suborder comprises 3 families: (1) the Ixodidae, (2) the Argasidae, and (3) the Nuttalliellidae, the latter represented by a single species, *Nuttalliela namaqua*. The family Ixodidae, or hard ticks, is by far the largest and economically most important family, with 13 genera and approximately 645 species. The family Argasidae, or soft ticks, comprises 5 genera and approximately 170 species (Fig. 112–1).

Ixodidae. The Ixodidae (hard ticks) have a tough, sclerotized scutum, which covers the anterior part of the dorsum (entire dorsum in males) (Figs. 112–2 and 112–3). Elsewhere, the body cuticle is characterized by innumerable tiny surface folds, except in males of some species where it is covered by sclerotized ventral plates. Eyes, when present, occur on the posterolateral margins of the scutum. The palps have 4 segments (i.e., articles), but the terminal fourth segment is retractible and is recessed into segment 3. Females bear a pair of porose areas and a pair of remarkable, eversible sacs (termed Gené's organ) that wax the eggs during oviposition. The spiracle is located posterior to coxa IV and situated within a prominent spiracular plate. On the tarsi of the walking legs, padlike pulvilli occur adjacent to the claws in all life stages, enabling these ticks to climb virtually any surface. The nymphal and larval stages resemble the adults but lack the external genital pores and porose areas. Sexual dimorphism is pronounced in the adults, but absent in the immature forms. Larvae bear only 3 pairs of walking legs. A discussion of some of the more important genera follows.

Genus Ixodes. This is the largest genus of hard ticks, with approximately 245 species (Figs. 112–2 and 112–5). These ticks are readily recognized by the anal groove, which curves anterior to and encloses the anus. In the males, the ventral surface is covered by sclerotized ventral plates. Most species of the genus are nest- or burrow-inhabiting parasites with cryptic, nonfeeding males. Several species, however, are non-nidiculous, distributed widely throughout wooded or grassy environments. All are 3-host ticks; each life stage drops off after feeding to molt on the ground or in the nest. Important species include (1) *I. persulcatus*, an important vector of Russian spring-summer encephalitis (RSSE) in the Soviet Union (Chapter 21.5); (2) *I. ricinus*, the major vector of tick-borne encephalitis (i.e., RSSE) in most of Europe, as well as louping ill, erythema chronicum migrans (similar to Lyme disease), and other maladies; (3) *Ixodes dammini*, the primary vector of Lyme disease in the eastern and central United States (Chapter 36) and babesiosis in the northeastern United States (Chapter 77); (4) *I. pacificus*, the vector

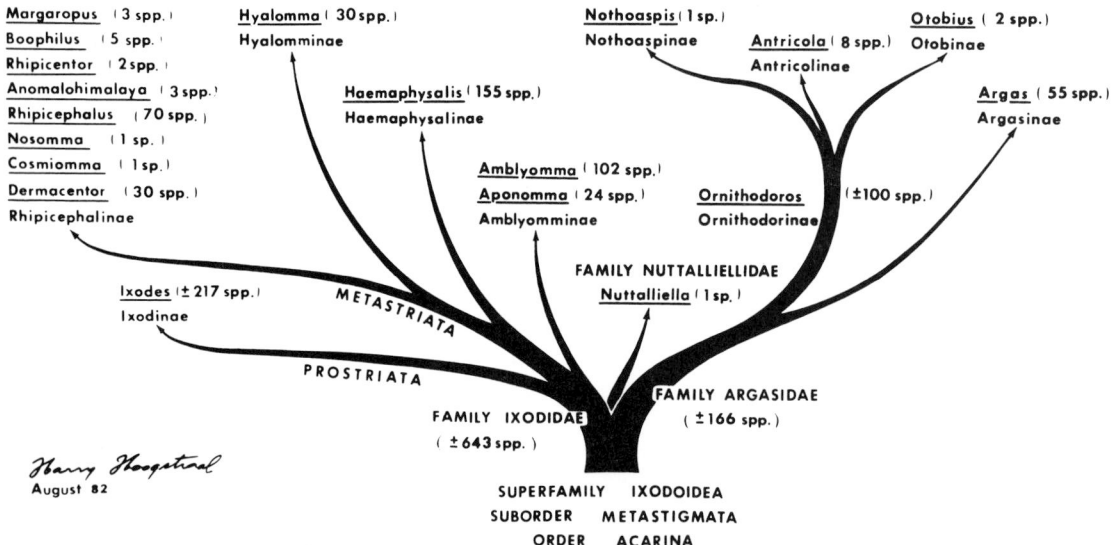

FIGURE 112–1. Dendrogram of the suborder Ixodida showing families, subfamilies, genera, and number of species.

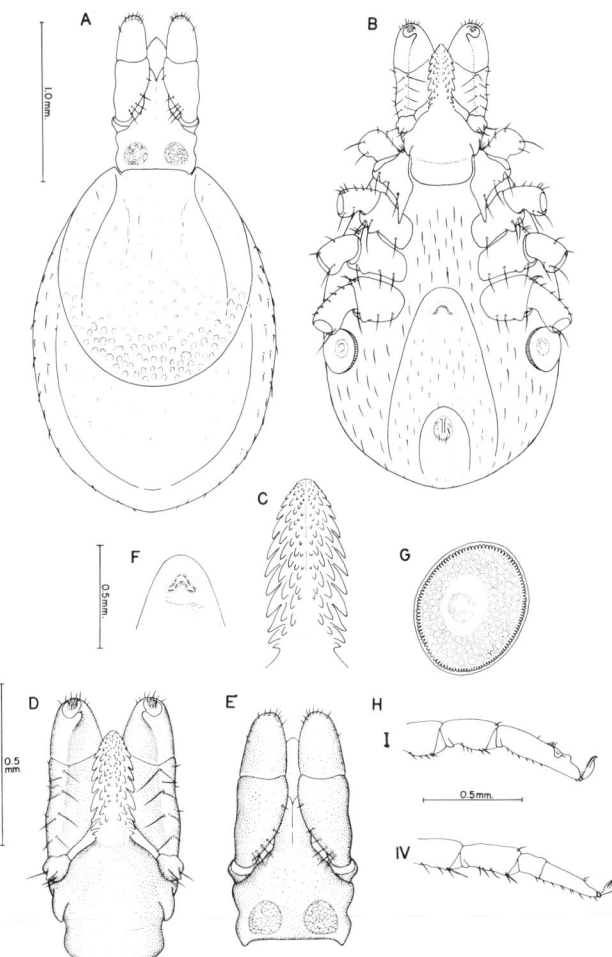

FIGURE 112–2. The structure of a representative ixodid tick, a female of the bird tick, *Ixodes dentatus*. *A*, Entire tick, dorsal aspect. *B*, Entire tick, ventral aspect. *C*, Hypostome. *D*, Capitulum, showing the relationships of the palps, hypostome, and the basis capituli; ventral aspect. *E*, Capitulum, dorsal aspect. *F*, Genital pore. *G*, Spiracular plate. *H*, Tarsal segments of legs I and IV; tarsus I bears Haller's organ.

of Lyme disease in the western United States; (5) *I. petaurista* and *I. ceylonensis*, vectors of Kyasanur Forest disease in India (Chapter 22.7); and (6) *I. holocyclus*, responsible for severe or fatal paralytic symptoms in Australia. The genus is worldwide in distribution.

Genus Dermacentor. Species of this genus typically have an ornate scutum with eyes (absent in *D. dissimile*) and short, thick palps. All are 3-host ticks. The genus is widespread, with species in many localities throughout the world. Important species include *D. variabilis*, the American dog tick, the predominant vector of Rocky Mountain spotted fever (RMSF) in the eastern United States (Chapter 24.1) and (2) *D. andersoni*, the Rocky Mountain wood tick, the vector of RMSF and Colorado tick fever (Chapter 20.12) in the Rocky Mountain region. The distribution is Holarctic, Oriental, and African.

Genus Haemaphysalis. According to Hoogstraal and Aeschlimann (1982), this large and varied genus contains about 155 species. These ticks are easily recognized by the characteristic lateral projection of palpal article II beyond the margins of the basis capituli. All are 3-host ticks. The distribution is predominantly Old World, with only 5 species in the Nearctic and Neotropical regions. *H. spinigera* and other species in India transmit Kyasanur Forest disease. In the Soviet Union, *H. longicornis* has been reported to be infected with Powassan virus and to transmit fatal meningoencephalitis and RSSE. An unusual association occurs in India, where *H. intermedia* and *H. wellingtoni* transmit Ganjam virus, an agent identical with that causing Nairobi sheep disease in East Africa.

Genus Amblyomma. This is one of the largest of the ixodid tick genera, found mostly in tropical and subtropical regions of the world. These ticks are easily recognized by their remarkably ornate multicolored scutum and their unusually long mouthparts, particularly palpal article two, which is about twice as long as article three (Fig. 112–3). All species are 3-host ticks. In Africa, *A. hebraeum* and *A. variegatum* are important vectors of animal disease, especially heartwater, and are also important as pests of livestock. Congo-Crimean hemorrhagic fever (CCHF) has also been recovered from *A. variegatum* on many occasions, and specimens have also been found to be infected with the yellow fever virus. In the United States, *A. americanum*, an important pest of livestock, deer, and humans, is a known vector of *Rickettsia rickettsii*, the agent of RMSF. These ticks parasitize a wide variety of hosts, including reptiles and even amphibians. Their distribution is worldwide, but they are found predominantly in humid tropical and subtropical regions.

Genus Hyalomma. These ornamented medium-sized to large ticks have festoons (rectangular demarcations along the posterior end of the body), eyes, and elongated palps. The males have distinctive adanal shields. *Hyalomma* species frequently parasitize a diversity of wild and domesticated mammals and birds. They are found almost entirely in savanna, semiarid or arid deserts, and grassy steppes in southern and eastern Europe, Asia, and Africa. The most important human disease transmitted by these ticks is CCHF (Chapter 22.5). Other pathogens, especially tick-borne arboviruses, are disseminated by these and other *Hyalomma* species during the spring and fall migrations of vast flocks of migratory birds. *H. dromedarii* and *H. anatolicum excavatum* are adapted to extremely dry environments and survive for long periods in the sand and dust along camel paths and caravansaries.

Genus Rhipicephalus. These inornate ticks are easily recognized by the distinctive shape of the basis capituli. This structure bears protruding, pointed lateral margins, which present a hexagonal shape when viewed from the dorsal aspect. Males have adanal shields. These ticks are widely distributed throughout Africa, Europe, and Asia. The brown dog tick, *R. sanguineus*, has spread to North America and Australia and is now a major pest of pet animals in many homes. Few authentic records of North American brown dog tick's attacking humans have been recorded. Nevertheless, it has also been incriminated in the transmission of *Ehrlichia* (Chapter 27.2) to humans. These pathogens, especially *E. canis*, were previously regarded as pathogens of dogs and other carnivores. In the United States, cases of human ehr-

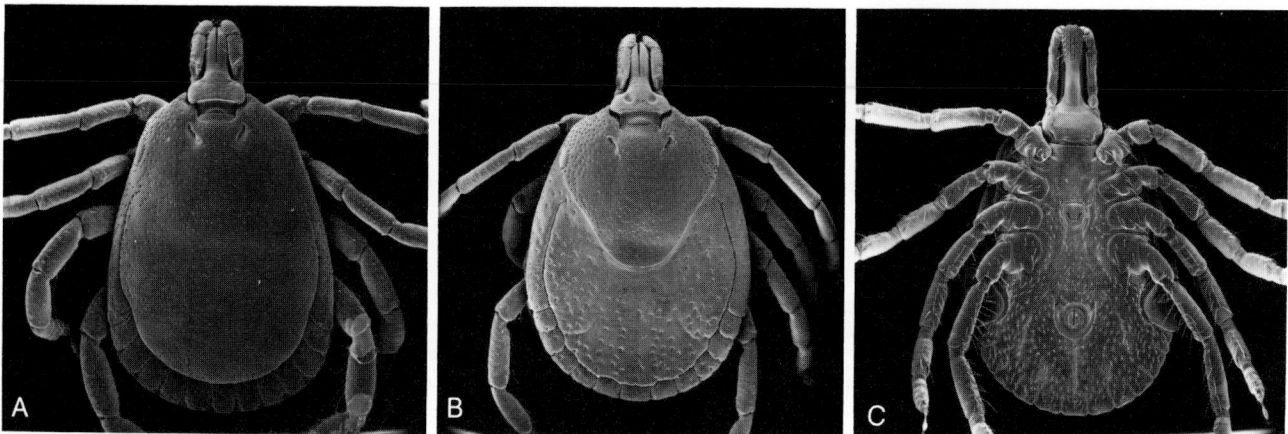

FIGURE 112–3. Scanning electron micrographs illustrating the characteristic features of the genus *Amblyomma (A. americanum)*. *A*, Male, dorsal aspect. Note 11 festoons visible beyond the scutum. *B*, Female, dorsal aspect. *C*, Female, ventral aspect.

lichiosis have been reported in recent years, presumably transmitted by the brown dog tick. In southern and southeastern Africa, *Rhipicephalus appendiculatus* is the predominant vector of East Coast fever, caused by *Theileria parva,* a highly fatal disease of cattle in that region. *R. sanguineus* is also responsible for transmission of Mediterranean spotted fever (i.e., fièvre boutenneuse), caused by *Rickettsia conorii,* a rickettsial disease similar to RMSF, in the Mediterranean region and throughout large areas of Africa and western Asia (Chapter 24.2).

Argasidae. The Argasidae (soft ticks) have a tough leathery integument (except in the larval stage, which has a minutely folded cuticle reminiscent of ixodids) (Fig. 112–4). There is no scutum, but a pseudoscutum is present in the obscure bat ticks of the genus *Nothoaspis.* A dorsal shield occurs in the larva (not a true scutum). The capitulum is ventral, near the anterior end, and is not visible from the dorsal aspect. Eyes, when present, occur on the ventral surface of the body, usually on the ventrolateral folds. The spiracles occur on the ventrolateral folds between the coxae of legs III and IV, but never on large plates and never behind the leg coxae as in the Ixodidae. Coxal pores, the openings

of the coxal glands, are located between the paired coxae of legs I and II. The walking legs lack prominent padlike pulvilli. Sexual dimorphism is slight. A brief description of *Argas* and *Ornithodoros,* the two medically important genera, follows.

Genus Argas. This genus comprises those ticks in which the adults and nymphs have a leathery folded cuticle and a distinct sutural line separating the dorsal and ventral margins. There are distinct marginal plates or marginal striae. The flattened margins are evident even when the tick has fed. Eyes are absent in this genus. Although the hosts vary and may include many mammals, most species are parasitic on birds and bats. The genus is worldwide in distribution.

Genus Ornithodoros. This includes species that lack a distinct sutural line separating the dorsal and ventral body margins (Fig. 112–4). The body margin is rounded or flattened, but never marginated, and lacks marginal plates or striae. Adults and nymphs have a leathery cuticle with innumerable minute elevations termed mammillae. There is no sutural line separating the dorsal and ventral margins. Typically, the anterior end of the body is more or less pointed and hoodlike in appearance. The hosts are varied, including reptiles, birds, and

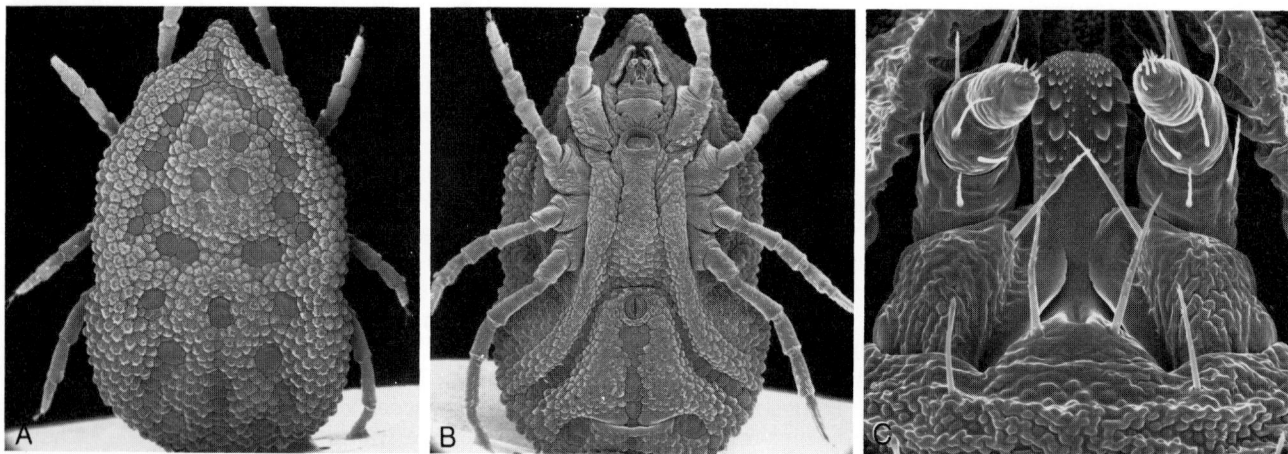

FIGURE 112–4. Scanning electron micrographs illustrating the characteristics of the genus *Ornithodoros (O. capensis)*. *A*, Male, dorsal aspect. *B*, Male, ventral aspect. *C*, Male, ventral aspect. Enlargement showing detail of the capitulum recessed in the camerostomal cavity and the adjacent cheeks.

mammals. The genus is worldwide in distribution. Some examples of important species include (1) *O. moubata*, an important vector of relapsing fever in eastern and southern Africa (Chapter 34), and (2) *O. coriaceus*, the vector of epizootic bovine abortion in the western United States and Mexico. Most *Ornithodoros* species shelter in dry caves, rodent burrows, birds nests and rookeries, or human-constructed shelters. Aside from a few species that are parasitic on bats or tortoises in humid areas, most *Ornithodoros* occur in dry climates. Hosts include a diverse array of birds and mammals and, occasionally, even reptiles. The genus is worldwide in distribution.

LIFE CYCLE AND FEEDING HABITS

Ixodid Ticks. Metamorphosis is incomplete in ixodid ticks. The larval and nymphal stages resemble the adults, although larvae have only 3 pairs of legs. There is only 1 nymphal instar in ticks of this family. In most ixodid species, larvae, nymphs, and adults feed and drop off to molt in the natural environment; each instar feeds on a separate host. Such species are known as 3-host ticks. In some other species, the immature stages remain and molt on the same host, reattaching to feed again. Such species are known as 2-host ticks when only the immatures remain on the same host (e.g., *Hyalomma dromedarii*) and 1-host ticks when both immatures and adults feed on that host (e.g., *Boophilus annulatus*). Ixodid ticks feed slowly, usually requiring several days or even weeks to complete their blood meal. New cuticle is secreted to accommodate the enormous blood meal, often hundreds of times the parasite's prefeeding weight. Digestion proceeds relatively slowly when compared with that of blood-feeding insects. Digestion is almost entirely intracellular, an unusual phenomenon that allows pathogenic organisms greater opportunities for survival and may, perhaps, contribute to the remarkable diversity of tick-borne disease agents. Mating, guided by sex pheromones, takes place on the host, except in species of *Ixodes*. In all Ixodidae, replete, mated females drop and oviposit thousands of eggs before they die. In contrast to the case with the Argasidae, there is only 1 gonotrophic cycle, i.e., females feed, mate, and oviposit only once. Because of their extended feeding periods, species that attach to wide-ranging hosts may spread rapidly, providing a mechanism for dissemination of disease to distant foci.

Argasid Ticks. The life cycle of argasid ticks is considerably different from that of their ixodid relatives. Metamorphosis is also incomplete in this family, but there are more nymphal instars; 2 to 4 are common, but as many as 6 or 7 instars have been recorded in some species. Virtually all argasid ticks are multihost parasites, but there are notable exceptions, e.g., the 2-host tick *Ornithodoros lahorensis* and the 1-host ticks *Otobius megnini* and *Otobius lagophilus*. Except in larvae, which may require several days for their blood meal, feeding is rapid in virtually all argasid nymphs and adults. Often, only 30 to 60 minutes is required to complete the meal. Following feeding, the engorged parasite leaves to molt and seek another host. The integument is deeply folded, allowing the body the opportunity for extensive stretching without additional cuticle growth. These ticks can consume several times their original body weight at each feeding. The meal is concentrated rapidly by elimination of water during or after feeding (coxal fluid). Adults mate in the nest or burrow or, occasionally, while feeding. Females feed and oviposit many times, i.e., there are many gonotrophic cycles. This pattern of multiple nymphal instars and frequent meals in the adult stages contributes to an unusually long existence. Argasid ticks may survive for months or even years between blood meals, and many individuals live for years. The implications of this remarkable longevity for human and animal health are obvious. Pathogens transmitted by these vectors may survive unnoticed for years or even decades, emerging periodically in isolated foci when humans or animals encounter the ticks.

BEHAVIOR AND HOST RANGE

Habitats. Most ixodid ticks are dispersed in vegetation in forests, brushy habitats, meadows, or other grassy habitats; in deserts or semidesert environments, they may even occur in sand, in gravel, or under shale and rocks. While questing for hosts, they climb emergent stems or outcroppings and wait for passing hosts. This is the "ambush" or non-nidiculous mode of host-seeking behavior. When desiccated, they retreat and seek shelter at the base of the vegetation or other protected moist microhabitats. In these more favorable microclimates, they take up water by direct sorption from the hydrating atmosphere. Atmospheric water condenses on hygroscopic salt solutions secreted on the hypostome and the diluted solutions are imbibed, restoring the tick to its normally hydrated state. In all but the nest-inhabiting species of *Ixodes*, host-seeking behavior is seasonal and is usually limited to the warmer periods of the year. Daylength (photoperiod) and incident solar radiation are important factors influencing the onset and termination of this activity. At other times, 1 or more life stages remain in diapause, and the ticks survive from 1 year to the next until stimulated to commence the next seasonal cycle of host-seeking activity.

Argasid ticks and most species of the genus *Ixodes* are nidicoles, living in the nests, burrows, or other shelters made by their hosts. These ticks depend on the return of their hosts to the nest or burrow to feed. Nest-, burrow-, or cave-inhabiting argasids avoid bright light and settle in the more humid zones of their microenvironments, habits that minimize wandering from these shelters. Argasids adapted to migratory birds or bats may exhibit ovipositional diapause, delaying egg deposition and hatching until the hosts return and commence the nesting season.

These patterns of periodic host-seeking activity interspersed with diapause ensure the coincidence of tick population expansion with the periods when host population and weather conditions are most favorable for species survival.

Host Range. Host range varies greatly among the different species of ixodid ticks. Most species have a well-defined, restricted range of hosts. According to Hoogstraal and Aeschlimann (1982), host specificity is an important factor contributing to confining tick species within narrow ecologic niches and geographic ranges. For example, the American dog tick, *Dermacentor var-*

iabilis, the major vector of RMSF, occurs primarily in areas of the eastern and central United States dominated by deciduous forest communities. This species feeds almost exclusively on small mammals in the juvenile stages and on larger mammals in the adult stage. Other species, e.g., the lone star tick, *Amblyomma americanum,* are opportunistic and attack a wide range of vertebrate hosts. Argasid ticks also exhibit well-defined host-selection patterns. Many feed exclusively on the bats or birds that inhabit the nests they infest. A few species are less discriminating and attack virtually any warm-blooded vertebrate that enters the niche. In general, the opportunistic species are more likely to attack human than are those with a highly restricted host range.

MEDICAL AND VETERINARY IMPORTANCE OF TICKS.

Ticks transmit a greater diversity of disease-causing agents than any other group of arthropod vectors. These include protozoan parasites, e.g., the babesias and theilerias affecting livestock, bacterial agents such as the borrelias, numerous rickettsiae, and an even greater variety of arboviruses. In addition, some ticks cause severe toxemias and fatal paralysis of their hosts.

Disease Relationships of the Ixodidae (Hard Ticks)

Lyme Disease. In the United States, the most prevalent tick-borne disease is Lyme borreliosis, also known as Lyme disease (Chapter 36). This disease is caused by a spirochete and is transmitted by certain species of the genus *Ixodes.* The disease was first described from the vicinity of Old Lyme, Connecticut, United States, but has spread and is now reported in 43 states throughout the country. Approximately 5000 cases were reported in 1988, especially in southeastern New York state and eastern Connecticut. The disease is now regarded as epidemic. In the eastern and central United States, the major vector is the deer tick, *Ixodes dammini* (Fig. 112–5). First described in 1979, the deer tick is now widely distributed in New England, the northeastern United

States, and the north central United States, especially where white-tailed deer (*Odocoileus virginiana*) are abundant. Ticks acquire the spirochete when larvae feed on spirochetemic mice, especially white-footed mice. The fed larvae molt and the hungry, spirochete-infected nymphs attack a variety of hosts, including humans. The nymphs transmit the spirochetes in their saliva when they feed. Thus, the nymphal stage is the primary vector of the disease to humans and other animals. Fed nymphs molt to adults, which are usually spirochete free. Occasionally, disease-free nymphs may acquire the spirochetes and transform into spirochete-infected adults. The incidence of infection in the tick population is remarkably high; in some localities well over 50% of the nymphal *I. dammini* collected have been infected. Thus, the major attributes of the epizootiology of Lyme disease are (1) it is zoonotic, with transmission occurring trans-stadially (i.e., from stage to stage) rather than transovarially (i.e., from the female parent); (2) small mammals, especially mice and occasionally other vertebrates, are the reservoir hosts; (3) the disease is most commonly found in areas where deer are abundant. A similar disease is known in Europe and Asia (Siberia, China, Japan), namely, *Erythema Chronicum Migrans* (also caused by *Borrelia burgdorferi*) with similar symptoms, transmitted by the European sheep tick, *Ixodes ricinus,* or the east Asian tick, *Ixodes persulcatus.*

Other animals, including dogs, may also serve as reservoir hosts for Lyme borreliosis. Considerable attention also needs to be directed to the possible role of migratory birds in its spread. The role of other tick species and other human-biting arthropods has not been excluded in the dissemination of this disease.

Rocky Mountain Spotted Fever. Until the epidemic rise of Lyme disease, RMSF was the most prevalent tick-borne disease in the United States. This disease is caused by *Rickettsia rickettsii.* Despite its name, most

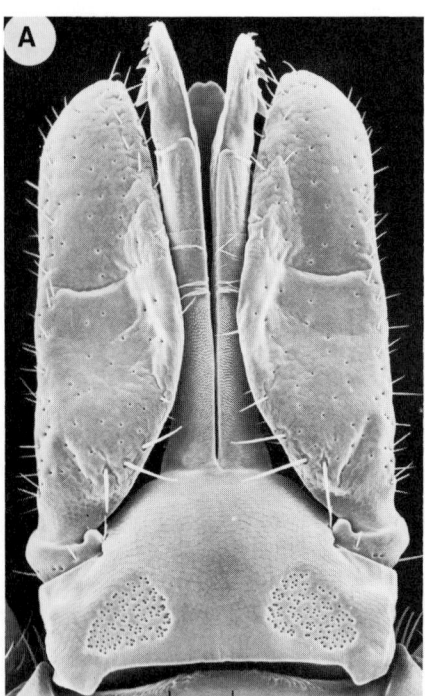
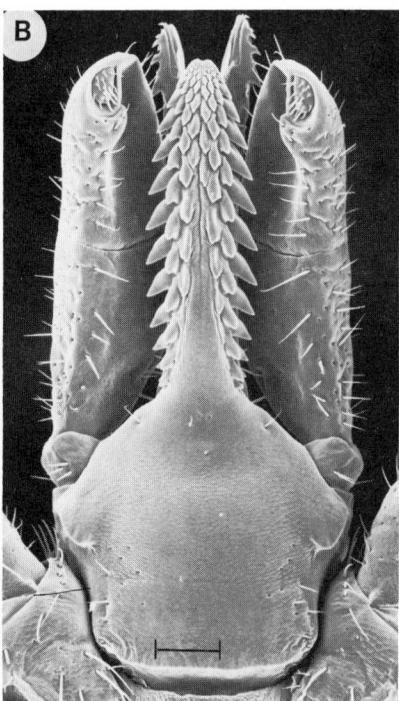
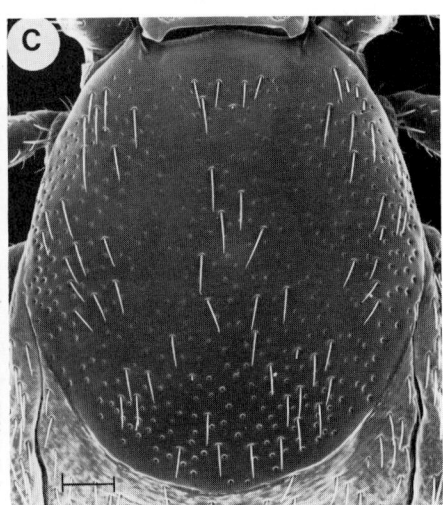

FIGURE 112–5. Scanning electron micrographs illustrating the mouthparts and scutum of a female deer tick, *Ixodes dammini. A,* Capitulum, ventral aspect. *B,* Capitulum, dorsal aspect. *C,* Scutum, dorsal aspect. (Measurement bars 200 μm. Photos prepared by Drs. Richard Robbins and James E. Keirans, U.S. Public Health Service.)

cases of RMSF occur in the eastern regions of the country (Chapter 24.1). The primary vector is the American dog tick, *Dermacentor variabilis,* although a variety of other species can also transmit the rickettsiae. Ticks are the reservoir hosts, and the organism persists in the vector ticks from generation to generation by transovarial transmission. Thus, rickettsia-infected ticks inoculate mice and other small mammals on which they feed, spreading the disease and providing opportunities for uninfected ticks to acquire the infection by simultaneous blood feeding on rickettsemic hosts. Humans acquire the disease when biten by rickettsia-infected, human-biting ticks.

Congo-Crimean Hemorrhagic Fever. CCHF is a viral disease that is widespread throughout large areas of central and western Asia, Europe, and Africa (Chapter 22.5). CCHF is a true tick-borne arbovirus, because it passes trans-stadially and transovarially within the tick population and survives interseasonally in these vectors. At least 25 tick species and subspecies have been reported to serve as vectors and/or reservoirs for this virus. The 2-host vectors *Hyalomma marginatum rufipes* and other subspecies are especially important because the immatures may feed on migratory birds as well as hares and hedgehogs, whereas the adults select artiodactyls and, when available, humans. Thus, these ticks are important in disseminating the virus intercontinentally along the migratory routes followed by migratory birds. The vast numbers in these flocks ensure repeated inundation of host populations along the bird flyways with virus-infected ticks. The *H. marginatum* complex and other human-biting *Hyalomma* species contribute to the periodic epidemics and epizootics of CCHF because of their aggressiveness in attacking human hosts and their large numbers. These ticks serve as the reservoirs as well as the vectors of the pathogens. Immatures of these ticks, especially *H. marginatum rufipes,* feed readily on migratory birds, providing a means of long-range dispersal of the disease agents between Europe and Asia or Africa. Major epidemics of CCHF have occurred in the recent past. One of the most notable of these outbreaks occurred in the Crimea (Soviet Union) in 1944 to 1945, when hundreds of Soviet soldiers were infected while assisting the war-devasted population of the region.

Omsk Hemorrhagic Fever (OHF). This is an acute, febrile disease with a distinct hemorrhagic syndrome (Chapter 22). It is caused by a virus of the genus *Flavivirus,* family Togaviridae. This virus is in the same category as the causative agents of the closely related tick-borne encephalitis (TBE) (i.e., RSSE), Powassan, Louping ill, and Kyasanur Forest disease and other tick-borne Togaviridae. These agents were formerly known as group B viruses. Typical OHF foci are lowland steppe forest and grassland communities in western Siberia (Soviet Union). Ticks, especially *Ixodes persulcatus* and *I. apronophorus,* maintain the virus in nature, whereas *Dermacentor reticulatus* is regarded as primarily responsible for spread of the agent (amplification) within the wild host community and to humans.

Disease Relationships of the Argasidae (Soft Ticks). Species of *Argas* are important as vectors of several viral and bacterial diseases.

Quaranfil Virus Disease. This is found in Egypt and, possibly, adjacent countries, where the heron tick, *Argas arboreus,* infests herons and similar roosting birds. The virus is circulated among nestling birds in heron rookeries and is transmitted from bird to bird by the nest-infesting ticks. Occasionally, humans are infected, resulting in severe illness. However, these ticks rarely if ever bite humans; thus, the route of infection to people is enigmatic.

Relapsing Fever. Perhaps the most important human disease transmitted by argasid ticks is relapsing fever, a spirochetal disease caused by species of *Borrelia* (Chapter 34). In East Africa, relapsing fever is transmitted by species of the *Ornithodoros moubata* complex (sensu Walton). Relapsing fever outbreaks have also occurred in the western United States, particularly in rodent- and tick-infested cabins or similar shelters for hikers or campers. *O. morocanus,* a tick of southern Europe and northwest Africa, when infected by *Borrelia hispanica* can transmit this agent to burrowing mammals, as well as humans and domestic animals, when it infests buildings and other constructed shelters. In California and adjacent states of the western United States, the "pajaroello" tick, *Ornithodoros coriaceus,* is greatly feared because of its vicious bites, but this tick also transmits epizootic bovine abortion, a viral pathogen affecting livestock and wildlife.

112.2. MITES

CHARACTERIZATION. In contrast to the ticks, mites exhibit much greater diversity in their body structure and biology. Most mites are small when compared with ticks, although a few reach sizes as great as 7 mm long. This vast assemblage of tiny arthropods consists of more than 200 families and over 30,000 species; thousands, perhaps tens of thousands, more species remain to be described. In contrast to the ticks, the chelicerae of mites are quite variable, but usually scissor-like, with their cutting edges most often located on the medial facets. Mites lack Haller's organ, although various types of leg sensilla are present, and the hypostome, when present, lacks retrorse teeth. The genital pore is located in the podosomal region in the parasitiform mites but in the opisthosomal region in the acariform mites (Figs. 112–7 and 112–9).

CLASSIFICATION. Mites are subdivided into 2 main taxonomic groupings, the order Parasitiformes and the order Acariformes. The dendrogram (Fig. 112–6) illustrates this divergence and the suborders associated with these 2 orders. Parasitiform mites have 1 to 4 pairs of stigmata posterior to coxae II; the coxae are distinct and freely movable; the setae are not birefringent and are characterized as not optically active, i.e., isotropic. Acariform mites usually have propodosomal sensory organs and podocephalic canals; the coxae are fused with the body wall. Often, there is a distinct separation between the propodosomal (body region bearing the first 2 pairs of walking legs) and the metapodal portions (last 2 pairs of walking legs) of the body. Typically, the

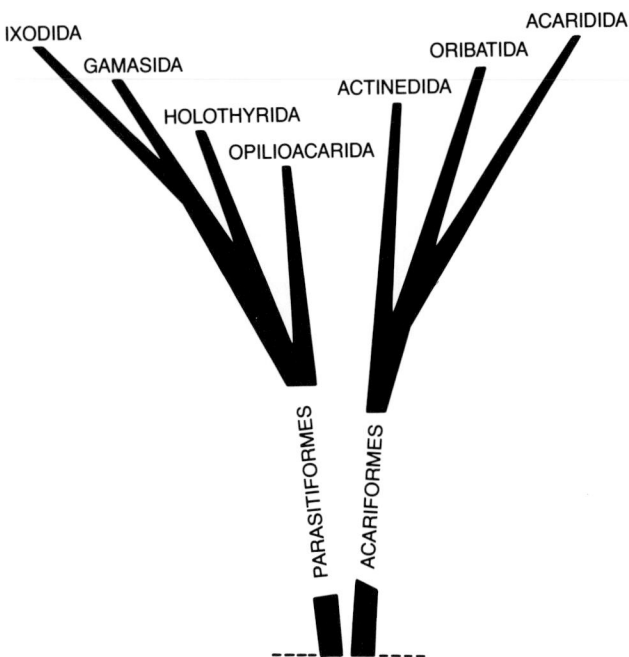

FIGURE 112–6. The systematic and evolutionary relationships among the orders and suborders of the subclass Acari. (From Krantz G.W.: A Manual of Acarology. Corvallis, Oregon State University Press, 1978.)

setae are anisotropic (optically active) and birefringent. Brief descriptions of some of the suborders of mites that cause or transmit disease to humans and animals follow.

Tetrastigmatid Mites (Suborder Holothyroidea). These are relatively large (2 to 7 mm long), heavily sclerotized mites. There is a pair of stigmata lateral to coxae III and another on the lateral margins of the dorsal shield posterior to the ventral stigmata. These mites are believed to be carnivorous. Although not known to be responsible for transmission of any pathogenic agents, some mites of this group have been reported to cause ill effects when swallowed.

Mesostigmatid Mites (Suborder Gamasida). This suborder contains numerous species that transmit diseases to humans or animals. These mites are closest to the ticks in general appearance. Mesostigmatid mites are generally robust, with sclerotized body plates. They have a single pair of stigmata located just posterior to and adjacent to the third pair of coxae (Fig. 112–7). Extending anteriorly from each stigmatal opening is a curved tube, the peritreme, of uncertain function. The chelae of the chelicerae are normally chelate-dentate, but many modifications occur; in males of some species, the chelae may be modified for spermatophore transfer (spermatodactyl). The pedipalps have 5 distinct segments and an apotele with a 2- to 4-tined seta-like structure on the medial surface of the tarsal segment. An elongated bristle-like structure, the tritosternum, occurs on the ventral surface of the gnathosoma. The body bears a prominent peritreme on either side. Most mesostigmatid mites are free living, especially in soil and on the ground. Many are parasitic, either on insects or on vertebrates. An example is the tropical rat mite, *Ornithonyssus bacoti,* which parasitizes various rodents and birds

throughout the world. These mites are intermittent feeders, sucking blood within minutes when exposed to a host. Females produce up to 100 eggs, which hatch into nonfeeding larvae and molt into protonymphs. The protonymphs feed, molt to nonfeeding deutonymphs, and then molt to adults.

Prostigmatid Mites (Suborder Actinedida). This is a large, diverse group of mites, including many species that transmit (or cause) human and animal diseases. The group is characterized by the presence of a pair of stigmata at the base of chelicerae. The chelicerae show many modifications, including modification into piercing stylets, hooklike structures, or even fusion. The pedipalps are simple, or with fangs or claws. Genital suckers occur in both sexes. A tracheal system occurs in the majority of families. Typically, prostigmatid mites are only weakly and incompletely sclerotized. This group includes several disease-transmitting species, especially those that include the chigger mites (family Trombiculidae) responsible for transmission of scrub typhus (*Rickettsia tsutsugamushi*) (Fig. 112–8).

Astigmata (Suborder Acaridida). These are mostly small (i.e., less than 1 mm), slow-moving mites. Many are fungivorous; others are saprophagous or feed on detritus. Few are predaceous. Several species are exclusively parasitic. The body is soft, with little or no sclerotization. The palpi are distinct, though small, with only 2 segments. True claws are lacking on the walking legs, although a terminal clawlike spine may be present. Females have a terminal or posterodorsal *bursa copulatrix,* whereas males frequently have anal suckers. As in other Acariformes, the idiosoma is subdivided by a furrow into an anterior propodosoma and a posterior

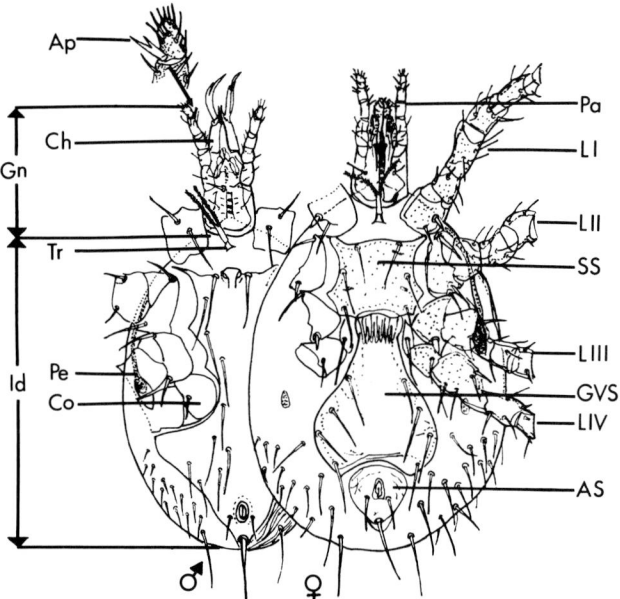

FIGURE 112–7. The major body structures of a representative mesostigmatid mite, as found in *Laelaps echidninus*. The male and female are shown in ventral view. *Ap,* Apotele; *AS,* anal shield; *Ch,* chelicera; *Co,* coxa (of leg IV); *Gn,* gnathosoma; *Id,* idiosoma; *L,* leg (I–IV); *Pa,* palp; *pe,* peritreme; *Tr,* tritosternum; *SS,* sternal shield; *As,* anal shield; *GVS,* genitoventral shield. (Redrawn from various sources, including Azad AF, 1986.)

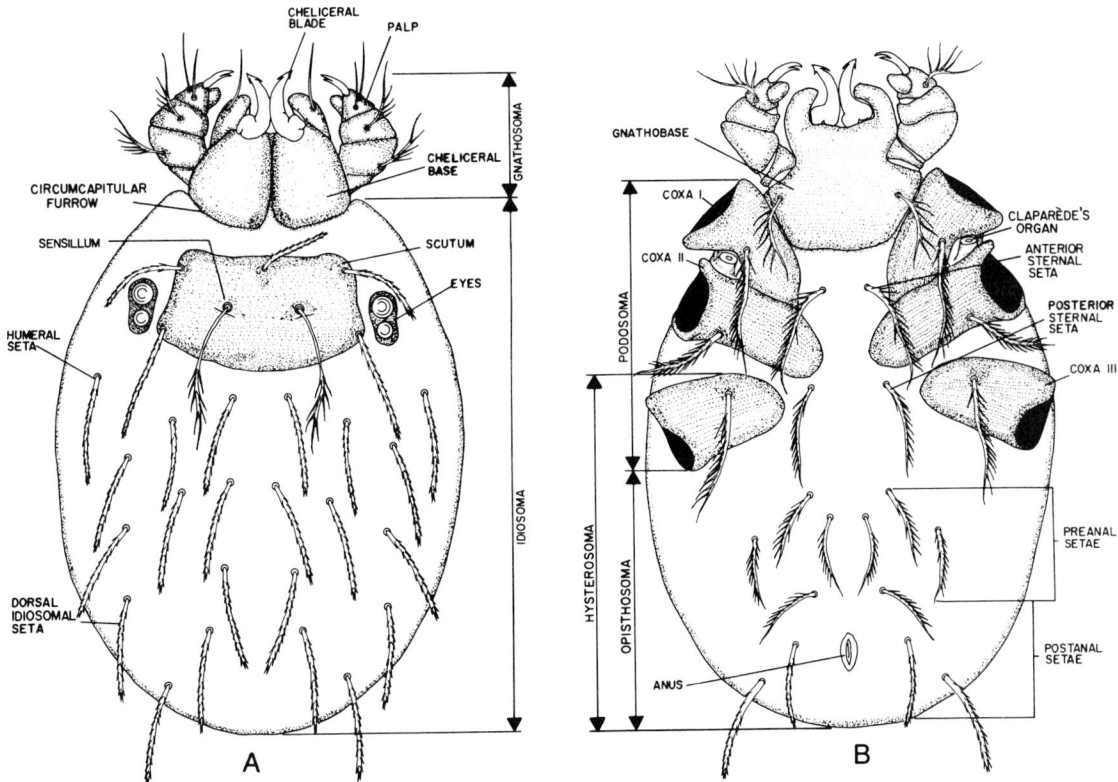

FIGURE 112–8. The idiosoma and gnathosoma of a representative chigger mite (larva of the Trombiculidae), *Eutrombicula alfreddugesi. A,* Dorsal aspect; *B,* ventral aspect. (From Goff ML, et al.: J Med Entomol 19:221, 1982.)

hysterosoma. This group includes many disease-causing or disease-transmitting mites, especially (1) skin-infesting *Sarcoptes scabei;* (2) the allergy causing house dust mites, *Dermatophagoides farinae* (Fig. 112–9), *D. pteronyssinus,* and others; (3) the dog mange mite, *Demodex canis,* which is similar to the human mite, *D. folliculorum;* and (4) the straw itch mite, *Pyemotes tritici,* and many others.

HABITATS AND LIFE CYCLES. Mites occupy an exceptionally diverse array of habitats. Numerous species live entirely in the soil, feeding on fungi, bacteria, other microorganisms, or decomposing organic matter. Others live on the ground, especially in the upper layers of the soil, at the interface with the duff, detritus, and/or leafy layer that characterizes the top of the root zone of the vegetation. These may include predaceous species, dung-feeding species, and others feeding on vegetation. Numerous species are phytophagous, feeding on a wide variety of plants or stored foods. Many mites are parasitic, including some that have obligate parasitic life cycles. Many are parasitic on insects, others on vertebrates. Some, such as the itch mite, *Sarcoptes scabei,* live their entire lives in the tissues of their host (Chapter 105.2). Although most could be classified as ectoparasites, living in the skin, in feathers, or in the fur of their hosts, others, such as the nasal mites (Halarachnidae), are endoparasitic, living in the nasal passages of seals and walruses or in the lungs, bronchi, tracheae, or sinuses of various mammalian hosts.

The typical life cycle includes the egg, protonymph, deutonymph, tritonymph, and the adult. Often, one or more of the immature stages is omitted as development

is accelerated. In the insect-parasitizing "hay itch mite," *Pyemotes ventricosus,* the female does not lay eggs but reproduces viviparously. The opisthosomal region of the female swells during feeding, forming a balloon-like structure. Young mites develop within this sac and emerge when they are sexually mature adults.

BEHAVIOR, LIFE CYCLES, AND HOST RANGE. The enormous diversity of disease-causing and disease-transmitting mites makes it difficult to generalize regarding their behavior and host range. In the Mesostigmata, most of the parasitic mites are nidicoles, living in the nest or burrow environment of their mammal or bird hosts. Typically, they are intermittent feeders, attacking hosts when present, feeding for brief periods and returning to the shelter of the nest material to molt or lay eggs. The chicken mite, *Dermanyssus gallinae,* is an example of this parasitic habit. These mites live in cracks, crevices, detritus, or fibrous material and usually leave their shelters only at night. Others are permanent ectoparasites, e.g., *Ornithonyssus silvarium,* which lives out its entire life cycle on the host. A closely related parasite, *Ornithonyssus bursa,* has a similar parasitic habit but leaves its host to lay eggs. Many parasitic mites are true hematophages, piercing the host skin and sucking blood. Others, such as spiny rat mite, *Echinolaelaps echidninus,* feed on bloody exudates from abrasions and skin lesions; they cannot penetrate the unbroken skin. Although numerous mesostigmatid mites are opportunistic, i.e., feeding on virtually any hosts that they encounter, other species exhibit varying degrees of host specificity, e.g., the snake mite, *Ophionyssus natricis.*

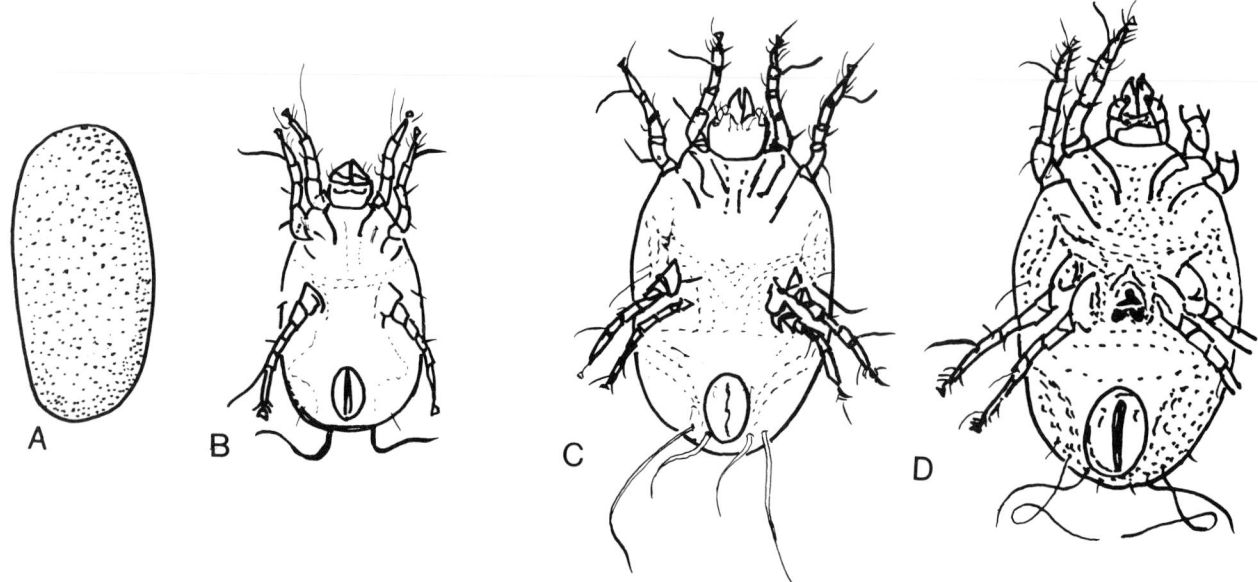

FIGURE 112–9. The developmental stages of the house dust mite, *Dermatophagoides farinae. A*, Egg; *B*, larva; *C*, nymphal stage (protonymph-tritonymph); *D*, adult. (Modified from Wharton GW, J Med Entomol 12:577, 1976.)

Examples of parasitism are also numerous among the acariform mites. Among the prostigmatid mites, one of the most important parasites is the chigger mite (family Trombiculidae). In these species, only the larva is parasitic. The larval mite burrows into the skin, forming a cavity (stylostome) in which it feeds and shelters, avoiding host grooming. When satiated, the mite escapes to continue its development on the ground. Nymphs and adults are predaceous. Other prostigmatid mites are obligate parasites in all stages, spending their entire lives on the same host, e.g., feather mite, *Syringophilus bipectinatus*. These tiny mites live inside the quill feathers, feeding on desquamated cells and sebaceous secretions from which they derive necessary nutrients. Not only are these mites highly species specific, they are even specialized for specific feather groups. Among the astigmatid mites, one finds similar examples of highly adapted obligate ectoparasitic life cycles. Thus, fur mites spend their entire lives on and among the hairs of their mammalian hosts, commonly on rodents. These mites bear special adaptations for this habitat, e.g., a somewhat laterally compressed body and modification of the palps and legs to form claspers for clinging to the hairs. In *Listrophorus* spp., the endites of the palpal coxae form an apparatus for attaching to hair. As a result of these adaptations, these mites are relatively host specific.

MEDICAL AND VETERINARY IMPORTANCE OF MITES

Mesostigmatoid Mites. These mites transmit a variety of human and animal diseases. Some transmit rickettsial diseases, e.g., rickettsialpox, caused by *Rickettsia akari,* and transmitted by the house mouse mite, *Liponyssus sanguineus* (Chapter 24.3). Others are serious pests of domestic fowl, such as the chicken mite, *Dermanyssus gallinae;* the northern fowl mite, *Ornithonyssus sylviarum;* and the tropical fowl mite, *O. bursa,* which are serious pests of chickens, turkeys, and other domestic

fowl in various parts of the world. In infested buildings, these mites may proliferate in such enormous numbers that they kill many birds. Other parasitized birds become extremely irritable, their skin becomes inflamed and scabby, and the birds become progressively anemic and emaciated; as might be expected, weight gain and egg production diminish precipitously. *O. sylviarum* also bites humans, resulting in erythema, induration, and pruritus around the wound sites. *D. gallinae* may also bite humans, leading to painful urticaria.

Rodent mites may also constitute a problem. *O. bacoti,* the tropical rat mite, parasitizes small mammals and other vertebrates. It occasionally attacks humans, with severe and painful dermatitis resulting from these bites. In contrast to these ectoparasitic mites, some mesostigmatid mites are endoparasites, e.g., species of the genus *Halarachne* that live in the respiratory system of seals or the nasal mite, *Pneumonyssus caninum,* that inhabits the nasal passages and sinuses of dogs. Mite-infested dogs develop inflammation of the nasal passages, excessive production of mucus, rhinitis, sinusitis, sneezing, and violent head-shaking behavior.

Prostigmatid Mites. These include the chigger mites, the vectors of scrub typhus. This disease, caused by *Rickettsia tsutsugamushi,* is the most important mite-borne disease of humans (Chapter 25). Scrub typhus is prevalent in eastern Asia, especially Japan, eastern China, Taiwan, Vietnam, India, the Philippines, and many islands of the South Pacific and Australia. It does not occur in the Americas, Europe, or Africa, even though trombiculid mites (i.e., chigger mites) occur in those regions. Even where the mites do not carry disease, the attacks of chigger mites are serious and cause intense itching and severe dermatitis, even to the point of requiring hospitalization (Fig. 112–10).

Astigmatid Mites. These include many species that are serious pests or causative agents of disease and allergy. Among the best known are the mange mites,

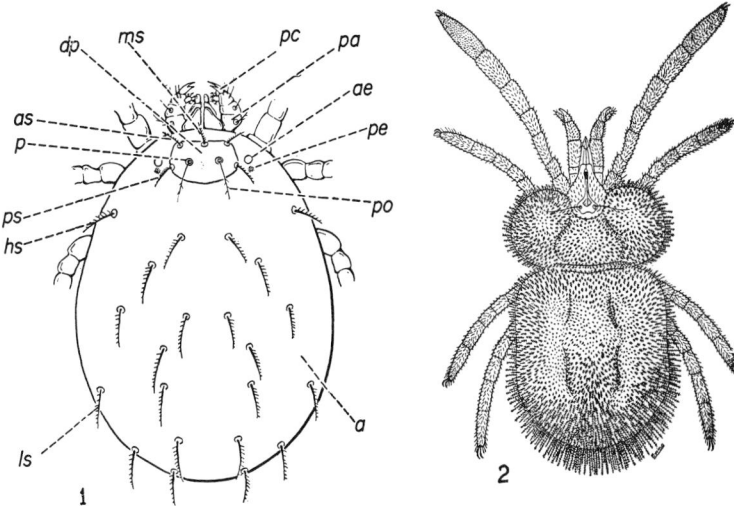

FIGURE 112–10. *Eutrombicula alfreddugesi. 1,* Larva (North American chigger), greatly enlarged (*a*, abdomen; *ae*, anterior eye; *as*, anterolateral seta; *dp*, dorsal plate; *hs*, humeral seta; *ls*, lateral seta; *ms*, median seta; *p*, pseudostigma; *pa*, palpus; *pc*, palpal claw; *pe*, posterior eye; *po*, pseudostigmatic organ; *ps*, posterolateral seta). *2,* Adult.

especially the families Psoroptidae, Sarcoptidae, and Demodicidae. Species of *Psoroptes* pierce the skin and suck fluids, which congeal to induce scabbing and related growths; the scabs provide shelter for the mites, which reproduce rapidly in the protected environment. In rabbits, the rabbit ear mite, *P. cuniculi,* proliferates deep in the ear canal and can penetrate into the brain; the mites eventually kill these animals unless the patient is treated. In humans, females of the human itch mite, *Sarcoptes scabei,* tunnel into the stratum corneum of the skin. These burrows fill with eggs, hatched larvae, excrement, ecdysed cuticles, and other debris, which induce an intense irritation in the affected host (Chapter 105.2). Transmission occurs by direct physical contact between infected and uninfected individuals. In addition, transfer experiments show that canine mites can infect humans. Fortunately, human and animal cross-infestations are self-limiting.

Dust Mite Allergy. An increasingly recognized mite-associated illness is dust mite allergy. Proteins in mite feces, rather than the mites themselves, are regarded as the primary allergen responsible for the allergic reactions (Chapter 105.1). In the United States, after pollen or hay fever, house dust is the most common cause of allergic reactions. The problem may be seasonal in northern temperate climates, declining during the heating season, but is perennial in more mild, humid climates. Common symptoms resemble allergies to pollen and other dustlike substances, with upper respiratory distress, swellings of nasal membranes and sinuses, sneezing, tearing, and related symptoms. Dust mite allergies occur worldwide but are most commonly associated with warm, humid environments. In households, mattresses, pillows, stuffed furniture, carpets, and other household objects where human or animal dander accumulates in large quantities may provide optimal environments where the mites find food.

BIBLIOGRAPHY

Azad AF: Mites of public health importance and their control. WHO/VBC/86.931. Geneva, World Health Organization, 1986.
Hoogstraal H, Aeschlimann A: Tick-host specificity. Bull Soc Entomol Suisse 55:5, 1982.
Knulle W, Rudolph D. Humidity relationships and water balance of ticks. *In* Galun R, Obenchain FD (eds.): Physiology of Ticks. Oxford, Pergamon Press, 1982, pp. 43–70.
Krantz GW: A Manual of Acarology. Corvallis, Oregon State University, 1978.
Oliver JH Jr: Chromosomes, genetic variance and reproductive strategies among mites and ticks. Bull Entomol Soc Am 29:9, 1983.
Savory, T: Arachnida. New York, Academic Press, 1977.

113. INSECTS IN DISEASE TRANSMISSION

Duane J. Gubler

HISTORY. Although early scholars recognized a relationship between certain arthropods and illness in humans and animals, the concept of disease transmission by insects is relatively new. The first actual demonstration that a parasite of humans required a developmental phase in an insect to complete its life cycle occurred more than 100 years ago. Sir Patrick Manson, working in China in 1877, showed that the human filarial parasite *Wuchereria bancrofti* required an obligatory period of development in the mosquito *Culex pipiens fatigans (C. pipiens quinquefasciatus).* Since that time, many important disease pathogens of humans have been shown to depend on insects to complete their transmission cycles.

The pathogens transmitted to humans by insects fall into 5 main categories of microorganisms: nematodes or roundworms, protozoa, bacteria, rickettsiae, and viruses. Some are true parasites of humans, e.g., *W. bancrofti,* but most are zoonotic, with other primary vertebrate hosts (reservoirs). Humans in this case become an incidental host, and although they may contribute to the transmission cycle on a temporary basis, they are not required for survival of the pathogen in nature.

DISEASE TRANSMISSION. An arthropod may transmit a disease agent from 1 person or animal to another in 1 of 2 basic ways.

Mechanical Transmission. This consists of a simple transfer of the organism on contaminated mouth parts or feet or by regurgitation or defecation. There is no multiplication or developmental change of the pathogen on or in the insect during this type of transmission. Examples include a variety of enteroviruses, bacteria, and protozoa of humans that have a direct fecal-oral transmission cycle. Insects such as houseflies may become contaminated with these pathogens while feeding on feces and transport them directly to the food of people.

Biologic Transmission. The second and most important type of transmission by insects is biologic. As the name implies, the pathogen must undergo some type of development in the body of the insect vector in order to complete its life cycle. There are 3 types of biologic transmission.

Propagative Transmission. This type occurs when the organism ingested with the blood meal undergoes simple multiplication in the body of the insect. Examples are the arboviruses, which replicate extensively in the tissues of the insect.

Cyclopropagative Transmission. In this type of transmission, the pathogen undergoes a developmental cycle (changes from 1 stage to another) as well as multiplication in the body of the insect. The best example of this type is malaria, in which a single zygote may give rise to over 200,000 sporozoites.

Cyclodevelopmental Transmission. In this third type of biologic transmission, the pathogen undergoes developmental changes from 1 stage to another but does not multiply. With the filariae, for example, a single microfilaria ingested by a mosquito may result in only one infective larva.

Extrinsic Incubation Period. In all types of biologic transmission, time is required for development of the pathogen to the infective stage that can be transmitted. With arboviruses, this means infection and replication in the salivary glands; with the malaria parasite, it means invasion of the salivary glands by the infectious sporozoites; and with filariae, it means development of the juvenile worms to the active stage III larvae. This period of time is called the extrinsic incubation period and is generally 7 to 14 days in duration, depending on the pathogen, the vector, and a variety of environmental factors.

Transovarial Transmission. Some viral and rickettsial diseases are transmitted from the female parent arthropod through the eggs to the offspring. This is termed transovarial transmission. The newly hatched insect larval stages are infected with the pathogen, which is then transmitted to subsequent developmental stages of the arthropod (trans-stadial transmission). Finally, venereal transmission of certain viruses has been documented. Thus, male mosquitoes that become infected transovarially can transfer the infective virus to uninfected female mosquitoes in the seminal fluid during copulation. These latter types of transmission have obvious epidemiologic importance in the ultimate infection of humans or other animals and in the maintenance of the pathogen in nature.

Factors Influencing Transmission. The ability of insects to transmit a disease agent is dependent on many factors. Successful mechanical transmission depends on the degree of contact insects have with humans and on

feeding behavior. For example, the domestic housefly has been incriminated as a mechanical vector of a variety of intestinal pathogens, primarily because this insect breeds in large numbers, lives in intimate contact with humans and has the bad habit of feeding on both feces and food. Tabanid flies are efficient mechanical vectors of both viruses and protozoa because of frequent interrupted feeding.

The ability to transmit a pathogen biologically varies greatly among species of insects and even among geographic strains within a species. Significant variation in susceptibility to become infected and to subsequently transmit an etiologic agent has been demonstrated in a number of insect vectors. Most work, however, has been done with mosquitoes, and variation in vector competence has been documented with all of the major diseases they transmit, i.e., malaria, filariasis, and arbovirus infections. Thus, within a single mosquito species, it is common to find geographic strains that are good vectors and other strains of that same species that are poor vectors. Because this general susceptibility to infection and growth of the pathogen in the tissues of the insect are genetically controlled, it may be expected to change with time.

In addition to innate susceptibility to infection, the overall vector competence of an insect is influenced by other biologic and behavioral characteristics of the insect population. The degree of contact the species has with humans is influenced by the host preference, the intrinsic blood-feeding behavior of the insect, and the population density of both insect and humans. Longevity, flight behavior, and breeding habits of the insect population are important intrinsic factors, which are influenced by extrinsic environmental factors such as temperature, humidity, wind, and rainfall.

Finally, other extrinsic factors may influence whether an individual insect becomes infected with a pathogen. For example, it has been shown that mosquitoes ingesting blood containing both microfilaria and Rift Valley fever virus have a higher viral susceptibility because disseminated virus infection is facilitated by microfilaria escaping from the midgut into the hemocoel. There may also be other factors that influence this "leaky gut" phenomenon and thus susceptibility to infection.

In temperate regions, insect transmission of disease is usually seasonal and can be correlated with temperature. In the tropics, transmission generally occurs year round and is most frequently correlated with rainfall.

Systematics. Table 113–1 outlines the orders and lower taxa of the class Insecta that are known to transmit disease pathogens of humans. Other arthropods such as mites and ticks are not included, as they are discussed elsewhere (Chapter 112). It will be noted that the order Diptera is by far the most important, primarily because of the family Culicidae (mosquitoes).

Importance. Collectively, the insects are responsible for millions of cases of disease each year. In the past 15 years, the world has experienced a resurgence of vector-borne diseases such as malaria, leishmaniasis, yellow fever, Japanese encephalitis, and dengue hemorrhagic fever. A major problem is that the most important vector-borne diseases occur in the tropics, usually in the

TABLE 113–1. Taxonomic Groups of the Class Insecta That Transmit Human Disease

Order	Family	Important Genera
Siphonaptera	Pulicidae	*Pulex*
		Xenopsylla
		Ctenocephalides
	Ceratophyllidae	*Nosopsyllus*
		Diamanus
	Leptopsyllidae	*Leptopsylla*
Anoplura	Pediculidae	*Pediculus*
Hemiptera	Cimicidae	*Cimex*
	Reduviidae	*Triatoma*
		Rhodnius
		Panstrongylus
Diptera	Ceratopogonidae	*Culicoides*
	Psychodidae	*Phlebotomus*
		Lutzomyia
		Sergentomyia
	Simuliidae	*Similium*
		Prosimulium
		Austrosimulium
	Culicidae	*Aedes*
		Anopheles
		Culex
		Mansonia
		Haemogogus
		Psorophora
		Sabethes
	Tabanidae	*Tabanus*
		Chrysops
	Glossinidae	*Glossina*
	Muscidae	*Musca*
		Fannia
		Muscina
	Chloropidae	*Hippelates*
		Siphunculina
	Calliphoridae	*Calliphora*
		Lucilia
		Phaenicia
		Phormia
		Chrysomyia
		Cochliomya
	Sarcophagidae	*Sarcophaga*
Dictyoptera	Blattidae	*Blatta*
		Periplaneta
		Blattella

areas where resources are most limited. With the highly increased human mobility, however, these diseases are not just problems of the tropics but present the world community with possibly its greatest health problem today. For example, in 1980, more than 2000 cases of malaria were imported into the United States, and there are several fatalities, mainly due to late diagnosis, every year. Many areas of the United States still have the anopheline vectors of this parasite, and local transmission has been documented in California. Similarly, many cases of dengue fever are imported into the United States each year. The principal vector mosquito, *Aedes aegypti,* still occurs in most Gulf Coast states, and in 1985, another important vector mosquito, *A. albopictus,* was found in Texas. This species subsequently spread throughout the Southeast and into some North Central states. The first indigenous dengue transmission since 1945 was documented in Texas in 1980 and again in 1986. This underscores how important it is for physicians in nonendemic areas to be aware of these diseases and knowledgeable as to where they occur and how to recognize and treat them.

The resurgence of some insect-borne viral diseases has become more acute in the 1980s. The incidence of dengue has increased dramatically in all major regions of the tropics, occurring not only as larger and more frequent epidemics but also in countries where the disease had not occurred before. Moreover, the severe and fatal form of disease, dengue hemorrhagic fever, has moved out of Southeast Asia and is now occurring in many American countries. Other viruses such as yellow fever and Japanese encephalitis virus have caused major epidemics in Africa and Asia, respectively. The latter disease has also moved into areas where it was previously unknown.

DISEASE TRANSMISSION BY MAJOR INSECT GROUPS

FLEAS (ORDER SIPHONAPTERA)

Biology. Fleas make up the order Siphonaptera. The adults are small, wingless, laterally flattened, obligate bloodsuckers that parasitize a wide variety of vertebrate hosts (Fig. 114–11). The larvae are normally free living, legless, eyeless, and wormlike. They generally live in the nest or habitat of the host and feed on organic matter. There are over 2000 species of fleas, with representatives on all continents, including the Arctic and Antarctic. The majority (94%) of species parasitize mammals, with the remainder parasitizing birds. Only a relatively few species are of importance in transmitting disease to humans (Table 113–2 and Fig. 110–1).

The developmental cycle of fleas from egg to adult normally takes place in the nest of the host. Eggs are generally laid in the nest, where the elongate larvae feed on organic material such as scales, dried blood, and feces deposited by the adults. After 2 to 3 weeks, the fully grown larvae spin a cocoon and pupate. The pupal stage may last from 1 to 2 weeks, after which the adult emerges, often after the stimulus of movement or vibration caused when a host enters the nest. The entire period of development may last 3 to 4 weeks or longer, depending on temperature in the nest. The larvae require high humidity.

Most fleas are not strictly host specific and therefore attempt to feed on almost any animal. Adults can go without feeding for considerable periods, which allows them to search for new hosts after the nest has been vacated or the hosts have died.

Disease Transmission. Fleas are important natural vectors of 2 diseases of humans—plague and murine typhus. In addition, they have been implicated as, but not proved to be, vectors of a variety of other diseases such as tularemia, pseudotuberculosis, erysipeloid, hemorrhagic nephrosonephritis, boutonneuse fever, and Q fever and are known intermediate hosts for at least 2 tapeworms (Table 113–2).

Plague. Caused by *Yersinia pestis,* plague is a typical zoonosis of rodents and small mammals that exists in much of the world in a flea-rodent-flea transmission cycle (Chapter 47). Large epidemics of plague, which in the past caused millions of deaths, no longer occur. However, sporadic human cases continue to occur each year in many parts of the world where plague exists in

TABLE 113–2. Important Species of Fleas That Transmit Human Diseases

Flea	Principal Host	Geographic Distribution	Diseases
Xenopsylla cheopis	Rats	Tropicopolitan	Plague, murine typhus, rat tapeworm
X. brasiliensis	Rats	Africa, South America, India	Plague
X. astia	Rats	Asia	Plague
Nosopsyllus fasciatus	Rats, mice, swine, domestic animals	Europe, North America	Plague, murine typhus, rat tapeworm
Pulex irritans	Humans, domestic animals	Cosmopolitan	Plague
P. simulans	Humans	North and South America	Plague
Leptopsylla segnis	Rats, mice	Cosmopolitan	Plague, murine typhus
Ctenocephalides canis	Dogs, cats	Cosmopolitan	Dog tapeworm
C. felis felis	Dogs, cats	Cosmopolitan	Dog tapeworm
Diamanus montanus	Ground squirrels	Western United States, Mexico	Plague

enzootic foci. This is called sylvatic or rural plague and is maintained in nature by over 200 species of rodents that are known hosts of plague bacilli and by many species of fleas that normally feed on these rodents. People become involved accidentally when they invade the plague focus, usually for hunting, trapping, or recreational purposes.

Occasionally, epidemics still occur. For example, in Kenya, after an absence of plague for 10 years, 166 cases with 9 deaths were reported in 1978. Factors responsible for periodic epizootics and/or epidemics are not well understood and are peculiar to each natural plague focus.

Urban plague usually occurs during the course of an epizootic when commensal rodents become involved. The infection is then maintained in the urban rat population by several species of fleas that parasitize these rodents (Table 113–2). Humans may become involved when urban rats begin to die of plague and infected fleas search for new hosts (Fig. 110–1).

Transmission of plague by fleas can occur in several ways, most importantly by the bite of an infected flea. Fleas become infected by ingesting plague bacilli with the blood meal taken from a rodent with bacteremia. The bacteria undergo multiplication in the stomach of the flea and frequently move forward to the proventriculus, resulting in partial or complete blockage. Fleas with a blocked proventriculus can take blood only with difficulty and frequently regurgitate in an attempt to get blood past the blocked area. In the process, plague bacilli are inoculated into the host. Because of the difficulty in getting blood past the proventricular obstruction, infected fleas become starved and biting frequency increases, making these fleas important in transmission. Factors that influence proventricular blockage include strain of pathogen, species of flea, temperature, and type of blood ingested.

Although it is a less important means of transmission, fleas have also been known to transmit plague bacilli in their feces. In this case, the organism is rubbed into the bite wound, other skin abrasions, or mucous membranes. Transmission has also been reported when infected fleas are crushed between the teeth. Finally, pneumonic plague is transmitted from person to person by aerosol.

Murine Typhus. Murine or flea-borne typhus is a rodent zoonosis caused by *Rickettsia typhi (mooseri)* (Chapter 23.2). This is a disease primarily of rats and mice and has a worldwide distribution, mainly in the tropics. Clinically, it is similar to epidemic or louse-borne typhus, but somewhat milder. The rash is the same.

The infection is maintained in nature by a rat-flea-rat cycle. The usual vertebrate reservoirs are *Rattus rattus* and *R. norvegicus,* and the principal insect vector is the tropical rat flea *Xenopsylla cheopis,* although other species of fleas can become infected (Table 113–2).

Humans become infected incidentally by a flea that has strayed from its host. Rickettsiae are ingested by the flea with a blood meal from an infected rat. The organisms multiply within the gut and are passed in the feces of the flea. The mechanism of transmission is by rubbing infected feces into skin abrasions or by transfer to mucous membranes. Transmission may also occur by inhalation of dust contaminated with infected flea feces.

Cestode Infections. In addition to serving as vectors, fleas also act as intermediate hosts for at least 2 tapeworms that may infect humans, *Dipylidium caninum* of dogs (Chapter 100.4) and *Hymenolepis diminuta* of rats (Chapter 100.3). Eggs of both parasites are passed in the feces of their respective vertebrate hosts and are ingested by larval fleas feeding on detritus in the nest. They hatch, and the cysticeroids develop in the body cavity of the immature flea. The adult flea is thus infected at the time of emergence from the pupa, and transmission occurs when the flea is ingested or crushed between the teeth of a dog, rat, or person.

The dog and cat fleas, *Ctenocephalides canis* and *C. felis,* are the most important intermediate hosts of *D. caninum,* whereas *X. cheopis* and *Nosophyllus fasciatus* are important intermediate hosts for *H. diminuta* (Table 113–2).

SUCKING LICE (ORDER ANOPLURA)

Biology. Sucking lice are small, wingless, obligate ectoparasites of mammals belonging to the order Anoplura. The body is flattened, and the legs, in part, are adapted for clinging to hairs and feathers. Most species are very host specific, and the entire life cycle is spent on one host.

There are about 225 species of Anoplura, but only 3 are parasites of humans. These are the human body louse, *Pediculus humanus corporis* (Fig. 114–1); the head louse, *P. humanus capitis;* and the crab or pubic louse, *Phthirus pubis* (Fig. 114–2). All have a worldwide distribution.

The life cycle of all 3 species is incomplete, takes about 3 weeks, and is completed on the human host. The head and crab lice glue their eggs to hairs, whereas the body louse lays eggs in the seams of clothing.

Disease Transmission. Only the body louse is of known importance in the transmission of human disease. This species lives in the clothing of humans, where it makes close contact with the skin. Heavy infestations of up to 10,000 lice can build up on individuals during cold months and times of poor hygiene. In general, all louse-borne diseases described in the following sections require the same epidemiologic conditions and are seen only when conditions are favorable for maintenance of large louse populations.

There has been considerable discussion in the popular press about insect transmission of acquired immunodeficiency syndrome (AIDS) or human immunodeficiency virus (HIV), including speculation about lice. Although no field or experimental work has been done to implicate lice in transmission, it is generally agreed that this insect should be investigated. Both head and pubic lice are common in areas where AIDS is prevalent. Of interest is that pubic lice are only found on adult humans and are transmitted from person to person during intimate sexual contact. Both species have biologic and behavioral characteristics that would allow transmission either mechanically or biologically.

Epidemic (Louse-Borne) Typhus. Epidemic typhus is caused by *Rickettsia prowazekii* (Chapter 23.1). The disease has a wide distribution in Europe, Africa, Asia, and the Western Hemisphere. Large epidemics are generally associated with cooler temperatures during times of war, famine, and natural disasters where people are crowded together in conditions of poor sanitation and hygiene.

Epidemic typhus has a human-louse-human cycle. A person is usually infectious for the lice during the febrile period, and lice become infected when taking a blood meal at that time. The rickettsiae enter the epithelial cells of the midgut and multiply to such an extent that the cells rupture in 3 to 5 days, releasing large numbers of rickettsiae into the lumen of the intestine, from which they are then passed in the feces of the louse. People become infected when infectious feces are rubbed into abrasions of the skin caused by scratching or into mucous membranes. Less commonly, infectious rickettsiae can be released from lice by crushing. Lice feces may dry in the clothing and can remain infectious for 60 to 90 days. As a result, the feces may become airborne, causing transmission by inhalation. Transmission of *R. prowazekii* does not occur by the bite of lice.

Epidemic transmission of louse-borne typhus is facilitated by the fact that lice are sensitive to changes in temperature. They immediately abandon hosts with high fevers and those who have died, seeking out other hosts and thus transferring the infection with them. Unlike many insect-borne diseases, *R. prowazekii* infection is also fatal to the lice, which eventually succumb to the damage caused by ruptured midgut epithelial cells.

Humans are apparently the principal reservoir of *R. prowazekii*. Asymptomatic carriers of the agent may remain infective to lice for many years and thus may provide sources of infection in areas where the rickettsiae have been absent. Another characteristic of louse-borne typhus is that it has a tendency to recrudesce, producing a disease known as Brill-Zinsser disease as many as 50 years after the initial infection. Evidence suggests that certain tree squirrels in Virginia may also be reservoir hosts of *R. prowezekii*.

Trench Fever. Trench fever is caused by *Rickettsia quintana*. It takes its name from the trenches of World War I, where it was first described and where it was a major problem. It was reported again in Eastern Europe during World War II. Trench fever has been reported from Europe, Africa, Mexico, and Central and South America but is an uncommon disease today (Chapter 27.1).

Lice become infected with *R. quintana* when taking a blood meal from an infective person. The rickettsiae do not enter the midgut epithelial cells but, rather, multiply in the lumen of the louse intestine. As a result, this infection is not fatal to the lice. Like epidemic typhus, however, transmission to humans is via infected louse feces, with the rickettsiae entering the body through abrasions in the skin or mucous membranes or by inhalation.

Epidemic (Louse-Borne) Relapsing Fever. Epidemic, or louse-borne, relapsing fever is caused by a spirochete, *Borrelia recurrentis* (Chapter 34). There are a variety of other species of *Borrelia* associated with certain species of soft ticks that cause endemic, or tick-borne, relapsing fever. It is likely that *B. recurrentis* originated from one of the tick-borne strains of *Borrelia,* because some of these can infect and be transmitted by lice.

Relapsing fever has been known clinically since the days of Hippocrates, who called it ardent fever. It has a worldwide distribution in its various forms, but *B. recurrentis*, once widespread, now appears to be limited primarily to East Africa.

Transmission of epidemic relapsing fever is strictly by a human-louse-human cycle. Lice become infected by taking a blood meal from an infected person. The spirochetes enter the hemocoel of the louse and multiply there instead of in the intestine. Transmission occurs only when an infected louse is crushed, releasing infective spirochetes, which may then enter the human host via skin abrasions or mucous membranes. In some areas, lice are frequently crushed with the teeth, resulting in transmission. The louse feces are not infective. Because *B. recurrentis* can be transmitted only by crushing infected lice, large louse populations are required before epidemic transmission can occur.

BUGS (ORDER HEMIPTERA). Medically important bugs belong to 2 families in the order Hemiptera. These are the families Cimicidae (bedbugs) and Reduviidae (triatome bugs). Members of the order Hemiptera are the true bugs and are recognized by the characteristic forewing, the basal half of which is membranous. The mouth parts are of the piercing-sucking type and are segmented. The proboscis is attached anteriorly and is kept folded back between the coxae of the first pair of legs. The life cycle is simple, with all instars requiring a meal of blood, hemolymph, or plant juices, depending on whether the species is hematophagous, predaceous on other insects, or phytophagous.

Family Cimicidae (Bedbugs). Of the many species of bedbugs that are obligate ectoparasites primarily of birds, poultry, and bats, only 2 are parasites of humans.

These are *Cimex lectularius,* the common bedbug, and *C. hemipterus,* the tropical bedbug (Figs. 113–1 and 114–10). The former has a cosmopolitan distribution but is more common in temperate regions, whereas the latter has a wide distribution in the tropics.

Disease Transmission. Bedbugs meet all the criteria for human disease transmission, i.e., they are obligate bloodsucking parasites that have close and frequent contact with humans. They are most commonly found in hotels and public places such as transportation terminals, where they have contact with many different hosts. Experimentally, they become infected with a variety of pathogens, but to date, they have not been incriminated in transmission of any human disease. Work has shown that the swallow bug, *Oeciacus vicarius,* is a vector of Fort Morgan virus in swallows in the western United States. Mechanical transmission of hepatitis B virus by *C. lectularis* has been demonstrated experimentally. Considering the epidemiology of hepatitis B virus in the tropics, the stability of the virus outside the host, the high viremia levels associated with this infection in humans, and the biting habits of bedbugs, it is possible that bedbugs play a role as mechanical vectors of this virus. The bedbug has been considered as a possible vector of AIDS virus (HIV). Experimental studies in at least two laboratories, however, have shown that HIV does not replicate in bedbug tissues and that mechanical transmission is unlikely. Moreover, HIV has not been detected in the feces of bedbugs, making it unlikely that transmission could occur by scratching fecal material into the bite wound.

Family Reduviidae (Triatome Bugs)

Biology. The family Reduviidae consists of a large number of species that are primarily entomophagous and thus feed on other insects (assassin bugs). One predominantly American subfamily, Triatominae, feeds only on the blood of a variety of vertebrate animals, including humans.

The triatome bugs are relatively large (1 to 4 cm) and can be recognized by the elongate, cylindrical, or cone-shaped head bearing a pair of long 4-segment antennae situated apically and bulging compound eyes situated laterally (Fig. 114–9). The proboscis, consisting of 3 segmented mouth parts, is carried flexed beneath the head, projecting posteriorly when at rest but projecting forward when feeding.

Most species of bugs are sylvatic and live in close association with a variety of wild animals, e.g., armadillos, opossums, mice, rats, bats, and squirrels. Others live in close association with humans and their domestic animals. The bugs usually lay their eggs in or near the habitation of the host. The eggs hatch in 10 to 30 days, depending on the temperature and species. The life cycle is incomplete with 5 nymphal instars, each requiring a blood meal before molting occurs. There is usually only 1 generation per year. Overwintering can occur in any stage, depending on the species. The adults can fly considerable distances in search of new hosts. The nymphs cannot fly.

Disease Transmission

CHAGAS' DISEASE (AMERICAN TRYPANOSOMIASIS). The etiologic agent of Chagas' disease is a protozoan, *Trypanosoma cruzi.* This is a disease only of the American tropics and subtropics, with a wide distribution in South and Central America. It occurs sporadically in the southwestern United States (Chapter 75).

The bugs become infected with *T. cruzi* when they take a blood meal from a person or from a reservoir host with parasitemia. They may also become infected by cannibalism. The trypanosomes remain in the gut of the bugs and develop into infective metacyclic forms in 7 to 14 days. The infective trypanosomes are located in the hindgut and are passed in the feces. Transmission is usually associated with the bite of the bug, which often takes 10 to 20 minutes to engorge and frequently defecates during or shortly after the feeding process. Infection of the new host is usually accomplished by scratching the infective trypanosomes into the bite wound or into other skin abrasions or, most commonly, by transferring the agents on fingers to the highly receptive conjunctiva of the eye or to the mucosa of the mouth or nose.

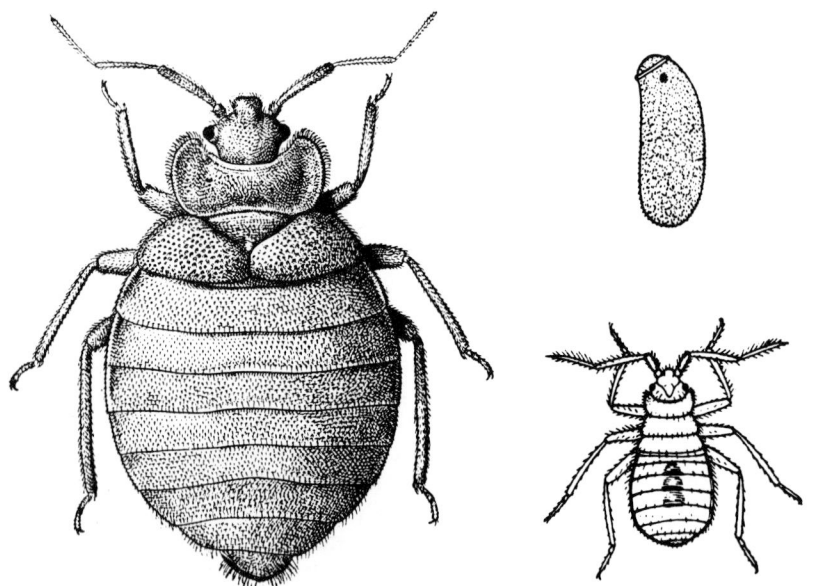

FIGURE 113–1. The bedbug. *Cimex lectularius–* egg, nymph, and adult. (Courtesy of the Wellcome Foundation.)

TABLE 113–3. Important Species of Known Triatome Vectors of Human American Trypanosomiasis

Species	Geographic Distribution
Panstrongylus megistus	Brazil
Rhodnius prolixus	Venezuela, Colombia, Central America
R. pallescens	Panama
Triatoma maculata	Venezuela, Colombia
T. infestans	Southern Brazil, Uruguay, Chile, Paraguay, Argentina, Bolivia
T. dimidiata	Central America, Mexico
T. barberi	Mexico

There are many species of triatome bugs that are susceptible to infection by *T. cruzi,* and over half of these species from the Americas have been found naturally infected. However, relatively few species are associated with people and their domestic animals, an essential condition for efficient transmission of this parasite. Those known to be vectors of human infection are listed in Table 113–3.

Factors that influence the evolution of domesticity on the part of triatome bugs include physiologic and ecologic adaptability of the insects, availability of alternate hosts (domestic animals), climate, and location and type of construction of houses. The last is important, because the bugs are nocturnal and seek out cracks and crevices for hiding during the day. The triatomes that are most highly domesticated are associated with poorly constructed houses that provide adequate daytime resting places.

Trypanosoma rangeli INFECTION. *Trypanosoma rangeli* is another parasite of humans and other mammals transmitted by triatome bugs. It is often found in the same areas as *T. cruzi,* and because of similar morphology in both human and insect stages, it may cause some confusion. However, it is apparently nonpathogenic to humans (Chapter 75.1). *Rhodnius prolixus* is the most important vector of *T. rangeli,* but unlike the case with *T. cruzi,* development in the insect occurs in the hemolymph after a period in the gut. The infective trypomastigotes eventually invade the salivary glands, and transmission occurs through the bite of the triatome.

FLIES (ORDER DIPTERA)

Biology. The flies constitute the largest and single most important group of insects that cause or transmit human disease. They make up the order Diptera, which is characterized by having only 1 pair of wings instead of 2 like most other insects. The second pair of wings are called halters, small knob-like structures situated behind the functional wings and used for stability during flight. Most species have large compound eyes and 3 simple eyes, or ocelli, arranged in a triangular formation at the top of the head. Mouth parts are always of the sucking type, having undergone considerable evolution in the bloodsucking or hematophagous groups, with stylets used for piercing or lacerating the flesh of animals.

All Diptera undergo a complete metamorphosis with egg, larval, pupal, and adult stages. Eggs, depending on the species, are laid in a variety of places, including all types of water, decaying vegetation, soil, feces, and both dead and live animal tissues. The term myiasis is given to the invasion of human and animal tissues by fly larvae (Chapter 105.2)

Systematics. It is convenient to divide the large number of species of the order Diptera into smaller groups of more closely related species (Table 113–4). The most commonly used classification divides the Diptera into 3 suborders. The Nematocera are the most primitive and are most important medically. This suborder includes the midges, gnats, sandflies, black flies, and mosquitoes, and all members are characterized by a simple filamentous type of antennae, represented by the Culicidae in Figure 113–2. Only the females of Nematocera are hematophagous; the males feed on nectars and other plant juices. The suborder Brachycera are generally large flies and include the medically important horseflies and deer flies (family Tabanidae). This suborder is characterized by shorter 3-segment antennae, the last segment of which is largest and may be annulated (Fig. 113–2). The last suborder, Cyclorrhapha, includes the higher Diptera. Members of this suborder are generally what most laypersons consider to be flies and include houseflies, stable flies, blowflies, and tsetse flies. They are characterized by having short 3-segment antennae, the last segment of which bears a bristle called the arista, as represented by the Muscidae in Figure 113–2. The larvae of Cyclorrhapha are headless, usually having a pair of mouth hooks in the head's place.

Family Ceratopogonidae (Biting Midges)

Biology. The biting midges are among the smallest hematophagous flies (Fig. 114–16). There are approximately 50 genera of Ceratopogonidae, of which only 4—*Culicoides, Forcipomyia, Leptoconops,* and *Austroconops*—feed on humans and other vertebrates and are therefore of medical importance. *Culicoides* is by far the most important genus and is the only one incriminated in disease transmission to humans.

Ceratopogonids have worldwide distribution, with over 800 species described. Most species lay their eggs in batches in mud, wet soil, decaying leaves or other vegetation, manure, rotting banana stumps, or similar sites. The eggs usually hatch within a week or 10 days. The larvae, which may be aquatic or terrestrial, develop to the pupal stage in 2 to 3 weeks, feeding on a variety of decaying organic debris. There are 4 larval instars. The pupal stage usually lasts 3 to 4 days but may last as long as 10 days. In temperate regions, ceratopogonids may overwinter in the egg or larval stages, depending on the species.

TABLE 113–4. Taxonomic Subdivisions of Medically Important Diptera

Suborder	Family	Common Name
Nematocera	Ceratopogonidae	Biting midges, gnats
	Psychodidae	Sandflies
	Simuliidae	Black flies
	Culicidae	Mosquitoes
Brachycera	Tabanidae	Horseflies, deer flies
	Rhagionidae	Snipe flies
	Athericidae	Athericids
Cyclorrhapha	Glossinidae	Tsetse flies
	Muscidae	Houseflies, stable flies, face flies
	Calliphoridae	Blowflies
	Sarcophagidae	Blowflies
	Chloropidae	Eye gnats

ANTENNAE OF DIPTERA

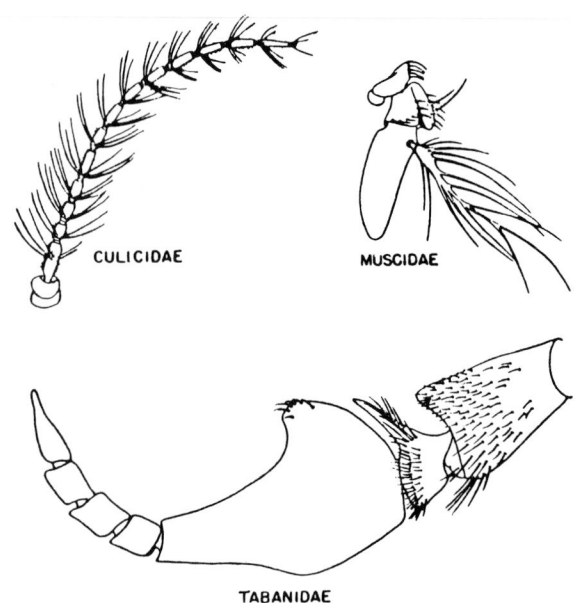

CULICIDAE

MUSCIDAE

TABANIDAE

FIGURE 113–2. Types of antennae of the suborders of Diptera: Nematocera (Culicidae). Brachycera (Tabanidae), and Cyclorrhapha (Muscidae).

The adults feed on plant juices and nectars, and females also require blood. They frequently occur in swarms, biting around the head and other unprotected parts of the body. The blood-feeding periodicity varies with the species. Many feed throughout the day, some feed in the early evening and night, and others feed primarily during early morning hours. Most species are exophilic and are not strong fliers, and adults remain within the vicinity of the breeding sites.

Disease Transmission. Ceratopogonidae are generally not important vectors of human disease. Although they are vectors of a variety of animal filariae, protozoa, and arboviruses, few of these are pathogens of humans.

VIRUSES. Ceratopogonids are documented vectors of arboviruses of animals such as blue tongue. A total of 34 viruses have been isolated from *Culicoides* sp. Only recently, however, has there been evidence that these flies transmitted a viral disease of humans. Oropouche virus has been recognized as a major cause of febrile illness in Brazil, with periodic epidemics occurring in the Amazon region. This virus apparently exists in a sylvatic cycle with primates and sloths as the vertebrate hosts. The sylvatic vector is unknown. Epidemiologic evidence during recent epidemics suggested that *Culicoides paraensis* was involved in urban transmission of this virus. Successful experimental transmission of oropouche virus by this species has now been documented.

FILARIAL INFECTIONS. Flies of the genus *Culicoides* are the principal vectors of 3 filarial parasites of humans. *Mansonella ozzardi* occurs in Central and South America and some Caribbean islands. The principal vector is *C. furens.* Filariae that are indistinguishable from *M. ozzardi* have also been described from *Simulium* (black flies) in Africa. *Mansonella perstans* is a common filarial parasite of humans in tropical Africa and certain coun-

tries of South America. It is transmitted by *C. grahami* and *C. milnei (austeni)* in Africa and by other *Culicoides* species in the Americas. A third filarial parasite, *Mansonella streptocerca,* occurs primarily in West and Central Africa and is also transmitted by *C. grahami* and *C. milnei.*

All 3 of the aforementioned filarial parasites are generally considered nonpathogenic to their human host. They are essentially nonperiodic, with the microfilariae present in the peripheral blood at all times of the day. Microfilariae ingested with the blood meal invade the thoracic muscles of the fly and undergo 2 molts to become active third-stage larvae in 10 to 12 days. These infective larvae eventually migrate to the head and are deposited on the skin of humans when the midge takes a subsequent blood meal.

Family Psychodidae (Sandflies)

Biology. The family Psychodidae contains 1 major subfamily, Phlebotominae, which is important in human disease transmission (Fig. 114–7). There are over 600 species in the subfamily, but most of the important vectors of human pathogens belong to 3 genera. *Phlebotomus* is an Old World genus containing many important vectors of leishmaniasis and the phlebotomus fever group of viruses. *Sergentomyia* is also an Old World genus but is less important in the transmission of human disease. The genus *Lutzomyia* is found only in the Western Hemisphere.

Phlebotomine sandflies lay their eggs in small batches in protected places with high humidity and a high content of organic matter. Examples are cracks in walls, rodent burrows, tree buttresses, and under dead leaves on the forest floor. Depending on the temperature, the eggs hatch in 6 to 17 days or longer. The larvae are scavengers and feed on a variety of organic matter. There are 4 instars, and larval development may last 3 to 6 weeks. The pupal stage may last another 8 to 10 days, and the entire life cycle requires from 5 to 12 weeks. In temperate regions, the flies overwinter in the larval stage.

Only females suck blood, which is taken from a variety of vertebrate animals, including amphibians, reptiles, and mammals. The genera *Phlebotomus* and *Lutzomyia* most commonly feed on humans. Most species are nocturnal feeders, but some may feed during the day in dark rooms or in forests on dark days. Phlebotomine sandflies are weak fliers; they rarely fly more than a few meters from their breeding sites. Most fly in short hopping motions and can be repelled with the use of a good fan.

Disease Transmission. Phlebotomine sandflies are important vectors of *Leishmania*, the phlebotomous fever group of arboviruses, and bartonellosis.

LEISHMANIASIS. Leishmaniasis is a disease of man caused by species of *Leishmania* that are natural parasites of a variety of animals, both wild and domestic. *L. donovani* causes visceral leishmaniasis or kala-azar; *L. tropica* causes oriental sore; and *L. braziliensis* causes different types of mucocutaneous leishmaniasis. The type of disease, parasite, geographic distribution, reservoir hosts, and principal phlebotomine sandfly vectors are presented in Table 76–1. It will be noted that leishmaniasis is primarily a zoonosis, although there are some areas of the world, e.g., India, where there is no known reservoir host and the parasite is thought to exist in a human-sandfly-human cycle.

The principal mode of transmission of leishmaniasis is by the bite of infective sandflies. The amastigote stage of *Leishmania* is found in macrophages of the host and ingested when the sandfly takes a blood meal. The amastigotes are released from the cells into the lumen of the sandfly gut, where they elongate and become promastigotes, which then multiply in the insect intestine by asexual reproduction. These infective promastigotes eventually move forward to the esophagus and mouth parts of the sandfly and are injected into a new host when a subsequent blood meal is taken. The injected promastigotes are then phagocytized by macrophages of the new human host. The salivary glands of sandflies are not involved in the transmission of leishmaniasis.

SANDFLY FEVER. Sandfly fever (phlebotomus or papatasi fever) is caused by arboviruses belonging to the genus *Phlebovirus,* family Bunyaviridae (Chapter 20.11). Natural hosts for these viruses probably include a variety of rodents and wild animals, but 7 viruses have been isolated from humans or have been implicated in causing disease in humans. These include SF-Naples and SF-Sicily, the original sandfly fever viruses that are transmitted by phlebotomine sandflies. Two other viruses, Chagres and Punta Toro, have been isolated from both humans and sandflies in Panama and are probably arboviruses. A fifth member of this virus group has been isolated in Brazil from persons with an illness compatible with sandfly fever, but the vector is not known.

SF-Naples and SF-Sicily viruses are the most widespread; isolation records suggest that they are endemic around the Mediterranean, the Middle East, central Asia, and the Indian subcontinent, in arid areas that have suitable breeding habitats for phlebotomine sandflies. The disease is generally mild in endemic areas. Epidemics usually occur only when a large population of susceptible individuals, such as an army, moves into the endemic area. Transmission generally occurs during the spring and summer months in the northern latitudes. *Phlebotomus papatasi* is the principal vector in most endemic areas, although the Naples virus has also been isolated from flies of the genus *Sergentomyia*. The sandflies become infected while taking a blood meal from a viremic animal or person, usually in the first 4 days of illness. The extrinsic incubation period has been shown to be as short as 7 days but probably is 10 to 14 days, depending on the temperature.

The viruses have been isolated from male sandflies of the genera *Phlebotomus* and *Sergentomyia* that were collected in endemic areas. This, plus experimental work, suggests that the viruses are transmitted transovarially from the female fly to her offspring, thus making the flies reservoir hosts. There is suggestive epidemiologic evidence that this mechanism is important in the maintenance of the viruses in nature.

The phlebotomine sandflies also are important vectors of other arboviruses in Central and South America. Six viruses of the Changuinola group (family Reoviridae, genus *Orbivirus*) have been isolated from sandflies, and

one of these, Changuinola, has also been isolated from humans. Serologic evidence suggests that some of the other viruses of this group also infect humans, although illness associated with these viruses is not known. A total of 42 viruses belonging to 7 antigenic groups have been isolated from phlebotomine sandflies.

BARTONELLOSIS. Bartonellosis (Chapter 51) is caused by a bacterium, *Bartonella bacilliformis,* and is a disease of humans in the mountainous areas of Peru, Ecuador, and Colombia. The disease has 2 forms—the highly fatal visceral form known as *Oroya fever* and the milder cutaneous form known as *verruga peruana*. There are no other known hosts of this bacterium, and because it can be isolated from asymptomatic individuals, humans are the likely reservoir host.

Bartonellosis is transmitted by sandflies of the genus *Lutzomyia*. *L. verrucarum* is the principal vector throughout its geographic range. Other species are also probably involved, but the mechanism of transmission has not been well studied. The bacteria are associated with the red blood cells of the host and are ingested when the fly takes a blood meal. It is not known whether multiplication occurs in the fly or whether transmission occurs as a result of proboscis contamination.

Family Simuliidae (Black Flies)

Biology. The Simuliidae are small, stout-bodied, humped-back flies, and more than 1300 species have been described worldwide (Fig. 114–15). They are fierce biters and, in addition to disease transmission, are important as pests in many areas of the world, especially in temperate regions, where they occur in large swarms (Chapter 105.2).

The breeding habitat of all known species is flowing water, usually a river or stream. Fast-flowing "white" water is preferred by many species, whereas others prefer slow-moving water. In either case, female flies deposit masses of eggs just below the waterline on objects protruding from the water. Frequently, female flies are attracted to small sections of the stream for oviposition, resulting in a concentration of large numbers of larvae in a small area. The eggs hatch within a few days, and larvae attach to objects in the water by means of a posterior sucker. There are 6 to 8 larval instars, which may last 7 to 14 days. Pupation takes 2 to 6 days, and adults emerge to the water surface in protective bubbles of gas.

Adults are strong fliers and may travel considerable distances from the breeding site in search of a blood meal. Only the female fly feeds on blood, and most species are zoophilic. Of the 12 or more genera described, only 3 are important in human disease transmission, mainly because of their human-biting habits. These are *Simulium, Prosimulium,* and *Austrosimulium,* the first being the most important.

Disease Transmission. The black flies are important vectors of only 1 major human disease, onchocerciasis, but are also important vectors of both protozoan and filarial infections of animals. In addition, they are important pest insects over much of their geographic range.

ONCHOCERCIASIS. Onchocerciasis, or river blindness, is caused by the filarial worm, *Onchocerca volvulus,* and is characterized by 3 cardinal features: subcutaneous nodules containing adult worms, pruritic dermatitis, and blindness (Chapter 87). It occurs in tropical Africa and in South and Central America and affects an estimated 40 million people. In some savanna areas of West Africa, blindness due to onchocerciasis affects the majority of older adults in entire villages.

The adult worms live in the skin and subcutaneous tissue of humans. They produce microfilariae that migrate throughout the body, primarily in the skin. Black flies, being pool feeders, tear or cut the skin of the host to rupture the blood vessels. Microfilariae are ingested with the blood meal, penetrate the gut wall, and migrate to the thoracic muscles (Fig. 87–5). They enter the muscle cells and develop to third-stage infective larvae over a period of 7 to 14 days. The infective larvae break out of the muscle cells, migrate to the head and proboscis of the fly, and escape onto the skin when a subsequent blood meal is taken. They enter the human host, generally through the bite wound, and develop to the adult stage.

The localization of the subcutaneous nodules (onchocercomas) containing adult worms varies with geographic region and with the species of black fly vector. In Africa, where members of the *Simulium damnosum* complex are the principal vectors (Fig. 87–3), nodules are localized in the lower parts of the body, primarily around the pelvis and, occasionally, on the lower legs. In Venezuela, the onchocercomas are also located on the lower part of the body. Both *S. metallicum*, the principal vector in Venezuela, and *S. damnosum* prefer to feed on the lower part of the body. In Central America, however, nodules are primarily on the upper part of the body, and the principal vector, *S. ochraceum*, also feeds on the upper part of the body. This species breeds in streams at relatively high altitudes (1000 to 1500 m), and persons there, e.g., coffee plantation workers, generally are well covered, in contrast to people in Africa, who usually wear less clothing.

Table 113–5 lists the major black fly vector species and their distribution. The *S. damnosum* complex now consists of 9 sibling species, the distribution of which closely coincides with the distribution of onchocerciasis in West and Central Africa. The *S. neavei* group has 9 species, but only 3, *S. neavei, S. woodi,* and *S. ethiopiense* are important vectors. *S. neavei* and *S. woodi* have an interesting biology in that they have an obligatory phoretic relationship with river crabs, with the larvae and pupae completing development while attached to the crabs.

Family Culicidae (Mosquitoes). Mosquitoes are by far the most important group of insects in terms of human disease transmission; more people die each year from mosquito-borne diseases than from any other single cause. There are over 3000 described species in 34 genera, but only relatively few are important in disease transmission. The most important genera, *Aedes, Culex,* and *Anopheles,* contain vector species for viruses, protozoa, and filariae of humans. Diseases transmitted by mosquitoes are worldwide and affect millions of people each year.

Biology. Mosquitoes belong to the family Culicidae, suborder Nematocera. Taxonomically, the family is bro-

TABLE 113–5. Principal Onchocerciasis Vector Species of *Simulium* and Their Geographic Distribution

Species	Geographic Distribution
S. damnosum Group	
S. damnosum	Widespread in West, Central, East, and South Africa
S. sirbanum	Mali, Ivory Coast, Guinea, Burkina Faso, Ghana, Nigeria
S. sudanense	Mali, Ivory Coast, Guinea, Burkina Faso, Ghana, Nigeria
S. squamosum	Cameroon, Burkina Faso, Ivory Coast
S. soubrense	Benin, Guinea, Ivory Coast, Liberia
S. sanctipauli	Ivory Coast, Liberia
S. yahense	Guinea, Ivory Coast, Liberia
S. kilibanum	Burundi, Zaire, Tanzania, Uganda
S. dieguerense	Mali
S. neavei Group	
S. neavei	Angola, Zaire, Uganda, Kenya
S. woodi	Malawi, Tanzania
S. ethiopiense	Ethiopia
S. ochraceum	Bolivia, Colombia, Ecuador, Guatemala, southern Mexico, Panama
S. metallicum	Widespread in Central, North, and South America
S. callidum	Colombia, Guatemala, Mexico
S. exiquum	Colombia, Ecuador, Venezuela
S. gulanense	Venezuela, Brazil

ken into 3 subfamilies: Toxorhynchitinae, large non-blood-feeding mosquitoes; Anophelinae, the anopheline mosquitoes that transmit malaria (Fig. 114–4); and the Culicinae, by far the largest subfamily with 30 genera (Fig. 114–6).

Most mosquitoes are small and slender (Fig. 113–3) and may vary in color from a drab brown to black and white to metallic colors. They inhabit nearly every part of the globe, being limited only by the availability of breeding sites. All species are aquatic in the larval stage. Some breed in tundra or alpine pools, others in collections of water in desert areas, and still others in nearly all conceivable natural and artificial containers holding water in between these two environmental extremes.

The majority of adult female mosquitoes are obligate bloodsuckers, requiring blood to develop their eggs. Both sexes feed on plant juices and nectars. Some species have evolved the capability of developing the first batch of eggs without a blood meal (autogenous development), an obviously advantageous survival mechanism. Animals that provide blood for mosquitoes include all major groups, e.g., fish, amphibians, reptiles, birds, and mammals. Many species of mosquito have evolved strict host requirements and feed only on a certain group of animals. Others have broader host ranges and feed on a variety of animals, including humans. Those that feed exclusively on animals are called *zoophilic,* whereas those that prefer to feed on humans are called *anthropophilic.* The degree of anthropophilic behavior in zoophilic species is a major factor in human disease transmission because it allows for the transfer of animal diseases to humans (zoonoses).

After the adult female has taken a blood meal, eggs begin to develop, and within 3 to 7 days she seeks a breeding site, which is generally quite specific to the species. Eggs, laid individually or in batches, may be deposited directly on the water, just above the waterline,

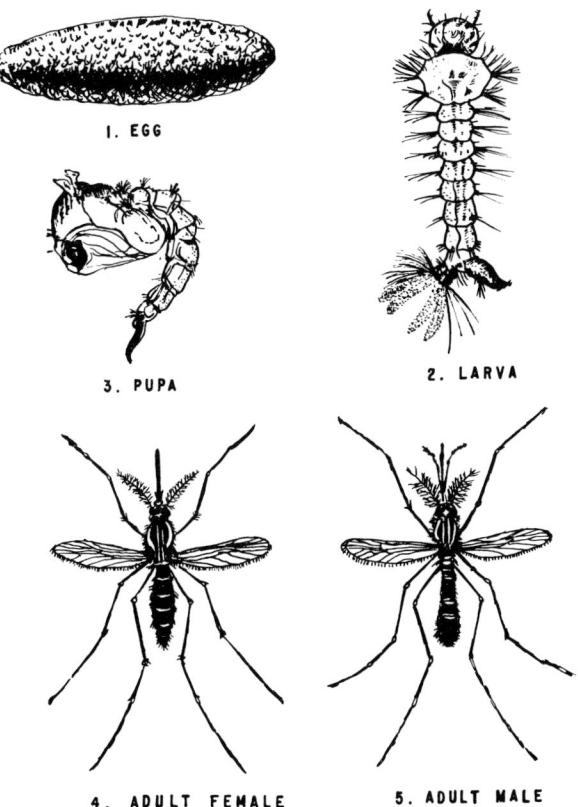

FIGURE 113–3. The yellow fever mosquito. *Aedes aegypti.*

or in damp soil on a flood plain. Hatching usually occurs in 24 to 72 hours after contact with water, and first-stage larvae emerge. There are 4 larval stages, with the larvae feeding on a variety of microorganisms in the water. Pupation occurs in 5 to 14 or more days, and the adults emerge 2 to 5 days later, depending on the species and environmental conditions. The newly emerged adults usually mate and begin to feed. If hosts are available, most female mosquitoes take their first blood meal within 1 to 4 days of emergence. Adult mosquitoes have survived in the laboratory for over 4 months, but in nature, they are generally short lived, with the majority not surviving the 10- to 14-day extrinsic incubation period required for transmission of most pathogens. Survival obviously depends on the species and environmental conditions.

In temperate regions, mosquitoes overwinter in the egg, larval, or adult stage, depending on the species. Depending on the location, there may be one generation per year (tundra), or there may be a new generation every 10 to 14 days (tropics). In temperate regions, the cycle usually continues as soon as the ice melts; adult blood-feeding mosquitoes are usually present from about March to October. In the tropics, mosquitoes are present year round, but in some areas where the dry season is extended, mosquitoes may estivate as adults or in the egg stage.

Disease Transmission

VIRUSES. At least 265 viruses have been isolated from mosquitoes, mostly from culicines. Of these, 109 have also been isolated from humans, and there is serologic evidence that many more infect humans in nature. Most of these viruses are natural pathogens of other animals. People usually become involved in the transmission cycle accidentally and are a dead-end host for most of these viruses. Nevertheless, they can cause serious illnesses when people become infected.

There are a few viruses that cause serious endemic and epidemic disease in humans, primarily because the mosquito vectors are closely associated with the domestic habitats. Table 113–6 lists the most important mosquito-borne viral diseases of humans, their distribution, and the principal vectors. Details of the systematics and biology of these viruses are presented in Chapters 20 to 22.

Alphaviruses. Chikungunya virus is undoubtedly the most widespread and one of the most important alphaviruses in terms of human health. This virus, first described in Africa, probably exists there in a mosquito-primate-mosquito cycle involving forest mosquitoes. Humans are also susceptible and may carry the virus back to the village where a person—*Aedes aegypti*—person transmission cycle may exist. The virus is presently widespread in the large urban areas of Asia, where it exists in this type of cycle. Periodically, transmission may occur in epidemic form.

Another alphavirus, Ross River virus, which may eventually have a similar epidemiology, causes a disease known as epidemic polyarthritis in humans and has been limited to the Australia–New Guinea area. This virus has been known clinically for over 50 years in Australia but was not isolated until 1963 and then only from mosquito pools. The mosquito vectors were *Culex annulirostris* and *Aedes vigilax.* Although many attempts were made, only a single isolate was made from human sera, leading to speculation that the polyarthritis was caused by virus-antibody complexes and that humans generally had low viremia. In 1979 and 1980, major epidemics of polyarthritis occurred on several South Pacific islands. During these epidemics, it was shown that humans did have viremia high enough to infect mosquitoes, and epidemiologic and experimental evidence suggested that *Stegomyia* mosquitoes, especially *Ae. polynesiensis, Ae. albopictus,* and *Ae. aegypti,* were efficient vectors of the virus. Furthermore, it has been demonstrated by Australian workers that *Ae. vigilax* can experimentally transmit Ross River virus transovarially. With these new developments and with increased air travel by people, epidemic polyarthritis may move west into Asia and east into the Caribbean and Central and South America.

Other alphaviruses have more complex cycles involving several mosquito species as vectors and both avian and mammalian reservoir hosts. Examples are the equine encephalitis viruses in North and South America (Table 113–6 and Fig. 21–7). The cycle of western equine encephalitis (WEE) (Fig. 113–4) is an example. The virus is maintained with spring and summer amplification in a *Culex tarsalis*–nestling and juvenile bird–*Cx. tarsalis* cycle in the western United States. Occasionally, for reasons that are not fully understood, epidemic WEE occurs, and humans and horses may become involved. However, both are dead-end hosts that contribute nothing to the maintenance cycle of the

TABLE 113–6. Important Mosquito-Borne Viral Diseases of Humans and Known Vectors

Virus	Geographic Distribution	Vectors
Alphaviruses		
Chikungunya	Africa, Asia	*Aedes aegypti*, other *Aedes* species
Eastern equine encephalitis	North America, South America, Europe	*Culiseta melanura* *Aedes taeniorhynchus* *Aedes sollicitans*
O'nyong-nyong	Africa	*Anopheles funestus* *Anopheles gambiae*
Ross River	Australasia, Pacific Islands	*Culex annulirostris* *Aedes vigilax* *Aedes polynesiensis* *Aedes aegypti*
Sindbis	Africa, Asia, Australasia, Europe	*Culex univittatus* *Culex tritaeniorhynchus*
Venezuelan equine encephalitis	North and South America	*Culex melanacom* species
Western equine encephalitis	North and South America	*Culex tarsalis* *Culiseta melanura*
Flaviviruses		
Japanese encephalitis	Asia	*Culex tritaeniorhynchus* group *Culex annulus*
Murray Valley encephalitis	Australia	*Culex annulirostris* *Culex bitaeniorhynchus*
Rocio	South America	*Aedes scapularis*
St. Louis encephalitis	North and South America	*Culex pipiens* complex *Culex tarsalis* *Culex nigripalpus* *Culex restuans* *Culex salinarius*
West Nile	Africa, Asia	*Culex univittatus* *Culex pipiens* complex *Culex vishnui* subgroup
Dengue	Tropicopolitan	*Aedes aegypti* *Aedes albopictus* *Aedes polynesiensis*
Yellow fever	Africa	*Aedes aegypti* *Aedes africanus* *Aedes simpsoni* *Aedes furcifer-taylori*
	Americas	*Aedes aegypti* *Haemagogus janthinomys* *Haemagogus spegazzinii* *Haemagogus leucocelaenus* *Sabethes chloropterus*
Zika	Africa, Asia	*Aedes aegypti* *Aedes africanus*
Bunyaviruses		
La Crosse	North America	*Aedes triseriatus*
Tahyna	Africa, Asia, Europe	*Aedes vexans*
Oropouche	South America	*Culex* species
Phleboviruses		
Rift Valley fever	Africa	*Culex pipiens* complex

virus. The overwintering mechanism is not known but possibly involves migrating birds, persistence of the virus in overwintering mosquitoes, or even transovarial transmission.

Flaviviruses. Flaviviruses are considerably more important to human health than any other group of arboviruses. Important viruses that collectively infect millions of persons each year include dengue, yellow fever, and Japanese encephalitis viruses. All have a wide distribution and are transmitted by species of mosquitoes that may have close human contact.

Dengue fever: Dengue fever is an acute infection characterized by sudden onset of fever and a variety of nonspecific symptoms in its classic form. These viruses also have the potential to cause severe and fatal disease in humans, and large epidemics of dengue hemorrhagic fever (DHF) are not uncommon in several countries of Southeast Asia. This form of disease primarily affects younger age groups and is one of the 10 leading causes of hospitalization and death among children in Southeast Asia. Epidemic dengue associated with hemorrhagic disease has also become a major health problem in the South and Central Pacific and the Caribbean basin (Chapter 20.1).

There are 4 serotypes of dengue viruses (types 1, 2, 3, and 4), all closely related antigenically. The viruses have a tropicopolitan distribution that is closely linked to the distribution of the principal vector, *Ae. aegypti.* Today, there are more people (approximately 2 billion) at risk for dengue virus infection than for any other arbovirus infection.

The viruses probably originated in the jungles of the Malay peninsula and/or in Africa. In Malaysia they exist in a mosquito-monkey-mosquito cycle involving species of the *Ae. niveus* complex of mosquitoes and leaf monkeys. Evidence obtained by French workers suggests that a similar cycle exists in Africa. The importance of these jungle cycles in the maintenance of the viruses is not considered great, because all 4 dengue serotypes coexist in most of the large urban centers of Southeast Asia in an *Ae. aegypti*–human–*Ae. aegypti* cycle. In rural and some urban areas of Asia and the Pacific, 2 other *Stegomyia* species, *Ae. albopictus* and *Ae. polynesiensis,* are important vectors. Transovarial transmission of these viruses has been demonstrated in all 3 species of mosquito, with vertical transmission being least efficient in the domestic *Ae. aegypti.* Mosquitoes become infected with dengue virus by feeding on a viremic human host and, depending on the species and strain of mosquito, the strain of virus, and environmental factors, can transmit the virus to a new host after an extrinsic incubation period of about 10 to 14 days.

Studies have shown that not all geographic strains of *Ae. aegypti* or *Ae. albopictus* are efficient vectors of dengue viruses. Some strains are refractory to oral

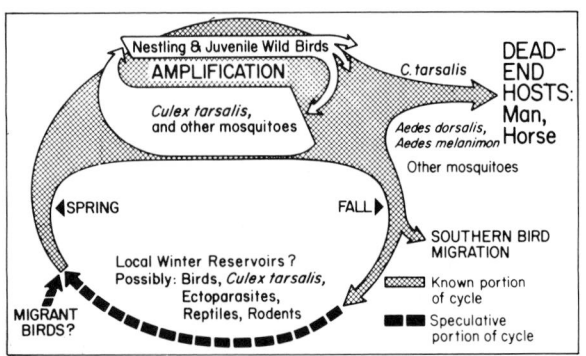

FIGURE 113–4. Maintenance cycle of western equine encephalitis virus in the western United States. (Courtesy of the Centers for Disease Control.)

infection with dengue viruses, a trait that is apparently genetically controlled. Other work has shown that there is also variation among strains of dengue viruses in their epidemic potential. This variation among different strains of mosquito and dengue viruses could help explain why some areas or cities that appear to be permissive to dengue virus transmission do not have large epidemics of either dengue fever or DHF, whereas others do.

Yellow fever: Yellow fever is a flavivirus that is closely related to the dengue viruses ecologically, antigenically, and clinically. Antigenically, there is considerable cross-reaction between dengue and yellow fever viruses, although there is not complete cross-protective immunity. Clinically, yellow fever is characterized by sudden onset of fever and a variety of nonspecific symptoms similar to those of dengue fever. This may be followed by a more severe disease involving jaundice, hemorrhagic manifestations, and death (Chapter 22.1).

The virus is maintained in the jungles of Africa and Central and South America in a mosquito-monkey-mosquito cycle. In Africa, species of cercopithecid monkeys are the vertebrate hosts, and transmission is generally by forest canopy mosquitoes, *Ae. africanus* and *Ae. furcifer-taylori*. It has been shown that transovarial and trans-stadial transmission of yellow fever virus occurs in both forest species and in *Ae. aegypti* (Fig. 114–5). This may be an even more important maintenance mechanism during long dry periods.

In Africa, humans can become infected with jungle yellow fever in 2 ways: Infected canopy dwelling mosquitoes may transmit the virus to people when they are working in the jungle (Fig. 110–2). These workers may not get sick until they are back in the village or city where *Ae. aegypti* is present. Probably, a more common way yellow fever gets out of the jungle is by the monkeys themselves. They may frequent banana groves where another mosquito, *Ae. simpsoni*, breeds in the banana leaf axils. These mosquitoes feed on the monkeys when they raid the banana plantations and can subsequently transmit the virus to people when they visit the plantation to harvest bananas and work.

In Central and South America, a similar cycle exists involving forest monkeys and canopy mosquitoes belonging to the genus *Haemagogus*. Forest workers may be infected as in Africa and carry the virus back to the village or city where *Ae. aegypti* is present. In both Africa and the Americas, major urban epidemics may be transmitted by *Ae. aegypti*.

Yellow fever virus is found only in Africa, where it probably originated, and in Central and South America, where it was most likely introduced with the slave trade in the 1500s. The virus has never been documented in Asia and the Pacific, where *Ae. aegypti* is widespread and abundant. The reasons for this lack of spread is not known but is probably due to the cross-protective immunity provided by the high endemicity of other closely related flaviviruses such as dengue, Japanese encephalitis, and West Nile viruses. Other studies have suggested that the Asian strains of *Ae. aegypti* are not good vectors of yellow fever. Thus, even though the virus is probably introduced on occasion, the combination of cross-pro-

tective immunity from other flaviviruses and low vector susceptibility probably prevent subsequent transmission and spread.

Large urban epidemics of yellow fever have not occurred in Central and South America for many years as a result of combined *Ae. aegypti* control programs and yellow fever vaccination in many countries of the region. Although the mosquito was not eradicated, it was controlled in many cities, and yellow fever now occurs only in the jungle and in a few rural areas. In recent years, however, *Ae. aegypti* has reinvaded many urban areas of South and Central America, putting them at high risk for epidemic transmission. Africa still experiences large epidemics transmitted by *Ae. aegypti*. Moreover, for the first time in over 40 years, major epidemics of urban yellow fever occurred in West Africa in 1986 to 1987.

Japanese encephalitis virus: Japanese encephalitis (JE) virus is another important flavivirus that is related antigenically to dengue viruses. It is strictly an Asian virus, ranging from India in the west to Japan and Siberia in the east. The illness in humans ranges from inapparent infection to severe viral encephalitis and death. It is primarily a rural disease, but in Asia, where dense human populations occur, large epidemics occur periodically. Thousands of cases have occurred in India, especially in West Bengal and Bihar State, and in Nepal.

Transmission of JE virus is seasonal in the northern part of its range. Thus, it only occurs during the summer months in areas such as Japan, Korea, and China. In tropical areas, e.g., Indonesia, the virus appears to be transmitted sporadically year round. Most of the large epidemics of JE virus have occurred in the northern part of its geographic range.

The exact maintenance cycle of JE virus is not known but most likely involves birds as the principal reservoir hosts (Fig. 21–8). The principal vectors are members of the *Cx. tritaeniorhynchus* complex of mosquitoes, which breed in rice fields, barrow pits, and other standing water. The virus overflows from this maintenance cycle to farms, where pigs may act as amplification hosts. Humans usually become involved as a result of contact with farm areas where there are pigs, and large epidemics of Japanese encephalitis are usually associated with areas with large pig populations.

Humans are apparently a dead-end host for JE virus because it has been infrequently isolated from human sera. Human viremia may occur, however, before onset of symptoms, when it would not be detected. Mosquitoes are most likely infected by feeding on viremic birds or pigs, although it has been documented experimentally that transovarial transmission of JE virus can occur in *Cx. tritaeniorhynchus*. This could be an important maintenance mechanism for the virus, especially in northern temperate regions of Japan, Korea, and China, where overwintering would be a problem.

Control of JE virus is difficult because it is a rural disease. In Japan, Korea, People's Republic of China, and Taiwan, however, epidemic JE has been reduced considerably by a combination of vaccination and water management practices.

St. Louis encephalitis virus: St. Louis encephalitis (SLE) virus is the most important arbovirus in North

America and has caused major epidemics periodically since it was first described in 1933. This is strictly an American virus and has been documented in Central and South America as well as North America. As with JE, epidemics of SLE occur primarily in the temperate areas of its distribution.

SLE virus is maintained in nature in a bird–*Culex* mosquito–bird cycle (Fig. IX–1). Depending on the area, the species of birds and mosquitoes may change. In the central and eastern United States, for example, a variety of domestic and peridomestic birds, such as house sparrows, pigeons, blue jays, and robins, are the important maintenance and amplifying hosts. *Culex pipiens pipiens* and *Cx. pipiens quinquefasciatus,* which breed in storm drains, sewage treatment ponds, and other polluted water, are the principal mosquito vectors. Both vertebrate and mosquito hosts bring the virus into the human habitat, where transmission to humans may occur. Other *Culex* species such as *Cx. restuans* and *Cx. salinarius* have been shown to be efficient vectors of SLE virus and are probably important maintenance hosts in locations such as the Ohio-Mississippi River basin, where they are involved in enzootic transmission. In Florida, *Cx. nigripalpus* is the important epidemic vector. In the western United States, however, SLE is primarily a rural infection. The principal vector there is *Cx. tarsalis,* which breeds in a variety of clear or foul water, irrigation ponds, ditches, and other sources of ground water in areas fed by irrigation systems. Although mosquitoes of the *Cx. pipiens* complex are common in the western United States and may transmit SLE virus, they are not the principal vectors in that part of the country.

An important question that remains to be answered is how the virus survives the cold winter season, when mosquitoes do not feed. Studies have demonstrated repetitive foci in the central United States where SLE virus transmission occurs every year, even during interepidemic periods, suggesting that the virus is indigenous, and not introduced. Other work has demonstrated that this virus is also transmitted transovarially in *Culex* species and also that it can survive the winter months in hibernating *Culex* mosquitoes. Thus, there may be more than one mechanism for the virus to overwinter and be available for spring amplification. Furthermore, biologic and biochemical work on the viruses suggests that there are epidemic strains of SLE virus that produce higher viremia in birds. Thus, a combination of factors are probably involved in maintenance of the virus in nature and its subsequent epidemic transmission (Fig. IX–1).

Mosquitoes have also been considered by some workers as potential vectors of AIDS virus. Limited experimental work, however, suggests that HIV does not replicate in mosquito tissues. More important, the current epidemiologic disease pattern is not compatible with biologic transmission of HIV by mosquitoes. Finally, the low viremia in humans infected with HIV make it unlikely that mechanical transmission would occur.

PROTOZOA. Of the protozoan parasites of humans transmitted by insects, the malarial parasites are by far the most important. Although malaria was nearly under control by 1970 in many parts of the tropics, it is again the most important vector-borne disease in the world. A combination of insecticide resistance in the mosquito vectors and drug resistance by the malarial parasites has resulted in a resurgence of malaria in most major endemic areas of the tropics (Fig. 73–1).

Malaria is a disease of humans caused by 4 species of *Plasmodium. P. falciparum* is widespread in the tropics and causes the most severe disease in humans (malignant tertian malaria). *P. vivax,* which causes benign tertian malaria, is also widespread in the tropics but occurs in temperate regions as well. *P. malariae,* the cause of quartan malaria, is relatively rare but is found in temperate regions and subtropics. *P. ovale,* which causes benign tertian malaria, is uncommon, occurring primarily in Africa, but has also been reported in South America and Asia. In addition, there are many other species of *Plasmodium* that are natural parasites of primates. Some of these are indistinguishable morphologically from the parasites of humans and, in fact, can infect humans.

All malarial parasites of humans and lower primates have *Anopheles* mosquitoes as vectors. Table 113–7 lists the major geographic areas of the world and the principal malaria vectors found in each. In addition, there are many more species of anophelines that are important vectors locally. Malaria has been controlled or eradicated from some of these areas, and therefore, transmission may no longer occur. The mosquito species listed, however, are documented vectors and could transmit malaria in the future if the parasite should be reintroduced.

The life cycle of all malarial parasites is similar and involves a human-*Anopheles*-human transmission cycle (Fig. 73–2). There is an exogenous sexual phase with multiplication in the mosquito and an endogenous asexual phase with multiplication in humans. Mosquitoes become infected when they ingest microgametocytes and macrogametocytes while taking a blood meal from a person with parasitemia. After exflagellation and fusion of the gametes, the zygote makes its way through the gut epithelium and encysts on the outside wall of the mosquito midgut. The oocyst forms, and in 10 to 14 days, over 200,000 sporozoites may develop, break out of the oocyst, and migrate to all parts of the body, including the salivary glands. The parasites in the salivary glands can then be transmitted to a new person when the mosquito takes a subsequent blood meal. The exogenous or sexual phase of the cycle in the mosquito is termed sporogony. The infecting sporozoites enter the blood, and some eventually invade the liver parenchyma cells. There they multiply asexually, with each sporozoite giving rise to 10,000 to 15,000 progeny called merozoites. Liver merozoites are discharged and enter the blood system and penetrate erythrocytes. In the latter cells, they multiply asexually, producing more merozoites, the number being characteristic for each malarial parasite. This asexual or endogenous part of the cycle is termed schizogony. For reasons that are not fully understood, some tropozoites in the erythrocytes do not undergo schizogony but, instead, develop into a gametocyte; when these are ingested by a mosquito, the

TABLE 113–7. The More Important Vectors of Malaria by Geographic Region

Geographic Region	Vector Species
North America	*Anopheles quadrimaculatus*
	An. freeborni
Central America	*An. albimanus*
	An. aquasalis
	An. bellator
	An. pseudopunctipennis
South America	*An. albimanus*
	An. darlingi
	An. nuneztovari
	An. pseudopunctipennis
Northern Europe	*An. aquasalis*
	An. atroparvus
	An. claviger
	An. labranchiae
Mediterranean and North Africa	*An. sacharovi*
	An. sergenti
	An. stephensi
	An. pharoensis
Africa (south of Sahara)	*An. gambiae* complex (6 species)
	An. funestus
	An. moucheti
	An. nili
Indo-Persian region	*An. stephensi*
	An. culcifacies complex
	An. fluviatilis
	An. hyrcanus
	An. pulcherrimus
Indo-Chinese region	*An. dirus* complex
	An. minimus minimus
	An. lesteri anthropophagus
	An. sinensis
Southeast Asia	*An. balabacensis*
	An. dirus complex
	An. minimus minimus
	An. aconitus
	An. campestris
	An. letifer
	An. sundaicus
	An. barbirostris
Australasia	*An. farauti*
	An. koliensis
	An. punctulatus

cycle begins again. The incubation period in malaria coincides with the prepatent period. Some *P. vivax* and *P. ovale* infections, however, may have a protracted incubation period of 9 months or more (Chapter 73).

There are many factors that influence the transmission of malarial parasites. These include those associated with the mosquito population, such as susceptibility to infection, longevity, feeding and resting behavior, population density, breeding habits, and flight range; factors associated with the human population, such as susceptibility to infection, occupation, type of housing, population density, and migrations or movement of people; and factors associated with the environment, such as topography of the area and climate. The combination of these factors that exists in malarious areas determines the extent of interactions among parasite, humans, and vector, and this interaction in turn determines whether an area has stable or unstable malaria.

Most malaria transmission occurs indoors because of the feeding and resting behavior of the mosquitoes. This single factor made malaria controllable with residual insecticides and was responsible for the control successes of the 1960s. However, it also produced selection pressures that resulted in insecticide resistance in many species of *Anopheles* and in behavioral changes in some species. These changes in the mosquito populations, along with drug resistance, are the main factors responsible for the resurgence of malaria in the 1970s.

FILARIASIS. There are 3 species of filaria of humans that are transmitted by mosquitoes. These are *Wuchereria bancrofti*, *Brugia malayi*, and *Brugia timori*. In addition, there are many other mosquito-borne filariae parasitizing other animals. These include some species in monkeys that can also infect humans, the common heartworm of dogs, and other species that infect a variety of mammals, birds, reptiles, and amphibians.

Mosquito-borne human filariasis is widely distributed throughout the tropics and subtropics of the world. *W. bancrofti*, the most widely distributed, is basically a tropicopolitan species (Fig. 85–2). *B. malayi* is widespread in Asia from India and Sri Lanka in the west to Indonesia, the Philippines, and Japan in the east (Fig. 85–9). *B. timori* has a limited distribution and has been documented only from several eastern Indonesian islands from Timor to Sumba (Fig. 85–9). Table 113–8 lists the 3 species of filarial parasites and the different strains of each along with the geographic distribution and important mosquito vectors.

The basic life cycle is the same for all filarial parasites (Fig. VI B–1). The embryonic microfilariae circulating in the peripheral blood (Fig. 85–1) are ingested by the mosquito when they take a blood meal. The microfilariae immediately exsheath, penetrate the midgut wall, and migrate to the thorax of the mosquito, where they enter a muscle cell and begin to develop. The juvenile filariae molt twice during a development period of 10 to 14 days and emerge from the muscle cells as active third-stage or infective larvae. These larvae migrate throughout the body of the mosquito, including the proboscis or mouth parts. When the infective mosquito takes a subsequent blood meal, the larvae escape from the labium onto the skin of the person and penetrate the skin.

Unfortunately, little is known of that part of the life cycle in humans from invasion by the third-stage larvae to maturation in the lymphatics. Apparently *W. bancrofti* larvae can reach sexual maturity in as little as 3 months, and therefore, under ideal conditions, patent infections can occur as early as 3 to 4 months after exposure. However, most infections take longer to become patent, even in highly endemic areas.

The epidemiology of mosquito-borne filariasis varies with the strain and species of parasite and with the species of mosquito vector. Filariasis caused by *W. bancrofti* in Asia is essentially an urban disease. The parasite is the nocturnally periodic form, which means that the microfilariae are found circulating in the peripheral blood only at night. This strain of *W. bancrofti* is transmitted in most urban areas by the night-biting common house mosquito, *Cx. pipiens quinquefasciatus*. This mosquito breeds in sewage-contaminated water that

TABLE 113–8. Mosquito-Borne Filarial Parasites of Humans

Parasite	Distribution	Rural	Urban
Wuchereria bancrofti (periodic form)	Tropicopolitan (except Polynesia)	*Anopheles gambiae* *An. funestus* *An. flavirostris* *An. punctulatus* group *An. barbirostris* *An. balabacensis* *Aedes niveus* *Ae. kochi* *Ae. poecilius* *Ae. togoi*	*Culex pipiens quinquefasciatus* *Cx. pipiens pallens*
W. bancrofti (subperiodic form)	Polynesia, New Caledonia	*Ae. polynesiensis* *Ae. tabu* *Ae. vigilax*	
Brugia malayi (periodic form)	Asia—India to Japan	*Mansonia annulifera* *M. indiana* *M. uniformis* *Ae. togoi* *Ae. barbirostris* *An. lesteri anthropophagus* *An. sinensis* *Anopheles* species	
B. malayi (subperiodic form)	Swamp forests of Southeast Asia	*M. dives* *M. bonneae* *M. annulata* *M. uniformis*	
B. timori	Indonesia—Timor to Sumba	*An. barbirostris*	

can be found in drains, tanks, and other ground water close to human habitations. It is a highly domesticated species and lives in intimate contact with humans. In tropical America, *W. bancrofti* is also transmitted by *Cx. pipiens quinquefasciatus,* but in Africa, the principal vectors are *An. gambiae* and *An. funestus,* which also transmit malaria. In rural rain forest communities of Asia, this parasite may be transmitted by forest mosquitoes of the genus *Aedes* or *Anopheles.*

Another strain of *W. bancrofti* found only in the South Pacific shows little or no microfilarial periodicity. This form, known as subperiodic or aperiodic *W. bancrofti,* has microfilariae circulating in the peripheral blood with little variation throughout the 24-hour period. Nearly coincident with subperiodic bancroftian filariasis is the distribution of *Ae. (Stegomyia) polynesiensis,* the principal vector throughout its range. Transmission by this species is associated with the peridomestic environment and coconut plantations on most islands. *Ae. polynesiensis,* which breeds in a variety of natural and artificial containers, e.g., coconut shells, crab holes, and stored water containers, feeds by day on people working in these areas. On some islands, such as Tonga, Rotuma, and Niue, other *Stegomyia* species that are closely related to *Ae. polynesiensis* transmit filariasis, and in New Caledonia, *Ae. vigilax* is the principal vector.

B. malayi is the most common filaria of humans throughout most of rural Southeast Asia. It is most frequently associated with mosquitoes of the genus *Mansonia,* immature stages of which are associated with water plants of the genera *Pistia, Eichornia,* and *Salvinia.* The subperiodic form of *B. malayi* is found primarily associated with swamp forests in Southeast Asia, where it occurs in macaques, leaf monkeys, and wild and domestic cats as well as in humans. Transmission

thus occurs, via mosquito bite, from person to person, from humans to monkeys and cats, and from these animals to humans. *Mansonia* mosquitoes may feed during the day, but most blood feeding occurs in the evening and may take place indoors or outdoors.

The periodic form of *B. malayi* is also transmitted by *Mansonia* species, but certain species of *Aedes* and *Anopheles* are the principal vectors in some areas. Therefore, the epidemiology varies considerably from area to area. In India and Sri Lanka, *M. uniformis* is the principal vector, and transmission is associated with coconut plantations; in areas of Indonesia, *An. barbirostris* is the vector, and transmission is associated with rural village areas and rice culture; and in Japan and Korea, *Ae. togoi* is the vector, and transmission is associated with coastal areas, where this mosquito breeds in rock pools. The periodic form of *B. malayi* is not known to have any vertebrate host other than humans. The extent to which animal reservoirs influence the epidemiology of brugian filariasis and the extent to which they complicate the problem of control remain to be determined.

The epidemiology of *B. timori* is similar to that of periodic *B. malayi* in certain areas of Indonesia because both parasites are transmitted by *An. barbirostris. B. timori* is a newly described parasite, and reservoir hosts other than humans are not yet known.

Family Tabanidae (Deer Flies)
Biology. The Tabanidae are large, robust flies belonging to the suborder Brachycera (Fig. 114–14). They are divided taxonomically into 4 subfamilies, of which only 2, *Chrysopsinae* and Tabaninae, are of medical importance. There are more than 3000 species of tabanids described worldwide. Only 3 genera (*Chrysops, Tabanus,* and *Haematopota*) contain species of medical

importance, and only 1 of these, *Chrysops,* is important in the transmission of disease to humans.

As with the mosquitoes, only the females take blood meals from a wide variety of animals. The mouth parts are the cutting-lacerating type and thus produce pooled blood on which flies feed. The female flies deposit their eggs on the underside of leaves, rocks, and branches over the larval habitat, which may be a pond with clear or brackish water, or over muddy or semiaquatic sites. The eggs hatch in 7 to 14 days; the larvae drop to the underlying mud or water and usually burrow into the mud and begin to feed on organic matter, including other insect larvae. Tabanid larvae are commonly found along the edges of ponds, marshes, rice fields, and ditches and in rotting vegetation. Depending on the species, the temperature, and other environmental factors, larval development may last as long as 2 to 3 years. Most species, however, produce one generation or more per year. The mature larvae move to drier soil to pupate, usually an inch or two below the surface. The pupal period may last 1 to 3 weeks, after which the emerging adults make their way to the surface.

Most species are diurnal and thus feed during the day. They are strong fliers and may be found a considerable distance from their breeding sites. Because of the type of mouth parts these flies have, their bite is painful, and they are frequently interrupted from feeding. This facilitates mechanical transmission, because the flies may bite several hosts in a short period of time before completing the blood meal.

Disease Transmission. Two bacteria may be transmitted mechanically by species of Tabanids. These are *Bacillus anthracis* and *Francisella tularensis.* The former has been documented only on rare occasions, but experimental and circumstantial evidence suggests that horseflies may be an important mechanical vector of this bacillus. The other bacterium, which causes tularemia, exists in natural cycle involving rabbits, mice, squirrels, beavers, and a variety of other animals, including birds. The natural transmission cycle in the western United States involves ticks, but both field and experimental evidence implicates several species of *Chrysops* as mechanical vectors in outbreaks of tularemia (deer fly fever) in humans. Important species are *C. discalis, C. fulvaster,* and *C. aestuans.*

Deer flies of the genus *Chrysops* are most important as biologic vectors of *Loa loa,* the African eye worm of humans (Chapter 86). This filaria occurs in the tropical rain forests of West and Central Africa and is transmitted from person to person by *C. dimidiata* and *C. silacea.* The adult worms live in the subcutaneous tissues of humans and migrate to various parts of the body, including the eye. They produce microfilariae that have a dirunal periodicity in the peripheral blood. The microfilariae are ingested with the blood meal of the day-feeding flies, after which they penetrate the gut wall, migrate to the thoracic muscles, enter a muscle cell, and develop to third-stage infective larvae, much like the other filariae in mosquitoes. Transmission may occur in 10 to 14 days.

Another filaria that is morphologically identical to *L. loa* but that is found in monkeys and has a nocturnal microfilarial periodicity is transmitted by the night-biting tabanids *C. centurionis* and *C. langi.* Whether this is a new species or just a variant of *L. loa* and whether it can infect humans are not yet known.

No human viral diseases are known to be transmitted by tabanid flies. There are some retrovirus diseases of animals, however, that are transmitted mechanically by tabanids, including equine infectious anemia virus and bovine leukosis virus. Human AIDS virus is also a retrovirus and there has been speculation, therefore, that this virus could also be transmitted mechanically by tabanids. However, there is no experimental or epidemiologic evidence to support this speculation. Mechanical transmission of HIV is also considered unlikely because of the low HIV human viremia and low infection rate in lymphocytes.

Muscoid Flies. The muscoid flies represent the most specialized Diptera. They belong to the suborder Cyclorrhapha and are readily distinguished from the other suborders by the adult antennae (Fig. 113–2), the presence of the frontal (ptillinial) suture, and larvae that have no distinct head capsule. The muscoid flies have a worldwide distribution and breed in feces, decaying vegetation, or dead animal tissues. There are 3 families that are important in the transmission of human disease.

Family Glossinidae (Tsetse Flies). The tsetse flies are considered part of the family Muscidae by some authors, but biologic as well as morphologic differences justify their elevation to family status. *Glossina* is the only genus in the family. They occur only in Africa but are widely distributed between 14 degrees north and 29 degrees south latitudes.

BIOLOGY. The tsetse flies are medium sized, robust, and strong fliers. They are readily identifiable by the saber-like proboscis that projects forward and the cleaver-shaped cell in the wing (Fig. 114–13). Both male and female flies suck blood and bite humans as well as a variety of other animals. Although most species have preferred hosts, tsetse flies generally have broad host ranges and feed on several kinds of animals.

Unlike most other Diptera, tsetse flies do not have a free-living larval stage in their development. Instead, after a blood meal, the inseminated female fly produces a single egg, which is fertilized and hatches in the uterus. The egg shell is passed, and the young larva feeds on fluid from accessory glands. Regular blood meals must be taken every 2 to 5 days for the female to support development of the larva. After 3 molts during an 8- to 12-day development period, the mature third-stage larva is deposited by the female in loose, shaded soil. The larva immediately burrows into the soil, and the larval skin begins to harden and forms a reddish-brown puparium.

The pupation period generally lasts 3 to 5 weeks, depending on the temperature, but during cool periods, this time may be extended to 8 to 10 or more weeks. After pupation is complete, the adult emerges, crawls through the soil to the surface, and is ready to fly within 15 to 20 minutes.

There are 3 groups of tsetse flies, which are separated on the basis of morphology and ecology. The *Glossina fusca* group is the largest but is the least important medically. These are primarily forest species that rarely feed on humans and therefore do not transmit disease. The *Glossina morsitans* group of species prefers the thornbush and myombo type of vegetation associated with the savanna and its edges in East and Central Africa. The *Glossina palpalis* group of species is found in wetter regions, primarily in the fringing woodland along rivers in West and Central Africa. The ecology of each of these groups has led to the commonly used terms forest tsetses *(G. fusca)*, savanna tsetses *(G. morsitans)*, and riverine tsetses *(G. palpalis)* when discussing African trypanosomiasis. The distribution of all of the aforementioned groups of tsetse flies expands and contracts during the rainy and dry seasons, respectively, as favorable and adverse conditions occur.

DISEASE TRANSMISSION. The only disease of humans transmitted by tsetse flies is African trypanosomiasis. This disease alone, however, has probably had a greater negative impact on the economic development of Central Africa than any other. African trypanosomiasis (African sleeping sickness) is caused by protozoan parasites belonging to the genus *Trypanosoma*. There are 2 species that affect humans, *T. brucei rhodesiense* and *T. brucei gambiense*, and another species, *T. brucei brucei*, does not infect humans but causes a disease called nagana in animals. All 3 species of *Trypanosoma* are morphologically identical but are biologically distinct. All have a similar developmental cycle in *Glossina*.

The tsetse fly ingests the trypanosomal form of the parasite with the blood meal (Fig. 74–3). In the midgut, the parasites multiply by binary fission. From the midgut, the parasites migrate forward again to the proboscis, enter the salivary duct, and finally reach the salivary glands, where the infective metacyclic forms develop. Alternatively, it has been shown that the parasites can also penetrate the gut wall and enter the salivary glands from the hemocoel. The extrinsic incubation period is about 20 days but may be as long as 30 days, depending on the species and environmental conditions. Transmission occurs when the tsetse fly takes a blood meal after metacyclic forms are present in the salivary glands.

The ecology and distribution of African sleeping sickness are closely tied to the tsetse fly (Fig. 74–2). Thus, the distribution of disease also expands and contracts along with that of the flies. Rhodesian sleeping sickness, caused by *T. brucei rhodesiense*, is primarily an East African disease and is transmitted by species of the *Glossina morsitans* group. These flies and the disease are associated with the savanna, where human populations are sparse. The principal animal reservoir for the parasite is a variety of game animals and domestic ungulates. Since *G. morsitans, G. swynnertoni,* and *G. pallidipes,* the principal vectors, prefer to feed on animals rather than on people, human disease is more sporadic and seldom occurs in epidemic form.

West African sleeping sickness, caused by *T. brucei gambiense*, is found in West and Central Africa. The disease is associated with river ecologies, where human population density is usually highest and where the principal vectors, *G. palpalis, G. tachinoides,* and *G. fuscipes,* occur. The disease is more chronic, and persons with parasitemia are seldom bedridden during the early stages of infection. Therefore, transmission may be more intense, and epidemics of this form are common. There are no known animal reservoirs of *T. brucei gambiense*, although there is some evidence that domestic pigs may play a role.

Family Muscidae (Houseflies). The family Muscidae contains the common housefly, *Musca domestica* (Fig. 113–5 and 114–8), and a number of other synanthropic species that live in intimate association with humans. Although the family contains several species that have evolved the bloodsucking habit, none of them have been incriminated in biologic transmission of human disease agents. The importance of houseflies lies in their indiscriminate feeding habits, which may include feces of humans and animals and the food of humans. They are thus capable of mechanically transmitting many organisms, primarily enteric pathogens belonging to a number of taxonomic groups (Table 113–9).

Their success in the mechanical transmission of organisms is directly related to the behavior of the housefly

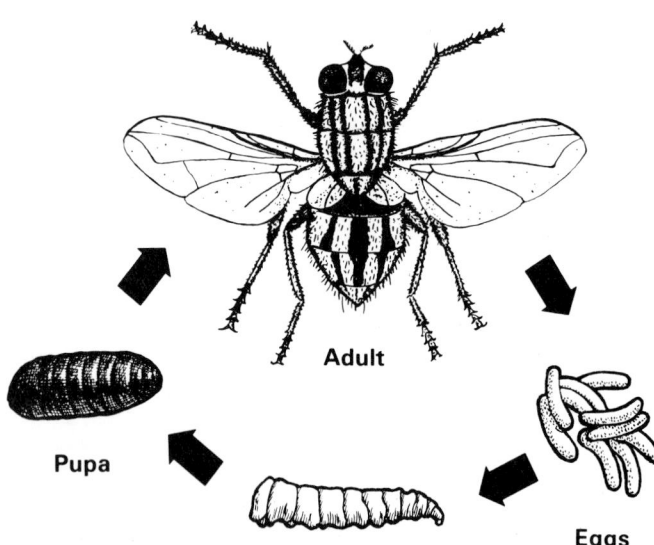

Adult

Pupa

Larva

Eggs

FIGURE 113–5. Life cycle of the housefly, *Musca domestica.*

TABLE 113–9. Human Pathogens Mechanically Transmitted by Houseflies and Their Relatives

Classification	Agent	Source
Virus	Poliomyelitis	Feces
	Coxsackievirus	Feces
	Hepatitis A	Feces
	Enteroviruses	Feces
Rickettsia	*Coxiella burnetii*	Milk
Bacterium	*Chlamydia trachomatis*	Conjunctiva
	Shigella species	Feces
	Salmonella species	Feces
	Salmonella typhi	Feces
	Escherichia coli	Feces
	Vibrio cholerae	Feces
	Bacterial conjunctivitis	Conjunctiva
Spirochete	*Treponema pertenue*	Skin ulcers
Protozoon	*Entamoeba histolytica*	Feces
	Entamoeba coli	Feces
	Giardia lamblia	Feces
	Toxoplasma gondii (oocyst)	Feces
Cestode (eggs)	*Taenia solium*	Feces
	Dipylidium caninum	Feces
	Diphyllobothrium latum	Feces
Nematode (eggs)	*Ascaris lumbricoides*	Feces
	Trichuris trichiura	Feces
	Enterobius vermicularis	Feces

and its relatives and the type of feeding that occurs. These flies are strong fliers and may be feeding or resting on uncovered food only moments after having fed on or visited feces. Transfer of the organisms can be by simple contamination of the mouth parts, feet, and body hairs or by ingestion and subsequent regurgitation or defecation on food. Although there is little doubt that houseflies play a role in the transmission of a variety of human pathogens, their actual importance in the epidemiology of the diseases is hard to assess, because most of the evidence is circumstantial.

Family Chloropidae (Eye Gnats). These are small, robust flies that are attracted to a variety of body secretions and sores of humans and animals. They are strong fliers and are persistent in their feeding habits, continuing to return after being brushed away. Breeding sites are usually loose, sandy soil that has a high content of organic material.

There are 2 genera that are of medical importance. The genus *Hippelates* is American, ranging from Canada in the north to Argentina in the south. *Siphunculina* is similar in biology and habits but is an Asian genus, ranging from India through Southeast Asia.

The medical importance of both genera is mechanical transmission of conjunctivitis and yaws. Although these flies are not bloodsuckers, their habits of frequenting sores, wounds, the eye, and other secretions make them ideal for mechanical transmission. Again, most evidence is circumstantial, but it seems highly probable that *Hippelates* and *Siphunculina* species play important roles in the transmission of both bacterial and viral conjunctivitis, outbreaks of which usually occur during the fly season. Chloropid flies have also been implicated in the transmission of streptococcal and staphylococcal skin infections and yaws. The latter is a rural disease caused by the spirochete *Treponema pertenue* (Chapter 32.2).

It is widespread in the tropics and results in large ulcerating sores. Both *Hippelates* and *Siphunculina* feed on sores of this kind and may ingest *T. pertenue*. It has been demonstrated that *Hippelates flavipes* may regurgitate active spirochetes during subsequent feedings within 2 days of the original infection. It should be noted that, although these flies may be involved in mechanical transmission of all of these agents, they are not necessary. Most of the diseases have a broader geographic distribution than the flies, and all can be transmitted directly by contact and by fomites.

COCKROACHES (ORDER DICTYOPTERA). Other insects, such as cockroaches (Fig. 114–12), are also capable of mechanical transmission of a variety of organisms, but in general, the evidence for this is, again, circumstantial. Furthermore, they are probably not as important as flies in this respect because of their habits and less frequent contact with feces.

BIBLIOGRAPHY

Beige TO (ed): International Catalogue of Arboviruses, Including Certain Other Viruses of Vertebrates, 2nd ed. Bethesda, MD, Department of Health, Education and Welfare, DHEW Pub. No. (CDC) 75–8301, 1975.

Bruce-Chwatt LJ: Essential Malariology. New York, John Wiley & Sons, 1985.

Busvine JR: Insects and Hygiene. The Biology and Control of Insect Pests of Medical Importance, 2nd ed. London, Methuen & Co, 1966.

Greenberg B: Flies and Disease, Vol II (Biology and Disease Transmission). Princeton, Princeton University Press, 1971.

Harwood RF, James MT: Entomology in Human and Animal Health, 7th ed. New York, Macmillan, 1979.

Hawking F: The Distribution of Human Filariasis Throughout the World, Parts I–IV. WHO Working Document Series, WHO/FIL/ 71.94, 73.114, 74.124, and 75.136. Geneva, World Health Organization, 1971–1975.

Horsfall WR: Medical Entomology, Arthropods and Human Disease. New York, Ronald Press, 1962.

Horsfall WR: Mosquitoes: Their Behavior and Relation to Disease. New York, Ronald Press, 1955.

Hubbert WT, McCulloch WF, Schnurrenberger PR (eds): Diseases Transmitted from Animals to Man, 6th ed. Springfield, IL, Charles C Thomas, 1975.

Jamnback H: Simuliidae (Blackflies) and Their Control. WHO/VBC 6.653, Geneva, World Health Organization, 1976.

Knight KL, Stone A: A Catalog of the Mosquitoes of the World (Diptera: Culicidae). College Park, Thomas Say Foundation, Entomological Society of America, 1977.

Lewis DJ: The biology of Phlebotomidae in relation to leishmaniasis. Annu Rev Entomol 19:363, 1974.

Monath TP (ed): St. Louis Encephalitis. Washington, DC, American Public Health Association, 1980.

Monath TP (ed): Arboviruses: Epidemiology and Ecology. Vols I, II, III, IV, V. Boca Raton, FL, CRC Press, 1988.

Poland JD, Barnes AM: Plague. *In* Steele JH (ed): CRC Handbook Series in Zoonoses. Boca Raton, FL, CRC Press, 1979.

Pollitzer R: Plague, WHO Monograph Series, No. 22, Geneva, World Health Organization, 1954.

Sandosham A: Malariology. Kuala Lumpur, University of Malaya Press, 1965.

Service MM: A Guide to Medical Entomology. London, Macmillan Press, 1980.

Shelly AJ: Vector aspects of the epidemiology of onchocerciasis in Latin America. Annu Rev Entomol. 33:337, 1988.

Smith KGV (ed): Insects and Other Arthropods of Medical Importance. London, British Museum of Natural History, 1973.

World Health Organization: Epidemiology of Onchocerciasis. Report of a WHO Expert Committee. WHO Tech Rep Ser 597, 1976.

Zahar AR: Studies on Leishmaniasis Vectors/Reservoirs and their Control, Parts I–V. WHO Working Document Series, WHO/VBC/79.749 and WHO/VBC/81.812. Geneva, World Health Organization, 1979.

114. CONTROL OF ARTHROPODS OF MEDICAL IMPORTANCE

George Davidson

GENERAL PRINCIPLES. Some of the most common diseases in the world are vector borne. Most of them, transmitted by insects, ticks, and mites, are predominantly tropical and most common in underdeveloped countries with limited health services. In many cases, there is no simple cure for the disease or preventive vaccine. Often, these diseases could be controlled by simple changes in the habits and customs of the people or by community efforts to create conditions unfavorable for transmission. Personal protective measures, e.g., suitable clothing and footwear, screening for houses, and mosquito nets, are available only to the minority. Adequate housing, water supply, and sanitation can only come from a buoyant economy, as can major environmental preventive measures. Thus, it is easy to conclude that the control method giving the greatest benefit to the greatest number of people in the shortest period of time is control of the vector.

Control methods may be aimed at vector eradication or reduction to low numbers or at disease eradication. Eradication is for vectors that are mechanical carriers of disease pathogens, e.g., flies and cockroaches. When the pathogen undergoes a cycle of development in the vector, control is directed toward reducing life expectancy to less than the time needed for the completion of this extrinsic cycle and before the vector is capable of passing on the infection. For eradication, methods with a maximum effect on insect numbers, usually an integration of antilarval and antiadult measures are necessary. This may combine source reduction methods with chemical control. Therefore, efficient housefly control may comprise the proper disposal of refuse, the use of insecticides to spray garbage collections, and the use of residual spot sprays or space sprays against adult flies. Transmission control generally involves the application of residual insecticides onto the surfaces where the insect usually rests. On a few occasions when the vector rests predominantly indoors, e.g., *Anopheles darlingi,* the malaria vector in coastal Guyana, and *A. funestus* in tropical Africa, this has led to vector eradication, but in most cases, it interrupts the transmission of the disease, eradicating the pathogen.

COLLECTING AND TRAPPING. Two simple, direct methods of vector control are collecting and trapping, which are seldom used separately because they only rarely contribute significantly to control by themselves. Thus, the search for and collection of the larger venomous arthropods, e.g., scorpions and spiders, in households may be helpful if the points of entry are dealt with at the same time. The removal of ticks causing paralysis is an obvious remedy once the symptoms are recognized. Using sticky fly papers to collect flies accidentally entering screened premises may be preferable to the use of insecticides. A combined attractant and trapping device may be useful, both indoors, e.g., for the control of cockroaches, and outdoors, e.g., to catch houseflies and tsetse flies. The potential of specific attractants has long been recognized, but few have been isolated for use against pests of medical importance. Bait-trapping of rodents has long been practiced as a supplement to flea control measures to combat plague outbreaks.

ENVIRONMENTAL CONTROL. Environmental control methods aimed at the breeding and assembly areas of pests can produce long-lasting effects and, in some cases, permanent solutions. These were the methods of choice before modern chemicals, which almost invariably need repeated applications. Good environmental sanitation is a prerequisite for the prevention of insects that breed in refuse and sewage, e.g., houseflies and mosquitoes such as *Culex quinquefasciatus.* Proper storage, collection, and disposal of garbage and sewage are the only ways to avoid these pests. The removal or prevention of unnecessary water collections will help a great deal to control mosquito-borne and certain other vector-borne diseases. Such measures, include drainage, canalization, filling in, water-level fluctuation, flushing, salinity change, pollution, and induced sunshine or shade. With a thorough knowledge of the life history and biology of the pest, it may be possible to produce habitat changes unfavorable to survival. Removal of vegetation may result in the disappearance of some species, e.g., tsetse flies, whereas its growth and the concomitant production of shade may be detrimental to others, e.g., some mosquito species. However, one must be certain that what is unfavorable to the pest in question does not encourage another.

INSECTICIDES. Chemical methods of control, especially those involving the use of residual insecticides, form a convenient and rapid means of destroying vectors. Used indoors, they have a minimal effect on the environment and nontarget organisms. It is their widespread, often indiscriminate use outdoors in controlling agricultural pests that may cause environmental damage. This has produced some of the resistance in human disease vectors by the contamination of breeding and resting places.

Types of Insecticides. Insecticides are of 3 main types: those that act as stomach poisons, e.g., Paris green or copper acetoarsenite (sometimes used for the control of mosquito larvae); those that act as fumigants, e.g., ethyl formate (used for the delousing of clothing); and those that act through external contact with the arthropod exoskeleton, e.g., the nonresidual pyrethrum flowers and the true residuals, e.g., dichlorodiphenyltrichloroethane (DDT). Some compounds can act in all 3 ways. Dichlorvos is an organophosphorus compound that is volatile and can therefore act as a fumigant. Applied in solution or emulsion to water, it can act as a stomach poison to mosquito larvae, and applied to solid surfaces, it can act through contact. The contact insecticides are particularly useful in vector control.

The active ingredients of pyrethrum flowers, mainly pyrethrins, and now some synthetic relatives, e.g., bioresmethrin and bioallethrin, produce extremely rapid knockdown effects through contact but have little or no residual effect. They make safe space sprays for domestic use, with almost immediate alleviation of biting nuisances in closed spaces, and are often combined with residuals to flush out hiding pests. Dissolved in propellant liquefied gases they form the basic ingredient of the modern aerosol dispenser ("fly spray"). They are also constituents of aerosols used outdoors for the containment of epidemics of fly-borne diseases and mosquito-borne viral infections.

Four main groups of chemicals make up the residual insecticides: organochlorines, organophosphates, carbamates, and pyrethroids. The organochlorines DDT, hexachlorocyclohexane (HCH), and dieldrin transformed the control of vectors after World War II and were responsible for saving millions of people from malaria and other vector-borne diseases. Unfortunately, many vectors have become resistant to this group of compounds, and it is now necessary to use the less efficient and more expensive organophosphates (e.g., malathion), carbamates (e.g., propoxur), and pyrethroids (e.g., permethrin).

Table 114–1 presents a list of compounds that have been used against arthropods of medical importance, classified according to their general chemical grouping.

Application Methods. All the modern residual insecticides are effective in minute quantities. Usually, dilution is necessary in a formulation suitable for a particular method of application. Formulations and application methods differ for different pests and situations.

Surface Spraying. Insecticide is most frequently applied to internal surfaces of human dwellings and other buildings, usually walls and roofs, but sometimes floors as well. Three formulations are available: (1) solutions,

which usually require special solvents such as kerosene for their dilution; (2) emulsions; and (3) wettable powders, which require water for dilution. Solutions and emulsions are normally used only where the surfaces should not be marked, but they are too readily absorbed (and lost from action) by some surfaces for general use. The most common formulation is the wettable powder, which, on dilution, produces a suspension of solid particles that remains on the surface of absorbent materials. Application is by a direct spray coarse enough to thoroughly wet the surface, delivered at a pressure low enough to give maximum adherence. The machine generally used for the application is the cylindrical, pneumatic, knapsack-type sprayer having a capacity of 9 to 14 L, operating at 40 lb/in² (2.8 bar), and delivering 760 ml of spray per minute through a fan-jet nozzle with a 0.8-mm diameter. Held 45 cm from the surface to be sprayed, with a flat fan-spray with a spray angle of 80 degrees, this produces a swath 75 cm wide. Spraying is done in bands slightly less than this width to ensure uniformity, and those performing the spraying are trained to cover 19 m² in 1 minute (or 40 ml/m²). Dilution of 75% DDT wettable powder at the rate of 67 gm/L of water will result in a deposit of 2 gm/m², which will give a persistently high kill on most surfaces for about 6 months. γ HCH (lindane) diluted at a quarter of this rate may produce comparable results on absorbent surfaces but not on nonabsorbent ones. The organophosphates and carbamates are usually applied at 2 gm/m², although some may be applied at 1 gm/m². Their persistence on nonabsorbent surfaces is usually about 3 months but is considerably shorter on absorbent ones.

These details apply to the spraying of houses for malaria control. Such spraying will, of course, kill other insects, e.g., other mosquito species, sandflies, houseflies, bedbugs, triatomine bugs, cockroaches, fleas, and ticks. If these, rather than anopheline mosquitoes, are the main pests, spraying can be concentrated on those areas where insects congregate, e.g., beds (bedbugs), the bases of walls (cockroaches), and the floor (fleas).

Other Formulations and Applications. In addition to the formulations used to spray buildings with residual insecticides, numerous other methods of dispersion of residual insecticides exist.

Dusts. These are mixtures of insecticides and finely ground, light inert diluents such as china clay, talc, or even locally sieved road dust or wood ash. DDT dusts usually contain 5% to 10% of the insecticide; 10% DDT in talc is commonly used for the control of body lice. HCH dusts contain 0.5% of the gamma isomer, and malathion dust contains 1% of the insecticide. Dusts are commonly used in the control of agricultural pests and against cockroaches, fleas (especially in rodent burrows), fly maggots, and lice whose precise location is known. Dusts are also useful as mosquito larvicides on breeding waters containing emergent or floating vegetation, where control by oil films is not possible. Various methods of dust distribution are employed, ranging from the simplest, by hand, to the use of aircraft.

Aerosols or Fogs. These are dispersions of solutions

TABLE 114–1. Residual Insecticides

Organo-chlorines	Organo-phosphates	Carbamates	Pyrethroids
aldrin	bromophos	bendiocarb	allethrin*
chlordane	chlorfenvinphos	carbaryl	bioallethrin*
chlordecone	chlorphoxim	dimetilan	bioresmethrin*
dicofol	chlorpyrifos	propoxur	cypermethrin
dieldrin	chlorpyrifos-		deltamethrin
DDT	methyl		fenvalerate
endosulfan	diazinon		natural
endrin	dichlorvos		pyrethrins*
heptachlor	dimethoate		permethrin
HCH	dioxathion		phenothrin*
lindane	fenchlorphos		resmethrin*
(γ HCH)	fenitrothion		tetramethrin*
toxaphene	fenthion		
	jodfenphos		
	malathion		
	naled		
	parathion		
	parathion-methyl		
	phoxim		
	pirimiphos-methyl		
	temephos		
	tetrachlorvinphos-		
	trichlorphon		

*Nonpersistent.

of insecticides in fine droplet form (usually less than 50 μm in diameter) that remain suspended in the atmosphere for a considerable time. They are produced in a variety of ways from several kinds of machines:

1. *Atomizer,* in which a stream of air is made to impinge on a stream of insecticide solution, as in the ordinary Flit gun.

2. *Aerosol dispenser,* in which the insecticide is dissolved in or mixed with liquefied gases under pressure. When the pressure is released, the carrier liquid boils off, dispersing a cloud of insecticide solution droplets.

3. *Fogging machines,* in which larger machines produce aerosols. In the Todd Insecticide Fog Applicator (TIFA), an atomized spray is introduced into a hot (the usual) or cold blast of air and further fractionated. The TIFA is a large vehicle-mounted machine, but smaller, backpack, internal combustion engine–powered machines also use similar principles, e.g., Fontan.

4. *Aircraft,* in which the insecticide may be gravity- or pump-fed into a boom beneath the aircraft wings bearing nozzles at intervals along its length. The spray is further broken up in the slip stream of the aircraft. Insecticide solution may also be distributed by introduction into the exhaust system of an aircraft, similar to the production of a thermal aerosol from a fogging machine.

Ultra-low-volume (ULV) application is a development in aerosol dispersion involving the distribution of low volumes of high insecticide concentration with a narrow range of droplet size. The concentration depends on the activity level of the insecticide and the ease of dispersion of small volumes. Special ground machinery exists for this dispersion, or it can be applied from slow-flying aircraft.

Aerosols are primarily used where rapidity and good penetration are required and where residual effect is not of major importance. The persistent suspension of fine droplets is effective against flying insects; pyrethrins are often added to residual insecticides dispersed in this form to stimulate resting insects to fly. Aerosols have been effective in controlling insect pests of stored products, e.g., grain, tobacco, and hides, as well as in controlling insects resting in dense vegetation, e.g., mosquitoes, black flies, and tsetse flies. They have also proved efficient for the control of epidemics of fly-borne infections and plague where rapid applications both indoors and outdoors are considered more essential than the slower methods of applying residual deposits.

Smoke Generators. In smoke generators, the insecticide is mixed with a slow-burning chemical that, when ignited, produces a smoke bearing fine particles, droplets, or vapor of insecticide. Smokes have similar uses to liquid aerosols, without the elaborate production, but usually are not as effective. One reason is that a proportion of the insecticide is decomposed by the heat producing the smoke. The pyrethrum coil is a smoke generator designed to burn for an entire night and repel biting insects in bedrooms.

Vapors. Naturally volatile insecticides can be used in the vapor phase. Plastic strips impregnated with dichlorvos, an organophosphate, can be used in houses and in closed sewage systems to control houseflies, cockroaches

and mosquitoes. In addition, less volatile compounds may be deliberately vaporized by heating.

Insecticidal Whitewashes, Distempers, Resins, and Paints. Mixing of insecticides with whitewashes and distempers has no advantage over the spraying of the insecticides onto such surfaces, because the insecticide is diluted and masked by the whitewash or distemper. In addition, lime causes a slow decomposition of many insecticides. With oil-bound paints, the insecticide is lost in solution in the paint and thus is not available to affect the insect. However, with a high concentration of insecticide, i.e., more than sufficient to saturate the paint oils, "blooming" crystals of insecticide occur on the surface, which are highly toxic to alighting insects. This principle of blooming from supersaturated solution has been successful in surface coatings of urea-formaldehyde resins. Blooming from such surfaces continues over long periods and withstands the usual methods of cleaning (in fact, rubbing the surface encourages blooming). This method is favored for the "band treatment" of cockroach runs in hospital and restaurant kitchens.

Slow-Release Formulations. Mostly used as mosquito larvicides, these formulations take the form of combinations of insecticide in sand granules, clay pellets, briquettes, or capsules that disintegrate slowly in water, prolonging the insecticide's effect.

High-Spreading Oils. The control of mosquito larvae by a continuous film of ordinary oil required some 20 to 25 gal/acre (more than 200 L/ha) in the past. The addition of spreading agents, e.g., certain resins, increases the oil's spreading pressure and allows a reduction in the quantities to cover a given area. The addition of small amounts of residual insecticides greatly increases the toxicity of such thin films. The dispersion of such small quantities over large areas presents problems, however. Spraying from the air can be the answer only where large areas of water are involved and where economically feasible. For small collections of water such as rainwater pools, a small oiler is more satisfactory.

Baits. A combination of insecticide with some substance that will attract the pest makes a useful method of control. Specific attractants derived from the pests themselves are ideal. At present, most baits are animal protein or sugar in one form or another. Bait-insecticide combinations are commonly used to control synanthropic flies and cockroaches.

Toxic Hazards. All insecticides are poisonous to humans to some extent. Persons most at risk are those handling the undiluted formulations and the applicator and those who are continuously exposed to dusts or droplets, often within the confines of dwellings. Dermal penetration is of greater importance than inhalation or swallowing; hence, the need for protective clothing. In tropical climates, this must be simple; must cover most of the skin, e.g., lightweight overalls and a broad-brimmed hat; and must be able to be easily washed after each spraying occasion. The mixer of undiluted formulations should wear gloves and an apron. Facilities for washing with soap and water should be on hand at all times.

An arbitrary classification of toxicities has been made

by the World Health Organization (WHO), based on LD_{50} values (mg/kg body weight) when the insecticide is administered to rats orally or dermally and depending on whether it is a solid or liquid. The classification is by hazard, which is defined as "the acute risk to health" (Table 114–2).

Insecticide Resistance. One major effect of the widespread use of chemicals for pest control has been the selection of those arthropods genetically endowed with protective mechanisms against the chemicals used. The persistence of these arthropods and their offspring results in the eventual replacement of a mixed population (one with some members susceptible to insecticides) by a resistant one. Among arthropods of medical importance, more than 150 species have shown resistance of one kind or another. In fact, the only major group of species not yet showing resistance is tsetse flies.

The protective mechanisms vary from enzymes that break the insecticide down into harmless metabolites, to reduced sensitivity of the target site of action of the insecticide (usually the central nervous system), to reduced penetration, or to an increased excretion rate of the insecticide. Some of these mechanisms are specific for particular groups of chemicals and others protect against more than 1 group. The enzyme carboxylesterase metabolizes those organophosphates with a carboxylester band in the molecule, e.g., malathion, but not those without it, e.g., nearly all the other organophosphates. An insensitive acetylcholinesterase enzyme, on the other hand, imparts cross-resistance to a wide range of organophosphates and carbamates. Another group of enzymes, the mixed function oxidases, are the principal enzymes involved in pyrethroid metabolism and may be involved in the metabolic breakdown of some organophosphates and carbamates.

Standard susceptibility tests designed to detect and monitor the spread of resistance for most of the major arthropod vectors of disease are distributed by the WHO. The pests are exposed to standard concentrations of the various insecticides known to normally kill the species (discriminating or diagnostic dosages), and their survival rate is monitored. New biochemical tests are now being developed, however, which will virtually eliminate all the ambiguities of the current, somewhat crude, WHO susceptibility tests. Eventually they should be able to identify actual resistance mechanisms in single insects and indicate directly what cross-resistance is likely to be shown and to what alternative compounds they will still be susceptible.

When resistance first appears as a mutation in the population, it is rare and in the heterozygous state. Only if heterozygotes survive the field dosage of insecticide and mate can a homozygote appear. Therefore, the degree of resistance imparted by the gene and its dominance characteristics are important in the process of resistance selection, because resistance is dependent on survival of the heterozygote. Leaving part of the environment unsprayed and using more than 1 (independently acting) insecticide either in mixture or in rotation encourage the survival of susceptible genes. The rationale for the use of mixtures of insecticides is that when resistance genes are rare, the likelihood of finding an individual insect with 2 genes affecting 2 differently acting insecticides is remote. The rationale for using insecticides in rotation is that resistance genes are less fit than their susceptible counterparts; thus, without insecticide selection, they tend to decline in the population.

OTHER CHEMICALS. A number of alternatives to conventional residual insecticides are now under investigation, mainly as mosquito larvicides.

Monolayers. These are substances that produce thin, continuous films over open water, denying mosquito aquatic stages access to the air. High-molecular-weight alcohols such as lauryl alcohol, lipids such as lecithin, and semisynthetic surfactants such as Monoxci are bio-

TABLE 114–2. WHO Classification of Insecticide Toxicities

Extremely Hazardous	Highly Hazardous	Moderately Hazardous	Slightly Hazardous	Unlikely to Present an Acute Hazard in Normal Use
chlorfenvinphos	aldrin	bendiocarb	allethrin	bioresmethrin
parathion	dichlorvos	bioallethrin	bromophos	borax
parathion-methyl	dieldrin	carbaryl	dicofol	chlorphoxim
	dimetilan	chlordane	malathion	chlorpyrifos-methyl
	dioxathion	chlordimeform	pirimiphos-methyl	diflubenzuron
	endrin	chlorpyrifos	resmethrin	jodfenphos
	fenthion	cypermethrin	trichlorphon	methoprene
	Paris green	DDT		permethrin
		deltamethrin		phenothrin
		diazinon		temephos
		dimethoate		tetrachlorvinphos
		endosulfan		tetramethrin
		fenchlorphos		
		fenitrothion		
		fenvalerate		
		γ HCH		
		heptachlor		
		naled		
		phoxim		
		propoxur		
		pyrethrins		
		toxaphene		

degradable and nontoxic. They are also harmless to those organisms that do not have to penetrate the water surface film to breathe air, i.e., gill-breathers.

Insect Growth Regulators

Juvenile Hormones. Juvenile hormones and their synthetic counterparts, of which methoprene (Altosid) is the best-known example, act by affecting or preventing the molt from the last larval instar to pupa or that from pupa to adult. Because they affect only these late developmental stages, they have to be either applied repeatedly or delivered from some slow-release formulation. Methoprene is biodegradable and functional against mosquito larvae at 0.1 parts per million or less and has little effect on other organisms. Houseflies and *Culex quinquefasciatus,* however, have already developed resistance to it.

Chitin Inhibitors. Diflubenzuron (Dimilin) is the most widely used substance that affects the fundamental processes of chitinization and melanization. Unlike juvenile hormones, they operate against all life stages, causing almost complete inhibition of adult emergence.

Precocines. These substances antagonize the synthesis of natural juvenile hormones and thus interfere with metamorphosis from larva to pupa to adult. Precocines cause premature metamorphosis, producing "precocious" sterile adults with incompletely developed reproductive systems.

ALTERNATIVES TO CHEMICALS.

Chemicals require extensive tests for biologic activity and safety. Such evaluations involve direct toxicity tests on laboratory animals and extended tests for mutagenicity, teratogenicity, and carcinogenicity. Even after expensive testing, the end product may have only a short marketable life because of the development of resistance. The increase in the frequency, extent, and complexity of chemical resistance, the reluctance to pollute the environment with long-lasting chemicals, and the rising cost of developing new chemicals have led to alternatives to chemicals for vector control.

The 3 main alternatives to chemical control are environmental management measures (which have already been discussed), biologic control agents, and genetic control methods.

Biologic Control. This consists of the use of 1 plant or animal to control another, thus exploiting predator-prey and parasite-host relationships either by introducing new predators and parasites or by artificially increasing the proportions of existing ones.

Through the special program for research and training in tropical diseases, the WHO is promoting research on biologic control agents. It lists 2 agents likely to be widely used in the near future, a larvivorous fish, *Gambusia affinis,* and a bacterium, *Bacillus thuringiensis.*

G. affinis is a small (4 to 6 cm long) top-feeding minnow that originated in the United States and has been used for many years to control mosquito larvae. It breeds rather rapidly; a single female may produce 200 to 300 offspring in 1 year, and its mass production and distribution present few difficulties. It is most efficient at a density of about 5000/acre. However, where vegetation is dense, as favored by mosquito larvae, it may not gain access to its prey. Other limitations are that it

will not thrive everywhere, is subject to diseases and predation itself, and may produce undesirable changes in the ecosystem by eating desirable organisms. However, where mosquito breeding places are suitable, *G. affinis* has produced useful control.

B. thuringiensis israelensis is a spore-forming bacterium that produces a crystal of toxic protein (δ-endotoxin). When spores and crystals are ingested by mosquito larvae, the mouth parts and gut are paralyzed and the gut epithelium destroyed. The crystal itself appears to be most important, but death due to bacterial septicemia can also occur. Because the crystals are insoluble in water, it is a particulate insecticide, usually formulated as a wettable powder or emulsion. Mass production in culture with isolation and extraction of endotoxin is now possible. Thus, *B. thuringiensis israelensis* is a biologic larvicide. Trials against both culicine and anopheline mosquito larvae, as well as those of the black fly (*Simulium* species), have produced favorable results.

Numerous other predators and pathogens (viruses, bacteria, protozoa, fungi, and nematode worms) are under investigation, with the following ready for field evaluation: *Poecilia reticulata* and *Aplocheilus* species (fish); *Toxorhynchites* species (nonbiting mosquitoes whose larvae prey on other mosquito larvae); *Bacillus sphaericus* (another spore-forming bacterium); *Culicinomyces clavosporus* (a fungus); and *Romanomermis culicivorax* (a nematode worm).

Genetic Control

Sterility. The genetic manipulation of arthropods to render them sterile, partially sterile, more susceptible to conventional methods of control, or harmless to humans has been the subject of laboratory and field research since the early 1950s. The impetus came from the successful eradication of the screwworm fly (*Cochliomyia hominivorax*) by the mass rearing of the insect and the sterilization of male and female pupae by γ irradiation. These pupae were then introduced into the wild population just before adult emergence. The emerging sterile adults mated with the wild ones to produce dramatic reductions in fly numbers and eventual eradication in certain areas.

Sterility of arthropods can also be achieved by exposure to chemosterilants and, in some mosquito complexes, by crossing closely related species to produce sterile hybrid offspring. In the *Culex pipiens* and *Aedes scutellaris* complexes, cytoplasmic incompatibility between certain populations of mosquitoes is evident, with the sperm of one dying in the cytoplasm of the other before fertilization. Such matings produce only sterile eggs; thus, the release of incompatible males into a wild population could lead to elimination of that population. Partial sterility can be achieved by the production of chromosome translocations from irradiation at lower dosages than those causing complete sterility. When this occurs in only 1 of a pair of homologous chromosomes, the resulting individual produces a proportion of chromosomally imbalanced gametes, which, when mated with normal individuals, produce eggs of which only a portion hatch. If this inherited sterility is high enough, population depression follows. Another phenomenon, known only in the yellow fever mosquito, *Aedes aegypti,* and in *Culex quinquefasciatus,* the tropical house mosquito, is sex ratio distortion in favor of the male sex. When strains producing more than 9 males to every female are released, the numbers of females (the biting and disease-transmitting sex) and the reproductive potential of the population will be reduced.

Population Replacement. For effective population suppression of highly reproductive pests (nearly all arthropods of medical importance with the exception of tsetse flies), large releases of sterile or partially sterile insects over considerable time and areas will be necessary. Therefore, more attention is being paid to genetic control techniques resulting in population replacement, in particular the introduction of strains that are not carriers of disease or that are more amenable to control by other means. In its simplest form, population replacement can be achieved by the prolonged release of fertile males carrying the gene or genes considered desirable to introduce into the population. The release of both sexes of a bidirectional, cytoplasmically incompatible strain or of those with a homozygous translocation (involving both chromosomes of a homologous pair) to produce nonviable matings could be used.

Desirable genes could be those affecting the continued existence of the pest population, e.g., temperature-sensitive lethal genes or insecticide-susceptibility genes, or those that can render the pest incapable of supporting and transmitting disease agents. Temperature-sensitive lethal genes have been isolated in both the housefly and *Culex tritaeniorhynchus,* the vector of Japanese encephalitis. They have not yet been used for field control purposes. The release of males carrying genes for susceptibility to insecticides has been advocated in areas of insecticide resistance so that inexpensive, safe, and efficient compounds such as DDT can continue to be used. Examples of strains of insects no longer capable of supporting development of the pathogen are to be found in the mosquito vectors of viruses, malarial parasites, and filarial worms. No one has yet tried replacing wild populations with the strains, although some long-term population cage trials have been done.

Requirements for Genetic Control Systems. The success of any genetic control system is dependent on a number of requirements. It must be possible to rear the pests in large numbers, and they must survive, disperse, and mate competitively with their wild counterparts. Fitness and competitiveness may be affected by the sterilization procedure or by the genetic manipulation to produce the particular control system. γ Irradiation and chemosterilants attempt to achieve a high degree of sterility without serious effect on fitness, a goal less easily obtained with radiation. The developmental stage of the insect at which sterilization is most conveniently performed is a consideration, as is the maturity of the gonads.

Sexing Techniques. With most pests of medical importance, the female sucks blood and transmits disease; therefore, for genetic control purposes, it is preferable to release only the male sex, because even a sterile female transmits disease. Thus, an efficient sexing technique is essential. With some pests, size differences between the sexes can be utilized as well as a sieving process. However, these seldom result in perfect separation of the sexes. In several mosquito species, much greater accuracy is obtained from actual genetic sexing techniques in which insecticide-resistant genes or temperature-sensitive lethal genes are translocated by irradiation onto the male sex chromosomes. Dieldrin resistance has been used in *Anopheles gambiae, A. arabiensis,* and *A. culicifacies,* and propoxur resistance has been used in *A. albimanus.* The partially resistant male carrying translocated chromosomes survives a small amount of the appropriate insecticide placed into the water where the eggs are laid. When these males mate with females, they transmit resistance at the heterozygous level to their sons, but their daughters remain susceptible. Thus, a partially resistant male could be released into a sprayed area where resistance is present and survive to introduce susceptibility into the population.

Arthropod Ecology. For their efficient application, genetic control methods demand a detailed knowledge of pest ecology. A knowledge of flight range, longevity, population size, reproductive potential, and seasonal changes in these variables is essential for decisions on when and where to release genetically manipulated arthropods, how many to release, and over what area and period. It might be thought that the best time for release is when the target population is at its lowest level and least able to expand. However, the adverse conditions responsible for this low level may be even more adverse to the pest population being released, which, in the interests of mass production, has been reared under optimal conditions. The ideal might be to integrate the release with some other method of population reduction at the time of year when the release material is most likely to be effective. The other method of suppression could be conventional insecticide use, in which case it would be an advantage if the released arthropods were resistant to the particular insecticide.

THE CONTROL OF SPECIFIC ARTHROPODS OF MEDICAL IMPORTANCE.
The following are descriptions of methods employed for the control of insects and mites living on humans and those commonly found in people's houses and in outdoor situations.

Lice (Order Anoplura). Three different kinds of lice parasitize humans—body, head, and crab lice. The last 2 stay on the body continuously. The first, except when feeding, is found in the clothing. Infections pass from person to person through social and sexual contact.

Body Lice (Fig. 114–1). Regular laundering and changing of clothing minimize the likelihood of body lice infestations, which are usually associated with poverty or with mass congregations and migrations of people, e.g., during wars, famines, and other disasters. The old methods of clothing decontamination by heat or fumigants have been replaced by the use of dusts containing residual insecticides. These can be distributed by plunger-type dust guns with long nozzles for insertion beneath clothes without the need for undressing. During World War II, 10% DDT in talc was used in this way to combat typhus epidemics. Alternatively, sifter-top cans can be issued for individual use. A 1% lindane

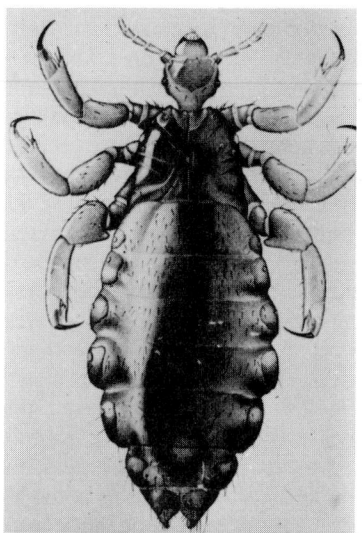

FIGURE 114–1. Body louse.

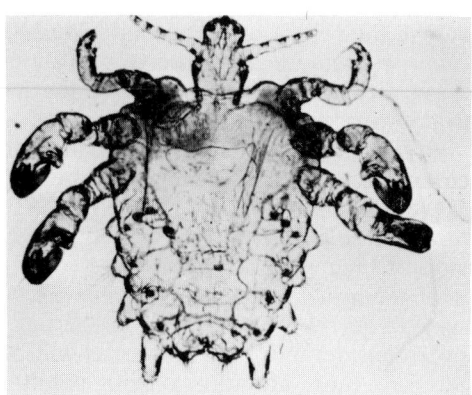

FIGURE 114–2. Crab louse.

(γ HCH) powder may be used where DDT resistance is evident, although a second application of lindane within 7 to 10 days of the first may be necessary. Where resistance to both DDT and lindane has arisen, 1% malathion, 2% temephos, 1% propoxur, or 5% carbaryl dusts can be used. Resistance to malathion is now evident in Burundi, Ethiopia, and Egypt.

Head Lice. These are best controlled with insecticide lotions rubbed into the hair. Those containing malathion (0.5%) or carbaryl (0.5%) kill eggs as well as nymphs and adults. If 1% lindane lotion is used, a weekly treatment for 3 weeks is recommended. Although resistance to the organochlorines is known in head lice, no resistance to organophosphates or carbamates has yet been recorded. Shampoos are less effective than lotions.

Crab Lice (Fig. 114–2). These are controlled in the same way as head lice. Although usually confined to the pubic region, they can extend to other parts of the body, i.e., the axillae, chest hair, and even beards and eyelashes. Manual removal from eyelashes is preferable to insecticidal treatment. No resistance has yet been found in this species.

Scabies Mite (Order Astigmata, Family Sarcoptidae) (Fig. 114–3). A lotion containing 1% lindane applied to the entire body from the neck down is the favored method of treatment for scabies. The lotion should not be washed off for 12 hours, and if the hands are washed, the lotion should be reapplied. A second application 3 days later is desirable. Commonly used is 25% benzyl benzoate emulsion, which should be applied after a bath and left on the body for 24 hours. A repeat treatment on the third day is essential, and another on the fifth day is desirable.

Scabies is so highly contagious that it is essential to treat all members of a family or closely associated group; otherwise, reinfestation will soon occur.

Mosquitoes (Order Diptera, Family Culicidae). Most mosquitoes feed on blood, constituting a major biting nuisance; many transmit diseases as well. Individual control may alleviate the biting problem, but communitywide control is necessary to reduce disease transmis-

sion (Fig. IX–2). Personal protection using repellents, mosquito nets, space sprays, and the screening of houses provide individual control. Other personal protective methods are the use of residual house sprays and perhaps attacking breeding places if these are few in number, small enough, and localized.

On a community basis, the use of residual insecticides, either in houses or in and around breeding sites, is the usual method of control, along with environmental measures directed against the breeding places. The following sections present methods adopted for the control of diseases carried by 4 groups of mosquitoes.

Anopheles Species (Fig. 114–4). Some 60 species of *Anopheles* are malaria vectors. The normal method of control is by spraying the walls and roofs or ceilings of the houses where they rest with a specific, uniform dose of a residual insecticide. Where the species are partly zoophilic, animal shelters should be sprayed as well. Other control measures must be adopted for some species that spend little or no time in houses. For example, anophelines of the Kerteszia group, e.g., *A. bellator* and *A. cruzii* of South America, whose larvae breed in water held in the axils of the leaves of epiphytic bromeliad plants, bite predominantly outdoors. The removal or treatment of these plants is the method of attacking these vectors. *A. balabacensis* of the Far East spends little time indoors, although the control of malaria transmitted by this species in Vietnam is claimed

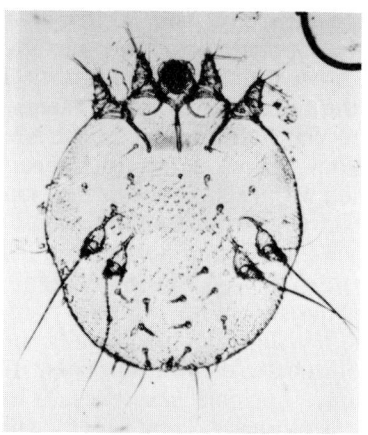

FIGURE 114–3. Scabies mite.

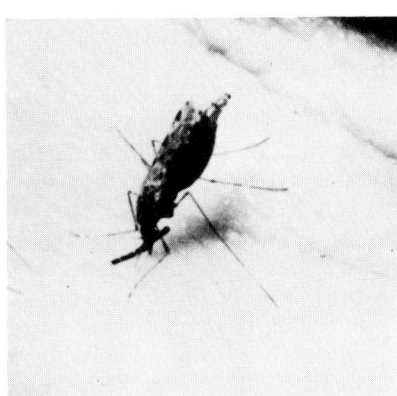

FIGURE 114–4. Anopheline mosquito.

to have been achieved by spraying both the inside and outside (around the eaves) of houses with DDT.

DDT is still the insecticide of choice if the local vector mosquitoes remain susceptible. It is irritating to most insects, however, and causes some to depart from a treated surface before they receive a lethal dose. HCH is an alternative but is volatile and has a shorter persistence on nonabsorbent surfaces. For safety reasons, dieldrin is no longer recommended for house spraying. When organochlorine resistance is evident, malathion is the popular alternative, with fenitrothion, pirimiphos-methyl and chlorphoxim being other possibilities among the organophosphates, propoxur among the carbamates, and deltamethrin and permethrin among the synthetic residual pyrethroids. DDT can be expected to remain active for at least 6 months; the other compounds remain active for up to 3 months.

Smoke generators, cold aerosols, thermal fogs, and ULV sprays have all been used for exterior space treatments, especially during malaria epidemics produced by partially exophilic vectors and in large temporary gatherings of people such as religious pilgrimages. Malathion or some of the pyrethroids are usually favored as exterior space sprays.

Larvae. Larvicides may be added where indoor residual insecticide spraying is insufficient to interrupt disease transmission. It is also used in urban or semiurban areas where indoor residual insecticide spraying is not practical or where breeding sites are relatively limited in number and size. If both adult and larval chemical control is being used against the same species, it is advisable to use differently acting insecticides for each control method to avoid the appearance of resistance. Organochlorine insecticides are not recommended as larvicides because of possible environmental toxicities attributable to their stability and persistence. The organophosphates temephos, malathion, fenthion, chlorpyrifos, jodfenphos, fenitrothion, and pirimiphos-methyl and the pyrethroids permethrin and deltamethrin have all been recommended for use against anopheline larvae. They may be applied in solution with oils, as emulsions, wettable powders, or dusts, or in a special slow-release formulation. Various types of ground and aerial equipment are used for their distribution. The treatment cycle is usually every 10 to 14 days, but longer effect has been recorded. Temephos has proved to be

particularly efficient and safe, but all larvicides present some hazard to fish and other aquatic life. The insect growth regulators methoprene and diflubenzuron have also been used as anopheline larvicides; they affect only arthropods.

Resistance. More than 50 anopheline species are resistant to 1 insecticide or another in 1 or more parts of their distribution. Nearly 30 of them are resistant to 3 of the 4 chemical groupings to which the common insecticides belong, viz., organochlorines, organophosphates, carbamates, and pyrethroids. Eleven of them are major malaria vectors. Of particular concern are multiple resistances in *A. albimanus* in most of the Central American states, *A. sacharovi* in Turkey, *A. culicifacies* in the Indian subcontinent (now known to be a complex of at least 3 sibling species), *A. sinensis* in China, and *A. stephensi* in Iraq, Iran, Pakistan, and India. These complicated resistances have been attributed in some instances, particularly in *A. albimanus*, *A. sacharovi*, and *A. sinensis*, to the contamination of the mosquito breeding places, by drift, with the numerous different insecticides used for agricultural purposes (mainly against pests of cotton and rice).

Other Control Measures. Environmental measures, such as water management aimed at the removal or alteration of existing breeding places, are alternatives to chemicals. Biologic control agents and genetic control methods have also been used. Of the biologic methods, the greatest emphasis has been on the use of larvivorous fish and the bacterial agent *Bacillus thuringiensis israelensis*. Various fish have been tried, of which *Gambusia affinis* is the best known. Where breeding places are suitable for the fish and are the main or only sources of the mosquitoes, they have proved useful. Some 30 countries are using fish alone or as part of an integrated program of mosquito control. *B. thuringiensis israelensis* has proved efficient in the laboratory against anophelines, but a major field trial has yet to be undertaken. Two trials of genetic control of anophelines have been done. The first involved the release of sterile hybrid males produced by crossing 2 sibling species of the *Anopheles gambiae* complex against a third species of the same complex in an isolated village in Upper Volta in West Africa. It was unsuccessful because the sterile males failed to mate with the wild females. A larger trial with *A. albimanus* in Central America had some success. Sterilization was achieved by immersing pupae in the chemosterilant bisazir. At the peak of the trial, more than 1 million sterile males were released daily in an area of 150 km². Eradication was not achieved, however.

Aedes Species. *Aedes aegypti* (Figs. 113–3 and 114–5) is the most important vector and has been responsible for nearly all urban epidemics of yellow fever, dengue, and dengue hemorrhagic fever. *Ae. albopictus* is mainly involved with dengue transmission in Southeast Asia and the western Pacific. *Ae. simpsoni* is widespread in Africa and is a vector of yellow fever. *Ae. polynesiensis*, *Ae. pseudoscutellaris*, *Ae. vigilax*, *Ae. niveus*, and *Ae. togoi* are all vectors of filariasis (bancroftian and brugian) in the Far East. All breed in small collections of water, natural, e.g., leaf axils or crab holes, or artificial,

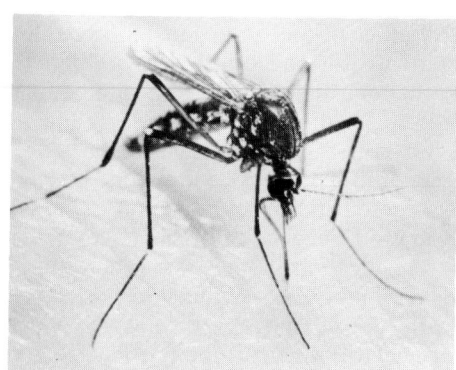

FIGURE 114–5. *Aedes aegypti.*

e.g., tin cans or discarded tires. The adults are largely day feeders and have a limited flight range.

Chemical Control. These measures are directed more toward larval breeding places and their vicinity (perifocal spraying in the case of the domestic *Ae. aegypti*) or toward exterior space spraying rather than house spraying. Nonpotable water may be treated with malathion, fenitrothion, fenthion, temephos, pirimiphos-methyl or methoprene applied as solutions, emulsions, or granules. For potable water, only temephos in the form of 1% sand granules is used at a dosage of 1 mg/L. Hand or power sprayers are used to apply the insecticides as a peripheral spray in and around nonpotable water containers and adjacent surfaces. The resulting insecticide residue is supposed to destroy present and subsequent larval infestations as well as adults that frequent the sites. A syringe or pipette can be used for treating indoor or outdoor flowerpots and ant traps. Exterior space treatments may be from the ground or from the air and are justifiable where epidemic conditions prevail. Malathion, naled, fenitrothion and pirimiphos-methyl have all been used from thermal fog and ULV machines and are best applied up to a 400-m radius from houses.

Many of the common *Aedes* species show resistance to both organochlorines and organophosphates, while pyrethroid resistance occurs in *Ae. aegypti* in Thailand.

Biologic Control. Most biologic control methods operate against the larval stages of mosquitoes. The problem in the case of *Aedes* species, which inhabit small collections of water, is delivering the agent to the breeding place. The larva of the large nonbiting *Toxorhynchites* mosquito occurring naturally in some *Aedes* habitats is an efficient predator.

Genetic Control. These methods, some highly sophisticated, have been tried in limited field trials against *Ae. aegypti* in India and Africa. They have included the release of males sterilized by irradiation and chemosterilants and the release of males carrying translocated chromosomes and meiotic-drive sex-ratio distortion systems.

The obvious solution to control of *Aedes* species that breed in small, usually synthetic containers is the proper disposal of such containers. A piped water supply to houses eliminates the necessity for water storage in pots.

There are other *Aedes* species, e.g., *Ae. nigromaculis, Ae. sollicitans,* and *Ae. taeniorhynchus* in the United States and *Ae. caspius, Ae. detritus,* and *Ae. cantans* in

Europe, that breed in extensive marshy sites, often coastal, brackish, and subject to periodic drying and flooding. Eggs laid in the dry season remain viable until the following rainy season. Insecticides or insect growth regulators must be delivered in a form, e.g., granules, that will remain active and release the compound when flooding occurs.

Culex Species (Fig. 114–6). The common tropical house mosquito *Culex quinquefasciatus,* which is found all over the world, is a vector of bancroftian filariasis in many urban areas. Its near relative of more temperate climates, *C. pipiens,* has been linked with the transmission of epidemic Rift Valley fever. Other vectors include *C. tritaeniorhynchus,* which transmits Japanese encephalitis in the Far East; *C. tarsalis,* which transmits St. Louis encephalitis in the United States; and *C. annulirostris,* which transmits Murray Valley encephalitis and Ross River fever in Australia.

Insecticides. Methods for the control of *Culex* species are usually directed against the aquatic stages rather than the adult. Many species that habitually bite humans breed in well-defined waters, often heavily polluted and quite near habitations, e.g., cesspools and open drains. Control by prevention of access to or by removal or treatment of these breeding places is often relatively simple; the difficulty lies in locating them. In general, insecticidal emulsions, suspensions, and pellets are better larvicides than oil solutions, especially where organic matter in the water prevents the spread of oil. Higher dosages than those used for the control of anopheline larvae are usually required, and allowance must be made for the effects of dilution in deep water, because culicines are not as confined to surface feeding as anophelines. Organophosphates, especially chlorpyrifos, are particularly good for highly polluted water. In addition, tetramethrin among the pyrethroids, methoprene and diflubenzuron, Flit MLO, malariol, gas oil, and Paris green have all been used successfully against *C. quinquefasciatus* in polluted drains and pit latrines.

For those species that occupy extensive breeding areas, e.g., *C. tritaeniorhynchus,* typically a rice field breeder, and *C. tarsalis,* dusts, fogs, and ULV applications are used from ground-based equipment or from the air.

Organochlorine and organophosphate resistances are common in all the *Culex* species except *C. annulirostris. C. pipiens* and *C. quinquefasciatus* also show resistance

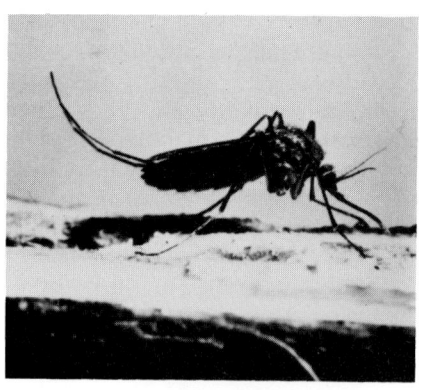

FIGURE 114–6. Culicine mosquito.

to many organophosphates and carbamates, and resistance to methoprene and pyrethroids has been produced in the laboratory. Organophosphate resistance also occurs in *C. tritaeniorhynchus* and *C. tarsalis*.

Environmental Control. Environmental measures against *C. pipiens* and *C. quinquefasciatus* involve the proper construction of sewage systems and the prevention of access to them by gravid female mosquitoes. Pit latrines should have tight-fitting lids and screened vent pipes. Soakage pits and roadside drains should also be covered; a useful safeguard in such closed systems is the hanging at intervals of plastic strips impregnated with the volatile organophosphate dichlorvos. Expanded polystyrene beads in sufficient quantity to completely cover the water surface have proved an extremely efficient way of preventing pit-latrine breeding and a single application can last for years. Small collections of water near houses should always be discouraged.

Biologic Control. Biologic control methods have included the use of predatory fish. *Poecilia reticulata* can survive high degrees of pollution. Pathogens tried on a small scale include *Bacillus thuringiensis israelensis,* microsporidia, and the mermithid worm *Romanomermis culicivorax.*

Genetic Control. Many attempts have been made to control *C. quinquefasciatus* by genetic means. The phenomenon of cytoplasmic incompatibility is exhibited in this species and *C. pipiens* and consists of different strains of the Rickettsia *Wolbachia pipientis* occurring in the cytoplasm of the different populations. Sperm die in the cytoplasm of the ovum of incompatible females. Control can be achieved by the release of incompatible males. The release of males sterilized by irradiation or chemosterilants has also been tried with some success, as has the release of males carrying translocated chromosomes. A combination of the latter with cytoplasmic incompatibility (an "integrated" strain) has shown great promise.

Mansonia Species. Several species of *Mansonia* are important vectors of filariasis, transmitting both *Wuchereria bancrofti* and *Brugia malayi*. *M. uniformis* is the most widely distributed species. The larvae and pupae of this genus attach themselves to the roots of aquatic plants, e.g., *Pistia, Eichornia, Scirpus,* and *Salvinia* and breathe through the air system of the plant. Control is usually directed toward the destruction of the plants with herbicides, which are generally applied from ground equipment, with the spray directed vertically onto the plants. In the case of *Pistia,* treatment should be done prior to seed formation. Two annual applications usually suffice.

The adults of some species, e.g., *M. uniformis* and *M. annulifera,* rest in houses and can be controlled by house spraying in the same way as endophilic anophelines. Organochlorine resistance is known in *M. indiana, M. annulifera,* and *M. uniformis* in Thailand.

Sandflies (Order Diptera, Family Psychodidae) (Fig. 114–7). These delicate moth flies, the vectors of leishmaniasis, bartonellosis, and viral sandfly fever, either may be outdoor feeders and resters or may frequent the indoors. The latter type are readily controlled when houses are sprayed with residual insecticides, although

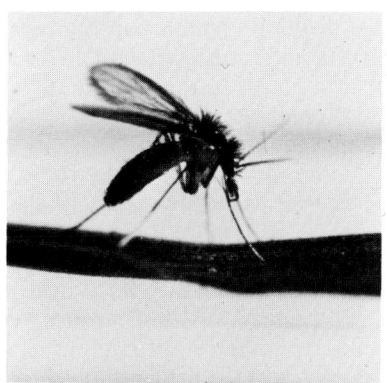

FIGURE 114–7. Sandfly.

this is seldom done specifically for sandfly control. Where outside resting places are well known, e.g., termite hills in the case of *Phlebotomus martini*, a vector of kala-azar in Kenya, these may also be treated with residual insecticides. The larval habitat is often difficult to identify, and measures against it are seldom attempted. The use of mosquito repellents and sandfly nets (which have smaller holes than mosquito netting and are more uncomfortable in hot climates) provide personal protection. Larger mesh that has been treated with repellents is more comfortable and works well.

Resistance to DDT, the first example of insecticide resistance in sandflies, has been established in *P. papatasi* in North Bihar. However, *P. argentipes* is the vector of kala-azar in this area.

Houseflies, Related Flies, and Stable Flies (Order Diptera, Family Muscidae). The synanthropic (associated with humans) flies include not only species in the family Muscidae but also some of those species in the families Calliphoridae and Sarcophagidae that breed on carrion and that cause myiasis. The Muscidae include the common housefly (*Musca domestica*) (Figs. 113–5 and 114–8), the greater housefly (*Muscina stabulans*), the lesser housefly (*Fannia canicularis*), the latrine fly (*Fannia scalaris*), and the bloodsucking stable fly (*Stomoxys calcitrans*). Because of their habits of visiting both excreta and food and their regurgitatory feeding methods, these flies may be mechanical vectors of viral, bacterial, protozoan, and helminthic diseases.

Breeding Sites. These flies prefer the excreta of humans or their domestic animals, decomposing animal or vegetable matter, and farm manure for egg laying and larval breeding. Control measures, e.g., construction of

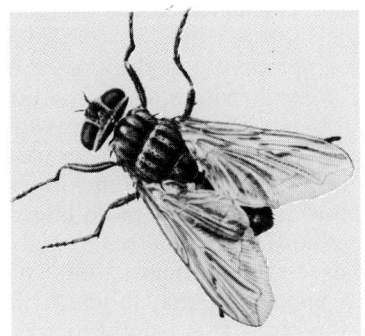

FIGURE 114–8. Housefly.

closed sewage disposal systems and the correct disposal of animal excreta and refuse, are largely directed toward the prevention of access to this excreta or refuse so that it is no longer available for breeding. Good standards of hygiene and sanitation are basic to fly control and are becoming more important because these insects have developed resistance to a wide variety of chemicals. The common housefly has more resistant populations to more groups of insecticides than any other insect species. Populations present in both the Old World and the New World are resistant to organochlorines, organophosphates, carbamates, pyrethroids, and insect growth regulators. A particularly disturbing feature is cross-resistance between a certain type of DDT resistance and the new synthetic residual pyrethroids.

Indoor Control. Screening denies flies access to both food and potential breeding areas. A 10-mesh net from 32 s.w.g. wire or plastic with an aperture of 2.17 mm is adequate. Particularly attractive items of foodstuffs, e.g., milk and sugar, may need their own gauze protection. Occasional invaders of screened premises can be dealt with by insecticidal space sprays, sticky traps (fly papers), electrocution traps (usually an ultraviolet lamp behind an electrified grid), electric vaporizers (a small electrically heated surface to which insecticide can be added), or residual fumigants (PVC strips impregnated with a volatile insecticide, usually dichlorvos). There may, however, be objection to the last two methods on the grounds of overconcentration of toxic insecticide in small enclosed domestic premises. Space sprays are usually composed of 0.035 to 0.1% pyrethrins in deodorized kerosene with a residual insecticide added. A simple contribution that the householder can make to the prevention of fly breeding is the addition every week or two of 60 gm of paradichlorobenzene to the garbage can.

Surface spraying of residual insecticides is directed against those areas where flies tend to congregate, rather than against the entire insides of houses, as is usually done for the control of endophilic mosquitoes. Places sprayed to control adult flies include doors, windows, sills and some of the outside surfaces of houses, kitchens, porches, latrines, animal shelters, and fences as well as around the grids of drains. Larval control is aimed at refuse dumps and accumulations of animal excrement and their vicinity. The spraying of such dumps will not always kill breeding fly larvae but will kill flies attempting to lay their eggs and new adults as they emerge. It must be emphasized, however, that no insecticidal treatment can replace efficient methods of rubbish and excrement disposal.

At present, emphasis is on the use of organophosphates for fly control, with some restrictions on their use in milk rooms (dairy barns), restaurants, food-processing plants, and food stores. There are no restrictions on the use of bromophos, fenchlorphos, fenitrothion, jodfenphos, trichlorphon, pirimiphos-methyl, diazinon, or malathion. Dimethoate and naled (Dibrom) should not be used in milk rooms, although the latter is considered safe enough to spray in poultry houses without removing the birds. It is helpful to add attractants, e.g., sugar or molasses, to these insecticides.

Cords and strips impregnated with insecticide and hung high in infested buildings are an accepted form of control. Five-mm cords dipped in 25% diazinon-xylene solution and installed at the rate of 1 m of cord/m² of floor area are effective for several months. Care is needed in the handling and preparation of these cords (gloves are essential). They should be marked to show what they are and to prevent their being used for other purposes.

Both organophosphates and carbamates have been incorporated in liquid and dry baits for spot treatments against flies. Dichlorvos and trichlorphon are the most widely used insecticides for this purpose, with the bait being some form of sugar or perhaps the housefly pheromone muscalure. Viscous paint-on baits are also used and are composed of an insecticide (2 to 6%), a binder, and sugar. These are applied by paintbrush as spot treatments to posts and walls.

Outdoor Control. Outdoor space treatments may be necessary where fly populations are excessive, especially during epidemics of enteric diseases. They are also useful in market areas where foods are on display and in large human assemblies. Power units are usually used to produce ULV mist sprays or thermal aerosols. The latter have the disadvantage of reducing visibility in traffic areas. Often, the equipment is mounted on vehicles that move at 8 to 16 km/hour and dispense the formulations at 24 to 48 L/km. Application rates of organophosphates vary from 200 to 700 gm/ha. The synthetic pyrethroids are also effective in ULV applications.

Triatomine Bugs (Order Hemiptera, Family Reduviidae) (Fig. 114–9). Variously known as cone-nose bugs, assassin bugs, barbeiros, kissing bugs, or vinchucas, several species are carriers of Chagas' disease in Mexico and Central and South America. The main genera concerned in the transmission of the disease to humans are *Triatoma, Panstrongylus,* and *Rhodnius.* Numerous animal species such as armadillos, opossums, domestic and wild rodents, birds, dogs, and squirrels act as reservoirs of the disease.

These bugs dwell in cracks and crevices in human

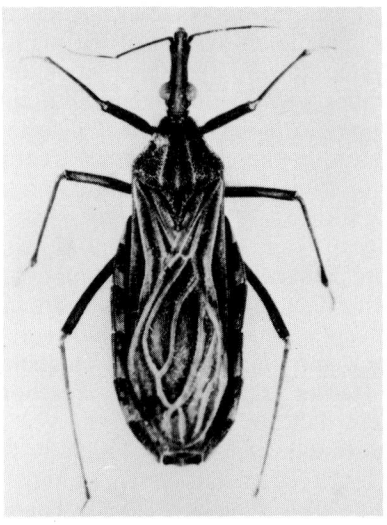

FIGURE 114–9. Triatomine bug.

habitations and in animal haunts and bird nests. House spraying with residual insecticides with special attention to cracks and crevices (pyrethroids may be added to flush them out) is the usual method of control. This is often combined with treatment of peridomestic sites of infestation, e.g., chicken houses, pigeon lofts, and piggeries. HCH and dieldrin, at dosages used for malaria control, have been employed rather than DDT. Dieldrin is no longer recommended for domestic use, and resistance to it and to HCH has been recorded in Venezuela. Organophosphates, carbamates, and residual pyrethroids are all possible alternatives. The plastering of wall cracks is encouraged.

Bedbugs (Order Hemiptera, Family Cimicidae) (Figs. 113–1 and 114–10). Strictly nocturnal, these bloodsucking insects spend their daylight hours in cracks and crevices in walls, floors, and roofs, behind pictures, and in bed springs, slats, mattresses, and furniture. Sprays of residual insecticides directed at these daytime resting places constitute the best method of control. The addition of 0.1 or 0.2% pyrethrins or synthetic pyrethroids, e.g., bioresmethrin, flushes the bugs from their hiding places, causing them to come into contact with the residuals. Resistance to the original residual, a 5% DDT emulsion or solution, has forced a change to 0.5% lindane or, where resistance to both groups of organochlorines is evident, to 2% malathion, 1% pirimiphos-methyl, fenchlorphos, carbaryl, or propoxur, or 0.5% diazinon. Some *Cimex lectularius* have developed organophosphate resistance, but control is still satisfactory with the carbamates carbaryl and propoxur. Infant beds and bedding should not be treated with residual insecticides. Care must be taken in applying these chemicals to adult bedding.

Fleas (Order Siphonaptera) (Fig. 114–11). Adult fleas are transient ectoparasites of animals, whereas the immature stages live in the nests, burrows, or other resting places of the animals. Control is directed more against the latter than the former, preferably with dusts containing residual insecticides. While killing the fleas, the dusts also contaminate the animal host; in sufficient concentration, they may kill the animal. In plague and murine typhus control, it is important to kill the fleas before the rats. The killing of rats by rodenticides alone may cause disease-carrying fleas to move from rodent to humans. Dust commonly used are 2% concentrations

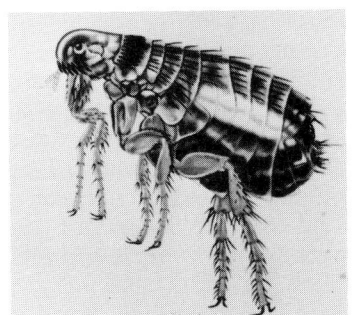

FIGURE 114–11. Flea.

of diazinon, fenitrothion, and pirimiphos-methyl, 3% γ HCH, 5% carbaryl, malathion, and propoxur, and 10% DDT. They are directed against the resting places and "runs" of the animals. Resistance to the organochlorines is known in several species, including 3 species of *Xenopsylla.*

The fleas of domestic pets are a "modern" nuisance, especially where there is central heating and fitted carpets. Regular vacuum cleaning helps to reduce infestations, but the application of insecticides to the animal and to its kennel and bedding may be necessary. Care must be taken in applying insecticides to pets, however, especially cats, which lick their fur, and young animals. Pyrethrum dust (0.2% pyrethrins + 2% synergist) is safer than the synthetic residual insecticides for this purpose. Plastic collars impregnated with the volatile organophosphate dichlorvos have proved useful for both cats and dogs.

Cockroaches (Order Dictyoptera). Cockroaches are habitually associated with dirt, human excrement, and human food and have been suspected of transmitting diseases. An estimated 16 species are involved in different parts of the world. The 3 most common ones in temperate climates are the Oriental *(Blatta orientalis),* the German *(Blatella germanica)* (Fig. 114–12), and the American *(Periplaneta americana)* cockroaches. The tropical cockroaches include some large species in the genus *Blaberus.* Those of most concern to humans are associated with sewage systems, food stores, and home and restaurant kitchens.

Control should be directed toward denying the insects access to food, sewage, and dirt, including strict cleanliness of food stores and kitchens and the proper sealing of service ducts supplying these premises. Insecticides should be used with care to prevent food contamination.

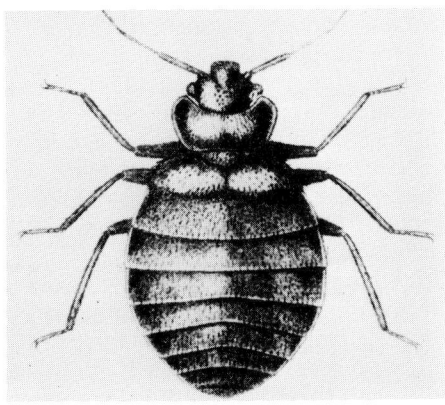

FIGURE 114–10. Bedbug.

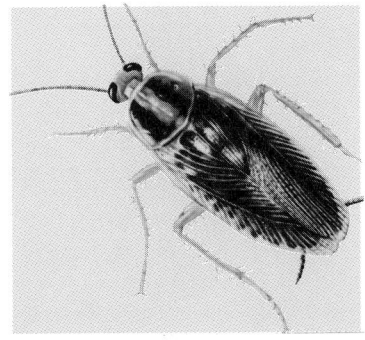

FIGURE 114–12. German cockroach.

Chemical control is usually directed at the specific "runs" and resting places of the insects, i.e., around baseboards and door frames; under fixed furniture, sinks, stoves, and refrigerators; in cupboards and drawers; around and beneath dustbins and drain grids; and in and around cracks and crevices. The formulations used may be liquid sprays, lacquers, or gels; dusts; or baits. Sprays and dusts are favored for good penetration into small spaces; sprays are less unsightly, whereas dusts require less elaborate machinery to apply. Lacquers or gels include insecticide dissolved in urea-formaldehyde resins or methylcellulose and are painted in bands on appropriate places, e.g., on baseboards and around door frames, where insects are likely to cross. Baits are usually combinations of insecticide, cereal, and some form of sugar. Jodfenphos (an organophosphate) is the favored insecticide for baits, but boric acid seems to be equally popular. Organophosphates, carbamates, and the pyrethroid permethrin are also used for roach control. Organochlorine resistance is common in all 3 main species of cockroaches *(B. orientalis, B. germanica,* and *P. americana),* with some species also resistant to organophosphates, carbamates, and the pyrethroids.

Alternatives to chemical control are under investigation. Pheromone attractants used in trapping devices seem particularly promising. Genetic control methods involving chromosome translocations that produce partial sterility are being developed in *B. germanica.*

Tsetse Flies (Order Diptera, Family Glossinidae) (Fig. 114–13). Tsetse flies are confined to tropical Africa, where 5 species are responsible for the transmission of human sleeping sickness and 10 for the transmission of trypanosomal diseases of animals. The adult fly is the only stage amenable to vector control measures; the transient larval stage buries itself in the soil to pupate. Fortunately, all species remain susceptible to insecticides, which, distributed from the air or the ground, have led to control and even complete eradication of tsetse flies from large areas. DDT, HCH, dieldrin, and endosulfan have been used, with the last 2 being preferred. The use of organophosphates, carbamates, and pyrethroids is now being considered to alleviate the fear

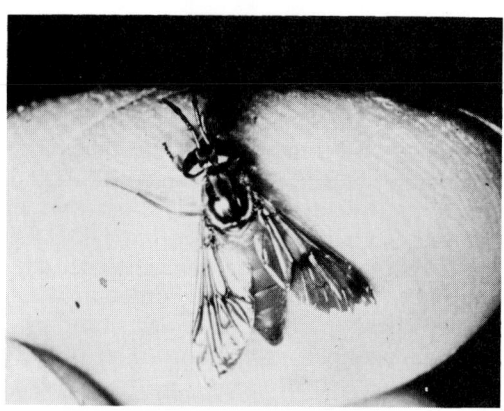

FIGURE 114–14. *Chrysops dimidiata* (tabanid).

of environmental pollution from the widespread use of organochlorines.

Spraying. Two spraying techniques have been developed. One aims at producing residual deposits of insecticides on the known resting sites of adult flies. The vegetation bordering rivers and streams favored by the sleeping sickness vectors, *Glossina palpalis* and *G. tachinoides,* can be sprayed with the conventional knapsack sprayer. For the control of the savanna-type species, e.g., the *G. morsitans* group responsible for animal trypanosomiasis, those parts of trees and bushes that the flies favor as resting places are selectively sprayed. Thus, in northern Nigeria, only certain branches of the "doka" tree at certain heights and angles are sprayed with residual insecticides. A more indiscriminate spraying technique utilizes aerial application as either an aerosol or a ULV spray. Repeated applications by this method are necessary because the pupal stage, which can last as long as 5 weeks, is not affected. In Botswana, for example, endosulfan has been applied from fixed-wing aircraft 5 times at 21-day intervals at a total cost for fly eradication of 70 to 75 dollars/km².

Trapping. The use of trapping devices impregnated with insecticide has had success in the control of riverine tsetse fly species in West Africa, where biconical traps impregnated with deltamethrin have reduced fly populations by more than 99%. Costs are low, and there are no harmful environmental effects.

Genetic Control. Genetic control by the release of mass-reared male flies sterilized by irradiation or by exposure to chemosterilants has been tried against both savanna and riverine tsetse fly species with some success, but difficulties in mass production of these male flies pose problems for large-scale application.

Environmental Control. Vegetation clearance can also lead to the disappearance of tsetse flies, especially when followed by human occupation and use of reclaimed land.

Horseflies, Deer Flies, and Clegs (Order Diptera, Family Tabanidae). Control of these biting flies, including the vectors of tularemia and loiasis (Fig. 114–14), is seldom attempted because of their extensive and often ill-defined breeding places, usually in marshy areas, but sometimes in environments with relatively dry soil. Effective trapping devices can catch adults, but significant control with them is doubtful. Diethyltoluamide is fairly effective as a repellent.

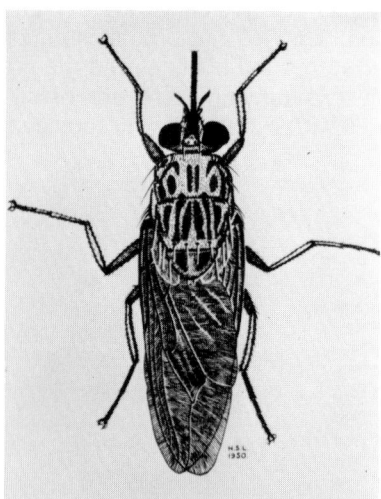

FIGURE 114–13. Tsetse fly.

Black Flies (Figs. 87–3 and 114–15) **or Buffalo Gnats (Order Diptera, Family Simuliidae).** The immature stages of these flies characteristically breed in rapidly flowing water. The adults, which are outdoor daytime biters, often occur in large numbers. They are a tremendous nuisance to humans and animals not only in the tropics, where they may be vectors of onchocerciasis, but also in colder parts of the world, e.g., northern Canada and Siberia.

Control is usually directed against the aquatic stages, using insecticides delivered at the water head in quantities sufficient to give concentrations downstream of 0.01 to 5 parts per million for periods of 5 to 30 minutes. The actual quantities required depend on the depth and flow rate of the water. Delivery may be by drip feed, from fixed-wing aircraft flying across the water source, or from helicopters. DDT, which was used initially, has been largely replaced by the environmentally safe methoxychlor and temephos (Abate).

The onchocerciasis control program of the Volta River basin in West Africa, which was started in 1975, covers an area of 700,000 km². Of the 10 million inhabitants there, about 1 million were afflicted with onchocerciasis, with some 70,000 being either blind or nearly so. Resistance to temephos and to the substitute chlorphoxim has been shown in some parts of the area in some species of the *Simulium damnosum* complex but has so far been satisfactorily dealt with by a change to permethrin in the rainy season and to serotype H14 of *B. thuringiensis israelensis* in the dry season. This program must be continued for as many years as it takes for the adult worm *(Onchocerca volvulus)* to die out in the human population. Some success in control of the adult flies has been obtained from the use of aerosols and ULV sprays applied to vegetation bordering breeding areas.

Black flies are less easily repelled by diethyltoluamide than mosquitoes, but considerable relief has been obtained by those wearing special jackets impregnated with the repellent.

Biting Midges (Order Diptera, Family Ceratopogonidae). The true biting midges, including the genera *Culicoides* (Fig. 114–16), *Leptoconops,* and *Styloconops,* are not known to be of great importance as disease vectors. However, they constitute severe biting nuisances because they occur in large numbers and are

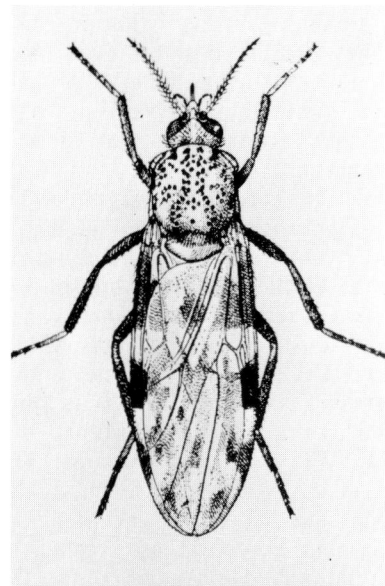

FIGURE 114–16. *Culicoides.*

small enough to pass through the finest of house screening and sandfly netting. Because these midges do not rest indoors for long periods, house spraying with residual insecticides does not contribute to their control, although painting screens with insecticides is useful. The treatment of nets with repellent may also be helpful.

Breeding grounds, almost invariably extensive swampy areas, can be controlled by drainage or insecticide treatment. This is extremely expensive, as is the repetitive use of thermal fogs or ULV applications in attempts to kill adult midges resting in vegetation.

Ticks (Order Metastigmata, Families Argasidae and Ixodidae). Ticks are vectors of many viral, rickettsial, and bacterial diseases. Most ticks parasitize a wide range of host animals. Each stage, the larva, nymph, and both sexes of adult, requires a blood meal. They often remain attached to the host animal for long periods and are usually difficult to remove because their mouth parts become fully embedded. Simple pulling often leaves

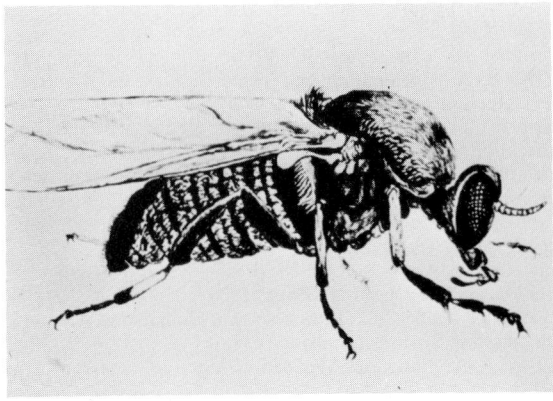

FIGURE 114–15. Black fly *(Simulium).*

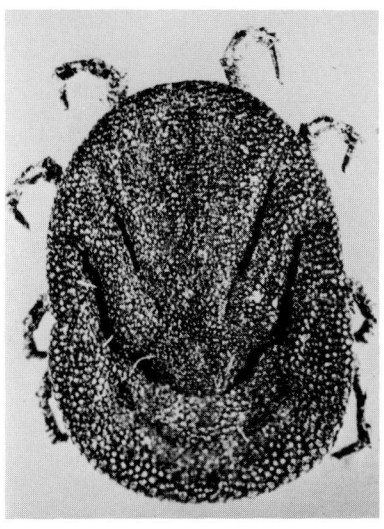

FIGURE 114–17. Soft tick *(Ornithodoros).*

these parts behind, causing irritation and secondary infection. They can be best removed carefully using tweezers. Repellents such as dimethyl phthalate, dibutyl phthalate, and diethyltoluamide can prevent infestation and are strongly recommended for those exposed to infested vegetation.

Soft Ticks. The soft ticks (Argasidae) include the vectors (*Ornithodoros* species [Fig. 114–17]) of relapsing fever caused by *Borrelia (Treponema) duttonii.* These ticks live in the earthern floors of houses and manmade or natural shelters for animals. Control can be achieved by spraying or dusting infested areas with residual insecticides. γ HCH is a favored one, and the highest dosage (3 gm/m²) is claimed to last as long as 1 year. There is no evidence as yet of resistance in this genus.

Hard Ticks. The hard ticks (Ixodidae) (Fig. 114–18) include vectors of Colorado tick fever, Rocky Mountain spotted fever, the tick-borne encephalitis of Central Europe, Kyasanur Forest disease, certain hemorrhagic fevers, and tularemia. The genera *Ixodes, Dermacentor, Haemaphysalis, Hyalomma, Amblyomma, Rhipicephalus,* and *Boophilus* are involved in their transmission. Primarily ectoparasites of domestic animals and pets, particularly dogs, these ticks can be controlled by treating the animals with insecticide washes, sprays, dips, or dusts or by treating the tick haunts, e.g., pasture vegetation or animal sleeping areas. Large-scale exterior treatments with ground and aerially produced fogs or ULV sprays are sometimes necessary. Tick invasion of houses may also necessitate spot applications to baseboards, floors, and wall cracks.

Organochlorines, organophosphates, carbamates, chlordimeform, and pyrethroids have all been used for tick control, with resistance to the first 3 of these groups now common in a number of genera and species. Some of the new synthetic pyrethroids, especially deltamethrin, permethrin, and cypermethrin, are proving to be efficient alternatives, although cross-resistance between DDT and pyrethroids has been established in *Boophilus microplus* in Australia.

Scrub Typhus Mites (Order Prostigmata, Family Trombiculidae). The medically important species belong to the genus *Leptotrombidium,* e.g., *L. akamushi* and the *L. deliense* group of species. They are vectors of

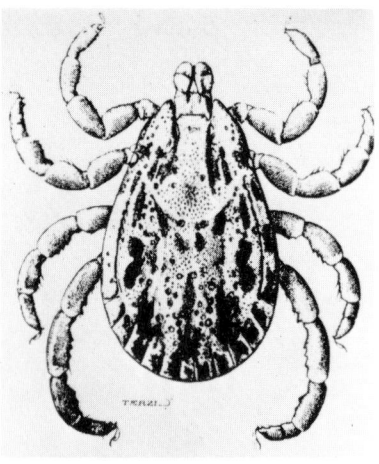

FIGURE 114–18. Hard tick.

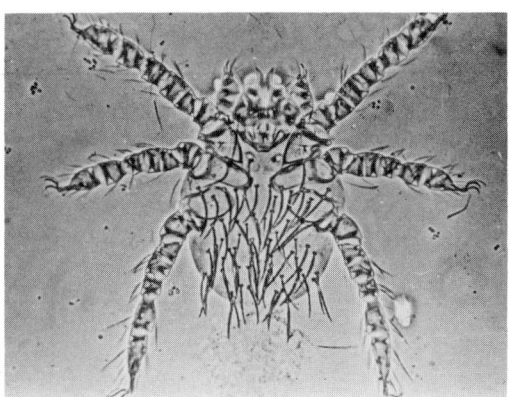

FIGURE 114–19. Scrub typhus mite larva.

scrub typhus caused by *Rickettsia tsutsugamushi,* a disease restricted to Southeast and East Asia, northern Australia, and most of the islands located between these areas. Only the larval stage (Fig. 114–19) is parasitic, and normally it feeds only once in its life.

Control is directed against infested terrain, usually by spraying with a residual insecticide such as HCH, malathion, or propoxur. Dieldrin is extremely effective but is generally proscribed because of environmental toxicity. Personal protection against these and related mites is afforded by repellents, particularly dibutyl phthalate, diethyltoluamide, and benzyl benzoate, applied either to the skin or to the clothing of areas likely to be bitten, e.g., the legs.

BIBLIOGRAPHY

Burges HD, Fontaine RE, Nalim S, et al: World Health Organization research on the biocontrol of vectors of disease: present status and plans for the future. *In* Laird M (ed): Biocontrol of Medical and Veterinary Pests. New York, Praeger Publishers, 1981.

Busvine JR: Insects and Hygiene, 3rd ed. London, Chapman & Hall, 1980.

Chemical Methods for the Control of Arthropod Vectors and Pests of Public Health Importance. Geneva, World Health Organization, 1984.

Davidson G: Genetic Control of Insect Pests. London, Academic Press, 1974.

Davidson G: Insecticides. Bulletin No. 1. London, The Ross Institute, London School of Hygiene and Tropical Medicine, 1988.

Davidson G: Overview of genetic mechanisms as an alternative to chemical control. Misc Pub Entomol Soc Am 11:12, 1980.

Davidson G: Developments in malaria vector control. Br Med Bull 38:201, 1982.

Environmental Management for Vector Control. Fifth report of the WHO Expert Committee on Vector Biology and Control. WHO Tech Rep Ser 649, 1980.

Equipment for Vector Control, 2nd ed. Geneva, World Health Organization, 1974.

Gratz NG: Problems and developments in the control of flea vectors of disease. *In* Traub RL, Starcke H (eds): Fleas. Proceedings of the International Conference on Fleas. Ashton, England, June 1977. Rotterdam, A.A. Balkema, 1980.

Gunn, DL, Stevens JGR (eds): Pesticides and Human Welfare. Oxford, Oxford University Press, 1976.

Harwood RF, James MT: Entomology in Human and Animal Health, 7th ed. New York, Macmillan, 1979.

Matthews GA: Pesticide Application Methods. London, Longman, 1979.

Resistance of Vectors and Reservoirs of Disease to Pesticides. Tenth report of the WHO Expert Committee on Vector Biology and Control. WHO Tech Rep Ser 737, 1986.

Safe Use of Pesticides. Fifth report of the WHO Expert Committee on Vector Biology and Control. WHO Tech Rep Ser 634, 1979.

Service MW: A Guide to Medical Entomology. London, Macmillan Press, 1980.

Specifications for Pesticides used in Public Health, 5th ed. Geneva, World Health Organization, 1979.

The WHO Recommended Classification of Pesticides by Hazard and Guidelines to Classification 1988–1989. Division of Vector Biology and Control, WHO/VBC/88.953. Geneva, World Health Organization, 1988.

PART X

TROPICAL DISEASE IN A TEMPERATE CLIMATE

GENERAL PRINCIPLES

Jay S. Keystone

Increasing numbers of North Americans and Europeans are embarking on travel to the developing world for business purposes or in the pursuit of sun, sand, surf, and sex. It has been estimated that more than 8 million Americans travel to the developing world each year, many of whom are exposed to infectious diseases that occur infrequently, if at all, in North America. For health care providers to advise on appropriate vaccinations and precautions for international travelers, it would be worthwhile for them to know the health risks that their patients are likely to encounter overseas (Chapter 121).

HEALTH RISKS FOR TRAVELERS. Steffen and colleagues in Switzerland have compiled the most comprehensive data on health problems encountered during travel to developing countries. A summary of the results of their 1984 study of more than 10,000 short-term travelers and a review of the medical literature up to 1987 is depicted in Figure X–1. What is notable about the data in this figure is the absence of "exotic" tropical infections, e.g., filariasis, leishmaniasis, and schistosomiasis. The message here is that helminth infections and other diseases of rural life are rarely acquired by short-term travelers to the developing world. On the other hand, temporary residents such as Peace Corps volunteers and missionaries are at greater risk of acquiring infections endemic in nationals of developing countries.

Traveler's Diarrhea. Traveler's diarrhea affects some 30 to 50% of visitors to developing countries. The highest risk appears to be in Latin America, Asia, the Middle East, and Africa (Chapter 117). Although enterotoxigenic *Escherichia coli* is the most common cause of traveler's diarrhea, recent studies have shown that enteroadherent and enteroinvasive *E. coli*, *Aeromonas*, *Plesiomonas*, and *Cryptosporidium* may also play small, but important, roles. As new causes of traveler's diarrhea are discovered, so are new remedies being made available for prevention and treatment. For instance, the quinolone group of antibiotics has now been shown to be effective in treatment courses as short as 1 dose when combined with an antimotility agent such as loperamide.

Typhoid Fever. The risk of typhoid fever for travelers varies from 0.035/1000 short-term (1 month) visitors to developing countries to as high as 12/100,000 in travelers

to India and Pakistan. Although the efficacy of the new typhoid vaccines approximates that of the older killed vaccines, they are more convenient to administer and have fewer adverse effects. The live, attenuated vaccine using the Ty21a mutant of *S. typhi* can be administered orally, whereas the purified Vi-capsular-polysaccharide of *S. typhi* can be given in 1 intramuscular dose (Chapters 38 and 116).

Hepatitis. The risk of hepatitis of all types has been shown by Steffen and associates to be 1 to 3/1000 visitors for a 2- to 3-week stay in a developing country. Another study from Sweden quotes a risk of 6 to 10/1000 travelers, exclusively for hepatitis A for a mean stay of 2 weeks. With the declining incidence of hepatitis A in developed countries it is estimated that less than 20% of children born now will have natural antibodies to this disease by the time they are 50 years of age. In spite of the relatively high risk of acquiring hepatitis, some

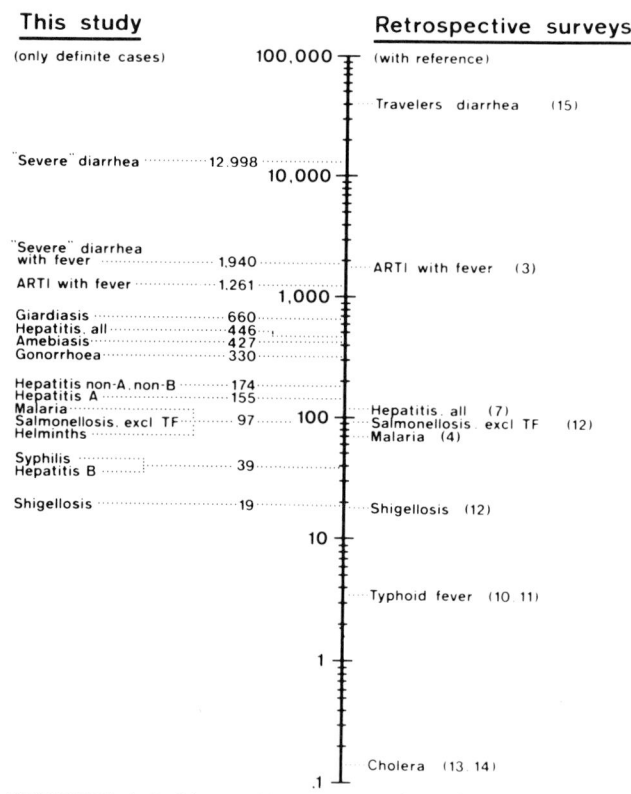

FIGURE X–1. Incidence of infections per 100,000 travelers for a stay of 1 month in a developing country. ARTI = acute respiratory tract infection; TF = typhoid fever. (From Steffen R, et al.: J Infect Dis 156:84–91, 1987. Reprinted by permission.)

travelers refuse gamma globulin or hepatitis B vaccine because of unfounded fears of developing acquired immunodeficiency syndrome (AIDS) from these products (Chapters 19 and 115).

Human Immunodeficiency Virus (HIV) Infection and AIDS. The risk of AIDS for visitors to the developing countries has not yet been ascertained, but it is certainly a concern for the traveling public. Acquisition of HIV by blood transfusion following a motor vehicle accident or by injection with contaminated needles and syringes or during sexual activity with nationals are the most likely routes of infection. As of October 1990, over 300,000 cases of AIDS have been reported worldwide. By the end of 1991, the World Health Organization estimates that over 1 million persons will have AIDS and 5 to 10 million persons will be infected with the virus. The infection rate among some prostitute groups currently ranges from 27 to 88% in Africa and is increasing steadily in parts of Southeast Asia, notably Thailand (Chapter 15.1).

Malaria. The dramatic spread of drug-resistant *Plasmodium falciparum* malaria to almost all areas of the world where the infection is endemic has increased the risk of malaria for travelers. In 1988, the number of malaria cases in US civilians exceeded, for the first time since 1974, the number of cases among foreign civilians. Imported *P. falciparum* malaria in US civilians infected in Africa has increased each year since 1981, with an overall increase of 410% by 1988. In long-term residents, such as Peace Corps volunteers working in Africa, the attack rate for *P. falciparum* malaria was reported in 1987 to be 15 cases/100 volunteers per year. Figures from the United Kingdom show that the attack rate for malaria has remained relatively stable over the years. For instance, in 1986 an attack rate of 279/100,000 was calculated for British residents returning from short-term visits to Africa and Asia (Chapters 73 and 116).

Although mefloquine appears to be the new hope for malaria prevention, adverse drug effects and well-documented widespread in vitro *P. falciparum* resistance have thrown some doubt on the potential usefulness of the drug. Unfortunately, initial evaluations of candidate malaria vaccines have proved disappointing. Personal protection measures against mosquito bites will continue to play an important role in the prevention of malaria.

Motor Vehicle Accidents. Assessment of health risks for the traveler to the developing world would be incomplete unless the causes of fatalities during overseas travel were considered. Hargarten and Baker have shown, in a 20-year analysis of Peace Corps volunteers, that 70% and 24% of fatalities were due to unintentional injury and illness, respectively. Motor vehicle accidents accounted for almost 50% of the injury deaths, whereas malaria, rabies, and pneumonia were the most frequent causes of fatal illness. In a broader study looking at deaths of all American travelers during the years 1975 and 1984, the same authors showed that cardiovascular disease accounted for almost 50% of deaths. Unintentional injury was responsible for 22% and infectious disease for only 1% of deaths. Motor vehicle accidents caused almost one-third of the injury deaths. Although the risk of serious injury in a motor vehicle accident is

relatively small for most travelers, it is likely to approximate that of serious infectious disease.

INTRODUCTION. The chapters in Part X provide the reader with current guidelines for providing pretravel health advice (Chapter 115) and a problem-oriented approach to illness in immigrants (Chapter 120) and travelers arriving from the developing world (Chapters 116 to 119). The chapter on global epidemiology of infectious disease should assist the practitioner in advising travelers of their risks of infectious disease and help in the diagnosis of illness in returning travelers and immigrants (Chapter 121). Because the geographic distribution of diseases in the developing world is constantly changing, as are the drugs and vaccines used to control them, it is wise to have up-to-date information when preparing international travelers for departure and when attending those who return ill.

BIBLIOGRAPHY

Bernard KW, Graitcher PL, Van der Vlugt T, et al: Epidemiological surveillance in Peace Corps volunteers: A model for monitoring health in temporary residents of developing countries. Int J Epidemiol 18:220, 1989.

Chin J, Mann J: Global surveillance and forecasting of AIDS. Bull WHO 67:1, 1989.

Hargarten SW, Baker SP: Fatalities in the Peace Corps: A retrospective study: 1962 through 1983. JAMA 254:1326, 1985.

Hill DR, Pearson RD: Health advice for international travel. Ann Intern Med 108:839, 1988.

Lange WR: Viral hepatitis and international travel. Am Fam Physician 36:179, 1987.

Levine MM, Ferreccio C, Black RE, et al: Progress in vaccines against typhoid fever. Rev Infect Dis 11 (Suppl 3): S552, 1989.

Phillips-Howard PA, Radalowicz A, Mitchell J, Bradley DJ: Risk of malaria in British residents returning from malarious areas. Br Med J 300:499, 1990.

Steffen R, Rickenbach M, Wihelum U, et al.: Health problems after travel to developing countries. J Infect Dis 156:84, 1987.

115. ADVICE TO TRAVELERS

Elaine C. Jong

International travel has become an increasingly common activity among diverse segments of the population. The spectrum of motivation for travel, ranging from tourism, education, sports, politics, and business to missionary and volunteer efforts, means that the population of travelers seeking health advice includes people of many ages, people in variable states of health, and people traveling under markedly different standards of accommodation.

The basic body of health advice applicable to all travelers covers three main areas: (1) vaccine-preventable diseases, (2) malaria, and (3) traveler's diarrhea. The health advice given in each of these areas must be personalized for each traveler, taking into account age, underlying health, and anticipated level of geographic risk. Other areas of health advice that may be of concern to travelers include traveling with chronic health conditions, insect precautions, high-altitude sickness, jet lag, motion sickness, pregnancy, birth control, safe sexual practices, blood transfusions, personal injury prevention, and environmental hazards. A comprehensive discussion of these other health concerns is beyond the scope of this chapter, but information on specific topics may be found in the bibliography at the end of this chapter.

VACCINE-PREVENTABLE DISEASES

Standard Routine Immunizations. The routine immunizations that all adults should be up to date on include tetanus, diphtheria, poliomyelitis, measles, mumps, and rubella.

Tetanus/Diphtheria. The tetanus/diphtheria (Td) vaccine that is used for immunization of patients 7 years of age and older needs to be boosted every 10 years to maintain immunity after the primary series is completed.

Poliomyelitis. Although primary immunization against poliomyelitis with oral poliomyelitis vaccine (OPV), a live attenuated viral vaccine, is recommended for healthy persons younger than 18 years of age, enhanced potency inactivated poliovirus vaccine (eIPV) is recommended for unimmunized adults (18 years and older) (Chapter 18.1). If travel plans do not permit at least 2 doses of eIPV given 4 weeks apart to be received by a traveler departing for a poliomyelitis endemic or epidemic area, a single dose of OPV or eIPV should be given. In either case, primary immunization with eIPV should be completed after the trip. If primary immunization with OPV or the old-type inactivated polio vaccine (IPV) was incomplete, the primary series can be completed with OPV or eIPV regardless of the interval since the last dose or the type of vaccine previously used. If a primary vaccine series with either OPV or IPV was completed more than 5 years before anticipated travel into an area with epidemic or endemic poliomyelitis, a single additional dose of OPV or eIPV should be used to boost immunity in travelers of all ages. Persons who should not receive OPV include patients with altered immunity or those living in households with such patients. Pregnancy is a relative contraindication.

Measles/Mumps/Rubella. The primary immunization with measles/mumps/rubella (MMR) vaccine is customarily given as a single injection at 15 months of age or older. A booster dose of MMR or single-antigen measles vaccine is recommended at 5 to 12 years of age. However, if the MMR vaccine was given before 15 months of age, or if the patient received an early version of this vaccine (before 1967), or if the patient never received the vaccine and did not contract the natural viral infections, MMR vaccine may be recommended for adults prior to travel in developing areas.

Other Immunizations. In subsets of the general population at risk because of underlying medical conditions, occupation, or age, the viral influenza vaccine, the pneumococcus vaccine, the *Hemophilus* b conjugate vaccine, and the hepatitis B vaccine should be given prior to travel. These vaccines, with the exception of hepatitis B vaccine, are not discussed in this chapter, as they are covered in many standard references.

Special Immunizations for Travelers. The vaccines traditionally given for travel may be divided into two groups: those regulated by the World Health Organization (WHO) and those that are recommended but not required for travel.

Yellow Fever. Yellow fever vaccine is the only vaccine currently regulated by the WHO that may be required. Yellow fever is a virus transmitted by the bites of *Aedes aegypti* mosquitoes in equatorial Africa and South America (Chapter 22.1). The virus can cause a severe and often fatal hepatitis. Many countries in the yellow fever endemic zones do not require the vaccination of travelers arriving from nonendemic areas. However, if there are not medical contraindications, a prudent traveler might get the vaccine prior to going to an endemic area, regardless of official requirements, as an outbreak of yellow fever could occur at any time without warning in endemic zones. In addition, valid proof of yellow fever vaccination is often required when travelers enter a tropical country after travel in other countries in the yellow fever endemic zones, even if there was no stated requirement for travelers entering directly from nonendemic temperate climates. A single injection of this attenuated live virus vaccine will stimulate protective immunity lasting 10 years.

Receipt of the vaccine from an Official Vaccination Center (designated by the public health department at the state, provincial, or national level) must be documented by an Official Stamp on the yellow fever certificate page contained in the International Certificates of Vaccination. Yellow fever vaccine is purified from chick embryo cultures, so people with a history of anaphylactic reaction to eggs or egg products may not be able to tolerate this vaccine. If the history is questionable, a test dose of the vaccine (according to manufacturer's directions) can be given. If the reaction to the test dose is positive, or if the history is unequivocal for serious egg allergy, the standard vaccine dose should not be given, and WHO member countries will accept a signed letter on letterhead stationery from the physician stating that, for medical reasons, vaccination with yellow fever vaccine is contraindicated in that traveler. Unless there are time constraints, cholera and yellow fever vaccines should be administered at a minimal interval of 3 weeks. Live virus vaccines are generally contraindicated during pregnancy. However, if travel to a known yellow fever zone were unavoidable by a pregnant woman, the remote theoretical risk to the fetus from the vaccine might be outweighed by the expected protection derived by immunization against this life-threatening disease. The vaccine can be given to infants 6 months of age or older.

Smallpox and Cholera. Smallpox vaccine and cholera vaccine are no longer regulated by the WHO. There has been no natural transmission of smallpox virus anywhere in the world in over a decade (Chapter 16.2). Although the cholera pandemic still involves native populations of Asia and Africa, the cholera vaccine in current use is thought to offer little protection to the routine healthy traveler, whose risk of cholera acquisition is negligible in any case (Chapter 40). The primary cholera vaccine series of 2 injections given a week or more apart may be considered for travelers with known risk factors that promote cholera infection in otherwise healthy people: achlorhydria, gastric resection, or any other condition decreasing gastric acidity. However, advice on selection of safe food and water while traveling and self-treatment with oral rehydration salts and antibiotics would probably be reasonable alternatives to the vaccine for prevention of cholera in travelers at risk.

Typhoid Fever. The injectable typhoid fever vaccine in current use is a purified bacterial vaccine, which causes inflammation and tenderness at the site of injection in many people (Chapter 38). Some people get a more severe reaction to this vaccine, consisting of fever, headache, and malaise. The primary series consists of 2 injections 1 month apart. Booster doses are given if 3 years or more have elapsed since the last dose. If a person has an unusually severe local or systemic reaction to the vaccine, further doses should not be given, and the person should follow advice for selection of safe food and beverages. Alternatively, the booster dose might be administered by the intradermal route (except when acetone-killed and dried vaccine is used) because less reaction has been shown to occur with this method of vaccination.

A new oral typhoid vaccine, which may be more efficacious and have fewer side effects than the present vaccine, has been recently released. The oral typhoid vaccine is made from attenuated *Salmonella typhi* Ty21a bacteria, and the taking of an enteric-coated capsule on days 1, 3, 5, and 7 will give protection commencing 2 weeks after the fourth dose and lasting for at least 5 years.

Immune Globulin. Immune globulin purified from pooled human serum and given as an intramuscular injection can provide protection against hepatitis A for a period of 3 to 5½ months depending on the dose given (Chapter 19.1). This vaccine can be given at the same time as most travel vaccines at a separate injection site, but should be given at least 3 to 4 weeks after a dose of MMR, OPV, eIPV, or *Hemophilus influenzae* type vaccine.

Only about 1 of 3 adults tests seropositive for hepatitis A antibody in studies of North American and Western European populations, thus the majority of adult travelers in these populations are susceptible to hepatitis A infection. It appears that at least one-half of reported cases of hepatitis A in American travelers occurred in people on standard tourist itineraries. This implies that the risk of hepatitis A exposure for the individual traveler cannot be predicted on the basis of quality of accommodations, rural versus urban itineraries, or food preferences. Immune globulin is therefore recommended for all travelers going to destinations where sanitation may be a problem.

Owing to concern about the safety of blood products with regard to human immunodeficiency virus (HIV) transmission, many people express reluctance to receive immune globulin prophylaxis for travel. Concerned travelers need to be reassured about the safety of immune globulin: Unlike the fresh blood used for transfusion of cells or clotting factors, immune globulin is a highly purified blood product and the purification process would destroy any HIV theoretically present in the original serum pool. This is borne out by a long record of product safety in clinical practice.

Hepatitis A vaccines are currently in use in the People's Republic of China and are undergoing evaluation elsewhere, but not in general use as yet.

Meningococcal Vaccine. Meningococcal Polysaccharide Vaccine (quadrivalent groups A/C/Y/W-135) vaccine is a purified polysaccharide vaccine that is given as a single injectable dose to people 3 years of age and older (Chapter 42). The vaccine is recommended for people going to live or work in the Sahel region of Africa, in Brazil, and in other areas where epidemics of meningococcal meningitis recur. Since 1985, there have been reports of meningococcal meningitis among travelers trekking in Nepal, and the vaccine is highly recommended for travelers in this category. More recently, immunization has been recommended for travelers to Kenya and Tanzania.

Hepatitis B Vaccine. Hepatitis B vaccine is available as a human serum–derived antigen vaccine or as a recombinant DNA yeast antigen product (Chapter 19.2). Both types of vaccine involve a primary series of 3 injections, the first 2 given 1 month apart, and the third given 6 months after the first dose. An alternative schedule for the Engerix recombinant hepatitis B vaccine is four doses at 0, 1, 2, and 12 months. Hepatitis B vaccination has had widespread use in the United States among health care workers and intimate contacts of known hepatitis B–infected persons. Travelers who plan to live or work among native populations in Africa and Asia, or people who may be involved in high-risk activities in these countries (sexual contact, acupuncture, tattoos, ear-piercing, etc.), should be advised to get hepatitis B vaccine. However, because activities that involve a high risk of hepatitis B acquisition are also a risk for HIV transmission, travelers should be advised to avoid these activities if possible, regardless of their hepatitis B vaccination status.

Rabies. Travelers going to Mexico, Central and South America, Africa, and Asia need to be warned about rabid dogs and the need to avoid contact with stray animals (Chapter 21.1). Other animals such as bats, monkeys, foxes, wolves, and livestock in these countries may also be rabid. If an animal bite inadvertently occurs, travelers need to know that this could be an emergency situation requiring specific postexposure treatment with rabies immune globulin (RIG) and rabies vaccine. They should ask for help from their nearest consulate or embassy. In some cases, emergency evacuation may be appropriate, as the most effective treatments may not be available in the locale of the animal bite.

Travelers anticipating extensive trips or residence in rural areas of rabies endemic countries or whose work involves animal contact should receive the pre-exposure series of the human diploid cell vaccine (HDCV) for rabies, which consists of 3 injections given on days 0, 7, and 21 or 28. A small intradermal dose (0.1 ml) can be used if the series can be completed before chloroquine prophylaxis for malaria is instituted. If the time period is not adequate, a larger dose (1.0 ml) of HDCV given intramuscularly on the same schedule should be used. The receipt of the pre-exposure rabies vaccine series will obviate the need for RIG after a high-risk bite and decrease the number of postexposure HDCV doses given (2 over 1 week instead of 5 over 1 month).

Japanese Encephalitis Vaccine (JEV). This is a purified killed virus vaccine prepared from brain tissue of infected laboratory mice. The vaccine manufactured in Japan has been efficacious and safe in the first decade of its widespread use. The JEV (Biken, Japan) was available through an investigational protocol sponsored by the United States Centers for Disease Control Arbovirus Research Branch in the mid 1980s. However, this program is not now active owing to complex legal and administrative problems.

Although many travelers are going to areas in Asia where epidemics of Japanese encephalitis (JE) routinely cause morbidity and mortality among native populations (Korea, People's Republic of China, Philippines, Indonesia, Malaysia, Thailand, India, Sri Lanka, and Burma), most short-term travelers going on the usual tourist routes are not at risk for infection through the bites of *Culex* mosquitoes (Chapter 21.3). However, students, educators, missionaries, agricultural advisors, and others doing intensive travel or residence in rural areas where JE is a risk should try to obtain 2 or 3 doses of JEV given 1 week apart prior to travel. The vaccine is not currently available for civilian use in most western countries. If travel is likely to constitute a significant risk for JE, the traveler might want to consider routing through Canada, Japan, Hong Kong, or Sri Lanka to get this vaccine.

Plague and Typhus. Immunization against plague is rarely recommended, except for travelers planning to camp in rural, mountainous, or upland areas in Africa, Asia, and the Americas where plague is reported, and persons whose occupations may lead them to direct or indirect exposure to wild animals (Chapter 47). Two injections are given at 4-week intervals, and the third dose is given 3 to 6 months after the second dose. Typhus is rarely seen in North American travelers (Chapter 23). The vaccine is no longer available in the United States.

Bacille Calmette-Guérin (BCG) Immunization. Tuberculosis is common in developing countries (Chapter 61). Persons who intend to live and work there are at an increased risk of exposure. BCG, a live vaccine derived from a strain of *Mycobacterium bovis,* has been recommended by some for persons with a negative tuberculin skin test who are planning an extended stay in a developing country. The efficacy of currently available BCG vaccine is questionable, as exemplified by the negative results in the recent BCG trial in India. Side effects, ranging from draining abscesses at the site of immunization (common) to disseminated infection (rare), must be weighed against the individual's risk of active tuberculosis—a risk that varies directly with the intimacy of contact with the indigenous population. BCG vaccination usually results in a positive tuberculin skin test; the size of the reaction decreases over years. BCG vaccine is contraindicated in patients with altered immunity.

Instead of BCG, most North American consultants recommend that long-stay travelers should have a tuberculin skin test prior to departure and, if negative, every 1 to 2 years during exposure.

MALARIA. Selection of the itinerary and the local climate at the time of the trip are primary malaria risk determinants (Chapter 73.1). Advice to travelers on malaria prevention falls into three categories: personal behavior, mosquito repellents, and chemoprophylaxis.

Personal Behavior and Mosquito Repellents. Travelers in malarious areas should try to stay indoors in screened rooms between dusk and dawn when anopheline mosquitoes, which transmit malaria, are most likely to bite. When outdoors during these hours, clothing that covers the arms and legs and the use of insect repellent on exposed body areas will decrease the risk of mosquito bites. Before going to sleep, the room should be inspected for mosquitoes on the walls and ceilings: the use of a spray insecticide or the burning of insect coils will usually reduce the number of mosquitoes. Recent field studies suggest that sleeping under bed nets impregnated with permethrin (an insecticide) greatly reduces the likelihood of bites by mosquitoes as well as other insects and ectoparasites (Chapter 73.1).

Malaria Chemoprophylaxis. This has become an increasingly complex issue because of the emergence of Chloroquine-resistant *Plasmodium falciparum* (CRPF) malaria (Chapter 73.1). In some areas, the CRPF mosquitoes are also resistant to sulfadoxine-pyrimethamine (Fansidar). In addition to receiving a malarial chemoprophylaxis regimen appropriate for a given geographic area, successful prevention of malaria depends on the traveler's compliance in taking the recommended medications. No matter which chemoprophylactic regimen is being used, breakthrough attacks of resistant malaria can occur: travelers to remote areas may be required to self-diagnose malaria by clinical symptoms and to initiate treatment when medical services are not available.

Table 115-1 gives major geographic areas where malaria is endemic and suggests regimens that might be appropriate. Regimens 1 through 5 summarize the malaria chemoprophylaxis in current use (late 1990) throughout the world. Some antimalarial drugs may be unavailable or contraindicated in a given traveler. Alternatively, an acceptable strategy in most situations is to take standard chloroquine phosphate prophylaxis and carry a treatment dose of drugs with efficacy against CRPF for emergency self-treatment of a suspected attack. Regimens 6 through 9 outline drugs useful for emergency self-treatment should a traveler elect to take the weekly chloroquine regimen in a CRPF area.

Several antimalarial drugs and drug combinations being used by international travelers from Western Europe, Australia, and Southeast Asia in areas of drug-resistant falciparum malaria are not available to the North American traveler. In some cases, it may be appropriate for travelers to obtain and use these alternative drugs for malaria prevention in the areas of risk, even though the drugs are not licensed and approved for use in the United States or Canada. As with any medication, the relative benefits and risks of a given drug must be carefully reviewed by the physician with the patient. Recently, mefloquine has become the drug of choice for the prevention of CRPF malaria in most endemic areas of the world. (See Chapter 73.1 for further details.)

Although Table 115-1 lists recommended antimalarial regimens by country, the actual risk of malaria and of drug resistance may be quite variable within each country (Table 121-1). For example, there is no malaria risk in most urban centers of Southeast Asia or South

TABLE 115–1. Malaria Chemoprophylaxis Regimens

Geographic Area	Suggested Regimen(s)*					
	1	2	3	4	5	6
Mexico	X					
Central America, Haiti	X					
South America		X	X		X	X
North Africa, Turkey, Middle East	X					
Sub-Saharan Africa		X	X	X	X	X
Nepal					X	X
India	X				X	X
People's Republic of China	X	X			X	X
Thailand (rural and border), Laos, Cambodia, Vietnam, rural Philippines, Indonesia, Malaysia, Papua New Guinea		X	X		X	X

*See text in this chapter and Chapter 73.1 for discussion; see Table 121–1 for more exact description of geographic locations of drug-resistant plasmodia.

1. Chloroquine phosphate (Aralen), 500 mg orally once a week, beginning 1 week before travel, continuing once a week on the same day during travel and for 4 weeks after travel in a malaria risk area.

2. Doxycycline (Vibramycin), 100 mg orally every day of the trip and daily for 4 weeks after travel, in a CRPF risk area.

3. Chloroquine phosphate (1); plus dapsone, 100-mg tablet; plus pyrimethamine (Daraprim), 12.5-mg tablet: take both latter medications at the same time once a week, beginning 1 week before travel, continuing on the same day weekly during travel and for 4 weeks after travel. This combination of dapsone and pyrimethamine is sold as Maloprim in some countries.

4. Chloroquine phosphate (1) plus daily proguanil (Paludrine), 100-mg tablet: 2 tablets (200 mg) of proguanil orally every day during the trip and for 4 weeks after in addition to weekly chloroquine phosphate.

5. Mefloquine (Lariam), 250-mg tablets: 1 tablet (250 mg) orally once a week beginning 1 week before travel and continuing up to and including 4 weeks after departure from a malarious area.

6. Chloroquine phosphate (1) plus a treatment dose of sulfadoxine, 500 mg–pyrimethamine, 25 mg (Fansidar): adults should take 3 Fansidar tablets as a single oral dose to treat an attack of suspected CRPF malaria.

America, and in rural areas travelers are at risk only if they remain overnight. However, in other regions such as sub-Saharan Africa and Haiti, malaria transmission occurs in both urban and rural areas. In some countries, China for example, CRPF is located in certain regions, whereas in other areas, only chloroquine-sensitive strains are transmitted.

Self-Treatment for Malaria. Because no present-day drug regimen guarantees protection against malaria, travelers, particularly those to remote areas, should be instructed about self-diagnosis of malaria. Any illness with high fever associated with headache, muscle aches, nausea, and abdominal discomfort occurring during or after travel in a malarious area must be considered to be malaria until proved otherwise. Although there are other important causes of fever in the tropics, urgency of therapy is often not as crucial as it is for malaria. Prompt self-treatment of malaria could be lifesaving if medical care is not readily accessible (Chapter 73.1). On the other hand, in case of fever on return home, travelers should be reminded to inform their health care providers that they have been exposed to malaria and that their antimalarial prophylaxis may not have provided complete protection.

CHEMOPROPHYLAXIS FOR OTHER SYSTEMIC PARASITES

African Trypanosomiasis. Chemoprophylaxis against trypanosomiasis has rarely been used in the past for workers living in endemic areas in rural West or Central Africa, where they may be exposed to Gambian trypanosomiasis (Chapter 74). A single intramuscular injection of 250 mg of pentamidine protects an adult for about 6 months. Pentamidine may not be available in parts of Africa where it is needed and is not available for preventive use in the United States. Chemoprophylaxis is not recommended for the usual safari visitor,

who will have very low exposure and is more likely to be exposed in East and South Africa to Rhodesian trypanosomiasis.

Filariasis. Most travelers to areas endemic for filariasis will not have sufficient exposure to acquire disease. For some persons planning an extended stay, e.g., Peace Corps volunteers, prophylactic diethylcarbamazine (DEC) may be recommended (Chapter 85). Untoward drug effects are rare in uninfected persons. The dosage is 5 mg/kg taken once each month for up to 12 months. For prophylaxis for human Loa loa infections in equatorial West and Central Africa, the DEC dosage is 300 mg orally once a week for up to 2 years. Ivermectin may replace DEC for these purposes in a few years.

TRAVELER'S DIARRHEA. Up to 50% of travelers going to a tropical climate will experience a form of acute infectious diarrhea called traveler's diarrhea. Although the illness is usually self-limited, lasting an average of 3 to 5 days, the frequent watery bowel movements and abdominal cramps associated with this condition can cause significant discomfort and interfere with travel plans. The majority of cases of traveler's diarrhea are thought to be caused by toxigenic strains of the bacteria Escherichia coli (Chapter 41.1). Other bacteria, viruses, and parasites cause traveler's diarrhea, but are detected less frequently.

Preventive strategies for avoiding traveler's diarrhea include: food and water precautions, daily doses of bismuth subsalicylate (BSS), or daily doses of a broad-spectrum antibiotic such as doxycycline, trimethoprim-sulfamethoxazole (TMP/SMX), ciprofloxacin, and others.

Food and Water Precautions. Although following the food and water precautions listed in Table 115–2 probably decreases the transmission of enteric pathogens and the occurrence of food poisoning in areas where unsan-

TABLE 115–2. Food and Water Precautions

Eat foods that are thoroughly cooked and served piping hot.
Avoid raw or undercooked fish, shellfish, and meat.
Avoid green salads and other salads served cold.
Avoid dairy products, such as milk, ice cream, cheese, and yogurt, which may be unpasteurized in some countries or improperly stored.
Drink bottled carbonated beverages, canned fruit juices, or beverages such as tea, coffee, or bouillon that have been prepared with boiled water. Beer and wine are usually safe.
Avoid ice cubes in cold beverages, including alcoholic beverages.
Use a water purification method when in doubt about tap water.
Use safe water for brushing teeth and for taking medications.

itary food preparation and storage may be a problem, there is no evidence that strict adherence to the precautions will guarantee prevention of traveler's diarrhea.

Chemoprophylaxis. Prophylaxis against traveler's diarrhea by taking daily doses of BSS (Pepto-Bismol) or antibiotics has been shown to be effective. In 1 study, 2 tablets of BSS by mouth 4 times a day decreased the incidence of traveler's diarrhea by 60% in American students in Mexico. Doxycycline, taken orally as one 100-mg capsule once a day, significantly decreased the incidence of diarrhea among Peace Corps volunteers in Africa. However, increasing tetracycline resistance has been shown to reduce the efficacy of this antibiotic for traveler's diarrhea in some countries. Trimethoprim-sulfamethoxazole double-strength tablets; ciprofloxacin, 500-mg tablets; or norfloxacin, 400-mg tablets, taken once a day also appear to be effective for traveler's diarrhea prophylaxis. These drugs should be started prior to arrival in the tropics and continued for 2 days after departure.

However, the National Institutes of Health (USA) National Travelers' Diarrhea Consensus Conference did not endorse the prophylactic use of BSS or antibiotics against traveler's diarrhea for the usual traveler. The effectiveness of the various prophylactic routines was studied for relatively short periods of 3 weeks or less. The prophylactic routines may cause problems for some travelers owing to salicylate intolerance or adverse effects related to broad-spectrum antibiotics (drug allergy, skin rashes, yeast infections, antibiotic-associated diarrhea). Some of the drugs are not FDA approved for use in children or during pregnancy and are potentially toxic in these groups. However, some experts in travel medicine do recommend antibiotic or BSS prophylaxis for individuals who are at particularly high risk for traveler's diarrhea or its sequelae. Such groups of individuals include persons with achlorhydria, diabetes, inflammatory bowel disease, or immunosuppressive disorders or those with a history of frequent gastrointestinal problems associated with travel.

Suitable drugs are not available at present for the chemoprophylaxis of the common intestinal parasites causing diarrhea, such as amebiasis and giardiasis.

Patients need to be warned about buying antibiotics for prevention or treatment of diarrhea in foreign countries; in some countries, potentially dangerous drugs, such as chloramphenicol and iodochlorhydroxyquin, are available from pharmacies without a prescription.

Self-Treatment of Diarrhea with Antibiotics. The al-

ternative to antibiotic prophylaxis is the empiric self-treatment of diarrhea that develops during travel. If a traveler is stricken by a typical case of traveler's diarrhea, the use of an agent for symptomatic relief (BSS) or antiperistaltic drugs (loperamide, diphenoxylate, paregoric, etc.) and empiric self-treatment with an antibiotic (tetracycline, doxycycline, double-strength TMP/SMX, ciprofloxacin, norfloxacin) for 3 to 5 days at appropriate therapeutic doses (usually twice daily) may contribute to a rapid recovery. The use of antiperistaltic drugs is contraindicated in diarrhea accompanied by a high fever and/or bloody or mucoid stools. These cases require the care of a physician, although travelers in remote areas may need to initiate antibiotic treatment if access to medical care is not possible.

The selection of the antibiotic for the treatment (or prevention) of diarrhea depends on the geographic location of the trip: drug-resistant strains of diarrhea-causing bacteria are present in areas where there has been widespread use of a given drug. For instance, TMP/SMX-resistant strains of bacteria are an increasing problem in Mexico and the Middle East. Tetracycline resistance is widespread among bacterial enteric pathogens in Central and South America and the Middle and Far East.

Oral Rehydration. No matter what drugs are employed by the traveler for self-treatment of traveler's diarrhea, prevention of dehydration by increasing the usual oral fluid intake to approximate the volume lost through watery bowel movements is of prime importance. Canned fruit juices, carbonated beverages, clear soups, and other drinks made with boiled or purified water can be used. If available, reconstituted powdered oral rehydration salts (formulated according to the WHO recipe) or the CDC oral fluids program provides replacement of fluid and electrolytes closely matching intestinal losses due to diarrhea. However, it is good to remember that rehydration with impure water is better than no rehydration at all!

HEALTH CARE ABROAD. Medical emergencies can occur at home and abroad. The prudent traveler should carry, in addition to the International Certificates of Vaccination, a summary of the health history, a list of current medications (including generic or chemical name and dosage), and pertinent data if an underlying medical condition is under treatment (allergies; cardiovascular problems, including hypertension, ischemic heart disease, artificial heart valves, and artificial pacemakers; pulmonary problems, including emphysema and asthma; diabetes mellitus; malignancies; etc.) Should the need for medical treatment arise while a person is traveling, such information would be invaluable to the treating physician. The traveler should also check with his or her health insurance provider to find out provisions for illness abroad. Even a traveler in perfect health could accidentally break a leg.

HEALTH CARE AFTER RETURN HOME. Travelers should be advised to consult a knowledgeable physician on return home if they have experienced any significant change in their health while abroad. The development of a high fever in the weeks to months after a trip in a malarious area, even if malaria chemoprophylaxis was taken, should raise the possibility of malaria since no chemoprophylactic regimen can be considered to be 100% protective. Changes in gastrointestinal function and skin lesions are other post-trip health problems that often require medical care.

SUMMARY. Although the traveler going on a trip to urban areas of developed countries may need only general advice for maintenance of health, the traveler planning to visit rural areas, especially in tropical and developing countries, may need extensive preparation. Physicians who advise travelers must help them tread the thin line between caution and neurosis. The advice given and the emphasis with which it is presented should be weighed according to the personality of the patient and the anticipated health risks of the trip.

BIBLIOGRAPHY

Barrett-Connor E: Chemoprophylaxis of amebiasis and African trypanosomiasis. Ann Intern Med 77:797, 1972.

Centers for Disease Control: Health Information for International Travel, 1990 (HHS Publication No. (CDC) 90-8280). Atlanta, GA, US Department of Health and Human Services, Public Health Service, 1990 (updated annually).

Dupont HL, Ericsson CD, Johnson PC, et al: Antimicrobial agents in the prevention of travelers' diarrhea. Rev Infect Dis 8:S167, 1986.

Dupont HL, Ericsson CD, Johnson PC, et al: Prevention of travelers' diarrhea by the tablet formulation of bismuth subsalicylate, JAMA 257:1347, 1987.

Ericsson CD, Johnson PC, Dupont HL, et al: Ciprofloxacin or trimethoprim-sulfamethoxazole as initial therapy for travelers' diarrhea: A placebo-controlled, randomized trial. Ann Intern Med 106:216, 1987.

Hoke CH, Nisalak A, Sangawhipa N, et al: Protection against Japanese encephalitis by inactivated vaccines. N Engl J Med 319:608, 1988.

Johnson PC, Ericsson CD, Dupont HL, et al: Comparison of loperamide with bismuth subsalicylate for treatment of acute travelers' diarrhea. JAMA 255:767, 1986.

Jong EC (ed): The Travel and Tropical Medicine Manual. Philadelphia, W.B. Saunders, 1987.

Keystone JS: Advantages and disadvantages of antimalarials for chemoprophylaxis. In Steffen R (ed): International Travel Medicine. Berlin, Springer-Verlag, 1989, pp 102–110.

Levine MM, Black RE, Ferreccio C, et al: Large-scale field trial of Ty21A live oral typhoid vaccine in enteric-coated capsule formulation. Lancet 1:1049, 1987.

McMullen R, Jong EC: Incidence of antibody to hepatitis A among employees of a multinational corporation: Implications for immunoglobulin prophylaxis. In Steffen R (ed): Travel Medicine. Berlin, Springer-Verlag, 1989, pp 265–269.

Nutman TB, Miller KD, Mulligan M, et al: Diethylcarbamazine prophylaxis for human loaiasis. N Engl J Med 319:752, 1988.

Sack DA, Kaminsky DC, Sack RB, et al: Prophylactic doxycycline for travelers' diarrhea: Results of a prospective double-blind study of Peace Corps volunteers in Kenya. N Engl J Med 298:758, 1978.

Travelers' Diarrhea Consensus Conference. JAMA 253:2700, 1985.

World Health Organization: Vaccination Certificate Requirements and Health Advice for International Travel, 1990. Geneva, World Health Organization, 1990 (updated annually).

116. FEVER IN TRAVELERS

G. Thomas Strickland

With the marked increase in international travel during the past 20 to 30 years, practitioners in the United States, Europe, and other temperate areas are seeing many more patients with diseases of tropical climates. This increase in tropical diseases in temperate climates is due not only to the increased numbers of patients exposed to tropical diseases but also to the increased speed of air travel. Travelers are returning home within the incubation period of infectious diseases. A febrile patient in his or her physician's office could have been on an East African camera safari 3 or 4 days previously. Therefore, the differential diagnosis must include falciparum malaria, African trypanosomiasis, Rift Valley fever, and other exotic infections.

Individuals who have traveled or lived in the tropics are liable not only to all of the usual causes of fever seen in temperate climates, e.g., influenza, pneumococcal pneumonia, and streptococcal pharyngitis, but also to other infectious conditions endemic to the tropics or subtropics, e.g., malaria, visceral leishmaniasis, amebiasis, dengue, and yellow fever. Furthermore, other fever-causing infectious diseases, e.g., tuberculosis, one of the hepatitis virus infections, and salmonellosis, are far more prevalent in developing countries. There have been recent outbreaks of influenza in cruise ship passengers visiting China and Alaska.

It is not necessary to travel outside the country to be infected with exotic microbes. Recently, a textile worker in North Carolina had fever and chills from cutaneous anthrax. He was believed to have been infected from *Bacillus anthracis*–contaminated West Asian cashmere used in the mill's yarn production. Two clusters of vivax malaria involving 27 patients were identified near San Diego, California, in the summer of 1986. All but 2 of those infected were Mexican migrant workers who slept in the open on a hillside bordering a marsh where *Anopheles freeborni,* a local mosquito that is an excellent malaria vector, was breeding. A migrant worker infected local mosquitoes, which were then able to transmit malaria to others.

In general, the risk of acquiring febrile illness during international travel depends on the area of the world visited (Chapter 121). Travelers to underdeveloped countries are at greater risk than those traveling in more developed areas. Within each area, the risk of acquiring disease can vary greatly. Travelers who venture to smaller cities off the usual tourist routes and those who spend time in villages or rural areas for extended periods are at greater risk of acquiring infectious diseases because of greater exposure to the disease-transmitting insect vectors and to contaminated water and food and closer contact with local residents who could harbor infectious organisms. Therefore, it is not sufficient to ask, "Where have you been?" The physician must also ask, "Where did you go in the country?" and "How long did you stay?" and "What did you do?"

EVALUATION OF FEVER IN A TRAVELER. A history of recent travel in the tropics complicates and extends the differential diagnosis of fever and makes it more imperative that the patient be evaluated. Malaria, typhoid fever, meningococcemia, and other infectious diseases can be rapidly fatal if not quickly diagnosed and treated. Others, e.g., tuberculosis, Marburg virus infection, Lassa fever, and Ebola fever, are highly contagious if not detected and if the patient is not isolated.

Useful Points in Diagnosis. The majority of febrile illnesses, even in recent travelers to the tropics, are self-limiting and undiagnosed. Most are caused by infectious agents, more than half of which are viruses. Points useful in reaching a diagnosis are the incubation period, the vaccination and prophylaxis history, the length of patient's stay and living conditions, the fever pattern, the associated signs and symptoms, and the geographic location of exposure (Fig. 116–1).

Incubation Period. Knowledge concerning the time of exposure to communicable diseases helps in making the correct diagnosis (Table 116–1). Some diseases can be excluded if the time when the patient left the endemic area is known. In the case of malaria, this time ranges from 12 days for falciparum malaria to 1 month for *Plasmodium malariae* infection. However, this interval can be prolonged if the patient has received antimalarial suppressive therapy or has partial immunity. Some strains of *P. vivax* can also have prolonged incubation periods (Chapter 73). Exposure does not have to be recent. (I had my first symptoms from a *P. vivax* infection approximately 1 year following the last exposure. The diagnosis was made by detecting parasites on a Giemsa-stained blood film taken on the fifth day of elevated temperature.) The incubation period for visceral leishmaniasis and hepatic amebiasis can be years, and because of the prolonged time for development of the parasite, "filarial fevers" seldom develop before 8 to 10 months following exposure. The incubation periods for hepatitis A (15 to 45 days) and hepatitis B (45 to 160 days) have been well documented. Symptoms due to arboviral infections usually occur within 1 week of the infecting bite, whereas the incubation period for the hemorrhagic fevers is usually longer.

Vaccination History. A history of being vaccinated for yellow fever or hepatitis B virtually rules these out. Immunization with the currently available typhoid vaccines only provide partial protection—usually quoted as between 50 and 70%. Childhood immunization for po-

TABLE 116–1. Incubation Periods for Tropical Infectious Diseases

Incubation Period	Infection
Short (less than 10 days)	Arboviral infections, including dengue and yellow fever Typhus fevers Plague Paratyphoid fever
Intermediate (10 to 21 days)	*Plasmodium falciparum* infections *P. vivax, P. ovale,* and *P. malariae* infections Hemorrhagic fevers, including Lassa fever Scrub typhus African trypanosomiasis Enteric fever Brucellosis
Prolonged (greater than 21 days)	Viral hepatitis Human immunodeficiency virus (HIV) infection Rabies Tuberculosis *P. vivax, P. ovale,* and *P. malariae* infections Visceral leishmaniasis Amebic abscess of the liver Filariasis

liomyelitis, diphtheria, and tuberculosis (bacille Calmette-Guérin [BCG]) may not provide protection in adults unless they received boosters or had natural exposure. Individuals coming from developing countries may not have received routine immunizations.

Prophylaxis History. Immune globulin provides partial protection for hepatitis A, which decreases as the time following administration increases, e.g., protection is much better during the first month than during the third month following the inoculation. Malaria chemoprophylaxis is complicated (Chapter 73.1). A history of faithful use of chloroquine is likely to prevent malaria in Central America and the Caribbean. However, in other areas where chloroquine-resistant *P. falciparum* is common, chloroquine (or most other antimalarials) often does not prevent illness due to malaria.

Length of Patient's Stay and Living Conditions. The degree and type of exposures are heavily influenced by living conditions and length of stay. Tourists who stay for brief periods in first-class hotels in the capital city or tourist centers have different and much less exposure than do backpackers or volunteer workers who live on the economy with the local population—often for longer periods and in rural areas. These latter groups have a higher likelihood of acquiring diseases such as tuberculosis, filariasis, visceral leishmaniasis, and schistosomiasis, as well as malaria, diarrheal illness, and intestinal parasites.

Temperature Pattern. The height of temperature and the type of temperature curve can assist in the differential diagnosis. Infections that characteristically have high fever spikes, frequently in the 105 to 106F (40.5 to 41.0C) range, are falciparum malaria, pneumococcal pneumonia, encephalitis, measles, and meningococcemia. The maximum fever in other infections, e.g., influenza, typhoid fever, tuberculosis, vivax malaria, African trypanosomiasis, pyelonephritis, brucellosis, re-

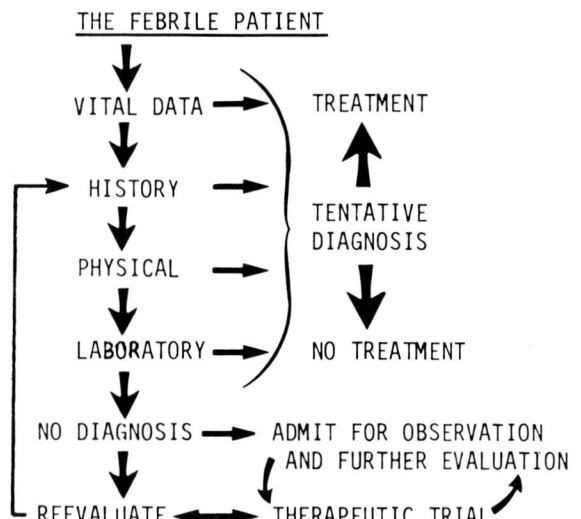

THE FEBRILE PATIENT

FIGURE 116–1. An algorithm for evaluation of a febrile patient who has been in the tropics.

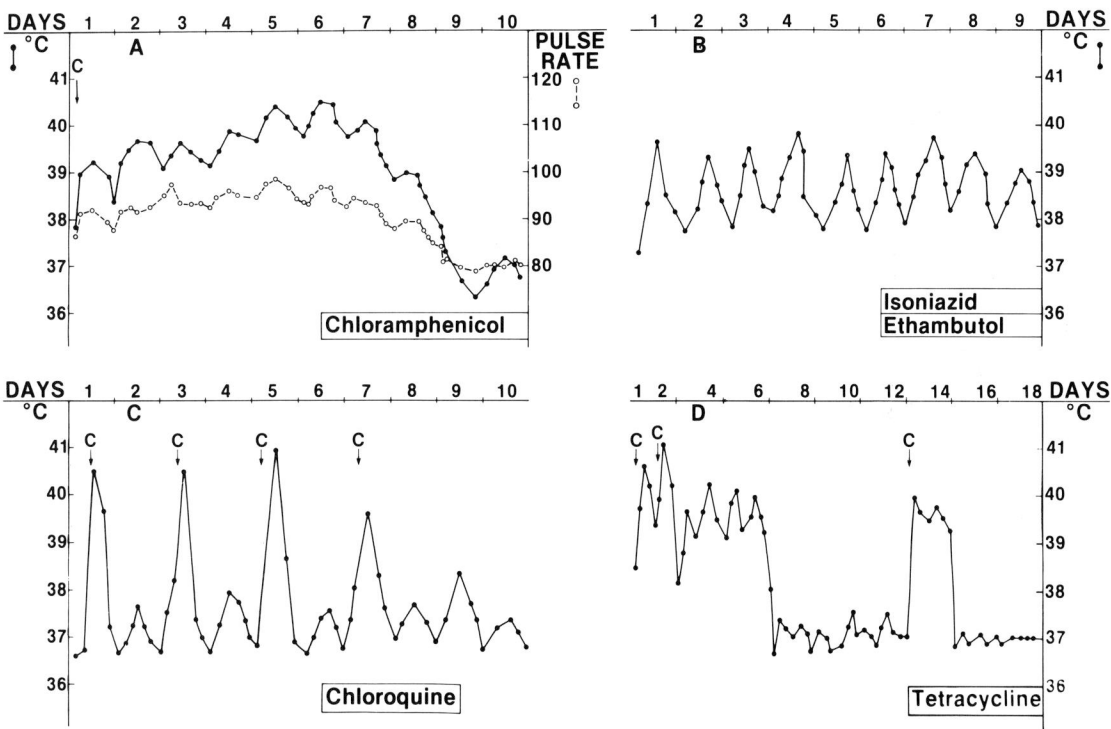

FIGURE 116–2. Four examples of fever patterns. *A, Continuous fever.* Temperature and pulse curve in a 26-year-old Indonesian male with typhoid fever who had a single chill (c) and clinical response to chloramphenicol therapy. *B, Remittent fever.* Temperature curve in a 27-year-old Indian woman with pulmonary tuberculosis who was treated with isoniazid and ethambutol. She was chilly every afternoon during the temperature elevation but did not have a rigor. *C, Intermittent fever.* Temperature curve of a 14-year-old Filipino female with established vivax malaria. She had shaking chills (c), each time associated with temperature elevations, and had an excellent response to chloroquine therapy. *D, Relapsing fever.* Temperature curve of a 22-year-old Ethiopian man with *Borrelia recurrentis* infection. He had chills (c) associated with temperature elevations and was treated with tetracycline.

lapsing fever, leptospirosis, dengue, and the viral hemorrhagic fevers, is usually in the 103 to 104F (39.5 to 40.0C) range. Lower fever spikes (101 to 102F [38.5 to 39.0C]) are usually noted in most other viral infections, diphtheria, nontyphoidal *Salmonella* infections, and familial Mediterranean fever.

The type of fever pattern is sometimes helpful in making the correct diagnosis (Fig. 116–2). A *continuous fever* (Fig. 116–2A) is one in which the temperature curve remains elevated without significant diurnal variation. Untreated typhoid fever and typhus often have this type of pattern. A *remittent fever* (Fig. 116–2B) has a curve with daily fluctuations of more than 2C, with the low point in the day approaching but not reaching the normal level. This is the most common fever pattern and is characteristically found in pulmonary tuberculosis, bacterial septicemias, and African trypanosomiasis. An *intermittent fever* (Fig. 116–2C) is one in which the temperature drops to normal or below normal each day, with a large variation between the peak and nadir. This pattern is often seen in malaria, pyogenic abscesses, and miliary tuberculosis. A *relapsing fever* (Fig. 116–2D) is one in which febrile periods alternate with several days of normal temperature. This pattern is sometimes seen in quartan malaria, dengue fever, and relapsing fever caused by *Borrelia recurrentis.*

Associated Signs and Symptoms. There are signs and symptoms that are suggestive of an infectious etiology. These are an abrupt onset of pyrexia, high temperature (102F [39.5C] or greater), and chills. Other nonspecific

but common symptoms are malaise, myalgia, arthralgia, headache, and photophobia. Others that may help in pinpointing the site of infection and/or agent(s) are nausea, vomiting, diarrhea, lymphadenopathy, splenomegaly, dysuria, urinary frequency, flank pain, sore throat, coryza, cough, pleuritic pain, and nuchal rigidity. Fever with diarrhea suggests a bowel pathogen, e.g., *Shigella, Campylobacter,* invasive *Escherichia coli, Entamoeba histolytica,* or rotavirus infection. Frequent loose stools may occur with malaria, dengue, scrub typhus, leptospirosis, and enteric fever. However, constipation is frequently present in the latter. The viral hemorrhagic fevers can cause bloody diarrhea, as can the bowel pathogens. Chills occur occasionally in many infectious diseases. However, they are quite common in some. These diseases (Table 116–2) are those in which a rapid proliferation of the agent is characteristic. Lymphadenopathy occurs so frequently that it is often not a useful diagnostic finding. Malaria and the enteric pathogens seldom cause lymph node enlargement. Splenomegaly can be a useful finding in the differential diagnosis (Table 116–3). Although often difficult to detect in dark-skinned individuals, a rash can assist in the diagnosis (Table 116–4). Jaundice suggests viral hepatitis, malaria, leptospirosis, yellow fever and other viral hemorrhagic fevers, and louse-borne relapsing fever.

Geographic Location of Exposure. There are areas of the world where exposures to specific infectious agents are rather common (Table 116–5 and Chapter 121).

TABLE 116–2. Infectious Diseases Characteristically Associated with Chills

Malaria	Plague
Lobar pneumonia	Typhus fever
Influenza	Pyelonephritis
Typhoid fever	Bacterial abscess
Bacterial septicemia	Dengue
Cholangitis	Chikungunya

Malaria, typhoid fever, and infectious hepatitis are widespread throughout the tropics and must be considered in every febrile patient. However, the geographic distribution of many other infectious diseases is quite localized. For example, Ebola fever, Marburg disease, Lassa fever, and African trypanosomiasis are limited to certain locations in Africa.

Work-Up of Fever. A patient complaining of fever with a recent history of travel should have at least an abbreviated evaluation (Fig. 116–1). This is done even though there is an excellent chance that the cause of the fever is nontropical and self-limiting.

History. As noted previously, the usual historical questions, as well as a travel history, are important. There are some short febrile illnesses that are not caused by infections. A careful history should assist in ruling out allergic reactions to drugs or serum, an exaggerated circadian temperature rhythm, factitious fever, and other noninfectious causes of fever. A travel history can help to focus the diagnostic possibilities, and the associated symptoms can lead toward the correct diagnosis. For example, a Cambodian refugee who has had fever and night sweats for 2 weeks, along with cough and weight loss for the past month, has a good chance of having pulmonary tuberculosis.

Travelers who stay abroad for short periods rarely develop tuberculosis or filariasis, whereas long-stay travelers and recent immigrants are more at risk for such infection. Similarly, travelers who confine their stay to urban areas are at little or no risk for African hemorrhagic fevers, schistosomiasis, and scrub typhus and are unlikely to acquire leptospirosis or yellow fever. A good exposure history can often assist in the diagnosis (Table 116–6).

Physical Examination. During the initial screening examination for fever, the following are the minimal requirements: temperature (to confirm the pyrexia); pulse rate; auscultation of the chest and heart; palpation of the liver, spleen, and lymph nodes; visual inspection of the skin for rash; and more extensive examination of any organ system associated with symptoms.

Laboratory Tests. Minimal laboratory tests to be

TABLE 116–3. Infections Causing Splenomegaly and Fever

Viruses	Bacteria	Parasites
Infectious mononucleosis	Enteric fever	Malaria
	Typhus	Visceral leishmaniasis
Cytomegalovirus (CMV)	Endocarditis	African trypanosomiasis
	Tuberculosis	
HIV infection	Brucellosis	Acute schistosomiasis
	Leptospirosis	Toxoplasmosis
	Relapsing fever	Acute American trypanosomiasis

TABLE 116–4. Infections Causing Fever and Rash

Infection	Cutaneous Manifestations
Measles	Maculopapular
Rubella	Maculopapular
Dengue	Diffuse erythematous or scarlatiniform; petechiae and ecchymoses in a few
Viral hemorrhagic fevers	Petechiae, ecchymoses
Infectious mononucleosis	Maculopapular
Monkey pox	Maculopapular, vesicular, pustular
HIV infection	Morbilliform
Spotted fever	Diffuse macular or maculopapular; petechiae
Epidemic typhus	Diffuse macular or maculopapular
Scrub typhus	Eschar; diffuse macular or maculopapular
Secondary syphilis	Papular (copper penny)
Lyme disease	Maculopapular, erythematous
Typhoid fever	Rose-colored papules on trunk
Gonococcemia	Pustular, hemorrhagic, necrotic
Meningococcemia	Maculopapular, petechiae, ecchymoses
Plague	Macules, pustules, vesicles, petechiae
Bartonellosis	Erythematous papules
Scarlet fever	Maculopapular
Visceral leishmaniasis	Dark pigmentation, papule or ulcer
African trypanosomiasis	Chancre; erythematous

performed include complete blood count, urinalysis, malaria blood film (if the patient was potentially exposed to malaria), and chest radiograph (if chest disease is a possibility). Other tests that should be performed, if historical, physical, or other laboratory findings suggest that they are indicated, include blood, stool, and urine cultures for bacteria, sputum smears and cultures for acid-fast bacilli, determinations of serum enzymes and alkaline phosphatase, and selected serologic tests.

If an African hemorrhagic fever is suspected on clinical or epidemiologic grounds, the communicable diseases branch of the Department of Health should be informed and all nonessential laboratory tests should be withheld until the situation has been thoroughly reviewed. In addition, the patient should be managed using strict barrier nursing techniques (e.g., gown, gloves, mask, separate room) until these highly contagious and serious infections have been ruled out.

Follow-Up. If the preceding findings are inconclusive and it is not believed that the patient has a serious illness, he or she may be sent home with the recommendation that the patient chart his or her temperature and return in 2 or 3 days if the fever persists (sooner if the patient becomes sicker). If there are positive or suspected positive findings, the patient should be hospitalized and/or treated. A young college student with an unremittent fever of 103F, a pulse of 90, headache, chills, cough, constipation, and splenomegaly who had been working on a ranch in Mexico until 2 weeks before the onset of symptoms may have typhoid fever. This patient should be hospitalized, and blood, stool, and urine cultures should be performed. Not everyone who has a diagnosis established needs to be hospitalized. For example, most patients with vivax malaria can be treated as outpatients.

Most patients sent home following the initial evaluation have a spontaneous resolution of their illness, because the majority of short febrile illnesses are self-limiting viral infections. However, some will remain

**TABLE 116–5. Selected Diseases Causing
Fever in the Tropics**

Common with Wide Distribution
Malaria
Tuberculosis
Arboviral infections
   Dengue
Enteric fevers
   Typhoid fever

Less Common with Wide Distribution
Amebic liver abscess
Infectious hepatitis
Brucellosis
Poliomyelitis
Toxoplasmosis
Schistosomiasis
Filariasis

Less Common with Limited Distribution
Visceral leishmaniasis
Leptospirosis
Scrub typhus
Louse-, flea-, and tick-borne typhus
Relapsing fever
African trypanosomiasis
Hemorrhagic fevers
   Ebola hemorrhagic fever
   Lassa fever
   Marburg disease
Plague
Melioidosis
Yellow fever
HIV infection

Noninfectious Conditions
Rheumatic fever
Sickle cell anemia
Familial Mediterranean fever
Rheumatoid arthritis
Systemic lupus erythematosus
Factitious conditions

febrile. If they have been keeping a temperature chart, this could be of diagnostic assistance. On the return visit, the initial history and physical examination should be repeated, and this time the examination should be performed in detail. Both a thick and thin Giemsa-

**TABLE 116–6. Exposures Suggesting Specific
Infectious Agents**

Ingestion of Unpasteurized Milk	*Ticks or Mites*
Brucellosis	Congo-Crimean hemorrhagic fever
Salmonellosis	Colorado tick fever
Tuberculosis	Kyasanur Forest disease
Fresh Water	Russian spring-summer encephalitis
Leptospirosis	Spotted fevers
Schistosomiasis	Typhus
Dracontiasis	Scrub typhus
	Q fever
Animal Contact	Rickettsial pox
Rabies	Tularemia
Viral hemorrhagic fevers	Lyme disease
Q fever	Relapsing fever
Leptospirosis	Babesiosis
Tularemia	
Plague	*Injections or Transfusions*
Brucellosis	Hepatitis B and C
Babesiosis	HIV infection
	Malaria
	Chagas' disease
	Toxoplasmosis

stained blood film for malarial parasites should be done. It is the physician's responsibility to see that these are prepared and read by someone experienced in the diagnosis of malaria. If this cannot be ensured and malaria is a diagnostic possibility, the patient or his or her blood smears should be sent to an institution where the reading of malaria blood films is reliable. Laboratory tests as noted for the first visit are repeated or performed for the first time. Any procedure that is clinically indicated is performed at this time, and most physicians would order some screening tests, e.g., chest radiograph, febrile agglutinins, tuberculin skin test, liver scan, and/or sonogram.

Depending on the clinical status and the length of the febrile period, the undiagnosed patient may be sent home to continue to chart his or her fever and to return if the condition worsens or if the fever persists, or the patient may be hospitalized and evaluated for prolonged fever.

Inpatient Studies. Persistent undiagnosed fever and/or progression of illness would lead to hospitalization. A complete history and physical examination would be repeated. Routine laboratory tests would be performed, including a complete blood count, urinalysis, liver function tests, and chest radiograph. Blood, urine, and stool cultures would be obtained. Appropriate serologic and skin tests would be ordered. Noninvasive procedures, e.g., liver and spleen scans, sonography and computed tomography (CT) scan of the abdomen and any suspicious sites, would be performed.

Bone marrow aspirations and biopsies could be performed for smears and cultures. Biopsy of other available suspicious sites, e.g., liver, lymph nodes, and spleen, could be performed for histologic examination and cultures.

A laparotomy is seldom required to establish the diagnosis, and careful consideration should be given before performing a splenectomy in someone who will be returning to the tropics, because individuals who have had splenectomies have less satisfactory immune responses to infections, particularly to malaria.

In rare cases, a diagnosis will not be made following the aforementioned procedures, in which circumstance a therapeutic trial is indicated. Chemotherapy can be started for tuberculosis if this is suspected. Often, a patient may become afebrile and have considerable improvement in clinical symptoms within 2 weeks of institution of specific antituberculosis therapy. Patients with bacterial endocarditis, typhoid fever, and other bacterial septicemias who have previously received antibiotics may have repeatedly negative blood cultures. These individuals should be treated with the most appropriate antibiotic(s), with a therapeutic response suggesting that the presumptive diagnosis was correct. Rarely, patients with malaria (particularly individuals with *P. malariae* infections and those receiving incomplete treatment), visceral leishmaniasis, and amebiasis might need to be treated before the diagnosis is confirmed. Again, a response to therapy suggests that the clinical impression was correct.

CAUSES OF FEVER IN TRAVELERS
Conditions That Cause Fever in a Temperate Climate.
It must be stressed that people who have visited or lived

in the tropics can have all of the usual causes of fever that occur in temperate climates, and the majority of febrile episodes will have nonexotic etiologies.

Infections. The majority of febrile episodes are not diagnosed and are caused by viruses. Infectious mononucleosis is a rather common cause of fever in adolescents. Influenza commonly attacks all age groups. Bacterial infections in most sites of the body can cause fever, e.g., abscesses, endocarditis, pneumonia, osteomyelitis, pyelonephritis, and infections of the biliary tract. Systemic fungal infections, including histoplasmosis and cryptococcosis, can be causes of fever of unknown origin (FUO).

Malignancies. The malignancies usually associated with FUO are Hodgkin's disease, non-Hodgkin's lymphomas, leukemia, and cancer of the colon, liver, pancreas, and kidney. Atrial myxomas, although rare, have been manifested as FUO.

Collagen Vascular Disease. Systemic lupus erythematosus is the most common autoimmune disease causing FUO. However, rheumatoid arthritis (particularly juvenile rheumatoid arthritis), idiopathic vasculitis, and polymyalgia rheumatica can all present as fever.

Miscellaneous Conditions. The granulomatous diseases, i.e., sarcoidosis, granulomatous hepatitis, inflammatory bowel disease, and temporal arteritis, may all cause an unexplained fever. Drug fever and serum sickness would be more common in travelers because of greater exposure. Other nontropical causes of fever include pulmonary embolization, cirrhosis of the liver, alcoholic hepatitis, central nervous system tumors or vascular lesions, septic thrombophlebitis, cyclic neutropenia, and familial Mediterranean fever (FMF). The collagen vascular diseases and granulomatous diseases are rare in residents of the tropics. However, cirrhosis of the liver and primary hepatoma are common. Other associated signs and symptoms should suggest these problems. Liver function tests and hepatic scanning and sonography should focus on the lesion, and a liver biopsy would confirm the diagnosis.

Infectious Diseases Associated with Tropical Exposure. There is a group of diseases that are almost exclusively associated with exposure in the tropics, diseases rarely transmitted in temperate climates today.

Malaria. Malaria is widespread in the tropics and is the most common cause of pyrexia in the returning traveler when a cause is documented. *Fever in a traveler from a malarious area is malaria until proved otherwise.* Malaria must be suspected as a potential etiology of fever in a traveler, and thick and thin Giemsa-stained blood films must be made and read by a knowledgeable technician. Mortality is minuscule when the diagnosis is rapidly confirmed and appropriate treatment given. However, when there is delay in diagnosis and treatment, preventable deaths occur (Chapter 73).

Some useful points are as follows: (1) The careful taking of prophylactic drugs does not always prevent drug-resistant falciparum malaria. (2) Vivax and ovale malaria may occur and may be difficult to diagnose in individuals who have received suppressive prophylaxis with chloroquine but not causal prophylaxis with primaquine. (3) These individuals and others, who have

partial immunity and/or have received incomplete prophylaxis, may develop clinical malaria after returning from the tropics. Three-fourths of patients with falciparum malaria have the onset of symptoms within 1 month of return from the tropics, whereas only 45% of those with vivax and the other forms of malaria have symptoms within the first month. With falciparum malaria, there is almost never onset of symptoms 6 months or more after exposure, whereas 1 of 4 patients with vivax and ovale malaria has initial symptoms 6 months or more following return from the tropics. (4) Malaria often causes signs and symptoms in paroxysms; therefore, it should be suspected in patients with intermittent fever and symptoms. However, falciparum malaria is less likely to be paroxysmal and it usually takes several days for infection with the other species to develop a rhythm. Therefore, continuous or minimal fluctuation in fever is also compatible with malaria.

Arboviral Infections. Viruses transmitted by arthropods are more common in the tropics or are limited to the tropics. Dengue is the most prevalent of those occurring in Asia and is now common in Latin America and the Caribbean Islands. Dengue caused by 3 serotypes is particularly prevalent in Brazil, Mexico, Puerto Rico, and Colombia, where it is a hazard to tourists who are bitten by mosquitoes (Chapter 20.1). There was an epidemic of Rift Valley fever in Egypt and northeastern Africa 10 to 15 years ago. Some excellent serologic studies have shown that dengue and chikungunya are common causes of fever in nonimmune adults in Southeast Asia.

Clinical features that suggest the diagnosis of dengue are chills, headache, malaise, anorexia, backache, myalgia, lymphadenopathy, and leukopenia. Generally, fever and other symptoms occur 5 to 8 days after exposure and then subside within 5 days. The classic "saddleback" relapsing fever curve, when it occurs, is a helpful diagnostic sign. Chikungunya infection is characterized by chills, arthralgias, malaise, myalgia, headache, arthritis, lymphadenopathy, and a macular rash.

There are many arboviruses that cause brief undiagnosed febrile illnesses in travelers who have recently returned from the tropics (Chapter 20).

Amebic Liver Abscess. A history of a recent visit to the tropics is not essential to make the diagnosis of amebic abscess of the liver (Chapter 68). Cases have occurred in individuals who have not been in the tropics for 5 years or more and, in rare cases, in persons who have never left a temperate climate. Associated symptoms and signs that suggest amebic liver abscess are anorexia, weight loss, right upper quadrant abdominal pain, hepatomegaly, hepatic tenderness, and leukocytosis. Hepatomegaly without splenomegaly is a helpful clue. The patient is often a male who drinks alcohol. Amebic serologic tests and a hepatic scan or sonography and a chest radiograph showing right-sided pleural effusion or elevation of the diaphragm help in making a presumptive diagnosis. Sometimes, hepatic aspiration is required to rule out a bacterial abscess.

Visceral Leishmaniasis. Visceral leishmaniasis can rarely cause fever in a traveler or expatriate from the tropics, especially in the Mediterranean area (Chapter

76.1). The incubation period can be prolonged. The commonly associated findings, e.g., weight loss, hepatosplenomegaly, anemia, leukopenia, and elevated IgG, suggest the diagnosis. The diagnosis is best made by demonstration of the organisms in a Giemsa-stained smear or in culture from a bone marrow aspirate. To demonstrate the organism, splenic aspiration or liver biopsy is sometimes necessary.

Miscellaneous Viral Illnesses. The hemorrhagic fevers, although rare, are important because of their high mortality and infectivity (Chapter 22). Recent small epidemics of Korean hemorrhagic fever have been occurring in US military troops during training exercises in Korea. The infection, also called hemorrhagic fever with renal syndrome (HFRS) is caused by *Hantavirus* and is acquired during exposure to infectious rodent urine and feces. The troops were bivouacked in areas inhabited by infected rodents (Chapter 22.6). Visitors to West, Central, and South Africa could be exposed to Ebola hemorrhagic fever, Lassa fever, or Marburg disease. Yellow fever can be prevented by vaccination. Rarely, immigrants or travelers from developing countries have symptomatic rabies in the United States or Europe. Rabies should always be suspected in febrile patients with unexplained encephalitis who have been exposed to dogs in countries where canine rabies still occurs.

Rickettsial Infections. The typhus infections are transmitted by mites, fleas, ticks, and lice. Scrub typhus was one of the more common causes of fever in American military personnel during the Vietnam conflict (Chapter 25). Characteristic findings were exposure to the mites in the jungles, eschar, a high incidence of malaise, chills, headache, myalgia, backache, macular rash, lymphadenopathy, and a dramatic response to tetracycline therapy. The diagnosis can be confirmed by use of serologic tests. Scrub typhus has a wide distribution in South and East Asia.

Louse-, flea-, and tick-borne typhus infections must also be suspected in travelers who have had appropriate exposure (Chapters 23 and 24). High temperature, rash, and constitutional symptoms are the usual manifestations. Serologic tests are the best method of establishing the diagnosis.

Diarrheal Illnesses. Fever in association with diarrhea is common in returning travelers (Chapter 117). Although bacterial pathogens, e.g., *Shigella, Salmonella,* and *Campylobacter,* are the most frequent etiologic agents, malaria and systemic viral infections must be considered, especially in children who often develop diarrhea with febrile illnesses.

Sexually Transmitted Diseases. Sexually transmitted diseases have a very high prevalence in some areas of the tropics. An individual with lymphadenopathy and/ or rash with fever and a homosexual or heterosexual exposure a few weeks to a few months previously could have primary human immunodeficiency virus (HIV) infection (Chapter 15.1) or secondary syphilis (Chapter 32.1). HIV and hepatitis B and C viruses can also be parenterally transmitted by injections, transfusions of blood or blood products, and the sharing of needles for the intravenous injection of drugs. In these circumstances, an accurate and candid medical history becomes important.

Miscellaneous Bacterial Infections. Brucellosis is uncommon but should be suspected in someone who has eaten unpasteurized dairy products. The organisms are difficult to culture, but attempts should be made if the disease is suspected. Serologic tests demonstrating a rising antibody titer are helpful. Granulomas can be demonstrated in tissue biopsy specimens (Chapter 50). Brucellosis is a frequent cause of fever in Southwest Asia, particularly in Saudi Arabia and Kuwait.

Melioidosis has been associated with prolonged fever and generalized infection in individuals who have been to Southeast Asia. The incubation period can be prolonged (Chapter 56.2). Plague is another cause of fever and severe illness. With the most common bubonic form, the patient has the characteristic fluctuant lymph nodes, which can be aspirated. The organisms may be seen on smear or culture (Chapter 47).

Miscellaneous Parasitic Infections. *Schistosoma mansoni* and *S. japonicum* can cause fever during the acute invasive stage. This is usually associated with diarrhea, blood in the stool, and eosinophilia. The diagnosis may be difficult because often ova are not present in the stools. This syndrome is more likely to occur in a nonimmune expatriate than in a national of the endemic country (Chapter 96). There is an increased incidence of pyelonephritis in patients with *S. haematobium* infections, and *Salmonella* enteric fever has been associated with schistosomiasis.

Filariasis has a wide distribution in the tropics. Febrile episodes lasting about a week and associated with lymphadenitis and lymphangitis occur frequently in subjects with bancroftian and Malayan filariasis (Chapter 85). The incubation period is almost never less than 6 months. Eosinophilia and perhaps some chronic changes of elephantiasis are also found. The diagnosis can be established by demonstrating the microfilariae on a Giemsa-stained blood smear. Serologic tests can be helpful.

African trypanosomiasis, although rare, can be a serious cause of fever in a tourist to or emigrant from Africa who has been bitten by the vector, the tsetse fly. There may be a chancre at the site of the bite, and skin rash, lymphadenopathy, hepatosplenomegaly, anemia, and elevated serum or cerebrospinal fluid IgM levels are characteristic. The diagnosis is confirmed by demonstrating the trypanosome in the blood, in a lymph node aspirate, or in the spinal fluid (Chapter 74).

Infectious Diseases with Increased Prevalence in the Tropics. There are diseases that, although present in countries with temperate climates, are much more common in the tropics. Therefore, travel to the tropics increases the chance of exposure to these infections.

Tuberculosis. Tuberculosis is rare in Americans, but when it occurs, it does so more frequently in elderly males. However, it is a common cause of fever in immigrants and should be suspected in individuals of all age groups who have prolonged fever, weight loss, and cough (Chapter 61). In Asian immigrants to the United States tuberculosis is recognized in 40% within the first year of arriving and in almost half by the end of the second year. Half are under the age of 35 years. Tourists to the tropics seldom are infected with *Mycobacterium tuberculosis*. Chest radiographs are essential when tuberculosis is suspected. Tuberculin skin tests can be helpful in children not previously given BCG immunization. The diagnosis is confirmed by demonstrating acid-fast bacilli in sputum smears or by culturing the organism in sputum, urine, gastric washings, or other specimens. Sometimes, the patient must be treated without bacteriologic confirmation of the diagnosis. Granulomas in tissue biopsy specimens are helpful, and a clinical response to chemotherapy gives a presumptive diagnosis.

Salmonellosis. Enteric fever is most commonly associated with infection with *Salmonella typhi, S. paratyphi A,* and *S. paratyphi B* (Chapters 38 and 39). Over half of patients diagnosed in temperate climates have a history of recent travel in the tropics. Nineteen of 27 patients reported from a single hospital in Montreal had traveled in the tropics during the month prior to the onset of symptoms. Typhoid fever should be suspected in a febrile overseas traveler or immigrant who has many of the following symptoms and signs: headache, chills, cough, constipation, diarrhea, nausea, abdominal pain, unremittent fever (Fig. 116–2*A*), splenomegaly, elevated hepatic enzymes, and anemia. Serologic tests are sometimes helpful, but the diagnosis is confirmed by a positive blood, stool, or urine culture.

Infectious Hepatitis. Hepatitis caused by hepatitis A, B, C, D, or other non-A, non-B hepatitis viruses is common in the developing world, and nonimmune individuals can be heavily exposed during their travels. Non-A, non-B hepatitis can be transmitted by either the parenteral or the fecal-oral route. The attack rate was 42% in Somalia refugee camps during an epidemic of enterically transmitted non-A, non-B hepatitis in 1985 and 1986. Hyperimmune globulin gives passive immunity, and a hepatitis B vaccine is available, although expensive.

Hepatitis can present as FUO. Other nonspecific associated symptoms are anorexia, nausea, malaise, and arthralgias. Jaundice, dark urine, hepatomegaly, hepatic tenderness, and abnormal liver function tests suggest the correct diagnosis, which can be confirmed by serologic tests (Chapter 19).

Toxoplasmosis. Toxoplasmosis can cause an acute febrile illness that is often associated with lymphadenopathy, myalgia, leukopenia, and anemia and that is difficult to differentiate from infectious mononucleosis or cytomegalovirus (CMV) infection (Chapter 78). It is more prevalent in the tropics, where food and water are more likely to be contaminated with cat feces containing the highly contagious oocyst. A history of exposure to cats or the ingestion of rare or raw meat helps in establishing the diagnosis. The organism can be isolated in laboratory animals inoculated with suspensions containing lymph node tissue. However, excellent serologic tests are readily available.

Miscellaneous Infections. Since the development of vaccines, poliomyelitis is rare in the temperate climates. However, people from the developing world frequently have not been immunized, and poliomyelitis should be suspected in a febrile immigrant with neurologic symptoms (Chapter 18.1). Rarely, an adult immunized as a child may develop acute poliomyelitis following exposure in the tropics. This is believed to be due to waning immunity following an incomplete immunization or no booster from natural exposure to wild viruses. Most specialists working in travelers' clinics give booster poliomyelitis immunizations to adult travelers to developing countries (Chapter 115). Viral encephalitis, including Japanese B encephalitis, must also be considered. Leptospirosis is more common in the tropics. Helpful points suggesting leptospirosis are severe headache, myalgia, nausea, abdominal pain, conjunctivitis, an abnormal urine sediment, proteinuria, polymorphonuclear leukocytosis, and abnormal liver function tests. A history of exposure to water that could have been contaminated by infected rats is helpful in the diagnosis. Serologic testing is the easiest method to confirm the diagnosis (Chapter 35). People who have eaten undercooked meat and who have fever, myalgia, and eosinophilia may have trichinosis (Chapter 90). There were 2 outbreaks of horsemeat-associated trichinosis in France in 1985.

Noninfectious Causes of Fever in the Tropics. Fever is not always caused by infection. Fever caused by malignancies, collagen vascular diseases, and granulomatous diseases is infrequently diagnosed in the tropics. However, there are some noninfectious diseases associated with fever that have a higher prevalence in the tropics and subtropics than in temperate climates.

Rheumatic Fever. Acute rheumatic fever is more prevalent in developing countries than in developed countries. Fever is characteristic. The diagnosis should be suspected when carditis and migratory polyarthritis are also present. Subcutaneous nodules, erythema marginatum, chorea, and positive throat cultures for β-hemolytic streptococcus are reported less frequently than in descriptions of the classic disease in temperate climate. Valvular heart disease is common, occurs at an early age, and is often rapidly progressive (Chapter 2).

Sickle Cell Anemia. Fever is a common complication of sickle cell anemia (Chapter 5). Homozygotes for SS hemoglobin have an increased incidence of infections and multiple pulmonary embolizations, accounting for their pyrexia. Sickled erythrocytes cause microthrombi and macrothrombi, leading to recurrent vaso-occlusive phenomena. Occasionally, the resulting pulmonary, bone, and other infarcts are secondarily infected. Patients with sickle cell disease have a higher incidence of pneumococcal infection and are more likely to have a *Salmonella* osteomyelitis. Repeated infarcts of the spleen impair splenic function. This, along with a defect in opsonin antibodies, interferes with the immune response to some bacteria. The diagnosis of sickle cell anemia can be easily established in a febrile black child (Chapter 5).

Familial Mediterranean Fever. FMF is a syndrome manifested by recurrent, self-limited attacks of fever along with abdominal, chest, and joint pains. Almost all individuals with FMF are of Mediterranean or Middle Eastern ethnic origin, i.e., Jewish, Armenian, Turkish, and Arab. It is believed to be inherited as a single autosomal recessive trait with an incidence in homozygotes of 1:2000 in Israel.

The cause of FMF remains unknown. However, a genetic predisposition is present and involvement of the vascular system with immunologic abnormalities has been clearly established. Recurrent polyserositis appears to be the principal pathophysiologic finding. FMF is clearly polymorphic, with several phenotypes and the inheritance has some variables that are not fully discernible. In addition, cases of a similar disease have been described among non-Mideastern families. However, a physician working with travelers would most likely see fever caused by FMF in immigrants or visitors from the Middle East.

Pathologic findings are nonspecific. Peritonitis, pleuritis, and arthritis are manifested by exudates containing a predominance of polymorphonuclear leukocytes. Biopsies demonstrate acute inflammatory changes.

The age of onset of symptoms is usually between 5 and 15 years. There is a 20% incidence of consanguinity, and a 50% incidence of positive family history; 60% of the patients are male. The duration and frequency of attacks vary. The usual attack lasts 24 to 72 hours but sometimes is prolonged for 7 to 10 days. From 1 to 52 attacks per year occur, with the usual frequency being every 2 to 4 weeks. Spontaneous remissions lasting for years have been reported. During the acute attack, the temperature is usually between 100 and 102F (38 and 39C) and is often associated with symptoms and signs of peritonitis, pleuritis, arthritis, and, occasionally, erysipelas-like skin rashes on the dorsum of the foot and the anterior aspect of the lower leg or the thighs. The peritonitis varies in severity. The pain sometimes involves the entire abdomen and is associated with nausea, vomiting, and abdominal distention, rigidity, rebound tenderness, and evidence of paralytic ileus. Many patients have undergone exploratory laparotomy before the diagnosis of FMF was suspected and confirmed.

Other complications include amyloidosis, which is progressive and usually leads to death from renal failure. This is more common in Israel than elsewhere, including the United States. Narcotic addiction and emotional disturbances are problems that occur frequently. Splenomegaly is the most common physical abnormality found between attacks.

Laboratory abnormalities during attacks include elevation of the erythrocyte sedimentation rate, white blood cell counts, and acute phase reactants, e.g., C-reactive protein and IgM.

The diagnosis is suspected in individuals of appropriate ethnic origin with the characteristic self-limited attacks, particularly if they have a positive family history. The rare patient who has only fever requires a complete work-up for FUO and prolonged observation.

Febrile Egyptian patients with FMF were rapidly diagnosed by their characteristic history and physical findings and their response to colchicine. Thirty-five of 299 patients (12%) admitted to an Abassia Fever Hospital–NAMRU-3 study for fever from 1971 to 1975 had FMF.

A multitude of therapeutic measures, including corticosteroids and a low-fat diet, have been used to prevent and treat the acute attacks of FMF. Colchicine can reduce the number of acute attacks and abort attacks in some patients. It is usually given in a dosage of 0.6 mg 3 times daily. If this dosage causes gastrointestinal symptoms, it is reduced to 0.6 mg 2 times daily. To abort attacks, the dosage used is 0.6 mg every hour for 4 hours starting at the first prodromal symptom. This is followed by the same dose every 2 hours twice, and then every 12 hours for 2 days. Colchicine probably interferes with the inflammatory response and thus reduces or prevents symptoms. Recent studies have shown that it prevents the development of amyloidosis.

BIBLIOGRAPHY

Anderson KE, Joseph SW, Nasution R, et al: Febrile illnesses resulting in hospital admission: A bacteriological and serological study in Jakarta, Indonesia. Am J Trop Med Hyg 25:116, 1976.

Barakat MH, Karnik AM, Majeed HWA, et al: Familial Mediterranean fever (recurrent hereditary polyserositis) in Arabs—a study of 175 patients and review of the literature. Q J Med 60:837, 1986.

Berman SJ, Irving GS, Kundin WD, et al: Epidemiology of the acute fevers of unknown origin in South Vietnam: Effect of laboratory support upon clinical diagnosis. Am J Trop Med Hyg 22:796, 1973.

Centers for Disease Control: *Plasmodium vivax* malaria—San Diego County, California, 1986. MMWR 35:679, 1986.

Cook GC: Periodic disease, recurrent polyserositis, familial Mediterranean fever, or simply 'FMF.' Q J Med 60:819, 1986.

Deller JJ, Russell PK: An analysis of fevers of unknown origin in American soldiers in Vietnam. Ann Intern Med 66:1129, 1967.

MacLean JD, Lalonde RG: Fever from the tropics. Medicine NA 8:734, 1984.

Rees GH: Fevers of hot climates. Br J Hosp Med 17:38, 1977.

Schwabe AD, Peters RS: Familial Mediterranean fever in Armenians. Analysis of 100 cases. Medicine 53:453, 1974.

Wise M, Walter A: Fever in the returning traveller. Diagnosis, May, 1986, pp. 30–41.

Wolfe MS: Disease of travelers. Clin Symp 36:1, 1984.

World Health Organization: Dengue Hemorrhagic Fever: Diagnosis, Treatment, and Control. Geneva, World Health Organization, 1986.

117. DIARRHEA IN THE RETURNING TRAVELER

Richard L. Guerrant and Jay S. Keystone

INTRODUCTION AND EPIDEMIOLOGY. Diarrhea is probably the commonest illness found in the 300 million international travelers each year. Although it is not the most serious threat to the traveler, diarrhea causes some of the greatest preoccupation and requests for medications and doubtless influences where the $100 billion of international tourism dollars are spent each year.

Traveler's diarrhea is but the tip of the iceberg of endemic diarrheal illnesses in tropical developing areas. Indeed, the major pathogens that plague immunologically virgin travelers are those that dehydrate, malnourish, and kill more than 4 million children each year in Asia, Africa, and Latin America. The attack rate of traveler's diarrhea is determined by where the traveler is from, where he or she is going, and probably when he or she is there. By far, the greatest rates occur in the 16 million people (8 million from the United States) who travel from industrialized countries to developing

**TABLE 117–1. Causes of Traveler's Diarrhea
(Median [Range] from 26 Studies)**

	Latin America (15 Studies)	Africa (3 Studies)	Asia (8 Studies)
Duration of stay (days)	21 (2–42)	28 (28–35)	(28–42)
Attack rate (%)	52 (21–100)	54 (36–62)	(39–57)
Percentage with			
ETEC	46 (28–72)	36 (31–75)	(20–34)
Shigella	0 (0–30)	0 (0–15)	(4–7)
Salmonella	0 (0–16)	0 (0–0)	(11–15)
C. jejuni	—	—	(2–15)
V. parahemolyticus	—	—	(1–13)
Rotavirus	23 (0–36)	0 (0–0)	—

countries. Although reported attack rates vary widely, travelers from a temperate, industrialized region to a tropical, developing area for 2 weeks or more face a 20 to 50% risk of acquiring traveler's diarrhea. Rates appear to be highest in young adults and decrease with age after 25 years old. Indeed, traveler's diarrhea was documented to be the most common health problem encountered by Swiss travelers to developing countries.

ETIOLOGY AND PATHOGENESIS. The bacterial etiology of most cases of traveler's diarrhea was first suggested in the early 1960s by the effective reduction in attack rates by the prophylactic use of a wide range of antimicrobial agents, e.g., the sulfonamides. Since 1970, numerous studies have shown a consistent predominance of enterotoxigenic *Escherichia coli* (ETEC) as the leading cause of traveler's diarrhea throughout Latin America, Africa and Asia (Table 117–1). Given the relative insensitivity of nonselective methods for identifying ETEC, the 28 to 72% recovery rates doubtless show that ETEC constitutes the major cause of traveler's diarrhea. ETEC may produce the heat stable toxin (ST), the heat-labile toxin (LT), or both ST and LT (Chapter 41.1). After colonization via one of several specific colonization traits, ETEC causes net water and electrolyte secretion, primarily in the upper small bowel, by activating adenylate cyclase (by LT acting much like cholera toxin) or by activating guanylate cyclase (by ST) to produce the characteristic, noninflammatory watery diarrhea.

Other causes include *Salmonella* (Chapter 39), *Shigella* (Chapter 37), and *Campylobacter jejuni* (Chapter 41.2) (that characteristically cause inflammatory enteritis or dysentery) and *Vibrio* (usually *V. parahemolyticus* or other non-O1 cholera vibrios (Chapters 40.2 and 40.3), especially in Asia with the consumption of inadequately cooked seafood). The parasites *Giardia lamblia* (Chapter 69), *Cryptosporidium* (Chapter 70), *Strongyloides stercoralis* (Chapter 84.2), and *Entamoeba histolytica* (Chapter 68) may cause prolonged illnesses characterized by weight loss (with *Giardia* or *Cryptosporidium*), vague abdominal symptoms, perianal itching, occasional wheezing and eosinophilia (with *Strongyloides*), or rarely, invasive amebic colitis. Although Norwalk-like viruses and rotaviruses (Chapter 18.2) are often acquired in travel, their roles in causing traveler's diarrhea remain unclear.

CLINICAL MANIFESTATIONS. The onset of diarrhea in travelers is usually between 5 and 15 days after arrival, with illnesses usually characterized by malaise, anorexia, nausea, occasional vomiting, and watery diarrhea that may be explosive and profuse. Fever, if present, is usually low grade. Reflecting the predominant small bowel pathogens noted above, the vast majority of traveler's diarrhea is noninflammatory, without blood or pus in the stools. Illnesses are usually self-limited, lasting 2 to 5 days, but some may extend beyond 10 to 14 days. Patients with prolonged diarrhea after travel to developing areas present special problems.

It is important to consider and recognize potentially serious systemic infections such as malaria and typhoid fever that may be acquired in tropical areas and present with diarrhea. These life-threatening infections usually present with higher fevers and must be evaluated by blood smears and cultures and treated promptly when suspected. Other considerations may include plague, typhus, melioidosis, and arboviral hemorrhagic fevers.

DIAGNOSIS. The appropriate diagnostic approach to acute traveler's diarrhea requires careful history for a typical noninflammatory, watery diarrheal illness (Table 117–2). Although new gene probes for enterotoxins are becoming increasingly available, most immunologic, tissue culture, and animal assays for ETEC remain research tools and are not necessary in sporadic cases of traveler's diarrhea. Clues to other, inflammatory processes (Table 117–2) that may warrant bacterial culture or parasite examinations include high fever, tenesmus, bloody dysentery, and prolonged illnesses with weight loss. If there is any suspicion of an inflammatory, bloody, or prolonged diarrheal illness, a prompt microscopic examination of fresh samples for fecal leukocytes (with methylene blue or Gram's stain) and for parasites should be done. Although one may see motile trophozoites of *Giardia lamblia* or *Entamoeba histolytica,* special stains for amebae (e.g., trichrome stain, with micrometer measurements of parasite size), *Cryptosporidium* and *Isospora belli* (with modified acid-fast stain), or *Strongyloides* (with Baermann's funnel gauze concentration) may be necessary (Chapter 122). A history of recent antibiotic use, especially if inflammatory diarrhea follows, should prompt a consideration of colitis caused by *C. difficile* cytotoxin (Chapter 55.4). The increasing frequency of acquired immunodeficiency syndrome (AIDS) should also broaden the considerations

TABLE 117–2. Infectious Causes of Acute and Prolonged Diarrhea in Travelers

Acute Diarrhea	Prolonged Diarrhea (>10–14 days)
Noninflammatory	
Enterotoxigenic *E. coli* (ETEC)	*Giardia lamblia*
Vibrio (*V. parahemolyticus,*	*Cryptosporidium*
non–O1 *V. cholerae*)	*Strongyloides stercordis*
Norwalk-like viruses, rotaviruses	Prolonged bacterial colonization (? tropical sprue)
Inflammatory (with fecal leukocytes in mucus)	
Shigella	*Entamoeba histolytica***
Salmonella	Prolonged or postinfectious
Campylobacter jejuni	enteritis

**Fecal leukocytes may be pyknotic or destroyed by the parasite in invasive amebic colitis.

of diarrhea causes to include additional viruses (e.g., cytomegalovirus or herpesvirus) as well as parasites (especially *Cryptosporidium* and *I. belli*), bacteria (e.g., *Salmonella, Campylobacter, Mycobacteria,* and others) and even fungi (e.g., *Candida*) agents.

TREATMENT

Oral Rehydration. The mainstay of therapy for traveler's diarrhea is the adequate fluid and electrolyte replacement that can usually be accomplished with oral glucose (or sugar)–containing electrolyte rehydration solutions (General Principles, III D).

Antibiotic Therapy. Although traveler's diarrhea is rarely life-threatening and is usually limited to within 3 to 5 days with oral rehydration, several studies have documented the effect of trimethoprim (200 mg twice daily for 3 to 5 days), trimethoprim-sulfamethoxazole (1 double strength tablet twice daily for 3 to 5 days), ciprofloxacin (500 mg twice daily for 3 to 5 days), and other agents in reducing the duration of illness to 1 to 1½ days. Ciprofloxacin may also be effective in treating the common causes of inflammatory diarrhea, including *Shigella, Campylobacter,* and *Salmonella* infections (Table 117–3). Increasing antibiotic resistance to commonly used antimicrobial agents (such as tetracyclines or trimethoprim-sulfa) continues to emerge and limit effective options for antimicrobial therapy.

Antimotility Agents. Some use bismuth subsalicylate, 30 ml or 2 tablets every ½ to 1 hour if needed to maximum of 8 doses/24 hours, or an antimotility agent such as loperamide (Imodium), 2 or 4 mg, then 2 mg after each unformed stool up to 8 capsules/day, and diphenoxylate with atropine (Lomotil), 1 tablet every 4 to 6 hours, to provide relief of abdominal cramps and frequent bowel movements. However prolonged (longer than 3 days) or inflammatory symptoms (such as fever with blood or pus in the stools) may be worsened by antimotility agents, which should be avoided in those settings.

PREVENTION.
The prevention of traveler's diarrhea includes the avoidance of salads, raw vegetables, and untreated or unboiled water or ice, which can reduce risk, even in highly endemic areas. Even bottled, noncarbonated water or beverages may not be safe, as outbreaks of cholera and typhoid fever have been traced to bottled drinks. The intense desire to avoid bothersome traveler's diarrhea has led to inappropriate use of potentially toxic drugs such as iodochlorhydroxyquine (Entero-Vioform, clioquinol), which is ineffective and may cause subacute myelo-optic atrophy. Likewise, an-

timotility agents, cautiously used by some in treating noninflammatory, nonbloody diarrhea, have no role in prophylaxis. Bismuth subsalicylate has been shown to inhibit enterotoxin activity in experimental animals, may have some antimicrobial activity, and has been used for prophylaxis and early treatment. However, salicylate toxicity with bismuth subsalicylate should be carefully avoided, especially in children and in patients already receiving salicylate therapy. Although a number of antimicrobial agents have been shown to be effective, the potential side effects (such as photosensitivity with doxycycline), increasing antibiotic resistance, and ease of treating traveler's diarrhea are the reasons that most experts do not recommend or use prophylactic antibiotics themselves, but prefer cautious eating and drinking habits and early treatment for traveler's diarrhea.

APPROACH TO PATIENTS WITH CHRONIC DIARRHEA AFTER FOREIGN TRAVEL.
Some travelers return with the troubling and perplexing problem of protracted and disabling diarrhea. Such illnesses may persist for weeks, months, or even years after return from foreign travel. Although this syndrome is well recognized, its frequency, etiology, and pathogenesis are unclear.

Persistent Infection. Chronic traveler's diarrhea may result from a variety of different conditions. The first of these is a persistent infection with one of the pathogens responsible for acute illnesses. *Salmonella, Shigella, Campylobacter,* and *Yersinia* may produce chronic diarrhea in some individuals. Recently, enteroadherent strains of *E. coli* have been implicated as a cause for chronic diarrhea in children from developing countries. Strongyloidiasis, giardiasis, and amebiasis classically have extended courses when untreated.

Intestinal Mucosal Damage. Microbial pathogens may cause widespread damage to the intestinal mucosa, which may require extended periods of time for complete repair. The resulting temporary malabsorption is most often associated with intestinal disaccharidase deficiency, the most common being hypolactase deficiency. This enzyme deficiency may be temporary, resolving after several weeks, or may become permanent. The latter may be the result of a patient's genetic predisposition to lactase deficiency, which was unmasked by an infectious agent. Typically, the condition presents with bloating, excessive flatulence, lower abdominal cramps, and watery diarrhea, which follows the ingestion of milk or dairy products.

In addition to causing mucosal damage, intestinal pathogens may be responsible for producing a constellation of symptoms identical to an irritable bowel syndrome. Patients usually have prolonged symptoms of intermittent diarrhea, crampy abdominal pain, excessive flatulence, and occasionally nausea. Typically, weight loss and nocturnal diarrhea are absent. The problem may develop in individuals who prior to travel give no history of gastrointestinal problems even under stress. Although the mechanism for this postinfectious syndrome is as yet undefined, alteration in gut motility is a possible explanation.

In practice, the least common causes for chronic traveler's diarrhea are tropical sprue (Chapter 3) and

TABLE 117–3. Antimicrobial Treatment of Bacterial Diarrheas

	Duration of Diarrhea (days)		
	Placebo	Trimethoprim-Sulfamethoxazole	Ciprofloxacin
Shigella	3.4	0.7	1.2
ETEC	3.5	1.1	1.4
No agent (turista)	3.2	0.5	1.1
Salmonella	3.4		1.9
Campylobacter	2.2		1.1

Data from DuPont and colleagues (1987) and Pichler and associates (1987).

the unmasking of an underlying, previously asymptomatic gastrointestinal disorder such as celiac sprue or inflammatory bowel disease. Although relatively rare, these conditions must be considered, particularly when weight loss accompanies protracted diarrhea.

Clinical Evaluation. The work-up for a patient with chronic traveler's diarrhea while traveling parallels that for the acute illness. The history should include particular attention to several points: (1) Were antibiotics taken at any time in the recent past? (2) Has weight loss been associated with the chronic symptoms? (3) Does the patient have an intolerance to lactose-containing foods? (4) Is there a history to suggest malabsorption (e.g., frequent, bulky, foul-smelling stools)? (5) Was there a history prior to travel of gastrointestinal disease or surgery on the gastrointestinal tract?

To exclude the presence of a persistent infection, several stool cultures and parasite examinations should be obtained, with particular attention to *Giardia, Cryptosporidium, Isospora belli,* and *Strongyloides* (with trichrome and acid-fast stains and Baermann's funnel gauze concentration). If the patient has been exposed to antibiotics, stool should be studied for *C. difficile* cytotoxin or cultured for cytotoxigenic *C. difficile.*

The diagnosis of postinfectious lactose intolerance requires only an accurate history or an assessment of symptom response to a lactose-free diet. A lactose tolerance test is usually unnecessary. When a more complete malabsorption picture is present, a work-up is required to exclude tropical sprue, giardiasis, and underlying celiac sprue. Although tests for fat and carbohydrate malabsorption may be helpful as screening tests, small bowel aspiration (for *Giardia* and quantitative bacterial culture) and mucosal biopsy are usually required to exclude these entities.

When blood and pus persist in the stools of individuals with chronic diarrhea, sigmoidoscopy and mucosal biopsies should be considered to diagnose amebic colitis, pseudomembranous colitis, or inflammatory bowel disease. Amoebic antibody determination may be helpful in this situation. If studies for infectious processes are nonrevealing, barium enema may define the extent of inflammatory bowel disease.

Management. In the experience of many clinicians, a diagnostic work-up is unrevealing in many patients with chronic diarrhea after travel, and the long-term outcome in such patients is difficult to predict. Some individuals experience spontaneous remission after many weeks or months, while others continue to be chronically ill. In cases where no specific cause is found, treatment is often empirical. Some physicians prefer a trial of antibiotics or metronidazole therapy in case a bacterial or parasitic pathogen has been missed. Other practitioners try dietary alteration, consisting initially of a lactose-free period, followed, if there is no response, by a high-fiber diet to which a synthetic fiber substitute is added (e.g., 2 tbs of psyllium hydrophilic mucilloid [Metamucil] per day).

Until more studies are carried out to examine the long-term consequences of traveler's diarrhea, advice to the clinician who is faced with this problem will consist largely of personal opinion based on experience rather than firmly established fact.

BIBLIOGRAPHY

Black PE: Pathogens that cause traveler's diarrhea in Latin America and Africa. Rev Infect Dis 8(Suppl 2):S131, 1986.

Blake PA, Rosenberg ML, Florencia J, et al: Cholera in Portugal, 1974. II. Transmission by bottled mineral water. Am J Epidemiol 105:344, 1977.

Blaser MJ: Environmental interventions in the prevention of traveler's diarrhea. Rev Infect Dis 8(Suppl 2):S142, 1986.

Consensus Development Conference Statement on Traveler's Diarrhea. JAMA 253:2700, 1985 or Rev Infect Dis 8(Suppl 2):S227, 1986.

DuPont HL, Ericsson CD, Robinson A, Johnson PC: Current problems in antimicrobial therapy for bacterial enteric infection. Am J Med 82:324, 1987.

DuPont HL, Reves RR, Galindo E, et al: Treatment of traveler's diarrhea with trimethoprim/sulfamethoxazole and with trimethoprim alone. N Engl J Med 307:841, 1982.

Ericsson CD, DuPont HL, Sullivan P, et al: Bicozamycin, a poorly absorbable antibiotic effectively treats traveler's diarrhea. Ann Intern Med 98:20, 1983.

Ericsson CD, Johnson PC, DuPont HL, et al: Ciprofloxacin compared with trimethoprim-sulfamethoxazole as initial treatment for acute traveler's diarrhea. Ann Intern Med 106:216, 1987.

Giannella RA: Chronic diarrhea in travelers: Diagnostic and therapeutic considerations. Rev Infect Dis 8(Suppl 2):S223, 1986.

Gonzales-Cortez A, Gangarosa EJ, Parrilla C, et al: Bottled beverages and typhoid fever: The Mexican epidemic of 1972–3. Am J Public Health 72:844, 1982.

Gorbach SL, Hoskins DW: Traveler's diarrhea. Disease-a-Month 27:1, 1980.

Guerrant RL, Rouse JD, Hughes JM: Turista among members of the Yale Glee Club in Latin America. Am J Trop Med Hyg 29:895, 1980.

Harris JR: Are bottled beverages safe for travelers? Am J Public Health 72:787, 1982.

Kean BH: The diarrhea of travelers to Mexico. Summary of five-year study. Ann Intern Med 59:605, 1963.

Klipstein FA: Tropical sprue in travelers and expatriates living abroad. Gastroenterology 80:590, 1981.

Lowenstein MS, Balows A, Gangarosa EJ: Turista at an international congress in Mexico. Lancet 1:529, 1973.

Merson MH, Morris GK, Sack DA, et al: Traveler's diarrhea in Mexico, a prospective study of physicians and family members attending a congress. N Engl J Med 294:1299, 1976.

Pichler HET, Diridl G, Stickler K, Wolf D: Clinical efficacy of ciprofloxacin compared with placebo in bacterial diarrhea. Am J Med 82:329, 1987.

Rosenberg MI, Koplan JP, Wachsmuth IK, et al: Epidemic diarrhea at Crater Lake from enterotoxigenic *Escherichia coli*. A large, waterborne outbreak. Ann Intern Med 86:714, 1977.

Sack DA, Kaminsky DC, Sack RB, et al: Enterotoxigenic *Escherichia coli* diarrhea of travelers. A prospective study of American Peace Corps volunteers. Johns Hopkins Med J 141:63, 1977.

Steffen R: Epidemiologic studies of traveler's diarrhea, severe gastrointestinal infections, and cholera. Rev Infect Dis 8(Suppl 2):S122, 1986.

Steffen R, Rickenbach M, Wilhelm V, et al: Health problems after travel to developing countries. J Infect Dis 156:84, 1987.

Taylor DN, Echeverria P: Etiology and epidemiology of traveler's diarrhea in Asia. Rev Infect Dis 8(Suppl 2):S136, 1986.

Tjoa W, DuPont HL, Sullivan P, et al: Location of food consumption and traveler's diarrhea. Am J Epidemiol 106:61, 1977.

118. DERMATITIS IN TRAVELERS

Evan R. Farmer

With the increasing use of foreign travel for both business and pleasure, there will be an increase in the number of patients returning home with cutaneous diseases that have appeared while traveling or shortly after returning home. These patients will present for examination with the fear of having contracted an "exotic disease" that is going to cause disfigurement or death and for which there is no satisfactory therapy. This fear, although usually exaggerated, is based on the patients' experiences in tropical countries, particularly the frequent occurrence of deformed beggars and the obvious physical results of malnutrition and poverty on the indigenous population. This fear must be treated in addition to providing therapy for the cutaneous disorder and can best be handled by an accurate diagnosis.

After the details of a patient's trip have been ascertained, it may be classified as one of the following:
1. Short-term visit abroad (less than 1 month).
2. Long-term visit abroad (greater than 1 month) or multiple visits abroad.
3. Immigration to this country.

These categories may be further subdivided into whether the patient has spent most of his time in a rural or urban environment. This information, coupled with the countries visited, provides a rough probability of the patient having a specific skin disease. For example, the likelihood of having contracted leprosy during a 2-week visit to a major city is essentially zero, but the probability would be higher in a missionary who has worked in the countryside for 4 years. To reiterate a significant point, the fear of this disease may be the same in both patients.

The most common cutaneous diseases that are encountered in the traveler are (1) insect bites and their sequelae, especially secondary bacterial infection; (2) superficial fungal infections, especially tinea pedis, tinea cruris, and tinea corporis; (3) miliaria rubra (prickly heat); and (4) exacerbation of chronic dermatoses that were present prior to traveling but were aggravated by the change in climate. Other disorders are discussed in the chapter on dermatologic diseases (Chapter 7) and under specific diseases throughout the text.

INSECT BITES. Insect bites, by far, constitute the most frequent complaint of patients returning from the tropics to a temperate environment (Chapter 105.2). The body sites involved, distribution, number of lesions, and morphology of the lesions vary widely from patient to patient. The morphology of the lesion in large part is the result of the patient's inflammatory response directed against the bite and the foreign material injected by the insect.

The patient usually notes the onset of skin lesions during the trip or shortly after returning home. The lesions are usually described as pruritic, although in rare cases no pruritus may be experienced. The pruritus is usually more pronounced at night, but this is not specific for insect bites. At times, only one individual traveling in a group may develop lesions and symptoms of insect bites, but this does not negate the diagnosis. Body odor,

personal habits, unremembered activities, and immune response to the insect bite may account for the difference.

On physical examination, the patient may have only excoriations without primary lesions, or the lesions may present as small erythematous, edematous papules; occasionally, vesicles and bullae may form (Fig. 118–1). These lesions, in turn, may be excoriated, and a careful search is required to identify a primary lesion. Some bites, such as that of a spider, may cause tissue necrosis, leaving areas of ulceration.

Secondary bacterial infection of insect bites is a common complication and is characterized clinically by the presence of yellow to yellow-brown crusts and erythema extending beyond the border of the primary bite lesion. The infection may spread to involve areas of the skin not affected by the arthropod bites, and associated lymphadenopathy may develop. Fever rarely occurs unless the infection extends deep into the skin as a cellulitis. The individual lesions may be painful, but itching is usually the predominant symptom with the secondary infection. The patient characteristically describes generalized itching and an increase in the intensity of the itching over that noted when the insect bites first appeared. A Gram stain will usually demonstrate gram-positive cocci, and cultures usually grow *Staphylococcus aureus* or a mixture of *Staphylococcus* and *Streptococcus* species.

The diagnosis of insect bites is based on the history of an acute disorder, the presence of pruritus, and the morphology of the lesions. Isolation of the insect from the patient confirms the diagnosis, but this usually is not achieved except in the cases of scabies, lice, or ticks. A skin biopsy of a lesion may show the characteristic pattern of inflammatory response, but the pattern is not specific for a given insect. In the differential diagnosis, vasculitis, pityriasis lichenoides et varioliformis acuta, dermatitis herpetiformis, lichen planus, and irritant contact dermatitis should be considered. These entities can be excluded by a skin biopsy.

Treatment is usually best accomplished by simply

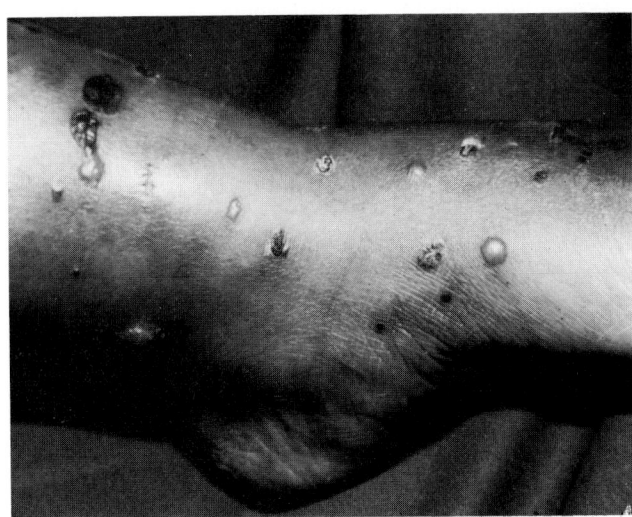

FIGURE 118–1. Insect bites. Discrete papules and vesicles with crust formation are present on the leg and dorsum of the foot.

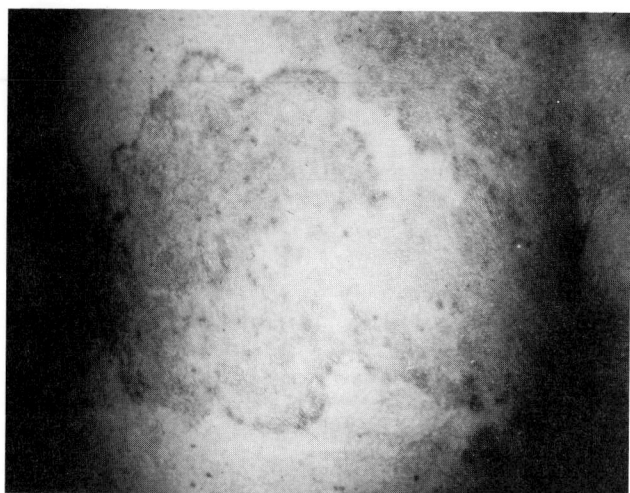

FIGURE 118–2. Tinea corporis. Annular and polycyclic erythematous lesions typical of dermatophyte infection are present on the buttocks.

removing the patient from the environment and by reassurance. Symptomatic relief may be provided by shake lotions such as calamine lotion or lotions containing menthol or phenol. Cool showers or baths will provide quick but short-term relief. Topical or intralesional corticosteroids may be helpful in more severe cases. Systemic antihistamines, especially at bedtime, may provide some relief from the itching. If secondary bacterial infection is present, a systemic antibiotic such as penicillin, dicloxacillin, or erythromycin is indicated. If the insect is still suspected to be on the patient, as in cases of scabies, lice, or fleas, an insecticide, e.g., 1% hexachlorobenzene, 10% crotamiton, 12% benzyl benzoate, or 6% sulfur ointment, should be used.

SUPERFICIAL CUTANEOUS FUNGAL INFECTIONS. By definition, these fungal infections are restricted to the outer layers of the epidermis, including the nails, hair shafts, and hair follicles (Chapter 64). These infections are widely distributed throughout the world, with involvement of both sexes and all age groups. In general, the infections are caused by three groups of fungi—dermatophytes, *Candida* species, and *Pityrosporum* species. Most patients are chronically infected with these organisms, and the infections clinically wax and wane in response to changes in immune status of the host or environmental conditions. Traveling from the temperate zone to the heat and humidity of the tropics will aggravate latent infections, and they will become clinically manifest during the trip or shortly after return home. Many patients will assume, however, that the infection was acquired in the tropics. In all cases of superficial cutaneous fungal infections, the diagnosis may be established by demonstration of the fungus by KOH examination of scrapings from the infected area. In cases of dermatophyte infection or infection with *Candida* species, the diagnosis may also be confirmed by culture of the organism on appropriate media. *Pityrosporum* is difficult to grow in the laboratory, and in general, culture of the organism is not successful.

Dermatophyte Infections. Dermatophyte infections of the skin, hair, and nails are generally categorized ac-

cording to body site involved rather than the specific species of fungus that is causing the eruption (Chapter 64.1). For example, infection of scalp hair is designated tinea capitis (Fig. 64–4), infection of the nails is labeled tinea unguium, and that of the body surface is called tinea corporis (Fig. 64–3). Many of these infections also possess common and local names, including ringworm, athlete's foot, and jock itch (Fig. 64–2). The hallmark of all these infections is erythema with associated scaling. Annular, polycyclic, and diffuse lesions may all be present (Figs. 64–1 and 118–2). In general, a good rule to follow is that if scaling is present, a KOH examination should be performed. Itching, burning, pain, or other symptoms may or may not be present. Infection of the hair follicles usually results in alopecia, whereas infection of the nail results in nail dystrophy to include either thickening of the nail plate, thickening of the subungual region, or extreme friability.

Localized disease of the skin may be treated successfully with a variety of topical agents, including Whitfield's ointment, tolnaftate (Tinactin), miconazole, or clotrimazole. These agents may be applied twice daily. Decreasing moisture and heat to the infected area such as by wearing cool porous clothing or sandals and the use of drying powders may also be helpful. For widespread infection, infections of the hair, and infections of the nail, systemic antifungal agents are required for the best results. Griseofulvin and ketoconazole are both effective but usually require several months of daily therapy.

There is a subset of patients who seem to have an immune defect permitting the establishment of widespread, chronic dermatophyte infections. Many of these patients have an atopic background that includes a personal or family history of asthma, hay fever, or atopic dermatitis. Control of the infection may be achieved in these patients, but complete cures are rather difficult, if not impossible.

***Candida* Infections.** Most infections with *Candida* species involve the oral mucosa, genitalia, or perianal region. These infections are generally caused by *Candida albicans,* but other species may be involved. Most cases

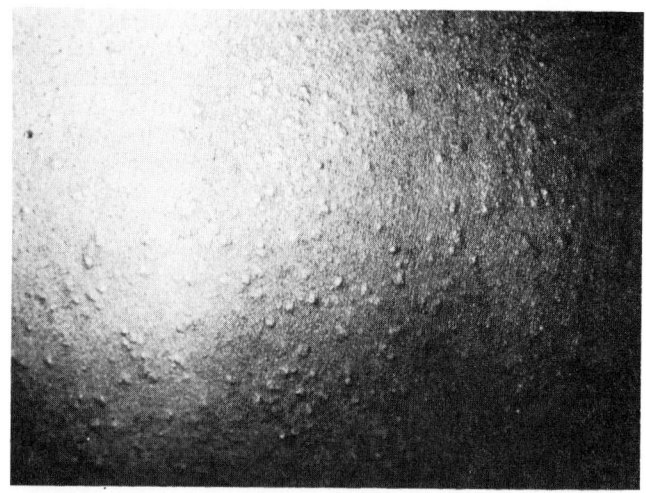

FIGURE 118–3. Miliaria rubra. Discrete erythematous papules are diffusely distributed over the back of this patient.

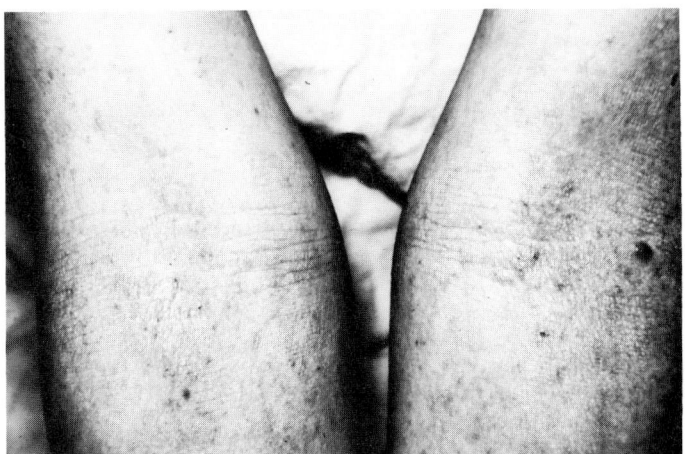

FIGURE 118–4. Atopic dermatitis (eczema). The antecubital fossae show lichenification, erythema, and excoriations.

occur in patients with diabetes mellitus or in those using systemic antibiotics, allowing the overgrowth of *Candida* in the gastrointestinal tract, bladder, or vagina (Chapter 64.3). The clinical features of *Candida* infection include beefy-red erythema in association with a whitish membrane on the mucosal surfaces (Fig. 64–6) and small pustules on the skin.

Treatment is best accomplished by using both systemic and local therapy. At present, oral nystatin is the drug of choice, but ketoconazole may also play a role in the future. Topical clotrimazole may be used twice daily on the affected areas.

Pityrosporum **Species Infections.** The most common infection caused by *Pityrosporum* species is tinea versicolor, which is an infection of the skin generally involving the trunk and proximal aspects of the extremities (called *Malassezia furfur* in Chapter 64.4). Occasionally, infection of the hair follicles on the trunk occurs. The infection is characterized by hypopigmented, slightly scaling, tan macules without erythema (Fig. 64–8). It is most frequently perceived by the patient after exposure to sunlight, because the involved areas fail to tan, in contrast to uninfected skin. The diagnosis is established by the demonstration of short hyphae and numerous spores on KOH examination of scales (Fig. 64–7). The extent of the infection may be demonstrated by examination of the patient in a darkened room under Wood's light, which will highlight the hypopigmented areas.

If the disease is localized, topical therapy with 2.5% selenium sulfide or 1% clotrimazole may be used. For topical treatment failures, extensive disease, or follicular infection, a 5- to 7-day course of systemic ketoconazole is usually effective.

MILIARIA RUBRA. Miliaria rubra, or prickly heat, is a common disorder in tropical environments and particularly affects people traveling to these areas from temperate zones. It is characterized by an erythematous, papular to vesicular eruption that is usually confined to the covered areas of the body (Fig. 118–3). The lesions are pruritic or stinging and are usually exacerbated at times of sweating. On clinical examination, the lesions are quite discrete, sparing the hair follicles, and do not tend to become confluent unless secondarily infected.

Treatment is accomplished by removal of excessive

clothing, by the use of cool showers or tap water compresses, and by application of shake lotions that include menthol or phenol. Secondary bacterial infection should be treated with systemic antibiotics.

EXACERBATION OF CHRONIC DERMATOSES. Chronic dermatoses, excluding superficial fungal infections, are quite common and may be exacerbated by traveling in the tropics. For example, acne vulgaris, especially in teenage males, may be transformed into what is termed tropical acne, with the development of large inflammatory nodules with draining sinuses on the trunk and buttocks. Secondary infection with *Staphylococcus aureus* is quite common, and systemic antibiotics are required for control of the disorder. Many of the patients must be removed from the tropics to stop or control the process. Other dermatoses such as atopic dermatitis (eczema) (Fig. 118–4), psoriasis, and lichen planus may all be adversely affected by traveling. If the patient had minimal or unrecognized disease prior to traveling, this exacerbation may be interpreted as the development of new disease rather than an exacerbation of a previously existing condition. It is important that the diagnosis of the disease and the reason for its exacerbation be correctly established, not only to provide the best therapy but for psychologic support as well.

BIBLIOGRAPHY

Goodman PH, Kurtz KJ, Carmichael J: Medical recommendations for wilderness travel. 2. Field management of illness and injury. Postgrad Med 78:253, 1985.

Jopling WH: Tropical dermatoses likely to be encountered in Britain. Br J Hosp Med 17:14, 1977.

Marshall J: Tropical dermatoses. Practitioner 211:620, 1973.

Pearson RD, Hewlett EL, Guerrant RL: Tropical diseases in North America. Dis Mon 30:1, 1984.

Tapia A: Perspectives in dermatology: Central America. 1974–1979. Int J Dermatol 18:623, 1979.

Walker E, Williams G: Infections on return from abroad—II. Br Med J 286:1197, 1983.

Wolfe MS: Diseases of travelers. Clin Symp 36:2, 1984.

119. EOSINOPHILIA IN TRAVELERS AND IMMIGRANTS

Jay S. Keystone
and J. Philpott

Eosinophilia in returning travelers and newly arrived immigrants from developing countries is one of the more common problems encountered by clinicians who practice travel medicine. Although eosinophilia in itself is rarely harmful, it is often a clue to an underlying parasitic infection that may cause significant morbidity or even death. The challenge for the clinician is to determine, if possible, the cause of the eosinophilia, thereby ensuring that a potentially harmful illness does not go untreated. The approach to the diagnosis of eosinophilia in returning travelers and immigrants should be a stepwise process that hinges on the answers to several questions: (1) Is the absolute eosinophil count elevated? (2) Is the eosinophilia associated with the patient's travels or present symptoms? (3) If travel related, which parasitic infections are likely? (4) What are the most appropriate diagnostic steps? (5) What should one do if the cause of the eosinophilia cannot be determined?

IS THE ABSOLUTE EOSINOPHIL COUNT ELEVATED?

The clinician must first determine whether there is a significant elevation of the eosinophil count. Eosinophils normally constitute 3 to 6% of the granulocytes in peripheral blood. Contrary to what is observed in many scientific papers, the absolute eosinophil count should be considered in determining the presence or absence of eosinophilia. Using the relative eosinophil count (percentage of eosinophils) alone is fraught with error. For example, an individual with 10% eosinophils does not have eosinophilia if the total white blood cell count is below 4000/mm³. Normally, there are up to 350 eosinophils/mm³ in the peripheral blood. As a general rule, the absolute count should be greater than 450/mm³ to be considered a significant elevation.

With the introduction of electronic white blood cell counters, which have a high degree of accuracy, the absolute eosinophil count is most readily and cost effectively determined by multiplying the percentage of eosinophils detected in the differential count by the total white blood cell count. The degree of eosinophilia may be arbitrarily classified as being low (less than 1000 eosinophils/mm³), moderate (1000 to 3000 eosinophils/mm³), or high (greater than 3000 eosinophils/mm³).

Eosinophil counts exhibit a diurnal variation, with the highest levels occurring at midnight and the lowest at mid-day. Levels are known to be affected by glucocorticoids, epinephrine, and estrogen. Studies have shown that individuals with parasite-induced eosinophilia may have counts that vary from day to day by as much as 100 to 200%.

IS THE EOSINOPHILIA RELATED TO THE PATIENT'S TRAVEL OR PRESENT SYMPTOMS?

After eosinophilia has been confirmed, the next problem is to determine if the eosinophilia is related to the patient's travel or present complaints. It may be helpful to review pretravel differential white blood cell counts, if they are available, to ascertain whether the patient's eosinophilia was present prior to the trip abroad. Does the patient have any pre-existing medical conditions (e.g., hay fever and asthma) that could account for the present eosinophilia? It is crucial to keep an open mind and consider the possibility that the patient's signs and symptoms may be unrelated to the eosinophilia. This is likely to occur in a national from a developing country where a significant proportion of the population is infected with intestinal helminths. Thus, an immigrant may have a light helminth infection causing eosinophilia that is unrelated to his or her complaints.

Parasitic causes of eosinophilia are emphasized, as these are the most important considerations in a traveler or immigrant arriving from the tropics. However, there are many other situations in which the eosinophil count may be elevated (Table 119–1). Eosinophilia associated with allergies (e.g., hay fever and asthma) is usually low. However, high eosinophilia may occur in those with drug allergy, patients with the pulmonary infiltrates with eosinophilia (PIE) syndrome, and aspirin-sensitive asthmatics.

IF TRAVEL RELATED, WHICH PARASITIC INFECTIONS ARE LIKELY TO CAUSE EOSINOPHILIA?

In a returning traveler or immigrant with eosinophilia, a parasitic cause is most frequent. A few general guidelines should help focus on the most likely possibilities.

Protozoan infections. Malaria, amebiasis or giardiasis, and most protozoan infections are not associated with eosinophilia. The 3 exceptions generally quoted in the literature include isosporosis, toxoplasmosis, and dientamebiasis (*Dientamoeba fragilis*). Unfortunately, those who have reported such findings have usually not ruled out other causes of eosinophilia.

Helminth Infections. On the other hand, helminth infections are the primary cause of parasite-related eosinophilia. It is important to remember that the degree of eosinophilia is a function of the extent of tissue invasion by the parasite. For example, tapeworms and adult roundworms, which do not invade the intestinal mucosa and remain in the bowel lumen, are associated with little or no eosinophilia. In contrast, migrating larval ascarids (*Toxocara canis*) or filaria may give rise to marked eosinophilia because these organisms have in their life cycle a significant degree of tissue invasion.

TABLE 119–1. Nonparasitic Causes of Eosinophilia

Allergy: asthma, seasonal rhinitis, atopic dermatitis, pulmonary aspergillosis, drug allergy, organic dust hypersensitivity, eosinophilia-myalgia syndrome (L-tryptophan consumption)
Skin disorders: pemphigus, pemphigoid, herpes gestationis
Pulmonary disorders: Löffler's syndrome, pulmonary infiltrates with eosinophilia
Gastrointestinal disorders: inflammatory bowel disease, eosinophilic gastroenteritis
Neoplastic disorders: lymphoma, carcinomas, acute lymphoblastic leukemia, immunoblastic lymphadenopathy
Rheumatic disorders: Churg-Strauss vasculitis, rheumatoid arthritis, Wegener's granulomatosis, polyarteritis nodosa
Immunodeficiency syndromes
Hereditary eosinophilia
Miscellaneous: hypereosinophil syndrome, angiolymphoid hyperplasia with eosinophilia, Kimura's disease

However, clinicians should keep in mind that some infections, such as ascariasis and clonorchiasis, may produce significant degrees of eosinophilia transiently during their initial larval migration phase, with subsequent resolution when adult worms are fully developed. Figure 119–1 provides a graphic outline of the magnitude of eosinophilia usually associated with various parasitic infections. This is meant only as a guideline to degree of eosinophilia because the range is wide and many exceptions occur. It is most important to know those infections that cause extremely high eosinophilia and those that are not usually associated with eosinophilia.

WHAT IS THE BEST APPROACH TO DETERMINE THE ETIOLOGY OF TRAVEL-ASSOCIATED EOSINOPHILIA?

History. The medical history should take into consideration both parasitic and nonparasitic causes of eosinophilia. Patients should be questioned in detail about their history of drug ingestion, atopy, and immune disorders, (e.g., rheumatoid arthritis and inflammatory bowel disease). A particular note of the countries visited, as well as the duration and extent of exposure to parasitic infections, should be made. Many parasitic infections (e.g., filariasis and schistosomiasis) have well-defined distributions, whereas others (e.g., hookworm, whipworm, and roundworm) have little geographic specificity. For the geographic history to have any relevance, a knowledge of the distribution of parasitic infections is required (Chapter 121).

In addition to places where the individual has traveled, the exposure history is often crucial. Individuals who travel to tropical areas, but remain in resorts or urban areas and stay in first-class accommodation, are not likely to acquire soil or arthropod-transmitted nematode infections. For example, if they have not walked in their bare feet in soil contaminated with human excrement, travelers are unlikely to acquire hookworm or *Strongyloides* infections. The possibility of schistosomiasis should be entertained only if there was exposure to fresh water in endemic areas. Parasitic infections, e.g., loiasis, Guinea worm, onchocerciasis, hydatid disease, and schistosomiasis can usually be excluded in the absence of a history of travel to rural areas. Dietary history may be helpful in making or excluding a diagnosis of trichinosis, toxocariasis, or tapeworm infections.

The duration of stay in the tropics can help to establish or rule out some parasitic infections. For example, short-term travelers (less than 3 months) rarely acquire filaria (bancroftian filiariasis, onchocerciasis), larval tapeworms (hydatid disease, cysticercosis), and most trematodes (paragonimiasis, clonorchiasis) with the exception of schistosomiasis. Prolonged stay or travel in the tropics should raise the index of suspicion for infections that are usually found in the indigenous population, having been acquired with extensive exposure.

Physical Examination. In asymptomatic individuals with eosinophilia, results of examination most often are normal. Some filariae (*Loa loa, Onchocerca volvulus, Mansonella streptocerca*) can cause subcutaneous swellings or dermatitis. Examination of the liver and spleen may be helpful in the diagnosis of schistosomiasis, hydatid disease, or toxocariasis (Table 119–2).

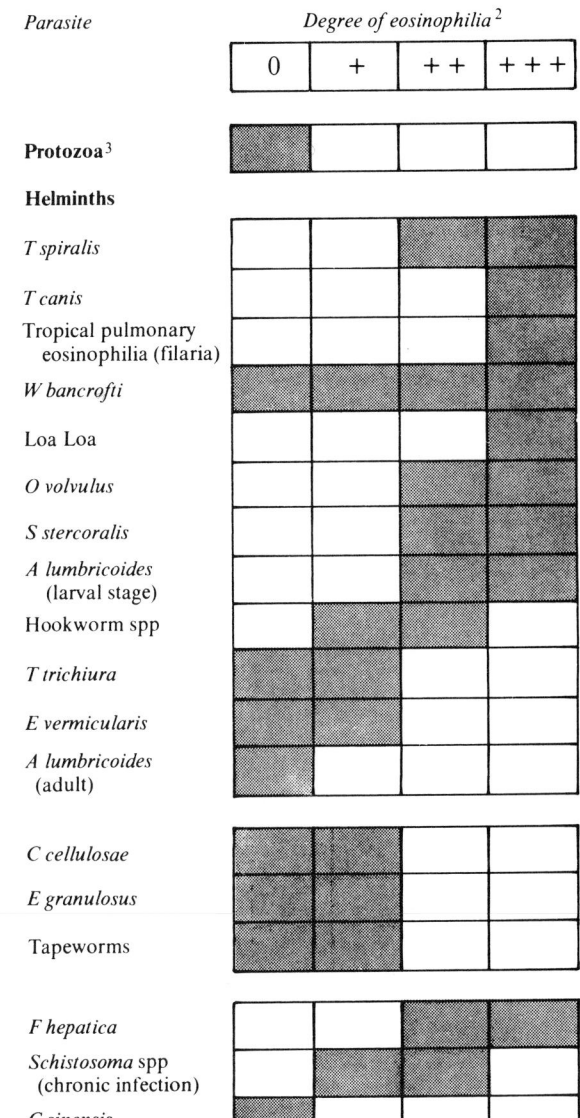

[1]Since eosinophilia in parasitic infections may be quite variable, the information given on the degree of eosinophilia is intended as a 'rule of thumb'
[2]+ = Mild (450–1,000 eosinophilis/mm³); + + = Moderate (1,000–3,000/mm³); + + + = Marked (>3,000/m³).
[3]Eosinophilia has been described very occasionally with *Isospora, Toxoplasma* and *D fragilis* infections.

FIGURE 119–1. Eosinophilia associated with selected parasitic infections.

Laboratory Investigations. Laboratory investigations should proceed in a stepwise manner. A recommended approach to the investigation of eosinophilia is summarized in Table 119–3 and detailed below.

Before initiating investigations, the incubation period of various helminth infections must be considered. Eosinophilia in travelers who have recently returned from the tropics might be due to the migrating larval stage of an intestinal nematode infection that could not be diagnosed for several months, until eggs are present in the stool. Similarly, eosinophilia might occur during the

TABLE 119–2. Parasite-Induced Eosinophilia by Tissue Involved

Location in Host	Helminth
Skin	Onchocerca volvulus
	Mansonella streptocerca
	Strongyloides stercoralis
	Ancylostoma brasiliense
Subcutaneous tissue	Loa loa
	Onchocerca volvulus
	Spirometra spp. (sparganum)
	Cysticercus cellulosae
	Gnathostoma spinigerum
	Dracunculus medinensis
Blood/lymphatics	Wuchereria bancrofti
	Brugia malayi
	Mansonella ozzardi
	Mansonella perstans
Gastrointestinal tract	Strongyloides stercoralis
	Ancylostoma duodenale
	Necator americanus
	Taenia solium
	Taenia saginata
	Trichuris trichiura
	Enterobius vermicularis
	Capillaria philippensis
	Fasciolopsis buski
	Schistosoma mansoni, Schistosoma japonicum, Schistosoma mekongi (venules of bowel)
Lung	Paragonimus westermani
	Larvae of
	Strongyloides stercoralis
	Ascaris lumbricoides
	Necator americanus
	Ancylostoma duodenale
	Toxocara canis
	Echinococcus granulosus, Echinococcus multilocularis
Liver	Echinococcus granulosus
	Echinococcus multilocularis
	Fasciola hepatica
	Schistosoma mansoni, Schistosoma japonicum, Schistosoma mekongi
Urinary tract	Schistosoma hematobium (venules of lower urinary tract)
Muscle	Trichinella spiralis
Central nervous system	Angiostrongylus cantonensis
	Cysticercus cellulosae
	Multiceps multiceps
	Schistosoma mansoni, Schistosoma japonicum
	Paragonimus westermani
	Echinococcus granulosus, Echinococcus multilocularis
	Trichinella spiralis

incubation period of a filarial infection that would not produce symptoms or microfilaria in skin or blood for at least 6 months after exposure. On the other hand, because *Strongyloides stercoralis* infection may last for the lifetime of the host, eosinophilia may be related to an infection that was acquired in the tropics many years before its discovery.

Initial investigations for patients with eosinophilia include the following:

1. A total white blood cell count, differential count, and hemoglobin and platelet count. The eosinophil count should be repeated if it is elevated initially to confirm whether the elevation is reproducible and significant.

2. Examination of 3 stool specimens for ova and parasites. Because most parasite eggs and larvae are excreted intermittently, at least 3 specimens collected 48 hours apart should be examined by direct smear and a concentration technique (e.g., formalin-ether, zinc flotation) (Chapter 122). Negative stool examinations do not exclude a parasitic cause of eosinophilia. Helminths invade a variety of tissues, including blood and subcutaneous tissue (e.g., filariasis), muscle (e.g., trichinosis), and liver (e.g., visceral larva migrans) (Table 119–2). As noted above, most helminth infections have a prepatent period of several weeks to months before eggs or larvae are detectable in body fluids or excreta.

3. Urinalysis and examination of 3 mid-day urine specimens for parasites and ova. The latter should be performed only on individuals with a history of freshwater exposure who have traveled to *Schistosoma hematobium* endemic areas (Middle East or Africa).

The following additional investigations for specific parasites might be included in the initial evaluation of a patient who has had significant exposure to these parasites in endemic areas (e.g., indigenous population, long-term residents, or adventurous travelers).

TABLE 119–3. Approach to Investigation of Eosinophilia in a Returning Traveler

History	Allergy
	Drugs and vitamins (L-tryptophan)
	Geographic and exposure
Physical examination (areas of concentration)	Skin, subcutaneous tissues
	Liver/spleen
Investigations	*Baseline:*
Step 1	Complete blood count and differential white blood cell count
	Stool examination for ova and parasites ($\times$ 3)
	Urinalysis
	Examination of mid-day urine for ova and parasites ($\times$ 3) (Africa, Middle East)
Step 2	*Assuming appropriate geographic and exposure history:*
	Strongyloides culture and serology
	Duodenal aspirate/Entero-Test (strongyloidiasis, hookworm)
	Serology (*Schistosoma*, filaria, etc.)
	Day/night bloods (filariasis)
Step 3	*If history and physical examination suggest a specific diagnosis:*
	Skin snips (onchocerciasis)
	Mazzotti test (onchocerciasis)
	Liver biopsy (schistosomiasis, fascioliasis)
	Chest x-ray (hydatid, tropical pulmonary eosinophilia, paragonimiasis)
	Soft tissue x-ray (cysticercosis)
	Sputum examination for ova and parasites (paragonimiasis)
	Abdominal ultrasound (hydatid)
	Cystoscopy with or without biopsy (schistosomiasis)
	Rectal snips (schistosomiasis)

1. *Strongyloides* culture: This procedure concentrates the living strongyloides larvae and is best accomplished by the Baermann technique (Chapter 122).

2. *Strongyloides* serology (enzyme-linked immunosorbent assay [ELISA]): This has moderate sensitivity (70%) and high specificity (80%) (Chapter 125):

3. *Schistosoma* serology (indirect fluorescent antibody test [IFA], indirect hemagglutination [IHA], ELISA): This test has a high degree of sensitivity but is not specific for human schistosomiasis (Chapter 125). It may be positive in those with swimmer's itch or cercarial dermatitis from exposure to bird schistosomes.

4. Filaria serology (IHA, IFA, ELISA): This test is usually not specific because filaria antibodies are elevated in a variety of different helminth infections (Chapter 125). However, high titers (1:1024 or greater) may be more predictive of infection, and more species-specific antigens are being used in some research laboratories.

5. Day and night bloods for filaria: Concentrated midday bloods should be examined for *Loa loa, M. perstans,* or *M. ozzardi* (Chapter 123). Blood should be taken at midnight for *Wuchereria bancrofti.* If a night blood specimen is difficult to obtain, a single 100-mg dose of diethylcarbamazine (DEC) may be administered and the blood examined for microfilaria 1 hour later. For bancroftian filariasis, this challenge test significantly increases the yield from daytime blood specimens.

A number of other diagnostic procedures that are parasite specific may be helpful if the clinical picture suggests a particular diagnosis. These will be dealt with in turn.

1. Duodenal aspirate, Entero-Test, and/or biopsy: Examination of the small bowel and its contents may be helpful in making a diagnosis of *Strongyloides stercoralis, Trichostrongylus,* hookworm, *Clonorchis sinensis,* or *Fasciola hepatica* infections (Chapter 123).

2. Rectal and bladder biopsy (snips): In the diagnosis of *Schistosoma mansoni* or *S. japonicum,* a rectal biopsy is one of the most sensitive diagnostic tests (Chapter 123). Approximately 40% of cases of *S. hematobium* also can be diagnosed by this method, and ova can also be detected in bladder biopsies taken during cystoscopy (Fig. 96–23). The biopsy specimen should be crushed in a drop of saline between 2 glass slides and microscopically examined for eggs under low power.

3. Plain radiography: A chest x-ray film may be helpful during the larval migration phase of *Ascaris lumbricoides* or in the diagnosis of tropical pulmonary eosinophilia. In ascariasis, pulmonary infiltrates on the chest x-ray film associated with bronchospasm and eosinophilia constitute Löffler's syndrome, of which parasites are only one cause. *Echinococcus granulosus* may show up as one or more well-defined spherical masses (Fig. 101–8) or as a calcified liver cyst on chest x-ray (Fig. 101–10). On the other hand, *Echinococcus multilocularis* may presumptively be diagnosed by finding a pathognomonic "Swiss cheese" pattern of calcification in the liver, which may be detected on a flat plate of the abdomen. Typical coin lesions may be seen in dirofilariasis. Paragonimiasis can cause hilar masses and pulmonary infiltrates (Figs. 99–4 and 99–5).

Occasionally, soft tissue x-rays of the arms and thighs are helpful in the diagnosis of cysticercosis.

4. Sputum for ova and parasites: Sputum examination may be helpful by detecting ova of *Paragonimus westermani.* Rarely, one might find larval stages of *Toxocara canis* or *A. lumbricoides* or hooklets of *E. granulosus.* Larvae of *S. stercoralis* may be seen in sputum during hyperinfection (Chapter 123).

5. Skin snips: If onchocerciasis is suspected, a diagnosis may be made by finding microfilariae in the epidermis and upper dermis (Chapter 87 and 123).

6. Mazzotti test: This test may be helpful in making a presumptive diagnosis of onchocerciais when microfilariae are too few to be found in skin snips (Chapter 87). An intense pruritic reaction occurs within 24 hours of the administration of a 50-mg dose of DEC and is considered to be diagnostic of infection. Skin snips should always precede a Mazzotti test because in heavy infections anaphylaxis may result from drug-induced killing of microfilaria.

7. Muscle biopsy: Although a diagnosis of trichinosis can be confirmed by muscle biopsy, serodiagnosis has replaced this invasive test except early on in infections (Chapters 82.2, 123, and 125).

8. Other serologic tests: Blood tests for hydatid disease, cysticercosis, trichinosis, toxocariasis, and fascioliasis are sometimes available and may be useful in specific situations (Chapter 125).

WHAT SHOULD BE DONE IF THE CAUSE OF EOSINOPHILIA CANNOT BE DETERMINED?

Even after extensive investigations, it is not unusual for the cause of eosinophilia in a returning traveler or immigrant to remain elusive. If the clinical picture does not warrant further investigations, a 3- to 6-month waiting period might prove useful because the eosinophil count may return to normal during observation. If eosinophilia persists, stool, urine, and, if indicated, blood examinations for parasites should be repeated. Recent studies in refugees from Southeast Asia have documented hookworm and *Strongyloides* infections to be the most common causes of cryptic eosinophilia.

If the patient remains asymptomatic, 2 options exist. Some tropical disease specialists recommend a course of thiabendazole (or albendazole) for strongyloidiasis to prevent hyperinfection should the patient become immunocompromised at a later date (Chapter 84.2). If a treatment trial is not instituted, patients should be informed of the possibility that they might be harboring a parasite that has the potential to create health problems. They should be warned of the need to have their eosinophil count checked before receiving immunosuppressive therapy. If eosinophilia is present in such cases, an empiric course of treatment for strongyloidiasis should be given.

Morbidity is directly proportional to worm burden, and helminth infections are usually self-limited. Therefore, a lightly infected individual with eosinophilia caused by parasites is not likely to come to harm if the infection remains untreated, except in the case of strongyloidiasis. Long-term clinical follow-up of these patients has shown that undiagnosed travel-related eosinophilia is not a significant health hazard for the returning traveler.

Challenging Problem. The problem of eosinophilia in a returning traveler is certainly challenging. After initial basic investigations, the approach requires knowledge of the geographic distribution of disease and the epidemiology and clinical presentations of helminth infections. Nontropical causes of eosinophilia are part of the differential diagnosis and influence decisions for more extensive investigations.

BIBLIOGRAPHY

Cohen SG, Ottesen EA: The eosinophil, eosinophilia and eosinophil-related disorders. *In* Middleton E, Reed CE, Ellis EF (eds): Allergy—Principles and Practice. St Louis, CV Mosby, 1983.

Fauci AS, Harley JB, Roberts WC, et al: NIH conference on the idiopathic hypereosinophilic syndrome. Clinical, pathophysiologic, and therapeutic considerations. Ann Intern Med 97:78, 1982.

Kay AB: The eosinophil in infectious diseases. J Infect Dis 129:606, 1984.

Kelbourne EM, Swygert LE, Philen RM, et al: Interim guidelines on the eosinophilia-myalgia syndrome. Ann Intern Med 112:85, 1990.

Nutman TB, Ottesen EA, Ieng S, et al: Eosinophilia in South East Asian refugees: Evaluation at a referral centre. J Infect Dis 155:309, 1987.

Spry CJF: Eosinophilia. Practitioner 226:79, 1982.

Teo CG, Singh M, Ting WC, et al: Evaluation of the common conditions associated with eosinophilia. J Clin Pathol 38:305, 1985.

Weller PF: Eosinophilia. J Allergy Clin Immunol 73:1, 1984.

Wolfe MS: Eosinophilia from the tropics. Med Clin North Am 8:797, 1984.

120. DISEASES OF IMMIGRANTS

Herbert B. Tanowitz, Louis M. Weiss, and Murray Wittner

Immigration into North America and Western Europe has increased in the past decade. Many of these immigrants have arrived from Asia, Africa, and Latin America, including the Caribbean basin. In the United States, immigration patterns have changed. At the beginning of the twentieth century the majority of immigrants were unskilled laborers from Europe. However, since 1975 nearly 1.5 million Vietnamese and other Southeast Asians have fled their homelands and nearly 900,000 have come to the United States. It is expected that by the end of this decade 9 million immigrants, mainly Asians and Hispanics, will have entered the United States legally.

Immigrants often bring illnesses, usually chronic infectious diseases (Chapter 121), with them, whereas travelers from developed to developing countries are more at risk for acute infectious diseases (Chapters 116 through 119 and 121). Imported tropical diseases, with the exception of hepatitis, tuberculosis, salmonellosis, and the acquired immunodeficiency syndrome (AIDS), do not usually represent a significant person to person risk. In addition, transfusion-acquired malaria, hepatitis B and non-A, non-B, AIDS, and Chagas' disease represent a potential risk to the population at large.

Immigrants to developed countries are often subjected to a medical history, physical examination, and basic laboratory tests, including chest radiography and stool examination for ova and parasites. The physical examination should include an assessment of the nutritional status of the patient. In addition, careful evaluation of the eyes and skin should be included. Moreover, the abdominal examination should assess the size of the liver and spleen.

In spite of these examinations, many diseases remain undiagnosed and the process often needs to be repeated. The history should include details of immunizations, including bacille Calmette-Guérin (BCG) vaccination. A complete blood count should be performed to detect anemia and eosinophilia. A second chest x-ray film may be indicated. Blood chemistries and urinalysis are important in evaluating renal and liver function. Even if the initial stool examination did not yield a pathogen, the presence of diarrhea or eosinophilia requires that it be repeated.

REPRESENTATIVE CAUSES OF FEBRILE ILLNESSES IN IMMIGRANTS. Fever is a common manifestation of infectious diseases acquired in tropical and subtropical areas of the world.

Malaria. Malaria represents a serious and common disease of immigrants and should always be considered in the differential diagnosis of febrile illness (Chapter 73). The increase in cases of imported malaria in the United States in recent years has been among immigrants from Asia, Africa, and Central and South America. Many of the Indochinese refugees have contracted the disease in camps along the Thai-Kampuchea border or in refugee camps in Indonesia and the Philippines. *Plasmodium vivax* was the most common species causing infection. However *Plasmodium falciparum* acquired on the Thai-Kampuchea border is often multidrug resistant. Among African immigrants, *P. falciparum* is the leading cause of malaria. Because immigrants from malaria endemic areas may lose their immunity after prolonged residence in the United States, they should receive prophylaxis when they return home.

Tuberculosis. In the late 1970s and early 1980s, Indochinese refugees accounted for nearly 6% of cases of active tuberculosis in the United States (Chapter 61). More than 50% of Indochinese immigrants were skin test positive, which may be due, in part, to the use of BCG immunization. Immigrants who are skin test positive may reactivate their disease at some later date. For example, in the United States, there is a high rate of both pulmonary and extrapulmonary tuberculosis among Haitians with AIDS. Infections with atypical mycobacteria and *Mycobacterium bovis* are also present in this population.

Because *Mycobacterium tuberculosis* acquired in Southeast Asia may be resistant to isoniazid (INH), it is imperative that all isolates be subjected to drug sensitivity testing. Initial therapy should include 3 drugs, pending results of these tests.

Enteric Fevers. The differential diagnosis of febrile illnesses in immigrants from Latin America and Asia should include enteric fever. Classic typhoid fever due to *Salmonella typhi* (Chapter 38), as well as enteric fevers due to nontyphoidal *Salmonella* (Chapter 39), are endemic in many Third World countries. Depending on the stage of the illness, blood and stool cultures can assist in the diagnosis. Bone marrow culture may be required in difficult cases, especially in those individuals who were started empirically on antibiotics. Drug sensitivity testing should be done because *Salmonella* species from Asia and Latin America often exhibit multiple antibiotic resistance.

Brucellosis. Brucellosis has become rare in the United States (Chapter 50). However, each year a number of imported cases occur in immigrants from Asia, Latin America, and the Mediterranean basin. Infected individuals often give a history of having ingested unpasteurized milk or milk products or of exposure to cattle. This infection may present as adenopathy and fever of unknown origin.

Trypanosomiasis. African trypanosomiasis has only rarely been diagnosed in immigrants (Chapter 74). American trypanosomiasis (Chagas' disease) in its chronic form is now being diagnosed with increasing frequency (Chapter 75). The latter often presents with cardiomyopathy and arrhythmias and/or "mega" syndromes, e.g., megacolon and megaesophagus. Serologic tests are usually positive. These patients, as well as asymptomatic seropositive patients, may be the source of transfusion-transmitted Chagas' disease. Recently, an 11-year-old with Hodgkin's disease acquired acute Chagas' disease after a platelet transfusion. The platelet donor was a 70-year-old asymptomatic woman from a highly endemic area in Bolivia. This case underscores the potential hazard to the blood supply from immigrants with asymptomatic *Trypanosoma cruzi* infection.

Visceral Leishmaniasis. Visceral leishmaniasis has been reported among immigrants from endemic areas, e.g., the Middle East, Mediterranean littoral, East Africa, Latin America, and South Asia (Chapter 76.2). When individuals from these areas have fever and hepatosplenomegaly, a diagnosis of visceral leishmaniasis should be considered. In such cases, if bone marrow aspirates are negative, splenic puncture may yield the organism. Several cases of visceral leishmaniasis have recently been reported in AIDS patients from endemic areas.

Melioidosis. This disease, caused by *Pseudomonas pseudomallei,* is prevalent throughout Southeast Asia (Chapter 56.2). During the Vietnam War, more than 300 cases were reported among U.S. military personnel, with a mortality of 10%. Patients with melioidosis often have fever associated with focal suppuration, septicemia, and/or an acute or chronic pulmonary infection mimicking tuberculosis. Because there may be a prolonged latent period, manifestations may occur months to years after emigration from endemic areas.

Diphtheria. Cutaneous and nasopharyngeal diphtherias have been reported in the United States and England among Southeast Asian immigrants (Chapter 57). Although immunizations are required on entry into the United States and other developed countries, a full series is not always given. Therefore, the diphtheria immunization status of all child immigrants should be carefully reviewed.

Rickettsial Infections. Fever and rash, with or without an eschar, in immigrants should raise the suspicion of rickettsial diseases. Louse-borne typhus remains a public health problem in Africa and parts of Latin America (Chapter 23.1). Brill-Zinsser disease or recrudescent typhus fever may occur years after the primary attack in immigrants from former endemic areas of Europe (Chapter 23.2). Scrub typhus occurs in Southeast Asia, and the Pacific (Chapter 25), and tick-borne rickettsial fevers are common in Africa, Asia, and the Middle East (Chapter 24.2).

Relapsing Fever. Louse and tick-borne relapsing fever continues to be a problem in many parts of the developing world (Chapter 34). Louse-borne relapsing fever caused by *Borrelia recurrentis* is a major disease in Ethiopia. A number of refugees from Ethiopian camps have been diagnosed as having relapsing fever.

Leptospirosis. Infections with *Leptospira* cause fever, hepatitis, and meningitis (Chapter 35). This infection is acquired by contact with water that has been contaminated with urine of infected animals. It would be a rare cause of fever in immigrants.

Viral Diseases. Measles and rubella continue to be problems among nonimmune individuals from developing countries (Chapter 16.1). Japanese encephalitis, the most common cause of epidemic viral encephalitis in the world, occurs in many parts of Asia (Chapter 21.3). A variety of other arboviral diseases are endemic in many parts of the world. Dengue fever is endemic in the Caribbean basin, Africa, Asia, and areas of the South Pacific (Chapter 20.1). Yellow fever is still endemic in areas of South America and Africa (Chapter 22.1). Other important viral diseases include Lassa fever and Marburg virus, Ebola, and Rift Valley fevers (Chapters 20.1, 22.2, and 22.4). These are found in areas of the African continent. All have shorter incubation periods and are not unique problems in immigrants.

Filarial Diseases. Filarial infections may, on occasion, cause a febrile illness in immigrants from endemic areas (Chapter 85). Acute bancroftian or Malayan filariasis is rarely encountered among tourists or immigrants. However, chronic filariasis manifested by lymphedema or frank elephantiasis is not infrequently encountered by physicians in the United States and Europe. These patients occasionally have episodic fever associated with lymphadenitis or lymphangitis. An occasional case of loiasis is diagnosed among tourists or life-long residents that have emigrated from endemic areas (Chapter 86).

Trichinosis. Several hundred cases of trichinosis are reported annually in the United States, but several thousand sporadic cases go undetected because of the mildness of the signs and symptoms (Chapter 90). Several immigrant groups in the United States traditionally eat undercooked pork or pork products. In recent years, Asians , e.g., Thais and Laotians, have had outbreaks of trichinosis caused by consuming pork. In this regard, it should be noted that a stringent trichinosis inspection program does not exist in the United States.

Familial Mediterranean Fever (FMF). Fever, abdominal pain, joint pain, and general signs and symptoms of polyserositis in immigrants from the Mediterranean area and the Middle East should always suggest to the physician that the patient may have FMF (Chapter 116).

DIARRHEAL DISEASES AND ABDOMINAL PAIN. Diarrhea in recently arrived immigrants may have many causes. Carriers of *S. typhi*, *Entamoeba histolytica*, and *Giardia lamblia* among immigrants employed as food handlers or in child care represent a public health hazard.

Bacterial. Typhoidal and nontyphoidal *Salmonella*, *Shigella*, and *Campylobacter* are all important causes of acute bacterial diarrhea (Chapters 37 to 39 and 41.2). Many *Shigella* and *Salmonella* strains from Central America and Asia may be resistant to multiple antibiotics. Cholera, enterotoxigenic *Escherichia coli*, and rotavirus, common causes of traveler's diarrhea, are rare among immigrants. Abdominal pain, diarrhea, and blood in the stools may accompany infection with *M. tuberculosis* (Chapter 61) and intestinal parasites.

Intestinal Parasites

Protozoa. *G. lamblia* is a common cause of subacute and chronic diarrhea among immigrants from developing countries and has been the most frequent cause of protozoan diarrhea among Indochinese refugee children (Chapter 69).

Intestinal amebiasis and amebic liver abscess are not uncommon among several immigrant populations, e.g., Mexicans (Chapter 68). Other intestinal protozoa that immigrants frequently harbor include *Dientamoeba fragilis*, *Entamoeba coli*, *Endolimax nana*, *Entamoeba hartmanni*, *Iodamoeba butschlii*, and *Blastocystis hominis* (Chapter 71). In addition, *Cryptosporidium* (Chapter 70) and *Isospora belli* (Chapter 71.2) are being increasingly recognized as a cause of diarrhea in normal hosts as well as in patients with AIDS. *Balantidium coli* occasionally causes diarrhea in immigrants, especially in individuals with a history of exposure to swine (Chapter 71.1).

Helminths. *Strongyloides stercoralis* is found throughout the tropics and subtropics (Chapter 84.2). As a result of its unique internal and external autoinfectious cycle, chronic infection occurs, and can persist many years after the patient leaves the endemic area. Immigrants may have chronic diarrhea, larva currens, or midepigastric "ulcer-like" pain associated with moderate eosinophilia. In immunosuppressed hosts, receiving corticosteroids or those with AIDS, this infection may cause a hyperinfection syndrome, usually without eosinophilia.

Other intestinal nematodes commonly seen in immigrant populations include whipworm (*Trichuris trichiura*) (Chapter 82.2), roundworm (*Ascaris lumbricoides*) (Chapter 83), and hookworm (*Necator americanis* or *Ancyclostoma duodenale*) (Chapter 84.1). These do not have an autoinfectious cycle and consequently the worm burden gradually decreases after affected immigrants have several years of residence in a nonendemic area. Young children are more likely to have clinically significant illnesses.

Tapeworm infections with *Taenia* sp. are common among certain immigrant groups from Africa, Asia, and Latin America (Chapter 100.2). These infections may be associated with abdominal pain and diarrhea. *Hymenolepis nana* is often diagnosed in individuals from Central America and the Middle East, India, and Pakistan (Chapter 100.3). Entire families may be infected because an intermediate host is unnecessary for transmission. Young children are often more severely affected. Diarrhea may also be associated with infections with trematodes such as *Schistosoma* (Chapter 96) and *Clonorchis* (Chapter 98.2), particularly the former.

LIVER DISEASE

Viral Hepatitis. Viral, protozoan, and helminthic diseases affect the liver. Hepatitis A, B, and non-A, non-B are common in developing countries (Chapter 19). Chronic hepatitis B carriage is extremely common in many underdeveloped areas and represents a significant cause of chronic liver disease in immigrant groups (Chapter 19.2). These chronic carriers may potentially infect others. In addition, primary hepatoma of the liver, often associated with the HB$_s$Ag carrier state, is seen with high frequency among certain African and Asian groups. Wilson's disease, a cause of cirrhosis of the liver, is common among Taiwanese.

Helminth Infections. Periportal fibrosis of the liver occurs among certain immigrant groups, e.g., Puerto Ricans, Africans, and Brazilians who are infected with *S. mansoni* (Chapter 96). Those from the Far East may be infected with *S. japonicum*, whereas those arriving from Southeast Asia may be infected with *S. mekongi*. Immigrants from Africa may occasionally be infected with *S. intercalatum*.

Clonorchis sinensis is a common liver fluke, which is endemic in the Far East, particularly among the Chinese population (Chapter 98.2). Often, these patients are asymptomatic but can have signs and symptoms of acute or chronic biliary tract disease. Among immigrants from Thailand, a related liver fluke, *Opisthorchis viverrini*, causes a similar spectrum of clinical disease (Chapter 98.1). Therefore, liver or biliary tract disease in an Asian from an endemic area should indicate the possibility of infection with these liver flukes.

The liver is the most common site of hydatid cysts. The majority of cases are from immigrants from the Mediterranean basin and elsewhere in the Middle East. With the increase in immigrants with hydatid cysts in recent years, physicians in developed countries should be aware of recent advances in diagnosis and medical-surgical management of hydatid liver disease (Chapter 101.2).

Protozoan Infections. Amebic liver abscess represents another cause of liver disease among immigrants (Chapter 68). Over two-thirds of those with amebic liver abscess do not have amebae in their stool. Consequently, serology remains the most reliable method of diagnosis.

SPLENOMEGALY. Splenomegaly is common in the tropics. It is often a sign of the involvement of the reticuloendothelial system by an underlying disease process: chronic malaria, enteric fever, leishmaniasis, brucellosis, schistosomiasis, tuberculosis, cirrhosis, or myeloproliferative disorders. In some geographic areas, more than 70% of patients have splenomegaly without an apparent cause.

Hyperactive malarial syndrome (HMS) has been most widely used to describe this entity. It is thought that HMS is the result of an aberrant immunologic response to malaria (Chapter 73.2).

PULMONARY DISEASE

Bacterial and Fungal Infections. Pulmonary and extrapulmonary tuberculosis continues to be a serious public health concern among immigrant groups (Chapter 61). With the advent of the AIDS epidemic, the incidence of tuberculosis has risen, especially among Haitians. Similarly, in the setting of AIDS, histoplasmosis in now reported among Caribbean groups living in the United States (Chapter 66.1). Coccidioidomycoses (Chapter 66.2) and South American blastomycosis (paracoccidioidomycosis) (Chapter 66.4) are seen in the United States among immigrant groups from Central and South America. North American blastomycosis occurs in immigrants from Central and South America (Chapter 66.3).

Melioidosis may have a clinical and radiographic picture indistinguishable from that of tuberculosis among immigrants from Southeast Asia (Chapter 56.2). In addition, penicillin-resistant pneumococcal disease may be present in newly arrived immigrants from the South Pacific and South Africa.

Parasitic Infections. Transient eosinophilic pneumonias, seen among recent arrivals from endemic areas, may be due to the pulmonary migration of several helminths, such as *Ascaris, Strongyloides,* and hookworm (Chapters 83 and 84). Tropical pulmonary eosinophilia (TPE), a manifestation of bancroftian filariasis, may cause nocturnal asthmatic bronchitis, peripheral eosinophilia, and bilateral infiltrate on chest x-ray film (Chapter 85.4). This is more likely to occur in immigrants from Guyana and the Indian subcontinent.

Immigrants from East Africa and East Asia, especially Korea, may have pulmonary paragonimiasis (Chapter 99). The clinical and radiologic picture consisting of hemoptysis, pulmonary infiltrates, nodules, or cysts is similar to tuberculosis from which it must be differentiated.

Amebic liver abscess may rupture through the diaphragm and cause pleural effusion or pericarditis (Chapter 68). In addition, the lung is the second most common site for hydatid disease (Chapter 101.2).

CARDIOVASCULAR DISEASES.

Chronic chagasic cardiomyopathy (i.e., cardiomegaly, heart failure, and arrhythmias) is the most important cause of heart disease in parts of Latin America (Chapter 75). It is seen with increasing frequency among immigrants from endemic areas. Although extremely rare, cysticercosis of the heart may also be associated with arrhythmias and heart block (Chapter 101.1). Pericarditis may be caused by amebiasis and tuberculosis as well as by African and South American trypanosomiasis. Schistosomiasis may cause pulmonary hypertension and cor pulmonale (Chapter 96) and hydatid disease may involve the heart and pericardium. High-output heart failure may develop as a consequence of anemia due to several causes, including iron deficiency (from hookworm disease) and hemoglobinopathies (Chapter 5).

Endomyocardial fibrosis is a progressive disease of the connective tissue network of the heart of unknown etiology (Chapter 2). This may be found among immigrants from Africa, although cases from South America and Asia have been reported.

HEMATOLOGIC DISORDERS

Peripheral Blood Count Changes. Eosinophilia in newly arrived immigrants suggests helminthic infection; multiple stool examinations should be performed (Chapter 119). Leukopenia and lymphopenia in an immigrant, especially from Central Africa or Haiti, should raise the possibility of human immunodeficiency virus (HIV) infection and AIDS (Chapter 15.1). Residents of the Caribbean and Japan may have the human T-cell leukemia virus (HTLV-1) (Chapter 15.2), and natives of the African continent may have Burkitt's lymphoma and HIV-related malignancies such as Kaposi's sarcoma (Chapter 11).

Anemia. Nutritional disorders and iron deficiency, especially as a result of heavy hookworm infection, may lead to severe anemia (Chapter 108.1). Bartonellosis may present as a hemolytic anemia (Chapter 51). Malaria may cause a chronic hemolytic state (Chapter 73). Hemolytic anemia in immigrants is frequently the result of a hemoglobinopathy or enzyme deficiency (Chapter 5). These include forms of thalassemia, especially in those of Mediterranean basin extraction; glucose-6-phosphate dehydrogenase deficiency, sickle cell disease, and hemoglobin C disease and its variants encountered in African immigrants; and hemoglobin E disease in those from Southeast Asia.

NUTRITIONAL DISORDERS AND MALABSORPTION.

Although rarely encountered, tropical sprue is a cause of malabsorption among immigrants from the Caribbean areas (Chapter 3). Lactose intolerance is not uncommon among certain African and Asian immigrant groups. This entity is also common after treatment of intestinal protozoan infections, e.g., giardiasis. Rickets and other vitamin and mineral deficiencies may be seen in immigrant children who are severely malnourished, including those with protein-calorie malnutrition (Chapters 106 to 108). Endemic goiter may be found throughout the world.

GENITOURINARY TRACT DISEASE.

Among immigrants from Africa and the Middle East, infection with *Schistosoma hematobium* may lead to a variety of urinary tract signs and symptoms, including suprapubic pain and hematuria and recurrent urinary tract infection (Chapter 96). Squamous cell carcinoma of the urinary bladder is a complication of infection with this parasite. Schistosomiasis occasionally involves the female genital tract, causing vaginal papillomas and endometritis.

Chyluria is a complication of chronic bancroftian filariasis (Chapter 85.1). Disorders of the female genital tract such as pelvic inflammatory disease and trichomoniasis are common, especially among refugee groups (Chapter 6). Rarely, amebiasis may involve the male or female genital tract. In the male, it may cause a penile ulceration as a result of vaginal or anal intercourse.

SEXUALLY TRANSMITTED DISEASES (STD).

STD continue to be important among certain immigrant groups (Chapter 10). Penicillinase-producing *Neisseria gonorrhoeae* (PPNG) were originally reported from Asia (Chapter 44). Therefore, suspected gonococcal disease in immigrants from these areas should be empirically treated as PPNG with appropriate antibiotics. In addition, syphilis is highly prevalent among immigrants from certain areas, e.g., the Dominican Republic and Haiti (Chapter 32.1). Chancroid is endemic in Africa, South America, and the Far East (Chapter 45), whereas granuloma inguinale is endemic in Africa, West Indies, South America, South India, and New Guinea (Chapter 46). Lymphogranuloma venereum is endemic in areas of Asia and South America (Chapter 29). In addition, the prevalence of HIV infection among Africans and Haitians is a continuing source of concern (Chapter 15.1).

SKIN DISEASES. Skin lesions are common among residents in the tropics. They are caused by infectious agents, as well as by environmental conditions (Chapter 7). Organisms capable of causing skin lesions include parasites, rickettsiae, fungi, bacteria, mycobacteria, and viruses (Table 120–1).

Bacterial Infections. Leprosy, a chronic infection with *Mycobacterium leprae,* is endemic in most developing countries (Chapter 62). It is estimated that there are 15 million patients with leprosy worldwide. The highest prevalence is in Africa. Of the 100 to 200 new cases reported annually in the United States, the majority are from Mexico, Puerto Rico, and Asia. In England, the majority of cases come from Asia, Africa, and the Mediterranean basin. However, different forms of this disease occur in different geographic areas. For example, 90% of cases imported from India and Africa are borderline-tuberculoid or tuberculoid. Cases from Mexico are 90% lepromatous, whereas those from China and Southeast Asia are equally divided between the 2 types. Although leprosy may be diagnosed clinically, it should always be confirmed histopathologically on skin biopsy and by slit skin smears.

Bacterial infections are common in newly arrived immigrants from the tropics and subtropics. Skin infection caused by *Staphylococcus aureus* is more common in the tropics than in temperate climates. Myiasis rarely occurs in immigrants and returning travelers from Africa and South America (Chapter 105.2). Cutaneous anthrax (Chapter 53) and cutaneous diphtheria (Chapter 57) may be seen in immigrant children.

Protozoan Infections. Cutaneous leishmaniasis is one of the most important parasitic dermatologic diseases of the tropics. American or New World leishmaniasis is composed of two main forms: *Leishmania mexicana* complex and the *Leishmania braziliensis* complex (Chapter 76.3). *L. mexicana mexicana,* usually causing a single, self-limited, nonmetastasizing cutaneous lesion ("chicle ulcer"), is found in Mexico, Belize, and Guatemala. *L. mexicana amazonensis* mostly causes a mild and self-limited skin lesion in immigrants from the Amazon basin and Trinidad. *L. braziliensis braziliensis*

TABLE 120–1. Ulcerative Lesions of the Skin in Immigrants and Refugees

Cutaneous leishmaniasis	Syphilis
Dracontiasis	Sickle cell anemia
Amebiasis cutis	Cutaneous tuberculosis
Yaws	Buruli ulcer (*Mycobacterium*
Tropical phagedenic ulcer	*ulcerans*)
Cutaneous diphtheria	
Cutaneous anthrax	

often causes mucocutaneous leishmaniasis (espundia) in areas of Brazil and in the forest areas east of the Andes. *L. braziliensis guyanensis* occurs in Guyana, Surinam, Brazil, and Venezuela. It usually causes single or multiple cutaneous ulcers associated with lymphatic spread. *L. braziliensis panamensis* is found in Panama and may cause several superficial ulcers that may metastasize along the lymphatics much like sporotrichosis. *L. braziliensis peruviana* (uta), acquired in Peru and on the western elevated slopes of the Andes, causes self-healing ulcers.

Post–kala-azar dermal leishmaniasis is a complication of unsuccessfully treated kala-azar (visceral leishmaniasis) and may occur weeks to many years after appropriate therapy (Chapter 76.1). It often heals spontaneously within a few months. Nodular lesions, which may be hypopigmented or erythematous, appear on the face, chest, neck, and buttocks.

Cutaneous or "Old World" leishmaniasis usually has self-limited lesions and is prevalent throughout the Middle East, Asia, and Africa (Chapter 76.2). A few patients who are unable to mount a suitable cell-mediated immune response may develop diffuse cutaneous leishmaniasis (DCL).

Both acute American (Chapter 75) and African (Chapter 74) trypanosomiasis may be accompanied by a maculopapular eruption. A chagoma (trypanosomal chancre) at the inoculation site is present only in patients with acute infections with these parasites. Amebiasis of the skin (ameba cutis) is a complication of amebic liver abscess and peritonitis as well as a postsurgical complication (Chapter 68). Penile and vulvar lesions and perianal fistulas from colorectal involvement are uncommon complications of amebiasis.

Helminth Infections. These are often associated with urticaria or maculopapular eruptions, which can occur during any stage of the infection. Moreover, during the treatment of helminth infections, skin manifestations may develop, presumably as a result of antigens released from dying worms.

Chronic filariasis is manifested by recurrent lymphangitis and lymphadenitis, usually of the lower extremities and may eventually lead to chronic lymphedema and finally elephantiasis (Chapter 85). The poorly nourished overlying skin may become scaly and hyperkeratotic, partly as a result of frequent episodes of streptococcal and staphylococcal cellulitis. Patients with *Loa loa* may experience urticaria or papular dermatitis. The most common skin manifestation is Calabar swelling (Chapter 86). Onchocerciasis, common in Africa and Central and South America, is associated with a variety of dermatologic manifestations in immigrants from endemic areas (Chapter 87). These manifestations include subcutaneous nodules, pruritus, and areas of hypo- and hyperpigmentation. Dracontiasis (Chapter 89), cysticercosis (Chapter 101.1), and cutaneous larva migrans (CLM) (Chapter 94) are other helminthic infections associated with dermatologic manifestations. Larva currens is a form of CLM caused by *S. stercoralis* seen on the perineum, thigh, and lower abdomen.

NEUROLOGIC AND OPHTHALMOLOGIC DISEASES. A variety of viral, bacterial, mycobacterial, fungal, and parasitic organisms are capable of causing infections of the eye (Table 120–2) and nervous system (Table 120–3) in immigrant populations.

Ophthalmic Diseases. Trachoma remains an important cause of blindness in Africa, the Middle East, and Southeast Asia; relapses may occur after the patient leaves the endemic area (Chapter 26). Viral conjunctivitis among refugee children from developing countries is common (Chapter 9). "River blindness" is caused by *Onchocerca volvulus* (Chapter 87). When immigrants from West and Central Africa have visual disturbances the possibility of onchocerciasis should be considered. Another filarial worm that causes ocular manifestations is *Loa loa;* adult worms can be found in the conjunctiva (Chapter 86). Ocular involvement is also a complication of cysticercosis (Chapter 101.1) and toxocariasis (Chapter 91). *Toxoplasma* chorioretinitis is a common complication of congenital disease and occurs frequently in children and young adults from highly endemic tropical areas (Chapter 78). Xerophthalmia, as a result of severe vitamin A deficiency, is often present in young refugee children (Chapter 107.1).

Infections of the Nervous System

Bacteria and viruses. Bacterial meningitis due to *Streptococcus pneumoniae, Neisseria meningitidis,* and *M. tuberculosis* is common in immigrant populations (Chapter 43). Meningoencephalitis may be due to arboviruses (Chapter 21) and *Rickettsia.*

Paralytic poliomyelitis and tetanus are seen in immigrants from developing countries. Some adult immigrants may exhibit sequelae of the former disease manifested as postpoliomyelitis syndromes (Chapter 18.1).

Tuberculosis and fungal infections can be associated with granulomas and other space-occupying lesions of the central nervous system (CNS). In immigrants from the Caribbean basin and Japan, tropical spastic paraparesis due to HTLV-1 is occasionally seen.

Protozoa. The clinical signs of cerebral malaria may vary from subtle behavior changes to frank psychosis (Chapter 73). Disturbances in consciousness from obtundation to deep coma, movement disorders, and seizures have been reported. Meningoencephalitis due to African trypanosomiasis is infrequently encountered (Chapter 74). Patients with invasive amebiasis may rarely have hematogenous dissemination to the CNS, with a resulting brain abscess.

Helminths. Schistosomiasis of the CNS is a fairly common complication of infections with *S. mansoni* and *S. japonicum* (Chapter 96). The latter usually affects the brain, whereas the former may affect the spinal cord. Transverse myelitis has been reported with both *S. mansoni* and *S. hematobium. S. mekongi,* however, has not been associated with CNS involvement. Cerebral

TABLE 120–2. Ophthalmologic Conditions Among Recent Immigrants and Refugees

Injuries	Loiasis
Cataracts	Cysticercosis
Viral infections	Gnathostomiasis
Xerophthalmia	Angiostrongyliasis
Trachoma	Toxoplasmosis
Onchocerciasis	Toxocariasis

TABLE 120–3. Central Nervous System Infections in Immigrants and Refugees

Bacterial	***Protozoan***
Pneumococcal meningitis	Amebic brain abscess
Meningococcal meningitis	Malaria
Tuberculous meningitis	Toxoplasmosis
	African trypanosomiasis
Fungal	
Histoplasmosis	***Helminthic***
Cryptococcosis	Angiostrongyliasis
	Cysticercosis
Viral	Echinococcosis
Arboviruses	Gnathostomiasis
HIV-related	Paragonimiasis
HTLV-1	Schistosomiasis
	Strongyloidiasis
Rickettsial	Toxocariasis
	Trichinosis
Spirochetal	
Leptospirosis	
Relapsing fever	

and spinal cord involvement in infections with the lung fluke *Paragonimus* is a well-recognized complication in Koreans, Japanese, and Southeast Asians (Chapter 99).

Cysticercosis is an infection caused by the larval stage of *Taenia solium* (Chapter 101.1). Space-occupying lesions of the head caused by cysticercosis are readily diagnosed by computed tomography (CT) (Fig. 101–5) or magnetic resonance imaging (MRI) scans and may be confirmed by serodiagnosis. CNS involvement is associated with headache and seizures in most cases. Anyone from an endemic area with these symptoms should be investigated for this possibility.

Intracranial hydatid disease is most often seen in children (Chapter 101.2). Hydatid disease in vertebrae may gradually erode the bone, causing spontaneous fractures with compression of adjacent spinal cord and roots.

The presence of nematodes in the CNS usually results from accidental human infection by larval stages of nonhuman parasites that migrate aimlessly in human tissues. Gnathostomiasis, caused by *Gnathostoma spinigerum,* is endemic in Thailand, the Philippines, Taiwan, and Japan (Chapter 92). The gnathostome larvae wander in the skin but frequently reach the brain, spinal cord, or eye, causing severe ocular damage, seizures, and ataxia. Examination of the cerebrospinal fluid (CSF) in some cases may reveal an eosinophilic pleocytosis. Eosinophilic meningoencephalitis caused by the nematode *Angiostrongylus cantonensis* has occurred sporadically in outbreaks in the Pacific islands of Tahiti, Samoa, and New Caledonia and in Thailand, Taiwan, Vietnam, and Central America (Chapter 93.1). The larval worms migrate to the brain, causing a meningoencephalitis or meningitis accompanied by a CSF eosinophilic pleocytosis. On occasion, the eye may be invaded, leading to blurred vision and ocular pain.

Visceral larva migrans due to *Toxocara canis* and *T. cati* may cause a meningoencephalitis or a chorioretinitis and should be suspected in children with pica (Chapter 91). The neurologic complications of trichinosis are uncommon, but during the acute phase of illness a meningoencephalitis may occur (Chapter 90).

Psychiatric Disorders. Immigrant groups have always been stressed by changes in life style, culture, language, and separation from family and friends. In some ethnic groups, criminal behavior has been a problem. Since the 1970s there have been reports of sudden deaths among healthy Southeast Asian males. There were similar deaths reported in young Asian males, supporting the notion that this resulted from terrifying dreams. Post-traumatic stress disorder is seen in immigrants from war-torn areas of the world. Some patients may benefit from counseling, whereas others may require more formal psychiatric care. Ideally, one should seek mental health professionals that speak the native language and/ or have experience in the treatment of patients from that particular area of the world.

BIBLIOGRAPHY

Barrett-Connor E: Latent and chronic infections imported from Southeast Asia. JAMA 239:1901, 1978.

Centers for Disease Control: Sudden unexplained death syndrome in South East Asian refugees: A review of CDC surveillance. MMWR 36:43SS, 1987.

Gordon S, Brennessel DJ, Goldstein JA, Rosner F: Malaria: A city hospital experience. Arch Intern Med 148:1569, 1988.

Grant IH, Gold JWM, Wittner M, et al: Transfusion-associated acute Chagas' disease acquired in the United States. Ann Intern Med 111:849, 1989.

Hewlett D, Pitchumoni CS: Tropical splenomegaly syndrome (TSS). Baillieres Clin Gastroenterol 319, 1987.

Hofstetter M, Nash TE, Cheever A, et al: Infection with *Schistosoma mekongi* in Southeast Asian refugees. J Infect Dis 144:420, 1981.

Lin KM, Tazuma L, Masuda M: Adaptional problems of Vietnamese refugees: I. Health and mental health status. Arch Gen Psychiatry 36:955, 1979.

Monath TP: Japanese encephalitis—a plague of the orient. N Engl J Med 319:641, 1988.

Neill MA, Hightower AW, Broome CV: Leprosy in the United States, 1971–1981. J Infect Dis 152:1064, 1985.

Nutman TB, Miller KD, Mulligan, M, et al: *Loa loa* infection in temporary residents of endemic regions: Recognition of a hyperresponsive syndrome with characteristic clinical manifestations. J Infect Dis 154:10, 1986.

Nutman TB, Ottesen EA, Jeng S, et al: Eosinophlia in South East Asian refugees: Evaluation at a referral center. J Infect Dis 155:309, 1987.

Pearson RD, Hewlett EL, Guerrant RL: Tropical Diseases in North America. Dis Mon 30:1, 1984.

Sandler RH, Jones TC (eds): Medical Care of Refugees. New York, Oxford University Press, 1987.

121. GLOBAL EPIDEMIOLOGY OF INFECTIOUS DISEASES*

Charles B. Beal
and William H. Lyerly, Jr.

The purpose of this chapter is to (1) offer both a quick reference and a comprehensive guide for the recommendation of appropriate preventive measures to international travelers; (2) facilitate the differential diagnosis of illness acquired in a particular region; and

---

*All material in this chapter is in the public domain, with the exception of any borrowed figures or tables.

(3) provide a compendium of the occurrence of infectious disease in a particular geographic location.

The chapter is divided into three sections: (1) *Quick Reference Guide to Disease Risk Assessment* in broad geographic regions of the world; (2) *Gazetteer of the Regional Distribution of Infectious Disease,* with maps; and (3) *Drug-Resistant Falciparum Malaria Registry.*

The gazetteer omits opportunistic infections and detailed lists of cosmopolitan agents such as staphylococci, sexually transmissible diseases, other genitourinary tract infections, childhood exanthems, and many of the respiratory and enteric viruses. In certain cases disease sequelae are included, such as for areas known to have a very high incidence of rheumatic heart disease following streptococcal pharyngitis.

Precise information regarding disease occurence is not available from many parts of the world, and even in technically advanced countries, sporadically or rarely occurring infections may be overlooked. Further, changing disease patterns may make current data rapidly obsolete. Additional information and periodic updating are available from the following sources:

Weekly Epidemiological Record

Published by World Health Organization and available from WHO Distribution and Sales, 1211 Geneva 27, Switzerland.

Morbidity and Mortality Weekly Report (MMWR)

Published by Centers for Disease Control, Atlanta, GA 30333, and available from Superintendent of Documents, U.S. Government Printing Office, Washington, D.C. 20402, USA.

Reference also can be made to the publications emanating from the Ministries of Health of the various countries.

Finally, the Centers for Disease Control (USA) can provide current information by phone. The number is (404) 639–3311. The night, weekend, and emergency number is (404) 639–2888.

QUICK REFERENCE GUIDE TO DISEASE RISK ASSESSMENT

Considerations Needed for Proper Disease Risk Assessment for Individual Travel

1. Incidence and prevalence of endemic diseases
   a. Endemic diseases recognized in local populations
   b. Recent outbreaks of diseases in the region
   c. Diseases encountered during previous travel to area
   d. Diseases encountered during similar types of activities in similar areas
   e. Diseases in long-term visitors/travelers to area
2. Morbidity and mortality of specific diseases
   a. Symptomatic vs. asymptomatic infections
   b. Severity of illness and medical complications
   c. Length of illness and disability
   d. Incubation period and potential impact on accomplishing travel objectives

e. Hospitalization and medical evacuation requirements
3. Risk factors associated with specific travel activity
   a. Climate factors
   b. Seasonality of diseases
   c. Topographic considerations
   d. Level of sanitation
   e. Urban vs. rural exposures
   f. Contact with local populations
4. Environmental conditions
   a. Intensity and duration of exposure to vectors or etiologic agents
   b. Animal hosts in the area
5. Preventive measures
   a. Field sanitation and personal hygiene
   b. Immunizations for specific diseases
   c. Chemoprophylaxis against specific diseases
   d. Vector control and personal protective measures

Disease Risk Assessment by Geographic Region

UNITED STATES, CANADA, GREENLAND, AND ICELAND. Viral and bacterial respiratory infections are the most common illnesses experienced by travelers to these countries. Some gastroenteritis is also reported. Campers, particularly in the Sierra and Rocky Mountain ranges, who drink directly from streams frequently contract giardiasis. Sexually transmissible infections, including HIV/AIDS, are common.

MEXICO, CENTRAL AMERICA, AND CARIBBEAN ISLANDS. The most common infections acquired by travelers are enteritis and gastroenteritis due to pathogenic *E. coli, Campylobacter* spp, and occasionally *Giardia lamblia.* Hepatitis A, amebiasis, shigellosis, salmonellosis (including typhoid), and the enterovirus group are highly prevalent in areas where hygiene is poor. Beef and pork tapeworms, ascariasis, and trichuriasis are common. Arthropod-borne viruses such as dengue are widespread but less commonly encountered. Malaria is present in tropical areas of Mexico, Central America, and some islands, especially Haiti. Viral respiratory infections are cosmopolitan. The longer term visitor also should be concerned about rabies, hepatitis B and C, sexually transmissible diseases, leptospirosis, tuberculosis, and toxoplasmosis. Depending upon the specific areas visited, cutaneous leishmaniasis, onchocerciasis, tick-borne relapsing fever, and brucellosis also are of concern.

SOUTH AMERICA. The most common infections acquired by travelers are enteritis and gastroenteritis due to pathogenic *E. coli, Campylobacter* spp. and, occasionally *Giardia lamblia.* Hepatitis, the enteroviruses, amebiasis, and shigellosis are prevalent, as is typhoid fever. Beef and pork tapeworms, ascariasis, and trichuriasis are common. Sexually transmissible diseases are widespread. Schistosomiasis is endemic in eastern Brazil, coastal Venezuela, and Surinam. Arthropod-borne viruses are widespread but not frequently diagnosed. Malaria is present in most rural areas (except the Andean highlands) in the central and northern thirds of the continent. American trypanosomiasis (Chagas'

disease) is widely found in rural and suburban areas north of 42°S latitude but not often encountered unless contracted while sleeping in traditional mud or grass dwellings. Both visceral and cutaneous leishmaniasis sometimes occur, particularly in those residing in forested areas. Longer term visitors also should be concerned about tuberculosis, brucellosis, onchocerciasis, rickettsial diseases, relapsing fever, and bartonellosis, depending upon specific areas visited.

EUROPE AND ASIAN USSR. This moderately to highly industrialized continent within a temperate to cold climatic zone exposes the traveler to relatively few arthropod- and soil-borne diseases. With some exceptions (for example, Lyme disease and tick-borne encephalitis) these infections are seen mostly in countries bordering the Mediterranean Sea. The common respiratory and sexually transmissible diseases are present throughout the continent. Most tourist accommodations, including hotels and camping facilities, provide safe drinking water and food, although outbreaks of waterborne or food-borne salmonellosis, shigellosis, and hepatitis A as well as typhoid fever and giardiasis have been reported in recent years, particularly in the southern areas.

EASTERN MEDITERRANEAN AND NORTHERN AFRICA. The most common infections acquired by travelers are due to enteritis agents, particularly pathogenic *E. coli* and *Campylobacter* spp. Hepatitis A, the enterovirus group, shigellosis, and salmonellosis also are prevalent. In the major hotels and restaurants in the more industrialized countries the risk is minimal to moderate and certainly less than purchasing food from street merchants. Malaria is focally present in Egypt and in some of the North African oases. Schistosomiasis is present in the Nile Valley and along some of the waterways of North Africa. Sexually transmissible diseases are common. Longer term residents are at increased risk for rabies, hepatitis B and C, tuberculosis, leptospirosis, and both cutaneous and visceral leishmaniasis, depending upon specific areas visited.

AFRICA SOUTH OF THE SAHARA. Taking this large portion of the continent as a whole, the most common infections acquired by travelers are due to enteritis agents, particularly the enteroviruses pathogenic *E. coli* and *Campylobacter* spp. Hepatitis and shigellosis are prevalent. The risk of exposure varies considerably, however, depending upon both the economic development of the country visited and the climate. In the major hotels and restaurants of the Republic of South Africa, for instance, the risk is similar to that in other industrialized countries. Malaria is present in most countries but in general does not extend farther south than the northern border areas of South Africa. Drug-resistant malaria has become widespread in the region. Schistosomiasis is present in waterways in nearly all countries. Trypanosomiasis has a spotty distribution in rural savanna areas and game forests. Other common diseases include the respiratory viruses, amebiasis, and various intestinal worms. Sexually transmissible diseases, including HIV/AIDS, are highly prevalent. Longer term visitors also may encounter tuberculosis, rabies, hepatitis B and C, onchocerciasis and other filarial infections, as well as dengue and viral hemorrhagic fevers, depending upon specific areas visited.

EASTERN, CENTRAL, AND SOUTHEAST ASIA. In eastern Asia, viral and bacterial respiratory infections are the most common illnesses experienced by travelers. Traveler's diarrhea and other forms of enteritis also occur, particularly in the more rural areas. Tick and scrub typhus are fairly common in rural areas. Japanese encephalitis is widespread but infrequently encountered by the traveler. Malaria is present in rural areas in southern China. In central and southeast Asia, enteroviruses, typhoid fever, and hepatitis A are very common. In the warmer regions one must include a significant risk for malaria (including drug-resistant malaria), amebiasis, and the arthropod-borne viruses, particularly dengue. Sexually transmissible diseases are common. Longer term visitors to Asia are at increased risk for tuberculosis, rabies, clonorchiasis, tapeworm and other intestinal helminths, leptospirosis, relapsing fever, rickettsial diseases, and in the warmer areas, filariasis. Hepatitis A, B, and C are highly prevalent throughout.

OCEANIA, INCLUDING AUSTRALIA AND NEW ZEALAND. The environmental conditions in this area vary from the temperate climate and modern cities of Southeastern Australia to the dense tropical rain forests of Papua New Guinea. Thus, risk of infection depends greatly on the region visited. The common respiratory viruses and bacteria are endemic throughout. The common intestinal viral agents, protozoa, and helminths are widespread in the warmer zones. Drug-resistant malaria is present in Papua New Guinea, Vanuatu, and the Solomon Islands. Arthropod-borne viruses, particularly dengue, are prevalent. Tick typhus and scrub typhus are endemic on some of the islands and in northern Australia. Sexually transmissible diseases are found throughout, and tuberculosis and hepatitis A, B, and C are common in rural areas. Some islands have a high leprosy transmission rate.

GAZETTEER OF THE REGIONAL DISTRIBUTION OF INFECTIOUS DISEASE

Area 1—United States, Canada, Greenland, Iceland

Enteric Infections

VIRUSES. Enterovirus group; hepatitis A, B, and C; rotavirus; Norwalk and Norwalk-like viruses.

BACTERIA. Diarrhea-producing *Escherichia coli;* shigellosis; salmonellosis.

Rare. Typhoid fever; *Campylobacter* sp.; *Vibrio* sp.; *Yersinia pseudotuberculosis* (particularly Vancouver, Canada); *Y. enterocolitica; Edwardsiella tarda; Plesiomonas shigelloides;* botulism; cholera (SE and SC USA).

PROTOZOA. Amebiasis (*Entamoeba histolytica* and *Dientamoeba fragilis, E. polecki* [very rare]); giardiasis; isosporosis (rare); cryptosporidiosis.

HELMINTHS. Pinworm; fish tapeworm—C and W Canada, USA (W Alaska), elsewhere from imported fish, and previously, Great Lakes area.

Uncommon. Ascariasis, whipworm, hookworm (*Ne-*

cator americanus); strongyloidiasis; trichinosis; beef and dwarf tapeworms.

Rare. Anisakiasis—primarily Hawaii; fascioliasis—Hawaii; gongylonemiasis—particularly SE USA; *Dipylidium caninum; Stellantchasmus falcatus* and *Diorchitrema pseudocirratum*—Hawaii; *Troglotrema salmincola*—USA and Canada (Pacific Northwest); pork tapeworm.

Skin and Subcutaneous Infections

VIRUSES. Molluscum contagiosum.

BACTERIA. *Pasteurella multocida*—more common in warmer areas; mycobacterial ulcer and erythrasma—unusual but more common in warmer areas; erysipeloid—more common in warm coastal areas; cutaneous diphtheria—uncommon, mostly rural.

Rare. *Vibrio* sp. wound infection—usually coastal areas; anthrax—particularly in SC USA; *Erysipelothrix rhusiopathiae* (including endocarditis)—USA; leprosy—mostly imported, rare reports of endemic disease from Louisiana, Texas, Hawaii, California.

FUNGI. Common dermatomycoses.

Rare. White piedra—SE USA; sporotrichosis; mycetoma.

PROTOZOA. *Leishmania mexicana*—rare reports from S Texas.

HELMINTHS. Cutaneous larva migrans—particularly SE USA; cercarial dermatitis—particularly in freshwater lakes; sparganosis—SE USA (rare reports); subcutaneous dirofilariasis—N USA, S Canada (rare reports); gongylonemiasis—rare reports.

ARTHROPODS. Scabies; pediculosis.

UNCERTAIN ETIOLOGY. Ainhum—SE USA (rare reports).

Meningitis, Encephalitis, and Viral Fevers

ARTHROPOD-BORNE VIRUSES

Undifferentiated Fevers. Rio Bravo—SW USA; Tamiami—Florida; Tensaw—S Florida.

Dengue-like Fevers. Dengue—intermittent reports from SE Texas eastward and, rarely, Great Lakes area; Colorado tick fever—W Canada, USA (Rocky Mountains and probably N California) from 1200 to 3300 m altitude.

Meningoencephalitis. California encephalitis—USA W of Ohio, Alaska, Canada (coastal provinces); La Crosse—USA and S Canada westward to Rocky Mountains; infrequent reports of related viruses snowshoe hare and Jamestown Canyon; Eastern equine (EEE)—SE Canada, eastern half of USA; Powassan—S Canada and northern USA, rare reports in humans; St. Louis (SLE)—all USA northward to S Canada and SE Alaska, usually rural but occasional small urban outbreaks; Venezuelan equine (VEE)—S Florida and S Texas; Western equine (WEE)—S Canada, USA (except New England, and particularly W states and C California).

OTHER VIRUSES. Lymphocytic choriomeningitis; rabies—all areas except Greenland and Iceland.

BACTERIA. Bacterial meningitis and abscess—throughout.

PROTOZOA. Amebic meningoencephalitis—rare reports.

Oropharyngeal and Respiratory Tract Infections

VIRUSES. Common respiratory agents; condyloma acuminatum (extragenital).
Rare. Vesicular stomatitis (Indiana and New Jersey serotypes)—USA (Arizona northward and eastward except New England), Canada (SW Ontario, S Manitoba).
CHLAMYDIAE. Psitticosis.
BACTERIA. Common respiratory agents; tuberculosis; diphtheria—throughout but uncommon and mostly rural; *Haemophilus parainfluenzae*—rare reports in children; legionellosis.
FUNGI. Coccidioidomycosis—SW USA (Fig. 66–4); histoplasmosis—Canada (SE and W Manitoba), USA (particularly midwest, Appalachia, S and E Texas, S Arizona, C California); *Blastomyces dermatitidis*—USA (Mississippi River Valley eastward, except New England); rhinosporidiosis—SE USA (rare reports).

Other Parasitic Infections

PROTOZOA. Toxoplasmosis—throughout.
Rare. Babesiosis—USA (primarily NE coast islands); malaria—no endemic foci, occasional transmission by other means and rare outbreaks from imported cases (Texas and California); *Trypanosoma cruzi*—very rare reports S Texas, S California.
HELMINTHS. *Echinococcus g. granulosus*—S USA and lower Mississippi; *E. g. canadensis*—Canada (except E area), USA (Alaska); *E. multilocularis*—Canada (Hudson Bay area), USA (W Alaska, NC states); trichinosis; visceral larval granulomatosis (including ocular larva migrans)—particularly SE USA.
Rare. *Brugia* sp.—NE USA (rare reports); thelazia conjunctivitis—California; *Angiostrongylus cantonensis*—Hawaii; *A. costaricensis*—Texas.

Other Infections

VIRUSES. Cytomegalovirus; Epstein-Barr; herpes simplex and zoster; HIV/AIDS; retrovirus-associated myelopathy; rabies—cosmopolitan except Hawaii and Iceland; acute hemorrhagic conjunctivitis—occasional outbreaks.
CHLAMYDIAE. Lymphogranuloma venereum—particularly SE USA; trachoma—occasional reports.
RICKETTSIAE: American spotted fever—W Canada, USA (particularly SE and E coast, including small urban focus in New York City [Bronx]).
Rare. Endemic typhus—SE USA; epidemic typhus—E USA; Q fever—throughout except Iceland; rickettsialpox—no recent reports but probably present.
BACTERIA. Brucellosis (particularly *B. abortus*)—occasional reports; cat scratch disease; leptospirosis; relapsing fever (tick-borne)—primarily W USA to British Columbia, Canada; Lyme disease—USA (primarily NE coastal, NC states, N Montana, S Oregon, NW Nevada, N California), Canada (British Columbia); tularemia—30°N to 71°N latitude; chromobacteriosis—SE

USA, particularly Florida; plague—W USA (rare) (Fig. 47–1).
UNCERTAIN ETIOLOGY. Mucocutaneous lymph node (Kawasaki) disease—Canada, USA (particularly Hawaii); Behçet's syndrome—rare reports; restrictive cardiomyopathy (endomyocardial fibrosis)—SE USA; chronic fatigue syndrome (epidemic neuromyasthenia)—sporadic cases and outbreaks.
NONINFECTIOUS BUT SIMULATING INFECTION. Ciguatera fish poisoning—S coastal regions and islands except Iceland and Greenland.

Area 2—Mexico, Central America, and Caribbean Islands

(Mexico; Belize, Costa Rica, El Salvador, Guatemala, Honduras, Nicaragua, Panama; Anguilla, Antigua, Aruba, Bahamas, Barbados, Bermuda, Cayman, Cuba, Curaçao, Dominica, Dominican Republic, Grenada, Guadeloupe, Haiti, Jamaica, Martinique, Montserrat, Puerto Rico, St. Kitts and Nevis, St. Lucia, St. Maarten, St. Vincent and the Grenadines, Trinidad and Tobago, Turks and Caicos, Virgin Islands)

Enteric Infections

VIRUSES. Enterovirus group; hepatitis A, B, C, delta; E—reported from Mexico.
BACTERIA. Diarrhea-producing *E. coli;* shigellosis; salmonellosis (including typhoid and paratyphoid fevers); *Campylobacter* sp.; *Edwardsiella tarda*—rare reports from Cuba, Panama.
PROTOZOA. Amebiasis (invasive disease particularly common in Mexico); giardiasis; balantidiasis; isosporosis.
HELMINTHS. Ascariasis; hookworm; trichuriasis; strongyloidiasis; beef tapeworm; dwarf tapeworm; pork tapeworm (including cysticercosis)—particularly Mexico and Central America; fascioliasis—Mexico, Central America, Cuba; *Schistosoma mansoni*—Puerto Rico, E Dominican Republic, Antigua, Guadeloupe, Martinique, St. Lucia, St. Maarten (Fig. 96–9).
UNCERTAIN ETIOLOGY. Tropical sprue—particularly E Mexico, E Central America.

Skin and Subcutaneous Infections

VIRUSES. Molluscum contagiosum—cosmopolitan.
BACTERIA. Erysipeloid; erythrasma; cutaneous diphtheria; chancroid; leprosy—mainland and islands (particularly St. Lucia and Trinidad and Tobago); anthrax—particularly Haiti, Central America; mycobacterial ulcer—Cuba, Mexico, Dominican Republic; pinta—SE Mexico, Cuba, Dominican Republic, Guadeloupe, Haiti; yaws—Dominican Republic, Haiti.
FUNGI. Common dermatophytoses; sporotrichosis; chromomycosis; mycetoma; white piedra; tinea nigra and imbricata—Central America; Lobo's disease—Central America (rare reports).
PROTOZOA. *Leishmania b. braziliensis*—Mexico (S Yucatan), Central America (particularly Atlantic sea-

board and C Panama) (Fig. 76–3); *L. panamensis*—SE Panama; *L. mexicana mexicana*—Mexico (Monterrey, Yucatan), Belize, Guatemala; *L. donovani chagasi* skin lesions—reported from Honduras; diffuse cutaneous leishmaniasis—Dominican Republic, Belize, Panama.

HELMINTHS. *Onchocerca volvulus*—SW Mexico, Guatemala, El Salvador (minimal focus) (Fig. 87–2*B*); *Mansonella ozzardi*—Trinidad, most other islands, Guatemala, Panama; *Mansonella (Dipetalonema) perstans*—Mexico (Yucatan), SE Panama, Trinidad, St. Vincent, St. Lucia, Guadeloupe, St. Kitts and Nevis, Dominican Republic; cutaneous larva migrans; cercarial dermatitis—particularly Cuba, Haiti, El Salvador, Mexico; sparganosis—rare.

ARTHROPODS. Scabies; pediculosis; tungiasis and myiasis—particularly tropical areas of Central America and Mexico.

UNCERTAIN ETIOLOGY. Ainhum—occasional reports.

Meningitis, Encephalitis, and Viral Fevers

ARTHROPOD-BORNE VIRUSES
Undifferentiated Fevers. At least 14 viruses isolated, particularly in Panama and Trinidad, but rarely clinically identified.

Dengue-like Fevers. Dengue—Mexico (particularly E coast) and throughout, usually in intermittent epidemic waves.

Hemorrhagic Fevers. Dengue hemorrhagic fever—recent reports in Dominican Republic, El Salvador, Nicaragua, St. Lucia; yellow fever—S Central America, Trinidad and Tobago.

Meningoencephalitis. Eastern equine (EEE)—rare reports have come from E Mexico, Guatemala, Honduras, Panama, Trinidad (1972); St. Louis (SLE)—prior reports from Mexico, Belize, Guatemala, Panama, previously on larger islands; Venezuelan equine (VEE)—E and SW Mexico, subtropical areas of Central America, Trinidad and Tobago; recent reports in Costa Rica; Western equine (WEE)—epizootic incidence in Mexico (no human cases documented).

OTHER VIRUSES. Lymphocytic choriomeningitis; rabies—present on mainland and the following islands: Cuba, Dominican Republic, Grenada, Haiti, Puerto Rico, Trinidad.

BACTERIA. Bacterial meningitis and abscess.

Oropharyngeal and Respiratory Tract Infections

VIRUSES. Common respiratory agents; vesicular stomatitis—Mexico.

CHLAMYDIAE. Psitticosis—throughout.

BACTERIA. Tuberculosis; nocardiosis; diphtheria—particularly Barbados and Dominican Republic; rhinoscleroma—Mexico, Guatemala, El Salvador; streptococcal pharyngitis with rheumatic heart disease—particularly Mexico City, Mexico.

FUNGI. Aspergillosis; cryptococcosis—Cuba; mucormycosis; coccidioidomycosis—NW Mexico, Guatemala (rare), Honduras (Comayagua Valley); paracoccidioidomycosis—Mexico, Central America; histoplasmosis—Central America, Mexico, Cuba, Jamaica, and probably other islands; *Blastomyces dermatitidis*—Mexico; rhinosporidiosis—Cuba, Guadeloupe, Mexico (rare reports); rhinoentomophthoromycosis—Costa Rica, Jamaica.

PROTOZOA. Pneumocystis pneumonia—occasional reports.

HELMINTHS. Syngamosis—rare reports from Martinique, St. Lucia, Trinidad.

Other Parasitic Infections

PROTOZOA. Malaria—Haiti, Dominican Republic, Mexico (W coast, central lowlands, and southern third but no risk in major tourist resorts and urban areas). Risk in all Central America except urban areas in Costa Rica, El Salvador, Honduras, Nicaragua, and Panama. Guatemala City, risk-free; Belize, hyperendemic; occasional outbreaks on smaller islands, often involving *Plasmodium malariae* (Fig. 73–1).

Drug-resistant falciparum malaria—see Table 121–1.

Toxoplasmosis—throughout; American trypanosomiasis (*Trypanosoma cruzi*)—Mexico, Central America, Trinidad and Tobago (no recent cases); *Trypanosoma rangeli* (nonpathogenic; may coexist with *T. cruzi*)—S Mexico, Central America; babesiosis—Mexico (rare).

HELMINTHS. *Wuchereria bancrofti*—Costa Rica (Puerto Limon), Panama (contiguous to Puerto Limon), all islands except Jamaica, Grenada, St. Vincent; rare in Cuba (Fig. 85–2); *Mansonella ozzardi*—Haiti and several other islands; *Echinococcus granulosus*—Mexico, Central America (rare reports); *E. vogeli*—Panama (rare reports); visceral larval granulomatosis (including ocular larva migrans)—particularly Mexico, Puerto Rico; tropical pulmonary eosinophilia—islands where *W. bancrofti* is present; paragonimiasis—Costa Rica, Honduras, Panama; trichinosis—Mexico, Bahamas, rare in Central America; lagochilascariasis—islands (rare); *Angiostrongylus costaricensis*—S Mexico, Central America; *A. cantonensis*—Cuba (Havana area).

Other Infections

VIRUSES. Acute hemorrhagic conjunctivitis—occasional outbreaks; cytomegalovirus; acute epidemic conjunctivitis, Epstein-Barr; herpes simplex and zoster; HIV/AIDS; retrovirus-associated myelopathy.

CHLAMYDIAE. Trachoma.

RICKETTSIAE. Q fever; American spotted fever—Mexico, Panama; endemic typhus—particularly Mexico and Central America; epidemic typhus—Guatemala (mountainous areas); tick typhus—Mexico, Guatemala, Honduras, Panama; trench fever—Mexico (rare).

PROTOZOA. Visceral leishmaniasis (*L. d. chagasi*)—SC Mexico, Central America (Atlantic side), possibly Guadeloupe and Martinique (Fig. 76–3).

BACTERIA. Cat scratch disease; tetanus; tularemia—N Mexican border; tetanus; relapsing fever (tickborne)—Mexico, Central America; brucellosis; leptospirosis—mainland and probably all islands; well recognized in Cuba, Barbados, Jamaica, Puerto Rico, and Trinidad; melioidosis—rare in Central America, Aruba, Bahamas; listeriosis; rat-bite fever.

UNCERTAIN ETIOLOGY. Hypertrophic cardiomyopathy—several islands; restrictive cardiomyopathy (endomyocardial fibrosis)—Mexico; congestive cardiomyopathy—rare reports; endemic elephantiasis—Guatemala (probably soil-related, not infectious).

NONINFECTIOUS BUT SIMULATING INFECTION. Ciguatera fish poisoning—islands; recent reports in Cuba and Dominican Republic.

Area 3—South America

(Argentina, Bolivia, Brazil, Chile, Colombia, Ecuador, French Guiana, Guyana, Paraguay, Peru, Surinam, Uruguay, Venezuela, Falkland [Malvinas] Islands, South Georgia Island)

Enteric Infections

VIRUSES. Enterovirus group; hepatitis A, B, C, delta.

BACTERIA. Diarrhea-producing *E. coli;* shigellosis; salmonellosis (including typhoid and paratyphoid fevers); *Campylobacter* sp.; cholera.

PROTOZOA. Amebiasis (invasive disease particularly common in Colombia); giardiasis; balantidiasis; isosporosis (frequently reported in Santiago, Chile).

HELMINTHS. Ascariasis; hookworm; trichuriasis; strongyloidiasis; *Schistosoma mansoni*—E and S Brazil (Santa Catarina north to Belém, particularly coastal areas [focus at Manaus]), coastal Venezuela and Surinam (Fig. 96–3); fascioliasis—particularly Argentina, Brazil, Chile, Uruguay; beef and dwarf tapeworms; pork tapeworm (including cysticercosis)—particularly Peru; fish tapeworm—Argentina, S Chile, coastal Peru; anisakiasis—along Pacific coast (rare); *Angiostrongylus costaricensis*—Brazil, Colombia, Venezuela; dicroceliasis—Brazil; heterophyiasis—Brazil.

Rare. *Bertiella* sp.—Guyana, Ecuador; lagochilascariasis—Surinam; *Inermicapsifer* sp.—Venezuela; *Gastrodiscoides hominis*—Guyana; esophagostomiasis—Brazil.

OTHER. Pentastomiasis—warmer areas.

Skin and Subcutaneous Infections

VIRUSES. Molluscum contagiosum—cosmopolitan.

BACTERIA. Erysipeloid; erythrasma; cutaneous diphtheria; chancroid; granuloma inguinale; tropical ulcer; leprosy—not reported in Chile; anthrax—particularly Chile; mycobacterial ulcer—reported from Bolivia, French Guiana, Peru; pinta—N coastal areas, particularly Colombia; yaws—sporadic reports from Guyana, Surinam, French Guiana, Colombia (Pacific coastal region).

FUNGI. Common dermatophytoses; tinea nigra and imbricata; chromomycosis; mycetoma; sporotrichosis; black piedra—particularly forested areas; Lobo's disease—Brazil (particularly Amazon), Colombia, Surinam, Venezuela.

PROTOZOA. *Leishmania b. braziliensis*—N of 28°S latitude (not reported in Chile), particularly in N Argentina, E Bolivia, Brazil, Colombia, Paraguay, E Peru and Venezuela (Fig. 76–3); *L. b. guyanensis*—primarily N of Amazon river; *L. b. panamensis*—northern Colombia; *L. peruviana*—Peru (C Andes valley); *L. mexicana amazonensis*—N of 23°S latitude (including N Bolivia and NE Peru; rare in French Guiana); *L. m. garnhami*—NW South America; *L. m. pifanoi*—N Venezuela; diffuse cutaneous leishmaniasis—uncommon but widespread in *Leishmania* endemic areas.

HELMINTHS. Dracunculiasis—possibly Surinam; cercarial dermatitis—reported from Argentina; sparganosis—occasional reports, warmer areas.

ARTHROPODS. Scabies; pediculosis; tungiasis—N three quarters of continent; myiasis—particularly tropical areas.

UNCERTAIN ETIOLOGY. Brazilian pemphigus foliaceus (fogo selvagem)—Brazil, rare reports in bordering countries; ainhum—Brazil.

Meningitis, Encephalitis, and Viral Fevers

ARTHROPOD-BORNE VIRUSES

Undifferentiated Fevers. About 20 viruses widely distributed, particularly in N half of continent; rarely identified (Oropouche and Mayaro viruses probably most important of the group).

Dengue-like Fevers and Dengue. N border of Brazil and northward.

Hemorrhagic Fevers. Dengue hemorrhagic fever—reports in Colombia; yellow fever—Amazon River basin (Brazil, Bolivia, Colombia, Peru, Surinam), Orinoco River Basin (Venezuela, Colombia), Atrato and Magdalena River Basins (Colombia, prior reports from Ecuador and Paraguay).

Meningoencephalitis. Eastern equine (EEE)—Argentina (Buenos Aires), Brazil (Belém), Colombia, Ecuador, N Peru, Venezuela (E and W border areas), Guyana; Ilheus—N South America; St. Louis (SLE)—prior rare reports from Brazil, Argentina, Surinam; Venezuelan equine (VEE)—N and NW coastal areas of continent, plus a few foci in N tropical forests; Western equine (WEE)—epizootic occurrences documented in Colombia, Brazil, Guyana, Uruguay, Argentina but no recent human cases; Rocio—Brazil (coastal São Paulo State), no recent cases recorded.

OTHER VIRUSES. Lymphocytic choriomeningitis; rabies; Argentinian hemorrhagic fever (Junin virus)—C Argentina (between 33–37°S and 59–64°W); Bolivian hemorrhagic fever (Machupo virus)—Bolivia.

BACTERIA. Bacterial meningitis and abscess—throughout.

PROTOZOA. Amebic meningoencephalitis—reported from Brazil.

Oropharyngeal and Respiratory Tract Infections

VIRUSES. Common respiratory agents; vesicular stomatitis; vesicular stomatitis Algoas (Indiana serotype)—Brazil (Algoas and Bahia).

CHLAMYDIAE. Psitticosis.

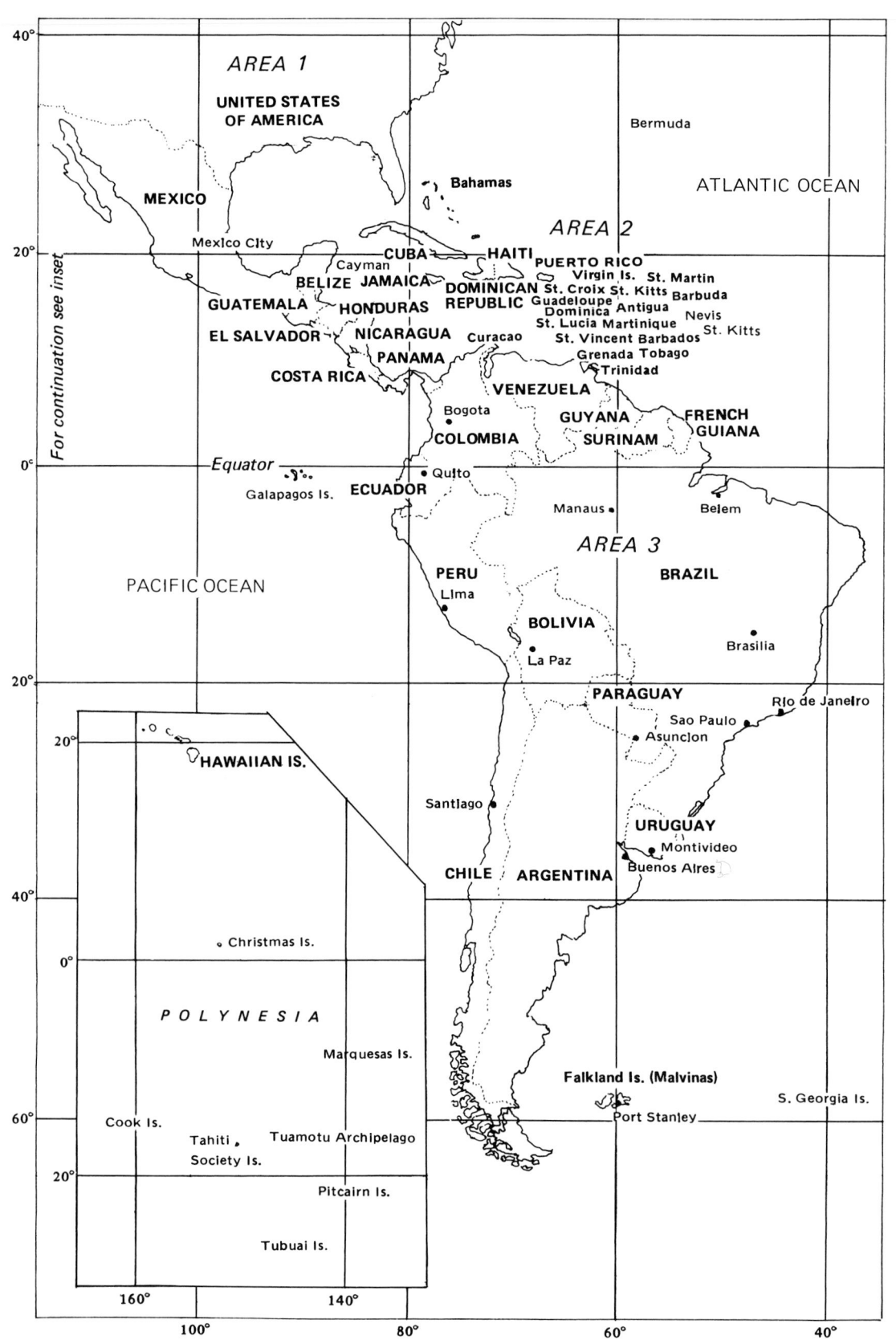

FIGURE 121–1. Geographic regions 1–3.

BACTERIA. Tuberculosis; nocardiosis; rhinoscleroma (Venezuela); diphtheria; streptococcal pharyngitis with rheumatic heart disease—particularly La Paz, Bolivia.

FUNGI. Coccidioidomycosis—N Argentina, W Paraguay, S Bolivia, NW Venezuela; histoplasmosis—particularly NW countries, Argentina, S Brazil, and Uruguay; infrequent in S one quarter of continent; paracoccidioidomycosis—throughout to 32°S latitude and particularly São Paulo area of Brazil; rhinosporidiosis—Argentina, Brazil, Ecuador, Paraguay; rhinoentomophthoromycosis—Brazil, Colombia.

PROTOZOA. Pneumocystis pneumonia.

HELMINTHS. Paragonimiasis—particularly N Peru, coastal Ecuador, Venezuela; syngamosis—rare reports from Brazil and Guyana.

Other Parasitic Infections

PROTOZOA. Malaria (*P. falciparum, P. vivax,* and rarely, *P. malariae*)—no risk in urban areas in Colombia, Brazil (except in greater Amazon basin), Guyana, Surinam, Venezuela; no risk in Argentina except at Bolivian and Paraguayan borders; no risk in Chile and Uruguay; no risk in Paraguay except along Bolivian and Brazilian borders; in Bolivia, no risk in Provinces of La Paz, Oruro, and Potosi; in Ecuador, no risk in vicinity of Quito, Andean highlands, and Galápagos Islands; in French Guiana, no risk in Cayenne City; in Peru, no risk in urban areas and Andean highlands (Fig. 73–1). Drug-resistant *P. falciparum*—see Table 121–1.

American trypanosomiasis (Chagas' disease)—particularly E Brazil; reported from all countries except Surinam; not present S of 42°S latitude; *Trypanosoma rangeli* (nonpathogenic; may coexist with *T. cruzi*)—Colombia, Peru, Venezuela, probably Paraguay; toxoplasmosis—cosmopolitan; visceral leishmaniasis (*L. d. changasi*)—Brazil, particularly N Brazil (Amazon mouth), E Brazil (hyperendemic); Paraguay; E Bolivia; sporadic in NE Argentina; foci in N Colombia and N Venezuela; sporadic in Ecuador; Surinam (Fig. 76–3).

HELMINTHS. *Wuchereria bancrofti*—NE coast of Brazil, NW Venezuela, N Guyana, French Guiana, Surinam (Fig. 85–2); *Onchocerca volvulus*—Venezuela (Orinoco River Basin, including Amazonas Territory), W Colombia (Cauca), Ecuador (Cayapas River, Esmeraldas), small foci in N Brazil and Surinam (Fig. 87–2*B*); *Mansonella (Dipetalonema) perstans*—E Colombia, French Guiana, Guyana, Surinam, S and NE Venezuela; *Mansonella ozzardi*—greater Amazon basin extending to N Argentina; *Wuchereria lewisi*—Brazil (Recife); tropical pulmonary eosinophilia—similar distribution to *W. bancrofti*; *Echinococcus granulosus*—W coast and S half of continent; *Echinococcus vogeli*—Brazil, Colombia, Ecuador, Venezuela; trichinosis—particularly W Argentina, Chile, Uruguay; visceral larval granulomatosis (including ocular larva migrans)—particularly warmer areas; lagochilascariasis—Brazil, Surinam.

Other Infections

VIRUSES. Cytomegalovirus; Epstein-Barr; herpes simplex and zoster; HIV/AIDS particularly Brazil; retrovirus-associated myelopathy; acute hemorrhagic conjunctivitis—occasional outbreaks.

CHLAMYDIAE. Lymphogranuloma venereum and trachoma.

RICKETTSIAE. Epidemic typhus—mountainous areas of Bolivia, Ecuador, Peru; American spotted fever—Brazil, Colombia; endemic typhus—particularly Argentina and Chile; Q fever—occasional reports.

BACTERIA. Brucellosis—particularly Argentina, Peru; leptospirosis; rat-bite fever; bartonellosis—Peruvian Andes, Ecuador, and Colombia near Peruvian borders; plague—Bolivia (La Paz and central areas), N Argentina, E Brazil (Ceara to Bahia), C Ecuador (particularly Chimborazo, NE Peru (Fig. 47–1); relapsing fever; louse-borne—particularly Peruvian Andes; tick-borne—widespread; melioidosis—Ecuador (rare).

UNCERTAIN ETIOLOGY. Tropical sprue—French Guiana, Guyana, Surinam, Venezuela; restrictive and hypertrophic cardiomyopathies—Brazil, Colombia, Venezuela; congestive cardiomyopathy—rare reports; annular subvalvular aneurysm—Brazil (rare reports); endemic elephantitis—Ecuador (probably not infectious but soil-related).

Area 4—Europe and Asian USSR

(Albania, Andorra, Austria, Belgium, Bulgaria, Crete, Czechoslovakia, Denmark, Finland, France, Germany, Hungary, Ireland, Italy, Liechtenstein, Luxembourg, Malta, The Netherlands, Norway, Poland, Portugal, Romania, Spain, Sweden, Switzerland, United Kingdom [UK], Union of Soviet Socialist Republics [USSR], Yugoslavia)

Enteric Infections

VIRUSES. Enterovirus group; hepatitis A, B, C, delta and E (reported from USSR); Norwalk.

BACTERIA. Diarrhea-producing *E. coli;* shigellosis; salmonellosis (including typhoid and paratyphoid fevers); *Campylobacter* sp.—particularly warmer climates; *Yersinia enterocolitica*—particularly Belgium, Finland, Sweden; *Y. pseudotuberculosis*—not reported in Greece, Italy, Portugal, Spain; *Plesiomonas shigelloides*—occasional reports; *Edwardsiella tarda*—Spain (rare reports).

PROTOZOA. Amebiasis; giardiasis; isosporosis; balantidiasis—occasional reports from continent.

HELMINTHS. Ascariasis; hookworm; trichuriasis; strongyloidiasis—present in warmer climates, plus foci in NW Italy, Romania, Czechoslovakia, Hungary, Belgium, Switzerland; beef tapeworm—particularly USSR (Caucasian area), Yugoslavia; pork tapeworm (including cysticercosis)—reported from Portugal, Spain, Italy, Poland; dwarf tapeworm—particularly S Europe; fish tapeworm—particularly Finland, Romania, USSR (NW area, Volga basin, Siberia); fascioliasis—sheep- and cattle-raising areas; dicroceliasis—C Europe, France, Spain, USSR (Caucasian area); echinostomiasis—Romania, USSR; heterophyiasis—Greece, USSR (maritime provinces); metagonimiasis—SE Europe, Spain,

USSR (Ukraine); opisthorchiasis—C, E, and S Europe; paragonimiasis—USSR (maritime provinces); trichostrongyliasis—SE USSR, rare reports from France, Greece.

Rare. *Capillaria hepatica*—Czechoslovakia; *Dipylidium caninum;* gongylonemiasis—S and SE Europe; anisakiasis—UK, Netherlands, Norway, Sweden; *Gastrodiscoides hominis*—USSR (Kasakstan).

UNCERTAIN ETIOLOGY. Tropical sprue—Italy (Sicily).

Skin and Subcutaneous Infections

VIRUSES. Molluscum contagiosum—cosmopolitan.

BACTERIA. Anthrax—particularly SC areas; erysipeloid; erythrasma; cutaneous diphtheria; leprosy; *Pasteurella multocida;* mycobacterial ulcer—all unusual and more common in warmer areas; chancroid—particularly Scandinavian countries.

FUNGI. Common dermatophytoses; sporotrichosis—particularly warmer areas; chromomycosis—Finland, USSR.

PROTOZOA. *Leishmania tropica* and *L. infantum*—Mediterranean areas including S Portugal, Italy (Abruzzi region), islands, SE USSR (Turkmania, Usbek) (Fig. 76–3); *L. major*—SE Turkey.

HELMINTHS. Cutaneous larva migrans—southern areas; cercarial dermatitis—C Europe, France, Switzerland, UK; gongylonemiasis—rare reports; subcutaneous dirofilariasis—rare reports, particularly Italy, SE France.

ARTHROPODS. Scabies; pediculosis; myiasis—occasional reports from more southern areas.

UNCERTAIN ETIOLOGY. Ainhum—rare reports, warmer areas.

Meningitis, Encephalitis, and Viral Fevers

ARTHROPOD-BORNE VIRUSES
Undifferentiated Fevers. Calovo—Czechoslovakia, Austria, Yugoslavia; Inkoo—Finland (serologic evidence only), Kemerova—USSR; phlebotomus fever—S Italy, including Sicily.

Dengue-like Fevers. Sindbis—Czechoslovakia, USSR; West Nile—S France (Rhone delta, Corsica) and countries eastward; Tahyna—Portugal, France eastward to W USSR.

Hemorrhagic Fever. Crimean-Congo—S Europe and S USSR, rarely in C Europe and Scandinavia; Omsk—USSR.

Meningoencephalitis. Central European—Balkans to S Sweden; louping ill—UK (SE England, Scotland), Ireland; Kumlinge—Finland; Russian spring-summer (tick-borne encephalitis)—Europe (except Norway, Italy, UK, Ireland, Spain, Portugal), and primarily USSR; Powassan—E USSR; Thogoto—Italy (Sicily); California encephalitis–related—Norway (serologic positives only).

OTHER VIRUSES. Lymphocytic choriomeningitis; rabies—not reported from UK, Ireland, Finland, Norway, Sweden, Portugal, Spain, Cyprus, Corsica (France); hemorrhagic fever with renal syndrome (nephropathia epidemica)—Scandinavia, particularly Finland (Lake Finland area), C and E Europe, USSR (Siberia N of Manchuria).

BACTERIA. Bacterial meningitis and abscess.
PROTOZOA. Amebic meningoencephalitis—UK, Belgium, Czechoslovakia.

Oropharyngeal and Respiratory Tract Infections

VIRUSES. Common respiratory agents.
BACTERIA. Diphtheria; tuberculosis; legionellosis; rhinoscleroma—Poland, USSR.
CHLAMYDIAE. Psitticosis.
FUNGI. Histoplasmosis—sporadic reports, particularly C Italy; rhinosporidiosis—UK, Italy.
PROTOZOA. Pneumocystis pneumonia.
HELMINTHS. *Capillaria aerophila* bronchopneumonia—USSR fox farms; gongylonemiasis—rare reports, particularly USSR.

Other Parasitic Infections

PROTOZOA. Babesiosis—UK, Ireland, France, USSR, Yugoslavia; malaria—USSR (Iranian and Chinese borders); (imported—areawide); toxoplasmosis—widespread, particularly France; visceral leishmaniasis *(L.d. infantum)*—Mediterranean coastal regions, including Portugal, islands, France (maritime Alps), N Turkey, Bulgaria, S Romania, S Hungary, Greece (Corfu), SE Austria, S USSR to 65°E (Fig. 76–3).

HELMINTHS. *Wuchereria bancrofti*—Spain (rare reports); trichinosis—particularly Hungary, Poland, Spain, USSR; Cyprus probably is risk-free; visceral larval granulomatosis (including ocular larva migrans)—reports from Netherlands, UK, France (S Pyrenees); *Echinococcus g. granulosus* ("European" strain)—S half of continent, including islands; ("Northern" strain)—N half of continent; *E. multilocularis*—C Europe, USSR, and rare reports from UK and Italy (Sardinia); trichinosis.

Other Infections

VIRUSES. Acute hemorrhagic conjunctivitis—occasional outbreaks; cytomegalovirus—particularly warmer areas; HIV/AIDS; retrovirus-associated myelopathy; Epstein-Barr; herpes simplex and zoster; swine vesicular disease—rare reports from UK, Italy.

CHLAMYDIAE. Lymphogranuloma venereum and trachoma—particularly warmer areas.

RICKETTSIAE. Epidemic typhus—rare reports from E Europe; Q fever—throughout except Denmark, Finland, Sweden, Norway, Belgium; particularly frequent in Great Britain and NE Spain (Basque); rickettsialpox—USSR (Ukraine); scrub typhus—USSR (particularly S of 45°N latitude—foci in Primorsk area, Tadzhik USSR, Kuril Island); Mediterranean spotted fever, boutonneuse fever *(R. conorii)*—Mediterranean, Black, and Caspian Sea areas; recent reports in Spain, France, and Switzerland; Asian tick typhus—USSR; trench fever—continental Europe.

BACTERIA. Brucellosis—particularly France, Germany, Portugal, Italy, Spain, Greece, Malta; cat scratch disease; Lyme disease—throughout except N Scandinavia and Mediterranean coastal areas; relapsing fever (tick-borne)—particularly Mediterranean area; leptospirosis; listeriosis and rat-bite fever—occasional reports; plague—SE USSR (Fig. 47–1); tularemia—particularly USSR (Ukraine), not reported in UK, Ireland, Spain, Portugal.

OTHER. Pentastomiasis—rare reports, warmer areas.

UNCERTAIN ETIOLOGY. Kaposi's sarcoma—N Italy, Poland, USSR, S Greece; mucocutaneous lymph node (Kawasaki) disease—W Europe; Behçet's syndrome—rare reports from UK and Mediterranean basin; chronic fatigue syndrome (epidemic neuromyasthenia, myalgic encephalomyelitis)—sporadic cases and outbreaks; congestive cardiomyopathy—rare reports.

Area 5—Eastern Mediterranean and Northern Africa

Bahrain, Cyprus, Gaza Strip, Iran, Iraq, Israel, Jordan, Kuwait, Lebanon, Oman, United Arab Emirates, Qatar, Saudi Arabia, Syria, Turkey, Yemen, West Bank; *Northern Africa:* Algeria, Egypt, Libya, Morocco, Tunisia, Western Sahara)

Enteric Infections

VIRUSES. Enterovirus group; hepatitis A, B, C, delta—present throughout; delta is most commonly reported from Egypt and Algeria, often in sporadic outbreaks; hepatitis E—reported from Egypt; Norwalk—reported from Israel.

BACTERIA. Diarrhea-producing *E. coli; Campylobacter* sp.; shigellosis; salmonellosis (including typhoid and paratyphoid fevers); cholera—reported intermittently from various countries.

PROTOZOA. Amebiasis; giardiasis; isosporosis; balantidiasis—particularly Egypt.

HELMINTHS. Ascariasis; hookworm; trichuriasis; strongyloidiasis; beef tapeworm—particularly Lebanon, Syria; fish tapeworm—particularly Israel (Lake Tiberias); dwarf tapeworm; clonorchiasis—Turkey, Israel; fascioliasis—N Africa, C Iran (Isfahan); opisthorchiasis—E Mediterranean; trichostrongyliasis—particularly Egypt, Iran, Iraq; *Schistosoma mansoni*—Saudi Arabia (particularly, in the SW coastal plain), Egypt (lower Nile Valley), Yemen, Oman, Libya (coastal focus in Misnatah area).

Rare. Dicroceliasis—C Iran (Isfahan), Egypt; heterophyiasis—particularly Egypt (Nile delta); pork tapeworm—Egypt, Lebanon; *Stellantchasmus falcatus*—Egypt; *Capillaria philippinensis*—Iran, Egypt.

OTHER. Pentastomiasis—particularly Egypt.

UNCERTAIN ETIOLOGY. Tropical sprue—particularly Syria, Mediterranean coast.

Skin and Subcutaneous Infections

VIRUSES. Molluscum contagiosum.
BACTERIA. Cutaneous diphtheria; chancroid; trop-

ical ulcer; anthrax—particularly Iran, Iraq; endemic syphilis—particularly NW and SW Saudi Arabia.

FUNGI. Common dermatophytoses; tinea nigra—particularly warmer areas; chromomycosis—occasional reports; mycetoma.

PROTOZOA. *Leishmania tropica, L. major,* and *L. infantum*—Mediterranean border, N and SW Saudi Arabia, Iraq, C, N, and SE Iran.

HELMINTHS. Cutaneous larva migrans; dracunculiasis—Egypt (Nile Valley), C and S Iran, Arabian Peninsula.

ARTHROPODS. Scabies; pediculosis.

UNCERTAIN ETIOLOGY. Kaposi's sarcoma—particularly Israel.

Meningitis, Encephalitis, and Viral Fevers

ARTHROPOD-BORNE VIRUSES

Undifferentiated Fevers. Phlebotomus—particularly Egypt, Iran; Dugbe and Quaranfil—most frequently isolated in Egypt.

Dengue-like Fevers. West Nile—widespread; Sindbis and Zika—most frequently isolated in Egypt.

Hemorrhagic Fevers. Crimean-Congo—probably throughout Middle East and Egypt; not documented in S half of Arabian Peninsula; Rift Valley—Egypt and probably Sinai peninsula; Thogoto—Egypt.

OTHER VIRUSES. Lymphocytic choriomeningitis; rabies—reported from all countries except Cyprus.

BACTERIA. Bacterial meningitis and abscess.

Oropharyngeal and Respiratory Tract Infections

VIRUSES. Common respiratory agents; vesicular stomatitis—Iran (Ishfahan).

CHLAMYDIAE. Psitticosis.

BACTERIA. Tuberculosis; rhinoscleroma—scattered foci; streptococcal sore throat with rheumatic heart disease—particularly Algeria, Egypt, Morocco; diphtheria—occasional reports; legionellosis—reported from Israel, Bahrain.

FUNGI. Histoplasmosis—Algeria, Egypt; positive skin tests in Iran, Saudi Arabia, Turkey; *Blastomyces dermatitidis*—Israel and N Africa (rare reports).

PROTOZOA. Pneumocystis pneumonia.

HELMINTHS. Fascioliasis (halzoun).

Other Parasitic Infections

PROTOZOA. Malaria (*P. vivax, P. malariae,* and some *P. falciparum* in warmer areas).

Present as follows: Iran (particularly W and S, but major cities risk-free), Iraq (N and E below 1500 m), Jordan (rural areas of Jordan River Valley and Kerak lowlands), Oman, United Arab Emirates, Saudi Arabia (coastal areas except Qatar and northward), Syria (N and NW primarily), Turkey (S and SE, with no risk in major cities), Yemen (except Aden, Hajja and Sada Provinces); recent outbreaks at Suez canal.

Risk-free: Kuwait, Lebanon, Cyprus, Israel, Bahrain.

In N Africa, present as follows: Algeria (residual focus in Blida and perhaps Annaba), SW Libya, S Egypt and lower half of Nile, Fayoum, and oases (Cairo risk-free), Morocco (W half and N).

Risk-free: Tunisia.

Drug-resistant *P. falciparum*—Iran (see Table 121–1).

Visceral leishmaniasis, including lymph node involvement *(L. d. infantum)*—coastal areas to N border of W Sahara, Iraq, Iran (except SE), S Yemen, N, E, and S Arabian Peninsula, rare in Libya; toxoplasmosis—particularly Egypt.

HELMINTHS. *Schistosoma haematobium*—SW Iran, Iraq (Tigris and Euphrates Valleys), Saudi Arabia (primarily W area), N Syria, SE Turkey, Yemen, S Lebanon (probably no recent transmission), Algeria (N oases and Algiers area), Egypt (Nile Valley, coast), C Tunisia (Chott Djerid), Libya (SW and NE coastal focus); *Wuchereria bancrofti*—Turkey (Mediterranean coast opposite Cyprus), N Africa (particularly Egypt, Algeria, Tunisia); *Onchocerca volvulus*—Yemen in localized foci; *Mansonella (Dipetalonema) perstans*—Algeria, Tunisia; *Echinococcus granulosus*—throughout, but particularly N Africa; probably no recent transmission in Cyprus; *E. multilocularis*—rare reports from Turkey; trichinosis—occasional reports from Egypt, Lebanon, otherwise rare; *Angiostrongylus cantonensis*—Egypt (rare reports); visceral larval granulomatosis (including ocular larva migrans).

Other Infections

VIRUSES. Cytomegalovirus; Epstein-Barr; herpes simplex and zoster; HIV/AIDS; retrovirus-associated myelopathy.

CHLAMYDIAE. Lymphogranuloma venereum and trachoma—particularly N Africa.

RICKETTSIAE. Epidemic typhus—occasional reports from Iraq, Kuwait, Sinai Peninsula, and desert regions of N Africa; Mediterranean spotted fever; endemic typhus; Q fever.

BACTERIA. Brucellosis—particularly Iran; plague—Iran, Iraq, SW Saudi Arabia (Asir), NW Yemen, Libya, Western Sahara; endemic syphilis—particularly SW Saudi Arabia; relapsing fever (tick-borne); rat-bite fever; melioidosis—occasional reports from Turkey, Iran; tularemia—Turkey.

UNCERTAIN ETIOLOGY. Behçet's syndrome—frequent reports; mucocutaneous lymph node (Kawasaki) disease—Turkey, Kuwait; congestive cardiomyopathy—rare reports.

NONINFECTIOUS BUT SIMULATING INFECTION. Familial Mediterranean fever and familial paroxysmal polyserositis.

Area 6—Western and Central Africa and Adjacent Islands

(*Western:* Benin, Burkina Faso, Côte d'Ivoire [Ivory Coast], Gambia, Ghana, Guinea-Bissau, Guinea Republic, Liberia, Mali, Mauritania, Niger, Nigeria, Senegal, Sierra Leone, Togo; *Central:* Angola, Cameroon, Central African Republic [CAR], Chad, Congo, Equatorial Guinea, Gabon, Zaire; *Islands:* Azores, Canary, Cape Verde, Madeira, São Tomé and Principe)

Enteric Infections

VIRUSES. Enterovirus group; hepatitis A, B, and C; delta hepatitis—present throughout but particularly prevalent in Ivory Coast.

BACTERIA. Diarrhea-producing *E. coli; Campylobacter* sp., shigellosis; salmonellosis (including typhoid and paratyphoid fevers); cholera—intermittently in most countries; *Vibrio parahaemolyticus*—coastal areas; *Aeromonas hydrophila*—reported from coastal Ivory Coast; *Edwardsiella tarda*—reported from Mali, Chad, Zaire.

PROTOZOA. Amebiasis (hepatic involvement more common in humid climates); giardiasis; balantidiasis.

HELMINTHS. Ascariasis; hookworm; trichuriasis; *Strongyloides stercoralis; S. fulleborni*—particularly rain forests between 2° and 4° N latitude; *Schistosoma mansoni*—all countries except Mauritania, Equatorial Guinea; present in S Angola, S Niger, S Chad, E Guinea-Bissau; beef tapeworm—common; pork tapeworm (including cysticercosis)—rare in Muslim areas; fish tapeworm—Madeira, CAR.

Rare. Dicroceliasis—Ghana, Sierra Leone, CAR; echinococcosis—Mauritania, Senegal; *Fasciola gigantica;* esophagostomiasis; *Schistosoma intercalatum*—foci in S Cameroon, Gabon, C Zaire, E and N Congo, S CAR, and probably S Chad; *S. matthei*—particularly S areas; *S. rodhaini*—Zaire.

OTHER. Physalopteriasis—tropical areas; pentastomiasis (including halzoun)—particularly Zaire, Nigeria.

UNCERTAIN ETIOLOGY. Tropical sprue—Nigeria (occasional reports).

Skin and Subcutaneous Infections

VIRUSES. Molluscum contagiosum; monkeypox—rare reports from Zaire, Liberia, Nigeria, and Sierra Leone.

BACTERIA. Anthrax—particularly W and N areas of subcontinent; leprosy; chancroid; tropical ulcer; mycobacterial ulcer—particularly Ghana, Nigeria; cutaneous diphtheria—particularly C Africa; yaws—particularly Ghana and in the pygmies in Central Africa.

FUNGI. Common dermatophytoses; *Malassezia tropica;* mycetoma; mucormycosis; chromomycosis; *Histoplasma capsulatum* var. *duboisii*—throughout to 10°N latitude; subcutaneous phycomycosis—occasional reports.

PROTOZOA. *Leishmania major*—generally between 16°N and 8°N latitude; rare reports from Liberia and S Ivory Coast; none in islands.

HELMINTHS. Dracunculiasis—all countries except Sierra Leone, Guinea-Bissau, Angola, Congo, and Equatorial Guinea; none in islands (Fig. 89–3); *Loa loa*—all countries except Guinea-Bissau, Liberia, Mauritania, Senegal, Sierra Leone, Burkina Faso, Gambia, CAR, Equatorial Guinea; none in islands; hyperendemic in Congo River basin; coenurosis—particularly Gabon, Angola, Zaire.

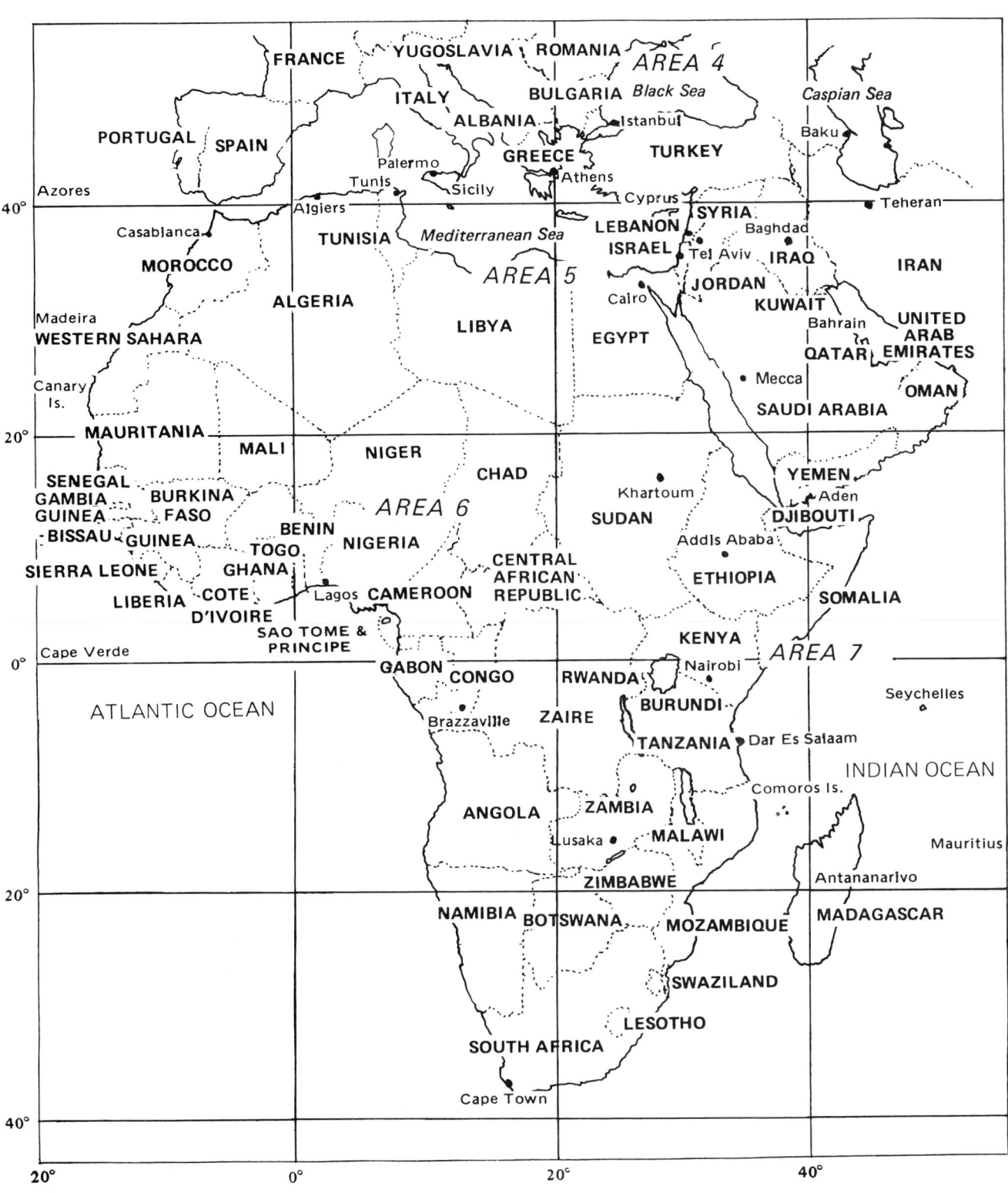

FIGURE 121–2. Geographic regions 4–7.

ARTHROPODS. Tungiasis and myiasis—particularly tropical areas; scabies; pediculosis.

UNCERTAIN ETIOLOGY. Ainhum; granuloma multiforme—Cameroon, Nigeria, Zaire; tumoral calcinosis—occasional reports; onyalai (a thrombocytopenic purpura)—C Africa 0°–30°S latitude; endemic elephantiasis—Cameroon highlands (soil-related, probably not infectious).

Meningitis, Encephalitis, and Viral Fevers

ARTHROPOD-BORNE VIRUSES

Undifferentiated Fevers. About 10 viruses (including phlebotomus fever) widely distributed, rarely identified.

Dengue. Tropical and subtropical areas, particularly Nigeria.

Dengue-like Fevers. About 10 viruses (including Bunyamwera, chikungunya, O'nyong-nyong, Sindbis, and West Nile) widely distributed, rarely identified.

Hemorrhagic Fevers. Yellow fever—Angola, Gambia, Guinea (Siguiri region), N Ghana, SE Burkina Faso, E Ivory Coast, Nigeria, Zaire (N of 10°S latitude), N Senegal, S Mauritania, SW Mali; Crimean-Congo—rare reports from Nigeria, Zaire, CAR, Senegal, Gambia, Mauritania, Burkina Faso; Rift Valley—present throughout; recent epidemic in S Mauritania; Hantaan (hemorrhagic fever with renal syndrome)—rare reports from CAR.

Meningoencephalitis. Thogoto—Nigeria; Semliki Forest—reported in Senegal, Nigeria, Cameroon, CAR; very rarely documented human cases; tick-borne—occasional reports.

OTHER VIRUSES. Rabies—throughout except Azores, Canary, Madeira; Makola and Lagos bat (rabies-like)—Nigeria; Lassa—Sierra Leone, Liberia, Guinea, Ivory Coast, Mali, Nigeria; Ebola hemorrhagic fever—border of Zaire, Sudan, and Uganda; Marburg—Cameroon and CAR (rare reports), positive serologies in Nigeria; simian orthopox—SW CAR (rare reports).

BACTERIA. Epidemic meningitis—intermittently and generally between 15°N and 8°N latitude from Burkina Faso eastward and also in C Africa extending southward to N Zaire; bacterial meningitis and abscess.

PROTOZOA. Trypanosomiasis—one or more foci in all countries except Senegal, Gambia, Mauritania, between 15°N and 9°S latitude; not in islands (Fig. 74–2).

Oropharyngeal and Respiratory Tract Infections

VIRUSES. Common respiratory agents.

CHLAMYDIAE. Psittacosis.

BACTERIA. Tuberculosis; diphtheria—probably throughout; rhinoscleroma—isolated foci, particularly Burkina Faso.

FUNGI. *Histoplasma capsulatum*—throughout but infrequent; *H.c.* var. *duboisii*—throughout to 10°N latitude, particularly Cameroon, Congo, Zaire.

Rare. *Blastomyces dermatitidis*—Zaire; rhinoentomophthoromycosis—Nigeria, Cameroon; very rare elsewhere.

HELMINTHS. Paragonimiasis—W Cameroon and E Nigeria; rare reports from Liberia and Guinea.

Other Parasitic Infections

PROTOZOA. Malaria (*P. falciparum* with some *P. ovale* and *P. malariae*)—all countries including urban areas. *Islands:* Cape Verde (São Tiago), São Tomé and Principe.

Drug-resistant *P. falciparum*—see Table 121–1.

Toxoplasmosis—probably cosmopolitan; visceral leishmaniasis (*L. d. donovani*)—S of 16°N latitude to Zaire and NW Angola (Fig. 76–3).

HELMINTHS. *Wuchereria bancrofti*—all countries. *Islands:* Cape Verde, São Tomé and Principe (Fig. 85–2); *Onchocerca volvulus*—all countries except Gambia, Mauritania, Senegal; none in islands (Fig. 87–2*A*); *Mansonella (Dipetalonema) streptocerca*—SE Ghana, S Ivory Coast, Cameroon, Nigeria, Zaire, E CAR; *M. perstans*—all countries except Mauritania and Guinea-Bissau; rare in southern C Africa. *Islands:* Cape Verde, São Tomé and Principe; *Microfilaria rodhaini*—Gabon; *Schistosoma haematobium*—all countries except Equatorial Guinea; small foci only in S Congo, S Zaire (Fig. 96–8); trichinosis—occasional reports from W Africa; echinococcosis—rare reports.

Other Infections

VIRUSES. Acute hemorrhagic conjunctivitis—occasional outbreaks; cytomegalovirus; herpes simplex and zoster; Epstein-Barr; HIV/AIDS; retrovirus-associated myelopathy—particularly C Africa.

CHLAMYDIAE. Lymphogranuloma venereum and trachoma.

RICKETTSIAE. Tick typhus (*R. conorii*); epidemic typhus—rare reports from Nigeria, Gabon, E Angola; unidentified rickettsia—high percentage of positive serologies in CAR; Q fever—rare reports.

BACTERIA. Plague—NE Zaire; endemic syphilis—northern areas; brucellosis (particularly *B. abortus*); leptospirosis; relapsing fever (louse-borne)—Chad; (tick-borne)—throughout; rat-bite fever—occasional reports; tularemia—W Africa and Cameroon (rare reports); melioidosis—reported from Chad.

UNCERTAIN ETIOLOGY. Kaposi's sarcoma—particularly NE Zaire; congestive cardiomyopathy—particularly Nigeria; restrictive cardiomyopathy (endomyocardial fibrosis)—occasional reports; hypertrophic cardiomyopathy—rare reports; annular subvalvular aneurysm—Nigeria (rare reports).

Area 7—Eastern and Southern Africa

(*Eastern:* Burundi, Djibouti, Ethiopia, Kenya, Malawi, Mozambique, Rwanda, Somalia, Sudan, Tanzania, Uganda, Zambia; *Southern:* Botswana, Lesotho, Namibia, South [S.] Africa, Swaziland, Zimbabwe; *Islands:* Comoros, Madagascar, Mauritius, Réunion, Seychelles)

Enteric Infections

VIRUSES. Enterovirus group; hepatitis A, B, C, delta.

BACTERIA. Diarrhea-producing *E. coli;* shigellosis; salmonellosis (including typhoid and paratyphoid fevers); *Campylobacter* sp.; *Clostridium perfringens* type C—reported from Uganda; cholera—intermittent reports from most countries; *Edwardsiella tarda*—reported from Madagascar.

PROTOZOA. Amebiasis—throughout (hepatic involvement more common in humid parts of continent); giardiasis; balantidiasis; isosporosis.

HELMINTHS. Ascaris; hookworm; trichuriasis; *Strongyloides stercoralis; S. fulleborni*—S Ethiopia, E Rwanda, Zambia, Zimbabwe, and particularly rain forests between 2° and 4°N latitude; *Schistosoma mansoni*—all countries except Somalia, Djibouti, and Lesotho; NE Namibia only (Fig. 96–9); beef tapeworm—particularly Ethiopia, Kenya; pork tapeworm including cysticercosis)—particularly S. Africa; fascioliasis—particularly Uganda, Kenya; *Inermicapsifer* sp.—Kenya, Rwanda, Burundi, Tanzania; *Ternidens deminutus*—S Tanzania, southern Africa.

Rare. Esophagostomiasis—tropical areas; *Raillietina* sp.—Mauritius; visceral larval granulomatosis (including ocular larva migrans)—reports from S. Africa; *Schistosoma matthei*—S. Africa (Port Elizabeth, Durban areas, and Mozambique border); *S. margrebowiei*—S. Africa, Zambia; *S. rodhaini*—Uganda; *Bertiella* sp.—Mauritius.

OTHER. Pentastomiasis (including halzoun)—particularly C E Africa; physalopteriasis—tropical areas.

UNCERTAIN ETIOLOGY. Tropical sprue—occasional reports from Sudan, Uganda.

Skin and Subcutaneous Infections

VIRUSES. Molluscum contagiosum; tanapox—rare reports from Kenya.

BACTERIA. Anthrax—particularly Burundi, Kenya, Rwanda, Tanzania; leprosy; chancroid; tropical ulcer; mycobacterial (Buruli) ulcer—particularly Uganda, S Sudan, probably Mozambique; cutaneous diphtheria—particularly tropical areas; yaws—tropical areas.

FUNGI. Common dermatophytoses; tinea nigra and *Malassezia tropica*—particularly tropical zones; mycetoma; mucormycosis; chromomycosis; sporotrichosis—particularly S. African miners; subcutaneous phycomycosis—particularly Uganda, Kenya; *Histoplasma capsulatum* var. *duboisii*—Zimbabwe northward.

PROTOZOA. *Leishmania major*—C Sudan, Kenya; *L. aethiopica*—Ethiopia, W Kenya, E Uganda; *Leishmania* sp.—SC Sudan, W Tanzania, S Namibia.

HELMINTHS. Dracunculiasis—S Sudan, S Ethiopia, N Kenya, N Uganda (Fig. 89–3); *Loa loa*—SW Sudan, W Uganda; *Onchocerca volvulus*—E Africa: all countries except Djibouti, Somalia. In Sudan, present in S and E river valleys; single case report from Zambia. Southern Africa: Swaziland. *Islands*: Madagascar, Comoros, Mauritius (Fig. 87–2*A*); coenurosis—particularly in sheep-raising areas; cercarial dermatitis—reported from S. Africa; sparganosis—occasional reports.

ARTHROPODS. Scabies; pediculosis; tungiasis and myiasis—particularly tropical areas.

UNCERTAIN ETIOLOGY. Ainhum; granuloma multiforme—Kenya, Tanzania, Uganda; tumoral calci-

nosis—rare reports; onyalai (a thrombocytopenic purpura)—0°–30°S latitude; myospherulosis—rare reports from Kenya, Uganda; endemic elephantiasis—Ethiopia, SW Burundi, Kenya (mountainous areas), Rwanda, Uganda, NW Tanzania (soil-related, probably not infectious).

Meningitis, Encephalitis, and Viral Fevers

ARTHROPOD-BORNE VIRUSES

Undifferentiated Fevers. At least 6 viruses, widely distributed, rarely identified.

Dengue. Tropical areas and particularly Somalia and coastal Kenya.

Dengue-like Fevers. About 10 viruses, including chikungunya, Sindbis, O'nyong-nyong, Bunyamwera, and West Nile, widely distributed, rarely identified.

Hemorrhagic Fevers. Yellow fever—Sudan (S of 12°N latitude); Crimean-Congo—rare reports from E and S Africa, Namibia; Rift Valley—all countries and Madagascar but not other islands.

Meningoencephalitis. Thogoto—Kenya; tick-borne—occasional reports.

OTHER VIRUSES. Lymphocytic choriomeningitis; rabies; Duvenhage (rabies-like)—S. Africa; Ebola hemorrhagic fever—border of Sudan, Uganda, Zaire; Lassa complex—Zimbabwe, Mozambique; Marburg—reported in S. Africa in 1975, Kenya (twice in the 1980s).

BACTERIA. Bacterial meningitis and abscess—throughout; epidemic meningitis—intermittently in C and S Sudan, W Ethiopia, Kenya, S Egypt.

PROTOZOA. Amebic meningoencephalitis—reported from Zambia; trypanosomiasis *(T. b. gambiense)*—S Sudan, N Uganda, W Kenya; *(T. b. rhodesiense)*—one or more foci in all countries between 10°N and 20°S latitude except Kenya, Somalia, and Namibia (Fig. 74–2).

HELMINTHS. *Angiostrongylus cantonensis*—Madagascar and Réunion (rare reports).

Oropharyngeal and Respiratory Tract Infections

VIRUSES. Common viral agents.

CHLAMYDIAE. Psittacosis—occasional reports.

BACTERIA. Tuberculosis; diphtheria—probably cosmopolitan; legionellosis—reported from S. Africa; rhinoscleroma—scattered foci, particularly Uganda.

FUNGI. *Blastomyces dermatitidis*—particularly Zimbabwe, S. Africa; *Histoplasma capsulatum*—rare reports throughout; *H. c.* var. *duboisii*—Zimbabwe northward; rhinosporidiosis—particularly Uganda; also Tanzania, Kenya, Sudan.

Other Parasitic Infections

PROTOZOA. Malaria *(P. falciparum, P. ovale, P. malariae, P. vivax)*—present in all countries and islands except Lesotho, Réunion, Seychelles; minimal risk in Nairobi, Kenya; risk in N Namibia only; no risk in S. Africa except areas bordering Botswana, Mozambique, Zimbabwe; risk in N Swaziland only; no risk in Harare, Zimbabwe (Fig. 73–1).

Drug-resistant *P. falciparum*—see Table 121–1.

Visceral leishmaniasis *(L.d. donovani)*—S Sudan, S and W Ethiopia, Kenya, E Uganda, with occasional reports from Zimbabwe and Mozambique (Fig. 76–3); toxoplasmosis—probably cosmopolitan.

HELMINTHS. *Wuchereria bancrofti*—E Africa: all countries except Somalia, Djibouti; southern Africa: N of 20°S latitude; all islands (Fig. 85–2); tropical eosinophilia—throughout, and particularly Tanzania; *Mansonella (Dipetalonema) perstans*—Burundi, W Kenya, Rwanda, Malawi, W Tanzania, W Mozambique, SW Sudan, Uganda, Zambia, Zimbabwe; *Mansonella streptocerca*—SW Sudan; echinococcosis—particularly SW Ethiopia and NW Kenya; *Schistosoma haematobium*—all islands and countries except Lesotho; present in N Namibia and S Somalia only; in Ethiopia, SW border and Awash and Webi Shebele River basins (Fig. 96–8); trichinosis—occasional reports, particularly from Kenya and Tanzania.

Other Infections

VIRUSES. HIV/AIDS—particularly E Africa; retrovirus-associated myelopathy; cytomegalovirus; herpes simplex and zoster; Epstein-Barr; acute hemorrhagic conjunctivitis—occasional outbreaks.

CHLAMYDIAE. Lymphogranuloma venereum and trachoma.

RICKETTSIAE. Tick typhus *(R. conorii);* epidemic typhus—particularly Ethiopia; also Burundi, Kenya, Rwanda, Uganda, Lesotho; endemic typhus—particularly Ethiopia; Q fever—occasional reports; trench fever—Ethiopia.

BACTERIA. Brucellosis—particularly Kenya, Tanzania; leptospirosis; plague—particularly S. Africa; also Lesotho, Madagascar, Namibia, Botswana, Zimbabwe, Zambia, Kenya, Tanzania, Sudan; relapsing fever (tickborne)—particularly S. Africa; (louse-borne)—Ethiopia, Sudan, Somalia; endemic syphilis—particularly N areas; rat-bite fever—occasional reports; melioidosis—reported from Madagascar.

UNCERTAIN ETIOLOGY. Kaposi's sarcoma—particularly Burundi, Rwanda, W Uganda; chronic fatigue syndrome (epidemic neuromyasthenia)—reported from S. Africa; restrictive cardiomyopathy (endomyocardial fibrosis)—particularly Uganda; congestive cardiomyopathy—particularly tropical areas; hypertrophic cardiomyopathy—rare reports; annular subvalvular cardiac aneurysm—rare reports.

Area 8—Eastern Asia

(China [including Manchuria], Hong Kong, Japan, Macao, Mongolia, North and South Korea, Taiwan)

Enteric Infections

VIRUSES. Enterovirus group; hepatitis A, B, C, delta; Izumi fever—Japan; Norwalk—Japan.

BACTERIA. Cholera—intermittently reported primarily from Korea and China; diarrhea-producing *E. coli; Campylobacter* sp.; shigellosis; salmonellosis (including typhoid and paratyphoid fevers); *Yersinia* sp.; *Vibrio parahaemolyticus*—particularly Japan, Korea; *Plesiomonas shigelloides*—occasional reports.

PROTOZOA. Amebiasis; giardiasis; isosporosis; balantidiasis (reported rarely from China).

HELMINTHS. Ascariasis; hookworm; trichuriasis; strongyloidiasis; beef tapeworm; dwarf tapeworms (*Hymenolepis nana*, rarely *H. diminuta*)—cosmopolitan; pork tapeworm (including cysticercosis)—particularly N China, Manchuria, and mountainous areas of Taiwan; fish tapeworm—particularly Manchuria, Korea, Japan, Taiwan; clonorchiasis—China (particularly Kwangtung; not present in NW China); Japan (particularly Okinawa and Miyagi Prefectures; not present in Hokkaido); Korea; Taiwan (particularly S and C), Hong Kong, Macao; fasciolopsiasis—particularly E and S China, S Taiwan; heterophyiasis—C and S China, S Japan, Korea, Taiwan; metagonimiasis—Japan, Korea, Taiwan; trichostrongyliasis—particularly Korea, N Japan, N China; *Schistosoma japonicum*—China (between 22°25′N and 33°N latitude, and E of 99°E longitude, particularly in Yangtze Valley and Szechwan); Japan (rare cases in Kofu and Tone River areas but no recent transmission) Fig. 96–8).

Rare. Anisakiasis—Japan, coastal China; dicroceliasis—Taiwan, Japan; echinostomiasis—China (particularly W Szechwan), Japan, Taiwan; *Echinochasmus japonicus;* opisthorchiasis—Japan, Korea; *Raillietina* sp.—Taiwan; *Stellantchasmus falcatus*—particularly Japan; *Schistosoma spindale*—China, Yunan Province (no human cases reported); *Capillaria philippinensis*—Japan.

UNCERTAIN ETIOLOGY. Tropical sprue—E China, S Japan, Taiwan.

Skin and Subcutaneous Infections

VIRUSES. Molluscum contagiosum.

BACTERIA. Anthrax; erysipeloid; erythrasma; leprosy; yaws; chancroid—particularly Korea.

FUNGI. Common dermatophytoses; sporotrichosis; mycetoma; tinea imbricata—coastal areas; chromomycosis—particularly Japan (especially Kanto, Chuba).

PROTOZOA. *Leishmania* sp.—Taiwan.

HELMINTHS. Cutaneous larva migrans—particularly warmer areas; cercarial dermatitis—reports from Japan, Taiwan; sparganosis—particularly S China and S Japan; gongylonemiasis—China (rare reports).

ARTHROPODS. Scabies; pediculosis.

Meningitis, Encephalitis, and Viral Fevers

ARTHROPOD-BORNE VIRUSES

Dengue-like Fevers. Kunjin, Sindbis, Tembusu—widely distributed, rarely identified.

Hemorrhagic Fevers. Xinjiang—China; Crimean-Congo—China (southwestern border).

Meningoencephalitis. Japanese encephalitis (JE)—particularly China (except for western Xinging and Shanxi), Japan, Korea, Taiwan.

OTHER VIRUSES. Rabies—not reported from Japan, Hong Kong, Taiwan; hemorrhagic fever with renal syndrome (HFRS, muroid virus nephropathy)—E and NE China, Japan, Korea, probably E Mongolia.

BACTERIA. Bacterial meningitis and abscess.

HELMINTHS. *Angiostrongylus cantonensis*—particularly Taiwan.

Oropharyngeal and Respiratory Tract Infections

VIRUSES. Common respiratory agents.

BACTERIA. Streptococcal sore throat with rheumatic heart disease—particularly Mongolia; legionellosis—reported from China; tuberculosis; diphtheria.

FUNGI. Histoplasmosis—rare reports from Japan; *Penicillium marneffi*—rare reports from S China (Guangxi, Zhuang).

HELMINTHS. Paragonimiasis—widespread.

Other Parasitic Infections

PROTOZOA. Malaria (*P. falciparum* [primarily warmer areas], *P. vivax*, rarely *P. ovale,* and *P. malariae*)—China: no risk west of a line drawn from Tientsin in the north to the tip of India in the south, except at USSR border; risk-free regions include Xinjing, Gansu, Shaunxi, Xizang (Tibet); main cities and rural tourist attractions are free of risk; Hainan Island is infected. Risk-free: Hong Kong, Japan, Taiwan, Mongolia; no recent reports from Korea (Fig. 73–1).

Drug-resistant *P. falciparum*—see Table 121–1.

Toxoplasmosis—widespread and particularly Japan, rare in Taiwan; visceral leishmaniasis, including superficial lymph node involvement *(L.d. donovani)*—China (N and far W including central highlands), SW Mongolia (Fig. 76–3).

HELMINTHS. Filariasis—China (S coast including Hainan), Japan (S islands including Amamio and Ryukus but probably no recent transmission in Okinawa) (Fig. 85–2); tropical eosinophilia—China (S coast); dirofilariasis—Japan; *Echinococcus g. granulosus*—southern areas of subcontinent; *E.g. canadensis*—northern areas of subcontinent; *E. multilocularis*—China (mainly Xinjiang, Quing Rai, Ningxia, Gansu, and Sichven), Mongolia, C and N Japan (particularly Rebun Island in Hokkaido); gnathostomiasis—Japan (Kyushu, Shikoku, Honshu); thelazia conjunctivitis—rare reports from China, Japan, S. Korea; trichinosis—occasional reports, mostly from China; *Rhabditis* sp. (urinary tract)—rare reports, particularly from China.

Other Infections

VIRUSES. Cytomegalovirus; herpes simplex and zoster; Epstein-Barr; HIV/AIDS; retrovirus-associated myelopathy; swine vesicular disease—rare reports from Hong Kong; acute hemorrhagic conjunctivitis—occasional outbreaks.

CHLAMYDIAE. Lymphogranuloma venereum and trachoma.

RICKETTSIAE. Asian tick typhus (spotted fever); epidemic typhus—China (rare at present); scrub typhus—generally S of 45°N latitude in Japan, Taiwan, Korea; S and SE China; murine (flea-borne) typhus; rickettsialpox—Korea; Q fever—occasional reports; *Rickettsia sennetsu*—W Japan.

BACTERIA. Brucellosis (particularly *B. abortus*); leptospirosis; rat-bite fever; listeriosis—rare reports; plague—C China, Manchuria, Mongolia; melioidosis—Korea (Fig. 47–1); relapsing fever—W China (rare reports); tularemia—Japan; glanders—China (Manchuria), Mongolia.

UNCERTAIN ETIOLOGY. Idiopathic arteritis—particularly China, Japan; mucocutaneous lymph node (Kawasaki) disease—Japan, occasionally Korea; Behçet's syndrome—frequent reports from Japan (particularly Hokkaido); congestive cardiomyopathy—occasional reports.

Area 9—Central and Southeast Asia

(*Central:* Afghanistan, Bangladesh, Bhutan, Cambodia, India, Maldive Islands, Nepal, Pakistan, Sri Lanka; *Southeast:* Brunei, Burma, Indonesia, Laos, Kampuchea, Malaysia, Philippines, Singapore, Thailand, Vietnam)

Enteric Infections

VIRUSES. Enterovirus group; hepatitis A, B, C, delta; hepatitis E— reported from India.

BACTERIA. Cholera—intermittent reports from most countries; diarrhea-producing *E. coli; Campylobacter* sp.; shigellosis; salmonellosis (including typhoid and paratyphoid fevers); *Yersinia* sp; *Plesiomonas shigelloides*—particularly Bangladesh; *Vibrio parahaemolyticus*—particularly Thailand (Bangkok), India; *Clostridium perfringins* type C—rare reports from Indonesia, Thailand, Malaysia; *Edwardsiella tarda*—W Malaysia, rare elsewhere.

PROTOZOA. Amebiasis; giardiasis; balantidiasis; cryptosporidiosis; isosporosis—particularly Philippines.

HELMINTHS. Ascariasis; hookworm; trichuriasis; *Strongyloides stercoralis; Strongyloides* sp.—Indonesia (Irian Jaya); beef and dwarf tapeworms; pork tapeworm (including cysticercosis)—particularly India; fish tapeworm—particularly Bangladesh; clonorchiasis—particularly Indonesia and N Vietnam; opisthorchiasis—particularly N and E Thailand, SW Laos, Malaysia, Vietnam, India; *Schistosoma japonicum*—Indonesia (Napu and Lundu Valleys in Celebes, with single report from N Java), Philippines (S Luzon, NE Leyte, SE Mindanao, Mindoro, Samar), Malaysia Peninsula (C Perak and C Phang) (Fig. 96–8); *Schistosoma* sp. (resembling *S. japonicum*)—Malaysia (Malay area); *S. mekongi*—Mekong River Valley (Kampuchea, W Laos [Khong Island], E Thailand); trichostrongyliasis—C Asia, particularly Assam in India, Indonesia; heterophyiasis—W India, Malaysia, N Thailand, Philippines; fasciolopsiasis—Bangladesh (Dacca District), E India, E Pakistan, Kampuchea, Laos, N Vietnam, C Thailand, Indonesia (Kalimantan, Sumatra); echinostomiasis—In-

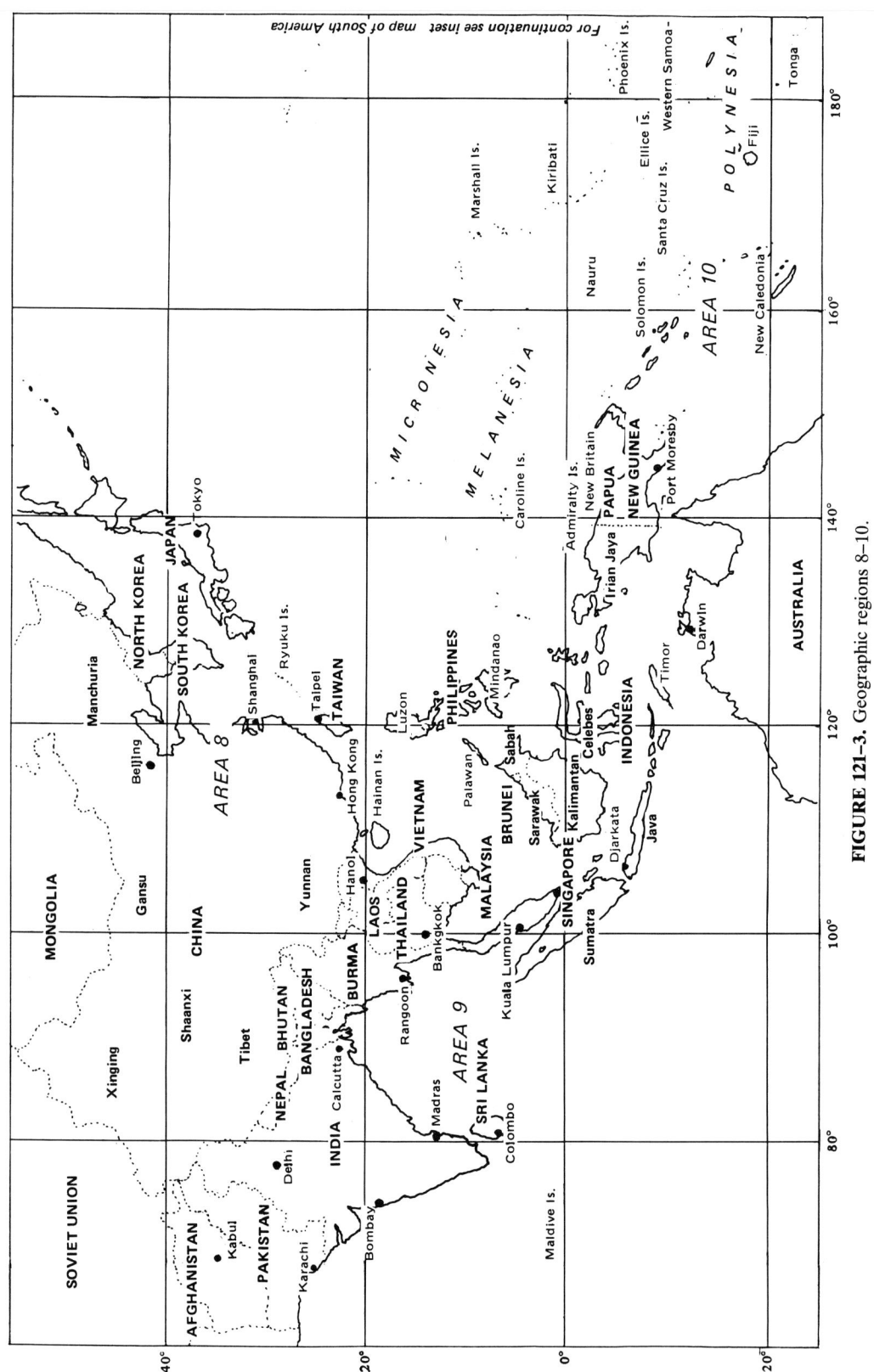

FIGURE 121-3. Geographic regions 8–10.

dia (Madras, Assam), Indonesia (C Sulawesi, Java), Malaysia, Singapore, NE Thailand, Philippines (particularly Ilocos Sur); gastrodisciasis—E India, Kampuchea, Laos, Vietnam, Malaysia; gnathostomiasis—particularly Burma; also India (Bengal), C Thailand.

Rare. Esophagostomiasis—tropical areas; *Inermicapsifer* sp.—Malaysia, Philippines, Thailand; *Ternidens deminutus*—India, Indonesia; *Bertiella* sp.—India, SE Asia, Philippines; *Capillaria philippinensis*—Philippines (N and W Luzon, NE Mindanao), S Thailand; *metagonimiasis*—Philippines; *Raillietina* sp.—Philippines, Thailand; *Poikilorchis congolensis*—Malaysia (Sarawak); *Stellantchasmus falcatus*—India, Philippines; *Phaneropsolus bonnei*—N Thailand, Indonesia (Java).

OTHER. Pentastomiasis—particularly Malaysia.

UNCERTAIN ETIOLOGY. Tropical sprue—particularly India, Sri Lanka, Burma, Vietnam, Laos, Kampuchea, Indonesia, Philippines.

Skin and Subcutaneous Infections

VIRUSES. Molluscum contagiosum.

BACTERIA. Anthrax; erysipeloid; erythrasma; leprosy; yaws—particularly W Burma, Indonesia (except Java), Malaysia, Sri Lanka; chancroid—common; cutaneous diphtheria; mycobacterial ulcer—particularly Malaysia; granuloma inguinale—particularly India, Indonesia.

FUNGI. Common dermatophytoses; tinea nigra; *Malassezia tropica;* tinea imbricata—particularly S India, Sri Lanka, and SE Asia; black piedra—particularly forested areas; subcutaneous phycomycosis—particularly Indonesia; sporotrichosis—occasional reports; chromomycosis; mycetoma; rhinosporidiosis—particularly India and Sri Lanka.

PROTOZOA. Cutaneous leishmaniasis—India (Pakistan border areas), Afghanistan (Fig. 76–3).

HELMINTHS. Cutaneous larva migrans; cercarial dermatitis—reported from India, Malaysia, Philippines; dracunculiasis—S and W India, S and C Pakistan, Afghanistan, Bangladesh; sporadic foci in Indonesia (Fig. 89–3); sparganosis—occasional reports.

ARTHROPODS. Tungiasis—particularly Pakistan, W coast of India; scabies; pediculosis.

UNCERTAIN ETIOLOGY. Granuloma multiforme—Indonesia (Sumba); endemic elephantiasis—India (soil-related and probably not infectious); ainhum—C Asia.

Meningitis, Encephalitis, and Viral Fevers

ARTHROPOD-BORNE VIRUSES
Undifferentiated Fevers. Phlebotomus—Pakistan.
Dengue (Serotypes 1, 2, 3, 4). Region-wide.
Dengue-like Fevers. Region-wide and particularly Philippines, Thailand; chikungunya—particularly Burma, S India; Sindbis—particularly India, Indonesia (Kalimantan), Malaysia, Brunei, Philippines; West Nile—India, Pakistan, Malaysia, Indonesia (Kalimantan).
Hemorrhagic Fevers. Dengue hemorrhagic fever—reported in Vietnam, Thailand, Singapore, Malaysia,

Laos, Indonesia; Crimean-Congo—infrequent reports from W Pakistan, India (Tamil Nadu and Rajasthan); Hazara—W Pakistan; chikungunya—hemorrhagic cases recently in Indonesia; Kyasanur Forest disease—India (Shimoga, N and S Kanara, Chickamagaloor districts in Karnataka State).

Meningoencephalitis. Japanese encephalitis (JE)—throughout region, especially Thailand, Burma, Nepal, Bangladesh, Sri Lanka, and India (West Bengal, Assam, Tamil Nadu, Andhra Pradesh, Arunachal Pradesh, Rajasthan).

OTHER VIRUSES. Rabies—all areas except Singapore, Timor and Irian Jaya in Indonesia, and Palawan, Philippines; epidemic hemorrhagic fever (hemorrhagic fever with renal syndrome, HFRS)—C Asia (northern areas).

BACTERIA. Bacterial meningitis and abscess.

PROTOZOA. Amebic meningoencephalitis—C Asia (rare reports).

HELMINTHS. *Angiostrongylus cantonesis*—particularly Thailand; also Indonesia, Philippines, Vietnam, SW India.

Oropharyngeal and Respiratory Tract Infections

VIRUSES. Common respiratory agents.

CHLAMYDIAE. Psittacosis.

BACTERIA. Streptococcal sore throat with rheumatic heart disease—particularly common in N and C Asia, Sri Lanka, Philippines; tuberculosis; diphtheria.

FUNGI. Histoplasmosis—occasional reports from Bangladesh, India, S Malay Peninsula, Indonesia (Java and W Irian Jaya), Philippines; rhinosporidiosis—India, Sri Lanka, Indonesia, Malaysia, Philippines.

PROTOZOA. Pneumocystis pneumonia.

HELMINTHS. Paragonimiasis—widespread.

Other Parasitic Infections

PROTOZOA. Malaria (*P. falciparum, P. vivax,* and rarely, *P. malariae*)—throughout except risk-free areas as follows: higher altitudes of NC Asia, including Katmandu, Nepal; Colombo, Sri Lanka; Malé, Maldive Islands; Brunei; Singapore (Fig. 73–1); *P. ovale*—particularly N Vietnam, Thailand.

Drug-resistant *P. falciparum*—see Table 121–1.

Visceral leishmaniasis (*L. b. donovani*)—Bangladesh, India (Bihar, Assam, Tripura, West Bengal, Sikkim), S Nepal, NE Pakistan, and occasionally Malaysia; (*L. b. infantum*)—W Burma (Fig. 76–3); *Trypanosoma* sp.—rare reports from C India, Malaysia.

HELMINTHS. Filariasis (*W. bancrofti, B. malayi*)—all countries and islands; high altitudes risk-free (Fig. 85–2); Timore microfilaria—Indonesia (Timore, Flores, Sunda) (Fig. 85–2); tropical eosinophilia—particularly S India, Sri Lanka, Malaysia, Philippines; *Schistosoma haematobium*—India (Bombay area) (Fig. 96–8); *Echinococcus granulosus*—particularly C India, N Pakistan, Laos, Philippines, N Vietnam; *E. multilocularis*—single report from N India (Kashmir); *trichinosis*—particularly N Thailand, rare elsewhere; visceral larval granulomatosis (including ocular larva migrans)—reported from Philippines; thelazia conjunctivitis—rare reports from Thailand.

Other Infections

VIRUSES. Acute hemorrhagic conjunctivitis—occasional outbreaks; cytomegalovirus; herpes simplex and zoster; Epstein-Barr; HIV/AIDS; retrovirus-associated myelopathy; hand, foot, and mouth disease—Singapore (1981).

CHLAMYDIAE. Lymphogranuloma venereum and trachoma.

RICKETTSIAE. Epidemic typhus—particularly NC Asian highlands; endemic typhus—widespread, particularly Burma; scrub typhus—throughout, including islands, to 3800 m altitude; tick typhus *(R. conorii)*—India; probably Malaysia, Pakistan, and Thailand; Q fever.

BACTERIA. Plague—N Afghanistan, India (N tip and NW of Madras), Nepal, N Pakistan, Indonesia (C Java), Malaysia (Sarawak), Vietnam, probably Bhutan; brucellosis (primarily *B. abortus*)—particularly India; chromobacteriosis—SE Asia (rare reports); leptospirosis; rat-bite fever; relapsing fever (tick-borne)—C Asia; melioidosis—SE Asia, India, Sri Lanka, Philippines, rarely Pakistan; glanders—probably present; chromobacteriosis—rare reports, tropical and subtropical areas.

UNCERTAIN ETIOLOGY. Indian cor pulmonale—N India (including Delhi); restrictive cardiomyopathy (endomyocardial fibrosis)—S India and Delhi area; congestive cardiomyopathy—occasional reports; hypertrophic cardiomyopathy and idiopathic arteritis—rare reports.

Area 10—Oceania

(Australia, New Zealand; *Micronesia:* Caroline, Ellis, Mariana [including Guam], Marshall; *Melanesia:* Admiralty, Fiji, New Britain, New Caledonia, Vanuatu, Loyalty, Papua New Guinea [PNG], Santa Cruz, Solomon; *Polynesia:* Cook, Marquesas, Phoenix, Pitcairn, Samoa, Society [including Tahiti], Takelau)

Enteric Infections

VIRUSES. Enterovirus group; hepatitis A, B, C; Norwalk—particularly Australia.

BACTERIA. Diarrhea-producing *E. coli; Campylobacter* sp.; salmonellosis (including typhoid and paratyphoid fevers); shigellosis; *Vibrio parahaemolyticus; Yersinia* sp.; *Clostridium perfringens* type C (pig-bel)—PNG highlands; cholera—Caroline Islands (Truk) (1983).

PROTOZOA. Amebiasis; giardiasis; isosporosis; balantidiasis—particularly PNG.

HELMINTHS. Ascariasis; hookworm; trichuriasis; *Strongyloides stercoralis; Strongyloides* sp. causing swollen belly syndrome—W PNG; beef and pork tapeworms; dwarf tapeworms *(Hymenolepis nana)*—widespread; *H. diminuta*—particularly PNG highlands; fish tapeworm—

Australia, PNG; trichostrongyliasis—particularly NW Australia; fascioliasis—Australia.

Rare. *Raillietina* sp.—N Australia; *Stellantchasmus falcatus*—N Australia.

Skin and Subcutaneous Infections

VIRUSES. Molluscum contagiosum.

BACTERIA. Anthrax—Australia, PNG, Polynesia; cutaneous diphtheria—islands; mycobacterial ulcer—C Australia, PNG; yaws—PNG; previously reported from N Australia and islands; leprosy—throughout; rare in New Zealand; chancroid—particularly tropical areas; granuloma inguinale—particularly PNG; *Vibrio parahaemolyticus* wound infection—Australia.

FUNGI. Common dermatophytoses; tinea imbricata—particularly warmer areas; *Microsporum distortum*—particularly S New Zealand.

HELMINTHS. Cercarial dermatitis—reported from Australia, New Zealand; cutaneous dirofilariasis—Australia.

ARTHROPODS. Scabies; pediculosis.

UNCERTAIN ETIOLOGY. Tumoral calcinosis—particularly PNG.

Meningitis, Encephalitis, and Viral Fevers

ARTHROPOD-BORNE VIRUSES

Dengue. Widespread (NE Australia only, not in New Zealand).

Dengue-like Fevers. Ross River (epidemic polyarthritis)—particularly E Australia, Samoa, Cook, Fiji, PNG, Solomon, Vanuatu, Tonga; Sindbis—Australia.

Hemorrhagic Fevers. Dengue (occasional manifestation); Murray Valley—E Australia, PNG, and E Indonesia (New Guinea); Kunjin—Australia.

OTHER VIRUSES. Barmah Forest—Australia; rabies is not reported from Oceania; encephalomyocarditis—particularly islands; kuru—PNG (probably no recent transmission).

BACTERIA. Bacterial meningitis and abscess.

PROTOZOA. Amebic meningoencephalitis—reports from Australia, New Zealand.

HELMINTHS. *Angiostrongylus cantonensis*—Australia (particularly Cherbourg area), most islands (particularly New Caledonia, Tahiti, Vanuatu).

Oropharyngeal and Respiratory Tract Infections

VIRUSES. Common respiratory agents.

CHLAMYDIAE. Psittacosis.

BACTERIA. Diphtheria—probably cosmopolitan; tuberculosis; streptococcal sore throat with rheumatic heart disease—particularly Cook Islands and French Polynesia.

FUNGI. Histoplasmosis—Australia.

HELMINTHS. Paragonimiasis—PNG; gongylonemiasis—rare reports from Australia and New Zealand.

Other Parasitic Infections

PROTOZOA. Malaria (*P. falciparum, P. vivax, P. malariae*, and drug-resistant *P. falciparum*)—PNG, Solomon group, Vanuatu (Fig. 73–1); see Table 121–1; toxoplasmosis.

HELMINTHS. *Echinococcus granulosus*—SE Australia (except Tasmania); New Zealand (little or no recent transmission); *E. multilocularis*—Australia (rare reports); *Wuchereria bancrofti*—NE Australia, most islands (particularly Cook), rarely New Zealand (Fig. 85–2); tropical eosinophilia—particularly Samoa, Cook.

Rare. Trichinosis—New Zealand; visceral larval granulomatosis (including ocular larva migrans) reported from Australia; *Raillietina* sp.—N Australia; *Stellantchasmus falcatus*—N Australia.

UNCERTAIN ETIOLOGY. Tropical sprue—N Australia, probably PNG.

Other Infections

VIRUSES. Acute hemorrhagic conjunctivitis—occasional outbreaks; cytomegalovirus; HIV/AIDS—Australia, New Zealand, PNG, and probably most other islands; retrovirus-associated myelopathy.

CHLAMYDIAE. Lymphogranuloma venereum and trachoma—particularly warmer areas.

RICKETTSIAE. Queensland tick typhus—Australia (N and S Queensland); scrub typhus—particularly Australia (N coastal Queensland), PNG, E Solomon, Vanuatu; generally does not occur S of 20°S latitude; Q fever, including endocarditis.

BACTERIA. Leptospirosis—recent reports in French Polynesia and Australia; melioidosis—particularly N Australia, PNG, rarely Guam; brucellosis—Australia, New Zealand, Polynesia; Lyme disease—Australia (coastal area N of Sydney).

UNCERTAIN ETIOLOGY. Peripartum cardiomyopathy—rare reports; chronic fatigue syndrome (epidemic neuromyasthenia, myalgic encephalomyelitis).

NONINFECTIOUS BUT SIMULATING INFECTION. Ciguatera fish poisoning—particularly New Caledonia, New Zealand, Polynesia.

TABLE 121–1. DRUG-RESISTANT FALCIPARUM MALARIA REGISTRY

Users of this registry should be aware of the following limitations or caveats: (1) for many countries, the reported geographic distribution of drug-resistant strains, particularly for drugs other than chloroquine, may be more indicative of the distribution of researchers than of the organism(s): (2) the number and frequency of reports in themselves do not always equate to the overall importance of resistance strains in a given country; and (3) terminology usage is not consistent.

Africa

The rapid spread of chloroquine-resistant falciparum malaria westward across sub-Saharan Africa has been well documented. However, the geographic distribution of resistance to other antimalarials is more difficult to assess, with the few published studies often consisting of surveys of small numbers of travelers returning from Africa with clinical malaria. These isolated reports may or may not accurately reflect the actual distribution of strains resistant to these antimalarials.

Country	Malaria Endemic Areas	Drug Resistance[1]	Reported Area of Resistance/Remarks
Angola	Countrywide, including urban areas	chloroquine (in vivo)	Northwest provinces of Cuanza Sul, Luanda, and Malanje
		Fansidar (in vivo)	Northern coastal province of Luanda
		proguanil (suspected)	Origin of infection unspecified/based on study of Namibian refugees
Benin	Countrywide, including urban areas	chloroquine (in vivo)	Southern provinces of Zou and Atlantique (Cotonou region)
		Fansidar (suspected)	Unspecified
		mefloquine (in vitro)	Southern provinces of Zou (Dassa Zoume) and Atlantique (Cotonou region)
		quinine (in vitro)	Unspecified
Botswana	Primarily northern areas (north of 21° S latitude); sporadic along southeastern border with South Africa	chloroquine (unspecified)	Presumed to occur, but original documentation not available for confirmation
Burkina Faso	Countrywide, including urban areas	chloroquine (in vitro) mefloquine (in vitro) quinine (in vitro)	Centre Province Unspecified Unspecified
Burundi	Countrywide, including urban areas	amodiaquine (in vivo) chloroquine (suspected)	Western border area (Ruzizi plain) Western border area (including Bujumbura)

Table continued on following page

TABLE 121–1. DRUG-RESISTANT FALCIPARUM MALARIA REGISTRY Continued

Africa

Country	Malaria Endemic Areas	Drug Resistance[1]	Reported Area of Resistance/Remarks
		chlorproguanil (suspected)	Western border area (Ruzizi Valley)
		quinine (in vitro)	Unspecified
Cameroon	Countrywide, including urban areas	amodiaquine (in vivo)	Coastal (Doula) and south central (Yaounde)
		chloroquine (in vivo)	Coastal, southwest, south central, and northern
		Fansidar (suspected)	Coastal (Doula)
		mefloquine (in vivo)	Northern (Garoua), Maroua and eastern (Bertoua)
		quinine (in vitro)	Coastal and northern (Garoua)
Central African Republic	Countrywide, including urban areas	amodiaquine (in vitro)	Unspecified
		chloroquine (in vivo)	Southern (Bangui, Bouar, Bambari, Bangassou)
		Fansidar (suspected)	Southwest (Berberati) prophylactic-therapeutic breakthrough
		quinine (in vitro)	Unspecified
Chad	Countrywide, including urban areas, especially southern half of the country	chloroquine (in vitro)	Southwestern corner (N'djamena)
		mefloquine (in vitro)	Southwestern corner
Comoros	Countrywide, including urban areas	chloroquine (in vivo)	Primarily reported from Njazidja (Grande Comora)
Congo	Countrywide, including urban areas	amodiaquine (in vivo)	Southern (Pointe-Noire, Brazzaville)
		chloroquine (in vivo)	Southern (Pointe-Noire, Brazzaville) and forest mountains of Mayombe and Chaillu
		quinine (in vitro)	Unspecified
Côte d'Ivoire	Countrywide, including urban areas	chloroquine (in vivo)	Coastal and central (including Abidjan and Bouake)
		Fansidar (suspected)	Unspecified
		mefloquine (in vivo)	Origin of infection unspecified/individual also traveled to Senegal
		quinine (in vitro)	Unspecified
Equatorial Guinea	Countrywide, including urban areas	chloroquine (in vitro)	Bioko Island
		mefloquine (in vitro)	Unspecified
Ethiopia	Countrywide, below 2000 m, including urban areas (Addis Ababa is risk-free)	chloroquine (in vivo)	Along southern and western borders
Gabon	Countrywide, including urban areas	amodiaquine (in vitro)	Unspecified
		chloroquine (in vivo)	Western (including Port Gentil and Libreville), southeast (Franceville), south central (Lebamba), and northeast (Makokou)
		Fansidar (suspected)	Western (Lambarene)
		quinine (in vitro)	Western and eastern (including Libreville and Franceville)
Gambia	Countrywide, including urban areas	chloroquine (in vitro)	West central (Farafenni)
		chlorproguanil (in vitro)	Farafenni vicinity
Ghana	Countrywide, including urban areas	chloroquine (in vivo)	Coastal (Accra)
		Fansidar (suspected)	Unspecified
		proguanil (suspected)	Unspecified
		quinine (suspected)	Unspecified/concomitant with Fansidar treatment failure
Guinea	Countrywide, including urban areas	chloroquine (in vitro)	Coastal region (Conakry, Boke)
		mefloquine (in vitro)	Southern coast (Conakry)
		quinine (in vitro)	Southern coast (Conakry)
Guinea-Bissau	Countrywide, including urban areas	chloroquine (unspecified)	Presumed to occur, but original documentation not available for confirmation
Kenya	Countrywide below 2500 m, including urban areas and game parks	amodiaquine (in vitro)	Unspecified
		chloroquine (in vivo)	Coastal, southern, and Lake Victoria region/presumably all malarious areas
		chlorproguanil (in vitro)	Coastal
		Fansidar (in vitro)	Coastal and Lake Victoria region

TABLE 121–1. DRUG-RESISTANT FALCIPARUM MALARIA REGISTRY *Continued*

Africa

Country	Malaria Endemic Areas	Drug Resistance[1]	Reported Area of Resistance/Remarks
		Maloprim (suspected)	Coastal
		mefloquine (in vitro)	Unspecified/additional presumptive prophylactic-therapeutic breakthroughs
		quinine (in vitro)	Unspecified
Liberia	Countrywide, including urban areas	chloroquine (in vitro)	Northwest (Zorzor)
		chlorproguanil (suspected)	Northeast (Yekepa)
		Fansidar (in vitro)	Northwest (Zorzor)
		mefloquine (in vitro)	Unspecified
		quinine (suspected)	Northwest (Zorzor)
Madagascar	Countrywide, including urban areas, particularly eastern coastal areas	amodiaquine (in vivo)	Eastern coast
		chloroquine (in vivo)	Presumably all malarious areas/widely reported
		quinine (suspected)	Central highlands/possible therapeutic breakthrough
Malawi	Countrywide, including urban areas	amodiaquine (in vivo)	Central (including Lilongwe)
		chloroquine (in vivo)	Presumably all malarious areas/widely reported
		Fansidar (suspected)	Concurrent Fansidar-quinine resistance
		proguanil (suspected)	Unspecified
		quinine (in vitro)	Unspecified
Mali	Countrywide, including urban areas, primarily in the southern half	chloroquine (in vitro)	South central (Bamako)
		mefloquine (in vitro)	Unspecified
Mauritania	Countrywide, except in the following northern areas: Dakhlet-Nouadhibou, Inchiri, Adrar, and Tiris-Zemour	chloroquine (unspecified)	Presumed to occur, but original documentation not available for confirmation
Mozambique	Countrywide, including urban areas	amodiaquine (in vivo)	Southern coast (Maputo), extreme northeast
		chloroquine (in vivo)	Primarily coastal (including Maputo, Beira, and inland as far as Nampula), Tete Southern coast (Maputo)
		Fansidar (in vivo)	Southern coast (Maputo)
		quinine (in vitro)	Unspecified
Namibia	Primarily in the northern areas of Ovamboland and Caprivi Strip, but now extending into central and southern areas	chloroquine (suspected)	Primarily northern
		proguanil (suspected)	See *Angola*
Niger	Countrywide, including urban areas	chloroquine (in vivo)	Southwest (including Niamey vicinity)
Nigeria	Countrywide, including urban areas	chloroquine (in vivo)	North central (Zaria) and southern (including Ibadan, Benue State, Anambra State)/suspected in Lagos, Port Harcourt, and Jos
		Fansidar (in vivo)	North central (Zaria) and southern (Benue State)/ based on a modified WHO 7-day in vivo test
		mefloquine (in vitro)	Southwest (Ibadan)
		quinine (suspected)	Unspecified/concomitant with Fansidar treatment failure
Rwanda	Countrywide, including urban areas	amodiaquine (in vivo)	Central, northwest, southeast (Kigali and Kibungo), and extreme south
		chloroquine (in vivo)	Central, northwest, southeast, and extreme south/presumably all malarious areas
		Fansidar (in vivo)	Central, northwest, and southeast (Kigali and Kibungo)
Senegal	Countrywide, including urban areas	chloroquine (in vivo)	West central (Dakar, Thies, Kaolack)
		mefloquine (in vivo)	Unspecified/see *Côte d'Ivoire*
		quinine (in vitro)	Central coast (Thies)
Sierra Leone	Countrywide, including urban areas	chloroquine (in vitro)	Unspecified/additional presumptive prophylactic breakthroughs
		mefloquine (in vitro)	Unspecified/treatment failure concomitant with halofantrine treatment

Table continued on following page

TABLE 121–1. DRUG-RESISTANT FALCIPARUM MALARIA REGISTRY Continued

Africa

Country	Malaria Endemic Areas	Drug Resistance[1]	Reported Area of Resistance/Remarks
Somalia	Countrywide, including urban areas	chloroquine (in vitro)	Southern coast (including Balcad, north of Mogadishu)
South Africa	Northeastern (Transvaal) low-altitude areas bordering Botswana, Zimbabwe, and Mozambique (including game parks), and the Natal coast north of 28°S latitude (Richard's Bay)	chloroquine (in vitro)	Coastal areas north of Richard's Bay (Natal-Kwazulu), northern Transvaal (including Venda)/reported as in vivo in Kwazulu
Sudan	Countrywide, including urban areas; possibly excluding desert areas of extreme north and northwest	chloroquine (in vivo)	Central and east central (including Khartoum vicinity)
Swaziland	Lowveld areas	chloroquine (in vivo)	Primarily eastern lowveld region
Tanzania	Countrywide below 1800 m, including urban areas; risk reportedly increasing in high plateau areas	amodiaquine (in vitro) chloroquine (in vivo) chlorproguanil (suspected) Fansidar (in vivo) mefloquine (in vivo) quinine (in vitro)	Northwest (Lake Victoria), Zanzibar, northeast (Tanga Region) Coastal, southeast, northeast, north central, Lake Victoria region, Zanzibar/presumably all malarious areas Central coast (Dar es Salaam) Lake Victoria, coastal, north central, northeast Northeast (Tanga Region) Northeast (Tanga Region)
Togo	Countrywide, including urban areas	chloroquine (in vivo) mefloquine (suspected) quinine (in vitro)	Central (Sokode) and south Unspecified (Benin/Togo) Unspecified
Uganda	Countrywide, including urban areas	chloroquine (unspecified)	Presumed to occur, but original documentation not available for confirmation
Zaire	Countrywide, including urban areas	amodiaquine (in vitro) chloroquine (in vivo) Fansidar (suspected) mefloquine (in vitro) quinine (in vitro)	Unspecified Presumably all malarious areas (including Kinshasa)/widely reported Unspecified Unspecified Unspecified
Zambia	Countrywide, including urban areas	amodiaquine (in vivo) chloroquine (in vivo) Fansidar (in vivo) quinine (in vivo)	Luapula (Lubwe), Northwestern (Kalene), Northern, and Copperbelt Provinces Luapula, Northern, Eastern, Central, Northwestern, and Copperbelt Provinces/presumably all malarious areas Copperbelt and Northern Provinces Copperbelt Province/additional presumptive treatment failure
Zimbabwe	Countrywide below 1200 m, including urban areas (city of Harare is risk-free)	chloroquine (in vivo) Fansidar (suspected) quinine (suspected)	Northern (including Zambezi Valley bordering Zambia) Zambezi Valley/based on alleged treatment failure Northern/based on alleged treatment failure

TABLE 121–1. DRUG-RESISTANT FALCIPARUM MALARIA REGISTRY Continued

Americas

The majority of reports of confirmed drug-resistant strains have been from Brazil, particularly in the Amazonian lowlands. Information from some other countries is more limited, and the status of drug-resistant falciparum malaria is therefore less certain. However, if strains resistant to an antimalarial appear to be well established in Brazil, the presence of similar strains in border areas of neighboring countries may be anticipated, even if not reported. Some strains of *Plasmodium vivax* in Colombia reportedly have exhibited resistance to chloroquine and amodiaquine.

Country	Malaria Endemic Areas	Drug Resistance[1]	Reported Area of Resistance/Remarks
Bolivia	Rural areas below 2500 m, east of the Andes	chloroquine (in vitro)	North central lowlands (Beni Dependency)/may be more widespread in areas adjacent to Brazil
Brazil	All areas of Acre, Amapa, Rondonia, and Roraima States; rural areas of Amazonas, Bahia, Espirito Santo, Goias, Maranhao, Mato Grosso do Sul, Para, Parana, Piaui, and Santa Catarina States	amodiaquine (in vivo)	Acre and Maranhao States/problem most severe in western Amazon region
		chloroquine (in vivo)	Likely present in all malarious areas/particularly severe in the Amazonian lowlands
		Fansidar (in vivo)	Acre and Maranhao States/may occur throughout the Amazonian lowlands
		mefloquine (in vitro) quinine (in vitro)	North central lowlands/likely present in Rondonia State Western, northern, and central/reduced sensitivity more common than actual resistance
Colombia	Rural areas below 800 m, except for the Caribbean islands of Providencia and San Andres	amodiaquine (in vitro)	Most malarious areas, except for Pacific and Caribbean coasts/relatively few cases reported
		chloroquine (in vivo)	Presumably all malarious areas /resistance found in nearly all patients tested in 1985
		Fansidar (in vivo)	Most malarious areas except for Pacific coast/less common than chloroquine resistance
		mefloquine (in vitro)	Extreme south central/not common
Ecuador	Rural and urban areas below 1500 m (Galápagos Islands are risk-free)	chloroquine (in vitro)	Extreme northwest and northeast
French Guiana	Countrywide, including urban areas	amodiaquine (in vitro) chloroquine (in vitro)	Unspecified/presumed countrywide Probably countrywide/more than 90% of recent isolates demonstrated resistance
		quinine (in vitro)	Unspecified
Guyana	All rural areas below 900 m, except for the coastal strip; risk exists in the outskirts of Georgetown	chloroquine (in vivo)	Unspecified/presumably all malarious areas
		Fansidar (in vivo)	South Guyana (Area IX)/may be more widespread, based on reported treatment failures
Mexico	Rural areas below 1000 m, including Pacific coast, from Guaymas south to Guatemala border; Gulf coast, from Tampico through the Yucatán Peninsula, and valleys of central Mexico	Chloroquine (suspected)	Northeastern Chiapas State, near border with Guatemala
Panama	All rural areas below 800 m, east of the Panama Canal, including the San Blas Islands, rural coastal areas west of the Panama Canal, and the periphery of Lake Gatun	chloroquine (in vitro)	Northern coast east of the Canal/unconfirmed reports from extreme western Bocas del Toro Province/present in all malarious areas east of the Canal
		Fansidar (in vitro)	North coast of Colon Province, east of the Canal/some strains resistant to pyrimethamine but susceptible to sulfadoxine
Peru	Rural areas below 1500 m in Amazonas, Cajamarca, Loreto, San Martin, and Ucayali Departments; rural coastal areas below 1500 m in Libertad, Lambayeque, Piura, and Tumbes Departments	chloroquine (undetermined, original document not available)	Extreme northeast/believed to be present in all northeastern malarious areas adjacent to Brazil

Table continued on following page

TABLE 121–1. DRUG-RESISTANT FALCIPARUM MALARIA REGISTRY *Continued*

Americas

Country	Malaria Endemic Areas	Drug Resistance[1]	Reported Area of Resistance/Remarks
Surinam	Countrywide except for the city of Paramaribo, a narrow coastal strip, and areas of the interior over 1300 m of altitude	chloroquine (in vivo)	Presumably all malarious areas/majority of studies done in eastern half of country
		Fansidar (in vivo)	Central and eastern areas/may be more widespread
Venezuela	Rural interior areas, especially in states bordering Brazil, Colombia, and Guyana. Foci exist in northern rural areas below 800 m	chloroquine (in vivo)	Southeastern area adjacent to Brazil/suspected to exist in all malarious areas
		mefloquine (in vitro)	South central areas, adjacent to Colombia/mefloquine had not been used as an antimalarial in Venezuela at the time the study was conducted
		Fansidar (suspected)	South central area adjacent to Colombia/reported as "in vivo," but lacking documentation

Asia and Oceania

Multiple drug–resistant falciparum malaria is common in this region, especially in southeast Asia. The large number of studies from Thailand reflects their research impetus. Similar drug resistance probably occurs in other South Asian countries but is unreported. **Recently published information indicates that strains of *Plasmodium vivax* in Papua New Guinea and the Solomon Islands have exhibited resistance to chloroquine.**

Country	Malaria Endemic Areas	Drug Resistance[1]	Reported Area of Resistance/Remarks
Afghanistan	Countrywide below 1500 m, including urban areas, except central highland (Kabul is risk-free)	chloroquine (in vivo)	Southeast border/low prevalence
Bangladesh	Countrywide, including urban areas (except Dhaka)	chloroquine (in vivo)	Eastern and northern borders/may be countrywide
		Fansidar (suspected)	Unspecified/clinical data unavailable; suspected along Burma border
Bhutan	Southern rural areas below 1700 m (Thimbu is risk-free)	chloroquine (in vivo)	Unspecified/probably widespread
		Fansidar (suspected)	Unspecified/clinical data unavailable
Burma (Myanmar)	Rural areas below 1500 m	amodiaquine (in vivo)	Unspecified/clinical data unavailable
		chloroquine (in vivo)	Widespread
		Fansidar (in vivo)	Widespread
		Fansimef (in vivo)	Central (Pegu Division)
		proguanil (in vivo)	Unspecified/clinical data unavailable
		quinine (in vivo)	Central (Pegu Division) and northeast (Shan State)
Cambodia	Countrywide below 1500 m, including urban areas	amodiaquine (in vivo)	Sporadic (west border)
		chloroquine (in vivo)	Widespread
		Fansidar (in vivo)	West border/may be more widespread
		Maloprim (in vivo)	Widespread (west border)
		mefloquine (suspected)	West border
		quinine (in vivo)	Southwest, northwest
		quinine-tetracycline (in vivo)	Sporadic (west border)
China, People's Republic of	Rural areas in southwestern and south central provinces below 1500 m	amodiaquine (in vivo)	Hainan Island
		chloroquine (in vivo)	Widespread (southern provinces and Hainan Island)
		Fansidar (in vivo)	Hainan Island/may be more widespread
		piperaquine (in vivo)	Hainan Island
		qinghaosu (in vivo)	Unspecified/clinical data unavailable
		quinine (suspected)	Hainan Island

TABLE 121–1. DRUG-RESISTANT FALCIPARUM MALARIA REGISTRY *Continued*

Asia and Oceania

Country	Malaria Endemic Areas	Drug Resistance[1]	Reported Area of Resistance/Remarks
India	Countrywide below 1350 m, including urban areas	amodiaquine (in vivo) chloroquine (in vivo) Fansidar (suspected)	Punjab/single clinical case Widespread in the east, sporadic in the south, central, and west/prevalence spreading west Central and south/infrequently used compound
Indonesia	Rural areas countrywide (including urban areas in Irian Jaya) below 1500 m	chloroquine (in vivo) Fansidar (in vivo) Fansimef (in vivo) mefloquine (in vivo) quinine (in vivo)	Widespread Irian Jaya/may be more widespread Irian Jaya Irian Jaya Irian Jaya
Laos	Countrywide, including urban areas (except Vientiane)	chloroquine (in vivo)	Widespread
Malaysia	Countrywide, including urban areas	chloroquine (in vivo) Fansidar (in vivo) mefloquine (in vitro) proguanil (in vivo)	Widespread Sabah and peninsula Peninsula Peninsula/clinical data outdated
Nepal	Southern rural areas below 1300 m (Katmandu is risk-free)	chloroquine (in vivo)	Central and western malarious areas/probably widespread
Pakistan	Countrywide below 1500 m, including urban areas	amodiaquine (in vivo) chloroquine (in vivo) Fansidar (in vivo)	East (Punjab) East Punjab/probably widespread East Punjab/limited reports, protocol undetermined
Papua New Guinea	Countrywide below 1500 m, including urban areas	amodiaquine (in vivo) chloroquine (in vivo) Fansidar (in vivo) Maloprim (suspected) proguanil (in vivo) quinine (suspected)	West Province Widespread Widespread Vivigandi/single clinical case Seak District Unspecified
Philippines	Rural areas below 1500 m (except provinces of Bohol, Catanduanes, Cebu, and Leyte)	amodiaquine (in vivo) chloroquine (in vivo) Fansidar (in vivo) mefloquine (in vitro) quinine (in vivo)	Luzon Luzon, Basilan, Samar, Mindanao, Palawan, Mindoro Islands, and Sulu Archipelago Luzon Unspecified/based on single published report Luzon
Solomon Islands	Countrywide, including urban areas	chloroquine (in vivo) Fansidar (suspected) quinine (suspected)	Widespread Unspecified/single clinical case Unspecified/single clinical case
Sri Lanka	Countrywide below 760 m, including urban areas (except Colombo)	chloroquine (in vivo) Fansidar (suspected)	Eastern province (Dambulla)/may be widespread Unspecified/single clinical case
Thailand	Rural areas below 1500 m (except coastal resort areas of Pattaya and Phuket)	amodiaquine (in vivo) chloroquine (in vivo) Fansidar (in vivo) Fansimef (in vivo) halofantrine mefloquine (in vivo) proguanil (in vivo) quinine (in vivo)	South (Yala) Widespread Widespread East and west borders West border/during clinical trials East and west borders West border South and east borders
Vanuatu	Countrywide, including urban areas (except Futuna Island)	chloroquine (in vivo) Fansidar (suspected) quinine (in vivo)	Widespread Unspecified/reported as "strongly suspected" Sporadic (Epi and Malakula Islands)
Vietnam	Countrywide below 1500 m, including urban areas (except Red and Mekong Deltas)	chloroquine (in vivo) Fansidar (in vivo) mefloquine (in vivo) proguanil (in vivo) quinine (in vivo)	Widespread Widespread Unspecified/clinical data unavailable Unspecified/clinical data unavailable Unspecified/clinical data unavailable

Table continued on following page

TABLE 121–1. DRUG-RESISTANT FALCIPARUM MALARIA REGISTRY Continued

Middle East

The spread of drug-resistant falciparum malaria has been delayed in this region because, except for the southwestern area of the Arabian Peninsula, *Plasmodium falciparum* is uncommon *(Plasmodium vivax* is the predominant species). Drug-resistant falciparum malaria has been reported only recently, and the majority of reports pertain to chloroquine. Since chloroquine remains largely effective, other drugs have not been widely used and only sporadic resistance has been reported.

Country	Malaria Endemic Areas	Drug Resistance[1]	Reported Area of Resistance/Remarks
Iran	Rural and possibly urban areas in south and southeast; rural areas in north below 1500 m	chloroquine (in vivo)	Southeast (Sistan-Baluchestan and Hormozgan) provinces/low prevalence
		mefloquine (in vitro)	Southeast/single published report
Oman	Inland areas of north-central Oman below 2000m, and the central plain north of Seeb, including urban areas	chloroquine (in vitro)	The first two confirmed cases of chloroquine-resistance were detected in Ibri district
Saudi Arabia	Rural and urban areas in southwest; rural areas in west below 2000 m	chloroquine (suspected)	No country-specific data/unconfirmed report from "southwestern Arabian peninsula."
Yemen	All areas in foothills (Tihama) and coastal areas below 1500m, including urban areas; rural ares in the highlands (Sana and Aden are risk-free)	chloroquine (suspected)	No country-specific data/unconfirmed report from "southwestern Arabian peninsula."

[1]Terms used in this column reflect the highest level of confidence that resistance for a particular drug exists in a country and do not imply that that particular evidence exists for the entire geographic extent of resistance. Also, the studies or reports themselves are not always consistent in the usage of terms—for example, reports citing on in vivo evidence do not always clearly differentiate between standard WHO protocol and extended clinical observations on malaria patients. Likewise, many reports on in vitro procedures do not clearly distinguish between resistance and decreased sensitivity. "Suspected" indicates that the report was based on alleged treatment or prophylactic failure.

PART XI

LABORATORY DIAGNOSIS OF PARASITIC DISEASES

GENERAL PRINCIPLES

In the majority of cases, parasitic diseases cannot be diagnosed on clinical grounds alone. Clinical signs and symptoms, together with the patient's travel history, may enable the clinician to use laboratory and other diagnostic aids more judiciously, but confirmation of a suspected diagnosis usually depends on the results of appropriate laboratory studies. The physician in practice in North America and Europe is increasingly confronted with exotic infections as a result of increased international travel and immigration from developing countries. The AIDS pandemic has brought with it an increased prevalence of many of the more common parasitic infections as well as some (e.g., cryptosporidiosis, microsporidiosis, pneumocystosis) that seldom cause symptomatic infections in immunocompetent persons.

Thus, competence of the laboratory becomes important. The techniques described (Chapters 122 and 123) should be available in the clinical parasitology laboratory, and many can be performed by the clinician in the field or in an emergency when technical assistance may not be at hand. A few of the techniques listed are not in general use in the clinical laboratory but have applicability in the field. At times it is not possible to make a diagnosis by isolation and identification of the parasite. Other techniques, such as x-ray, ultrasound, and magnetic resonance imaging, may be helpful in specific instances, such as in neurocysticercosis and hydatid disease. Serologic tests, which in recent years have become increasingly sensitive and selective, are often utilized to make the diagnosis or follow the results of treatment (Chapter 125). Many serologic tests can be performed successfully in the clinical laboratory or the field, whereas others require referral to specialized laboratories.

122. EXAMINATION OF STOOL SPECIMENS

Edward K. Markell

Many methods, some of general applicability, others serving only limited purposes, have been described for examination of stool specimens. For routine examination, it is best to employ standard techniques in order to become familiar with their advantages and limitations.

Time may be lost by using methods for purposes for which they were not intended, and identification of a parasite becomes difficult or impossible unless the correct method of examination is employed.

PHYSICAL CHARACTERISTICS OF THE SPECIMEN. The consistency of an unpreserved stool specimen is important, giving an indication of the organisms that it may contain. Trophozoites of the intestinal protozoa are usually found in liquid or soft stools but almost never in fully formed ones. Protozoan cysts are rarely seen in liquid stools, unless these are the result of administration of a cathartic, in which case both trophic and cystic forms may be present. Cysts will usually be found in fully formed specimens. Helminth eggs may be present in either liquid or formed stools, but as the liquid stool is usually very dilute, they may be difficult to detect in such specimens.

If the unpreserved specimen is available, its surface should be examined for macroscopic parasites. Pinworms may be seen on the surface, and tapeworm proglottids may be found there or in its interior. The stool should be broken up with applicator sticks to check for helminths. If bright red blood is seen on the surface of formed stools, it is most frequently a sign of bleeding hemorrhoids; bloody mucus in loose or liquid specimens is suggestive of amebic ulcerations in the large intestine, though it may be due to other conditions. Patches of mucus on the surface of a specimen, particularly if blood-tinged, should always be examined carefully for trophic amebas. Occult blood in a stool may be a result of intestinal bleeding caused by parasites, but it is more likely to be indicative of other gastrointestinal disorders.

The age of an unpreserved specimen is of great importance. Freshly passed specimens are essential for the detection of trophic amebas or flagellates. All liquid or soft stools are best examined *within one-half hour of the time of passage.* If this is impossible, part of the specimen should be preserved within this time for subsequent examination. The immediate examination of fully formed specimens is not as critical, but when they cannot be examined within 3 to 4 hours they should be preserved.

Examination of a freshly passed stool specimen is impractical in the field and often difficult to accomplish in an urban laboratory setting. Many laboratories now rely exclusively on specimens preserved immediately after passage in various fixative solutions. The specimens may then be submitted to the laboratory for examination at a convenient time. Kits containing these solutions are commercially available or may be prepared by the laboratory for distribution to patients. Some kits also allow for submission of an unpreserved portion of the specimen.

TECHNIQUES OF STOOL EXAMINATION. Unfortunately, no single technique of stool examination will yield satisfactory results, as none of the methods is equally applicable to the detection of trophic protozoa, cysts, and helminth eggs. For this reason, a combination of two or more is desirable.

Direct Wet Film. This method is most useful for the detection of trophic forms of amebas and flagellates but should be reserved for the examination of freshly passed liquid or soft stools or the mucoid portion of formed specimens. It allows the study of motility of the organisms, which is often characteristic and of value in making a precise identification. Protozoan cysts and helminth eggs may also be seen on wet film if they are present in large enough numbers; however, concentration methods are more efficient for their detection.

In the preparation of a wet film, a small portion of feces is mixed with a drop of normal saline on a clean slide; a coverslip is placed on the preparation; and it is first examined unstained. In making the wet film, it is best to take small amounts of material from several parts of the stool specimen. The film should not be too thick. A convenient rule of thumb is to prepare the film just thin enough so that ordinary newsprint can easily be read through it. After the wet film has been thoroughly checked for trophic amebas and flagellates, under low power of the microscope and using a low intensity of illumination, an iodine stain may be prepared.

Iodine stains the cysts of amebas and other protozoa, revealing some details that cannot be seen in the unstained preparation. Trophozoites are rapidly killed and are sometimes unidentifiable after iodine staining; the stain should not be applied until after the specimen has been thoroughly examined in the unstained condition. Gram's iodine or Lugol's solution will give satisfactory results, but modified D'Antoni's iodine solution is preferable.

A separate iodine stain may be prepared by the addition of a small drop of this reagent to a wet film of fecal material before it is covered, or the iodine may be added to the edge of the coverslip so that it gradually diffuses into the saline mount. It should be borne in mind that a concentrate of the stool may also be stained with iodine and will reveal, in larger numbers, any organisms that may be seen by direct examination of the iodine-stained specimen. Organisms present in such small numbers that they may not be seen at all on direct examination can at times be detected with ease after concentration of the specimen. The MIF stain will fix and stain both trophozoites and cysts; iodine stains will shrink and distort trophic amebas or flagellates.

Concentration Techniques. Concentration methods attempt the separation of protozoan cysts and helminth eggs from the bulk of fecal matter through differences in specific gravity (Fig. 122–1). With the various sedimentation methods, eggs and cysts, which are heavier than the suspending liquid, become concentrated in the bottom of a tube. Flotation of eggs and cysts involves use of a heavy liquid, and the lighter parasites rise to

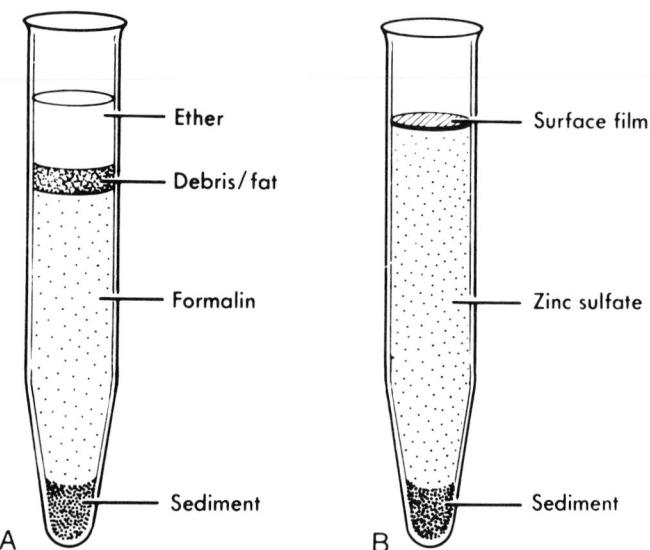

FIGURE 122–1. Fecal concentration procedures: various layers seen in tubes after centrifugation. *A,* Formalin-ether (or ethyl acetate). *B,* Zinc sulfate (the surface film should be within 2 to 3 mm of the tube rim). (Illustration by Nobuko Kitamura. From Garcia LS, Bruckner DA: Diagnostic Medical Parasitology. New York, Elsevier, 1988.)

its surface. The formalin-ether sedimentation technique of Ritchie is excellent for the concentration of both cysts and eggs and may be used with preserved specimens (Chapter 96). None of the sedimentation methods results in as good a separation of fecal debris from the eggs and cysts as can be achieved by a flotation method; the one recommended is a modification of the zinc sulfate centrifugal flotation method of Faust. The zinc sulfate flotation is also excellent for the recovery of protozoan cysts and most eggs, but it does not work well with trematode eggs or those of the broad fish tapeworm. Eggs of other types and protozoan cysts will be concentrated relatively free from fecal debris by this method. The laboratory worker should be familiar with both techniques.

After concentration, the diagnostic material is transferred to a microscope slide, and a drop of iodine is added to stain any protozoan cysts that may be present. Complete examination of every concentrate under low power of the microscope is required. A little practice will make it possible to recognize even the smaller protozoan cysts at this magnification, though for specific identification, high dry magnification may be necessary. Oil-immersion magnification serves no useful purpose, as the structural differentiation produced by iodine or MIF stains is not improved by higher magnification.

Stained Slides. Frequently it is impossible to make an exact identification of certain protozoa with a combination of the foregoing techniques. In such cases, the cytologic detail revealed by one of the permanent stains is essential. Such a stain will reveal significantly higher percentages of *Entamoeba histolytica* and other protozoan parasites than are detected when only direct examination and concentration methods are used. It is widely held that a report of *E. histolytica* infection should be made *only* when confirmed by a permanent stain.

When fresh stool specimens are used, a small quantity of feces is transferred to a clean slide with an applicator stick. The material is then streaked out in a thin uniform film. With a little practice, films of the correct thickness can be made regularly. Generally, formed stools are of the proper consistency for making films, but if the specimen is hard, it may be necessary to add a small amount of saline.

A liquid stool will sometimes fail to adhere to the slide; in such cases a thin layer of serum or of egg albumin, as used in mounting tissue sections, will increase adherence. When using fresh specimens, it is essential that the film be placed in fixative immediately after it is made; if it dries at any time, it will be useless.

When PVA-fixed material is used, slides are prepared as follows: The preserved specimen is again thoroughly mixed and may be strained through gauze to remove large particulate matter. After sedimentation, a portion of the fecal matter is removed with applicator sticks and placed on absorbent material, such as blotting paper, to remove the excess PVA. The material is then streaked onto slides, and the slides are allowed to dry for about 2 hours at room temperature or 1 hour at 37°C. They may then be stained or stored dry for subsequent staining.

Gomori's trichrome stain, originally intended for histologic use, has been adapted for use in staining intestinal protozoa and is the method most frequently used at present. It is not generally recognized that helminth eggs can be identified in the trichrome-stained fecal film, but with a little experience it is possible to recognize most by this method. More precise cytologic detail may be obtained with the use of iron hematoxylin, which may be preferable for staining SAF-preserved material. However, this stain requires considerable technical competence, whereas trichrome will give satisfactory results even in the hands of relatively inexperienced persons.

Artifacts. When examining stool specimens, it is possible to confuse some yeast, plant, or tissue cells or other commonly occurring objects with diagnostic forms of helminths or protozoa, especially with amebic cysts. A number of objects commonly found in the feces that may be mistaken for parasites are illustrated in Figure 122–2. The taxonomic status of *Blastocystis hominis*, illustrated in this figure, and its possible pathogenicity are still the subject of debate (Chapter 71.5).

NUMBER OF SPECIMENS TO BE EXAMINED. The number of stools that should be examined will depend on the purpose for which the examination is made. If one is interested only in determining the presence or absence of intestinal or hepatic helminth parasites, one or two examinations may be sufficient if concentration methods are used, as these methods are very efficient in the detection of small numbers of eggs. On the other hand, Sawitz and Faust (1942) stated that a single stool examination, even if a combination of techniques is used, will uncover somewhat under 50% of *Entamoeba histolytica* infections, and that at least six examinations are necessary if over 90% accuracy is to be obtained. This is shown graphically in Figure 122–3. These percentages apply to normally passed stools only. Many authorities recommend the routine use of purged

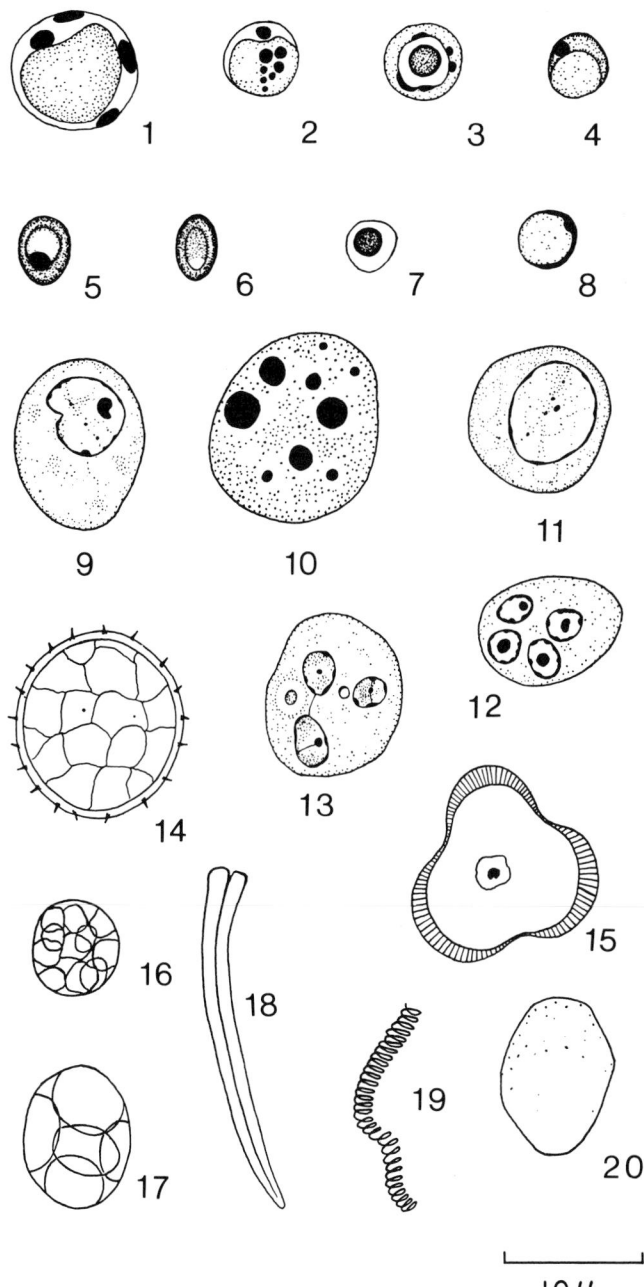

FIGURE 122–2. Various structures seen in stool preparations: *1, 2, 4, Blastocystis hominis; 3, 5, 6, 7, 8,* various yeasts; *9, 11,* squamous cells from rectal mucosa; *10,* deteriorated macrophage without nucleus; *12, 13,* polymorphonuclear leukocytes; *14, 15,* "pollen grains"; *16, 17,* aggregates of starch granules; *18,* plant hair; *19,* vegetable spiral; *20,* amorphous vegetable material, superficially resembling helminth egg or protozoan cyst. (From Markell EK, Voge M, John DT: Medical Parasitology. Philadelphia, W.B. Saunders, 1986.)

stools if one is searching for *Entamoeba histolytica*, since purged specimens may increase the chances of finding parasites. Purged specimens must be examined or placed in a fixative solution immediately, or they are worthless. If one has the facilities to collect purged specimens and *examine them immediately after they have been passed*, this procedure will probably increase the percentage of positive results. Castor and mineral oils must be

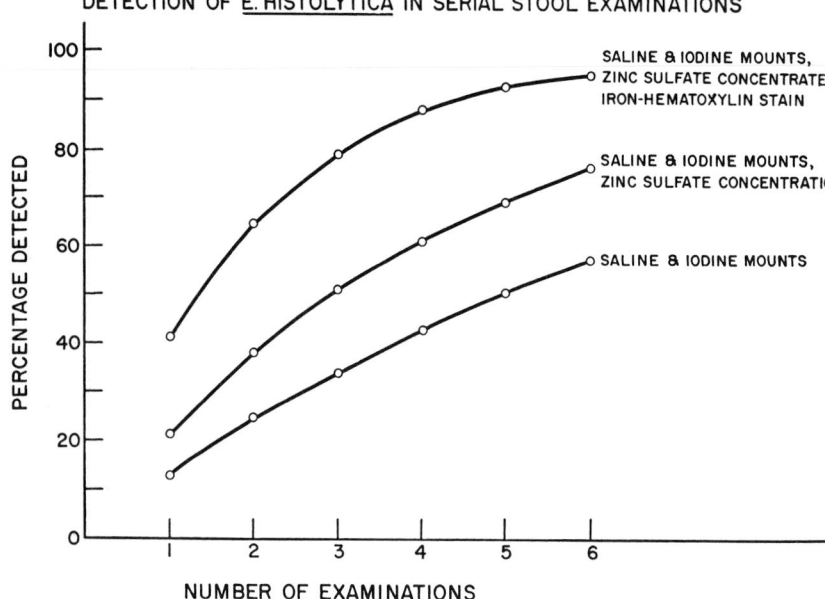

DETECTION OF E. HISTOLYTICA IN SERIAL STOOL EXAMINATIONS

FIGURE 122–3. Probability of detecting *Entamoeba histolytica* by successive stool examinations, using various techniques. (Based on figures from Sawitz and Faust, 1942. From Markell EK, Voge M, John DT: Medical Parasitology. Philadelphia, W.B. Saunders, 1986.)

avoided, as they will make examination of the specimen almost impossible. A saline purge of Epsom salts or Fleet's Phospho-Soda is recommended. Parasites in the first bowel movement will probably be distorted; those in the second and subsequent movements will most likely be recognizable.

SUBSTANCES THAT INTERFERE WITH STOOL EXAMINATIONS. Castor oil or mineral oil should not be administered prior to the collection of stool specimens. Antibiotics that affect the intestinal flora, administered within the preceding month, will decrease the chances of finding intestinal protozoa, as will antimalarials, e.g., chloroquine. Stools passed for about a week after the administration of barium cannot be examined for parasites, as the barium interferes with microscopy. Enemas of any type should be avoided. Compounds containing kaolin and bismuth, milk of magnesia, and antacids will also interfere with the examination for parasites, as will the presence of urine in the specimen.

PRESERVATION OF STOOL SPECIMENS. The trophic protozoa contained in a stool specimen begin to deteriorate almost as soon as the stool is passed. If the specimen cannot be examined promptly, a portion should be preserved for subsequent use. MIF solution will preserve the specimen for some months and also stain it for examination. A permanent preparation cannot be made from MIF-preserved material, and identification must be made on the basis of detail revealed by Merthiolate and iodine.

If one desires to make permanent stains at a later date, PVA or SAF fixative solutions should be used. PVA-preserved material retains excellent staining properties for at least a month, after which time it slowly deteriorates. SAF fixative has the advantage of not containing mercuric chloride but is technically a little more difficult to use. If a helminth infection is suspected, a portion of the specimen should be preserved in formol-saline.

STAINS FOR DIRECT SMEARS
Modified D'Antoni's Iodine

Distilled water	100 ml
Potassium iodide	1 gm
Powdered iodine crystals	1.5 gm

The potassium iodide solution should be saturated with iodine, with some excess remaining in the bottle. Store in brown, glass-stoppered bottles in the dark. The solution is ready for use after 4 days, and sufficient quantity for daily use is decanted into a brown glass dropping bottle and discarded after 1 day. The stock solution remains good as long as an excess of iodine remains in the bottle.

Lugol's Solution

Distilled water	100 ml
Potassium iodide	10 gm
Iodine crystals	5 gm

Gram's Iodine

Lugol's solution	1 part
Distilled water	14 parts

MIF Stain-Preservative Solution
Stock MF solution

Distilled water	250 ml
Tincture of Merthiolate	200 ml
Formaldehyde	25 ml
Glycerin	5 ml

This solution is stored in brown glass bottles. For use, it is combined with fresh Lugol's solution (not over 1 week old) in the following manner:

1. Measure 2.35 ml of stock MF solution into a small test tube, and stopper with a cork.

2. Measure 0.15 ml of Lugol's solution into a second tube, and close with a rubber stopper.

The two solutions are combined immediately before

addition of the fecal specimen. The amount of fecal material to be added to this volume of preservative should be about 0.25 gm. Break up the specimen in the MIF solution and mix thoroughly. The specimen may be examined immediately or stored in a well-stoppered tube; it will retain a good stain for some months. After storage, it will be found that most protozoa and helminth eggs occur in the upper layers of sedimented feces. A drop of mixed supernatant fluid and feces is withdrawn, placed on a slide, and covered with a coverslip.

PRESERVATIVE SOLUTIONS

PVA Fixative Solution.* This fixative, which consists of polyvinyl alcohol, glycerin, glacial acetic acid, and Schaudinn's solution, will keep indefinitely but must not be subjected to extremes of temperature. It is convenient to dispense the PVA fixative solution in screw-capped bottles, in approximately 5 ml quantities. To this volume of fixative, approximately 1 gm of feces may be added. It must be well broken up and thoroughly mixed with the preservative solution. The solution preserves both trophozoites and cysts of protozoa; most eggs are recognizable after PVA preservation. Protozoa remain stainable for at least 1 month. To prepare slides for staining, shake the preserved specimen well or mix contents with two applicator sticks. Pour some of the PVA mixture onto blotting paper and allow to stand for a few minutes. Apply stool material to slide in the manner described earlier, and dry for 2 hours at 37°C, or overnight at room temperature, before staining. The dry unstained slides may be mailed in this condition if necessary. This method is particularly useful because outpatients may be given vials containing PVA fixative and given instructions on how to fix their own stool specimens immediately after passage. If desirable, an entire series of specimens may be brought in at one time after all have been collected.

Schaudinn's Solution

```
Mercuric chloride, saturated aqueous .... 2 parts
Ethyl alcohol, 95% ........................ 1 part
```

Glacial acetic acid is added to Schaudinn's solution in the proportion of 1 part acetic acid to 19 parts of stock immediately before use.

SAF Fixative Solution (Yang and Scholten, 1977). Like PVA, the sodium acetate–acetic acid–formalin (SAF) fixative-preservative may be used for the preservation of material, which can then be concentrated by the formol-ether technique or made into permanent stained smears. The fixative is more liquid than PVA, and the preserved specimen must be centrifuged after straining through gauze and the sediment used to prepare smears for staining; adherence to the glass slide may be improved if the slide is coated with albumin. After drying, the slides may be placed in 70% alcohol.

---

*Obtainable from Medical Chemical Corporation, P.O. Box 445, Santa Monica, CA 90404; Scientific Products, 17111 Red Hill Ave., Irvine, CA, 92714; Marion Scientific, 30 Encore Ct., Newport Beach, CA 92663. However, many commercial stool-collection kits containing PVA fixative solution are now available.

The fixative solution is made up as follows:

```
Sodium acetate ........................... 1.5 gm
Acetic acid, glacial ...................... 2.0 ml
Formaldehyde, 40% ........................ 4.0 ml
Distilled water .......................... 92.5 ml
```

CONCENTRATION METHODS. Concentration of stool specimens to demonstrate cysts and eggs present in small numbers should be a routine part of the parasitologic examination. Special techniques have been devised for the concentration of nematode larvae in the stool. These are rather simple to perform and should be used whenever the presence of these parasites is suspected if they cannot be demonstrated by more direct forms of examination.

Modified Zinc-Sulfate Flotation

```
Zinc sulfate, USP ........................ 330 gm
Distilled water ................... to make 1 liter
```

This is only an approximation of the correct solution, which should have a specific gravity of 1.180. A reliable battery hydrometer must be used in adjusting to the correct specific gravity by the addition of zinc sulfate or water. Specific gravity is critical and must be checked frequently. The procedure is as follows:

1. Prepare a fecal suspension of approximately 1 ml of feces (more if dilute) in 10 to 15 times its volume of tap water.

2. Strain through two layers of wet gauze in a funnel, into a small test tube. Add 1 to 2 ml of ether, cork or use plastic wrap as stopper, shake (with caution), then fill with water to about 1 cm from top of tube.

3. Centrifuge for 45 seconds at approximately $2000 \times g$. Break up any "plug" that may have formed at the top, and decant supernatant.

4. Add 2 to 3 ml of tap water, shake or tap tube to resuspend sediment, and fill tube with tap water to 1 cm from top. Centrifuge as before.

5. Decant supernatant, add 2 to 3 ml zinc sulfate solution, resuspend, and fill tube with zinc sulfate solution to about 0.5 cm from top.

6. Centrifuge at $2000 \times g$ for 2 minutes. Do not "brake" the centrifuge or jar the tubes.

7. Without removing tubes from centrifuge, remove several loopfuls of material floating on surface (be careful not to go below surface film with wire loop), place on a slide with a drop of iodine solution, and cover with a coverslip.

Current's Modification of Sheather's Sugar Flotation for *Cryptosporidium*

Sheather's sugar solution:
```
Sucrose ....................... 500 gm
Tap water ..................... 320 ml
Phenol ........................ 6.5 gm
```

Boil sugar solution until clear. *Carefully* add phenol and stir. (Use fume hood.) Cool to room temperature.

1. Place 1 to 2 ml of fecal suspension in 12 ml conical centrifuge tube.

2. Add Sheather's sugar solution until tube is ¾ full.

3. Stir vigorously with applicator stick.

4. Fill tube to 1 to 2 cm from top.

5. Centrifuge at 300 × g for 5 to 10 minutes.

6. Transfer surface material to microscope slide by means of wire loop.

7. Cover with a coverslip and observe with phase-contrast microscopy.

The rounded oocysts, 4 to 6 μm in diameter, contain crescentic sporozoites that are best seen by this method.

STAINED SMEARS. For many years the somewhat laborious iron hematoxylin stain, in various forms, was the only one available for permanent stains of stool specimens. It is a very precise stain when properly used. The one recommended is the "short method" of the United States Naval Medical School.

Iron Hematoxylin
Hematoxylin stock solution:

Hematoxylin crystals, certified .... 10 gm
Ethyl alcohol, 95% .... 100 ml

The crystals are dissolved in the alcohol with gentle heating, after which the stock solution must be allowed to "ripen" for 6 to 8 weeks in a stoppered bottle no more than two-thirds filled. Exposure to sunlight as well as daily shaking will hasten the ripening process. When the solution is fully ripened, a drop added to 100 ml of tap water will produce a delicate violet color. The unripe solution will turn the water reddish or red-purple.

Hematoxylin working solution:

Hematoxylin stock solution .... 1 part
Distilled water .... 19 parts

Preparations to be stained with iron hematoxylin must be fixed in freshly prepared Schaudinn's fluid while still moist, if unpreserved stool specimens are used. If the specimen is preserved in PVA fixative, start with step 2 of the procedure given below; with SAF-preserved material, start with step 4:

1. Fix in Schaudinn's solution with acetic acid 30 minutes.

2. Dehydrate in 70% alcohol for 15 minutes.

3. Wash, to remove fixative, in 70% alcohol with iodine added sufficient to give a port-wine color for 3 minutes.

4. Wash in 70% alcohol for 3 minutes.

5. Rinse in tap water.

6. Mordant in 4% ferric ammonium sulfate 15 minutes.

7. Rinse in tap water.

8. Stain in hematoxylin working solution 10 minutes.

9. Rinse in tap water.

10. Decolorize in 0.25% ferric ammonium sulfate 12 minutes.

11. Wash in running water for at least 5 minutes.

12. Dehydrate in 70%, 95%, and two changes of 100% alcohol, each 5 minutes.

13. Place in xylol, two changes each 5 minutes.

14. Mount in Permount, or other mounting medium, for examination.

The trichrome stain has supplanted iron hematoxylin in most laboratories; the detail obtained is sufficient for diagnostic purposes, and the stain is easier to use.

Gomori's Trichrome Stain

Chromotrope 2R* .... 0.6 gm
Light green SF* .... 0.3 gm
Phosphotungstic acid .... 0.7 gm
Acetic acid, glacial .... 1.0 ml
Allow to stand for 30 to 60 minutes,
    then add distilled water .... 100.0 ml

Slides may be prepared from fresh or PVA- or SAF-preserved material. If PVA-preserved material is used, start with step 3 of the procedure; with SAF-preserved stools, start with step 4:

1. Fix in Schaudinn's solution with acetic acid added 30 minutes.

2. Wash in 70% alcohol 15 minutes.

3. Wash in 70% alcohol to which sufficient iodine has been added to produce a port-wine color 3 minutes.

4. Wash in 70% alcohol, two changes, each 1 minute.

5. Stain in Gomori's trichrome 8 to 15 minutes.

6. Rinse in 90% alcohol with 1% acetic acid 1 to 2 seconds.

7. Dip twice in 100% alcohol.

8. Dehydrate in second change of 100% alcohol 30 seconds.

9. Place in xylol 1 minute.

10. Mount in Permount or other mounting medium.

Although excellent for all other stool protozoa, neither of the foregoing methods will stain coccidia well. These organisms are acid-fast and stain well with a modified acid-fast stain (Garcia et al., 1983).

Cryptosporidium is a common pathogen in patients with HIV infection, and for this reason it is probably well to use formol-saline or formalin-preserved specimens in preparing the stained smears, although the technique works well on slides prepared from a fresh stool specimen. If the formalin-preserved material is used, approximately 1 ml of the preserved material should be added to 10 ml of 10% formalin in a centrifuge tube. The mixture is centrifuged at 300 × g for 2 minutes, the supernatant decanted, and the sediment spread in uniform thin layers on glass microscope slides.

Modified Acid-Fast Stain for *Cryptosporidium* and *Isospora*
Kinyoun's carbol-fuchsin:

Basic fuchsin .... 4 gm
Phenol (liquefied) .... 8 gm
Ethyl alcohol, 95% .... 20 ml
Distilled water .... 100 ml

Dissolve fuchsin in alcohol, add liquefied phenol and mix well, then add water.

---

*Manufactured by National Aniline Divison, Allied Chemical and Dye Corp., New York, NY.

Loeffler's alkaline methylene blue:

Methylene blue (90% dye content) ..... 0.3 gm
Ethyl alcohol, 95% .... 30 ml
KOH solution 0.01% by weight .... 100 ml

Dissolve methylene blue in alcohol, then add KOH.

1. Make fecal smears either from the sediment of a centrifuged formalinized specimen or from the unpreserved stool, and allow to air-dry.
2. Place slide on staining rack and flood with carbol-fuchsin.
3. Gently heat slide to steaming with Bunsen burner. Do not boil.
4. Stain for 5 minutes, adding more carbol-fuchsin if necessary, without additional heating.
5. Rinse slide with tap water.
6. Decolorize with 1% sulfuric acid for about 2 minutes. Do not overdecolorize.
7. Rinse with tap water. Allow to drain.
8. Flood slide with methylene blue and stain for 1 minute.
9. Rinse with tap water, drain, and air-dry.

Oocysts of *Cryptosporidium* and *Isospora* stain red. Yeasts and most other material stain blue.

SPECIAL DETECTION METHODS

Baermann Apparatus for Recovery of *Strongyloides* Larvae. *Strongyloides* larvae do not always concentrate well with either of the concentration techniques, though they may be detected by those methods. The Baermann technique yields a good concentration of the *living* larvae of *S. stercoralis*. It should be used when there is a high index of suspicion and routine stool examinations are negative, and for following the results of therapy.

1. A glass funnel with a diameter of 10 cm or greater is set up in a ring stand, with a short piece of rubber tubing attached to its stem and a pinchcock closing the tubing.
2. A wire circle, of slightly smaller diameter than the top of the funnel, is covered with two layers of gauze. The edges of the gauze are folded under the ring, which is fitted into the funnel.
3. The funnel is filled with lukewarm water to a level just covering the gauze, and a specimen of stool is placed on the gauze, partially in contact with the water.
4. Allow apparatus to stand at room temperature for 8 to 12 hours, then draw off a few drops of fluid through the tubing into a small glass dish.
5. Examine for larvae under low power of the microscope.

Filter Paper Strip Procedure for Recovery of *Strongyloides* or *Trichostrongylus* Larvae. This method takes too long for clinical usefulness but is well adapted for field or survey use, where quick results are not essential. The technique, originally described by Harada and Mori in 1955, requires minimal equipment.

A 20 × 13 mm filter paper strip, in the center of which is placed 0.5 to 1.0 gm of feces, is inserted into a 15 ml centrifuge tube containing 3 to 4 ml of distilled water. The tube is placed upright or in a slightly slanted position, such that the filter paper is kept moist by capillary flow. Water may be added as needed to maintain the original fluid level. After 10 days a small amount of fluid is withdrawn from the bottom of the tube and examined for larvae.

Cellophane Tape Swab for *Enterobius* and *Taenia* Eggs. A number of commercial pinworm detection kits are now available, but if cellophane is used, the procedure is as follows:

1. Fold together sticky surfaces of a piece of cellophane tape, 1 by 8 cm in length, for about 1 cm at each end.
2. Stretch tape, sticky side out, over butt end of a test tube, holding nonsticky ends firmly with thumb and forefinger.
3. Apply tape to anal area, rocking back and forth to cover as much of the mucosa and mucocutaneous area as possible.
4. Remove tape and apply to microscope slide, sticky side down. Press firmly into position.
5. Examine for eggs under low power of microscope. Pinworm eggs, which are generally deposited at night, will be found scattered around the perianal region. The tape should be used in the morning before the patient has washed or defecated.

Use of the clear type of cellophane tape is essential. That which has a frosted appearance obscures the eggs. A number of commercial kits are available.

Schistosomal Hatching Test. If feces containing viable schistosome eggs is diluted with approximately 10 volumes of water, the eggs will hatch within a few hours, releasing miracidia. The miracidia are positively phototropic. The following procedure takes advantage of this characteristic.

1. A stool specimen is homogenized by shaking in normal saline and is then strained through two layers of gauze.
2. The material is allowed to sediment, the supernatant is decanted and the sediment resuspended in saline. This process is repeated at least twice.
3. The saline is decanted and replaced with distilled water, and the suspension is placed in a side-arm or Erlenmeyer flask. The side-arm flask is covered with black paper, aluminum foil, or black paint, except for the side arm. If an Erlenmeyer flask is used, it is covered to 1 cm below the level of fluid in the neck of the flask. Additional water is added if necessary.
4. The flask is allowed to stand at room temperature for several hours in subdued light.
5. The side arm, or water in the neck of the flask, is then illuminated strongly from the side.
6. The illuminated area is examined with a magnifying glass to detect the presence of free-swimming miracidia.

Eggs of *Schistosoma haematobium* in the urine may also be hatched in this manner, but they are more easily concentrated by centrifugation or membrane filtration.

DUODENAL SAMPLING AND BIOPSY. Sampling and examination of duodenal contents is a reliable means of recovery of *Strongyloides* larvae and other small intestine parasites such as *Giardia, Isospora,* and *Cryptosporidium.* Specimens may be obtained by intubation or by use of the enteric capsule or string test (Enterotest). A No. 00 gelatin capsule containing a 90 cm line (Fig. 122–4), composed of a 20 cm silicon rubber–covered thread and a 70 cm soft nylon yarn, is swallowed by the patient while the thread, which protrudes from a hole in the capsule, is held firmly. To the

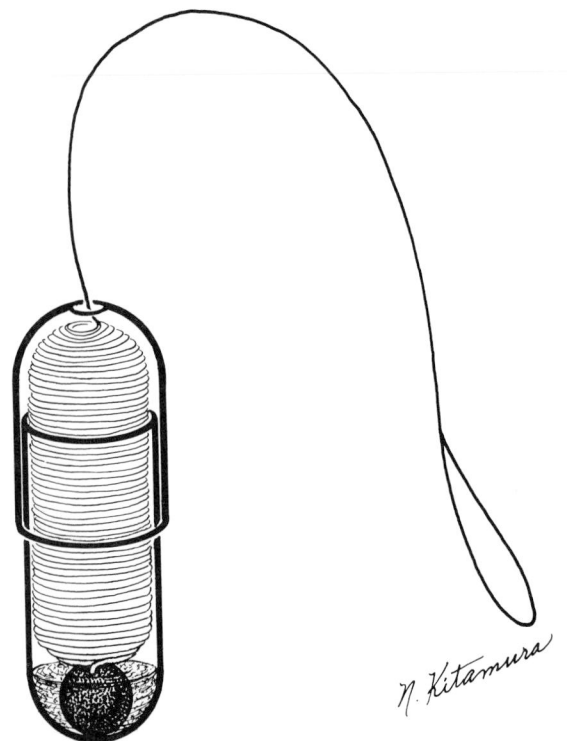

N. Kitamura

FIGURE 122–4. Enteric capsule for sampling duodenal content. (From Garcia LS, Bruckner DA: Diagnostic Medical Parasitology. New York, Elsevier, 1988.)

end of the nylon yarn is attached a 1 gm weight, which eventually helps carry the string into the duodenum. The free end of the line is taped to the patient's neck or cheek and may be pulled up after 4 hours. The bile-stained mucus adhering to its distal end is examined under the microscope. The weight becomes disengaged in the intestine at the time the thread is withdrawn.

Biopsy of the small intestinal mucosa may reveal *Giardia, Cryptosporidium,* and microsporidia as well as *Strongyloides* larvae.

CULTURE METHODS. Many of the intestinal protozoa have now been successfully cultured. Cultivation of the nonpathogenic amebas, the flagellates, and *Balantidium* falls into the category of research procedures, requiring too much material and time to be of diagnostic usefulness.

Entamoeba histolytica can be cultivated on a variety of media, some of which may be purchased in the dehydrated form and prepared with a minimum of effort. Various authorities advocate the use of *E. histolytica* cultures in the diagnostic laboratory as a screening procedure. Others suggest that the cultures be employed in every suspected case of amebiasis when the microscopic examination yields negative results. A third viewpoint is that expressed by certain workers who have determined the number of *E. histolytica* cysts that must be present per gram of feces to ensure a high percentage of successful cultures. Results of these studies indicate that the number of cysts necessary for viable cultures is so large as to be detectable by ordinary microscopic methods, and suggest that cultures are superfluous.

The success with which *E. histolytica* is cultivated will depend largely upon familiarity with the techniques involved. For this reason, sporadic use of culture techniques is not recommended; they should be undertaken only in laboratories where the number of specimens examined is sufficiently large to justify considerable time being spent on their maintenance and examination. Likewise, culture methods should never be used as a substitute for routine and thorough microscopic examination by the various methods outlined previously. Diamond's medium may be obtained freeze-dried for reconstitution as a liquid medium; Boeck and Drbohlav's L.E.S. medium is solid with a liquid overlay and can be prepared in the laboratory.

Diamond's Medium for Axenic Culture of *Entamoeba.* Now obtainable as TYI-S-33 Medium, freeze-dried, from the American Type Culture Collection.* It is prepared as follows:

TYI-S-33 broth base with 10%
        bovine serum................. 1 bottle
Distilled water.................... 55 ml

Dispense 13 ml of medium per tube into 16 × 125 mm screw-cap culture tubes. It may be stored at ambient temperature (± 25°C) for up to 90 days, but for longest shelf life it is recommended that it be stored at 2 to 8°C. Some strains of *E. histolytica* require 15% bovine serum, necessitating the addition of an extra 5% by volume of bovine calf serum, inactivated at 56°C for 30 minutes, prior to use.

Inoculate with a portion of stool the size of a small pea, adding to the medium before inoculation 100 units of penicillin and 100 µg of streptomycin/ml. Gentamicin 50 µg/ml may substitute for penicillin and streptomycin. Incubate at 37°C and examine after 2, 3, and 4 days of incubation by removing a small amount of sediment with a pipette. The sediment is transferred to a slide, covered, and examined under low power. Primary isolation may yield few organisms, whereas subsequent transfers show a considerable increase in numbers. It should be unnecessary to use antibiotics for successive transfers after primary isolation.

Boeck and Drbohlav's Locke-Egg-Serum (L.E.S.) Medium for Amebas
  Locke's solution:

NaCl........................... 9.0 gm
CaCl₂ .... 0.2 gm
KCl .... 0.4 gm
NaHCO₃........................ 0.2 gm
Glucose....................... 2.5 gm
Distilled water .... 1 liter

This solution should be autoclaved before storage. L.E.S. medium is prepared as follows:

1. Wash four eggs, brush with alcohol to sterilize, and break into a sterile flask containing glass beads.

2. Add 50 ml Locke's solution; shake until homogeneous.

*American Type Culture Collection, 12301 Parklawn Drive, Rockville, MD 20852.

3. Dispense in test tubes sufficient quantity to produce a 2½ to 3½ cm slant in bottom of tube.

4. Slant plugged tubes and place in inspissator at 70°C until slants are solidified. If an inspissator is not available, a substitute may be devised by leaving the door of the autoclave partly open.

5. When slants have become solidified, autoclave at 15 pounds pressure for 20 minutes. If any slants are badly broken, discard them.

6. Cover slants to a depth of about 1 cm with mixture of 8 parts of sterile Locke's solution to 1 part sterile inactivated human blood serum. Sterility of mixture of Locke's solution and serum should be ensured by filtration sterilization followed by incubation at 37°C for 24 hours or longer before use.

A loopful of sterile rice starch or powder is added to each tube before inoculation. Inoculate with a portion of stool the size of a small pea, break up well in medium, and incubate at 37°C. Examine as noted for Diamond's medium. Note that this is not an axenic medium and that antibiotics are not added.

METHODS FOR ESTIMATION OF WORM BURDEN. Estimates of daily egg output have been made for a number of hepatic and intestinal worms. If one can estimate the total number of eggs in a 24-hour stool specimen, it is possible to calculate the approximate number of adult worms present. This makes it possible to follow the results of therapy in a somewhat quantitative manner by periodic egg counts, affording a basis for comparison of the efficacy of various medications.

Estimates on numbers of eggs laid per female worm vary considerably and depend to some extent on the numbers of worms present. The Chinese liver fluke may lay 2400 or so eggs within 24 hours and an *Ascaris* female about 200,000 during the same period. Thus, from 1000 to 2000 eggs would be found per gram of feces in a 24-hour specimen from a patient infected with one pair of *Ascaris*. The egg-laying capacity of a single *Necator* female may vary from 12 to 44 eggs per gram of feces in a 24-hour period. *Ancylostoma* females lay about twice as many eggs as *Necator*. *Trichuris* females presumably lay about 14,000 eggs in 24 hours, but egg-laying capacity seems to vary inversely with total numbers of worms present.

Stoll Egg-Counting Technique

1. Save entire 24-hour stool specimen, and determine weight in grams.

2. Weigh out accurately 4 gm of feces.

3. Place feces in calibrated bottle or large test tube; add sufficient N/10 NaOH to bring volume to 60 ml.

4. Add a few glass beads and shake vigorously to make a uniform suspension. If specimen is hard, the mixture may be placed in a refrigerator overnight before shaking, to aid in its comminution.

5. With a pipette, remove immediately 0.15 ml of the suspension and drain onto a slide.

6. Do not use a coverslip; place slide on mechanical stage and count *all* the eggs on the slide.

7. Multiply egg count by 100 to obtain the number of eggs per gram of feces, and by weight of specimen to get total number of eggs per 24-hour specimen.

Kato Thick-Smear Technique. This technique has undergone a number of modifications since its introduction. Martin and Beaver (1968) suggest examination of a standard 50 mg sample of fresh feces, pressed between a microscope slide and a strip of wettable cellophane soaked in glycerin. After the fecal film has cleared, eggs in the entire film are counted (Fig. 96–22). The fecal sample may be weighed, but these investigators found that with some practice it was possible to estimate sample size with an acceptable degree of reliability. Samples taken from various portions of the specimen do not differ greatly in the number of eggs that they contain. Materials needed for this method are wettable, medium-thickness cellophane coverslips, 22 × 30 mm. They are soaked for at least 24 hours in a solution of 100 ml pure glycerin, 100 ml water, and 1 ml 3% malachite green (the last is optional).

Feces are transferred to a clean slide and covered with a presoaked cellophane coverslip. The slide is inverted and pressed against an absorbent surface until the fecal mass covers an area 20 to 25 mm in diameter. The preparation is left for 1 hour at room temperature to allow clearing of the fecal material (but *not* of the eggs); it should then be examined promptly.

Peters and Kazura (1987) have found that for eggs of *Schistosoma mansoni* longer periods of clearing (24 hours) are needed. To obtain 10, 20, or 50 mg samples they utilize metal templates containing holes calibrated to deliver those amounts of feces.

SPECIAL METHODS FOR INTESTINAL HELMINTHS

Platyhelminths. If gravid proglottids are found in a stool specimen or brought in for identification, *Diphyllobothrium* can usually be identified by the presence of a uterine rosette in the middle of each segment. If no rosette is seen, the segments are probably those of a *Taenia*. To differentiate between the two species, segments should be rinsed in tap water and placed between two microscope slides that are separated at the edges by thin pieces of cardboard. The preparation may then be fastened by means of rubber bands at each end of the slides so that the segments become somewhat flattened. The uterine branches should be clearly visible under the low power of a dissecting microscope.

Species identification on the basis of uterine structure of gravid segments may be greatly facilitated by injection of segments with India ink. A little ink is drawn into a 1 ml tuberculin syringe, a No. 26 hypodermic needle is inserted into the distal end of the proglottid or in the central uterine stem, and a small amount of ink is slowly injected. The branches of the uterus will become black and can be easily counted (Fig. 100–3). This procedure works best with fresh specimens but may at times be successful with formalin-fixed segments.

Nematodes. Generally, nematodes found in the feces can be readily recognized, but anisakids coughed up and brought to the laboratory or recovered by endoscopy must be identified by their internal structure (Fig. 95–4). This may be made visible by clearing in glycerin.

If the worms are still alive, they should be fixed by immersion in 70% alcohol heated to 75°C. Otherwise, transfer to a relatively large volume of 10% glycerin in 70% alcohol in a Petri dish. Leave the dish uncovered in a dust-free location, allowing the alcohol to evaporate over several days. The specimen may then be mounted on a slide in glycerin and covered with a coverslip for microscopic examination.

BIBLIOGRAPHY

Beal CB, Viens P, Grant RLG, Hughes JM: A new technique for sampling duodenal contents: demonstration of upper small-bowel pathogens. Am J Trop Med Hyg 19:349–352, 1970.
Brooke MM, Goldman M: Polyvinyl alcohol–fixative as a preservative and adhesive for protozoa in dysenteric stools and other liquid material. J Lab Clin Med 34:1554–1560, 1949.
Garcia LS, Bruckner DA: Diagnostic Medical Parasitology. New York, Elsevier, 1988.
Garcia LS, Bruckner DA, Shimizu RY: Techniques for the recovery and identification of *Cryptosporidium* oocysts from stool specimens. J Clin Microbiol 18:185–190, 1983.
Harada Y, Mori O: A new method for culturing hookworm. Yonago Acta Med 1:177–179, 1955.
Markell EK, Voge M, John DT: Medical Parasitology. 6th ed. Philadelphia, WB Saunders, 1986.
Martin LK, Beaver PC: Evaluation of Kato thick-smear technique for quantitative diagnosis of helminth infections. Am J Trop Med Hyg 17:382–391, 1968.
Peters PAS, Kazura JW: Update on diagnostic methods for schistosomiasis. Clin Trop Med Comm Dis 2:419–464, 1987.
Sapero JJ, Lawless DK: The MIF stain-preservation technique for the identification of intestinal protozoa. Am J Trop Med Hyg 2:613–619, 1953.
Sawitz WG, Faust EC: The probability of detecting intestinal protozoa by successive stool examinations. Am J Trop Med 22:131–136, 1942.
Yang J, Scholten T: A fixative for intestinal parasites permitting the use of concentration and permanent staining procedures. Am J Clin Pathol 67:300–304, 1977.

123. EXAMINATION OF BLOOD, OTHER BODY FLUIDS AND TISSUES, SPUTUM, AND URINE

Edward K. Markell

EXAMINATION OF FRESH BLOOD. Microscopic examination of fresh blood is not undertaken routinely but is useful for the detection of two types of parasites. Trypanosomes and microfilariae may be easily recognized by their characteristic motility in fresh blood. For specific identification of these organisms, however, a permanent stain is essential. When fresh blood is to be examined, it is important to make a sufficiently thin preparation so that the relatively small protozoan parasites are not masked by several layers of blood corpuscles. A small drop of blood is placed on a slide and covered with a coverglass to prevent clotting. If the preparation is too thick, it may be diluted with normal saline. For the detection of trypanosomes, the high-dry objective with reduced illumination is most suitable. During a search for microfilariae, the low power of the microscope should be employed. Whiplike motions of microfilariae and the rapid undulating and twisting movements of trypanosomes are usually seen before the precise shape of the organism is apparent. Organisms may quickly attract one's attention through their movements even when they are so few that a long search may be required to reveal them in fixed preparations.

STAINED PREPARATIONS. The preparation of good blood films will depend to a large extent upon the cleanliness of the microscope slides and coverglasses employed. All glassware must be free of dust and oil. It is essential that both slides and coverglasses be washed in alcohol and dried with a clean towel before a blood film is prepared. Even slides taken from a newly opened box may be covered with an invisible oily film that prevents proper adherence, particularly of thick blood films.

Many methods have been described for the preparation and permanent staining of blood films. Correct initial handling of the blood is essential if good stains are to be obtained, regardless of the specific methods used. It is preferable to use peripheral blood, from fingertip or ear lobe. The skin should be cleansed with alcohol before an incision is made, in order to remove all fatty substances, and the incision should be sufficiently deep so that blood flows freely. Blood that has been "milked" from the finger is mixed with tissue fluids, which dilute the parasites and make their detection more difficult. Films should be prepared as quickly as possible to prevent clotting. If venous blood must be employed, a small amount of heparin or other anticoagulant must be added, but preparations made from such blood will usually show some distortion.

The Thin Film. Thin blood films are used for the specific identification of malarial parasites, trypanosomes, and microfilariae. A thin film should consist of *one* layer of evenly distributed blood cells. Since malaria parasites are intracellular, a piling-up of red blood cells makes specific identification of these parasites difficult, if not impossible. Specific identification of blood parasites rests on their morphologic characteristics. The chief advantage of a thin film is that it preserves the structure of the parasites and red cells with a minimum of distortion.

There are several ways in which to make a thin blood film; although the procedure adopted will vary with individual preference, the following is recommended. Place a small drop of blood near one end of a microscope slide; raise the end of the slide farthest from the drop of blood by placing the end of the slide on your finger as your hand rests on a steady surface. Taking a second slide for a spreader, hold your hand so that the second slide makes an angle of approximately 30 degrees with the first. Draw back the supporting finger to move the slide back until the blood touches the spreader slide and begins to run out toward the edges. Before the blood has a chance to reach the edges of the spreader, move the finger that supports it forward in an even quick motion, so that the drop is drawn out into a thin film. Ideally, this should not reach the edges of the slide and should taper off into a "comet's tail" toward the end of the slide. After the film has been air-dried, it may be stained.

The stains commonly used are of two general types. One of these has the fixative incorporated in the staining solution so that fixation and staining of the dried film are accomplished simultaneously. An example is Wright's stain, in which methyl alcohol acts as a fixative. Wright's stain will give only fair results in staining malaria parasites and is *not* recommended for parasitologic use. More precise detail is seen in slides prepared with Giemsa's stain. Since this stain does not contain a fixative, thin films must be fixed in absolute methyl alcohol and air-dried before they are placed in the staining solution. It is important to dry slides in a vertical position after removal from either fixative or stain. As soon as the stained films are dry, they may be examined under oil immersion of the microscope. Immersion oil may be placed directly on the uncovered blood film and, when no longer needed, carefully removed with xylene and lens paper. Slides that one desires to keep for a permanent collection should always have the protection of a coverglass; a mounting medium, such as Permount, should be used.

Thick Blood Films. The thick film may also be used in identification of malaria parasites, trypanosomes, and microfilariae. As a thick layer of blood is used in this method, many more parasites will be present in each field. Increased distortion of the parasites is a disadvantage of this method, but experience enables one to recognize them readily.

To make a thick film, place three drops of blood, each of about the size that would be used to make a thin film, close together near one end of the slide. With one corner of another absolutely clean slide, stir the blood, mingling the three drops over an area 2 cm in diameter. Continue stirring for at least 30 seconds; this prevents the formation of fibrin strands, which otherwise tend to obscure the parasites. Allow the films to dry normally; do not heat, because this will fix the blood. After the films are thoroughly dry they must be laked to remove the hemoglobin. This can be done by immersion in buffer solution, prior to staining, or in Giemsa stain itself. Thick films that cannot be stained immediately should be laked in buffer solution before storage, because removal of hemoglobin becomes increasingly difficult with time. When Giemsa's stain is used for thick films, the procedure is exactly the same as that employed with thin films, except that fixation in methyl alcohol is omitted. Staining times for thick and thin films are similar, but if separate preparations are made, different staining times may be required for optimal results. Thick and thin films may, however, be made on the same slide and stained simultaneously with Giemsa. To accomplish this, the thin portion of the slide is fixed for 1 minute in methyl alcohol and then dried before staining.

Another method that may be used in the staining of thick films is that described by Field. It is very rapid and gives satisfactory, though not outstanding, results. Field's stain has been used extensively for survey purposes and when large numbers of slides must be prepared, but it is not recommended for routine use.

Blood Concentration Procedures. The thick film is itself a type of concentration technique and the only one applicable to the identification of parasites within the red cell. Buffy coat films serve to concentrate the white cells, in which *Leishmania* may be found, and are useful for detection of trypanosomes and microfilariae. A tri-ple-centrifugation technique is also used to check for trypanosomes when they are too sparse to be found even in thick blood films. The presence of small numbers of microfilariae in the blood can be detected by means of a membrane filtration technique.

EXAMINATION OF CEREBROSPINAL FLUID. Trophozoites of *Naegleria* (Chapter 80) and trypanosomes (Chapter 74) may be found in the cerebrospinal fluid (CSF). *Trichinella* larvae may be found in the CSF of patients with severe infections; they also may be isolated from the blood. CSF eosinophilia may be caused by parasites such as *Angiostrongylus* and *Gnathostoma*, which will not be found in the blood. Transverse myelitis caused by *Schistosoma mansoni* may result in an eosinophilic CSF pleocytosis. Ova are rarely seen in the CSF.

The CSF must be examined promptly, as trypanosomes will survive for only about 20 minutes, and *Naegleria* may become rounded and nonmotile. The CSF may be centrifuged ($7000 \times g$ for 10 minutes), the supernatant removed, and the sediment examined under reduced illumination. Motility of *Naegleria* may be enhanced by use of a warm stage, and culture of the CSF or its sediment may be effective in isolation of this organism. Examination of the CSF and blood (not a routine diagnostic procedure in suspected trichinosis) may reveal the migrating larvae in severe infections, and filtration of blood or CSF through a membrane filter (Chapter 90) will increase the chances of finding them.

TISSUE IMPRESSIONS. The detection of intracellular parasites such as *Leishmania* and *Toxoplasma* is greatly facilitated by examination of tissue impression smears stained with Giemsa's stain. Fresh lymph nodes, liver biopsy material, or bone marrow is lightly impressed on a clean microscope slide; the film is allowed to dry at room temperature and is stained in the manner of a thin blood film. Whole cells, with organisms showing little if any distortion, may be clearly distinguished in such preparations. When dealing with lymph nodes or other fairly solid tissue, it is best to prepare the smear from a freshly cut surface. The remaining tissue can then be fixed for conventional pathologic procedures or be used as desired.

BIOPSY AND ASPIRATION. Spleen, liver, and bone marrow biopsies are extensively used in the diagnosis of visceral leishmaniasis. Organisms may be demonstrated directly in the biopsy material, which also may be used for culture or animal inoculation. Sternal marrow aspiration is approximately as productive as the more hazardous splenic or hepatic biopsy. *Leishmania tropica* cannot be recovered from the surface of an oriental sore; if a hypodermic syringe is introduced through normal tissue at the side of the ulcer to the area below the ulcer bed, intracellular parasites may be demonstrated in the fluid that is withdrawn after instillation of a few drops of normal saline (Fig. 76–13). Aspiration of enlarged posterior cervical or other involved lymph nodes will at times reveal trypanosomes when the blood is apparently free of them. The lymph nodes are less often involved in Rhodesian sleeping sickness than in the Gambian form or in Chagas' disease. Biopsy of enlarged nodes from patients having the latter disease may reveal intracellular (amastigote) forms of the parasite.

Aspiration of fluid from a hydatid cyst (a dangerous procedure unless done as part of an open surgical operation or perhaps with ultrasonographic guidance) may reveal hydatid sand, but it must be remembered that certain hydatid cysts are sterile, so that the absence of scoleces or hooklets from the sediment, centrifuged or put through a membrane filter, is not evidence against the parasitic nature of the cyst. Aspiration of an amebic abscess will often demonstrate a thick reddish brown fluid, but amebas are seldom seen, as they occur chiefly in the tissue surrounding the abscess cavity (Fig. 68–15).

Eggs of *Schistosoma mansoni* may be found in tissue taken from the rectal mucosa when they cannot be recovered from the stool; mucosa from the bladder wall, taken at cystoscopy, may likewise reveal eggs of *S. haematobium* (Fig. 96–23). Larval *Trichinella spiralis* may be found in any voluntary muscle, but biopsies are usually taken from the gastrocnemius. Larvae may be most abundant in the diaphragm, and a search may be made for them in this muscle at autopsy (Fig. 90–1*B*). Microfilariae of *Onchocerca volvulus, Mansonella ozzardi,* and *M. streptocerca* may be demonstrated in skin snips (Figs. 87–1*A* and 88–3).

EXAMINATION OF THE SPUTUM. Examination of the sputum is indicated when there is a question of pulmonary paragonimiasis, although the swallowed eggs are often found in the feces. *Entamoeba histolytica* may appear in the sputum of patients with pulmonary abscesses. *Pneumocystis carinii* may be found in the sputum but is more readily seen in aspirates or in impression smears of lung biopsy material (Figs. 79–1 and 79–2). Migrating larvae of *Ascaris,* hookworm, and *Strongyloides* are rarely seen. *Entamoeba gingivalis* may multiply in bronchial mucus and like *Trichomonas tenax* is usually an oral contaminant. *Cryptosporidium* has been found in both sputum and lung biopsy material. Ruptured hydatid cysts may be recognized by the presence of hooklets in the sputum.

Sputum specimens should be induced, if possible. Early-morning specimens, uncontaminated with saliva, also are acceptable. They should be examined by wet mount while fresh, or preserved in PVA fixative for protozoa and formol-saline for other organisms or eggs. If the specimen is very viscid, it may be necessary to dilute with an equal quantity of 3% NaOH, mix thoroughly, and centrifuge before examination or preservation. Sodium hydroxide will, of course, destroy any amebas or flagellates that might be present.

EXAMINATION OF URINE AND VAGINAL SECRETIONS. Eggs of *Schistosoma haematobium* and, on occasion, microfilariae of *Wuchereria* and *Onchocerca* may be found in the urine. *Trichomonas vaginalis* may be found in the urinary sediment of both males and females and in prostatic and vaginal secretions.

Schistosome eggs and microfilariae may best be recovered by examination of centrifuged or membrane-filtered urine specimens. A fresh or midday urine specimen is preferred for *S. haematobium;* microfilariae of *Wuchereria* are found in the urine of patients exhibiting chyluria, while those of *Onchocerca* are usually seen immediately following treatment with diethylcarbama-

zine. The hatching test (Chapter 122) may demonstrate the presence of small numbers of schistosome eggs, if viable.

Trichomonas vaginalis may be recognized in a fresh specimen of urine or in vaginal or prostatic exudate by its jerky motility or (under high dry power) by the movement of its undulating membrane (Fig. 72–1). It may also be seen in Papanicolaou smears.

BLOOD FILMS AND TISSUE IMPRESSION SMEARS
Field's Stain

Solution A:
    Methylene blue .... 0.8 gm
    Azure I .... 0.5 gm
    Na_2HPO_4 anhydrous .... 5.0 gm
    KH_2PO_4 anhydrous .... 6.25 gm
    Distilled water .... 500 ml

Solution B:
    Eosin .... 1.0 gm
    Na_2HPO_4 anhydrous .... 5.0 gm
    KH_2PO_4............................. 6.25 gm
    Distilled water .... 500 ml

Dissolve salts first, then add the stains, after grinding the azure I in a mortar. Let the solutions stand for 24 hours, then filter. If a scum forms or dye precipitates, filter again. The same solutions may be used for many weeks, but the eosin should be renewed when it becomes greenish. The staining procedure is as follows:

1. Dip slides in solution A for 1 second.
2. Rinse by immersion in water, waving gently for a few seconds until stain ceases to flow from film.
3. Dip slides in solution B for 1 second.
4. Rinse as before for 2 to 3 seconds.
5. Place vertically against a rack to drain and dry.

Giemsa's Stain. Giemsa's stain is sold commercially as a concentrated stock solution. The product is quite variable, and each new lot should be thoroughly tested before being put into use. In general, if the coloration of the red and white cells seems satisfactory, it can be assumed that the stain will be adequate for the demonstration of malarial and other parasites. The procedure for use of Giemsa's stain with thin films is as follows:

1. Fix blood films in absolute methyl alcohol for 1 minute.
2. Allow slides to dry.
3. Immerse slides in a solution of 1 part of Giemsa stock to 30 to 50 parts of buffered water (pH 7.2). Stain 30 minutes to 1 hour.
4. Dip slides briefly in buffered water, drain quickly and thoroughly, and air-dry.

The procedure to be used with thick films is the same, except that steps 1 and 2 are omitted. If the slide has a thick film at one end and a thin film at the other, fix only the thin portion, then stain both parts of the film simultaneously.

Method for Estimating Numbers of Malaria Parasites in Blood. Determine the patient's white blood cell count. On a thick blood smear, count the number of parasites seen per 100 white blood cells; the total number per cubic millimeter of blood can then be determined.

Rapid Methenamine Silver Stain for *Pneumocystis carinii*. A number of stains, including periodic-acid–Schiff and Giemsa, have been utilized for the demonstration of *Pneumocystis* in sputum, brushings, and biopsy specimens. The best results are obtained by means of a methenamine silver impregnation technique. Modifications introduced by Mahan and Sale (1978) and by Shimono aand Hartman (1986) have reduced the processing time of what was formerly a long and laborious procedure to approximately 15 minutes. The solutions needed are as follows:

10% chromic acid (CrO_3) solution
5% silver nitrate ($AgNO_3$) solution
3% methenamine (hexamethylenetetramine, $[CH_3]_6N_4$)
5% borax (sodium borate, $Na_2B_4O_7 \cdot 10\ H_2O$)
1% gold chloride ($HAuCl_4 \cdot 3\ H_2O$)
1% sodium metabisulfite ($Na_2S_2O_5$)
5% sodium thiosulfate ($Na_2S_2O_3 \cdot 5\ H_2O$)

Each of these is made up separately as an aqueous solution by the addition of distilled water.

A working methenamine silver solution is made by adding 2 ml of 5% silver nitrate to 40 ml of 3% methenamine. A white precipitate forms but dissolves on shaking. To this is added 3 ml of 5% borax plus distilled water to a total of 80 ml of the working solution.

This working methenamine silver solution *must* be prepared fresh each time the stain is done. Do not reuse, even for consecutive runs. Control slides of *Pneumocystis* or fungi should be stained with each batch of slides.

The staining procedure is as follows:

1. Deparaffinize sections and hydrate to distilled water; air-dry smears.
2. Place in 10% chromic acid in Coplin jar for 10 minutes (discard solution after use).
3. Wash slides in tap water to remove excess chromic acid.
4. Place in 1% sodium metabisulfite for 1 minute.
5. Rinse in hot tap water for 1 minute (until Coplin jar is hot).
6. Place microscope slides on a 70°C electric hot plate (either directly on the plate or in a large Petri dish), and layer working methenamine silver solution on the slides. (A Corning model PC351 hot plate at a setting of 2 is suggested by Mahan and Sale (1978), but Yu et al. (1989) found that other heating units provide better temperature control.) In approximately 1 minute (4 to 5 minutes if slides are in Petri dish), when control tissue becomes a golden brown, rinse in warm tap water.
7. Place in Coplin jar and rinse in hot tap water, cooling gradually with tap water to avoid cracking jar.
8. Rinse in distilled water.
9. Tone in 1% gold chloride, approximately 10 seconds (solution can be reused).
10. Rinse in distilled water.
11. Place in 5% sodium thiosulfate solution for 3 minutes.
12. Wash thoroughly in tap water.
13. Counterstain with light green or other stain.
14. Dehydrate in successive changes of 95 and 100% alcohol, clear in xylol, and mount.

The results will be as follows: Fungi will be sharply delineated in black. *Pneumocystis carinii* will have a delicately stained wall, usually brownish or grayish, rather transparent. Structures described as "parentheses" are often seen and stain black. Mucin will be taupe to dark gray, the inner parts of mycelia and hyphae will be old rose, and the background will be pale green.

Membrane Filtration Method for Microfilariae. (Dennis and Kean, 1971)

1. Blood is collected in tubes containing 3.8% sodium citrate (20% by volume of blood specimen).
2. A Nuclepore* filter of 5 μm pore size is placed in a Swinney adapter; a 20 to 50 ml disposable plastic syringe is attached to the adapter.
3. Several milliliters of normal saline are added to the upright barrel.
4. About 2 to 4 ml of the blood specimen are added to the saline, and the mixture of blood and saline is forced through the filter.
5. Following several washes of small amounts of saline or distilled water, the filter may be removed from the adapter, placed on a microscope slide, and examined for living microfilariae; it can also be dried, fixed, and stained as for a thin blood film.

Gradient Centrifugation Technique for Concentration of Microfilariae. (Jones et al, 1975)

1. Thirty ml of 50% Hypaque is mixed with 14 ml of distilled water; 1 part of this mixture is added to 2.4 parts of 9% Ficoll.
2. Four ml of the Ficoll-Hypaque mixture is placed in a 17 × 100 mm plastic centrifuge tube and overlaid with 4 ml of heparinized venous blood.
3. The tube is centrifuged at 400 × *g* for 40 minutes.
4. Microfilariae will be found in the middle Ficoll-Hypaque layer, which separates the overlying plasma and white cell layers from the underlying red cells.

Buffy Coat Films for Leishmanias. This method is useful for the detection of *Leishmania donovani* if present in the circulation and will also reveal *Histoplasma capsulatum*. Microfilariae and trypanosomes also may be found in the buffy coat.

1. Obtain 5 ml of blood and deliver into a tube containing oxalate crystals (prepared as for the Wintrobe hematocrit method).
2. Transfer blood with a capillary pipette into a Wintrobe tube. Cap to prevent evaporation, and centrifuge for 30 minutes at 2500 × *g*.
3. With a fine capillary pipette, withdraw the cells of the buffy coat, which lies between the packed red cells and the overlying plasma.
4. Spread out as thin film, dry, and stain with Wright's or Giemsa's stain.

Triple Centrifugation Method for Trypanosomes.

1. Deliver 9 ml of blood, obtained by venipuncture, into a centrifuge tube containing 1 ml of 6% citrate solution.
2. Centrifuge at 300 × *g*.
3. Remove supernatant fluid to another centrifuge tube; recentrifuge at 600 × *g* for 10 minutes.

---

*This method is unsatisfactory for the isolation of *M. perstans* microfilariae because of their small size. Other filters of similar pore size are not as satisfactory as the Nuclepore.

4. Remove supernatant fluid once more to a clean centrifuge tube; centrifuge at 1800 × *g* for 10 minutes.

5. Examine sediment as a wet film, or make a thin film and stain with Giemsa's stain.

CULTURE METHODS. *Acanthamoeba* and *Naegleria* (Chapter 80), the leishmanias (Chapter 76), *Trypanosoma cruzi* (Chapter 75), and *Toxoplasma* (Chapter 78) can be cultured with relative ease. Cultivation of other blood and tissue parasites either has not been successful or (as in the case of the plasmodia) remains a research procedure.

Culbertson's Medium for *Acanthamoeba*. For the isolation of *Acanthamoeba* from tissues, Culbertson et al. (1965) recommend the following procedure:

Materials

1. Prepare a neomycin sulfate solution, 0.56% in sterile distilled water.

2. Prepare a sterile nystatin suspension in distilled water containing 1500 units per ml.

3. Prepare agar stock, 3 gm of Bacto-Agar per 100 ml of 1.7% NaCl.

4. Prepare suspension of *Enterobacter aerogenes* in trypticase soy broth, giving 40% transmission on a Coleman Junior spectrophotometer against uninoculated broth. Since both live and killed bacteria are to be used in medium preparation, place at least 5 ml of the suspension in a sealed ampule and immerse in a water bath at 65°C for 30 minutes to kill the organisms. Keep refrigerated until use.

Procedure

1. To a mixture consisting of 5 ml of each antibiotic solution, 5ml of killed bacterial suspension, and 85 ml of sterile distilled water, add 100 ml of melted and cooled 3% agar and combine all ingredients at 56°C in water bath.

2. Pour mixture into Petri plates, 8 ml per plate; allow excess moisture to evaporate by inverting bottom plate and resting it at a slight angle.

3. Place 0.05 ml of live *Enterobacter* suspension in center of plate and spread over an area 25 to 40 mm in diameter. Allow surface to dry at room temperature or at 4°C overnight.

Inoculation

Place drops of fluid or small pieces of tissue suspected of containing amebas near center of plate. Check for presence of amebas at edges of inoculum during the following 4 or 5 days.

Modified Nelson's Medium for *Naegleria*. The following procedure is for the isolation of *Naegleria* from the cerebrospinal fluid.

Materials

1. Make up the following in Page's saline solution: 0.1% liver infusion (Oxoid, Wilson 1:20, or Panmede) and 0.1% glucose.

Page's solution:

MgSO₄·7HOH	0.4 mg
CaCl₂·2HOH	0.4 mg
Na₂HPO₄	14.2 mg
KH₂PO₄	13.6 mg
NaCl	12.0 mg
Distilled water	100.0 ml

2. Prepare non-nutrient agar: Page's saline with liver and glucose, 100 ml, and Difco agar 1.5 gm. Dissolve agar in Page's saline with gentle heating. Aliquot 20 ml quantities into 20 × 150 mm screw-cap tubes. Autoclave at 15 psi for 15 minutes. Store in refrigerator.

Procedure

1. Prepare non-nutrient agar plates from above as needed, or store in refrigerator (up to 3 months) and warm to 37°C before use.

2. Add 2 or 3 drops of a suspension of *Escherichia coli* in Page's saline to the surface of the plate, and spread with a bacteriologic loop.

Inoculation. Inoculate a few drops of CSF sediment onto plate. Incubate at 35 to 37°C, and examine daily under low power. Cysts may appear within 4 to 5 days and trophozoites earlier.

Novy-Mac Neal-Nicolle (N.N.N.) Medium for *Leishmania* and *Trypanosoma cruzi*

Agar	14 gm
NaCl	6 gm
Distilled water	900 ml

The water is brought to the boiling point and the salt and agar added and dissolved in it. It is then distributed in test tubes filled to about one-third capacity. The test tubes are plugged and sterilized in the autoclave in the usual manner. Tubes containing the agar base may be stored in the refrigerator and used as needed.

For use, the tubes are placed in hot water to melt the agar, after which they are cooled to 48 to 50°C. To each tube is added approximately one third as much sterile defibrinated rabbit's blood as the volume of agar. The blood and agar are thoroughly mixed by rapid rotation of the tube, and the tube is then placed in a slanting position, on ice, and cooled. After the tubes are cool, they are placed in an upright position and incubated for 24 hours at 37°C to determine sterility.

Blood may be obtained from the rabbit by cardiac puncture, sterile precautions being observed. The blood so obtained is placed in a sterile flask containing glass beads and defibrinated by shaking.

Peripheral blood, or material obtained by biopsy or marrow aspiration or from cutaneous ulcers by aspiration from below the ulcer bed, may be cultured on this medium, which gives excellent results. The tubes are kept at room temperature, as close to 22°C as possible. The organisms develop in the water of condensation, which collects at the bottom of the slanted agar. Cultures should be examined every other day for a month before being discarded as negative. If leishmanias are present in the inoculum in some numbers, culture forms will usually be found within 2 to 10 days, but if scarce, may require much longer to develop in sufficient numbers to be detected. Leishmanias will not grow in the presence of bacterial contamination.

Tissue Culture of *Toxoplasma gondii*. A method for culture of *Toxoplasma* has been described by Shepp et al. (1985) and is applicable to blood, CSF, placental and presumably other tissues. The procedure for blood specimens is as follows:

1. Collect 10 ml of blood in preservative-free heparin tubes; allow to sediment by gravity.

2. Remove the buffy coat with aseptic precautions; centrifuge at 800 × g for 10 minutes.

3. Wash buffy coat cells three times with Eagle's minimal essential medium.*

4. Inoculate washed buffy coat material onto complete human foreskin fibroblast monolayers, and observe weekly for cytopathologic effects.

Other tissues may be inoculated directly onto the tissue culture. If more than 1 ml of CSF is available, it may be centrifuged at 500 × g for 10 minutes and the sediment used for the inoculum.

ANIMAL INOCULATION. *Trypanosoma brucei gambiense* and *T. b. rhodesiense* infections can be established in a number of laboratory animals. White rats, white mice, and guinea pigs are most useful for diagnosis and the maintenance of laboratory strains. Young animals are most readily infected, and *T. b. rhodesiense* is more virulent than *T. b. gambiense*. Rats infected with *T. b. gambiense* will survive for several months with a low-grade parasitemia; infected with *T. b. rhodesiense,* they die within a short time with an overwhelming parasitemia. *Trypanosoma rangeli* multiplies in the common laboratory animals but does not cause apparent disease. Young white rats and white mice can be infected with *T. cruzi;* the white mouse is best for diagnostic inoculation. When first isolated, this trypanosome is quite virulent, but after repeated animal passage it loses its virulence and may become noninfective. Intraperitoneal or subcutaneous inoculation should be used; amounts up to 2 ml of blood are injected, depending upon the size of the animal used. It is important to check rats for the presence of their common parasite, *T. lewisi,* before inoculation.

For isolation of leishmanias, the hamster is most satisfactory; other laboratory animals are infected only with difficulty. Following intraperitoneal or intratesticular inoculation, hamsters will develop a generalized infection with any form of *Leishmania,* and the organisms may be demonstrated in spleen impression smears or in testicular aspirates. This infection develops slowly, and culture methods are generally regarded as being superior for diagnostic use.

Toxoplasma gondii, a parasite that shows little host specificity, will infect all common laboratory animals. White rats and mice are generally used; rats develop a chronic infection and are good for maintenance of the strain, whereas intraperitoneal infection of mice results in tremendous proliferation of the organisms in the ascitic fluid and death of the mice within a few days. Mouse peritoneal fluid, rich in organisms, is used as a source of toxoplasmas for the dye test and other diagnostic procedures.

Xenodiagnosis may be considered a special case of animal inoculation; the term was originally applied to the diagnosis of Chagas' disease by feeding uninfected reduviid bugs on a patient suspected of having the disease. Subsequent examination of the bugs will reveal developmental stages of the parasites if the test result is positive. Recently the term "xenodiagnosis" has been used for the diagnosis of trichinosis by feeding rats with muscle tissue from patients suspected of having the infection.

BIBLIOGRAPHY

Culbertson CG, Ensminger PW, Overton WM: The isolation of additional strains of pathogenic *Hartmanella* sp. (*Acanthamoeba*). Proposed culture method for application to biological material. Am J Clin Pathol 43:383–387, 1965.

Dennis DT, Kean BH: Isolation of microfilariae: report of a new method. J Parasitol 57:1146–1149, 1971.

Mahan CT, Sale GE: Rapid methenamine silver stain for *Pneumocystis* and fungi. Arch Pathol Lab Med 102:351–352, 1978.

Markell EK, Voge M, John DT: Medical Parasitology. 6th ed. Philadelphia, WB Saunders, 1986.

Shepp DH, Mackman RC, Conley FK, et al: *Toxoplasma gondii* reactivation identified by detection of parasitemia in tissue culture. Ann Intern Med 103:218, 1985.

Shimono LH, Hartman B: A simple and reliable rapid methenamine silver stain for *Pneumocystis carinii* and fungi. Arch Pathol Lab Med 110:855–856, 1986.

Yu PKW, Uhl JR, Anhalt JP: Rapid methenamine silver stain. Arch Pathol Lab Med 113:111, 1989.

124. PRESERVATION AND SHIPMENT OF SPECIMENS

Edward K. Markell

At times it may be necessary or desirable to refer specimens to various experts for identification. Adequate preservation and shipment of such specimens is important and will facilitate subsequent examination.

PRESERVATION AND CONCENTRATION. If stool specimens containing cysts are to be preserved for more than a few weeks, a 10% formalin solution should be used for preservation. Specimens containing eggs should also be preserved in 10% formalin. When large amounts of stool containing cysts or eggs are to be preserved in formalin, it is advantageous to prepare a concentrate. To make a concentration of a large volume of fecal material, proceed as follows:

1. Make a homogeneous suspension of the specimen in several volumes of water.

2. Strain through two layers of gauze to eliminate large particulate material.

3. Place in large centrifuge tubes, add approximately 5% ether, and shake.

4. Centrifuge at 500 × g for 1 minute.

5. Loosen fatty material at top of tubes and decant, retaining only the sediment.

6. Preserve sediment in 10 volumes of 10% formalin.

After a few days the formalin may be changed and its volume reduced. The MIF stain preservation technique may also be used for preservation of fairly large quantities of stool. Preserved material is generally not optimal for identification. If protozoa found in a stool specimen are to be referred to a specialist for identification, it is best to send one or more slides stained with iron hematoxylin or trichrome as well as material preserved in PVA or SAF, if available.

---

*Grand Island Biological Co., Grand Island, NY.

Large adult roundworms may be fixed in 2% formalin, and transferred to 10% formalin for preservation, or fixed and preserved in 70% alcohol. Smaller roundworms are best fixed in hot 70% alcohol, as this will kill them in an extended condition. Identification of larval cestodes may depend upon recognition of the calcareous corpuscles, best preserved by fixation in buffered formalin.

Buffered Formalin. To a 10% formalin solution made by the addition of 100 ml of USP formaldehyde to 900 ml of 0.85% normal saline, add 0.8 gm of a combination of the following buffer salts:

$$Na_2HPO_4 .... 6.10 \text{ gm}$$
$$NaH_2PO_4 .... 0.15 \text{ gm}$$

The salts may be prepared in advance, mixed thoroughly, and stored in a tightly closed container.

Fly larvae, lice, fleas, and other arthropods may be fixed in 80 to 90% alcohol. Snails should be fixed and preserved in 70% alcohol but not in formalin. Snail shells may also be preserved dry for identification; species determination sometimes requires reference to the soft parts of the snail, and some whole specimens should be preserved.

SHIPMENT. Packages of clinical or laboratory specimens prepared for mailing must conform to postal regulations. Double mailing containers should be used, consisting of an inner screw-cap mailing tube and an outer screw-cap cardboard mailing container. Specimen bottles or tubes should be packed in cotton to lessen the chances of breakage or leaking. Information concerning the specimens may be wrapped around the metal container. Stained fecal smears or blood films or unstained PVA-fixed fecal smears do not require double mailers, but the slides should be individually wrapped in tissue and packed so as to prevent breakage.

125. PARASITIC IMMUNODIAGNOSIS

Irving G. Kagan and Shirley E. Maddison

For the parasitic diseases in which etiologic proof of infection is difficult to obtain, serology with a sensitive and specific assay is an aid to diagnosis. Serology, however, is not indicated for intestinal parasitic diseases for which parasitic eggs are easily detected in fecal specimens.

The demonstration of parasitic antibody and/or antigen suggests recent or past infection with the parasite. A variety of serologic tests, such as complement fixation (CF), agglutination reactions, indirect immunofluorescence (IIF), and agar gel tests, are used for laboratory diagnosis. Immunologic techniques, e.g., enzyme-linked immunosorbent assay (ELISA) including modifications such as FAST-ELISA, immunoelectrotransfer blot (Western blot) (EITB), and radioimmunoassay (RIA),

are being used in the detection of parasitic antibody and circulating antigen.

Tests vary in sensitivity, specificity, and reactivity. Sensitivity is defined as the percentage of positive responses in a group of patients with proven parasitic infection. Specificity is the percentage of negative responses in patients without parasitic infection. Reactivity is a threshold concept and is dependent on the amount of antigen and antibody needed for serologic interaction. RIA and ELISA have high levels of reactivity; these test assays can detect nanograms of antibody and antigen in the sera of infected patients. Tests of medium reactivity are IIF and indirect hemagglutination (IHA). Those with low levels of reactivity are CF, agglutination tests (latex, bentonite, charcoal, cholesterol), direct agglutination of organisms (DAT), and agar gel tests, e.g., double diffusion (DD), immunoelectrophoresis (IE), and counterelectrophoresis (CEP). The sensitivity, specificity, and diagnostic levels of reactivity may differ between laboratories and are influenced by the quality of the reagents. The diagnostic levels of reactivity given in the text are those used in the author's (I.G.K.) laboratory.

Since antibody can persist for many years after an acute parasitic infection (e.g., for as long as 5 years after an amebic infection), antibody levels can rarely differentiate between acute and chronic infection. In the case of toxoplasmosis, IgM antibody in the newborn is indicative of an acute infection. In the adult, IgM antibody resulting from infection can persist for at least a year. Antibody levels before and after chemotherapy give no indication of treatment efficacy. For these reasons there is a great deal of interest and research in the detection of parasite antigen in body fluids. Between 1983 and 1988 more than 50 publications appeared in the literature on the detection of parasite antigen in body fluids. A positive test for parasite amebic antigen in a liver aspirate or *Echinococcus* antigen in aspirated cyst fluid is an indication that the individual is infected with the parasite.

SERODIAGNOSTIC TESTS. The serodiagnostic tests used for 17 parasitic infections are listed in Table 125–1.

ANTIBODY DETECTION TESTS FOR SPECIFIC PARASITIC DISEASES. Serologic diagnosis should not replace etiologic diagnosis. For some parasitic infections, e.g., toxoplasmosis, trichinosis, echinococcosis, amebic liver abscess, Chagas' disease, leishmaniasis, and occult filarial and malarial infections, serologic tests are very useful in arriving at a differential diagnosis. Specific diagnosis, however, is made by finding eggs or life-cycle stages of the parasite in the stool, urine, blood, skin or other tissues, or biologic fluids. Diagnosis for ascariasis, cryptosporidiosis, hookworm, and patent malaria should be made by microscopic examination of stool or blood.

Serologic Tests of High Diagnostic Potential

Amebiasis. The diagnosis of amebiasis by stool examination may be difficult; e.g., in a lightly infected individual, amebas may not be found in the stool because of diet, drug intake, or inadequate experience on the part of the technician (Chapter 68). It is important to differentiate ulcerative colitis from amebic colitis,

TABLE 125–1. Serologic Tests Used for the Diagnosis of Parasitic Diseases

Disease	Antibody Tests of Choice	Tests for Antigen
African trypanosomiasis	ELISA, IIF	
Amebiasis	IHA, CEP, DD, LAT, ELISA	+
Chagas' disease	CF, DAT, IHA, IIF	+
Cysticercosis	IHA, IE, CF, EITB	+
Echinococcosis	IHA, IE, EITB	+
Fascioliasis	DD, ELISA	+
Filariasis	IHA, IIF, ELISA	+
Giardiasis	IIF, ELISA	+
Leishmaniasis	DAT, IIF, CF, CEP, ELISA	+
Malaria	IIF, ELISA, IHA	+
Paragonimiasis	ELISA, IB, CF, CEP, EITB	
Pneumocystosis	IIF, CF	+
Schistosomiasis	IIF, IHA, ELISA, COPT, CHR	+
Strongyloidiasis	IHA	
Toxocariasis	ELISA, IHA	+
Toxoplasmosis	IIF, IgM-IIF, C-IgM, ELISA, IHA, S-F dye	+
Trichinosis	BFT, CEP, LAT, IIF	

BFT = bentonite flocculation test; C-IgM = capture IgM ELISA; CEP = counterelectrophoresis; CF = complement fixation; CHR = cercarienhullenreaktion; COPT = circumoval precipitin test; DAT = direct agglutination test; DD = double diffusion in agar; EITB = immunoelectrotransfer blot (Western blot); ELISA = enzyme-linked immunosorbent assay; IB = immunoblot; IE = immunoelectrophoresis; IHA = indirect hemagglutination; IIF = indirect immunofluorescence; LAT = latex agglutination test; S-F dye = Sabin-Feldman dye test.

since treating an amebic infection with steroids may lead to deterioration of the clinical status of the patient and an exacerbation of the amebic infection. Tests for amebiasis are sufficiently sensitive to detect specific antibody in 85% of patients with amebic colitis. The sensitivity of serologic tests in the differential diagnosis of a hepatic abscess (the parasite is usually not demonstrable in the stool or hepatic abscess material) is in the order of 96% to 98%.

In addition to the IHA test, the CEP and DD tests are used extensively. In areas of high endemicity, e.g., Mexico, the CEP and DD tests give excellent results for both diagnosis and seroepidemiology. An IHA titer of 1:128 to 1:256 is considered a diagnostically positive test.

Chagas' Disease. Except in the acute stage of infection, detection of trypanosomes in the blood is difficult (Chapter 75). Serologic tests are sensitive and, except for cross-reactions with leishmania, are specific. CF, a DAT with trypsinized formalin-fixed organisms, IHA, and IIF tests are also used extensively for diagnosis. The reference test is CF, and a titer of 1:8 is diagnostic. For acute or early infections, the DAT titer (1:128) is more sensitive than the IHA test (titer 1:64) or the IIF test (titer 1:16).

Cysticercosis. Muscle infection can be diagnosed by biopsy (Chapter 101.1). A diagnosis of cerebral cysticercosis can be suggested by scans or x-rays of the brain. Serologic sensitivity is related to the severity of clinical involvement. Therefore, for patients with meningitis and increased intracranial pressure, the serologic sensitivity is 80% to 90%, and antibody can be detected in spinal fluid. Serum from patients with seizures or with cutaneous lesions has a sensitivity of only 40% to 50%, and spinal fluid findings are usually negative. Both ELISA and IHA tests are used in diagnosis, with a titer of 1:32 diagnostic for serum and an ELISA titer of 1:8 diagnostic for spinal fluid. In Mexico, IE is employed extensively for both diagnosis and seroepidemiologic surveys by employing a purified extract of *Taenia solium* as antigen in EITB (patterned after the Western blot method used in AIDS diagnosis). Sensitivity of 98% and specificity of 100% were obtained in neurologic and subcutaneous cysticercosis.

Echinococcosis. Echinococcosis is endemic in all areas of the world where sheep are raised (Chapter 101.2). Because of the occult locations of the cyst, serologic diagnosis is used extensively. The IHA test and LAT (latex agglutination test) are recommended for initial screening, with confirmation by immunoelectrophoresis. The demonstration of "arc 5" in IE is diagnostic, although some cross-reactions with sera from patients with cysticercosis have been reported. An IHA titer of 1:128 is diagnostic. Recently, screening by IHA and confirmation by EITB has resulted in an assay with 91% sensitivity and 100% specificity for surgically confirmed echinococcosis of the liver.

Leishmaniasis. A diagnosis of cutaneous leishmaniasis can be difficult if the organisms are scanty in the ulcerative lesion (Chapter 76). Until the use of IIF tests, serologic diagnosis of cutaneous leishmaniasis was insensitive. Visceral leishmaniasis due to *Leishmania donovani* has high serologic sensitivity and can frequently be difficult to diagnose by detection of the parasite. An IIF titer of 1:16 is diagnostic. A CF test with a *Mycobacterium* antigen has also been used. Cross-reactions with antibody from patients with Chagas' disease present a problem in areas where the diseases coexist. Testing the serum with homologous leishmania and heterologous Chagas' antigens will differentiate specific from cross-reacting antibody. A patient with leishmaniasis will have a higher titer with homologous antigen.

Paragonimiasis. Owing to the occult nature of the cyst in the lung and the paucity of eggs in the sputum in chronic cases, serologic diagnosis is useful in assessing the differential diagnosis (Chapter 99). Employing ELISA and EITB, the detection of antibodies in the serum of infected patients is both sensitive and specific.

Schistosomiasis. Although eggs can be found in the stool of a patient with acute schistosomiasis mansoni or japonica, finding eggs in the stool of patients with chronic disease often requires rectal biopsy or specialized concentration methods plus well-trained laboratory personnel (Chapter 96). *Schistosoma haematobium* eggs are frequently not detected in the urine of older patients with active infections. Serologic testing is helpful in chronic cases and in very early or light infections. IIF is used with cryostat sections of adult worms. An IIF titer of 1:16 is diagnostic. Limited use of RIA indicates that the technique is very sensitive. However, ELISA utilizing various antigens is rapidly becoming the test of choice. A crude Chaffee delipidized extract of adult worms of *S. mansoni* is employed as an antigen in the ELISA test, and a titer of 1:32 is considered diagnostically positive. Excellent diagnostic results have been obtained employing a purified adult worm microsomal antigen (MAMA) in the FAST-ELISA and speciation of the *Schistosoma* infection with species-specific EITB strips using homologous microsomal antigens of *S. mansoni, S. haematobium,* and *S. japonicum.*

Toxocariasis. Infection of a young child with eggs of *Toxocara canis* leads to the clinical syndrome known as visceral larva migrans (VLM) (Chapter 91). When the larvae of *T. canis* invade the eye (OLM), the resulting inflammation mimics retinoblastoma. Employing a sensitive and specific ELISA for toxocariasis has prevented unnecessary enucleation for suspected tumor. When crude *Toxocara* egg antigens were used, the serum had to be absorbed with *Ascaris* antigen. Employing specific secretory/excretory antigen obtained from *T. canis* larvae maintained in culture medium, an ELISA titer of 1:32 is diagnostic for VLM and 1:8 for OLM.

Toxoplasmosis. Infection with *Toxoplasma gondii* early in pregnancy may damage or destroy the fetus (Chapter 78). IIF is used routinely for screening. A titer of 1:1024 or greater suggests recent infection. Because of the high prevalance of antibody in the general population, to determine whether an infection is of recent origin one can use a capture ELISA (C-ELISA) for IgM antibody modified to use peroxidase-labeled soluble *Toxoplasma* antigen as conjugate. An IIF-IgG titer of 1:1024 or greater combined with a capture IgM ELISA titer of 1:256 or greater is indicative of infection probably acquired within the past year.

Trichinosis. Serologic tests are important tools in the differential diagnosis of trichinosis (Chapter 90). With the development of more specific antigens, CEP has been evaluated for enhanced sensitivity and specificity. Bentonite flocculation (BF) will detect acute infections; however, depending on the infective dose of larvae consumed by the patient, the time between infection and serologic detection can be several weeks. An IHA titer of 1:32 or greater is diagnostic.

Serologic Tests with Fair to Low Diagnostic Potential

African Trypanosomiasis. The diagnosis of African trypanosomiasis is normally made by finding organisms in the blood (Chapter 74). A marked polyclonal increase in IgM antibody (only a minor component of which is specific for *Trypanosoma*) is suggestive of infection with these parasites. The serologic tests being used are IIF, ELISA, a capillary IHA, an immunoprecipitation test for IgM estimation, a capillary flocculation test, and a card-agglutination test with fixed trypanosomes (CATT). All these tests, with the exception of IIF and ELISA, are adapted for field use.

Fascioliasis. Infection with *Fasciola hepatica* can usually be diagnosed by finding eggs in the stool or in the biliary drainage (Chapter 98.3). A gel diffusion test has been developed. The presence of a band that links with a positive control serum is indicative of an infection. More recently, an ELISA test has also been developed.

Filariasis. The serologic tests routinely used for filariasis are not species-specific (Chapter 85). In addition to IHA, IIF and ELISA are used. Until specific antigens are isolated for human filarial infection, cross-reactivity of heterologous antigens must be relied on. The use of antigens prepared from *Brugia malayi,* which can be maintained in the laboratory in Jirds, and microfilariae of *Wuchereria bancrofti* isolated from human blood have enhanced the specificity of the test. Preliminary studies with these antigens in ELISA show promise. In both Malayan and bancroftian filariasis an IHA titer of 1:128 is diagnostic in a test that uses *Dirofilaria immitis* as antigen.

Giardiasis. An IIF test has been developed for serologic evaluation employing *G. lamblia* from axenic culture as antigen. It has a sensitivity of only 76% (Chapter 69). A titer of 1:32 is diagnostic. Giardiasis should be diagnosed by microscopically visualizing the protozoa in stool or duodenal aspirate.

Malaria. Diagnosis of malaria is normally made by examination of a blood smear (Chapter 73). However, in transfusion malaria or in patients with low parasitemias, e.g., *Plasmodium malariae* infections, and in epidemiologic studies, serologic tests are used. IIF is the test of choice because species of malaria can be determined by using homologous antigens of the various plasmodia that infect humans. ELISA and IHA tests are also used. The availability of human malaria species infection in *Aotus* and *Ateles* monkeys has greatly enhanced the use of serologic testing for malaria. The in vitro culture of *P. falciparum* has been a signal advance in the preparation of malaria antigen. An IIF titer of 1:64 is diagnostic.

Pneumocystosis. Serologic diagnosis for antibody against *Pneumocystis carinii* has proved to be nonspecific (Chapter 79). The detection of cysts in sputum can be made by an immunofluorescent test with the patient's sputum as antigen and an anti–*P. carinii* monoclonal or polyclonal antibody that binds to the cysts in the sputum and is detected by an anti-mouse or anti-rabbit serum labeled with fluorescein. Because of the scarcity of cysts, liquefaction and concentration of sputum enhances the sensitivity of the test. A commercial kit is available in the United States.

Strongyloidiasis. For positive diagnosis, an ELISA test prepared from filariform larvae of *Strongyloides stercoralis* is used. The diagnostic titer is 1:32 or higher. The test, however, has not been extensively evaluated for sensitivity and specificity, although it has become more valuable in diagnosing superinfection in patients with AIDS and other immunosuppressive conditions (Chapter 15.1).

SKIN TESTS. Because of lack of specificity of antigens, particularly in terms of cross-reactivity between the helminths, physicians have become reluctant to use diagnostic skin testing. Skin test antigens have not been available either commercially or for experimental studies in the United States since 1982. Despite a frequent lack of specificity, skin tests have been used by some investigators in Europe and the tropics as quantitative tools for case diagnosis and for epidemiologic studies of parasitic diseases. To obtain reproducible results, antigens of known nitrogen or protein concentrations should be used, and the technique of administering and measuring the test should be standardized. For the schistosome skin test, for example, an antigen of adult worm extract should contain between 30 and 40 μg of N/ml, and exactly 0.05 ml must be injected intradermally with a 26- or 27-gauge needle. After 15 minutes, for the immediate skin response, the area of the wheal (but not the erythema) is measured with a template (Fig. 125–1). Following this procedure, highly reproducible results can be obtained.

The criterion of a positive test may differ for different segments of a population. The skin test for schistosomiasis is not as sensitive in children as in adults. For this reason, two levels of positivity can be used. For individuals less than 14 years of age, a positive skin test is a wheal measuring 1.0 cm or greater, and for individuals 15 years and older, it is a wheal measuring 1.2 cm^2 or greater.

Skin Test Reactions. The responses to skin tests are classified as immediate, Arthus, and delayed reactions.

The Immediate Reaction. The immediate wheal and flare reaction develops rapidly after antigen injection, reaching a peak in 15 to 30 minutes and subsiding within a few hours. Immediate reactions to skin tests are mediated by immunoglobulin of the IgE class. The predominant cell type is the eosinophil. Almost all helminth antigens elicit an immediate response in the skin. Immediate skin reactions have not been extensively evaluated in protozoan infections.

The Arthus Reaction. An Arthus reaction develops 3 to 5 hours after antigen injection, peaks at 6 to 8 hours, and generally subsides by 24 to 48 hours. The Arthus reaction is mediated by antigen-antibody complexes that are deposited on the capillary walls in the area of antigen injection. The antibody is of the IgG class. The deposited complexes attract polymorphonuclear neutrophils, which are able to extravasate through the damaged vessel walls.

The Delayed Reaction. In the tuberculin-type delayed response, which is an in vivo manifestation of cellular immunity, the antigen reacts with sensitized lymphocytes in the area of injection, stimulating the release of lymphokines, including a chemotactic factor for monocytes. An accumulation of small lymphocytes and monocytic cells occurs 12 to 72 hours after antigen injection and, in severe reactions, may assume a granulomatous character, with the transition of monocytes to epithelioid macrophage-type forms with the appearance of giant cells. The classic delayed response has been recognized in parasitic infections for many years. The early workers who used hydatid fluid as antigen measured the delayed response because they believed it to be more specific than the immediate response. In leishmaniasis and toxoplasmosis, the skin test response is of the delayed type. Delayed responses have been described for many helminth infections, but these tests are not readily performed in epidemiologic studies because of the necessity for a 24- to 48-hour follow-up.

Pitfalls in Skin Testing. Intradermal tests are useful as tools in epidemiologic studies but may lack specificity when crude antigens are used. Skin tests cannot differentiate between present and past infection. However, a *Toxoplasma* serologic titer in a skin test–positive pregnant woman suggests past exposure to the parasite and little danger to the fetus because the woman has been infected long enough to have developed some degree of acquired immunity. On the other hand, a serologic titer in a skin test–negative pregnant woman points to recent exposure to the parasite, with possible injury to the fetus.

Reference standards for parasitic skin test antigens and for performance, including reading of the test, have not been developed. There is a danger of stimulating an anaphylactic response when *Ascaris* or *Toxocara* antigens are used. Skin tests may induce serologically detectable antibody that could interfere with subsequent serologic evaluation of the individual.

Clinically Useful Skin Tests. For the skin tests listed in Table 125–2, the schistosome, leishmania, and hydatid skin test antigens are available commercially in various countries other than the United States. The other antigens are experimental.

Schistosomiasis. The schistosome skin test antigen has been extensively evaluated for epidemiologic and diagnostic purposes. A positive test in a Peace Corps volunteer in an endemic area suggests exposure to cercariae and should be followed up with stool and urine examinations to determine whether the infection is patent. A delayed skin test response in a person living in an endemic area suggests that he or she may have some degree of immunity. The prevalence of delayed responses is higher in individuals who continue to reside in endemic areas than in those who move to urban areas and presumably lose their immunity with time. Arthus

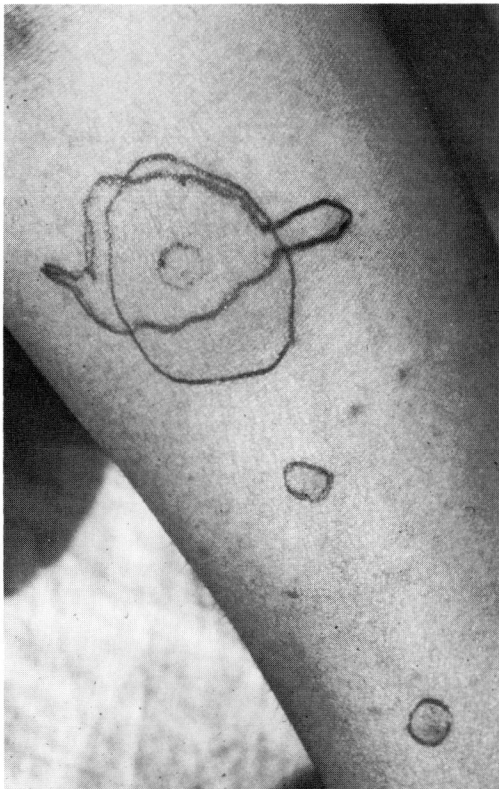

FIGURE 125–1. An intradermal test for schistosomiasis. Note the 2 small control responses: the outline of the immediate 15-minute skin responses with the ameboid irregular outline, and the outline of the larger Arthus 5-hour response with the smooth edge.

TABLE 125–2. Skin Test Antigens for Parasitic Diseases

Disease	Antigen	Remarks
Leishmaniasis	Promastigote stages from culture	Commercially available in Europe
Filariasis	Extract of filarial worms	Experimental antigen
Trichinosis	Extract of larvae of *Trichinella spiralis*	Experimental antigen
Schistosomiasis	Extract of adult worm of *Schistosoma mansoni*	Commercially available in Europe
Echinococcosis	Hydatid fluid of *Echinococcus granulosus*	Commercially available in Europe
	Extract of cysts of *E. multilocularis*	Experimental antigen
Toxoplasmosis	Extract of trophozoites of *Toxoplasma gondii*	Commercially available in Europe

responses occur in 40% to 60% of individuals with positive skin tests. Because of the overlap in time intervals of Arthus and delayed hypersensitivity reactions, skin biopsies are required to unequivocally identify Arthus responses. However, the sensitivity of the Arthus reaction is significantly lower than that of the immediate skin reaction, and thus, negates the use of Arthus reactions with biopsy as a diagnostic tool.

Leishmaniasis. *Leishmania* skin test antigens are used for both epidemiologic and diagnostic purposes. Positive skin test responses of the delayed type may be caused by sensitization by nonhuman *Leishmania* promastigote stages in bites of the intermediate sandfly host. Such false-positive reactions can provide misleading information in epidemiologic surveys. For clinical diagnosis of cutaneous or mucocutaneous leishmaniasis, the skin test will often be positive in infected individuals; however, a positive reaction should not serve as a substitute for identification of the parasite by biopsy or aspiration of the lesion. Patients with untreated visceral leishmaniasis usually are anergic to the skin test. In those with early or occult asymptomatic disease or those undergoing successful chemotherapy, the delayed intradermal test is usually positive.

Echinococcosis. With antigens of low nitrogen content (in the range of 10 to 20 µg N/ml), skin test results of the immediate and delayed type have been used for diagnosis and epidemiologic studies of hydatid disease. Crude undiluted hydatid fluid should not be used because of high levels of protein, which cause nonspecific positive reactions. Because the skin test antigen is thermostable, highly specific antigens have been prepared by boiling hydatid fluid and precipitating nonspecific protein. *Echinococcus* skin tests cross-react in patients with cysticercosis. Arthus responses have been documented in echinococcosis, but their significance has not been fully evaluated. For clinical diagnosis, the immediate skin test reaction is routinely used.

Trichinosis. At one time, *Trichinella* skin tests were available commercially in the United States, as they had been used in epidemiologic studies in Alaska with good results with 17 µg N/ml of antigen. A positive skin test

suggested exposure to the parasite. Such reagents are no longer being sold.

Filariasis. Filarial skin test antigens have been extensively used for epidemiologic studies. The antigens are nonspecific and give positive tests in individuals exposed to other nematode infections. Nonhuman filarial species are commonly used for antigen. The availability of a *Brugia malayi* animal model and relatively simple methods to separate microfilariae of *Wuchereria bancrofti*–infected human blood by column chromotography have provided specific antigens. They have been evaluated in endemic areas in India and Asia with promising results.

Toxoplasmosis. The *Toxoplasma* skin test antigen has been used extensively in Europe for epidemiologic studies as an adjunct to serologic diagnosis in pregnant women. The antigen is not available in the United States.

Skin tests have a great deal of appeal to the clinician and the epidemiologist. With the development of more specific antigens, the usefulness and reliability of the skin test must be re-evaluated.

ANTIGEN DETECTION. Owing to the persistence of antibody following infection and cure (either spontaneously or following chemotherapy) the detection of antigen in serum and other body fluids is a better measurement of active infection and possibly of parasite load. At the present time, diagnostic kits for the detection of *Entamoeba histolytica*, *Giardia lamblia*, and *Cryptosporidium* are available but require further study to determine whether their sensitivity is invariably higher than microscopic examination for the detection of the parasite. Specificity may also be a problem with some of the available tests.

The sensitivity of the commercial kits, most often an ELISA, for antigen detection is usually based on the use of monoclonal antibodies with very high specificity for the parasitic life cycle stages found in the stool.

There are reports of the detection of circulating antigen in serum of patients with toxoplasmosis. In individuals who are immunosuppressed, pregnant women, and congenital cases the detection of antigen would be useful. To date no commercial kit is available. Research papers have been published on the detection of many parasite antigens (e.g., for *Plasmodium falciparum*, *P. vivax*, *E. histolytica*, *S. mansoni*, *W. bancrofti*) in the blood and urine of infected persons. Some of these may prove clinically useful when they become more readily available.

NEW DEVELOPMENTS IN DIAGNOSIS

DNA Probes and Synthetic Antigens. A number of DNA probes that employ molecular biologic technology to map the genome of parasitic organisms have been developed for diagnostic and epidemiologic purposes. These have been reported for all four malaria species that infect humans and for the leishmania. In the near future, recombinant DNA technology will be used to produce highly sensitive and specific antigens for diagnostic antibody tests. There are reports in the literature of such antigen's having been developed for echinococcosis, schistosomiasis, and malaria.

Diagnostic Kits. Immunodiagnostic technology is making rapid strides. Today the clinician can perform sensitive diagnostic procedures in the office using kits with a degree of sensitivity and specificity that was formerly available only in a clinical laboratory. The new technologies are rapidly being incorporated into the parasitic diagnostic laboratory. Great strides are being made, and with the introduction of DNA probes, synthetic peptide antigens, and new and technically simple diagnostic technologies, the immunodiagnosis of parasitic infection has a bright future.

BIBLIOGRAPHY

Campbell GH, Aley SB, Ballou WR, et al: Use of synthetic and recombinant peptides in the study of host-parasite interactions in malaria. Am J Trop Med Hyg 37:428–449, 1987.

Candolfi E, Derouin F, Kein T: Detection of circulating antigens in immunocompromised patients during reactivation of chronic toxoplasmosis. Eur J Clin Microbiol 6:44–48, 1987.

El Raziky EH, Khalil HM, El Kaluby A, et al: Gross and histological studies of immediate, Arthus, and delayed skin test responses to schistosome antigens, and of delayed responses to ubiquitous antigens in Egyptians. Am J Trop Med Hyg 30:373, 1981.

Flisser A, Perez-Montfort R, Larralde C: The immunology of human and animal cysticercosis. A review. Bull WHO 57:839, 1979.

Fortier B, Delplace P, Dubremetz JF, et al: Enzyme immunoassay for detection of antigen in acute *Plasmodium falciparum* malaria. Eur J Clin Microbiol 6:596–598, 1987.

Hillyer GV, Ruiz Tiben E, Knight WB, et al: Immunodiagnosis of infection with *Schistosoma mansoni:* Comparison of ELISA, radioimmunoassay and precipitin tests performed from eggs. Am J Trop Med Hyg 28:661, 1979.

Huijun Z, Zhenghou T, Reddy MV, et al: Parasitic antigens in sera and urine of patients with bancroftian and brugian filariasis detected by sandwich ELISA with monoclonal antibodies. Am J Trop Med Hyg 36:554–560, 1987.

Houba V (ed): Immunological Investigation of Tropical Parasitic Diseases. New York, Churchill Livingstone, 1980, pp 148–156.

Kagan IG: Serodiagnosis of parasitic diseases. *In* Rose NR, Friedman H (eds): Manual of Clinical Immunology. Washington, DC, American Society of Microbiology, 1980, pp 573–604.

Kagan IG, Pellegrino J, Memoria JMP: Studies on the standardization of the intradermal test for the diagnosis of bilharziasis. Am J Trop Med Hyg 10:200, 1961.

Kovacs JA, Valerie LNG, Masur H, et al: Diagnosis of *Pneumocystis carinii:* Improved detection in sputum with use of monoclonal antibodies. N Engl J Med 318:589–593, 1988.

Maddison SE: Parasitic infections. *In* Wicher K (ed): Microbial Antigen Diagnosis. Vol II: Practical Application. Boca Raton, FL, CRC Press, 1987, pp 109–123.

Maddison SE, Slemenda SB, Schantz PM, et al: A specific diagnostic antigen of *Echinococcus granulosus* with apparent molecular weight of 8 kDa. Am J Trop Med Hyg 40:377–383, 1989.

Marrero CA, Santiago N, Hillyer GV: Evaluation of diagnostic antigens in the excretory-secretory products of *Fasciola hepatica*. J Parasitol 74:646–652, 1988.

Schantz PM, Glickman LT: Toxocariasis. *In* Walls KW (ed): Immunology of Parasitic Diseases. New York, Marcel Dekker, 1982.

Slemenda SB, Maddison SE, Jong EC, et al: Diagnosis of paragonimiasis by immunoblot. Am J Trop Med Hyg 39:471–473, 1988.

Tsang VC, Brand JA, Boyer AE, et al: Enzyme-linked immunoelectrotransfer blot assay and glycoprotein antigens for diagnosing human cystic cysticercosis *(Taenia solium)*. J Infect Dis 159:50–59, 1989.

Ungar BL, Yolken RH, Quinn TC: Use of a monoclonal antibody in an enzyme immunoassay for the detection of *Entamoeba histolytica* in fecal specimens. Am J Trop Med Hyg 34:465–472, 1985.

Visvesvara GS, Smith PD, Healy GR, Brown WR: An immunofluorescence test to detect serum antibodies to *Giardia lamblia*. Ann Intern Med 93:802, 1980.

Williams JF: An evaluation of the Casoni test in human hydatidosis using an antigen solution of low nitrogen concentration. Trans R Soc Trop Med Hyg 66:160, 1972.

Wirth DF, Rogers WO, Barker R, et al: Leishmaniasis and malaria: New tools for epidemiologic analysis. Science 234:975–979, 1986.

INDEX

Note: Page numbers in *italics* refer to illustrations; page numbers followed by (t) refer to tables.